SARRAFIAN'S
Anatomy of the Foot and Ankle

Descriptive, Topographic, Functional

FOURTH EDITION

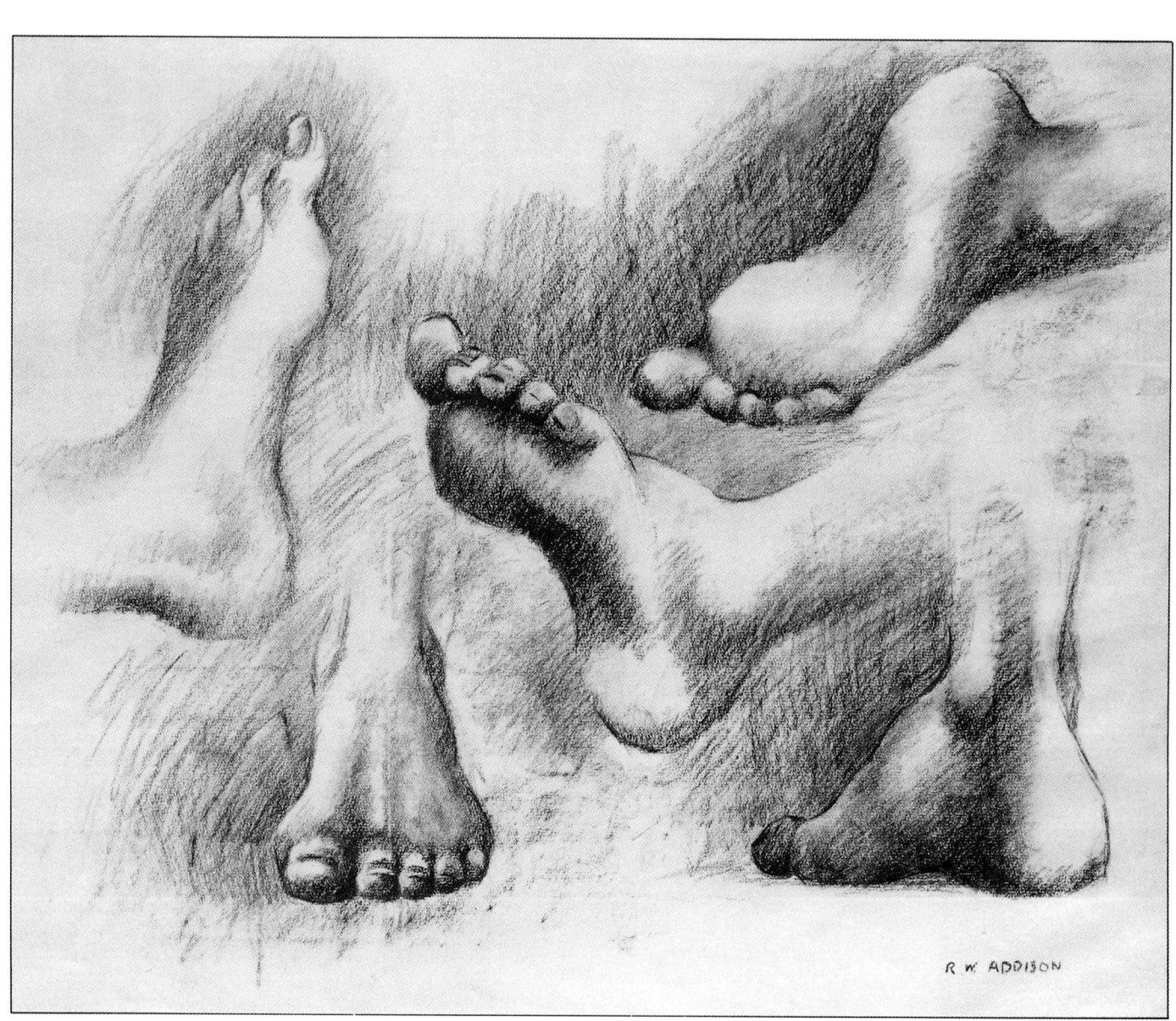

SARRAFIAN'S Anatomy of the Foot and Ankle

Descriptive, Topographic, Functional

FOURTH EDITION

EDITOR

Armen S. Kelikian, MD, FACS

Professor of Orthopedic Surgery
Northwestern University Medical Center
Clinical Instructor
University of Chicago
University of Illinois
NorthShore Orthopedics
Chicago, Illinois

Shahan K. Sarrafian, MD, FACS, FAOS, ABOS

Emeritus Associate Professor of Orthopedic Surgery
Northwestern University Medical School
Chicago, Illinois

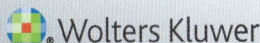

Philadelphia • Baltimore • New York • London
Buenos Aires • Hong Kong • Sydney • Tokyo

Executive Editor: Brian Brown
Senior Developmental Editor: Stacey Sebring
Editorial Coordinator: Vinodhini Varadharajalu
Marketing Manager: Phyllis Hitner
Senior Production Project Manager: Catherine Ott
Manager, Graphic Arts & Design: Stephen Druding
Manufacturing Manager: Beth Welsh
Prepress Vendor: TNQ Technologies

Fourth Edition
Copyright © 2024 Wolters Kluwer.

Copyright © 2011 by Lippincott Williams & Wilkins, a Wolters Kluwer business | Copyright © 1993, by J.B. Lippincott Company Copyright © 1983, by J.B. Lippincott Company. All rights reserved. This book is protected by copyright. No part of this book may be reproduced or transmitted in any form or by any means, including as photocopies or scanned-in or other electronic copies, or utilized by any information storage and retrieval system without written permission from the copyright owner, except for brief quotations embodied in critical articles and reviews. Materials appearing in this book prepared by individuals as part of their official duties as U.S. government employees are not covered by the above-mentioned copyright. To request permission, please contact Wolters Kluwer at Two Commerce Square, 2001 Market Street, Philadelphia, PA 19103, via email at permissions@lww.com, or via our website at lww.com (products and services).

9 8 7 6 5 4 3 2 1

Printed in Mexico

Library of Congress Cataloging-in-Publication Data

ISBN-13: 978-1-975160-63-0

Cataloging in Publication data available on request from publisher

This work is provided "as is," and the publisher disclaims any and all warranties, express or implied, including any warranties as to accuracy, comprehensiveness, or currency of the content of this work.

This work is no substitute for individual patient assessment based upon healthcare professionals' examination of each patient and consideration of, among other things, age, weight, gender, current or prior medical conditions, medication history, laboratory data and other factors unique to the patient. The publisher does not provide medical advice or guidance and this work is merely a reference tool. Healthcare professionals, and not the publisher, are solely responsible for the use of this work including all medical judgments and for any resulting diagnosis and treatments.

Given continuous, rapid advances in medical science and health information, independent professional verification of medical diagnoses, indications, appropriate pharmaceutical selections and dosages, and treatment options should be made and healthcare professionals should consult a variety of sources. When prescribing medication, healthcare professionals are advised to consult the product information sheet (the manufacturer's package insert) accompanying each drug to verify, among other things, conditions of use, warnings and side effects and identify any changes in dosage schedule or contraindications, particularly if the medication to be administered is new, infrequently used or has a narrow therapeutic range. To the maximum extent permitted under applicable law, no responsibility is assumed by the publisher for any injury and/or damage to persons or property, as a matter of products liability, negligence law or otherwise, or from any reference to or use by any person of this work.

shop.lww.com

To my wife Suzanne, whose love and constant support made the fourth edition possible.
Shahan K. Sarrafian

To Hamparzoum Kelikian, MD, my mentor, teacher, hero, and father.
Armen S. Kelikian

Acknowledgments

The completion of the fourth edition of Sarrafian's Anatomy of the Foot and Ankle came at the height of a worldwide pandemic in 2020. It was a challenge for the Wolters Kluwer team working remotely. To that end, I would like to extend a special thank you to Brian Brown, Medical Practice Director, and Stacey Sebring, Senior Development Editor of the Wolters Kluwer publishing team, as well as Barath Balasubramanian, Senior Proof Analyst, at TNQ Technologies.

Finally, I would also like to thank Armen B. Sarrafian for the outstanding original illustrations he created for the new chapter, Neuro Control of Stance and Gait, and Amara Kelikian for her patience in editing and organizing that chapter, as well as the chapter on Arthroscopy of the Talocrural and Subtalar Joints for Armen C. Kelikian's literature search.

Armen S. Kelikian, MD

Foreword to the Fourth Edition

It is a great honor for me to write this foreword.

I have met Dr. Shahan Sarrafian many many years ago when I started my academic life at Northwestern University, and then more recently. What an outstanding physician, passionate for anatomy and detail.

In adding even more pleasure to this foreword, Dr. Armen Kelikian was my resident years and years ago, and seeing him become one of the leading foot and ankle surgeons in the world is a great pleasure for me.

A new chapter has been introduced, "Neuro Control of Stance and Gait." It is a quite in-depth description of the neuro control of stance and gait. The illustrations are unique, elegant, and beautiful. There is no question that this chapter adds further strength to this book.

This book was born to be a great anatomy of foot and ankle, and the fourth edition is becoming a "bible" that every foot and ankle surgeon should utilize in their day-to-day practice.

Sincerely,
Dr. Luciano Dias
Emeritus Professor of Orthopedic Surgery
Northwestern University

Foreword to the Third Edition

The third edition of Dr. Shahan Sarrafian's definitive *Anatomy of the Foot and Ankle* is substantially enhanced with the clinical insights of editor Dr. Armen Kelikian. As in the previous editions, human foot and ankle anatomy and its many variations are beautifully described in exquisite detail with remarkable illustrations. The section on functional anatomy is expanded with greater development of the concepts of tibiotalar column's influence on the anatomic basis of remodeling and stability of the lamina pedis during locomotion. The treatment of this complex subject is elegant and clear. Four new chapters integrate anatomic fundamentals with clinical applications in the domains of (1) arthroscopy of the ankle and subtalar region, (2) angiosomal anatomy and surgical decision making, (3) radiographic and magnetic resonance imaging, and (4) ultrasound anatomy. For the clinical practitioner, these additions complete the original book, providing the bridge from the dissecting table to the bedside. Simply put, this book is a treasure and a "must have" for all those serious about care of patients with foot and ankle problems.

Charles Saltzman, MD
Chairman, Department of Orthopedics
Louis S. Peery, MD Presidential Endowed Professor
University of Utah

Foreword to the Second Edition

The second edition of *Anatomy of the Foot and Ankle* deserves H. Kelikian's epithet "classical" even more than did the first. It is unique in today's world for an entire medical book to be written by a single author; the obvious reason is the dedication needed for such a monumental task. In effect, books tend to be compilations of vignettes, interesting but without continuity. Dr. Sarrafian's book is solid from cover to cover.

It is a lover of anatomy who has compiled such great details of the bones, ligaments, and tendons of the foot and ankle. It is a surgeon who has given us his tool to do better surgery. Anatomy is truly the basis of all surgery. Within this book, caveats abound for the surgeon; for instance, the vascular anatomy of the base of the first metatarsal and the wonderful descriptions of the tibiotalo-calcaneal tunnel.

Perhaps the real gems of the second edition are the beautifully expanded chapters on topographical anatomy and functional anatomy. The cross-sectional specimens and diagrams truly contribute a third dimension to our understanding of anatomy. These plates alone serve as the keystone for MRI interpretations of this anatomical zone. Clinically, I know it was the basis for Dr. Sarrafian's ankle block anesthetic technique, which I have used with great success.

D'Abord la clarté puis encore la clarté et enfin la clarté. This remonstrance of Anatole France obviously applies to the entirety of Sarrafian's *Anatomy of the Foot and Ankle*; but above all, for me, a surgeon, it applies to the functional anatomy chapter. He has given us an invaluable tool to help in the quest for better diagnoses and solutions to problems of the foot.

> Gerard M. Goshgarian, MD
> Associate Professor of Orthopedic Surgery
> Northwestern University Medical School
> Chicago, Illinois

I have the honor of expressing my opinion and appreciation of Dr. Sarrafian's second edition of *Anatomy of the Foot and Ankle*. The text has been expanded 30%; most of the additional material involves more recent information on the kinesiology, functional anatomy, compartments, and biomechanics of the foot and ankle, as well as enhancement of cross-sectional anatomy. Once again, Dr. Sarrafian augmented the text with his own personal dissections as well as cities of the world literature. This classic anatomic book, with its added cross-sectional studies, provides the basis for the correlations with CAT scans and MRI of the foot and ankle.

Dr. Sarrafian is to be congratulated on this comprehensive, accurate, and most original work.

> Melvin H. Jahss, MD
> Chief, Orthopaedic Foot Service
> Hospital for Joint Diseases
> Orthopaedic Institute
> New York, New York

Foreword to the First Edition

The study of the foot has long been regarded as the stepchild of anatomical teaching. As medical students we began dissecting the head and ended with the foot. At the end of 3 or 6 months (in my time it was 6 months), when we reached the foot we found it dried out, gnarled, and so hard that it could not be cut with a scalpel, to say nothing about dissecting it. For some reason, standard textbooks of anatomy devote relatively limited space to the foot, and what is written hardly benefits the practicing surgeon; Dr. Sarrafian mentions the text, *Structure and Function as Seen in the Foot*. The author of this book, following the tradition of his predecessor, Sir Arthur Keith, gave surgeons a friendly wink and went on meandering in his wanted territory: comparative anatomy. Wood Jones said very little of value practicing surgeons who need detail and no pontifical remarks or generalizations.

I am aware of no book in anatomy that has supplied as much detail about the structure of the ankle and foot than the present one by Dr. Sarrafian. He has not taken the words of his predecessors for granted. He has put their findings to test by numerous dissections of fetal as well as postnatal ankles. I have seen him virtually compare 100 tali, measure their facets, note their configuration, and their disposition or axis as he prefers to call it. Besides his section about the talus, I am fascinated by his discussion of collateral ligaments of the ankle (especially the medial or deltoid ligament), Lisfranc's articulation, and the first metatarsophalangeal joint. There are only few nuggets. *Anatomy of the Foot and Ankle* abounds with equally brilliant ones. If any book deserves the epithet "classical," this one does. It will be read and used for reference for many years to come.

Hampar Kelikian, MD
Emeritus Professor of Orthopedic Surgery
Northwestern University Medical School
Chicago, Illinois

Preface to the Fourth Edition

Over my past 41 years of practice in orthopedics, the subspecialty of foot and ankle has grown in leaps and bounds. Functional and applied anatomy remain the foundation for the clinician for physical exam, analysis, and treatment, correlating topographic, cross-sectional, and surgical anatomy is essential.

I have known Dr. Sarrafian since I was a child. As a junior medical student he was influential in directing my career toward orthopedics. I remember seeing him dissecting fresh cadaveric specimens meticulously and with precision prior to the first edition in 1983. It was a valuable reference for a young orthopedist. By the second edition (1993) he expounded on functional anatomy and supported the functional concept of MacConaill. The foot is seen as the lamina pedis loaded by the tibiotalar column and converted into a loose pack or close pack unit through external or internal rotation of the column.

Unfortunately, the second edition went out of print. Future generations would not be exposed to this wealth of information.

On Christmas Eve in 2006—while I was carving a roast—he asked me to help him edit and revise the third edition of *Anatomy of the Foot and Ankle*. Without hesitation or a second thought I accepted. We set forth to update the first 10 chapters (Part I) with pertinent international literature from 1992 through 2008. Special attention was paid to Chapter 10 to emphasize the lamina pedis changes through the gait cycle. Though anatomy has not changed in the past decade from the 2010 publication, there have been advances in understanding the applied anatomical principles to our locomotion and gait.

Part II begins with a new Chapter 11, Neuro Control of Stance and Gait. Dr. Sarrafian spent 5 years of extensive research into the neurological basis of human locomotion. The four chapters (12-15) added to the third edition have been updated relative to applied anatomy: diagnostic imaging techniques, ultrasound anatomy, angiosomes, and arthroscopic anatomy are emphasized and correlated.

A bonus is included when we came upon some color photographs of dissections and original drawings of Dr. Sarrafian's, that will replace prior black-and-whites as well as few new photos.

We hope the fourth edition will aid the clinician—whether surgeon, radiologist, regional anesthesiologist, physiatrist, or physical therapist—in the application of anatomic basics to the treatment of the foot and ankle.

Armen S. Kelikian, MD, FACS

Preface to the Third Edition

Over my past 30 years of practice in orthopedics, the subspecialty of foot and ankle has grown in leaps and bounds. Functional and applied anatomy remain the foundation for the clinician for physical exam, analysis, and treatment, correlating topographic, cross-sectional, and surgical anatomy is essential.

I have known Dr. Sarrafian since I was a child. As a junior medical student he was influential in directing my career toward orthopedics. I remember seeing him dissect fresh specimens meticulously and with precision prior to the first edition in 1983. It was one of the most valuable references for a young orthopedist. By the second edition (1993) he expounded on functional anatomy and supported the functional concept of MacConaill. The foot is seen as the lamina pedis loaded by the tibiotalar column and converted into a loose pack or close pack unit through external or internal rotation of the column.

Unfortunately, the second edition went out of print. Future generations would not be exposed to this wealth of information.

On Christmas Eve in 2006—while I was carving a roast—he asked me to help him edit and revise *Anatomy of the Foot and Ankle*. Without hesitation or a second thought I accepted. We set forth to update the first 10 chapters (Part I) with pertinent international literature from 1992 through 2008. Special attention was paid to Chapter 10 to emphasize the lamina pedis changes throughout the gait cycle.

Four additional chapters (Part II) were added relative to applied anatomy. Normal arthroscopic anatomy, radiology, and angiosomes are emphasized and correlated.

We hope the third edition will aid the clinician—whether diagnostician, radiologist, regional anesthesiologist, or surgeon—in the application of anatomic basics to the treatment of the foot and ankle. As Dr. Sarrafian has taught me well after his retirement, one needs to "water his mind with knowledge to allow it to grow."

Armen S. Kelikian, MD, FACS

Preface to the Second Edition

The first edition of *Anatomy of the Foot and Ankle* offered a new platform of knowledge. The warm and supportive reception given by my colleagues encouraged me to expand the horizons of this work, guided by the clinical and surgical necessities requiring "further clarifications." The benchmark of the knowledge of anatomy is the cross-sectional anatomy. A complete, systematic, cross-sectional study of the distal leg-ankle-foot was done and added in Chapter 9 under the title "Cross-Sectional and Topographic Anatomy." The methodology used to prepare the fresh-frozen sections was as described in the first edition. Once more, I performed all anatomic dissections myself. The cross-sectional study made it possible to demonstrate the formation and the continuity of the compartments from the leg into the ankle-foot. Great emphasis was given to the tibiotalocalcaneal tunnel, which communicates with the intermediate compartment of the sole of the foot. This unified concept of the topographic anatomy is of prime importance for the clinical correlations. Clarification was provided to the concept of compartments and spaces in the foot as exemplified by the adductor compartment and adductor space. In lieu of surgical approaches, surgically oriented, topographic dissections were conducted, bringing forth the pertinent anatomical relationships and possible pitfalls.

The excellent anatomic work of Hidalgo and Shaw provided the basis for the rational approach to the sole of the foot. In this edition, the anatomy of the peripheral nerves was further emphasized with new dissections. Chapter 10, "Functional Anatomy," was completely revised with the goal of providing a unified source for the enormous contributions made in the field of functional anatomy from the early 1980s to the present. A great effort was made to integrate the results of the excellent investigative works of Van Langelaan and Lundberg and colleagues using the innovative x-ray photogrammetric methodology. The works of Kjaersgaard-Anderson and coworkers, Rasmussen, Stormont and associates, Attarian and colleagues, and Harper, to name but a few, were analyzed in relation to the problems of stability of the ankle and hindfoot.

Quantitative functional kinesiologic data confirmed the multiaxial nature of the motion of the ankle, hindfoot, and midfoot. The participation of the anatomic sites in pronation and supination twist of the forefoot (midfoot) was clarified by Ouzounian and Sliereff.

Finally, the unified concept of functional anatomy as presented by MacConaill and Hicks has been greatly expanded in this second edition.

The foot-ankle is and should be considered as a functional unit. The synarthrodial concept of MacConaill, integrating the ligamentous function with the osseo-geometric anatomy, is of prime importance. In the biomechanical understanding of the foot-ankle unit, unless the ligaments are taken into consideration, the truth may forever remain evasive.

Shahan K. Sarrafian, MD, FACS, FAOS, ABOS

Preface to the First Edition

Also we can affirm, without fear of being taxed for exaggeration, that it is at the school of anatomy, particularly in topographic anatomy, that the best surgeons are formed.
                                          TESTUT AND JACOB*

The knowledge of anatomy is essential for the treating surgeon and physician. As stated by Testut and Jacob, for the surgeon "the human body should be transparent like crystal" and the study of the topographic or surgical anatomy determines the regional knowledge to guide the scalpel, avoiding vital structures and interfering with other structures as specifically indicated. The practical concept of "down to bone" without due attention to the surrounding fine soft tissue structures is a primitive one and invites complications in foot and ankle surgery.

Five years ago I was invited to write a book on the anatomy and function of the foot. After 6 weeks of soul searching I accepted the great responsibility of undertaking the gigantic project. The excellent book of F. W. Jones, *Structure and Function as Seen in the Foot*, was then 28 years old. Thus, it became evident that there was a great need to update the knowledge in the field, particularly, since the advent of the rapid progress in the surgery of the foot and ankle.

A unified source of anatomical knowledge was set as a goal, bringing forth the classic and often forgotten works of giants of anatomy, combined with the recent comprehensive anatomical investigations. At no time was this approach intended to be encyclopedic but remained highly selective. This phase of the work required the translation of French, German, and Japanese works, the latter when written in German.

The personal investigative interest of the anatomy of the foot dates back to 1961. It was triggered by Dr. J. Boyes as he was explaining—at the end of a working day—the anatomy of the transverse lamina of the finger and retention of the common extensor tendon. The explanation and his diagrams were lucid and I decided to investigate, on my return to Chicago, the same retention mechanism in the toes. I undertook the anatomical investigation of the intrinsic muscles of the toes with my best friend and colleague, Dr. L.K. Topouzian and the data were presented as an exhibit in 1965 and published in 1969. My personal anatomical and functional studies of the foot and ankle continued as dictated various teaching responsibilities. The dissections were carried out primarily on the ankle and the hindfoot.

For the past 5 years all the dissections were personally done in a systematic manner. All specimens were fresh or preserved as fresh-frozen. No embalmed material was used. Each anatomical dissecting session was carried out in a continuous fashion for a period of 8 to 10 hours. Occasionally, the same foot and ankle were used a second time for another 6 to 8 hours. The documentation was done at each significant step through immediate photography, supplemented by pencil diagram during or immediately after the dissection. The pertinent phases were further documented by dictation and recording while dissecting. This methodology allowed me to remain as accurate as possible.

The cross sections of the foot and ankle were obtained by slicing the frozen specimens, followed by thawing and dissection. The latter was done under magnification and lasted 4 to 5 hours for each section. The arterial dissections were done after injecting the arterial tree with micropaque. The measurements on the tali and the calcanei were obtained from 100 dry tali and 50 dry calcanei from my own collection.

The osteo-anatomy and the syndesmology were emphasized as it became apparent that the knowledge of the geometry of the articular surfaces and the direction and tension of the various binding ligaments are essential to the understanding of the functional behavior of the joints. Skeletal coalition was added to the study of osteology because of its important clinical implications. I did not economize energy in bringing forth data related to variations. Unifying such information from many rare sources under one cover may be beneficial to colleagues, especially if they are not versed in other languages. The advent of microsurgery as related to the foot necessitated obtaining details on the vascular anatomy, and the works of Adachi, Huber, Edwards, and more recently, the works of Gilbert, Murakami, Man, and Acland were referred to extensively. The arterial blood supply of the skeletal element was dealt with in a comprehensive manner.

The topographic or surgical anatomy was presented in four regions. The first region includes the anterior aspect of the ankle and the dorsum of the foot. The second region includes the posterolateral aspect of the ankle and foot. The third region incorporates the posteromedial aspect of the ankle and the tibiotalocalcaneal tunnel. The subdivision of the latter into two distinct neurovascular compartments is emphasized. The fourth region is represented by the sole of the foot. Practical landmarks and guidelines are provided to localize the neurovascular bundles and the compartments. The ball of the foot and the big toe are dealt with separately.

In the study of the functional anatomy of the foot, the contributions of Hicks and MacConaill are enormous in the appreciation of the functional relationship of the forefoot and hindfoot. Most of the recent orthopedic literature refers to Hicks' windlass mechanism of tightening of the plantar aponeurosis through the hyperextension of the big toe, but I think that his explanation of the interrelationship of the forefoot and hindfoot deserves as much, if not more, attention. MacConaill's concept of the foot as a twisted plate—supination meaning untwisting and pronation meaning more twisting of the plate—is expressing the same relationship as defined by Hicks from a different angle. This also deserves much attention especially when untwisting or supination (forefoot supination and hindfoot valgus) renders the foot plate rigid and subject to fracture, and twisting or pronation (forefoot pronation and hindfoot varus) renders the foot pliable. These facts, very easily verifiable on one's own foot or on specimens, seem contrary to the present, common understanding of the relationship of the hindfoot and forefoot as presented in the orthopedic biomechanical literature. The works of Elftman and Huson deserve due consideration. The subluxation of the talus at the midtarsal joint during supination, immediately reduced by midtarsal combined motion of adduction supination—flexion, as described by Huson, is expressing Elftman's explanation that in supination the major axes of the calcaneocuboid and the talonavicular joints do not coincide and require the intervention of the subtalar axis for adjustment. The recent anatomical and functional investigations of Bojsen-Møller are also most interesting and are referred to extensively.

The effort invested in the preparation of this book has been gigantic but the learning process has been a most rewarding experience. If *Anatomy of the Foot and Ankle* offers useful information to my colleagues and provides a new platform of knowledge from which others can advance the frontier of knowledge of the anatomy and function of the foot and ankle, I will have then reached my goal.

Shahan K. Sarrafian, MD, FACS, FAOS, ABOS

Contributors

Gregory A. Dumanian, MD
Chief of Plastic Surgery
Stuteville Professor of Surgery
Northwestern University Feinberg School of Medicine
Chicago, Illinois

Thomas Grant, DO, FACR
Professor of Radiology
Northwestern University Feinberg School of Medicine
Chicago, Illinois

Armen S. Kelikian, MD, FACS
Professor of Orthopedic Surgery
Northwestern University Medical Center
Clinical Instructor
University of Chicago
University of Illinois
NorthShore Orthopedics
Chicago, Illinois

Imran M. Omar, MD
Chief, Musculoskeletal Radiology
Associate Professor of Radiology
Northwestern University Feinberg School of Medicine
Chicago, Illinois

Shahan K. Sarrafian, MD, FACS, FAOS, ABOS
Emeritus Associate Professor of Orthopedic Surgery
Northwestern University Medical School
Chicago, Illinois

Contents

Foreword to the Fourth Edition vi
Preface to the Fourth Edition x
Contributors xv

I Anatomy 1

1 Development of the Foot and Ankle 1
Shahan K. Sarrafian and Armen S. Kelikian

2 Osteology 38
Shahan K. Sarrafian and Armen S. Kelikian

3 Retaining Systems and Compartments 119
Shahan K. Sarrafian and Armen S. Kelikian

4 Syndesmology 162
Shahan K. Sarrafian and Armen S. Kelikian

5 Myology 222
Shahan K. Sarrafian and Armen S. Kelikian

6 Tendon Sheaths and Bursae 294
Shahan K. Sarrafian and Armen S. Kelikian

7 Angiology 304
Shahan K. Sarrafian and Armen S. Kelikian

8 Nerves 383
Shahan K. Sarrafian and Armen S. Kelikian

9 Cross-Sectional and Topographic Anatomy 430
Shahan K. Sarrafian and Armen S. Kelikian

10 Functional Anatomy of the Foot and Ankle 509
Shahan K. Sarrafian and Armen S. Kelikian

II Applied Anatomy 647

11 Neuro Control of Stance and Gait 647
Shahan K. Sarrafian

12 Angiosomes of the Calf, Ankle, and Foot: Anatomy, Physiology, and Implications 702
Gregory A. Dumanian

13 Diagnostic Imaging Techniques of the Foot and Ankle 713
Imran M. Omar

14 Ultrasound Anatomy of the Ankle and Foot 770
Thomas Grant

15 Arthroscopy of the Talocrural and Subtalar Joints 782
Armen S. Kelikian

Index 805

I Anatomy

Development of the Foot and Ankle

1

Shahan K. Sarrafian and Armen S. Kelikian

PRENATAL DEVELOPMENT

The embryonic period is divided into 23 horizons or stages. Each horizon corresponds to a developmental stage of the embryo based on a system of point scores. This method of classification and identification of the embryo advocated by Streeter has brought greater precision to embryologic descriptions.[1] Embryos of different crown-rump (C-R) lengths might belong to the same horizon. The growth curve of the embryo, correlating the C-R length with the fertilization or menstrual age of the embryo, as presented by Patten (Fig. 1.1), is used throughout this study.[2] The use of a growth curve in terms of one linear measurement correlated with age is still of value for the interpretation of embryologic information predating Streeter's classification.

▶ Morphogenesis of the Feet

Morphogenesis of the feet is illustrated in Figures 1.2 and 1.3.[1] The embryo of 2 weeks post fertilization is curved irregularly in a semicircle and presents no external evidence of a lower limb bud in the caudal area (Fig. 1.4).

Horizons or Stages of Development

At 3 weeks, a slight longitudinal swelling is discernible opposite the five lumbar and first sacral myotomes. Once initiated, the ontogeny of the lower limb progresses in a rapid sequential fashion, and definite morphologic changes are recognizable at 2-day intervals. At 4 weeks, in horizon 13 (3-6 mm), a minute lower limb bud germinates at the site of the previous swelling. Within the next 2 days, in horizon 14 (5-7 mm), the bud increases in size and springs laterally from the trunk. It exhibits a flat ventral and a rounded dorsal surface united by a convex margin (see Figs. 1.2 and 1.5). In horizon 15 (6-9 mm), the bud extends its base distally toward the sacral myotomes and further increases in length. The lumbar segment retains a round contour, whereas the sacral part tapers. A differentiation is initiated and is well evident in horizon 16 (8-11 mm). Three regions are visible, corresponding to the thigh, the leg, and the foot anlage. All three regions are more or less located in the same transverse plane, which is perpendicular to the plane of the lower trunk.

A rounded foot disk is recognized in horizon 17 (11-13.5 mm) at the fifth embryonic week. The surface of the foot plate is located in the transverse plane, and the ventral surface,

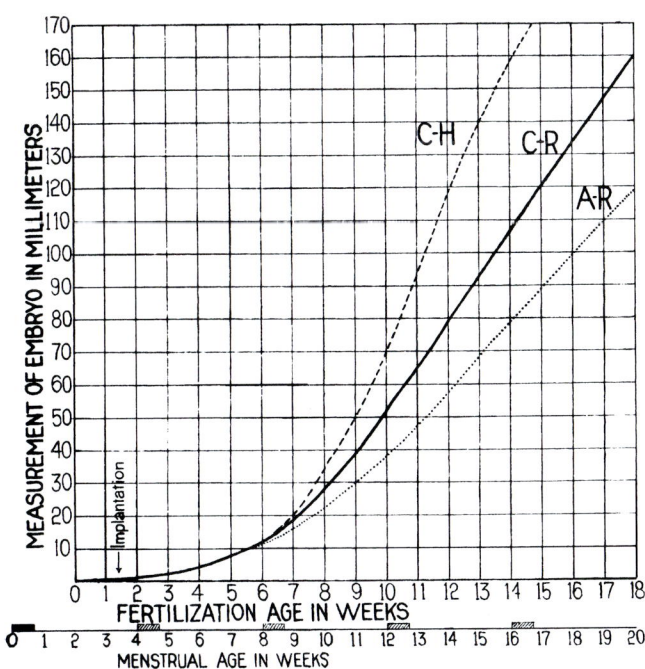

Figure 1.1 Crown-to-rump (C-R) length as compared with age of embryo. (After Patten BM. *Human Embryology.* 2nd ed. McGraw-Hill; 1953:185.)

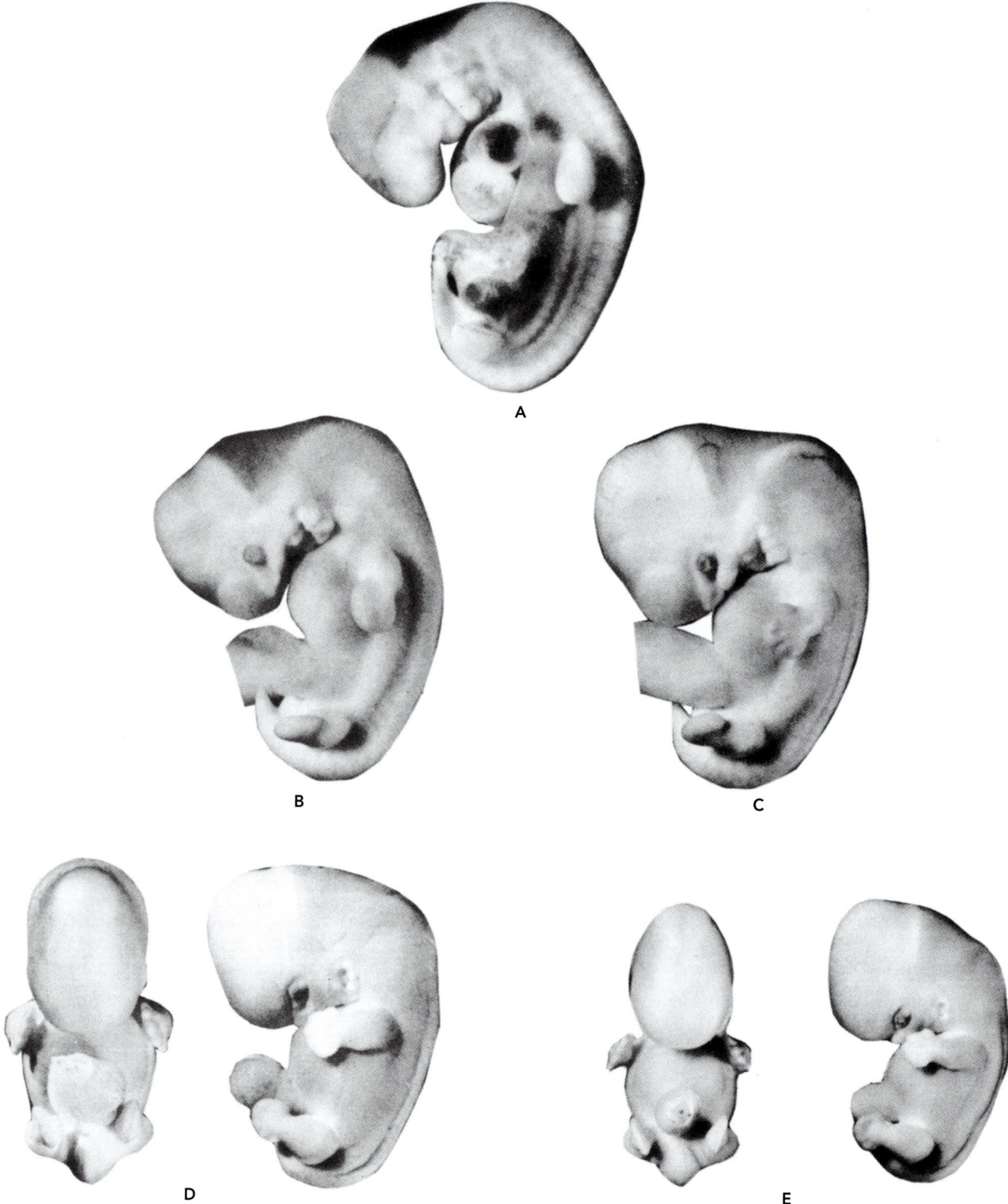

Figure 1.2 **Embryos.** **(A)** Horizon 14 (4.9-8.2 mm). **(B)** Horizon 16 (8-11 mm). **(C)** Horizon 17 (11-13.5 mm). **(D)** horizon 18 (14-16 mm). **(E)** horizon 19 (16.5-20 mm). (Assembled after Streeter GL. Developmental horizons in human embryos. *Contrib Embryol*. 1945;21, 1948;32, 1951;34.)

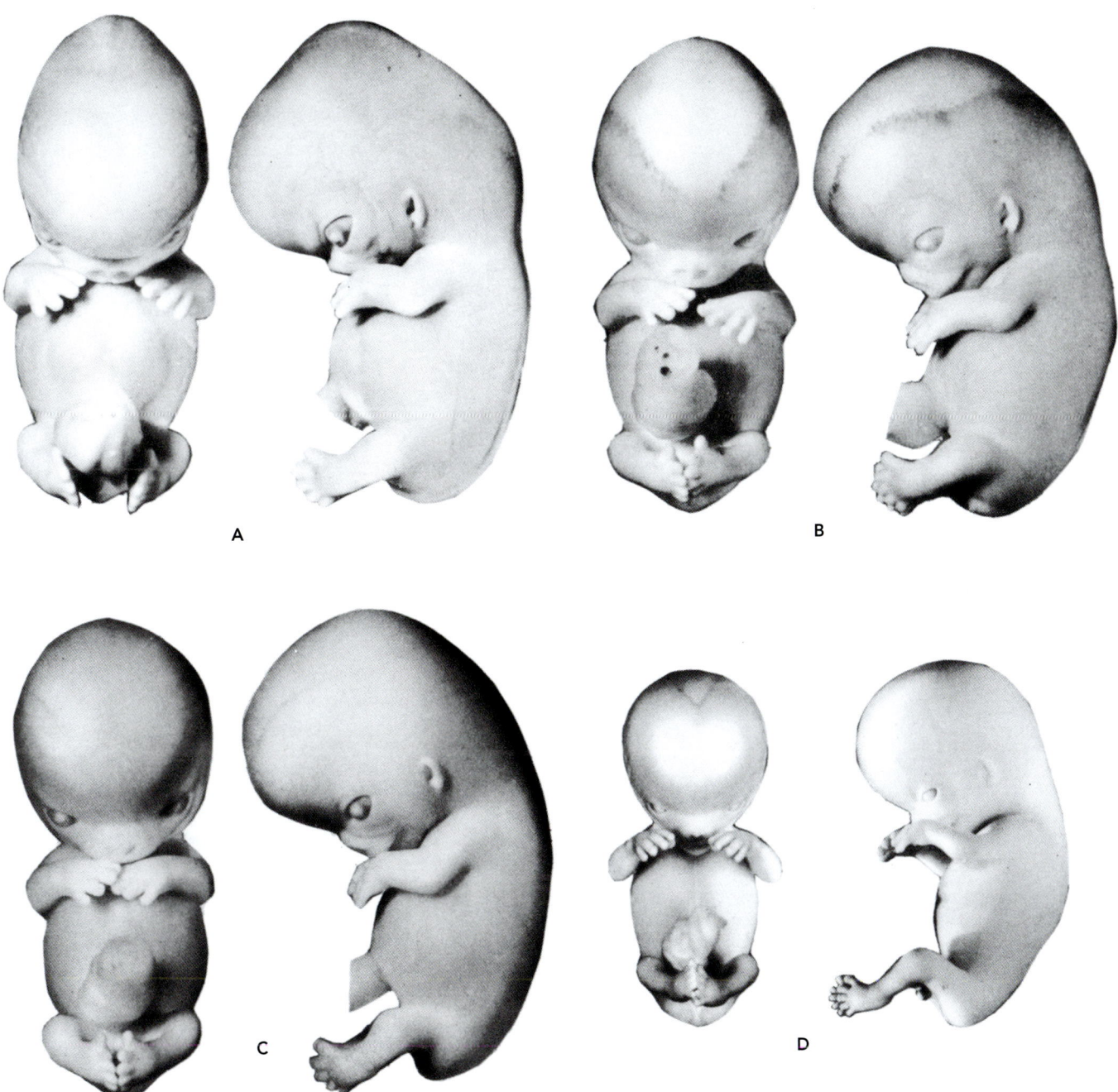

Figure 1.3 **Embryos. (A)** Horizon 20 (21-23 mm). **(B)** Horizon 21 (21-24 mm). **(C)** Horizon 22 (25-27 mm). **(D)** horizon 23 (28-30 mm). (Assembled after Streeter GL. Developmental horizons in human embryos. *Contrib Embryol.* 1945;21, 1948;32, 1951;34.)

the future plantar surface, faces the head. An inward rotation occurs, and the future flexor surface obliquely faces the median sagittal plane of the trunk (see Figs. 1.2 and 1.6). When viewed from the ventral aspect of the embryo, the rotation of the foot plate—a fundamental change—is counterclockwise on the left and clockwise on the right; the leg segment participates in this inward rotation. Morphologically, no toe rays are present in the foot plate. However, older embryos of this group have an indication of the great toe on the tibial or preaxial border. Within the next 2 days, in horizon 18 (14-16 mm; see Fig. 1.2), the sixth embryonic week, the inward rotation of the foot-leg segment continues. The medial surface of the foot plate faces more toward the median plane of the trunk, and this surface, when extended distally, makes with its counterpart an acute angle, open proximally. When the embryo is viewed from the lateral aspect, the future dorsal surface of the foot plate can be seen. An inward rotation of nearly 90° has occurred. The preaxial or tibial border is cephalad, and the postaxial or peroneal border is caudad. Digital rays are clearly visible, and some interdigital notching is present. In horizon 19 (16.5-20 mm), the features of the previous stage are accentuated. The digital notching is deeper (see Figs. 1.2 and 1.7). The foot plates are converted to a more recognizable foot structure in horizon 20 (21-23 mm; see Figs. 1.3 and 1.8), and by horizon 21 (22-24 mm; see Fig. 1.3),

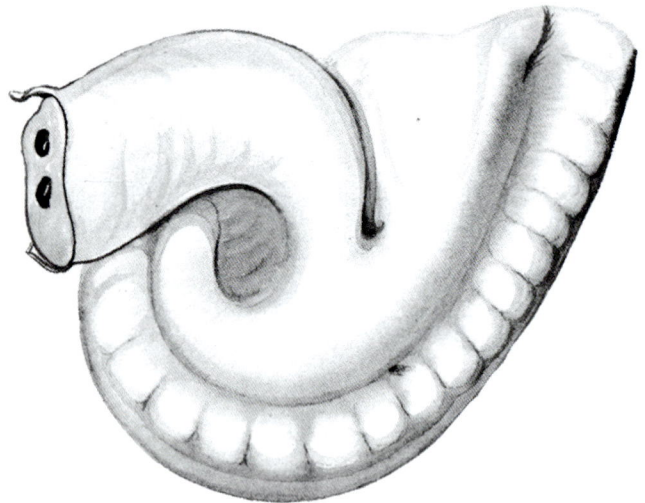

Figure 1.4 Embryo of 4.2 mm.

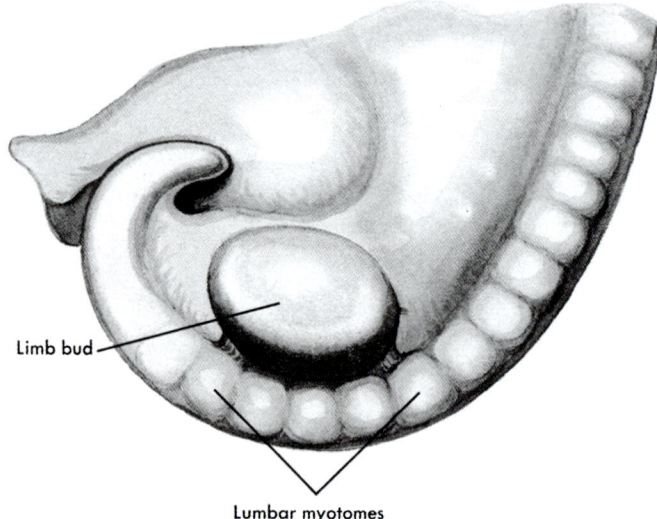

Figure 1.5 Embryo of horizon 14 (6.3 mm).

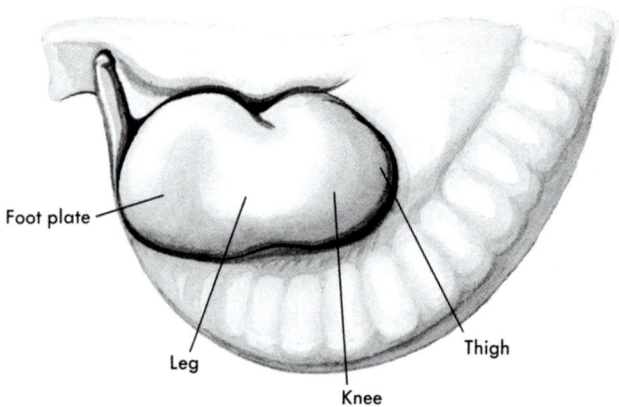

Figure 1.6 Embryo of horizon 17 (11-13.5 mm).

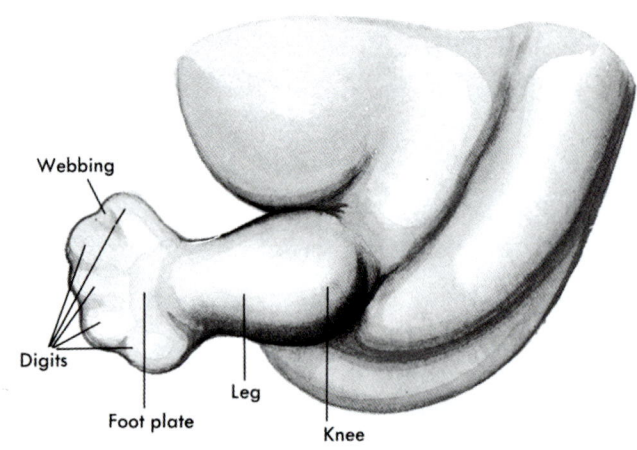

Figure 1.7 Embryo of horizon 19 (17.5 mm).

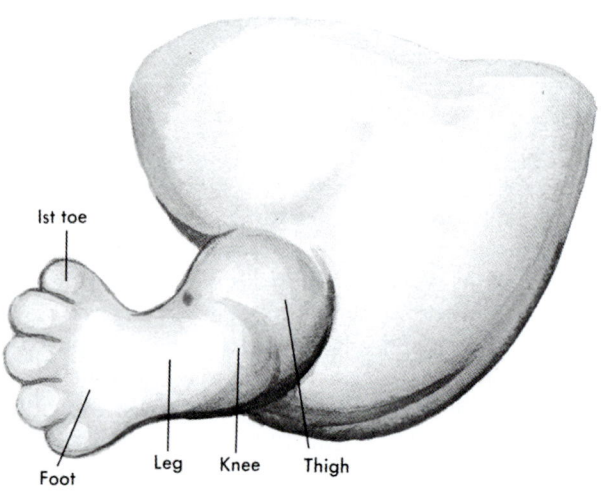

Figure 1.8 Embryo of horizon 20 (20 mm).

the seventh embryonic week, the orientation of the parts is as follows:

- Both feet face each other and are located in a nearly sagittal plane.
- The preaxial or tibial border of the leg-foot is cephalad.
- The postaxial or fibular border of the leg-foot is caudad.
- The extensor surface (future anterior surface of the leg and dorsum of the foot) faces laterally.
- The flexor surface (future posterior surface of the leg and plantar of the foot) faces medially.
- The toes are well delineated and spread apart. The big toe is on the tibial border of the foot.
- The foot surface is in continuity with the leg surface.
  - There is no dorsal angulation of the foot relative to the leg.
  - The foot is in an equinus position relative to the leg.
- The entire lower extremity is in a position of marked external rotation.

Horizon 23 marks the end of the embryonic period proper (see Figs. 1.3 and 1.9). It corresponds to the end of the eighth embryonic week and an average C-R length of 30 mm. The feet touch each other at their soles or medial aspects and are in a praying position. The toes are still fanning out.

During the fetal period, important rotational changes take place that alter the leg-foot relationship. Initially the feet, their soles facing each other, are in equinus relative to the leg. A progressive internal rotation of the thigh-leg occurs, and the foot is then in equinus, supination, and external rotation relative to the leg. Subsequently, the foot dorsiflexes and pronates, bringing the foot close to the adult neutral position; the toes do not diverge.

Böhm, describing the developmental phases of the foot in the embryo-fetus, ascribes four stages to the morphologic determinism.[3]

- Stage one (second month): The foot is in 90-degree equinus and adducted.
- Stage two (beginning of third month): The foot is in 90-degree equinus, adducted, and markedly supinated.
- Stage three (middle of third month): The foot dorsiflexes at the ankle but a mild degree of equinus is still present. The marked supination persists. The first metatarsal remains adducted. This stage corresponds to the fetal period of development.
- Stage four (beginning of fourth month): The foot pronates and reaches a position of midsupination. A slight metatarsus varus remains. The equinus is not present.

The pronation "continues during the remainder of fetal development and is not yet complete in the newborn."[3]

The division of the development of the foot into four stages brings schematic clarity, but in reality, as Böhm states, "the changes do not actually occur within the exact limits of four stages but by means of gradual, continuous transformations."[3]

Digital Formula

The study of the position and relative length of the toes presents another interesting aspect of the morphogenesis of the foot (Fig. 1.10).

The pedal digits make their clear appearance in horizon 20 (21-23 mm). They diverge from the convex border of the foot plate. The third toe arises from the apex of the convexity and is therefore the longest. Within a few days, the preaxial side of the foot grows more rapidly, and the second toe surpasses the third.[4] It is later in fetal life that the first toe might take the lead. According to Jones, in the very early embryo, the pedal digit formula may be 3 > 2 > 1 > 4 > 5 or 3 > 2 > 4 > 1 > 5 for a brief period.[4] When the embryo reaches horizon 22 (25-27 mm), the second toe takes the lead with a 2 > 3 > 1 > 4 > 5 distribution; later, the adult formula is reached in the form of 1 > 2 > 3 > 4 > 5 or its variant 2 > 1 > 3 > 4 > 5.

I have analyzed the pedal digital formula in 29 embryo feet. The feet were classified according to length into three developmental groups: group 1, feet up to 5 mm in length; group 2, feet 5 to 9 mm in length; group 3, feet 10 mm in length. The following distribution was present:

- Group 1 (5 feet total):
  - Four feet (3 mm, 4 mm, 4 mm, 4.5 mm): 3 > 2 > 4 > 1 > 5
  - One foot (4 mm): 2 > 3 > 4 > 1 > 5
- Group 2 (19 feet total):
  - One foot (5.5 mm): 3 > 4 > 2 > 1 > 5
  - Seven feet (5 mm, 5.5 mm, 5.5 mm, 6 mm, 6 mm, 6 mm, 6 mm): 3 > 2 > 4 > 1 > 5
  - Six feet (6 mm, 6 mm, 6 mm, 7 mm, 8 mm, 8 mm): 2 > 3 > 4 > 1 > 5
  - Four feet (5 mm, 6.5 mm, 7 mm, 9.5 mm): 2 > 3 > 1 > 4 > 5
  - One foot (8 mm): 2 > 1 > 3 > 4 > 5

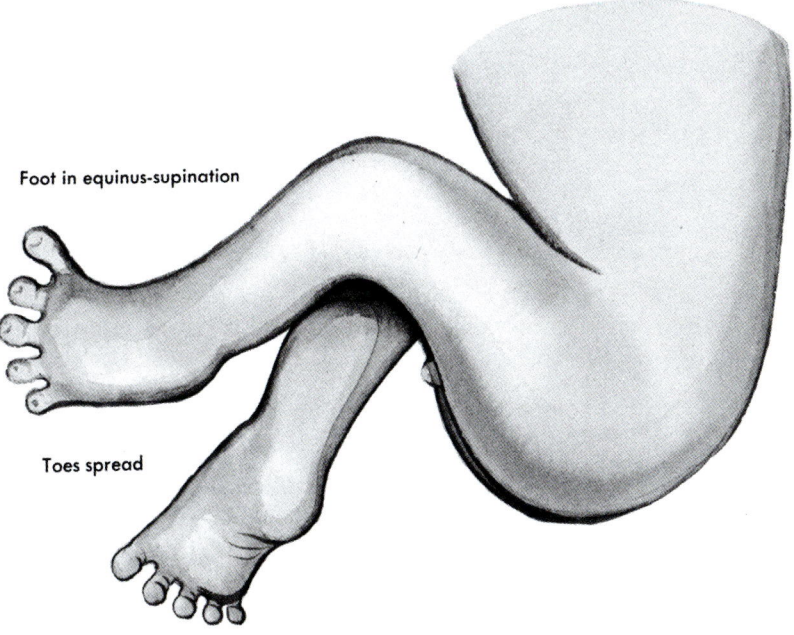

Figure 1.9 Embryo of horizon 23 (28-33 mm).

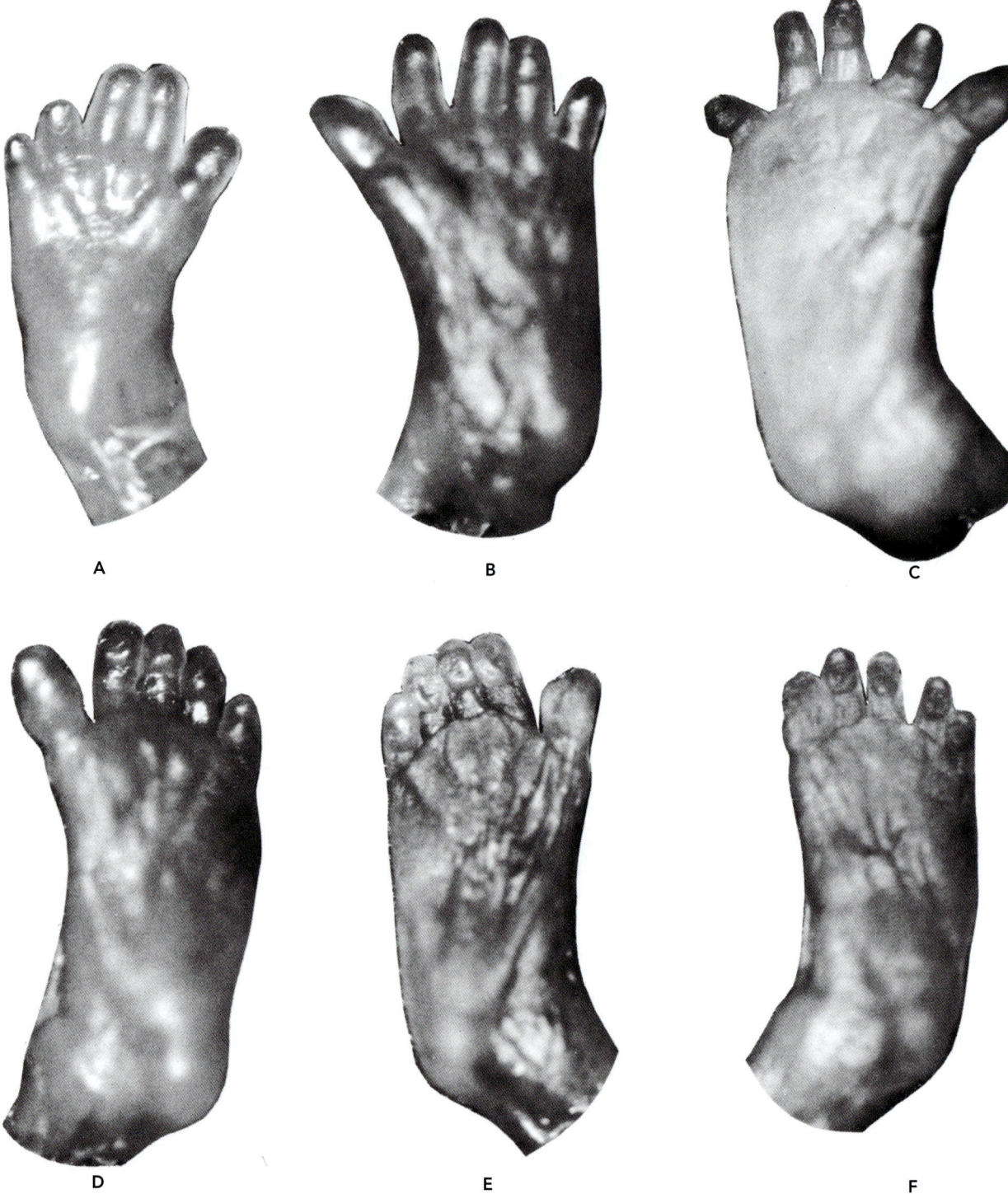

Figure 1.10 **Feet of embryos.** *Length*: **(A)** 3.5 mm; **(B)** 4 mm; **(C)** 5.5 mm; **(D)** 5 mm; **(E)** 6 mm; and **(F)** 6 mm.

Digital formula
2 > 3 > 4 > 1 > 5
3 > 2 > 4 > 1 > 5
3 > 4 > 2 > 1 > 5
2 > 3 > 1 > 4 > 5
2 > 3 > 4 > 1 > 5
2 > 3 > 1 > 4 > 5.

- Group 3 (5 feet total):
  - Two feet (11 mm, 12 mm): 2 > 1 > 3 > 4 > 5
  - One foot (10 mm): 2 > 3 > 1 > 4 > 5
  - Two feet (11 mm, 14 mm): 1 > 2 > 3 > 4 > 5

It is apparent, based on these measurements, that the third toe is the longest in the very young embryo. As the embryo grows, the third toe loses its place to the second. Later, the first toe moves next to the second, thus reaching one variation of the adult digital formula (2 > 1 > 3 > 4 > 5), and in the oldest embryos of this group (11 and 14 mm), the first toe took the lead with the common adult distribution (1 > 2 > 3 > 4 > 5).

Metatarsal Formula

In the embryo, the metatarsal formula initially is 3 > 2 > 1 > 4 > 5 or 3 > 2 > 4 > 5 > 1. In the fourth and fifth month of fetal life, the rule is 2 > 3 > 1 > 4 > 5, already resembling the common adult formula. From the sixth to the ninth month, the metatarsal formula is 2 > 1 > 3 > 4 > 5 or the occasional variant 2 > 3 > 1 > 4 > 5.[5]

Plantar or Walking Pads

Plantar or walking pads are soft-tissue elevations produced by localized accumulation of subcutaneous connective tissue and fat (Fig. 1.11).[6]

In the embryo of horizon 20, four distal plantar pads appear, corresponding to the interdigital spaces. A tibial pad and a fibular pad are also separately indicated. The proximal region of the sole of the foot shows no distinct pads. By horizon 22, five apical pads appear on the plantar aspect of the toes distally. The distal interdigital pads become more prominent in horizon 23, and on the tibial side, the first interdigital pad and the tibial pad merge to form the "hallucal pad." The interdigital pads are reduced to three. A central sole pad now makes its appearance, and the heel region is also slightly elevated. In the embryo of 40 mm, the central pad is nearly level. A general regression of the pads occurs when the fetus is 100 mm in C-R length or older. The pads become gradually lower and discrete. These pads persist during the remaining period of gestation in discrete regressed form.

In the last fetal weeks, the feet are swollen and the pads are temporarily masked. In the postnatal phase, the hallucal and interdigital pads are demonstrable, and the fibular pads are not noticeable.

Foot Growth

Foot measurement is possible only after the embryo reaches a C-R length of 24 mm, that is, after horizon 21.[7,8]

In the early fetal stage (30-60 mm), the foot grows less rapidly than the body (sitting height). After 70 mm, until term,

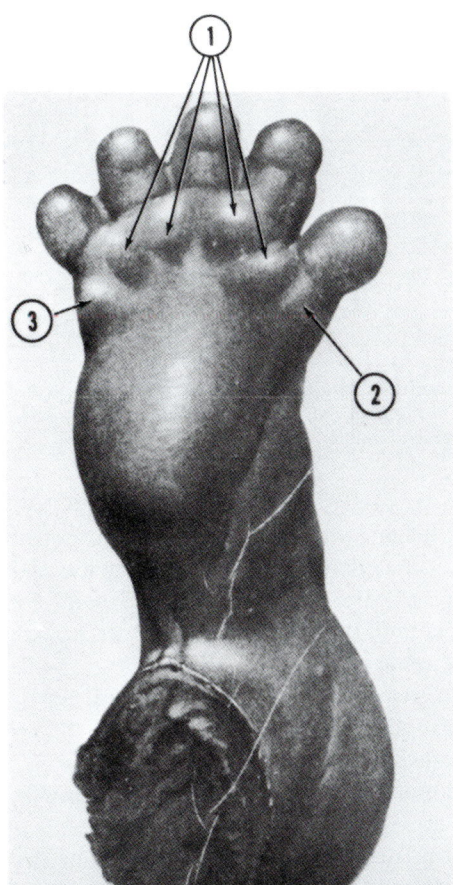
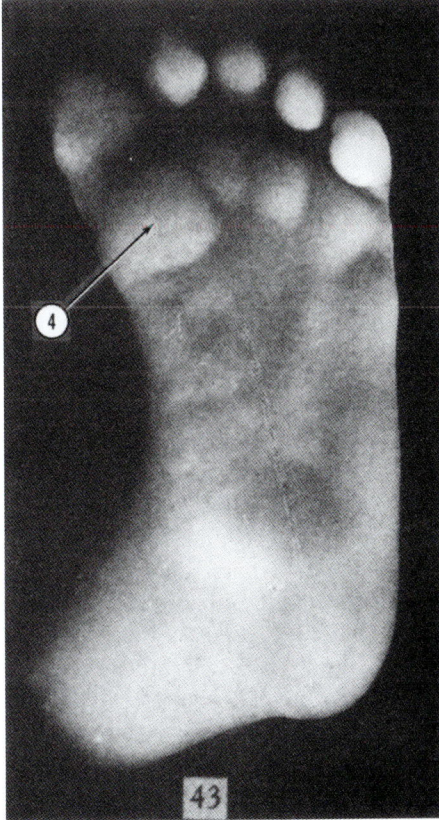

Figure 1.11 Plantar pads. **(A)** Foot of 24-mm embryo (*1*, interdigital pads; *2*, tibial pad; *3*, fibular pad). **(B)** Foot of 62.5-mm embryo (*4*, hallucal pad formed by fusion of tibial pad and first interdigital pad). (After Cummins H. The topographic history of the volar pads [walking pads, Tastballen] in the human embryo. *Contrib Embryol.* 1929;20:105.)

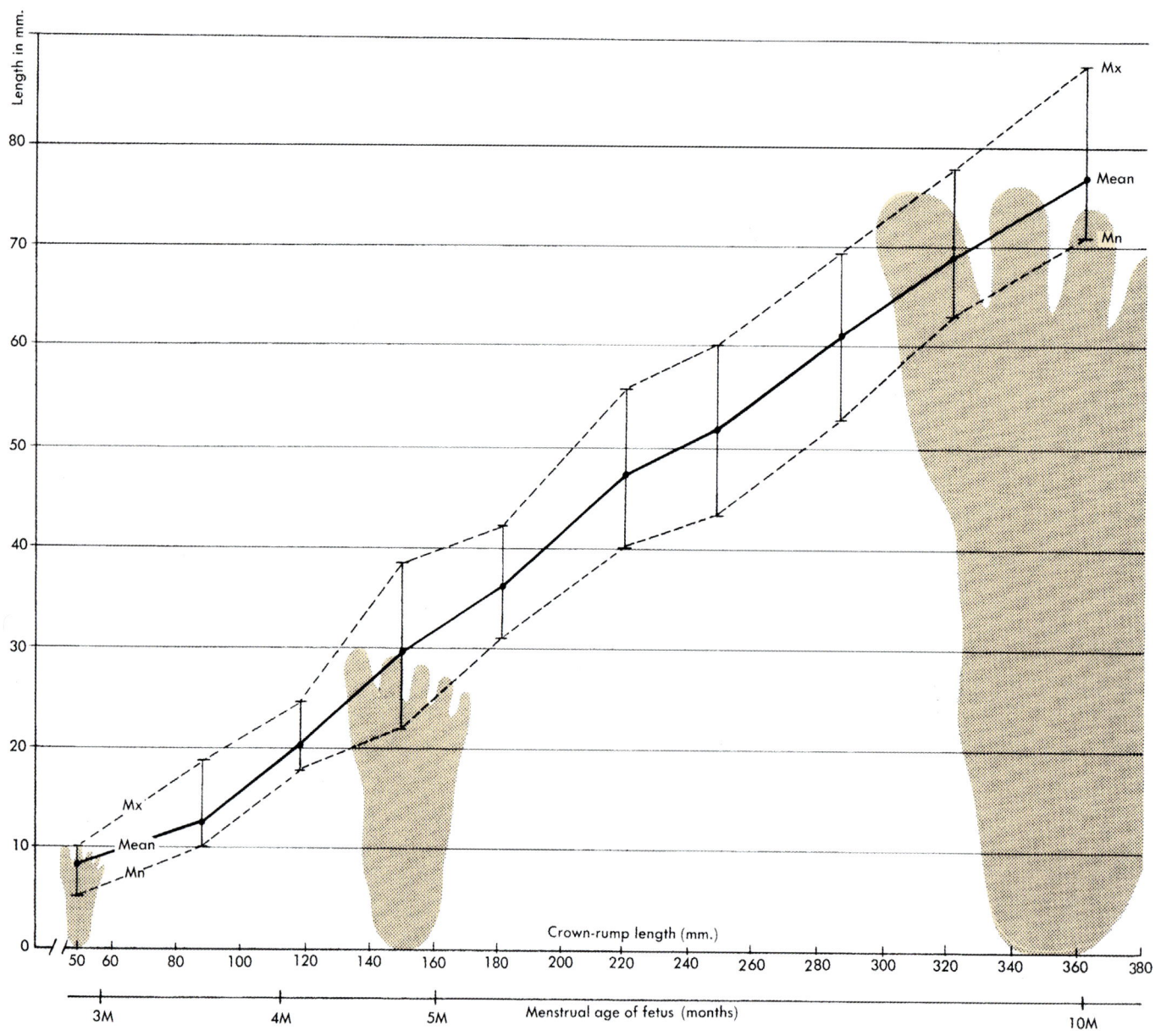

Figure 1.12 Prenatal foot growth and length. (Curves based on data from Scammon RE, Calkings LA. *The Development and Growth of the External Dimensions of the Human Body in the Fetal Period.* University of Minnesota Press; 1929:245-246.)

there is retardation in the increase of sitting height, whereas the foot maintains its growth rate and displays a relative acceleration of growth. This increase in foot length is slow from the 8th to the 14th week, then becomes more rapid until the 26th week, then slows down slightly until term. The average increase in length from the 14th week on is about 3 mm per week, with only slight variation.[7] The tabulated data of Scammon and Calkins, when converted into a growth curve, give the pattern shown in Figure 1.12.[8] At the end of the third month, the foot measures on average 0.8 cm, and at term, the average length is 7.6 cm (maximum, 8.7 cm; minimum, 7.1 cm). These dimensions are measured as a straight line from the posterior margin of the heel to the tip of the extended big toe.

The fetal foot narrows gradually with growth and remains longer than the adult foot when compared with the corresponding tibia length. The ratio of greatest foot length/tibia length is 1.41 at 8 weeks, 0.9 at birth, and 0.6 in the adult.[5]

▶ Internal Structures

Skeleton

The lower limb bud makes its appearance in horizon 13 (3-6 mm) at 4 weeks postfertilization. The bud is filled with blastemic tissue. An ectodermal thickening forms on the ventral aspect, and within 4 days, (horizon 15) it is converted into an ectodermal ridge on its lateral part. This ridge is transient and

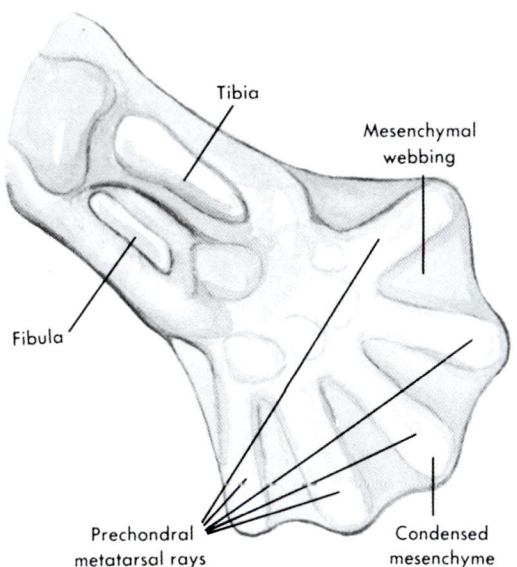

Figure 1.13 **Foot plate of embryo in horizon 18 (14-16 mm).** Skeleton in mesenchymal stage. (After Bardeen CR. Studies of the development of the human skeleton. *Am J Anat.* 1905;4:265.)

Mesenchymal. The mesenchymal stage is illustrated in Figure 1.13.[10,11] In horizons 17 (11-13 mm) and 18 (14-16 mm), the foot plate is already present. The axial mesenchyme condenses, differentiates, and forms the anlage of the foot. The metatarsals differentiate later. When the phalangeal models are formed, for a short time a thick web remains between the digital rays. The metatarsal rays are spread apart but they will gradually approximate.

The differentiation of the tarsus follows that of the metatarsals. Within the areas of condensation tissue, procartilage soon makes its appearance. The lower ends of the tibia and fibula are still formed of condensed blastemic tissue in horizon 20.

Cartilaginous. The cartilaginous stage is illustrated in Figure 1.14. Cartilage cells form in the mesenchymal-prochondral anlage. As the process of chondrification advances, the skeletal elements become clearly identifiable; morphogenesis, aiming toward the adult form, occurs. The chronologic sequence of chondrification was reported by Senior.[12] The process occurs in 14 stages (Fig. 1.15). The central three metatarsals chondrify first, followed by the fifth metatarsal and the cuboid. The chondrification of the tarsus continues with the calcaneus, the talus, and the third and second cuneiforms. The first cuneiform and the first metatarsal follow. The navicular is the last tarsal element to chondrify. The phalanges are next, and the process occurs in a proximodistal sequence.

The proximal phalanges of the second, third, and fourth toes chondrify, followed by the proximal phalanx of the fifth toe. The proximal phalanx of the big toe is next, to be followed by the middle phalanges of central toes two, three, and four. Next, in sequence is the chondrification of the middle phalanx of the little toe, the distal phalanx of the big

disappears within a week (horizon 19). Its importance seems primordial because it induces the differentiation of the future limb components and determines their directional (proximodistal) formation.[9]

Stages of Skeletal Development

There are three stages in the formation of skeletal elements: mesenchymal, cartilaginous, and osseous.

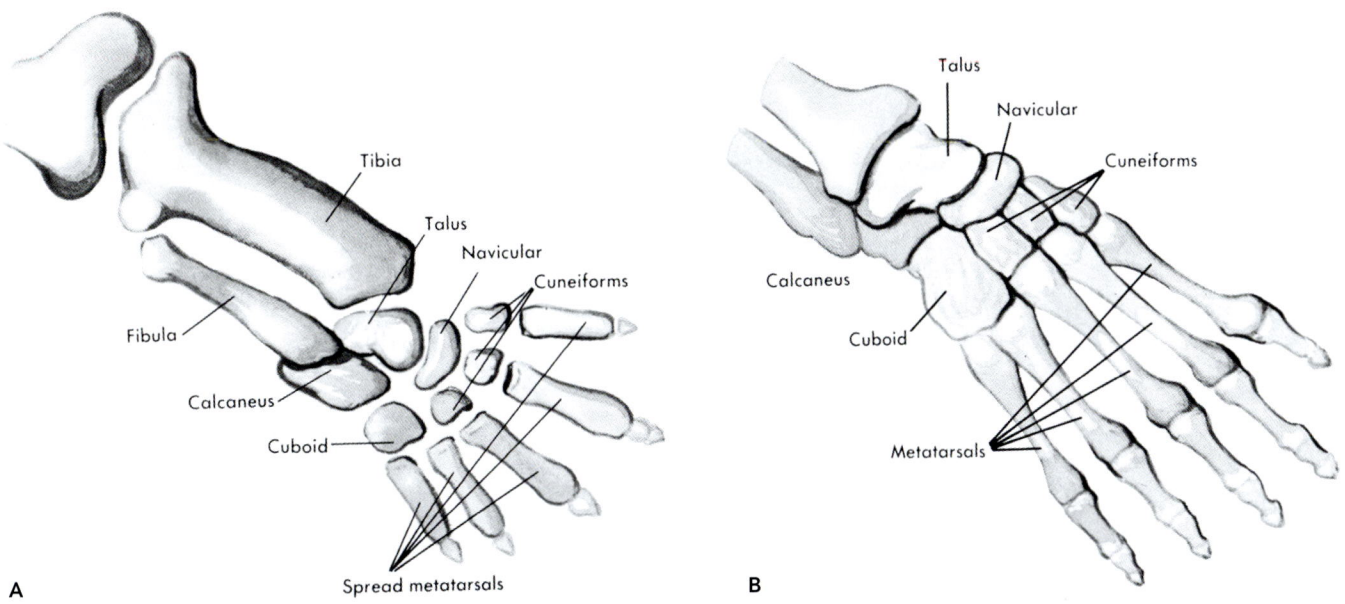

Figure 1.14 **(A) Foot and leg of embryo in horizon 19 (20 mm).** Skeleton in cartilaginous stage. **(B) Foot and ankle of 33-mm fetus.** Skeleton in cartilaginous stage. (After Bardeen CR. Studies of the development of the human skeleton. *Am J Anat.* 1905;4:265.)

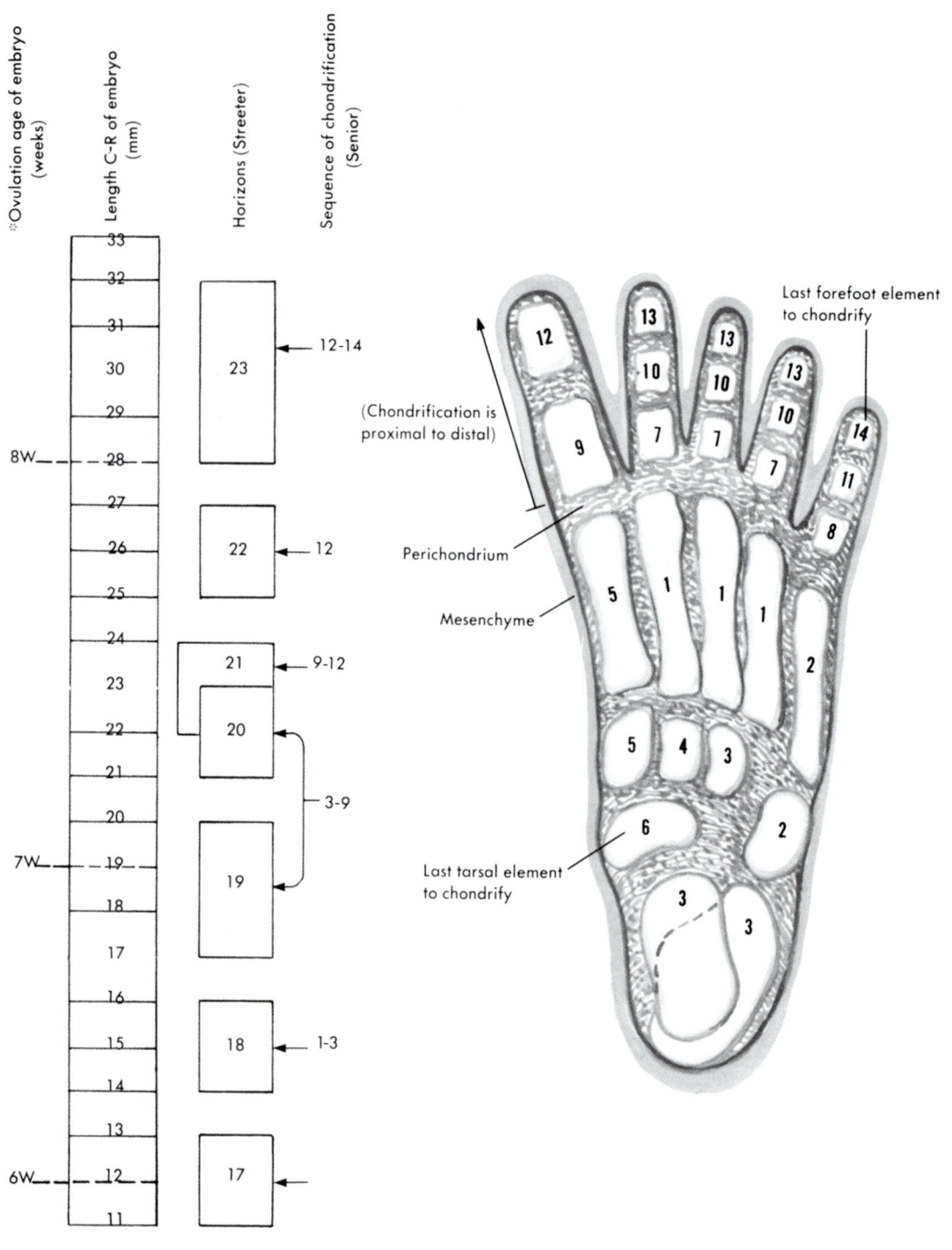

Figure 1.15 **Chronologic sequence of chondrification of the foot in the embryo.** (Based on data from Senior HD. The chondrification of the human hand and foot skeleton [abstr]. *Anat Rec.* 1929;42:35. Correlation between sequence of chondrification and Streeter's horizons based on O'Rahilly R, Gray DJ, Gardner E. Chondrification in the hands and feet of staged human embryos. *Contrib Embryol.* 1957;36:185.)

toe, and the distal phalanges of the second, third, and fourth toes. The last element to chondrify is the distal phalanx of the little toe.

The chondrification of the foot is initiated in horizon 18 (14-16 mm), and the last element, except for the sesamoids chondrifies in horizon 23 (28-32 mm), which represents the end of the embryonic period proper.

The relationship between Senior's sequence of chondrification and Streeter's horizons (see Fig. 1.15) has been reported by O'Rahilly and coworkers.[11]

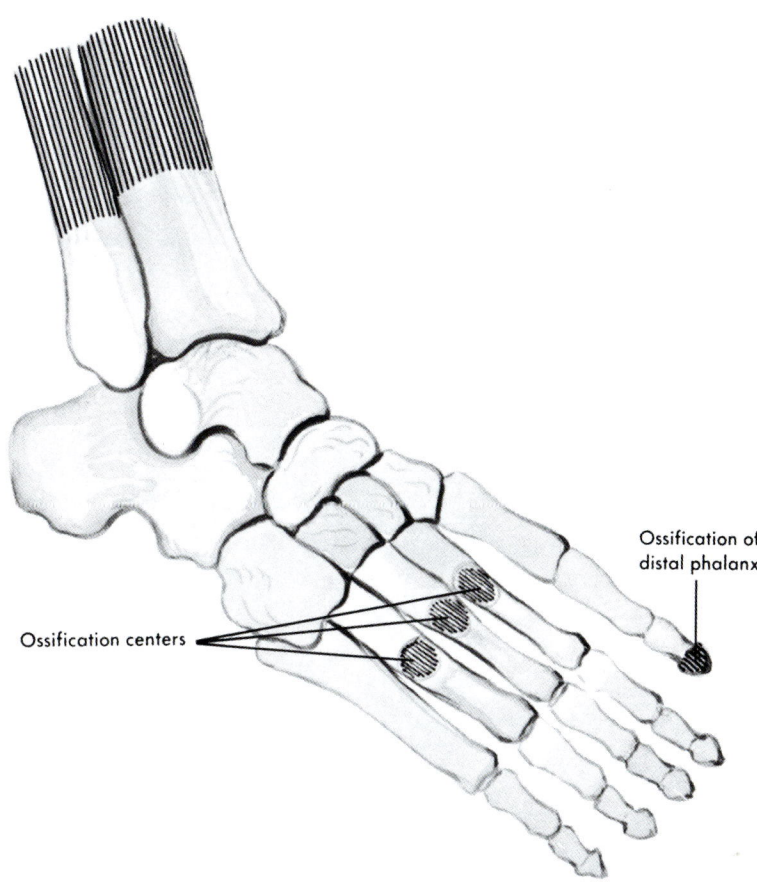

Figure 1.16 Foot of 50-mm fetus. Skeleton at onset of ossification. (After Bardeen CR. Studies of the development of the human skeleton. *Am J Anat.* 1905;4:265.)

Within a given condensed mesenchymal unit, chondrification of the future anatomic components occurs at different times. The body of the calcaneus begins to chondrify centrally in horizon 18, the tuber calcanei in horizon 21, and the sustentaculum tali in horizon 23.[13]

By the end of the embryologic period proper, the morphology and relationship of the cartilaginous skeletal components are determined and resemble closely those of the adult. The future articular surfaces acquire their definite contour at this early stage, prior to the formation of a joint space.[10]

Chondrification is present in the distal tibia and fibula in horizon 21.

Osseous. The osseous stage is shown in Figures 1.16 and 1.17.[10,13,14] The forefoot ossifies before the hindfoot. The general sequence of ossification is distal phalanx of the big toe, metatarsals, distal phalanges of lesser toes, proximal phalanges, and finally middle phalanges. The last element to ossify in the forefoot is the middle phalanx of the little toe. The ossification of the forefoot takes place between the third and fifth prenatal lunar months.

In the hindfoot, the calcaneus is the first to ossify. Gardner and associates describe periosteal bone formation on the inferolateral aspect of the calcaneus in a 93-mm fetus.[13] At 125 mm, the endochondral center of ossification appears. The talus may begin to ossify during the eighth lunar month but an ossification center is not always present at birth. An extensive study correlating roentgenographic findings with body weight in the newborn indicates that regardless of the weight of the newborn, the calcaneus is always ossified; the talus is also ossified except in infants weighing less than 2000 g.[15] In this low–birth-weight group, talar ossification was absent at birth in an average of 13.3% of infants. The cuboid is the last tarsal element that can exhibit prenatal ossification.

The histologic process of ossification is periosteal and endochondral in the metatarsals and proximal and middle phalanges. A bone collar forms first around the middle of the cartilaginous diaphysis, followed by invasion of the cartilaginous shaft by a periosteal bud, thus initiating the endochondral ossification that extends in a proximal and distal direction.

The distal phalanx differs in this regard from the other phalanges. The intramembranous and endochondral ossification starts at the tip and extends proximally. Dixey clearly describes the process as a "cap" of intramembranous bone formed at the distal end of the cartilaginous phalanx.[16] This cap is then converted into a bony "thimble fitting over the cartilaginous phalanx and enclosing it almost up to its base."[16]

Morphologic Development of the Skeletal Elements of the Foot

Embryonic Phase and Early Fetal Phase

Bardeen and, more recently, Olivier provided a detailed morphologic study of the skeletal elements of the foot in the embryonic phase.[10,17] In the 13.5-mm embryo, Olivier describes a

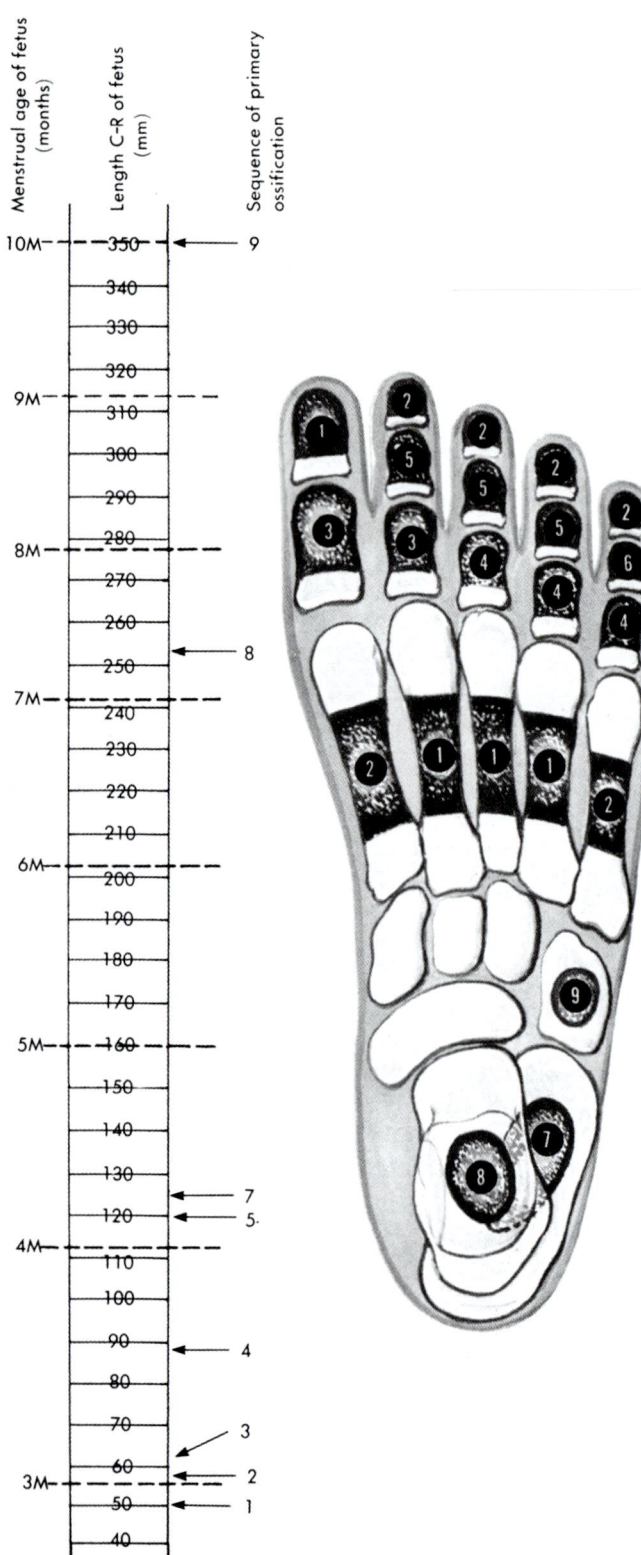

Figure 1.17 Chronologic sequence of ossification of fetal foot. (Correlation of menstrual age and C-R length based on Arey LB. *Developmental Anatomy.* 7th ed. WB Saunders; 1965:104.)

foot with three rays: a principal median ray and two lateral rudimentary rays.[17] This tridactylic stage suggests a fanlike growth from the median axis. This primitive foot is digitigrade and in acute plantarflexion, and there is no evidence of angulation of the foot relative to the leg.

The interosseous slit of the leg is extended onto the ventral aspect by a groove and divides the foot into two parts: preaxial (cranial), comprising the second ray, a rudiment of the first ray, the tarsal elements corresponding to the talus, the navicular, and the cuneiforms; and postaxial (caudal), comprising the third ray, the beginning of the fourth ray, and the tarsal elements corresponding to the cuboid and the calcaneus.[17] The fibula is extended by the calcaneus and the three lateral rays.

In embryos measuring 14.2 and 17 mm (horizon 18), the foot presents five rays separated fanlike from each other. The foot is sagittal in orientation, with the medial border cranial and the lateral border caudal. The mesenchymal anlages of the distal end of the tibia and fibula in horizon 18 (14 mm) are separated, and the talar element is wedged in between.[17] The distal end of the tibia is oblique and concave. Because of the obliquity of the tibial surface, the medial malleolus projects more distally than the end of the fibula (Fig. 1.18). In horizons 19 (17 mm) and 20 (21 mm), the malleoli are at the same level; it is only after horizon 22 (27 mm) that the lateral malleolus extends more distally than the medial. The fibulocalcaneal contact is established early and is clearly present at horizon 20 (21 mm). The tip of the lateral malleolus loses contact with the calcaneus at horizon 22 (27 mm). It is during this period that the distal tibia and fibula come close and establish contact for the formation of a distal tibiofibular joint; this is a relatively late occurrence in the embryonic developmental period.

The talus is delineated at horizon 18 (14.2 mm; see Fig. 1.18).[17] The contour is irregular. The element is angled at 90°, with a transverse segment corresponding to the body and future trochlea, and a sagittal segment located inward and inferiorly, corresponding to the neck and head. The superior surface is located between the tibia and the fibula. The element of the talar neck is directed toward the second metatarsal. Only the lateral third of the lower surface establishes contact with the calcaneus (Fig. 1.19). The anterior surface is in continuity with the navicular. The posterior part of the lateral surface has a surface corresponding to the lateral malleolus. The posterior part of the medial surface presents a convex surface (see Fig. 1.18) corresponding to the tibial plafond and the medial malleolus. At this stage "the talus is low, large, and located on the medial flank of the calcaneum over which it overlaps slightly; there is yet no torsion of the head nor clear declination of the neck."[17]

Sudden rapid changes occur in horizon 22 (27 mm). The sustentaculum tali appears, and the talus passes nearly entirely over the calcaneus (see Fig. 1.19). The talus "narrows transversely, elongates but does not elevate yet."[17] The superior talar surface is flat, descending medially and articulating with the tibia. No true trochlea is present yet. At 34 mm, the talus more or less resembles the adult structure (see Fig. 1.19). The foot has pronated. The declination angle of the talar neck-head has increased to 25°. The cephalic torsion has not occurred. The trochlea is narrow; the lateral process is well developed,

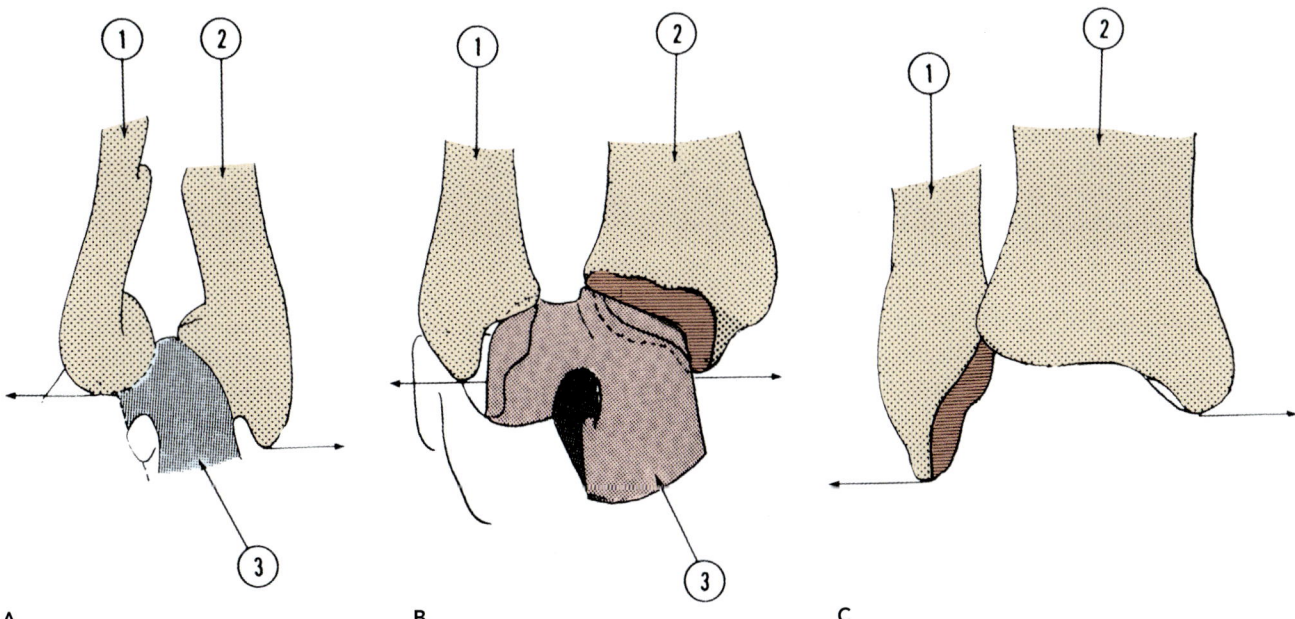

Figure 1.18 **(A) Ankle of embryo in horizon 18 (14 mm).** The talus is wedged between the tibia and the fibula. The distal end of the tibia is oblique and concave. The distal ends of the fibula and tibia are separated, and the former is proximal to the medial malleolus. **(B) Ankle of embryo in horizon 19 (17 mm).** The distal tibia and fibula are still separated, and the talus is wedged between the two. The fibular and tibial malleoli are at the same level. The talus is angled at 90°. **(C) Ankle of embryo in horizon 22 (27 mm).** The lateral malleolus is more distal than the medial malleolus (*1*, fibula; *2*, tibia; *3*, talus). (Adapted from Olivier G. *Formation du Squelette des Membres*. Vigot Frères; 1962.)

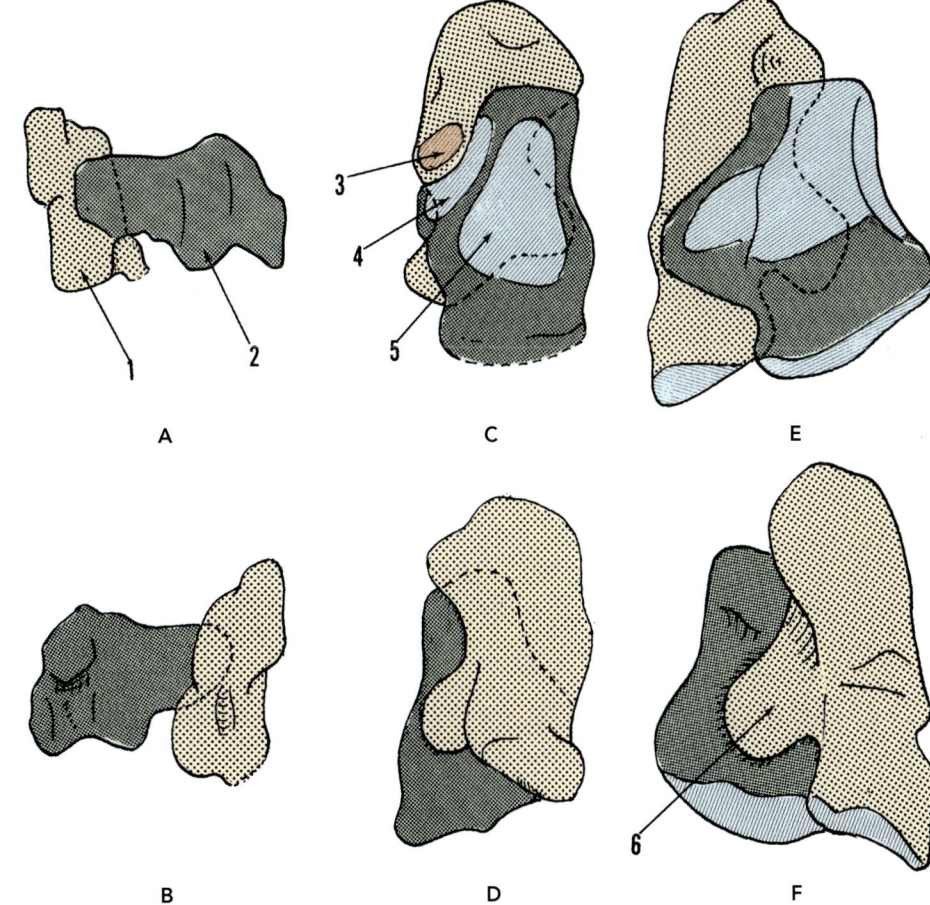

Figure 1.19 **Talocalcaneal formation and relationships.** Dorsal **(A, B)** plantar views of an embryo of 21 mm. Dorsal **(C, D)** plantar views of an embryo of 27 mm. The talus and the calcaneus overlap. The sustentaculum tali is initiated. The calcaneus presents an articular facet to the distal end of the fibula. The talus is narrower and longer. The lateral and superior talar articular surfaces are initiated but separated. **(E)** Dorsal and **(F)** plantar views of a fetus of 34 mm. The sustentaculum tali is well developed. The dorsal, lateral, and medial articular surfaces of the talus have merged. The calcaneal facet for the distal fibula has disappeared (*1*, calcaneus; *2*, talus; *3*, calcaneal articular facet for the distal fibula; *4*, lateral articular facet of talus; *5*, superior trochlear articular facet of talus; *6*, sustentaculum tali). (Adapted from Olivier G. *Formation du Squelette des Membres*. Vigot Frères; 1962.)

supporting the articular surface for the lateral malleolus. The talus is still a relatively flat structure. The navicular has separated from the talar head.

The calcaneus is initially short, with a narrow superior surface.[17] The anteromedial segment of this surface corresponds to the talar overlapping segment; the posterolateral segment gives support to the distal end of the fibula. This small fibular supportive surface, still seen early in horizon 22 (27 mm), fades away, with the lateral malleolus retaining only the talar relationship. The sustentaculum tali, clearly present at horizon 22, extends further medially, and by 34 mm, it nears the medial border of the talus. The inferior calcaneal surface presents a large posterolateral tuberosity in horizon 19 (17 mm), and by horizon 20 (21 mm), a posteromedial tuberosity emerges.

McKee and Bagnall[18] studied the skeletal relationship of the ankle, hindfoot, and forefoot in six human embryos with a C-R length ranging from 21.7 to 34.0 mm, representing horizon 20 to horizon 23. Three-dimensional reconstruction was used to recreate the skeletal elements of the embryonic foot. The sections were made in three different views of the embryonic foot. When observations were made with the sole of the foot directed downward, as if the foot were in the standard anatomic position, the embryonic calcaneus appeared to be located on the fibular side of the talus with the calcaneus exposed (Fig. 1.20). The tibia extended further plantarward than the fibula, and the medial malleolus was longer than the fibular malleolus. When the relationship of the skeletal elements was reconsidered with the embryonic first metatarsal directed cranially, a completely different relationship was evident. With the forefoot thus inverted, the study of the hindfoot skeletal elements as seen in the coronal sections indicated clearly the calcaneus situated below the talus and the fibula extended further than the tibia, as in the adult foot (Fig. 1.21).

The navicular is isolated at horizon 20 (21 mm).[17] It is flat and enters in contact laterally with the cuboid.

The cuboid is slightly distinct at horizon 20.[17] An anteromedial extension wedges between the bases of the third and fourth metatarsals. A medial extension meets the navicular. At 34 mm, the cuboid resembles the cuneiforms and articulates obliquely with the anterior surface of the calcaneus.

The lateral and middle cuneiforms are not distinct at horizon 20.[17] The medial cuneiform is present and voluminous, and the anterior surface is oriented anteriorly and medially.[17] Cuneiforms 2 and 3 appear in horizon 22 (27 mm). The second cuneiform is the smallest and the highest; "the anterior surface is at the level of the lateral cuneiform and even of the fourth metatarsal, therefore without any evidence of posterior retreat."[17]

Fetal Phase

During the fetal period of development, morphologic changes continue. A comprehensive study has been conducted by Straus.[5]

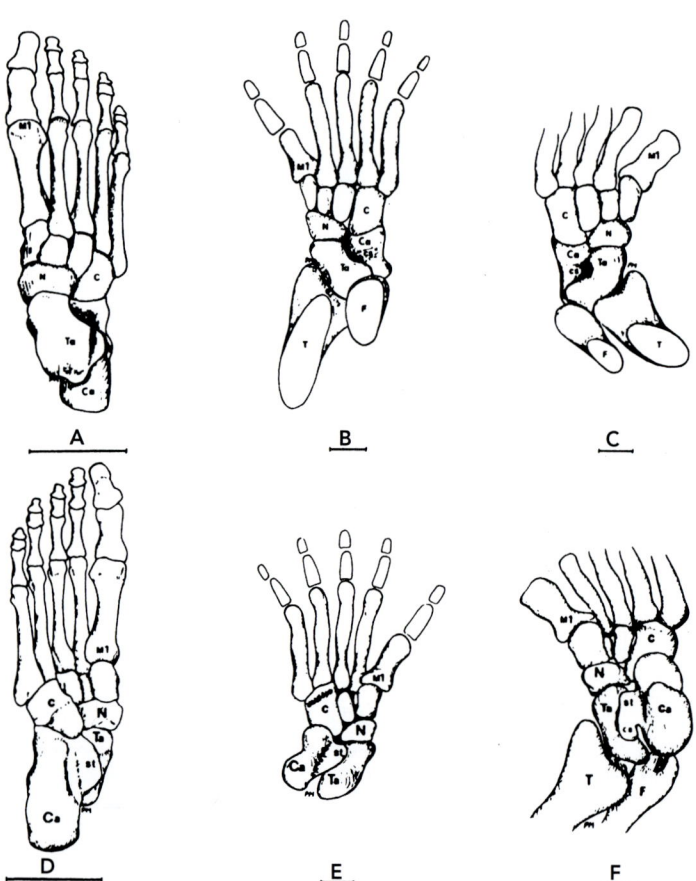

Figure 1.20 Embryonic skeletal elements compared to the adult foot. **(A, D)** Adult, right foot. **(B, E)** Embryo XXIIa, right foot. **(C, F)** Embryo XXIII, left foot. **(A–C)** Dorsal views. **(D–F)** Plantar views. C, cuboid; C1, medial/first cuneiform; C2, intermediate cuneiform/second; C3, lateral/third cuneiform; Ca, calcaneus; cs, calcaneal sulcus; F, fibula; M1, first metatarsal; M2, second metatarsal; M3, third metatarsal; M4, fourth metatarsal; M5, fifth metatarsal; N, navicular; st, sustentaculum tali; T, tibia; Ta, talus). **(A, D)** Bar = 5 cm. **(B, F)** Bar = 0.5 mm. **(C, F)** Bar = 0.5 mm. (After Mckee PR, Bagnall KM. Skeletal relationships in the human embryonic foot based on three-dimensional reconstructions. *Acta Anat.* 1987;129:34.)

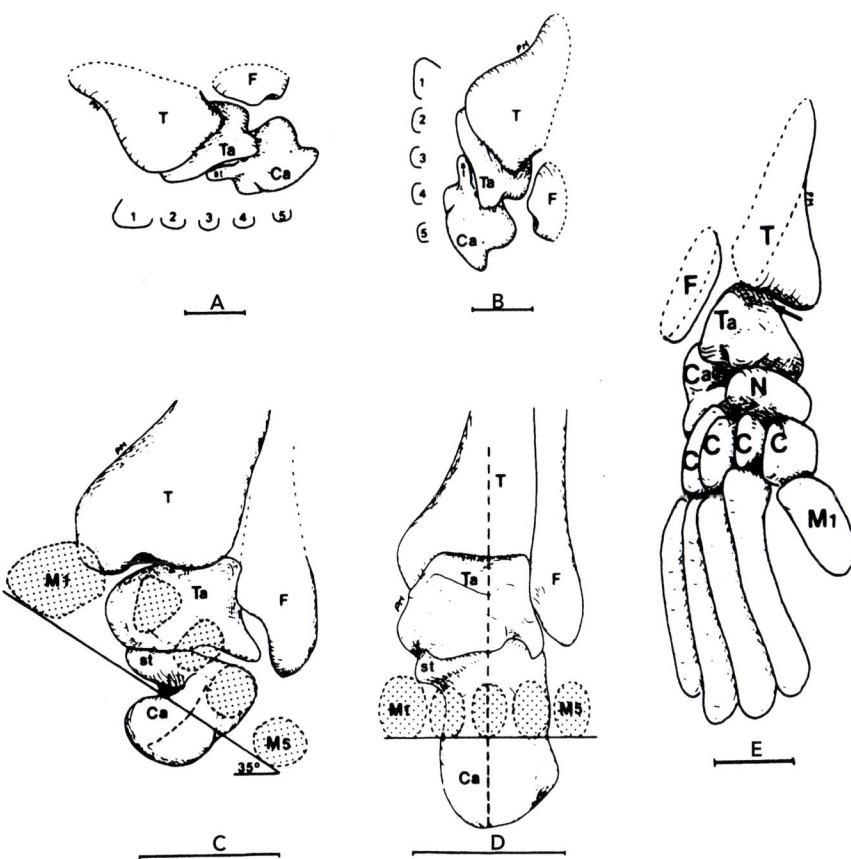

Figure 1.21 Hindfoot-forefoot relationships, comparing the embryonic and the adult foot (Abbreviations as in Fig. 1.20.). **(A)** Embryo XXIIa. Posterior view of right foot, drawn from the wax-plate model (developed from horizontal sections), oriented with the sole of the foot directed downward and with the metatarsal heads (1-5) in the horizontal plane, as in the standard anatomic position. **(B)** Embryo XXIIa. Posterior view of right foot, drawn from the wax-plate model, oriented with the sole of the foot facing medially and the first metatarsal (1) directed cranially, as in the embryonic position. **(C)** Embryo XXI. Posterior view of right foot, drawn from the transparency reconstruction (developed from coronal sections). A tracing through the metatarsal shafts (M1–M5, darkly shaded) has been superimposed in its aligned position onto the bones of the hindfoot. **(D)** Adult. Posterior view of right foot in the anatomic weight-bearing position. The broken line represents the vertical orientation of the long axis of the leg. The solid line represents the orientation of the metatarsal heads (M1–M5, shaded), which is perpendicular to the long axis of the leg. **(E)** Embryo XXIIa. Anterodorsal view, drawn from the wax-plate model, which has been oriented by placing the forefoot in approximately 35° of inversion. The *arrow* points to the trochlear surface of the talus. **(A–C, E)** Bars = 0.5 mm. **(D)** Bar = 5 cm. (After McKee PR, Bagnall KM. Skeletal relationships in the human embryonic foot based on three dimensional reconstructions. *Acta Anat.* 1987;129:34.)

Bones. The talus does not grow uniformly in all directions (Fig. 1.22). The talar body increases more rapidly in height than in length. The width of the posterior talar segment increases slightly more rapidly than the length.

The talar neck-trochlea declination angle narrows steadily during fetal development (see Fig. 1.22). Furthermore, the angle formed by the long axis of the talar head and the transverse axis of the talar body increases gradually as the head turns more and more laterally (Fig. 1.23). The lateral shift and the lateral torsion of the talar head-neck are some of the factors explaining the correction of the pedal supination.

The calcaneus of the fetus has a very short body, but subsequent to the initial stage, this segment grows faster relative to the total calcaneal length. A gradual increase of the posterior segment of the calcaneus results, contributing to the mechanical efficiency of the triceps surae (Fig. 1.24). It is also of interest to note that at 3 months the calcaneus of the fetus represents an average of 25.3% (range, 22.7%-27.9%) of the total foot length; in the adult, its contribution is 35% (range, 33.2%-38.5%).

The long axes of the calcaneal tuber and of the tibial diaphysis determine the angle of torsion of the calcaneus (see Fig. 1.24). At 3 months, the supination-varus angle of the calcaneus is 36.8° (range, 35°-38°). This angle decreases gradually; by 9 months, it is 26.3° (range, 24.5°-29.5°), and in the adult, it measures 3.5° (range, 1°-6°).[5] The calcaneus is overlapped by the talus, and during fetal growth, the collum tali and calcaneal angle narrows from 42° at 4 months to 30° at birth. The talar trochlear-calcaneal angle diminishes from 9° at 4 months to 1° at 9 months (Fig. 1.25).

De Palma et al[19] studied the development of the talocalcaneal joint in embryos at 8 weeks and in fetuses from 9 to 20 weeks. At 8 weeks, the talus and the calcaneus "appear as cartilaginous areas separated by mesenchymal tissue" (Fig. 1.26A). There is no talocalcaneal cavitation. At 9 weeks, cavitation of the subtalar joint is present and proceeds faster at the posterior talocalcaneal joint area (Fig. 1.26B). At 10 weeks, the "posterior surface of the subtalar joint is well formed." The anterior talocalcaneal joint and the spring ligament are visible (Fig. 1.26C). At 11 weeks, "the cavitational process of the subtalar joint is shown to be developing differentially in three regions, anterior, middle, and posterior" (Fig. 1.27A,B). The sinus tarsi and tarsal canal are well developed. At 14 weeks, "all the articular and capsuloligamentous structures of the subtalar joint and the sinus tarsi are clearly evident" (Fig. 1.27C,D).

In the fetus, the first metatarsal is shorter and thicker than the second metatarsal (Fig. 1.28).[5] Until birth, the first metatarsal grows faster than the second metatarsal; subsequently, they develop at about the same rate. The metatarsal 1 to metatarsal 2 length ratio is 0.73 (range, 0.63-0.81) at 3 months, 0.33 (range, 0.80-0.85) at 9 months, and 0.83 (range, 0.79-0.88) in the adult. The angle of divergence of the first two metatarsals is 32° at 2 months. Gradually, the divergence of the first metatarsal

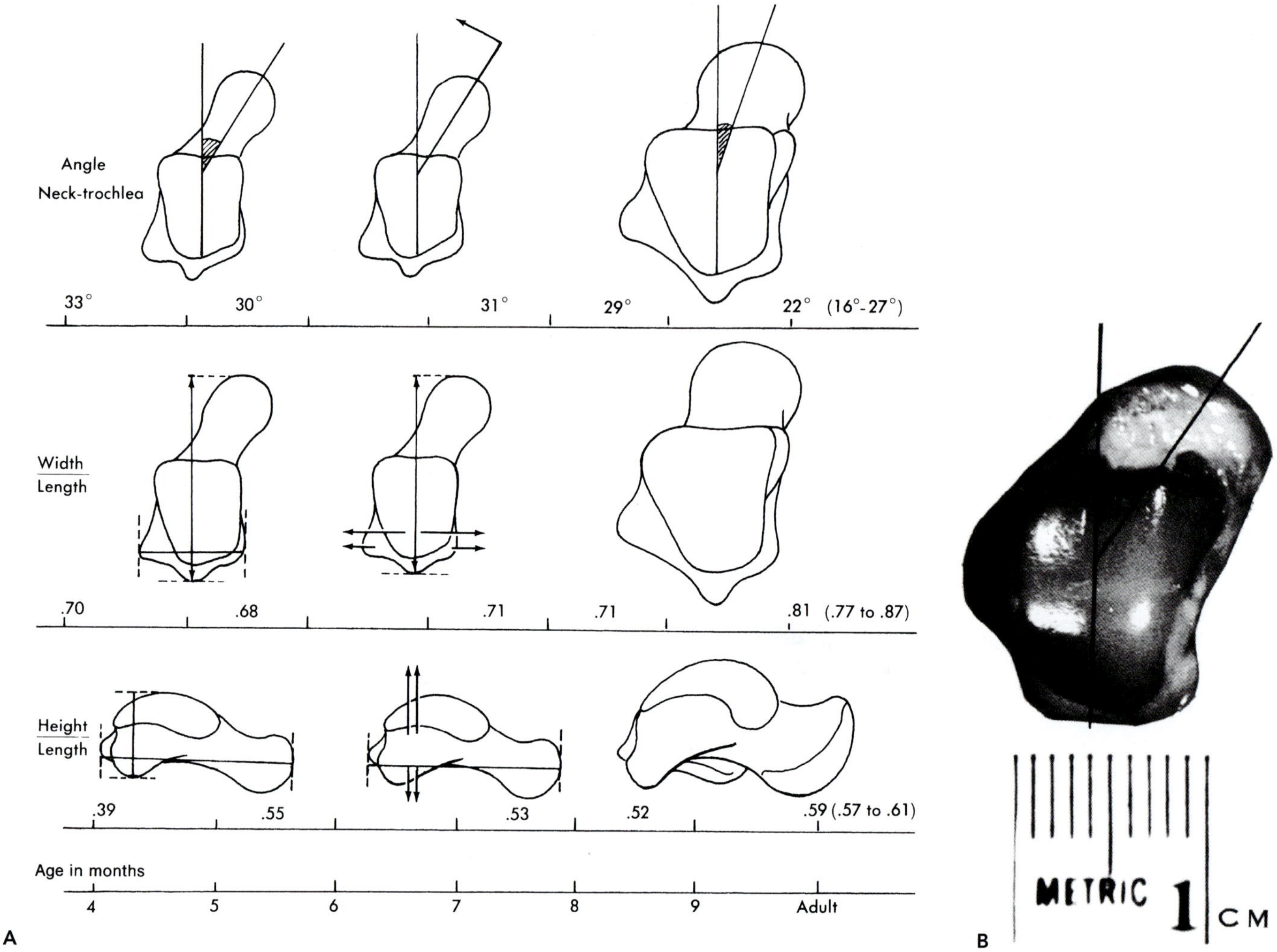

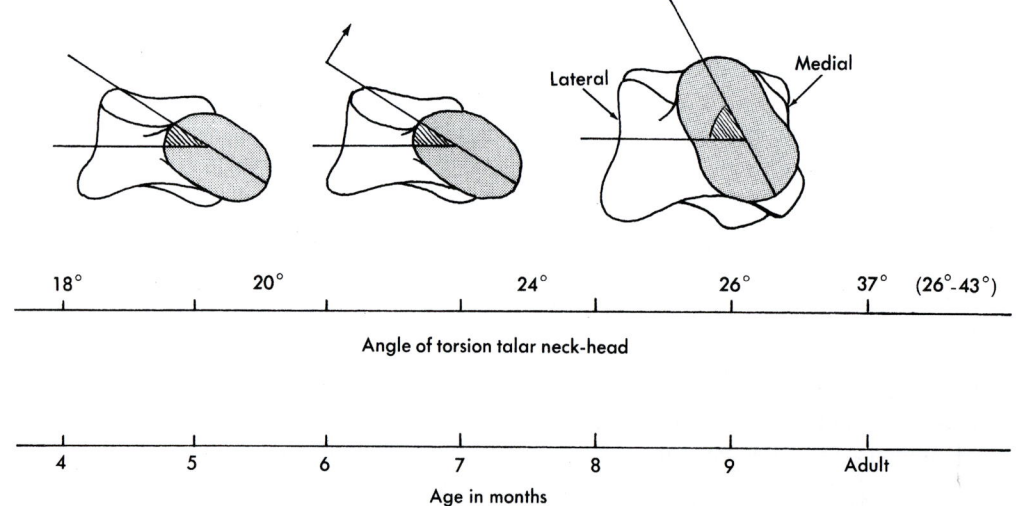

Figure 1.22 **(A) Morphologic changes and growth of the talus in fetus. (B) Declination angle between the trochlea and the neck of the talus in 7-month fetus.** ([A] Diagrammatic representation based on data from Straus WL Jr. Growth of the human foot and its evolutionary significance. *Contrib Embryol.* 1927;19:95.)

Figure 1.23 **Lateral rotation of the talar head in the fetus and in the postnatal phase.** The rotation contributes to the prone position of the foot. (Diagrammatic representation based on data from Straus WL Jr. Growth of the human foot and its evolutionary significance. *Contrib Embryol.* 1927;19:95.)

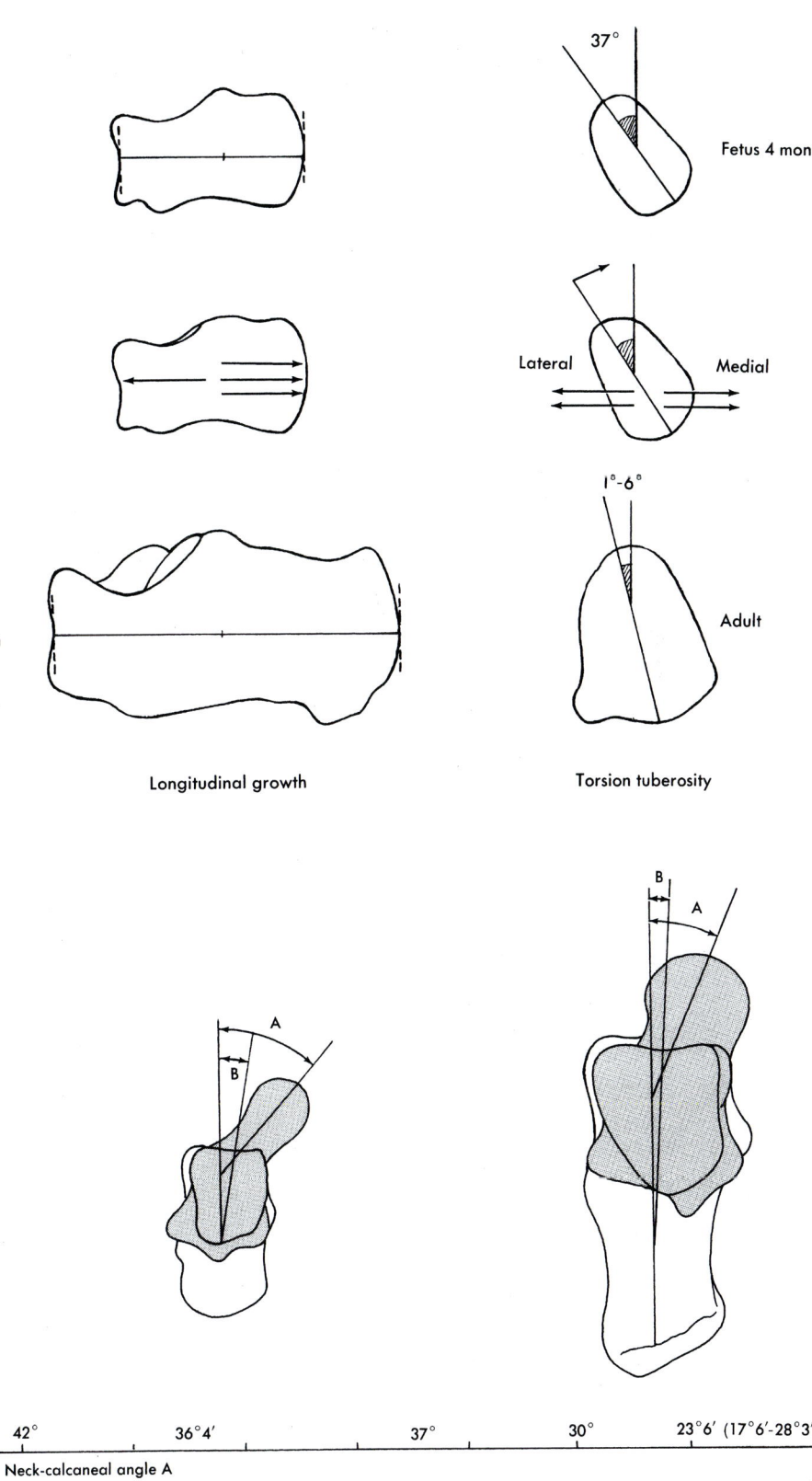

Figure 1.24 **Morphologic changes and growth of the calcaneus.** The posterior aspect of the calcaneal body grows faster than the anterior segment. In the fetus, the os calcis is in varus torsion, which gradually diminishes. (Diagrammatic representation based on data from Straus WL Jr. Growth of the human foot and its evolutionary significance. *Contrib Embryol.* 1927;19:95.)

Figure 1.25 **Talar neck and calcaneal angle (A) and talar trochlear and calcaneal angle (B) in the fetus and in postnatal phase.** Both angles diminish with growth, and this contributes to the correction of the adducted position of the forefoot. (Diagrammatic representation based on data from Straus WL Jr Growth of the human foot and its evolutionary significance. *Contrib Embryol.* 1927;19:95.)

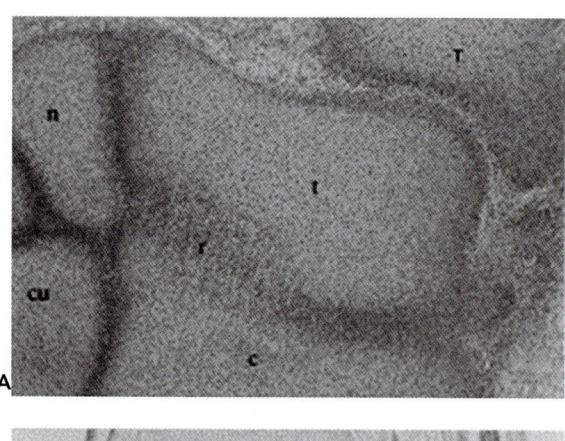
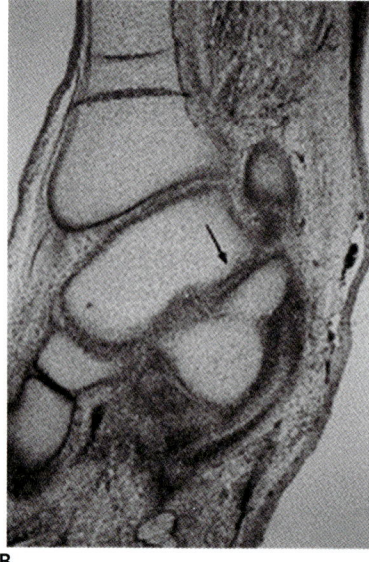
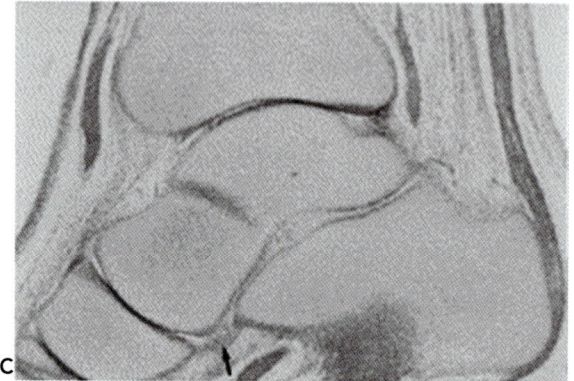

Figure 1.26 (A) **Embryo, 8 weeks: sagittal section.** Cavitational patterns of the talocalcaneal joint are absent (*c*, calcaneus; *cu*, cuboid; *n*, navicular; *r*, subtalar mesenchymal tissue; *T*, tibia; *t*, talus). (B) **Fetus, 9 weeks: frontal section.** Cavitation of the talocalcaneal joint is evident and proceeds more quickly in the posterior aspect of the joint (*arrow*). (C) **Fetus, 10 weeks: sagittal section.** The posterior and anterior surfaces of the talocalcaneal joint are well defined. The plantar calcaneonavicular ligament (*arrow*) is maturing. (Reprinted from de Palma L, Santucci A, Ventura A, et al. Anatomy and embryology of the talocalcaneal joint. *Foot Ankle Surg.* 2003;9:7-18, Figure 1, with permission from Elsevier.)

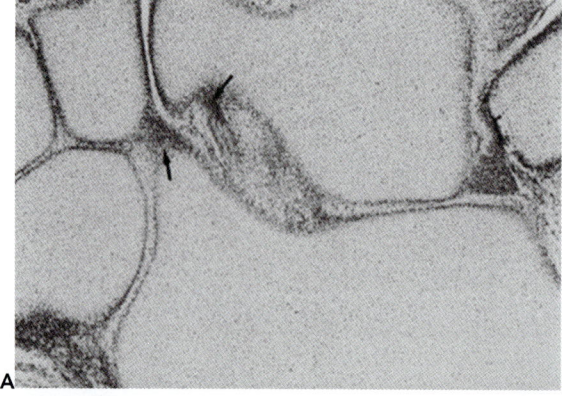
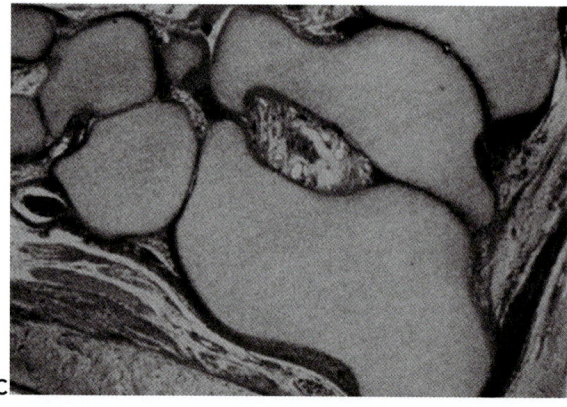
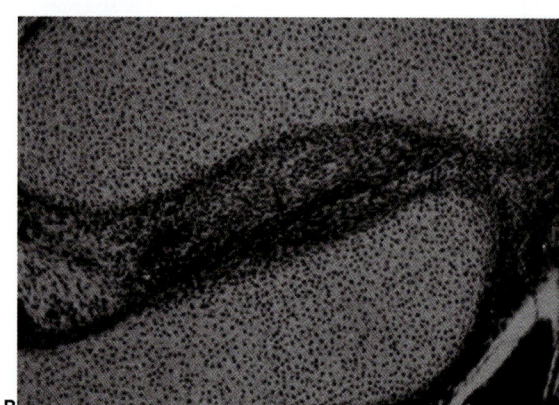
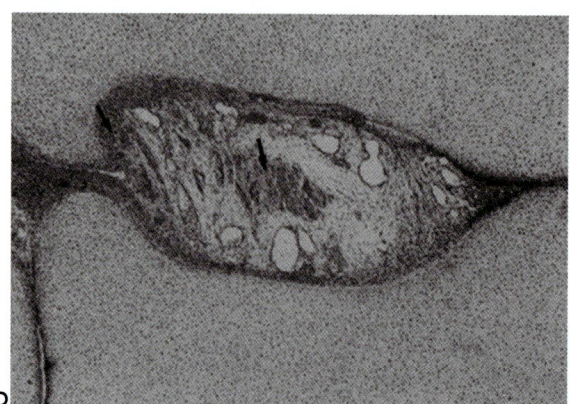

Figure 1.27 (A) **Fetus, 11 weeks: sagittal section.** Cavitational process of the subtatalar joint. The sinus tarsi and tarsal canal are well developed. The precursor of the calcaneonavicular ligament can be seen (*arrow*). (B) **Fetus 11 weeks: frontal section at the level of the sinus tarsi and canalis tarsi.** The precursor of the interosseous ligament can be detected. (C) **Fetus 14 weeks: sagittal section.** The articular and capsuloligamentous structures are recognized. (D) **Fetus 13 weeks: sagittal section (higher magnification).** Sinus tarsi ligament (*arrow*) with well-vascularized connective tissue. (Reprinted from de Palma L, Santucci A, Ventura A, et al. Anatomy and embryology of the talocalcaneal joint. *Foot Ankle Surg.* 2003;9:7-18, Figure 2, with permission from Elsevier.)

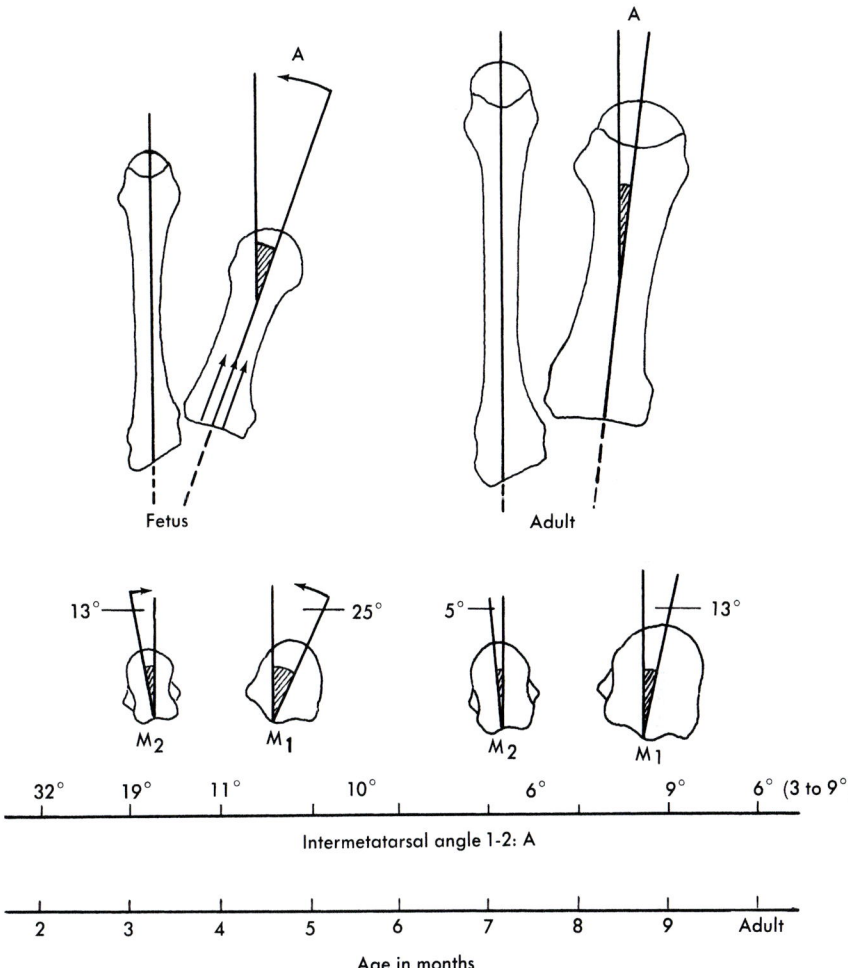

Figure 1.28 Intermetatarsal M1–M2 angle and rotation of the metatarsal heads M1 and M2 during growth. The intermetatarsal angle (A) decreases with time. The first metatarsal grows faster than the lesser metatarsals to reach its adult length. (Diagrammatic representation based on the lesser metatarsals to reach its adult length). (Diagrammatic representation based on data from Straus WL Jr. Growth of the human foot and its evolutionary significance. *Contrib Embryol.* 1927;19:95.)

decreases, and at 9 months, the angle is 8.9° (range, 3°-19.5°); it is 6.2° (range, 3°-9°) in the adult.

Early in fetal life there is torsion of the first and second metatarsals, which gradually decreases and reaches 13° for the first metatarsal and 5° for the second metatarsal in the adult. The first metatarsal presents a lateral twist and the second a medial twist.

During early fetal life, the lateral phalanges are longer than they are in the adult, indicating a phalangeal reduction.[5] Simultaneously, as the lesser toes reduce, the hallux reaches its dominant position. The reduction in the lesser toes occurs at the distal phalanges; the middle phalanges retain the same proportionate length, whereas the proximal phalanges become relatively longer with growth.

Fusion of the distal and middle phalanges of the little toe is common. Hasselmander reports this symphalangia to be present in 50% of fetuses and children; Straus reports a 9.4% occurrence in a corresponding group.[5,20] Pfitzner gives a figure of a 37% occurrence in the adult, whereas Adachi reports an 80% occurrence in the Japanese.[5]

The sesamoids appear as condensed blastemic tissue at 8 weeks and as definite cartilage at 12 weeks.[21] They remain cartilaginous during the entire prenatal period.

Two sesamoids are regularly present at the metatarsophalangeal joint of the big toe. The lateral sesamoid appears first in the third month, followed in a week by the medial sesamoid, which may be bipartite.[22]

Sesamoids are also found sometimes at the metatarsophalangeal joint of the little toe but rarely at the other metatarsophalangeal joints. Interphalangeal sesamoids are frequently seen in the big toe and are occasionally present in the little toe.[13]

A cartilaginous anlage of the os trigonum has been demonstrated in the 2-month fetus by Bardeleben.[23] Harris has described a cartilaginous anlage for the same skeletal element in a 12-week embryo (80.5 mm).[24] At birth, the development center of the os trigonum is cartilaginous.[25]

Joints. A joint is formed initially by a homogenous cellular condensation in the interzone, which then becomes a three-layered zone, followed by the apparition of a cavity in its middle.[13] Synovial tissue then lines the cavity.

The homogenous interzones appear in the foot in horizon 20 at the metatarsophalangeal joint. By the end of the embryonic period (horizon 23), most of the interzones are still homogenous. The three-layered interzones occur subsequently during the fetal period of development. Cavitation is present in most of the joints between the seventh and ninth postovulation

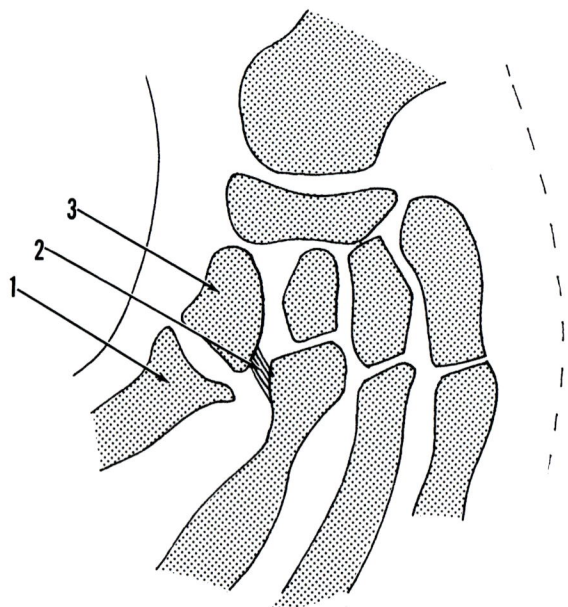

Figure 1.29 **First metatarsocuneiform joint and ligament of Lisfranc in a cross-section of an embryo foot measuring 2.3 mm.** The embryo measures 21 mm. The distal surface of the first cuneiform makes a 45° angle with the frontal plane, and this contributes to the adducted position of the first metatarsal (*1*, first metatarsal; *2*, ligament of Lisfranc; *3*, first cuneiform). (Adapted from Leboucq H. Le développement du premier metatarsien et de son articulation tarsienne chez l'homme. *Arch Biol.* 1882;3:335.)

weeks. The time of initial appearance of the three-layered interzone and of the process of cavitation is, however, variable. Cavitation of the ankle occurs earlier, at horizon 23, 8 weeks postovulation.

Leboucq attributes the abduction of the big toe in the embryo not only to the tibial deviation of the talar head but also to the obliquity of the distal articular surface of the first cuneiform.[26] "This surface, rather than to be located sensibly in the frontal plane, makes an angle of more than 45° (Fig. 1.29). As the evolution progresses, the tibial surface of the cuneiform develops more rapidly than the peroneal surface and the position of the distal articular surface approximates that of the adult. The obliquity of the facet has nearly completely disappeared already in the fetus of 40 mm in length."[26]

Barlow, in a cross-sectional study of the first metatarsocuneiform joint in 52 embryos and fetuses, indicates that the curvature of the joint is different in the upper and lower halves.[21] He makes, more specifically, the following observations (Fig. 1.30): In the upper part of the joint, the articular surface of the metatarsal is always larger than that of the cuneiform, and in the majority of the sections, it is flatter than the corresponding cuneiform surface. The joint faces anteromedially up to 48 mm in stage and slightly anteromedially at 75 mm, but at 86 mm, it faces anteriorly. In the lower part of the joint, the articular surface of the metatarsal coincides in size and curvature with that of the cuneiform, and the obliquity is not noticeable after 48 mm in stage.

Leboucq reports on a calcaneonavicular fusion in an embryo of 25 mm and a talocalcaneal fusion in a fetus of 80 mm.[27] Harris describes the occurrence of a talocalcaneal bridge in 4 (25 mm, 27.8 mm, 60.9 mm, and 72.3 mm) of 20 embryos.[24] The union extends from the posterior aspect of the sustentaculum tali to the talus. This bridge could be bilateral or unilateral. According to Harris, the talocalcaneal bridge could resorb, remain cartilaginous, or ossify.[24] When the center ossifies only, an os sustentaculi results. Instances of calcaneonavicular fusion in fetuses are reported by O'Rahilly and coworkers.[28] Fusions involving the plantar aspect of the third metatarsal and third cuneiform or that of the fourth metatarsal with the cuboid are also reported by Harris.[24]

Ligaments and Tendon Sheaths. Ligaments differentiate during the fetal period of development prior to the formation of the joint space or the capsule. Specific studies are reported relative to the ligaments of the ankle and subtalar joints, extensor retinaculum or anterior annular ligament, medial annular ligament or flexor retinaculum, interosseous ligaments of Lisfranc joint, fibrous tunnel of peronei, long plantar ligament, and transverse metatarsal ligament.[21,29-34]

Beau studied the sequential development of the ligaments of the ankle and subtalar joints in fetuses from 33 to 85 mm.[29]

In the 33-mm fetus, the posterior talofibular ligament is first to appear and extends transversely from the inner surface of the lateral malleolus to the posterior border of the talus. The posterior tibiofibular ligament is present as a layer of fibrous tissue uniting the tibia and fibula. Slightly below, another tibiofibular ligament differentiates; this represents the future ligamentum transversum or inferior transverse tibiofibular ligament. This ligament is triangular and originates from the lower fibular extremity. Directed transversely, it inserts along the posterior border of the tibia, reaching its inferomedial corner. The calcaneofibular ligament is clearly recognized. The anterior tibiofibular ligament is formed, but the anterior talofibular ligament is hardly seen. The deep layer of the deltoid or posterior talotibial ligament is already present and differentiates prior to the superficial layer, which is not clearly distinguishable at this stage. No ligaments are visible in the subtalar joint. With subsequent development, the posterior talofibular ligament bulges into the posterior ankle joint, depressing the capsule, and thus forming two transverse cul-de-sacs. This arrangement gives the appearance of an intra-articular ligament.

In the 40-mm fetus, the superficial layer of the deltoid is well delineated. It originates from the medial malleolus, partly covers the posterior talotibial ligament, and inserts on the superomedial corner of the calcaneus, the sustentaculum tali, and the tuberosity of the navicular, forming a continuous fibrous envelope. Ligaments now also appear in the sinus tarsi. With further development, the origin of the extensor digitorum brevis is seen in the sinus tarsi. The heads of this muscle are separated by three fibrous septa. The most lateral septum enters in contact with the sheath of the peronei. The inner septum extends to form the sling for the extensor digitorum communis in front of the talus, and the deep surface of this sling attaches to the perichondrium of the talus.

In the 85-mm fetus, a well-organized talocalcaneal interosseous ligament is present, located in the middle portion between the articular capsules of the two subastragalar joints.

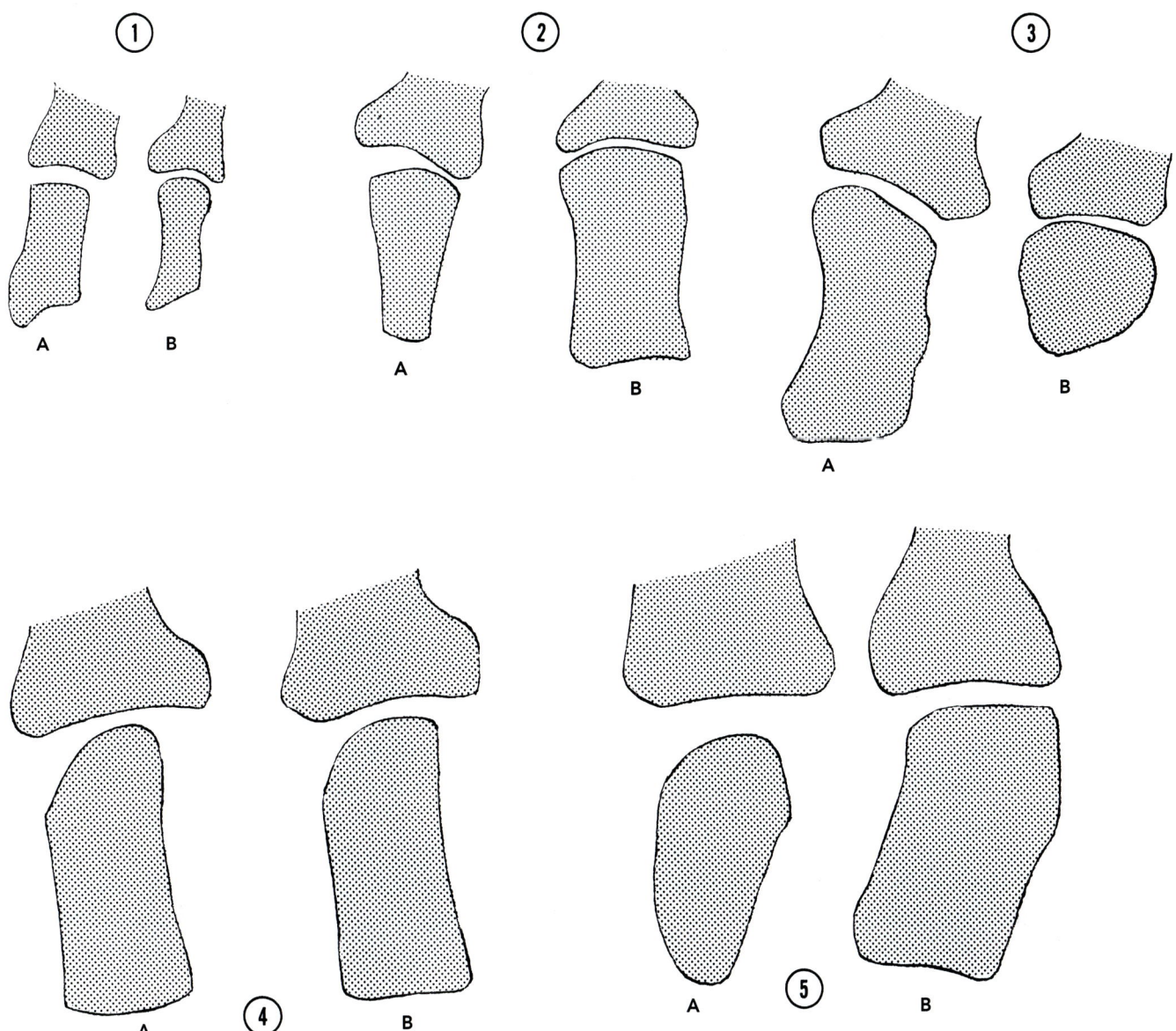

Figure 1.30 **Cross-section through the first cuneiform and metatarsal joint in the embryo and the fetus.** **(A)** Cross-section at the level of the ligament of Lisfranc. **(B)** Cross-section at the level of the peroneus longus tendon. The curvatures of the surfaces are different in the upper **(A)** and lower **(B)** sections. In the upper part of the joint, the articular surface of the first metatarsal is larger and flatter than that of the first cuneiform. The first cuneiform surface in the upper part is initially inclined anteromedially up to 48 mm in stage and faces anteriorly by 86 mm in stage. In the lower segment, the articular surfaces of the first metatarsal-first cuneiform coincide in size and curvature (*1*, 25-mm embryo; *2*, 30-mm embryo; *3*, 48-mm fetus; *4*, 90-mm fetus; *5*, 200-mm fetus). (Adapted from Barlow TE. *Some observations on the development of the human foot.* Thesis, University of Manchester; 1943. Data from Straus WLJr. Growth of the human foot and its evolutionary significance. *Contrib Embryol.* 1927;19:95.)

The peroneotalocalcaneal ligament of Rouvière and Canela Lazaro, the superomedial calcaneonavicular ligament (ligamentum neglectum), and the cervical talocalcaneal ligament have been demonstrated in the foot of a 7-month fetus (Fig. 1.31).

Lucien analyzed the development of the anterior annular ligament (extensor retinaculum) in fetuses measuring 30 to 70 mm (Fig. 1.32).[30]

In the 30-mm embryo, the superior extensor retinaculum is recognized as a narrow cellular band extending from the inner border of the tibial epiphysis to the anterior border of the fibula. In this chondrocellular tunnel, the tendons of the tibialis anterior, extensor hallucis longus, and extensor digitorum longus are united with embryonic connective tissue. In the 40-mm fetus, the inferior extensor retinaculum differentiates. The two extremities of this retinaculum arise (vaguely at this stage) from the sinus tarsi and form a distinct sling or frondiform ligament surrounding the extensor digitorum communis tendons. A second sling corresponding to the extensor hallucis longus is also recognized, but its limits are less precise. In the 65-mm fetus, the two extremities of the inferior extensor retinaculum are clearly seen arising from the sinus tarsi. The sling of the extensor hallucis longus, which arises from the medial

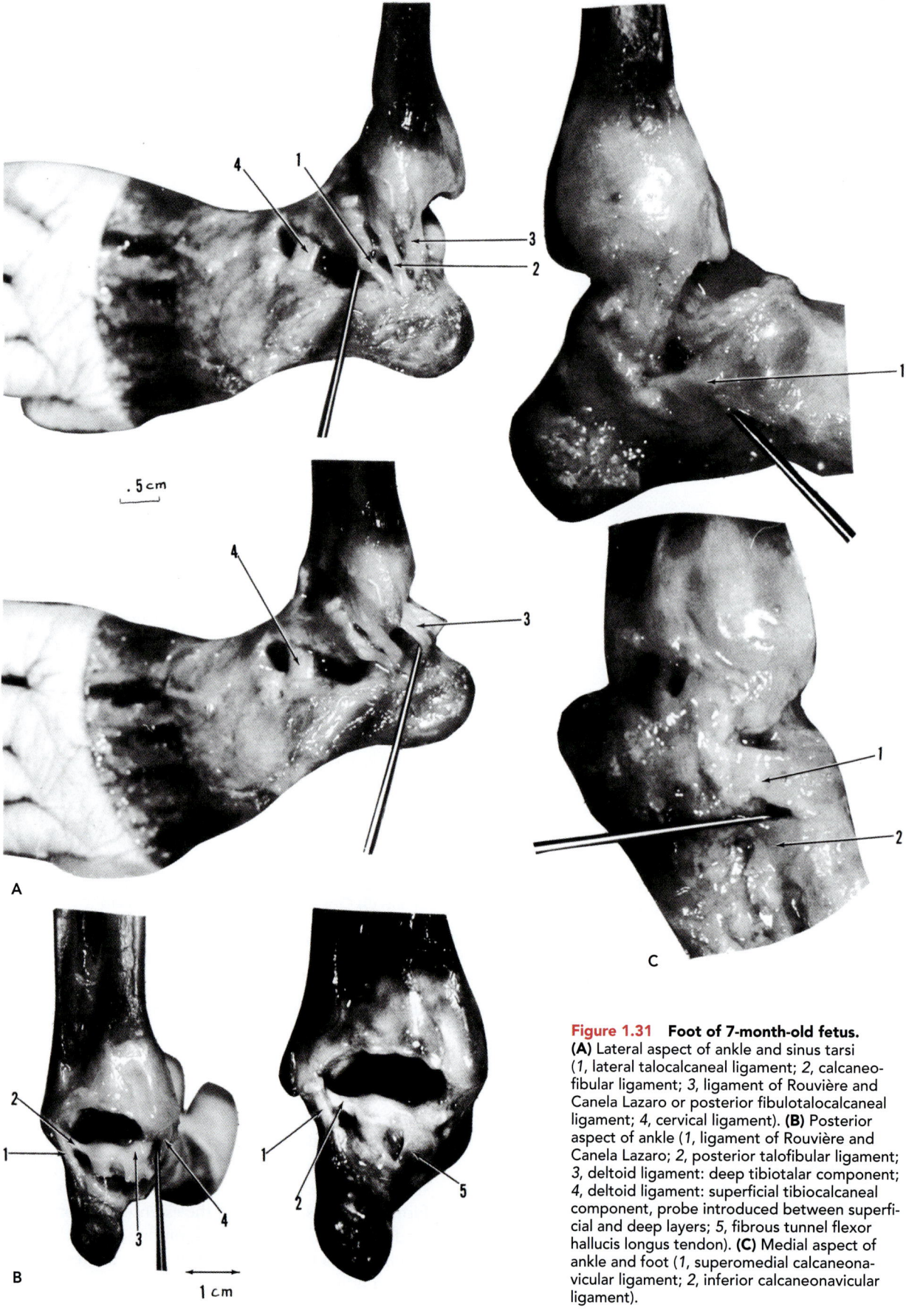

Figure 1.31 Foot of 7-month-old fetus. (A) Lateral aspect of ankle and sinus tarsi (*1*, lateral talocalcaneal ligament; *2*, calcaneofibular ligament; *3*, ligament of Rouvière and Canela Lazaro or posterior fibulotalocalcaneal ligament; *4*, cervical ligament). (B) Posterior aspect of ankle (*1*, ligament of Rouvière and Canela Lazaro; *2*, posterior talofibular ligament; *3*, deltoid ligament: deep tibiotalar component; *4*, deltoid ligament: superficial tibiocalcaneal component, probe introduced between superficial and deep layers; *5*, fibrous tunnel flexor hallucis longus tendon). (C) Medial aspect of ankle and foot (*1*, superomedial calcaneonavicular ligament; *2*, inferior calcaneonavicular ligament).

Figure 1.32 Morphogenesis of the extensor retinaculum. (A) Embryo of 30 mm. **(B)** Fetus of 40 mm. **(C)** Fetus of 65 mm. The extensor retinaculum is formed in a proximodistal direction. The superior extensor retinaculum is the first to differentiate, followed by the frondiform ligament; this is followed by formation of the tunnel for the extensor hallucis longus. The tunnel of the tibialis anterior is the last to form at the level of the inferior extensor retinaculum (*1*, superior extensor retinaculum; *2*, inferior extensor retinaculum-frondiform ligament of extensor digitorum communis [*6*]; *3*, tunnel for extensor hallucis longus [*7*]; *4*, tunnel for tibialis anterior tendon [*8*]; *5*, distal extensor retinaculum for [*7*] and [*8*]). (Diagrammatic representation based on data from Lucien M. Notes sur le développement du ligament annulaire antérieur du tarse. *Comptes Rendus Hebd Soc Biol.* 1908;2:253.)

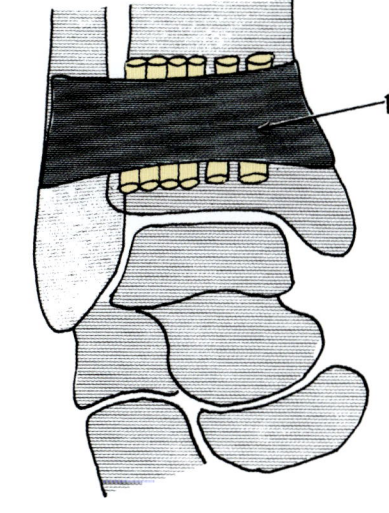

A

malleolus, fuses with the sling of the extensor digitorum communis. A third fibrous band is recognized distally over the second row of the tarsal bones. This retinaculum extends from the medial border of the scaphoid to the third cuneiform. It passes over the tendons of the tibialis anterior and extensor hallucis longus and enters in close relationship with the aponeurosis of the extensor digitorum brevis.

The three fibrous bands sequentially determined in a proximodistal direction are completely independent initially from the superficial aponeurosis of the leg and the foot. Ultimately, these structures blend and determine the architecture of the extensor retinaculum in the adult. The frondiform ligament is demonstrated in the dissected foot of a 7-month fetus in Figure 1.33.

The medial annular ligament, also known as the laciniate ligament or flexor retinaculum, was also studied by Lucien in embryos measuring 30 to 70 mm.[31]

The deep component of the medial annular ligament forms first. Initially, three fibrous semirings appear around the tendons of the tibialis posterior, flexor digitorum longus, and flexor hallucis longus, anchoring the tendons against the skeletal elements (Fig. 1.34). Subsequently, the fibrous tunnels of the tibialis posterior and flexor digitorum longus are united by an expansion from the inferior extensor retinaculum. The leg aponeurosis differentiates next and unites the previous two tunnels to the aponeurosis of the abductor of the big toe. A fourth tunnel is thus formed through which passes the neurovascular bundle. The tunnel of the flexor hallucis longus is deep in location and does not participate in the architecture of the annular ligament (see Fig. 1.34). It thus becomes apparent that the laciniate ligament has a deep layer formed by arciform fibers representing the vestiges of the primitive peritendinous sheaths. These fibers correspond to the frondiform ligaments of the peronei and extensors. The superficial layer of this ligament is formed by oblique fibers arising from both the anterior annular ligament and the aponeurosis of the leg.

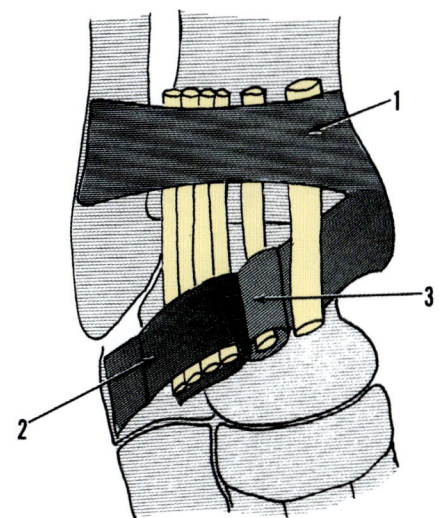

B

Thomas described the development of the interosseous ligaments of the joint of Lisfranc in fetuses measuring 15.6 to 47 cm crown to heel.[32]

Initially, a transverse lamina formed of connective tissue is present, extending proximally from the cuneoscaphoid interline to the intermetatarsal zone at the base. In each intercuneiform, intermetatarsal region, the continuous layer of fibrous tissue is transversely oriented (Fig. 1.35). With subsequent growth of the chondral elements, the intercuneiform ligaments and the intermetatarsal ligaments are formed and retain their transverse direction. The middle fibers are

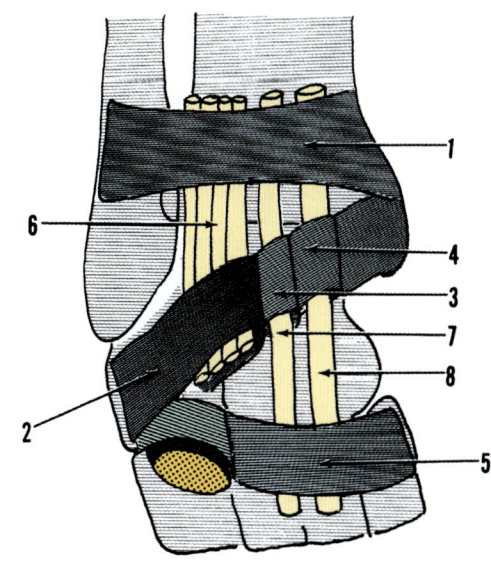

C

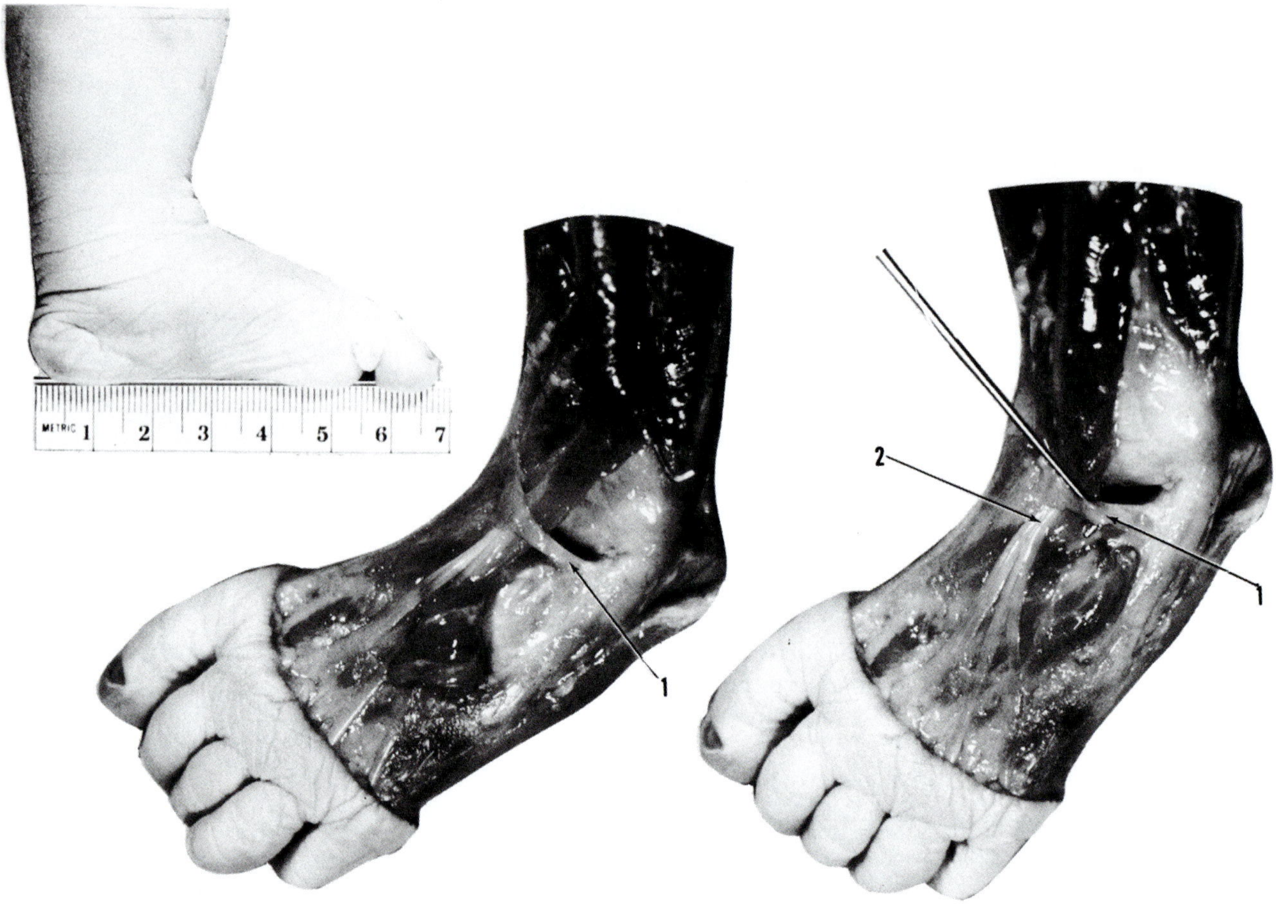

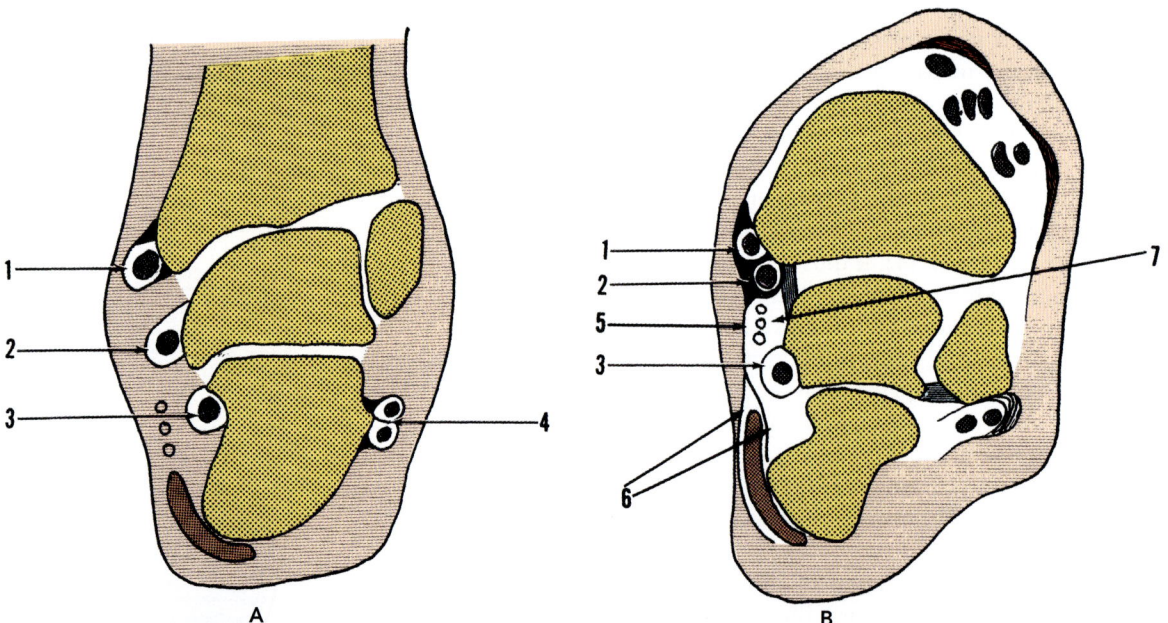

Figure 1.33 **Frondiform ligament of the inferior extensor retinaculum in the foot of a 7-month fetus** (*1*, frondiform ligament; *2*, extensor digitorum communis tendons).

Figure 1.34 **Morphogenesis of the flexor retinaculum or laciniate ligament.** Frontal cross-section of the ankle in a 49-mm embryo (**A**) and a 65-mm embryo (**B**). The tunnels of the tibialis posterior, flexor digitorum longus, and flexor hallucis longus are formed first. The flexor retinaculum appears subsequently, which adheres to the tunnels of the tibialis posterior and the flexor digitorum longus; splits into two layers, incorporating the abductor hallucis longus; unites with the extensor retinaculum; and forms the cover to the tarsal tunnel. It thus becomes apparent that the tendinous compartments at the level of the tarsal tunnel are not formed by deep expansions from the flexor retinaculum; instead, they antedate the latter (*1*, tunnel of tibialis posterior; *2*, tunnel of flexor digitorum longus; *3*, tunnel of flexor hallucis longus; *4*, tunnel of peronei longus, brevis; *5*, flexor retinaculum; *6*, split layers of flexor retinaculum covering abductor hallucis; *7*, medial neurovascular bundle). (Adapted from Lucien M. Développement et significantion anatomique du ligamet lateral interne du cou-du-pied. *Comptes Rend Assoc Anat.* 1908-1909;10-11:182.)

obliquely oriented. In the first space, the oblique fibers extend from the first cuneiform to the second metatarsal, forming the ligament of Lisfranc (see Fig. 1.35). Gradually, the transverse intermetatarsal ligament M^1-M^2 disappears. Only the superior fibers persist, and these blend with the oblique $cuneo_1$-$metatarsal_2$ ligament. The first interspace is thus occupied only by Lisfranc's ligament.

No interosseous ligament is present between the cuboid and the fourth and fifth metatarsals (see Fig. 1.35).

Lucien analyzed the formation of the fibrous tunnels of the peronei tendons in embryos and fetuses from 23 to 70 mm C-R length.[33]

The fibrous tunnel of the lateral peronei appears first in the form of a half-ring cellular structure attached to the outer and inner borders of the retromalleolar canal. One tunnel results from the two peronei. Next to be differentiated is a double tunnel at the level of the lateral aspect of the calcaneus. The fibers of the cellular rings originate from the external calcaneal apophysis, separately encircle each tendon, and return to their point of origin. These two structures form the superior and inferior peronei retinaculum but are in continuity without a precise line of demarcation. The intermediary portion, however, remains very thin.

At the level of the sole of the foot, the sheath of the peroneus longus appears, attached posteriorly to the posterior border of

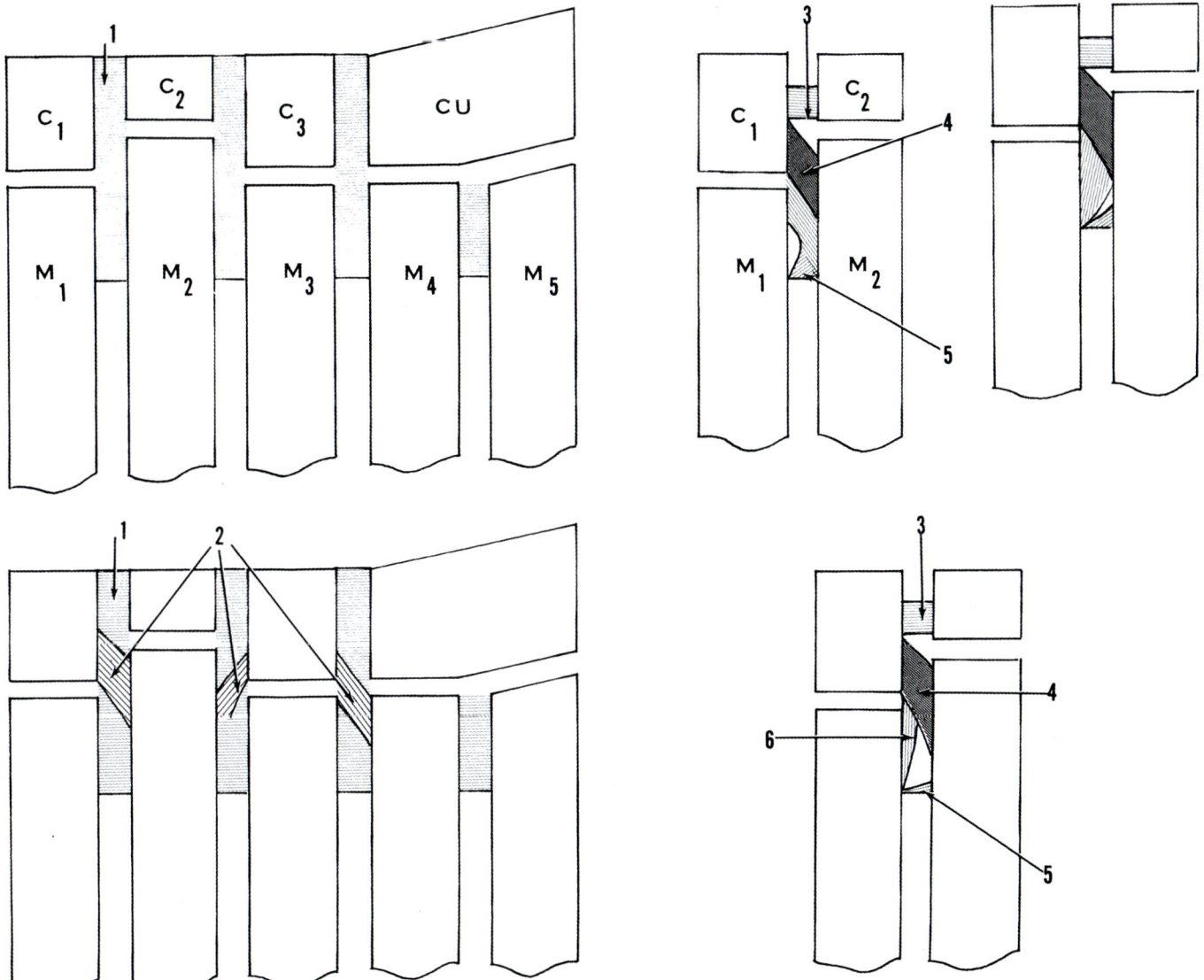

Figure 1.35 **Morphogenesis of the interosseous ligaments of the joint of Lisfranc.** A transverse homogenous lamina is formed initially. Within this lamina are next differentiated oblique cuneometatarsal ligaments. A regression of some fibers occurs and in the first space are delineated the intercuneiform C_1–C_2 ligament and ligament of Lisfranc. The intermetatarsal M_1–M_2 ligament becomes very atrophic or may disappear completely (C_1, first cuneiform; C_2, second cuneiform; C_3, third cuneiform; CU, cuboid; M_1–M_5, metatarsals one to five; *1*, homogenous transverse lamina; *2*, differentiation of oblique cuneometatarsal ligaments; *3*, intercuneiform C_1–C_2 ligament; *4*, Lisfranc's ligament; *5*, intermetatarsal M_1–M_2 ligament; *6*, longitudinal remnant of intermetatarsal ligament M_1–M_2). (Adapted from Thomas L. Recherches sur les ligaments interosseux de l'articulation de Lisfranc. *Arch Anat Histol Embryol.* 1926;5:104.)

the cuboid groove and anteriorly to the base of the last metatarsal.[34] This tunnel is independent of the inferior calcaneocuboid ligament.

The lateral annular ligament is the last to appear and results from the fusion of the fibrous tunnel of the lateral peronei to the superficial and middle aponeuroses of the leg.

The synovial sheath corresponding to the plantar segment of the peroneus longus tunnel differentiates first. A synovial cavity forms, with the mesotenon attached superiorly. Two synovial cavities are next formed, corresponding to the double portion of the peronei tendons, and these synovial cavities extend upward and penetrate the superior retromalleolar segment of the peronei tunnel. With further development in the fetus, all three synovial cavities fuse and establish continuity.

Lucien and Bleicher analyzed the development and anatomy of the long plantar ligament.[34] In the fetus prior to 6 months, the calcaneocuboid component of the long plantar ligament and the fibrous sheath of the peroneus longus are clearly separate. The inferior calcaneocuboid ligament inserts on the crest of the cuboid and is well developed as a fibrous lamina, whereas at this stage the sheath of the peroneus longus tendon is much thinner and transparent. After 6 months, the distinction between these two structures becomes even more evident.

The embryologic development of the transverse metatarsal ligament has been studied by Barlow.[21] At 22 mm, there is no evidence of this ligament in the region of the metatarsals (Fig. 1.36). At 23 mm, the beginnings of the transverse metatarsal ligament are seen. From 40 to 110 mm, the transverse metatarsal ligament is differentiated as an addition to the thick plantar portion of the capsule of the metatarsophalangeal joints. "There is no evidence in this series that there is a stage when the ligament includes the four lateral toes and not the great toe."[21]

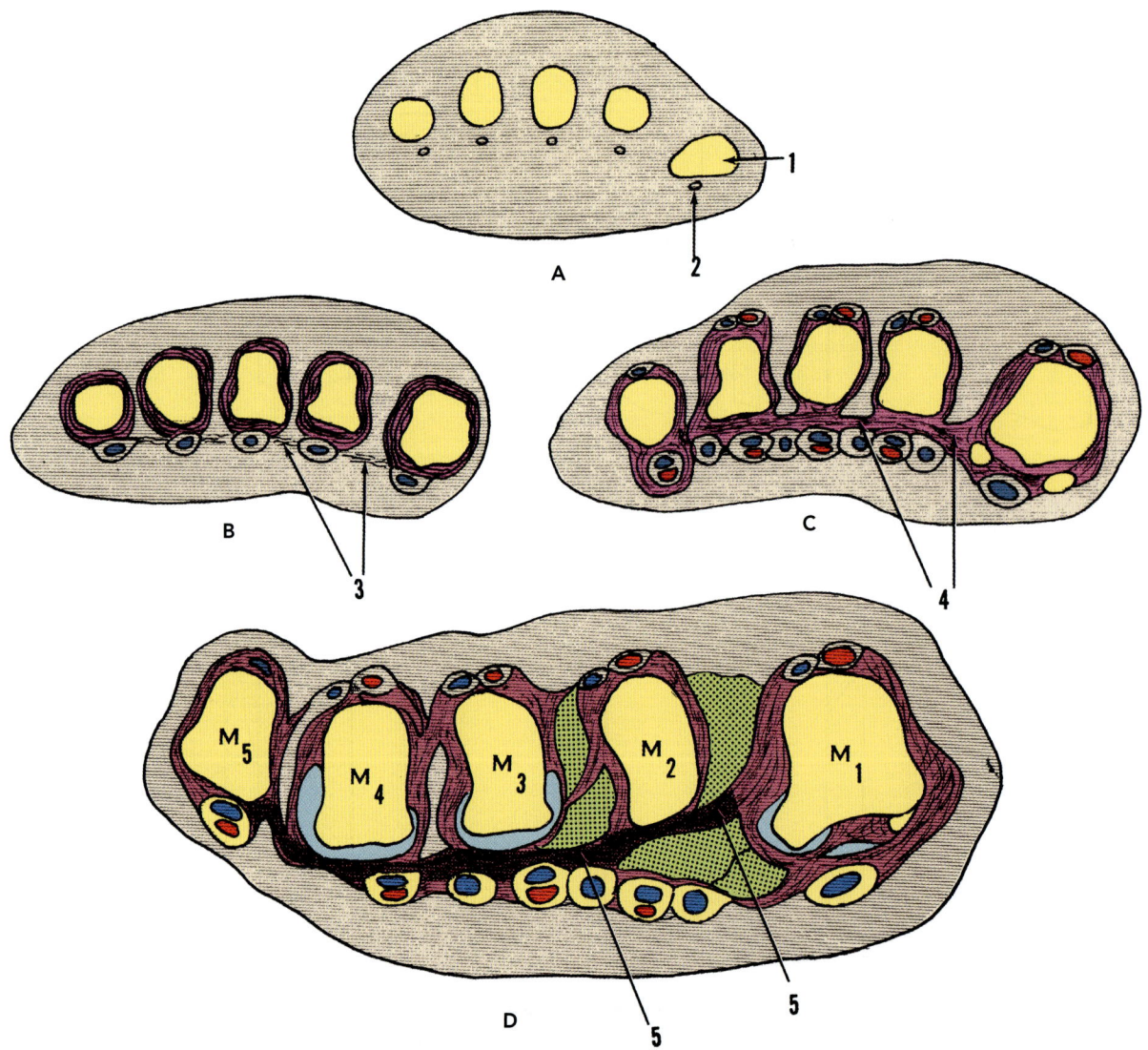

Figure 1.36 **Morphogenesis of the deep transverse metatarsal ligament—cross-section of the foot.** **(A)** Embryo of 22 mm. **(B)** Embryo of 32 mm. **(C)** Fetus of 40 mm. **(D)** Fetus of 110 mm (*1*, M_1–M_5, metatarsals one to five; *2*, flexor hallucis longus tendon; *3*, early formation of transverse metatarsal ligament; *4*, further structuring of transverse metatarsal ligament; *5*, transverse metatarsal ligament connecting plantar plates). (Adapted from Barlow TE. *Some observations on the development of the human foot.* Thesis, University of Manchester; 1943.)

Chapter 1: Development of the Foot and Ankle

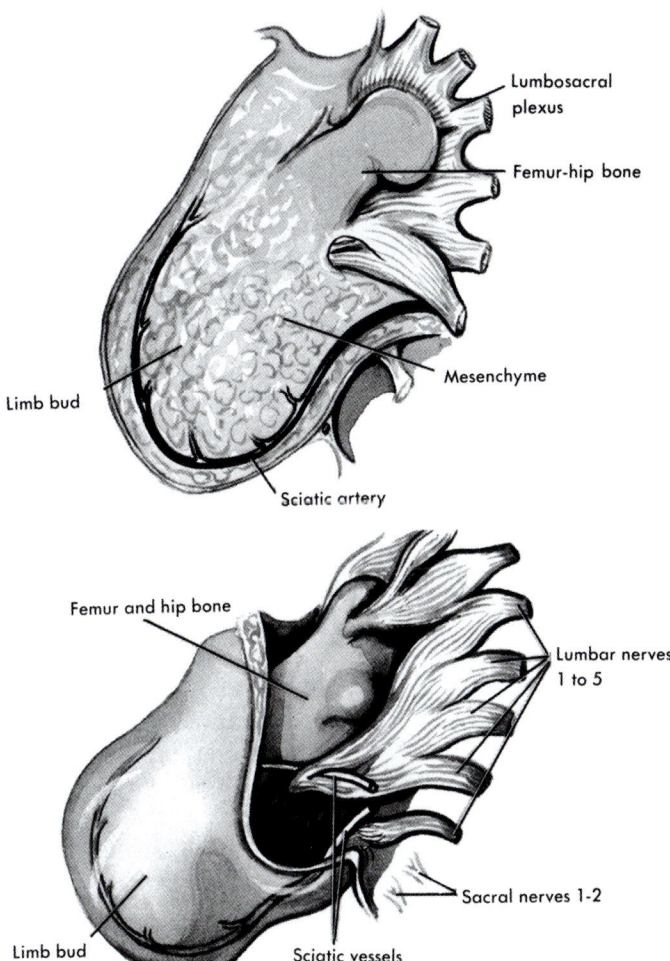

Figure 1.37 Limb bud in 9-mm embryo, about 4 weeks. The five lumbar and the first two sacral nerves form a plexus, and the main four nerves enter the limb. The sciatic vessels are present in the bud. (After Bardeen CR, Lewis WH. Development of the limbs, body wall and back in man. *Am J Anat.* 1901-1902;1:1.)

Muscles and Nerves. Bardeen and Lewis have researched the development of muscles and nerves.[35,36] At 9 mm, the limb bud is filled with mesenchymal tissue. A capillary network connected with the umbilical artery and the cardinal vein soon make their appearance (Fig. 1.37). The nerves to the limb arise from the lumbosacral plexus and penetrate the bud (see Fig. 1.37). During this process, the skeletal and muscular anlages begin to differentiate in situ. At 11 mm, the very condensed mesenchymal tissue or scleroblastema marks the development of the skeleton of the leg and, to a lesser degree, of the foot. An area of less-condensed tissue differentiates into a myogenous zone, which is the myoblastoma (Fig. 1.38). During this very early stage of development, the true muscle tissue cannot be clearly distinguished from the skeletal anlage or scleroblastema. The myoblastoma is not a homogenous zone. Anlages of muscle group are recognized early, separated more or less clearly from regions representing intermuscular spaces. The chief nerve trunks grow first in the regions where intermuscular spaces will develop. As the muscle group differentiates, the nerve trunk sends muscular branches into the muscle mass.

At 14 mm, the anlage of the ankle and foot is well differentiated. The main nerve trunks grow a considerable distance into the limb, and multiple muscular and cutaneous branches arise. The differentiation of muscular tissue from the skeletal anlage is well marked (Fig. 1.39A). The peroneal nerve extends over the dorsal aspect of the limb bud and ends in a slightly differentiated myogenous zone representing the anlage of the extensor muscles of the leg and foot. The anlage of the peroneal muscles is separated from the myogenous zone of the extensor group, and the superficial peroneal nerve runs between the two groups. The tibialis posterior nerve is recognized with the medial plantar nerve on the tibial side and the lateral plantar nerve on the fibular side (Fig. 1.39B). The former reaches the tarsus, whereas the latter does not yet reach as far distally. The muscles of the calf are very evident.

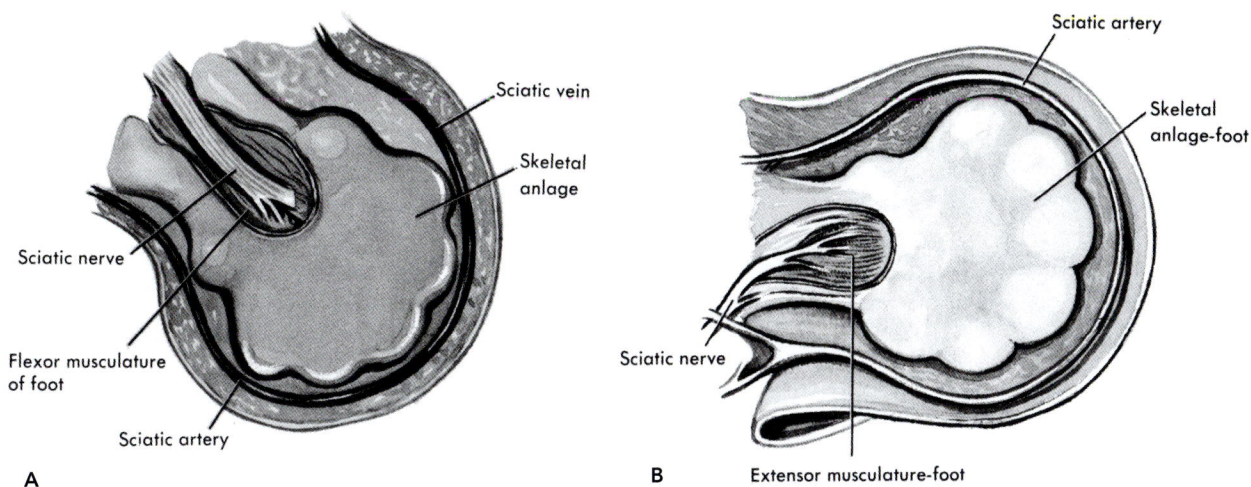

Figure 1.38 Limb bud in 11-mm embryo, about 5 weeks. **(A)** Flexor surface. Dense mesenchymal skeletal anlage is seen. The tibial nerve extends distally from the sciatic nerve and terminates in the flexor musculature anlage of the foot. The sciatic vessels are located at the periphery. **(B)** Extensor surface. Dense mesenchymal skeletal anlage is present. The extensor musculature anlage differentiates around the peroneal branches of the sciatic nerve. The peroneal musculature has not differentiated from the mesenchyme. (After Bardeen CR, Lewis WH. Development of the limbs, body wall and back in man. *Am J Anat.* 1901-1902;1:1.)

In the subsequent development, the muscle units are further delineated. Their anlages are often connected with the corresponding skeletal anlage at one end (less frequently, at both ends). The tendons are developed in continuity with the myogenous zones.

The peroneal nerve is divided into a superficial and a deep branch. The latter is clearly traced into the first intermetatarsal space.

The extensor muscle group of the leg and the foot is further differentiated. The anlage of the tibialis anterior is followed by a broad tendon that fades out over the first cuneiform and the first metatarsal base. From the central portion of the myogenous sheet, the extensor digitorum longus and the extensor hallucis longus differentiate simultaneously. An extensor tendon plate forms; initially, this plate is connected to the metatarsal scleroblastema, but it gradually separates from the scleroblastema. The extensor digitorum brevis differentiates beneath the extensor tendon plate, which gradually becomes segmented. The tendon of the extensor hallucis longus, fused to this tendinous plate, acquires its independence through further development.

The peroneus longus muscle anlage is continued into a tendon that fades out over the base of the fifth metatarsal. The peroneus brevis lies close to the extensor digitorum brevis, and the tendon is not connected to the extensor tendon plate but independently reaches the base of the fifth metatarsal.

The medial and lateral plantar nerves are seen separately in the foot plate. The medial plantar nerve spreads out superficially to the plantar aponeurosis; the lateral plantar nerve crosses underneath.

The gastrocnemius-soleus group of muscles unites broadly with the scleroblastema of the calcaneus. The anlage of the flexor hallucis longus is distinct, and the flexor digitorum longus differentiates more medially. The anlage of the latter covers that of the tibialis posterior. Both flexor groups end up distally in a flexor tendon plate, a rather flat aponeurosis from which tendinous processes extend to the blastema of the metatarsals and toes. The tibialis posterior is formed from the deep region of the tibial portion of the flexor anlage. The tendon differentiates early and independently and reaches the anlage of the navicular.

In the sole of the foot plate, the anlage of the quadratus plantae and abductor digiti quinti may be seen but the other intrinsic muscles are not defined.

At 20 mm, the nerves are well developed and the muscles of the foot are identifiable. The terminal branches of the common peroneal nerve are easily traced (Fig. 1.40). The superficial branch divides into two main terminal branches above the ankle. The medial branch reaches the tibial aspect of the first toe and the second web space. It also sends a small anastomotic branch to the cutaneous branch of the first web space arising from the deep branch of the common peroneal nerve. The lateral branch extends to the third and fourth web spaces and the corresponding contiguous surface of the toes dorsally. The sural nerve is visible and supplies the peroneal border of the foot and the fourth web space. The tendon of the peroneus longus, intimately fused to the scleroblastema of the foot, can be partially traced in the sole. The saphenous nerve is continued in one or two main trunks toward the ankle medially. The relationship of the musculotendinous units on the dorsum of the foot closely resembles that in the adult. Tendinous attachments extend from the extensor tendon plate to the digits. The tibialis anterior makes a firm attachment to the first cuneiform and the first metatarsal base. The Achilles tendon is well differentiated. On the plantar aspect, the long flexor muscles, continuous with the common plate, send extensions into the digits (Fig. 1.41).

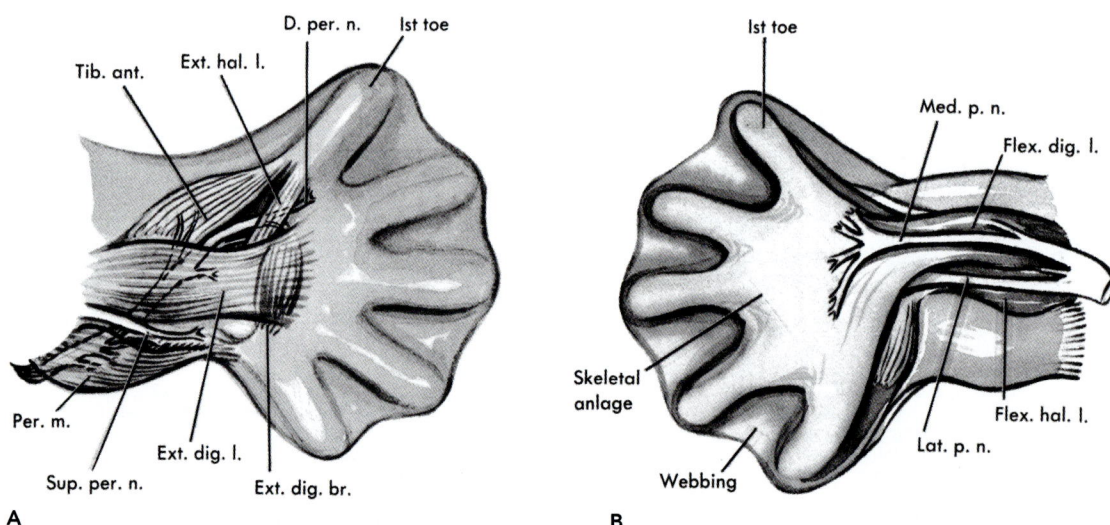

Figure 1.39 Foot plate in 14-mm embryo, 6 weeks. (A) Extensor surface. The peroneal and extensor muscles are differentiating. The superficial and deep peroneal nerves are recognized. The digital rays are well delineated with the connecting interdigital webbing. (B) Flexor surface. The medial and lateral plantar nerves are differentiated, including the flexor digitorum longus, the flexor hallucis longus, and the tibialis posterior muscles. (After Bardeen CR. Development and variation of the nerves and the musculature of the inferior extremity and of the neighboring regions of the trunk in man. Am J Anat. 1906;6:259-390.)

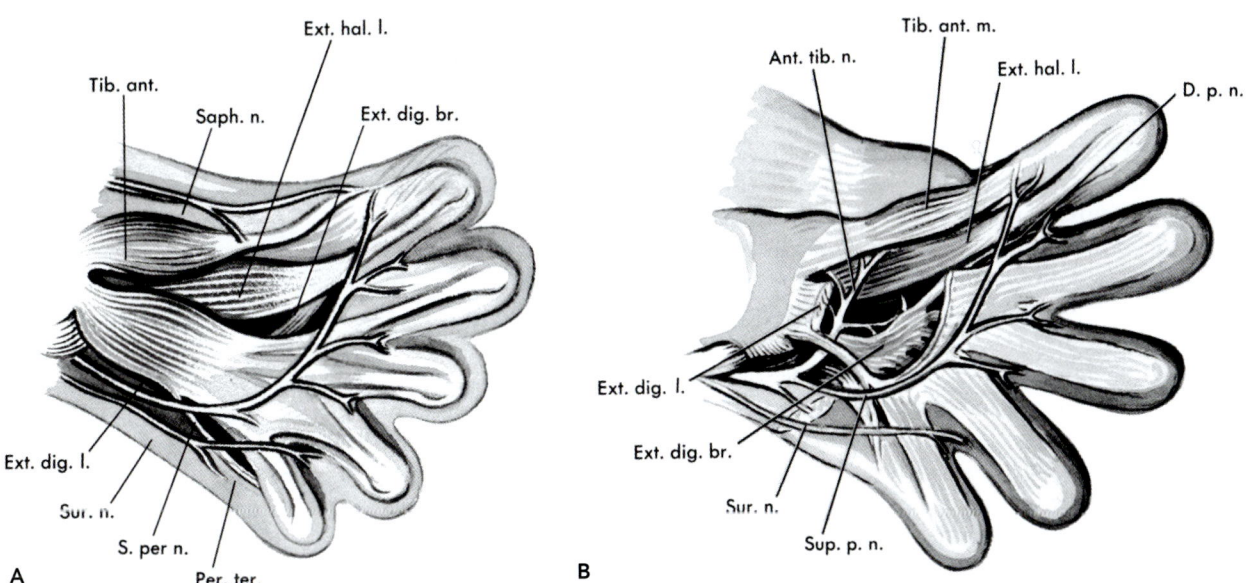

Figure 1.40 Foot in 20-mm embryo, about 7 weeks. **(A)** Extensor surface. The superficial peroneal nerve innervating the three medial digits, the sural nerve innervating the lateral two digits, and the saphenous nerve are well defined. The peroneus longus and brevis muscles, the tibialis anterior, the extensor digitorum longus, and the extensor hallucis longus are well delineated. The extensor digitorum brevis is also present. **(B)** Extensor surface, deep layer. The anterior tibial nerve and the deep peroneal nerve are demonstrated (*Ant.tib.n.*, anterior tibial nerve; **D**.p.n., deep peroneal nerve; *Sup.p.n*, superficial peroneal nerve; *Sur.n.*, sural nerve). (After Bardeen CR, Lewis WH. Development of the limbs, body wall and back in man. *Am J Anat.* 1901-1902;1:1.)

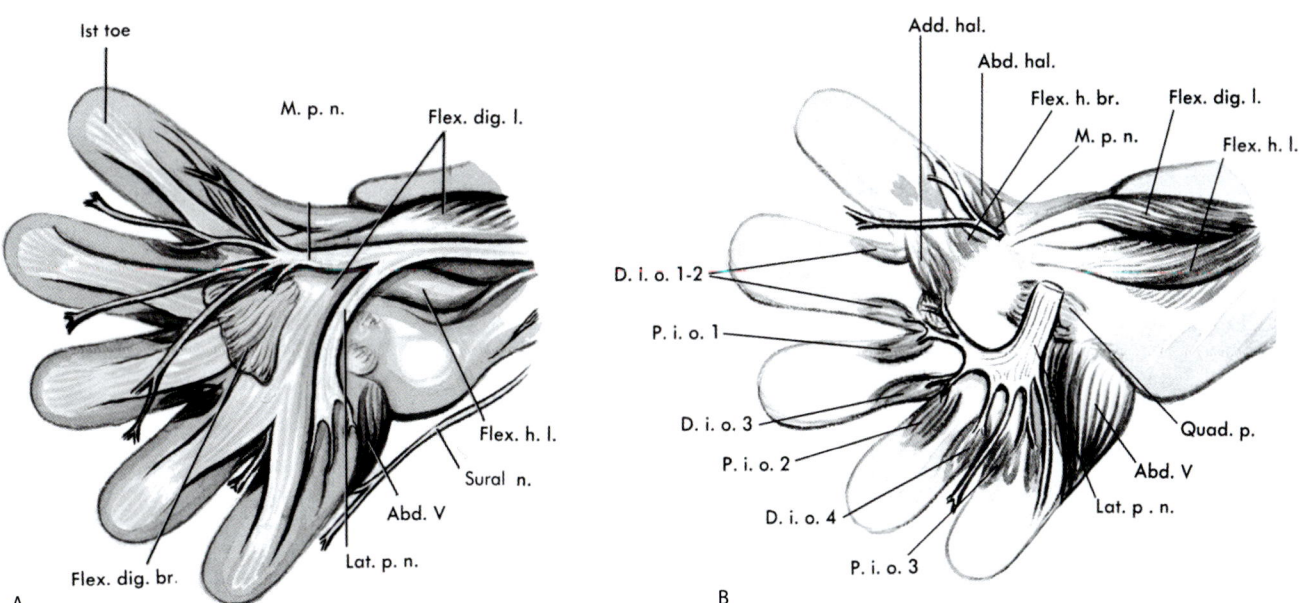

Figure 1.41 Foot in 20-mm embryo, about 7 weeks, flexor surface. **(A)** Superficial layer. The medial and lateral plantar nerves and the sural nerve are well delineated and in their definitive positions. The tibialis posterior muscle, the flexor digitorum longus, and the flexor hallucis longus muscles are well formed. The flexor digitorum brevis is differentiated. **(B)** Deep layer. The intrinsic muscles are delineated (*Abd.hal.*, abductor hallucis muscle; *Abd.V*, abductor digiti quinti; *Add.hal.*, adductor hallucis muscle; **D**.i.o. 1-4, dorsal interossei muscles, 1-4; *Flex.h.br.*, flexor hallucis brevis muscle; *Lat.p.n.*, lateral plantar nerve; *M.p.n.*, medial plantar nerve; *P.i.o. 1-3*, plantar interossei muscles 1-3; *Quad.p.*, quadratus plantae muscle). (After Bardeen CR. Development and variation of the nerves and the musculature of the inferior extremity and of the neighboring regions of the trunk in man. *Am J Anat.* 1906-1907;6:259-390.)

The anlages of most of the muscles can be distinguished but are incompletely differentiated (see Fig. 1.41). The quadratus plantae extends from the calcaneus to the deep surface of the plantar aponeurosis. The abductor digiti quinti reaches the base of the fifth metatarsal. The slightly differentiated anlages of the flexor brevis of the fifth toe and of the opponens digiti quinti are present. The interossei and lumbricals are ill defined.

The flexor digitorum brevis differentiates on the surface of the flexor plate, and with further development, tendons are extended to the toes. The adductor hallucis is present. The transverse and oblique heads arise from the same anlage. The abductor hallucis can be distinguished but is not well defined. The flexor hallucis brevis begins to appear. It is incompletely divisible into a lateral and a medial portion. With further development, the lateral head approaches the adductor hallucis, whereas the medial head is associated with the abductor hallucis.

The medial plantar nerve reaches the medial aspect of the big toe and the three medial web spaces; the lateral plantar nerve extends to the fibular border of the fifth toe and the fourth web space.

In horizon 23, when the big toe is gradually adducted and the foot is rotated, the peroneus longus tendon attaches to the first cuneiform and the deep transverse metatarsal ligament develops, with its fibers attaching to the soft tissues around the head of the first metatarsal. In this horizon or slightly later, the tendons of the flexor digitorum longus and flexor hallucis longus cross in the tarsal region and are surrounded by a common sheath at the crossing point; a slip of tissue unites them.[24]

Arteries (Fig. 1.42)[37,38]. In the 6-mm embryo, the axial artery arises from the dorsal root of the umbilical artery and ends up in two branches, each of which breaks up into a plexus.

At 8.5 mm, the axial artery passes distally into the posterior aspect of the skeletal anlage of the leg into the sole. Prior to ending in a plantar plexus, it gives origin to two or three branches, which perforate the mesenchymal skeleton and reach the dorsum of the foot, forming a dorsal plexus.

At 12 mm, the dorsal and plantar retia (plexuses) of the foot are richer. The axial artery is now connected to the dorsal rete of the foot through a single vessel of large size, the ramus perforans tarsi.

At 14 mm, major changes occur. The femoral artery participates in the blood supply of the leg and foot. A superior

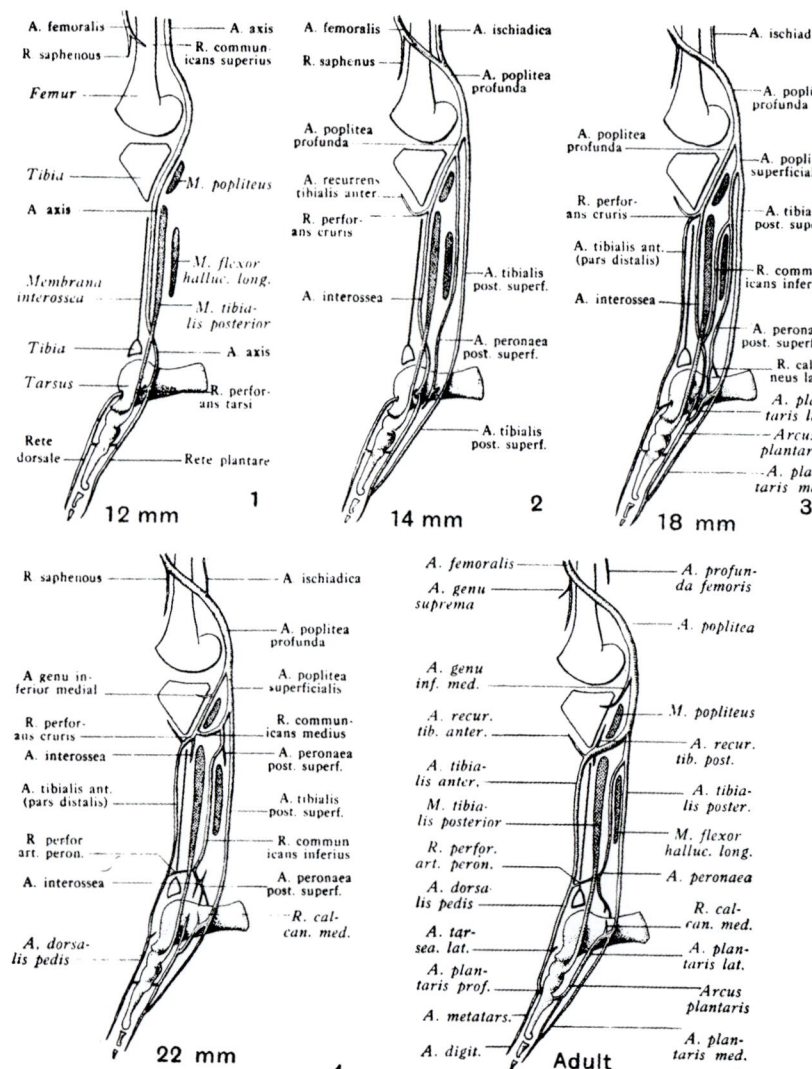

Figure 1.42 **Morphogenesis of the main arteries of the leg and foot at four stages of development and in the adult.** Labels in Roman type refer to embryonic arteries; italics are used for adult arteries and for all other structures. (From Senior HD. An interpretation of the recorded arterial anomalies of the human leg and foot. *J Anat.* 1919;53:130.)

communicating artery unites the femoral artery of the thigh with the axial or sciatic artery. An arterial branch, the ramus perforans cruris, passes through the proximal end of the tibiofibular interspace. The axial artery is now divided into three segments: the ischiatic artery (proximal to the superior communicating artery), the arteria poplitea profundus (between the superior communicating artery and the ramus perforans cruris), and the interosseous artery (distal to the perforans cruris). Two branches arise from the arteria poplitea profundus: the arteria tibialis posterior superficialis and the arteria peronea posterior superficialis. The former penetrates the sole, whereas the latter ends blindly in a medial and a lateral branch.

At 17.8 mm, the tibialis anterior artery appears, originating from the ramus perforans cruris and ending in the dorsal foot plexus. In this proliferative stage, four major arterial lines reach the foot: arteria tibialis posterior superficialis, arteria peronea posterior superficialis, arteria interossea (former arteria axis), and arteria tibialis anterior.

The arteria interossea is divided into two branches: plantar and dorsal. The dorsal branch is the arteria perforans tarsi. It passes dorsally through the talocalcaneal mass and is joined by the distal segment of the arteria tibialis anterior to form the dorsal arterial system. The plantar branch of the arteria interossea courses distally and forms the lateral plantar artery and the deep plantar arch after receiving the terminal branch of the arteria peronea superficialis. The latter unites the plantar branch of the arteria interossea with the arteria tibialis posterior superficialis. The medial plantar artery is the terminal branch of the latter (Fig. 1.43).

At 18 mm, the ischiatic artery becomes slender and the femoral artery enlarges. The arterial arrangement is similar to that in the preceding stage except for a new communicating branch, the ramus communicans inferiori, extending from the anterior arteria peronea superficialis to the interosseous artery.

At 22 mm, the ischiatic artery is interrupted, and the blood supply to the leg and foot is provided only by the femoral artery. Proximally, a new branch, the ramus communicans medius, connects the anterior tibial artery with the distal part of the anterior arteria poplitea profundus. Regressive changes now occur: The arteria interossea disappears, including the dorsal ramus perforans tarsi and a segment of its plantar branch up to the point of union with the anastomotic branch of the arteria peronea posterior superficialis. The lateral plantar artery is now only a branch of the arteria tibialis posterior superficialis. Also, the arteria peronea posterior superficialis, including its medial division branch, disappears. The lateral terminal branch of this artery unites with the ramus communicans inferioris. The latter now becomes the adult peroneal artery and sends a ramus perforans, the peroneal perforating artery, to the arteria tibialis anterior. The adult arterial pattern of the foot is achieved by the eighth week.

Cheng et al[39] investigated the intrachondral microvasculature of the growing talus in 16 fetuses aged from 15 to 44 weeks postgestation. They used celloidin-embedded serial microsections stained with hematoxylin and eosin and Van Gieson stains. Three fetuses were injected with Chinese ink, and additional thicker microslices were made for visualization of blood vessels. One intact talus was prepared according to the Spalteholz method to visualize the microvasculature. "In the 15- to 23-week-old fetuses, the cartilaginous model of the talus consisted of homogenously undifferentiated chondrocytes. Cartilage canals were well-developed throughout the cartilaginous model (Fig. 1.44). The talar body was supplied by four to five main branches originating from the sinus tarsi and the tarsal canal (see Figs. 1.44 and 1.45). A small portion of the talar neck and head was nourished by the vessels from the synovium in the superior aspect of the talar neck. The blood vessels of the cartilage canals were continuous with the perichondrial vessels (Fig. 1.46). They entered the cartilage model of the talus initially as a vessel bud; afterward, the bud divided into several branches, but the anastomoses were not observed between the vessels of the adjacent cartilage canals or between branches of the vessel within the cartilage canal. In essence, the cartilage

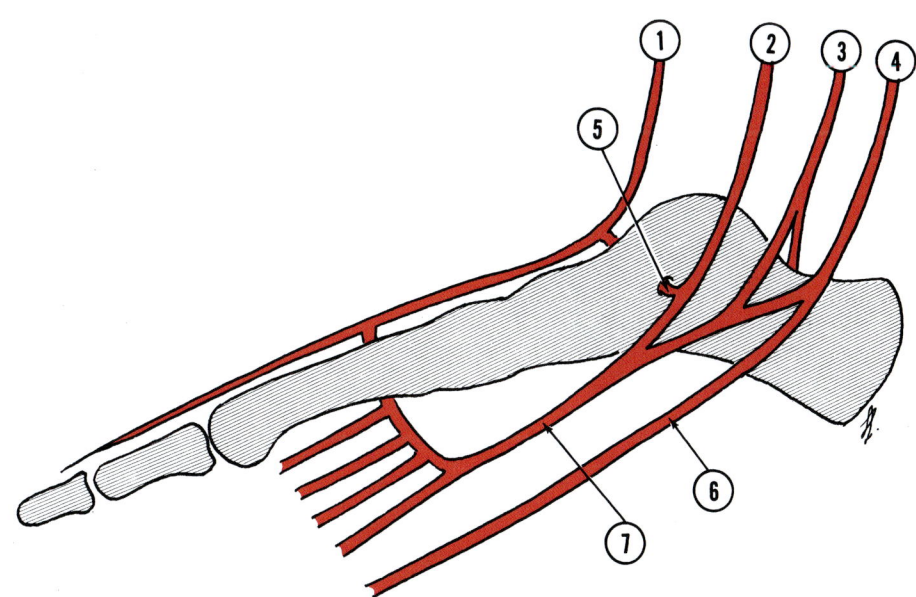

Figure 1.43 **Arteries supplying the foot in 17.8-mm embryo.** The medial branch of the artery peronea posterior superficialis divides into two branches and unites the artery tibialis posterior superficialis to the plantar branch of the artery interossea (1, artery tibialis anterior; 2, artery interossea dividing into two branches—dorsal, forming artery perforans tarsi [5], and plantar, contributing to formation of lateral plantar artery [7]; 3, artery peronea posterior superficialis dividing into two branches, lateral and medial; 4, artery tibialis posterior superficialis forming the medial plantar artery [6]). (Diagrammatic representation based on data from Senior HD. An interpretation of the recorded arterial anomalies of the human leg and foot. *J Anat.* 1919;53:130.)

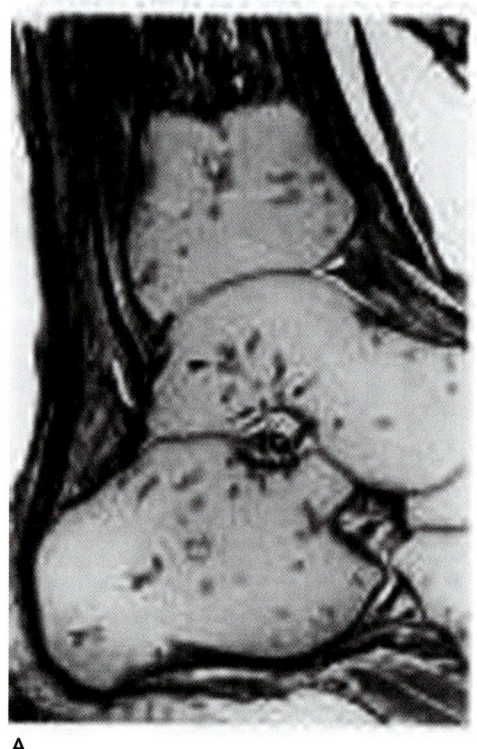
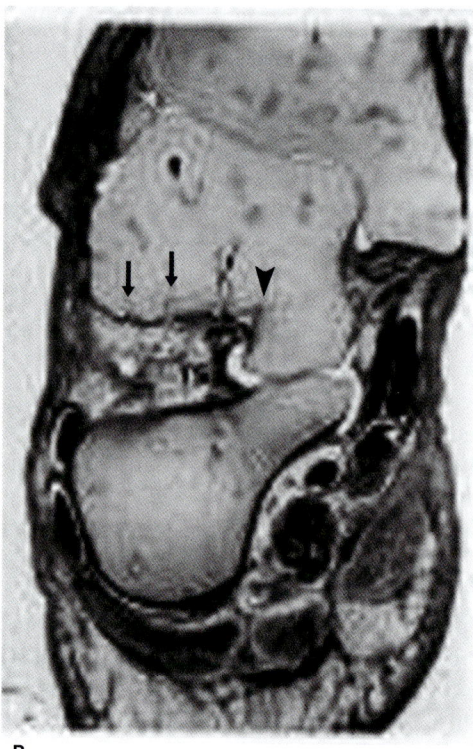

Figure 1.44 **(A) Photomicrograph of a sagittal section of the foot from a 17-week fetus. (B) The coronal view of the foot from a 23-week fetus** shows abundant cartilage canals (*arrowhead*) throughout the talar cartilage models; note several cartilage canals (*arrows*) from the tarsal canal (*TC*) and the tarsal sinus (*TS*) entering the talus. (From Cheng X, Wang Y, Qu H. Intrachondral microvasculature in the human fetal talus. *Foot & Ankle Inter.* 1997;18(6):335-338, Figure 1. Copyright ©1997. Reprinted by Permission of SAGE Publications.)

model of the talus was well vascularized before the appearance of the primary ossification center."

POSTNATAL DEVELOPMENT OF THE FOOT

▶ Growth of the Normal Foot

The length and growth pattern of the foot during childhood and adolescence, from age 1 to 18 years, has been studied by Anderson and coworkers and Blais and coworkers (Fig. 1.47).[40,41]

The length of the foot is measured from the back of the heel to the tip of the great toe in the standing position. The analyzed group consisted of 227 girls and 285 boys.

At age 1 year in girls and 1.5 years in boys, the foot achieves half the mature or adult dimension. The average annual increase in length is 0.9 cm from age 5 years through 12 years in girls and from 5 years through 14 years in boys, after which time the rate of growth markedly decreases. The mature foot length is reached at the average age of 14 years in girls and 16 years in boys. At all ages through 12 years, the average length of the foot

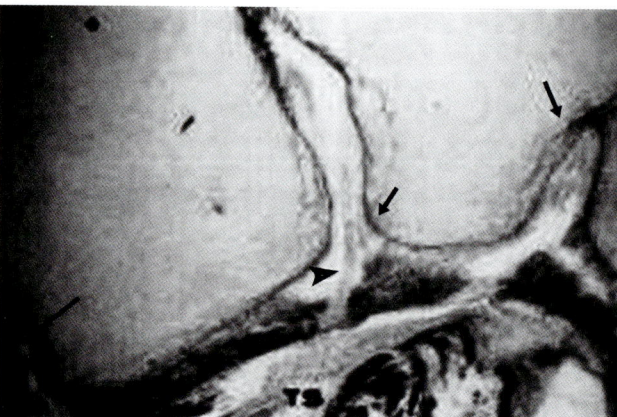

Figure 1.45 A photomicrograph of a top view of a 40-week talus that was injected with ink and cleared by Spalteholz method shows the primary ossification center (*POC*) in the middle, vessels and their branches (black) from the tarsal canal, and tarsal sinus supply to the talar body on the left and to the talar head on the right. No anastomoses were observed. (From Cheng X, Wang Y, Qu H. Intrachondral microvasculature in the human fetal talus. *Foot & Ankle Inter.* 1997;18(6):335-338, Figure 3.)

Figure 1.46 A magnified view of the sinus tarsi region of the talus shows three cartilage canals entering the talus from the tarsal sinus (*TS*). The walls of these cartilage canals were continuous with the perichondrium (*arrows*), and the blood vessels were connected with those of the perichondrium (*arrowhead*). (Cheng X, Wang Y, Qu H. Intrachondral microvasculature in the human fetal talus. *Foot & Ankle Inter.* 1997;18(6):335-338, Figure 5. Copyright ©1997. Reprinted by Permission of SAGE Publications.)

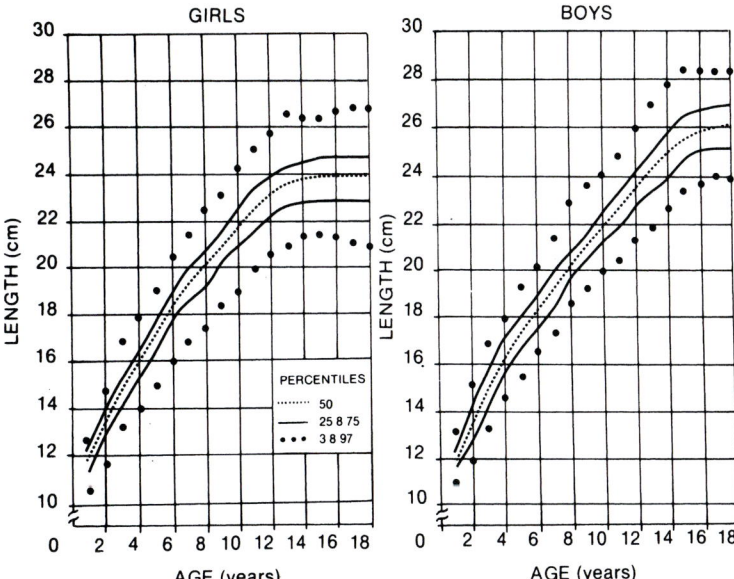

Figure 1.47 **Length of normal foot.** (After Blais MM, Green WT, Anderson M. Lengths of the growing foot. *J Bone Joint Surg Am.* 1956;38:998.)

is about the same for both girls and boys. At 12 years of age, the average foot length is 23.2 cm for girls and 23.5 for boys. After the age of 12, the foot grows slowly in girls for the next 2 years, with an average increase of 0.8 cm. The foot in boys continues to grow until age 16 and is an average of 2.2 cm longer than the female foot. The foot grows in synchrony with the body rather than with the lower extremity. Adult length is achieved first in the foot, next in the long bones, and last in stature.

In the female, the foot increases in size and width during and following pregnancy.[42]

▶ Primary and Secondary Ossification Centers and Epiphyseal Closures

Primary and secondary ossification centers and epiphyseal closures are shown in Figure 1.48. A comprehensive study of the postnatal appearance of the ossification centers and closure of the epiphyseal plates of the foot has been conducted by Hoerr and associates.[43] Variation ranges are evident when the available data from different sources are compared.[44-46] In the postnatal period, the primary ossification center of the lateral cuneiform is first to appear, followed by the secondary ossification center of the distal fibula. The sequence of ossification continues with the medial cuneiform, the intermediary cuneiform, and the navicular in the tarsus. At the level of the forefoot, the ossification center of the distal phalange epiphysis of the big toe is first to appear, followed by the ossification of the basal epiphyses of the proximal phalanges of toes two, three, and four. Subsequently, the epiphyseal ossification of the central lesser toes continues in a proximal distal direction. The epiphyseal ossification centers of the distal phalanges of the lesser toes are seen at 3 to 4 years. In the big toe, the secondary ossification centers appear in a distal to proximal direction. At the level of the metatarsal heads, the epiphyseal ossification centers appear in a medial to lateral direction (M_2-M_5). The ossification centers—primary or secondary—appear and close at the dates shown in Table 1.1.[43]

▶ Postnatal Structural Changes

The skeletal developmental changes initiated during the fetal period continue until adulthood; of interest are the structural changes occurring in the distal tibia, talus, os calcis, and metatarsals.

Distal Tibia

Le Damany, in an anatomic study of the distal tibia in the fetus, newborn, and adult, has demonstrated that the distal end of the tibia in the fetus and the newborn has no torsion.[47] External torsion of the distal end of the tibia is then acquired and increases gradually, reaching the adult degree of external torsion by the age of 5 years.

Le Damany's measurements of the external torsion of the distal tibia averaged 23.5° in 100 right adult tibias and 20° in 100 left adult tibias.[47]

Dupuis, in a comprehensive study of tibial torsion, provides more detail about the sequential acquisition of the torsion after birth.[48] In the newborn, there is a minimal degree (2°) of external torsion of the distal tibia in the majority; in about 40%, an internal torsion of 0° to 10° may be present. During the first 3 months of postnatal life, there is a rapid increase in the external torsion, which will reach an average of 10° and remain stationary during the second and third years of life. Between 3.5 and 4 years, there is again a sudden increase of the external tibial torsion, which will average 20°. From 4 to 5 years, the torsion reaches 23°, which is the average external tibial torsion seen in the adult (Fig. 1.49).

Talus

The declination angle between the axis of the trochlea of the talus and that of the talar neck is about 29° at birth and

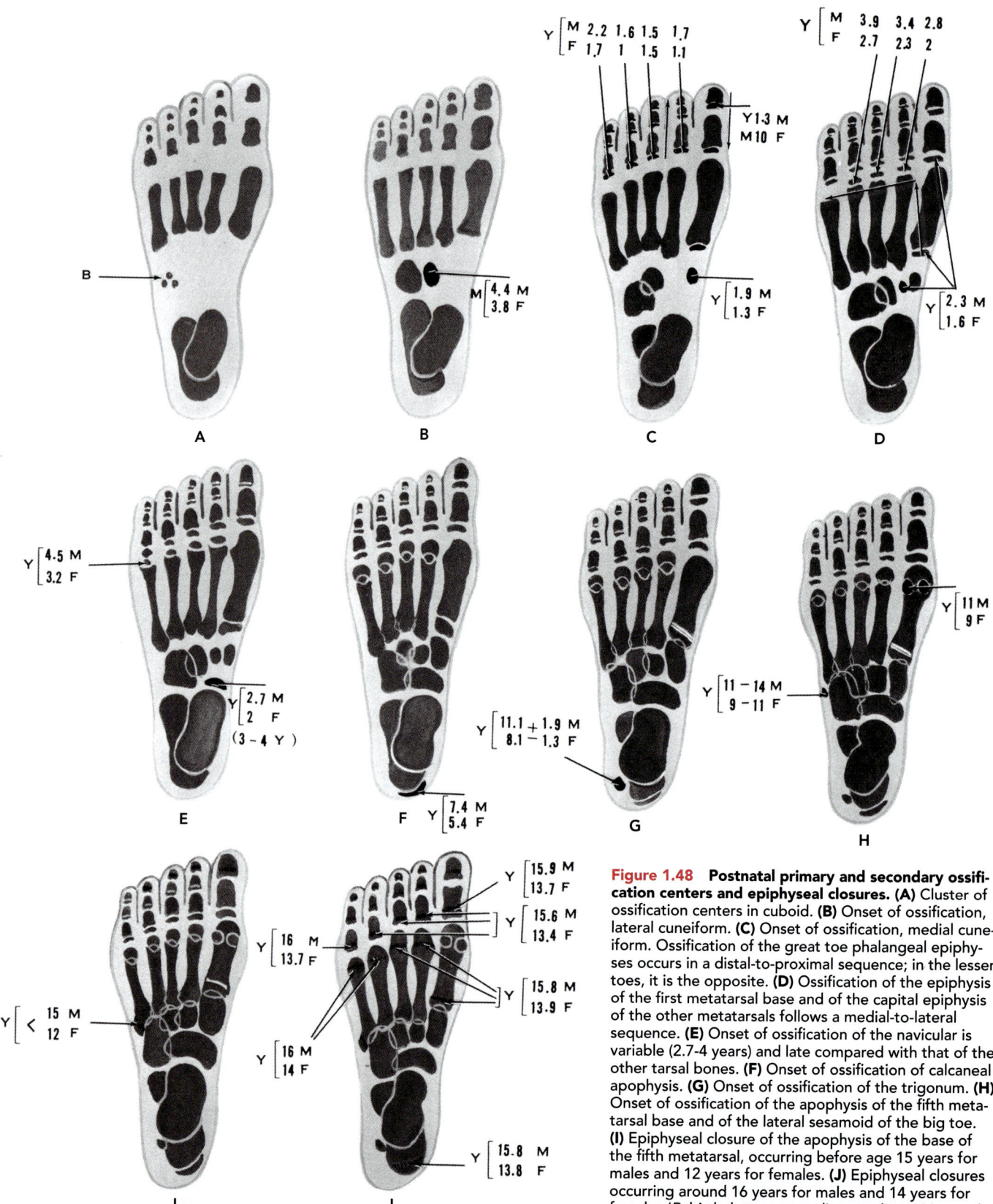

Figure 1.48 Postnatal primary and secondary ossification centers and epiphyseal closures. (A) Cluster of ossification centers in cuboid. (B) Onset of ossification, lateral cuneiform. (C) Onset of ossification, medial cuneiform. Ossification of the great toe phalangeal epiphyses occurs in a distal-to-proximal sequence; in the lesser toes, it is the opposite. (D) Ossification of the epiphysis of the first metatarsal base and of the capital epiphysis of the other metatarsals follows a medial-to-lateral sequence. (E) Onset of ossification of the navicular is variable (2.7–4 years) and late compared with that of the other tarsal bones. (F) Onset of ossification of calcaneal apophysis. (G) Onset of ossification of the trigonum. (H) Onset of ossification of the apophysis of the fifth metatarsal base and of the lateral sesamoid of the big toe. (I) Epiphyseal closure of the apophysis of the base of the fifth metatarsal, occurring before age 15 years for males and 12 years for females. (J) Epiphyseal closures occurring around 16 years for males and 14 years for females (B, birth; letters preceding numbers: M, month; Y, year; letters following numbers: M, male, F, female).

TABLE 1.1 Average Times of Appearance and Closure of Ossification Centers

Site	Ossification Center	
	Appearance	Closure
Distal Tibia-Fibula		
Distal tibial epiphysis	4.1 mo M, 3.7 mo F	16.4 yr M, 14.4 yr F
Distal fibular epiphysis	12.5 mo M, 9.1 mo F	16.4 y M, 14.1 y F
Separate Accessory Centers[a,b]		
Medial malleolus (20%) / Lateral malleolus (1%)	8.7 y M, 7.6 y F	12 y, M F
Tarsus		
Lateral cuneiform	4.4 mo M, 3.8 mo F	
Medial cuneiform	1.9 y M, 1.3 y F	
Intermediary cuneiform	2.3 y M, 1.6 y F	
Navicular	2.7 y M, 2 y F (ranges up to 3-4 y)	
Calcaneal apophysis	7¾ y M, 5.4 y F	15.8 y M, 13.8 y F
Secondary ossification center posterior border of talus	11.1 ± 1.9 y M, 8.1 ± 1.3 y F	12.9 ± 1.3 y M, 9.8 ± 1.3 y F
Os trigonum (14% M, 18% F)	11.1 ± 1.9 y M, 8.1 ± 1.3 y F	Remains unfused; ossification completed as in posterior border of talus
Forefoot		
Big Toe Ray		
Distal phalanx, epiphysis	1.3 y M, 10 mo F	16.3 y M, 13 y F
Proximal phalanx, epiphysis	2.3 y M, 1.6 y F	15.9 y M, 13.7 y F
Metatarsal 1, base epiphysis	2.3 y M, 1.6 y F	15.8 y M, 13.7 y F
Metatarsal 1, head epiphysis[c] (present in 96% of children 4-5 y)	2-3 y	10-11 y
Sesamoids metatarsophalangeal (lateral precedes the medial), lateral	11 y M, 9 y F	
Lesser Toe Rays		
Proximal phalanges, epiphysis		
Toe two	1.7 y M, 1.1 y F	15.6 y M, 13.4 y F
Toe three	1.5 y M, 1.5 y F	15.6 y M, 13.3 y F
Toe four	1.6 y M, 1 y F	15.6 y M, 13.4 y F
Toe five	2.2 y M, 1.7 y F	16 y M, 13.7 y F
Metatarsals, Capital Epiphysis		
Metatarsal 2	2.8 y M, 2 y F	15.8 y M, 13.9 y F
Metatarsal 3	3.4 y M, 2.3 y F	15.8 y M, 13.9 y F
Metatarsal 4	3.9 y M, 2.75 y F	15.9 y M, 14 y F
Metatarsal 5	4.5 y M, 3.2 y F	16 y M, 14.1 y F
Apophysis tuberosity of metatarsal 5[d]	11-14 y M, 9-11 y F	Before 15 y M, before 12 y F
Distal Phalanges, Epiphysis		
Toe two	4.7 y M, 2.9 y F	14.7 y M, 11.8 y F
Toe three	4.4 y M, 3.2 y F	14.7 y M, 11.7 y F
Toe four	4.2 y M, 2.5 y F	14.6 y M, 11.5 y F

F, female; M, male.

[a]Powell HDW. Extra center of ossification of the medial malleolus in children: incidence and significance. *J Bone Joint Surg Br*. 1961;43:107.
[b]Selby S. Separate centers of ossification of the tip of the internal malleolus. *Am J Roentgenol*. 1961;86:496.
[c]Vilaseca RR, Ribes ER. The growth of the first metatarsal bone. *Foot Ankle*. 1980;1:117.
[d]Dameron TB. Fractures and anatomical variations of the proximal portion of the fifth metatarsal. *J Bone Joint Surg Am*. 1975;57:788.

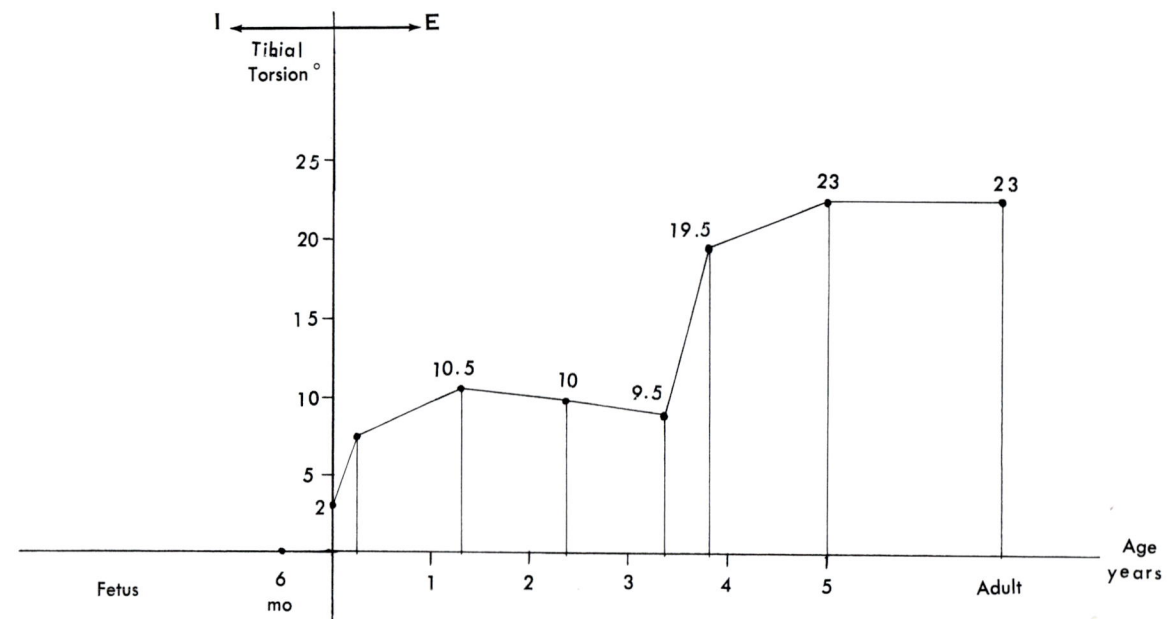

Figure 1.49 External torsion of the tibia during growth (*E*, external torsion; *I*, internal torsion). (After Dupuis PV. *La Torsion Tibiale: Sa Mesure—Son Intérêt Clinique, Radiologique et Chirurgical*. Dosoer et Masson; 1951.)

decreases until adulthood, reaching an average value of 22° (range, 16°-27°).[5] From birth to adulthood, the talus grows faster in width and height relative to the talar length. The relative values are as follows: talar width/length is 0.71 in the newborn and 0.81 (range, 0.77-0.87) in the adult; talar height/length is 0.52 in the newborn and 0.59 (range, 0.57-0.61) in the adult. The external rotation of the talar head continues and progresses from 23° at birth to 37° (range, 26°-43°) in adulthood.[5]

Os Calcis

The varus position of the os calcis diminishes after birth until cessation of bone growth.[5] The posterior segment of the calcaneal body maintains its increased rate of growth as compared with the anterior segment. The talar neck-calcaneal angle is 30° at birth and decreases to 23.6° (range, 17.6°-28.3°) in the adult.

Metatarsals

The intermetatarsal angle M_1-M_2 is 9° (average) in the newborn and decreases to 6° in the normal adult foot.[5]

The longitudinal arch of the foot is not clinically apparent in the newborn because it is hidden by adipose tissue. It does not shape before 12 to 16 months, and a definite longitudinal arch is present by 2 years. By 2.5 years, maximum longitudinal arching is attained, with the apex located at the junction of the posterior third and the distal two-thirds of the medial longitudinal arch; the apex corresponds to the tuberosity of the navicular.[42]

REFERENCES

1. Streeter GL. Developmental horizons in human embryos. *Contrib Embryol*. 1945;31.
2. Pattern BM. *Human Embryology*. 2nd ed. McGraw-Hill; 1953:185.
3. Böhm M. The embryologic origin of club-foot. *J Bone Joint Surg*. 1929;11(2):229.
4. Jones WF. *Structure and Function as Seen in the Foot*. 2nd ed. Baillière, Tindall & Cox; 1949:24.
5. Straus WL Jr. Growth of the human foot and its evolutionary significance. *Contrib Embryol*. 1927;19(101):95.
6. Cummins H. The topographic history of the volar pads (walking pads, Tastballen) in the human embryo. *Contrib Embryol*. 1929;20(113):105.
7. Streeter GL. Weight, sitting height, head size, foot length and menstrual age of the human embryo. *Contrib Embryol*. 1920;11(55):156.
8. Scammon RE, Calkins LA. *The Development and Growth of the External Dimensions of the Human Body in the Fetal Period*. University of Minnesota Press; 1929:245-246.
9. O'Rahilly R, Gardner E, Gray DJ. The ectodermal thickening and ridge in the limbs of staged human embryos. *J Embryol Exp Morphol*. 1956;4:256.
10. Bardeen CR. Studies of the development of the human skeleton. *Am J Anat*. 1905;4:265.
11. O'Rahilly R, Gray DJ, Gardner E. Chondrification in the hands and feet of staged human embryos. *Contrib Embryol*. 1957;36(250):185.
12. Senior HD. The chondrification of the human hand and foot skeleton (abstr). *Anat Rec*. 1929;42:35.
13. Gardner E, Gray DJ, O'Rahilly R. The prenatal development of the skeleton and joints of the human foot. *J Bone Joint Surg Am*. 1959;41(5):847.
14. Noback CR, Robertson GG. Sequences of appearance of ossification centers in the human skeleton during the first five prenatal months. *Am J Anat*. 1951;89(1):16.
15. Christie A. Prevalence and distribution of ossification centers in the newborn. *Am J Dis Child*. 1949;77:355.
16. Dixey FA. On the ossification of the terminal phalanges of the digits. *Proc R Soc Lond*. 1881;31:63.
17. Olivier G. *Formation du Squelette des Membres*. Vigot Frères; 1962:145-189.
18. McKee PR, Bagnall KM. Skeletal relationships in the human embryonic foot based on three-dimensional reconstructions. *Acta Anat*. 1987;129:34.

19. de Palma L, Santucci A, Ventura A, et al. Anatomy and embryology of the talocalcaneal joint. *Foot Ankle Surg.* 2003;9:7-18.
20. Hasselwander A. Growth of the human foot and its evolutionary significance. *Contrib Embryol.* 1927;19:95.
21. Barlow TE. *Some Observations on the Development of the Human Foot.* Thesis. University of Manchester; 1943.
22. Inge GAL, Ferguson AB. Surgery of sesamoid bones of the great toe. *Arch Surg.* 1933;27(3):466.
23. Bardeleben C. Das intermedium tarsi beim menschen. *Sitzungsberichte Jenaischen Gesellschaft Medicin Naturwissenschaft.* 1883;17:37.
24. Harris BJ. *Observations on the Development of the Human Foot.* Thesis. University of California; 1955.
25. Dwight T. *Clinical Atlas: Variations of the Bones of the Hand and Foot.* JB Lippincott; 1907:15.
26. Leboucq H. Le développement du premier metatarsien et de son articulation tarsienne chez l'homme. *Arch Biol.* 1882;3:335.
27. Leboucq H. De la soudure congénitale de certains os du tarse. *Bull Acad Royale Med Belgique.* 1890;4:103-112.
28. O'Rahilly R, Gardner E, Gray DJ. The skeletal development of the foot. *Clin Orthop.* 1960;16:7.
29. Beau A. Recherches sur le développement et la constitution morphologiques de l'articulation du cou-du-pied chez l'homme. *Arch Anat Histol Embryol.* 1939;26:205.
30. Lucien M. Notes sur le développement du ligament annulaire anterieur du tarse. *Comptes Rendus Hebd Soc Biol.* 1908;2:253.
31. Lucien M. Développement et signification anatomique du ligament lateral interne du cou-du-pied. *Comptes Rendus Assoc Anat.* 1908-1909;10-11:182.
32. Thomas L. Recherches sur les ligaments interosseux de l'articulation de Lisfranc. *Arch Anat Histol Embryol.* 1926;5:104.
33. Lucien M. Note sur le développement des coulisses fibreuses et des gaines synoviales annexées aux péroniers latéraux. *Comptes Rendus Assoc Anat.* 1908;148.
34. Lucien M, Bleicher M. Le grand ligament de la plante et ses constituants anatomiques. *Comptes Rendus Assoc Anat.* 1928;3:285.
35. Bardeen CR, Lewis WH. Development of the limbs, body wall and back in man. *Am J Anat.* 1901;1(1):1-35.
36. Bardeen CR. Development and variation of the nerves and the musculature of the inferior extremity and of the neighboring regions of the trunk in man. *Am J Anat.* 1906;6(1):259-390.
37. Senior HD. The development of the arteries of the human lower extremity. *Am J Anat.* 1919;25:55.
38. Senior HD. An interpretation of the recorded arterial anomalies of the human leg and foot. *J Anat.* 1919;53:130.
39. Cheng X, Wang Y, Qu H. Intrachondral microvasculature in the human fetal talus. *Foot Ankle Int.* 1997;18(6):335-338.
40. Anderson M, Blais M, Green TW. Growth of the normal foot during childhood and adolescence. *Am J Phys Anthropol.* 1956;14:287.
41. Blais MM, Green WT, Anderson M. Lengths of the growing foot. *J Bone Joint Surg Am.* 1956;38:998.
42. Giannestras JJ. *Foot Disorders.* 2nd ed. Lea & Febiger; 1973:70-84.
43. Hoer LN, Pyle SI, Francis CC. *Radiographic Atlas of Skeletal Development of the Foot and Ankle: A Standard of Reference.* Charles C. Thomas; 1962.
44. Coffey J. *Pediatric X-Ray Diagnosis.* Vol 2. 6th ed. Year Book Medical Publishers; 1972:884.
45. Lang J, Wachsmuth W. *Praktische Anatomie Erster Band Vierter Teil: Bein und Statik.* Springer-Verlag; 1972:31.
46. Paturet G. *Traité d'Anatomie Humaine. Volume 2, Membres Supérieur et Inférieur.* Masson et Cie; 1951:627-629.
47. Le Damany P. La torsion du tibia: normale, pathologique, expérimentale. *J Anat Physiol Normal Patholog.* 1909;45:598.
48. Dupuis PV. *La Torsion Tibiale: Sa Mesure. Son Intérêt Clinique, Radiologique et Chirurgical.* Dosoer et Masson; 1951.

Osteology

Shahan K. Sarrafian and Armen S. Kelikian

2

LOWER ENDS OF THE FIBULA AND TIBIA

The lower ends of the fibula and tibia form an anatomic and functional unit providing the osseoligamentous retention system to the talus and contributing to the ligamentous stabilization of the calcaneus at the subtalar joint. The bimalleolar retaining fork is rigid medially and movable laterally.

▶ Lower End of the Fibula

The lower end of the fibula is divided into the distal fibular shaft and the lateral malleolus.

Distal Fibular Shaft

The distal one-fourth of the fibular shaft terminates at the level of the tibial plafond. It has two surfaces, lateral and medial, separated by an anterior and a posterior border (Fig. 2.1).

Medial Surface

The interosseous crest divides the upper segment of the medial surface into an anterior narrow segment giving attachment to the peroneus tertius and a broader posterior part, flat or markedly convex, for the lower fibers of the flexor hallucis longus muscle. Where the anterior border and the interosseous crest merge, an oblique line originates and is directed downward and posteriorly, delineating a triangular area with a distal base and an anterosuperior apex. This triangular surface is covered by rugosities and gives insertion to the tibiofibular interosseous ligament, which is in continuity at the apex with the interosseous membrane. Distal to the insertion of the interosseous membrane is a triangular smooth surface with an anterior base and a posterior apex. The broader anterior part, which has an average height of 1 cm, corresponds to the tibioperoneal recess lined by periosteal synovium. The narrow posterior part gives insertion to a fatty synovial fringe that descends in the ankle joint (Fig. 2.2).

Lateral Surface

At the level of the distal fibula, the anterior border divides into two branches, anterior and posterior. The anterior branch remains anterior, merges with the interosseous crest, and continues into the anterior border of the lateral malleolus. The posterior branch or oblique crest is directed downward and posteriorly and continues with the posterior border of the lateral malleolus, forming the lateral border of the peroneal sulcus. This oblique crest delineates two surfaces: anteroinferior and posterosuperior. The anteroinferior segment is limited by the anterior and posterior divisions of the anterior border. The surface is laterally oriented, flat, and subcutaneous. The posterosuperior segment is initially posterolateral in orientation. Further down, through a twist, it becomes posterior and is in continuity with the posterior aspect of the lateral malleolus. The lower fibers of the peroneus brevis muscle originate from the upper segment of this surface. Both peronei muscle tendons, initially in a lateral position, follow the posterior shift of this segment. The anteroinferior and posterosuperior surfaces are slanted relative to each other along the oblique crest, and this must be taken into consideration during the application of a plate to a fractured fibular shaft at this level.

The anterior border was described previously. The posterior border is distinct proximally but loses its definition distally and dissipates toward the medial border of the peroneal groove.

Lateral Malleolus

The lateral malleolus is pyramidal in contour and presents three surfaces: lateral, medial, and posterior (Figs. 2.3 and 2.4). The lateral and medial surfaces converge toward the anterior border. The posterior surface is limited laterally by the oblique fibular crest and medially by the direct extension of the posterior border of the fibular shaft. The apex of the pyramid is inferoposterior. The lateral malleolus is projected outward and descends 1 cm further than the medial malleolus.

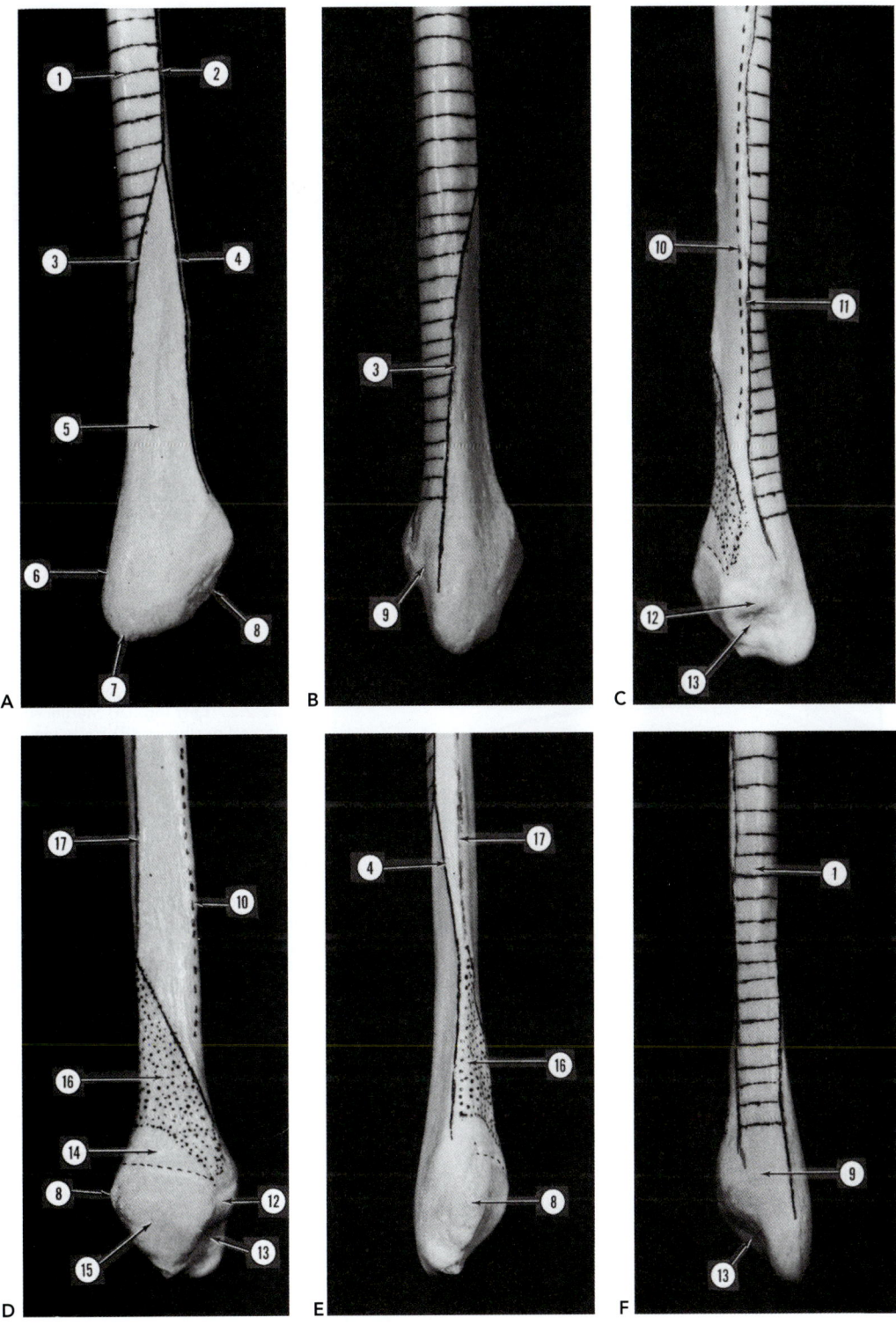

Figure 2.1 **Distal fibula and lateral malleolus. (A)** Lateral surface. **(B)** Posterolateral view. **(C)** Posteromedial view. **(D)** Medial surface. **(E)** Anterior surface. **(F)** Posterior surface. (*1*, surface of origin of peroneus brevis muscle—this surface becomes posterior distally and continues as posterior surface of lateral malleolus; *2*, anterior border of fibular shaft for insertion of anterior peroneal septum; *3*, posterior division branch of anterior border [*2*]—it forms a crest and continues as lateral border of posterior surface of lateral malleolus; *4*, anterior division branch of anterior border; *5*, subcutaneous surface; *6*, posterior border of lateral malleolus; *7*, tip of lateral malleolus; *8*, anterior border of lateral malleolus; *9*, sulcus of peronei tendons; *10*, line of insertion of deep transverse fascia of leg; *11*, line of insertion of posterior peroneal septum; *12*, posterior tubercle of medial surface of lateral malleolus; *13*, digital fossa; *14*, surface corresponding to peroneotibial recess; *15*, articular surface corresponding to lateral surface of talus; *16*, insertion of tibiofibular interosseous ligament; *17*, insertion line of the interosseous membrane.) The anterior division line[1] of the anterior fibular border and the line of the interosseous membrane[2] join distally.

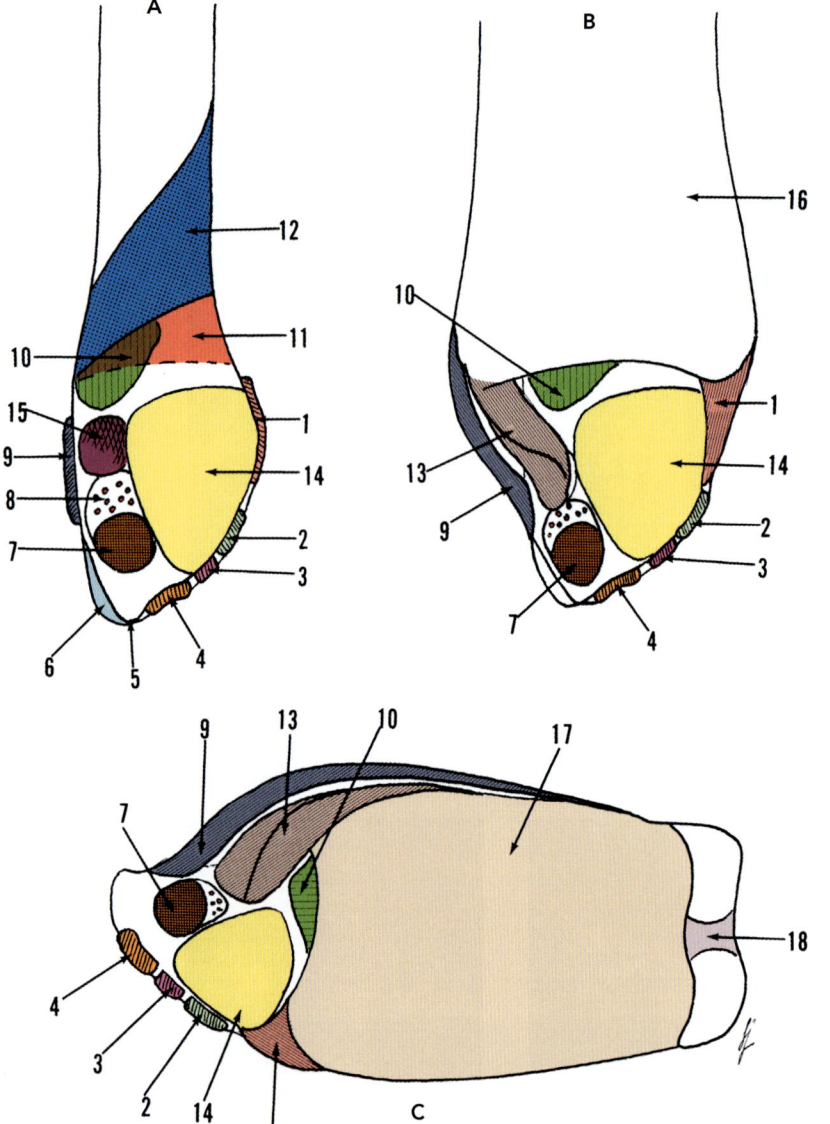

Figure 2.2 Left leg. (A) Medial surface of distal fibula and lateral malleolus. (B) Same view as in A. Distal tibia connected to fibula. (C) Inferior view of the distal tibiofibular complex. (1, anterior tibiofibular ligament; 2, main component of anterior talofibular ligament; 3, secondary band of anterior talofibular ligament; 4, calcaneofibular ligament; 5, tip of lateral malleolus, free of insertion; 6, gliding surface of peronei tendons; 7, posterior talofibular ligament; 8, cribriform fossa; 9, superficial component of posterior tibiofibular ligament; 10, synovial fringe; 11, peroneal surface corresponding to tibioperoneal recess; 12, insertion of tibiofibular interosseous ligament; 13, deep component of posterior tibiofibular ligament; 14, articular surface for the lateral surface of the talus; 15, posterosuperior tuberosity; 16, tibia; 17, tibia plafond; 18, medial malleolus.)

Lateral Surface

The lateral surface of the malleolus is smooth, convex, and subcutaneous and is in continuity with the anteroinferior segment of the fibular lateral surface.

Medial Surface

The medial surface is limited at a level corresponding to the incisura fibularis of the distal tibia. A large triangular articular surface occupies the anterosuperior aspect. The base of the triangle is proximal and convex. The apex is anteroinferior, located on the anterior border of the malleolus. The anterior border is inclined backward, whereas the posterior border is directed anteroinferiorly. The surface is convex along its long axis and corresponds to the lateral articular surface of the talus. Behind the posterosuperior angle of the triangular articular surface is the round posterior fibular tubercle, which gives origin to the deep component of the posterior tibiofibular ligament. Below the tubercle and behind the triangular articular surface is the digital fossa. The upper segment of the fossa is cribriform, with multiple vascular foramina. The lower segment gives origin to the posterior talofibular ligament. The superficial components of the posterior tibiofibular ligament originate from the posterior border of the peroneal tubercle and digital fossa (see Fig. 2.2).

The lateral malleolus is in contact with the incisura fibularis of the tibia through a minute crescentic cartilage-coated surface that is in continuity with the triangular articular surface of the fibula.

Posterior Surface

The posterior surface is broad proximally and tapers distally. The tendons of the peroneus brevis and peroneus longus

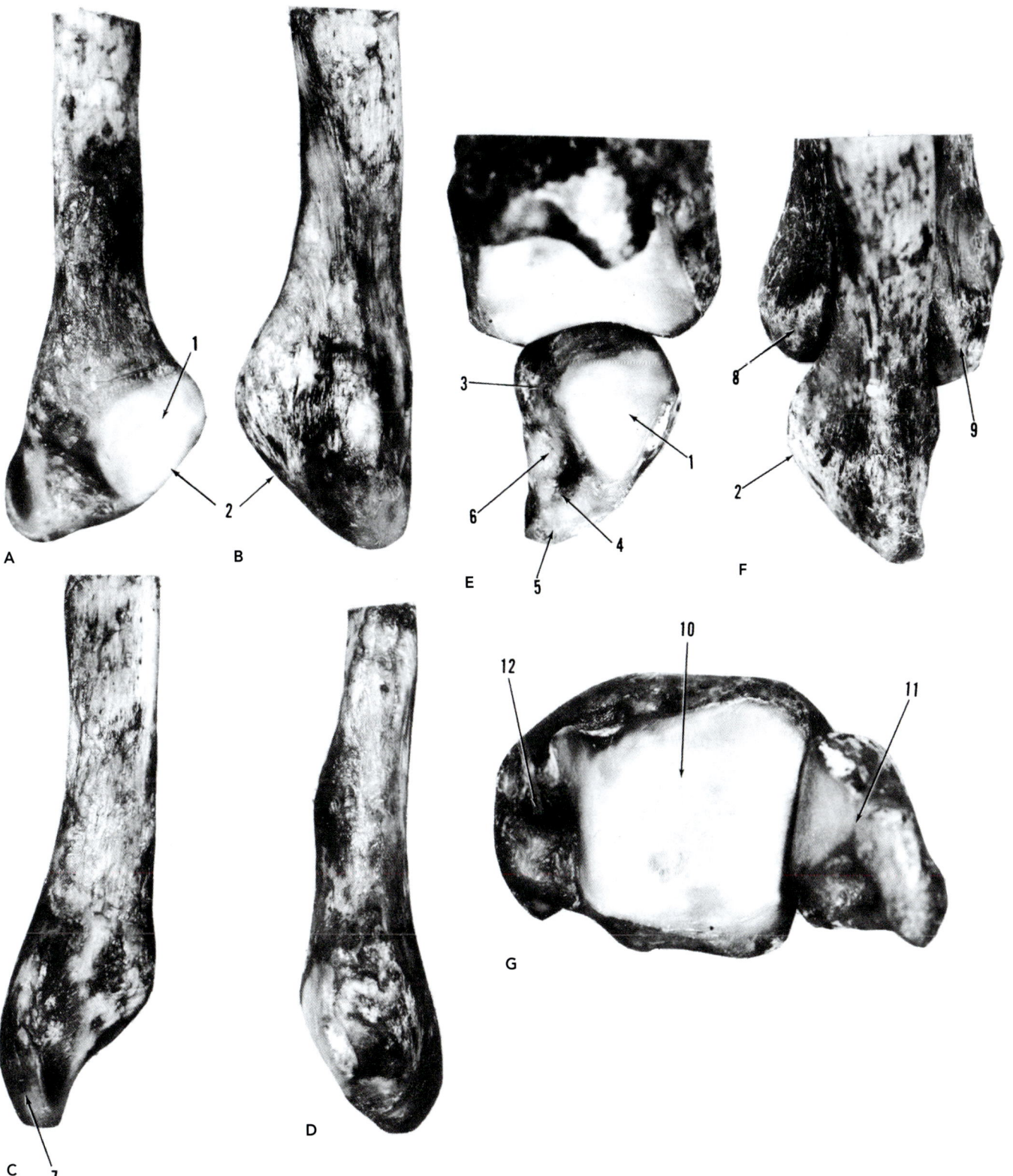

Figure 2.3 Left leg. (A), Medial view of fibula. (B) Lateral view of fibula. (C) Posterior view of fibula. (D) Anterior view of fibula. (E) Medial view of tibia-lateral malleolus. (F) Lateral view of distal fibula-tibia. (G) Inferior view of distal tibia-fibula. (*1*, articular surface; *2*, anterior border; *3*, posterosuperior tubercle; *4*, insertion tubercle of posterior talofibular ligament; *5*, tip of lateral malleolus; *6*, digital fossa; *7*, gliding surface for peronei tendon; *8*, anterior tibial tubercle; *9*, posterior tibial tubercle; *10*, tibial plafond; *11*, lateral malleolus; *12*, medial malleolus.)

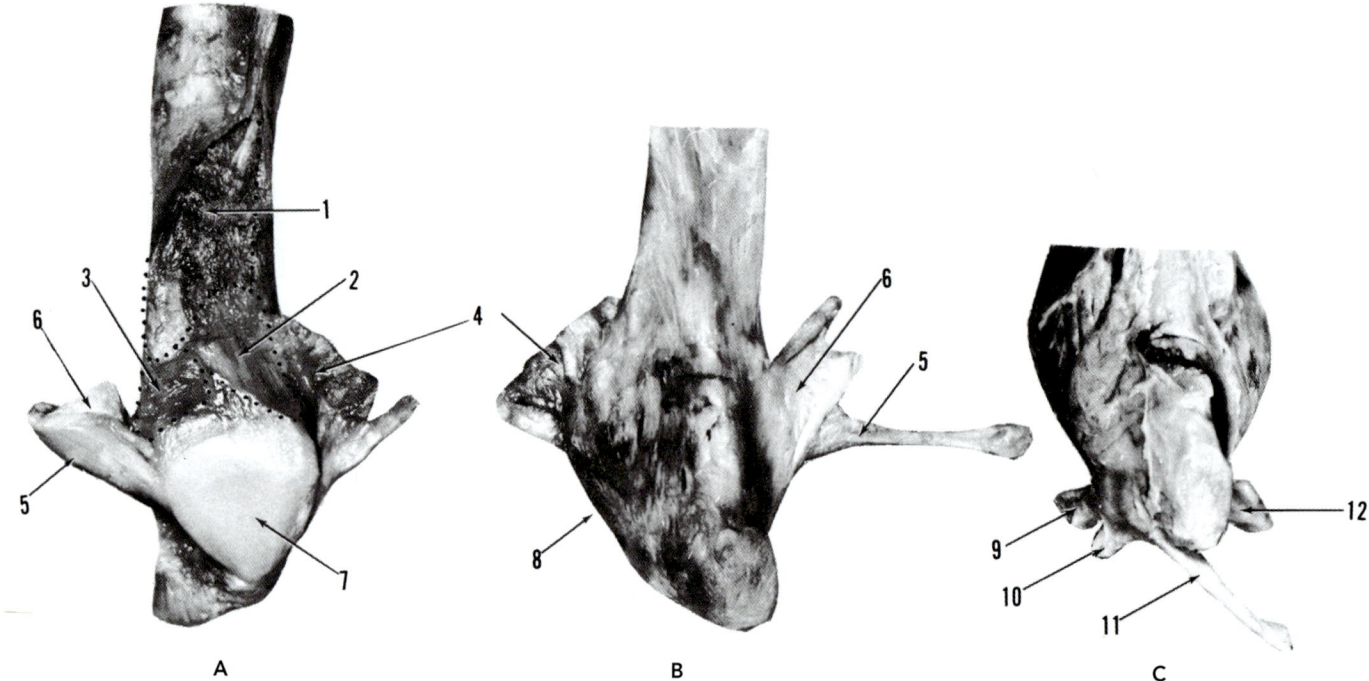

Figure 2.4 Left leg. (A) Medial view of distal fibula and lateral malleolus. (B and C) Lateral view of lateral malleolus. (1, insertion of tibiofibular interosseous ligament; 2, fibular component of tibiofibular recess; 3, insertion of synovial fringe; 4, anterior tibiofibular ligament; 5, 6, posterior tibiofibular ligament; 7, articular surface; 8, anterior border; 9, main component of anterior talofibular ligament; 10, secondary component of anterior talofibular ligament; 11, calcaneofibular ligament; 12, posterior talofibular ligament.)

follow the twist of the fibular corpus and lie on the posterior surface. The tendon of the peroneus brevis is against the bone, with the tendon of the longus on top of it. Usually, a sulcus is present on this surface. Edwards, in a study of 178 dry fibulas, gave the following data in regard to the contour of the posterior surface: definite sulcus present, 82%; flat surface, 11%; convex surface, 7%.[3] The width of the sulcus is given as the narrowest, 5 mm; the majority (62%), 6 to 7 mm; and the widest, 10 mm. The lateral border of the posterior surface may become prominent and form a lateral bony ridge. "It helps to form a flange against which the tendons of the peroneal muscles play, and it gives attachment to some of the fibers of the superior peroneal retinaculum."[3] The occurrence of this lateral bony ridge, based on Edwards' data, is as follows: well-developed lateral bony ridge, 22%; slightly developed lateral bony ridge, 48%; absence of a developed lateral bony ridge, 30%.[3] Most of the ridges are 2 mm high, but occasionally the ridges may reach an elevation of 4 mm. Cartilage covering may increase the ridge 1 to 2 mm, and often the ridge is formed by cartilage only.[3]

Edwards further reports on the presence of a prominence on the medial border on the posterior surface that forms a medial ridge in about 50% or, in the remaining half, a rounded tubercle.[3] In 4% of the fibulas, an intermediate low ridge is present between the lateral and medial ridges.

The peroneal sulcus, when present, is very shallow. Ozbag et al[4] investigated the morphometric features of the lateral malleolar groove in 93 specimens: 80 dry bones and 13 foot specimens. The malleolar groove was concave in 68% (63 specimens) and convex or flat in 32%. The mean groove width was 9.2 ± 1.6 mm and the groove depth was 1.0 ± 0.5 mm.

The anterior border of the lateral malleolus is thin above and thick below. The contour is strongly convex anteriorly. A longitudinal tubercle extending from the level of the anterosuperior angle of the articular surface to the midsegment gives insertion to the anterior tibiofibular ligament. Below this level, the anterior border bears flat tubercles corresponding to the insertion of the two bands of the anterior talofibular ligament. Further distally but still anterior in location is the insertion of the calcaneofibular ligament. The apex of the lateral malleolus is free of insertion.

The posterolateral and posteromedial borders of the lateral malleolus are covered in the descriptions of the posterior and medial surfaces.

▶ Lower End of the Tibia

The lower end of the tibia is formed by five surfaces: inferior, anterior, posterior, lateral, and medial (Fig. 2.5). The latter is prolonged distally by the medial malleolus.

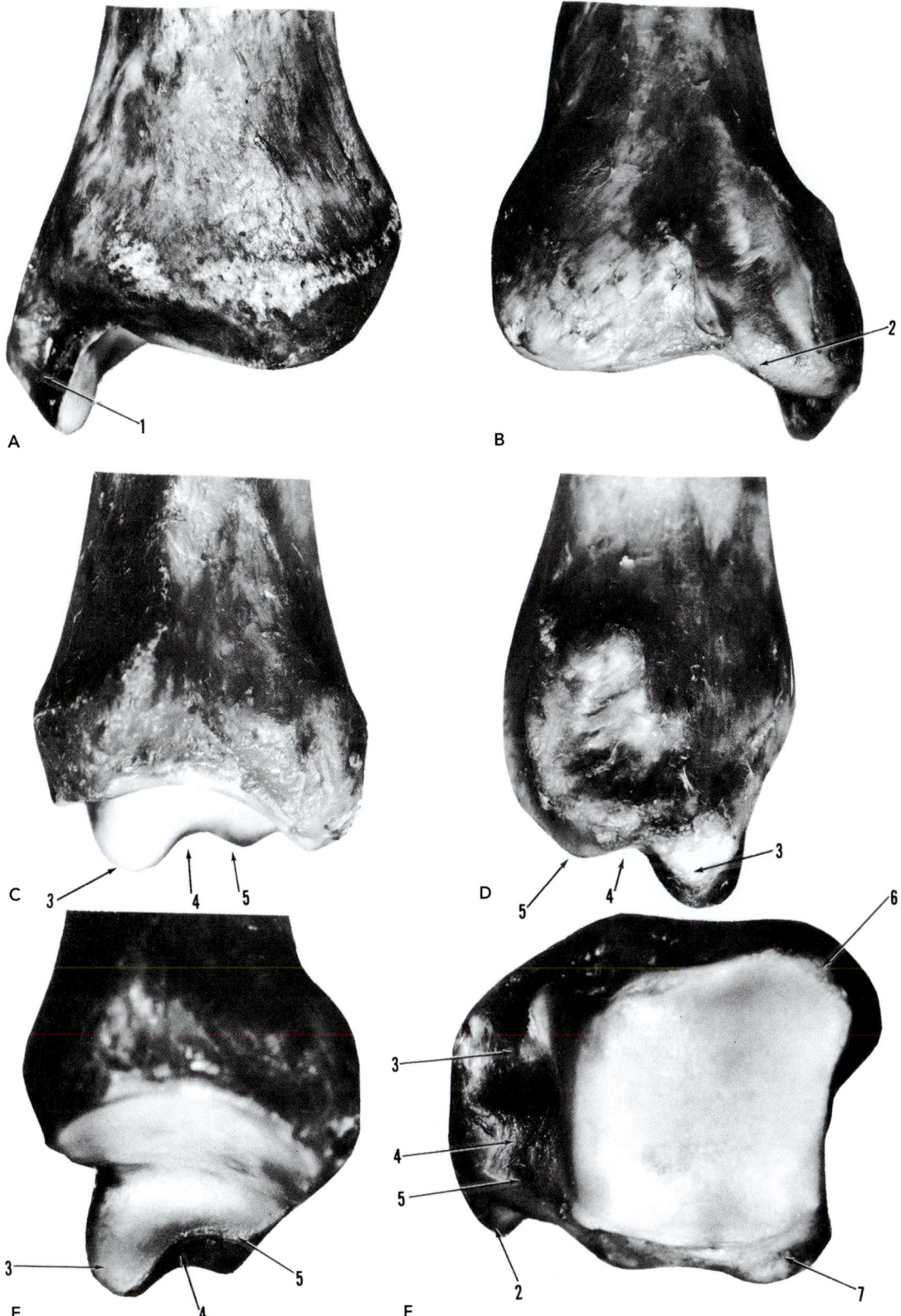

Figure 2.5 **Left leg.** **(A)** Anterior aspect of distal tibia. **(B)** Posterior aspect of distal tibia. **(C)** Lateral aspect of distal tibia. **(D)** Medial aspect of distal tibia and medial malleolus. **(E)** Lateral aspect of medial malleolus. **(F)** Inferior view of distal tibia. (*1*, medial malleolus; *2*, sulcus for tibialis posterior tendon; *3*, anterior colliculus; *4*, intercollicular groove; *5*, posterior colliculus; *6*, anterior tibial tubercle; *7*, posterior tibial tubercle.)

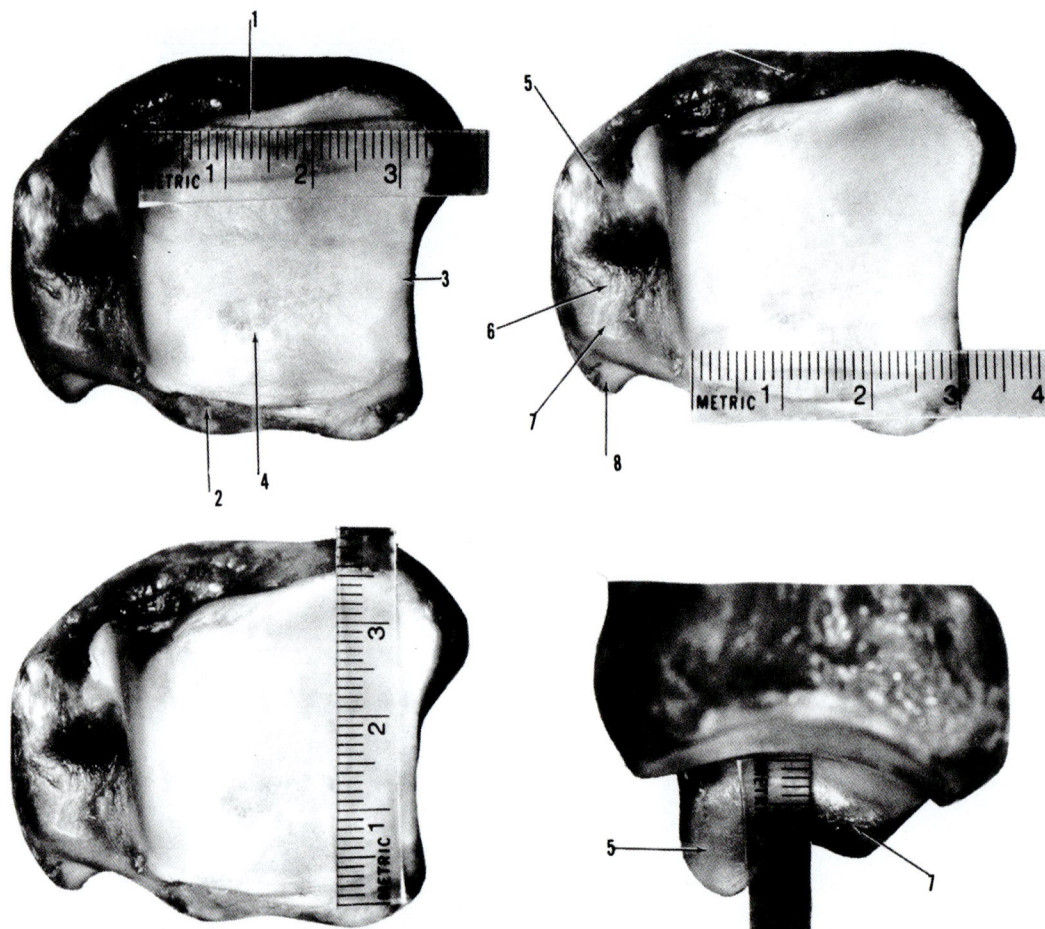

Figure 2.6 **Distal tibia and medial malleolus.** The anterior border of the distal tibia is longer than the posterior border, and the lateral border of the distal tibia is longer than the medial border. The anterior colliculus of the medial malleolus is 0.5 cm longer than the posterior colliculus. (*1*, anterior border of distal tibia; *2*, posterior border of distal tibia; *3*, lateral border of distal tibia—incisura tibialis; *4*, tibial plafond; *5*, anterior colliculus of medial malleolus; *6*, intercollicular groove of medial malleolus; *7*, posterior colliculus of medial malleolus; *8*, groove for tibialis posterior tendon.)

Inferior Surface

The inferior surface is articular and corresponds to the dome of the talus. It is concave anteroposteriorly and slightly convex transversely because of the presence of a slightly elevated ridge dividing the surface into a wider lateral and a narrower inner segment.

The lateral border is larger than the medial and the anterior border is longer than the posterior (Fig. 2.6). Geometrically, this surface is a section of a frustum of a cone with an average medial conical angle of 22° ± 4°.[5] This angle ranges from 0° to 35°.[5] An angle of 0° corresponds to a cylindrical surface. The radius of this cylinder is an average of 2 cm, and the corresponding articular arc measures 60°.[1] In any position of the talus, the tibial plafond covers only two-thirds of the talar surface, and one-third remains uncovered (Fig. 2.7). With the long axis of the tibia, the tibial plafond makes an angle of 93.3° ± 3.2°, with a range of 88° to 100°.[5]

The posterior border of the inferior articular surface is lower than the anterior. The direct implantation of the transverse component of the deep posterior tibiofibular ligament on the lateral half of this border forms a true labrum, thus increasing the depth of the containing surface (see Fig. 2.7).

Anterior Surface

The anterior surface is in continuity with the lateral surface of the tibial shaft. It is limited laterally by the interosseous border and medially by the anterior border. The surface is narrow proximally and enlarges distally, where it acquires a convexity in both the transverse and vertical directions.

A transverse ridge is present at 0.5 to 1 cm proximal to the anterior border and gives insertion to the anterior articular capsule. The transverse segment of the bone located between the articular border and the transverse ridge recedes posteriorly and

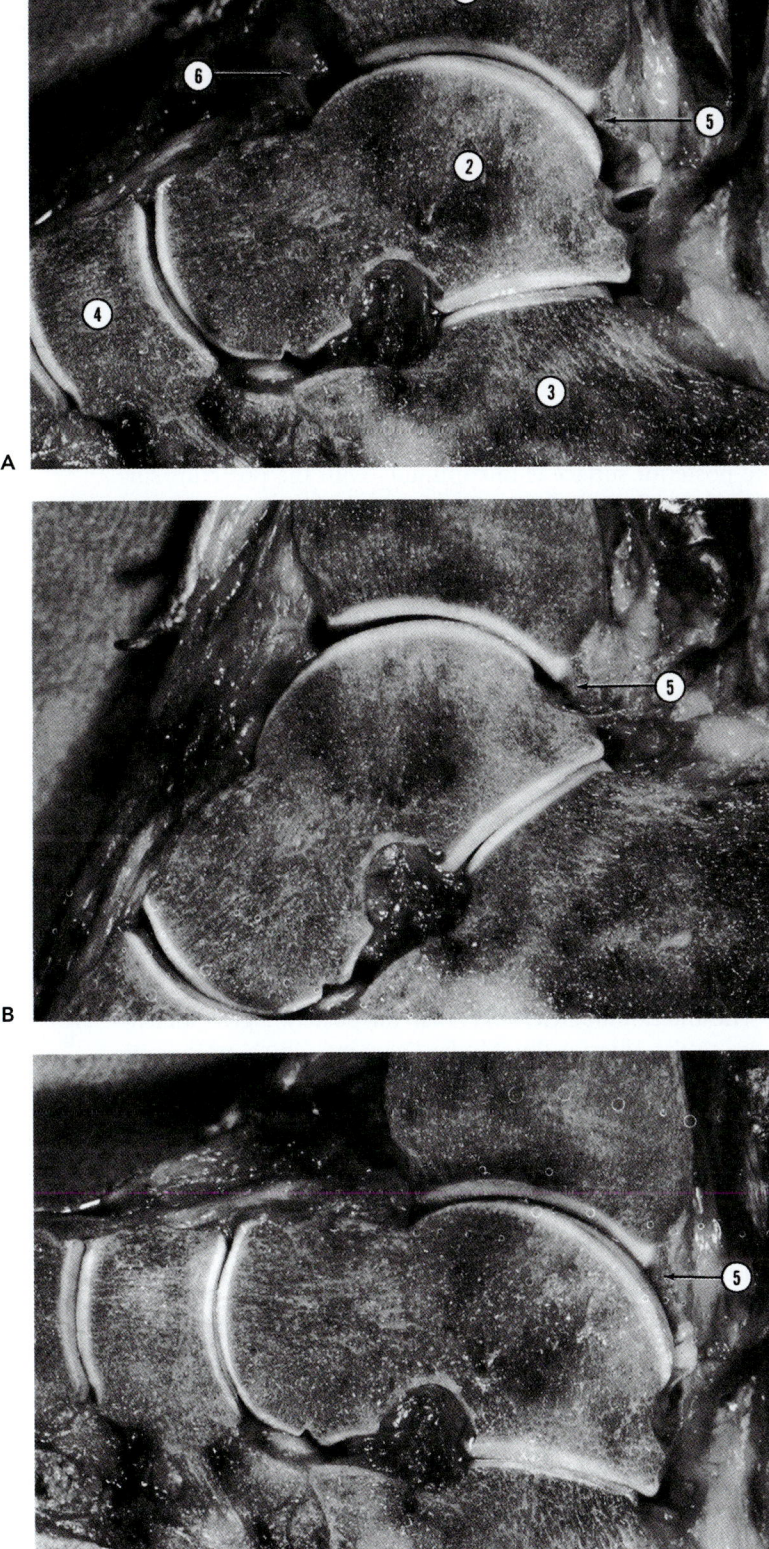

Figure 2.7 Sagittal cross-section of the ankle. (A) Ankle in neutral. **(B)** Ankle in plantar flexion. **(C)** Ankle in dorsiflexion. In any position, the articular surface of the distal tibia covers only two-thirds of the corresponding talar articular surface. (*1*, tibia; *2*, talus; *3*, calcaneus; *4*, navicular; *5*, deep component of tibiofibular ligament forming a labrum; *6*, anterior adipose body with large anterior joint cavity.)

TABLE 2.1 Distribution of Squatting Facets			
Author	Number of Tibias	Lateral Facet (%)	Medial Facet (%)
Wood[6]	118 European	17	1.7
	236 Australians	80.5	2.1
Singh[7]	292 Indian	77.4	1.7

is an intra-articular segment. This surface may bear a small articular surface (squatting facet), usually lateral in location and very occasionally medial and lateral. The distribution of these facets is as shown in Table 2.1.

Posterior Surface

The posterior surface is in continuity with the posterior surface of the tibial shaft. The proximal segment is smooth and slightly convex. The distal segment bears an oblique groove medially, directed downward and inward, corresponding to the tendon of the tibialis posterior. This segment is in continuity with the posterior surface of the medial malleolus. A second, much less delineated groove may be recognized corresponding to the tendon of the flexor digitorum longus (see Fig. 2.5).

Lateral Surface

The lateral surface is triangular with an inferior base and a superior apex. It has the contour of a vertical gutter. The apex continues with the lateral border of the tibial shaft. The anterior and posterior borders are continued distally by soft crests that terminate in an anterior and a posterior tubercle.

The anterior tubercle, larger than the posterior, gives attachment to the anterior tibiofibular ligament, which extends its fibers into the anterior surface of the distal tibia. The posterior tubercle gives attachment to the deep component of the posterior tibiofibular ligament, which extends its insertion through the transverse band onto the posterior border of the tibia. The superficial component of the posterior tibiofibular ligament has a broad attachment on the posterior tubercle and the posterior surface of the distal tibia, reaching the lateral border of the groove for the tibialis posterior tendon. The anterior tubercle overlaps the fibula, and this relationship is given interpretation in the radiologic study of the tibiofibular syndesmosis.

The tibiofibular interosseous ligament inserts on the rugosities of the upper segment of the lateral surface. The inferior segment presents a smooth, small triangular surface (base anterior, apex posterior), corresponding to the tibiofibular recess described previously. This segment is limited inferiorly by a minute crescentic cartilage-coated surface corresponding to a similar surface on the fibula.

Medial Surface

The medial surface is smooth, directed obliquely downward and inward. It is larger proximally, narrows progressively distally, and continues with the medial surface of the medial malleolus. It is limited by the anterior and posterior borders of the tibial shaft. This surface gives insertion to the upper arm of the inferior extensor retinaculum and to the flexor retinaculum.

Medial Malleolus

The medial malleolus (see Figs. 2.5 and 2.6) is a strong apophysis implanted at an obtuse angle into the medial aspect of the distal tibia. It is large at the base anteroposteriorly and flat and narrow transversely. It is formed by two segments or colliculi separated by the intercollicular groove. The anterior colliculus descends lower, usually 0.5 cm, than the posterior colliculus. The intercollicular groove is large and measures 0.5 to 1 cm in width. The deep talotibial component of the deltoid ligament inserts in the intercollicular groove, the anterior aspect of the posterior colliculus, and the posterior border of the anterior colliculus. The superficial deltoid ligament inserts on the medial surface and anterior border of the anterior colliculus and extends the attachment on the medial subcutaneous surface of the malleolus. The lateral surface of the malleolus is articular with the comma-shaped articular medial surface of the talus. The posterior border of the medial malleolus bears a groove and gives attachment to the fibrous tunnel of the tibialis posterior tendon.

The lateral malleolus, the tibial plafond, and the medial malleolus form a bony unit, the malleolar fork, covering and holding the talus on three sides. The long axis of the ankle mortise is directed posterolaterally in the transverse plane and makes an angle of 23° with the transverse axis of the tibial plateaus (Fig. 2.8). This torsion locates anatomically the medial malleolus anteromedially and the lateral malleolus posterolaterally.

TALUS

The talus is an intercalated bone located between the ankle bimalleolar fork and the tarsus. It is moored with strong ligaments but has no tendinous attachments.

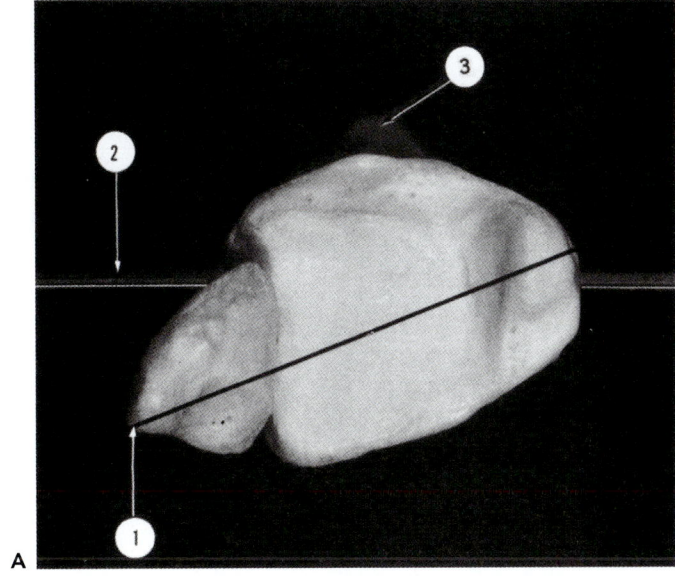

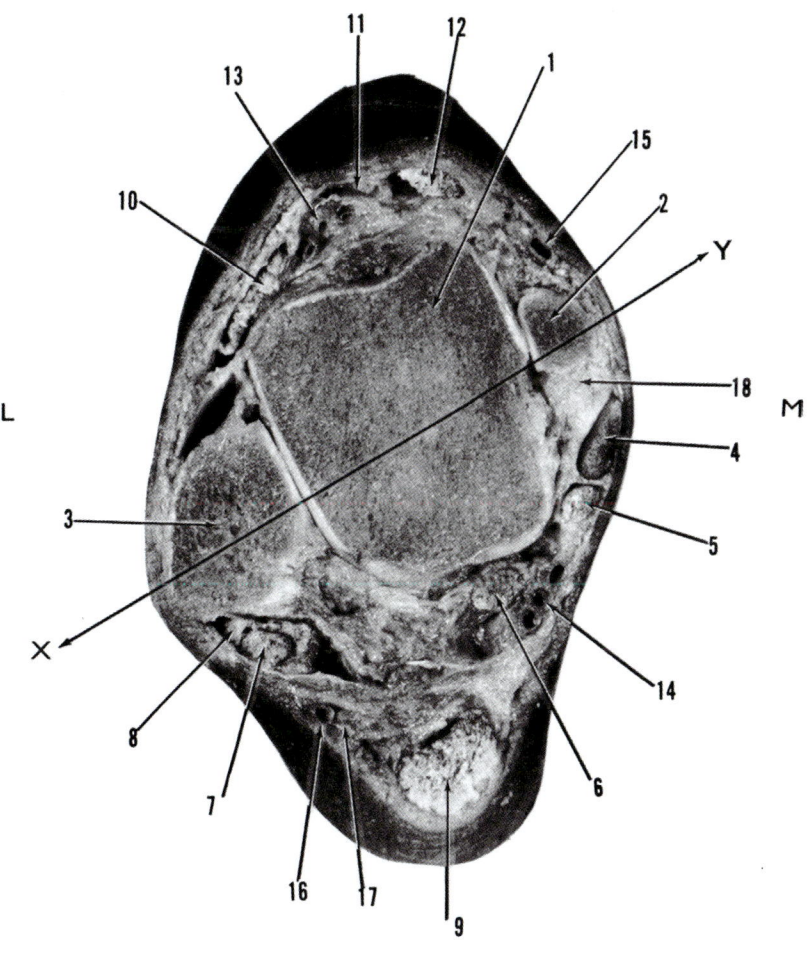

Figure 2.8 A) Distal tibia-fibula, right ankle, inferior view. (*1*, bimalleolar axis; *2*, transverse axis, transtibial plateau; *3*, anterior tibial tubercle.) The bimalleolar axis is oriented posterolaterally. The lateral malleolus is posterior, and the medial malleolus is anterior. **(B) Cross-section of left ankle, lower surface, passing 1 cm above the tip of the medial malleolus.** (*A*, anterior; *P*, posterior; *L*, lateral; *M*, medial; *1*, talus; *2*, anterior colliculus of medial malleolus; *3*, lateral malleolus; *4*,tibialis posterior tendon and tunnel; *5*, flexor digitorum longus tendon and tunnel; *6*, flexor hallucis longus tendon-muscle; *7*, peroneus longus tendon; *8*, peroneus brevis, inverted U-shaped tendon; *9*, Achilles tendon; *10*, extensor digitorum longus tendon; *11*, extensor hallucis longus tendon; *12*, tibialis anterior tendon; *13*, dorsalis pedis artery and veins; *14*, posterior tibial neurovascular bundle; *15*, greater saphenous vein; *16*, lesser saphenous vein; *17*, sural nerve; *18*, deltoid ligament, deep talotibial component [note relationship of tibialis posterior tendon and deltoid ligament]; *X-Y*, bimalleolar axis oriented posterolaterally.)

48 Sarrafian's Anatomy of the Foot and Ankle

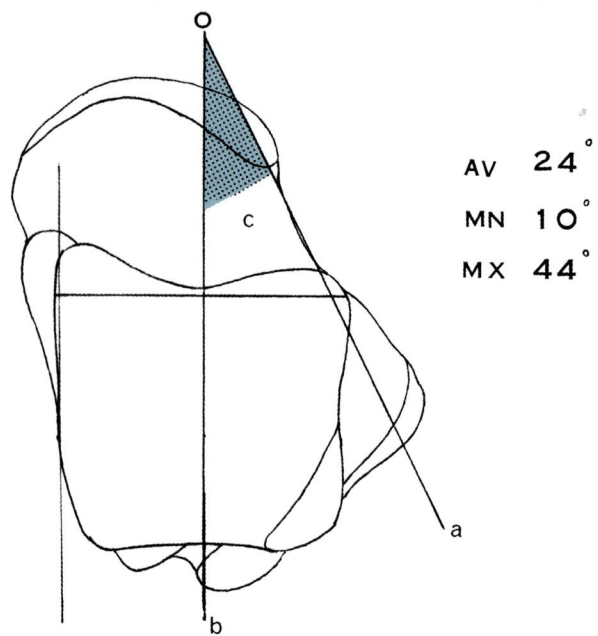

Figure 2.9 Declination angle (c) of the talar neck relative to the body. (a, Long axis of neck; b, long axis of body.)

Length: average, 48 mm; maximum, 60 mm; minimum, 40 mm.
Width: average, 37 mm; maximum, 45 mm; minimum, 30 mm.

▸ Body

The body (corpus tali) has five surfaces (Fig. 2.12): superior, lateral, medial, posterior, and inferior.

Superior Surface

The superior surface of the talar body is pulley shaped (Fig. 2.13) and articulates with the distal surface of the tibia and the transverse component of the inferior and posterior tibiofibular ligament. The groove of the pulley runs near the medial border, which makes the lateral segment of the surface wider than the medial. The surface is markedly convex anteroposteriorly, with a sagittal radius of convexity of 20 mm (average). It presents a mild concavity transversely. This concavity may be shallow or deep and is the norm in 80% of the tali; in the remaining 20%, the transverse curvature is more complex, with a medial concavity and a lateral convexity. These talar curvatures have their interlocking counterparts in the distal tibias.

The medial border of the trochlear surface is straight, slightly lower than the lateral, and soft in contour. The lateral border is oblique, directed posteromedially, and beveled in its posterior segment, thus forming a triangular facet (the facies articularis intermedia corporis tali). The lateral border is sharper than the medial in the midsegment. Because of the obliquity of the lateral border, the trochlear surface is wedge-shaped and is narrower posteriorly.

The difference in width between the anterior and posterior transverse diameters, including the triangular facet, is shown in Table 2.3.

The anterior border of the trochlear surface is variable in contour: it may be straight, slightly concave, convex in its entirety, or in the shape of an elongated "S." Extension facets from the superior articular surface onto the neck are seen both medially and laterally (see Fig. 2.12). A medial extension facet is always accompanied by a forward prolongation of the medial malleolar articular surface of the talus;

The talus is formed by three parts: the body (corpus tali), the neck (collum), and the head (caput). The body is defined as the part of the bone located posterior to an imaginary plane passing through the anterior border of the superior surface of the trochlea tali and the posterior calcaneal surface. The neck is the segment of bone anterior to this plane, located between the body and the head. *The body and the neck are not coaxial.* In the horizontal plane, the neck shifts medially and makes an angle of declination with the long axis of the trochlea tali. This angle is variable (Fig. 2.9), as indicated in Table 2.2.

In the sagittal plane, the neck is deviated downward relative to the talar body and makes an angle of inclination (Fig. 2.10; see Table 2.2).

The length and width of the bone measured on 100 dry tali are as follows (Fig. 2.11):

TABLE 2.2 Angles of Declination and Inclination in Talus			
Author	Number of Tali	Declination Angle	Inclination Angle
Testut[8]		22°	115°
Paturet[9]		20°-30°	115°
Sewell[10]	1006 Egyptian	18° average, 7° minimum, 43° maximum	112° average, 98° minimum, 127° maximum
Present series	100	24° average, 10° minimum, 44° maximum	114° average (24° plantar tilt), 95° minimum (5-degree plantar tilt), 140° maximum (50° plantar tilt)

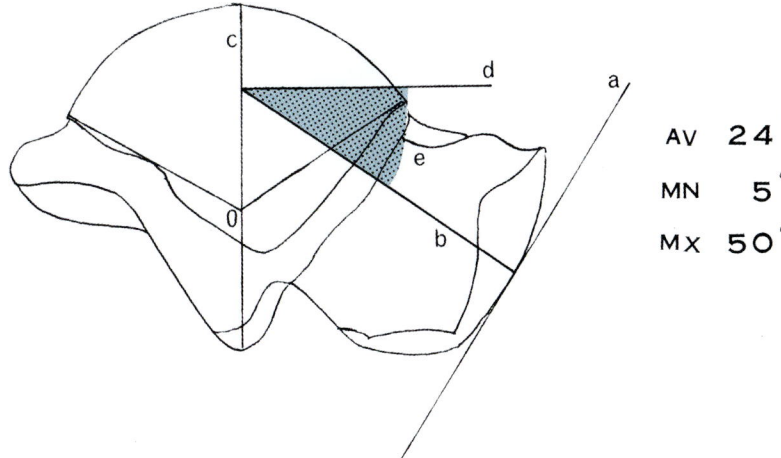

Figure 2.10 Inclination angle (e) of the talar neck relative to the body. The center O of the lateral trochlear arc is determined. The arc is bisected by the radius OC. A tangent is drawn at the apex of the navicular articular surface. A perpendicular line b is drawn at the tangential point. The line b gives the direction of the talar neck and intersects the radius OC of the talar trochlear arc. At this point of intersection, a perpendicular line d is traced, determining the inclination angle e.

however, the reverse is not true. The frequency of occurrence of a medial extension facet from the trochlear surface is shown in Table 2.4.

A lateral extension surface is to be differentiated from a squatting facet. The criteria of differentiation are clearly stated by Singh.[7] A lateral extension surface continues the convexity of the trochlear surface. During dorsiflexion, this facet establishes contact with the lower end of the distal tibia and not with its anterior border. In contradistinction, a squatting facet, in continuity with the trochlear surface, is concave anteroposteriorly and is directed upward and occasionally backward. During dorsiflexion of the foot, it establishes contact with the anterior margin of the distal tibia.

The frequency of occurrence of these lateral prolongations is shown in Table 2.5.

Lateral Surface

The lateral surface of the talar body is mostly occupied by a large trigonal articular surface, the facies malleolus lateralis. The curved base of this articular surface corresponds to the lateral border of the trochlear surface. The lateral profile of the base is almost an arc of a true circle measuring 106° ± 13°.[5,13] The surface is concave in the vertical direction and slightly convex transversely. The convexity is more pronounced in the apical portion. Rarely, a concavity replaces the convexity in this

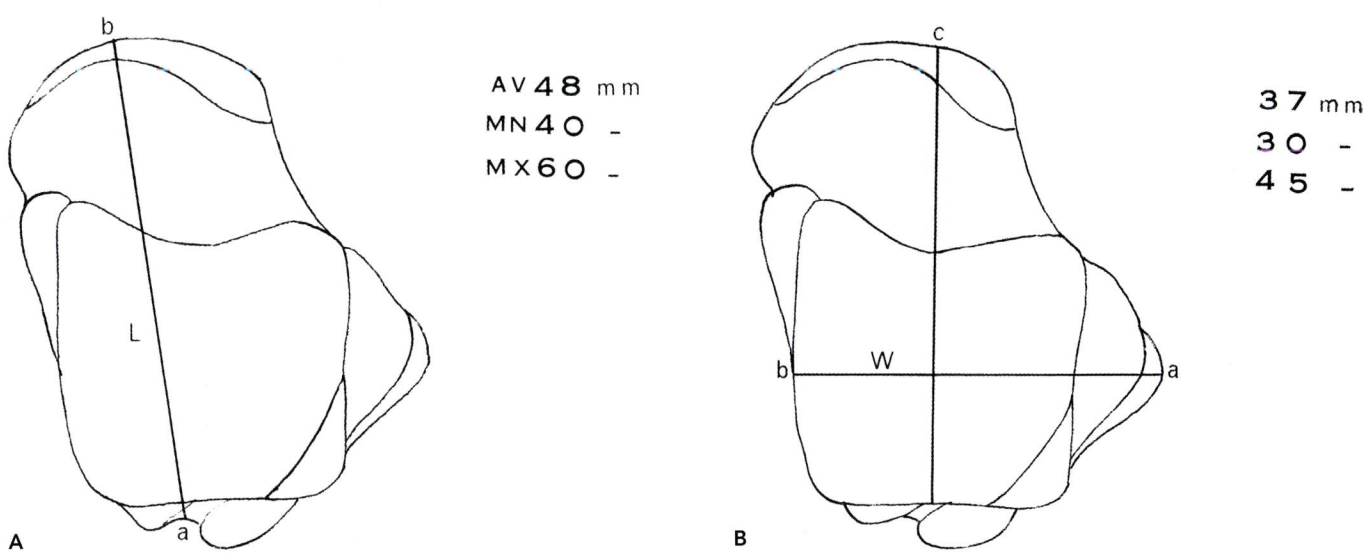

Figure 2.11 Measurements of talus. **(A)** Length of talus is (L) determined by a line joining the apex of the navicular articular surface to the flexor hallucis longus groove. **(B)** Width of talus (W) determined with caliper holding the talus at the tip of the lateral process and the middle of the medial trochlear line. The direction of the caliper is maintained perpendicular to the latter.

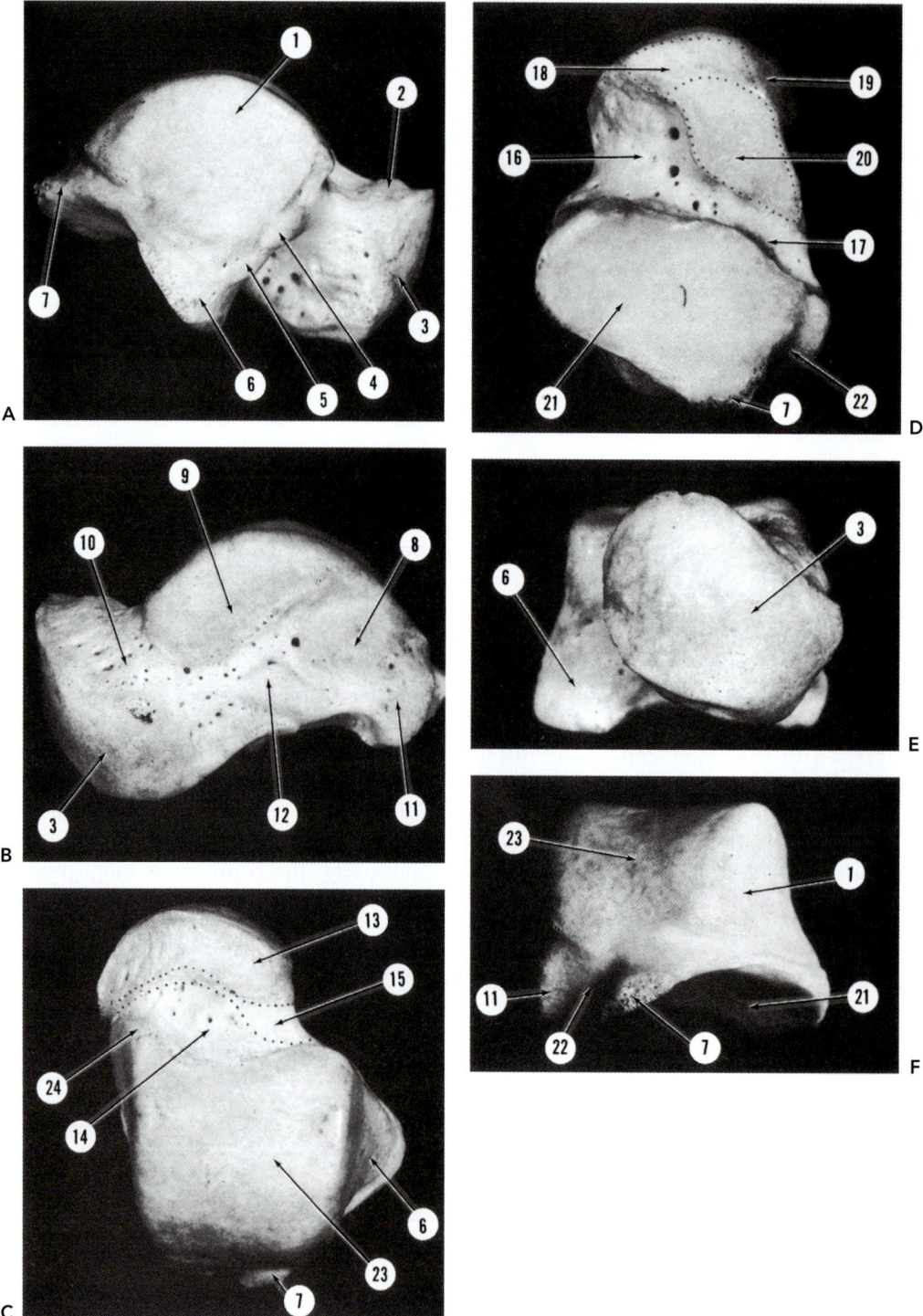

Figure 2.12 Talus. (A) Lateral aspect. **(B)** Medial aspect. **(C)** Superior aspect. **(D)** Inferior aspect. **(E)** Anterior aspect. **(F)** Posterior aspect. (*1*, articular surface—facies malleolus lateralis; *2*, cervical collar; *3*, articular surface—facies articularis navicularis; *4, 5*, tubercles for insertions of anterior talofibular ligaments; *6*, lateral process; *7*, posterolateral tubercle; *8*, oval surface for insertion of talotibial component of deltoid ligament; *9*, articular surface—facies malleolaris medialis; *10*, talar neck; *11*, posteromedial tubercle; *12*, tubercle of insertion of deltoid ligament; *13*, segment of talar neck located within talonavicular joint; *14*, segment of talar neck located within talotibial joint; *15*, extra-articular segment of talar neck where a bursa may be found against which glides medial root of inferior extensor retinaculum; *16*, sinus tarsi; *17*, canalis tarsi; *18*, anterior calcaneal articular surface of the talar head; *19*, articular segment of talar head corresponding to superomedial and inferior calcaneonavicular ligaments; *20*, middle calcaneal articular surface of talar neck; *21*, posterior calcaneal articular surface of the talar body; *22*, canal of the flexor hallucis longus tendon; *23*, trochlear surface; *24*, anteromedial extension of trochlear.)

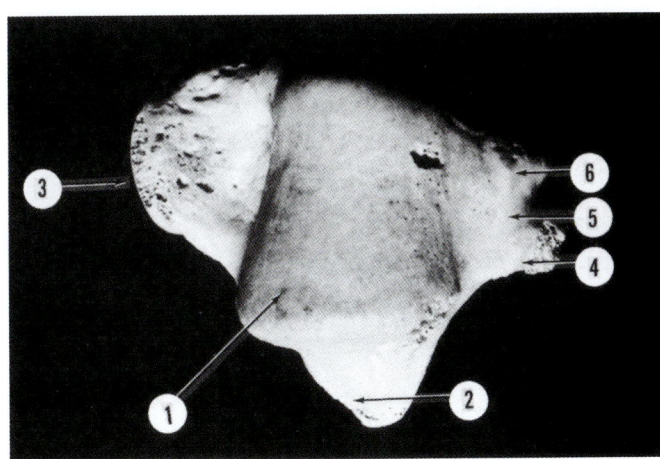

Figure 2.13 **Superior aspect of talus.** (1, talar pulley; 2, lateral process; 3, talar head; 4, posterolateral tubercle; 5, canal of flexor hallucis longus; 6, posteromedial tubercle.)

TABLE 2.4 Frequency of Occurrence of Medial Extension Facet		
Author	Number of Tali	Occurrence (%)
Singh[7]	300 Indian	55
Present series	100	36
Sewell[10]	1006 Egyptian	19
Barnett[12]	100 European	11

location. The vertical concavity is determined by the outward projection of the lateral talar process. The angle of projection as measured in 100 tali is 32° average, 55° maximum, and 15° minimum (Fig. 2.14).

The lateral talocalcaneal ligament inserts on the apex of the lateral process.

Along the anterior border of the trigonal articular surface are two tubercles for the insertion of the anterior talofibular ligament, the lower tubercle being less pronounced. Sometimes, the tubercles are replaced by a depression or notch. Occasionally, a small accessory articular surface is seen on the anterior segment of the lateral process. This surface, the facies externa accessoria corporis tali, is in continuity with the posterior calcaneal surface. When well developed, it is triangular with an inferior base and oriented anteroinferiorly (Fig. 2.15). In 100 Egyptian tali, this accessory surface was present in 10.15%.[10] In the present series of 100 tali, a large accessory surface was present in 4% and an accessory surface of variable size was present in 34%. Martus et al[14] surveyed 79 paired tali calcanei among 43 skeletons from individuals who had an average age of 13.4 years at the time of death. Skeletons of individuals less than 1 year had not been included. An accessory anterolateral facet of the talus was identified in 34% (27 specimens) and was large in 2.5% (2 specimens). The accessory anterolateral talar facet was significantly associated with dorsal talar beaking in 29% (Fig. 2.16).

Along the posteroinferior border of the lateral malleolar surface, there is a groove that gives attachment to the posterior talofibular ligament. This groove extends forward, usually up to the midsegment of the posteroinferior border, where it makes a notch. Rarely, it is continued forward to the apex of the facet.

Medial Surface

The medial surface is divided into two fields: superior and inferior.

The superior segment is occupied by the facies malleolaris medialis or the auricular facet. This articular surface is comma shaped, and the long axis is oriented anteroposteriorly. The anterior part is broad and circular; the tail is thin and posterior. The superior border of this surface forms the medial border of the trochlea. This border is convex anteroposteriorly. The anterior third of this curve is part of a circle with a radius smaller than that of the lateral surface. The posterior two-thirds is an arc of a circle, the radius of which is larger than that of the lateral profile.[13] Inman, contouring the trochlear surface in planes perpendicular to the functional axis of the ankle, found the medial side of the trochlea to be an arc of a circle in 80% of the tali and to deviate from it in the remaining 20%.[5] The average arc on the medial side is 103° ± 14°.[5]

The medial facet is often extended anteriorly over the medial aspect of the collum tali beyond the level of the anterior border of the trochlea. The frequency of occurrence of this extension was 96% in 300 Indian tali[7]; in the present series of 100 tali,

TABLE 2.3 Difference in Anterior and Posterior Transverse Diameters		
Author	Number of Tali	Difference
Testut[8]		5-6 mm
Poirier and Charpy[11]		4-5 mm
Inman[5]	100	2.4 ± 1.3 mm average
Present series	100	4.2 mm average, 2 mm minimum, 6 mm maximum

TABLE 2.5 Frequency of Occurrence of Lateral Extension and Squatting Facets				
		Occurrence (%)		
Author	Tali	Lateral Extension Facet	Squatting Facet	Total
Singh[7]	300 Indian	54.6	26.6	81.2
Present series	100	36	33	69
Barnett[12]	100 European	17	2	19

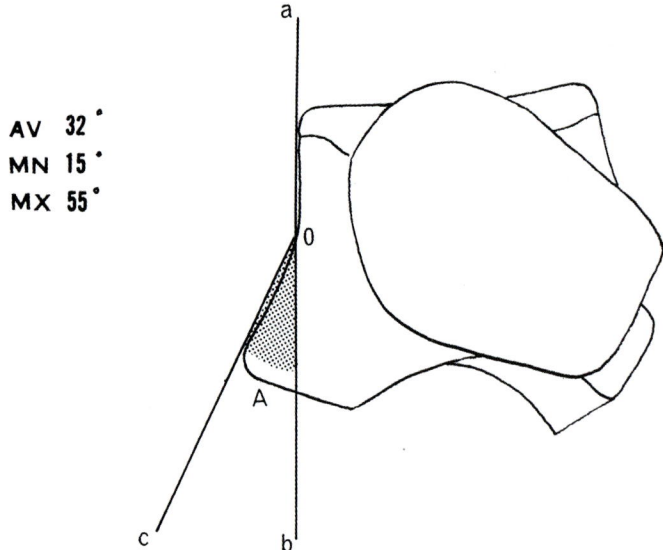

Figure 2.14 **Angle of lateral projection (A)** of talar lateral process. (*aob*, tangential line to lateral surface; *co*, tangential line to lateral process.)

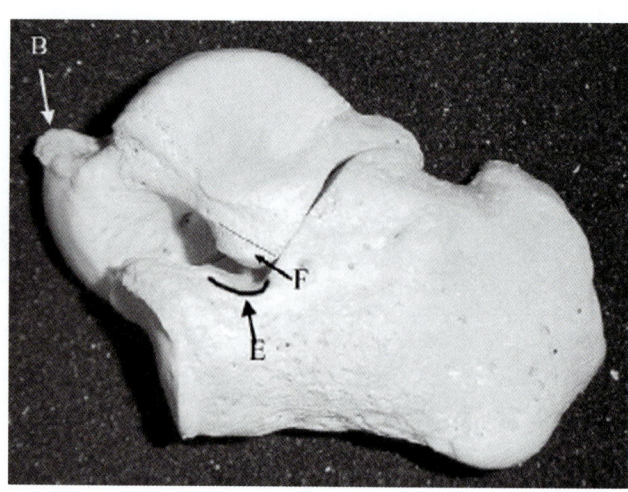

Figure 2.16 Lateral view of the talus and calcaneus, showing an accessory anterolateral talar facet (*F*), beaking of the dorsal aspect of the talar neck (*B*), and a calcaneal neck anterior extension facet (*E*). (From Martus JE, Fermino JE, Caird MS, et al. Accessory anterolateral facet of the pediatric talus: an anatomical study. *J Bone Joint Surg Am.* 2008;90:2453.)

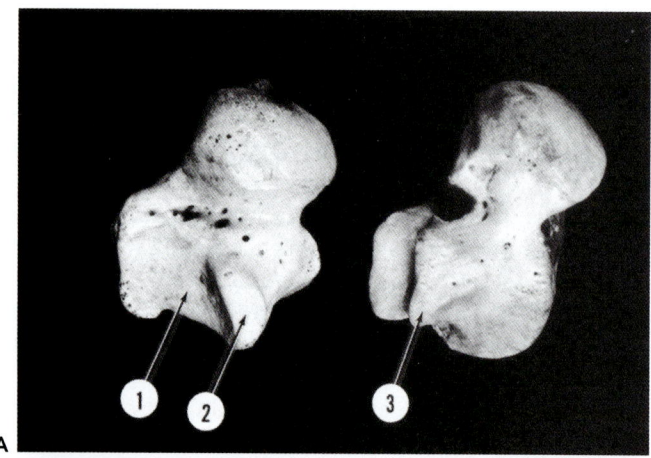

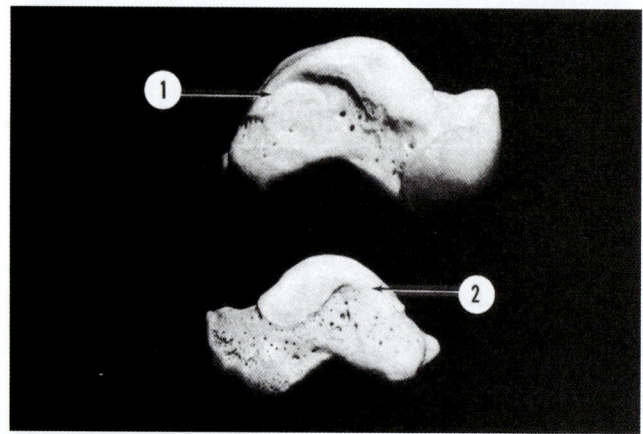

Figure 2.15 **(A) Inferolateral view of tali.** (*1*, posterior calcaneal articular surface with *2*, facies externa accessoria; *3*, absent accessory facet.) **(B) Medial view of tali.** (*1*, *2*, posterior extension of medial articular facet.)

it was 91% (55% isolated extension, 36% in association with anterior extension of trochlear surface).

When well developed, the anterior extension of the medial articular surface projects medially and downward and articulates in strong dorsiflexion with the corresponding anterior aspect of the medial malleolus, which is then covered with articular cartilage. A posterior extension of the medial articular surface behind the area of attachment of the deep portion of the deltoid ligament is also seen (see Fig. 2.15).

The inferior segment is occupied in the anterior half by a depressed surface perforated by numerous vascular foramina. Under the tail of the articular surface, the posterior half is occupied by a large oval surface, flat or elevated, which gives insertion to the talotibial deep component of the deltoid ligament.

Posterior Surface

The posterior surface or processus posterior tali comprises the posterolateral and posteromedial tubercles flanking the sulcus for the flexor hallucis longus tendon.

The posterolateral tubercle is large, more prominent than the medial tubercle. The size varies from a barely perceptible structure to a well-developed tubercle projecting posterolaterally from the talus (Fig. 2.17). This tubercle presents an inferior articular surface in continuity with the posterolateral corner of the posterior calcaneal surface of the talus. The superior surface is irregular and nonarticular and gives insertion on the lateral aspect to the posterior talofibular ligament and the talar component of the fibuloastragalocalcaneal ligament of Rouvière and Canela Lazaro.[15] The deep layer of the flexor retinaculum inserts on the medial aspect, whereas the posterior talocalcaneal ligament attaches to its inferior border.

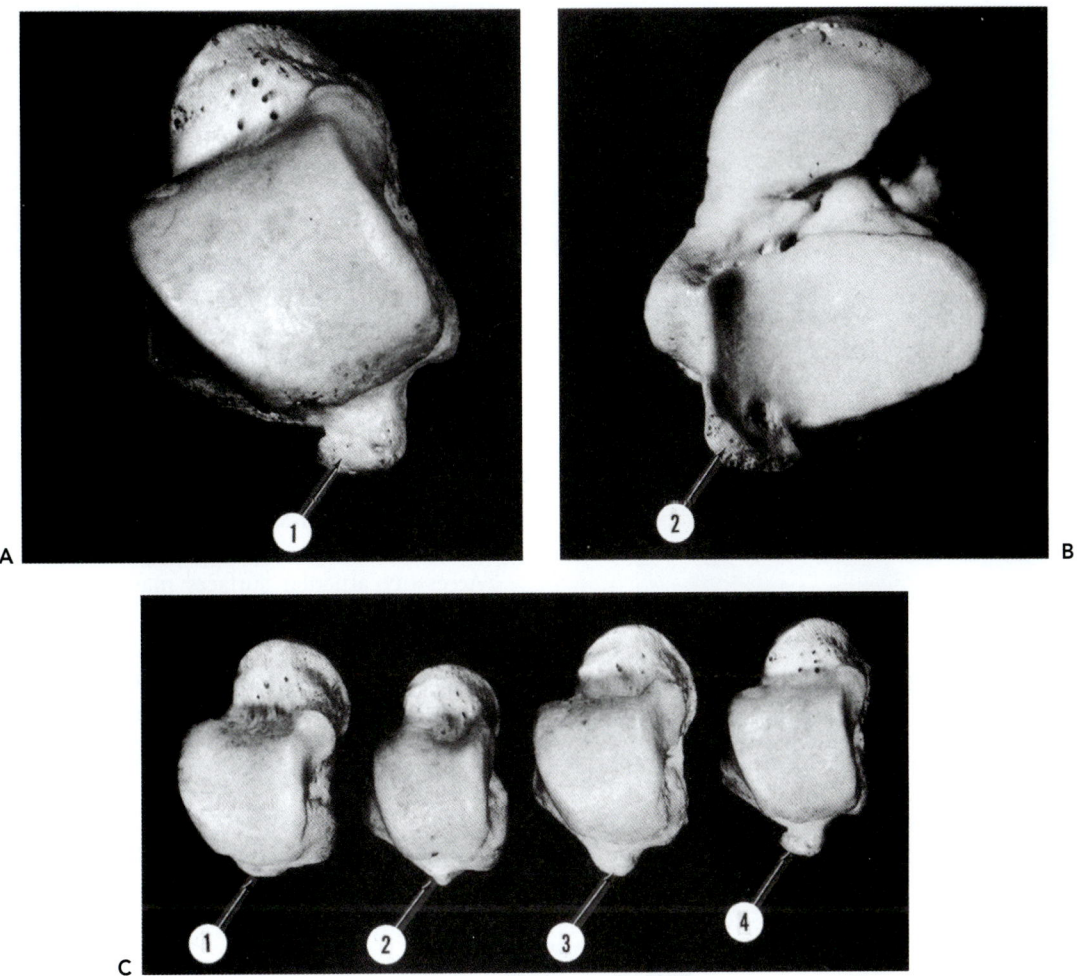

Figure 2.17 **(A)** Trigonal process, superior view. **(B)** Trigonal process, inferior view. Its articular surface is in continuity with that of the posterior calcaneal articular surface. **(C)** Variations in the size of the trigonal process. (*1*, absent; *2*, moderate; *3*, medium; *4*, large.)

An accessory bone, os trigonum (Figs. 2.18 and 2.19), may be found in connection with the posterolateral tubercle. This ossicle has three surfaces: anterior, inferior, and posterior. The anterior surface articulates with the posterolateral tubercle or is attached to the latter with fibrous, fibrocartilaginous, or cartilaginous tissue. The inferior surface articulates with the os calcis. The posterior surface is nonarticular. The capsuloligamentous structures attaching on the posterolateral tubercle extend their insertions on this surface. The frequency of occurrence of the os trigonum in adults is shown in Table 2.6.

Sewell found a percentage of "separation" of 10.9% in 1006 tali.[10] "Separation" includes the presence of a notch in the margin of the lateral process, a groove on the articular surface, a combination of both, or a frank separation. The last occurred in 24.1% of the separated group, which was 3% of the total group.

A fused os trigonum is called a trigonal process (see Fig. 2.17). The os trigonum is more often bilateral than unilateral. Very rarely, it is found in two equal or unequal parts. Distinct on one side, it may be present as a trigonal process on the other.

The medial tubercle is of variable size. It is in continuity with the medial talar surface and gives attachment to the deep and superficial layers of the talotibial components of the deltoid ligament, the medial talocalcaneal ligament, and the tunnel of the flexor hallucis longus tendon. Rarely, the tubercle may be very large and may extend downward over the os calcis, contributing to a talocalcaneal coalition (Fig. 2.20).

The sulcus of the flexor hallucis longus tendon is located between the posterolateral and the posteromedial tubercle. It is directed obliquely downward and inward and is curved anteriorly. The angle made by the long axis of the sulcus with the transverse trochlear axis in 100 tali is 68° average, 85° maximum, and 55° minimum (Fig. 2.21A).

Inferior Surface

The inferior surface is occupied by the facies articularis calcanea posterior. The long axis of this articular surface is directed anterolaterally. The angle made by this axis with the anterior border of the trochlea in 100 tali is 37° average, 50° maximum, and 26° minimum (Fig. 2.21B).

The articular surface is quadrilateral, rectangular medially, and more or less oval laterally. The surface is strongly concave in the long axis and usually flat or very minimally concave transversely. The anteromedial border is usually convex and forms the posterior

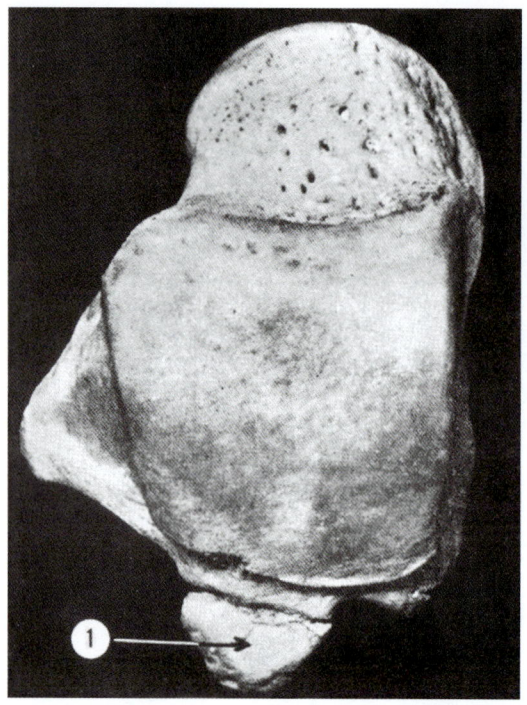

Figure 2.18 **Os trigonum (1).** (From Dwight T. *Variations of the Bones of the Hands and Feet: A Clinical Atlas.* JB Lippincctt; 1907:14-23.)

TABLE 2.6 Frequency of Occurrence of Os Trigonum in Adults		
Author	Number of Tali	Occurrence (%)
Thompson[16]	438	2.7
Stieda[17]	305	5.9
Pfitzner[18]	841	6.1
Storton[19]	558	7.7

border of the tarsal canal and the sinus tarsi. This border extends obliquely from the medial tubercle to the anterior surface of the lateral process of the talus. Occasionally, the border is straight or has a complex configuration (see Fig. 2.12). The posterolateral border is straight and parallel to the long axis. Of the two short sides, the medial is straight and directed posterolaterally and supports the posterior process of the talus; the lateral border is convex and supports the base of the lateral process of the talus.

Accessory articular surfaces may be present in continuity with the posterior calcaneal surface. Extending from the anterolateral corner is the facies externa accessoria corporis tali (see Fig. 2.15). A small facet may be present in the anteromedial corner, covering the undersurface of the medial tubercle. A trigonal process or a large lateral tubercle prolongs the articular surface posteriorly (see Fig. 2.17).

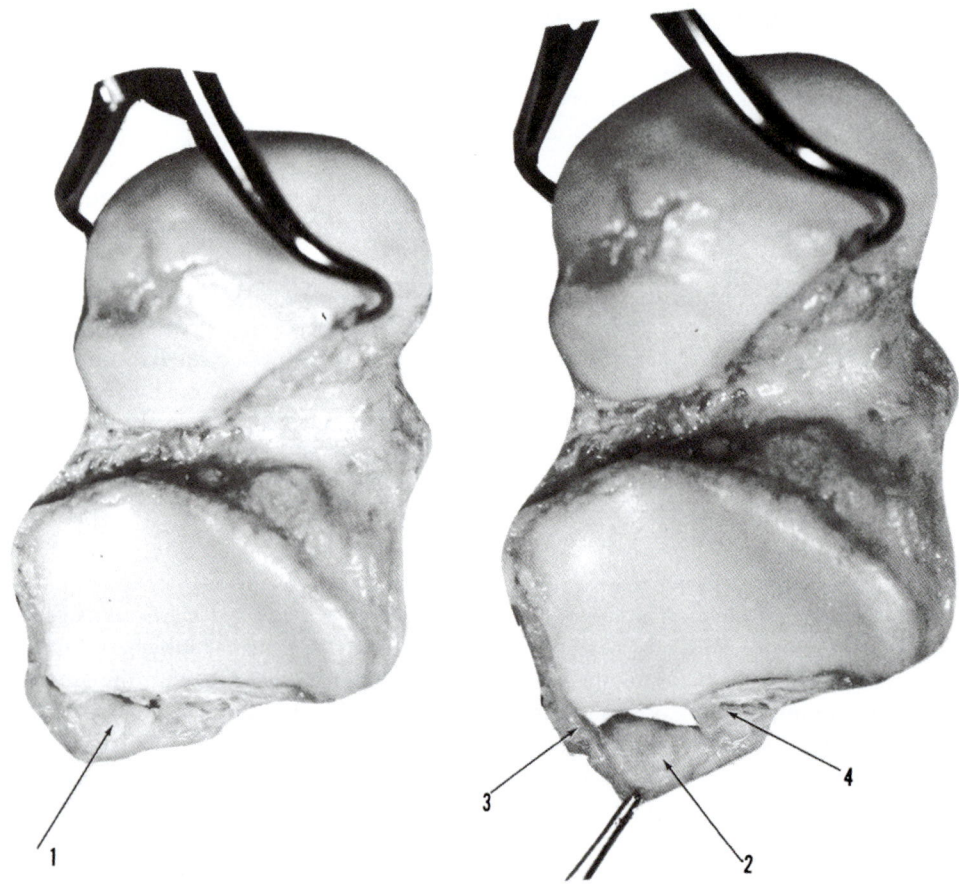

Figure 2.19 **Os trigonum.** (*1*, *2*, inferior articular surface; *3*, *4*, ligaments of attachment on each side: thin anterior capsular structure has been removed.)

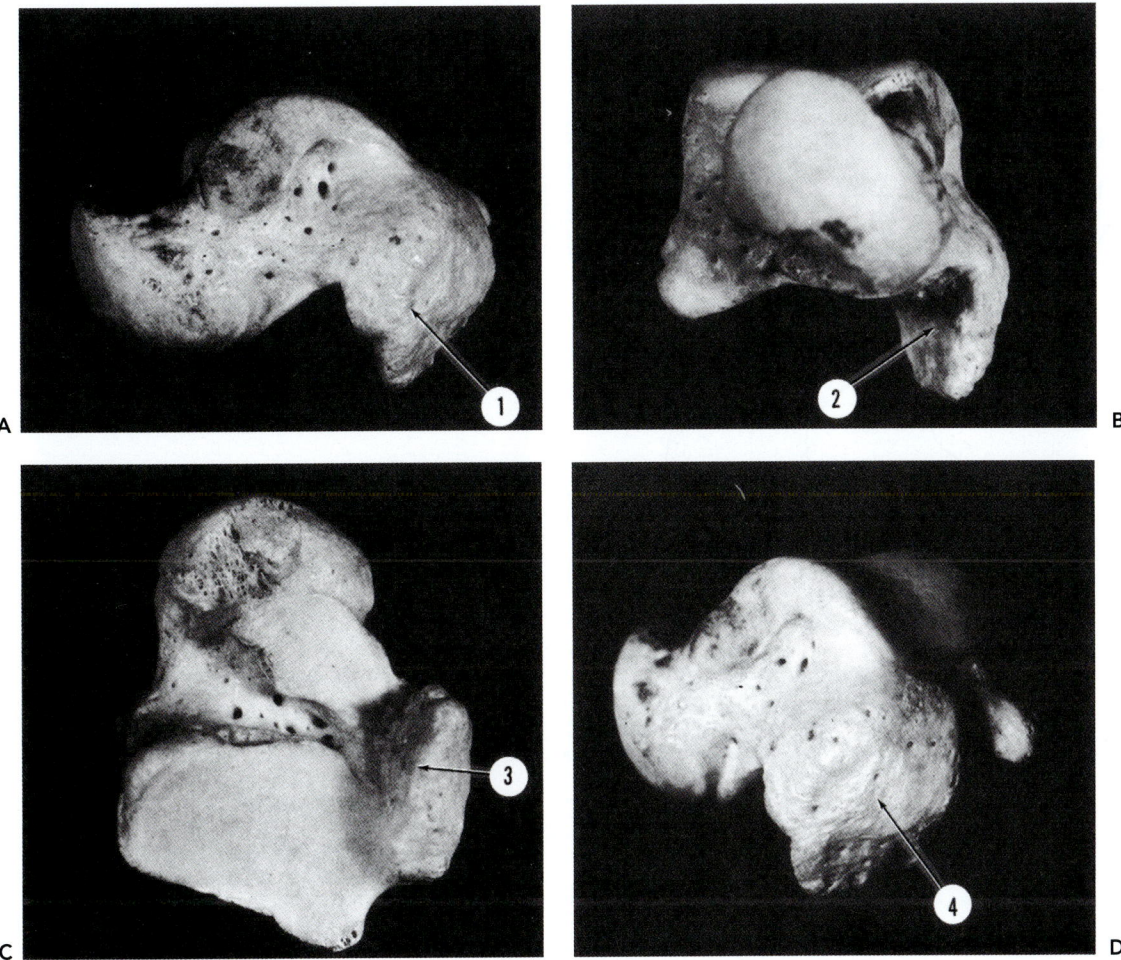

Figure 2.20 Talus. (A) Medial aspect. (B) Anterior aspect. (C) Inferior aspect. (D) Posteromedial aspect. Large posteromedial talar tubercle (1–4) probably forming a coalition with its corresponding calcaneus.

The posterior calcaneal surface may establish union with the facies articularis calcanea media, creating a single articulating surface running along the undersurface of the bone and closing the tarsal canal medially. In other instances, these two surfaces fuse through a direct anterior extension from the posterior calcaneal surface; without the medial detour, this extension completely obliterates the tarsal canal and a segment of the sinus tarsi (Fig. 2.22).

▶ Neck

The neck (collum tali) is the segment of the talus located between the body posteriorly and the head anteriorly (see Fig. 2.12). Its average length is 17 mm, with a maximum of 23 mm and a minimum of 12 mm (Fig. 2.23).

The neck is projected anteromedially and downward, as described previously. The lateral border is slightly concave and well delineated, whereas the medial border is round and at times not discernible. The neck presents four surfaces: superior, lateral, inferior, and medial.

Superior Surface

The superior surface is limited anteriorly by the articular surface corresponding to the navicular and posteriorly by the anterior border of the trochlea. The lateral half of the surface is mostly occupied by a deep, concave cribriform fossa. The remaining anterior part of this surface is occupied by a bony prominence or a smooth, flat bony segment. The medial half of the superior surface is inclined medially because of the rotation of the talar head. In certain tali, a transverse cervical ridge or collar runs parallel to the articular surface of the head.[20] The talotibial capsule inserts close to the malleolar facets laterally, medially, and distal to the cribriform fossa, which remains intra-articular. The talonavicular capsule inserts transversely along the articular surface of the head. On the lateral aspect of the neck, the capsules of the talotibial and talonavicular joints are separated by a bare extra-articular bony segment, over which glides the medial root of the inferior extensor retinaculum; a bursa may be found in this location. The superficial talotibial component of the deltoid ligament inserts on the medial aspect of the cervical

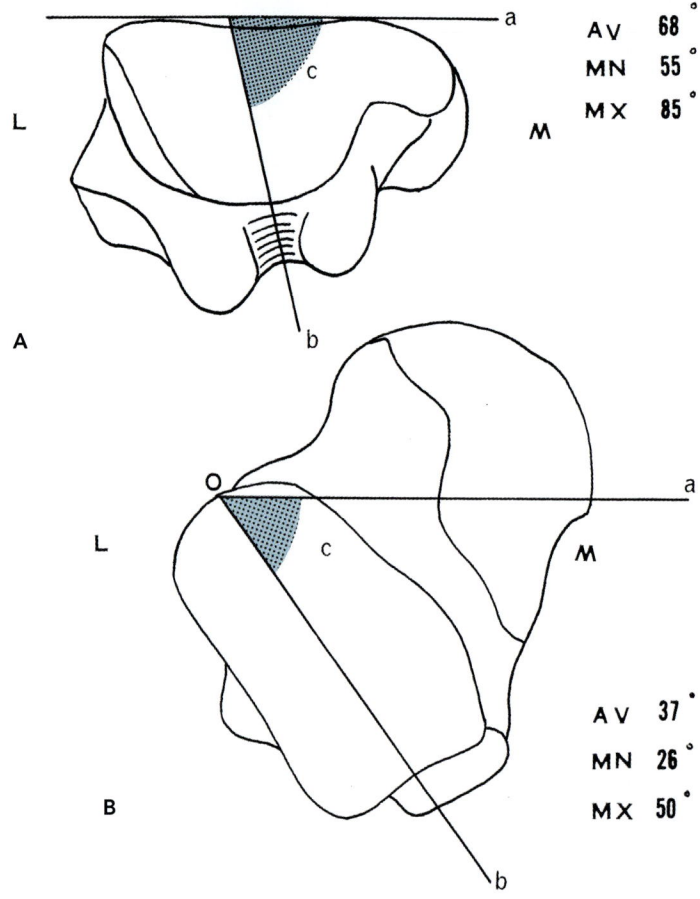

Figure 2.21 Angles of talus. **(A)** Posterior aspect of talus. Inclination angle (c) of the sulcus for the flexor hallucis longus tendon. **(B)** Inferior surface of talus. Angle (c) formed by the long axis *ob* of the posterior calcaneal surface with a line *oa* parallel to the anterior trochlear border. (L, lateral; M, medial.)

surface. The articular facets extending from the trochlear surface onto the superior aspect of the neck, the facies articularis interna and externa collae tali, including the squatting facet located laterally, were discussed previously.

Lateral Surface

The lateral surface of the neck is converted to a ridge extending from the anterolateral corner of the trochlea and talar body to the articular surface of the head. It is oriented anteromedially and presents a slight concavity. It may give insertion to the medial root of the inferior extensor retinaculum.

Inferior Surface

The inferior surface of the neck is formed by two nonarticulating segments, corresponding to the sinus tarsi and the tarsal canal, and an articular surface. The latter forms the facies articularis calcanea media, which occupies the anteromedial segment of the cervical surface. It has a variable contour and may be oval, elliptic, pyriform, or pentagonal. It is in continuity with the facies articularis calcanea anterior and the articular segment corresponding to the inferior calcaneonavicular ligament (Figs. 2.22 and 2.24). A ridge may delineate these surfaces. Occasionally, a separation notch is seen between the surfaces; if the notch is deep enough, a near-complete separation occurs between the middle and anterior calcaneal surfaces. In rare instances, a complete separation is present.

The bony segment corresponding to the sinus tarsi occupies the lateral half of the cervical surface. It is triangular, with a lateral base and a posteromedial apex continuing in the tarsal canal. Anteriorly, it bears a tubercle (tuberculum cervicis tali) that gives insertion to the cervical ligament.[21] In the present series of 100 tali, the tubercle was identified in 37%. Vascular foramina are distributed on the inner aspect of this surface. The lateral segment bears only a few vascular foramina.

The segment corresponding to the tarsal canal is located between the facies articularis calcanea media and the facies articularis calcanea posterior. It has a narrow, oblique surface oriented posteromedially. Laterally, it communicates with the sinus tarsi. Its medial opening is anterior to the talar posteromedial tubercle. Multiple vascular foramina are distributed along its longitudinal axis. A longitudinal crest may be present, giving insertion to the interosseous talocalcaneal ligament of the canalis tarsi and to the oblique calcaneotalar band of the inferior extensor retinaculum. As previously described, this sulcus interarticularis may be completely obliterated if a fusion occurs between the posterior and middle calcaneal articulating surfaces.

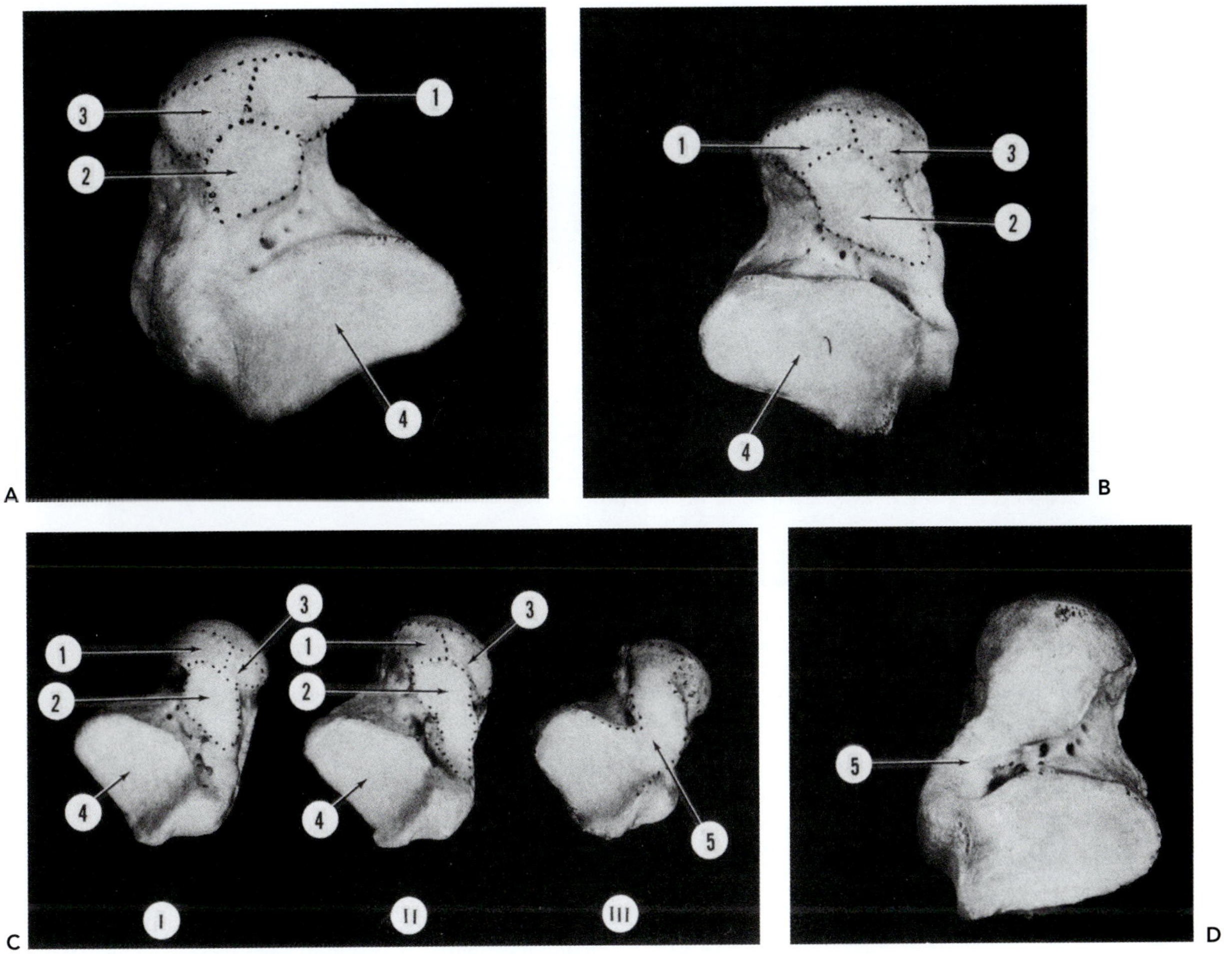

Chapter 2: Osteology   57

Figure 2.22 Variations in size and contour of the inferior articular surfaces of the talus. **(A)** Common configuration of the articular surfaces. **(B)** Posterior extension of the middle calcaneal surface. **(C)** (*I*) Moderate posterior extension of middle calcaneal surface. (*II*) Marked posterior extension of middle calcaneal surface. (*III*) Fusion (5) of all articular surfaces, obliterating the tarsal canal and a segment of the sinus tarsi. **(D)** Fusion (5) of the middle and posterior calcaneal surfaces on the medial aspect of the tarsal canal, which is still maintained. (*1*, anterior calcaneal articular surface of talar head; *2*, middle calcaneal articular surface of talar neck; *3*, articular segment of talar head corresponding to superomedial and inferior calcaneonavicular ligament; *4*, posterior calcaneal articular surface of talar body.)

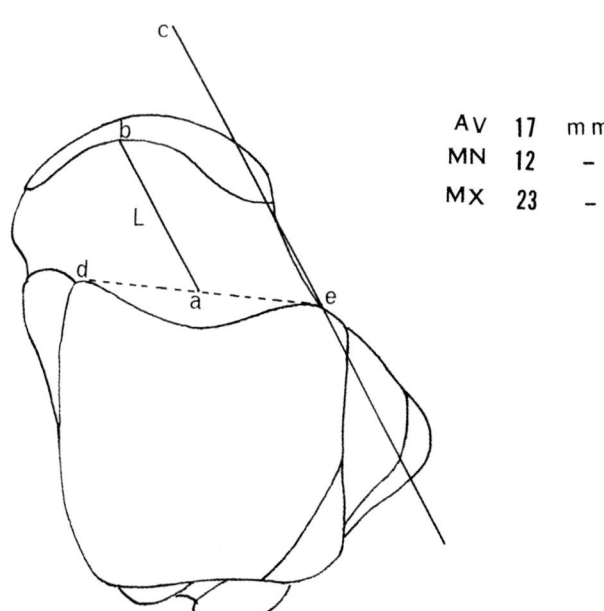

AV	17	mm
MN	12	–
MX	23	–

Figure 2.23 Length of talar neck (*L*). An anterior trochlear line *de* is drawn as indicated. The midpoint *a* is determined. A line *ec* is drawn along the talar neck. From the point *a*, a line *ab* is drawn, parallel to line *ec*. The segment *ab* is considered the length of the talar neck, and it terminates where the articular surface is encountered.

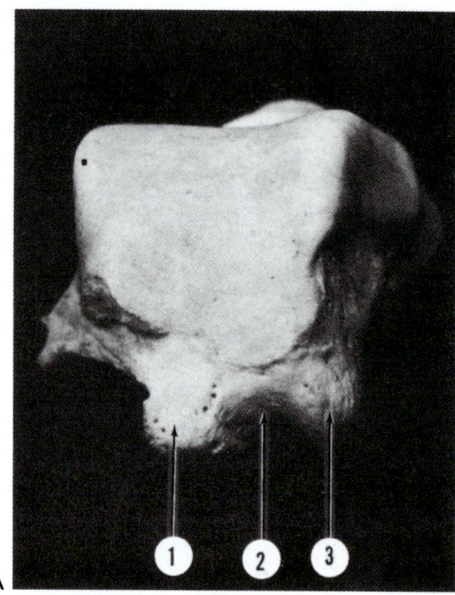
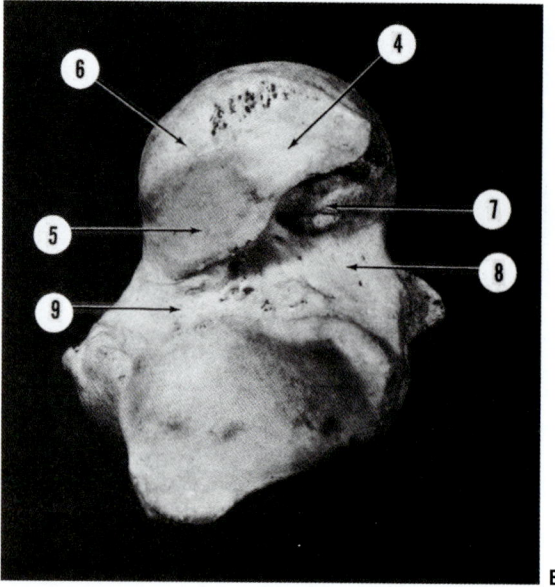

Figure 2.24 (A) Posterior aspect of talus. (B) Inferior aspect of talus. (1, posterolateral tubercle; 2, sulcus for flexor hallucis longus tendon; 3, posteromedial tubercle; 4, anterior calcaneal articular surface; 5, middle calcaneal articular surface; 6, articular segment of head corresponding to superomedial and inferomedial calcaneonavicular ligaments; 7, tubercle for cervical ligament; 8, sinus tarsi; 9, tarsal canal.)

Medial Surface

The medial surface of the neck is higher than the lateral surface. It represents the forward extension of the nonarticular segment of the medial surface of the talar body and provides insertion to the talonavicular capsule and ligaments. Occasionally, a posterior extension of the articulating surface of the head or an anterior extension of the medial malleolar articulating surface considerably narrows the medial surface of the neck.

▶ Head

The talar head (caput) articulates with the navicular, the calcaneus, and the calcaneonavicular ligaments. These articular fields are usually recognizable (see Fig. 2.22). The head is turned along a longitudinal axis relative to the talar body; the rotation is clockwise on the right and counterclockwise on the left. Because of this rotation, the navicular articular surfaces are higher laterally and lower medially, and its longitudinal axis is oriented upward and laterally. The longitudinal axis rotation relative to the transverse plane in 1006 Egyptian tali[22] was 45° average, 62° maximum, and 25° minimum; in the present series of 100 tali, it was 49° average, 65° maximum, and 30° minimum (Figs. 2.25 and 2.26).

The facies articularis navicularis is the largest of the three surfaces. It is convex along its long and short axes. The superolateral and lateral borders are sharply defined from the neck surface; the superomedial border, less defined, may be beveled. The navicular articular field is in continuity inferiorly with the facies articularis calcanea anterior and the facet for the inferior calcaneonavicular ligament (see Fig. 2.22). A low ridge or a change of direction of the surface demarcates the division.

The medial, inferior segment of the elliptic articular surface corresponds to the deep surface of the superomedial calcaneonavicular ligament and may have a more or less flat contour.

The anterior calcaneal articular surface is nearly quadrilateral or oval, and its surface curvature is clearly different from that of the navicular surface. It is flat and is continuous anteriorly with the navicular surface and posteriorly with the middle articular calcaneal surface, from which it may be separated by a ridge or a notch of variable depth. It is adjacent medially to the articular segment corresponding to the inferior calcaneonavicular ligament. This last surface is wedged between the navicular surface anteriorly and the middle calcaneal articular surface posteriorly.

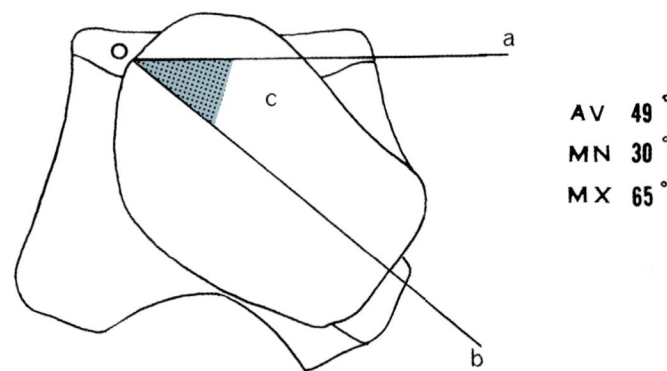

Figure 2.25 Angle (c) of lateral rotation of the talar head. (do, line parallel to trochlear surface; bo, long axis of head).

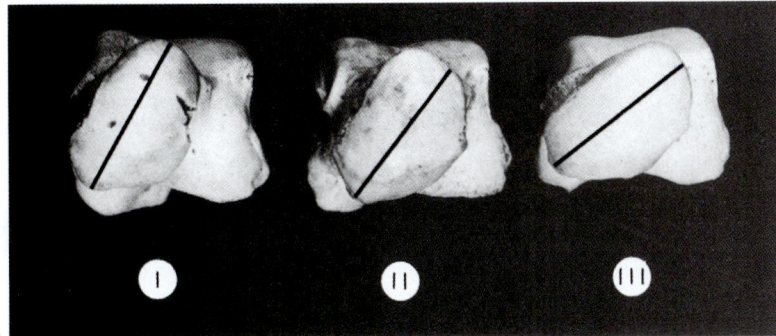
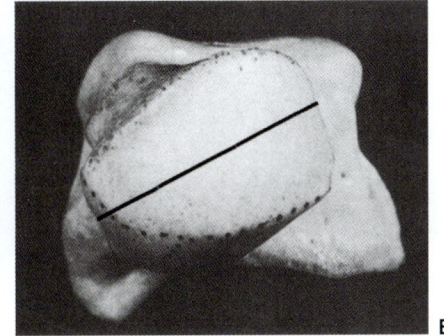

Figure 2.26 Variations in lateral rotation of talar head. (A) (I) Marked rotation. (II) Moderate rotation. (III) Minimal rotation. (B) Minimal rotation.

CALCANEUS

The calcaneus is the largest bone of the foot. The long axis is directed anteriorly, upward, and laterally. The upward tilt determines an angle of inclination relative to the horizontal plane—calcaneal pitch—and measures 10° to 30°.[23] The long axes of the calcaneus and of the talar neck normally make an angle of 30° to 35° in the horizontal plane (Fig. 2.27).[24]

The length and width of the calcanei vary (Fig. 2.28): in 750 calcanei, the length was 94 mm maximum and 48 mm minimum; the width was 53 mm maximum and 26 mm minimum.[25] In the present series of 50 calcanei, the length was 75 mm average, 83 mm maximum, and 65 mm minimum; the width was 40 mm average, 46 mm maximum, and 35 mm minimum. The average breadth × 100/length index in the present series is 53 and may range between 50 and 60.[25] The height of the os calcis is close to 50% of the length; in 50 calcanei, the average height was 40 mm, maximum 47 mm, and minimum 33.5 mm. The calcaneus is in the form of an irregular rectangle solid and presents six surfaces: superior, inferior, lateral, medial, posterior, and anterior.

▶ Superior Surface

The superior surface is divided into three parts: posterior, middle, and anterior (Fig. 2.29).

Posterior Third

The posterior third of the superior surface is nonarticular, narrow, transversely convex, and longitudinally concave. It is perforated by multiple vascular foramina, and the surface corresponds to the pre-Achilles corpus adiposum. Posterolaterally, it gives insertion to the calcaneal component of the ligament of Rouvière and Canela Lazaro.[15] The anterior segment gives attachment to the posterior talocalcaneal ligament and to the deep crural aponeurosis.

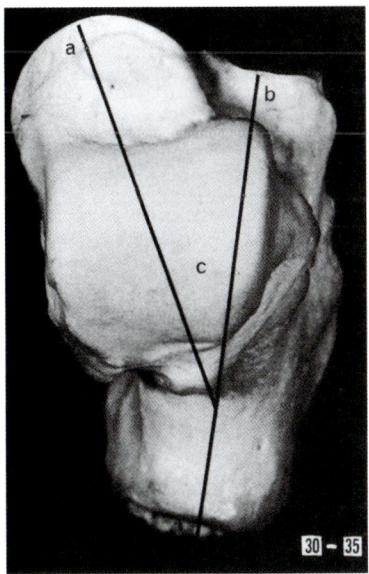
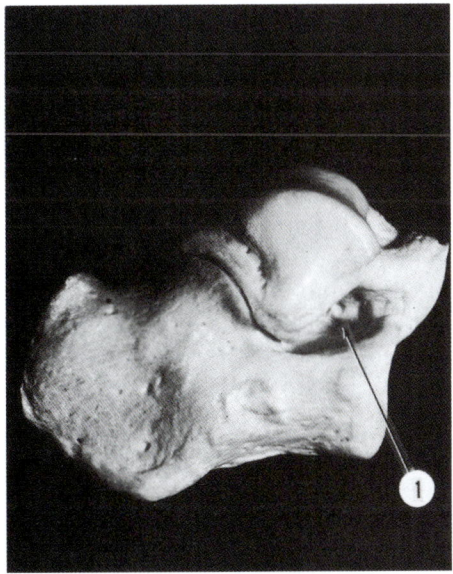
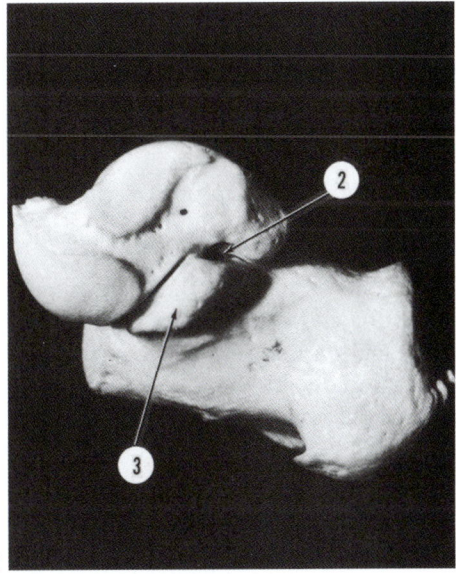

Figure 2.27 Talocalcaneal relationship. (A) Superior view—angle between long axis of calcaneus (b) and axis of talar neck (a), 30° to 35°. (B) Lateral view. (C) Medial view. (1, sinus tarsi; 2, medial opening of tarsal canal between posterior border of sustentaculum tali and anterior border of talar posteromedial tubercle; 3, sustentaculum tali.)

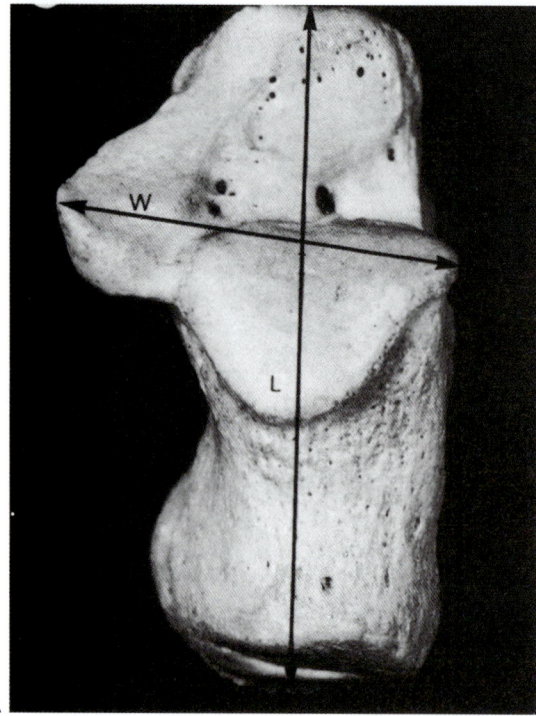
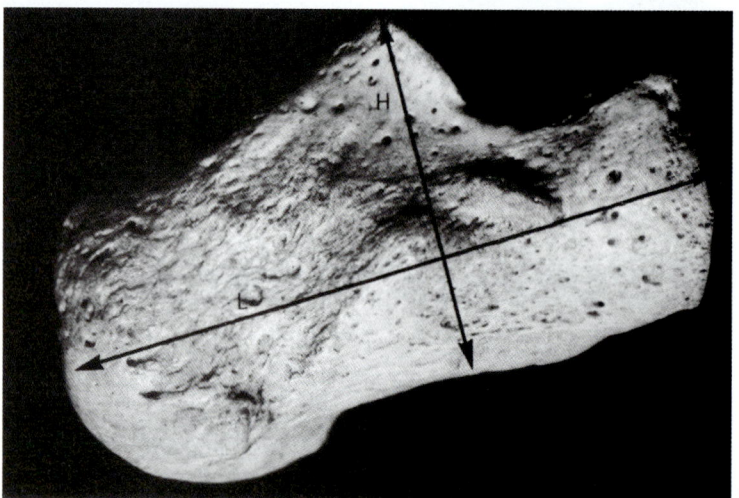

Figure 2.28 Dorsal (A) and lateral (B) views of calcaneus. (*H*, height; *L*, length; *W*, width.)

Middle Third

The middle third of the superior surface supports the large facies articularis talaris posterior. This articular surface makes a sharp change in orientation relative to the posterior segment. It inclines anteriorly and creates a step contour. The angle of inclination in 50 calcanei was average 65.5°, maximum 75°, and minimum 55° (Fig. 2.30, see Fig. 2.34).

Boehler has determined roentgenographically an angle expressing the height of the posterior talar surface.[26] This "tuber-joint angle" (see Fig. 2.30) measures 30° to 35°. This angle, measured anatomically, yields the following distribution in the present series of 50 calcanei: 17° to 20°, 2 calcanei; 21° to 30°, 25 calcanei; 31° to 40°, 20 calcanei; 41° to 44°, 3 calcanei; average 32°.

The long axis of the posterior articular surface is directed forward, downward, and outward. The surface is convex along the longitudinal axis and represents a segment of a cone. The apex of the cone is directed toward the sustentaculum tali, and the axis of the cone—the axis of revolution of the surface or the axis of motion along this surface—points anteromedially, intersecting the sustentaculum tali on the inner side at a nearly right angle in the adult.[1] The radius of the curvature along the greatest diameter (at the base of the cone) averages 30 mm, with a minimum of 12 mm and a maximum of over 40 mm.[25]

Manter considers the posterior talar articular surface as an oblique helicoid or screw-shaped surface in as much as sections made perpendicular to the joint surface axis reveal "spiral rather than circular arcs."[2] Inman, contouring the posterior talar articular surface with a dial indicator, demonstrated a screwlike behavior of the surface in only 58% of 42 specimens and concluded that "the remarkable variation is the important factor" in considering the geometry of this surface.[5]

Three accessory or extension facets may be present relative to the facies articularis talaris posterior: anterior, posterior, and medial. The anterior facet is seen in the anterolateral corner, extending onto the floor of the calcaneal fossa in a tonguelike projection. The counterpart to this surface on the talar side is the facies externa accessoria. The posterior facet is a trianglelike projection over the posterior third of the superior surface, corresponding to the presence of a trigonal process or to an os trigonum. The medial extension is directed toward the facies articularis talaris media and at times may succeed in establishing a union, thus obliterating the posterior end of the sulcus calcanei. The frequency of occurrence of these accessory facets is as shown in Table 2.7.

Anterior Third

The surface of the anterior third is formed by the sinus tarsi, the sulcus calcanei, and the facies articularis talaris anterior and media (see Figs. 2.27 and 2.29). The long axes of these last two articular surfaces and of the facies articularis talaris posterior make a diverging angle open anterolaterally.

The facies articularis talaris media and anterior form a continuous supportive surface located on the medial aspect of the sinus tarsi and sinus canal. The long axis of the surface is directed forward and laterally. These two surfaces form a concavity along the long axis, corresponding to the convexity of the talar head. The anterior surface is supported by the beak of the os calcis, and the middle surface is supported by the sustentaculum tali.

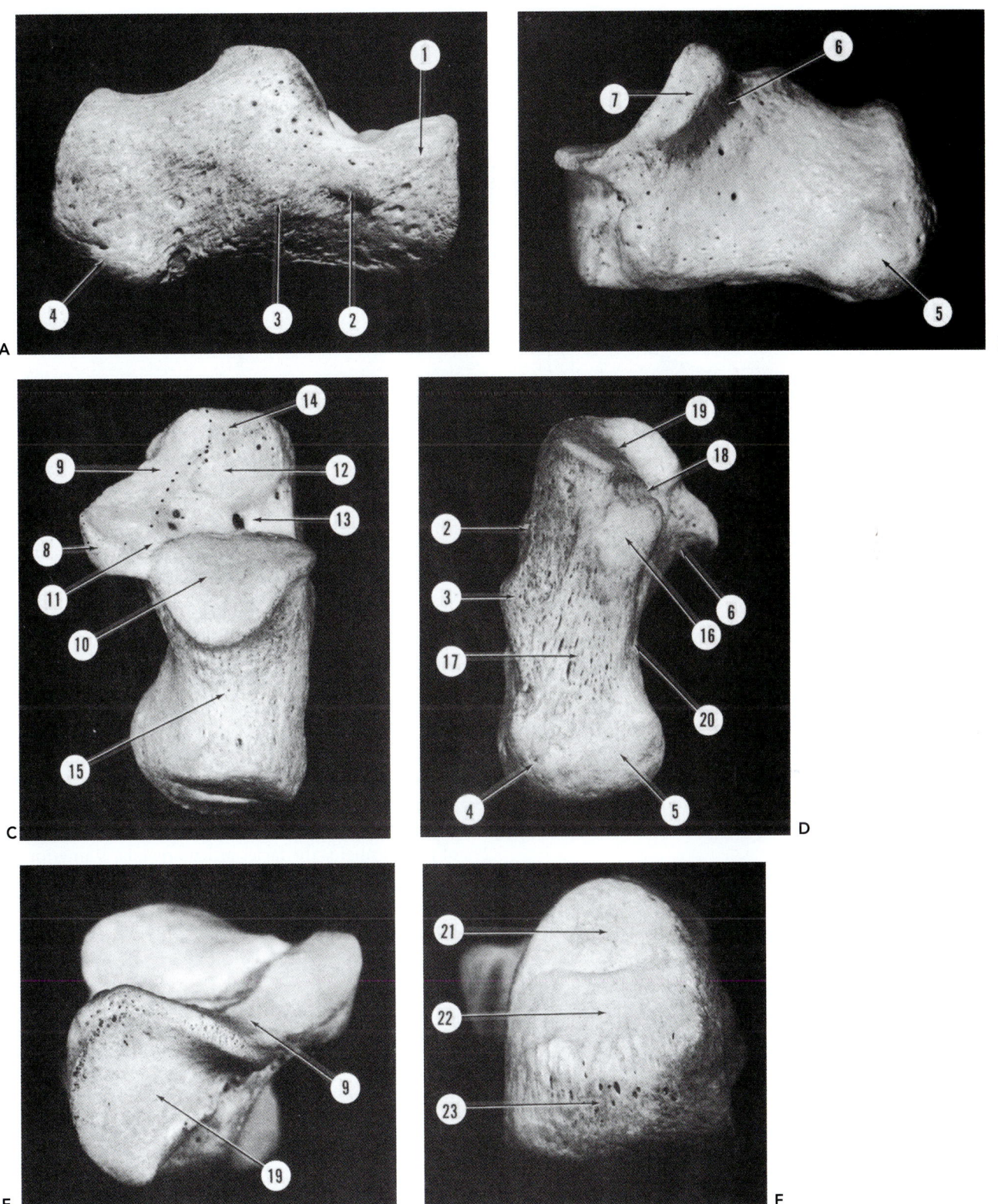

Figure 2.29 Calcaneus. **(A)** Lateral surface. **(B)** Medial surface. **(C)** Superior surface. **(D)** Inferior surface. **(E)** Anterior surface. **(F)** Posterior surface. (*1*, great apophysis; *2*, trochlear process; *3*, eminentia retrotrochlearis; *4*, lateral tuberosity; *5*, medial tuberosity; *6*, canal for flexor hallucis longus tendon; *7*, medial surface of sustentaculum tali; *8*, posterior border of sustentaculum tali; *9*, fused anterior and middle talar articular surfaces; *10*, posterior talar articular surface; *11*, canalis tarsi; *12*, sinus tarsi—bony eminence; *13*, sinus tarsi—fossa calcanei; *14*, sinus tarsi—insertion surface of bifurcate ligament; *15*, posterior third of superior surface; *16*, anterior tuberosity of inferior surface; *17*, longitudinally striated inferior surface; *18*, coronoid fossa; *19*, cuboidal articular surface; *20*, medial calcaneal canal; *21*, upper third of posterior surface, corresponding to pre-Achilles bursa; *22*, *23*, middle and lower thirds of posterior surface, corresponding to insertion of Achilles tendon.)

62 Sarrafian's Anatomy of the Foot and Ankle

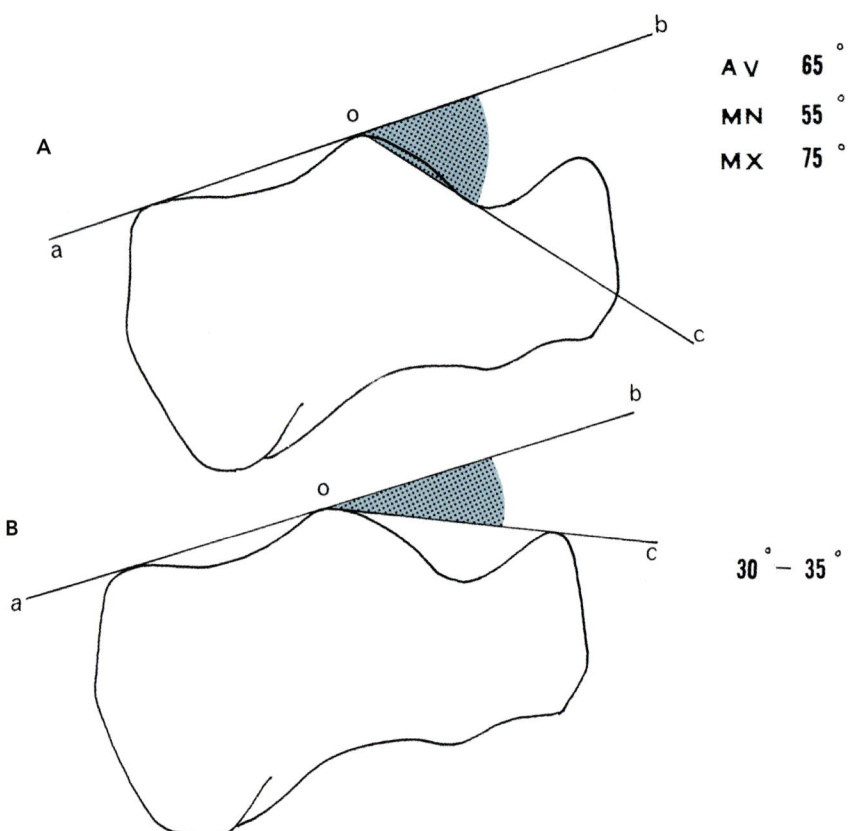

Figure 2.30 (A) Angle of inclination (boc) of the posterior talar articular surface. (B) Boehler tuber-joint angle (boc).

Variations are present in the contour and the degree of separation of these two surfaces. Bunning and Barnett classify the calcanei into three types: A, B, and C.[27] In type A, the anterior and middle surfaces are separate, and in type B, they are confluent. In type C, the anterior, middle, and posterior facets are united into a single surface. The distribution of these variations is shown in Table 2.8 (Fig. 2.31).

The degree of confluence of the anterior and middle facets is variable, being partial or complete. A constriction of the continuous surface determines two equal parts in 34% of the calcanei and a small anterior facet in association with a large middle surface in 18%. Trace of constriction is present in 12%, whereas nearly complete separation of the surfaces is seen in 2% of the calcanei of the present series. When a complete division of the surfaces is the norm, the two surfaces are of equal size in 12%, and in 20%, the middle facet is larger than the anterior; in only 2% of the calcanei is the facies articularis talaris anterior larger than the facies articularis talaris media.

Padmanabhan, in a study of 277 Indian calcanei, found the following distribution in regard to the anterior and middle talar facets: type A, 35%; type B, 65%.[28] In his series, there was no single case of type C.

TABLE 2.7 Frequency of Occurrence of Accessory Facets

	Laidlaw[25]		Present Series
Number of calcanei	750		50
Anterior extension facet			
	Tonguelike, 4%		6%
	Minor degree, 4.5%		
Posterior extension facet			
	Triangular area, 3.5%		
	Less definite triangular area, 5%		
Medial extension facet			5%
Union with middle surface	1.5%		2%

TABLE 2.8 Frequency of Occurrence of Variations in Calcanei

Author	Number of Calcanei	Occurrence (%)		
		Type A	Type B	Type C
Laidlaw[25],a	750	32	69	0
Bunning and Barnett[27]	Veddah 10	0	60	40
	African 492	36	63	1
	British 194	67	33	0
	Indian 78	22	78	0
Present series	50	34	64	2
Padmanabhan	Indian 272	35	65	0

[a]Laidlaw reports complete absence of the anterior facet in 0.9%.

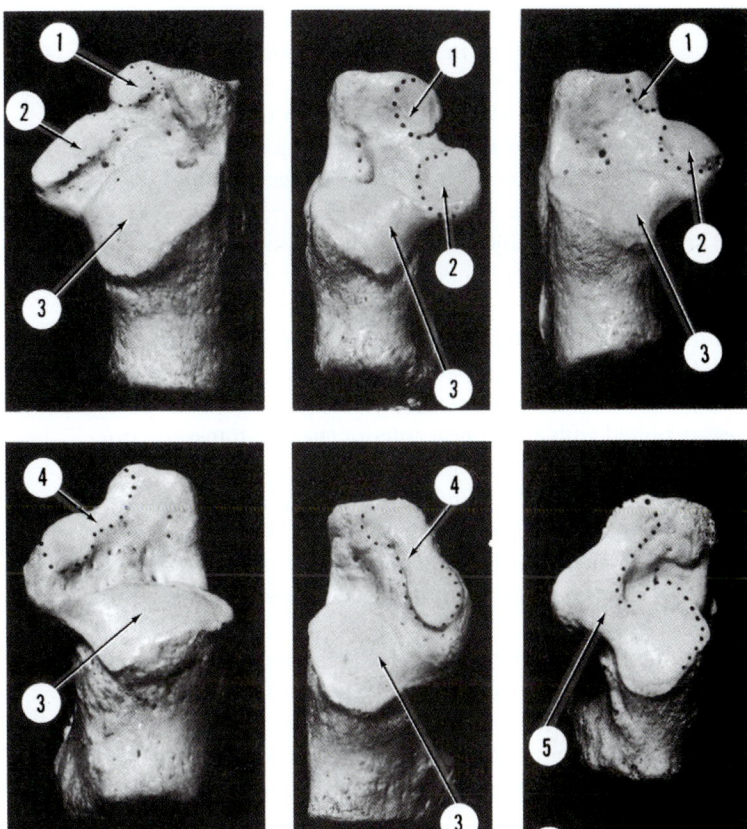

Figure 2.31 Variations of the articular surfaces on the superior aspect of the os calcis. (*1*, anterior talar articular surface; *2*, middle talar articular surface; *3*, posterior talar articular surface; *4*, fused anterior and middle talar articular surfaces; *5*, fused anterior, middle, and posterior talar articular surfaces.)

The canalis tarsus separates the middle and the posterior articular facets. It is narrow and oriented obliquely forward, laterally, and inferiorly. It is at a higher level than the floor of the sinus taris and has the same inclination as the sustentaculum tali. This angle of inclination relative to the lower border of the os calcis is 46° on average. This canal is not as deep as its counterpart on the talus, and it opens abruptly into the sinus tarsi. The interosseous talocalcaneal ligament or ligament of the tarsal canal makes its insertion on the floor of the canal, joined by the inward extension of the medial root of the inferior extensor retinaculum. Occasionally, a bony crest is seen in the canal, corresponding to this ligamentous insertion. The axis of motion of the talotarsal joint also passes through the canal. From both the anatomic and the physiologic point of view, the canalis tarsi and its contents are of prime importance.

The sinus tarsi, located on the anterior segment of the superior calcaneal surface, is limited posteriorly by the facies articularis talaris posterior and anteriorly by the anterior border separating the superior calcaneal surface from the anterior cuboidal articular surface. Laterally, the sinus tarsi is limited by the crista lateralis; medially, it is limited by the lateral border of the facies articularis talaris anterior. The posteromedial corner of the sinus tarsi continues with the calcaneal or tarsal canal.

In front of the posterior talar surface is the fossa calcaneus, perforated by multiple foramina leading to the antrum calcanei, an interior space free of cancellous trabeculae. Occasionally, a large, funnel-shaped foramen is seen in the fossa.

The anterolateral segment of the sinus tarsi is occupied by a bony eminence of variable configuration. This surface may be flat, covered only by rugosities, or it may be slightly elevated like a small plateau; occasionally, it is quite prominent in the form of a high tubercle. The sinus tarsi gives attachment to the following structures:

- The extensor digitorum brevis, arising from the anterolateral bony eminence and partially from the fossa calcanei
- The intermediate and medial roots of the inferior extensor retinaculum, located medial to the origin of the extensor digitorum brevis
- The cervical ligament, located between the anterior talar articular surface and the origin of the extensor digitorum brevis. A tubercle may indicate the origin
- The dorsal lateral calcaneonavicular and the medial calcaneocuboid ligaments, arising from the anteromedial corner of the surface
- The lateral calcaneocuboid ligament, originating from the anterolateral corner of the surface

The crista lateralis is a beamlike bony segment limiting the sinus tarsi laterally. It extends from the posterior articular surface to the anterolateral corner of the superior calcaneal surface, where it becomes less distinct.

▶ Inferior Surface

The inferior surface of the calcaneus is triangular, with the base posterior and the apex anterior (see Fig. 2.29). Two tuberosities occupy the base: the medial (which is the larger) and the lateral. The width of the bony heel as measured from the inner border of the medial tuberosity to the outer border of the lateral tuberosity is, on average, 3 cm in the present series of 50 calcanei (maximum, 3.5 cm; minimum, 2.5 cm).

The width of the posterior tuberosities in the present series of 50 calcanei is: medial—average 2 cm, maximum 2.4 cm, minimum 1.6 cm; lateral—average 1 cm, maximum 1.4 cm, and minimum 0.6 cm.

The medial tuberosity is the main weight-bearing bony segment. Rarely is the lateral tuberosity absent. In most of the calcanei, a triangular space separates the two tubercles; this space is directed anteromedially, with the apex located posterolaterally. At times, the apical separation takes the form of a groove. Occasionally, there is no intertubercular space and both tubercles are united with a common anterior (nearly) transverse border. Both tubercles have an anteroposterior convex contour.

The midsegment of the inferior calcaneal surface is covered by longitudinal bony striations. The lateral border is oblique and directed anteromedially and many times is less distinct than the rounder medial border, which presents a shallow medial concavity.

An anterior tuberosity is located near the apex of the triangular inferior surface. It is a round eminence measuring 1.5 cm in width on average (maximum 2 cm, minimum 1.2 cm).

On the posterior tuberosities, the aponeurosis plantaris and the flexor digitorum brevis muscle are inserted transversely in a posteroanterior sequence. The medial tuberosity gives origin to the abductor hallucis muscle and the lateral tuberosity to the abductor digiti minimi (which also reaches the medial tuberosity). The triangular surface interposed between the anterior and posterior tubercles gives attachments to the ligamentum plantaris longus. The anterior tuberosity provides insertion to the deep fibers of the longitudinal plantar ligament and to the short plantar calcaneocuboid ligament.

Between the anterior tuberosity and the anterior apex of the sustentaculum tali is a small depression, the coronoid fossa, that gives origin to the inferior calcaneonavicular ligament. A small articular surface in continuity with the anterior cuboidal articular surface is located on the lateral aspect of this fossa and receives the beak or coronoid process of the cuboid.

In the present series of 50 os calcis, a "heel spur" or shelflike anterior bony projection originating from the medial tubercle occurred in 36%.

▶ **Lateral Surface**

The lateral surface is shown in Figure 2.29. It is high posteriorly and low anteriorly. The posterior third is subcutaneous and is flat, except at the upper segment, where it is slightly convex in the vertical dimension. The middle third presents a tubercle, the eminentia retrotrochlearis, in its lower segment. This is nearly always present.[25] It is a large oval eminence of very variable dimensions. Edwards, in a study of 150 dry calcanei, found this eminence to be present in 98% and absent in only 2%.[3] Anterior to the retrotrochlear eminence is another tubercle, the processus trochlearis (Fig. 2.32). When present and well delineated, this process is a ridgelike structure located below the angle formed by the lateral border of the sinus tarsi and

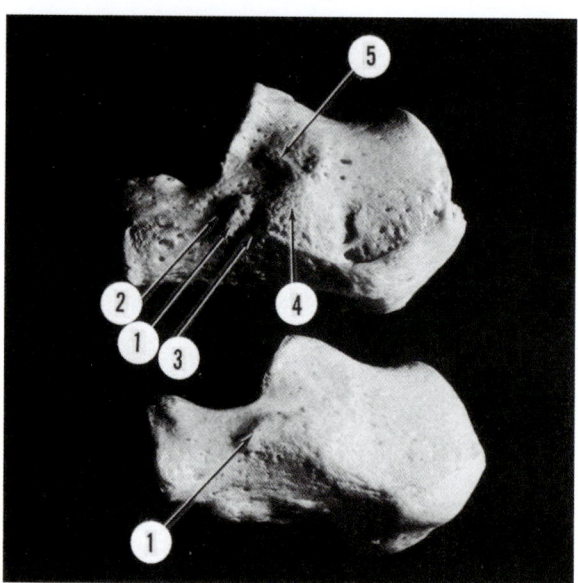

Figure 2.32 **Lateral aspect of calcanei.** (1, trochlear process; 2, sulcus for peroneus brevis tendon; 3, sulcus for peroneus longus tendon; 4, eminentia retrotrochlearis; 5, tubercle for calcaneofibular ligament.)

the lateral border of the facies articularis talaris posterior. This trochlear process is oriented downward and anteriorly, and the long axis makes an angle of 45° with the horizontal.[25]

The frequency of occurrence of the processes trochlearis in various series is as follows: Gruber,[29] 39.1%; Stieda and Der,[30] 33%; Pfitzner,[18] 39.9%; Laidlaw,[25] 36.5% (prominent, 20.5%; less marked, 16%); Edwards,[3] 44%; present series (50 calcanei), 32%.

Agarwal and colleagues reported on the variations of the peroneal tubercle in 1410 Indian calcanei from the regions of Agra and Lucknow.[31] They classified the calcanei into four types according to the pattern of the peroneal tubercles. Type I, with a single peroneal tubercle present anteroinferior to the tubercle for the attachment of the calcaneofibular ligament, occurred in 31.25% (Agra) and 60.11% (Lucknow). Type II, with a single peroneal tubercle incompletely divided into anterior and posterior parts by a smooth, shallow groove running obliquely from above downward occurred in 18.75% (Agra) and 23.66% (Lucknow). Type III, with two peroneal tubercles completely separated by a roughened area in the middle, occurred in 7.50% (Agra) and 13.76% (Lucknow). Type IV represented the absent peroneal tubercle and occurred in 42.5% (Agra) and 2.42% (Lucknow).

The dimensions of the trochlear process are as follows: length—maximum 17 mm, minimum 2 mm; breadth at base—maximum 10 mm, minimum 2 mm; height—maximum 7 mm, minimum 1 mm.[3]

On the inferior surface of this process glides the peroneus longus tendon. The superior surface is smooth and corresponds to the peroneus brevis tendon. The groove of the peroneus longus tendon leaves a landmark on the lateral aspect of the os calcis in 85%.[3] This groove may be present in the absence of a trochlear process, located then on the anterior aspect of the retrotrochlear eminence or on the lateral aspect of the os calcis.

A cartilage-covered gliding facet may be present on the os calcis along the course of the peroneus longus tendon. Edwards found such facets in 44% of his series, and of these, 10.6% were present in the absence of a trochlear process.[3] Those gliding facets are oval, usually not elevated, and located on the posterior slope of the trochlear process or partly on this slope and partly on the lateral surface of the calcaneus.

A definite groove for the peroneus brevis tendon is present in only 2.6%.[3] The inferior peroneal retinaculum, bridging both peroneal tendons, attaches to the os calcis above and below the trochlear process, and sends a septum to the crest of the process.

Hyer et al[32] investigated the occurrence and characteristics of the peroneal tubercle in 114 calcanei. The peroneal tubercles were "subjectively described as flat, prominent, concave, or tunnel."[32] The occurrence of the peroneal tubercle was then 90.4% with the following distribution: flat in 42.7% (44 specimens), prominent in 29.1% (30 specimens), concave in 27.2% (28 specimens), and tunnel in 1% (1 specimen) (Fig. 2.33). In our interpretation, if "flat" is considered by others as "no tubercle," then the data of occurrence of the peroneal tubercle are closer to the previously published data. The morphometric data in regard to the peroneal tubercle was reported as follows: length 13.04 mm (range 3.61-26.6 mm), height 9.44 mm (range 3.67-23.40 mm), and width 3.13 mm (range 1-10 mm).

The tuberculum ligamenti calcaneofibularis is a small tubercle situated behind the midsegment of the facies articularis talaris posterior and is posterosuperior to the eminentia retrotrochlearis. It is present as a well-defined tubercle in 43%.[25] The location of this tubercle for the insertion of the calcaneofibular ligament is typical in 64.5% and varies in the remaining 35.5% (anterior location, 25.5%; downward location, 4.5%; posterior location, 5.5%).[25]

The calcaneal component of the fibulocalcaneoastragalar ligament of Rouvière and Canela Lazaro extends its insertion on the superior aspect of the lateral surface behind the insertion of the calcaneofibular ligament in an oblique linear fashion; the lateral talocalcaneal ligament inserts anterior to it.[15] A tubercle (tuberculum ligamenti talicalcanei) may be present for this attachment. Occasionally, a small tubercle for the attachment of the lateral calcaneocuboid ligament is seen in the superior segment of the anterior third of the lateral surface. Morestin describes a second trochlear gliding facet for the tendon of the peroneus longus, located at the anteroinferior corner of the external calcaneal surface.[33] He recognizes two varieties: intra- and extra-articular. The intra-articular facet is at the extreme anterior portion of the calcaneus, and the capsule-synovium of the calcaneocuboid joint inserts at its periphery. The extra-articular type is at a distance from the calcaneocuboid articulation and is oval or circular, cartilage-covered, and somewhat elevated above the surrounding parts. When well developed, a sesamoid is found in the substance of the peroneus longus tendon; this sesamoid is different from the sesamoid found in the same tendon further distally as it passes over the tuberosity of the cuboid.

The frequency of occurrence of this second trochlear facet in various series is as follows: Morestin, 5%[33]; Edwards, 6.6%[3]; and present series (50 os calcis), 4%.

▶ Medial Surface

The medial surface of the os calcis, similar to the lateral surface, is high posteriorly and low anteriorly (Figs. 2.29 and 2.34). This surface forms a large oblique canal directed downward and anteriorly. It accepts the width of two fingers. The configuration is determined by the medial projection of the sustentaculum tali and the medial extension of the medial calcaneal tubercle. This calcaneal canal is the port of entry from the posteromedial aspect of the ankle to the plantar aspect of the foot.

The sustentaculum tali is a bracketlike projection, triangular with a posterior base and an anterior apex. This surface projects anteromedially and is inclined downward and anteriorly at an average angle of 46° (maximum 60°, minimum 30°) (see Fig. 2.34). The superior surface corresponds to the facies articularis talaris media, described previously. The inferior surface is carved into a groove for the gliding of the flexor hallucis longus tendon and provides attachment to the fibrous tunnel of the tendon. A crest may be present at the attachment site posteriorly. The medial surface of the sustentaculum tali is triangular, with a posterior base and an anterior apex. This surface corresponds to the flexor digitorum longus tendon and its fibrous tendon sheath. The tibiocalcaneal components of the deltoid ligament and the superomedial calcaneonavicular ligament insert on the upper border of the medial surface. The recurrent band of the tibialis posterior tendon inserts on the lower border of the same surface.

The posterior border of the sustentaculum tali corresponds to the medial entrance of the canalis tarsi and gives insertion to the medial talocalcaneal ligament. On rare occasions when the posterior talar articular surface extends medially over the superior

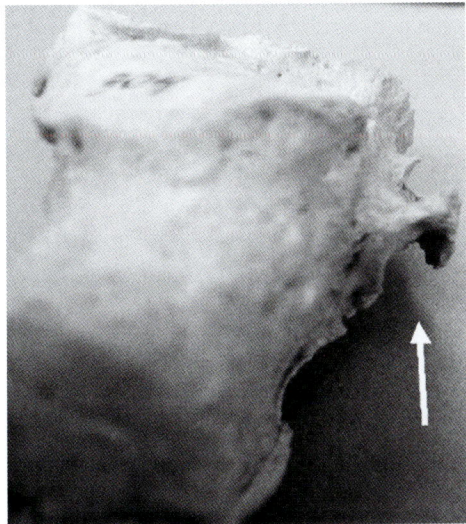

Figure 2.33 **Tunnel-type peroneal tubercle (*arrow*).** (Hyer CF, Dawson JM, Philbin TM, et al. The peroneal tubercle: description, classification, and relevance to peroneus longus tendon pathology. *Foot Ankle Int.* 2005;11:947-950, Figure 4. Copyright ©2005. Reprinted by Permission of SAGE Publications.)

surface of the sustentaculum, the opening of the canalis tarsi is on the medial border of the sustentaculum tali (see Fig. 2.31).

The width and length of the sustentaculum tali are variable. The width of the sustentaculum tali, as measured at the base (see Fig. 2.28), was on average 13 mm (maximum 18 mm, minimum 8 mm) in the present series of 50 dry calcanei. The ratio of the sustentacular width to the total width of the os calcis at the same level is on average 0.33 (maximum 0.47, minimum 0.23). These values may be correlated with the supportive function of the sustentaculum tali relative to the talar head. "Incompetent" sustentaculum tali may fall into a group with a minimum value or lower.

The sustentaculum tali may also be classified by length as long or short. A long sustentaculum is continuous through its medial border with the process anterior, which is then in association with a fusion of the facies articularis media and anterior. A short sustentaculum ends suddenly anteriorly, and a notch separates the two articular surfaces (see Figs. 2.31 and 2.34).[34] The frequency of occurrence of these varieties, including the intermediary forms, in Laidlaw series is long, about 40%; short, 32%; intermediary, 28%.[34] In the present series, the frequency is long, 60%; short, 34%; intermediary, 6%.

The medial surface of the os calcis gives insertion on its inferior two-thirds to the medial head of the quadratus plantae. This field of insertion is triangular, with the base posterior. The transverse interfascicular ligament inserts above the quadratus plantae and below the tunnel of the flexor hallucis longus.

▶ Posterior Surface

The posterior surface is triangular, with the apex superior and the base inferior (see Fig. 2.29). The medial and lateral borders are well delineated, but the inferior border is ill defined because the surface is continuous with the plantar aspect. The overall contour of the surface is convex. The upper segment is directed upward and anteriorly and is divided into two fields. The lower field is transverse and trapezoidal with an irregular, striated, crenated lower border and a soft and regular superior border. This surface corresponds to the insertion of the Achilles tendon. The upper field is free from tendinous insertion. It is triangular and smooth and corresponds to the pre-Achilles bursa. The lower surface is broad, directed downward and anteriorly; it is striated because of the insertion of the Achilles tendon.

▶ Anterior Surface

The anterior surface is almost entirely articular (see Fig. 2.29). It is saddle-shaped, convex transversely, and concave vertically. The contour of the surface forms a spiral-type groove directed downward and inward. At the posteromedial end of this groove is the calcaneal coronoid fossa, which receives the beak of the cuboid.

The superomedial corner of the articular surface makes a shelflike projection anteromedially. This beak or rostrum of the os calcis overhangs the cuboid.

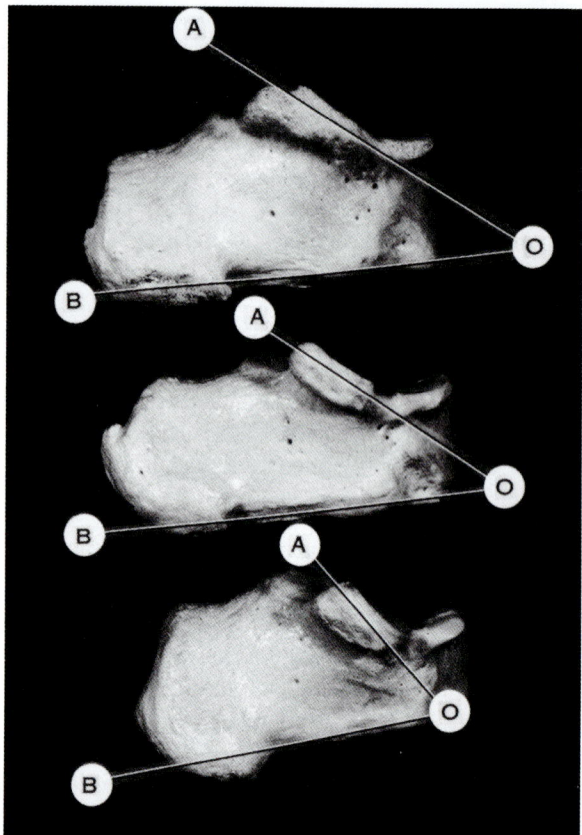

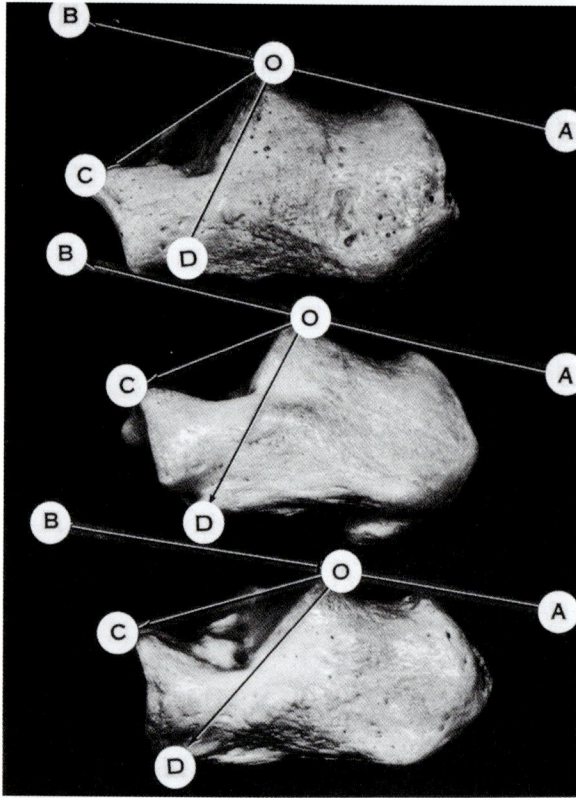

Figure 2.34 **(A) Variable inclination of sustentaculum-tali angle (*AOB*). (B) Variations of inclination angle (*BOD*) and of Boehler tuber-joint angle (*BOC*).** (*Top*, marked inclination; *center*, moderate inclination; *bottom*, minimal inclination.)

CUBOID

The cuboid is intercalated between the calcaneum and the base of metatarsals 4 and 5. It gives support to the lateral cuneiform and may enter in contact with the scaphoid.

The bone is wedge-shaped or cuneiform rather than cuboid, as the dorsal and plantar surfaces slope toward the narrow lateral surface or border (Fig. 2.35). It presents five surfaces: dorsal, plantar, medial or base, posterior, and anterior, as well as a lateral border or apex.

▶ Dorsal Surface

The dorsal surface is markedly inclined outward and is in continuity with the lateral surface of the calcaneum (Figs. 2.36 and 2.37). Transversely, it continues the curvature of the dorsal surface of the cuneiforms, contributing to the formation of the transverse arch of the midfoot (see Fig. 2.35).

The surface is trapezoidal, covered by rugosities, and crossed by the extensor digitorum brevis and the peroneus tertius tendon. This surface has four borders:

- Medial, which represents the base of the trapezoid. The distal segment has a medial projection. It corresponds to the navicular and the third cuneiform.
- Lateral, which represents the apex of the trapezoid. This border is short and slightly concave, corresponding to the crossing of the peroneus longus tendon.
- Proximal and convex, corresponding to the os calcis.
- Distal and obtuse, corresponding to the base of the fourth and fifth metatarsals.

The dorsal surface provides attachment to the following:

- Dorsomedial calcaneocuboid ligament, which attaches on a small tubercle located on the posteromedial corner of the surface
- Dorsolateral calcaneocuboid ligament, which attaches at least 0.5 cm distal to the proximal border and reaches the middorsal segment
- Lateral calcaneocuboid ligament, just above the lateral border
- Dorsal cubonavicular ligament, inserting on the medial side of the midsegment
- Dorsal cuneo$_3$-cuboid ligament, single or double, inserting in the distal half of the medial dorsal surface
- Dorsal cubometatarsal$_4$, cubometatarsal$_5$ ligaments, attached along the distal margin of the bone. The latter has a broader insertion area than the former

▶ Plantar Surface

The plantar surface faces inferiorly and medially (see Figs. 2.36 and 2.37). It is wider medially and narrower laterally. The medial border is oblique and is directed more posteriorly and slightly medially, while the posterior border is directed more medially and slightly posteriorly. At the junction of these two borders is the beak or coronoid process of the cuboid.

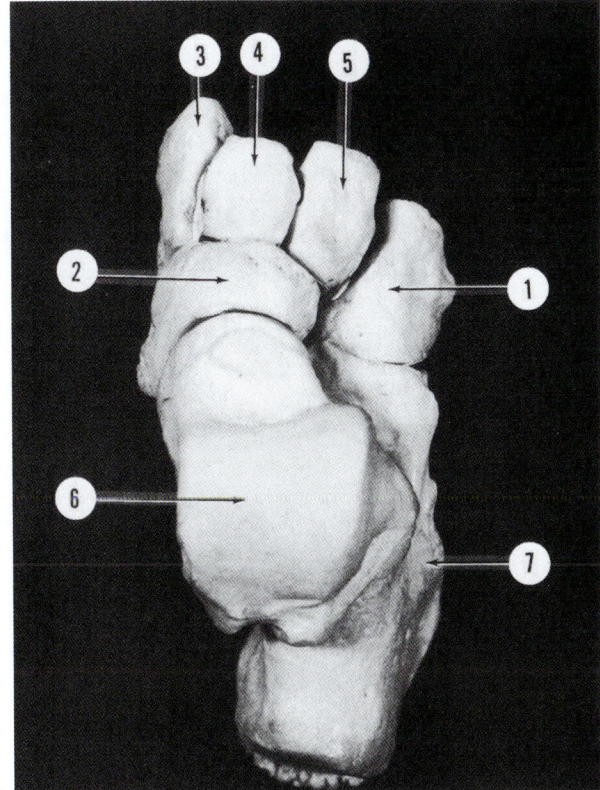

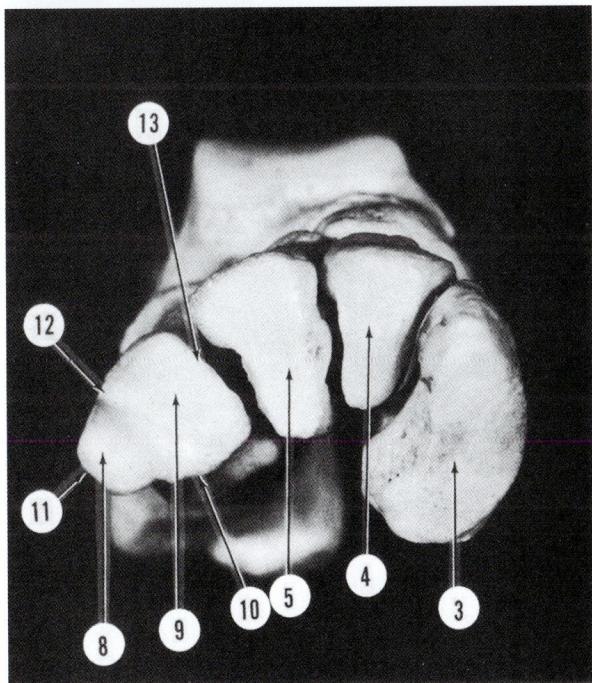

Figure 2.35 **(A) Dorsal aspect, tarsus. (B) Transverse arch formed by the cuneiforms and the cuboid,** which is also wedge-shaped. (*1*, cuboid; *2*, navicular; *3*, medial cuneiform; *4*, middle cuneiform; *5*, lateral cuneiform; *6*, talus; *7*, calcaneus. Cuboidal surfaces: *8*, *9*, lateral and medial aspect of anterior articular surface; *10*, inferior border; *11*, apex; *12*, dorsolateral border; *13*, medial border.)

The short lateral border is slightly concave. The anterior border is directed laterally and posteriorly and is divided into a short medial segment and a long lateral segment, which is more inclined posteriorly.

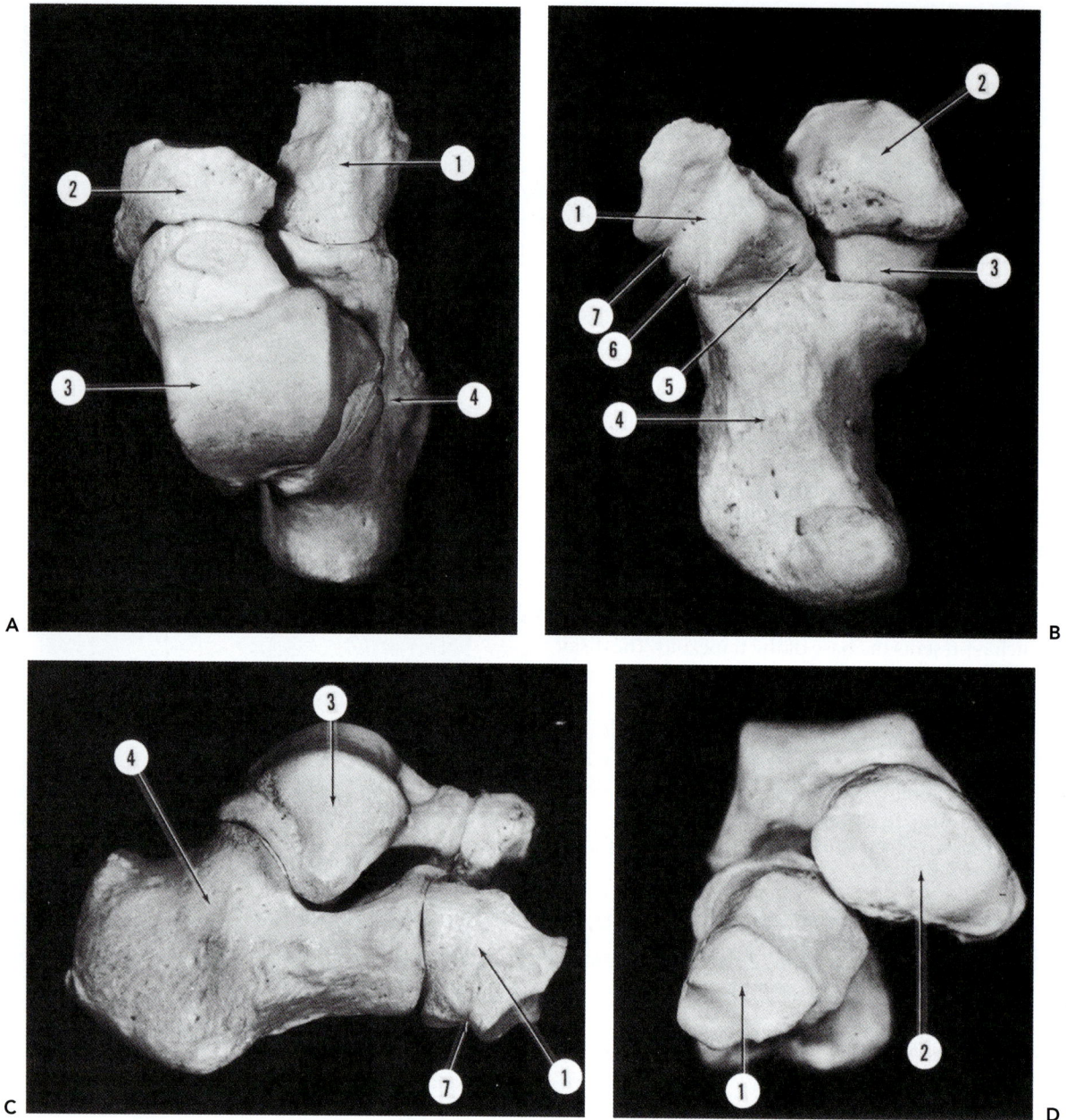

Figure 2.36 **Subtalar and midtarsal skeleton.** (A) Dorsal aspect. (B) Plantar aspect. (C) Lateral aspect. (D) Anterior aspect. (1, cuboid; 2, navicular; 3, talus; 4, calcaneus [elongated contour of Chopart joint is seen]; 5, beak of cuboid; 6, sesamoid facet of cuboid; 7, canal of peroneus longus.)

A strong ridge, the tuberositas ossis cuboidei, oriented obliquely anteromedially, divides the plantar surface into a small anterior and a large posterior area. A line extending in the direction of this tuberosity will reach the base of the first metatarsal.

As demonstrated by Stieda and Poirier, there is no cuboidal groove or peroneal groove on the anterior aspect of the plantar surface.[11,30] The tendon of the peroneus longus glides and is reflected over the anterior slope of the cuboidal tuberosity. Furthermore, a gliding facet corresponding to the sesamoid of the peroneus longus tendon is present on the anterolateral aspect of this tuberosity. The sesamoid facet or cuboid facet is present in 93%.[3] It is oval (77%), irregularly quadrilateral (18%), or triangular (5%) and is slightly convex.[3]

The anterior segment of the plantar surface is long and narrow. It is limited anteriorly by the anterior border corresponding to the base of the fourth and fifth metatarsals and posteriorly by the tuberosity of the cuboid. The surface is flat and may appear as a groove due to the elevation of the tuberosity and "to the presence of a slight ledge of bone which is thrown up along its anterior margin."[3]

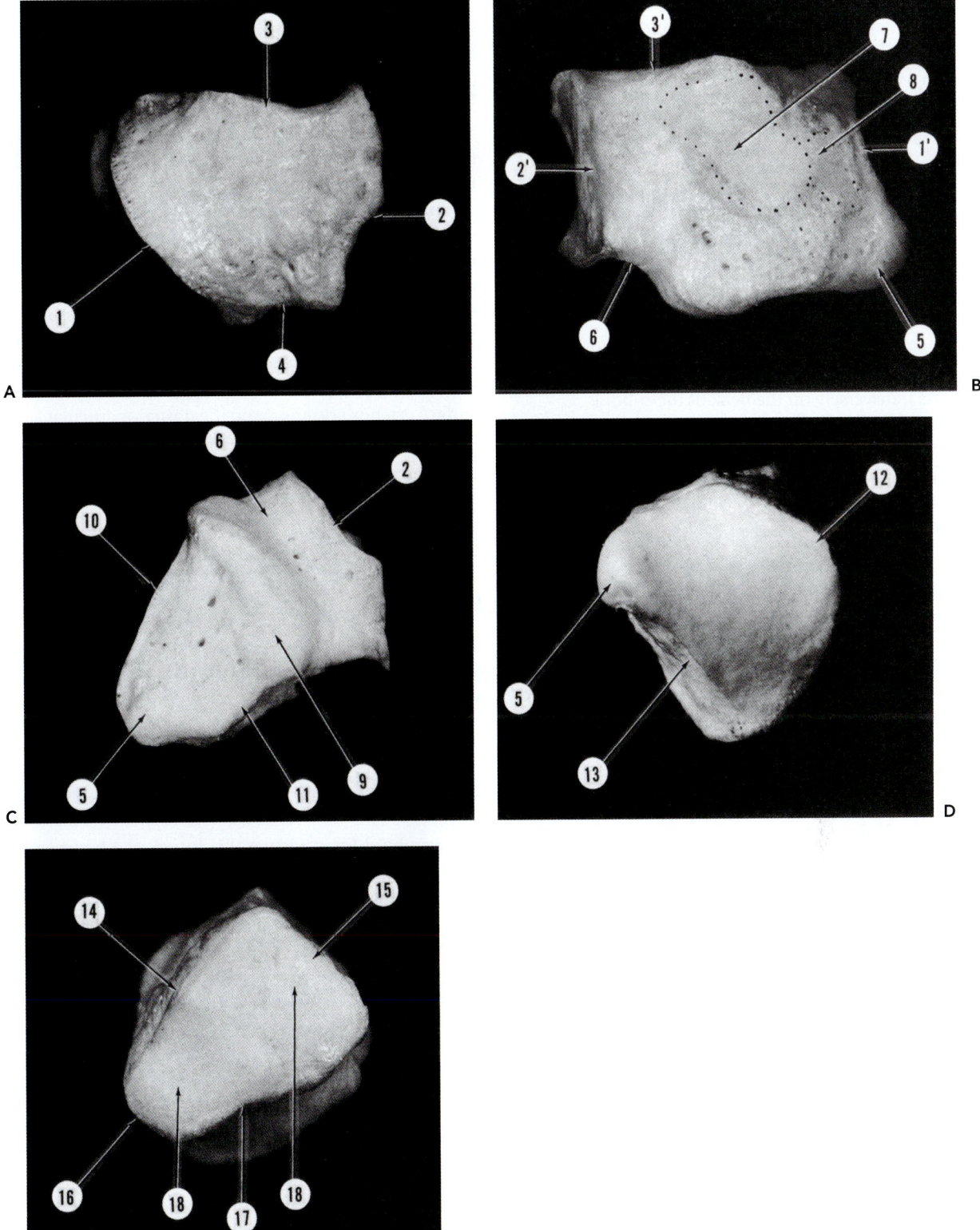

Figure 2.37 Cuboid, right. (A) Dorsal surface. (B) Medial surface. (C) Inferior or plantar surface. (D) Posterior surface. (E) Anterior surface. (1, posterior border of dorsal surface; 2, anterior border of dorsal surface; 3, medial border of dorsal surface; 1', posterior border of medial surface; 2', anterior border of medial surface; 3', superior border of medial surface; 4, lateral border of dorsal surface; 5, beak of cuboid; 6, groove for peroneus longus; 7, articular surface for third cuneiform; 8, articular surface for scaphoid; 9, tuberosity of cuboid; 10, posterior border of inferior surface; 11, medial border of inferior surface; 12, superior border of posterior surface; 13, inferior border of posterior surface; 14, superolateral border of anterior surface; 15, superomedial border or base of anterior surface; 16, apex of anterior surface; 17, inferior border of anterior surface; 18, articular surfaces corresponding to metatarsals 4 and 5.)

The posterior segment, located posterior to the ridge, is larger and triangular. The base corresponds to the tuberosity of the cuboid and the apex to the beak. It is a depressed surface and may form a deep concavity.

The plantar surface of the cuboid provides attachment to the following:

- Plantar cubometatarsal$_5$, cubometatarsal$_4$ ligaments, which are inserted along the margin of the anterior border
- Peroneus longus fibrous tendon sheath, which attaches to the anterior segment behind the cubometatarsal ligaments and over the crest of the cuboidal ridge
- Deep fibers of the longitudinal plantar ligament, inserting over the cuboidal tuberosity
- Short plantar calcaneocuboid ligament, which inserts on the entire triangular posterior aspect of the surface. A strong band inserts transversely on the beak of the cuboid
- Plantar cubonavicular ligament, which attaches to the medial border of the posterior segment and the beak of the cuboid
- Plantar cuneo$_3$-cuboid ligament, which inserts on the medial aspect of the cuboid crest and the segment of the medial border immediately behind it

An expansion from the tibialis posterior tendon may insert on the posteromedial corner in conjunction with the plantar cuboscaphoid ligament.

On the posterior aspect of the tuberosity of the cuboid are also attached, in a lateral to medial direction, the opponens and short flexor of the fifth toe, the oblique head of the adductor hallucis, and the flexor hallucis brevis. Some of these attachments are through their connection with the fibrous tunnel of the peroneus longus tendon.

▶ Anterior Surface

The anterior surface (see Figs. 2.35 to 2.37) articulates with the base of the fourth and fifth metatarsals. The long axis is directed downward and laterally. The surface is more or less triangular, with a medial base and a lateral apex. It is divided into two segments by a vertical smooth ridge. The lateral surface, which is triangular, has a long transverse axis and is larger than the medial; it is slightly concave in the center and corresponds to the base of the fifth metatarsal. The medial surface, which is rectangular, is smaller than the lateral and slightly concave, and its long axis is vertical; it corresponds to the base of the fourth metatarsal. The two segments of the surface join at an obtuse angle, forming an anterior angular convexity.

▶ Posterior Surface

The posterior surface articulates with the calcaneum. It is saddle-shaped, concave transversely, and convex vertically. The medial end of the surface bears the beak of the cuboid. This process (the pyramidal apophysis or coronoid of the cuboid) augments the concavity of the articular surface.[9] It lodges in a corresponding fossa of the calcaneum in flexion and adduction of the forefoot.[20] "The process 'undershoots' the os calcis, supporting it in a bracketlike way, in fact in a very similar manner to that in which the plantar point, on the navicular, supports the head of the astragalus."[35]

▶ Medial Surface

The medial surface faces medially and upward. It is quadrilateral and is narrower anteriorly. In the middle third, the articular surface for the third cuneiform is present. This articular surface is flat, round, oval, or triangular with a superior base. It is in touch with the superior margin and is separated from the inferior margin by a band of rugosities. The segment posterior to the cuneiform articular surface bears a small articular surface for the scaphoid. The contour of this segment is variable. The facet for the scaphoid occurs with the following frequency: in Gruber's series of 200 ft, it was present in 45.5%; in Pfitzner's series of 437 ft, it was present in 54.5%.[18,36] This surface extends posteriorly up the posterior articular surface but occasionally a depression separates the two. The rough surface below the scaphoid surface gives insertion to the plantar cuboscaphoid ligament. The anterior third of the medial surface is a rough area for the attachment of the interosseous cuneo$_3$-cuboid ligament.

▶ Lateral Border

The lateral border is the apex of the cuboid, formed by the junction of the dorsal and plantar surfaces. This border bears a concavity that corresponds to the beginning of the peroneal tunnel.

SCAPHOID

The scaphoid (os naviculare) is interposed between the head of the talus and the three cuneiforms (Figs. 2.38 and 2.39). It establishes minimal articular contact with the cuboid and is firmly bound with ligaments to the os calcis. It is an integral part of the talotarsal joint. The scaphoid is pyriform, with the long axis oblique, directed downward and medially. The round base is superolateral, and the enlarged apex is inferomedial. The bone is flattened anteroposteriorly and is thicker dorsomedially.

It presents four surfaces, posterior, anterior, dorsal, and plantar, and two extremities, lateral and medial.

▶ Posterior Surface

The posterior surface is oriented posteriorly and faces the talar head. It does not cover completely the navicular articular surface of the talus. It is biconcave and tear-shaped and has the same obliquity as the bone. The concavity of the surface is variable, and in a few cases, the surface is nearly flat.[37] Frequently, an inferior extension of the articular surface is present, corresponding to the beak of the navicular (Fig. 2.40). This projection gives a triangular or quadrangular outline to the scaphoid. Dwight considers this extension as a fused secondary cuboid.[38]

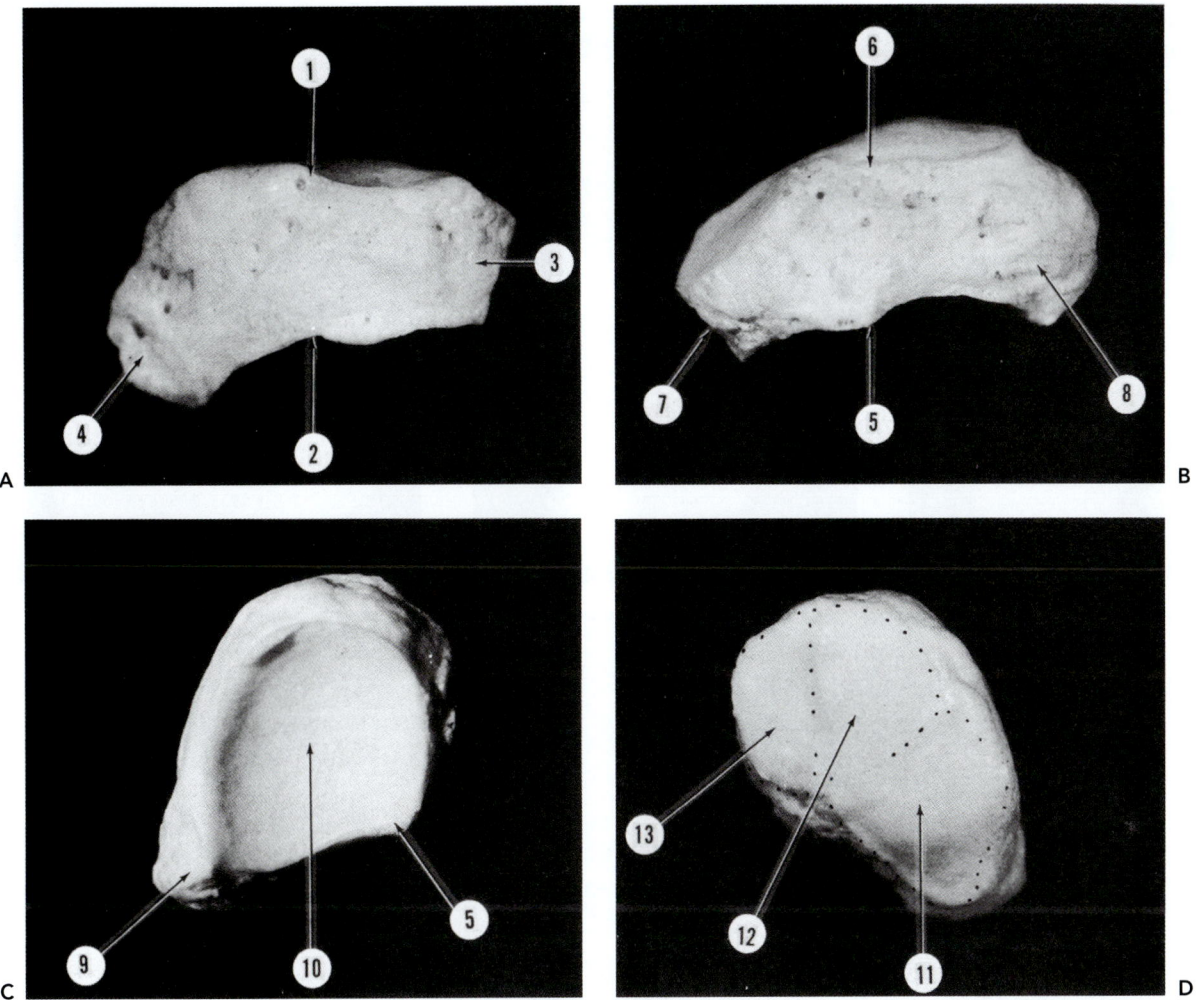

Figure 2.38 Navicular. (A) Dorsal surface. (B) Plantar surface. (C) Posterior surface. (D) Anterior surface. (1, anterior border of dorsal surface; 2, posterior border of dorsal surface; 3, lateral border of dorsal surface; 4, medial border of dorsal surface; 5, beak of navicular; 6, anterior border of inferior surface; 7, lateral border of inferior surface; 8, medial segment of inferior surface; 9, tuberosity of navicular; 10, talar articular surface; 11, articular surface for first cuneiform; 12, articular surface for second cuneiform; 13, articular surface for third cuneiform.)

▶ Anterior Surface

The anterior surface is reniform with inferior concavity. It is entirely articular and corresponds to the three cuneiforms. This surface is angular and faceted but yet is convex in its general contour. It is divided into three facets by two soft crests converging inferiorly, extending from the superior to the inferior border. The medial facet is the largest and corresponds to the first cuneiform. It is convex and triangular with a superolateral convex base and is oriented anteroinferiorly. The middle facet corresponds to the second cuneiform. It is triangular, with a superior base and an inferior apex. The surface is flat or slightly convex. It is oriented anteriorly with a minimal inferior tilt. The lateral facet is the smallest of the three. It is quadrilateral with rounded corners. This surface is flat or minimally concave and is oriented anterolaterally with a minimal inferior inclination.

When the general contour and the orientation of the anterior and posterior surfaces of the navicular are analyzed, it becomes evident that this bone induces a change of direction in the medial bony column. The talar head and neck initiate a medial deviation, whereas the navicular orients the column laterally and inferiorly. This zigzag arrangement maintains the overall axial alignment of the foot, overcoming the initial divergence (Fig. 2.41).

The inferior convergence of the articular facets on the anterior articular surface determines the formation of the transverse tarsal arch (see Fig. 2.39).

▶ Dorsal Surface

The dorsal surface is strongly convex, narrower laterally and larger medially. The apex of the convexity corresponds to the level of the middle articular facet of the anterior surface. The lateral one-fourth of the surface faces superolaterally and the medial three-fourths is oriented superomedially. The posterior border of the surface is concave. The anterior border is angular, formed by three segments united at an obtuse angle.

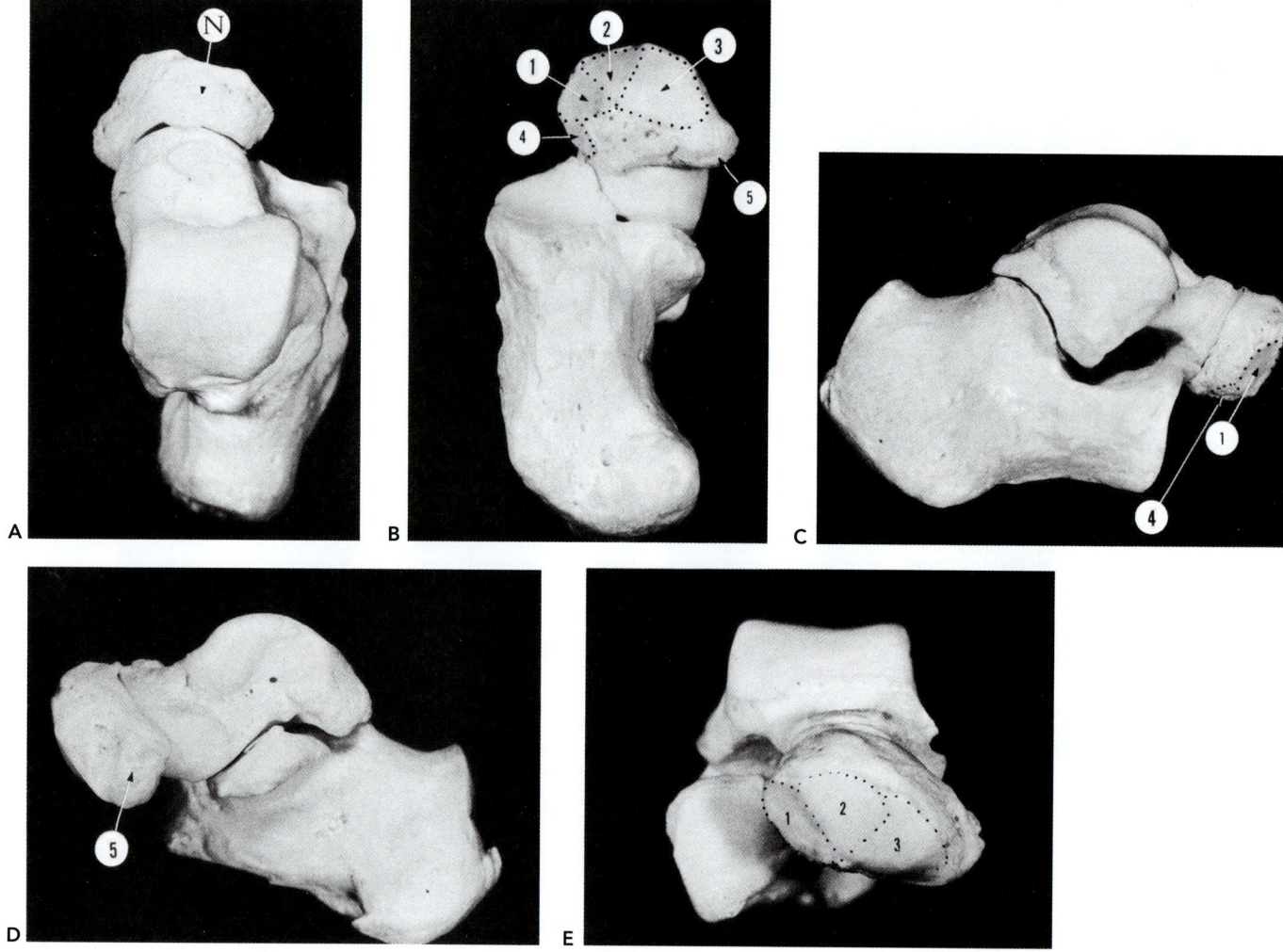

Figure 2.39 Navicular bone (N) in relation to hindfoot skeleton. (A) Dorsal view. (B) Plantar view. (C) Lateral view. (D) Medial view. (E) Anterior view. (1, articular surface with third cuneiform; 2, articular surface with second cuneiform; 3, articular surface with first cuneiform; 4, articular surface with cuboid; 5, tuberosity of navicular.)

The lateral segment is the shortest, oriented posterolaterally. The middle segment, nearly transverse, is longer. The medial segment is the largest; it is slightly convex and is oriented downward posteriorly. This segment is inferior to the other two.

The taloscaphoid capsule inserts at the periphery of the posterior articular surface.

The dorsal surface gives attachment to the following:

- Superomedial calcaneonavicular ligament, attaching along the superomedial aspect of the surface[39]
- Superficial and deep components of the dorsal talonavicular ligament
- Tibionavicular component of the superficial deltoid ligament, interlacing fibers with the superomedial calcaneonavicular ligament
- Dorsal cuneo$_{1,2,3}$-navicular ligament, originating from the distal segment of the dorsal surface
- Dorsal cubonavicular ligament inserting on the lateral segment of the surface

▶ Plantar Surface

The plantar surface is irregular and covered with rugosities and is in continuity medially with the tuberosity of the navicular. Frequently, an inferior bony projection—the beak of the navicular—is present in its midsegment.

The segment of the tibialis posterior tendon destined for the cuneiforms passes in a groove lateral to the tuberosity of the navicular and is oriented anterolaterally. The inferior calcaneonavicular ligament inserts on the inferior surface and posterior border, extending from the tuberosity of the navicular to the beak, where the insertion is most powerful.

The midsegment of the inferior surface gives attachment to the plantar cubonavicular ligament; further anteriorly, the second and third plantar cuneonavicular ligaments are inserted along the articular margin.

Manners-Smith mentions the rare occurrence (in 13 of 600) on the plantar surface of an articular facet for the os calcis close to the posterior surface, located between the beak of the navicular and the facet for the cuboid.[37]

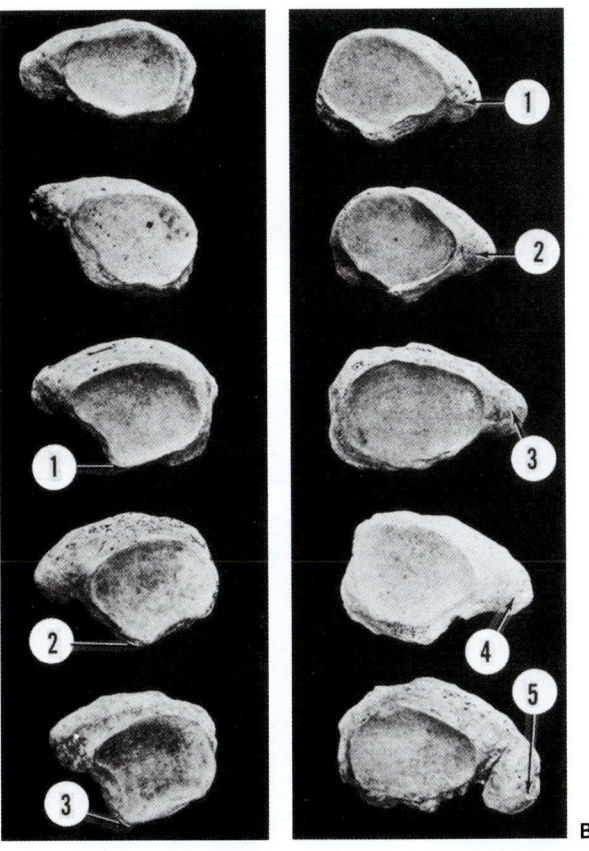

Figure 2.40 **(A) Variations in the size of the beak of the navicular,** more pronounced in 1, 2, and 3. **(B) Variations in the size of the tuberosity of the navicular.** (From Dwight T. *Variations in the Bones of the Hands and Feet: A Clinical Atlas.* JB Lippincott; 1907:14-23.)

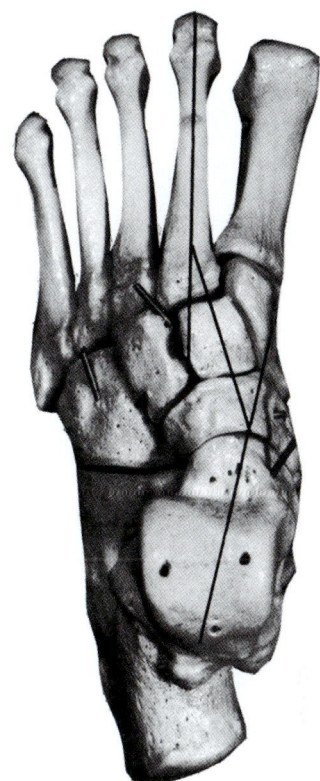

Figure 2.41 Zigzag pattern formed by the medial bony column—talus, navicular, cuneiform block, and metatarsals 2 and 3. The talar neck is deflected medially. The distal articular surface of the navicular deflects the cuneiforms laterally, neutralizing the medial deviation.

▶ **Medial End**

The medial end of the navicular is formed by a bony prominence, the navicular tuberosity. The size of this structure is variable (see Fig. 2.40). When separated from the main bone mass, it is called the *naviculare secundarium*. The tibialis posterior tendon inserts on the tuberosity.

The first plantar cuneonavicular ligament arises from the anterior aspect of the tubercle, and the medial cuneonavicular ligament arises from the medial aspect.

▶ **Lateral End**

The lateral end of the navicular is convex and presents two segments: inferior and superior. A small articular facet for the cuboid occupies most of the inferior surface. This surface is in continuity with the articular facet for the third cuneiform. As indicated by Manners-Smith, the cuboid facet is present in 70% of 600 naviculars and is variable in contour and size.[37] In some instances, it extends from the articular facet of the third cuneiform to the posterior articular surface. This cuboid surface not infrequently extends onto the beak of the navicular.

The superior segment of the lateral end gives insertion to the powerful lateral calcaneonavicular ligament, a component of the bifurcate ligament.

CUNEIFORMS

The cuneiforms are three in number and are interposed between the scaphoid proximally, the first three metatarsals distally, and the cuboid laterally. The three cuneiforms, in association with the cuboid, form an arcade or transverse arch that acts as a niche for the plantar musculotendinous and neurovascular structures. The cuneiforms are wedge-shaped. The first or medial cuneiform has a dorsal crest and plantar base; the second or middle cuneiform and the third or lateral cuneiform have a dorsal base and a plantar crest (see Fig. 2.35).

Proximally, on the dorsum of the foot, the bases of the cuneiforms form a polygonal line with two obtuse angles. The angle between the second and third cuneiforms is oriented posteromedially, and the angle between the bases of the first and second cuneiforms is directed posteriorly. Distally, the second cuneiform is in proximal recess, approximately 8 mm relative to the first cuneiform and 4 mm relative to the third cuneiform. This disposition creates the space necessary to receive and lock the base of the second metatarsal.

▶ **First Cuneiform**

The first cuneiform has five surfaces—anterior, posterior, medial, lateral, and inferior—and a crest (Fig. 2.42).

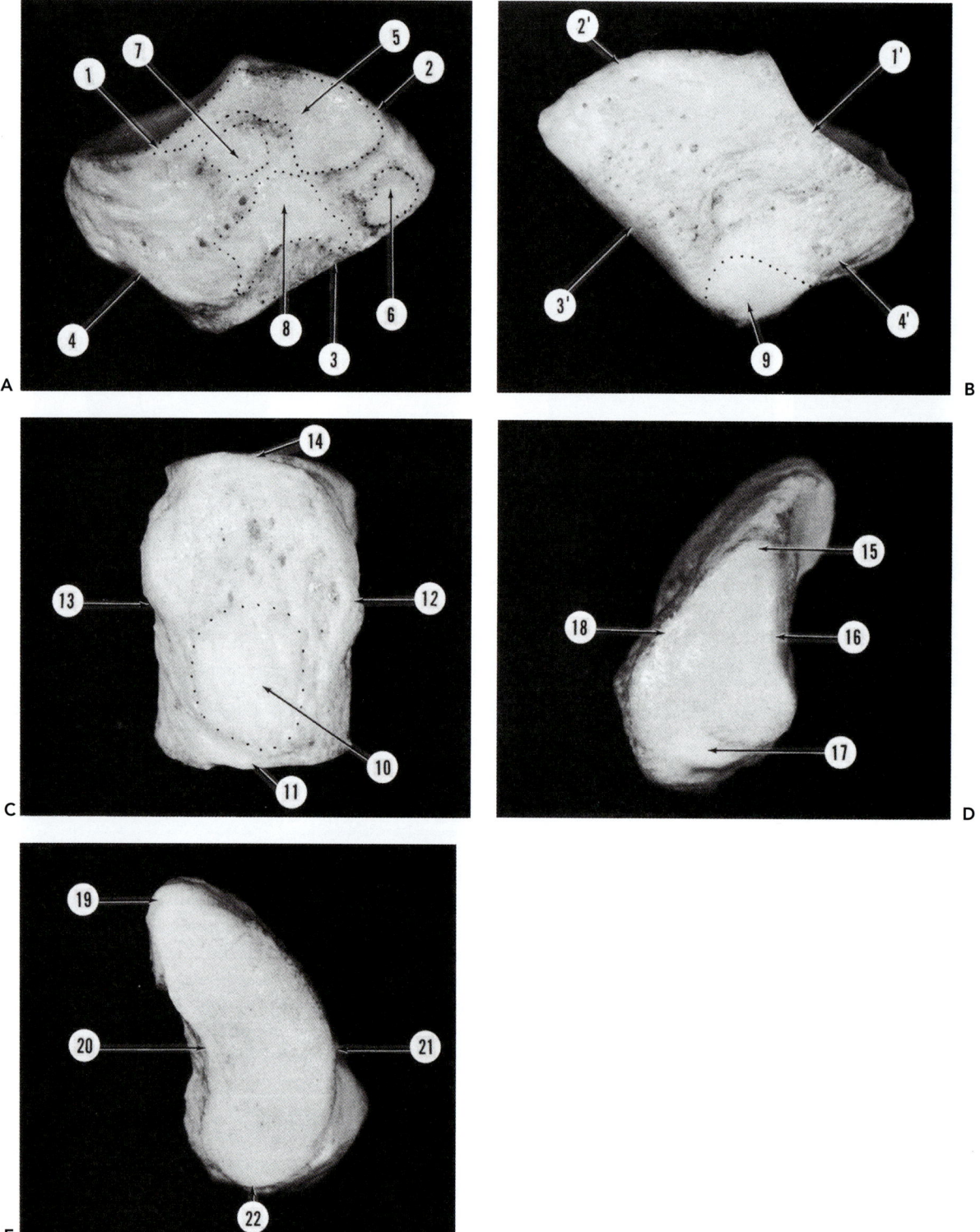

Figure 2.42 **First cuneiform, right. (A)** Lateral surface. **(B)** Medial surface. **(C)** Plantar surface. **(D)** Posterior surface. **(E)** Anterior surface. (*1, 1'*, posterior borders of lateral and medial surfaces; *2, 2'*, superior borders of lateral and medial surfaces; *3, 3'*, anterior borders of lateral and medial surfaces; *4, 4'*, inferior borders of lateral and medial surfaces; *5*, articular surface for second cuneiform; *6*, articular surface for base of second metatarsal; *7*, insertional zone of intercuneiform C_1-C_2 ligament; *8*, insertional zone of Lisfranc ligament C_1-M_2; *9*, oval smooth surface for tibialis anterior tendon, where a gliding bursa may be found; *10*, tubercle of inferior surface; *11*, posterior border of inferior surface; *12*, medial border of inferior surface; *13*, lateral border of inferior surface; *14*, anterior border of inferior surface; *15*, apex of navicular articular surface; *16*, lateral border of navicular articular surface; *17*, round base of navicular articular surface; *18*, medial border of navicular articular surface; *19*, apex of first metatarsal articular surface; *20*, concave lateral border of first metatarsal articular surface; *21*, convex medial border of first metatarsal articular surface; *22*, inferior border of first metatarsal articular surface.)

The posterior surface articulates with the scaphoid. It is triangular or pear-shaped, with an inferior base and a superior apex. The surface is concave in all directions.

The anterior surface articulates with the base of the first metatarsal. It is reniform, with a convex medial border and a concave lateral border. The surface is elongated in the vertical direction and is oriented anteriorly, with some inferior and medial inclination. The surface is minimally convex in the transverse direction and more or less flat in the vertical dimension. As mentioned by Jones, this facet is usually a single surface or (often) notched with a distinct constriction in its midsegment; not uncommonly, it is subdivided into two separate surfaces.[21]

The medial surface is pentagonal, higher distally, and lower proximally. The anteroinferior angle is occupied by an oval, smooth surface. The tibialis anterior takes insertion along the inferior and posterior margin of this oval surface. A bursa covers the smooth surface[40]; it corresponds to the cartilaginous sesamoid of the tibialis anterior tendon. The medial surface also provides attachment to the following:

- Dorsal cuneo$_1$-navicular ligament
- Dorsal intercuneiform$_{1,2}$ ligament, which occupies the lateral aspect of the surface
- Dorsal cuneo$_1$-metatarsal$_2$ ligament, arising from the anterolateral corner
- Dorsal cuneo$_1$-metatarsal$_1$ broad ligament, arising from the midsegment of the anterior margin
- Medial cuneo$_1$-navicular ligament, inserting on the lower and posterior aspect of the surface

The lateral surface, which is more or less rectangular, is limited along the posterior and superior borders by two articular surfaces. The articular surface corresponding to the second cuneiform is in the shape of an inferiorly reflected "L," the vertical arm running along the posterior border and the larger horizontal arm running along the posterior two-thirds of the superior border. The horizontal segment is concave anteroposteriorly, and the vertical is concave vertically. The anterior third of the surface along the superior border is occupied by an oval articulating surface, corresponding to the base of the second metatarsal. This surface reaches the anterior articulating surface but is separated from the superior border and the horizontal arm of the cuneiform surface by a small bony band. The angle formed by the two arms of the articulating surfaces is occupied by the insertion of the intercuneiform$_{1,2}$ ligament and anterior to it is located a bony eminence that gives attachment to the powerful cuneo$_1$-metatarsal$_2$ ligament (Lisfranc ligament).

The inferior or plantar surface is rectangular, large, and strongly convex transversely. It provides insertion to the following:

- Plantar cuneo$_1$-navicular ligament, attached to the tubercle located on the posterior aspect of the surface
- Plantar intercuneiform$_{1,2}$ ligament from the midsegment of the lateral border
- Cuneo$_1$-metatarsal$_1$ broad ligament, arising from the distal border of the surface
- Cuneo$_1$-metatarsal$_{2,3}$ ligament, which is very strong and originates from the posterolateral corner
- Peroneus longus tendon, inserting anterior to the tubercle and occupying the lateral half of the distal segment

The crest or superior border is round and smooth. The anterior one-fourth corresponds to the base of the second metatarsal and is directed posteriorly. The posterior three-fourths is directed downward, posteromedially, and corresponds to the second cuneiform.

Ajmani and colleagues reported on the variations of the articular facets in 100 medial cuneiforms.[41] The proximal articular surface was pear-shaped with the narrow end directed dorsally in 80%; it was oval-shaped in 14% and triangular with a plantar base in 6%. The distal articular surface was kidney-shaped with hilum on the lateral margin in 31%; two partially united upper and lower facets were present in 49%; two separate articular surfaces subdivided by a nonarticular segment were seen in 6%; there was a crescentic facet with concavity facing laterally in 14%. The lateral articular surface presented an inverted L-shaped facet in 67%. The horizontal arm of the latter was separated by a roughened ridge from the anteriorly located articular surface to the second metatarsal in 15%. The vertical articular surface was separated from the horizontal articular surface by a roughened area in 20%.

▶ Second Cuneiform

The second cuneiform is the smallest of the three and is in recess relative to the other two. The bone presents five surfaces—anterior, posterior, medial, lateral, and superior or dorsal—and a crest (Fig. 2.43).

The anterior surface articulates with the base of the second metatarsal. It is triangular, with a dorsal convex base and an inferior apex. The lateral border is slightly concave laterally. The surface is gently convex in its vertical dimension.

The posterior surface is also triangular, with a similar orientation. The lateral border is concave and the medial border is convex. This surface articulates with the scaphoid and presents vertical concavity.

The medial surface articulates with the first cuneiform, with a similar inferiorly reversed L-shaped articular surface. The vertical segment of this articular surface is narrower than the horizontal arm, which may overflow inferiorly. The surface of the bone located at the angle of the two articular arms gives insertion to the interosseous cuneiform$_{1,2}$ ligament. Jones describes a variant of the medial surface with an interosseous groove dividing the horizontal segment into two.[21]

The lateral surface, which is rectangular, bears also a reversed L-shaped articular surface occupying the superior and posterior borders. It articulates with the third cuneiform. A small tubercle located in the interarticular angle gives insertion to the interosseous cuneiform$_{2,3}$ ligament. From the anteroinferior segment of the surface originates the cuneo$_2$-metatarsal$_2$ or cuneo$_2$-metatarsal$_{2,3}$ ligament.

The dorsal surface is rectangular, minimally convex, and larger posteriorly. A small depression is often present near the posteromedial corner along its medial border. With a

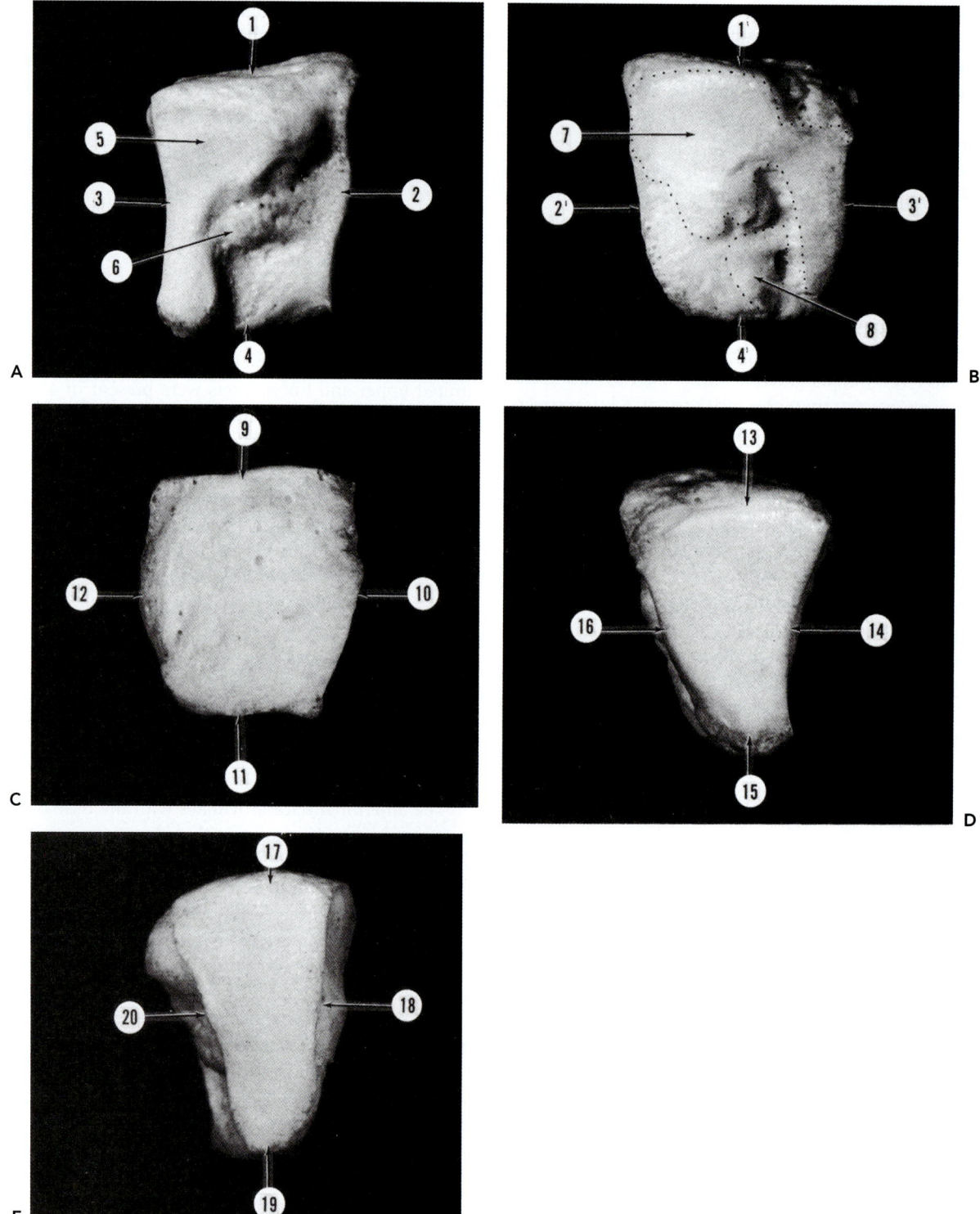

Figure 2.43 **Second cuneiform, right. (A)** Lateral surface. **(B)** Medial surface. **(C)** Plantar surface. **(D)** Posterior surface. **(E)** Anterior surface. (*1, 1′,* superior borders of lateral and medial surfaces; *2, 2′,* anterior borders of lateral and medial surfaces; *3, 3′,* posterior borders of lateral and medial surfaces; *4, 4′,* inferior borders of lateral and medial surfaces; *5,* articular surface for third cuneiform; *6,* tubercle for insertion of intercuneiform C_2-C_3 ligament; *7,* articular surface for first cuneiform; *8,* tubercle for insertion of intercuneiform C_1-C_2 ligament; *9,* posterior border of dorsal surface; *10,* medial border of dorsal surface; *11,* anterior border of dorsal surface; *12,* lateral border of dorsal surface; *13,* superior border of navicular articular surface; *14,* concave lateral border of navicular articular surface; *15,* apex of navicular articular surface; *16,* medial border of navicular articular surface; *17,* superior border of second metatarsal articular surface; *18,* medial border of second metatarsal articular surface; *19,* apex of second metatarsal articular surface; *20,* lateral border of second metatarsal articular surface.)

corresponding depression on the first cuneiform, a small pit is formed (the intercuneiform fossa).[21] The borders of the dorsal surface give insertion to the dorsal scaphocuneiform$_2$ ligament posteriorly, the dorsal cuneo$_2$-metatarsal$_2$ ligament anteriorly, the dorsal cuneiform$_{1,2}$ ligament medially, and the dorsal cuneiform$_{2,3}$ ligament laterally.

The crest or inferior border is thin and engulfed by the two other cuneiforms. It provides insertion to the plantar cuneo$_2$-navicular ligament and the plantar cuneiform$_{1,2}$ ligament, both masked by the insertion of the tibialis posterior tendon. The crest also gives attachment to the lateral fibrous arm of the Y origin of the flexor hallucis brevis muscle.

Ajmani and coworkers reported on the variations of the articular facets in 100 intermediary cuneiforms.[41] On the medial articular surface, an inverted L-shaped articular facet was present in 59%. The vertical limb was absent in 17%. The distal end of the horizontal limb was descending toward the plantar aspect in 18%. Two circular facets—one on the proximal and plantar corner and the other on the distal and dorsal corner—were seen in 6%. On the lateral surface, the long vertical articular facet with slight narrowing in the middle, located along the proximal border, was present in 65%. A vertical articular surface without indentation was seen in 8%, and the articular surface was triangular with a dorsal base in 27%. The proximal and distal articular surfaces were triangular, without variations.

▶ Third Cuneiform

The third cuneiform articulates with the scaphoid proximally, the cuboid laterally, the base of the third metatarsal distally, and the second cuneiform medially. The bone presents five surfaces—anterior, posterior, medial, lateral, and dorsal—and a plantar crest (Fig. 2.44).

The anterior surface articulates with the base of the third metatarsal. It is triangular, with the base dorsal and apex plantar. The surface is flat or has a minimal transverse concavity.

The posterior surface articulates with the scaphoid, with an oval surface occupying the upper three-fourths of the aspect, leaving the inferior one-fourth as a blunt pointed area. This surface is oriented posteriorly and medially and is flat.

The medial surface is rectangular. Articulating surfaces occupy vertically the anterior and posterior aspects, leaving the central segment for the insertion of the ligaments. The anterior articulating surface is a narrow band, corresponds to the base of the second metatarsal, and is divided into two segments by the interosseous ligament extending from the third cuneiform to the base of the third metatarsal or possibly to the third and second metatarsals. The intercuneiform$_{2,3}$ ligament inserts posterior to this ligament. The posterior articulating surface is also a vertical facet occupying most of the posterior aspect and leaving only a small, inferior, nonarticulating band. It is in continuity with the surface of the scaphoid and articulates with the second cuneiform. The anterior border of this surface is concave with a forward extension of the upper segment.

The lateral surface is quadrilateral. A large ovoid facet articulating with the cuboid occupies the posterosuperior corner extending just beyond the midlevels of the posterior and superior borders of the surface. Occasionally, a small articulating surface is present in the anterosuperior angle for the base of the fourth metatarsal. The remaining segment of the surface gives insertion to the cuneo$_3$-metatarsal$_3$, or cuneo$_3$-metatarsals$_{3,4}$, or cuneo$_3$-metatarsal$_4$ ligaments. The interosseous cuneo$_3$-cuboid ligament originates posterior to the previous ligament.

The dorsal surface is rectangular. The posterior border is oblique, directed laterally and slightly posteriorly. The medial border is beveled in the anterior segment in correspondence to the base of the second metatarsal and is followed proximally by a notch occupying the midsegment. The lateral border is oriented posteriorly and medially in the posterior half, whereas the anterior segment makes a gentle change in direction toward the medial aspect of the foot, thus announcing the direction of the third metatarsal. This surface gives insertion posteriorly to the scaphocuneiform$_3$ ligament, medially to the dorsal intercuneiform$_{2,3}$ ligament, and laterally to the cuneo$_3$-metatarsal$_3$ ligament and the cuneo$_3$-metatarsal$_2$ ligament.

The crest or inferior border is round and smooth and posteriorly bears a small tubercle. It provides insertion to the plantar cuneo$_3$-cuboid ligament, plantar cuneo$_3$-navicular ligament, plantar cuneo$_3$-metatarsals$_{3,4}$ ligament (one or both ligaments may be missing), tibialis posterior tendon, oblique head of the adductor hallucis, and lateral arm of the Y stem of the origin of the flexor hallucis brevis. The last three insertions cover the ligamentous attachments.

Ajmani and colleagues reported on the variations of the articular facets in 100 lateral cuneiforms.[41] On the medial surface, the articular facets were distributed proximally, and distally, they were separated by a nonarticular area. The proximal articular surface was present as a vertical strip, with slight indentation along the distal margin in 39%. A circular articular facet confined to the dorsal half was present in 35%, and a triangular facet with a distal base was present in 19%. A vertical articular strip without indentation was seen in 7%. In the distal articular half, two separate articular facets were present in 59%, a vertical strip was present in 18%, a single facet on the dorsal margin was present in 7%, and no facet was seen in 16%. On the lateral surface, a large triangular facet located proximally was present in 87%, corresponding to the cuboid. A vertical articular strip was present in 13%. No circular articular facet was observed. A small semioval facet was also present at the superodistal corner in 34% and was absent in 66%. The proximal articular surface, confined to the dorsal two-thirds, was square in 61% and triangular in 31%. The distal surface was completely covered with a triangular articular facet in 66% and a kidney-shaped facet with a lateral hilum in 34%.

METATARSALS

The five metatarsals articulate proximally with the three cuneiforms and the cuboid and form the tarsometatarsal or Lisfranc joint.

Proximally, the bases of the metatarsals are disposed in an arcuate fashion, forming a transverse arch high medially and low laterally (Fig. 2.45). The apex of this arch corresponds to the

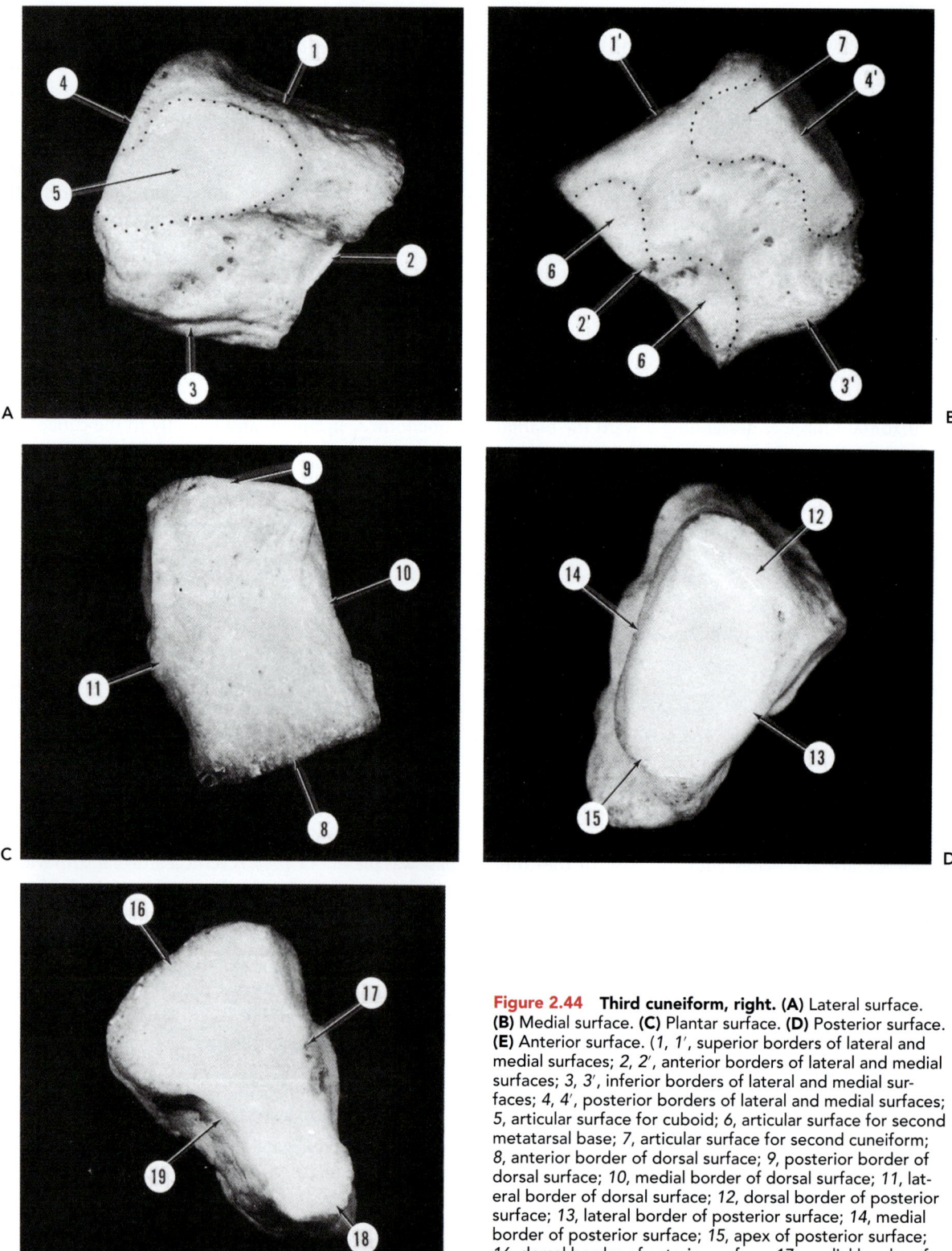

Figure 2.44 Third cuneiform, right. **(A)** Lateral surface. **(B)** Medial surface. **(C)** Plantar surface. **(D)** Posterior surface. **(E)** Anterior surface. (*1, 1′*, superior borders of lateral and medial surfaces; *2, 2′*, anterior borders of lateral and medial surfaces; *3, 3′*, inferior borders of lateral and medial surfaces; *4, 4′*, posterior borders of lateral and medial surfaces; *5*, articular surface for cuboid; *6*, articular surface for second metatarsal base; *7*, articular surface for second cuneiform; *8*, anterior border of dorsal surface; *9*, posterior border of dorsal surface; *10*, medial border of dorsal surface; *11*, lateral border of dorsal surface; *12*, dorsal border of posterior surface; *13*, lateral border of posterior surface; *14*, medial border of posterior surface; *15*, apex of posterior surface; *16*, dorsal border of anterior surface; *17*, medial border of anterior surface; *18*, apex of anterior surface; *19*, lateral border of anterior surface.)

base of the second metatarsal. The metatarsals are also flexed, thus contributing to the formation of longitudinal arches that are more pronounced medially and barely present laterally. Distally, the five metatarsal heads are located in the same plane horizontally, and no transverse arch is present at this level.

The first metatarsal diverges slightly from the second metatarsal. The intermetatarsal angle formed by the long axis of these two metatarsals is 2° to 8° in the adolescent and 3° to 9° in the adult.[42] Kelikian mentions that "any measurement in excess of 10° is indicative of varus deformity of the first metatarsal."[43]

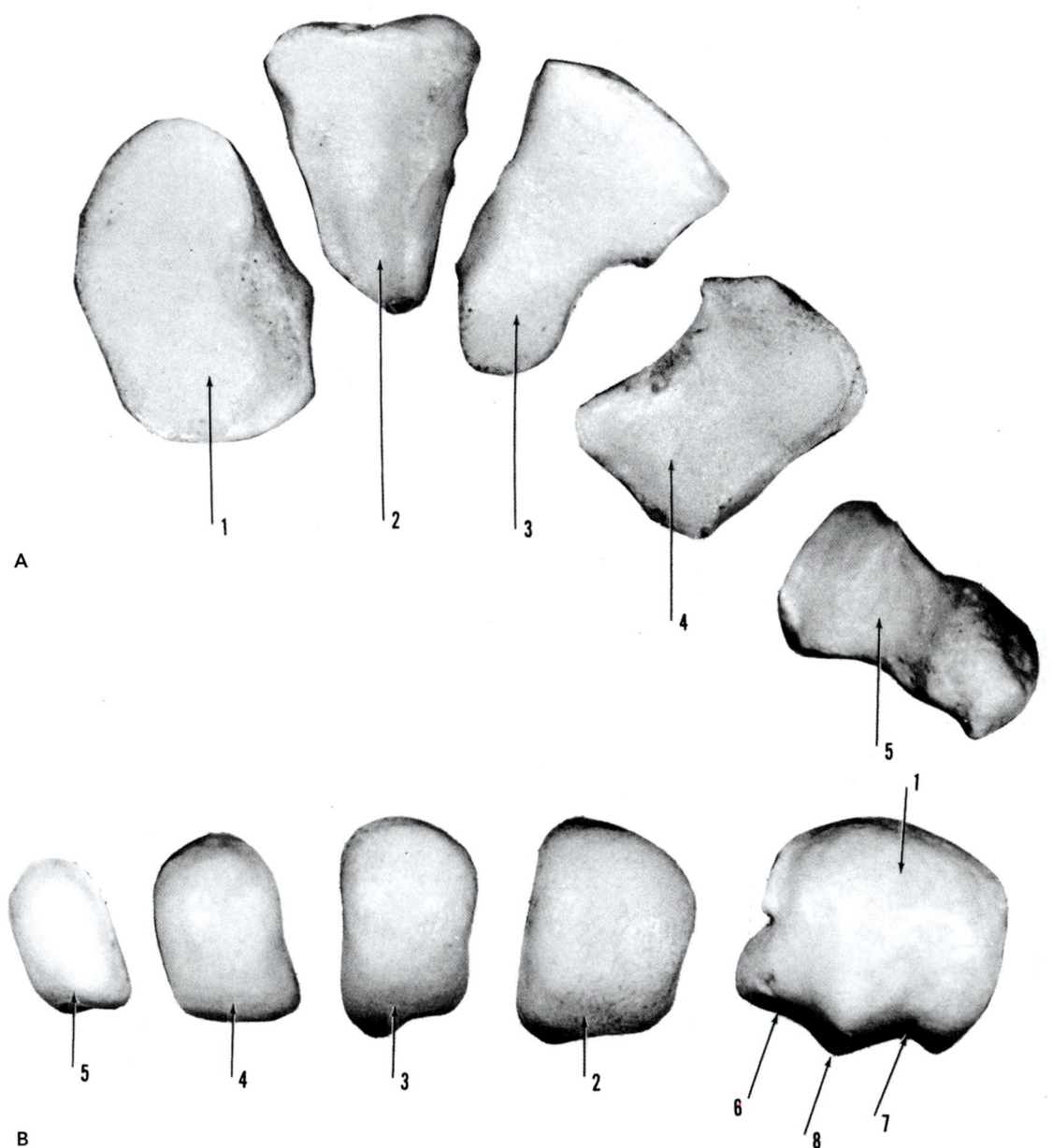

Figure 2.45 **(A) Bases of metatarsals 1 to 5 forming a transverse arch. (B) Heads of metatarsals 1 to 5; no arch is present.** (6, trochlear surface for lateral sesamoid; 7, trochlear surface for medial sesamoid; 8, crest of metatarsal head.)

In relationship to the axial alignment of the talar neck and the cuneiform block, the metatarsals contribute to the formation of an elongated Z arrangement (see Fig. 2.41).

The first metatarsal is shorter than the second metatarsal. Leboucq measured anatomically the length of these two metatarsals in the adult and the newborn-adolescent group.[44] In the adult, the average shortening of the first metatarsal is 10.5 mm (maximum 14 mm, minimum 7 mm), whereas in the newborn-adolescent group, the average shortening is 7.45 mm (maximum 10 mm, minimum 5.5 mm). Straus gives the following data concerning the length measurements of the first and second metatarsals: the average ratio of the greatest length of the metatarsal 1 × 100 to the greatest length of metatarsal 2 is 83 in the adult, 85 in the juvenile, and 86 in the newborn.[42] The metatarsal formula has been expressed in terms of the distal projections of the metatarsal heads relative to each other in mounted skeletons or on radiographs. Morton introduced the formula of 1 = 2 > 3 > 4 > 5 and stated that "one of the requirements for ideal foot function is an equidistance of the heads of the first and second metatarsal bones from the heel."[45] The metatarsal formula 2 > 3 > 1 > 4 > 5 is the one accepted by most anatomists; there are variations such as 2 > 1 > 3 > 4 > 5, 2 > 1 = 3 > 4 > 5, or other combinations, but "no anatomist appears to record a dominant first metatarsal."[21] The general alignment of the metatarsal baseline is oblique, oriented backward, and laterally from the base of the first metatarsal. This line and the corresponding tarsal line interlock in two locations: the base of the second metatarsal penetrates the tarsal line proximally at the level of the second cuneiform. The third cuneiform penetrates distally, to a much lesser degree, the metatarsal line at the level of the third metatarsal base. This arrangement secures the second and third metatarsals.

Each metatarsal is formed by a base, a head, and a shaft.

Base

First Metatarsal

The base of the first metatarsal is more or less triangular, with lateral, medial, and inferior surfaces supporting the articular surface for the first cuneiform (see Figs. 2.45 and 2.46). This articular surface has its long axis oriented downward and

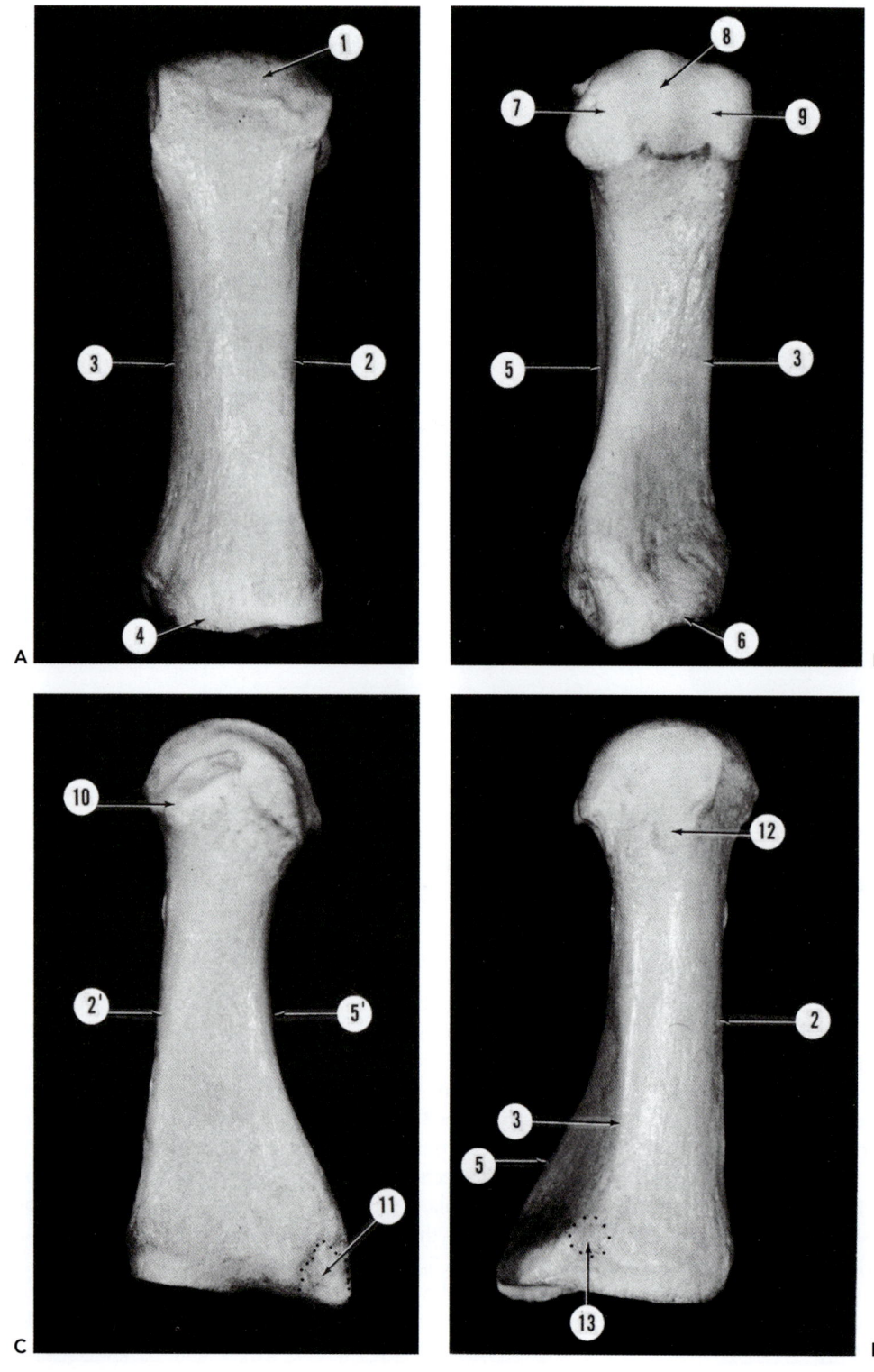

Figure 2.46 First metatarsal, right. **(A)** Dorsal surface. **(B)** Plantar surface. **(C)** Lateral surface. **(D)** Medial surface. (*1*, head; *2*, lateral border of dorsal surface; *2'*, superior border of lateral surface; *3*, medial border of dorsal surface and plantar surface; *4*, proximal border of dorsal surface; *5*, lateral border of plantar surface; *5'*, inferior border of lateral surface; *6*, proximal border of plantar surface; *7*, lateral trochlear surface; *8*, crest of metatarsal head; *9*, medial trochlear surface; *10*, tubercle for origin of lateral metatarsophalangeal ligament; *11*, tubercle for insertion of peroneus longus tendon; *12*, tubercle for origin of medial metatarsophalangeal ligament; *13*, insertion of tibialis anterior tendon.)

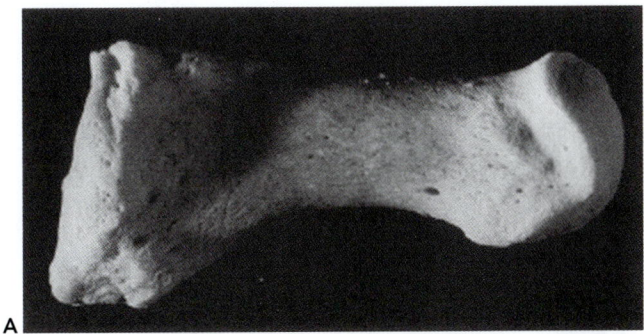
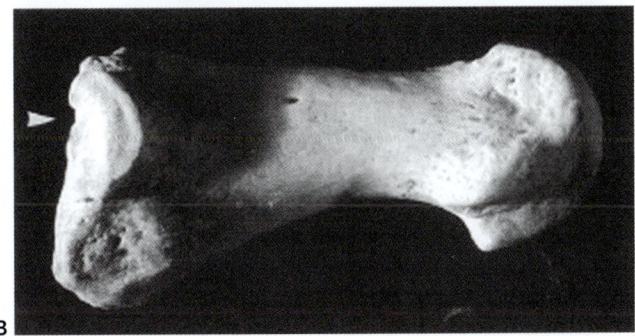

Figure 2.47 First metatarsal bone (lateral view of right bones). **(A)** Absence of the facet. **(B)** Presence of the intermetatarsal facet (*white arrow*). (Reprinted from Le Minor JM. The intermetatarsal articular facet of the first metatarsal bone in humans: a derived trait unique within primates. *Ann Anat.* 2003;185:360, Figure 1, with permission from Elsevier.)

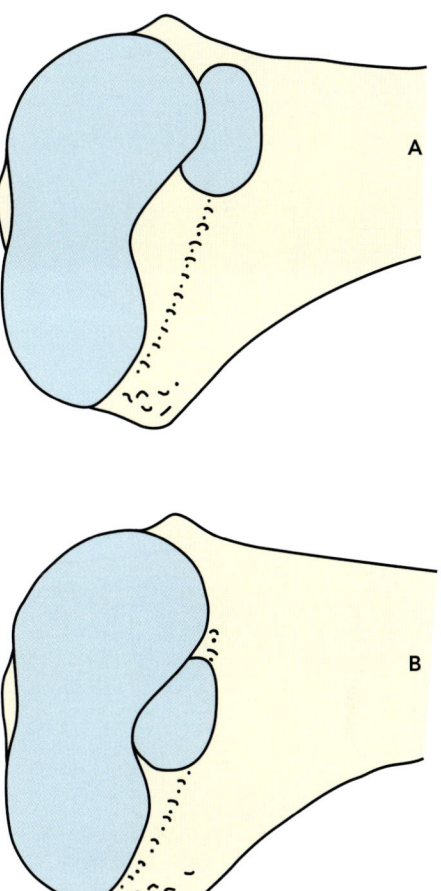

Figure 2.48 Location of intermetatarsal M1-M2 joint surface on lateral surface of M1 base. **(A)** Intermetatarsal facet located in the dorsal third of the lateral side. **(B)** Intermetatarsal facet located in the middle third of the lateral side. (Adapted from Le Minor JM. The intermetatarsal articular facet of the first metatarsal bone in humans: a derived trait unique within primates. *Ann Anat.* 2003;185:361.)

laterally. It is reniform, with the hilum on the lateral side, and presents a slight concavity transversely. It is flat in the direction of the long axis. This articular surface may be subdivided into partially united upper and lower segments.[46]

At the junction of the medial and inferior surfaces is a tubercle for the insertion of the tibialis anterior tendon; a more prominent tuberosity is present at the junction of the inferior and lateral surfaces for the insertion of the peroneus longus tendon. The medial surface provides attachment to the dorsal $cuneo_1$-$metatarsal_1$ ligament. The plantar $cuneo_1$-$metatarsal_1$ ligament inserts on the lateral half of the inferior surface. There is no intermetatarsal ligament between the first and second metatarsal bases.

The lateral surface of the base establishes variable contact with the second metatarsal. Singh gives the following distribution of areas of contact with the second metatarsal in 100 first metatarsals: smooth articular facet, 21; smooth area with indefinite margins, 40; no area of contact, 39.[46]

Romash and coworkers in a roentgenographic study of the feet in 118 subjects describe the presence of an articular facet between M_1 and M_2 in 27%, a transitional facet in 38%, and no articular facet in 35%.[47]

Wanivenhaus and Pretterklieber, in a study of 100 cadaveric feet, observed an intermetatarsal M_1-M_2 joint in 53%, mainly in the large male metatarsals.[48]

Le Minor and Winter[49] in a series of 412 human first metatarsal bones (dried bone) observed on the lateral side of the metatarsal base a well-defined intermetatarsal M_1-M_2 articular facet in 30.8% (see Fig. 2.47). The facet was elliptical in shape, measuring 10.7 mm in height and 6.1 mm in width on average. The long axis of the facet was perpendicular to the longitudinal axis of the metatarsal shaft. The surface was plane or slightly concave.

The intermetatarsal facet M_1-M_2 was located within the dorsal third of the lateral side in 81.1%; it was located in the middle third in 18.9%; it was not observed in the plantar third (see Figs. 2.48 and 2.49). The intermetatarsal M_1-M_2 articular surface connected with the articular surface of the M_1 base in 53.5%.

The proximal metatarsal M_1 articular angle (PMAA) was measured by ElSaid et al[50] in 478 first metatarsals. The PMAA ranged from −13.8° of lateral deviation to 12.7° of medial deviation (see Fig. 2.50) with an overall average of −1°.

A joint between the first and second metatarsal bases was present in 25% of the specimens. When present, it was located on the dorsal lateral aspect of the base of the first metatarsal (see Fig. 2.51).

Hyer et al[51] determined the obliquity of the first metatarsal base in 77 dry skeletal specimens. The mean medial obliquity angle (see Fig. 2.52) was 3.42° and the obliquity increased with age from 3.5° in the younger group to 5.13° in the older group.

82 Sarrafian's Anatomy of the Foot and Ankle

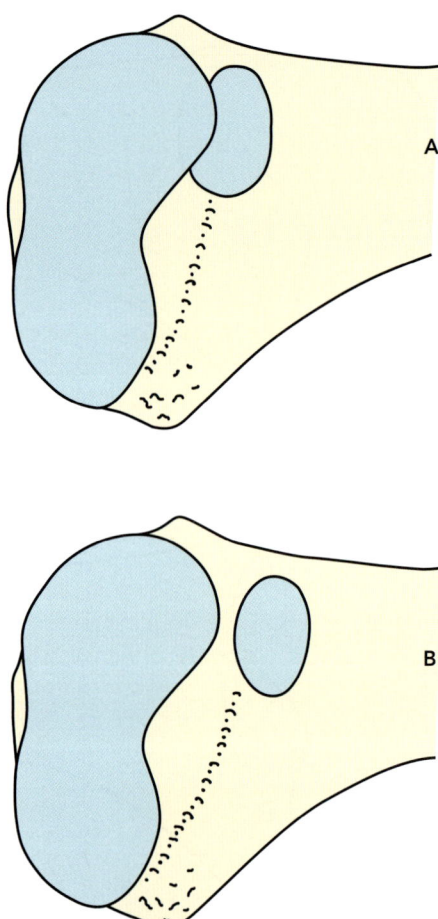

Figure 2.49 **Relations of the intermetatarsal facet of the first metatarsal with the proximal articular surface of the M1 base. (A)** Intermetatarsal facet in connection with the articular surface of the base. **(B)** Intermetatarsal facet separated from the articular surface of the base. (Adapted from Le Minor JM. The intermetatarsal articular facet of the first metatarsal bone in humans: a derived trait unique within primates. *Ann Anat.* 2003;185:361.)

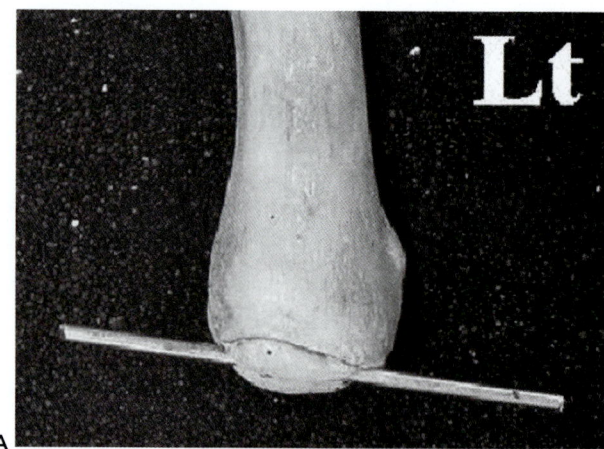

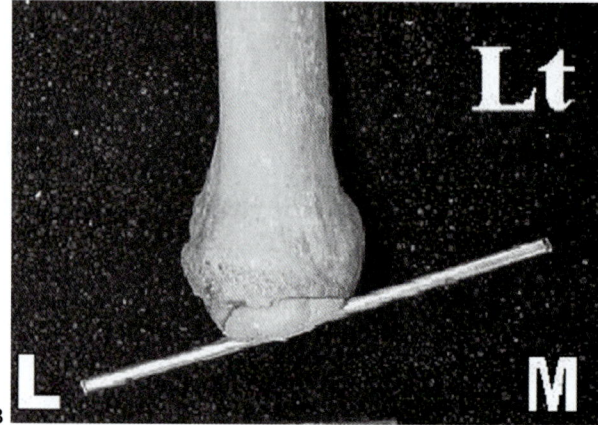

Figure 2.50 **Orientation of the proximal articular surface of the first metatarsal M1 base. (A)** The most medially deviated surface. **(B)** The most laterally deviated surface. (*L*, lateral; *Lt*, left bone; *M*, medial.) (ElSaid A, Tisdale C, Donley B, et al. First metatarsal bone: an anatomical study. *Foot Ankle Int.* 2006;12:1041-1048, Figure 6. Copyright ©2006. Reprinted by Permission of SAGE Publications.)

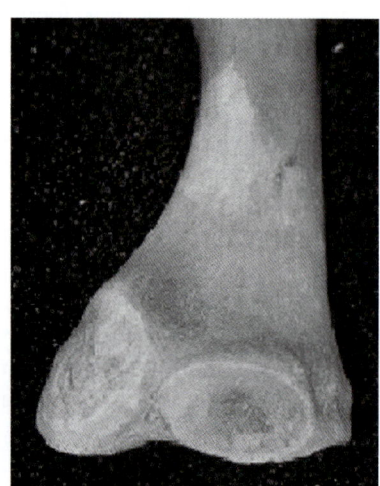

Figure 2.51 **Joint surface on base of M1 corresponding to the M1-M2 articulation.** (ElSaid A, Tisdale C, Donley B, et al. First metatarsal bone: an anatomical study. *Foot Ankle Int.* 2006;12:1041-1048, Figure 7. Copyright ©2006. Reprinted by Permission of SAGE Publications.)

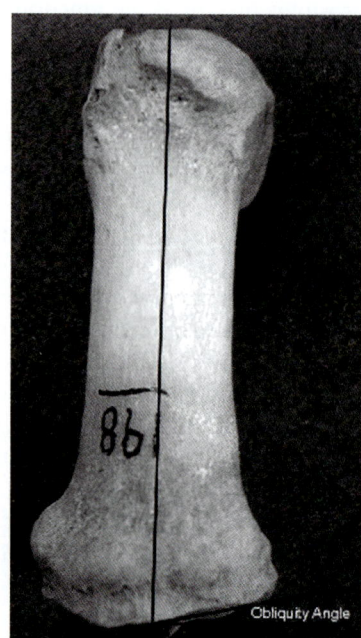

Figure 2.52 **The medial obliquity angle of the first metatarsal base.** (Hyer CF, Philbin TM, Berlet GC, et al. The obliquity of the first metatarsal base. *Foot Ankle Int.* 2004;8:728-732. Copyright ©2004. Reprinted by Permission of SAGE Publications.)

Second Metatarsal

The base of the second metatarsal is cuneiform (see Figs. 2.45, 2.53, and 2.54). The superior surface is flat. The lateral and medial surfaces converge on the plantar aspect to form a crest. These three surfaces support the triangular concave articular surface (base dorsal, apex plantar) for the second cuneiform. The base of the second metatarsal establishes contact with five bones: medially with the first cuneiform and possibly the base of the first metatarsal, laterally with the third metatarsal and the lateral cuneiform, and proximally with the middle cuneiform.

The dorsal surface provides insertion to the dorsal cuneometatarsal ligaments (C_1-M_2, C_2-M_2, and $C3$-M_2) and to the dorsal intermetatarsal ligament (M_2-M_3). The medial surface bears in the posterosuperior corner a small articulating oval surface that corresponds to a similar surface on the first cuneiform. The remaining segment of the surface provides attachment to the powerful cuneo$_1$-metatarsal$_2$ ligament (Lisfranc ligament). Two tonguelike articular surfaces, upper and lower, are present on the lateral surface of the base. They are both oriented longitudinally. The upper surface is longer than the lower and is separated from it by a small interval. These articular surfaces correspond anteriorly to the third metatarsal base and posteriorly to the third cuneiform. As reported by Singh, the configuration and distribution of the articular surface are very variable see (Fig. 2.60).[46] The nonarticular segment of the lateral surface provides attachment proximally to the cuneo$_2$-metatarsal$_2$ ligament and distally to the interosseous metatarsal ligament (M_2-M_3). On the crest are inserted the plantar cuneo$_1$-metatarsal$_2$ ligament, the plantar metatarsal$_{2,3}$ ligament, a slip from the tibialis posterior tendon, a slip from the long plantar ligament, and the adductor hallucis obliquum muscle.

Third Metatarsal

The base of the third metatarsal is also cuneiform, supporting a triangular flat articular surface (base dorsal, apex plantar) for the third cuneiform (see Figs. 2.45 and 2.55). The medial surface presents two articular surfaces for the base of the second metatarsal. These surfaces are plantar and dorsal, flat, and separated by an anteroposterior surface of rugosities giving insertion to the interosseous cuneometatarsal ligament (C_3-M_3).

On the distal segment of the medial surface inserts the interosseous metatarsal ligament (M_2-M_3). The distribution of these surfaces is also variable.[46] The lateral surface bears a large, oval, concave, or flat surface corresponding to the base of the fourth metatarsal. A deep groove limits this surface inferiorly and gives insertion to the interosseous cuneo$_3$-metatarsal$_3$ ligament. The interosseous metatarsal ligament (M_3-M_4) inserts anteriorly on a large segment of the lateral surface, which is covered by rugosities. The dorsal surface provides insertion to the dorsal intermetatarsal ligaments (M_2-M_3 and M_3-M_4) and to the dorsal cuneo$_3$-metatarsal$_3$ ligament. On the crest are attached the plantar cuneo$_1$-metatarsal$_3$ ligament, the plantar intermetatarsal ligaments (M_2-M_3 and M_3-M_4), a slip from the long plantar ligament, a slip from the tibialis posterior tendon, and the adductor hallucis obliquum.

Fourth Metatarsal

The base of the fourth metatarsal is quadrilateral (see Figs. 2.45D, 2.56, and 2.57)). The proximal surface, slightly convex, articulates with the cuboid. On the medial surface, there is a large dorsal oval facet corresponding to the base of the third metatarsal. The very posterior aspect of this surface corresponds to the third cuneiform. Variations are indicated in Figure 2.58. The nonarticulating segment provides insertion to the interosseous

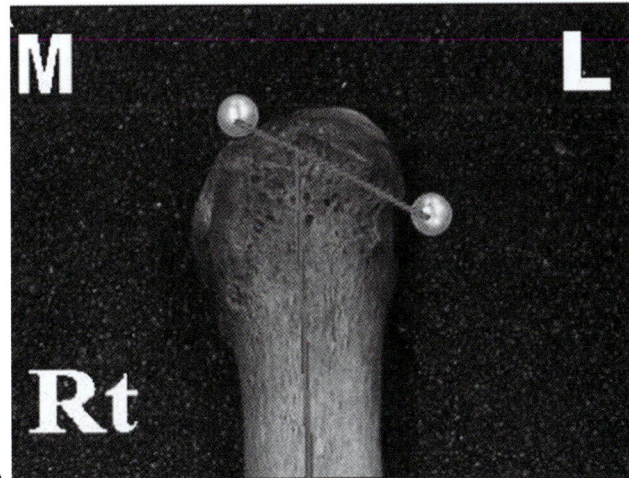
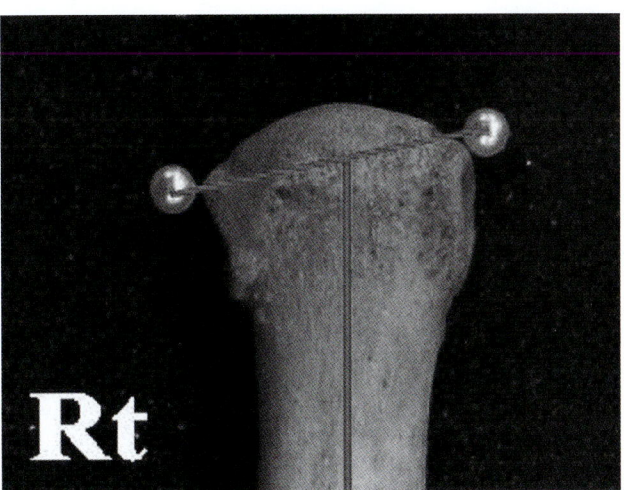

Figure 2.53 **The DMAA measured from a line connecting the two white beads intersecting a line lying along the metatarsal shaft. (A)** The most laterally deviated DMAA (maximum). **(B)** The most medially deviated DMAA (minimum). (*L*, lateral; *M*, medial; *RT*, right bone.) (ElSaid A, Tisdale C, Donley B, et al. First metatarsal bone: an anatomical study. *Foot Ankle Int.* 2006;12:1041-1048, Figure 3. Copyright ©2006. Reprinted by Permission of SAGE Publications.)

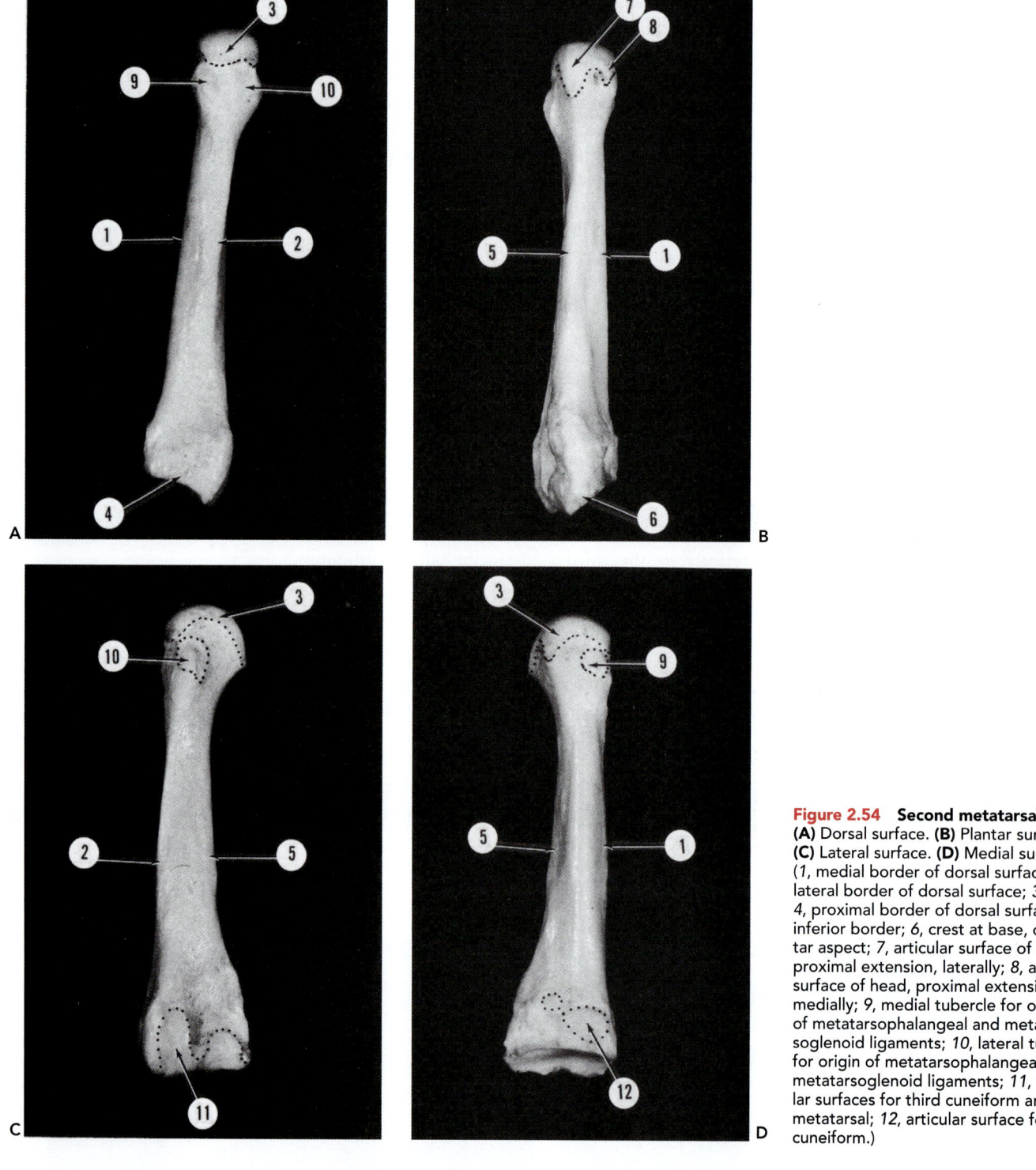

Figure 2.54 Second metatarsal, right. (A) Dorsal surface. (B) Plantar surface. (C) Lateral surface. (D) Medial surface. (1, medial border of dorsal surface; 2, lateral border of dorsal surface; 3, head; 4, proximal border of dorsal surface; 5, inferior border; 6, crest at base, on plantar aspect; 7, articular surface of head, proximal extension, laterally; 8, articular surface of head, proximal extension, medially; 9, medial tubercle for origin of metatarsophalangeal and metatarsoglenoid ligaments; 10, lateral tubercle for origin of metatarsophalangeal and metatarsoglenoid ligaments; 11, articular surfaces for third cuneiform and third metatarsal; 12, articular surface for first cuneiform.)

cuboideometatarsal$_4$ ligament or the cuneo$_3$-metatarsal$_4$ ligament and, further distally, to the interosseous metatarsal (M_3-M_4) ligament. The lateral surface gives support to a triangular articular surface (base dorsal, apex plantar), occupying the posterosuperior segment of the surface and articulating with the fifth metatarsal. A deep vertical groove limits this surface anteriorly. The interosseous metatarsal ligament M_4-M_5 inserts on the anterior aspect of the surface. The dorsal aspect of the metatarsal base provides insertion to the dorsal cuboideometatarsal$_4$ ligament and the dorsal intermetatarsal ligaments (M_3-M_4 and M_4-M_5). The inferior surface is rectangular and may bear a tubercle. It gives attachment to the plantar intermetatarsal ligaments (M_3-M_4 and M_4-M_5), the plantar cuboideometatarsal$_4$ ligament, the plantar cuneo$_3$-metatarsal$_4$ ligament, a slip from the longitudinal plantar ligament, a slip from the tibialis posterior tendon, and the adductor hallucis obliquum.

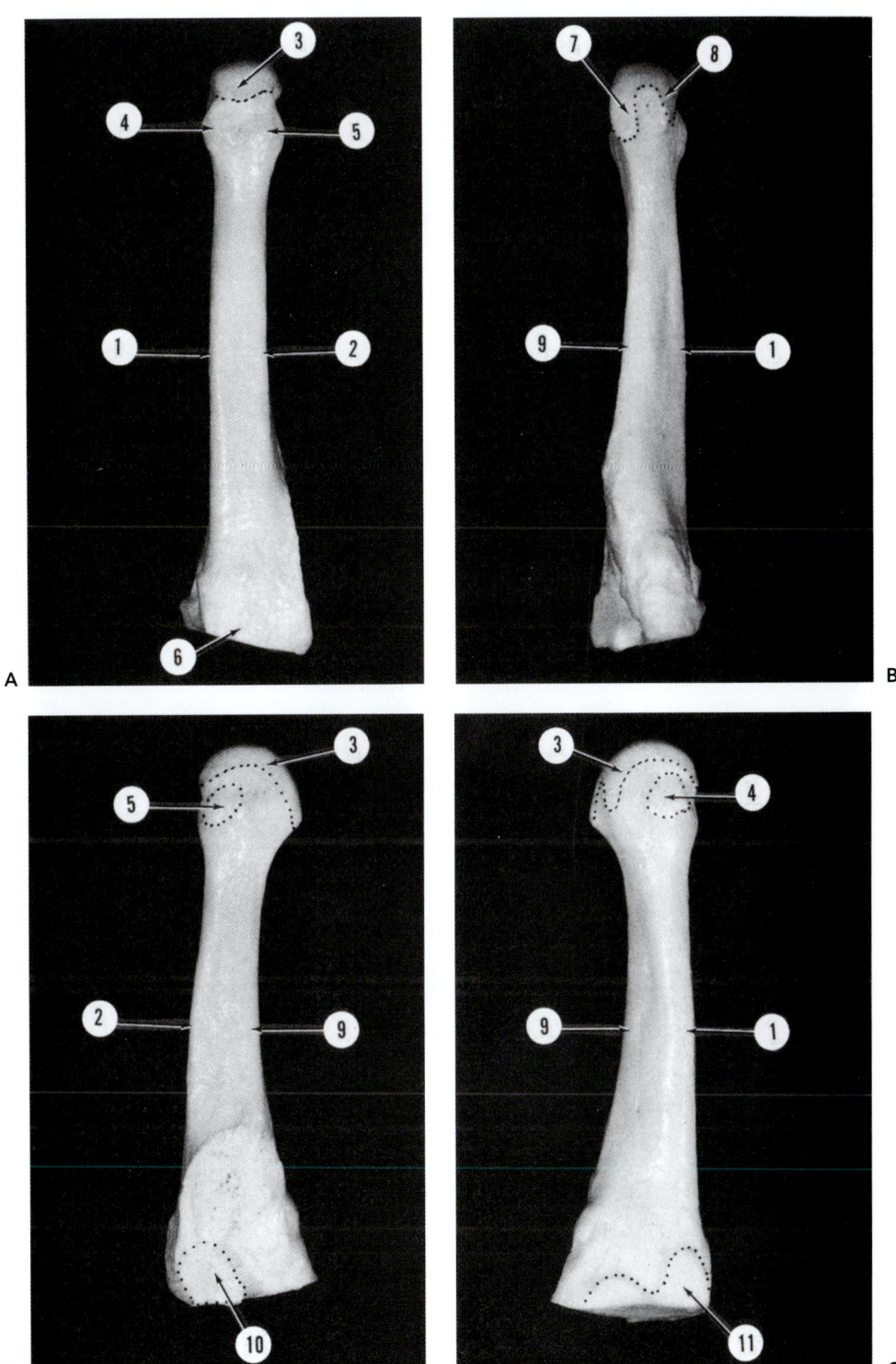

Figure 2.55 Third metatarsal, right.
(A) Dorsal surface. (B) Plantar surface. (C) Lateral surface. (D) Medial surface. (1, medial border of dorsal surface; 2, lateral border of dorsal surface; 3, head; 4, medial tubercle for origin of metatarsophalangeal and metatarsoglenoid ligaments; 5, lateral tubercle for origin of metatarsophalangeal and metatarsoglenoid ligaments; 6, proximal border of dorsal surface; 7, proximal extension of articular surface, laterally; 8, proximal extension of articular surface, medially; 9, inferior border; 10, articular surface with fourth metatarsal; 11, articular surface with base of second metatarsal.)

Batmanabane and Malathi,[52] in a study of 150 metatarsal bones, recognized a constant and distinct groove on the lateral surface of the base of the second, third, and fourth metatarsals, which helps identification in forensic medicine.

On the lateral surface of the second metatarsal base, the two articular facets are separated by a groove that starts just above the middle of the proximal border and runs almost at a right angle to the base, with an angular range of 85° to 111°.

On the lateral surface of M_3, the groove is located under the solitary articular facet; it starts from about the center of the lateral surface and runs obliquely upward. It may or may not reach the upper border. The angle of the groove with the base of M_3 ranges from 57° to 72°.

On the lateral surface of M_4, the groove is the deepest. It starts at the lower end of the surface just below the single articular facet and runs upward and obliquely, with a more acute angle averaging 37° to 54°, and it never reaches the upper border of the surface.

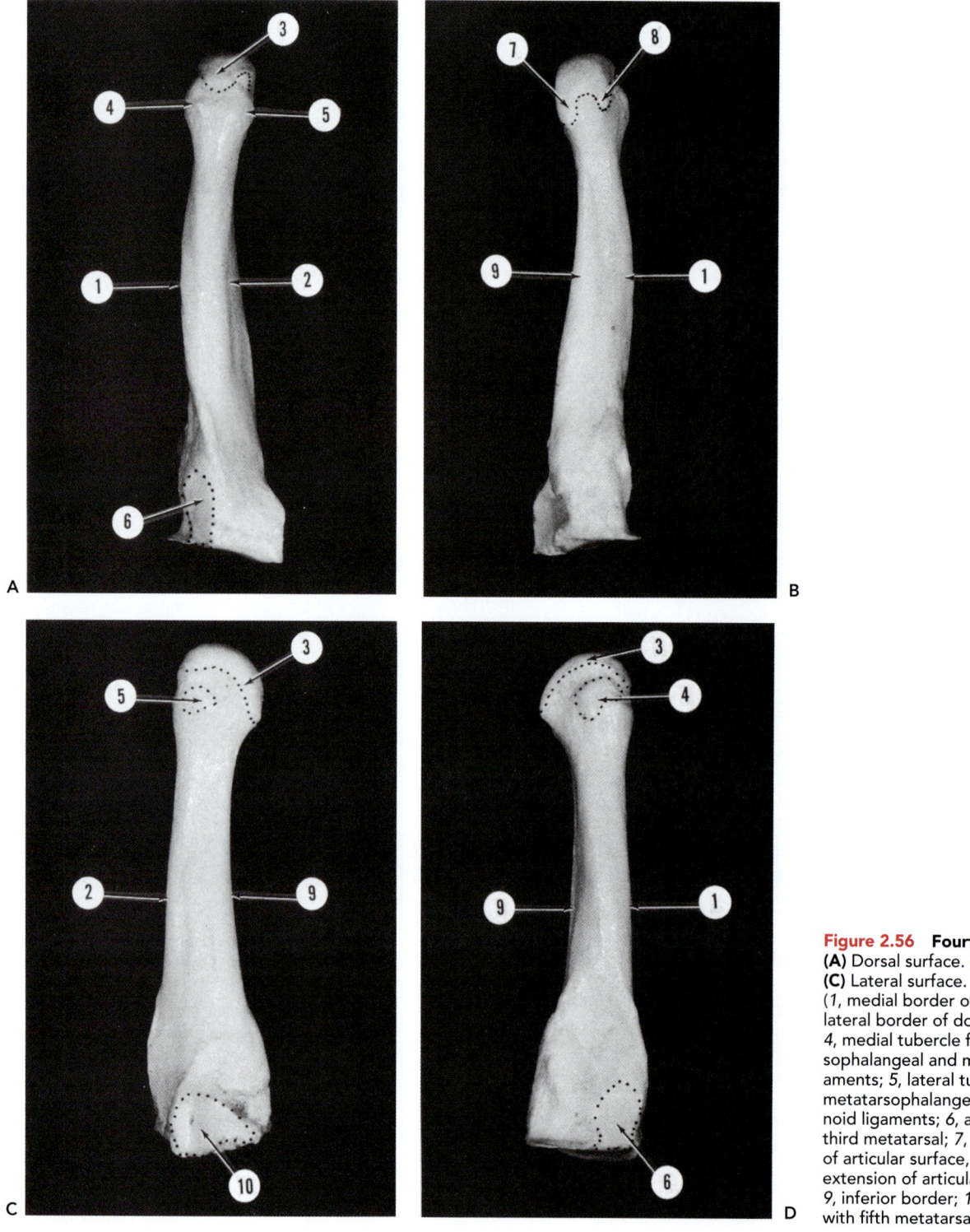

Figure 2.56 Fourth metatarsal, right. (A) Dorsal surface. (B) Plantar surface. (C) Lateral surface. (D) Medial surface. (1, medial border of dorsal surface; 2, lateral border of dorsal surface; 3, head; 4, medial tubercle for origin of metatarsophalangeal and metatarsoglenoid ligaments; 5, lateral tubercle for origin of metatarsophalangeal and metatarsoglenoid ligaments; 6, articular surface with third metatarsal; 7, proximal extension of articular surface, laterally; 8, proximal extension of articular surface, medially; 9, inferior border; 10, articular surface with fifth metatarsal.)

Fifth Metatarsal

The base of the fifth metatarsal is flat in a dorsoplantar direction and is projected laterally and posteriorly as the tubercle of the fifth metatarsal or styloid apophysis (see Figs. 2.45 and 2.57). The latter gives insertion to the peroneus brevis tendon.

The posterior surface presents an inner articulating field that is triangular (medial base, lateral apex) and corresponds to the cuboid. A smaller lateral field, irregular and nonarticular, contributes with the cuboid to the formation of the cubostyloid groove, which will lead to the cuboid canal for the peroneus longus tendon.

The medial surface bears an oval or triangular surface articulating with the base of the fourth metatarsal. The remaining segment provides insertion to the interosseous metatarsal M_4-M_5 ligament.

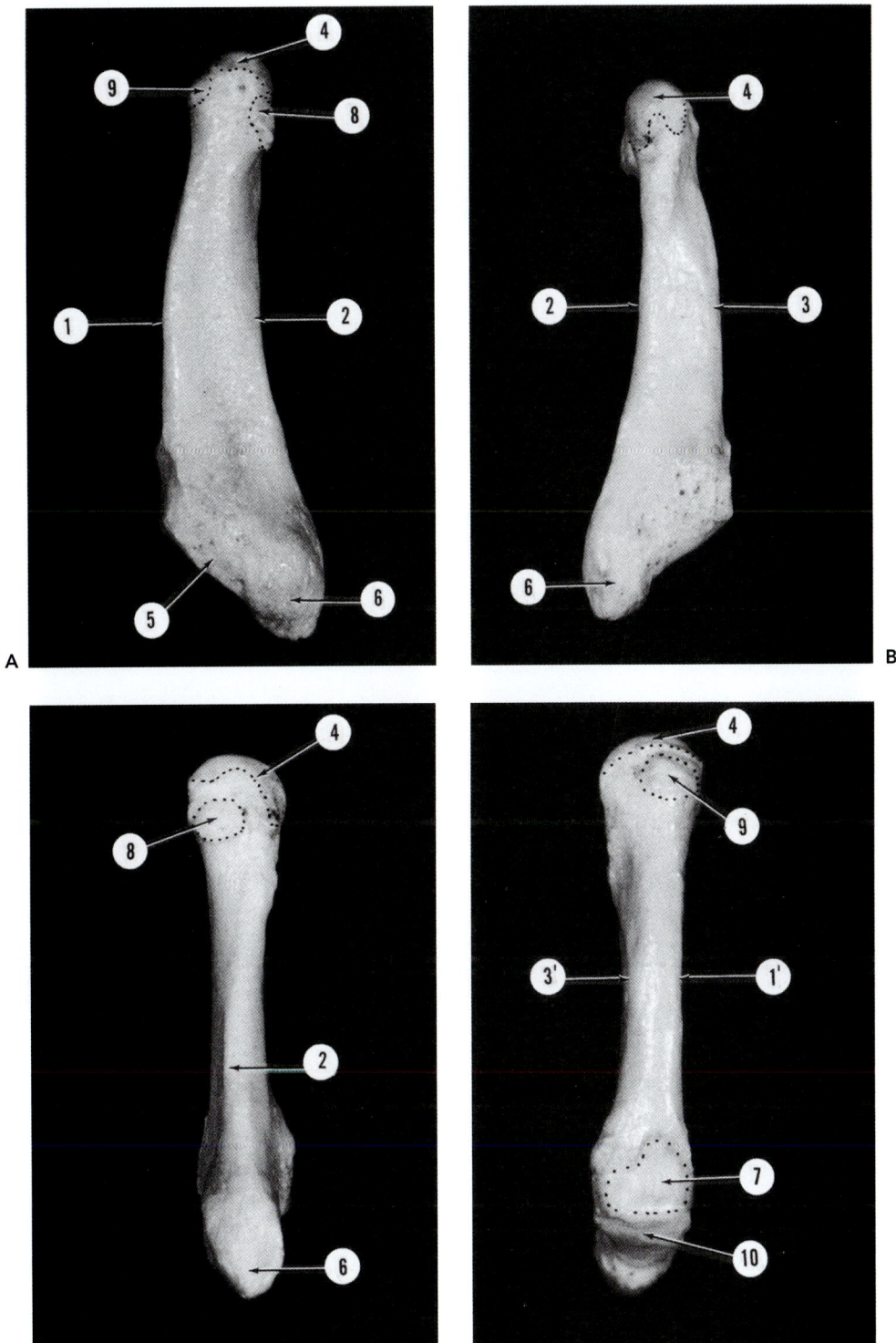

Figure 2.57 **Fifth metatarsal, right.**
(A) Dorsal surface. **(B)** Plantar surface. **(C)** Lateral surface. **(D)** Medial surface. (1, medial border of dorsal surface; 1', superior border of medial surface; 2, lateral border of dorsal and inferior surfaces; 3, medial border of inferior surface; 3', inferior border of medial surface; 4, head; 5, base; 6, tuberosity of base; 7, articular surface with fourth metatarsal; 8, lateral tubercle for insertion of lateral metatarsophalangeal and metatarsoglenoid ligaments; 9, medial tubercle for insertion of medial metatarsophalangeal and metatarsoglenoid ligaments; 10, articular surface with cuboid.)

The superior surface is flat and gives insertion to the peroneus tertius tendon, the dorsal cuboideometatarsal$_5$ ligament, and the dorsal intermetatarsal (M_4-M_5) ligament.

The inferior surface is broad and bears a medial bony prominence that gives insertion to the plantar intermetatarsal (M_4-M_5) ligament. The proximal segment provides attachment to the plantar short cuboideometatarsal$_5$ ligament and, further distally, to the broad slip from the long plantar ligament. In the central excavation of the surface inserts the short flexor of the fifth toe. The plantar aspect of the styloid apophysis occasionally gives insertion to the abductor of the fifth toe.

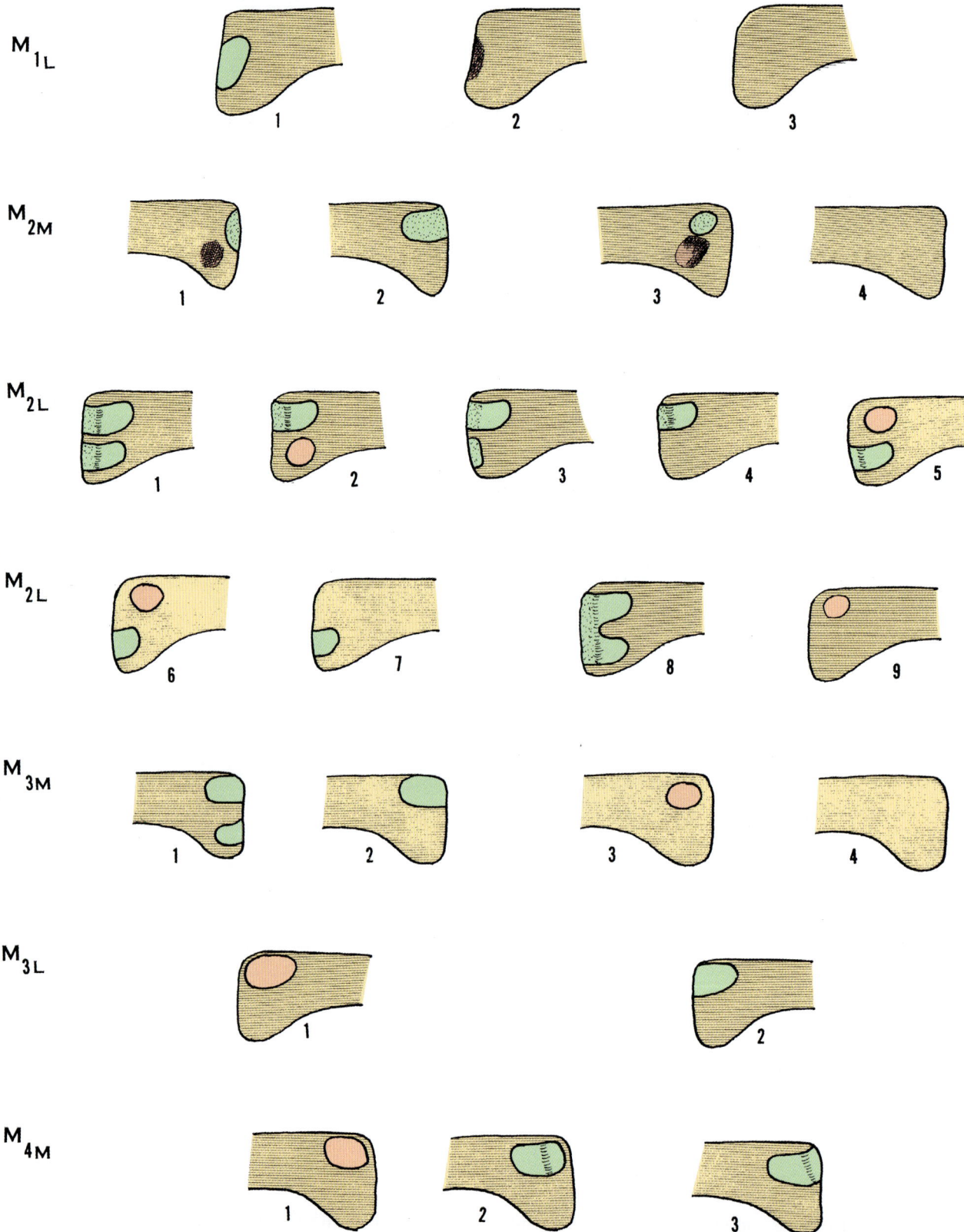

Figure 2.58 **Variations of the articular surfaces of the bases of the metatarsals.** (M_{1L}, base of metatarsal 1, lateral aspect; M_{2M}, base of metatarsal 3, medial aspect; M_{2L}, base of metatarsal 2, lateral aspect; M_{3M}, base of metatarsal 3, medial aspect; M_{3L}, base of metatarsal 3, lateral aspect; M_{4M}, base of metatarsal 4, medial aspect.) (Adapted from Singh I. Variations in the metatarsal bones. *J Anat.* 1960;94:345.)

▶ Shaft

First Metatarsal

The shaft of the first metatarsal is the shortest and the strongest of the metatarsals (see Fig. 2.46). It has a prismatic contour, mainly in the proximal two-thirds, and presents three surfaces: dorsomedial, lateral, and inferior. The three borders are superolateral, inferolateral, and inferomedial. The dorsomedial surface is convex and oriented dorsally in the distal third. The lateral surface is flat and smooth and provides insertion to the first dorsal interosseous muscle from its posterior third. The inferior surface has a longitudinally concave contour; this concavity is exaggerated by the plantar tubercles of the base.

Second, Third, and Fourth Metatarsal

The second, third, and fourth metatarsal shafts have a variable plantar concavity to their contour (see Figs. 2.54 to 2.56). They are prismatic and present three surfaces: dorsal, medial, and lateral. They have three borders: inferior, dorsolateral, and dorsomedial. The inferior border forms a smooth crest. The dorsal surface is flat and large posteriorly and convex and narrow distally. The medial and lateral surfaces converge toward the plantar crest; the medial surface is slightly convex and becomes more plantar in orientation distally. The fourth metatarsal has a recognizable twist to its shaft along the longitudinal axis, which orients the dorsal surface medially and brings the central plantar crest to a lateral position. The lateral surface then has a dorsolateral orientation.

Fifth Metatarsal

The fifth metatarsal shaft has the same longitudinal axial rotation, to a much greater degree, and this changes the general pattern of orientation of the three surfaces (see Fig. 2.57). The central plantar crest is now in a definite lateral position. The three surfaces of the general pattern—dorsal, lateral, medial—are now converted to dorsal, medial, *inferior* surfaces. The shaft is flat and prismatic, with a medial base and a lateral crest.

Ebraheim et al[53] investigated in 20 fifth metatarsals the cortical thickness (medial, lateral, plantar) and the intramedullary canal diameter (dorsoplantar and mediolateral) at three sectional sites (proximal, middle, distal) (Fig. 2.59). In six metatarsals, the contour of the medullary canal was determined radiographically after introducing lead wires in the medullary canal.

At the proximal site, the mean cortical thicknesses were as follows:

- Medial cortex: 2.86 mm
- Lateral cortex: 2.98 mm
- Dorsal cortex: 1.59 mm
- Plantar cortex: 1.48 mm

The medullary mean canal diameters were as follows:

- Dorsoplantar canal diameter: 6.01 mm
- Mediolateral canal diameter: 7.43 mm

At the middle site, the mean cortical thicknesses were as follows:

- Medial cortex: 2.56 mm
- Lateral cortex: 2.94 mm

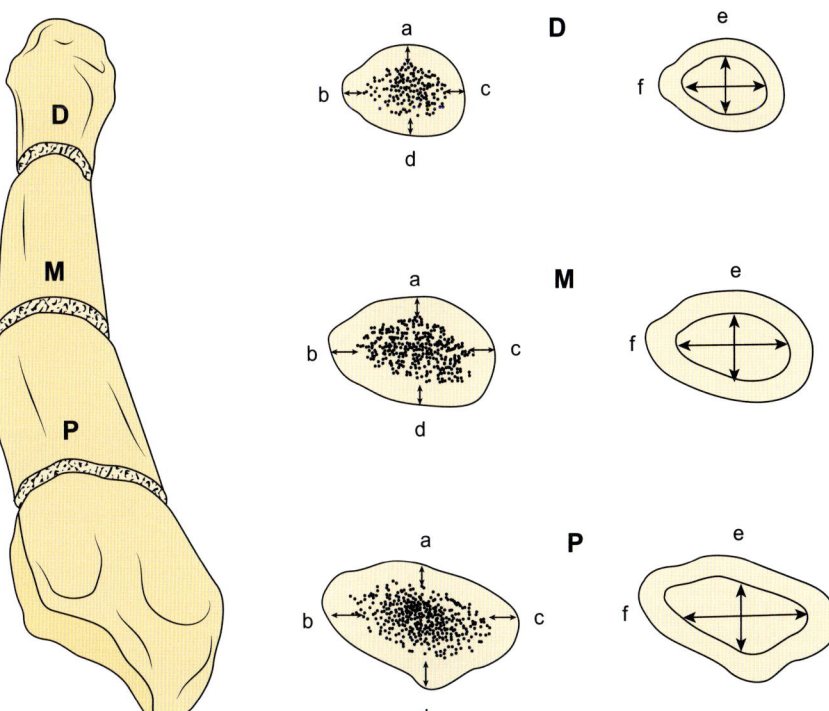

Figure 2.59 The fifth metatarsal was sectioned in three locations: *D* (distal), *M* (middle), and *P* (proximal). Thickness measurements were taken at *a* (dorsal cortex), *b* (medial cortex), *c* (lateral cortex), and *d* (plantar cortex). The canal diameter was measured from dorsal to plantar (*e*) and from medial to lateral (*f*). (Adapted from Ebraheim NA, Haman SP, Lu J, et al. Anatomical and radiological considerations of the fifth metatarsal bone. *Foot Ankle Int.* 2000;3:212-215.)

- Dorsal cortex: 1.38 mm
- Plantar cortex: 1.38 mm

The medullary mean canal diameter was as follows:

- Dorsoplantar canal diameter: 4.59 mm
- Mediolateral canal diameter: 5.88 mm

The canal decreased in diameter from proximal to distal in dorsoplantar measurement from 6.01 mm proximally to 4.59 mm in the middle to 4.02 distally. Mediolaterally, the canal diameter decreased from 7.43 mm proximally to 5.88 mm in the middle and to 5.71 mm distally.

The radiographic investigation of the medullary canal contour indicated the canal bowing laterally on the dorsoplantar view and being straight on the lateral view (Fig. 2.60).

The dorsal and plantar interossei muscles originate from the metatarsal shafts as follows (Fig. 2.61): first dorsal interosseous—posterior third lateral surface M_1, medial surface M_2; second dorsal interosseous—lateral surface M_2, upper segment medial surface M_3; third dorsal interosseous—lateral surface M_3, upper segment medial surface M_4; fourth dorsal interosseous—lateral surface M_4, medial surface M_5; first plantar interosseous—lower segment medial surface M_3, plantar crest M_3; second plantar interosseous—lower segment medial surface M_4, plantar crest M_4; third plantar interosseous—inferior surface M_5. The fifth metatarsal also provides origin to the opponens of the fifth from its lateral border.

▶ Head

First Metatarsal

The head of the first metatarsal is large and quadrilateral in general contour, with the transverse diameter exceeding the vertical dimension (see Figs. 2.45 and 2.46). This apparent superoinferior flattening is in contradistinction to the lesser metatarsal heads, which are flattened side to side transversely.

The articular surface covering the head presents two fields in continuity: superior phalangeal and inferior sesamoidal. The superior articular field is smooth and convex (more in the vertical direction than the transverse). This surface is larger than the corresponding articular surface of the proximal phalanx. Dorsally, this field is limited by a posteriorly convex border that is smooth and overhangs the dorsal surface of the shaft. The inferior articular surface is larger than the superior and is separated into two sloped surfaces by a rounded ridge or crest oriented anteroposteriorly. This crest is not central in location but passes at the junction of the outer third and inner two-thirds of the articular surface. The sloped surfaces are grooved, and each corresponds to a sesamoid. The inner groove is more pronounced than the outer groove. When the sesamoids are small, an intermediate groove is present over the ridge due to the pressure of the flexor hallucis longus tendon.[54]

Well-developed bony tubercles or epicondyles are located on the sides of the metatarsal head. They are in contact with or very close to the articular surface. The inner tubercle is more developed than the outer. These tubercles provide insertion to the metatarsophalangeal collateral ligaments and to the suspensory metatarsoglenosesamoid ligaments.

The distal metatarsal articular angle (DMAA) was measured by ElSaid et al[50] In 478 first metatarsals, the DMAA ranged from −14° of medial deviation to 30° of lateral deviation with an average of 8.21° (see Fig. 2.53).

Lesser Metatarsals

The heads of the lesser metatarsals are quadrilateral and flattened transversely (see Figs. 2.45 to 2.57). The articular surface is condylar, extending more on the plantar aspect than on the dorsal. The plantar articular segment has a proximal central concave border and two marginal articular proximal extensions. Usually, the lateral extension is more pronounced than the medial. On the sides of the metatarsal heads, a groove separates the articular surface from the pronounced tubercle for the origin of the metatarsophalangeal ligaments and for the metatarsoglenoid ligaments. When observed in the lateral profile, the metatarsal head has an elliptic articular contour and the lateral tubercle is superior. When viewed from the dorsum, the narrow neck is seen to flare up into the lateral tubercles.

PHALANGES

▶ Large Toe

The large toe has two phalanges: proximal and distal (Fig. 2.62).

Proximal Phalanx

The proximal phalanx has a large base directed transversely and bears an oval, concave articular surface, the glenoid cavity, smaller than the corresponding articular surface of the

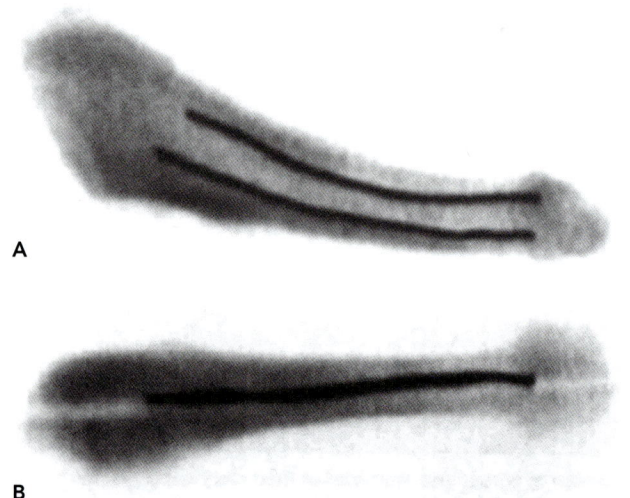

Figure 2.60 Dorsoplantar views of the fifth metatarsal with canal outlined with solder wire (lead wire) demonstrating lateral bow of the canal on the anteroposterior view **(A)** and straight canal contour on the lateral view **(B)**. (Ebraheim NA, Haman SP, Lu J, et al. Anatomical and radiological considerations of the fifth metatarsal bone. *Foot Ankle Int.* 2000;3:212-215, Figure 2. Copyright ©2000. Reprinted by Permission of SAGE Publications.)

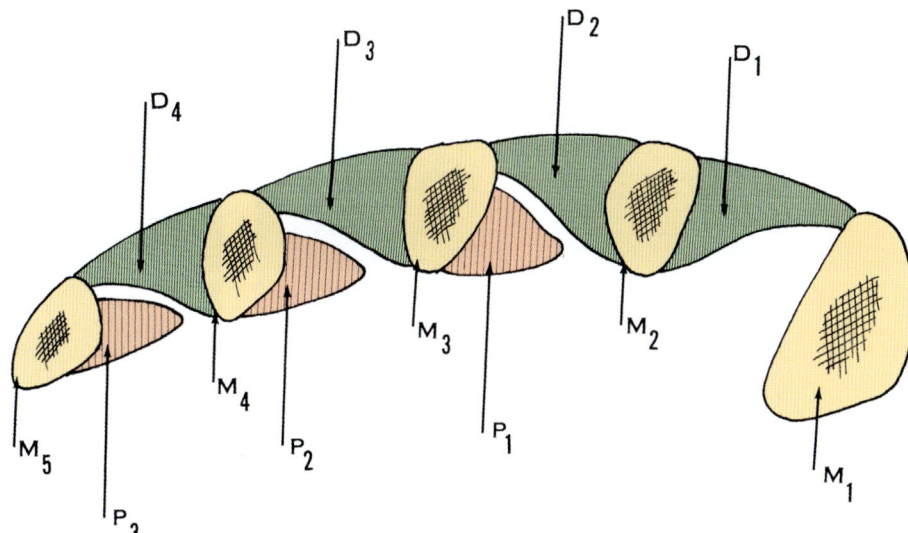

Figure 2.61 **Cross-section through metatarsal shafts M1 to M5—origin of interossei muscles.** (D_1 to D_4, dorsal interossei 1-4; P_1 to P_3, plantar interossei 1-3.)

metatarsal head. A transverse crest or bony prominence is present on the dorsum of the base at a small distance from the articular surface. The extensor hallucis brevis inserts on this tubercle. On the plantar aspect, two tubercles, lateral and medial, give insertion to the intrinsic muscles of the big toe. The larger medial plantar tubercle gives insertion to the medial head of the short flexor and to the abductor hallucis. The less prominent lateral plantar tubercle gives insertion to the lateral head of the short flexor and to the adductor hallucis. The plantar plate inserts firmly on the plantar border of the surface.

The shaft of the proximal phalanx is convex dorsally and flat on the plantar aspect, with slight grooving at each end for the flexor hallucis longus tendon. The head is flat vertically. The articular surface is trochlear and is larger and more concave on the plantar aspect. The surface is strongly convex in the dorsoplantar direction. A small fossa is present on the plantar aspect, just proximal to the articular surface. The collateral ligaments insert on small tubercles located on the head in a superolateral position behind the articular cartilage.

Distal Phalanx

The distal phalanx has a large, transversely oriented base bearing the articular surface corresponding to the trochlear surface of the proximal phalangeal head. This surface is convex centrally and concave laterally. The transverse tubercle on the dorsum of the base, close to the articular surface, gives insertion to the extensor hallucis longus tendon. This proximal position of the extensor tendon allows a large insertion of the ungual matrix on the dorsum of the phalanx. On the plantar aspect of the shaft, the flexor hallucis longus tendon inserts on a tuberosity directed toward the fibular side and strongly marked on the tibial side. This obliquely directed ridge may reach the distal tuberositas unguicularis in a bridge fashion on the fibular side, forming a "flying buttress."[55] Occasionally, a bony projection is present at the base, giving origin to side ligaments inserting on the base of the tuberositas unguicularis. The flexor hallucis longus thus makes a broad attachment over the oblique tuberosity, the side ligaments reaching the distal tuberosity.[55]

The shaft of the distal phalanx is not at right angles to the articular surface but deviates to the fibular side, and Wilkinson gives the deflection measurements as follows: mean, 14.7° (standard deviation 4.1°)—males 8° to 23°, females 10° to 22°.[55] A comparable figure was present in the big toes in 10 fetuses.

▶ Lesser Toes

The lesser toes (Fig. 2.63) have three phalanges: proximal, middle, and distal.

Proximal Phalanx

The proximal phalanx is the longest of the three, being slightly longer than the other two phalanges combined. The base is large and transverse, with an oval articular surface for the metatarsal head. Two plantar tubercles give insertion to the interossei muscles. The medial tubercles of the third, fourth, and fifth toes give insertion to the first, second, and third plantar interossei. The medial tubercle of the second toe gives insertion to the first dorsal interosseous. The lateral tubercles of the second, third, and fourth toes give insertion to the second, third, and fourth dorsal interossei. The lateral tubercle of the fifth toe gives insertion to its abductor and short flexor.

The shaft is convex dorsally and flat inferiorly, with slight concavity at both distal and proximal ends.

The head is flat and supports a trochlear type of articular surface that extends more on the plantar aspect. A small tubercle is present on each side of the head in a superolateral position for the origin of the collateral ligaments.

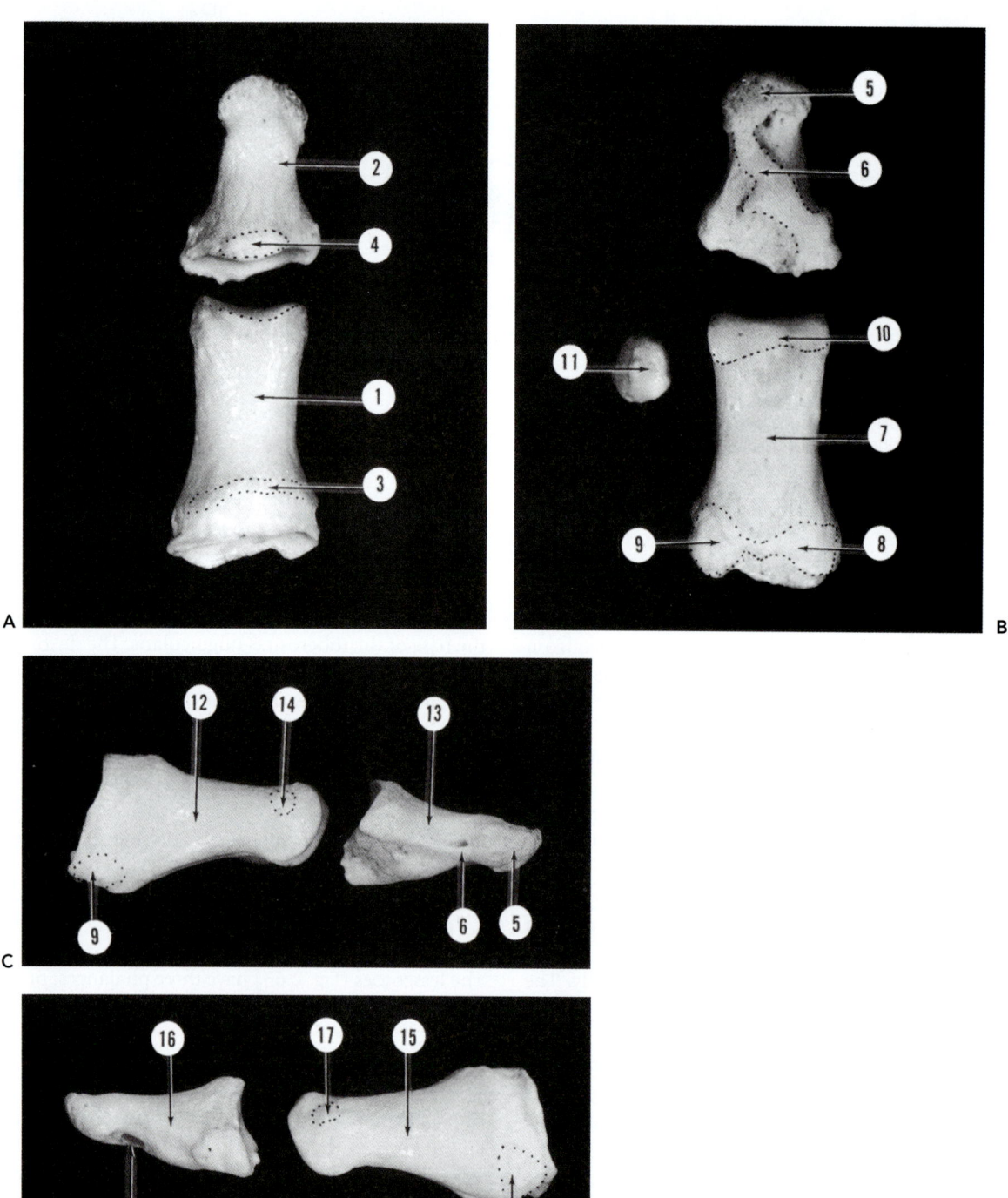

Figure 2.62 **Phalanges of the big toe, right.** **(A)** Dorsal aspect. **(B)** Plantar aspect. **(C)** Lateral aspect. **(D)** Medial aspect. (*1*, dorsal aspect of proximal phalanx; *2*, dorsal aspect of distal phalanx; *3*, insertion zone for capsule and extensor hallucis brevis; *4*, insertion zone for extensor hallucis longus; *5*, tuft of distal phalanx; *6*, bony ridge forming a "flying buttress" extending obliquely from the tibial side at the base to the fibular side at the level of the tuft—this is an insertion site for the flexor hallucis longus tendon; *7*, plantar aspect of proximal phalanx; *8*, medial tubercle for insertion of tendons of medial head of flexor hallucis brevis and abductor hallucis; *9*, lateral tubercle for insertion of tendons of lateral head of flexor hallucis brevis and adductor hallucis; *10*, head of proximal phalanx; *11*, sesamoid; *12*, lateral aspect of proximal phalanx; *13*, lateral aspect of distal phalanx; *14*, tubercle for insertion of lateral interphalangeal and phalangeoglenoid ligaments; *15*, medial aspect of proximal phalanx; *16*, medial aspect of distal phalanx; *17*, tubercle for insertion of medial interphalangeal and phalangeoglenoid ligaments.)

Chapter 2: Osteology

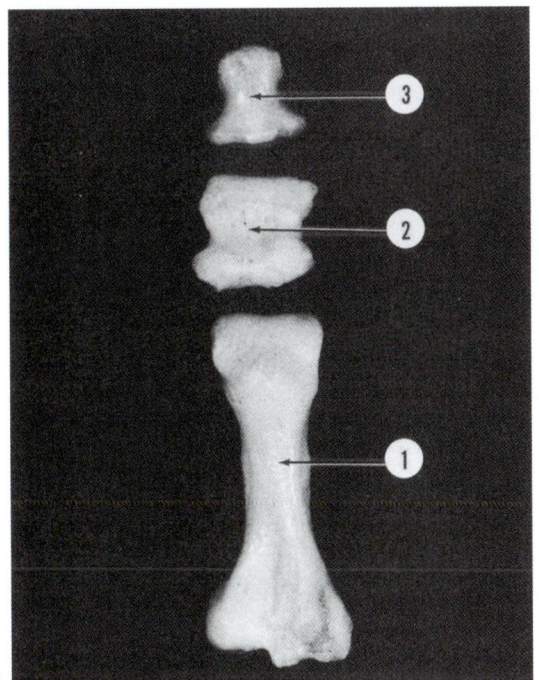
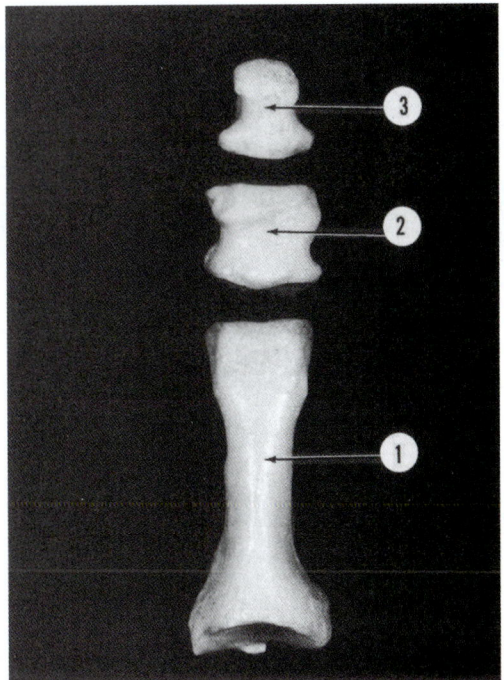
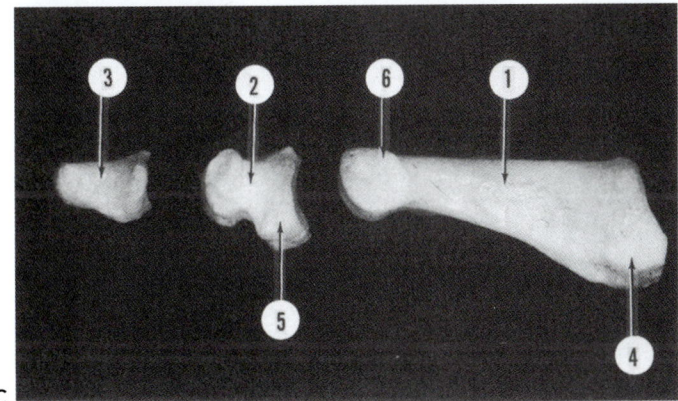

Figure 2.63 **Second toe, right.** (**A**) Plantar view. (**B**) Dorsal view. (**C**) Medial view. (*1*, proximal phalanx; *2*, middle phalanx; *3*, distal phalanx; *4*, tubercle for attachment of first dorsal interosseous tendon and metatarsophalangeal ligament; *5*, attachment site of medial collateral ligament of interphalangeal joint; *6*, tubercle of origin of medial collateral ligament of interphalangeal joint.)

Middle Phalanx

The middle phalanx is very short. The base bears a transverse articular surface corresponding to the trochlear contour of the proximal phalangeal head. The middle slip of the long extensor tendon inserts on the dorsum of the base. The shaft is convex dorsally. The flat plantar surface gives insertion to the two slips of the flexor brevis. The distal articular head is also transversely oriented but presents a strong convexity in the dorsoplantar direction.

Distal Phalanx

The distal phalanx is rudimentary. It is more or less triangular, with a crescent-shaped contour of the distal tuberositas unguicularis. The base supports an articular surface that is transverse, corresponding to the head of the middle phalanx. The extensor terminal tendon inserts on the dorsum of the base and the long flexor of the toe on the plantar aspect of the base and shaft. The dorsum of the shaft and the crescent-shaped distal tuberosity support the ungual matrix.

SESAMOIDS

The sesamoids are small, round bones deriving their names from the sesame seed. Their anatomic location is always the same even though certain sesamoids are not always present or occur infrequently.

The sesamoids are embedded, partially or totally, in the substance of a corresponding tendon. Structurally, some sesamoids always ossify, whereas others remain cartilaginous or fibrocartilaginous for life; this accounts for the discrepancies encountered in the studies reporting the frequency of occurrence of a

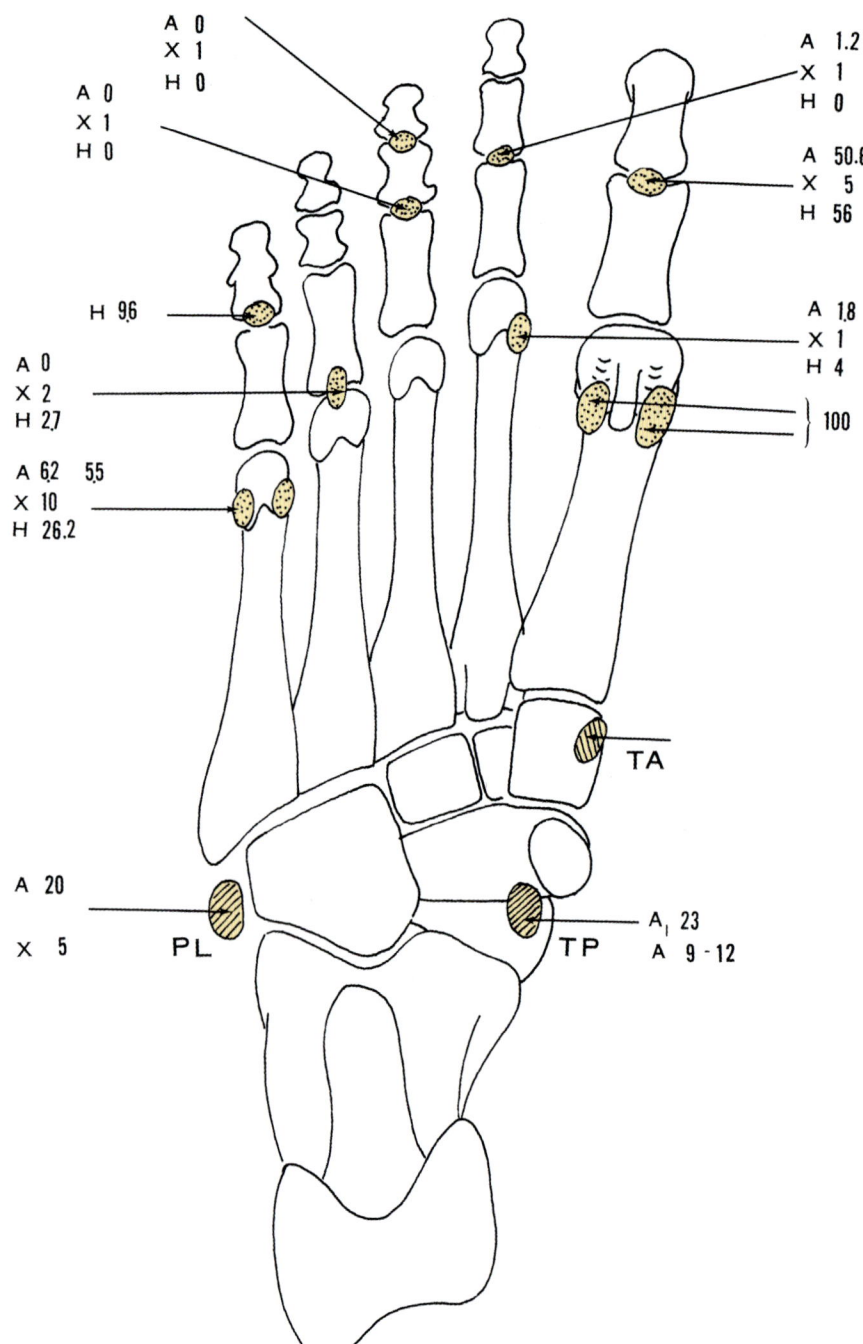

Figure 2.64 Sesamoids of the foot. Percentage of occurrence based on A, anatomic investigation; X, roentgenographic investigation; and H, histoembryologic investigation. (*PL*, os peroneum in peroneus longus tendon in ossified form; *TA*, sesamoid in tibialis anterior tendon; *TP*, sesamoid in tibialis posterior tendon.)

given sesamoid. Anatomically, the sesamoids are part of a gliding or pressure-absorbing mechanism and are located within the flexor hallucis brevis tendons, the plantar plates of the metatarsophalangeal and interphalangeal joints, the intrinsic tendons of the lesser toes, the peroneus longus tendon, the tibialis posterior tendon, and the tibialis anterior tendon (Fig. 2.64).

▶ Big Toe

The sesamoids of the big toe (Fig. 2.65) are three in number: two constant at the level of the plantar aspect of the metatarsophalangeal joint and one inconstant at the level of the plantar aspect of the interphalangeal joint.

Metatarsophalangeal Joint

The two sesamoids of the metatarsophalangeal joint (Figs. 2.66 and 2.67), lateral and medial, are plantar in location. They are embedded in the thick plantar plate and present two surfaces: inferior (convex, nonarticular, and insertional) and superior (articular with the metatarsal head).

The overall configuration of the sesamoids is variable, as they may be semiovoid, circular, or bean-shaped. The variations of contour are well depicted by Kewenter (Fig. 2.68).[56] The two sesamoids are not of the same size and configuration: the medial sesamoid is usually larger than the lateral and is ovoid and elongated, whereas the latter is smaller and more

Chapter 2: Osteology   95

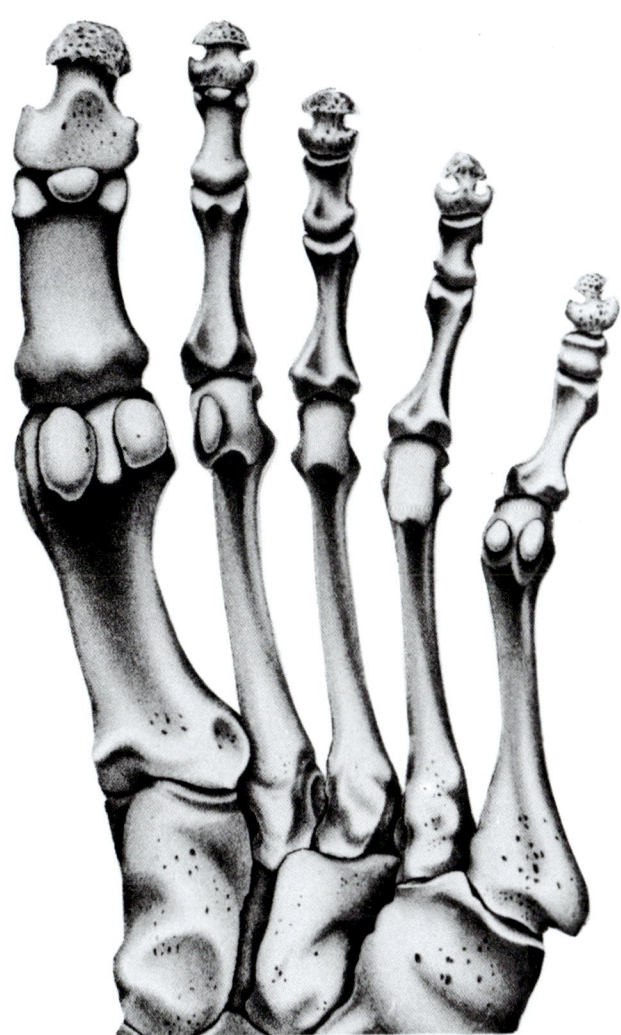

Figure 2.65 **Sesamoids of toes.** (From Pfitzner W. Die Sesambeine des Menschen. In: Schwalbe, ed. *Morphologische Arbeiten*. Vol I. Gustav Fischer; 1892:517-762.)

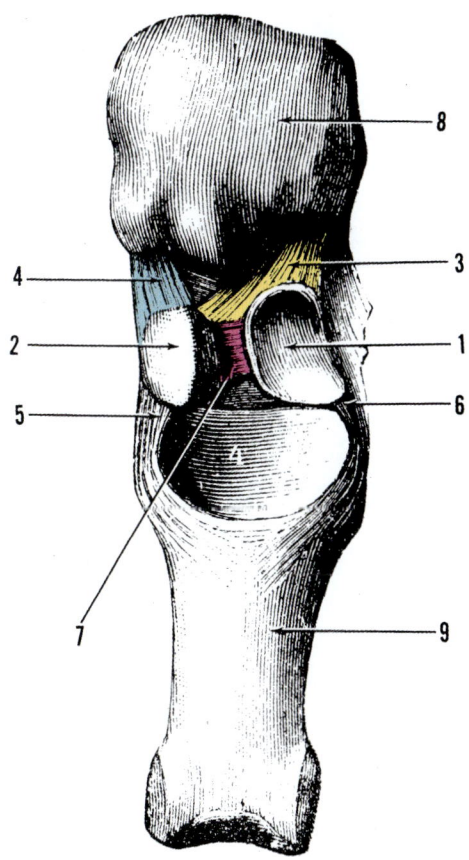

Figure 2.66 **Phalangeosesamoid apparatus of the big toe.** The dorsal capsule of the metatarsophalangeal joint has been excised and the first metatarsal head reflected backward. (*1*, medial sesamoid; *2*, lateral sesamoid; *3*, medial metatarsosesamoid ligament sending direct fibers to medial sesamoid and oblique fibers to lateral sesamoid; *4*, lateral metatarsosesamoid ligament; *5*, lateral short sesamophalangeal ligament; *6*, medial short sesamophalangeal ligament; *7*, intersesamoid transverse ligament; *8*, head of first metatarsal; *9*, proximal phalanx of big toe.) (Adapted from Gillette. Des os sésamoides chez l'homme. *Anat Physiol*. 1872;506-538.)

circular. Kewenter provides the following information on their size: medial sesamoid larger, 80%; both equal, 15%; lateral sesamoid larger, 5%.[56]

Gillette reports the most common dimensions of the nondeformed sesamoids as: length—lateral, 9 to 10 mm; medial, 12 to 15 mm; width—lateral, 7 to 9 mm; medial, 9 to 11 mm.[57]

Nonarticular Surface

The convex inferior surface and borders of the lateral sesamoid provide insertion to the following:

- Lateral head of the flexor hallucis brevis
- Three components of the oblique head of the adductor hallucis
- Transverse component of the adductor hallucis
- Deep transverse metatarsal ligament
- Suspensory lateral metatarsosesamoid ligament
- Lateral border of the flexor hallucis longus fibrous tunnel
- Lateral longitudinal septum of the plantar aponeurosis to the big toe
- Vertical and arciform fibrous fibers contributing to the formation of the preflexor tendon space

The convex inferior surface and borders of the medial sesamoid provide insertion to the following:

- Medial head of the flexor hallucis brevis
- Abductor hallucis tendon
- Suspensory medial metatarsosesamoid ligament
- Medial border of the flexor hallucis longus fibrous tunnel
- Medial longitudinal septum of the plantar aponeurosis of the big toe
- Vertical and arciform fibers contributing to the formation of the preflexor tendon space

The medial slope of the lateral sesamoid and the lateral slope of the medial sesamoid contribute to the formation of the proximal segment of the flexor hallucis longus tunnel. The preflexor tendon space retains an adipose cushion overlying both sesamoids and the flexor hallucis longus tendon.

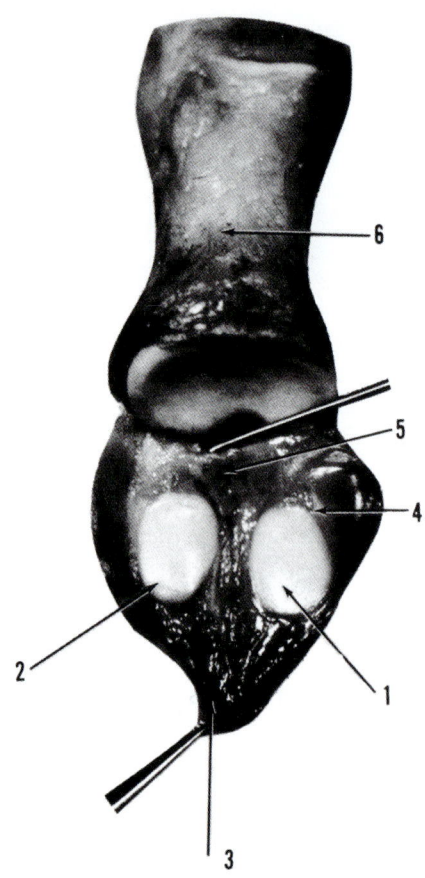

Figure 2.67 **Phalangeosesamoid apparatus of the metatarsophalangeal joint of the big toe, left.** (*1*, medial sesamoid; *2*, lateral sesamoid; *3*, capsule-synovial attachment to metatarsal neck inferiorly; *4*, metatarsoglenoid ligament; *5*, transverse ligament, lifted by probe, uniting lateral and medial sesamophalangeal ligaments—synovial pouch is present distal to this ligament; *6*, proximal phalanx of big toe.)

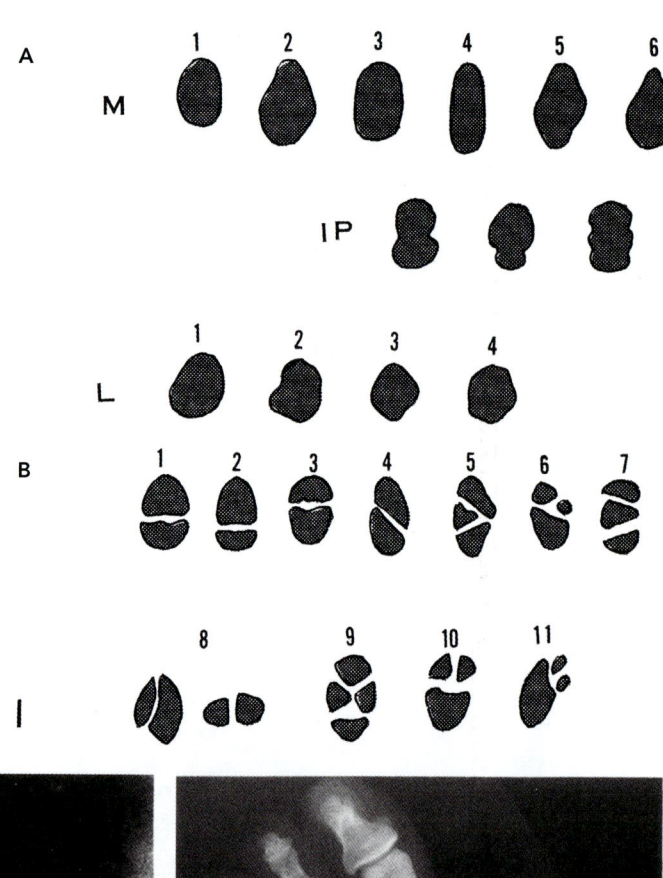

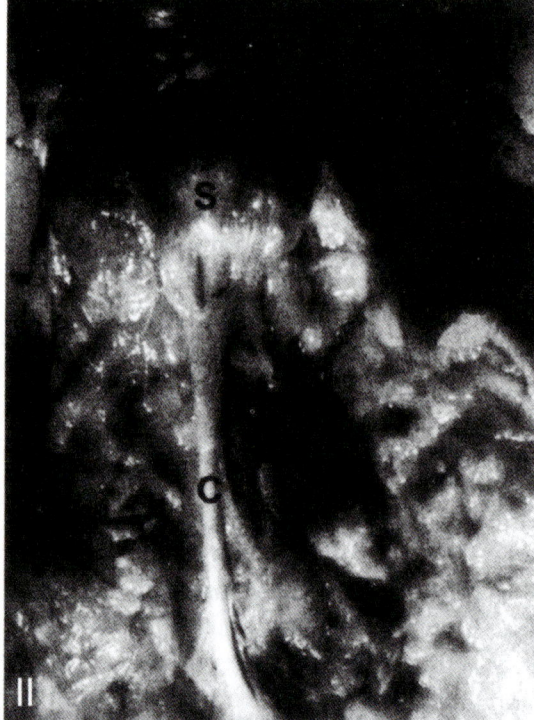

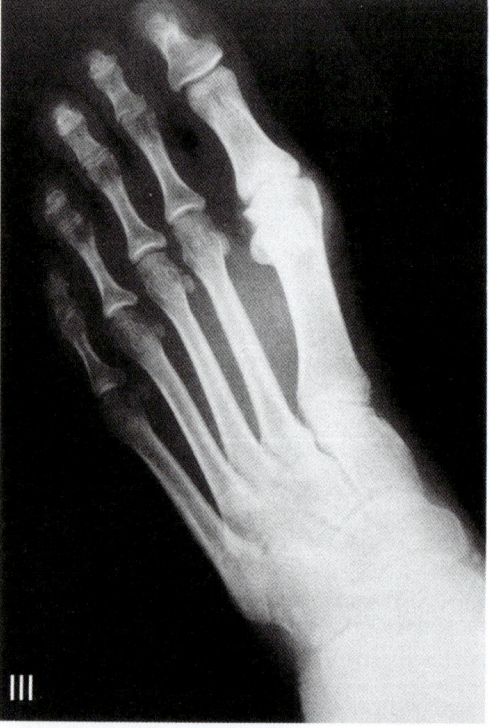

Figure 2.68 **(I) Variations in contour and partition of the sesamoids of the metatarsophalangeal joint of the big toe. (A)** *M*, medial sesamoid; *L*, lateral sesamoid; *IP*, intermediary partite. **(B)** Partite sesamoids. **(II) Interphalangeal hallucal sesamoid (S) and tendon of flexor hallucis capsularis interphalangeus (C). (III)** Roentgenogram demonstrating sesamoids of lesser toes at the metatarsophalangeal joints, tibial side, with two sesamoids to the metatarsophalangeal joint of the fifth toe. (**A and B,** Copyright © 1936 From Kewenter U. Die Sesambiene des I Metatarso-phalangeal-gelenks des Menschen. *Acta Orthop Scand* (Suppl). 1936;2:43. Reproduced by Permission of Taylor and Francis Group, LLC, a division of Informa plc. **C,** This figure was published in *JAPMA*, Vol 76, No 6, 1986, JD McCarthy, T Reed, N Abell, Interphalangeal hallucal sesamoid (S) and tendon of flexor hallucis capsularis inter-phalangeus (C). Copyright American Podiatric Medical Association. Used with permission.)

Articular Surface

The lower two-thirds of the large metatarsal head has a double trochlear contour: large medial and small lateral. The trochlear surfaces are separated by a central crest oriented anteroposteriorly. The articular surface of each sesamoid fits against the corresponding trochlear surface. In the well-developed sesamoid, the articular surface is concave longitudinally and bears a soft longitudinal crest corresponding to the trochlear groove. On each side, the surface is slightly convex in the transverse direction, adapting to the trochlear surface. This arrangement has brought forth the comparison of the sesamotrochlear joint to the patellofemoral joint or to the cubitohumeral joint.[57,58] In their anatomic position, the two sesamoids are not transverse but incline obliquely toward the central metatarsal ridge. They are firmly connected to each other and to the base of the proximal phalanx through the powerful plantar plate and form an anatomic and functional unit that moves relative to the metatarsal head; this unit is called the phalangeosesamoid apparatus.[57] It is suspended from the head of the metatarsal by the metatarsosesamoid and metatarsophalangeal ligaments. Normally, the sesamoids move with the proximal phalanx and follow the latter in the metatarsophalangeal dislocations.

The sesamoids are connected to each other mainly by their incorporation in the substance of the plantar plate. From within the joint, the following intrinsic connecting ligaments are recognized (see Figs. 2.66 and 2.67):

- An intersesamoid, thin fibrous transverse band
- Lateral and medial sesamophalangeal short ligaments inserting on the plantar tubercles of the proximal phalanx. These ligaments are also attached to a transverse band extending from one side of the phalanx to the other
- The metatarsosesamoid ligaments, which originate from the posteromedial and posterolateral aspects of the metatarsal head and insert on the corresponding sesamoid. The medial ligament is stronger and sends oblique fibers to the lateral sesamoid from the posterior aspect of the plate[57]

The sesamoids of the metatarsophalangeal joint may be partite; the frequency of occurrence is reported by Kewenter as male, 36.6% ± 2.3%, and female, 30.1% ± 2.3%.[56] The patterns of partition are shown in Figure 2.68.[56]

Interphalangeal Joint

This sesamoid is single and transversely oriented and has two surfaces: nonarticular and articular. The nonarticular surface is embedded in the plantar plate. The articular surface is divided by a transverse crest into two facets: anterior and posterior. The anterior surface is smaller and articulates with the distal phalanx; the posterior surface is larger and articulates with the trochlear surface of the proximal phalangeal head. The sesamoid is attached to the proximal phalanx with short plantar sesamoid ligaments and forms a distal phalangeal-sesamoid apparatus. The solitary sesamoid moves with the distal phalanx. Its occurrence is not constant and is reported as follows: Bizarro[59] (roentgenographic study), 5%; Pfitzner[60] (anatomic investigation), 50.6%; Trolle[61] (histoembryologic study), 56%.

Miller and Love described the presence of a cartilaginous sesamoid or nodule of the interphalangeal joint of the big toe in 50% of their operated 58 patients and "neither the osseous sesamoid nor the cartilaginous sesamoid is in the tendon of the flexor hallucis longus."[62] McCarthy and colleagues studied the interphalangeal hallucal sesamoid bone in cadaver specimens.[63] These sesamoids demonstrated most of the features of mature bone and were embedded in the substance of the plantar plate, as revealed by the microscopic section studies. Furthermore, they described an unidentified tendon, deep to the flexor hallucis longus tendon, originating at the level of the separation of the tibial and fibular heads of the flexor hallucis brevis. This tendon was about 2 cm in length and 2 mm in diameter. It coursed distally, enveloped the interphalangeal hallucal sesamoid, and inserted into the distal aspect of the plantar plate (see Fig. 2.68II). They named this structure the flexor hallucis capsularis interphalangeus tendon.

Masaki studied the interphalangeal sesamoid bone of the hallux in 144 adult cadaver feet, 32 fetal cadaver feet, and 958 patients.[64] In the adult cadaver feet, the sesamoid was present in 95.9% and was elliptic, located centrally, parallel to the interphalangeal joint space, and embedded in the plantar plate. It presented two cartilaginous surfaces, against the base of the distal phalanx and the head of the proximal phalanx. In the fetal feet, a cartilaginous sesamoid was present in 93.8%. In the 958 patients, the standard roentgenographic study detected the sesamoid in 56.3%; with the use of intensifying screen, the detection was 93%.

▶ Lesser Toes

The sesamoids of the lesser toes, when present, are connected to the intrinsic muscles (see Fig. 2.68III). Their occurrence is less frequent or rare. Pfitzner, in an anatomic study of 384 feet, provided the following frequencies of occurrence: second toe—metatarsophalangeal joint, tibial side, 1.8%, fibular side, 0%; distal interphalangeal, 0.8%; fifth toe—metatarsophalangeal joint, tibial side, 5.5%, fibular side, 6.2%.[60]

The roentgenographic investigations and the histoembryologic studies yield a different distribution, presented in Figure 2.68.[59,61]

▶ Peroneus Longus Tendon

This sesamoid (os peroneum, sesamum peroneum; Fig. 2.69) is located in the substance of the peroneus longus tendon at the level of the cuboid tunnel where it angulates to enter the sole of the foot. The articular surface glides along the anterior slope of the plantar oblique tuberosity of the cuboid. The sesamoid is always present in an ossified, cartilaginous, or fibrocartilaginous stage.[65] It may remain a fibrocartilaginous nucleus for life. The os peroneum occurs with the following frequency: anatomic study—fully ossified, 20%, not fully ossified, 75%[65]; radiographic investigation, 5%.[21] The os peroneum is frequently round but may be elongated or divided into several portions.[66]

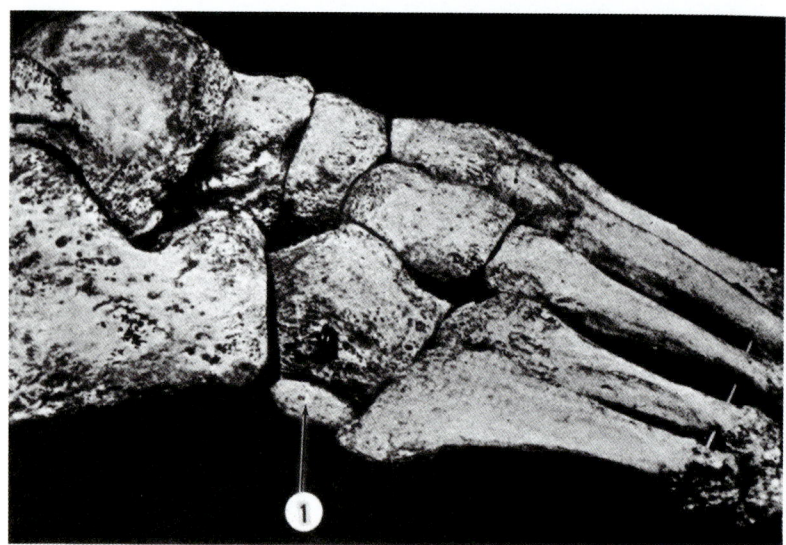

Figure 2.69 **Os peroneum (1).** (From Dwight T. *Variations of the Bones of the Hands and Feet: A Clinical Atlas.* JB Lippincott; 1907:14-23.)

▶ Tibialis Posterior Tendon

This sesamoid is located in the tibialis posterior tendon as it crosses the inferior calcaneonavicular ligament on the plantar aspect of the navicular tuberosity, and its occurrence is reported with the following frequency: Pfitzner (729 ft), before the age of 50 years, 9.2%, after the age of 50 years, 11.9%[18]; Storton (348 ft), 23% (paired, 52.5%, unpaired, 47.5%).[19]

▶ Tibialis Anterior Tendon

This sesamoid is located in the substance of the tibialis anterior tendon near its insertion at the level of the anteroinferior corner of the medial surface of the first cuneiform. An articular surface is found in this location on the cuneiform.

ACCESSORY BONES

The accessory bones are developmental anomalies.[67] They are "either normal parts or prominences of the ordinary tarsal bones that are abnormally separated from the main elements or they are subdivisions of the main elements."[21] They may, on the other hand, not only complete the canonical element in contour but also represent "a free element which appears to be additional to the adjacent portion of its canonical element."[67]

Multiple accessoria may be present in a single foot, and they are unilateral in about half or even more than half of the cases.[67] They may be multipartite. For a comprehensive account of the accessory bones of the foot, we refer to the classic work of Pfitzner and the studies of Dwight, Marti, Trolle, O'Rahilly, and Kohler and Zimmer.[18,38,61,66-69]

The more commonly occurring accessory bones are the os trigonum, the os tibiale, and the os intermetatarseum$_{1,2}$. The following accessory bones occur less frequently: os sustentaculi, os calcaneus secundarius, os cuboides secundarium, os talonaviculare dorsale, os intercuneiforme, os cuneometatarsale 1 plantare, os vesalianum, os subtibiale, and os subfibulare.

▶ Os Trigonum

The os trigonum (Fig. 2.70) has already been described in the study of the talus. It is located at the level of the posterolateral tubercle of the talus. Its reported occurrence ranges from 1.7% to 7.7%. It is to be differentiated from the trigonal process and its fracture (Shepherd fracture).

▶ Os Tibiale

The os tibiale (os tibiale externum, accessory navicular, naviculare secundarium; Figs. 2.71 and 2.72) is an accessory bone located on the posteromedial aspect of the tuberosity of the navicular. It is incorporated by the insertional fibers of the tibialis posterior tendon on the tuberosity of the navicular. It is to be differentiated from the sesamoid of the tibialis posterior tendon, which is located in the plantar portion of the tendon at the level of the inferior calcaneonavicular ligament. The sesamoid is located in the lateral aspect of the navicular tuberosity on the roentgenographic anteroposterior projection of the foot. A typical accessory navicular bone is pyramidal (see Fig. 2.71). The base is anterior and corresponds to the posteromedial aspect of the navicular tuberosity. The connection is fibrous or fibrocartilaginous. The apex is posterior. The contour of the os tibiale is very variable, and the roentgenographic morphologic variations are described by Mouchet and Moutier (Fig. 2.73).[70] The bone is at times semilunate, round, or ovoid and is rudimentary, not articulating with the tuberosity of the navicular. At times, it is partially or completely incorporated in the navicular tuberosity, which may then acquire the form of a bent hook.

The frequency of occurrence is as follows: Harris and Beath (roentgenographic), 4.1%[71]; Hoerr and coworkers (501 adolescents, roentgenographic), girls, 3% to 8%, and boys, 4% to 9%[72]; Bizarro (roentgenographic), 2%[59]; Holland (roentgenographic), 10% to 12%[73]; Pfitzner (425 ft, anatomic), 11.5%[18]; Trolle (histoembryologic), 6.4%[61]; Dwight (anatomic), about 10%.[38]

Zadek and Gold studied roentgenographically the fate of 14 accessory naviculars in children and adolescents.[74] Of 14

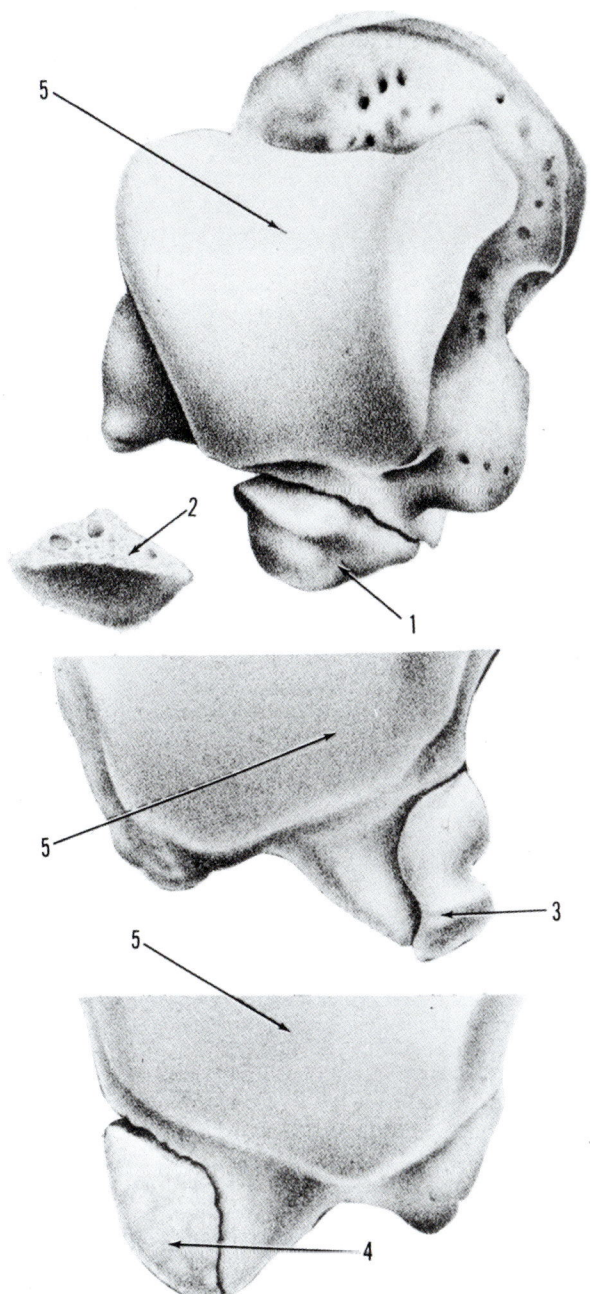

Figure 2.70 Os trigonum. (*1, 3, 4*, variations in contour; *2*, anterior talar connecting surface; *5*, talus.) (From Pfitzner W. Beiträge zur Kenntnis des Menschlichen Extremitätenskelets: VI. Die Variationen in Aufbau des Fussskelets. In: Schwalbe, ed. *Morphologische Arbeiten*. Gustav Fischer; 1896:245-527.)

accessory naviculars, five fused totally to the navicular, three fused partially to the navicular, and six remained as independent accessory bones.

The terminology of os tibiale *externum* is confusing because it relates to the phylogenetic concept of this accessory bone relative to the old representation of the primitive tetrapod foot. In the present concept of the primitive tetrapod foot and the development of the mammalian foot elements (Fig. 2.74), the head of the talus is formed by the two centrale proximale (fibulare and tibiale), the navicular is formed by the two centrale distale (fibulare and tibiale), and the tibiale, now medial to the talar head in this concept, forms the accessory navicular or os tibiale.[61] The tibiale is the third element participating in the formation of the navicular. The term *externum* is "only misleading and ought to be dropped."[61]

▶ Os Intermetatarseum[1,2]

The os intermetatarseum is found between the medial cuneiform and the base of the first and second metatarsals.[75] The bone has variable size and contour, and it may be free or fused. A comprehensive description of the variations is given by Pfitzner (Fig. 2.75), Dwight (Fig. 2.76), and Schinz.[18,38,76] The os intermetatarseum is usually spindle-shaped, fused to the distal dorsolateral corner of the medial cuneiform, and tapers distally while projecting between the first and second metatarsal bones. This accessory bone may fuse with the second metatarsal bone and then project anteriorly and medially. It may also fuse to the first metatarsal. When fused with one bone, the os intermetatarseum is in contact with the two others, and Dwight describes a case in which an articular surface is present with the three surrounding bones.[38] Friedl describes this bone as a sesamoid of the first dorsal interosseous muscle.[77] Henderson reports the association of hallux valgus and os intermetatarseum in both feet of a brother and sister[78]; a tendinous structure is described extending from the tip of the accessory bone through the belly of the first dorsal interosseous and attaching to the lateral aspect of the proximal phalanx of the big toe.

The frequency of occurrence of the os intermetatarseum is as follows: Pfitzner (anatomic), 8.2%[18]; Dwight (anatomic), 10%[38]; Gruber (anatomic), 8%[75]; Bizarro (roentgenographic), 0%[59]; Faber (roentgenographic), 1.2%[79]; Trolle (histoembryologic), 6.8%.[61]

▶ Os Sustentaculi

The os sustentaculi is an accessory bone located at the posterior aspect of the sustentaculum tali (Fig. 2.77).[18] It occurs rarely as a distinct bone (0.47%)[18] and is connected with fibrous tissue or fibrocartilage to the sustentaculum. Dwight has "never seen it separate."[38] Kohler and Zimmer have observed this bone on four occasions.[66] Hoerr and coworkers give a frequency of roentgenographic occurrence of 2% to 3% in boys and none in girls in a total adolescent population of 501.[72]

▶ Os Calcaneus Secundarius

The os calcaneus secundarius is located dorsally in the interval between the anteromedial angle of the os calcis, the cuboid, the navicular, and the head of the talus (Fig. 2.78).[80] The configuration is variable, being round or angular. According to Kohler and Zimmer, "a rounded form is an expression of underdevelopment; a triangular form is seen much more frequently."[66]

The reported frequencies of occurrence are as follows: Pfitzner (840 ft, anatomic), 2%[18]; Stieda (120 ft, anatomic),

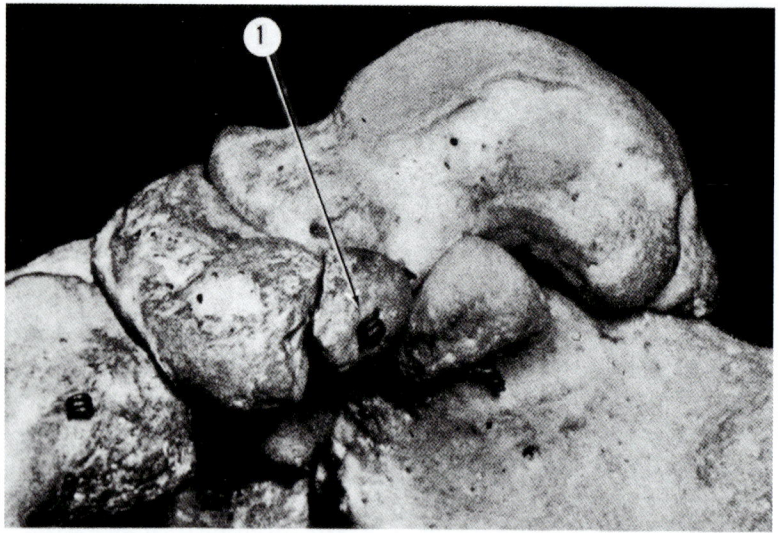
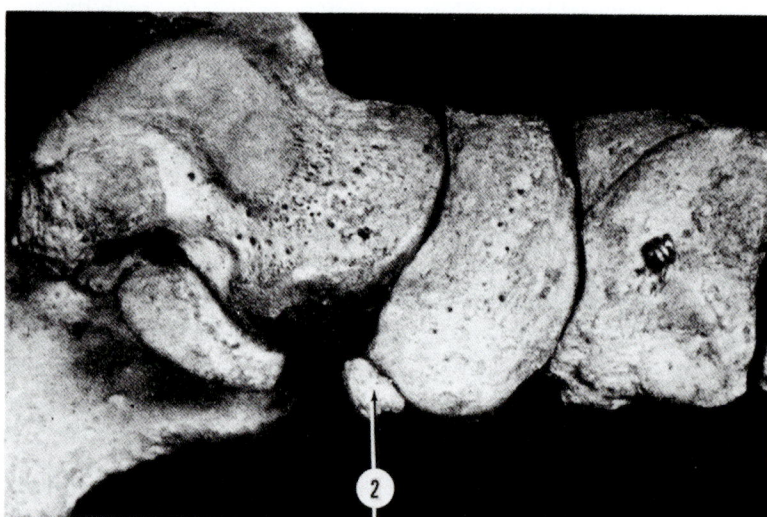

Figure 2.71 **Accessory navicular (1, 2).** (From Dwight T. *Variations of the Bones of the Hands and Feet: A Clinical Atlas.* JB Lippincott; 1907:14-23.)

2.5%[80]; Gruber (719 ft, anatomic), one case[81]; Laidlaw (750 ft, anatomic), three cases[34]; Hoerr and coworkers (510 adolescents, roentgenographic), boys, 7% to 11%, and girls, 6% to 7%.[72]

▶ Os Cuboides Secundarium

The os cuboides secundarium, an accessory bone, is of rare occurrence.[81] It is located on the plantar aspect of the foot between the cuboid, navicular, talus, and os calcis. Dwight gives the description of free cuboides secundarium.[82] Holland mentions having seen it once roentgenographically as a "small circular shadow."[73]

This bone is recognized as a process connected to the cuboid (Fig. 2.79) or "more frequently fused with the scaphoid" (Fig. 2.80).[38] Hoerr and associates give a roentgenologic occurrence of 1% to 3% in 501 adolescent feet.[72]

▶ Os Talonaviculare Dorsale

This accessory bone (os supranavicular, talonavicular ossicle, Pirie's bone) is located dorsally at the talonavicular joint near the midpoint.[83] Pfitzner considers it an avulsed exostosis and calls it *supranavicular spurium*.[18] Pirie describes this "normal ossicle" and reports subsequently on 14 cases, of which 4 were bilateral.[84,85] Kohler and Zimmer observed it in 20 cases over 2 years.[66] Hoerr and coworkers report a roentgenographic rate of occurrence of 15% in boys and 11% in girls in a group of 134 adolescents.[72]

▶ Os Intercuneiforme

The os intercuneiforme is located on the dorsum of the foot between the proximal segments of the internal and middle cuneiforms and in front of the navicular (Fig. 2.81).[86] It is wedge-shaped, and Dwight[86] mentions having seen this bone twice. Hoerr and coworkers report the frequency of occurrence of this accessory bone as 1% in boys and 1% in girls in a population of 367 adolescents.[72] Jones mentions the presence of "a little pit at the junction of the two tibial cuneiforms with the navicular that suggests that a very small free ossicle may have been present in the recent state."[21]

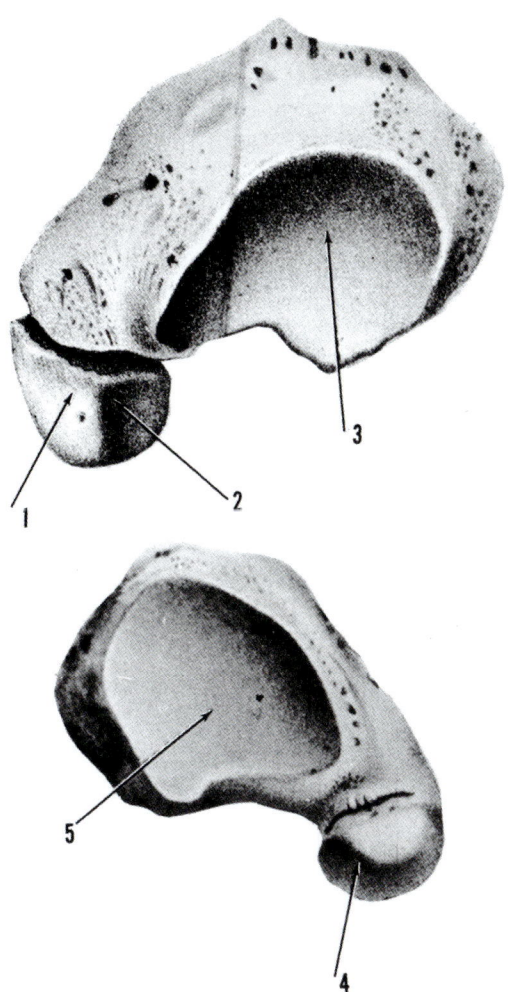

Figure 2.72 Accessory navicular. (Top: *1, 2,* Accessory navicular with two facets; *3,* navicular. Bottom: *4,* Accessory navicular attached to navicular [*5*].) (From Pfitzner W. Beiträge zur Kenntnis des Menschlichen Extremitätenskelets: VI. Die Variationen in Aufbau des Fussskelets. In: Schwalbe, ed. *Morphologische Arbeiten*. Gustav Fischer; 1896:245-527.)

▶ Os Cuneo$_1$-Metatarsale$_1$ Plantare

The os cuneo$_1$-metatarsale$_1$ plantare (pars peronea metatarsalis primi) is located on the plantar aspect of the foot between the base of the first metatarsal and the medial cuneiform (Fig. 2.82).[18] Its occurrence is rare.

▶ Os Vesalianum

The os vesalianum "has been the subject of much controversy and a good deal of confusion."[73] Holland reproduced two illustrations from the 1725 edition of *The Works of Vesalius* (edited by Boerhave) depicting a plantar and a dorsal view of the lateral tarsus and the fifth metatarsal.[73] The dorsal view shows a small bone located between the well-formed tuberosity of the fifth metatarsal and the cuboid. The plantar view shows a small bone at the tip of the same tuberosity. The original description of the os vesalianum, translated by Holland, is as follows: "a small bone, opposite to the outer

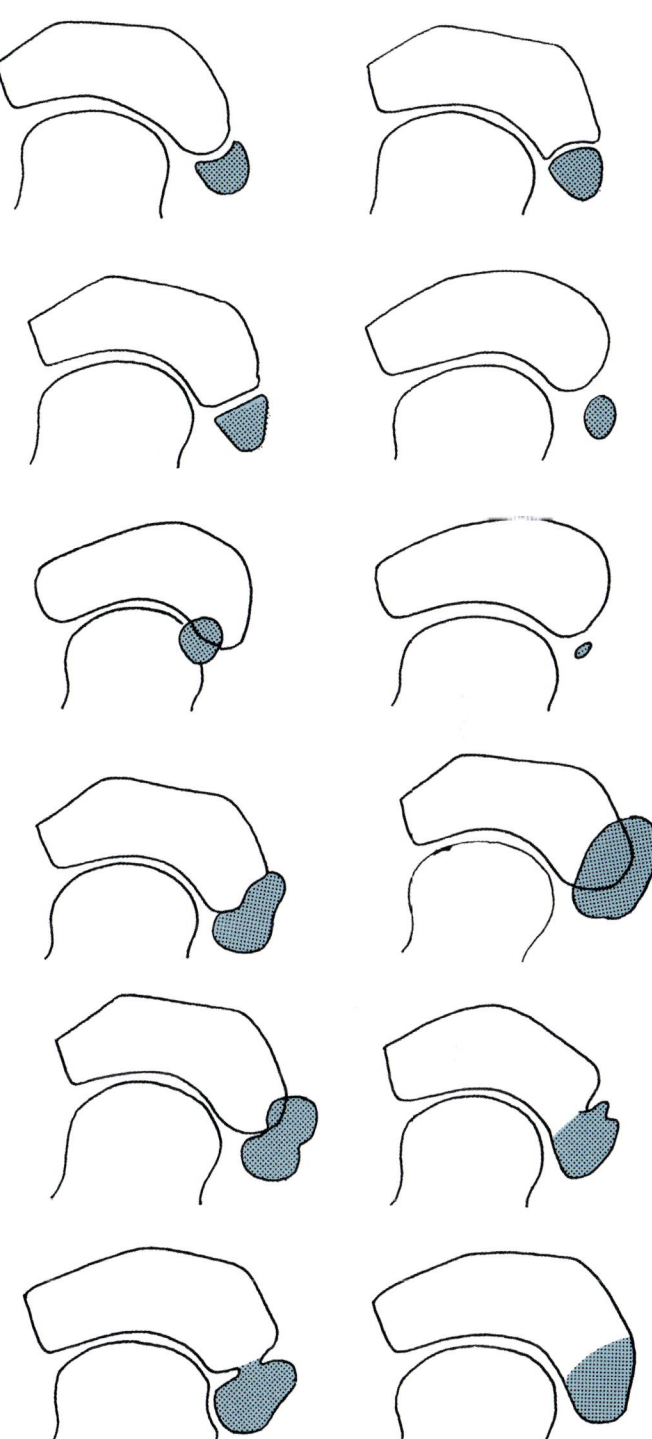

Figure 2.73 Variations in the roentgenographic forms of the accessory navicular. (Adapted from Mouchet A, Moutier G. Osselets surnuméraires du tarse [ossa tarsalia]. *Presse Médicale*. 1925;23:370.)

side of the joint, and placed proximately to the little toe, and probably articulating with the cuboid."[73]

This accessory bone is of rare occurrence. Dameron, in a roentgenographic study of 1000 ft, mentions its detection in one case.[87] Sporadic cases have been reported by Lequerrière and Drevon, Holland, and others.[73,88]

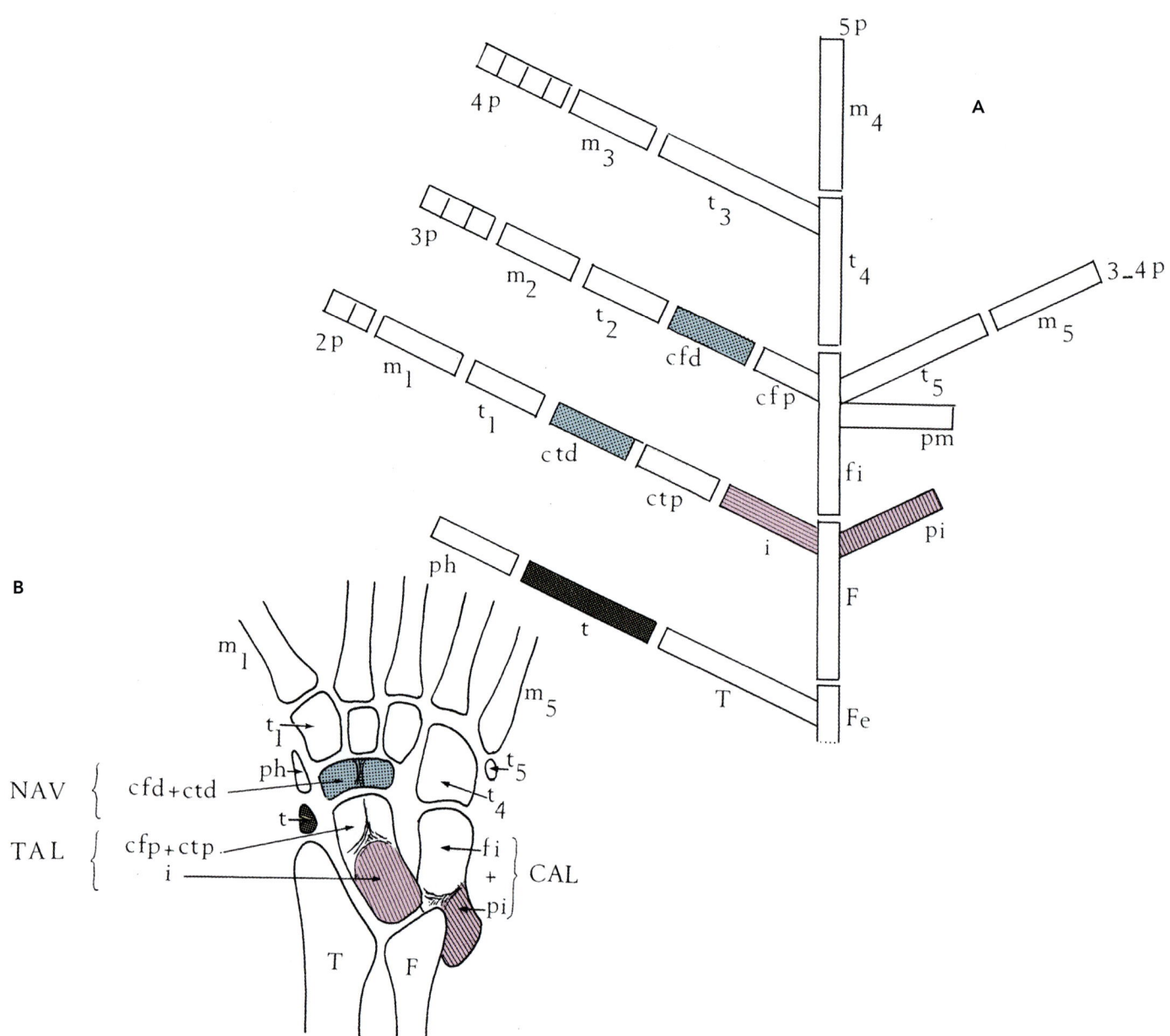

Figure 2.74 **(A) Development of the primitive tetrapod foot.** The basal cord is formed by the femur (Fe), the fibula (F), the fibulare (fi), the tarsale$_4$ (t$_4$), the metatarsale$_4$ (m$_4$), and five phalanges (5p). From the tibial side of the basal cord, four rays lead off. The first ray arises from the femur and is formed by the tibia (T), the tibiale (t), and the prehallux (ph). The second ray arises from the distal end of the fibula and is formed by the intermedium (i), the centrale tibiale proximale (cfp), the centrale tibiale distale (cfd), the tarsale$_1$ (t$_1$), the metatarsale$_1$ (m$_1$), and two phalanges (2p). The third ray takes off from the distal end of the fibulare and is formed by the centrale fibulare proximale (cfp), the centrale fibulare distale (cfd), the tarsale$_2$ (t$_2$), the metatarsale$_2$ (m$_2$), and three phalanges (3p). The fourth ray takes off from the tarsale$_4$ and is formed by the tarsale$_3$ (t$_3$), the metatarsale$_3$ (m$_3$), and four phalanges (4p). From the fibular side of the basal cord, the following take off: the pisiform, arising from the distal end of the fibula (pi), and a distal ray, arising from the distal end of the fibulare and formed by the tarsale$_5$ (t$_5$), the metatarsale$_5$ (m$_5$), and three or four phalanges (3–4p). The postminimus (pm) has a similar origin. **(B) The foot of the living mammal has developed in the following manner from the elements of the primitive tetrapod foot.** The tibiale (t) of the first ray forms the accessory navicular. The talus is formed by the intermedium (i) of the second tibial ray and the proximal tibial and fibular centrales (ctp + cfp) of the second and third tibial rays. The navicular is formed by the distal tibial and fibular centrale (ctd + cfd) of the second and third tibial rays. The cuneiform$_1$ is formed by the tarsale$_1$, the cuneiform$_2$ is formed by the tarsale$_2$, and the cuneiform$_3$ is formed by the tarsale$_3$. The calcaneus is formed by the fibulare (fi) of the basal cord and the pisiform (pi). The cuboid is formed by the tarsale$_4$ (t$_4$) of the basal cord. (Adapted from Trolle D. *Accessory Bones of the Human Foot: A Radiological, Histoembryological, Comparative Anatomical and Genetic Study.* Munksgaard; 1948:150-151.)

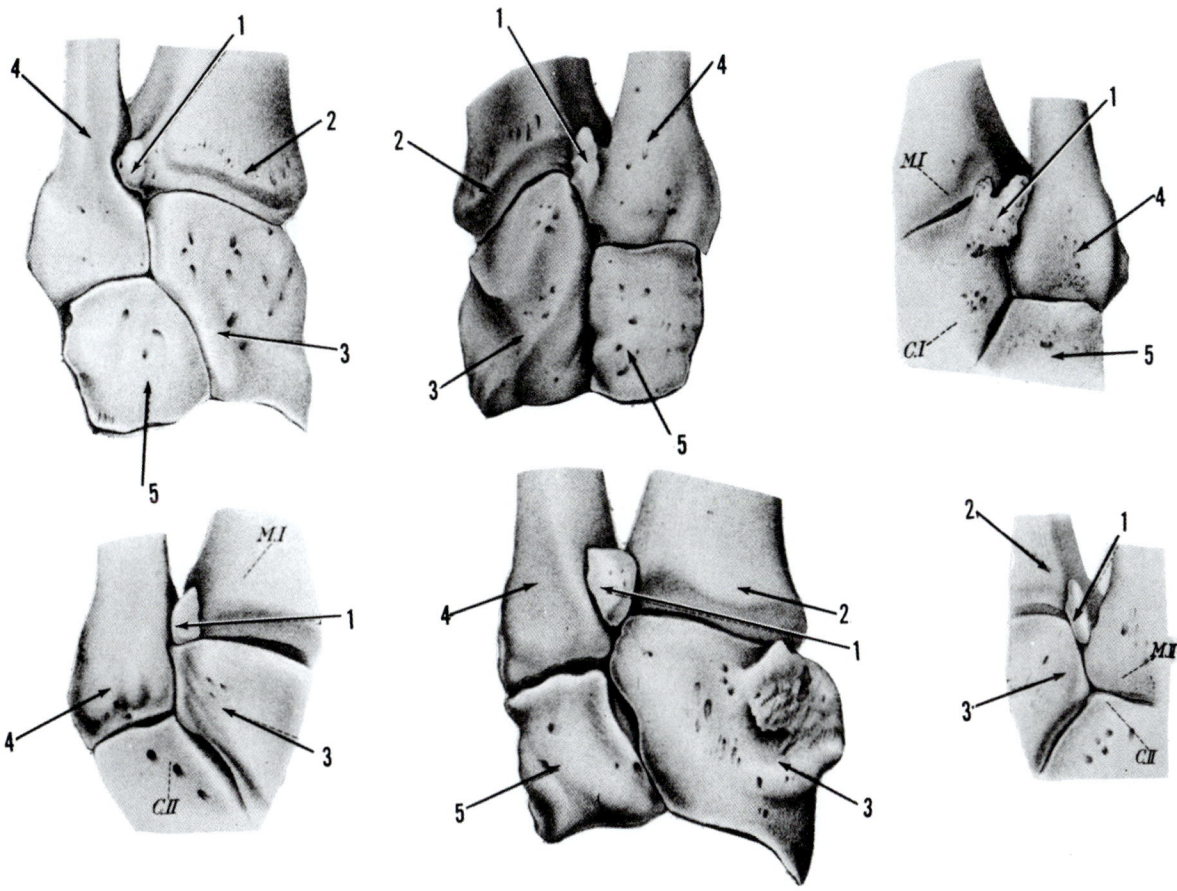

Figure 2.75 **Os intermetatarseum.** The os intermetatarseum is seen arising from the first or second metatarsal or from the first cuneiform. It may also present as an independent ossicle. (*1*, os intermetatarseum; *2*, first metatarsal; *3*, first cuneiform; *4*, second metatarsal; *5*, second cuneiform.) (From Pfitzner W. Beiträge zur Kenntnis des Menschlichen Extremitätenskelets: VI. Die Variationen in Aufbau des Fussskelets. In: Schwalbe, ed. *Morphologische Arbeiten.* Gustav Fischer; 1896:245-527.)

The os vesalianum is to be differentiated from the following (Fig. 2.83): the ossifying apophysis of the fifth metatarsal base, a fracture of the base of the fifth metatarsal bone or a nonunion of the same, an ununited apophysis of the fifth metatarsal base, and the sesamoid within the peroneus longus tendon. The following may help to differentiate the entities:[87]

- The os vesalianum is located just proximal to the tip of the well-developed tuberosity of the fifth metatarsal. The opposing surfaces may be sclerotic.
- The ossification center of the apophysis is linear initially and longitudinally oriented, parallel to the metatarsal shaft.
- The fracture of the apophysis or base of the fifth metatarsal is transverse in direction and may pass through the cubometatarsal joint or metatarsal M_4-M_5 joint.

▶ **Os Subtibiale and Os Subfibulare**

The os subtibiale is an accessory bone located under the medial malleolus. It may present as a round or angular ossicle. It is to be differentiated from a secondary ossification center of the medial malleolus or from a sequela of trauma. Powell, in a roentgenographic study of 100 healthy children aged 6 to 12 years, found an accessory ossification center to the medial malleolus in 20%.[89] Both ankles in 50 adults without history of injury were studied by the same author and separate submalleolar ossicles were found in 4% of the ankles.

The os subfibulare is an accessory bone located under the tip of the lateral malleolus in a posterior position. The ossicle may be round or comma-shaped or may present an articular facet facing the lateral malleolus. It is to be differentiated from a secondary ossification center of the lateral malleolus (which occurs in 1%) and from the sequela of trauma. The os fibulare was recognized by Leimbach and may be bilateral.[90] Kohler and Zimmer mention having seen several cases in adults.[66] Bjornson reported two cases in ankle injuries, recognizing the os fibulare in retrospect.[91] Griffiths described three cases of os fibulare in children aged 8 to 10 years seen for minor ankle injuries.[92]

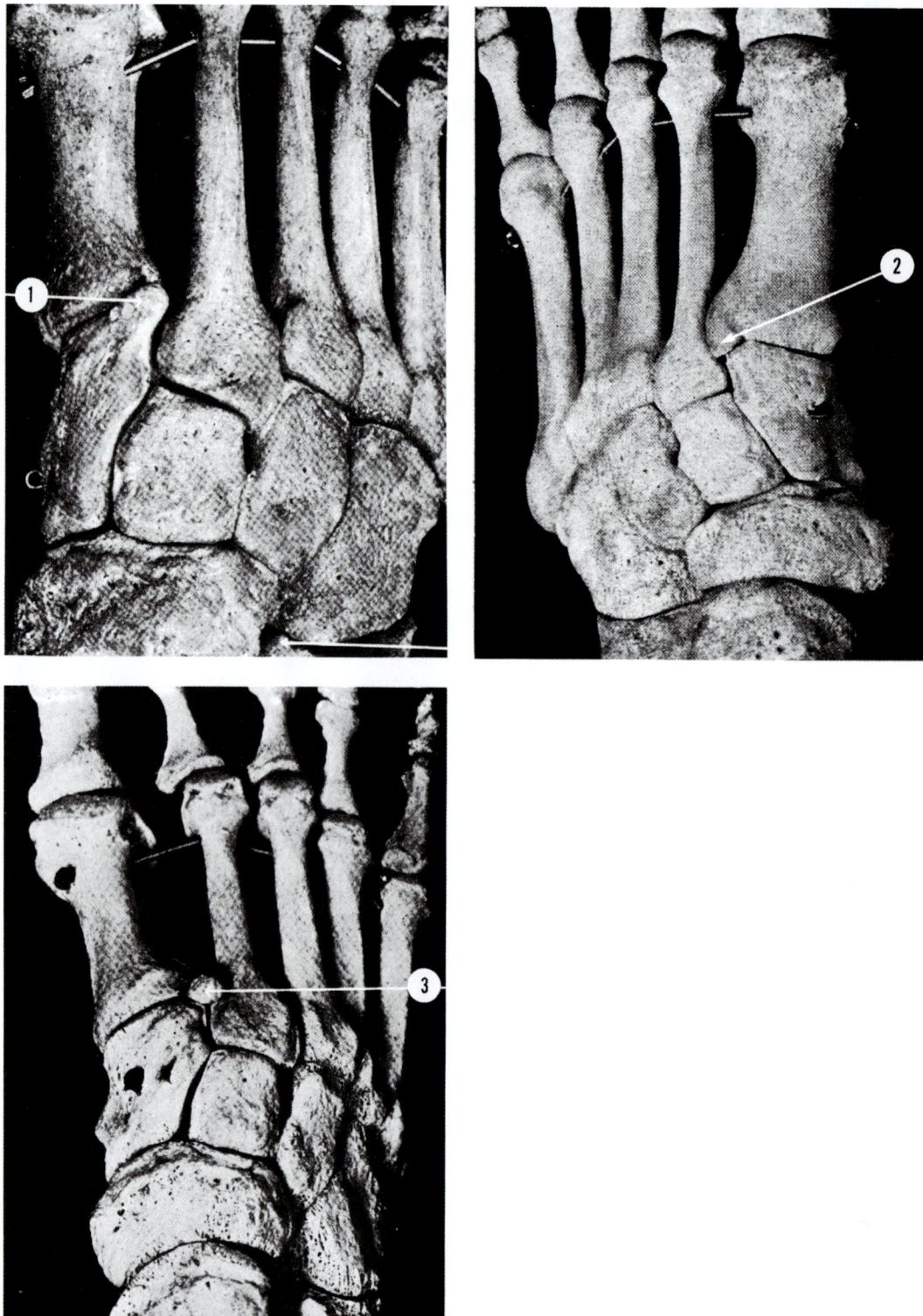

Figure 2.76 **Os intermetatarseum (1, 2, 3).** (From Dwight T. *Variations of the Bones of the Hands and Feet: A Clinical Atlas.* JB Lippincott; 1907:14-23.)

COALITION

Coalition is the union of two or more bony elements. It may be fibrous (syndesmosis), cartilaginous (synchondrosis), or osseous (synostosis) and may involve the tarsus, the tarsometatarsal elements, or the phalanges. Pfitzner, in an anatomic study of 750 ft, reported an overall occurrence of coalition in 2% with the following distribution[18]: talocalcaneal, 1; talonavicular, 1; calcaneonavicular, 15; cubonavicular, 3; intercuneiform$_{2-3}$, 1; cuneo$_3$-metatarsal$_3$, 15.

Harris reports the following anatomic sites involved in 102 patients with tarsal coalition[93]: talocalcaneal, 66 (medial 62, posterior 4); calcaneonavicular, 29; cubonavicular, 1; talonavicular, 1; calcaneocuboid, 1; multiple intertarsal, 4.

Stromont and Peterson,[94] based on the literature review from 1927 to 1981, reported the incidence of tarsal coalition of less than 1% with the following distribution: talocalacaneal 48.1%, calcaneonavicular 43.6%, talonavicular 1.3%, calcaneocuboid 1.3%, and others 5.7%. In their own group, they reported 53% calcaneonavicular and 37% talocalcaneal coalitions.

▶ Talocalcaneal Coalition

The talocalcaneal coalition occurs mainly on the medial side. Prior to the advent of roentgenographic investigation, the condition was recognized and reported by the anatomists.[95-98] Pfitzner described and gave a clear illustration of his only coalition occurring between the posterior end of the sustentaculum tali and the talus (Fig. 2.84).[18]

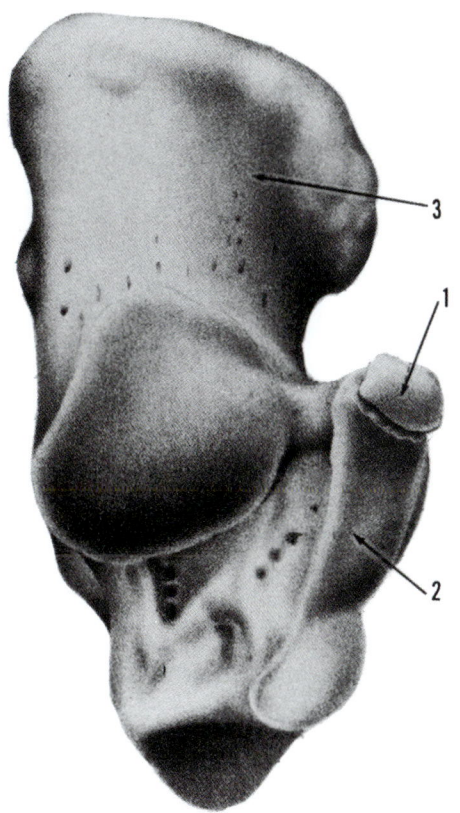

Figure 2.77 **Os sustentaculi.** (*1*, os sustentaculi; *2*, sustentaculum tali; *3*, calcaneus.) (From Pfitzner W. Beiträge zur Kenntnis des Menschlichen Extremitätenskelets: VI. Die Variationen in Aufbau des Fussskelets. In: Schwalbe, ed. *Morphologische Arbeiten*. Gustav Fischer; 1896:245-527.)

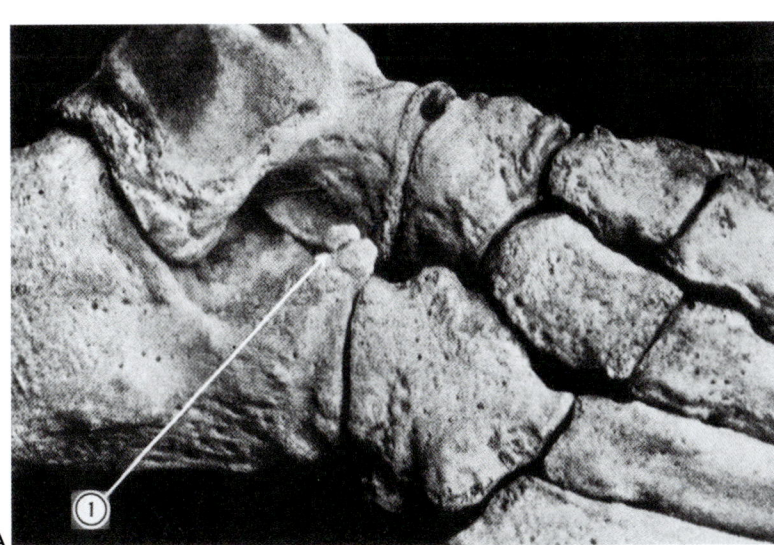
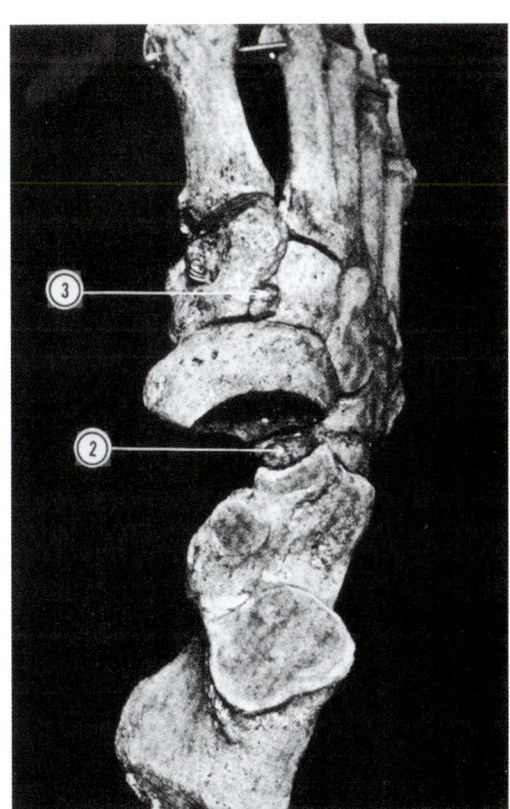

Figure 2.78 **Os calcaneus secundarius.** (*1*, os calcaneus secundarius; *2*, os calcaneus secundarius; *3*, os intercuneiform.) (From Dwight T. *Variations of the Bones of the Hands and Feet: A Clinical Atlas*. JB Lippincott; 1907:14-23.)

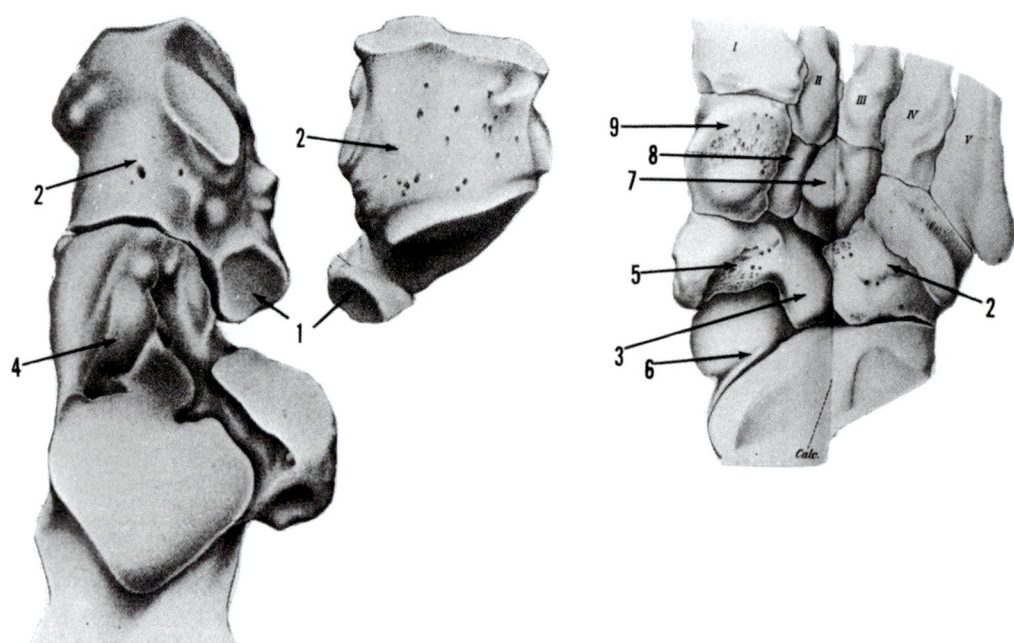

Figure 2.79 **Os cuboides secundarium.** (*1*, os cuboides secundarium arising from cuboid; *2*, cuboid; *3*, os cuboides secundarium arising from navicular; *4*, calcaneus; *5*, navicular; *6*, head of talus; *7, 8, 9*, cuneiforms *3, 2, 1*, respectively.) (From Pfitzner W. Beiträge zur Kenntnis des Menschlichen Extremitätenskelets: VI. Die Variationen in Aufbau des Fussskelets. In: Schwalbe, ed. *Morphologische Arbeiten*. Gustav Fischer; 1896:245-527.)

Few clinical reports[99-103] were available prior to the comprehensive study of the talocalcaneal coalition by Harris and Beath,[104] who correlated this anatomic variation with the etiology of peroneal spastic flatfoot. Harris described four anatomic types of medial talocalcaneal coalition[93]:

Complete (synostosis): a bony bridge unites the talus and the calcaneus at the level of the sustentaculum tali
Incomplete (synchondrosis, syndesmosis): a cartilaginous or fibrous bridge unites the talar and calcaneal projections on the posterior aspect of the sustentaculum tali
Rudimentary: a calcaneal sustentacular element extends from the posterior aspect of the sustentaculum tali and impinges on the medial aspect of the talus
Rudimentary: a talar element extends from the posteromedial talar tubercle toward the os calcis just posterior to the sustentaculum tali

The talocalcaneal coalition occurs more frequently at the level of the middle calcaneal facet or the posterior part of the sustentaculum tali; it sometimes occurs (but rarely) at the level of the posterior talocalcaneal joint.[99,105-107] It may involve the

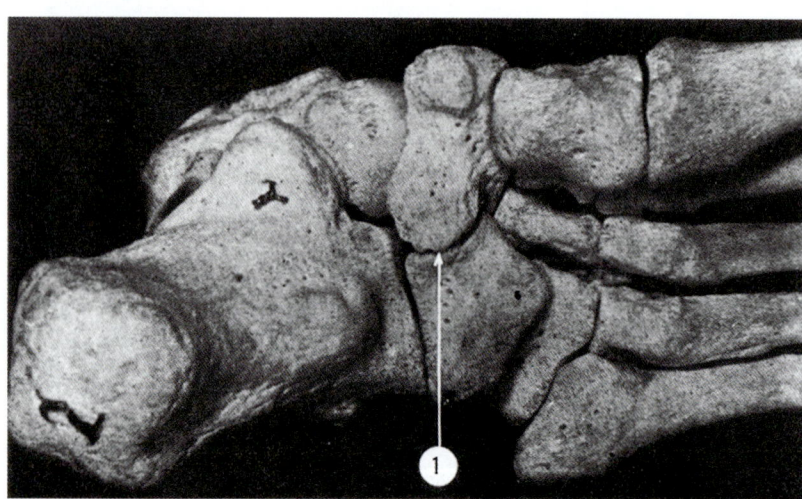

Figure 2.80 **Os cuboides secundarium (1) arising from navicular.** (From Dwight T. *Variations of the Bones of the Hands and Feet: A Clinical Atlas*. JB Lippincott; 1907:14-23.)

Chapter 2: Osteology

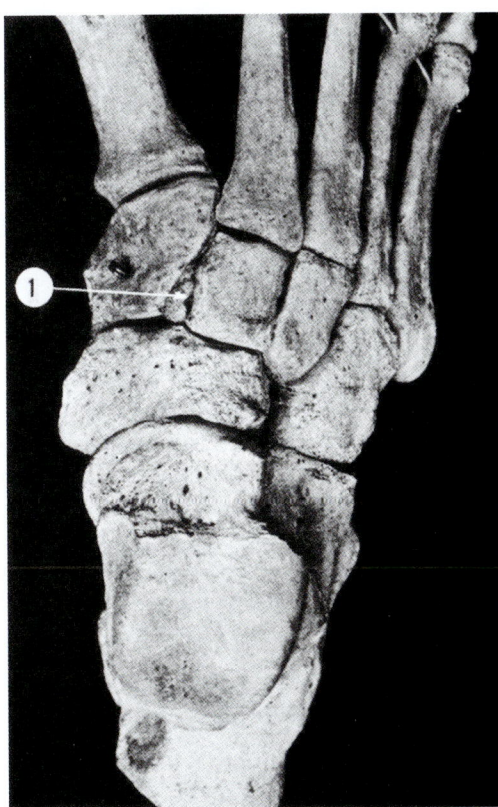

Figure 2.81 Os intercuneiform (1). (From Dwight T. Variations of the Bones of the Hands and Feet: A Clinical Atlas. JB Lippincott; 1907:14-23.)

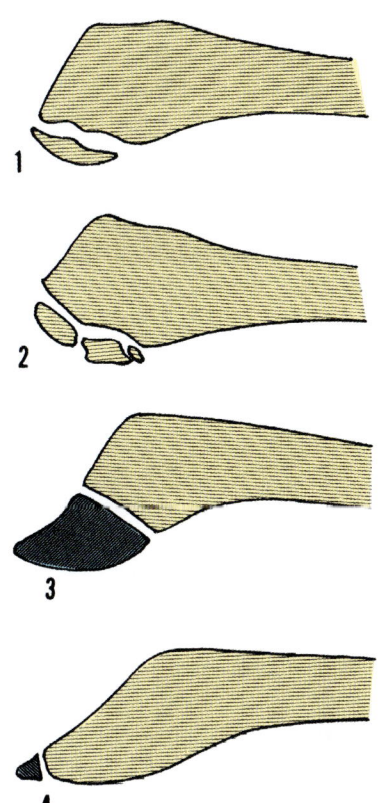

Figure 2.83 Fifth metatarsal base. (1, ossification within apophysis of base; 2, ossification within apophysis of base with fragmentation; 3, ununited apophysis of fifth metatarsal base; 4, position of os vesalianum.)

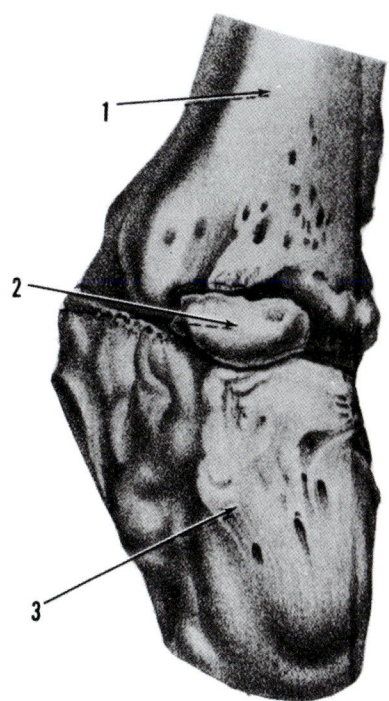

Figure 2.82 Os cuneo1-metatarsal1 plantare (2). (1, first metatarsal; 3, first cuneiform.) (From Pfitzner W. Beiträge zur Kenntnis des Menschlichen Extremitätenskelets: VI. Die Variationen in Aufbau des Fussskelets. In: Schwalbe, ed. Morphologische Arbeiten. Gustav Fischer; 1896:245-527.)

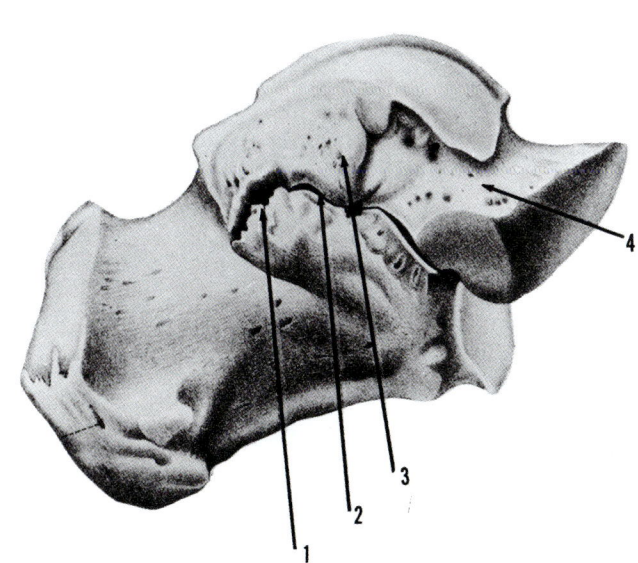

Figure 2.84 Talocalcaneal coalition. (1, coalition site, posteromedial; 2, posterior talocalcaneal segmental interline; 3, posteromedial talar tubercle; 4, medial aspect of talus.) (From Pfitzner W. Beiträge zur Kenntnis des Menschlichen Extremitätenskelets: VI. Die Variationen in Aufbau des Fussskelets. In: Schwalbe, ed. Morphologische Arbeiten. Gustav Fischer; 1896:245-527.)

anterior calcaneal facet, as reported by Conway and Cowell in their comprehensive study related to the roentgenographic demonstration of the tarsal coalitions.[108]

▶ Calcaneonavicular Coalition

Cruveilhier described and illustrated the first anatomic specimen of calcaneonavicular coalition (Fig. 2.85).[109] He mentioned that "this anatomic variety, which is certainly not a pathologic ossification, has already been seen many times."[109] This specimen was provided by Fischer, who encountered an unusual resistance while doing a Chopart disarticulation of the foot: "This resistance was an abnormal ossification but by no means pathologic, uniting the anterior facet of the os calcis to the scaphoid."[109]

Since then, many anatomists have reported on this union.[18,36,110-120] Pfitzner described 15 cases of calcaneonavicular coalition (Fig. 2.86A), and Dwight presented the photograph and roentgenogram of a calcaneonavicular synchondrosis (Fig. 2.86B).[18,38] The clinical recognition of this coalition and its correlation with flatfeet is attributed to Slomann, who described three forms[121,122]: abnormal projections between the two bones (amphiarthrosis); fibrous union between the bony projections (syndesmosis) and often containing one or more osseous nuclei (ossa calcanea secundaria) embedded in the fibrous tissues; and osseous union between the two bones (synostosis). Many clinical reports pertaining to the recognition and treatment of the condition confirmed the frequent occurrence of this coalition.[123-133]

When a synostosis is present, it is at least 1 cm wide, whereas in the amphiarthrosis, the width of the coalition is less than 0.5 cm.[133]

The reports in the literature indicate that this coalition is inherited.[134-136] Leonard reported a study of 31 patients with spastic flatfoot in association with tarsal coalition.[137] Ninety-eight first-degree relatives of these patients were studied; 39% of the relatives presented a tarsal coalition (25% calcaneonavicular; 14% talocalcaneal and other coalitions). In 80% of these patients and in 84% of their relatives, the coalition was bilateral. Leonard concluded that "tarsal coalitions are inherited, most probably as a unifactorial disorder of autosomal dominant inheritance, very nearly of full penetrance."[137] Interestingly, none of the relatives with tarsal coalition had any evidence of peroneal spastic flatfoot.

▶ Talonavicular Coalition

The first anatomic description of the talonavicular coalition was given by Anderson.[138] He described the synostosis in two anatomic specimens of a male subject, age 34 years, with "small and well-shaped" feet. The fusion was so complete that the skeletal element was called an astragaloscaphoid bone. The head of this coalesced bone articulates laterally and on the external segment of the inferior surface with the cuboid. The inner surface is nonarticular, and the anterior surface articulates with the cuneiforms. A small elevated articular surface on the inferior aspect of the head, located in the middle of a depression, articulates with the sustentaculum tali.

Chaput described a talonavicular synostosis in an adult, involving the right foot, and both feet were flat.[96] Pfitzner had only one specimen of such coalition in 750 ft (Fig. 2.87).[18] Only sporadic cases are described in the literature.[108,139-156]

Schreiber reported on five cases of talonavicular synostosis, three having the fusion bilaterally and two unilaterally.[157] Two patients had accompanying ball-and-socket ankle joint.

▶ Calcaneocuboid Coalition

Robert mentioned a bilateral calcaneocuboid synostosis attributed to Auzias.[158] Wagoner reported on a 9-year-old boy with bilateral and complete calcaneocuboid synostosis.[159] Both feet were flat and symptomatic. Few cases are reported in the literature.[160-166] A bilateral case of calcaneocuboid synostosis reported by Brobeck also featured a very prominent base of the fifth metatarsal bone articulating with the calcaneus[166]; this coalition seems to be in frequent association with other anomalies. Stern and coworkers, Poznanski and coworkers, and Kelikian mentioned the presence of the calcaneocuboid coalition in the hand-foot-uterus syndrome.[167-169]

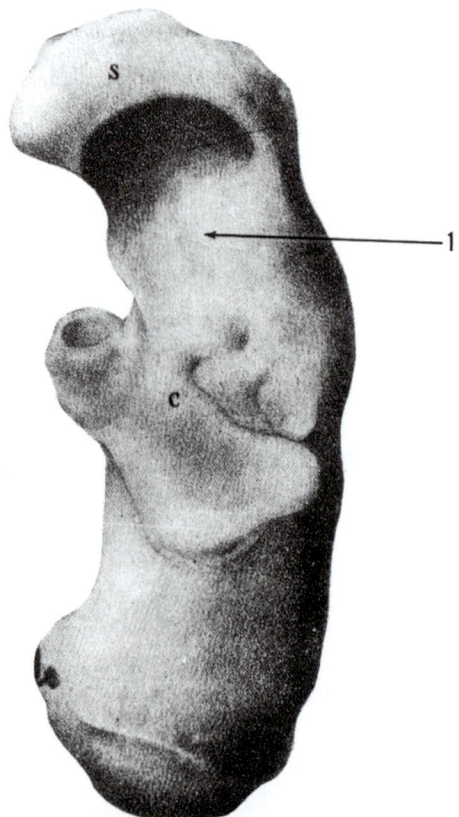

Figure 2.85 Calcaneonavicular coalition. (S, scaphoid; C, calcaneus; 1, calcaneonavicular coalition.) (From Cruveilhier J. Anatomie Pathologique du Corps Humain ou Descriptions avec Figures Lithographieés et Colorées des Diverses Altérations Morbides dont Le Corps Humain est Susceptible. Vol 1. Baillière; 1829-1835. Courtesy of Northwestern University Medical Library.)

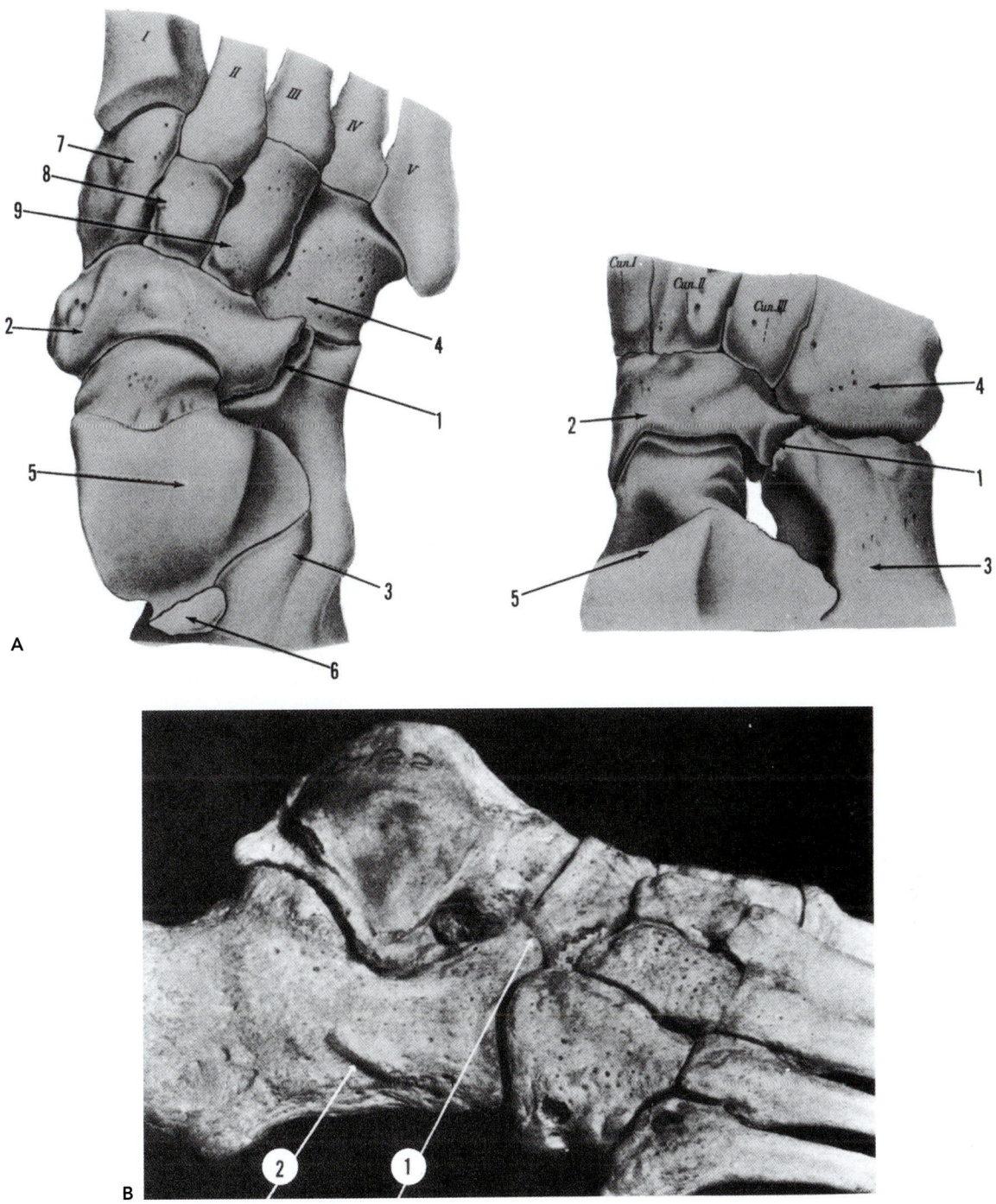

Figure 2.86 Calcaneonavicular coalition. (A) *1*, calcaneonavicular coalition; *2*, navicular; *3*, os calcis; *4*, cuboid; *5*, talus; *6*, os trigonum; *7, 8, 9*, cuneiforms *1, 2, 3*, respectively. (B) *1*, calcaneonavicular coalition; *2*, peroneal trochlear process, prominent. (A, From Pfitzner W. Beiträge zur Kenntnis des Menschlichen Extremitätenskelets: VI. Die Variationen in Aufbau des Fussskelets. In: Schwalbe, ed. *Morphologische Arbeiten*. Gustav Fischer; 1896:245-527. B, From Dwight T. *Variations of the Bones of the Hands and Feet: A Clinical Atlas*. Philadelphia: JB Lippincott; 1907:14–23.)

Kozlowski described a bilateral calcaneocuboid synostosis in a 14-year-old girl with bilateral hypoplasia of the distal ulna.[170] Schauerte and St. Aubin documented the occurrence of a sequential fusion of the tarsal joints in type I acrocephalosyndactyly (Apert syndrome), the calcaneocuboid coalition being stage 1, followed by the fusion of the lateral cuneiform and third metatarsal, and finally involving the navicular and the medial cuneiform.[171]

Craig and Goldberg reported on an 8-year-old girl with craniofacial dysostosis (Crouzon syndrome) and bilateral isolated calcaneocuboid coalition, with one foot symptomatic.[172]

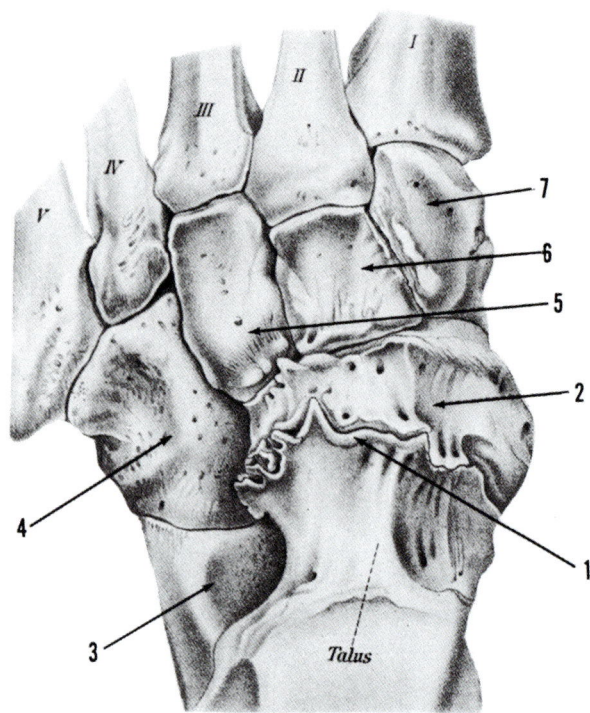

Figure 2.87 Talonavicular coalition. (*1*, talonavicular coalition; *2*, navicular; *3*, calcaneus; *4*, cuboid; *5, 6, 7*, cuneiforms 3, 2, 1, respectively.) (From Pfitzner W. Beiträge zur Kenntnis des Menschlichen Extremitätenskelets: VI. Die Variationen in Aufbau des Fussskelets. In: Schwalbe, ed. *Morphologische Arbeiten*. Gustav Fischer; 1896:245-527.)

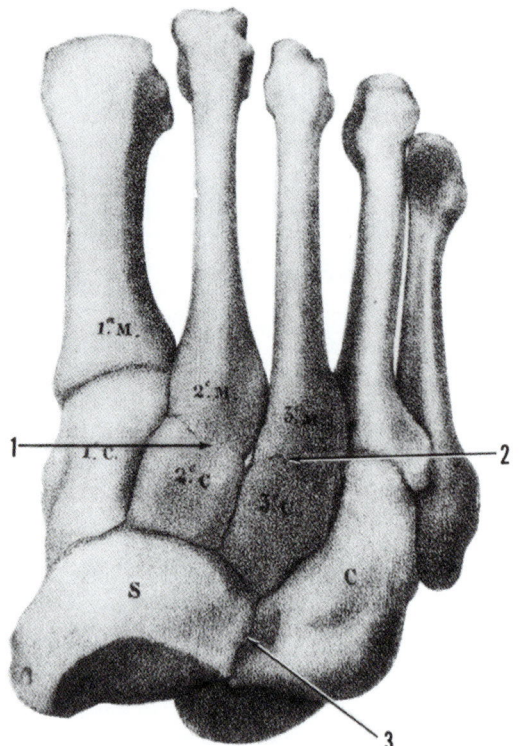

Figure 2.88 Cubonavicular coalition. (*S*, scaphoid; *C*, cuboid; *1*, cuneiform$_2$-metatarsal$_2$ coalition; *2*, cuneiform$_3$-metatarsal$_3$ coalition; *3*, cubonavicular coalition.) (From Cruveilhier J. *Anatomie Pathologique du Corps Humain ou Descriptions avec Figures Lithographieés et Colorées des Diverses Altérations Morbides dont Le Corps Humain est Susceptible.* Vol 1. Baillière; 1829-1835. Courtesy of Northwestern University Medical Library.)

▶ **Cubonavicular Coalition**

Cruveilhier illustrated a foot (Fig. 2.88) with cubonavicular coalition in association with synostosis between cuneiform$_2$-metatarsal$_2$ and cuneiform$_3$-metatarsal$_3$.[109] The text, however, does not carry a description of the cubonavicular union. Gruber presented four cases of cubonavicular coalition through the presence of a cuboides secundarium.[173] Pfitzner reported on three cases with a cuboides secundarius fused to the cuboid on the plantar side; in two specimens, they coalesced with the navicular, and the third specimen had a cuboides secundarius fused to the navicular and coalesced with the cuboid (Fig. 2.89).[18]

A true joint between the navicular and the cuboid is found frequently, as reported by the following anatomists: Gruber, in 200 ft, 45.5%[173]; Pfitzner, in 437 ft, 50.4%[18]; Dwight, in 200 ft, about 60%.[38]

When the joint is absent, normally the two bones are connected by ligaments. Dwight mentioned having "seen bony connection once and cartilaginous once or twice."[38]

The literature is very scarce in regard to the cubonavicular coalition.[174,175]

▶ **Cuneonavicular Coalition**

Lagrange described the foot of a 46-year-old woman with a bony fusion between the navicular and the three cuneiforms.[176] The coalition is, however, not limited to these skeletal elements, as the second and third metatarsals are fused to the cuneiforms. Furthermore, the cuboid and metatarsals$_{4,5}$ are also synostosed.

Lusby reported on the first isolated case of a cuneonavicular coalition.[177] The synostosis was present between the lateral cuneiform and the navicular; the patient was asymptomatic.

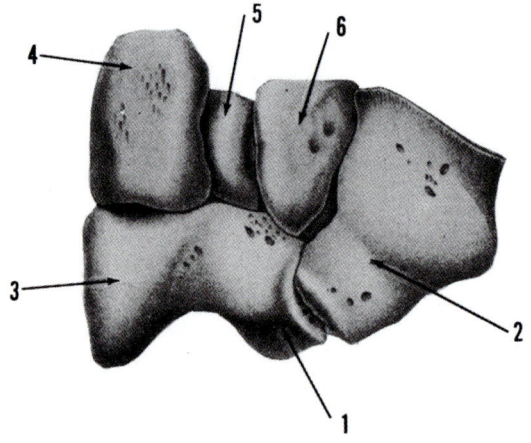

Figure 2.89 Cubonavicular coalition. (*1*, cubonavicular coalition; *2*, cuboid; *3*, navicular; *4, 5, 6*, cuneiforms 1, 2, 3, respectively.) (From Pfitzner W. Beiträge zur Kenntnis des Menschlichen Extremitätenskelets: VI. Die Variationen in Aufbau des Fussskelets. In: Schwalbe, ed. *Morphologische Arbeiten*. Gustav Fischer; 1896:245-527.)

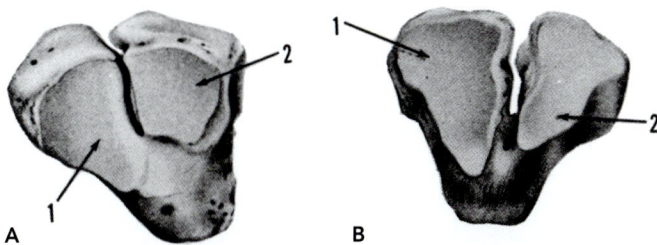

Figure 2.90 Intercuneiform2-3 **coalition. (A)** *1*, cuneiform$_2$; *2*, cuneiform$_3$. **(B)** *1*, cuneiform$_3$; *2*, cuneiform$_2$. Coalesced from plantar aspect. (From Pfitzner W. Beiträge zur Kenntnis des Menschlichen Extremitätenskelets: VI. Die Variationen in Aufbau des Fussskelets. In: Schwalbe, ed. *Morphologische Arbeiten*. Gustav Fischer; 1896:245-527.)

Gregersen reported on a bilateral cuneonavicular coalition in association with a bipartite navicular.[178] The medial half of the navicular was synostosed to the first cuneiform and the lateral half fused to the third cuneiform. The patient was 42-years-old and presented bilateral symptomatic flatfeet.

▶ Intercuneiform$_{2,3}$ Coalition

One case of synostosis between the second and third cuneiforms was described by Pfitzner.[18] The two cuneiforms were synostosed on the plantar aspect, and the joint between them was undisturbed (Fig. 2.90). The union occurred through the enlarged plantar aspect of the third cuneiform, corresponding to the processus uncinatus cuneiformis$_3$. Pfitzner also mentioned that he had never seen a coalition between the first and second cuneiforms.[18]

▶ Cuneo$_2$-Metatarsal$_2$ and Cuneo$_3$-Metatarsal$_3$ Coalitions

Cruveilhier described and illustrated one specimen with the second cuneiform fused to the second metatarsal bone and the third cuneiform to the third metatarsal (Fig. 2.91).[109] The synostosis was complete, and Cruveilhier stated also that "it is obvious that this union is not the result of a disease."[109] He furthermore advises that such a synostosis may create a surgical handicap, and "this inconvenience could also be encountered during the partial amputation of the foot at the tarsometatarso articulations, after the ingenious method of Lisfranc."[109]

Pfitzner found the coalition between the third cuneiform and the third metatarsal in 15 cases in 750 ft.[18] The synostosis was usually on the plantar aspect (Fig. 2.92) and included, in 14 cases, one-third to one-fourth of the joint surfaces. A complete synostosis was present in one case and a partial central synostosis in two others.

▶ Interphalangeal Coalition

The interphalangeal coalition or symphalangism involves mainly the middle and distal phalanges of the little toe (Fig. 2.93A).[18] It was first demonstrated by Leonardo da Vinci[179] (Fig. 2.93E). Pfitzner's monumental investigation yielded the following results: in 91 ft in embryos 5 months or older and

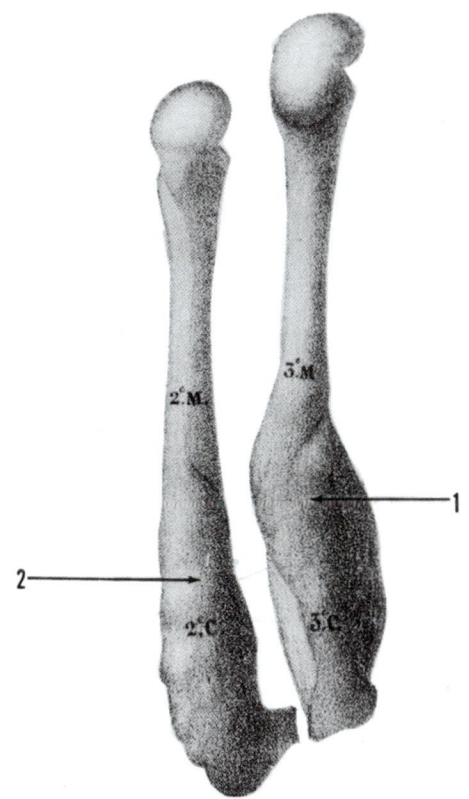

Figure 2.91 Cuneo3-metatarsal3 **coalition (*1*) and cuneo**2-**metatarso**2 **coalition (*2*).** (From Cruveilhier J. *Anatomie Pathologique du Corps Humain ou Descriptions avec Figures Lithographieés et Colorées des Diverses Altérations Morbides dont Le Corps Humain est Susceptible.* Vol 1. Baillière; 1829-1835. Courtesy of Northwestern University Medical Library.)

children up to 7 years, 37 coalitions (40.7%); in 838 adult feet, 310 coalitions (37%).[18] The coalition seems more frequent in females[73]: males, 35.5%; females, 40.2%. Coalition of the middle and terminal phalanges may involve toes other than the fifth, but this is relatively rare (see Fig. 2.93A to 2.93D). According to Pfitzner, when the other toes are involved, the progression is from lateral to medial and in an orderly fashion.[18] The fourth never shows a coalition when a coalition is

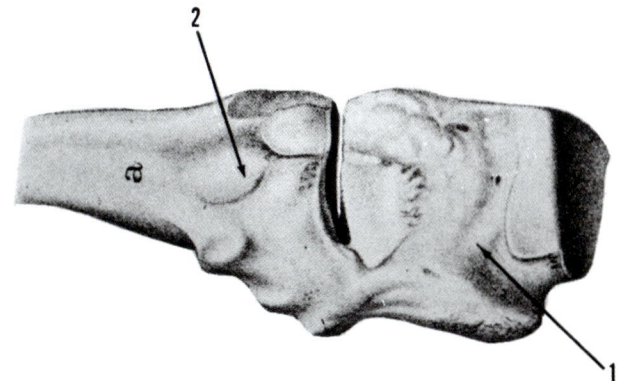

Figure 2.92 Cuneo3-**metatarsal**3 **coalition.** (*1*, third cuneiform; *2*, third metatarsal.) (From Pfitzner W. Beiträge zur Kenntnis des Menschlichen Extremitätenskelets: VI. Die Variationen in Aufbau des Fussskelets. In: Schwalbe, ed. *Morphologische Arbeiten*. Gustav Fischer; 1896:245-527.)

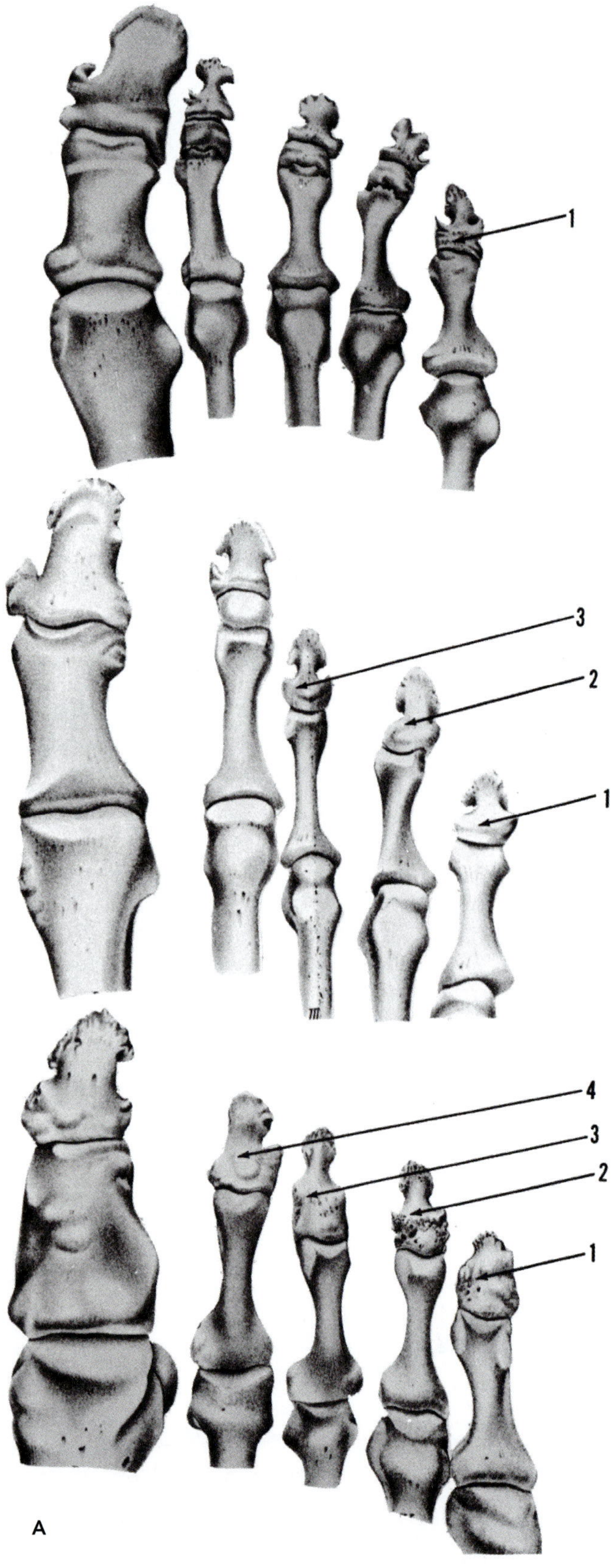

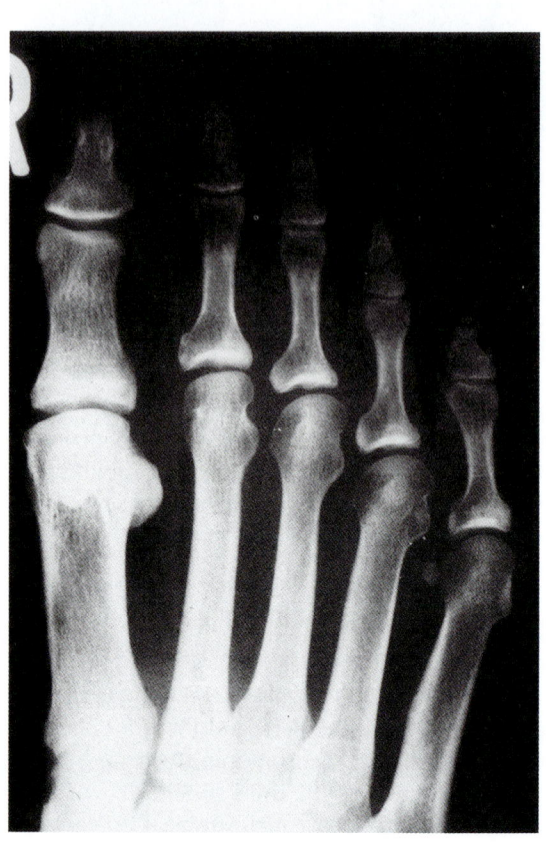

Figure 2.93 Middle and distal phalanges. (A) Interphalangeal coalition of middle and distal phalanges of toe 5 (*1*), toe 4 (*2*), toe 3 (*3*), and toe 2 (*4*). **(B)** Roentgenogram demonstrating coalition of middle and distal phalanges of all lesser toes. **(C)** Roentgenograms of coalition of middle and distal phalanges of toes 4 and 5 on the right and of toes 3, 4, and 5 on the left. **(D)** Dorsal aspect of little toe with coalition of middle and distal phalanges. **(E)** Symphalagism in the fifth toe. (**A**, From Pfitzner W. Beiträge zur Kenntnis des Menschlichen Extremitätenskelets: VI. Die Variationen in Aufbau des Fussskelets. In: Schwalbe, ed. *Morphologische Arbeiten*. Gustav Fischer; 1896:245-527. **E**, From Zollner F. *Leonardo da Vinci 1452-1519: The Complete Paintings and Drawings*. Kohn; 2003:433.)

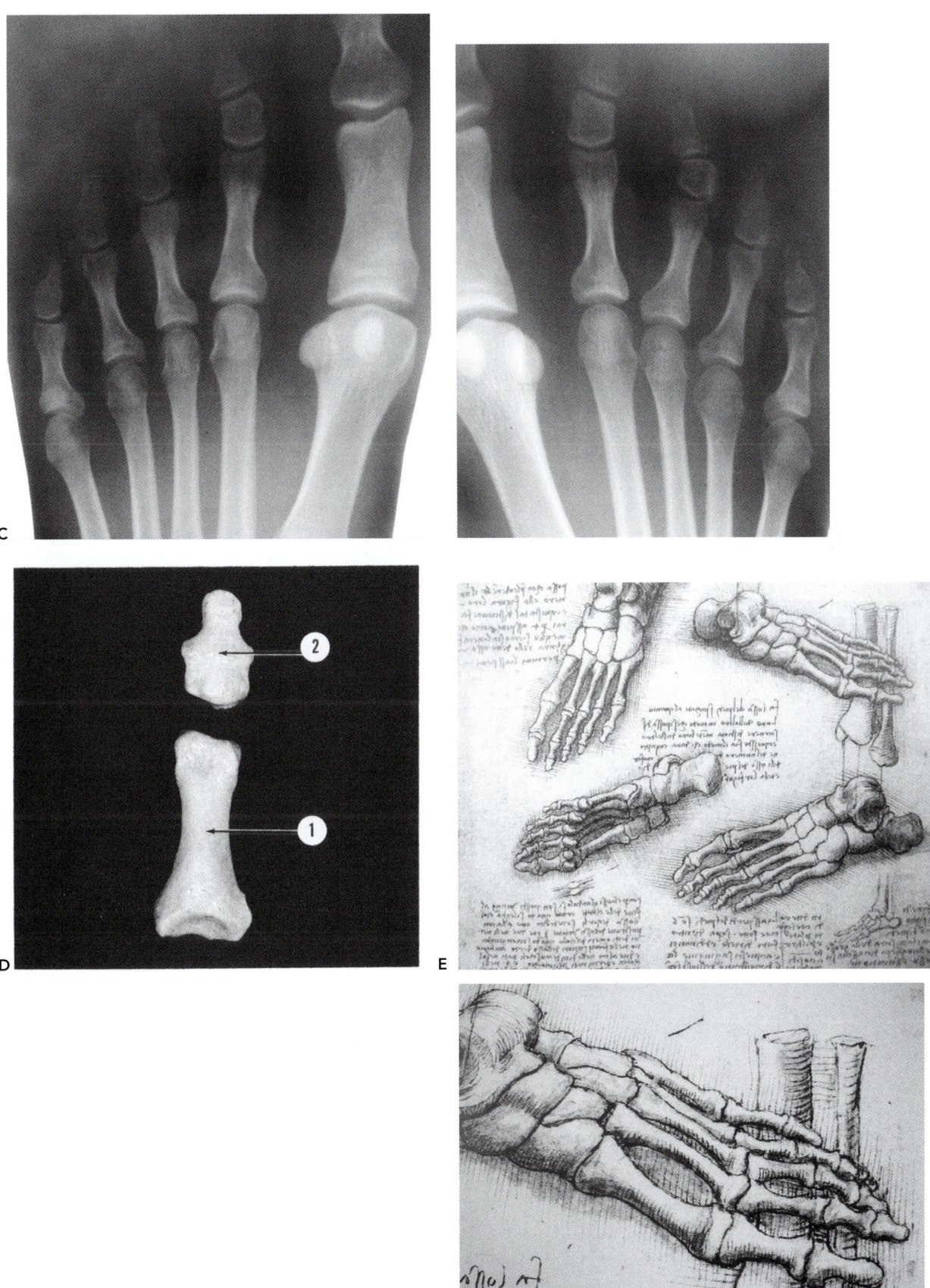

Figure 2.93 cont'd

not present in the fifth, nor the third if not present in the fourth and fifth, nor the second if not present already in the lesser three toes. The symphalangism in the Japanese population was reported as 72.5%.[180]

▶ Multiple, Massive, and Associated Coalitions

Cruveilhier, Lagrange, and Morestin have described multiple coalitions in the same foot.[44,109,176] Massive or multiple tarsal coalitions are recorded in the literature.[181-190]

Tarsal coalitions may also occur in association with other malformations: carpal fusions, carpal synostosis with radial head subluxation, symphalangism, and partial adactylia.[154,188-193] This may also occur in the following clinical entities: type I acrocephalosyndactyly (Apert syndrome),[171] hand-foot-uterus syndrome,[194] craniofacial dysostosis (Crouzon syndrome),[194] acropectorovertebral dysplasia (F syndrome),[194] arthrogryposis (occasionally),[194] and otopalatodigital syndrome.[194]

The occurrence of massive or multiple tarsal synostoses in Nievergelt-Pearlman syndrome is well established. Murakami, reporting 3 cases and reviewing the total of 13 cases in the literature, found tarsal fusions in 12.[195]

BIPARTITION

▶ Bipartite First Cuneiform

The bipartite first cuneiform was first described by Morel.[196] Four cuneiforms were present in the left foot, and a trace of partition was observed in the first cuneiform of the right foot.

The presence of this skeletal variation has been recorded by anatomists.[197-202] Gruber observed 10 complete and 5 incomplete bipartitions, and in a study of 2500 ft, the frequency of occurrence of a perfect bipartition was reported as 1 in 320.[203,204] Pfitzner, examining 750 ft, found and illustrated two bipartite first cuneiforms (Fig. 2.94).[18] Hartman and Mordret observed two such variations in 200 ft.[205] Roentgenographic recognition of the bipartition of this bone was reported early by many authors.[206-210] Barclay, after describing the roentgenographic recognition of this anatomic variation bilaterally in a jockey aged 34 years, mentioned that "cases of partial division seem to be fairly common, and several examples were found in the osteological collection here," and she produced diagrams of two such specimens.[208]

Barlow gave the following anatomic description of a bilateral bipartite first cuneiform in a male aged 82 years[211]:

The bone is divided by a horizontal cleft into a dorsal small and a plantar larger segment. A diarthrodial joint is present between these two segments on the medial half of the cleft. The *dorsal segment* articulates anteriorly with the dorsal part of the first metatarsal base. Its posterior surface articulates with the navicular. The superomedial surface gives attachment to ligaments connecting to the bones with which it articulates. The lateral surface is articular in the posterior half with the middle cuneiform. The anterior half of this lateral surface articulates with the second metatarsal base dorsally and gives insertion in its plantar half to the interosseous ligament. The inferior surface gives insertion laterally to a strong interosseous ligament uniting the dorsal plantar segments and the middle cuneiform. The *plantar segment* articulates anteriorly with the base of the first metatarsal and posteriorly with the navicular. The medial surface gives insertion to the tibialis anterior at the anteroinferior angle. The inferior surface has a prominent tubercle at its proximal end for the attachment of a portion of the tibialis posterior. A tubercle at the anteroinferior angle of the lateral surface gives insertion to the peroneus longus tendon. The two segments of the bipartite 1 cuneiform are together slightly larger than an undivided medial cuneiform.

▶ Bipartite Navicular

The bipartite navicular was not recognized prior to the roentgenographic era. In 1937, Volk reported on two cases of bipartite navicular.[212] Zimmer, in 1938, described roentgenographically

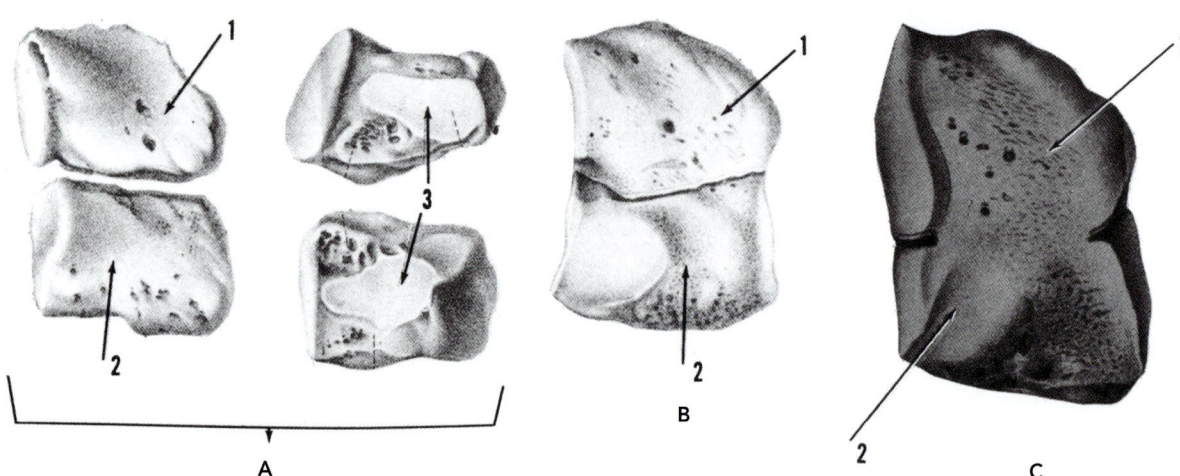

Figure 2.94 Bipartite cuneiform I. **(A)** Articulated. **(B)** Nonosseous union. **(C)** Fused. (*1*, dorsal; *2*, plantar; *3*, articular surface.) (From Pfitzner W. Beiträge zur Kenntnis des Menschlichen Extremitätenskelets: VI. Die Variationen in Aufbau des Fussskelets. In: Schwalbe, ed. *Morphologische Arbeiten*. Gustav Fischer; 1896:245-527.)

and histologically a case of bipartite navicular in a 19-year-old patient.[213] Roentgenographically, on the dorsoplantar view, the smaller fragment is a comma-shaped structure measuring 12 mm by 21 mm, superimposed on the first and second cuneiforms and the main navicular segment. On the lateral view, the smaller fragment is dorsal in location, triangular in contour, separated from the main navicular fragment by a cleft directed upward and anteriorly. No disease could be found histologically.

In 1941, Fine Licht reported on four cases, two of which were bilateral.[214] Typically, on the dorsoplantar projection of the roentgenogram, the smaller fragment is wedge-shaped, with the base directed medially and the apex laterally. On the lateral view, the same fragment is again wedge-shaped, and the apex is directed in a plantar direction.

Sporadic reporting of individual cases of bipartite navicular is further found in the literature.[215,216]

REFERENCES

1. Lang J, Wachsmuth W. *Praktische Anatomie Bein und Statik*. Vol 353. Springer-Verlag; 1972:361.
2. Manter JT. Movements of the subtalar and transverse tarsal joints. *Anat Rec*. 1941;80:397.
3. Edwards ME. The relations of the peroneal tendons to the fibula, calcaneus and cuboideum. *Am J Anat*. 1928;42(1):213.
4. Ozbag D, Gumusalan Y, Uzel M. Ercan cetinus morphometrical features of the human malleolar groove. *Foot Ankle Int*. 2008;1:77-81.
5. Inman VT. *The Joints of the Ankle*. Williams & Wilkins; 1976:2-97.
6. Wood WQ. The tibia of the Australian aboriginie. *J Anat*. 1920;52:232.
7. Singh I. Squatting facets on the talus and tibia in Indians. *J Anat*. 1959;93:540.
8. Testut L. *Traité d'Anatomie Humaine*. Vol 1. 7th ed. Doin; 1921:368.
9. Paturet G. *Traité d'Anatomie Humaine*. Vol 2. Masson; 1951:573.
10. Sewell RBS. A study of the astragalus, Part II. *J Anat Physiol*. 1904;38:423.
11. Poirier P, Charpy A. *Traité d'Anatomie Humaine*. Vol 1. Masson; 1899:263-264, 758.
12. Barnett CH. Squatting facets on the European talus. *J Anat Physiol*. 1954;88:509.
13. Barnett CH, Napier JR. The axis of rotation at the ankle joint in man: its influence upon the form of the talus and the mobility of the fibula. *J Anat*. 1952;86:1.
14. Martus JE, Fermino JE, Caird MS, et al. Accessory anterolateral facet of the pediatric talus. An anatomical study. *J Bone Joint Surg Am*. 2008;90:2452-2459.
15. Rouvière H, Canela Lazaro M. Le ligament péroneo-astragalo-calcanéen. *Ann Anat Pathol*. 1932;9(7):745.
16. Thomson A, Report of Committee of Collection Investigation of the Anatomical Society of Great Britain and Ireland for the year 1899-1890. *J Anat Physiol*. 1891;25:98.
17. Stieda L. Der Talus und das Os Trigonum Bardelebens beim Menschen. *Anat Anz*. 1899;4:305-351.
18. Pfitzner W. Beiträge zur Kenntnis des Menschlichen Eextremitätenskelets: VI. Die Variationen in Aufbau des Fussskelets. In: Schwalbe, ed. *Morphologische Arbeiten*. Gustav Fischer; 1896:245-527.
19. Storton CE. In: Grant JCB, ed. *Grant's Atlas of Anatomy*. 5th ed. Williams & Wilkins; 1962.
20. Farabeuf LH. In: Nouvelle, ed. *Précis de Manuel Opératoire*. Masson; 1889:80.
21. Jones FW. *Structure and Function as Seen in the Foot*. 2nd ed. Baillière Tindall & Cox; 1949:39-120.
22. Sewell RBS. A study of the astragalus. Part IV. *J Anat Physiol*. 1906;40:152.
23. Gamble FO, Yale I. *Clinical Foot Roentgenology*. Williams & Wilkins; 1966:153.
24. Steindler A. *Kinesiology of the Human Body*. 3rd ed. Charles C Thomas; 1970:405.
25. Laidlaw PP. The varieties of the os calcis. *J Anat Physiol*. 1904;38:133.
26. Boehler L. Diagnosis, pathology and treatment of fractures of the os calcis. *J Bone Joint Surg*. 1931;13:77.
27. Bunning PSC, Barnett CH. A comparison of adult and foetal talocalcaneal articulations. *J Anat*. 1965;99:71.
28. Padmanabhan R. The talar facets of the calcaneus. An anatomical note. *Anat Anz*. 1986;161:389.
29. Gruber W. Uber den eine Thierbildung Reprasentirenden Normalen, und uber den Exostotisch Gewordenen Processus Trochlearis Calcanei. *Virchows Arch [Pathol Anat]*. 1877;70:128.
30. Stieda L, Der M. Peroneus Longus und die Fussknochen. *Anat Anz*. 1889;4:600-661.
31. Agarwal AK, Jeyasingh P, Gupta SC, et al. Peroneal tubercle and its variations in the Indian calcanei. *Anat Anz*. 1984;156:241.
32. Hyer CF, Dawson JM, Philbin TM, et al. The peroneal tubercle: description, classification, and relevance to peroneus longus tendon pathology. *Foot Ankle Int*. 2005;11:947-950.
33. Morestin H. Note pour servir à l'étude de l'anatomie du calcaneum. *Bull Soc Anat Paris*. 1894;69:737.
34. Laidlaw PP. The os calcis: part II. *J Anat Physiol*. 1905;39:168.
35. Manners-Smith T. A study of the cuboid and os peroneum in the primate foot. *J Anat Physiol*. 1908;42:399.
36. Gruber W. Ueber den Fortsatz des Höckers des Kahnbeins der Fusswurzel—Processus Tuberositatis Navicularis—und dessen Auftreten als Epiphyse oder als Besonderes Arti-kulirendes Knochelchen. *Arch Anat Physiol Wiss Med*. 1871;8A:281.
37. Manners-Smith T. A study of the navicular in the human and anthropoid foot. *J Anat Physiol*. 1907;41:261.
38. Dwight T. *Variations of the Bones of the Hands and Feet: A Clinical Atlas*. JB Lippincott; 1907:14-23.
39. Barclay-Smith E. The astragalo-calcaneo-navicular joint. *J Anat Physiol*. 1896;30:399.
40. Breathnack AS, ed. *Frazer's Anatomy of the Human Skeleton*. 6th ed. Little Brown; 1965:149.
41. Ajmani ML, Ajmani K, Jain SP. Variations in the articular facets of the adult cuneiform bones. *Anthropol Anz*. 1984;42:121.
42. Straus WL Jr. Growth of the human foot and its evolutionary significance. *Contrib Embryol*. 1927;19(101):116-119.
43. Kelikian H. *Hallux Valgus Allied Deformities of the Forefoot and Metatarsalgia*. WB Saunders; 1965:102-112.
44. Leboucq H. Le développement du premier métatarsien et de son articulation tarsienne chez l'homme. *Arch Biol*. 1882;3:343.
45. Morton DJ. *The Human Foot: Its Evolution, Physiology and Functional Disorders*. Columbia University Press; 1935:179.
46. Singh I. Variations in the metatarsal bones. *J Anat*. 1960;94:345.
47. Romash MM, Fugate D, Yanklowit B. Passive motion of the first metatarso-cuneiform joint: preoperative assessment. *Foot Ankle*. 1990;10(6):293.
48. Wanivenhaus A, Pretterklieber M. First tarso-metatarsal joint: anatomical, biomechanical study. *Foot Ankle*. 1989;9(4):153.
49. Le Minor JM, Winter M. The intermetatarsal articular facet of the first metatarsal bone in humans: a derived trait unique within primates. *Ann Anat*. 2003;185:359-365.
50. ElSaid A, Tisdel C, Donley B, et al. First metatarsal bone: an anatomic study. *Foot Ankle Int*. 2006;12:1041-1048.
51. Hyer CF, Philbin TM, Berlet GC, et al. The obliquity of the first metatarsal base. *Foot Ankle Int*. 2004;10:728-732.
52. Batmanabane M, Malathi S. Identification of human second, third and fourth metatarsal bones. *Anat Rec*. 1983;207:509.
53. Ebraheim NA, Haman SP, Lu J, et al. Anatomical and radiological considerations of the fifth metatarsal bone. *Foot Ankle Int*. 2000;3:212-215.
54. Haines RW, McDougall A. The anatomy of hallux valgus. *J Bone Joint Surg [Br]*. 1954;36:272.
55. Wilkinson JL. The terminal phalanx of the great toe. *J Anat*. 1954;88:537.
56. Kewenter U. Die Sesambeine des I Metatarso-phalangeal-gelenks des Menschen. *Acta Orthop Scand Suppl*. 1936;2:43.
57. Gillette M. Des os sesamoides chez l'homme. *J Anat Physiol*. 1872;8:506-538.
58. Sabatier M. *Traité Complet d'Anatomie ou Description de toutes les Parties du Corps Humain*. Vol 1. Didot; 1775:231.
59. Bizarro AH. On sesamoids and supernumerary bones of the limbs. *J Anat*. 1921;55:258.

60. Pfitzner W. Die Sesambeine des Menschen. In: Schwalbe, ed. *Morphologische Arbeiten*, Vol I. Gustav Fischer; 1892:517-762.
61. Trolle D. *Accessory Bones of the Human Foot: A Radiological, Histoembryological, Comparative Anatomical and Genetic Study*. Munksgaard; 1948.
62. Miller WA, Love BP. Cartilaginous sesamoid or nodule of the interphalangeal joint of the big toe. *Foot Ankle*. 1982;2(5):291.
63. McCarthy DJ, Reed T, Abell N. The hallucal interphalangeal sesamoid. *J Am Podiatr Med Assoc*. 1986;76(6):311.
64. Masaki T. An anatomical study of the interphalangeal sesamoid of the hallux. *Nippon Seikeigeka Gakkai Zasshi*. 1984;58(4):419.
65. Anatomical Society. Collective investigation. Sesamoids in the gastrocnemius and peroneus longus. *J Anat Physiol*. 1897;32:182.
66. Kohler A, Zimmer EA. Borderlands of the Normal and Early Pathologic in Skeletal Roentgenology. 3rd ed. Grune & Stratton; 1968:460-507.
67. O'Rahilly R. Developmental deviations in the carpus and the tarsus. *Clin Orthop*. 1957;10:9.
68. Marti T. *Die Skelettvarietaten des Fusses ihre Klinische und Unfallmedizinische Bedentug*. Hans Huber; 1947:27-111.
69. O'Rahilly R. A survey of carpal and tarsal anomalies. *J Bone Joint Surg [Am]*. 1953;35:635.
70. Mouchet A, Moutier G. Osselets surnumeraires du tarse (ossa tarsalia). *Presse Med*. 1925;23:370.
71. Harris RI, Beath T. *Army Foot Survey*. Vol 1. National Research Council of Canada; 1947:52.
72. Hoerr NL, Pyle DI, Francis CC. *Radiographic Atlas of Skeletal Development of the Foot and Ankle, A Standard of Reference*. Charles C Thomas; 1962:41-44.
73. Holland CT. *The Accessory Bones of the Foot with Notes on a Few Other Conditions, the Robert Jones Birthday Volume*. Oxford University Press; 1928:160-170.
74. Zadek I, Gold AM. The accessory tarsal scaphoid. *J Bone Joint Surg [Am]*. 1948;30:957.
75. Gruber W. *Abhandlungen aus er Menschlichen und Vergleichenden Anatomie*. St. Petersburg University; 1852:111-113.
76. Schinz HR. In: Case JT, ed. *Roentgen-Diagnostics*. Grune & Stratton; 1951:124.
77. Friedl E. Das Os Intermetatarseum und die Epiphysenbildung am Processus Trochlearis Calcanei. *Dtsch Z Chir*. 1924;188:150.
78. Henderson RS. Os intermetatarseum and possible relationship to hallux valgus. *J Bone Joint Surg [Br]*. 1963;45:117.
79. Faber A. Ueber das Os Intermetatarseum. *Orthop Chir*. 1934;61:186.
80. Stieda L. Ueber sekundare fusswurzelknochen. *Arch Anat Physiol Wiss Med*. 1869;5:108.
81. Gruber W. Uber einen Neven Secundaren Tarsalknochen-Calcaneus Secundarius-mit Bemerkungen uber den Tarsus uber haupt. *Mém Acad Impériale Sci Saint-Petersbourg*. 1871;7:1.
82. Dwight T. Description of a free cuboides secundarium, with remarks on that element and on the calcaneus secundarius. *Anat Anz*. 1910;37:218.
83. Hyrtl J. Ueber die Trochlearfortsatze der Menschlichen Knochen. *Denkschrift Wiener Akad Math Naturaw*. 1860;18:141.
84. Pirie AH. A normal ossicle in the foot frequently diagnosed as a fracture. *Arch Radiol Electrother*. 1920;24:93.
85. Pirie AH. Extra bones in the wrist and ankle found by roentgen rays. *Am J Roentgenol*. 1921;8:573.
86. Dwight R. Os intercuneiforme tarsi, os paracuneiforme tarsi, calcaneus secundarius. *Anat Anz*. 1902;20:465.
87. Dameron TB Jr. Fractures and anatomical variations of the proximal portion of the fifth metatarsal. *J Bone Joint Surg [Am]*. 1975;57(6):788.
88. Laquerrière D. On the vesalian bone. *J Radiol Elec*. 1916;395.
89. Powell HDW. Extra centre of ossification for the medial malleolus in children: incidence and significance. *J Bone Joint Surg [Br]*. 1961;43(1):107.
90. Leimbach G. Beitrage zur Kenntnis der inkonstanten Skeletelamente des Tarsus (Akzessorische Fusswurzelknochen) (Untersuchunger an 500 rontgenbidern der Chir. Universitatsklinik zn Jen). *Arch Orthop Trauma Surg*. 1937;38:431.
91. Bjornson RGB. Developmental anomaly of the lateral malleolus simulating fracture. *J Bone Joint Surg [Am]*. 1956;38:128.
92. Griffiths JD. Symptomatic ossicles of the lateral malleolus in children. *J Bone Joint Surg [Br]*. 1987;69(2):317.
93. Harris RI. Follow-up notes on articles previously published in the J Retrospect: peroneal spastic flat foot (rigid valgus foot). *J Bone Joint Surg [Am]*. 1965;47(8):1657.
94. Stromont DM, Peterson HA. The relative incidence of tarsal coalition. *Clin Orthop Relat Res*. 1983;181:28-36.
95. Zuckerkandl E. Ueber einen Fall von synostose zwischen Talus und Calcaneus. *Allgem Wiener Med Z*. 1877;22:292.
96. Chaput. Etude anatomo-pathologique de deux pièces de pied plat valgus (tarsalgie des adolescents) guéris par ankylose, suivie de quelques considérations sur la pathogénie et le mécanisme de ces lésions. *Progres Med*. 1886;14:857.
97. Leboucq H. De la soudure congénitale de certains os du tarse. *Bull Acad Med Brux*. 1890;4:103.
98. Morestin H. De l'ankylose calcaneo-astragalienne. *Bull Soc Anat Paris*. 1894;69:985.
99. Bentzon PGK. Bilateral congenital deformity of the astragalo-calcaneal joint: bone coalescence between os trigonum and the calcaneus. *Acta Orthop Scand*. 1930;1:359.
100. Burman MS, Sinberg SE. An anomalous talocalcaneal articulation: double ankle bones. *Radiology*. 1940;34:239.
101. Gaynor SS. Congenital astragalocalcaneal fusion. *J Bone Joint Surg*. 1936;18:479.
102. Grashey R. Articulatio talo-calcanea (os sustentaculi). *Rontgenpraxis*. 1942;14:139.
103. Sutro C. Anomalous talo-calcaneal articulation: cause for limited subtalar movements. *Am J Surg*. 1947;74:64.
104. Harris RI, Beath T. Etiology of peroneal spastic flat foot. *J Bone Joint Surg [Br]*. 1948;30:624.
105. Maier K. Beitrage zur Verschmelzung des Os Trigonum mit dem Kalkaneus. *Fortschr Geb Rontgenst*. 1963;98:664.
106. Outland T, Murphy ID. Relation of tarsal anomalies to spastic and rigid flat feet. *Clin Orthop*. 1953;1:217.
107. Shands AR, Wentz IJ. Congenital anomalies, accessory bones and osteochondritis in the feet of 850 children. *Surg Clin*. 1953;33:1643.
108. Conway JJ, Cowell HR. Tarsal coalition: clinical significance and roentgenographic demonstration. *Radiology*. 1969;92:799.
109. Cruveilhier J. *Anatomie Pathologique du Corps Humain ou Descriptions, avec Figures Lithographiées et Colorées des Diverses Altérations Morbides dont le Corps Humain est Susceptible*. Vol 1. Baillière; 1829-1835.
110. Wedding CF. *Quaedam de Ancylosibus*. Berolinum; 1832:24.
111. Smith RW. Congenital malformation of the tarsus. *Dublin Q J Med Sci*. 1850;9:109.
112. Verneuil. In: Robert A, ed. *Des Vices Congénitaux de Conformation des Articulations*. Thesis; 1851.
113. Gurlt E. *Beiträge zur vergleichenden pathologischen Anatomie der Gelenkkrankheiten*. MV Medizen (Verlag); 1853:620.
114. Humphrey GM. *A Treatise on the Human Skeleton*. Macmillian and Company; 1858:80.
115. Gruber W. *Beobarhtungen aus der Menschlichen und Vergleichenden Anatomie*. Vol 1. 1879:15-18.
116. Zuckerkandl E. Neue Mittheilungen über coalition von Fusswurzelknochen. *Wien Med Jahrb*. 1880;125.
117. Holl M. Beiträge zur chirurgischen Osteologie des Fusses. *Langenbecks Arch Klin Chir*. 1880;25:211.
118. Weber M. Ober coalescentia calcaneo-navicularis. *Versl Med Kongl Acad Vmet Afd Naturk*. 1882;121.
119. Petrini P. *Articulation anomale entre le calcaneum et le scaphoide*. In: Atti del' XI Cong Med Internaz Roma. Vol 2. Anatomia; 1894:71-79.
120. Morestin H. Note sur un scaphoide s'articulant par de larges facettes avec le cuboide et le calcaneum. *Bull Soc Anat Paris*. 1894;69:798.
121. Slomann HC. On coalition calcaneo-navicularis. *J Orthop Surg*. 1921;19:586.
122. Slomann HC. On the demonstration and analysis of calcaneo-navicular coalition by roentgen examination. *Acta Radiol*. 1926;5:304.
123. Badgley CE. Coalition of the calcaneus and the navicular. *Arch Surg*. 1927;15:75.
124. Bentzon PG. Coalitio Calcaneo-navicularis, mit besonderes Bezungnahme auf die operative Behandlung des durch diese Anomalie bedingten Plattfusses. *Verh Dtsch Orthop Ges*. 1929;23:269.
125. Seddon HJ. Calcaneo-scaphoid coalition. *Proc Roy Soc Med*. 1933;26:419.
126. Herschel H, Von Ronnen JR. The occurrence of calcaneo navicular synostosis in pes valgus contracture. *J Bone Joint Surg [Am]*. 1950;32:280.
127. Hark FW. Congenital anomalies of the tarsal bones. *Clin Orthop*. 1960;16:21.
128. Kendrick JJ. Treatment of calcaneo-navicular bar. *J Am Med Assoc*. 1960;172:1242.
129. Braddock GTF. A prolonged follow-up of peroneal spastic flat foot. *J Bone Joint Surg [Br]*. 1961;43:734.

130. Rutt A. Zur genese der coalitio calcaneo-naviculare. *Z Orthop.* 1962;96:96.
131. Simmons EH. Tibialis spastic varus foot with tarsal coalition. *J Bone Joint Surg [Br].* 1965;47:533.
132. Mitchell GP, Gibson JMC. Excision of calcaneonavicular bar for painful spasmodic flat foot. *J Bone Joint Surg [Br].* 1967;49:281.
133. Heikel HUA. Coalitio calcaneo-navicularis and calcaneus secundarius. *Acta Orthop Scand.* 1961;31:78.
134. Webster FS, Roberts WM. Tarsal anomalies and peroneal spastic flat foot. *J Am Med Assoc.* 1951;146:1099.
135. Wray JB, Herndon CN. Hereditary transmission of congenital coalition of the calcaneus to the navicular. *J Bone Joint Surg [Am].* 1963;45:365.
136. Glessner JR Jr, Davis GL. Bilateral calcaneonavicular coalition occurring in twin boys. *Clin Orthop.* 1966;47:173.
137. Leonard MA. The inheritance of tarsal coalition and its relationship to spastic flat foot. *J Bone Joint Surg [Br].* 1974;56:520.
138. Anderson RJ. The presence of an astragalo-scaphoid bone in man. *J Anat Physiol.* 1879;14:452.
139. Holland CT. Two cases of rare deformity of feet and hands. *Arch Rad Elect.* 1918;22:234.
140. Blencke H. Ein seltner Fall von Synostosis talonavicularis. *Z Orthop Chir.* 1925-1926;47:594.
141. Esau P. Angeborene Missbildungen der Füsse (randdefekt). *Dtsch Z Cir.* 1925-1926;194:263.
142. Bullitt JB. Variations of the bones of the foot: fusion of the talus and navicular, bilateral and congenital. *Am J Radiol.* 1928;20:548.
143. Illievitz AB. Congenital malformations of the feet: report of a case of congenital fusion of the scaphoid with the astragalus and complete absence of one toe. *Am J Surg.* 1928;4:550.
144. Haglund P. Ein fall von vollständiger coalitio talo-navicularis. *Z Orthop Chir.* 1929;51:93.
145. Lapidus PR. Congenital fusion of the bones of the foot with a report of a case of congenital astragaloscaphoid fusion. *J Bone Joint Surg.* 1932;14:888.
146. Hayek W. Synostosis talonavicularis. *Z Orthop Chir.* 1934;60:231.
147. Rothberg AS, Feldman FW, Schuster OF. Congenital fusion of astragalus and scaphoid: bilateral, inherited. *NY Med.* 1935;35:29.
148. Lapidus PW. Bilateral congenital talonavicular fusion: report of a case. *J Bone Joint Surg.* 1938;20:775.
149. Jaubert de Beaujeu A, Benmussa. Synostose, astragaloscaphoidienne congénitale bilatérale et isolée. *J Radiol Elect.* 1939;23:348.
150. O'Donoghue DH, Sell LS. Congenital talonavicular synostosis: a case report of a rare anomaly. *J Bone Joint Surg.* 1943;25:925.
151. Boyd HB. Congenital talonavicular synostosis. *J Bone Joint Surg.* 1944;26:682.
152. Weitzner I. Congenital talonavicular synostosis associated with hereditary multiple ankylosing arthropathies. *Am J Roentgenol.* 1946;56:185.
153. Chambers CH. Congenital anomalies of the tarsal navicular with particular reference to calcaneo-navicular coalition. *Br J Radiol.* 1950;33:584.
154. Austin FH. Symphalangism and related fusions of tarsal bones. *Radiology.* 1951;56:882.
155. Sanghi JK, Roby HR. Bilateral peroneal spastic flat feet associated with congenital fusion of the navicular and talus: a case report. *J Bone Joint Surg [Am].* 1961;43:1237.
156. Challis J. Hereditary transmission of talonavicular coalition in association with anomaly of the little finger. *J Bone Joint Surg [Am].* 1974;56:1273.
157. Schreiber RR. Talonavicular synostosis. *J Bone Joint Surg [Am].* 1963;45(1):170.
158. Auzias. In: Robert A. *Des vices congénitaux de conformation des articulations.* Thesis; 1851:22.
159. Wagoner GW. A case of bilateral congenital fusion of the calcanei and cuboids. *J Bone Joint Surg.* 1928;10:220.
160. Bargellini D. Fusione calcaneo-cuboidea e piede piatto. *Arch Ital Chir.* 1928;21:386.
161. Esau P. Angeborene Synostose im Bereich des Carpus und Tarsus. *Rontgenpraxis.* 1933;5:235.
162. Rey. Angeborene Verschmelzung von Calcaneus und Kuboid. *Zentralbl Chir.* 1932;59:1666.
163. Mestern J. Erbliche Synostosen den Hand-eund Fusswurzelknochen. *Rontgenpraxis.* 1934;6:594.
164. Veneruso L. Unilateral congenital calcaneo-cuboid synostosis with complete absence of a metatarsal and toe. *J Bone Joint Surg.* 1945;27:718.
165. Mahaffey HW. Bilateral congenital calcaneo cuboid synostosis. *J Bone Joint Surg.* 1945;27:164.
166. Brobeck O. Congenital bilateral synosteosis of the calcaneus and cuboid and of the triquetral and hamate bones. *Acta Orthop Scand.* 1956;25:217.
167. Stern AM, Gall JC Jr, Perry BL, et al. The hand-foot-uterus syndrome. *J Pediatr.* 1970;77:109.
168. Poznanski AK, Stern AM, Gall JC Jr. Radiographic findings in hand-foot-uterus syndrome (HFUS). *Radiology.* 1970;96:129.
169. Kelikian H. *Congenital Deformities of the Hand and Forearm.* WB Saunders; 1974:131.
170. Kozlowski K. Hypoplasie bilatérale congénitale du cubitus et synostose bilatérale calcanéo-cuboide chez une fillette. *Ann Radiol.* 1965;1-2:389.
171. Schauerte EW, St Aubin PM. Progressive synosteosis in Apert's syndrome (acrocephalosyndactyly): with a description of roentgenographic changes in the feet. *Am J Roentgenol.* 1966;97:67.
172. Craig CL, Goldberg MJ. Calcaneo-cuboid coalition in Crouzon's syndrome. *J Bone Joint Surg [Am].* 1977;59:826.
173. Gruber W. Ueber einen neuen sekundären tarsalknochen—Calcaneus secundarius—mit Bemerkungen über den Tarsus über-haupt. *Mem Acad Sci St. Petersbourg.* 1871;17:6.
174. Waugh W. Partial cubo-navicular coalition as a case of peroneal spastic flat foot. *J Bone Joint Surg [Br].* 1957;39:520.
175. Del Sel JM, Grand NE. Cubo-navicular synostosis. *J Bone Joint Surg [Br].* 1959;41:149.
176. Lagrange M. Anomalie du pied, soudure des os du tarse et du métatarse. *Progr Med.* 1882;10:367.
177. Lusby JLJ. Naviculo-cuneiform synostosis. *J Bone Joint Surg [Br].* 1959;41:149.
178. Gregersen HN. Naviculocuneiform coalition. *J Bone Joint Surg [Am].* 1977;59:128.
179. Zollner F. *Leonardo da Vinci 1452-1519: The Complete Paintings and Drawings.* Kohn; 2003:433.
180. Nakashima T, Hojo T, Suzuki K, Ijichi M. Symphalangism (two phalanges) in the digits of the Japanese foot. *Ann Anat.* 1995;177:275-278.
181. Bersani FA, Samilson RL. Massive familial tarsal synostosis. *J Bone Joint Surg [Am].* 1957;39:1187.
182. Basu SS. Naviculo-cuneo-metatarso phalangeal synostosis. *Indian J Surg.* 1963;25:750.
183. Kadelbach G. Ein Beiträg zu den Fusswurzelsynostosen. *Arch Orthop Unfallchir.* 1940;40:363.
184. Sloane MWM. A case of anomalous skeletal development in the foot. *Anat Rec.* 1946;96:23.
185. Zock E. Ein Beiträg zu den synostosen der Fusswurzel. *Zentralbl Chir.* 1953;78:845.
186. Vizkelety T. Eine seltene Form der Synostose der Fusswurzelknochen. *Z Orthop.* 1963;97:245.
187. Rompe G. Ankylosen der Unteren Sprunggelenkes nach offenem Unterschenkelbruch. *Arch Orthop Unfallchir.* 1962;54:339.
188. Pearlman HS, Edkin RE, Warren RF. Familial tarsal and carpal synostosis with radial head subluxation. *J Bone Joint Surg [Am].* 1964;46:585.
189. Miller EM. Congenital ankylosis of joints of hands and feet. *J Bone Joint Surg.* 1922;4:560.
190. Lissoos I, Soussi J. Tarsal synostosis with partial adactylia. *Med Proc.* 1965;11:224.
191. Devoldere J. A case of familial congenital synostosis in the carpal and tarsal bones. *Arch Chir Neerl.* 1960;12:185.
192. Slater P, Rubinstein H. Aplasia of interphalangeal joints associated with synostoses of carpal and tarsal bones. *Q Bull Sea View Hosp.* 1942;7:429.
193. Harle TS, Stevenson JR. Hereditary symphalangism associated with carpal and tarsal fusions. *Radiology.* 1967;89:91.
194. Poznanski AK. *The Hand in Radiologic Diagnosis.* WB Saunders; 1974.
195. Murakami Y. Nievergelt-Pearlman syndrome with impairment of hearing. *J Bone Joint Surg [Br].* 1975;57(3):367.
196. Morel. *Diversités Anatomiques: Recueil Period d'Observ,* VII. 1757:432-434.
197. Jones S. A right foot showing two internal cuneiforms. *Trans Pathol Soc.* 1864;15:189.
198. Smith T. A foot having four cuneiforms. *Trans Pathol Soc.* 1866;17:222.
199. Turner W. Report on the progress of anatomy. *J Anat.* 1869;3:447.
200. Stieda L. Uber sekundare Fusswurzelknochen. *Mullers Arch, Arch F Anat Physio Wiss Med.* 1869;109:108-111.

201. Ledentu M. Anomalie du Squelette du pied: cunéiforme supplementaire. *Bull Soc Anat Ser.* 1869;14:13.
202. Friedlowsky A. Uber Vermehrung der Handwurzelknochen durch ein Os Carpale Intermedium und uber sekundare Fusswurzelknochen. *Sitzungsber Akad Wissensbh.* 1870;61:591.
203. Gruber W. Vorlänfige Mittheilung über die secundären Fusswurzelknochen des Mensche. *Arch Anat Physiol Wiss Med.* 1864;286-290.
204. Gruber W Monographie über das Zweigetheilte erste Keilbein der Fusswurzel—Os Cuneiforme I bipartitum Tarsi—beim Menschen. *Mem Acad Sci St. Petersbourg.* 1877;24(11):33.
205. Hartman H, Mordret J. Sur un point de l'anatomie du premier cunéiform. *Bull Soc Anat Paris.* 1889;71.
206. Hasselwander A. Studies on the ossification of the human foot. *Z Morphol.* 1903;5:466.
207. Haenisch GF. Die röntgenographie der Knochen und Gelenke und ihr Wert für die Orthopaedische Chirurgie. *Dtsch Med Wochenschr.* 1913;42:1039.
208. Barclay M. A case of duplication of the internal cuneiform bone of the foot. *J Anat.* 1932;67:175.
209. Friedl E. Divided cuneiform I in childhood. *Rontgenpraxis.* 1934;6:193.
210. Hiedsieck E. Os cuneiform I bipartitum. *Rontgenpraxis.* 1936;8:712.
211. Barlow TE. Os cuneiform I bipartitum. *Am J Phys Anthropol.* 1942;29:95.
212. Volk C. Zwei Fälle von Os naviculare pedis bipartitum. *Z Orthop Grenzgebiete.* 1937;66:396.
213. Zimmer EA. Krankheiten, Verletzungen und Varietäten des os Naviculare pedis. *Arch Orthop Unfallchir.* 1938;38:402.
214. Fine Licht E. On bipartite os naviculare pedi. *Acta Radiol.* 1941;22:377.
215. Hatoff A. Bipartite navicular bone as a cause of flat foot. *Am J Dis Child.* 1950;80:991.
216. Mau H. Zur Kenntnis des Naviculare bipartitum pedis. *Z Orthop.* 1960;93:404.

Retaining Systems and Compartments

Shahan K. Sarrafian and Armen S. Kelikian

GENERAL ORGANIZATION OF THE COMPARTMENTS

The study of the compartments of the distal leg in continuity with the compartments of the ankle and the foot provides a rational approach to their understanding.

The distal leg has four compartments: anterior, lateral, and posterior, the latter divided into superficial and deep compartments by the deep aponeurosis cruris (Fig. 3.1). The anterior compartment is formed by the anterior surfaces of the tibia and the fibula united by the interosseous membrane, the superficial aponeurosis cruris, and the anterior intermuscular septum. The lateral compartment is formed by the lateral surface of the fibula, the superficial aponeurosis cruris, the anterior intermuscular septum, and the lateral or posterior intermuscular septum. The deep posterior compartment is formed by the posterior surface of the tibia and the posteromedial surface of the fibula united by the interosseous membrane, the lateral intermuscular septum, and the deep aponeurosis cruris posteriorly and the overlapping, adherent segments of the deep and superficial aponeuroses cruris medially. The superficial posterior compartment is formed by the superficial and deep aponeurosis cruris.

Further distally, at 5 cm from the tip of the medial malleolus, the leg is divided into five compartments through the appearance of a subdivision of the deep posterior compartment on the posteromedial aspect.

At the level of the metaphysis and the ankle, the two deep posterior compartments of the leg are in continuity with the four posterior tunnels for the tibialis posterior tendon, the flexor digitorum longus tendon, the posterior tibial neurovascular bundle, and the flexor hallucis longus tendon. The lateral compartment of the leg now forms the tunnel of the peronei tendons and has shifted from a lateral to a posterior position relative to the fibula and the lateral malleolus. The superficial posterior compartment is in continuity with the tunnel of the Achilles tendon, and the anterior compartment of the leg remains as the anterior compartment in front of the distal tibia (see Fig. 3.1).

The anterior compartment is continued distally into the foot as the dorsal compartment of the foot. Posteriorly, the superficial compartment of the Achilles tendon terminates on the posterior aspect of the os calcis. In the deep posterior compartment, there is a diversion: the peroneal tunnel is directed laterally, whereas the tunnels of the tibialis posterior tendon, flexor digitorum longus, posterior tibial neurovascular bundle, and flexor hallucis longus are directed medially into the tibiotalocalcaneal tunnel, which then communicates with the sole of the foot. The tunnel of the peroneus longus tendon penetrates the sole from its lateral border.

▶ Anterior Compartment of the Distal Leg-Ankle and Dorsal Compartment of the Foot

The superficial aponeurosis cruris is reinforced at the level of the distal leg-ankle-tarsus by the superior extensor retinaculum and the inferior extensor retinaculum and continues on the dorsum of the foot as the dorsal aponeurosis reinforced on the dorsomedial aspect of the tarsometatarsal area by a transverse band.

▶ Superior Extensor Retinaculum

The superior extensor retinaculum (ligamentum transversum cruris) is a transverse aponeurotic band formed by the reinforcement of the distal segment of the superficial aponeurosis of the leg (Fig. 3.2). The proximal and distal borders are difficult to delineate and are more or less surgically created. This transverse ligament is attached laterally on the lateral crest of the lower fibula and the lateral surface of the lateral malleolus and medially on the anterior crest of the tibia and the medial malleolus. Laterally, the superior extensor retinaculum is in continuity with the superior peroneal retinaculum, and medially it is in continuity with the apical fibers of the flexor retinaculum.

The long digital extensors, the peroneus tertius tendon and the tibialis anterior tendon, pass under the ligament. In 25% of the cases, there is a separate tunnel for the tibialis anterior tendon, formed by the dissociation of the fibers into a superficial and a deep layer.[1] The apical fibers of the flexor retinaculum contribute to the formation of this tunnel by passing superficially and deep to the tibialis anterior tendon before inserting on the deep surface of the transverse ligament. The

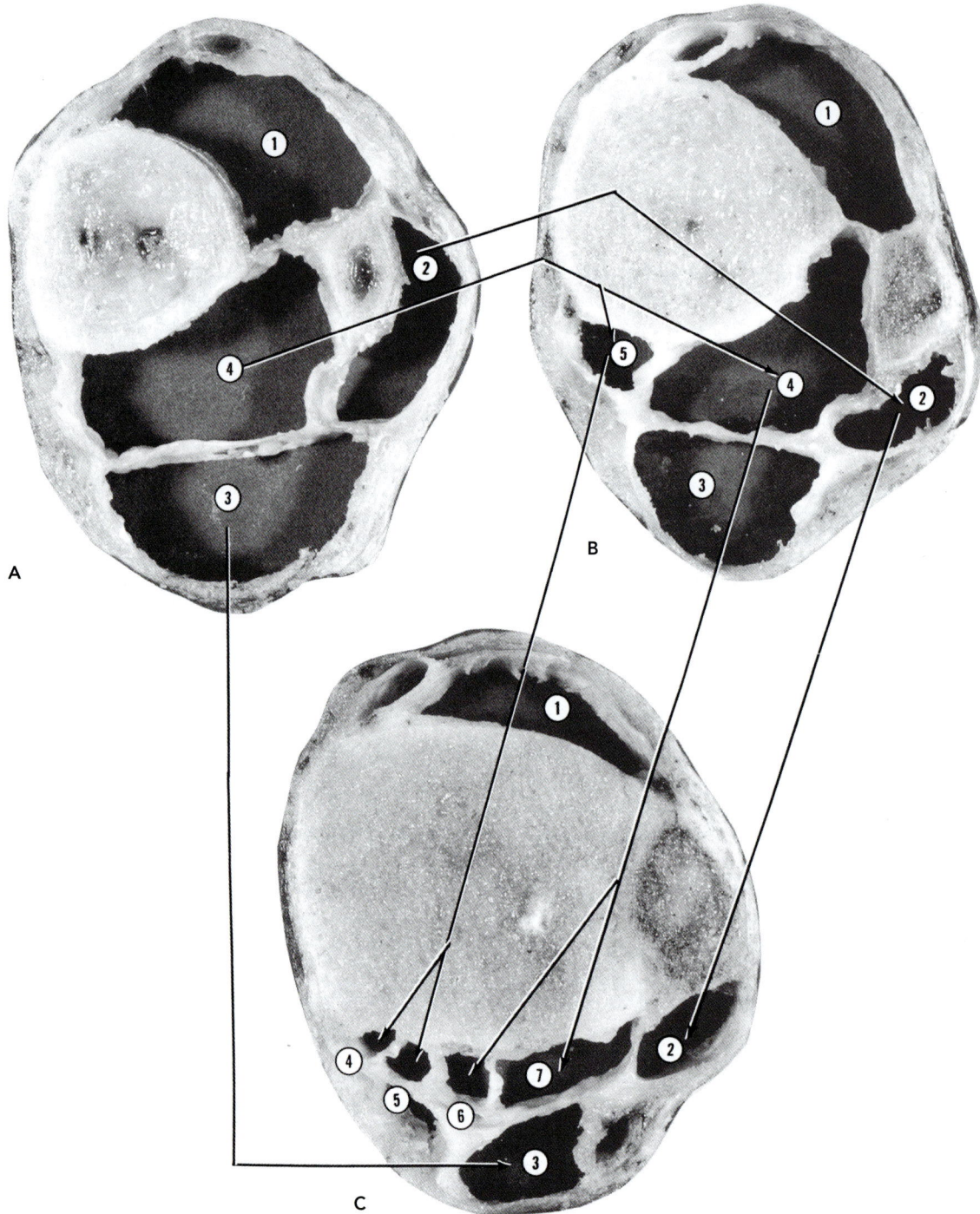

Figure 3.1 **General organization of the compartments of the distal leg.** Cross-sections of left leg at 8 cm (**A**), 5 cm (**B**), and 3 cm (**C**) from the tip of the medial malleolus. Distal surfaces of sections. (**A**) At 8 cm, four compartments are present. (*1*, Anterior; *2*, lateral; *3*, posterior superficial; *4*, posterior deep.) (**B**) At 5 cm, five compartments are present. (*1*, Anterior; *2*, lateral; *3*, posterior superficial.) The deep posterior compartment is divided now into two compartments (*4, 5*) by the appearance of an aponeurotic layer that originates from the posterior surface of the tibia medially, adheres to the deep intermuscular septum, and inserts on the posteromedial border of the tibia. Compartment 4 lodges the flexor hallucis longus muscle and the posterior tibial neurovascular bundle. Compartment 5 lodges the tibialis posterior and the flexor digitorum longus. (**C**) At 3 cm, seven compartments are present. (*1*, Anterior; *2*, lateral.) This compartment was initially (as shown in **A**) lateral and is now posterior to the lateral malleolus. The posterior superficial compartment (*3*) is getting smaller as the muscle is replaced by the Achilles tendon. The fifth compartment of **B** is subdivided into parts: 4 for the tibialis posterior tendon and 5 for the flexor digitorum longus. The deep posterior fourth compartment of **B** is also subdivided into compartment 6 for the posterior tibial neurovascular bundle and compartment 7 for the flexor hallucis longus. The deep intermuscular aponeurosis extends from the posteromedial border of the tibial metaphysis to the peroneal compartment.

Chapter 3: Retaining Systems and Compartments 121

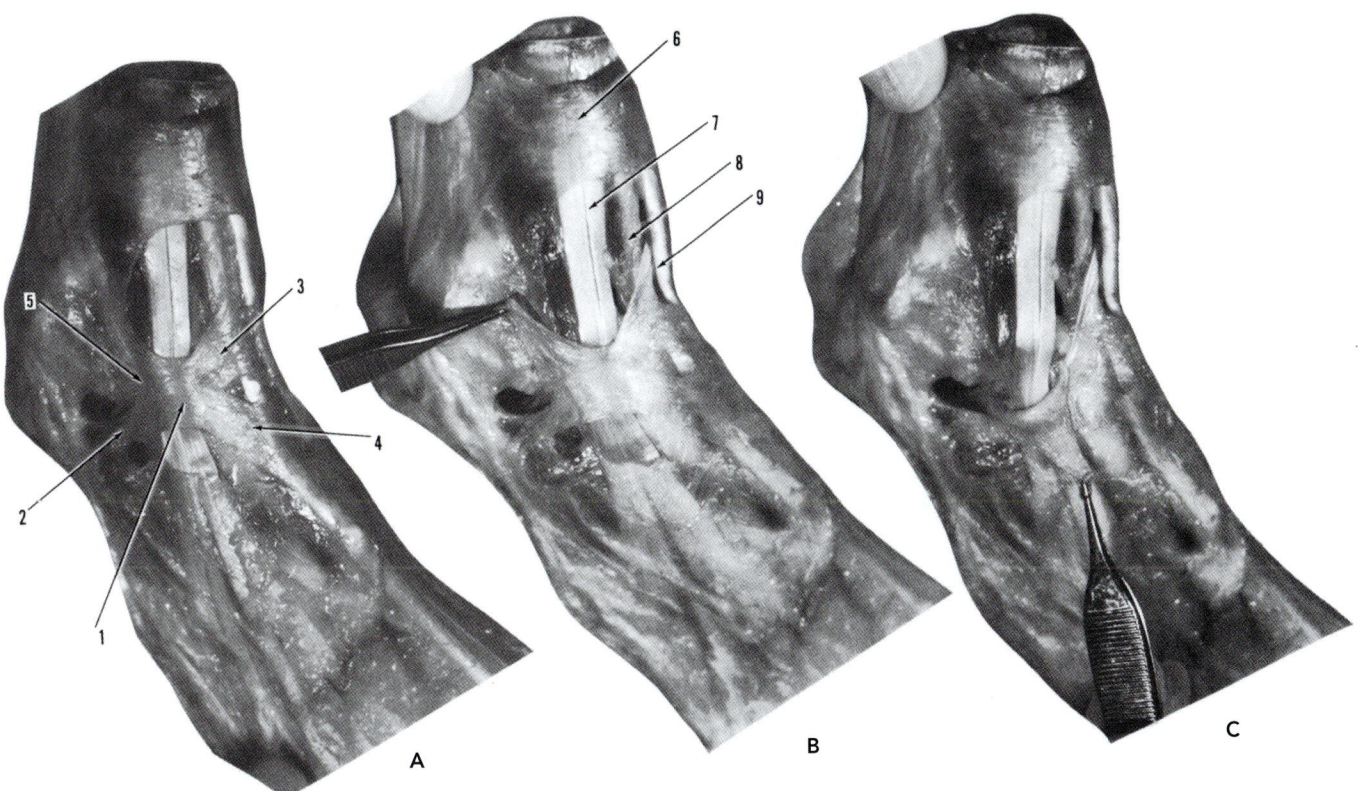

Figure 3.2 Inferior extensor retinaculum. **(A)** Inferior extensor retinaculum in situ. **(B)** Superolateral band of **A** detached. **(C)** Superolateral band of A reflected, demonstrating the frondiform or sling arrangement around the extensor digitorum longus tendons. (*1*, Inferior extensor retinaculum, cruciate form; *2*, stem of inferior extensor retinaculum; *3*, oblique superomedial band of inferior extensor retinaculum; *4*, oblique inferomedial band of inferior extensor retinaculum; *5*, oblique superolateral band of inferior extensor retinaculum; *6*, superior extensor retinaculum; *7*, extensor digitorum longus tendons; *8*, extensor hallucis longus tendon; *9*, tibialis anterior tendon.)

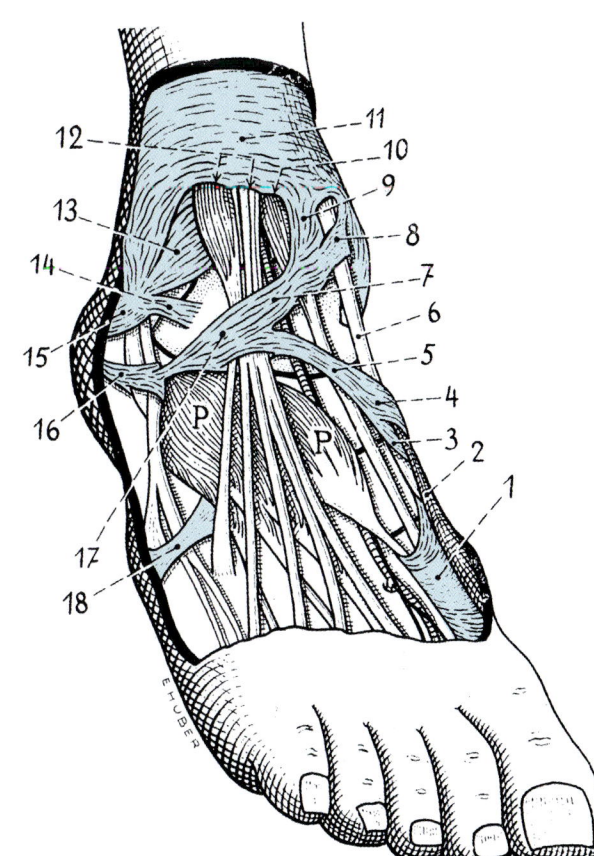

Figure 3.3 Inferior extensor retinaculum. (*1*, Medial transverse retinacular band of dorsum of foot; *2*, abductor hallucis muscle; *3, 4*, superficial and deep laminae of oblique inferomedial band of inferior extensor retinaculum; *5*, oblique inferomedial band of inferior extensor retinaculum; *6*, tibialis anterior tendon; *7*, oblique superomedial band of inferior extensor retinaculum; *8, 9*, superficial and deep components of oblique superomedial retinaculum forming tunnel of tibialis anterior tendon; *10*, extensor hallucis longus tendon; *11*, aponeurosis of leg; *12*, extensor digitorum longus and peroneus tertius tendons; *13*, anteroinferior tibiofibular ligament; *14*, anterior talofibular ligament; *15*, superior peroneal retinaculum; *16*, inferior peroneal retinaculum; *17*, stem of interior extensor retinaculum or frondiform ligament; *18*, lateral transverse band; *P*, extensor digitorum brevis muscle.) (Adapted from Meyer P. La morphologie du ligament annulaire antérieur du cou-de-pied chez l'homme. *Comptes Rendus Assoc Anat.* 1955;84:286.)

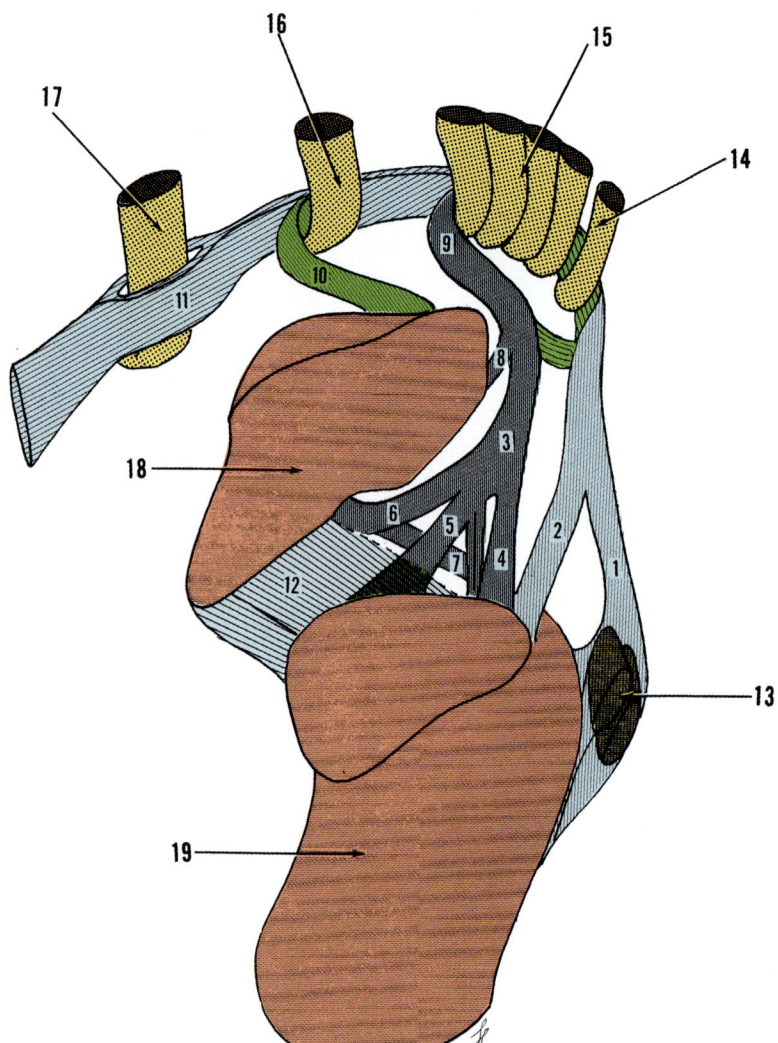

Figure 3.4 Diagram after dissection under magnification. The talus has been ostectomized obliquely in the direction of the canalis tarsi. The posterior half of the talus has been removed. Further exposure of the sinus tarsi and canal was obtained by removing bone from the talus with a rongeur. (*1*, Lateral root of inferior extensor retinaculum; *2*, intermediary root of inferior extensor retinaculum; *3*, medial root of inferior extensor retinaculum; *4*, lateral calcaneal component of medial root; *5*, medial calcaneal component of medial root; *6*, talar component of medial root attached into canalis tarsi; *7*, oblique talocalcaneal band of medial root; *8*, talar body attachment of medial root; *9*, loop formed by medial root of inferior extensor retinaculum turning around extensor digitorum longus tendon; *10*, reflected component of oblique superomedial band of inferior extensor retinaculum forming a sling for extensor hallucis longus tendon; *11*, tunnel for tibialis anterior tendon; *12*, interosseous ligament of canalis tarsi, oblique in direction, forming an "X" with medial calcaneal component of the medial root of inferior extensor retinaculum; *13*, tendons of peronei; *14*, peroneus tertius tendon; *15*, extensor digitorum longus tendons; *16*, extensor hallucis longus tendon; *17*, tibialis anterior tendon; *18*, talus; *19*, os calcis.)

superomedial band of the inferior extensor retinaculum also provides fibers to the deep layer of the same tunnel.

▶ Inferior Extensor Retinaculum

The inferior extensor retinaculum (anterior annular ligament of the tarsus, ligamentum cruciatum of Weitbrecht, frondiform ligament of Retzius, ligamentum lamboideum) is a Y- or X-shaped retaining structure located on the anterior aspect of the tarsus and the ankle (Figs. 3.2 to 3.6).[1-6] It is a complex structure that has four components: the stem or frondiform ligament, the oblique superomedial band, the oblique inferomedial band, and the oblique superolateral band.

Stem or Frondiform Ligament

The stem or frondiform ligament is a sling ligament retaining the tendons of the extensor digitorum longus and peroneus tertius against the talus and the calcaneus. This ligament has three roots: lateral, intermediary, and medial.

The lateral root is superficial, originates in the sinus tarsi lateral to the origin of the extensor digitorum brevis muscle, and blends with the deep fascia and the inferior peroneal retinaculum. The boundaries of this superficial root are difficult to delineate by dissection; tensing of the extensor tendons or inversion of the foot facilitates recognition of its borders.

The intermediary root arises from the sinus tarsi medial to the origin of the extensor digitorum brevis muscle and just posterior to the origin of the cervical ligament. At times, this root is fasciculated, and one large fascicle may divide the origin of the extensor hallucis brevis from that of the lesser toes.

The intermediary root extends upward and unites with the lateral root, forming the superficial component of the stem of the inferior extensor retinaculum. Once formed, the stem courses obliquely upward and inward across the neck of the talus. It passes over the peroneus tertius and extensor digitorum longus tendons and bifurcates into the oblique superomedial and inferomedial bands.

The medial root completes the formation of the retinacular sling for the extensor digitorum longus tendons and the peroneus tertius and forms the deep part of the stem. It has three components: two calcaneal (lateral and medial) and one talar.

The lateral calcaneal component is formed by vertical fibers and inserts in the sinus tarsi just posterior to the intermediary root and

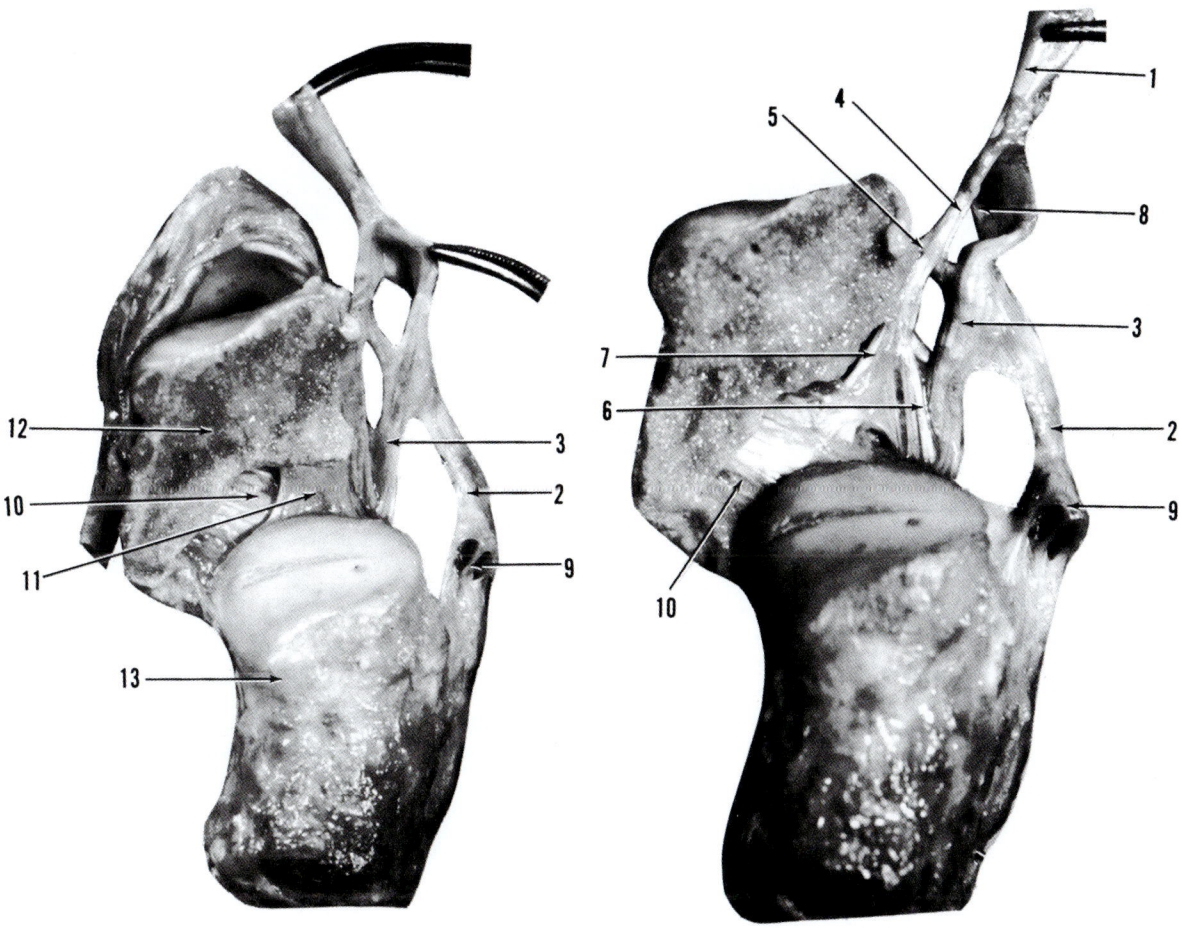

Figure 3.5 Anatomic preparation of the roots of the inferior extensor retinaculum. (*1*, Stem of inferior extensor retinaculum; *2*, lateral root inserting on the inferior retinaculum of peronei [9]; *3*, intermediary root of inferior extensor retinaculum; *4*, medial root of inferior extensor retinaculum; *5*, talar body attachment of medial root; *6*, lateral calcaneal attachment of medial root; *7*, oblique calcaneal component of medial root; *8*, sling or pulley for extensor digitorum longus and peroneus tertius tendons; *9*, inferior retinaculum of peronei tendons; *10*, interosseous ligament of tarsal canal; *11*, anterior capsule-ligament of posterior talocalcaneal joint; *12*, ostectomized talus, posterior half removed; *13*, calcaneus.)

establishes connection at this level. The major medial calcaneal component enters the tarsal canal very obliquely and inserts on the floor of the canal along its longitudinal axis, usually anterior to the ligament of the tarsal canal. The fibers of the ligament are oriented downward and laterally, whereas those of the medial calcaneal root are oriented downward and medially, forming an "X."

The talar component of the medial root attaches to the talus on the roof of the tarsal canal, joining the insertion fibers of the ligament of the tarsal canal. Arcuate fibers with inferior concavity unite the two calcaneal components of the medial root. An oblique band of the medial root originates at the calcaneal attachment of the intermediate root, extends medially upward, and joins the talar insertion of the ligament of the tarsal canal. This ligament has been described by Smith and, more recently, by Cahill, who named it the *oblique talocalcaneal band*.[3,4]

Jotoku et al,[7] in a study of 40 dissected feet, analyzed the variations of the ligaments of the sinus tarsi and canal. The anterior capsular ligament of the posterior talocalcaneal joint is present in 95%. The interosseous talocalcaneal ligament is present in 100%. In 92.5%, the ligament is bandlike: flat and thick. In 5%, the ligament is fanlike: broad at the origin in the tarsal canal and narrower at the insertion at the tarsal canal of the calcaneus. In 2.5%, the ligament is multiple type with three distinct bands (Fig. 3.7). In studying the components of the medial root of the extensor retinaculum, the lateral calcaneal branch is present in 100%, the medial calcaneal component is present in 100%, it is bandlike in 95%, and it is fanlike in 5%. The talar component is defined as the branch of the medial root attaching to the talus and is present in 90%. In type 1 (92%), it originates from the lateral calcaneal root of the inferior extensor retinaculum, and in type 2 (8%), it originates from the medial calcaneal root of the inferior extensor retinaculum. The ligament runs transversely or obliquely and inserts on the talus near the insertion of the interosseous talocalcaneal ligament (Fig. 3.8).

The medial root, ascending upward and medially, is applied against the lateral aspect of the talar neck. It passes anterior to the insertion of the anterior talofibular ligament. A bursa may be interposed between the two structures in 50% to 80% of the cases. Occasionally, instead of the bursa, one finds adipose tissue or even a fibrous band of attachment.

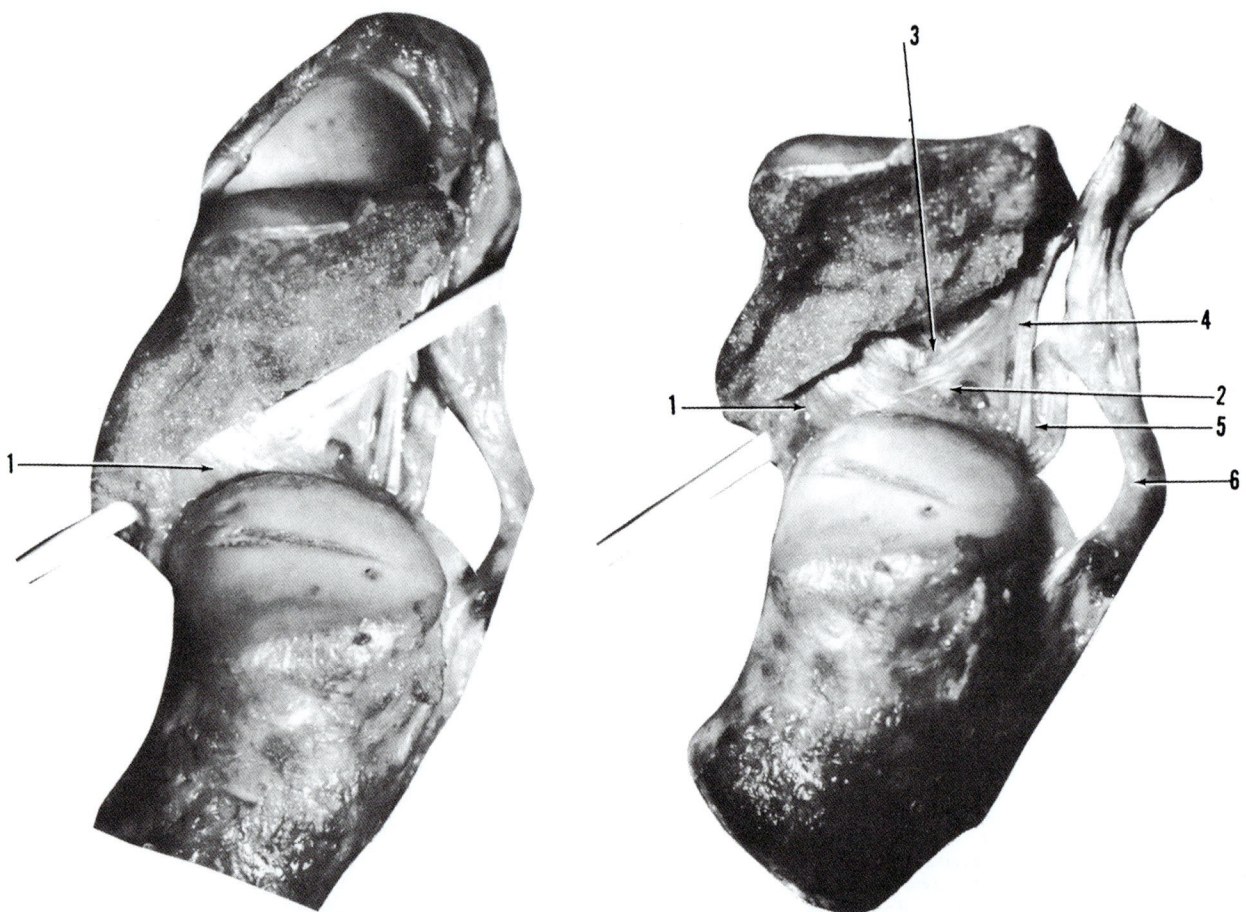

Figure 3.6 Anatomic preparation of the roots of the inferior extensor retinaculum. (*1*, Interosseous ligament of canalis tarsi [white rod passing anterior to the ligament]; *2*, medial calcaneal component of medial root of inferior extensor retinaculum crosses anteriorly; *3*, talar insertion of medial root; *4*, lateral calcaneal component of medial root; *5*, intermediary root of inferior extensor retinaculum; *6*, lateral root of inferior extensor retinaculum.)

After crossing the superior surface of the talar neck, the medial root forms a loop, joins the deep surface of the stem, and completes the sling for the extensor digitorum longus and peroneus tertius tendons. The internal architecture of the frondiform ligament and some of its variations are depicted in Figure 3.9.

Oblique Superomedial Band

The oblique superomedial band continues the direction of the stem, passes over the tendon of the extensor hallucis longus and under the tendon of the tibialis anterior, and inserts on the anterior aspect of the medial malleolus. Occasionally, the insertion fans out and reaches the anterior tibial crest and the medial surface of the medial malleolus, interchanging fibers with the superior extensor retinaculum and the flexor retinaculum (Fig. 3.10).

On the medial border of the extensor hallucis longus tendon, the deep fibers of the superomedial band loop around the tendon in a recurrent manner and have a variable insertion (Fig. 3.11). They insert on the apex of the lateral sling or on the deep surface of the medial root in 50% of cases, on the anterior aspect of the talar neck in 25% of cases (Fig. 3.12), or on the lateral sling and the anterior aspect of the talar neck in 25% of cases.[1] In the latter cases, the tendon of the extensor hallucis longus and the anterior neurovascular bundle are in the same compartment. Exceptionally, the deep layer of this segment of the retinaculum is absent.

Further medially, at the level of the tibialis anterior tendon, there is a bifurcation of the superomedial band, forming superior and inferior retention systems. The superior tunnel has a thick, deep wall and a very thin or even absent superficial wall. The inferior tunnel is well formed, with insertional fibers reaching the medial malleolus or occasionally blending with the fibers of the inferior arm of the extensor retinaculum.

Oblique Inferomedial Band

The oblique inferomedial band arises from the apex of the lateral sling, advances inferomedially, and reaches the medial border of the foot at the level of the $cuneo_1$-navicular joint. During its course, the 1- to 2-cm-wide band passes over the dorsalis pedis vessels, the deep peroneal nerve, and the extensor hallucis longus tendon. At the level of the tibialis anterior tendon, most of the fibers pass superficial to the tendon, and the remaining fibers slide under the tendon, forming a tunnel.

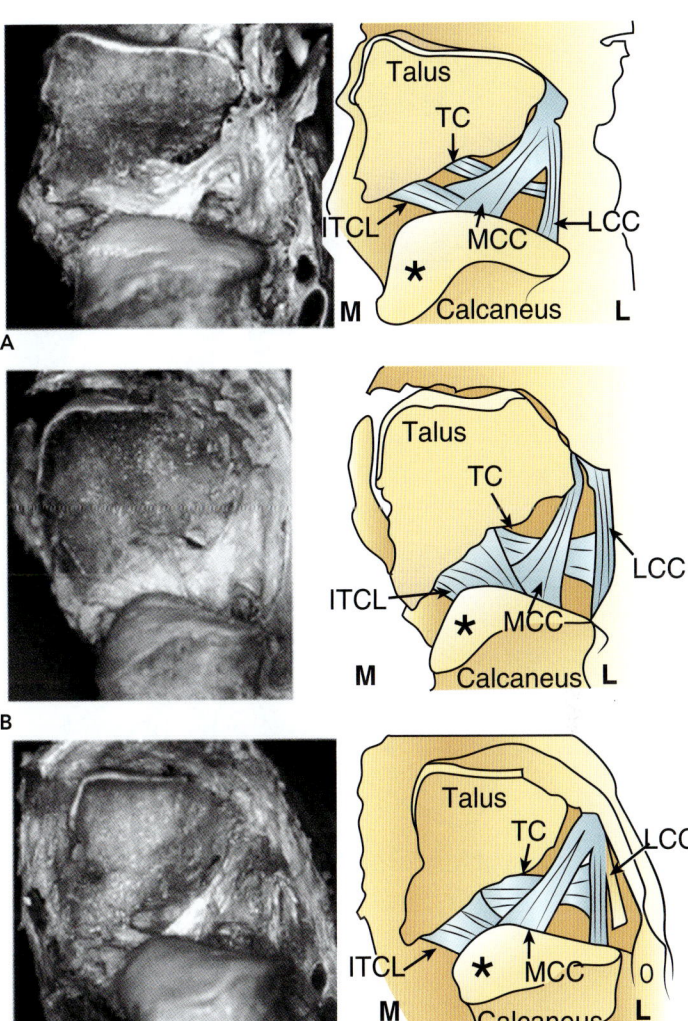

Figure 3.7 Variations of the interosseous talocalcaneal ligament and medial component of the extensor retinaculum (posterior view). (*, Posterior facet of the calcaneus; *ITCL*, interosseous talocalcaneal ligament; *L*, lateral; *LCC*, lateral calcaneal component; *M*, medial; *MCC*, medial calcaneal component.) **(A)** Band type ITCL and bandlike MCC. **(B)** Fanlike ITCL and fan type MCC. **(C)** Multiple type ITCL and band type MCC. (Adapted from Jotoku T, Kinoshita M, Okuda R, et al. Anatomy of ligamentous structures in the tarsal sinus and canal. *Foot Ankle*. 2006;7:5533-5538, Figure 4.)

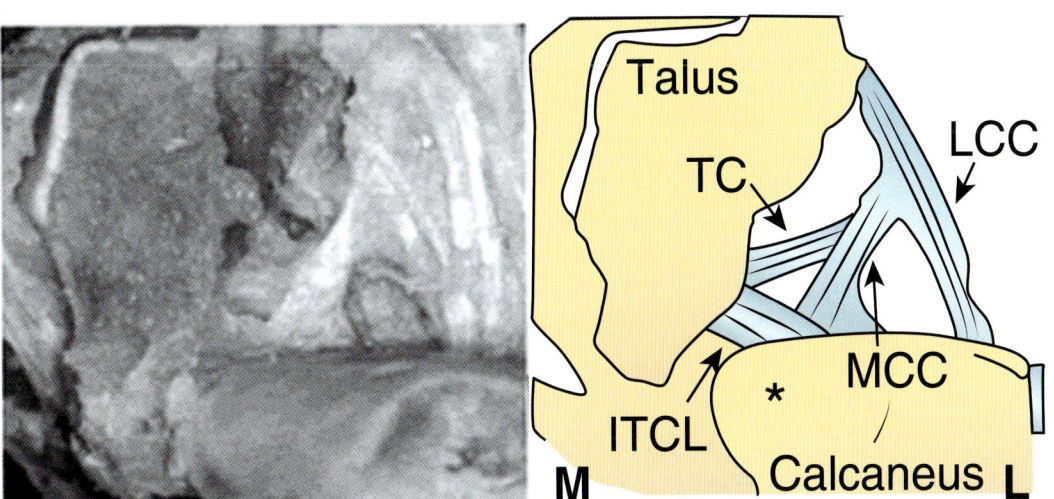

Figure 3.8 Talar component of the medial root diverged from MCC. (*, Posterior facet of the calcaneus; *ITLC*, interosseous talocalcaneal ligament; *L*, lateral; *LCC*, lateral talar component; *M*, medial; *MCC*, medial calcaneal component; *TC*, talar component.) (Adapted from Jotoku T, Kinoshita M, Okuda R, et al. Anatomy of ligamentous structures in the tarsal sinus and canal. *Foot Ankle*. 2006;7:5533-5538, Figure 5.)

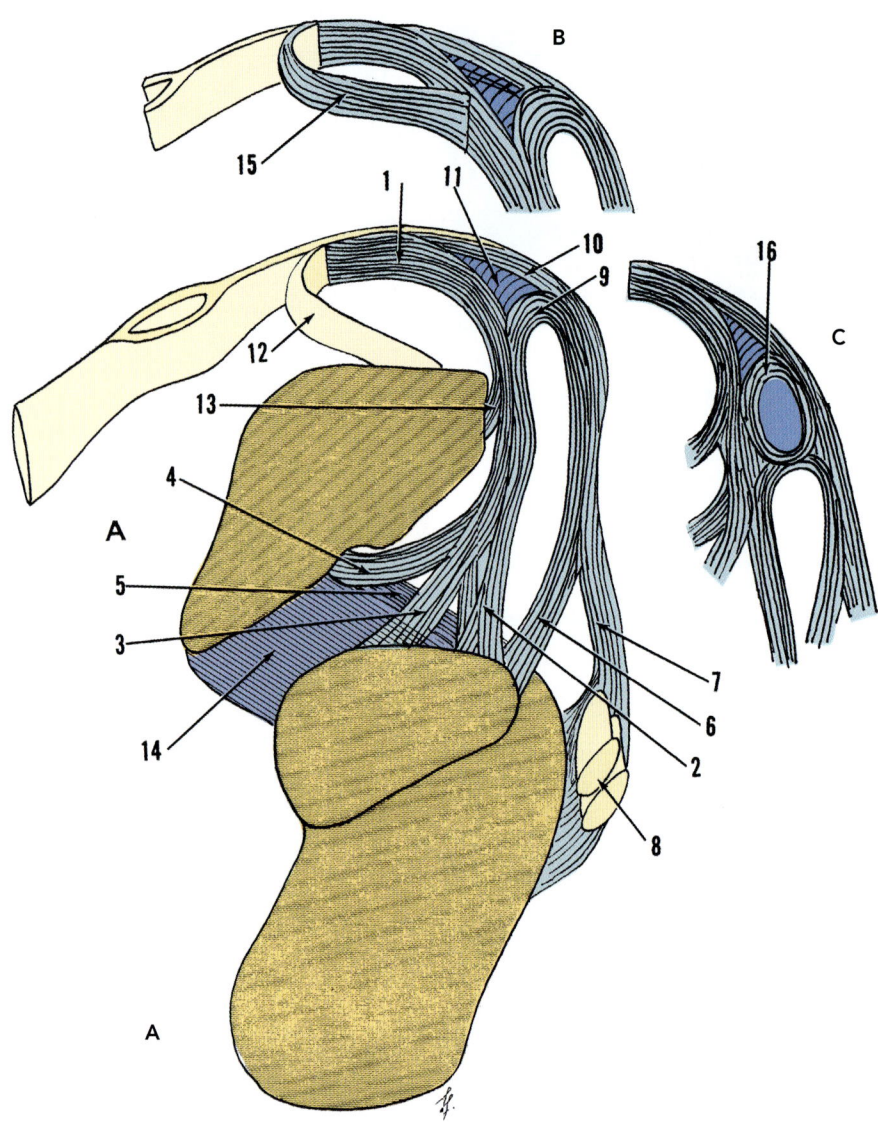

Figure 3.9 (A) Internal structure of the roots of the inferior extensor retinaculum. Sketch from dissection under magnification ×8. (1, Medial root of inferior extensor retinaculum with longitudinally oriented fibers continuing into 2, 3, 4, 13; 2, lateral calcaneal insertion of medial root; 3, medial calcaneal insertion of medial root; 4, talar insertion of medial root in canalis tarsi; 5, oblique talocalcaneal band; 6, intermediary root inferior extensor retinaculum; 7, lateral root inferior extensor retinaculum; 8, peronei tendons; 9, intermediary root 6 loops and continues as lateral calcaneal component of medial root; 10, lateral root continues mostly as the superficial fibers [10]; 11, triangular thinner component delineated by superficial [10] and deep components [1, 9]; 12, medial sling of extensor hallucis longus tunnel; 13, talar body attachment of medial root; 14, interosseous ligament of tarsal canal.) **(B) Variant with reflected band (15) of the extensor hallucis longus tendon tunnel attached to the medial root. (C) Variant with the extensor digitorum longus tunnel subdivided into a ring (16) medially and a sling laterally.**

The terminal segment splits to envelop the abductor hallucis muscle; deep fibers insert on the navicular and the medial cuneiform.

The level of division of the inferior extensor retinaculum into the oblique superomedial and inferomedial band is variable; it may be lateral to the extensor hallucis longus tendon, medial to the extensor hallucis longus tendon, or medial to the tibialis anterior tendon. The last is the least frequent, and when it occurs, the two division bands are in continuity except for a short distance on the medial aspect of the tibialis anterior tendon.[1]

Oblique Superolateral Band

The oblique superolateral band, when present, gives a cruciate configuration to the inferior extensor retinaculum, as described by Weitbrecht.[2] This band is present in 25% of cases, but the size varies considerably, from 2 to 25 mm.[1] It originates from the lateral sling, from the superomedial band, or from both. The band is directed upward and laterally, crosses the anterior tibiofibular ligament, and inserts on the lateral surface of the lateral malleolus and the lateral crest of the lower segment of the fibula. The fibers blend with those of the superior extensor and the superior peroneal retinacula.

DORSAL APONEUROSIS AND DORSAL COMPARTMENTS OF THE FOOT

A comprehensive study of the dorsal aponeurosis of the foot and the dorsal compartment (Fig. 3.13) is presented by Bellocq and Meyer.[8]

As one dissects the dorsum of the foot and removes the skin, a very thin layer of connective tissue is encountered—fascia superficialis—covering the superficial sensory nerves and veins. Next is a semitransparent, relatively thin fascia located under the superficial nerves and veins, investing all the musculotendinous units of the dorsum of the foot. This layer is the superficial

Chapter 3: Retaining Systems and Compartments 127

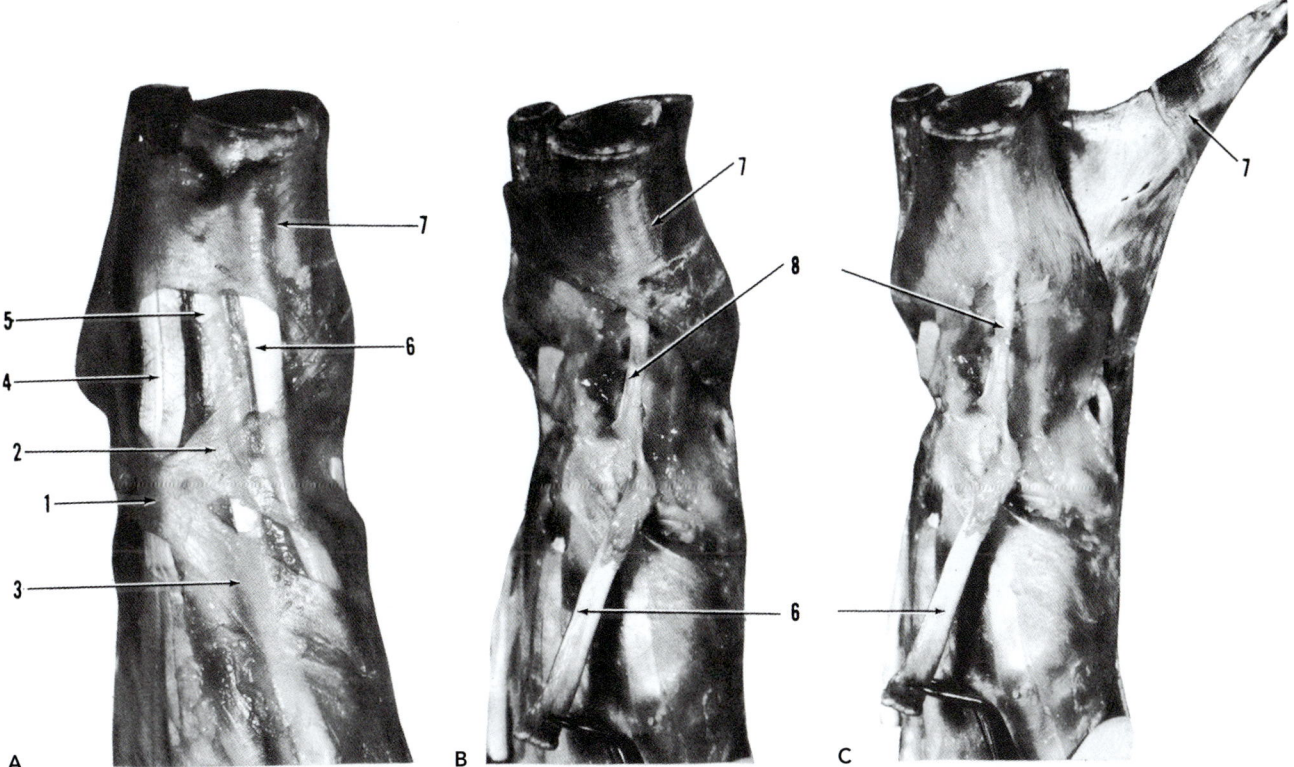

Figure 3.10 Anatomy of the oblique superomedial band of the inferior extensor retinaculum forming the pulleys for the tibialis anterior tendon. **(A)** The deep fibers of the oblique superomedial band of the inferior extensor retinaculum pass under the tibialis anterior tendon proximally, whereas the superficial fibers pass more distally. **(B)** Tibialis anterior tendon reflected downward exposing 8. **(C)** Superior extensor retinaculum reflected medially with the flexor retinaculum, which is in continuity and covers the medial aspect of the ankle. (*1*, Stem of inferior extensor retinaculum; *2*, oblique superomedial band of inferior extensor retinaculum. The deep component [*8*] of this band passes proximally under the tendon of the tibialis anterior, penetrates under the superior extensor retinaculum, and attaches to the tibia. The former is in continuity with the flexor retinaculum; *3*, oblique inferomedial band of inferior extensor retinaculum; *4*, extensor digitorum longus tendon; *5*, extensor hallucis longus tendon; *6*, tibialis anterior tendon; *7*, superior extensor retinaculum; *8*, deep tibial attachment of oblique superomedial band of the inferior extensor retinaculum.)

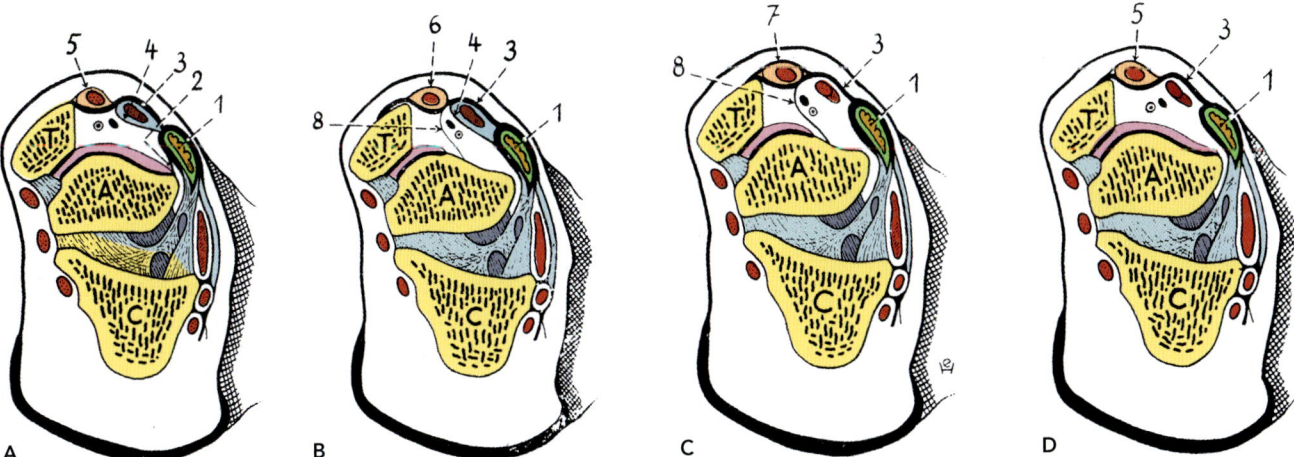

Figure 3.11 Cross-sections through the sinus tarsi and canal; variations of the insertion of the deep lamina or sling or reflected fibers of the extensor hallucis longus tunnel. **(A)** Deep fibers attached to the apex of the lateral sling of the extensor digitorum communis (50% occurrence). **(B)** Deep fibers attached to the deep surface of the lateral sling and to the anterior surface of the talus, forming a separate compartment to the neurovascular bundle (25% occurrence). **(C)** Deep fibers attached to the anterior aspect of the talus. The extensor hallucis longus tendon and the neurovascular bundle are in the same compartment (25% occurrence). **(D)** Absence of deep fibers and sling around the extensor hallucis longus tendon (rare). (*1*, Frondiform ligament; *2*, talar attachment of [*1*]; *3*, oblique superomedial band of inferior extensor retinaculum; *4*, deep lamina of the extensor hallucis longus sling; *5*, *6*, *7*, superficial lamina of tibialis anterior tunnel; *8*, talar attachment of extensor hallucis longus sling.) (Adapted from Meyer P. La morphologie du ligament annulaire antérieur du cou-de-pied chez l'homme. *Comptes Rendus Assoc Anat.* 1955;84:286.)

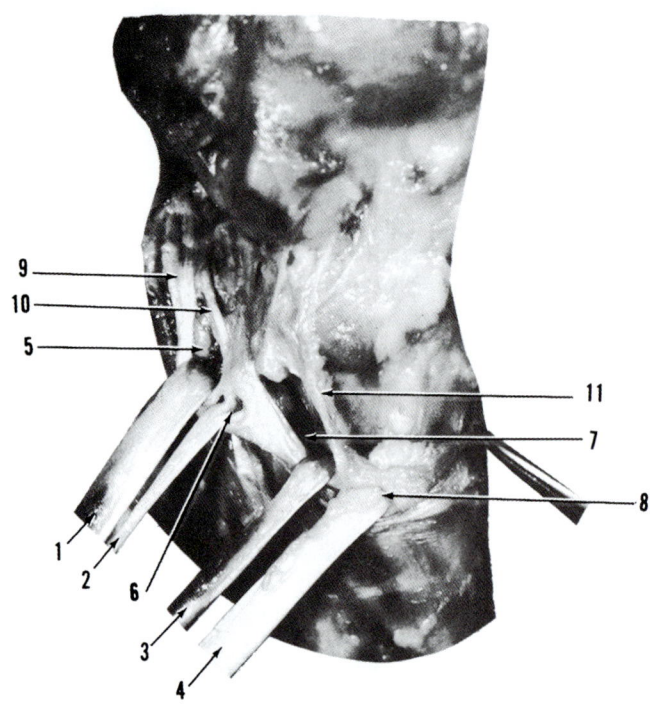

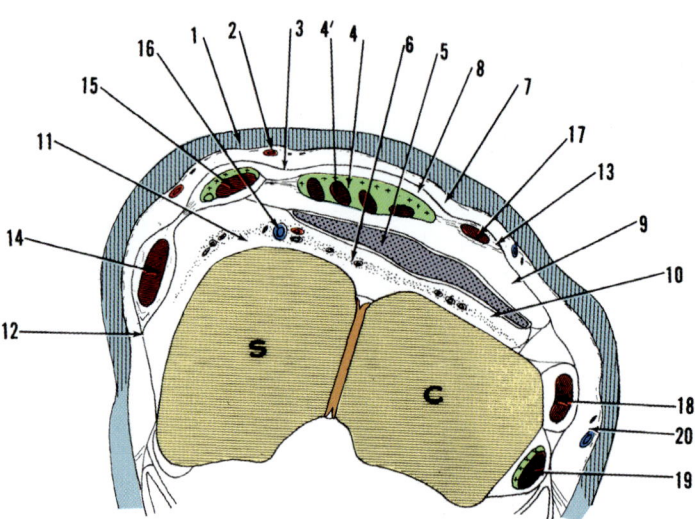

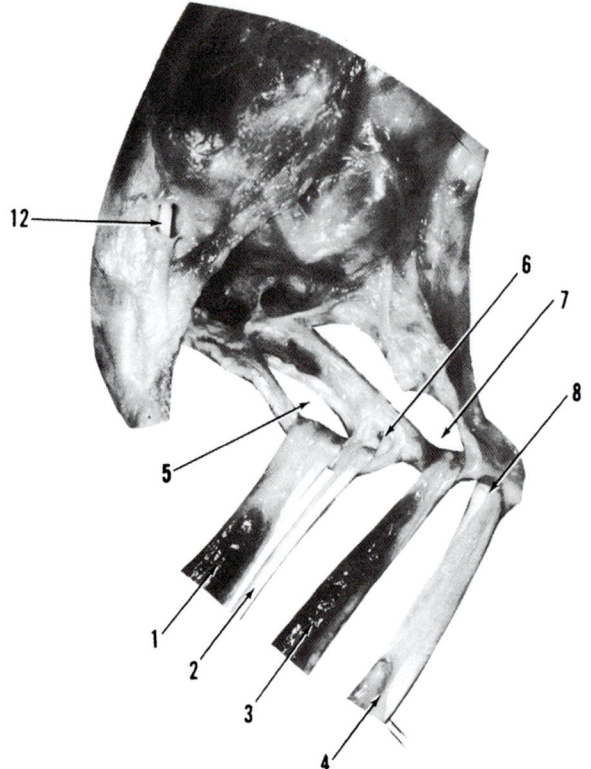

Figure 3.12 Inferior extensor retinaculum. (1, Extensor digitorum longus tendons, toes 5, 4, 3; 2, extensor digitorum longus tendon to second toe; 3, extensor hallucis longus tendon; 4, tibialis anterior tendon; 5, tunnel for extensor digitorum longus, toes 5, 4, 3; 6, tunnel extensor digitorum longus, toe 2; 7, tunnel for extensor hallucis longus; 8, tunnel for tibialis anterior; 9, stem of lateral and intermediary roots of inferior extensor retinaculum; 10, medial root of inferior extensor retinaculum; 11, talar attachment of extensor hallucis longus sling; 12, peronei tendons.)

Figure 3.13 Frontal cross-section of right foot passing through the anterior tarsus—view of anterior segment. (C, cuboid; S, scaphoid.) Layers: 1, Skin; 2, fascia superficialis covering the superficial veins and nerves; 3, superficial dorsal aponeurosis; 4, *first layer*, superficial tendinoconnective, formed by the tendons of the tibialis anterior (14), extensor hallucis longus (15), extensor digitorum longus (4′), peroneus tertius (17), and their fibrosynovial sheath connected with a layer of connective tissue. This layer attaches to the superficial dorsal aponeurosis on the medial border of the tibialis anterior tendon sheath and to the lateral border of the peroneus tertius tendon sheath. 5, *Second layer*, formed by the extensor digitorum brevis and its investing fascia, attaches to the superficial layer at the level of the deep surface of the extensor hallucis longus sheath, covering the underlying doralis pedis vessels. The lateral wing of this layer is attached to the cuboid and to the superficial aponeurosis medial to the peroneus brevis tendon (18). 6, *Third layer*, adipoconnective, carries the dorsalis pedis vessels and the deep peroneal nerve and its branches. Spaces: 7, subcutaneous space; 8, first fascial space between superficial dorsal aponeurosis and the superficial tendinoconnective layer; 9, second fascial space between the superficial tendinoconnective layer and the extensor digitorum brevis and its investing fascia; 10, third fascial space between the extensor digitorum brevis with its investing deep fascia and the neurovascular adipoconnective layer; 11, fourth fascial space between the neurovascular adipoconnective layer and the tarsal osteoarticular layer proximally and the dorsal interosseous aponeurosis distally; 12, connection of the superficial dorsal aponeurosis with the first layer, medially; 13, connection of the superficial dorsal aponeurosis with the first layer, laterally; 14, tibialis anterior tendon; 15, extensor hallucis longus tendon; 16, dorsalis pedis artery, veins, and deep peroneal nerve; 17, peroneus tertius tendon; 18, peroneus brevis tendon; 19, peroneus longus tendon; 20, sural nerve and short saphenous vein. (Adapted from Bellocq P, Meyer P. Contribution a l'étude de l'aponevrose dorsale du pied [fascia dorsalis pedis, P.N.A.]. *Acta Anat.* 1957;30:67.)

lamina or superficial dorsal aponeurosis. A true osteofascial space (the spatium dorsalis pedis) is created as this aponeurosis inserts on the foot skeleton at the lateral and medial margins. More precisely, the lateral insertion is on the os calcis, the cuboid, and the tuberosity and lateral border of the fifth metatarsal, and the medial insertion extends from the sustentaculum tali to the tuberosity of the scaphoid and the medial border of the first metatarsal.

This superficial dorsal aponeurosis extends fibers to the chorion of the skin, thus forming the retinacula cutis, and closes the subcutaneous space of the foot at its margins. Other connective fibers reach the sheath of the abductor of the big toe medially and the abductor of the little toe laterally.

The dorsal osteoaponeurotic space is subdivided into four gliding subspaces by three layers of tissue.

The first layer, located under the superficial dorsal aponeurosis, is formed by the tendons of the tibialis anterior, extensor hallucis longus, extensor digitorum longus, and peroneus tertius, surrounded by synovial sheaths or loose connective tissue united to each other. This superficial tendinoconnective layer unites with the superficial dorsal aponeurosis near the tibialis anterior medially and the outer aspect of the peroneus tertius laterally.

The second layer is formed by the extensor digitorum brevis and its investing fascia, the deep lamina of the dorsal aponeurosis. This aponeurosis attaches medially to the synovial sheath of the extensor hallucis longus. It courses laterally, passes over the dorsalis pedis vessels, and splits into two layers at the medial border of the extensor digitorum brevis. The thick superficial layer and the thin deep layer merge on the lateral border of the muscle and attach laterally on the superficial dorsal aponeurosis and the tarsus.

The third layer is adipoconnective, carrying the dorsalis pedis artery and the accompanying veins and the deep peroneal nerve and its branches. The dorsal interosseous aponeurosis is the last investing layer covering the metatarsals and the interossei muscles.

The four fascial spaces of the dorsal fibro-osseous compartment of the foot located between the previously described three soft-tissue layers and the dorsal aponeurosis are as follows:

- Space 1: Located between the superficial dorsal aponeurosis and the superficial tendinoconnective layer.
- Space 2: Located between the superficial tendinoconnective layer and the extensor digitorum brevis.
- Space 3: Located between the deep surface of the extensor digitorum brevis with its investing fascia and the neurovascular adipoconnective layer.
- Space 4: Located between the neurovascular adipoconnective layer and the tarsal osteoarticular layer proximally and the dorsal interosseous aponeurosis distally.

Space 2 has been investigated by Latarjet and Etienne-Martin with injection studies.[9] When distended, this space is well delineated, located under the layer formed by the long extensor tendons of the second, third, fourth, and fifth toes and the extensor digitorum brevis. This space is in the form of a trapezoid, with the small base proximal and the large base distal (Fig. 3.14). The proximal border does not reach the inferior extensor retinaculum, but variations are possible. The distal border is located in the middle of the dorsum of the foot and may send extensions under the tendons; this border has a variable location. Medially, the distended bursa reaches the tendon of the extensor hallucis longus but does not lift the latter.

In the distal segment at the level of the base of the metatarsals, the tendons are located in a fibrous sheath, with surrounding loose connective tissue or synovial sheaths. As the tendinoconnective superficial and deep layers are converted into fibrous sheaths, they adhere to the dorsal interosseous aponeurosis or remain separate from it, delineating fibroadipose small spaces (Fig. 3.15).

The superficial dorsal aponeurosis is reinforced along the medial and lateral borders of the foot by two aponeurotic transverse bands: medial and lateral (see Fig. 3.3).[1] The medial transverse band originates from the medial cuneiform and metatarsal$_1$-bones and may form a terminal fibrous tunnel for the tibialis anterior tendon. Directed laterally, the fibers pass under the inferior arm of the extensor aponeurosis but over the tendon of the extensor hallucis longus and occasionally over the tendon of the extensor hallucis brevis. The transverse fibers terminate on the cuneiforms and the first metatarsal. Occasionally, the metatarsal insertion may extend up to the level of the metatarsophalangeal joint and form an osteofibrous tunnel for the two extensor tendons.[1]

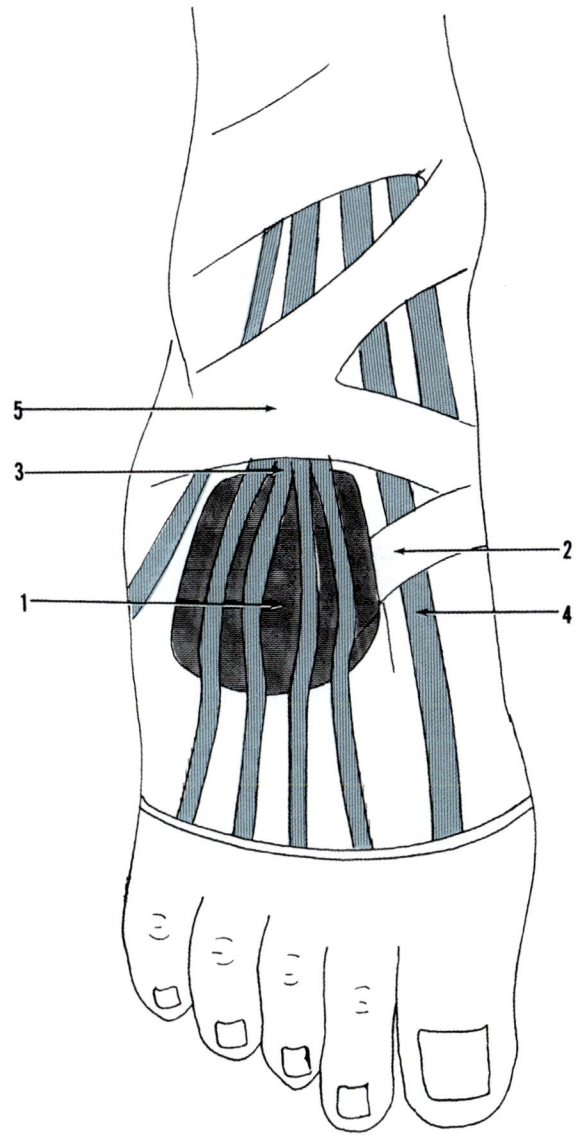

Figure 3.14 Gliding mechanism or cellular bursa or space located on the dorsum of the foot behind the extensor digitorum longus tendons. (1, Cellular space; 2, medial transverse retinacular band of dorsum of foot; 3, extensor digitorum longus tendons; 4, extensor hallucis longus tendon; 5, inferior extensor retinaculum.) (Adapted from Latarjet A, Etienne-Martin M. L'appareil de glissement des tendons extenseurs des doigts et des orteils sur le dos de la main et sur le dos du pied. Ann Anat Pathol Anat Normal. 1932;9:605.)

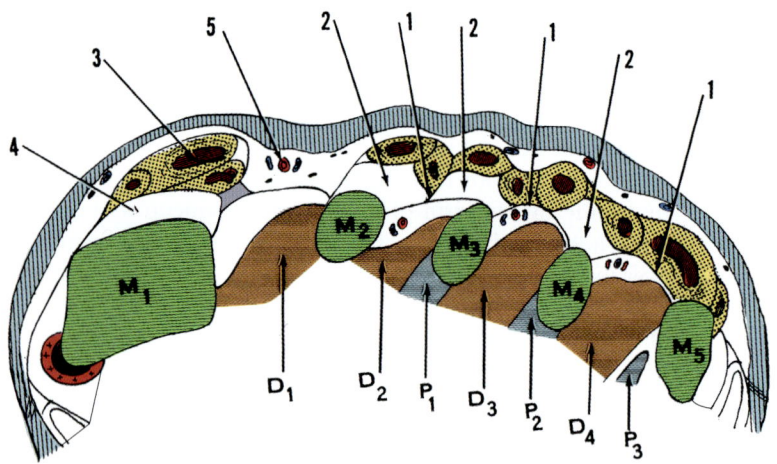

Figure 3.15 Coronal cross-section of right foot at the level of the distal segment of the metatarsal shafts: view of anterior segment. The extensor tendons and their sheaths adhere to the dorsal interosseous aponeurosis in certain locations and delineate with the latter fibroadipose small spaces. (1, Point or area of adhesion of the extensor tendon sheaths to the dorsal interosseous aponeurosis; 2, small spaces limited above by the extensor tendon sheaths and laterally and medially by their adhesion to the dorsal interosseous aponeurosis, which with the metatarsals forms the floor of the space; 3, extensor hallucis longus and brevis of the big toe with their sheaths, including an accessory tendinous band on the medial side; 4, premetatarsal$_1$ space; 5, dorsalis pedis artery and veins; M_1 to M_5, metatarsal shafts 1-5; D_1 to D_4, dorsal interossei muscles 1-4; P_1 to M_3, plantar interossei muscles.) (Adapted from Bellocq P, Meyer P. Contribution a l'étude de l'aponevrose dorsale du pied [fascia dorsalis pedis, P.N.A.]. Acta Anat. 1957;30:67.)

Kaneff and colleagues reported on the occurrence of the retinaculum musculorum imum in man.[10] This is a transverse or oblique extensor retinacular band that is present distal to the anteroinferior band of the inferior extensor retinaculum. It originates from the dorsum of the base of the second metatarsal, passes over the tendons of the extensor hallucis longus and brevis, and inserts on the medial side of the first cuneiform. It may also insert on a variant muscle of the first interspace. This retinaculum musculorum extensorium imum was present in 64.2% of 151 dissected specimens. The fibrous forms accounted for 52.3%, and the complete fibrous form accounted for 47%. In 5.3%, there was an incomplete fibrous form with the lateral or medial half missing. The musculofibrosum form—with muscular origin—occurred in 11.9% (Fig. 3.16).

The lateral transverse band is inconstant and located at the level of the base of the fifth metatarsal bone. It originates from the latter, bridges over the metatarsal or digital extensions of the peroneus tertius or the peroneus brevis tendon, and inserts on the fifth or the fourth metatarsal.

▶ Peroneal Tunnels and Retinaculum

Superior Peroneal Tunnel

The superior peroneal tunnel is the continuation of the lateral compartment of the leg, which gradually shifts from the lateral position in the distal leg to the posterior aspect of the fibula and remains as a tunnel on the posterior aspect of the lateral malleolus (see Figs. 3.1 and 3.17). The covering peroneal aponeurosis takes insertion on the medial and lateral retromalleolar surface or groove and forms a strong retaining aponeurotic ring. The deep aponeurosis of the posterior compartment takes insertion along the medial border of the peroneal tunnel, which may give origin at this junction to the peroneotalocalcaneal ligament of Rouvière and Canela Lazaro. The calcaneal arm of this ligament inserts nearly transversely on the entire width of the superior surface of the calcaneus and may reach the tip of the lateral malleolus and even the insertion of the calcaneofibular ligament.

Superior Peroneal Retinaculum

The superior peroneal retinaculum is a reinforcement of the aponeurosis cruris in the form of an obliquely oriented

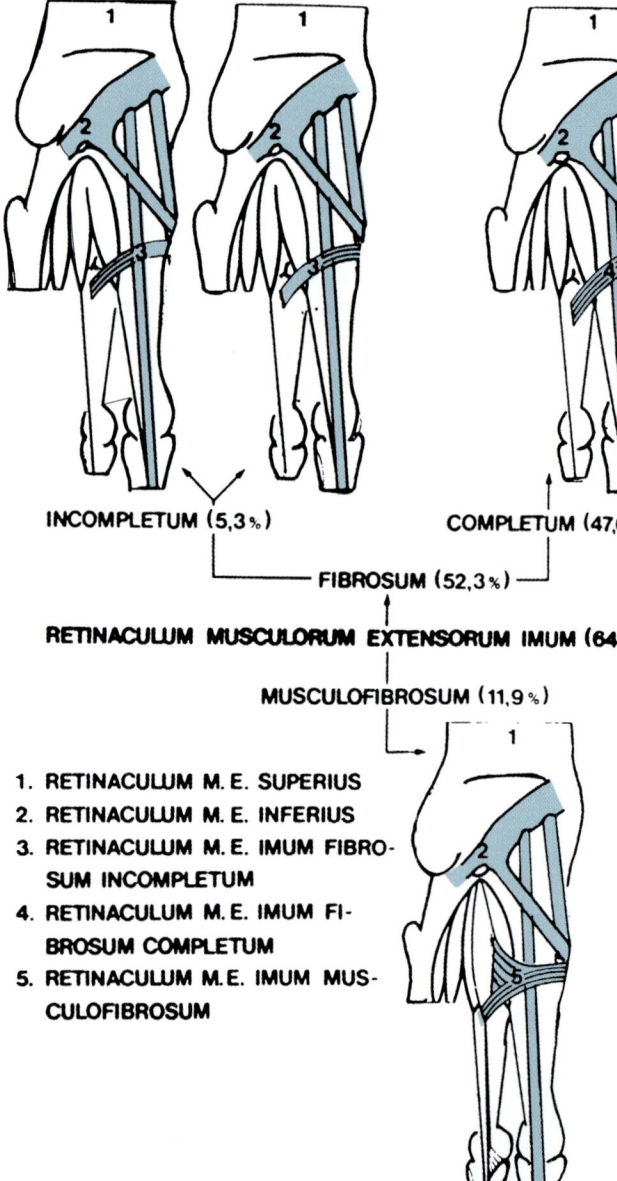

1. RETINACULUM M. E. SUPERIUS
2. RETINACULUM M. E. INFERIUS
3. RETINACULUM M. E. IMUM FIBROSUM INCOMPLETUM
4. RETINACULUM M. E. IMUM FIBROSUM COMPLETUM
5. RETINACULUM M.E. IMUM MUSCULOFIBROSUM

Figure 3.16 Retinaculum musculorum extensorum imum. (Adapted from Kaneff A, Mokrusch T, Landgraft P. Über die existenz eines retinaculum musculorum extensorum imum beim menschen. Occurrence of a retinaculum musculorum extensorum imum in man. Gengenbaurs Morph Jahrb Leipzig. 1984;130[6]:776.)

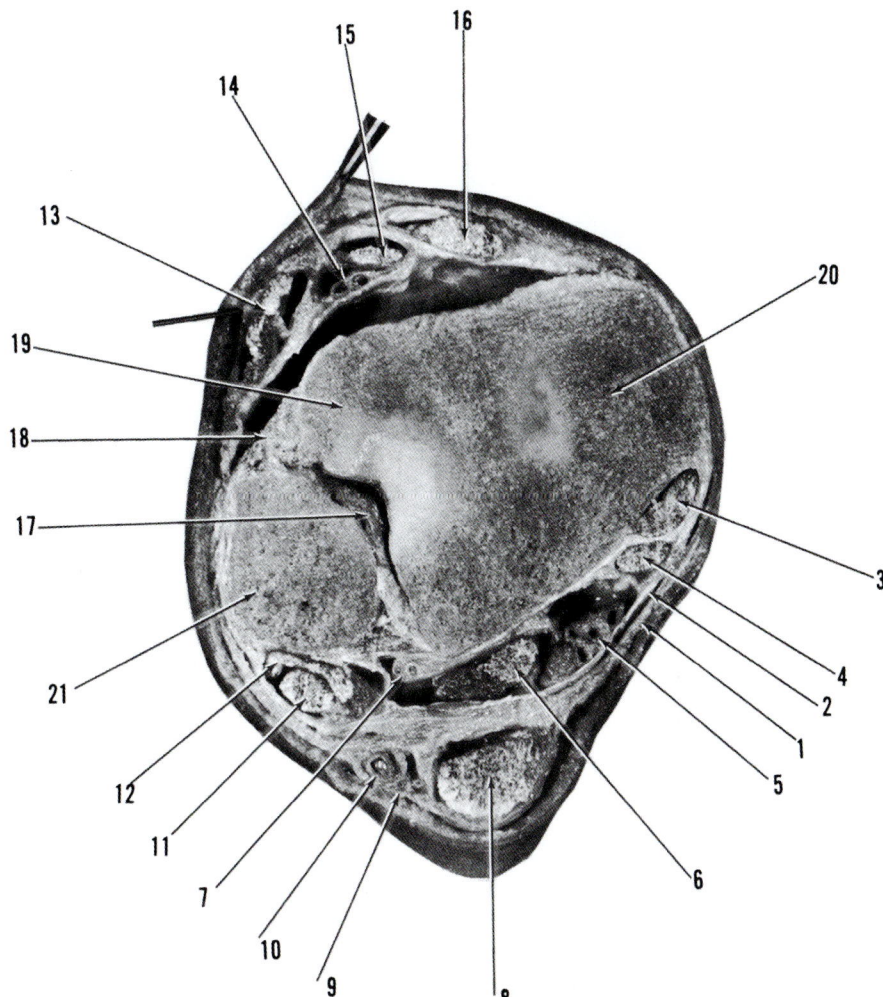

Figure 3.17 Cross-section of left ankle, 2 cm proximal to the tip of the medial malleolus, seen from lower surface of section. (*1*, Superficial aponeurosis of leg; *2*, deep aponeurosis of leg; *3*, tendon of tibialis posterior in its tunnel; *4*, tendon of flexor digitorum longus in its tunnel; *5*, posterior tibial artery and veins and posterior tibial nerve laterally in their compartment; *6*, flexor hallucis longus with tendon medially and low muscle fibers laterally in its compartment; *7*, posterior peroneal vessels in the same compartment as *6*; *8*, Achilles tendon covered by the split superficial aponeurosis [*1*]; the pre-Achilles space between the superficial and deep aponeuroses is filled with adipose tissue; *9*, sural nerve; *10*, lesser saphenous vein [*9* and *10* are in separate compartments]; *11*, peroneus longus tendon; *12*, peroneus brevis tendon, U shape [both peronei are located in a compartment]; *13*, extensor digitorum longus tendon and tunnel; *14*, dorsalis pedis, artery, and veins; *15*, extensor hallucis longus tendon and tunnel in common with *14*; *16*, tibialis anterior tendon and tunnel; *17*, synovial fringe of tibiofibular syndesmosis; *18*, anteroinferior tibiofibular ligament; *19*, anterolateral tubercle of distal tibia; *20*, distal tibia; *21*, lateral malleolus.)

quadrilateral lamina. It originates from the lateral border of the retromalleolar groove and the tip of the lateral malleolus. It is adherent to the underlying inferior segment of the superior peroneal tunnel and courses obliquely downward and posteriorly. It inserts on the aponeurosis of the Achilles tendon and the posterior aspect of the lateral calcaneal surface.

The sural nerve, the short saphenous vein, and the lateral calcaneal nerve and vessels are located under this superior peroneal retinaculum in their own compartment (see Fig. 3.17).

Intermediary Peroneal Tunnel

Below the tip of the lateral malleolus, the peroneal tunnel obliquely crosses the calcaneofibular ligament and is covered by a thin aponeurosis that is nearly transparent.

Inferior Peroneal Tunnel and Retinaculum

The inferior peroneal retinaculum is in continuity with the lateral root of the inferior extensor retinaculum (Fig. 3.18). It originates from the posterior segment of the lateral rim of the sinus tarsi. The superficial fibers are oriented downward and posteriorly, cross the trochlear process, and insert on the lateral surface of the os calcis just above the posterolateral tubercle. The deep layer attaches on the apex of the trochlear process. It provides superior and inferior arciform fibers and forms two fibrous tunnels over the superior and inferior surfaces of the trochlear process (Fig. 3.19). The upper tunnel lodges the peroneus brevis tendon, and the lower tunnel lodges the peroneus longus tendon.

Distal to the bony eminence, the inferior peroneal retinaculum forms two nearly circular separate fibrous tunnels for the peronei tendons.

The tunnel of the peroneus longus penetrates the sole of the foot through the lateral border and continues up to its insertion on the base of the first metatarsal and first cuneiform.

TIBIOTALOCALCANEAL TUNNEL

The tibiotalocalcaneal tunnel (Richet tunnel, tarsal tunnel, calcaneal tunnel), a major passageway, extends from the distal end of the tibia to the level of the plantar aspect of the navicular.[11-14] It is posteromedial in location and is concave anteriorly. The tunnel may be divided into two components: upper, tibiotalar, and lower, talocalcaneal.

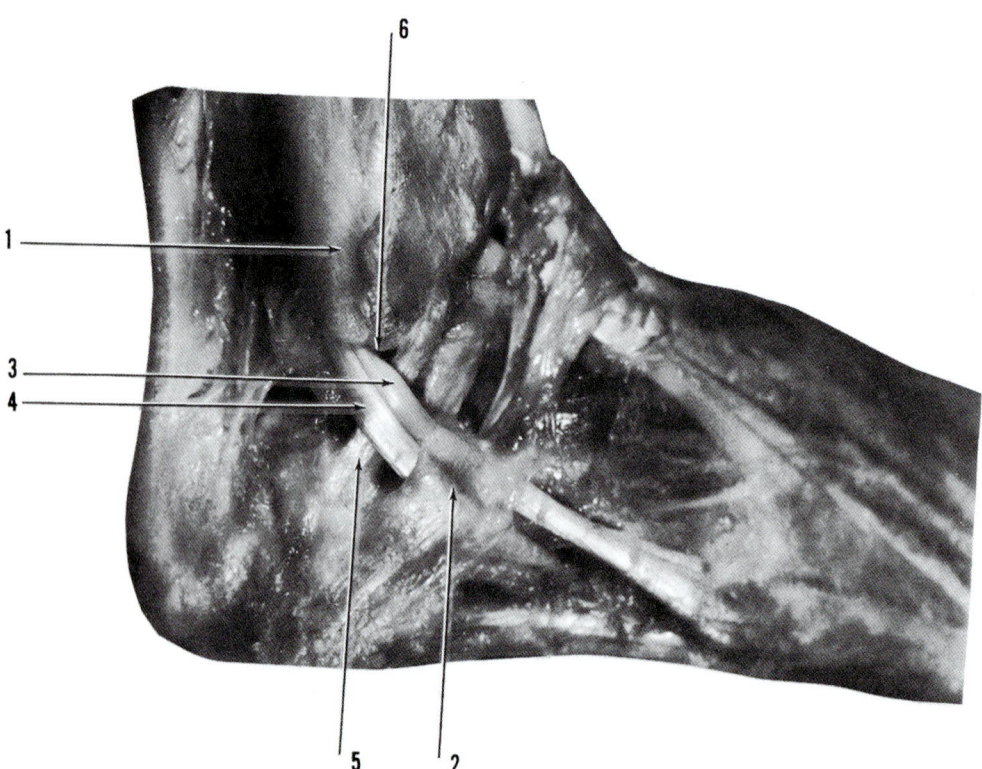

Figure 3.18 Peroneal retinaculum. The peronei tendons and the calcaneofibular ligament cross in an "X." (*1*, Superior peroneal retinaculum; *2*, inferior peroneal retinaculum; *3*, peroneus brevis tendon; *4*, peroneus longus tendon; *5*, calcaneofibular ligament; *6*, tip of lateral malleolus free of insertion.)

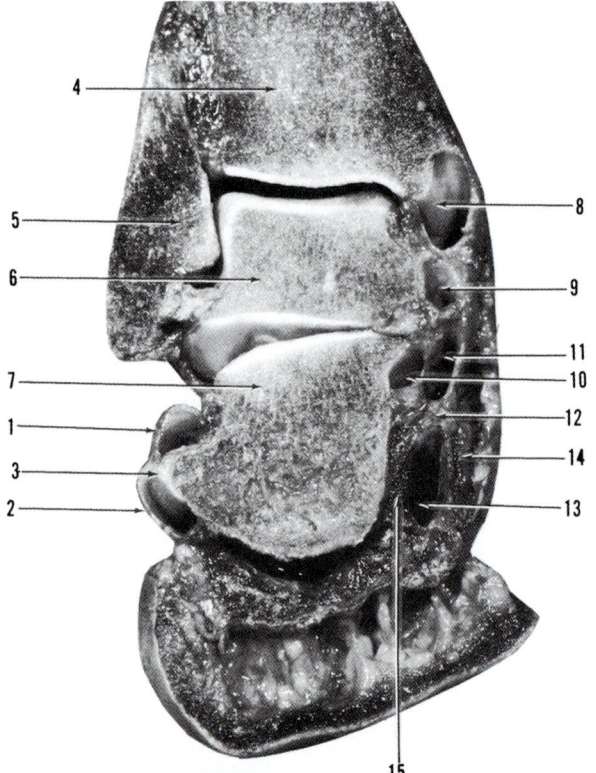

Figure 3.19 Frontal cross-section of the ankle and hindfoot. (*1*, Tunnel of peroneus brevis tendon; *2*, tunnel of peroneus longus tendon; *3*, peroneal trochlear process, well developed in this specimen; *4*, tibia; *5*, lateral malleolus; *6*, talus; *7*, calcaneus; *8*, tunnel of tibialis posterior tendon; *9*, tunnel of flexor digitorum longus tendon; *10*, tunnel of flexor hallucis longus tendon; *11*, upper chamber of tarsal tunnel for the medial plantar neurovascular bundle; *12*, interfascicular ligament; *13*, lower chamber of tarsal tunnel for the lateral plantar neurovascular bundle; *14*, abductor hallucis muscle covered by the split layers of the flexor retinaculum; *15*, quadratus plantae muscle.)

▶ Upper Tibiotalar Tunnel

The upper tibiotalar tunnel (Figs. 3.20 to 3.22) corresponds to the posterior aspect of the distal tibia, the retromedial malleolar surface, the posterior border of the talus with its central sulcus flanked by the posterior tubercles, and the posterior segment of the medial talar surface. The osseous canal is converted into a large tunnel or deep compartment by the covering deep aponeurosis of the leg. The latter is attached medially to the posteromedial border of the tibia and the posterior border of the medial malleolus and laterally to the fibrous sheath of the peronei tendons. Further distally, the deep aponeurosis attaches to the superomedial surface of the os calcis and continues anteriorly with the flexor retinaculum. Anteriorly, at the level of the tibiotalar tunnel, the deep aponeurosis is adherent to the covering superficial aponeurosis; in the posterior segment, the two aponeuroses part: the superficial aponeurosis courses toward the medial border of the Achilles tendon and the deep aponeurosis courses laterally toward the sheath of the peronei tendons (see Fig. 3.20).

In the proximal tibial segment of the tunnel are located, medially to laterally, the following structures: the fibrous tunnel of the tibialis posterior tendon; the fibrous tunnel of the flexor digitorum longus, adherent to the former; the superficial compartment for the posterior tibial neurovascular bundle; and the large loose compartment for the flexor hallucis longus muscle-tendon unit and the peroneal vessels laterally (see Fig. 3.20).

In the distal malleolar-talar segment of the tunnel, the same relationship is present, with some modifications. The flexor hallucis longus is all tendinous and passes through a strong fibrous tunnel on the posterior border of the talus (see Fig. 3.22). The peronei vessels have parted. The posterior tibial neurovascular

Chapter 3: Retaining Systems and Compartments 133

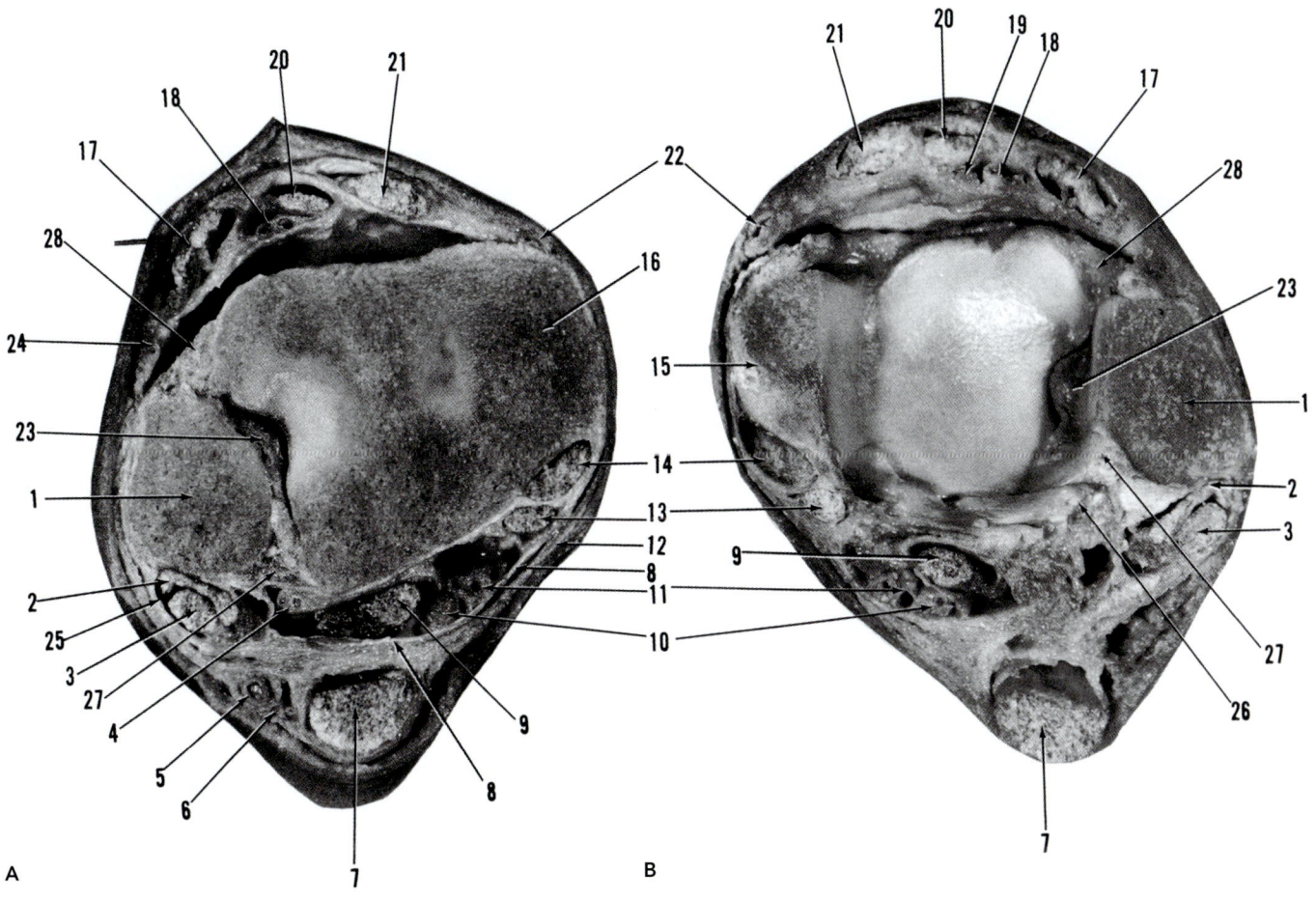

Figure 3.20 Cross-section of left ankle 2 cm proximal to medial malleolus. **(A)** Proximal surface of section. **(B)** Transmalleolar surface of section. (*1*, Distal fibula [**A**] and lateral malleolus [**B**]; *2*, frayed peroneus brevis tendon in the peroneal compartment; *3*, peroneus longus tendon in the peroneal compartment; *4*, posterior peroneal vessels; *5*, short saphenous vein; *6*, sural nerve; *7*, Achilles tendon and its compartment; *8, 25,* deep aponeurosis cruris; *9*, flexor hallucis longus and its tunnel; *10*, posterior tibial nerve; *11*, posterior tibial vessels; *12*, superficial aponeurosis cruris; *13*, flexor digitorum longus and tunnel; *14*, tibialis posterior and tunnel; *15*, medial malleolus; *16*, tibial metaphysis; *17*, extensor digitorum longus tendons and tunnel; *18*, anterior tibial vascular bundle; *19*, deep peroneal nerve; *20*, extensor hallucis longus tendon and tunnel; *21*, tibialis anterior tendon and tunnel; *22*, greater saphenous vein; *23*, tibiofibular syndesmotic synovial fringe; *24*, inferior extensor retinaculum; *26, 27,* inferior and posterior tibiofibular ligaments.)

compartment is superficial and overlies the tunnel of the flexor hallucis longus and the intertendinous interval between the flexor hallucis longus and flexor digitorum longus tunnels. The adherent segment of the superficial and deep aponeuroses is attached to the tibialis posterior and the flexor digitorum longus fibrous tunnel and forms the cover of the neurovascular compartment.

At this level, the tunnel of the tibialis posterior tendon crosses the posterior aspect of the deep deltoid ligament (see Fig. 3.21). The tunnels of the flexor hallucis longus, the posterior tibial neurovascular bundle, and the flexor digitorum longus cross obliquely the posteromedial aspect of the tibiotalar and posterior talocalcaneal joints (Figs. 3.23 and 3.24).

▶ Lower Talocalcaneal Tunnel or Tarsal Tunnel

The lower talocalcaneal tunnel or tarsal tunnel is the continuity of the deep posterior compartment of the leg-ankle, leading to the sole of the foot. The corresponding osseous canal is formed by the medial concave surface of the os calcis flanked anterosuperiorly by the posteromedial segment of the talus and the sustentaculum tali. It is flanked posteroinferiorly by the medial calcaneal tuberosity. This large canal is directed downward and anteriorly (Fig. 3.25). It is converted into a tunnel by the bridging flexor retinaculum above and the posterior segment of the abductor hallucis muscle below. The medial calcaneal surface is buttressed from within by the medial head of the quadratus plantae.

The flexor retinaculum (laciniate ligament, medial annular ligament) (Fig. 3.26) is formed by the juxtaposition of the superficial and deep aponeuroses cruris. It is trapezoidal with a proximal, anterior apex; an inferior base along the superior border of the abductor hallucis muscle; and an anterior and a posterior border.

At the apex, the flexor retinaculum corresponds to the anterior and medial segments of the medial malleolus. The deep aponeurotic component of the retinaculum inserts on the anterior aspect of the medial malleolus after passing under

134 Sarrafian's Anatomy of the Foot and Ankle

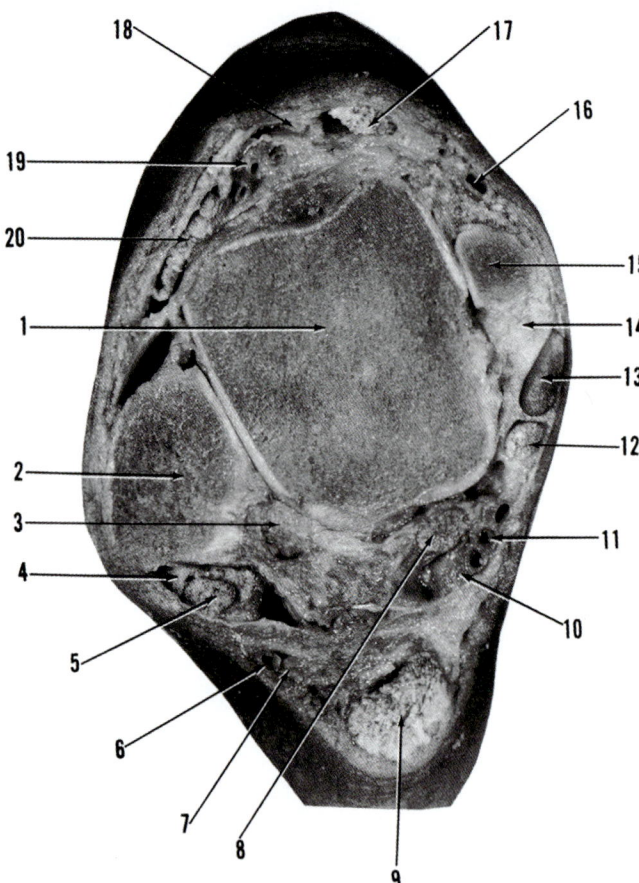

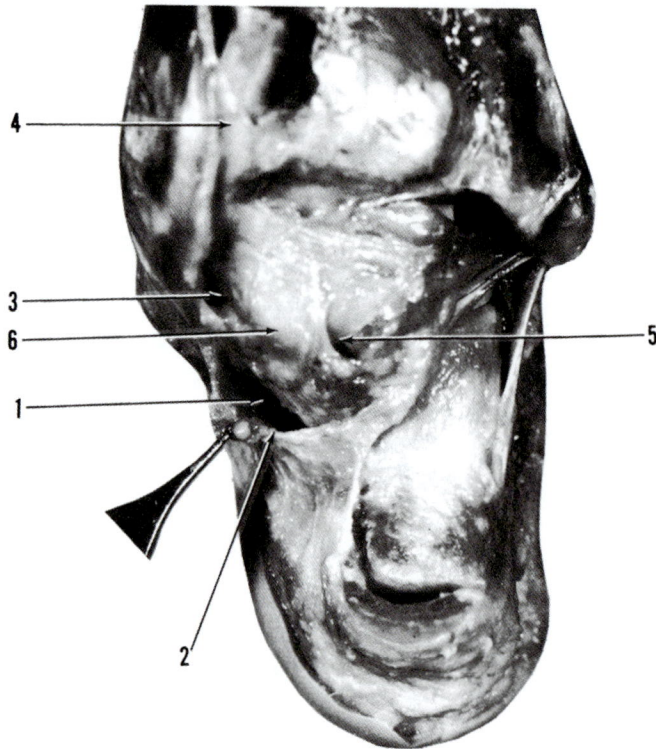

Figure 3.22 Posterior aspect of the ankle and hindfoot. Compartment of the posterior tibial neurovascular bundle (1) is covered by the adherent superficial and deep aponeuroses of the leg (2). This compartment is superficial to the tunnel of the flexor hallucis longus (5) and the intertendinous space (6) and posterior to the tunnel of the flexor digitorum longus (3) and the tibialis posterior tendon (4).

Figure 3.21 Cross-section of left ankle 1 cm from tip of medial malleolus. Proximal surface of section. (*1*, Talus; *2*, lateral malleolus; *3*, posterior talofibular ligament; *4*, frayed peroneus brevis tendon; *5*, peroneus longus tendon. Both peronei are in the superior peroneal tunnel. *6*, Short saphenous vein; *7*, sural nerve; *8*, flexor hallucis longus tendon; *9*, Achilles tendon; *10*, posterior tibial nerve; *11*, posterior tibial vascular bundle in its own tunnel; *12*, flexor digitorum longus and its tunnel; *13*, tibialis posterior tendon and its tunnel; *14*, deep component of deltoid ligament; *15*, medial malleolus, anterior colliculus; *16*, greater saphenous vein; *17*, tibialis anterior tendon and tunnel; *18*, extensor hallucis longus and tunnel; *19*, dorsalis pedis bundle and deep peroneal nerve; *20*, extensor digitorum longus tendons and tunnel.)

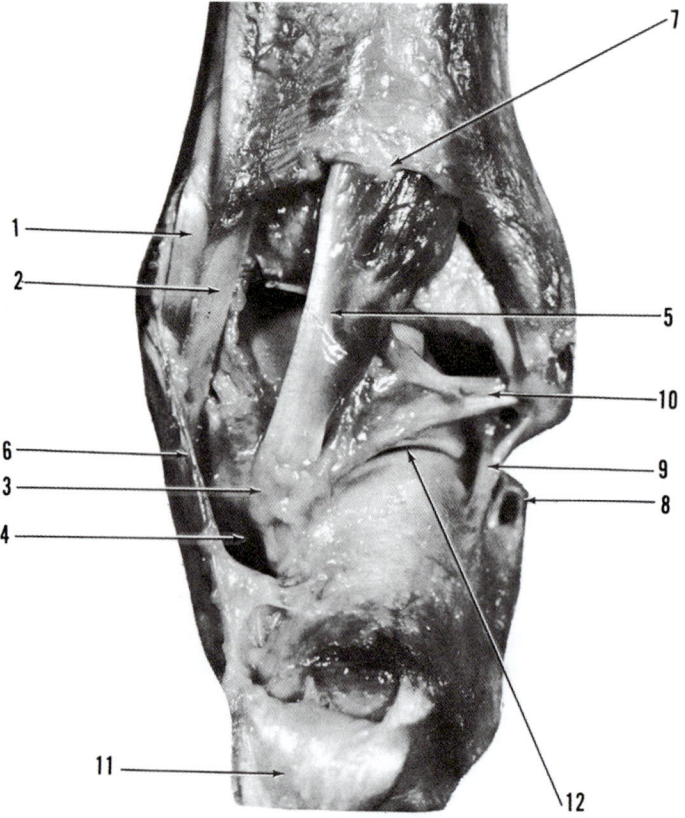

Figure 3.23 Posterior aspect of ankle and inferior talocalcaneal joint. (*1*, Tibialis posterior tendon with fibrous sheath excised; *2*, flexor digitorum longus tendon with fibrous sheath excised; *3*, flexor hallucis longus tendon in its tunnel on posterior border of talus; *4*, compartment for posterior tibial neurovascular bundle; *5*, flexor hallucis longus, which still has low descending muscle fibers at the level of the ankle on the lateral side; *6*, flexor retinaculum; *7*, intermediary aponeurosis of the leg; *8*, tunnel of peronei; *9*, calcaneofibular ligament; *10*, posterior talofibular ligament; *11*, reflected Achilles tendon; *12*, posterior talocalcaneal joint interline.)

Chapter 3: Retaining Systems and Compartments   135

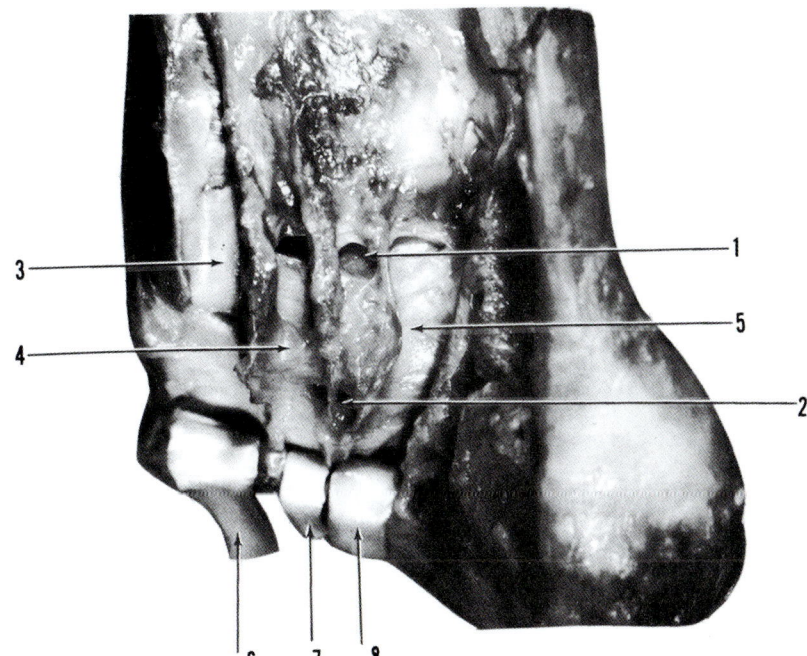

Figure 3.24 Anatomic preparation of the posteromedial aspect of the ankle and upper segment of the tibiotalar tunnel. The crossing tendons have been reflected downward after excision of their fibrous tendon sheaths; the implantations of the latter have been preserved. The joint levels are indicated by transverse partial incisions. The tendinous fibrous sheath as indicated in this preparation contributes to the reinforcement of the posterior capsuloligamentous complex. (*1*, Incisions indicating level of tibiotalar joint; *2*, incisions indicating level of posterior talocalcaneal joint; *3*, retromedial malleolar canal of tibialis posterior tendon; *4*, canal of flexor digitorum longus tendon; *5*, oblique canal of flexor hallucis longus tendon; *6*, tibialis posterior tendon, reflected; *7*, flexor digitorum longus tendon, reflected; *8*, flexor hallucis longus tendon, reflected. In the upper segment, the tunnels of the two flexors are separated by an intertendinous space.)

the tibialis anterior tendon. It crosses over the superomedial band of the inferior extensor aponeurosis (Figs. 3.27 and 3.28). The superficial aponeurotic component passes over the tibialis anterior tendon and inserts on the deep surface of the superior extensor retinaculum (see Fig. 3.27). The posterior border of the flexor retinaculum extends from the tip of the medial malleolus to the posterosuperior aspect of the os calcis medially. The anterior border corresponds to a vertical line drawn from the anterior border of the medial malleolus to the medial border of the foot. These last two borders are literally virtual because they are in continuity: the posterior border is in continuity with the superficial and deep aponeurosis cruris and the anterior border with the dorsal aponeurosis of the foot. The base of the flexor retinaculum corresponds to the superior border of the abductor hallucis muscle.

The proximal segment of the flexor retinaculum has obliquely oriented fibers. Anteriorly, the superficial and deep aponeurotic components are coalescent. Posteriorly, there is a dissociation of these two layers. The deep aponeurotic component of the flexor retinaculum inserts on the upper medial surface of the os calcis, whereas the superficial aponeurotic component envelops the lower segment of the Achilles tendon medially. This dissociation creates with the medial surface of the os calcis, a triangular

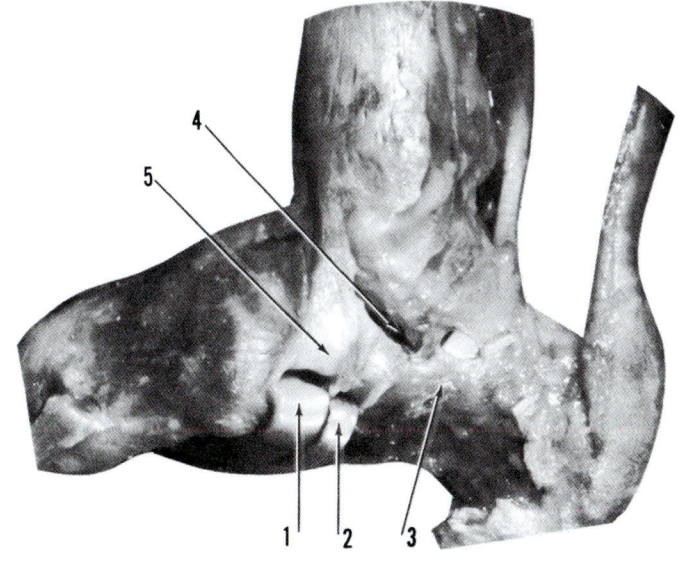

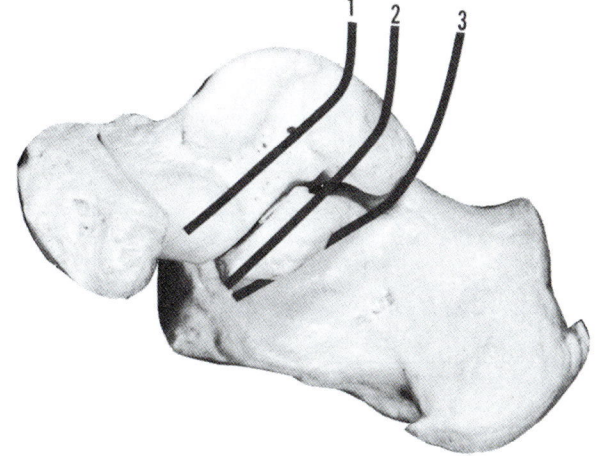

Figure 3.25 Anatomic preparation demonstrating the talocalcaneal canal, the crossing tendons and their relationship to the tibiotalar joint, the talus, and the calcaneus. The tibialis posterior tendon passes above the sustentaculum tali. The flexor digitorum longus tendon crosses the medial opening of the canalis tarsi and passes over the medial border of the sustentaculum tali. A longitudinal incision through the anterior border of its sheath leads to the sustentaculotalar interline, but this relationship varies. The flexor hallucis longus tendon passes under the sustentaculum tali. (*1*, Tibialis posterior tendon; *2*, flexor digitorum longus tendon; *3*, flexor hallucis longus tendon; *4*, medial opening of tarsal canal; *5*, medial calcaneonavicular ligament.)

space giving passage to the medial calcaneal vessels and nerve and filled with adipose tissue. Anteriorly, the coalesced segment of the flexor retinaculum is adherent to the fibrous tunnels of the tibialis posterior and flexor digitorum longus tendons. The deep aponeurotic segment of the flexor retinaculum, with its calcaneal attachment, forms the tunnel for the posterior tibial neurovascular bundle (Figs. 3.24, 3.29, and 3.30).

The distal segment of the flexor retinaculum has vertically oriented fibers anteriorly. At the level of the superior border of the abductor hallucis muscle, the coalesced aponeurotic layers split and envelop the muscle. The superficial layer is in continuity with the plantar aponeurosis. The deep layer adheres to the posterior segment of the medial intermuscular septum, thus reaching the trough between the abductor hallucis muscle and the flexor digitorum brevis. Posteriorly, the fibers take insertion on the calcaneal posteromedial tubercle.

A transverse triangular interfascicular lamina[11,14] appears in the lower segment of the intermuscular compartment of the calcaneal tunnel.

The lateral border of the lamina inserts on the medial surface of the os calcis between the upper border of the quadratus plantae muscle and the tunnel of the flexor hallucis longus. The medial border inserts proximally on the deep-covering aponeurosis of the abductor hallucis muscle at the level of the proximal

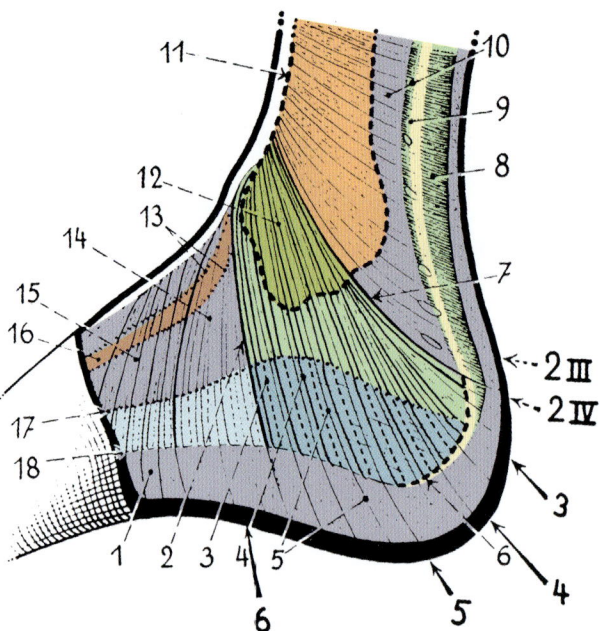

Figure 3.26 Medial aspect of the ankle and the flexor retinaculum. (1, Plantar fat; 2, anterior border of flexor retinaculum; 3, deep layer of sheath of abductor hallucis; 4, superficial layer of sheath of abductor hallucis; 5, superficial fibers of flexor retinaculum continued by retinaculum cutis; 7, posterior border of retinaculum; 8, sheath of Achilles tendon; 9, superficial aponeurosis cruris; 10, adherent superficial and deep aponeurosis cruris; 12, apex of flexor retinaculum; 13, projection of tibialis anterior tendon; 14, 16, superficial aponeuroses of foot; 15, oblique inferomedial band of inferior extensor retinaculum; 17, 18, superior and inferior borders of abductor hallucis muscle.) (Adapted from Bellocq P, Meyer P. Le ligament annulaire interne du cou-de-pied. Arch Anat Hist Embryol. 1954;37:23.)

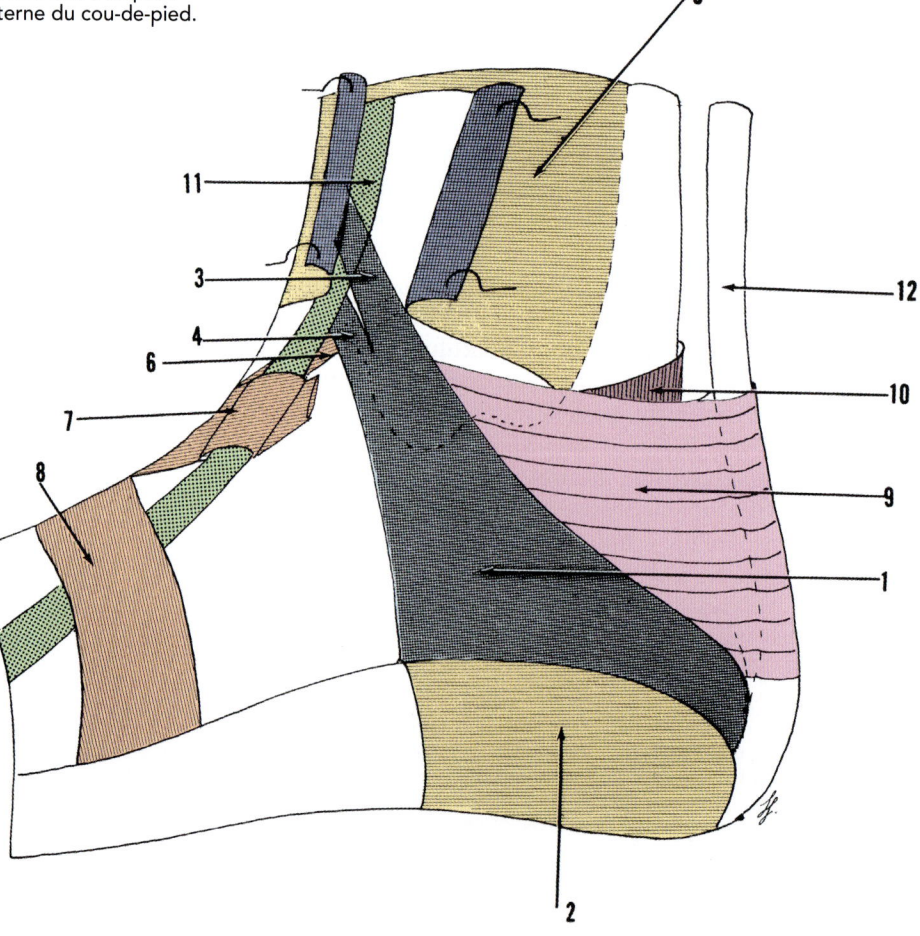

Figure 3.27 Diagram of the apical insertion of the flexor retinaculum, based on dissection under magnification. (1, Flexor retinaculum; 2, segment of flexor retinaculum covering abductor hallucis muscle; 3, 4, apical insertion of flexor retinaculum. One band passes over the tibialis anterior tendon and a deeper band passes under the same tendon. Both bands cross over the tibial insertion of the oblique superomedial band of the inferior extensor retinaculum and insert on the deep surface of the superior extensor retinaculum, creating continuity of the two. 5, Superior extensor retinaculum; 6, oblique deep component of superomedial band of inferior extensor retinaculum; 7, distal superficial component of the oblique superomedial band of inferior extensor retinaculum; 8, oblique inferomedial band of inferior extensor retinaculum; 9, superficial aponeurosis cruris; 10, deep aponeurosis cruris; 11, tibialis anterior tendon with its three retaining systems; 12, Achilles tendon incorporated within split layers of superficial aponeurosis cruris.)

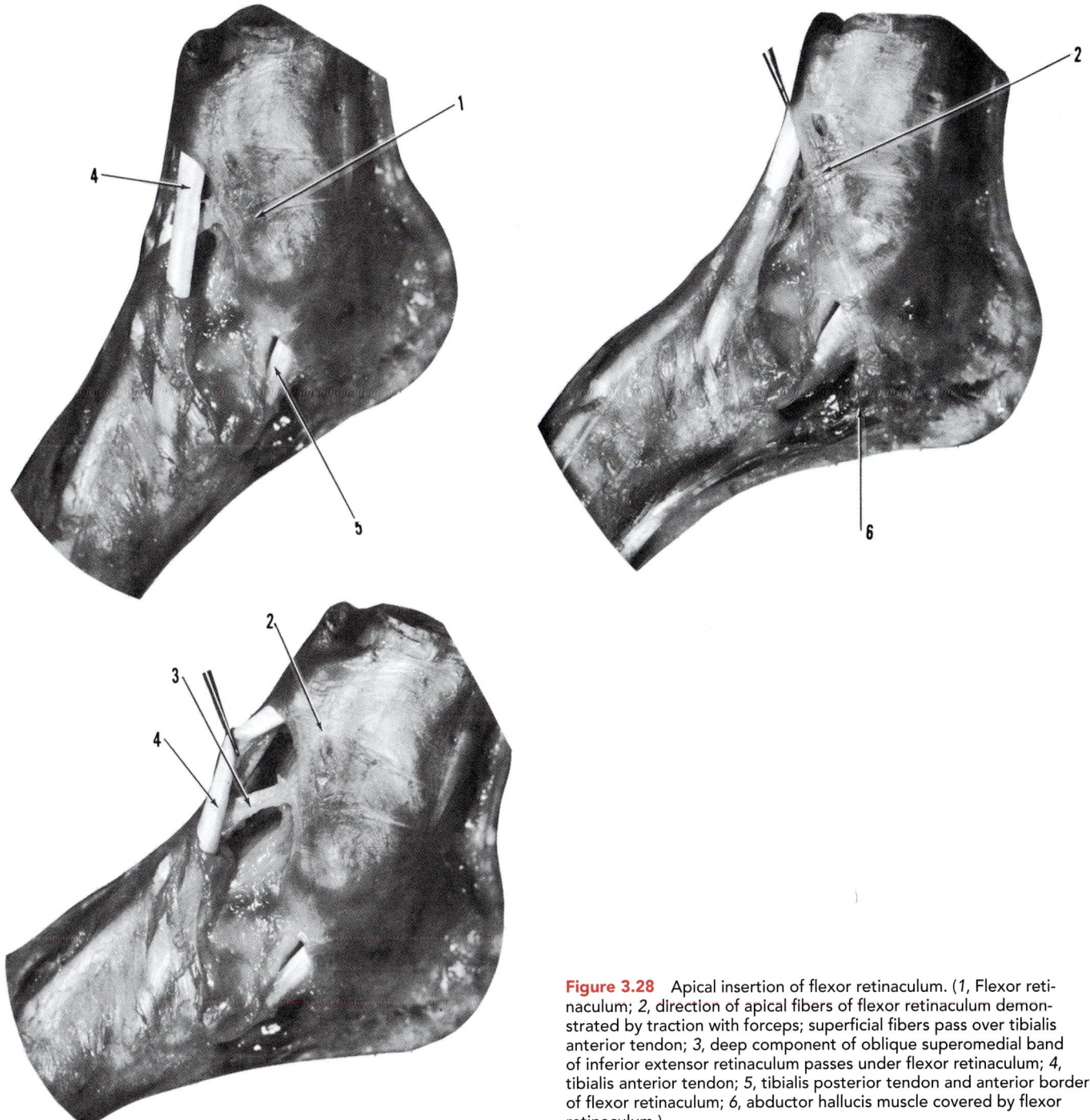

Figure 3.28 Apical insertion of flexor retinaculum. (*1*, Flexor retinaculum; *2*, direction of apical fibers of flexor retinaculum demonstrated by traction with forceps; superficial fibers pass over tibialis anterior tendon; *3*, deep component of oblique superomedial band of inferior extensor retinaculum passes under flexor retinaculum; *4*, tibialis anterior tendon; *5*, tibialis posterior tendon and anterior border of flexor retinaculum; *6*, abductor hallucis muscle covered by flexor retinaculum.)

border of the muscle; further distally, the insertion shifts to the midsegment and finally to the lower border of the same.

In its terminal portion, the interfascicular lamina is narrow and corresponds to the interval between the abductor hallucis muscle and the medial border of the flexor digitorum brevis. It is in continuity with the medial intermuscular septum of the sole of the foot.

The proximal border of the transverse interfascicular ligament forms a free, concave border. It divides the neurovascular tunnel into upper and lower calcaneal chambers (Figs. 3.31 to 3.33).

The lower chamber is limited laterally by the quadratus plantae muscle covering the medial calcaneal surface, medially by the abductor hallucis muscle covered by the deep aponeurosis, above by the interfascicular septum, and below by the space between the inferior borders of the abductor hallucis and the quadratus plantae. The upper chamber is limited medially by the flexor retinaculum, laterally by the tunnel of the flexor

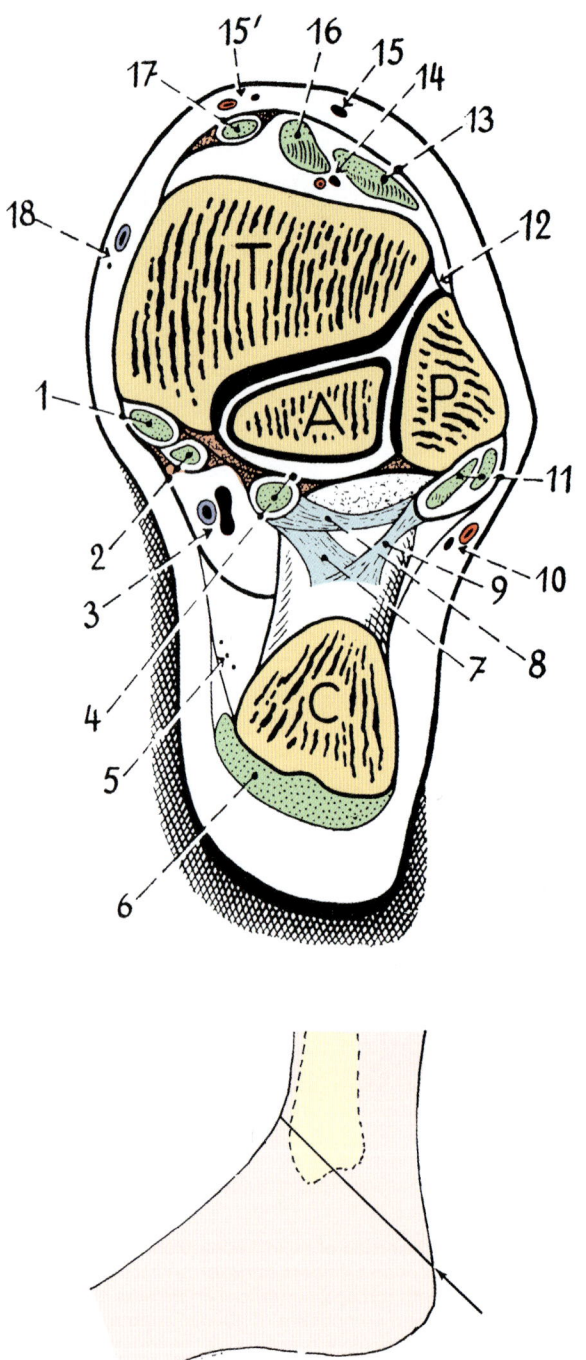

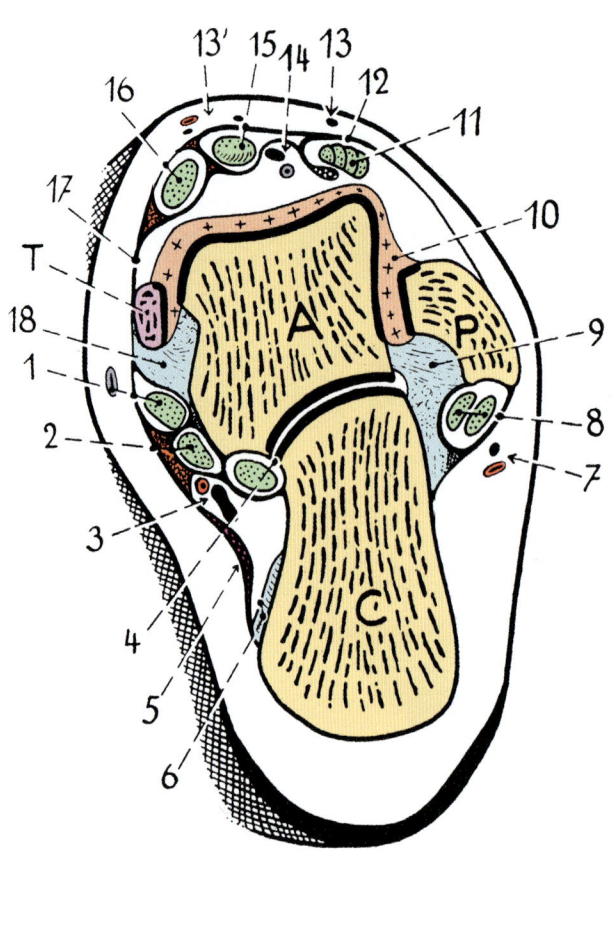

Figure 3.29 Cross-section through distal tibia, talus, and lateral malleolus as indicated by *arrow* in inset: distal surface of section. (*A*, Astragalus; *P*, peroneus; *T*, tibia; *1*, tunnel and tibialis posterior tendon; *2*, flexor retinaculum, tunnel, and tendon flexor digitorum longus; *3*, posterior tibial neurovascular bundle and its tunnel; *4*, tunnel and flexor hallucis longus tendon: tibiotalar capsule; *5*, medial calcaneal nerves; *6*, Achilles tendon; *7*, talocalcaneal posterosuperior ligament; *8*, talofibular fascicle; *9*, fibulocalcaneal fascicle of fibulotalocalcaneal ligament; *10*, sural nerve and short saphenous vein; *11*, tunnel and tendons of peronei muscles; *12*, anteroinferior tibioperoneal ligament; *13*, inferior extensor retinaculum, muscle-tendon extensor digitorum longus; *14*, tibialis anterior neurovascular bundle; *15, 15'*, superficial peroneal nerve; *16*, muscle-tendon extensor hallucis longus; *17*, fibrous tunnel and tendon tibialis anterior; *18*, saphenous nerve and long saphenous vein.) (Aapted from Bellocq P, Meyer P. Contribution a l'étude du canal calcanée. *Comptes Rendus Assoc Anat.* 1956;89:298.)

Figure 3.30 Cross-section through talus, calcaneus, and distal malleoli as indicated by *arrow* in inset: distal surface of section. (*A*, Astragalus; *C*, calcaneus; *P*, peroneus; *T*, tibia; *1*, greater saphenous vein, tunnel, and tibialis posterior tendon; *2*, flexor retinaculum, tunnel, and flexor digitorum longus tendon; *3*, posterior tibial neurovascular bundle and tunnel; *4*, tunnel and flexor hallucis longus tendon, posterior talocalcaneal articulation; *5*, flexor retinaculum with fibrous insertion site of abductor hallucis muscle; *6*, quadratus plantae and investing fascia; *7*, sural nerve and short saphenous vein; *8*, tunnel and tendons peronei; *9*, posterior talofibular ligament; *10*, tibiotalar articular cavity; *11*, tendon extensor digitorum longus; *12*, apex of frondiform ligament; *13, 13'*, branches of superficial peroneal nerve; *14*, tibialis anterior neurovascular bundle; *15*, tunnel and extensor hallucis longus tendon; *16*, fibrous tunnels and tibialis anterior tendon; *17*, superomedial band of inferior extensor retinaculum; *18*, deltoid ligament.) (Adapted from Bellocq P, Meyer P. Contribution a l'étude du canal calcanéen. *Comptes Rendus Assoc Anat.* 1956;89:300.)

Chapter 3: Retaining Systems and Compartments   139

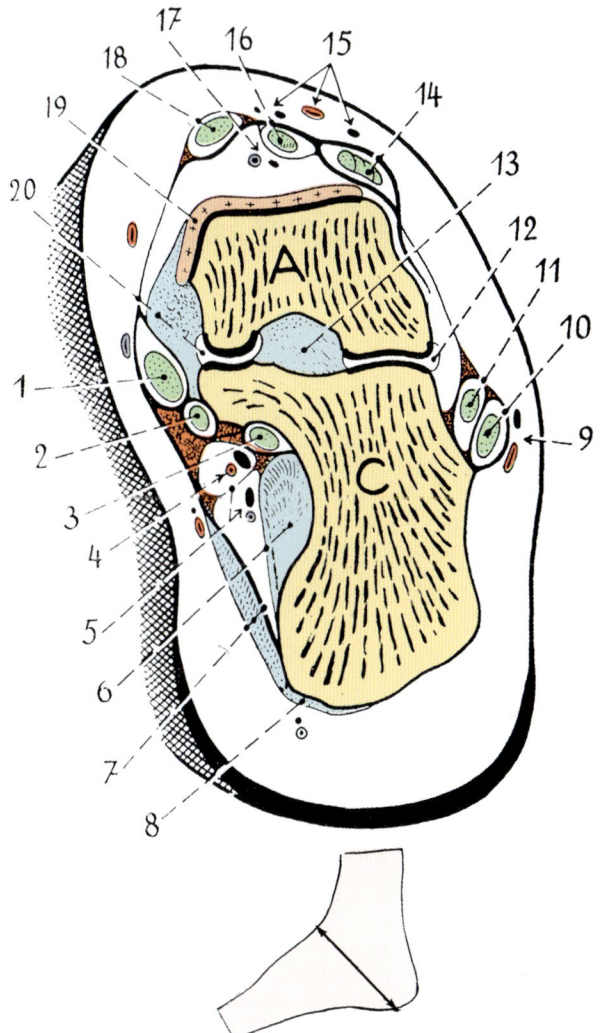

Figure 3.31 Oblique cross-section in direction of *arrow*; terminal section of calcaneal tunnel. (*1*, Tibialis posterior tendon and tunnel; *2*, flexor digitorum longus tendon and tunnel; *3*, flexor hallucis longus tendon and tunnel; *4*, upper chamber with medial neurovascular bundle; *5*, interfascicular lamina, lower chamber, and lateral plantar neurovascular bundle; *6*, quadratus plantae muscle and covering fascia; *7*, abductor hallucis muscle and investing fascia; *8*, middle segment of superficial plantar aponeurosis; *9*, sural nerve and short saphenous vein; *10*, tunnel and tendon of peroneus longus; *11*, tunnel and tendon of peroneus brevis; *12*, talocalcaneal posterolateral articulation; *13*, interosseous talocalcaneal ligament; *14*, frondiform ligament and extensor digitorum communis tendons; *15*, superficial peroneal nerve and superficial vein; *16*, sling and tendon of extensor hallucis longus; *17*, anterior tibial neurovascular bundle; *18*, fibrous tunnel of tibialis anterior tendon; *19*, tibiotalar joint cavity; *20*, superficial dorsal aponeurosis of foot and deltoid ligament.) (Adapted from Bellocq P, Meyer P. Contribution a l'éiude du canal calcanéen. *Comptes Rendus Assoc Anat.* 1956;89:292.)

Figure 3.33 The tibiotalocalcaneal tunnel (*TTC tunnel*). (*Abd. H*, abductor hallucis muscle; *CC*, calcaneal chamber, upper and lower; *FDL*, flexor digitorum longus; *FHL*, flexor hallucis longus; *FR*, flexor retinaculum; *IFL*, interfascicular lamina; *PTN*, posterior tibial nerve; *QP*, quadratus plantae; *TP*, tibialis posterior tendon.) The vascular tunnel is divided into two calcaneal chambers by the interfascicular lamina at the level of the upper border of the quadratus plantae and the abductor hallucis muscle. The upper calcaneal chamber lodges the medial plantar neurovascular bundle. The lower calcaneal chamber lodges the lateral plantar neurovascular bundle and communicates with the intermediary central plantar compartment.

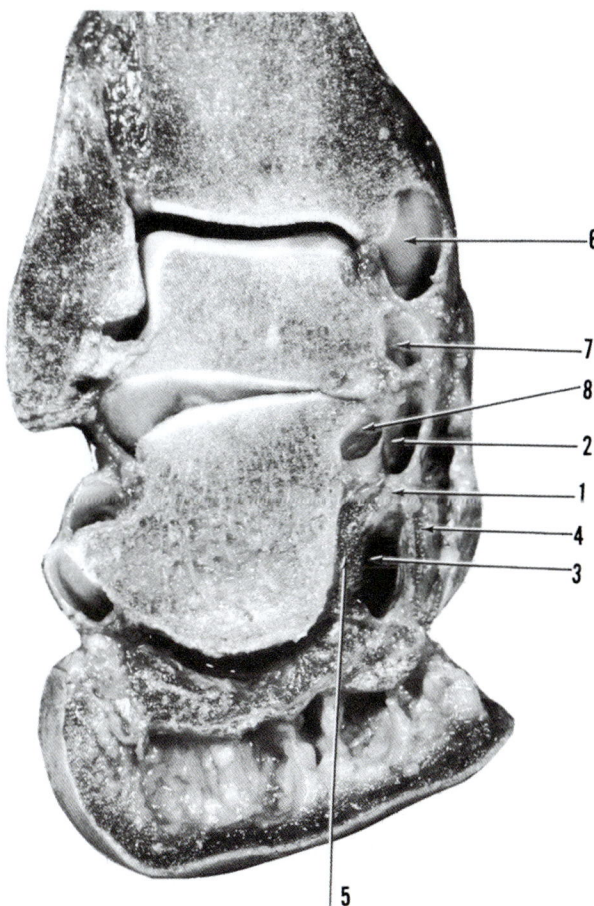

Figure 3.32 The compartments of tarsal tunnel as seen in a frontal cross-section of the ankle and hindfoot. (*1*, Interfascicular septum; *2*, upper chamber; *3*, lower chamber; *4*, abductor hallucis muscle with its investing fascia forming the medial wall of lower chamber; *5*, quadratus plantae muscle forming lateral wall of lower chamber; *6*, tibialis posterior tunnel; *7*, flexor digitorum longus tunnel; *8*, flexor hallucis longus tunnel.)

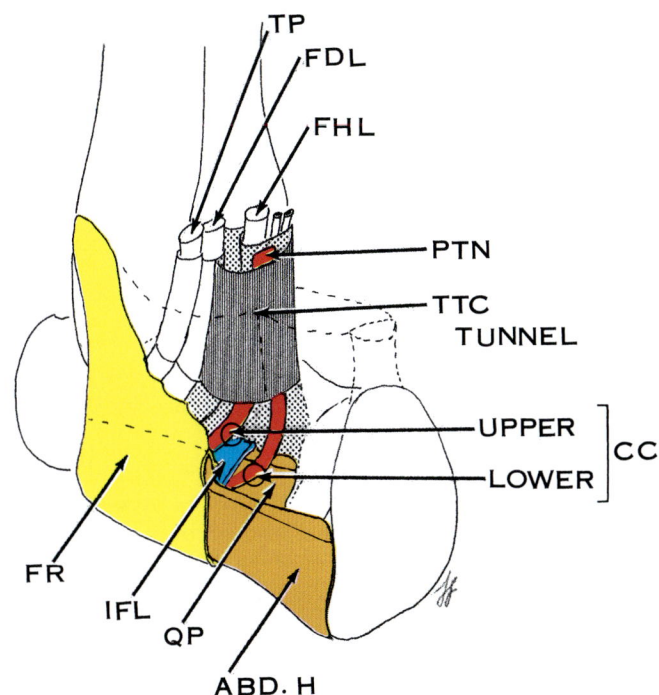

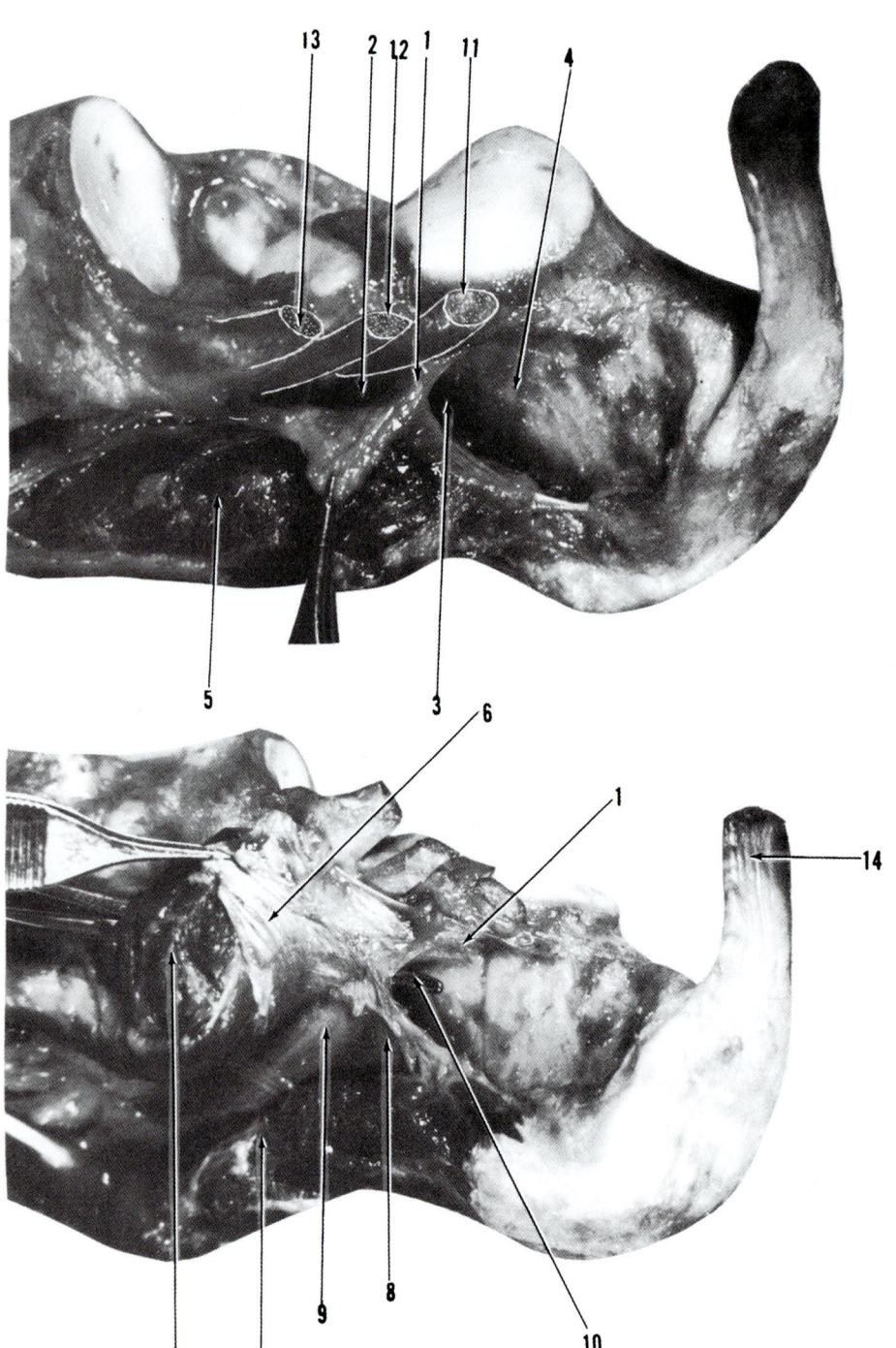

Figure 3.34 The lower calcaneal segment of the tarsal tunnel leading to the porta pedis. (*1*, Interfascicular ligament transversely oriented and inserting under flexor hallucis longus tendon and on the calcaneus, above the superior border, of the quadratus plantae [which has been removed in this specimen]; *2*, upper chamber of calcaneal canal for medial plantar neurovascular bundle; *3*, lower chamber of calcaneal canal for lateral plantar neurovascular bundle—this chamber leads to middle plantar space of sole of foot; *4*, medial calcaneal origin of quadratus plantae muscle; *5*, abductor hallucis muscle; *6*, medial investing fascia of abductor hallucis muscle reflected after detachment of its calcaneal insertion; *7*, flexor digitorum brevis muscle; *8*, medial intermuscular membrane; *9*, flexor hallucis longus tendon covered by its tenosynovial sheath; *10*, tip of hemostat emerging through lower chamber of calcaneal canal; *11*, flexor hallucis longus tendon; *12*, flexor digitorum longus tendon; *13*, tibialis posterior tendon; *14*, Achilles tendon.)

hallucis longus, above by the tunnel of the flexor digitorum longus, and below by the interfascicular septum (Figs. 3.34 and 3.35).

In the talocalcaneal tunnel, the tibialis posterior tendon with its fibrous sheath crosses the medial surface of the talus and passes over the posterior talotibial segment of the deltoid ligament, the tibiocalcaneal segment of the deltoid ligament, the superomedial calcaneonavicular ligament, and the inferior calcaneonavicular ligament (Figs. 3.36 and 3.37). Subsequently, the tibialis posterior tendon divides into three parts: navicular, plantar, and recurrent. The navicular segment terminates on the tuberosity of the navicular, the plantar segment continues under the inferior calcaneonavicular ligament and enters the planta pedis, and the recurrent portion inserts on the sustentaculum tali.

The tunnel of the flexor digitorum longus crosses the posteromedial talar tubercle and the posterior fibers of the deltoid ligament, passes over the medial border of the sustentaculum tali, and further distally shares a common tunnel with the flexor hallucis longus tendon.

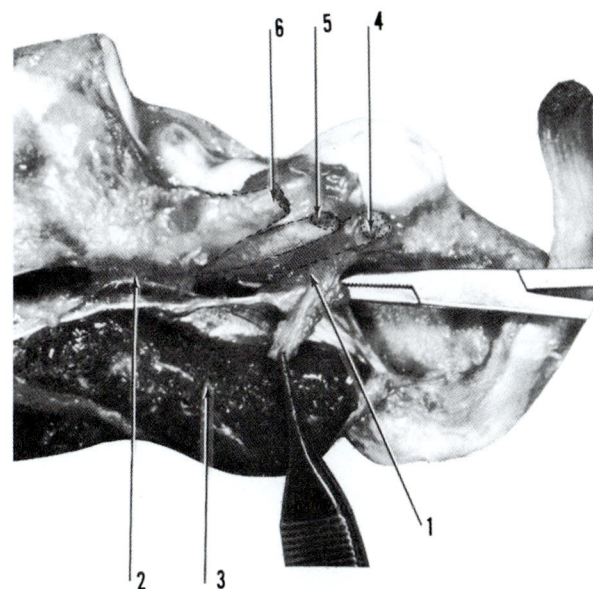

Figure 3.35 Lower chamber of the lower segment of the calcaneal canal. (*1*, Interfascicular ligament with hemostat underneath; *2*, second attachment site of investing sheath of abductor hallucis muscle; *3*, abductor hallucis muscle; *4*, flexor hallucis longus tendon; *5*, flexor digitorum longus tendon; *6*, tibialis posterior tendon.)

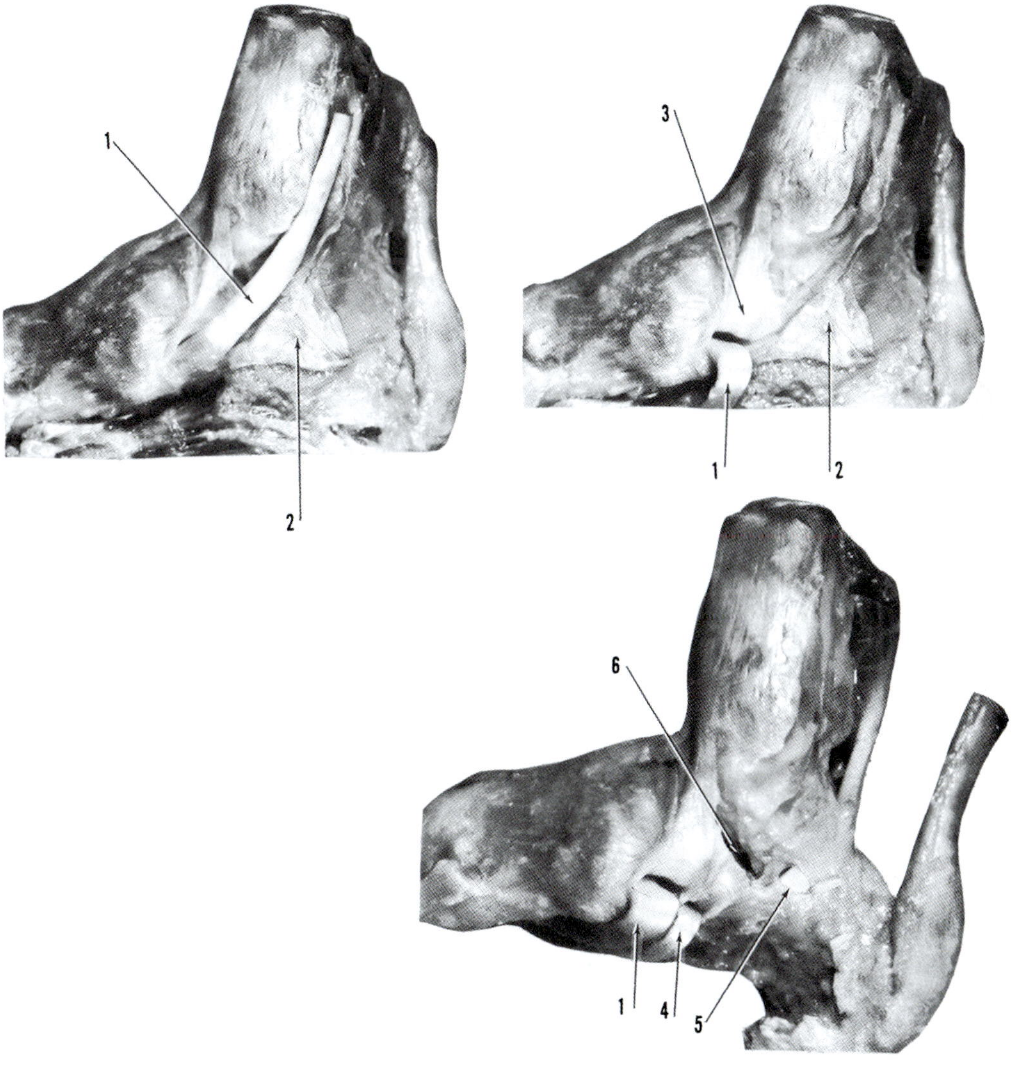

Figure 3.36 **Medial aspect of the tarsal tunnel with progressive reflection-excision of the flexor retinaculum.** In the bottom figure, the neurovascular bundle, the abductor hallucis muscle, and the medial calcaneal segment of the quadratus plantae muscle are removed. (*1*, Tibialis posterior tendon; *2*, reflected flexor retinaculum, which adheres to tunnel of tendon; *3*, superomedial calcaneonavicular ligament blending with anterior superficial fibers of deltoid ligament; *4*, tendon of flexor digitorum longus; *5*, tendon of flexor hallucis longus; *6*, medial opening of canalis tarsi.)

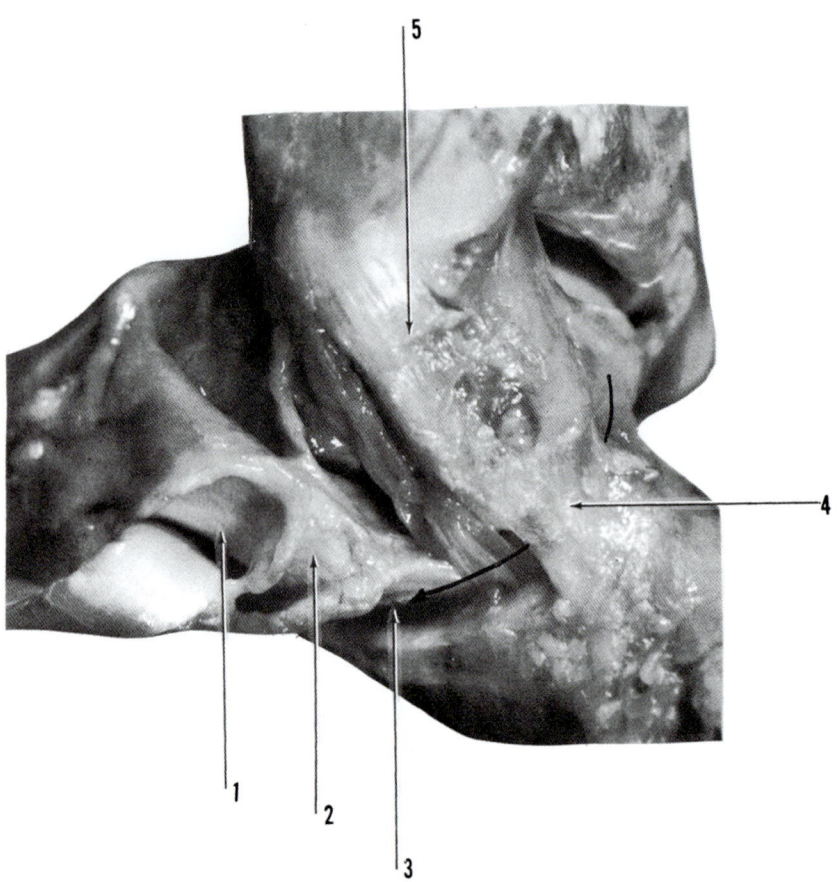

Figure 3.37 The canal of the lower surface of the sustentaculum tali is in direct continuity with the talocalcaneal flexor hallucis longus tunnel as indicated by the *arrow*. (*1*, Fibrocartilaginous canal of tibialis posterior tunnel; *2*, fibrocartilaginous canal of flexor digitorum longus passing over medial surface of sustentaculum tali and fibrous tunnel attached to its upper and lower borders; *3*, fibrocartilaginous tunnel of flexor hallucis longus tendon located on inferior surface of sustentaculum tali; *4*, fibrous talocalcaneal tunnel of flexor hallucis longus tendon; *5*, deltoid ligament.)

The tunnel of the flexor digitorum longus has a variable relationship with the sustentaculum tali.[11] The tunnel may extend above the sustentaculum tali, thus entering in contact with the anteromedial talocalcaneal joint, or it may shift inferiorly on the sustentaculum tali, thus covering partially the tunnel of the flexor hallucis longus, or it may extend simultaneously above and below the sustentaculum tali when the latter is underdeveloped.

The tunnel of the flexor hallucis longus, initially separated by an intertendinous space, crosses the posterior talocalcaneal joint and passes along the inferior surface of the sustentaculum tali; distally, the tendon shares a common sheath with the flexor digitorum longus tendon (see Figs. 3.36 and 3.37).

The common sheath of the long flexors extends nearly horizontally medial to the anterior end of the calcaneus.[11] It is attached laterally to the os calcis and medially to the deep investing aponeurosis of the abductor hallucis muscle. The thick ceiling of the common tunnel, in contact with the inferior calcaneonavicular ligament, is formed by a strong fibrous lamina uniting the calcaneus with the deep aponeurosis of the abductor hallucis muscle, reinforced by the recurrent fibers of the tibialis posterior tendon that are to insert on the os calcis. Contrary to the ceiling, the floor of this common tunnel is thin and formed also by a transverse fibrous lamina extending from the deep aponeurosis of the abductor hallucis to the os calcis, above the quadratus plantae (Fig. 3.38).[11]

The common sheath of the flexor digitorum longus and flexor hallucis longus tendons marks the end of the calcaneal tunnel. It represents the surgeon's knot of Henry.

The posterior tibial neurovascular tunnel is superficially located at the talocalcaneal level. It overlies the flexor intertendinous interval and the tunnel of the flexor hallucis longus (Fig. 3.39). Gradually, the latter converges toward the tunnel of the flexor digitorum longus and the intertendinous interval disappears. The neurovascular tunnel is then covered superficially by the coalesced layers of the flexor retinaculum. The deep surface of the tunnel corresponds to the tunnel of the flexor hallucis longus, the medial surface of the calcaneus with the quadratus plantae, and its covering aponeurosis (Fig. 3.40). At the next lower level, the calcaneal level, the neurovascular tunnel is divided into upper and lower calcaneal chambers by the interfascicular lamina of Raiga (see Figs. 3.31, 3.32, and 3.41).[14]

The medial plantar neurovascular bundle penetrates the upper calcaneal chamber, and the lateral plantar neurovascular bundle penetrates the lower calcaneal chamber. In both chambers, the nerve is anterior to the corresponding artery. The nerve to the abductor digiti quinti muscle arising from the lateral plantar nerve penetrates the lower calcaneal chamber (Fig. 3.42).

In the terminal segment of the calcaneal tunnel, at the level of the common tunnel of the long flexor tendons, the neurovascular tunnel remains subdivided into two tunnels (see Fig. 3.38). The fibrous tunnel of the medial plantar neurovascular bundle is now triangular. The base corresponds to the common sheath of both long flexors. The medial wall is formed by the deep aponeurosis of the abductor hallucis, and the lateral wall by the medial head of the quadratus plantae and its investing fascia. The apex of the tunnel corresponds to the very narrow portion of the interfascicular lamina that has joined the medial intermuscular groove septum.

The fibrous tunnel of the lateral plantar neurovascular bundle is now inferolateral and directed transversely. It is limited above by the medial head of the quadratus plantae and its investing fascia and further medially by the interfascicular lamina. The lateral wall of the tunnel corresponds to the inner segment of the calcaneocuboid ligament covered partially by the quadratus plantae. The medial wall is formed by the very lower segment of the abductor hallucis with its deep aponeurosis. The inferior wall corresponds to the flexor digitorum brevis muscle covered by its aponeurosis.[11] Laterally, the apex of this tunnel reaches the lateral intermuscular groove septum. The medial plantar neurovascular tunnel will remain in contact with the medial intermuscular septum and the medial compartment of the sole. The lateral plantar neurovascular tunnel is continued with the deep segment of the middle compartment of the sole.

PLANTAR APONEUROSIS

The plantar aponeurosis is the strong, fibrous, investing layer of the sole of the foot (Figs. 3.43 and 3.44). It is subcutaneous and extends from the heel to the ball of the foot. It is connected to the skin with retinacular vertical fibers proximally and transverse septa distally. Two longitudinally oriented intermuscular septa connect the plantar aponeurosis to the deep planta pedis. Smaller deep sagittal extensions bind the distal segment of the plantar aponeurosis to the depth of the ball of the foot.

In 1840, Maslieurat-Lagémard gave the first detailed description of the insertion of the plantar aponeurosis.[15] Henkel, in 1913, provided the most comprehensive study of the plantar aponeurosis.[16] The recent work of Bojsen-Møller and Flagstad confirmed and revived Henkel's work and brought further understanding of the insertions of the plantar aponeurosis and the anatomy of the ball of the foot.[17]

The plantar aponeurosis has three components: central, lateral, and medial.

▶ Central Component

The central or major component of the plantar aponeurosis is triangular, with a posterior apex and an anterior base. It originates from the plantar aspect of the posteromedial calcaneal

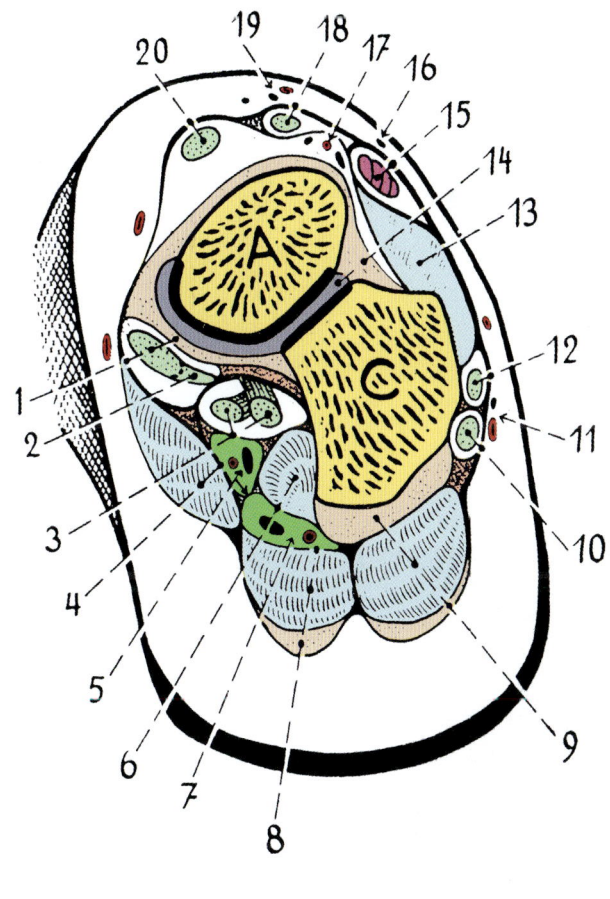

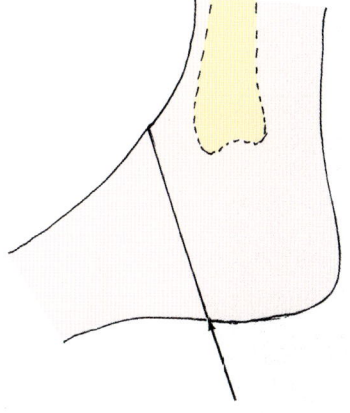

Figure 3.38 Cross-section through distal talus-calcaneus as indicated by the *arrow* in inset: distal surface of section. (*A*, Astragalus; *B*, calcaneum; *1*, tunnel and tibialis posterior tendon, inferior calcaneonavicular ligament; *2*, recurrent expansion of tibialis posterior tendon; *3*, common tunnel and flexor digitorum longus, flexor hallucis longus tendons; *4*, plantar aponeurosis inner portion, abductor hallucis muscle and its deep investing fascia; *5*, internal plantar neurovascular bundle, its fibrous tunnel and the interfascicular lamina; *6*, investing aponeurosis and quadratus plantae muscle; *7*, external plantar neurovascular bundle and its fibrous tunnel; *8*, plantar aponeurosis, middle portion, flexor digitorum brevis and its investing aponeurosis; *9*, plantar aponeurosis, lateral portion, muscle abductor digiti quinti, plantar calcaneocuboid ligament; *10*, tunnel and tendon of peroneus longus; *11*, sural nerve and short saphenous vein; *12*, tunnel and tendon of peroneus brevis; *13*, extensor digitorum brevis; *14*, talocalcaneal interosseous ligament; *15*, frondiform ligament and tendon, extensor digitorum longus; *16, 19*, branches of superficial peroneal nerve; *17*, dorsalis pedis bundle and deep peroneal nerve; *18*, tunnel and tendon of extensor hallucis longus; *20*, superomedial band of inferior extensor retinaculum and tibialis anterior tendon.) (Adapted from Bellocq P, Meyer P. Contribution a l'étude du canal calcanéen. *Comptes Rendus Assoc Anat.* 1956;89:304.)

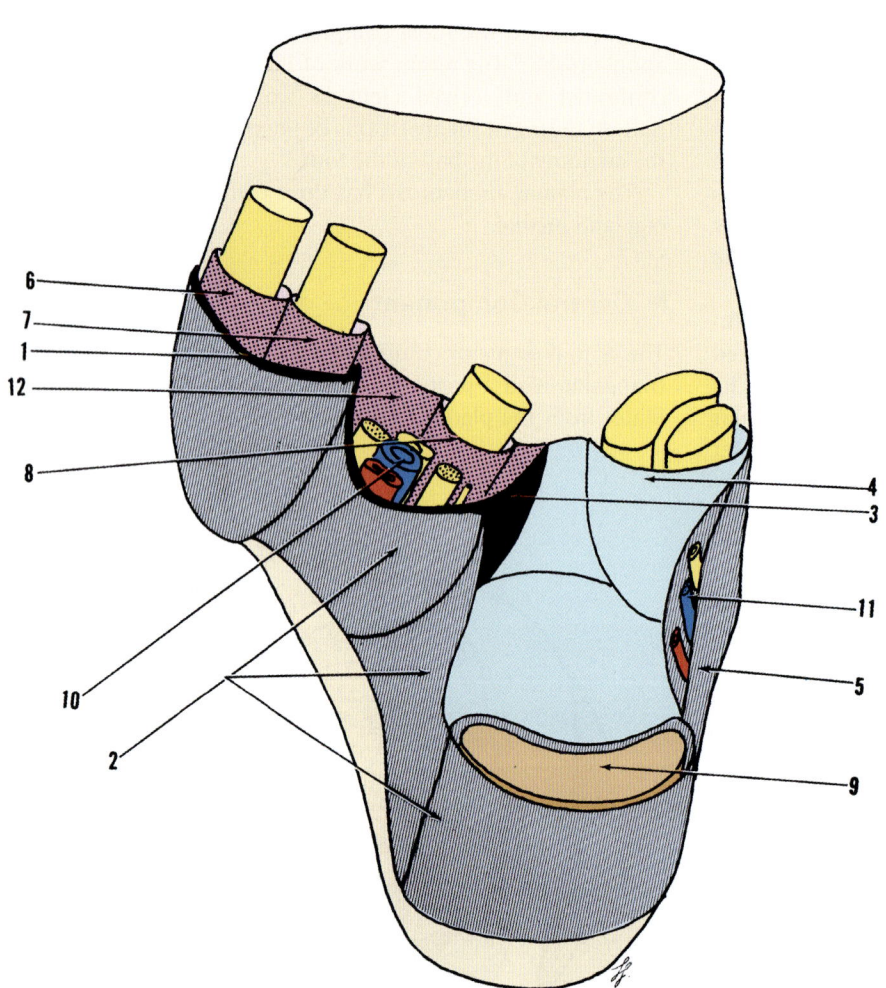

Figure 3.39 Posterior, posteromedial, and posterolateral compartments of the ankle and hindfoot. (*1*, Adherent superficial and deep layers of aponeurosis cruris contributing to formation of flexor retinaculum; *2, 5*, superficial aponeurosis cruris closing space between tarsal tunnel and medial border of Achilles tendon, then investing the latter and incorporating laterally the sural nerve and short saphenous nerve [*11*] before blending with peroneal retinaculum [*4*]; *3*, deep aponeurosis cruris, which covers the neurovascular bundle and inserts on intermedium aponeurosis lateral to tunnel of flexor hallucis longus tendon; *4*, tunnel of peronei tendons; *6*, tunnel of tibialis posterior tendon; *7*, tunnel of flexor digitorum longus tendon [both *6* and *7* are adherent to *1*]; *8*, tunnel of flexor hallucis longus tendon deep and nonadherent to deep aponeurosis cruris; *9*, Achilles tendon; *10*, neurovascular tunnel, superficial to flexor hallucis longus tunnel and to intertendinous space covered by intermediary aponeurosis [*12*] of leg. The neurovascular tunnel is covered by the superficial and deep aponeuroses cruris. It contains posterior tibial vessels and medial and lateral plantar nerves.)

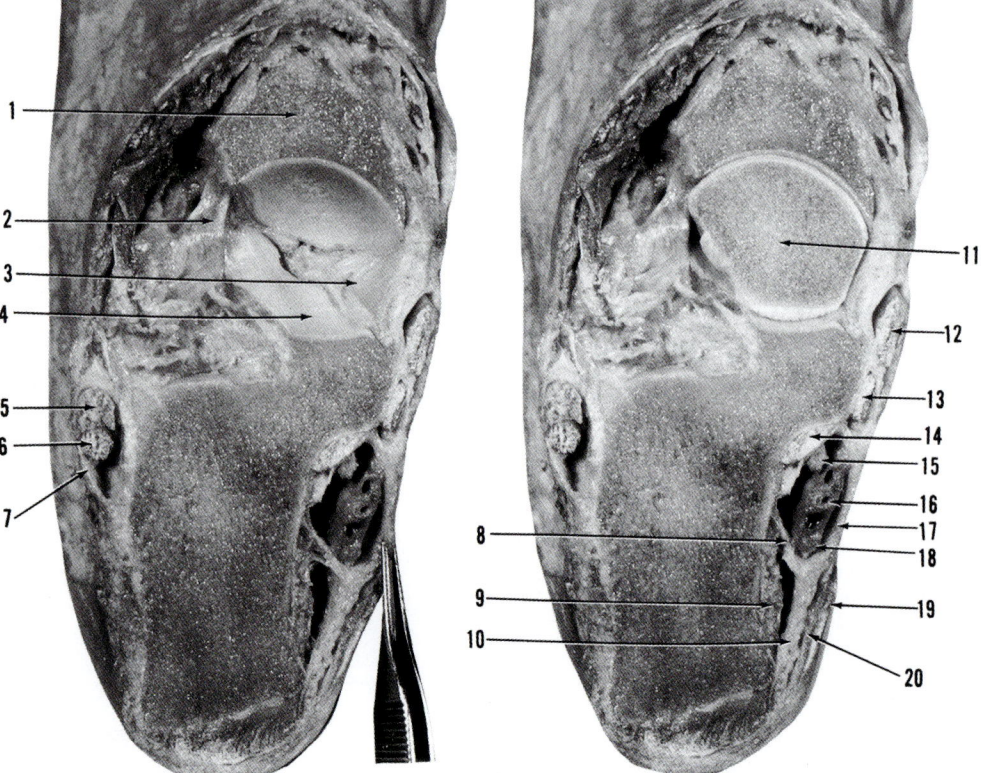

Figure 3.40 Cross-section of left foot, passing through the calcaneus, the lower segment of the talar head, and the navicular. Proximal surface of section. (*1*, Navicular; *2*, calcaneonavicular fascicle of bifurcate ligament; *3*, inferior calcaneonavicular ligament; *4*, anterior and middle calcaneal articular surfaces; *5*, peroneus brevis tendon; *6*, peroneus longus tendon; *7*, inferior peroneal retinaculum and tunnel; *8*, investing fascia of quadratus plantae; *9*, quadratus plantae; *10*, adherent investing fascia quadratus plantae, deep investing fascia of abductor hallucis muscle; *11*, talar head; *12*, tibial posterior tendon and tunnel; *13*, flexor digitorum longus tendon and tunnel; *14*, flexor hallucis longus tendon and tunnel; *15*, medial plantar nerve; *16*, posterior tibial artery and veins; *17*, flexor retinaculum; *18*, lateral plantar nerve; *19*, superficial investing aponeurosis of abductor hallucis muscle; *20*, abductor hallucis muscle.)

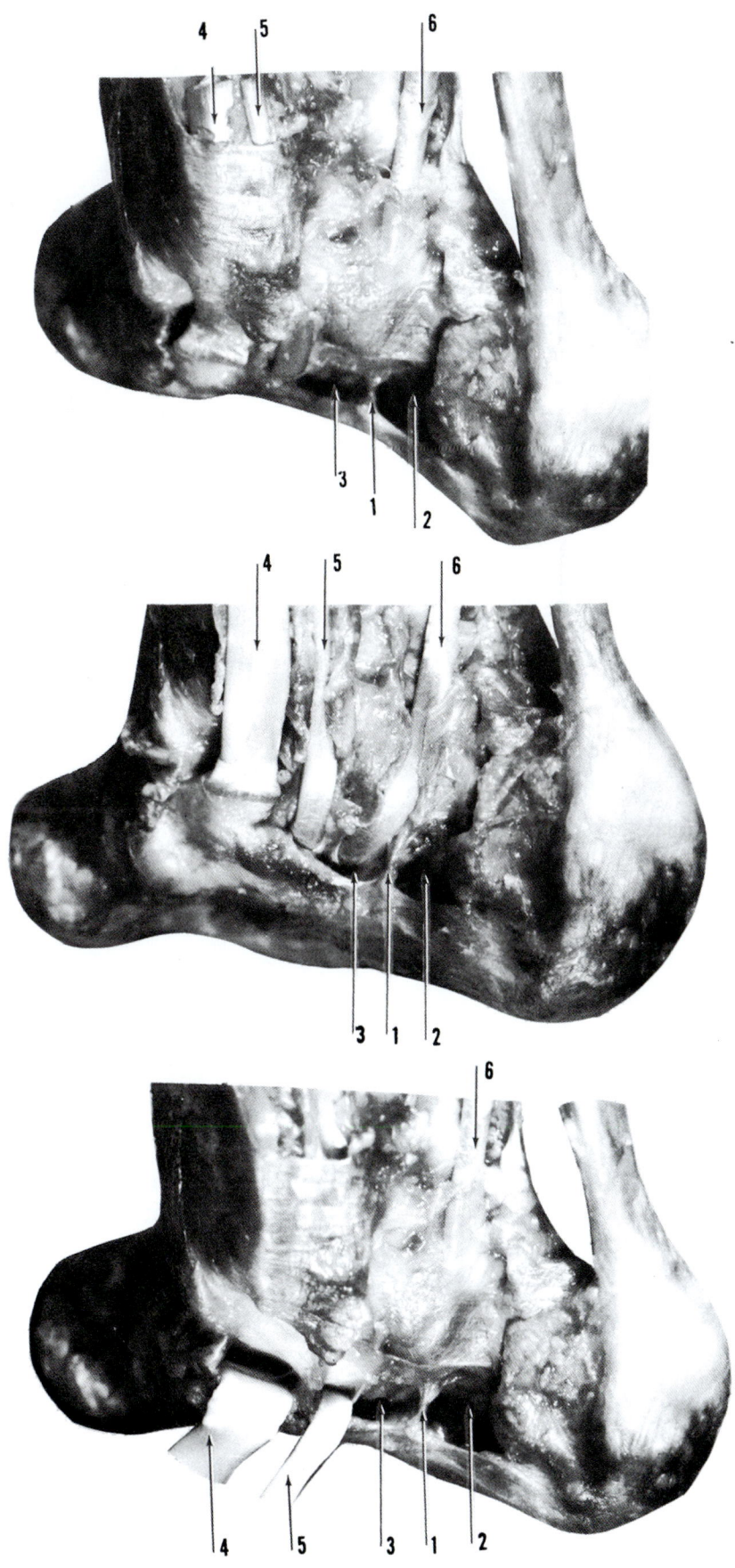

Figure 3.41 Compartments of the lower segment of the tarsal tunnel. In the top figure, the tendons are maintained in their fibrous tunnels. In the middle figure, a segment of the fibrous tunnels has been excised. (*1*, Interfascicular septum; *2*, lower chamber of tarsal tunnel for lateral plantar neurovascular bundle; *3*, upper chamber of tarsal tunnel for medial plantar neurovascular bundle; *4*, tibialis posterior tendon; *5*, flexor digitorum longus tendon; *6*, flexor hallucis longus tendon.)

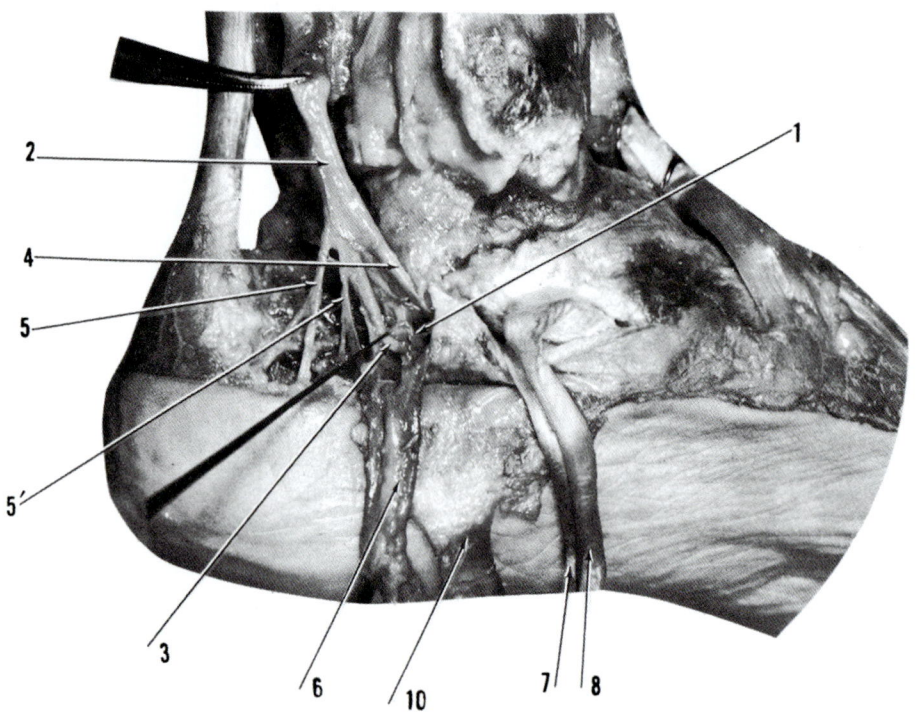

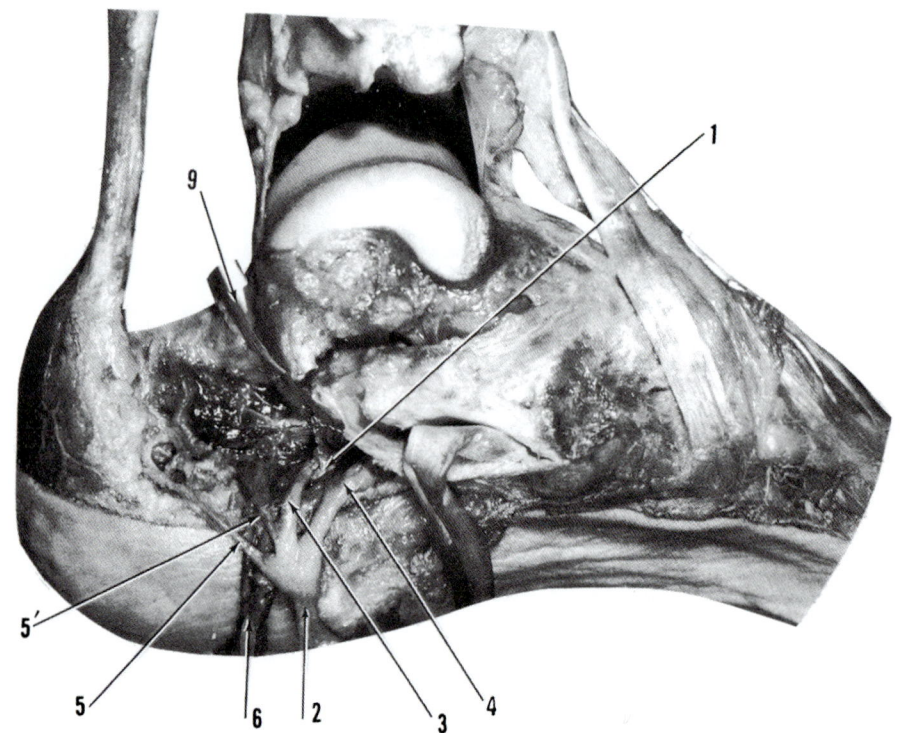

Figure 3.42 Medial aspect of tarsal tunnel. (*1*, Interfascicular ligament; *2*, posterior tibial nerve; *3*, lateral plantar nerve entering lower chamber; *4*, medial plantar nerve entering upper chamber; *5*, medial calcaneal nerve; *5′*, nerve to abductor digiti quinti; *6*, posterior tibial vessels reflected downward; *7*, flexor digitorum longus tendon reflected downward; *8*, tibialis posterior tendon reflected downward; *9*, flexor hallucis longus tendon, deep to neurovascular bundle; *10*, reflected flexor retinaculum.)

tuberosity. It conforms to the convexity of the tuberosity and may receive contributions from the Achilles tendon and especially from the plantaris tendon.

The origin of the central component of the aponeurosis is approximately 1.5 to 2 cm in width. The fibers group into a longitudinally oriented, thick, shiny, gently twisted band that gradually enlarges.

At the midmetatarsal level, the aponeurosis divides into five longitudinally oriented segments that gradually diverge. Proximal to the metatarsal heads, each longitudinally oriented

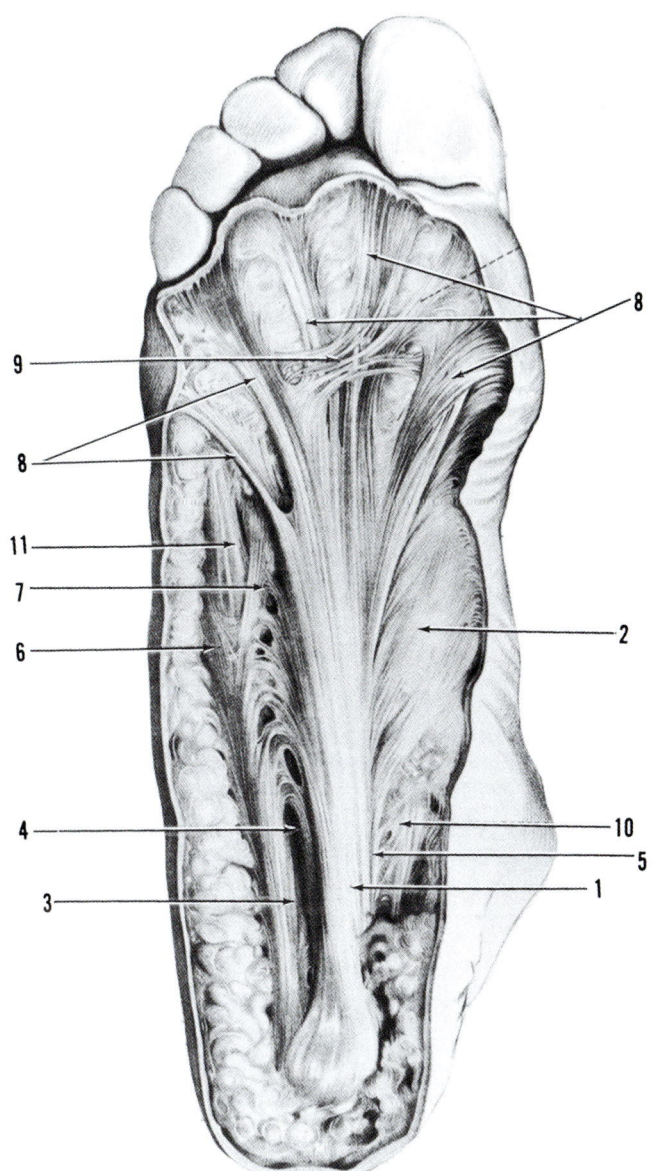

Figure 3.43 Plantar aponeurosis. (*1*, Central component of plantar aponeurosis; *2*, medial component of plantar aponeurosis; *3*, lateral component of plantar aponeurosis; *4*, lateral plantar sulcus; *5*, medial plantar sulcus; *6*, lateral crux of lateral plantar component; *7*, medial crux of lateral plantar component; *8*, superficial longitudinal tracts; *9*, transverse superficial tract; *10*, abductor hallucis muscle; *11*, abductor digiti quinti muscle.) (From Henkel A. Die aponeurosis plantaris. *Arch Anat Anat Ab Arch Anat Physiol.* 1913;113:113-123.)

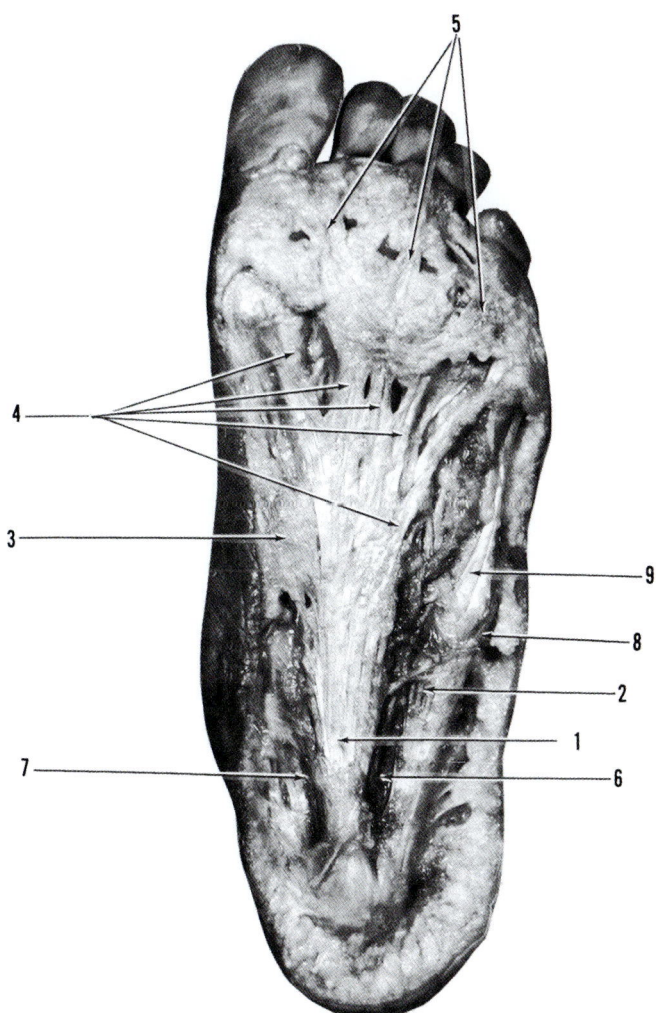

Figure 3.44 Plantar aponeurosis, dissection of superficial layer. (*1*, Central component of plantar aponeurosis; *2*, lateral component of plantar aponeurosis; *3*, medial component of plantar aponeurosis; *4*, superficial tracts; *5*, central superficial tracts at ball of foot; *6*, lateral sulcus; *7*, medial sulcus; *8*, lateral crux of lateral component; *9*, tendon of abductor digiti quinti.)

band divides into a superficial and a deep tract (lacertus aponeuroticus superficialis and profundus; Fig. 3.45).[16] The diversion of the deep tracts is completed as they reach the corresponding metatarsophalangeal complex.

The central three superficial tracts continue more or less in the direction of the toes. One tract reaches the interval between the first and second toes. The next tract is located at the base of the third toe or in the interval between the third and fourth toes. The third central superficial tract reaches the base of the fifth toe or the interval between the fourth and fifth toes. Anterior to the metatarsal heads, the three central superficial components insert into the skin and from their deep surfaces send transversely oriented fibers, contributing to the formation of the natatory ligament (Fig. 3.46).

The two marginal superficial tracts run to the margins of the foot. The medial tract continues in the direction of the big toe and the lateral tract that of the fifth toe, thus differing by their orientation from the central band. They contribute minimally to the formation of the transversely oriented natatory ligament.

Proximal to the metatarsal heads, the plantar aponeurosis is crossed superficially by transversely oriented retinacular bands separated by adipose tissue and forms the fasciculus aponeuroticum transversum (Fig. 3.47). Transversely oriented in the middle, the retinacular bands curve longitudinally at the margins and help form the ligamentum natatorium. At the level of the big toe, these fibers contribute to the medial longitudinal band. The subcutaneous transverse bands connect with the skin, and from their transverse segment, oblique fibers extend

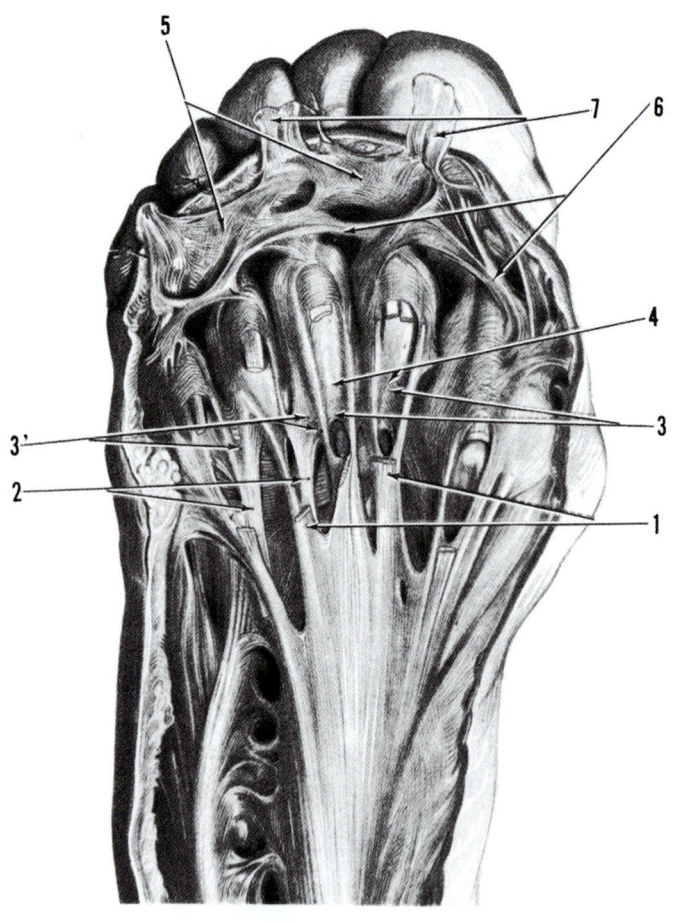

Figure 3.45 Deep components of plantar aponeurosis. (*1*, Superficial longitudinal tracts, transected and reflected distally [*7*]; *2*, sagittal septa of plantar aponeurosis; *3*, crossing fibers of the sagittal septa of the same ray at the level of the plantar plates [*4*]; *3′*, crossing fibers between sagittal septa of adjacent rays; *5*, natatory ligament; *6*, mooring ligament or deep transverse aponeurotic tract.) (From Henkel A. Die aponeurosis plantaris. *Arch Anat Anat Ab Arch Anat Physiol*. 1913;113:113-123.)

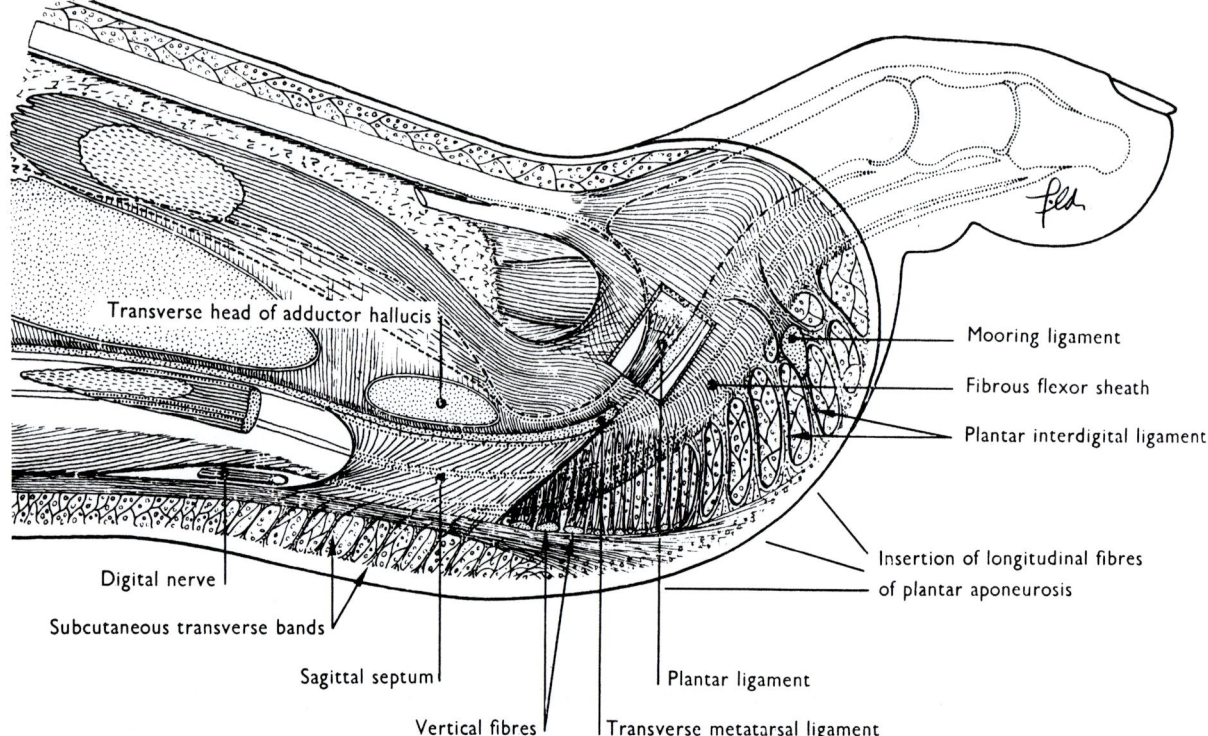

Figure 3.46 Drawing of a sagittal section through the second interstice showing the internal architecture of the three areas of the ball of the foot. The sagittal septum is attached to the proximal phalanx through the transverse metatarsal ligament and the plantar ligament of the joint. The vertical fibers and the lamellae of the plantar interdigital ligament are attached to the proximal phalanx through the fibrous flexor sheath. (Republished with permission of John Wiley, from Bojsen-Møller F, Flagstad KE. Plantar aponeurosis and internal architecture of the ball of the foot. *J Anat*. 1976;121:599; permission conveyed through Copyright Clearance Center, Inc.)

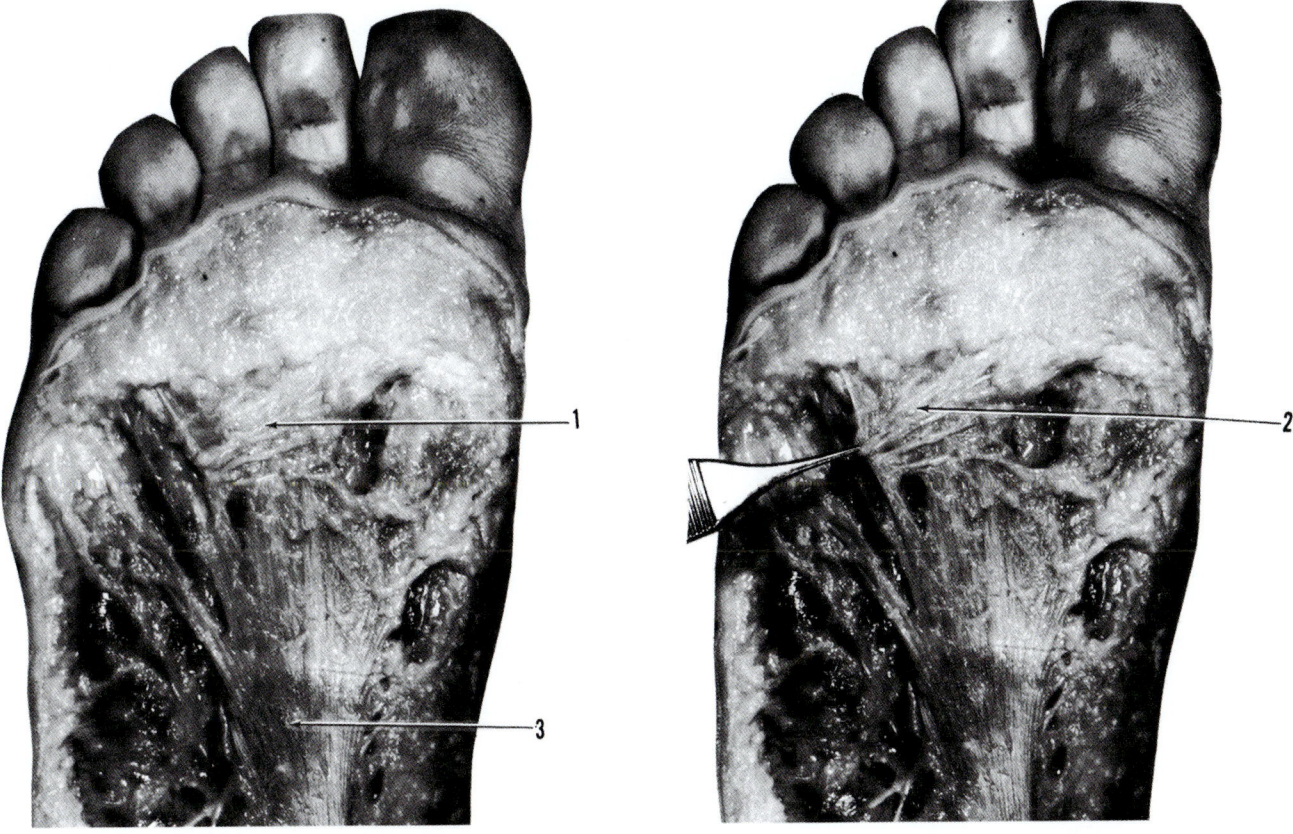

Figure 3.47 Plantar aponeurosis. (*1*, Superficial transverse tract of plantar aponeurosis; *2*, superficial transverse tract with side traction applied to emphasize direction of fibers; *3*, superficial central component of plantar aponeurosis.)

into the depth and connect with the longitudinal septa of the plantar aponeurosis and the bases of the proximal phalanges.[17]

Proximal to the metatarsal heads, sagittal septa extend from the deep surface of the longitudinal superficial aponeurotic bands (Fig. 3.48). These 10 septa arise in pairs from each of the five longitudinal bands (see Fig. 3.45).

The sagittal septa are oriented toward the corresponding metatarsophalangeal joint and pass on each side of the long flexor tendon, forming an arch of entrance for this tendon (Fig. 3.49). They insert sequentially on the interosseous fascia, the fascia of the transverse head of the adductor hallucis, the deep transverse metatarsal ligament, and the plantar plate and its junction with the accessory collateral ligament of the metatarsophalangeal joint.

The sagittal septa may cross fibers and form with the longitudinal band true foramina of entrance for the flexor tendons. Crossing fibers may also extend into the insertional fibers of the adjacent septum. Such a thick crossing band is seen in Figure 3.49, extending from the longitudinal septum of the big toe to the second toe, the plantar plate, and the deep transverse metatarsal ligament.

The medial septum of the aponeurotic band of the big toe inserts on the plantar plate and the medial sesamoid and connects with the fascia of the medial head of the flexor hallucis brevis.

The lateral septum of the same aponeurotic band inserts on the transverse metatarsal ligament, the plantar plate, and the lateral sesamoid and connects with the fascia of the lateral head of the flexor hallucis brevis muscle.

The proximal extension of the sagittal septa is limited by the origin of the lumbrical muscles.

At the level of the metatarsal heads, the sagittal septa are in continuity with vertical connective tissue fibers that arise from the sides of the fibrous flexor tendon sheath and the deep transverse metatarsal ligaments (see Fig. 3.46). The vertical fibers pass through the superficial aponeurosis and insert into the skin. Some of the vertical fibers cross over the flexor tendon sheath and form a pretendinous compartment retaining an adipose cushion (Fig. 3.50).[17]

At the level of the metatarsophalangeal joint, from the tibial side, a thin septum is extended, which forms a lumbrical compartment. In the intermetatarsal capitular space and over the plantar aspect of the deep transverse metatarsal ligament, an encapsulated fat body covers the common digital neurovascular bundle (Figs. 3.50 and 3.51).[17]

Distal to the metatarsal heads, a transverse retinacular system attaches to the fibrous flexor tendon sheaths and arches over the intertendinous spaces, forming the mooring ligament.

At the level of the web space, the distal segment of the ball of the foot is crossed by six to eight transverse bands or a weblike retinacular system forming the natatory ligament (Fig. 3.52).[16-18,*]

---

*Poirier and Charpy use the term *ligament palmant interdigital*, in which *palmant* should translate as *natatory*; *palmaire* would translate as *palmar* and *plantaire* as *plantar*.[17]

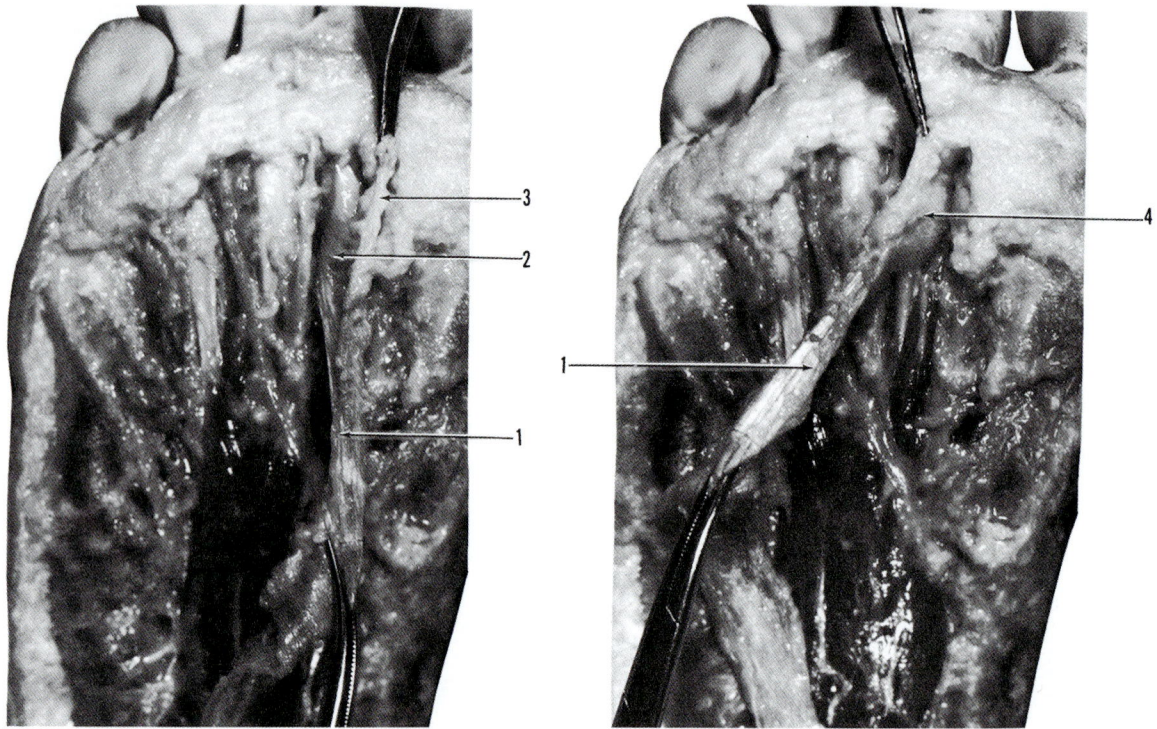

Figure 3.48 Plantar aponeurosis. (*1*, Superficial longitudinal tract continuing as *3*; *2*, lateral sagittal septum arising from superficial tract of second toe; *4*, medial sagittal septum to the second toe.)

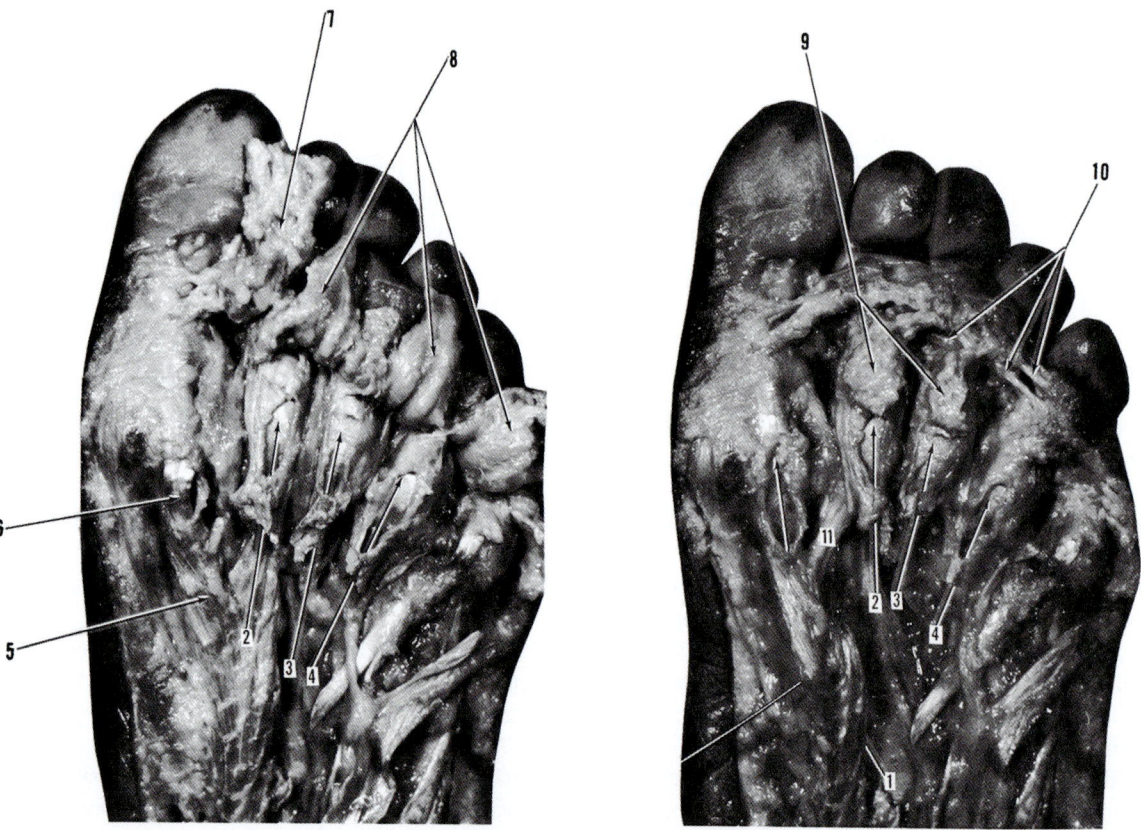

Figure 3.49 Plantar aponeurosis. (*1*, *Arrow* indicates direction of flexor hallucis longus [*6*] passing distally between the two sagittal septae arising from the longitudinal tract [*5*]; *2*, *3*, *4*, *arrows* indicating direction of long flexor tendons of toes *2*, *3*, *4*, passing through foraminae formed by septae of corresponding longitudinal aponeurotic tracts; *7*, reflected distal end of longitudinal aponeurotic tract; *8*, reflected intermetatarsal head fat bodies; *9*, preflexor tendon adipose cushions; *10*, transverse mooring ligament; *11*, connecting band between septae of first and second toes.)

Chapter 3: Retaining Systems and Compartments 151

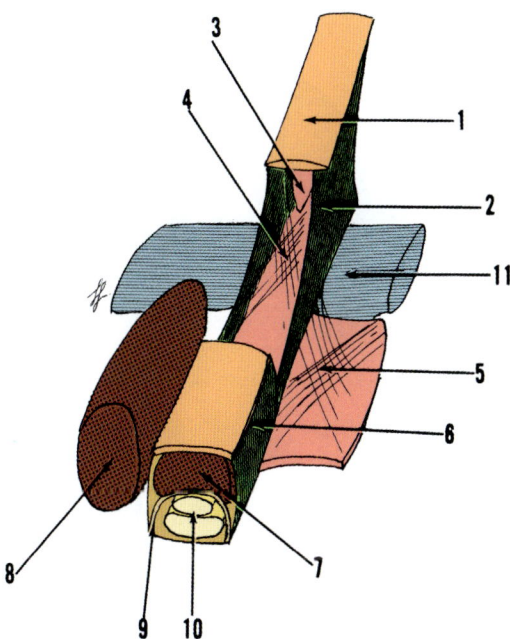

Figure 3.50 Diagram of deep insertion of plantar aponeurosis. (*1*, Superficial longitudinal tract; *2*, sagittal septa arising proximal to metatarsal heads; *3*, foramina for long flexor tendons formed by two septa of the ray; *4*, crossing fibers of two septa under long flexor tendons; *5*, oblique insertional fibers of sagittal septae on deep transverse metatarsal ligament; *6*, vertical fibers arising at level of metatarsal head from sides of fibrous tunnel [*9*] of long flexor tendons [*10*] and deep transverse metatarsal ligament. Some of these vertical fibers arch over the flexor tunnel and form a pretendinous space retaining an adipose cushion [*7*]; *8*, fat body that lies over plantar aspect of deep transverse metatarsal ligament; *11*, transverse component of adductor hallucis muscle.)

The fibers of the natatory ligament are deep to the longitudinally oriented terminal fibers of the superficial aponeurotic bands and originate from the fibrous flexor tendon sheaths and the mooring ligament. The proximal lamellae receive a contribution from the superficial longitudinal tracts of the plantar aponeurosis. The distal lamellae insert on the deep surface of the skin, but there is no insertion on the skin at the level of the plantodigital crease, where a transverse band of adipose tissue is interposed between the skin and the most frontal part of the natatory ligament. The digital neurovascular bundle passes under the bridging segment of the natatory ligaments.

On the superficial plantar aspect of the ball of the foot, the adjoining longitudinal superficial aponeurotic bands, crossed proximally by the transverse aponeurotic fibers and distally by the natatory ligaments, delineate a quadrilateral or oval space through which protrudes the fat body, forming the plantar monticuli. These adipose windows correspond to the common digital neurovascular bundles.

The medial border of the central component of the plantar aponeurosis is in continuity in the midsegment and distally with longitudinal thin fibers covering the abductor hallucis muscle; it blends with the dorsal aponeurosis. Proximally, a sulcus is present between the medial border of the plantar aponeurosis and the abductor hallucis. Superficially, this sulcus is bridged sparsely by oblique aponeurotic fibers (Fig. 3.53). The depth corresponds to the proximal segment of the medial intermuscular septum.

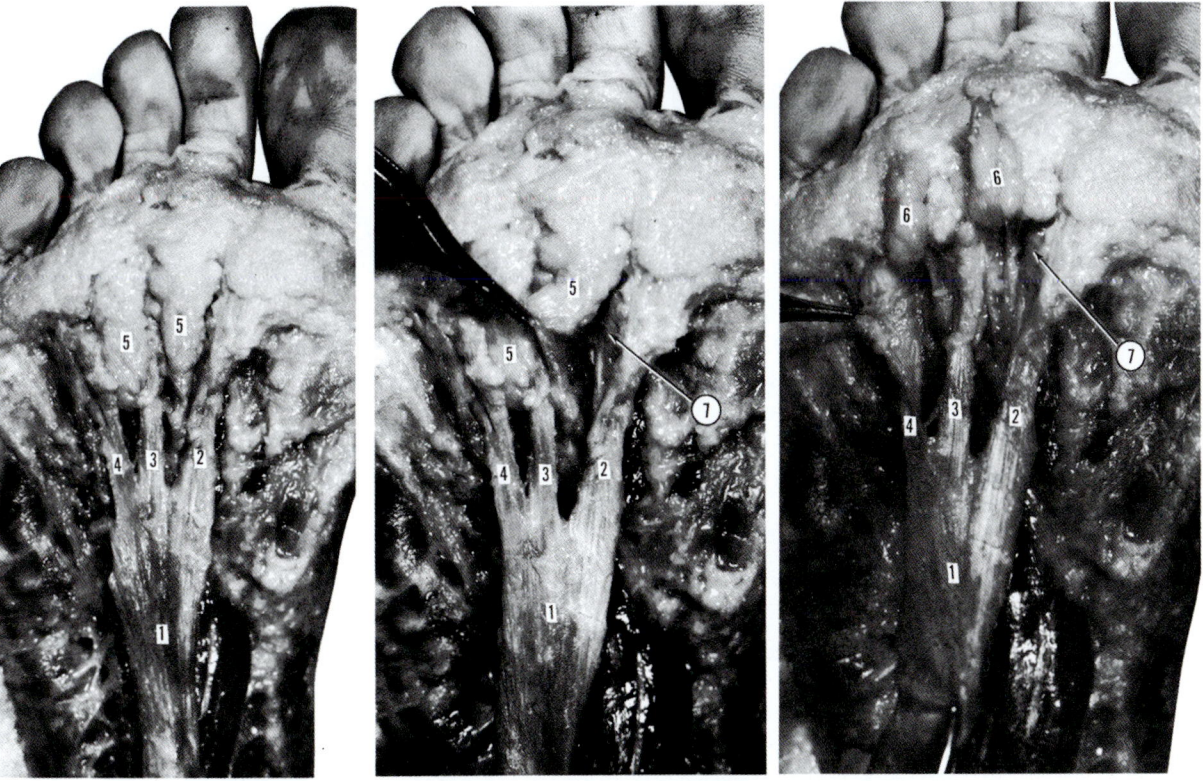

Figure 3.51 Plantar aponeurosis and ball of the foot. (*1*, Central component of plantar aponeurosis; *2*, *3*, *4*, superficial longitudinal tracts; *5*, fat bodies; *6*, reflected fat bodies exposing underlying neurovascular bundle; *7*, sagittal septum or deep insertion of plantar aponeurosis. The insertion of the septum is proximal to the metatarsal head.)

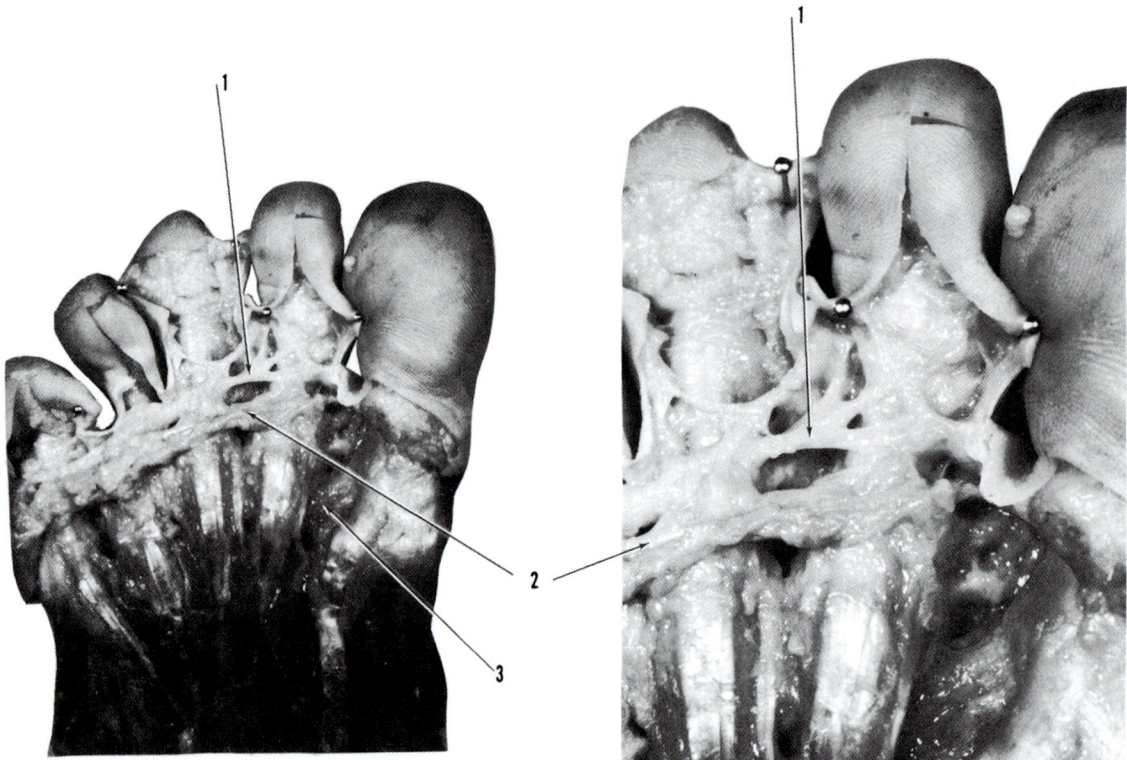

Figure 3.52 Natatory ligament. The fibers of the natatory ligament are deep to the longitudinally oriented terminal fibers of the superficial aponeurotic bands, which insert on the dermis of the ball of the foot. (*1*, Natatory ligament, crossing web space, with retinacular arrangement and general transverse orientation; *2*, transverse mooring ligament; *3*, deep transverse metatarsal ligament between first and second toes.)

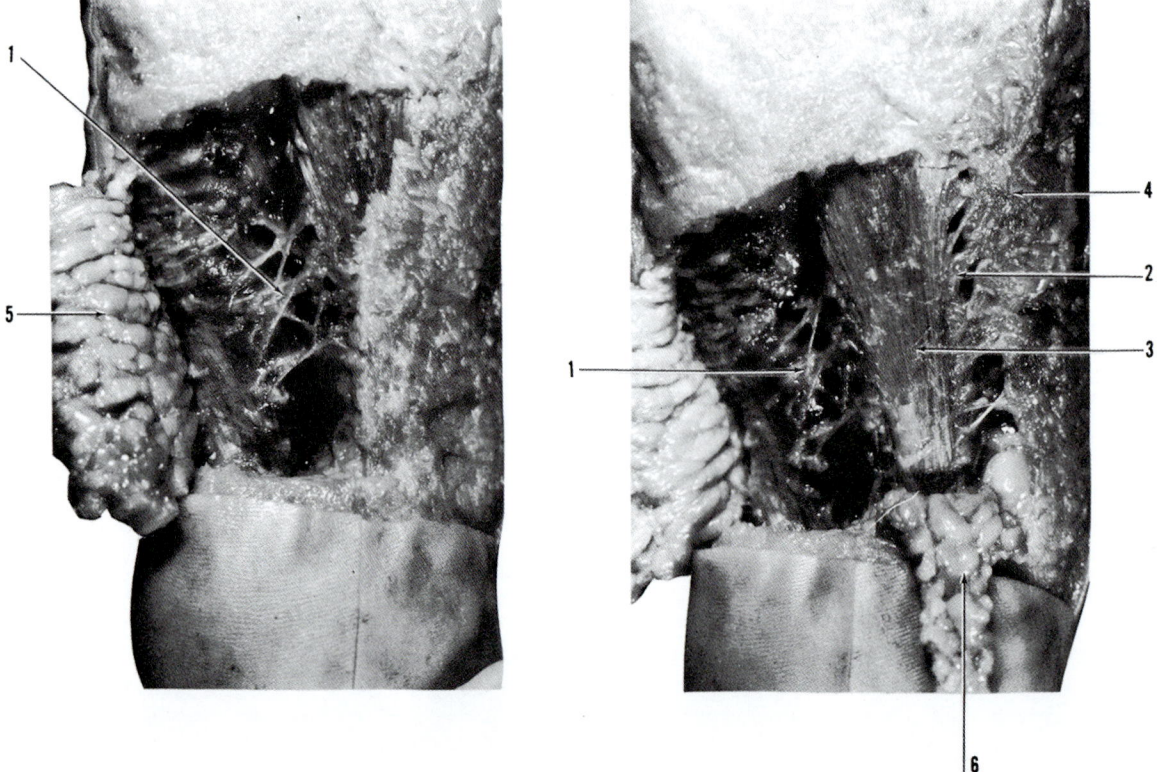

Figure 3.53 Anatomy of the lateral and medial sulci located between the components of the plantar aponeurosis. Specimen dissected under magnification ×8. (*1*, Lateral sulcus bridged by retinacular mesh-like connective retaining network for subcutaneous adipose tissue [5], which is reflected off interstices; *2*, medial sulcus bridged by less complex connective system; *3*, central component of plantar aponeurosis; *4*, medial component of plantar aponeurosis; *6*, adipose tissue reflected off central component.)

The lateral border of the central component of the plantar aponeurosis corresponds to the lateral sulcus. A fine network of aponeurotic fibers fills in the sulcus superficially, and fatty lobules are trapped in the intervals (see Fig. 3.53). The depth of the sulcus corresponds to the lateral intermuscular septum. The central segment of the plantar aponeurosis is connected laterally and medially to the intermuscular longitudinal septa of the planta pedis.[19]

The lateral intermuscular septum (Fig. 3.54) is attached to the medial calcaneal tubercle, the calcaneocuboid ligament, and the sheath of the peroneus longus. Distally, the septum splits, encloses the third plantar interosseous muscle, and inserts on the medial border of the fifth metatarsal shaft and on the base of the proximal phalanx at the insertion site of the tendon. At this level, it blends with the medial sagittal septum of the fifth deep aponeurotic tract of the plantar aponeurosis.

The medial intermuscular septum (see Fig. 3.54) is less well defined and is formed by a set of vertical fascicles arranged like a comb, leaving passages for the tendons and neurovascular structures. Posteriorly, the medial intermuscular septum is reinforced by the interfascicular lamina of the calcaneal tunnel. This lamina is attached to the medial surface of the os calcis, above the proximal border of the quadratus plantae. Distally, the medial longitudinal septum is attached to the navicular, the medial cuneiform, and the lateral aspect of the first metatarsal shaft after passing between the adductor hallucis and the flexor hallucis brevis, and it contributes to the formation of their sheaths.

▶ Peroneal or Lateral Component

The peroneal component of the plantar aponeurosis was extensively analyzed by Loth and Henkel.[16,20,21] This component is variable. It was present in 92% and absent in 7% in a study of 410 plantar aponeuroses.[20] This peroneal component may be of four types (Fig. 3.55): complete and well developed, complete and thin, incomplete with only partial distal extension, or absent distal segment.[20]

The well-developed peroneal component originates from the lateral margin of the medial calcaneal tubercle in close connection with the origin of the abductor digiti minimi muscle. The aponeurosis is 1 to 1.5 cm wide at the origin. It extends in the direction of the cuboid and bifurcates into a medial and a lateral component (Fig. 3.56). The lateral band or crux is the stronger component and inserts on the base of the fifth metatarsal and forms the calcaneometatarsal ligament. A longitudinal extension band may be present in close connection with the tendon of the abductor digiti minimi. Some fibers take a dorsal course and unite with the dorsal aponeurosis. The medial band or crux turns around the abductor digiti minimi muscle, passes into the depth under the neurovascular bundle to the fifth toe, and blends with the plantar plate of the fourth and, occasionally, the third metatarsophalangeal joints. This band gives origin to the transverse component of the abductor hallucis muscle.[21]

▶ Tibial or Medial Component

The medial component of the plantar aponeurosis is thin posteriorly and thicker anteriorly. It forms the covering fascia of the

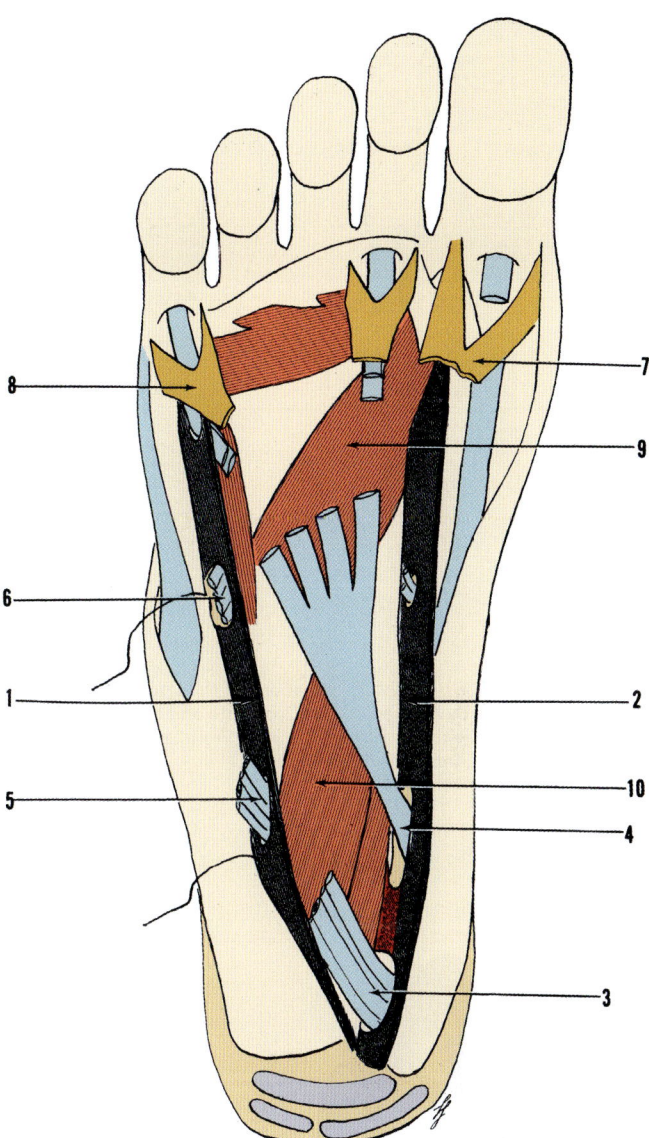

Figure 3.54 Intermuscular longitudinal septa. (1, Lateral intermuscular septum perforated twice by lateral plantar neurovascular bundle [5, 6] and by long flexor of fifth toe; 2, medial intermuscular septum perforated by lateral plantar neurovascular bundle [3] and flexor digitorum longus tendon [4]; 7, 8, longitudinal septae of plantar aponeurosis; 9, oblique head of adductor hallucis muscle; 10, quadratus plantae muscle.)

abductor hallucis muscle. The fibers are oriented distally and medially and are in continuity with the dorsal aponeurosis of the foot, the inferomedial arm of the inferior extensor retinaculum, and the flexor retinaculum.

PLANTAR COMPARTMENTS

The sole of the foot is divided into four compartments[22]: medial or tibial, lateral or peroneal, central, and interosseous (Figs. 3.57 and 3.58).

The medial compartment is limited superficially and medially by the medial segment of the plantar aponeurosis. In the

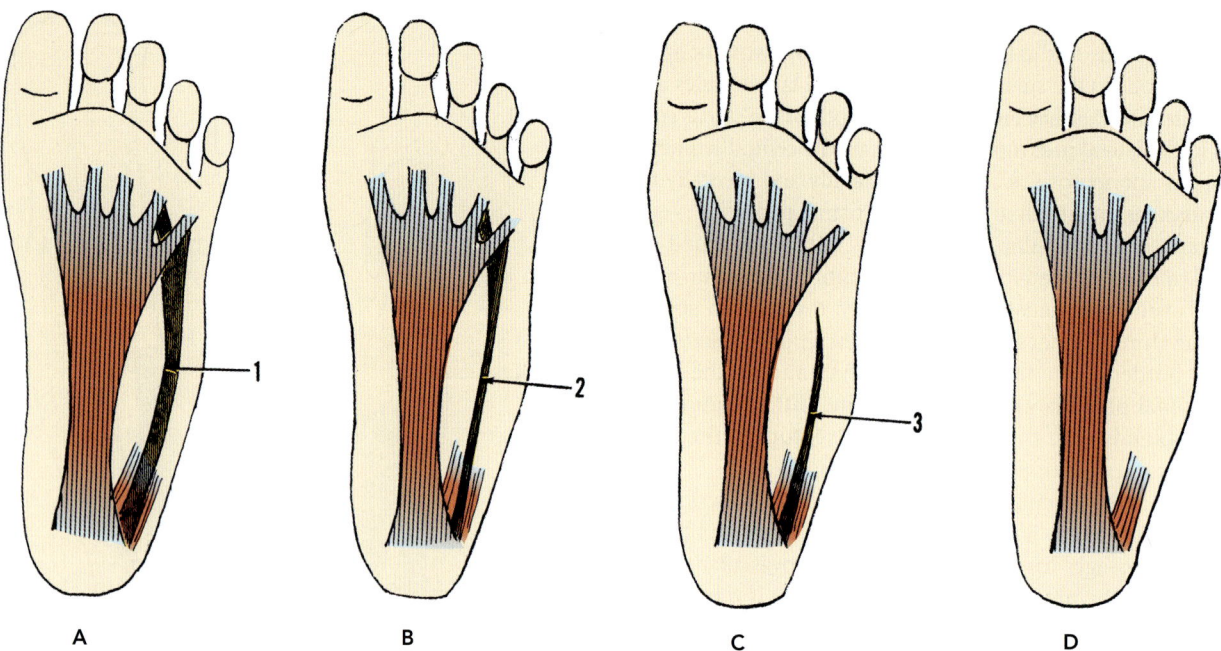

Figure 3.55 Variations of the lateral component of the plantar aponeurosis. **(A)** Complete and well developed (*1*). **(B)** Complete and thin (*2*). **(C)** Incomplete with partial distal extension (*3*). **(D)** Incomplete with no distal extension. (From Loth EM. Etude anthropologique sur l'aponévrose plantaire. *Bull Mem Soc Anthro Paris*. 1913;4:601.)

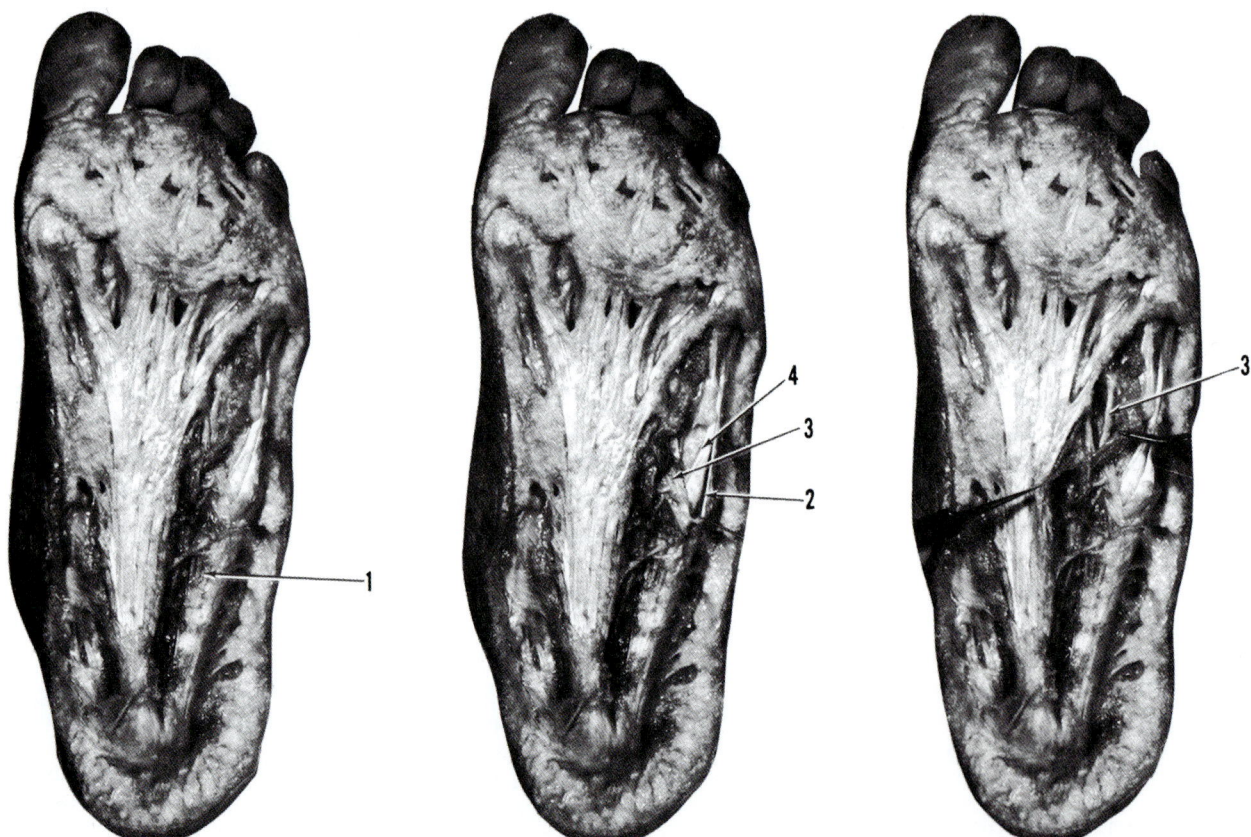

Figure 3.56 Plantar aponeurosis. (*1*, Lateral component; *2*, lateral crux of *1*; *3*, medial crux of *1*; *4*, tendon of abductor digiti quinti.)

Chapter 3: Retaining Systems and Compartments   155

proximal segment, the compartment is limited by the investing layers of the flexor retinaculum and is reinforced on its lateral side by the medial intermuscular septum and the vertical segment of the interfascicular lamina of the calcaneal tunnel (Fig. 3.59). The distal segment of the compartment corresponds to the first metatarsal shaft inferior surface, the first cuneiform, and the navicular and then bridges the calcaneal canal to insert on the medial calcaneal tuberosity: this determines the calcaneal component of the tibiotalocalcaneal tunnel. This compartment contains the abductor hallucis muscle, the flexor hallucis longus tendon, and the flexor hallucis brevis muscle distally. The medial compartment has no direct communication with

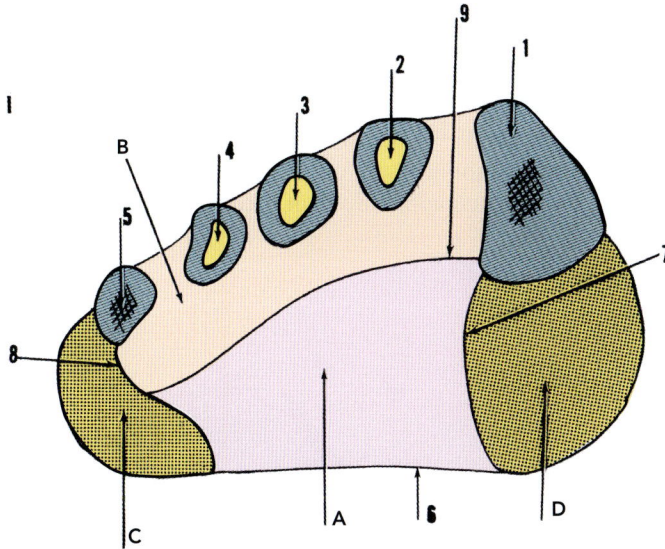

Figure 3.57 Plantar compartments of the sole of the foot, classic interpretation. (A, central compartment; B, interosseous compartment; C, lateral or peroneal compartment; D, medial or tibial compartment; 1-5, metatarsals 1-5; 6, central segment of plantar aponeurosis; 7, medial intermuscular septum; 8, lateral intermuscular septum; 9, interosseous fascia.)

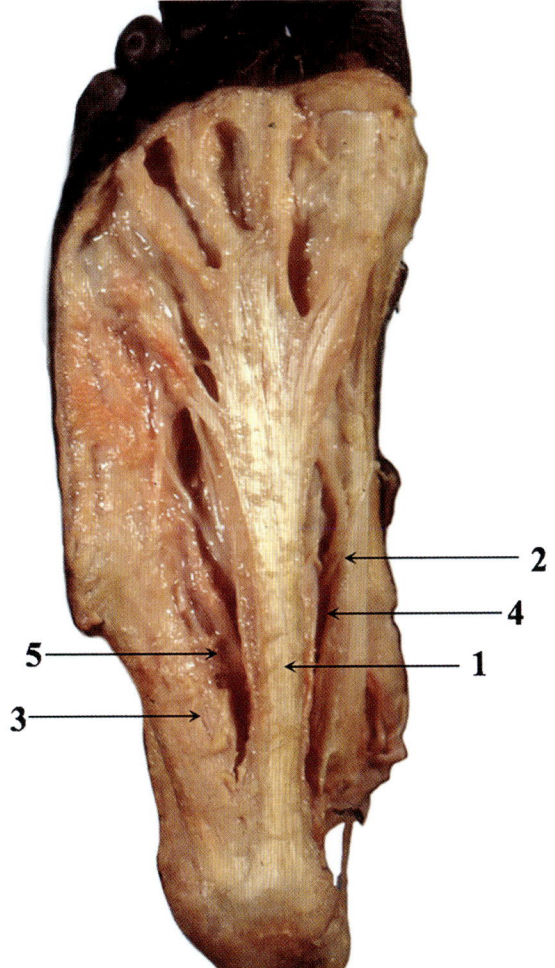

Figure 3.58 Plantar aspect of right foot. (1, Central compartment; 2, medial compartment; 3, lateral compartment; 4, medial intermuscular trough corresponding to medial intermuscular septum. Lodges fat wedge; 5, lateral intermuscular trough corresponding to lateral intermuscular septum. Lodges fat wedge.)

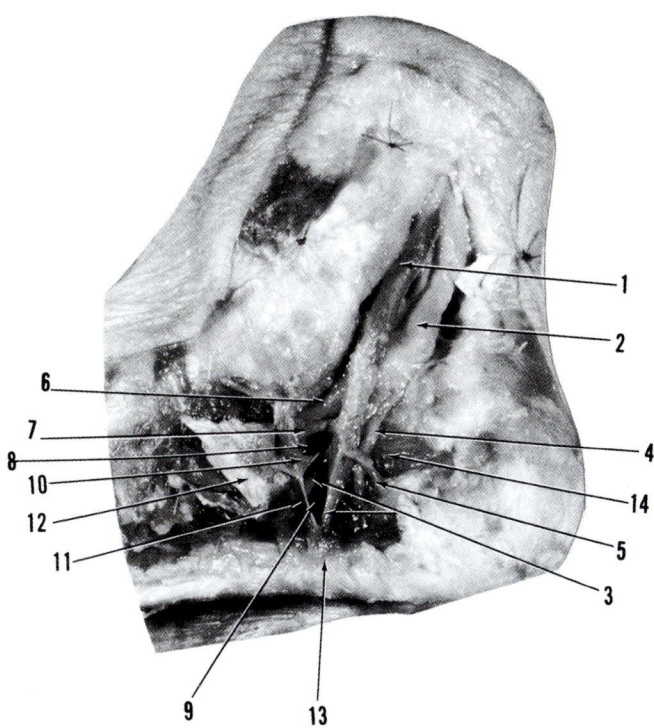

Figure 3.59 The upper and lower calcaneal chambers. The entire tibiotalocalcaneal tunnel has been exposed by opening the two adherent layers of the aponeurosis cruris (tagged with sutures), the flexor retinaculum, and by reflecting the insertion of the abductor hallucis muscle aponeurosis (12). The posterior tibial nerve (2) divides into the lateral plantar (3) and medial plantar (6) nerves at the level of the medial malleolus. The posterior tibial artery (1) divides into the medial plantar artery (7) and the lateral plantar artery (3) just prior to the free border of the transverse segment of the interfascicular ligament (10). The medial plantar neurovascular bundle penetrates the upper calcaneal chamber (8) and the lateral plantar neurovascular bundle penetrates the lower calcaneal chamber (9). This chamber represents the porta pedis and communicates with the intermediary central compartment of the sole of the foot. The lateral plantar neurovascular bundle (3) and the nerve to the abductor digiti quinti (4) course between the medial head of the quadratus plantae (14) and the abductor hallucis. The nerve to the abductor digiti quinti (4) is crossed by the medial calcaneal artery (5). (1, Posterior tibial artery; 2, posterior tibial nerve; 3, lateral plantar nerve [anterior] and artery [posterior]; 4, nerve to abductor digiti quinti; 5, medial calcaneal artery; 6, medial plantar nerve [anterior]; 7, medial plantar artery [posterior]; 8, upper calcaneal chamber; 9, lower calcaneal chamber; 10, interfascicular lamina, transverse section; 11, interfascicular lamina, vertical section; 12, reflected end abductor hallucis; 13, central segment of plantar aponeurosis in continuity with medial intermuscular septum; 14, quadratus plantae.)

the calcaneal tunnel or with the central compartment. It is separated from the latter by the medial intermuscular septum and trough proximally. Thick plantar adipose tissue is wedged into the trough.

The lateral compartment is limited superficially and laterally by the lateral segment of the plantar aponeurosis and medially by the lateral intermuscular septum. This compartment corresponds to the plantar aspect of the fifth metatarsal, the cuboid, and the calcaneus. The proximal segment of the compartment is attached to the lateral and medial calcaneal tuberosities, thus shifting medially. The lateral compartment contains the abductor, short flexor, and opponens muscles of the fifth toe and does not communicate with the calcaneal tunnel or the central compartment.

The central compartment is divided into three subcompartments: superficial, intermediary, and deep. The superficial and intermediary compartments extend from the heel to the middle and proximal segments of the central three metatarsals. The deep or adductor space compartment is present only in the forefoot.

The superficial central compartment contains the flexor digitorum brevis and a segment of the long flexors. It is limited superficially by the central segment of the plantar aponeurosis, laterally by the lateral intermuscular septum, and medially by the medial intermuscular septum. The dorsal investing layer of the compartment is complex. It has been well recognized by Liaras (Fig. 3.60)[23] and by Sarrafian (Fig. 3.61).[24] Liaras labels the dorsal aponeurosis of the superficial compartment as the middle plantar aponeurosis of Lacroix.[23] Proximally, the

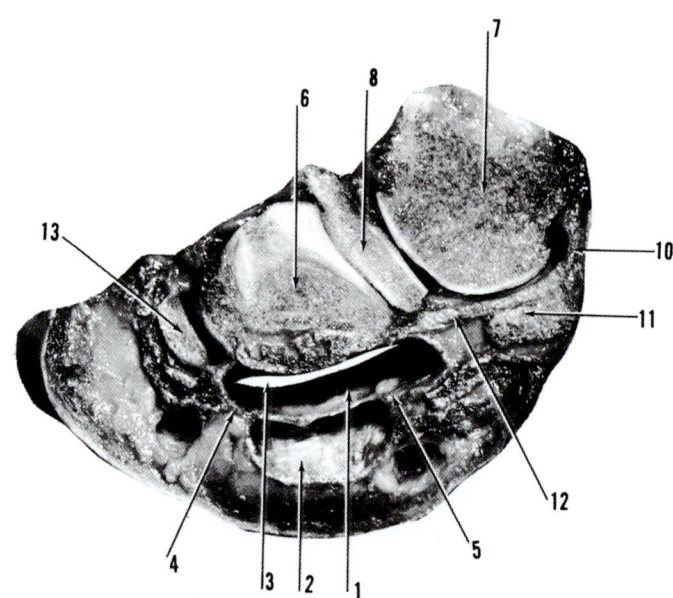

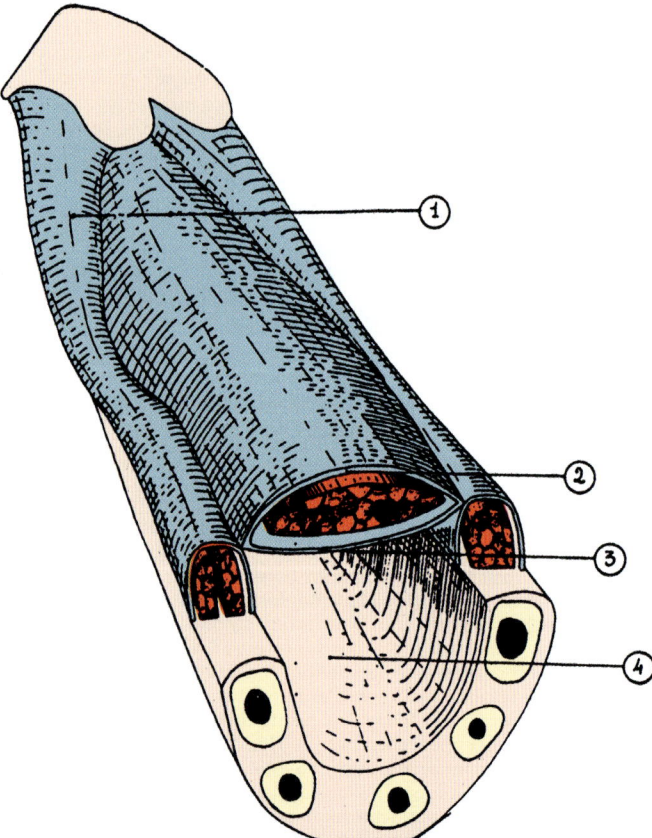

Figure 3.60 The osteoaponeurotic plantar canal. (*1,* Superficial plantar aponeurosis with its three segments: medial, middle, and lateral; *2,* middle superficial plantar compartment with the flexor digitorum brevis; *3,* middle plantar aponeurosis of Lacroix; *4,* osseous plantar canal.) (Adapted from Liaras H. Tissue cellulaire et topographie plantaire. Connexions de la plante et du mollet. *Ann Anat Path Anat Norm.* 1935;12:548.)

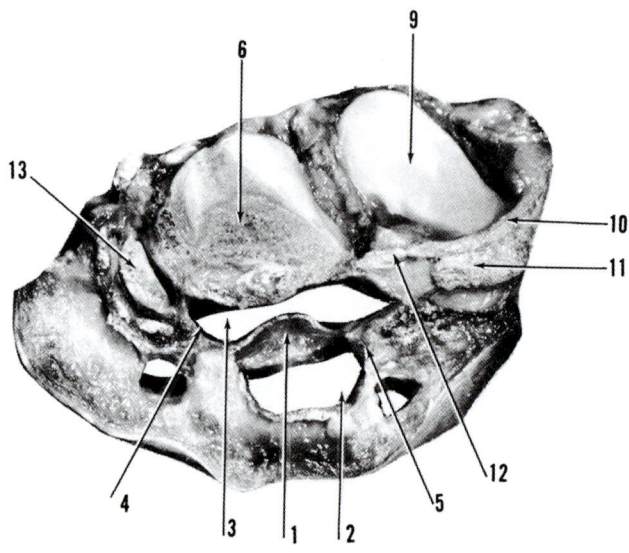

Figure 3.61 Distal view of transverse cross-section of the left foot, passing through the proximal segment of the cuboid, the beak of the os calcis, and the distal segment of the talar head. (*1,* Transverse septum dividing central compartment into compartment for flexor digitorum brevis [*2*] and compartment for quadratus plantae [*3*]. This septum extends from the lateral intermuscular septum [*4*] to the medial intermuscular septum [*5*]; *6,* cuboid; *7,* talar head supported by os calcis [*8*], inferior calcaneonavicular ligament [*12*], superomedial calcaneonavicular ligament [*10*], tibialis posterior tendon [*11*], and navicular [*9*]; *13,* peroneus longus tendon and tunnel.)

superficial central compartment extends to the medial calcaneal tuberosity; distally, it extends to the junction of the flexor digitorum brevis, with the long flexor tendons and the lumbricals reaching the level of the midsegment of the corresponding central metatarsals (Fig. 3.62). The superficial central compartment is independent from the surrounding compartments. This has been demonstrated with injection techniques by Liaras[23] and more recently by Manoli and Weber.[25] Liaras describes this compartment as "closed from all parts, appears thus as independent from the deep middle plantar compartment...as the lateral compartments."[23]

The intermediary compartment is deep or dorsal to the superficial central compartment. It lodges the quadratus plantae and the proximal segments of the flexor digitorum longus and of the lumbricals (Figs. 3.63 and 3.64). The compartment extends along the corresponding segments of the inferior calcaneal surface and its junction with the medial calcaneal surface, the inferior surface of the cuboid, the navicular, the middle lateral cuneiforms, and the proximal segments of the central three metatarsals. Dorsally, it is limited by the previously mentioned skeletal frame with its capsuloligamentous coverings, a segment of the peroneus longus tunnel, the proximal segment of the adductor hallucis oblique head, and the lateral origin of the flexor hallucis brevis muscle. Laterally and medially, it is walled off by the corresponding lateral and medial intermuscular septa. Superficially or plantarward, the intermediary central compartment is limited by the ceiling of the superficial central compartment. A transverse, thin aponeurotic layer arising from the calcaneal tuberosity and the intermuscular septa covers the plantar aspect of the crossing lateral plantar neurovascular bundle, the nerve to the abductor digiti quinti muscle, and the quadratus plantae, and terminates by thinning out over the long

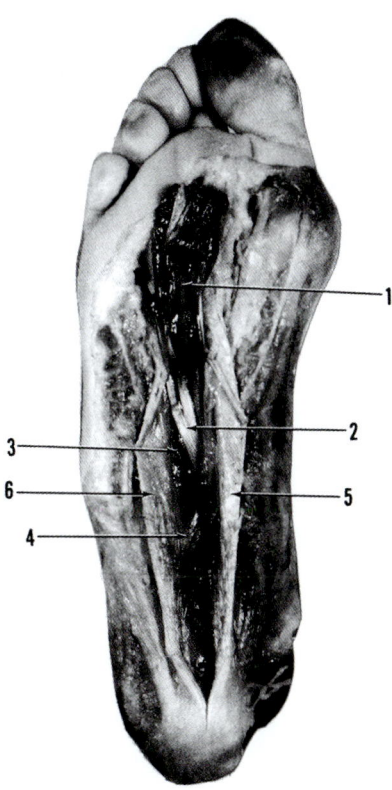

Figure 3.63 The central segment of the plantar aponeurosis is opened and the flexor digitorum brevis (*1*) is reflected distally, thus exposing the intermediary central compartment. An aponeurotic layer (*4*) covers the quadratus plantae (*3*) and forms the floor of this compartment, which extends distally through the flexor digitorum longus tendons (*2*) and the origin of the lumbricals. (*5,* Medial portion of central plantar aponeurosis in continuity with the medial intermuscular septum; *6,* lateral portion of central plantar aponeurosis in continuity with the lateral intermuscular septum.)

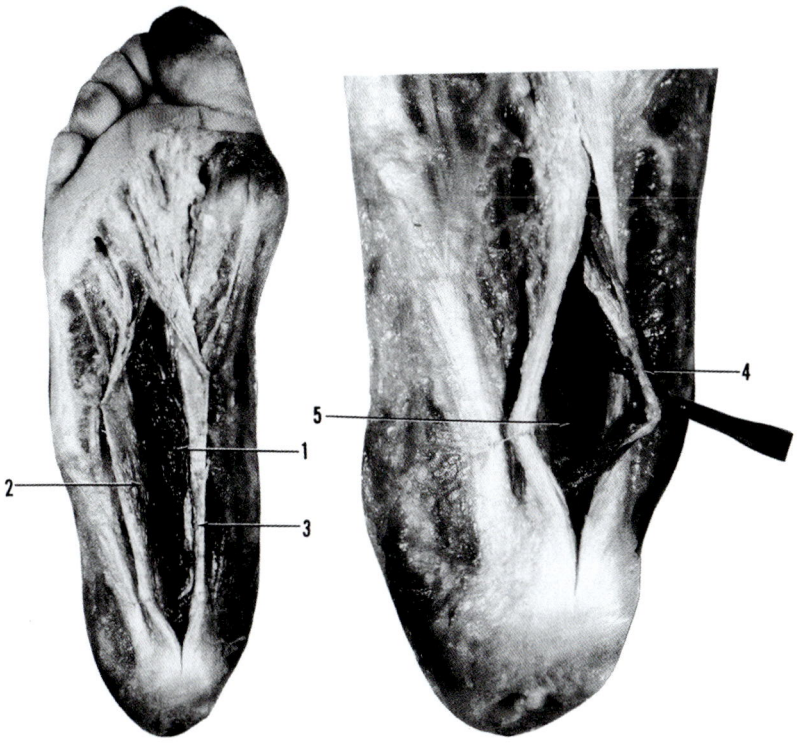

Figure 3.62 Superficial central compartment of the sole of the foot. The central segment of the plantar aponeurosis is opened longitudinally, thus exposing the superficial central compartment. (*1,* Flexor digitorum brevis muscle; *2,* lateral portion of central plantar aponeurosis in continuity with lateral intermuscular septum; *3,* medial portion of central plantar aponeurosis in continuity with medial intermuscular septum; *4,* reflected flexor digitorum brevis to reveal the floor [*5*] of the superficial central compartment covered by an aponeurotic layer.)

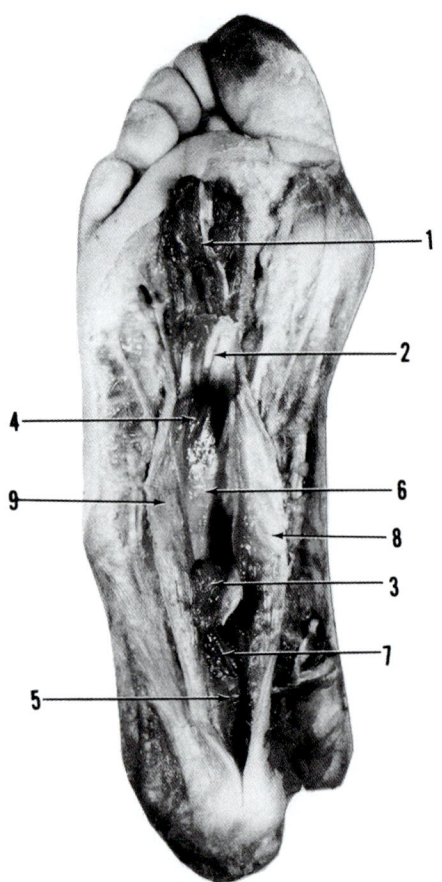

Figure 3.64 The central compartment is opened. The flexor digitorum brevis (1) is reflected distally. The flexor digitorum longus is transected and reflected distally (2). The quadratus plantae is reflected proximally (3). The deep surface or ceiling of the intermediary central compartment (6) is thus exposed. It is osseoligamentous proximally and corresponds to the adductor hallucis muscle distally (4). The lateral plantar neurovascular bundle (7) is covered proximally by a thick component of the investing fascia of the intermediary central compartment. (8) and (9) represent the lateral and medial sections of the central aponeurosis in continuity with the corresponding lateral and medial intermuscular septa.

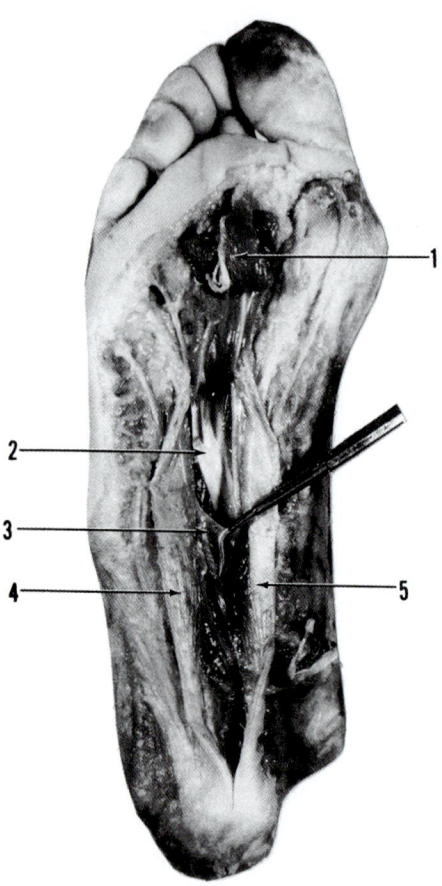

Figure 3.65 Intermediary central compartment exposed by incising the central segment of the plantar aponeurosis (4 and 5) and distal reflection of the flexor digitorum brevis (1). The distal border of the investing fascia of the intermediary central compartment is raised with a dental probe (3). This border reaches the flexor digitorum longus (2).

flexor tendons (Fig. 3.65). The proximal segment of this aponeurosis is thicker. A stronger transverse aponeurotic segment is located under the lateral plantar neurovascular bundle and covers the corresponding part of the quadratus plantae (Fig. 3.66). This strong aponeurotic layer extends from the medial to the lateral intermuscular septum and may continue as the investing fascia of the medial head of the quadratus plantae in the lower calcaneal tunnel. The latter fascia may be interpreted as the downward continuity of the intermediary aponeurosis of Baumann[13] of the tibiotalocalcaneal tunnel, interposed between the posterior tibial neurovascular bundle and the underlying tendons of the flexor hallucis, the flexor digitorum longus, and the tibialis posterior. The central intermediary compartment is in continuity proximally with the inferior calcaneal tunnel, which is located along the medial surface of the calcaneus (Fig. 3.67).

The deep component of the central compartment is the adductor compartment and space; it corresponds to the forefoot. The adductor space is located between the dorsal aspect of the oblique head of the adductor hallucis muscle and the plantar segment of the interosseous compartment with the corresponding metatarsals 2, 3, and 4 (Figs. 3.68 and 3.69). Kamel and Sakla[26] describe a horizontally oriented Y-shaped septum that originates from the medial side of the fifth metatarsal shaft and bifurcates at the level of the third metatarsal into an upper and lower limb (Fig. 3.70). The upper limb is directed upward and medially and attaches to the lateral side of the first metatarsal bone. The lower limb is directed downward and medially and blends with the medial border of the central segment of the plantar aponeurosis. The adductor hallucis muscle oblique head is contained in this compartment.

The interosseous compartment (see Fig. 3.68) is limited by the thin interosseous fascia that extends from the first to the fifth metatarsal. It is subdivided into four spaces by corresponding vertical septa. It is covered dorsally by the dorsal interossei aponeurosis. Each space contains the corresponding plantar and dorsal interossei.

Chapter 3: Retaining Systems and Compartments   159

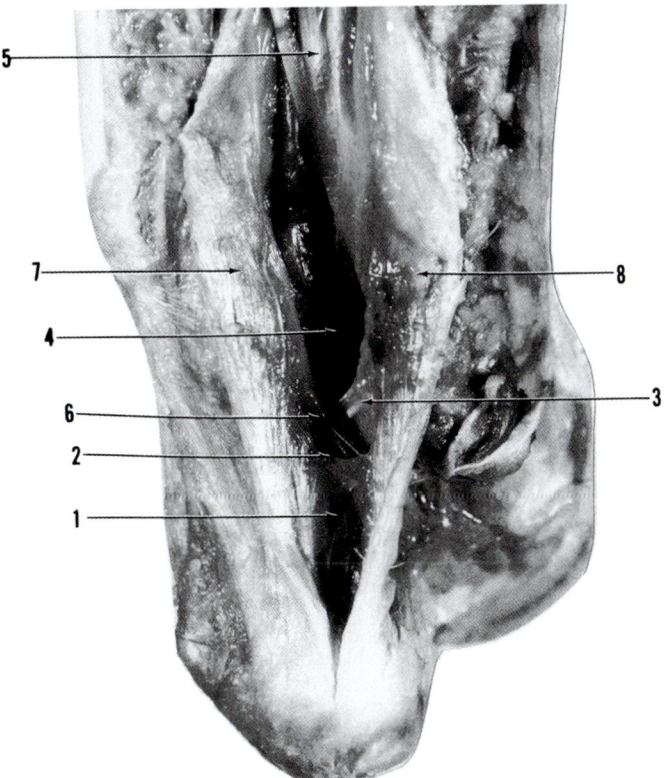

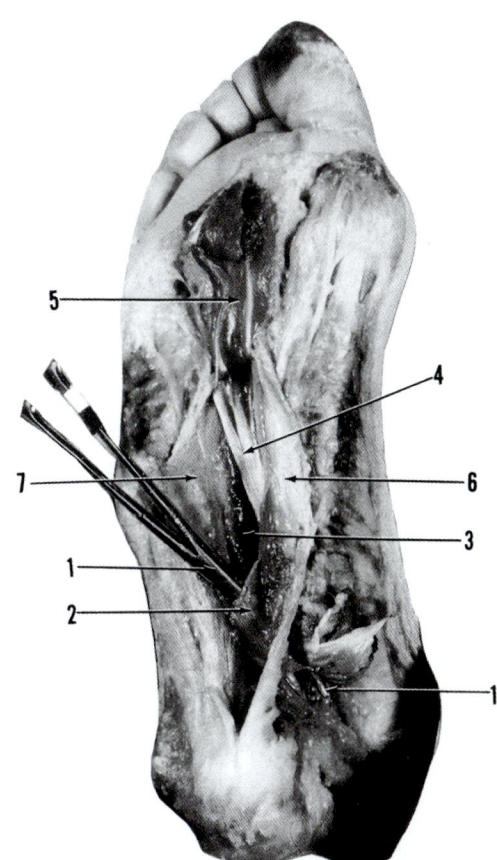

Figure 3.66 The proximal segment of the central intermediary compartment. The thin component of the investing fascia covering the distal segment of the lateral plantar neurovascular bundle (6) and the quadratus plantae (4) has been excised. Proximally, the investing layer forms a thick fascia (1) covering the proximal segment of the lateral plantar neurovascular bundle. A transverse aponeurosis (3) covers the proximal segment of the quadratus plantae muscle. The lateral plantar neurovascular bundle (6) is sandwiched between these two investing layers: (1) and (3). (2, Border of the superficial investing fascia; 5, flexor digitorum longus tendons; 7, 8, lateral and medial intermuscular septa in continuity with the corresponding portions of the central plantar aponeurosis.)

Figure 3.67 The central intermediary compartment is exposed. A hemostat (1) is introduced under the transverse aponeurosis (2), above the quadratus plantae (3), and exits in the lower calcaneal chamber (1). (4, Flexor digitorum longus tendons; 5, reflected flexor digitorum brevis; 6, 7, lateral and medial intermuscular septa in continuity with central segment of plantar aponeurosis.)

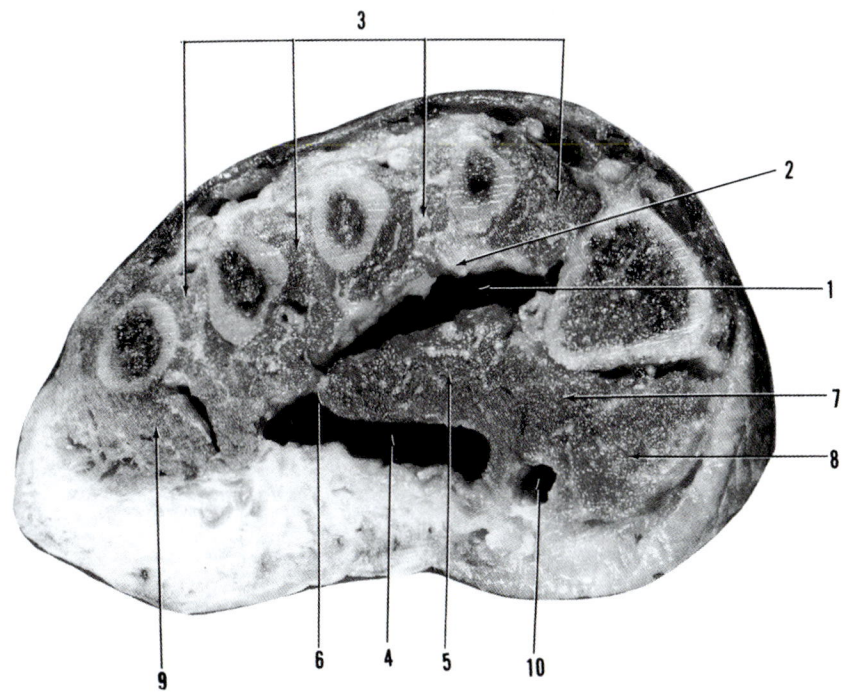

Figure 3.68 Cross-section of left foot through metatarsal shafts. Proximal surface of section. (1, Adductor space; 2, interossei investing fascia; 3, interossei muscles and four spaces; 4, continuity of central intermediary space; 5, adductor hallucis muscle, oblique component with investing thin fascia; 6, junction of adductor investing fascia with interossei fascia, thus separating the adductor space from the central intermediary space; 7, lateral head of flexor hallucis brevis; 8, medial head of flexor hallucis brevis and abductor hallucis; 9, lateral compartment with abductor, short flexor, and opponens of fifth toe; 10, tunnel of flexor hallucis longus tendon.)

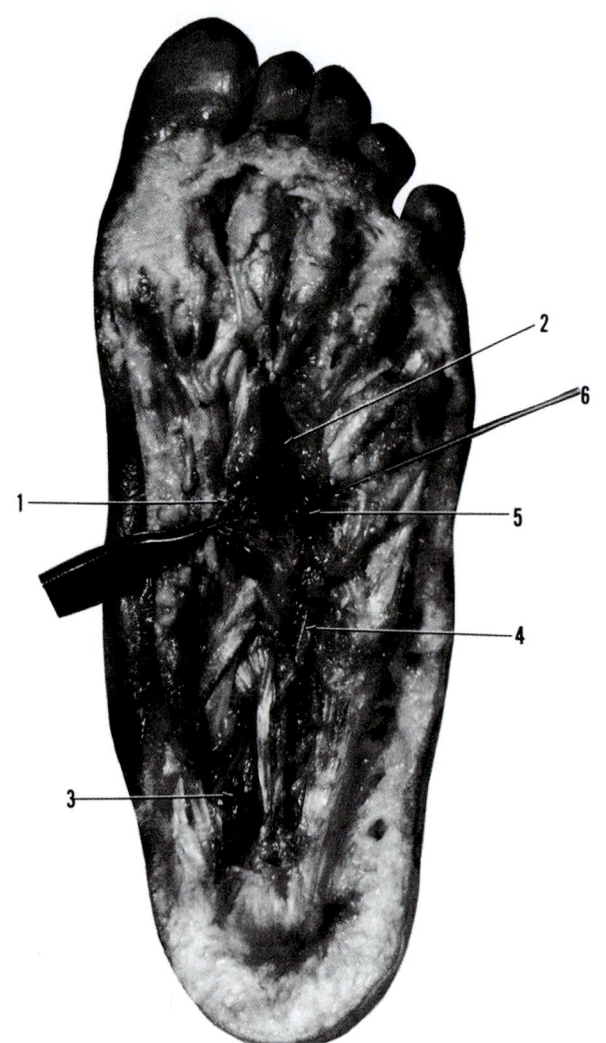

Figure 3.69 Lateral border of adductor hallucis is reflected medially (1), exposing the adductor space (2). The lateral plantar neurovascular bundle (3) is seen passing through the lateral intermuscular septum (4) to enter the deep adductor space (5). The probe (6) lifts the lateral plantar artery.

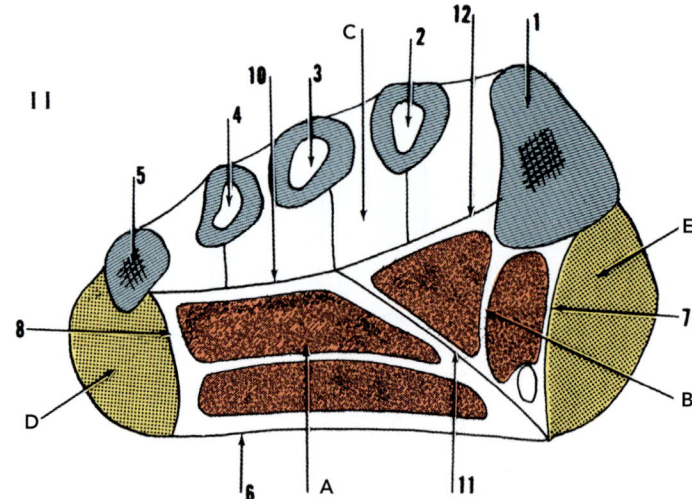

Figure 3.70 Plantar compartments of the sole of the foot. (*A*, superficial part of central or intermediary compartment; *B*, middle part of central or intermediary compartment; *C*, deep part of central or intermediary compartment; *D*, lateral compartment; *E*, medial compartment; *1, 2, 3, 4, 5*, refer to the corresponding metatarsals 1st, 2nd, 3rd, 4th, 5th metatarsals; *6*, refers to plantar skin; *7*, medial compartment fascia; *8*, lateral compartment fascia; *10*, horizontal stem of Y septum; *11*, inferomedial limb of Y septum; *12*, superomedial limb of Y septum.) (Adapted from Kamel R, Sakla BF. Anatomical compartments of the sole of the human foot. *Anat Rec.* 1961;140:57.)

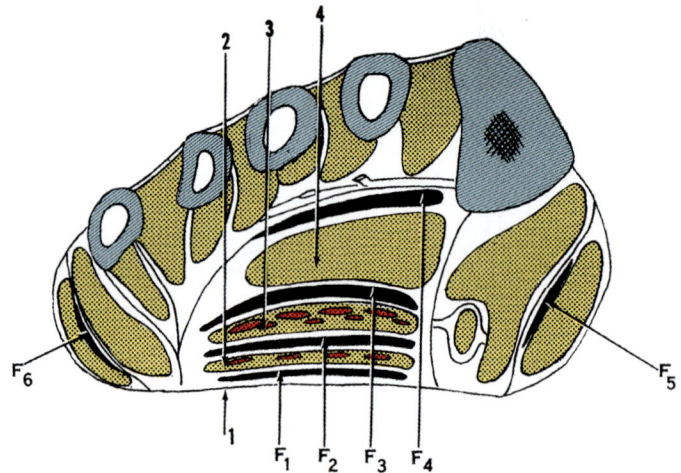

Figure 3.71 Fascial spaces of the sole of the foot: cross-section of foot at the level of the middle of the fifth metatarsal bone (proximal surface). *Central compartment:* F_1, fascial space between central plantar aponeurosis (1) and flexor digitorum brevis (2); F_2, fascial space between flexor digitorum brevis (2) and quadratus plantae (3); F_3, fascial space between quadratus plantae (3) and oblique head of adductor hallucis (4); F_4, fascial space between adductor hallucis (4) and interosseous fascia. *Medial compartment:* F_5, fascial space located between investing fascia of abductor hallucis and deep surface of muscle. *Lateral compartment:* F_6, fascial space located between investing fascia of abductor digiti quinti and deep surface of muscle. (Adapted from Grodinsky M. A study of the fascial spaces of the foot and their bearing on infections. *Surg Gynecol Obstet.* 1929;49:737.)

Anatomically, the plantar lateral compartment, the central superficial compartment, and the medial compartment form isolated closed spaces. The intermediary central compartment communicates with the lower calcaneal tunnel, thus leading to the tibiotalocalcaneal tunnel and further proximally to the posterior compartment of the leg. The forefoot adductor compartment is a relatively closed space. The interossei spaces are separate.

Grodinsky[19] described four fascial spaces in the central compartment of the foot (Figs. 3.71 and 3.72). Studies involving patterns of communication between compartments and/or fascial spaces have been conducted by Grodinsky,[19] Kamel and Sakla,[26] and recently Manoli and Weber.[25]

A subcutaneous space is described as located superficial to the posterior and plantar aspect of the os calcis.[27] In this location, a large calcaneal bursa is present.[28] However, Grégoire, in an anatomic study of the subcalcaneal bursa in 40 adult feet, found such a bursa in 1 foot.[29] In 19 ft, he detected a "considerable rarefaction of the fibrous tracts extending from the plantar aponeurosis to the deep surface of the skin."[29] A degenerative process may thus be responsible for this subcalcaneal space.

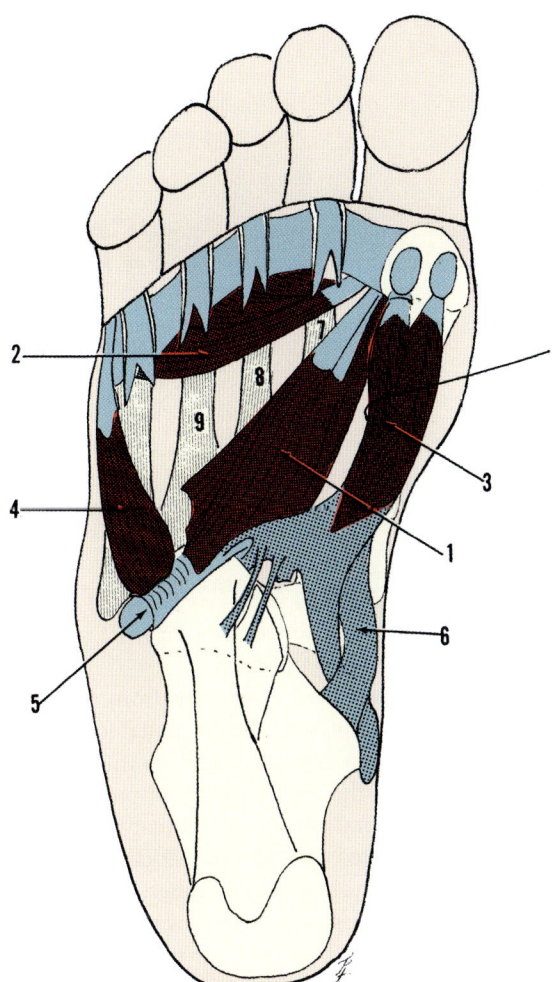

Figure 3.72 The fourth fascial space of the middle compartment is located under the oblique head of the adductor hallucis (*1*). This space extends along an oblique line drawn from the base of the fourth metatarsal to the lateral aspect of the base of the proximal phalanx of the big toe. (*2*, Transverse head of adductor hallucis muscle; *3*, flexor hallucis brevis, retracted; *4*, flexor digiti quinti; *5*, peroneus longus tendon and sheath; *6*, deep component of tibialis posterior tendon; *7*, *8*, *9*, metatarsal shafts 2, 3, 4.)

REFERENCES

1. Meyer P. La morphologic du ligament annulaire anterieur du coude-pied chez l'homme. *Comptes Rendus Assoc Anat*. 1955;84:286.
2. Weitbrecht J. *Syndesmology or a Description of the Ligaments of the Human Body: Arranged in Accordance with Anatomical Dissections and Illustrated with Figures Drawn from Fresh Subjects*. Vol 191. Translated by E. Kaplan. WB Saunders; 1969:1742.
3. Smith BE. The astragalo-calcaneo-navicular joint. *J Anat Physiol*. 1896;30:390.
4. Cahill DR. The anatomy and function of the contents of the human tarsal sinus and canal. *Anat Rec*. 1965;153:1.
5. Retzius A. Bemerkungen über ein schleuderformiges Band in dem Sinus Tarsi des Menschen und Mehrerer Thiere. *Arch Auat Physiol*. 1841:497.
6. Smith JW. The ligamentous structures in the canalis and sinus tarsi. *J Anat*. 1958;92:616.
7. Jotoku T, Kinoshita M, Okuda R, et al. Anatomy of ligamentous structures in the tarsal sinus and canal. *Foot Ankle*. 2006;7:5533-5538.
8. Bellocq P, Meyer P. Contribution a l'étude de l'aponevrose dorsale du pied (fascia dorsalis pedis, P.N.A.). *Acta Anat*. 1975;30:67.
9. Latarjet A, Etienne-Martin M. L'appareil de glissement des tendons extenseurs des doigts et des orteils sur le dos de la main et sur le dos du pied. *Ann Anat Pathol Anat Normal*. 1932;9:605.
10. Kaneff A, Mokrusch T, Landgraf P. Über die existenz eines retinaculum musculorum extensorum imum beim menschen. Occurrence of a retinaculum musculorum imum in man. *Gegenbaurs Morphol Jahrb*. 1984;130(6):769.
11. Bellocq P, Meyer P. Contribution a l'étude du canal calcanéen. *ComptesRendus Assoc Anat*. 1956;89:292.
12. Richet A. *Traite Pratique d'Anatomie Médico-Chirurgicale*. 5th ed. Lauwereyns; 1877:1311-1312.
13. Baumann J. La région de passage de la loge posterieure de la jambe à la plante du pied. *Ann Anat Pathol Anat Normal Medicochir*. 1930;7:201.
14. Raiga A. Le canal calcanéen. *La Presse Méd*. 1923;31:808.
15. Maslieurat-Lagémard. De l'anatomie descriptive et chirurgicale des aponevroses et des synoviales du pied: de leur appliction à la thérapeutique et à la médecine operatoire. *Gaz Med Paris*. 1840:274.
16. Henkel A. Die aponeurosis plantaris. *Arch für Anat und Physio Anat Abt*. 1913;113:113-123.
17. Bojsen-Møller F, Flagstad KE. Plantar aponeurosis and internal architecture of the ball of the foot. *J Anat*. 1976;121:599.
18. Poirier P, Charpy A. *Traité D'Anatomie Humaine*. Vol 2. Masson et Cie; 1901:300.
19. Grodinsky M. A study of the fascial spaces of the foot and their bearing on infections. *Surg Gynecol Obstet*. 1929;49:737.
20. Loth EM. Etude anthropologique sur l'aponévrose plantaire. *Bull Mem Soc Anthro Paris*. 1913;4:601.
21. Loth EM. Die Plantar aponeurose beim Menschen und den Übrigen primaten. *Korr Bl Deutsch Anthrop Ges*. 1907;38:169-172.
22. Wood Jones F. *Structure and Function as Seen in the Foot*. 2nd ed. Bailliére, Tindall & Cox; 1949:63.
23. Liaras H. Tissu cellulaire et topographic plantaire: connexions de la plante et du mollet. *Ann Anat Pathol Anat Normal*. 1935;12:537.
24. Sarrafian SK. *Anatomy of the Foot and Ankle. Descriptive, Topographic, Functional*. Vol 139. JB Lippincott; 1983:224.
25. Manoli A II, Weber TG. Fasciotomy of the foot: an anatomical study with special reference to release of the calcaneal compartment. *Foot Ankle*. 1990;10(5):267.
26. Kamel R, Sakla BF. Anatomical compartments of the sole of the human foot. *Anat Rec*. 1961;140:57.
27. Loeffler RD, Ballard A. Plantar fascial spaces of the foot and a proposed surgical approach. *Foot Ankle*. 1980;1:11.
28. Testut L, Jacob O. *Traité dAnatomie Topographique avec Applications Médico-chirurgicales*. Vol 2. 2nd ed. Doin; 1909:1075.
29. Grégoire R. Recherches sur la bourse sereuse sous-calcanéenne. *Bull Soc Anat Paris*. 1911;86:724.

Syndesmology

Shahan K. Sarrafian and Armen S. Kelikian

The distal segment of the fibular shaft and the lateral malleolus are firmly attached to the distal tibia and form a movable articulating system embracing the talar body. The inferior tibiofibular articulation is an integral part of the ankle joint. The subdivision of the ankle joint, as presented in the German literature, into an upper ankle joint (talocrural) and lower ankle joint (subtalar, talocalcaneonavicular) has merit from the anatomic and functional points of view.

LIGAMENTS OF THE INFERIOR TIBIOFIBULAR JOINT

The three ligaments uniting the distal fibular shaft and the lateral malleolus to the distal tibia are the anterior tibiofibular ligament, the posterior tibiofibular ligament, and the interosseous ligament. The lower segment of the interosseous membrane also participates in the stabilization of the distal fibular shaft.

▶ Anterior Tibiofibular Ligament

The anterior tibiofibular ligament (Figs. 4.1 and 4.2) is a flat, fibrous lamina. It originates from the longitudinal tubercle located on the anterior border of the lateral malleolus in front of the upper segment of the articulating surface of the talus and from the lower segment of the anterior border of the fibular shaft. The fibers are directed upward and medially and insert on the anterolateral tubercle of the tibia; some fibers reach the anterior surface of the distal tibia. The fibers increase in length from above downward, the lower fibers being the longest—close to 25 mm.

The anterior tibiofibular ligament is divided into two or three bands or may be multifascicular. Vessels from the anterior peroneal artery penetrate through the interlaminar spaces. During their oblique course, the most inferior fibers cover the tibiofibular corner of the joint and pass over the corresponding segment of the talus. The lowest fibers at their fibular site reach the origin of the anterior talofibular ligament.

▶ Posterior Tibiofibular Ligament

The posterior tibiofibular ligament (see Figs. 4.1 and 4.3) has two components: superficial and deep.

The superficial component originates from the posterior border of the tubercle located above the digital fossa of the lateral malleolus. The origin extends distally to the upper part of the posterior border of the digital fossa and proximally to the ridge separating the lateral and medial fibular surfaces posteriorly. The fibers are directed upward and medially and the major insertion is on the posterolateral tibial tubercle. The remaining fibers continue their course and insert on the distal tibia and they may reach the lateral border of the groove for the tibialis posterior tendon.

The deep component is the transverse ligament. This ligament is thick, strong, and conoid with a twist to its fibers; it originates from the round posterior fibular tubercle located above the digital fossa and from the upper segment of the digital fossa. The fibers are directed upward, medially, and posteriorly. At the posterior border of the tibial articular surface, the fibers change direction and become horizontal or transverse. This ligament inserts on the lower part of the posterior border of the tibial articular surface and reaches the medial border of the medial malleolus. The insertion is the strongest on the outer half. The transverse ligament descends below the posterior tibial margin and constitutes a true posterior labrum deepening the tibial articular surface (Figs. 4.1 and 4.4). The posterior half of the medial surface of the lateral malleolus is deficient in articular surface but is filled by the transverse ligament, which establishes contact with the talar surface and leaves its imprint as a beveled triangular facet on the posterior half of the lateral border of the superior talar surface.

▶ Interosseous Ligament

The interosseous ligament (Fig. 4.5) is a reddish ligament formed by a dense mass of short fibers intermingled with adipose tissue and vessels. These fibers form a vault over the underlying synovial recess and may be perforated in some specimens. The

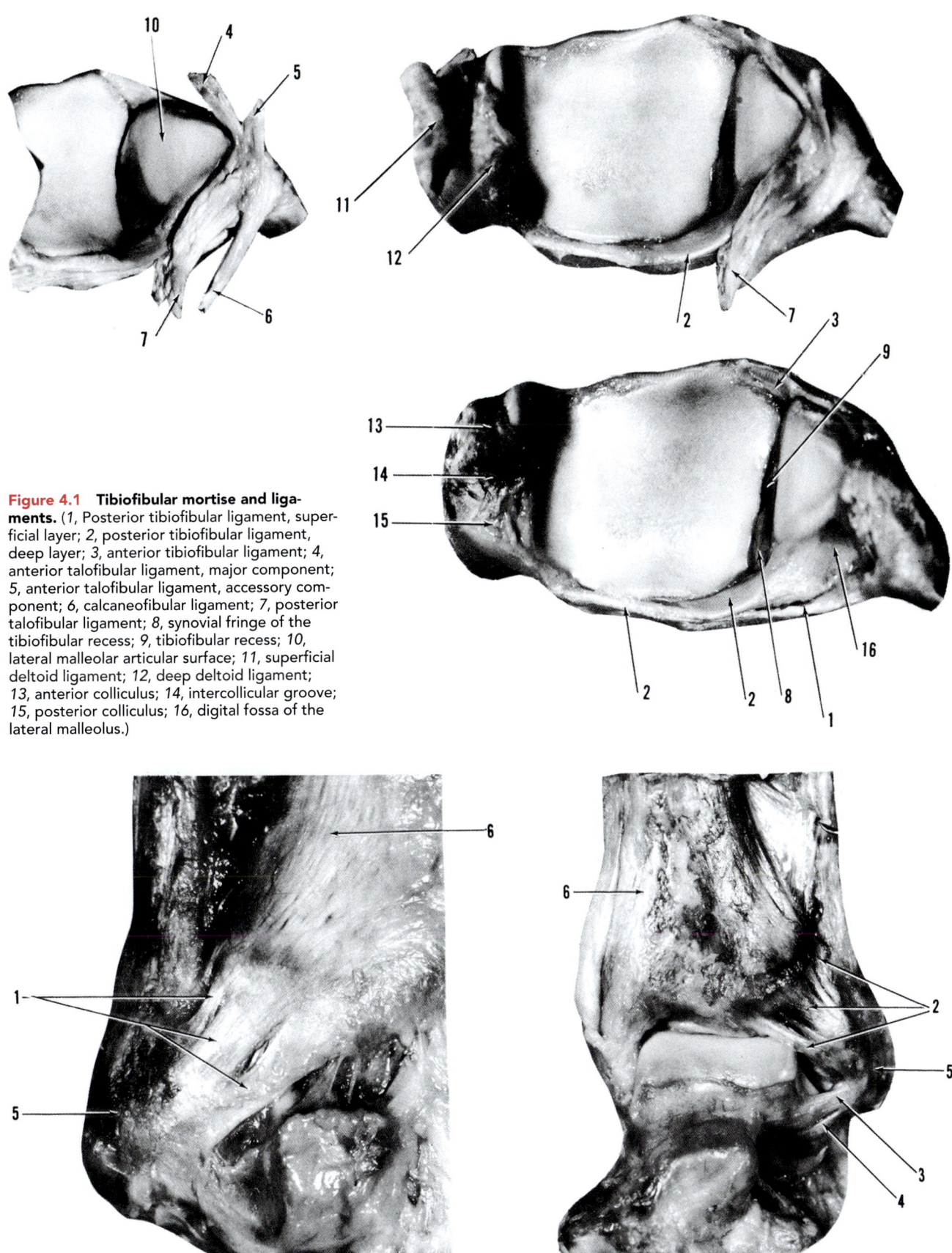

Figure 4.1 **Tibiofibular mortise and ligaments.** (*1*, Posterior tibiofibular ligament, superficial layer; *2*, posterior tibiofibular ligament, deep layer; *3*, anterior tibiofibular ligament; *4*, anterior talofibular ligament, major component; *5*, anterior talofibular ligament, accessory component; *6*, calcaneofibular ligament; *7*, posterior talofibular ligament; *8*, synovial fringe of the tibiofibular recess; *9*, tibiofibular recess; *10*, lateral malleolar articular surface; *11*, superficial deltoid ligament; *12*, deep deltoid ligament; *13*, anterior colliculus; *14*, intercollicular groove; *15*, posterior colliculus; *16*, digital fossa of the lateral malleolus.)

Figure 4.2 **Anterior tibiofibular ligament.** (*1*, Anterior tibiofibular ligament with three fascicles; *2*, anterior tibiofibular ligament with multiple fascicles; *3*, anterior talofibular ligament, major component; *4*, anterior talofibular ligament, accessory component; *5*, lateral malleolus; *6*, tibia.)

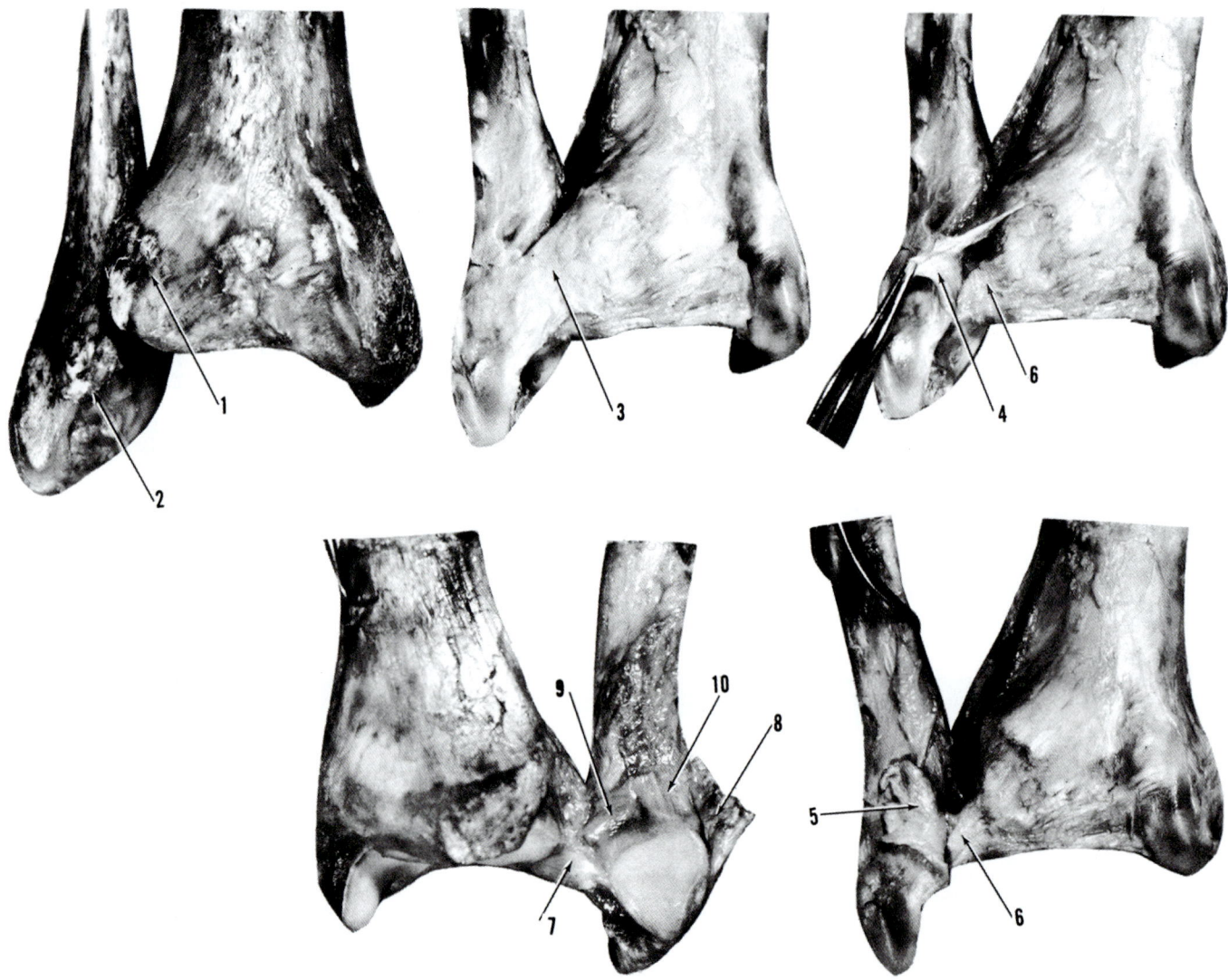

Figure 4.3 **Posterior tibiofibular ligament.** (*1*, Posterolateral tibial tubercle; *2*, lateral malleolus; *3*, posterior tibiofibular ligament, superficial layer; *4*, partially detached posterior tibiofibular ligament, superficial layer; *5*, completely detached posterior tibiofibular ligament, superficial layer; *6*, posterior tibiofibular ligament, deep layer, posterior aspect; *7*, posterior tibiofibular ligament, deep layer, anterior aspect; *8*, anterior tibiofibular ligament; *9*, synovial fringe of tibiofibular recess; *10*, tibiofibular synovial recess.)

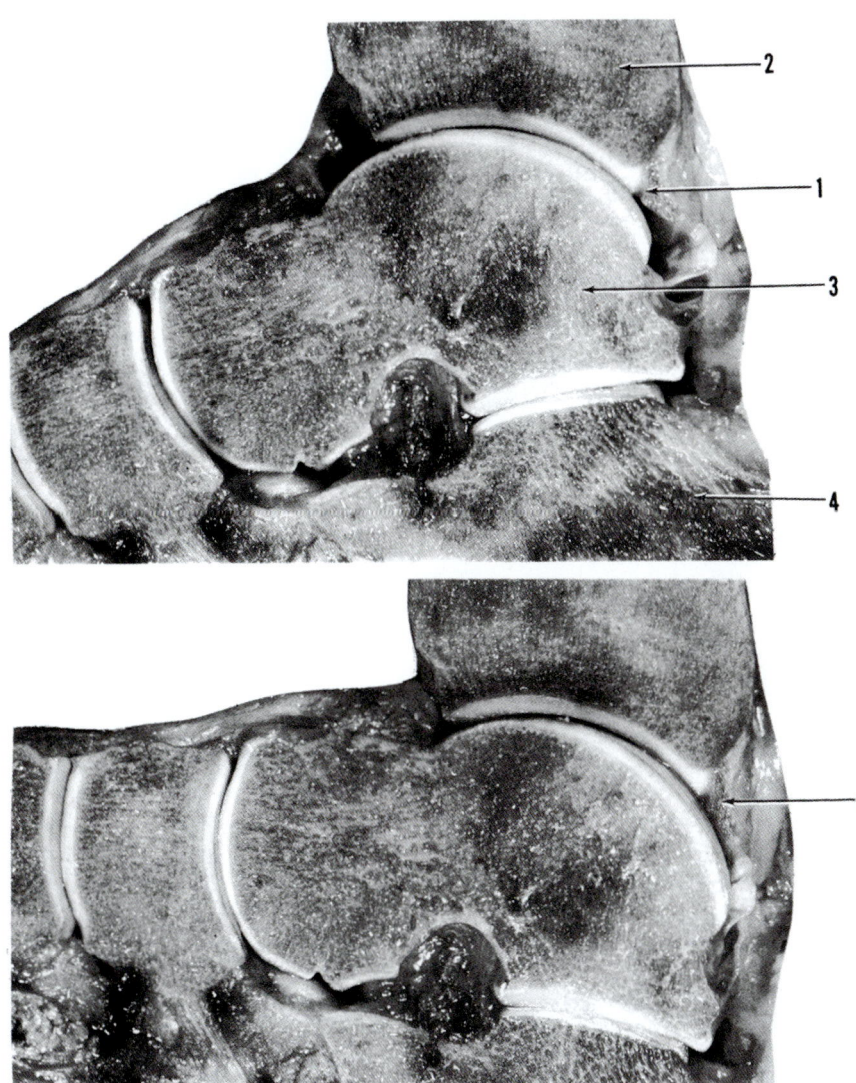

Figure 4.4 Sagittal cross-section of the ankle. (*1*, Tibial attachment of the deep component of the posterior tibiofibular ligament forming a labrum; *2*, tibia; *3*, talus; *4*, os calcis.)

ligament originates from the anteroinferior triangular segment of the medial aspect of the distal fibular shaft. This area of origin is higher anteriorly and lower posteriorly and the fibers insert on a similar corresponding area on the lateral surface of the distal tibia.

The fibula is in contact with the tibia only through a minute, crescent-shaped, cartilage-coated articular surface in continuity with the articular surface of the lateral malleolus.[1] A semilunar cavity is present above this tibiofibular interline and is limited proximally by the concave base of the interosseous ligament. The anterior segment of the cavity corresponds to a synovial recess communicating with the ankle joint through the linear opening. This synovial recess is about 1 cm in height. The posterior part of the semilunar cavity is smaller and occupied by a reddish synovial fringe that originates only from the peroneal surface and descends into the ankle joint between the fibula and the lateral talar surface (see Figs. 4.1 and 4.6). In dorsiflexion of the ankle, the synovial fringe retreats toward the upper chamber, and in plantar flexion, it descends into the ankle joint.[2,3]

Interosseous Membrane

The interosseous membrane is in continuity with the apex of the interosseous ligament (Fig. 4.7). The anterior fibers are oblique, directed downward and laterally, whereas the posterior fibers are nearly vertical.

LIGAMENTS UNITING THE DISTAL TIBIOFIBULAR COMPLEX TO THE TALUS, CALCANEUS, AND NAVICULAR

The distal tibiofibular complex is firmly connected to the talus and the os calcis. The talus is anchored to the fibula anteriorly and posteriorly and to the tibia medially. The calcaneus is anchored to the fibula laterally and to the tibia medially. The anterior connection of the tibia to the talus and to the navicular is of lesser magnitude.

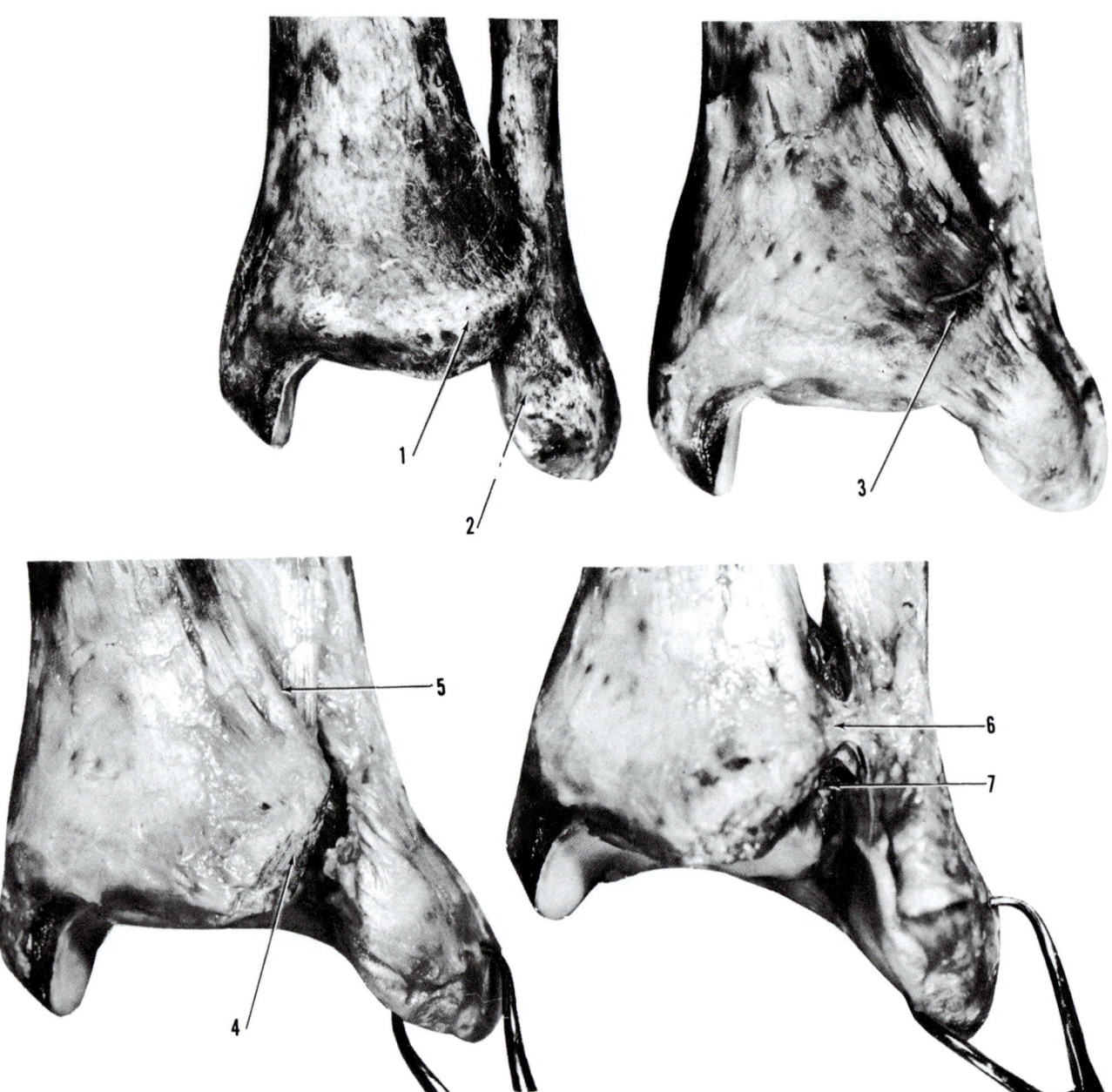

Figure 4.5 **Interosseous ligament.** (*1*, Anterolateral tibial tubercle; *2* lateral malleolus; *3*, anterior tibiofibular ligament; *4*, transected anterior tibiofibular ligament; *5*, interosseous membrane; *6*, interosseous ligament; *7*, tibiofibular synovial recess.)

▶ Lateral Ligament of the Ankle

Anterior Talofibular Ligament

The anterior talofibular ligament (Figs. 4.8 and 4.9) is a flat, quadrilateral, relatively strong ligament measuring approximately 15 × 8 × 2 mm, 20 × 6 × 2 mm,[4] or 12 × 5 × 2 mm.[5] This ligament is formed by two distinct bands separated by an interval that allows the penetration of vascular branches. The upper band is larger than the lower. A third band occasionally may be present. The ligament originates from the inferior oblique segment of the anterior border of the lateral malleolus. The upper band reaches the origin of the anterior tibiofibular ligament and the lower band that of the calcaneofibular ligament; in many specimens, these two ligaments are united with arciform fibers at their malleolar origin. The anterior talofibular ligament courses anteromedially and inserts not on the talar neck but on the talar body just anterior to the lateral malleolar articular surface. Two flat tubercles are occasionally seen, corresponding to the insertion of the two bands. The anterior talofibular ligament is in close connection to the capsule of the talofibular joint. In the neutral position of the talus, the ligament is horizontal. In dorsiflexion, the ligament is directed slightly upward. In plantar flexion, the ligament firmly braces the talar body as it stretches over the nearly right angle formed by the union of the anterior and lateral surfaces of the talar body (Fig. 4.10); in this position, the ligament is directed downward, medially, and anteriorly.

Chapter 4: Syndesmology 167

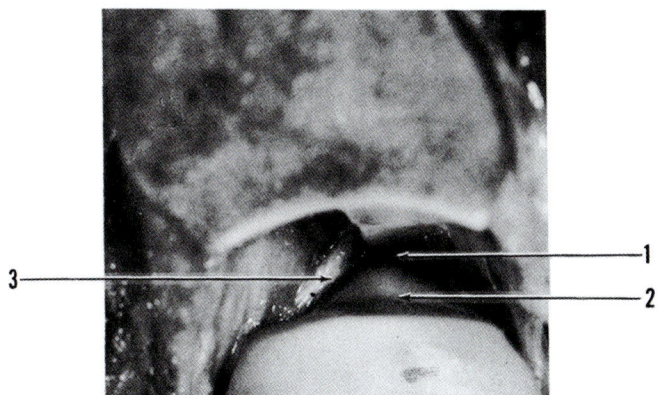
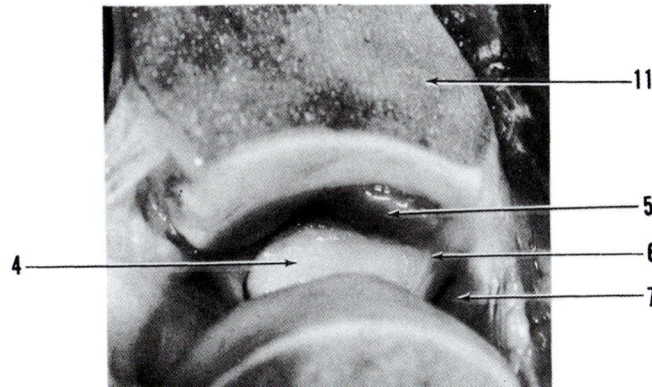

Figure 4.6 Sagittal section of the tibia and talus. (*1*, Talofibular joint; *2*, lateral talar articulating surface; *3*, anterior talofibular ligament; *4*, lateral malleolar articulating surface; *5*, tibiofibular synovial fringe; *6*, *7*, posterior tibiofibular ligament; *8*, posterior talofibular ligament; *9*, talus; *10*, posterior articular surface of calcaneus.)

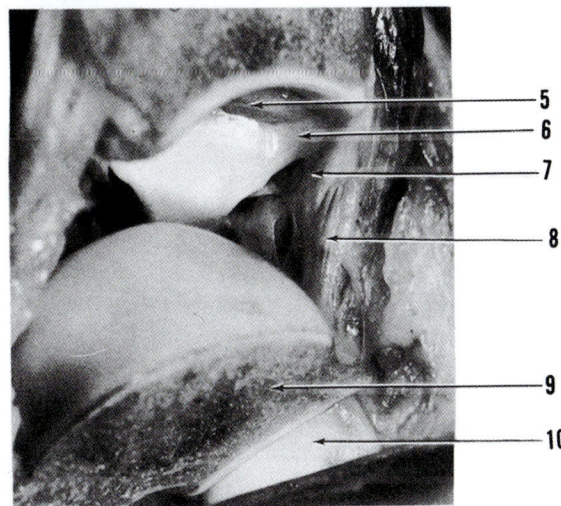

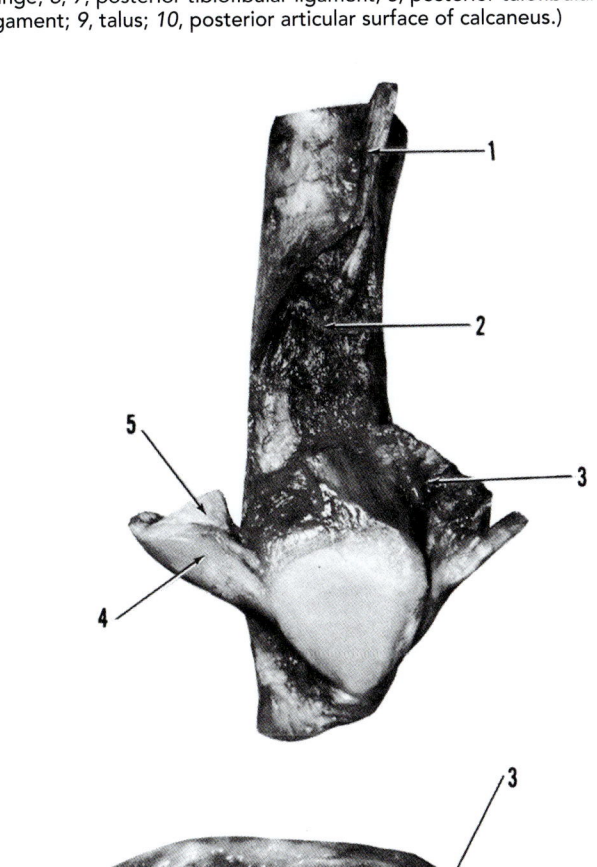

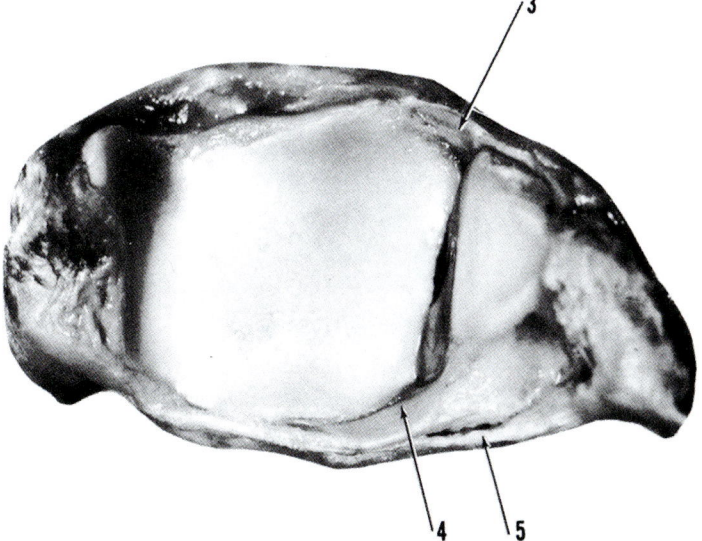

Figure 4.7 Interosseous membrane. (*1*, Insertion of interosseous membrane; *2*, insertion zone of tibiofibular interosseous ligament; *3*, anterior tibiofibular ligament; *4*, posterior tibiofibular ligament, deep component; *5*, posterior tibiofibular ligament, superficial component.)

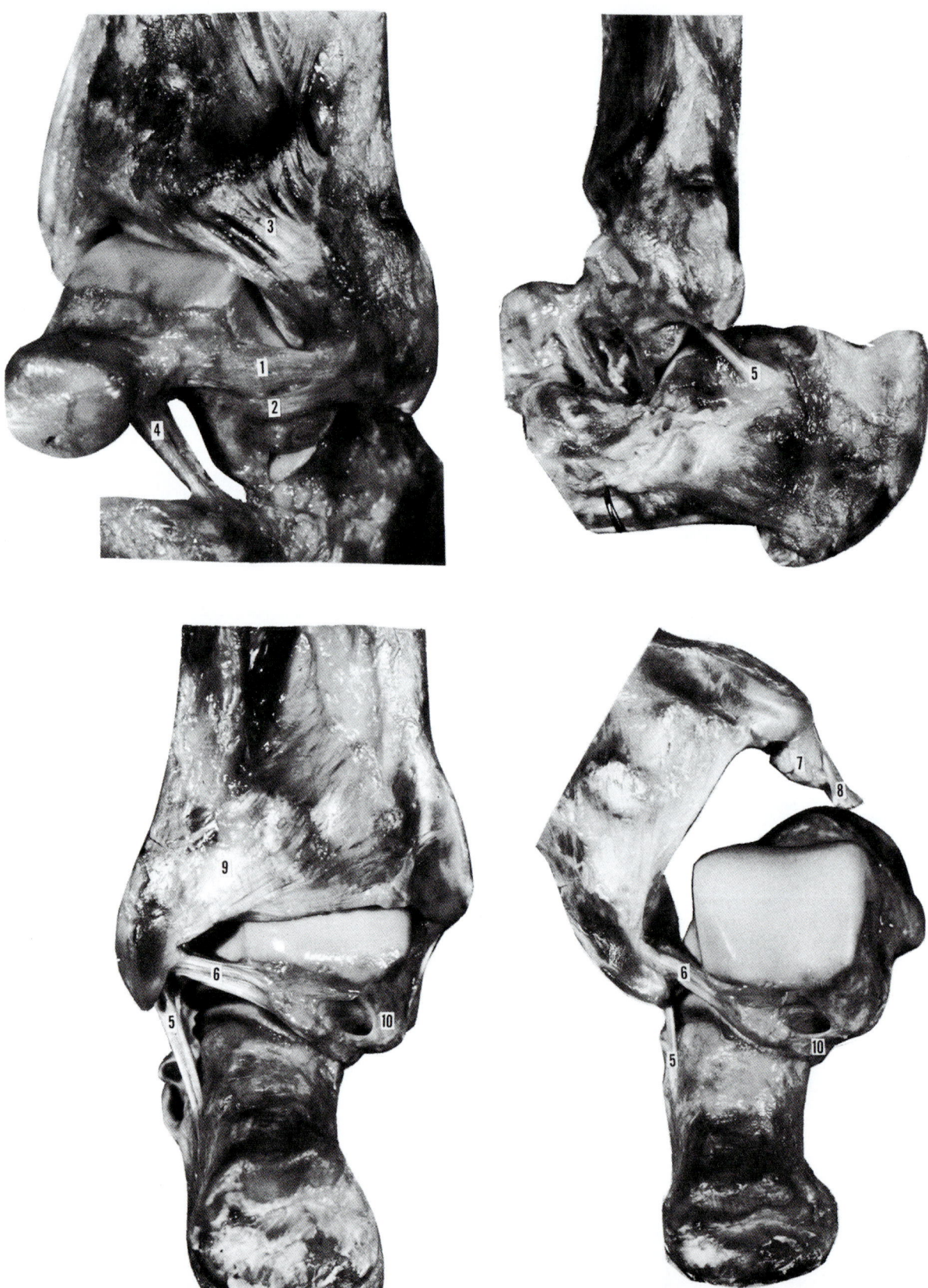

Figure 4.8 **Anterior talofibular ligament.** (*1*, Anterior talofibular ligament, main component; *2*, anterior talofibular ligament, accessory component; *3*, anterior tibiofibular ligament, fasciculated; *4*, cervical ligament; *5*, calcaneofibular ligament; *6*, posterior talofibular ligament; *7*, deltoid ligament, deep layer; *8*, deltoid ligament, superficial layer; *9*, posterior tibiofibular ligament; *10*, fibrous tunnel of flexor hallucis longus tendon.)

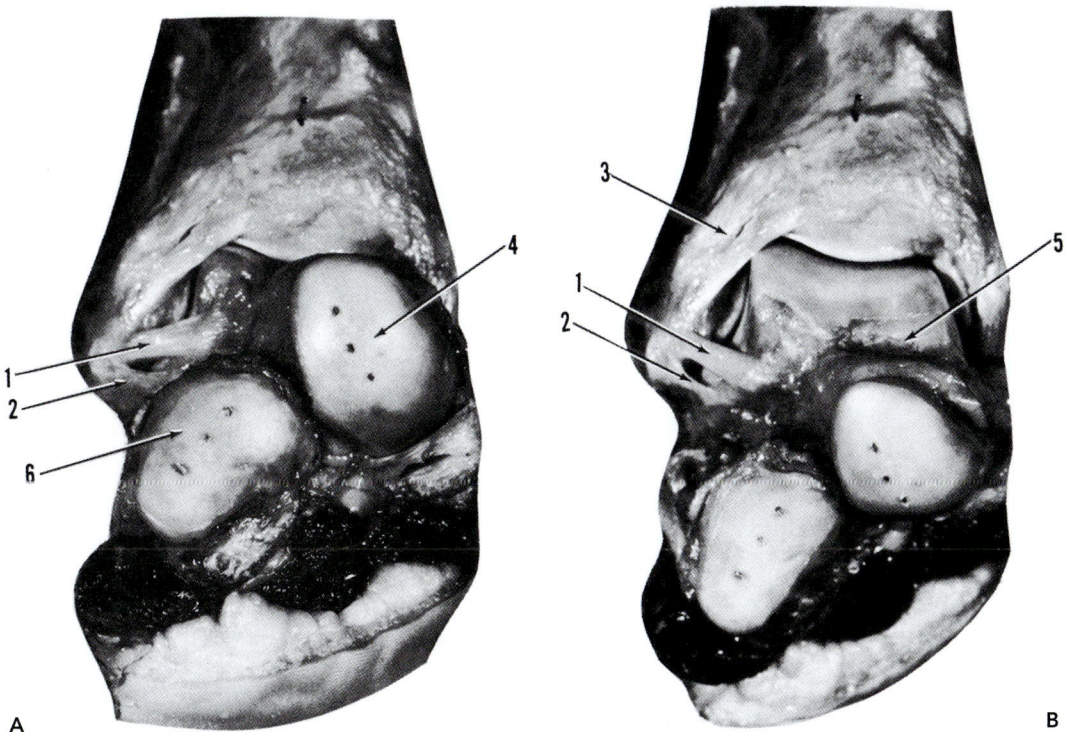

Figure 4.9 **Anterior talofibular ligament. (A)** Dorsiflexion. **(B)** Plantar flexion. (*1*, Anterior talofibular ligament, major component. The ligament is oriented upward, medially in dorsification [**A**], and downward, medially in plantar flexion [**B**]; *2*, anterior talofibular ligament, accessory component; *3*, anterior tibiofibular ligament; *4*, navicular articular surface of the talus; *5*, talus; *6*, cuboidal articular surface of the os calcis.)

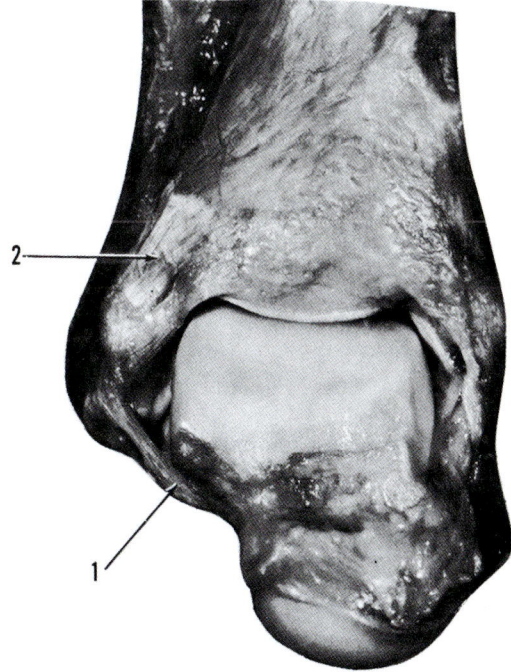

Figure 4.10 **Anterior talofibular ligament in plantar flexion.** (*1*, Anterior talofibular ligament inserting on the anterior surface of the talar body and under tension in plantar flexion; *2*, anterior tibiofibular ligament.)

Milner and Soames[6] investigated the anatomical variations of the anterior talofibular ligament (ATFL) in 26 ankle specimens. They observed single, bifurcate, and trifurcate forms of the ATFL. The single form occurred in 38% (10 occurrences with 8 bilateral and 2 unilateral), the bifurcate form in 50% (13 occurrences with 12 bilateral and 1 unilateral), and the trifurcate form in 12% (3 occurrences with all unilateral). "The overall width of the ATFL did not appear to vary greatly irrespective of the number of bands present."[6] In a subsequent study based on the dissection of 40 ankles, the same authors[7] provided the following mean measurements to the anterior talofibular ligament: length, 13 ± 3.9 mm; width, 11 ± 3.3 mm.

Calcaneofibular Ligament

The calcaneofibular ligament (see Figs. 4.8 and 4.11) is a strong cordlike or flat oval ligament and measures approximately 30 mm length, 5 mm width, and 3 mm thickness; *or* length of 20 mm with diameter of 4 to 8 mm[4]; *or* length of 30 to 40 mm with width of 4 to 5 mm.[3] It originates from the lower segment of the anterior border of the lateral malleolus just below the origin of the inferior band of the anterior talofibular ligament. The origin does not extend to the tip of the lateral malleolus, which is left free. Near the origin, arciform fibers may unite the calcaneofibular ligament and the inferior band of the anterior talofibular

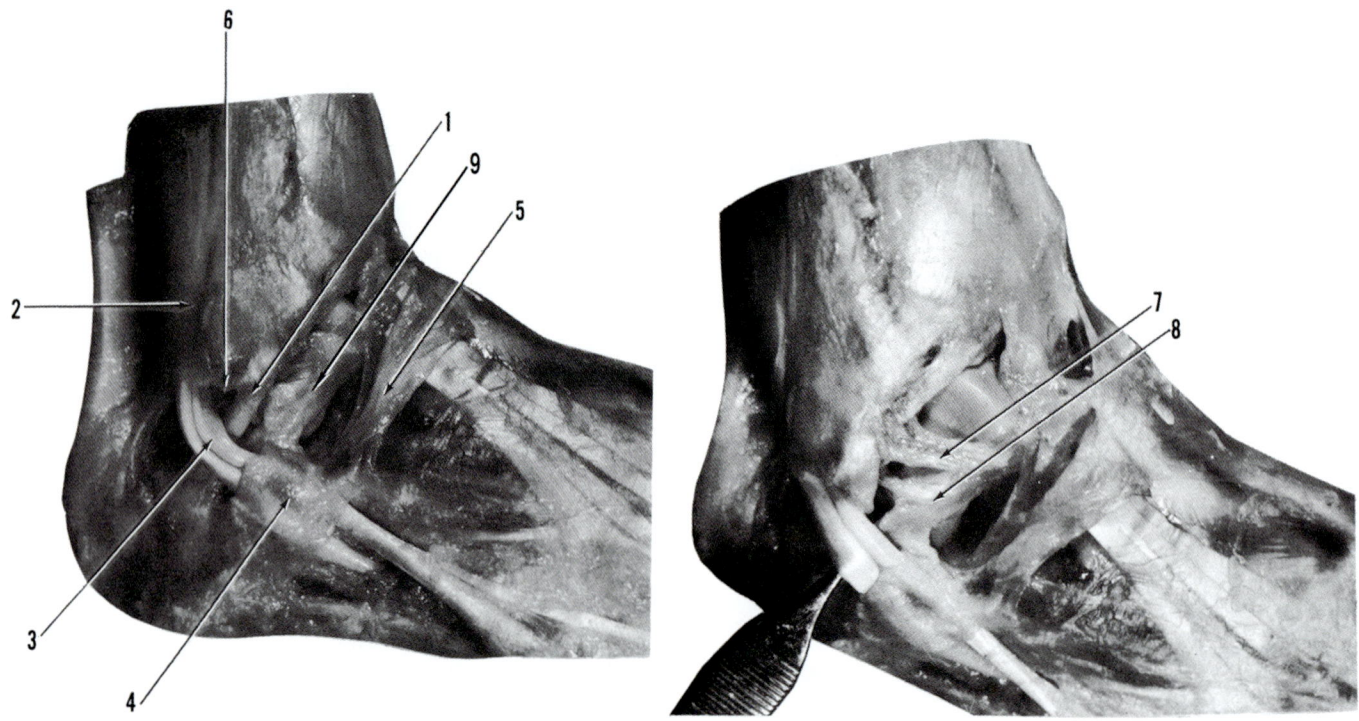

Figure 4.11 **Calcaneofibular ligament.** (*1*, Calcaneofibular ligament; *2*, superior peroneal retinaculum; *3*, peronei tendons, brevis anteriorly and longus posteriorly; *4*, inferior peroneal retinaculum; *5*, stem of inferior extensor retinaculum; *6*, tip of lateral malleolus, *free of insertion*; *7*, anterior talofibular ligament, major component; *8*, anterior talofibular ligament, accessory component; *9*, lateral talocalcaneal ligament.)

ligament. With the foot in neutral position, the ligament courses posteriorly, inferiorly, and medially and is crossed superficially by the peronei tendons and their sheaths, which may leave an imprint on the ligament (Figs. 4.12 to 4.14). Only about 1 cm of the ligament remains uncovered by the crossing peronei.

The calcaneofibular ligament inserts on a small tubercle (tuberculum ligamenti calcaneo fibularis) located on the posterior aspect of the lateral calcaneal surface, posterosuperior to the peronei processus trochlearis. The insertion of the ligament is variable. Laidlaw, in a study of 750 calcanei, gives the following location of the calcaneal insertion of the ligament: typical location, 64.5%; anterior location, 25.5%; posterior location, 5.5%; downward location, 4.5%.[8] The variable insertions result in variable obliquity of the ligament relative to the long axis of the fibula.

Ruth, in a study based on 30 dissected specimens and observations of 55 ankles during surgery, provides the following data with regard to the angle formed by the long axis of the calcaneofibular ligament and the long axis of the fibula (Fig. 4.15): 10° to 45°, 74.66%; 0°, 18.66%; 80° to 90°, 4%; fan-shaped, 2.66%.[5] The valgus or varus position considerably affects the direction of and the angle formed by the calcaneofibular ligament. The obliquity of the ligament is increased with valgus of the heel and decreased with varus (Fig. 4.16). The obliquity of the ligament is also variable with the position of the ankle joint (Fig. 4.17). The calcaneofibular ligament crosses the talocalcaneal joint and is separated from it by the lateral talocalcaneal ligament. The interval between the two ligaments is filled with adipose tissue.

Trouilloud and colleagues[9] reported on the variable relationship of the calcaneofibular ligament and the lateral talocalcaneal ligament in 26 ankles. They classified their findings into three categories: A, B, and C. In type A, 35%, the calcaneofibular ligament is reinforced by a lateral talocalcaneal ligament, attached to the former but diverging proximally or distally. In

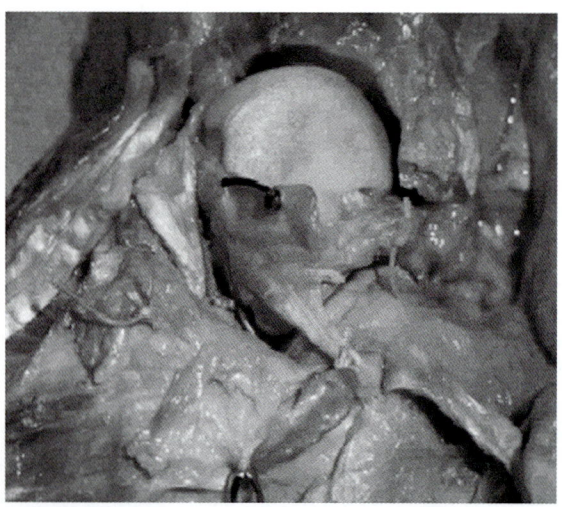

Figure 4.12 **Lateral talocalcaneal ligament.** (DiGiovanni CW, Langer PR, Nickish F, et al. Proximity of the lateral talar process to the lateral stabilizing ligaments of the ankle and subtalar joint. *Foot Ankle Int.* 2007;2:175-180, Figure 3A. copyright ©2007. Reprinted by Permission of SAGE Publications.)

Chapter 4: Syndesmology 171

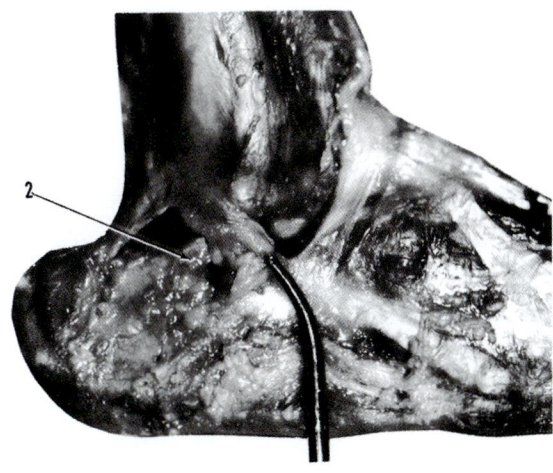
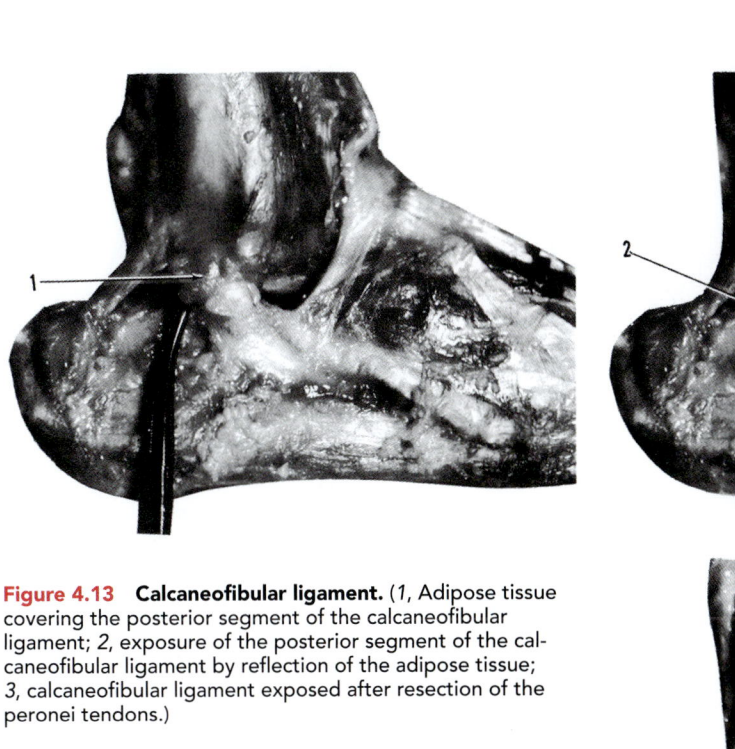
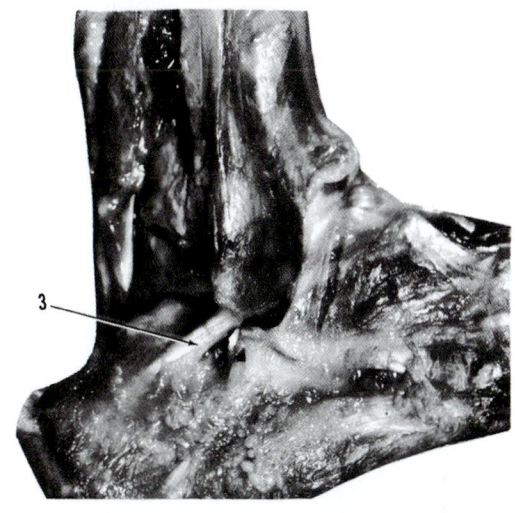

Figure 4.13 Calcaneofibular ligament. (*1*, Adipose tissue covering the posterior segment of the calcaneofibular ligament; *2*, exposure of the posterior segment of the calcaneofibular ligament by reflection of the adipose tissue; *3*, calcaneofibular ligament exposed after resection of the peronei tendons.)

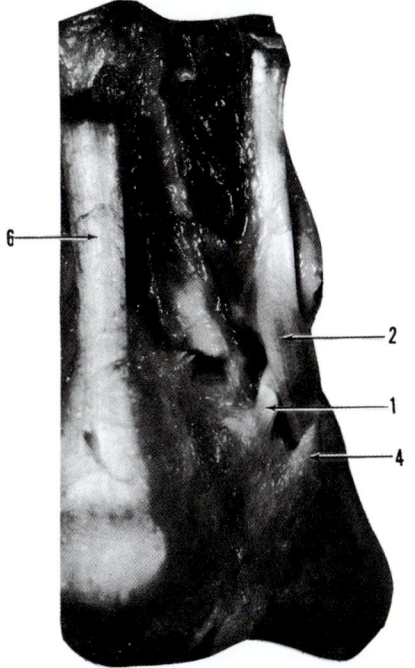
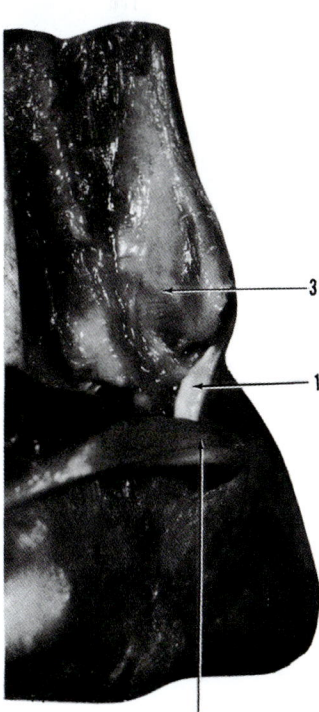

Figure 4.14 Posterolateral aspect of the ankle. (*1*, Calcaneofibular ligament and peronei tendons [*2*] crossing in X; *3*, sulcus of peronei tendons on posterior surface of lateral malleolus; *4*, inferior peroneal retinaculum; *5*, reflected peronei tendons; *6*, Achilles tendon.)

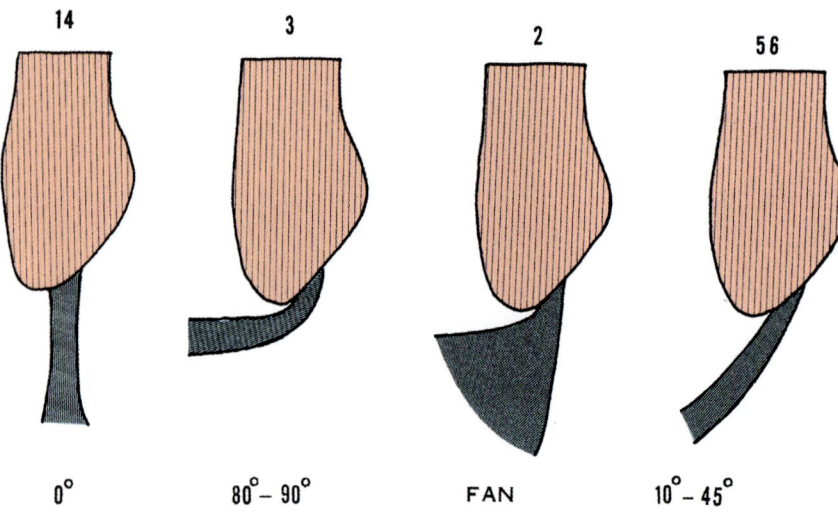

Figure 4.15 Anatomical variations of the calcaneofibular ligament in 75 ankles. *Left to right*: vertical, horizontal, fan shaped, oblique. (Adapted from Ruth CJ. The surgical treatment of injuries of the fibular collateral ligaments of the ankle. *J Bone Joint Surg [Am]*. 1961;43:233.)

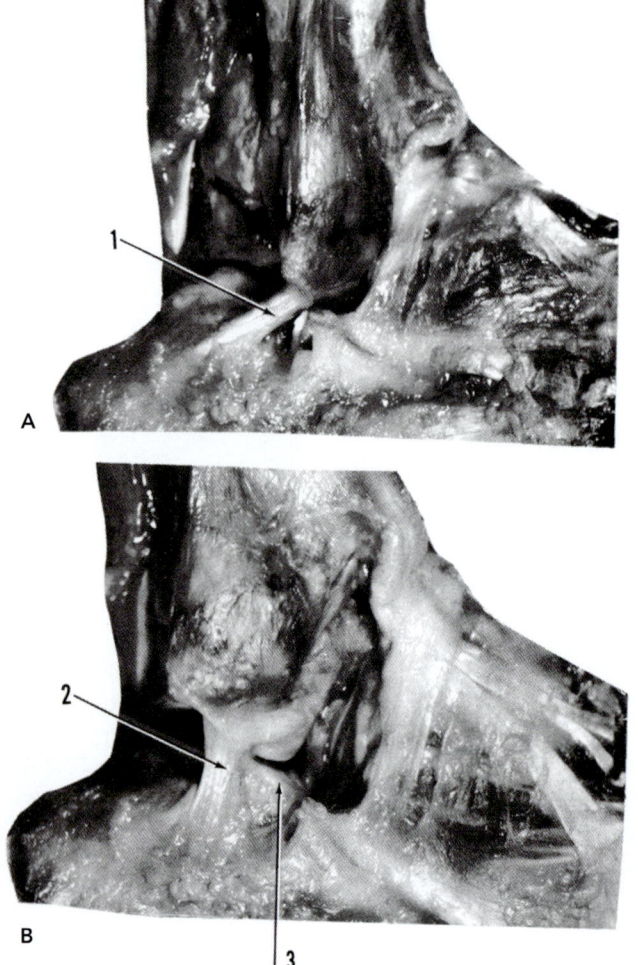

Figure 4.16 The heel in valgus and varus. (A) Heel in valgus; obliquity of calcaneofibular ligament (*1*) is increased. **(B)** Heel in varus, obliquity of calcaneofibular ligament (*2*) is decreased. In this specimen, the ligament is vertical. (*3*, Posterior calcaneal surface seen in varus.)

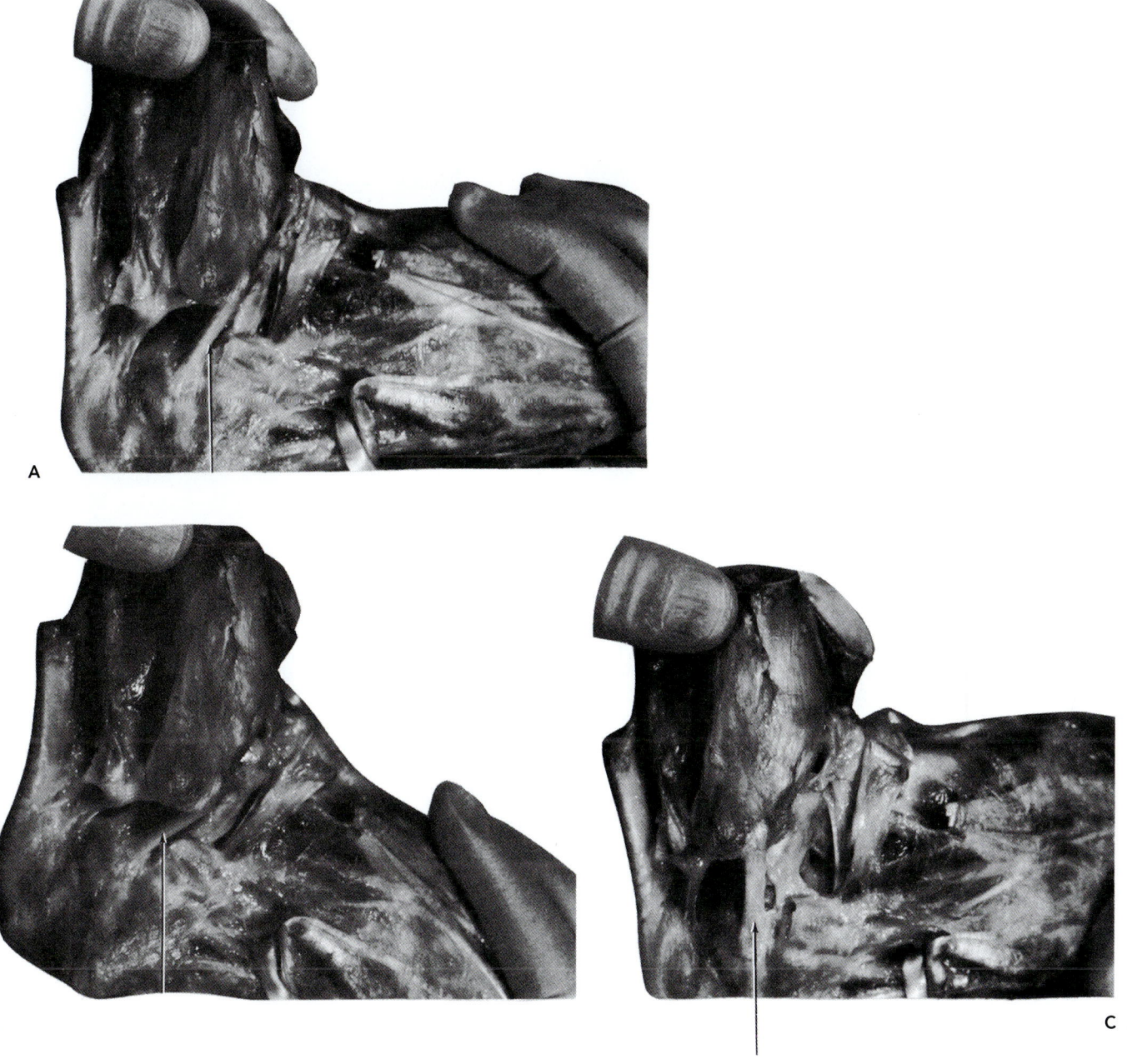

Figure 4.17 **Obliquity of the calcaneofibular ligament (*arrows*). (A)** In neutral position of the ankle. **(B)** In plantar flexion. **(C)** In dorsiflexion.

type B, 23%, a lateral talocalcaneal ligament exists anteriorly and independent of the calcaneofibular ligament. In type C, 42%, the lateral talocalcaneal ligament is absent and is replaced by an anterior talocalcaneal ligament, which is parallel now to the interosseous talocalcaneal ligament. In type C, the calcaneofibular ligament acquires more functional significance in providing stability to the subtalar joint.

Milner and Soames[7] in a study based on the dissection of 40 ankles provided the following measurements in regard to the calcaneofibular ligament: length, 19.5 ± 3.9 mm; width, 5.5 ± 1.6 mm.

Posterior Talofibular Ligament

The posterior talofibular ligament (Figs. 4.8 and 4.18) is a very strong ligament situated in a nearly horizontal plane. Trapezoidal in contour, the ligament measures approximately 30 mm in posterior length, 5 mm in width at the fibular origin, and 5 to 8 mm in thickness. The ligament originates on the medial surface of the lateral malleolus from the lower segment of the digital fossa (Fig. 4.19). Thick and fasciculated, it courses horizontally toward the lateral and posterior aspects of the talus. The short transverse and intermediary fibers insert along the lateral surface of the talus in a groove along the posteroinferior

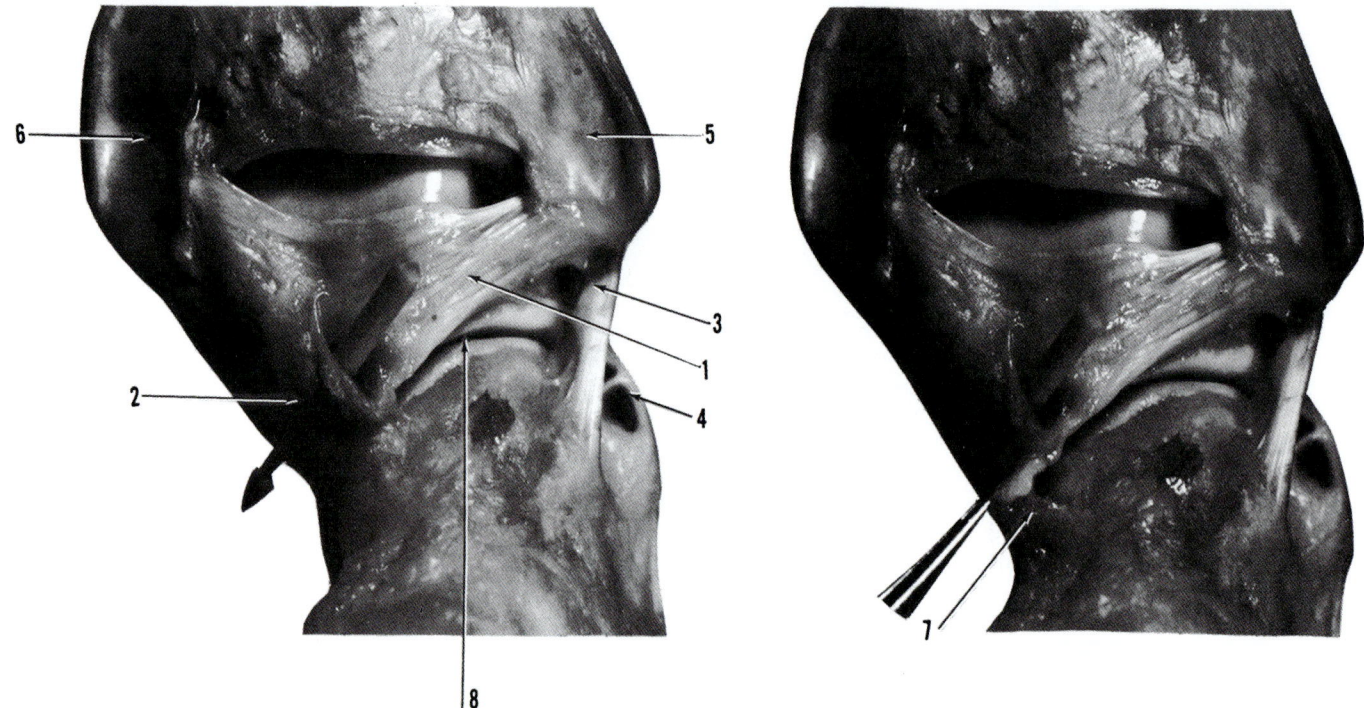

Figure 4.18 Posterior aspect of the ankle. (1, Posterior talofibular ligament; 2, fibrous tunnel of the flexor hallucis longus tendon; 3, calcaneofibular ligament; 4, inferior peroneal retinaculum; 5, sulcus of the peronei tendons on posterior surface of the lateral malleolus; 6, sulcus of tibialis posterior tendon on posterior aspect of the medial malleous; 7, posterior talocalcaneal ligament; 8, posterior calcaneal articular interline.)

border of the lateral malleolar articular surface up to its mid segment. The long fibers are directed posteromedially and insert on the posterior surface of the talus. The medial end expands and attaches on the posterolateral tubercle, the trigonal process, or the os trigonum (when present) and contributes to the formation of the floor of the flexor hallucis longus tunnel. When viewed posteriorly, the ligament is triangular, with a lateral apex and a medial base. The upper fibers of the posterior segment are in continuity medially with the superficial talotibial ligament, forming a posterior ligamentous sling.

Occasionally a band originates from the superior border of the posterior talofibular ligament near its origin, courses upward and medially, and inserts on the posterior tibial margin, blending with the fibers of the transverse component of the posterior tibiofibular ligament (Fig. 4.20); this insertion may reach the posterior surface of the medial malleolus. Paturet designates this ligament the posterior intermalleolar ligament.[10] The posterior talofibular ligament is intracapsular but extrasynovial. The fibular origin is covered by the peronei retinaculum (Fig. 4.21). The superomedial segment is crossed by the tendon of the flexor hallucis longus (Fig. 4.22).

Milner and Soames[7] in a study based on the dissection of 40 ankles provided the following measurements in regard to the posterior talofibular ligament: length, 23.0 ± 7.0 mm; width, 5.5 ± 2.5 mm.

Fibulotalocalcaneal Ligament

The fibulotalocalcaneal ligament of Rouvière and Canela Lazaro (Figs. 4.23 to 4.25) is an extrinsic ligament that occupies the posterolateral corner of the ankle and posterior subtalar joints. In 1924, Dujarier described briefly and produced a clear illustration of a posterior fibulocalcaneal ligament arising from the posterior aspect of the lateral malleolus and inserting on the

Figure 4.19 Tibiofibular mortise. (1, Posterior talofibular ligament; 2 calcaneofibular ligament; 3, anterior talofibular ligament, major component; 4, anterior talofibular ligament, accessory component.)

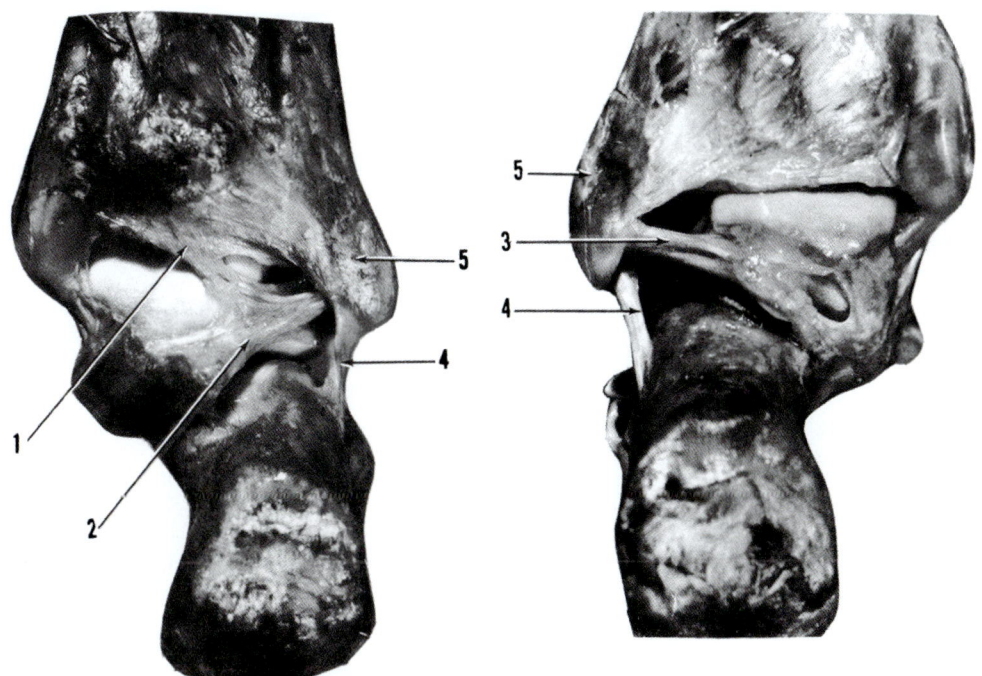

Figure 4.20 Posterior aspect of ankle. (*1*, Posterior intermalleolar ligament; *2, 3*, posterior talofibular ligament; *4*, calcaneofibular ligament; *5*, lateral malleolus.)

posterosuperior aspect of the calcaneus laterally.[11] He qualified this ligament as being abnormal and mentioned that, in certain clubfeet, this ligament is considerably developed, forming the posterior fibulocalcaneal ligament of Bessel-Hagen (Fig. 4.26).

In 1932, Rouvière and Canela Lazaro, in a comprehensive study, described the peroneotalocalcaneal ligament.[12] This ligament is independent of the capsules and ligaments of the neighboring joints. It originates from the medial border of the peroneal groove located on the posterior border of the lateral malleolus, in common with the origin of the posterior tibiofibular ligament. Inferiorly, the origin may descend to the tip of the lateral malleolus and quite frequently may reach the origin of the calcaneofibular ligament.

At the origin, the peroneotalocalcaneal ligament is in close connection with the fibrous sheath of the peronei but soon separates from it and is directed downward, medially and posteriorly. This flat structure then divides into two fibrous laminae: superomedial and inferolateral. The superomedial lamina or talar component inserts on the posterolateral tubercle of the talus and contributes to the formation of the flexor hallucis longus fibrous tunnel. The inferolateral or peroneocalcaneal lamina is the major component of the ligament. It is directed downward and posteriorly, enlarges, and inserts nearly transversely on the entire width of the superior surface of the calcaneus. At times the calcaneal insertion is oblique, directed forward and medially. In approximately two-thirds of the cases, the insertion remains localized to the superior surface of the calcaneus or reaches the lateral surface of the os calcis; the lateral border of the ligament is then separated by a small interval from the insertion of the calcaneofibular ligament. In the remaining one-third, the calcaneal insertion clearly extends to the lateral calcaneal surface and blends with the insertion of the calcaneofibular ligament.

The frequency of occurrence of this ligament is 60% present as a well-defined ligament, 20% present as a thin, weak structure but with ligamentous texture, and 20% absent and replaced by a thin fascia.[12] Occasionally both components of the ligament are united, forming a continuous lamina.

On close analysis and as described by Rouvière and Canela Lazaro, the fibulotalocalcaneal ligament is the very thick inferior and subcalcaneal portion of the deep aponeurosis of the leg between the tunnel of the flexor hallucis longus and the tunnel of the peronei.[12] This ligament limits the dorsiflexion of the foot.

▶ Medial Ligament or Deltoid Ligament

The medial malleolus provides attachment to the ligaments necessary to stabilize the talus and the naviculocalcaneal complex medially (Fig. 4.27A). The insertion of the talotibial fibers are concentrated on the posteromedial aspect of the talus, whereas the peritalar fibers insert mainly on the sustentaculum tali.

The remaining fibers of the ligament have received variable acceptance as ligaments because of the relative strength to qualify them; this applies particularly to the superficial anterior talotibial ligament.

The interpretation of the disposition of the fibers of the medial ligament as being one or two layers (superficial and deep) has brought forth a plethora of descriptions (Fig. 4.27B, E). On close examination, if one accepts the element of variability with regard to the lesser components of this ligament, the descriptions then fall into a harmonious pattern.

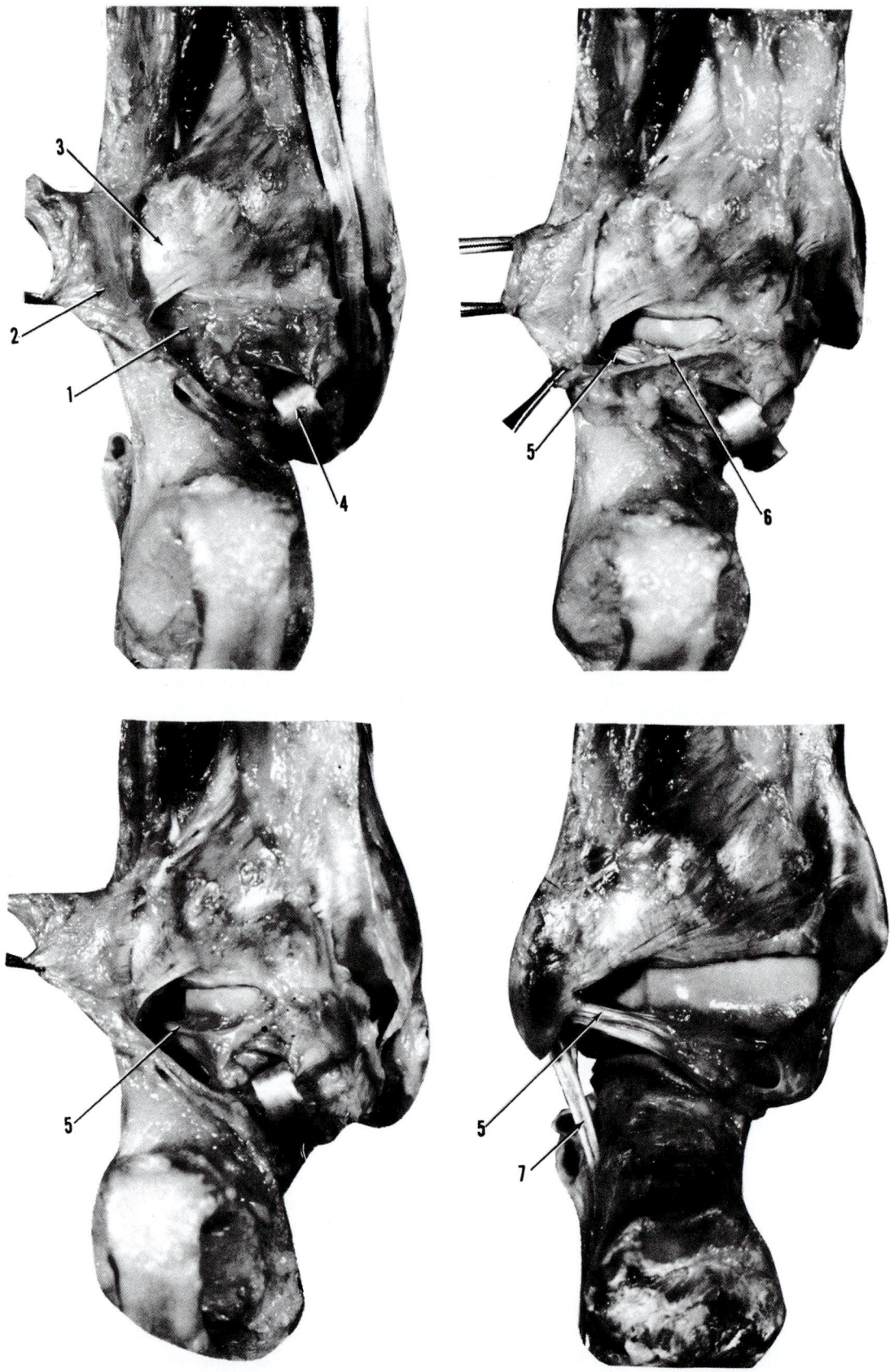

Figure 4.21 **Posterior aspect of ankle.** (*1*, Adipose tissue and capsule covering the posterior talofibular ligament; *2*, ligament of Rouvière and Canela Lazaro; *3*, posterior tibiofibular ligament; *4*, reflected tendon of flexor hallucis longus; *5*, posterior talofibular ligament; *6*, reflected posterior capsule; *7*, calcaneofibular ligament.)

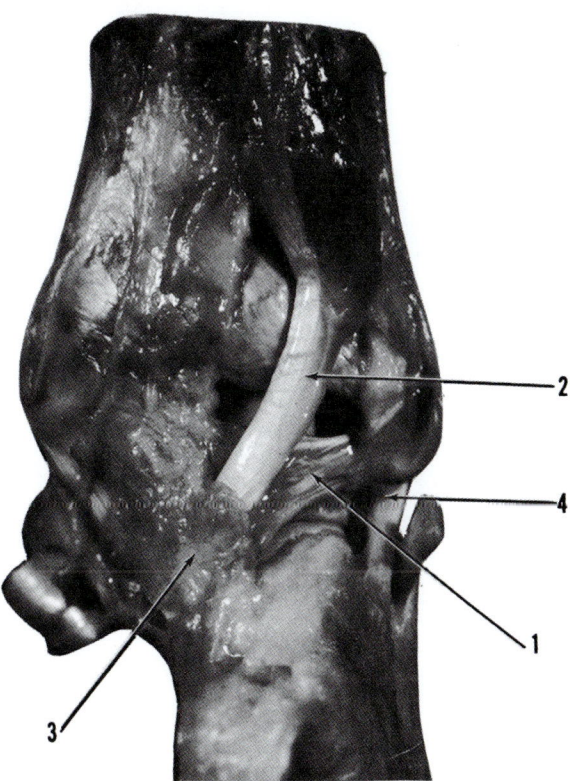

Figure 4.22 **Posterior aspect of ankle.** (*1*, Posterior talofibular ligament crossed by the flexor hallucis longus tendon [*2*]; *3*, tunnel of flexor hallucis longus; *4*, calcaneofibular ligament.)

A practical understanding of this ligament requires the consideration of a few points:

The entire medial ligamentous complex is invested, except in the very anterior part, by the deep crural fascia in continuity with the flexor retinaculum (Figs. 4.28 and 4.29).

The anterior border of the ligament is covered by the tibialis anterior tendon with its underlying adipose tissue. This anterior border is in continuity laterally with the thin anterior capsule.

A major segment—mid and posterior—of the ligament is covered by the obliquely crossing tibialis posterior and flexor digitorum longus tendons. The fibrosynovial floors of these tunnels blend with the underlying ligament (Figs. 4.30 and 4.31); minute dissection usually is necessary to separate the two.

The medial ligament, except for its deep talotibial component, is a continuous fibrous lamina and any division into components is usually artificial (Figs. 4.32 to 4.34). It is only by referring to the insertion of the fibers that descriptive differentiation is possible.

Posteriorly, the ligament is in continuity with the posterior capsule and the posterior talofibular ligament.

The medial ligament is divided into two layers, superficial and deep, each being formed by multiple fascicles. The superficial layer or deltoid ligament is broad and triangular. For the purpose of description, the following components are considered.

▶ Anterior Superficial Tibiotalar Fascicle and Tibionavicular Fascicle

The anterior superficial tibiotalar fascicle and tibionavicular fascicle (Fig. 4.35) have a common origin on the anterior border of the anterior colliculus. The fibers of origin extend to the medial corner of the anterior margin of the tibial quadrilateral inferior articular surface. As specified by Beau, the fibers delineate an anterolateral concave border and further distally divide into two layers.[13] The deep fibers insert on the dorsum of the talar neck slightly posterior to the talar head and to the talonavicular capsule; this component is the anterior and superficial tibiotalar ligament. The superficial fibers extend beyond the talonavicular interline and insert on the dorsomedial aspect of the navicular in a curvilinear fashion, extending medially a very short distance from the articular margin; this component is the tibionavicular ligament. The two ligaments overlap except at the most median site, where the talar fibers do not extend onto the navicular.

Tibioligamentous Fascicle

The tibioligamentous fascicle originates from the anterior segment of the anterior colliculus. The fibers present a gentle anterior concavity and insert on the superior border of the superomedial calcaneonavicular ligament. The anterior superficial tibiotalar fascicle, the tibionavicular fascicle, and the tibioligamentous fascicle constitute the broader but weaker component of the medial ligament (Fig. 4.36).

Tibiocalcaneal Ligament

The tibiocalcaneal ligament (Fig. 4.37) is the strongest superficial component. It originates from the medial aspect of the anterior colliculus, descends vertically, and inserts on the medial border of the sustentaculum tali after interlacing its fibers with those of the superomedial calcaneonavicular ligament.[14] This ligament is in continuity with the preceding tibioligamentous fascicle. In certain specimens, the origin of the latter overlaps the origin of the tibiocalcaneal ligament, and the interval is filled with adipose tissue. The tibiocalcaneal ligament measures approximately 1 cm in width at the origin and 1.5 cm at the insertion. The average length is 2 to 3 cm and the thickness 2 to 3 mm. It is a substantial structure.

Superficial Posterior Tibiotalar Ligament

The superficial posterior tibiotalar ligament originates from the posterior part of the medial surface of the anterior colliculus and the medial surface of the posterior colliculus (Fig. 4.38). The fibers are directed posteriorly, inferiorly, and laterally and insert on the posteromedial talar tubercle, reaching the flexor hallucis longus tunnel.[3,15-19] The posterior border of the tibiocalcaneal ligament is distinct from this ligament or the two may be in continuity; if they are in continuity, the superficial layer is represented as a large, fibrous, fan-shaped lamina deserving the "deltoid" denomination. The superficial posterior tibiotalar ligament is separated

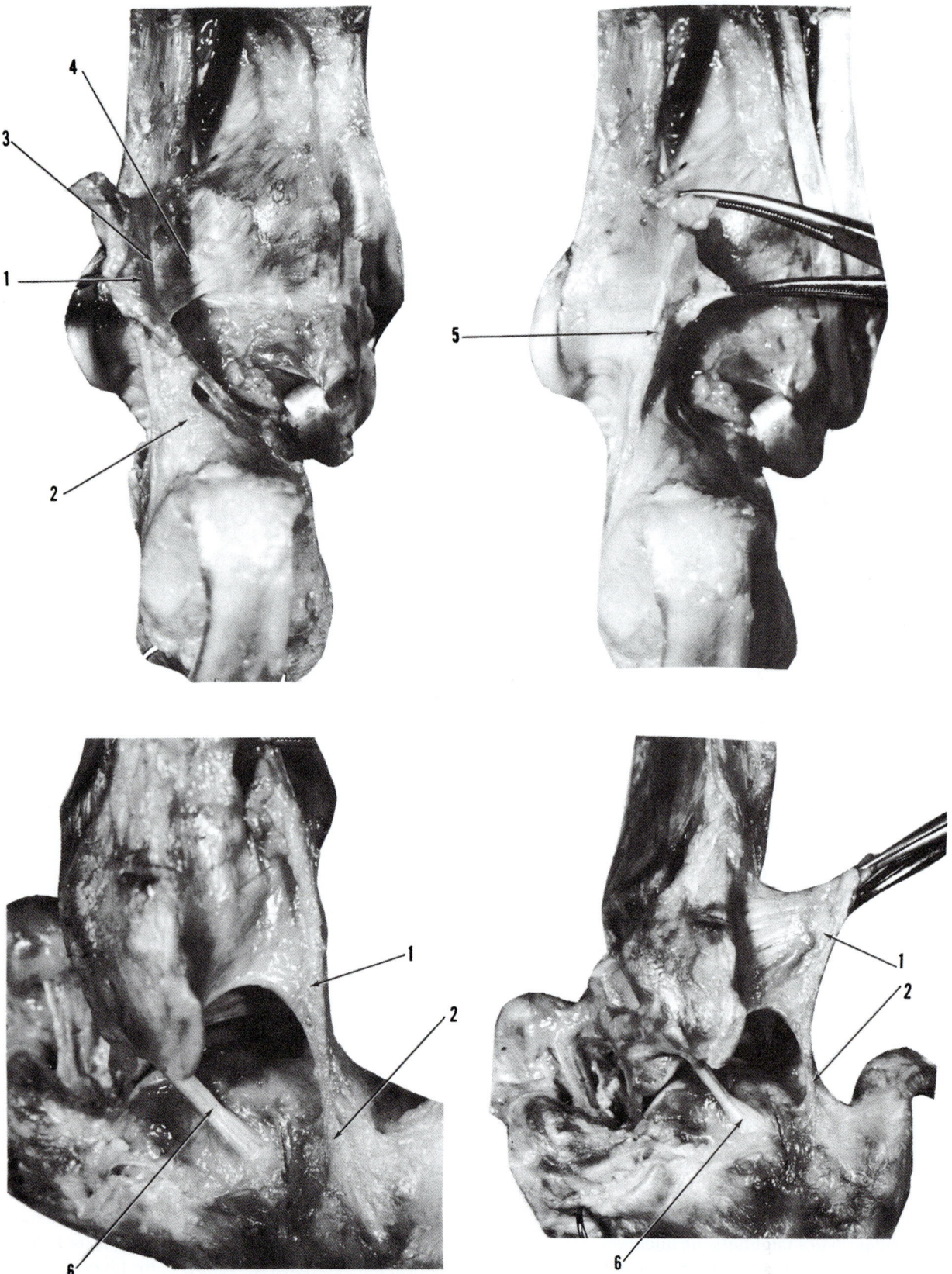

Figure 4.23 **Fibulotalocalcaneal ligament.** (*1*, Fibulotalocalcaneal ligament of Rouvière and Canela Lazaro; *2*, calcaneal insertion of *1*; *3*, common origin of *1* with the posterior tibiofibular ligaments [*4*]; *5*, connection of *1* with superior peroneal retinaculum; *6*, calcaneofibular ligament.)

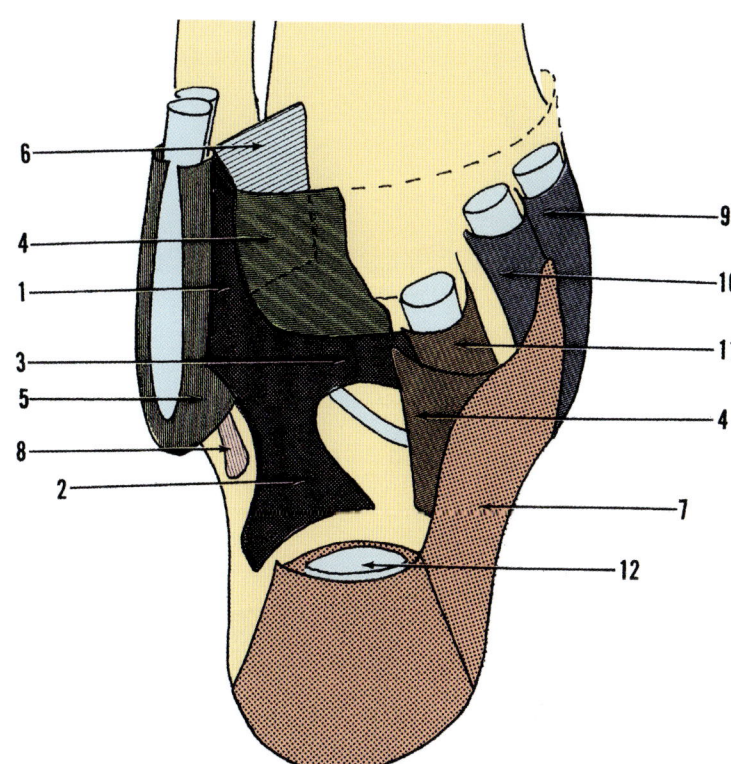

Figure 4.24 **Fibulotalocalcaneal ligament.** (*1*, Stem of fibulotalocalcaneal ligament of Rouvière and Canela Lazaro; *2*, calcaneal component, inferolateral, of *1*; *3*, talar component, superomedial of *1*; *4*, deep crural aponeurosis; *5*, retinaculum of peronei tendons; *6*, posterior tibiofibular ligament; *7*, superficial crural aponeurosis; *8*, calcaneal insertion of calcaneofibular ligament; *9*, tunnel of tibialis posterior tendon; *10*, tunnel of flexor digitorum longus; *11*, tunnel of flexor hallucis longus; *12*, Achilles tendon.)

from the underlying posterior deep tibiotalar ligament with adipose tissue (more so anteriorly) and is in continuity along its superolateral border with the posterior talotibial capsule and the posterior talofibular ligament. The occasional absence of this ligament or its fusion to the deep talotibial ligament accounts for some of the variations in description.

Deep Layer of Deltoid Ligament

The deep layer of the deltoid ligament (see Fig. 4.38) is short and strong. It is formed by a small anterior and a very strong posterior component.[9,16,18,19]

Deep Anterior Tibiotalar Ligament

The deep anterior tibiotalar ligament originates from the tip of the anterior colliculus and the anterior part of the intercollicular groove and inserts on the medial surface of the talus distal to the anterior segment of the comma-shaped talar articular surface. This ligament is "of variable size in different specimens, sometimes hardly discernible, and in some cases completely absent."[19]

Deep Posterior Tibiotalar Ligament

The deep posterior tibiotalar ligament is the strongest component of the entire medial ligament. In most cases, it is conical, with the base superior and the apex posteroinferior. The approximate measurements are 1.5 cm wide at origin, 1 cm wide at insertion, 1.5 cm long, and 1 cm thick at origin. The size of the ligament is variable. The thickness varies from 0.5 to 1.5 cm and the width from 1.5 to 2 cm.[2,20]

This ligament originates from the intermolecular fosse (which measures about 1 cm in width), the entire anterior surface of the posterior colliculus, and the upper segment of the posterior surface of the anterior colliculus. The fibers are directed downward, posteriorly, and laterally and insert on the medial surface of the talus on an oval elevation located under the tail of the comma-shaped articular surface. The insertion reaches the posteromedial talar tubercle. This intra-articular but extrasynovial ligament may be fasciculated (Fig. 4.39) or divided into two distinct bands.[18] Beau, in his comprehensive study of the ligaments of the ankle, considers this ligament as the homolog of the posterior talofibular ligament and describes it not as a medial ligament but as a posterior ligament of the ankle, bracing the talus posteriorly.[13]

Anterior Tibiotalar Fascicle, Capsule, and Fat Pad

The anterior capsule of the talotibial joint is thin and reinforced by an oblique fibrous band extending from the medial malleolus to the talar neck. This anterior tibiotalar fascicle (see Fig. 4.35) is narrow in the middle and broader at the origin and the insertion. The tibial attachment of the anterior capsule is 5 to 6 mm proximal to the articular margin (see Fig. 4.4). The talar insertion surrounds the cribriform fossa of the neck and is approximately 8 mm from the anterior trochlear margin. Laterally and medially, the anterior capsular insertion is close to the malleolar facets of the talus.

A prearticular fat pad is present anteriorly, extending transversely between the capsule and the tendons. This fat pad is thicker medially (see Fig. 4.27) and reinforces the anterior capsule.

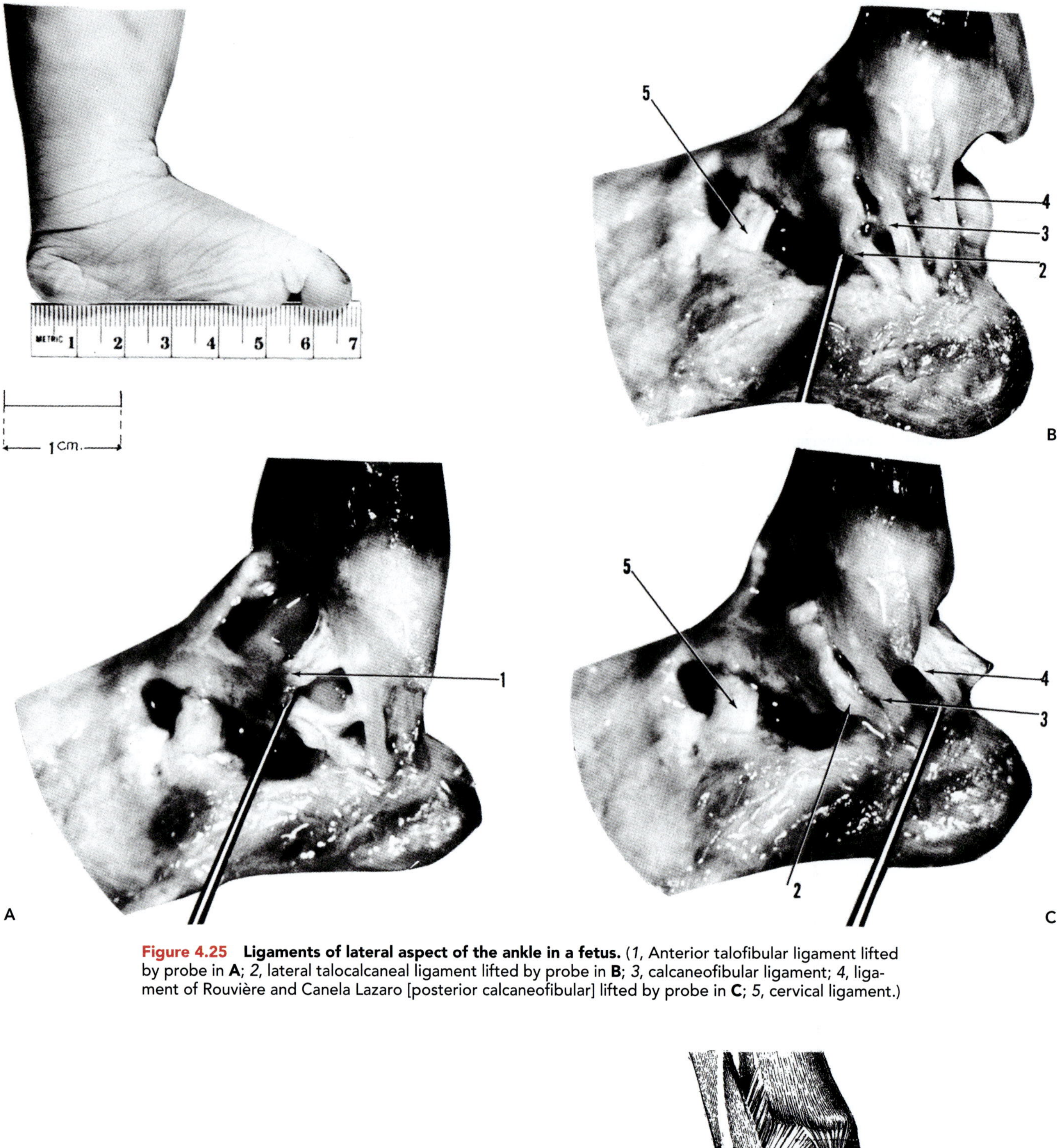

Figure 4.25 **Ligaments of lateral aspect of the ankle in a fetus.** (*1*, Anterior talofibular ligament lifted by probe in **A**; *2*, lateral talocalcaneal ligament lifted by probe in **B**; *3*, calcaneofibular ligament; *4*, ligament of Rouvière and Canela Lazaro [posterior calcaneofibular] lifted by probe in **C**; *5*, cervical ligament.)

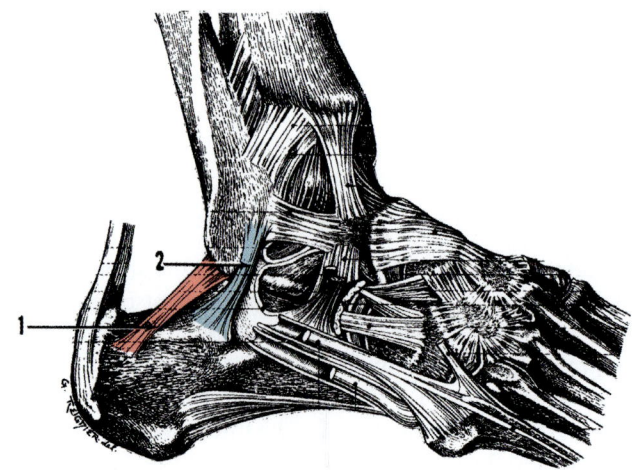

Figure 4.26 **Posterior fibulocalcaneal ligament.** (*1*, Posterior fibulocalcaneal ligament or ligament of Bessel-Hagen; *2*, fibulocalcaneal ligament.) (Dujarier CH. *Anatomie des Membres: Dissection—Anatomie Topographique.* 2nd ed. Masson; 1924:399.)

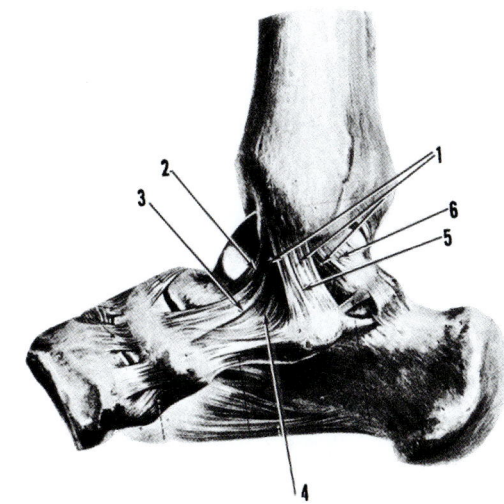

Figure 4.27 **(A) Medial or deltoid ligament.** (*1*, Deltoid ligament; *2*, anterior tibiotalar fascicle; *3*, tibionavicular fascicle; *4*, tibioligamentous fascicle [insertion on superomedial calcaneonavicular ligament]; *5*, tibiocalcaneal fascicle; *6*, posterior tibiotalar fascicle.) **(B) Interpretations of the deltoid ligament.** *Cloquet 1822:* Origin, apex of medial malleolus and its depression; insertion, medial aspect of talus (*2*), calcaneus (*1*); few fibers to fibrous tunnel of flexor digitorum longus. *Cruveilhier 1834:* (a) Superficial. Origin, apex and borders of medial malleolus; insertion, talus neck (*1*), scaphoid (*2*), inferior calcaneoscaphoid ligament (*2*), calcaneus (*3*). (b) Deep. Origin, apex and borders of medial malleolus; insertion, entire medial aspect talus under articular cartilage. *Sappey 1888:* (a) Superficial. Anterior: origin, anterior border of medial malleolus; insertion, scaphoid (*1*), inferior calcaneoscaphoid ligament (*1*). Posterior: origin, apex of medial malleolus; insertion, sustentaculum tali (*2*), tubercle of posterior aspect of talus (*3*) medial to tunnel of flexor hallucis longus. (a) Deep. (*4*) Origin, fossa occupying apex of medial malleolus; insertion, imprint on posterior extremity of medial talar surface.

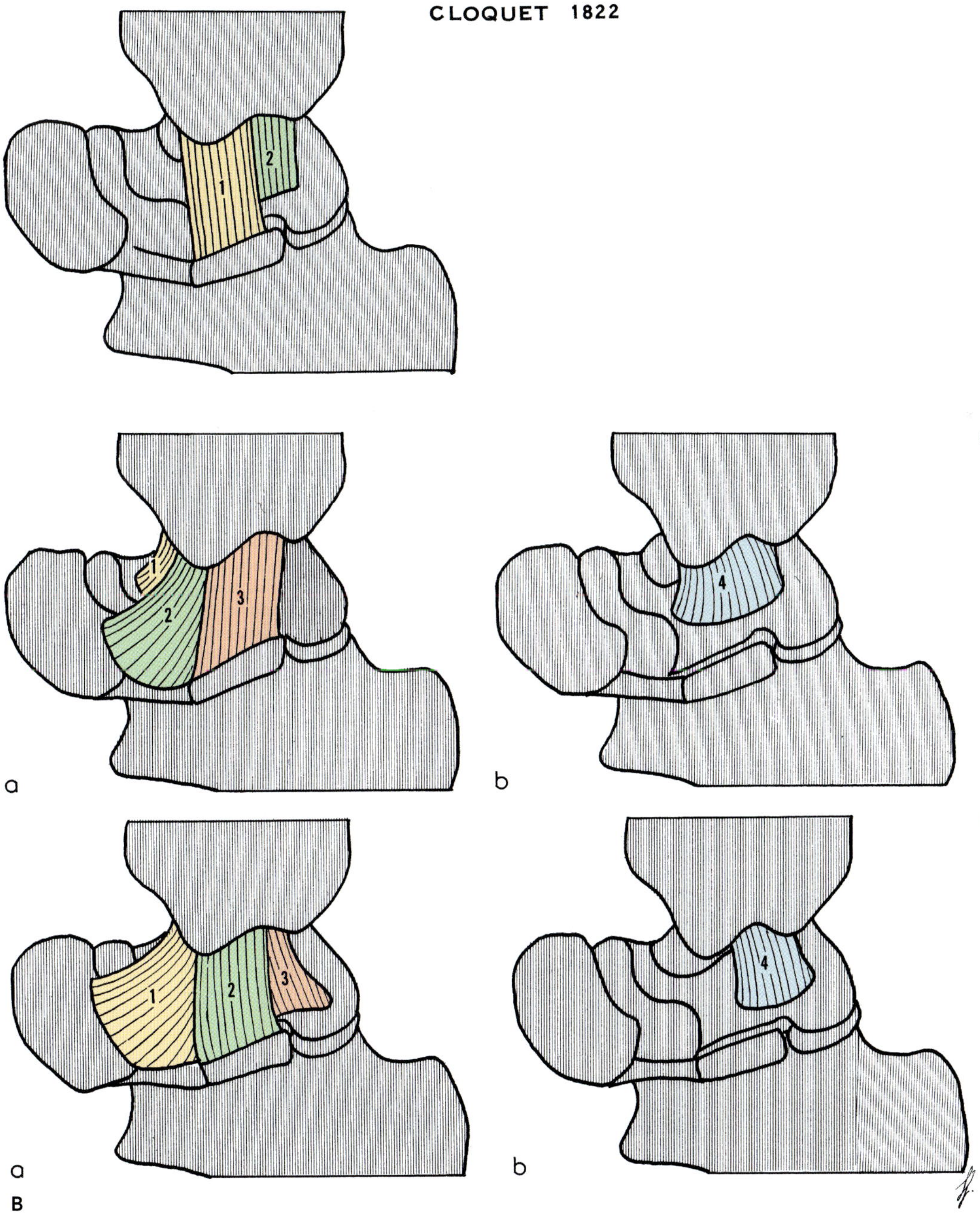

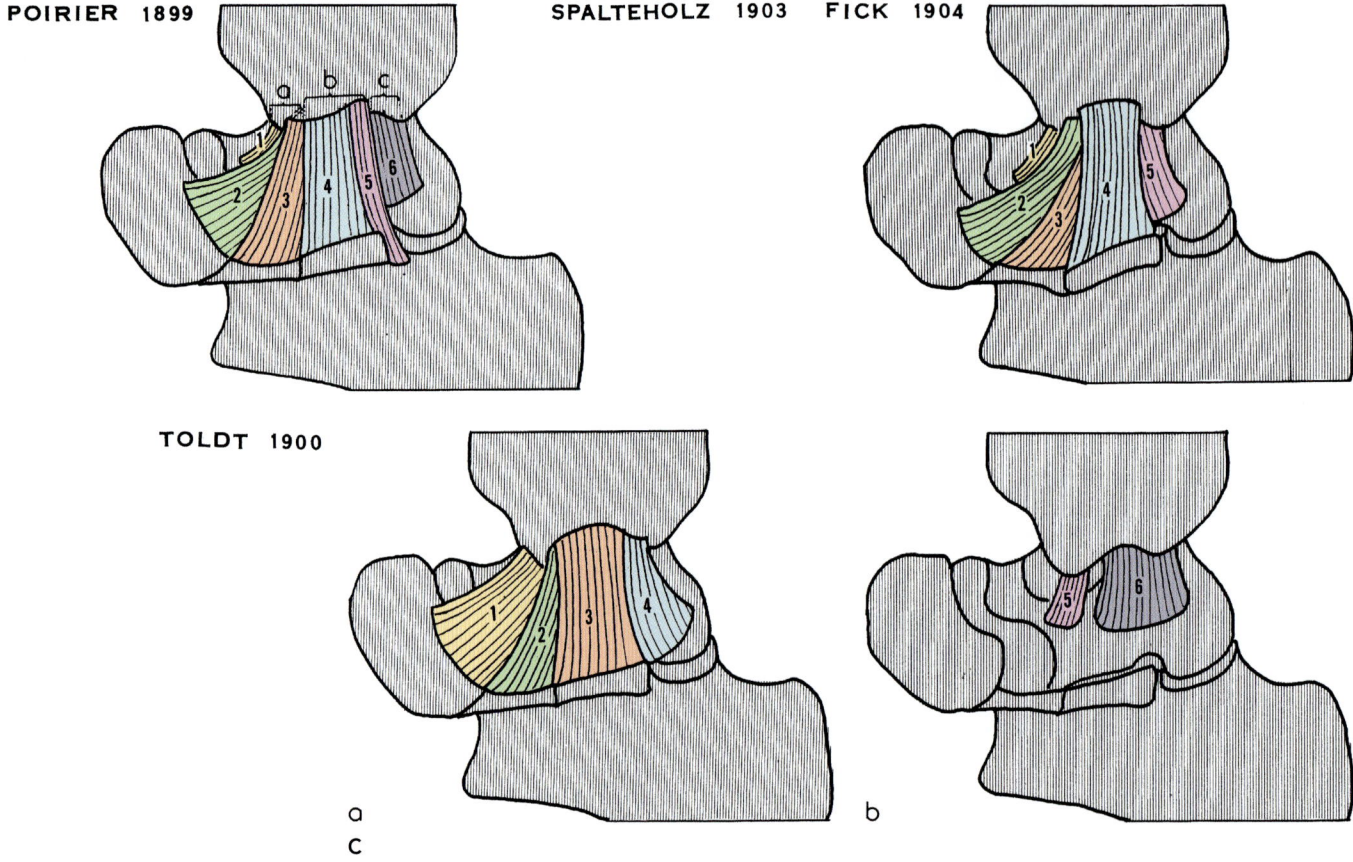

Figure 4.27 Cont'd **(C) Interpretations of the deltoid ligaments.** *Poirier 1899:* (a) Anterior fascicle or anterior tibiotalar. Origin, anterior border of medial malleolus; insertion, superficial fibers to superior surface of scaphoid (2), deep fibers to medial surface of talar neck (1), and on inferior calcaneonavicular ligament (3). (b) Middle fascicle or tibiocalcaneal. Origin, cutaneous surface of medial malleolus near its apex; insertion, middle fibers to sustentaculum tali (4), anterior fibers on inferior calcaneonavicular ligament (3), posterior fibers on calcaneal canal behind sustentaculum tali (5). (c) Posterior fascicle or posterior tibiotalar. Origin, at bifurcation of apex of medial malleolus; insertion, medial surface talus under tibial facet (6). *Toldt 1900:* (a) Superficial: Tibionavicular ligament: origin, anterior border of medial malleolus; insertion, navicular and dorsal calcaneonavicular ligament (1); calcaneotibial ligament: origin medial subcutaneous surface of medial malleolus; insertion, inferior calcaneonavicular ligament (2), sustentaculum tali (3), medial tubercle of talus (4). (b) Deep: Anterior talotibial ligament; origin, apex of medial malleolus; insertion, medial aspect of neck of talus under large segment of articular surface (5). Posterior talotibial ligament: origin, posterior border and fossa of medial malleolus; insertion, medial surface of talus, mid and posterior segment (6). *Spalteholz 1903/Fick 1904:* Several layers divisible according to the lower attachment. Anterior talotibial ligament: origin, tip of medial malleolus; insertion, below anterior portion of medial articular surface of talus (1). Most of ligament is hidden under tibionavicular and calcaneotibial ligaments. Tibionavicular ligament: origin, medial surface of medial malleolus just above origin of anterior talotibial ligament; insertion, dorsal and medial aspect of navicular (2), and medial margin of plantar calcaneonavicular ligament (3). At origin, ligament is partially hidden beneath calcaneotibial ligament. Calcaneotibial ligament (most superficial component): origin, medial surface of medial malleolus; insertion, sustentaculum tali (4). Posterior talotibial ligament: origin, behind tip of medial malleolus; insertion, on medial aspect of talus, mid and posterior segments reaching the posteromedial tubercle of talus (5).

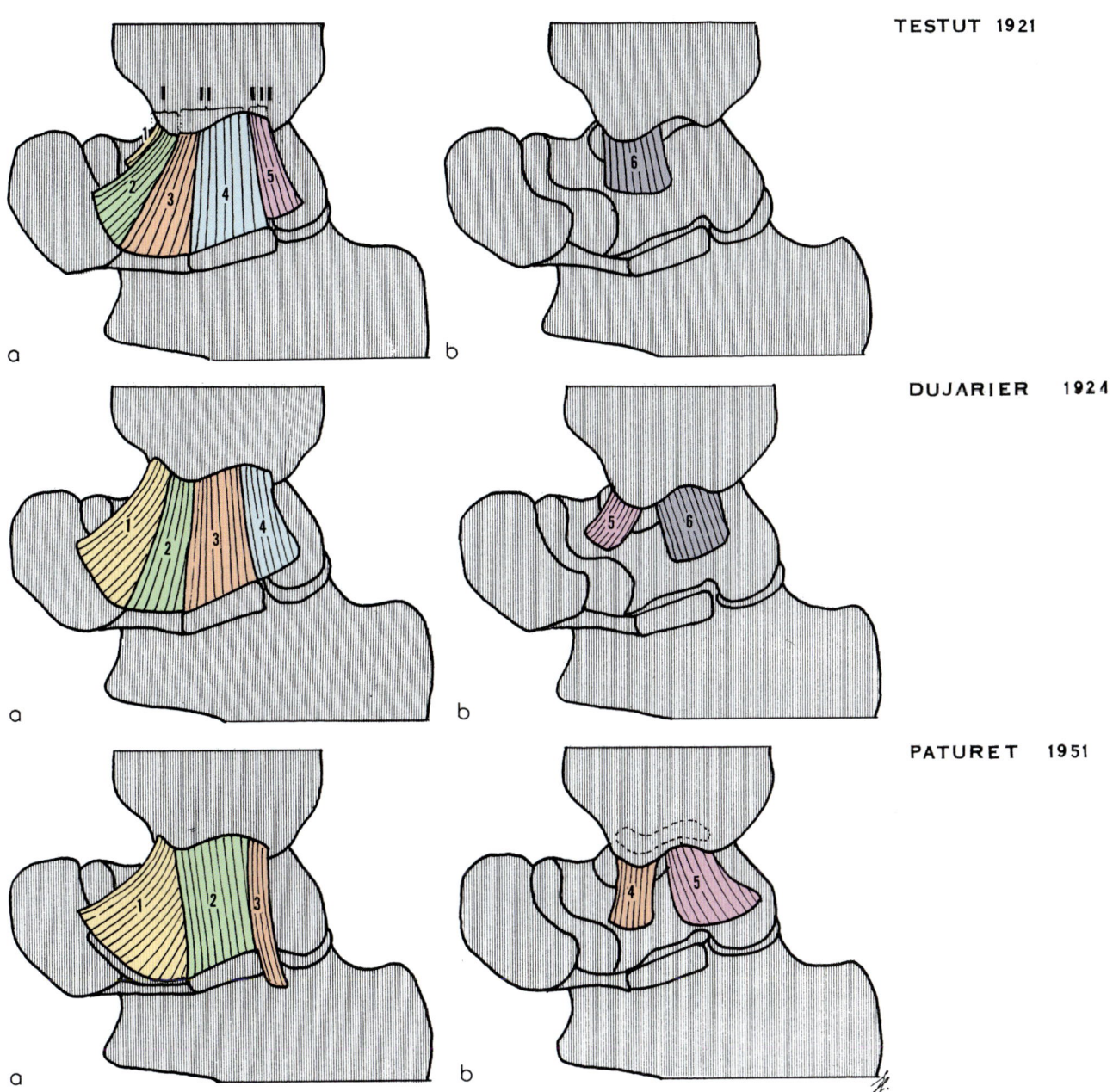

Figure 4.27 Cont'd **(D) Interpretations of the deltoid ligament.** *Testut 1921: (a)* Superficial: Origin, from inferior border and fossa of medial malleolus; insertion, *I*, anterior fibers; talar neck (*1*), superior surface of scaphoid (*2*). *II*, Middle fibers: inferior calcaneonavicular ligament (*3*), sustentaculum tali (*4*). *III*, Posterior fibers: posteromedial talar tubercle (*5*). *(b)* Deep: Origin, apex of medial malleolus; insertion, medial surface of talus below articular surface. *Dujarier 1924: (a)* Superficial: Origin, anterior and medial surfaces of medial malleolus; insertion, anterior fibers, navicular (*1*); middle fibers, inferior calcaneonavicular ligament (*2*), sustentaculum tali (*3*); posterior fibers, occasionally present and inserting on posteromedial tubercle of talus (*4*); *(b)* Deep: Anterior tibiotalar ligament (very thin, capsular): origin, anterior border and apex of medial malleolus; insertion, talar neck (*5*). Posterior tibiotalar ligament: origin, apex and sulcus of medial malleolus; insertion, round facet below and posterior to medial articular surface of talus (*6*). *Paturet 1951: (a)* Superficial: Origin, anterior border and medial surface of medial malleolus; insertion, anterior fibers, superior and medial surface navicular (*1*), medial surface of neck of talus, superior talonavicular ligament (*1*); middle fibers, inferior calcaneonavicular ligament, sustentaculum tali (*2*); posterior fibers (less numerous), medial surface of calcaneus, posterior to sustentaculum tali, reaching upper part of calcaneal canal (*3*). *(b)* Deep: Origin, apex and posterior part of medial malleolus; insertion, anterior fibers, medial surface of talus below comma-shaped articular surface (*4*); posterior fibers, on posteromedial tubercle, reaching tunnel of flexor hallucis longus (*5*).

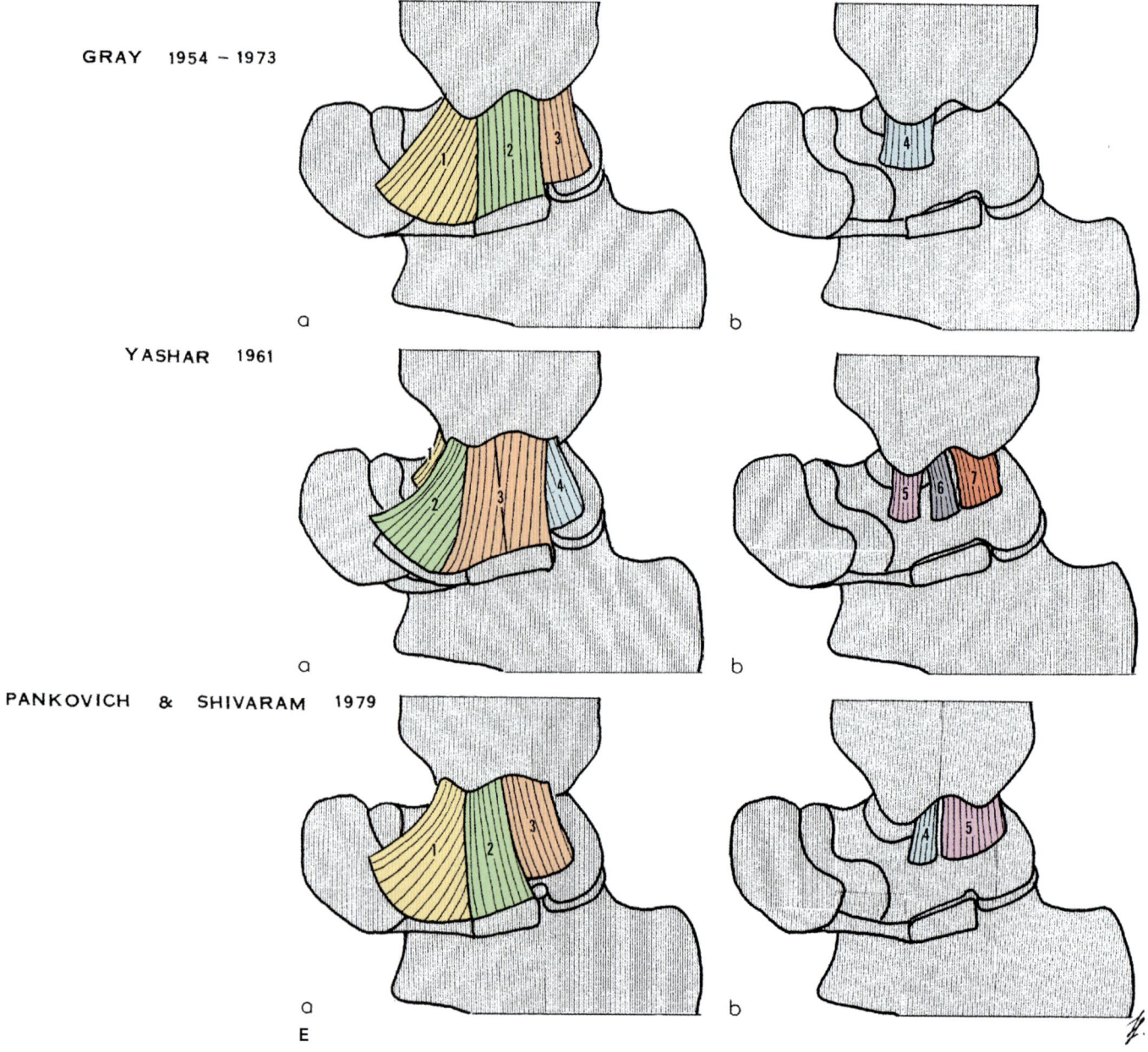

Figure 4.27 Cont'd **(E) Interpretations of the deltoid ligament.** *Gray 1954 to 1973:* (a) Superficial: Origin, apex. anterior and posterior borders of medial malleolus; insertion, tibionavicular, on navicular and plantar calcaneonavicular ligament (*1*); calcaneotibial, on sustentaculum (*2*); posterior talotibial, medial surface of talus and posterior medial tubercle (*3*). (b) Deep (anterior talotibial): Origin, tip of medial malleolus; insertion, medial surface of talus (*4*). *Yashar 1961:* (a) Superficial: Anterior and superficial tibiotalar fascicle (*1*): origin, anterior border of medial malleolus; insertion, inner surface of talar neck; tibioscaphoid fascicle, (*2*): origin, anterior border of medial malleolus; insertion, scaphoid superior surface and medial calcaneoscaphoid ligament; tibioligamentous ligament: origin, medial malleolus above apex; insertion, medial calcaneoscaphoid ligament and sustentaculum tali (*3*); tibiocalcaneal: origin, medial surface of medial malleolus; insertion, posterior segment of sustentaculum tali (*3*); posterior and superficial talotibial ligament: origin, medial surface of medial malleolus; insertion, medial aspect of talus, posteromedial talar tubercle (*4*). (b) Deep: Deep anterior tibiotalar ligament: origin, apex of medial malleolus; insertion, medial surface of talus (*5*); deep posterior tibiotalar ligament: origin (two portions): posterior border of anterior colliculus, intercollicular groove, posterior colliculus; insertion, medial surface of talus, posterior segment (*6* and *7*). *Pankovich and Shivaram 1979:* (a) Superficial: Tibionavicular: origin, anterior colliculus; insertion, dorsomedial aspect of navicular and plantar calcaneonavicular ligament (*1*); tibiocalcaneal ligament: origin, midportion of medial surface of anterior colliculus; insertion, medial border of sustentaculum tali (*2*); superficial talotibial ligament; origin, posterior part of medial surface of anterior colliculus and adjacent part of posterior colliculus; insertion, anterior portion of medial talar tubercle (*3*). (b) Deep: Deep anterior talotibial ligament: origin, intercollicular groove and adjoining anterior colliculus; insertion, medial surface of talus near its neck (*4*); deep posterior talotibial ligament: origin, intercollicular groove and inferior segment of posterior colliculus; insertion, medial surface of talus from medial tubercle to posterior third of articular surface of talar trochlea (*5*). (**A**, From Spalteholz W. *Hand Atlas of Human Anatomy.* Vol 1. B Lippincott; 1903:219.)

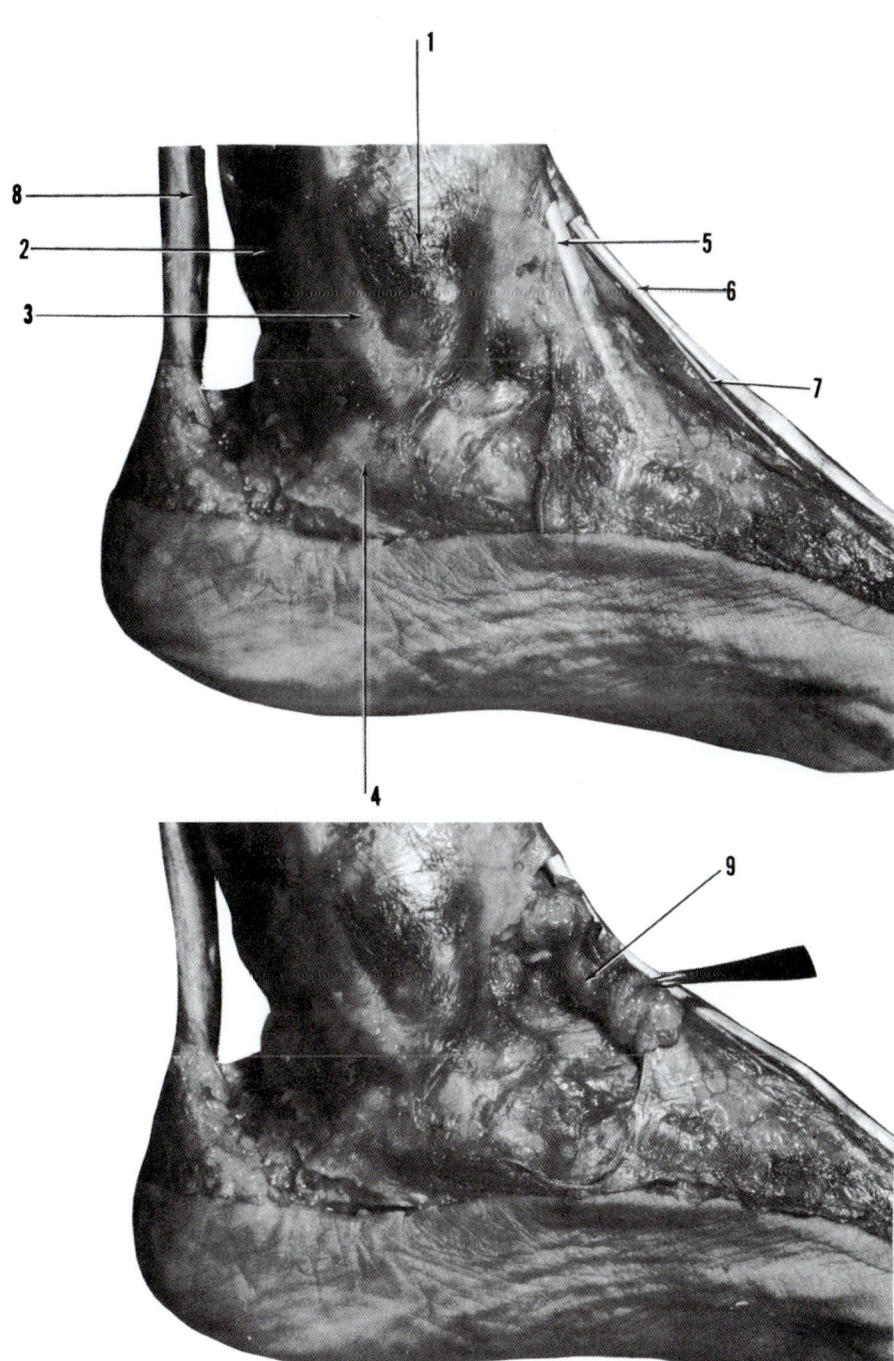

Figure 4.28 Medial aspect of ankle. (*1*, Medial malleolus covered by superficial aponeurosis cruris and flexor retinaculum; *2*, deep aponeurosis cruris covering the fibrous tunnel of the tibialis posterior tendon [*3*]; *4*, flexor retinaculum; *5*, tibialis anterior tendon; *6*, extensor hallucis longus tendon; *7*, accessory band of [*6*]; *8*, Achilles tendon; *9*, retrotibialis anterior tendon fat pad being reflected.)

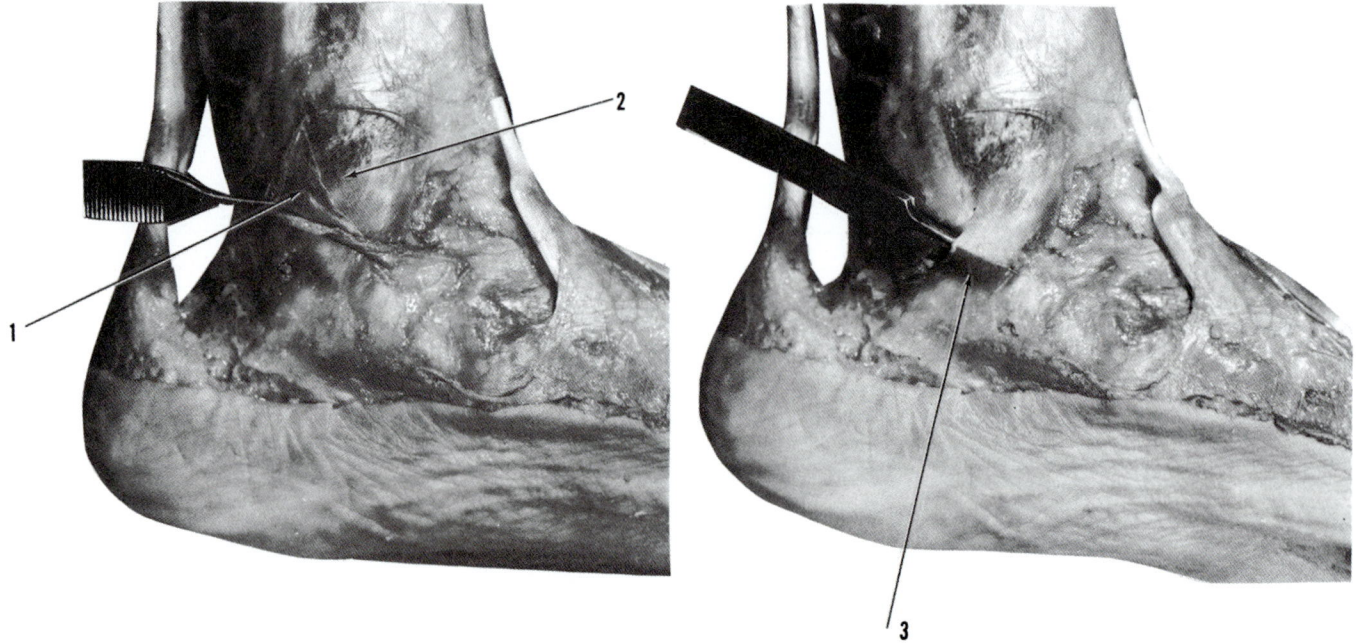

Figure 4.29 Medial aspect of ankle. (*1*, Reflected superficial aponeurosis cruris; *2*, medial aponeurosis and origin of flexor retinaculum; *3*, flexor retinaculum lifted with tissue forceps.)

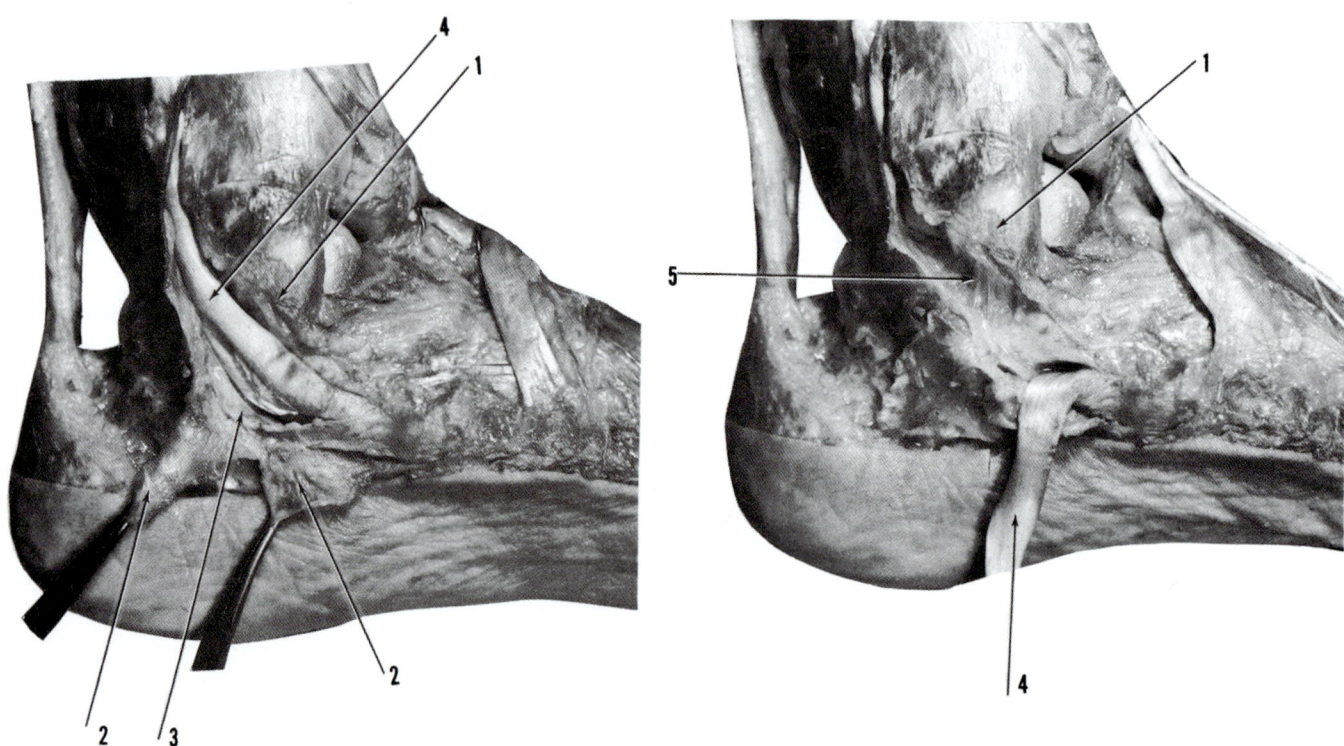

Figure 4.30 Medial aspect of ankle. (*1*, Deltoid ligament, superficial component; *2*, reflected flexor retinaculum; *3*, slit fibrous sheath of flexor digitorum longus tendon; *4*, tibialis posterior tendon; *5*, fibrocartilaginous bed of tibialis posterior tendon.)

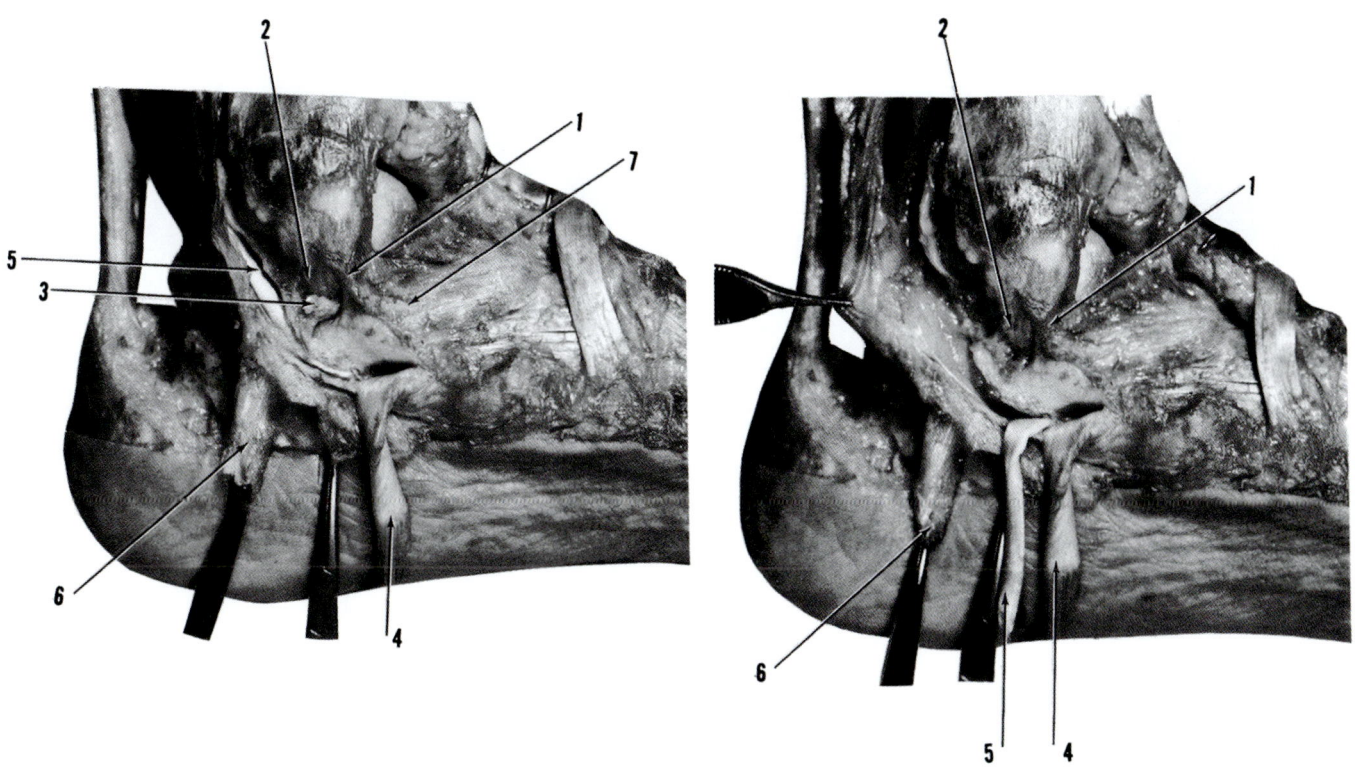

Figure 4.31 Medial aspect of ankle. (*1*, Deltoid ligament, talonavicular and taloligamentous component; *2*, deltoid ligament, talocalcaneal ligament separation from *1* with fat pad [*3*]; *4*, tibialis posterior tendon; *5*, flexor digitorum longus tendon; *6*, reflected flexor retinaculum; *7*, superomedial calcaneonavicular ligament.)

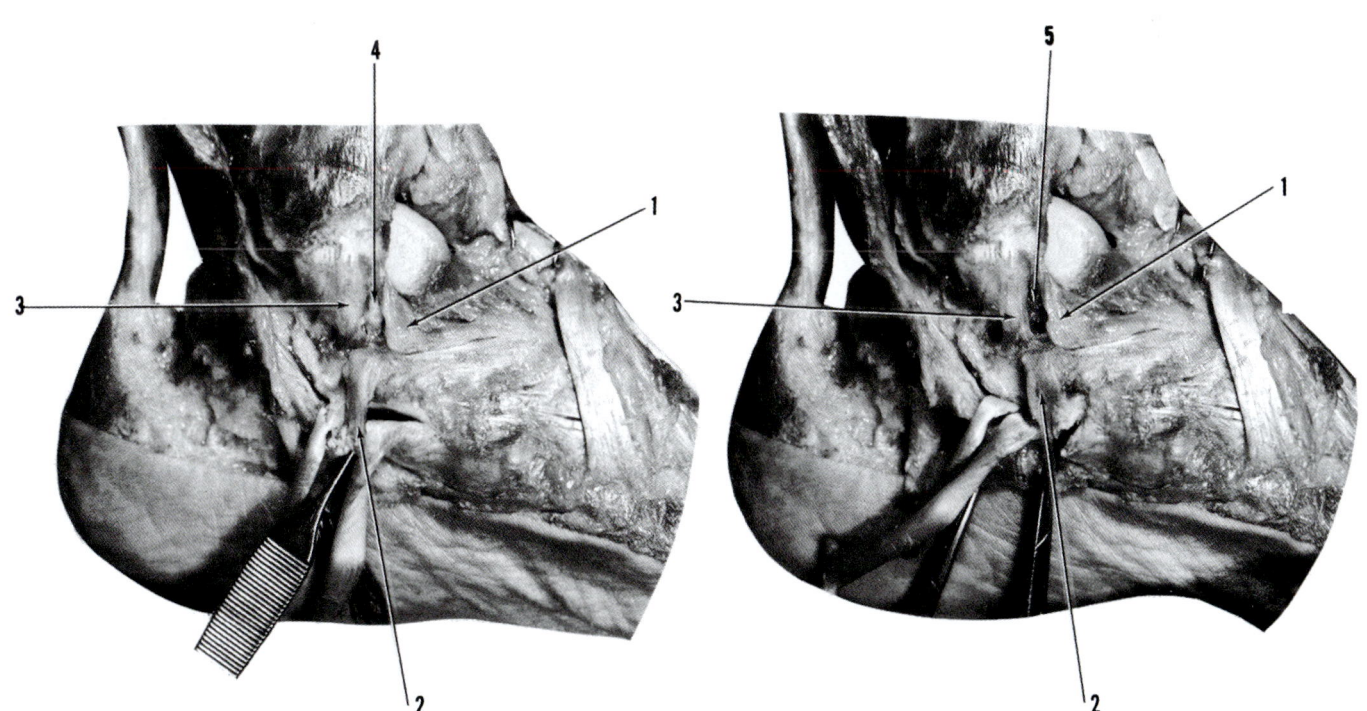

Figure 4.32 Medial aspect of ankle. (*1*, Deltoid ligament, tibionavicular component; *2*, deltoid ligament, tibioligamentous component, reflected; *3*, deltoid ligament, tibiocalcaneal component; *4*, interfascicular fat pad, *5*, interval occupied by *4*.)

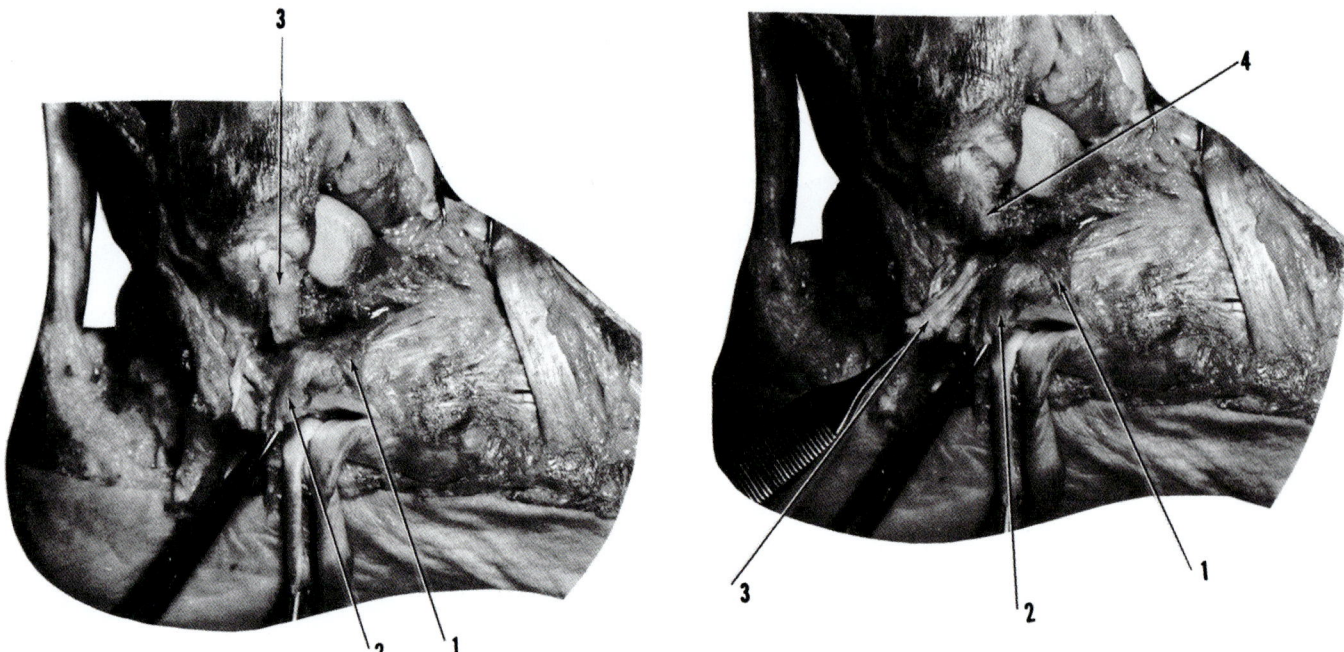

Figure 4.33 Medial aspect of ankle. (*1*, Deltoid ligament, talonavicular component, reflected; *2*, deltoid ligament, taloligamentous component reflected; *3*, deltoid ligament, talocalcaneal ligament; *4*, deltoid ligament, deep talotibial component.)

Milner and Soames,[7] based on the dissection of 40 ankles, describe six components to the medial collateral ligament complex: four superficial bands and two deep bands. The four superficial components are the tibiospring ligament (TSL), the tibionavicular ligament (TNL), the superficial posterior tibiotalar ligament (STTL), and the tibiocalcaneal ligament (TCL). The two deep components are the deep posterior tibiotalar ligament (PTTL) and the deep anterior tibiotalar ligament (ATTL). Only three ligaments are constant: PTTL, TSL, and TNL. In 52.5% (21 specimens), there was one additional band present; in 42.5% (17 specimens), there were no additional bands present; and, in 5% (two specimens), two additional bands were present.

LIGAMENTS OF THE CALCANEONAVICULAR JOINT AND ACETABULUM PEDIS

The head of the talus is received into a deep socket or acetabulum pedis formed by the navicular, the anterior and middle calcaneal articulating surfaces, the calcaneonavicular component of the bifurcate ligament, the superomedial calcaneonavicular ligament, and the plantar calcaneonavicular ligament (Figs. 4.40 and 4.41). The flexibility of the acetabulum pedis permits the adaptability in form and size of the containing socket as necessitated by the relative displacements of the talar head calcaneus and navicular.

▶ Superomedial Calcaneonavicular Ligament

The superomedial calcaneonavicular ligament (ligamentum neglectum; Fig. 4.42) is illustrated by Bourgery and Jacob, analyzed and illustrated as a component of a common tibiocalcaneonavicular ligament by Henle, and described as an individual ligament by Lane.[21-23] A comprehensive study of the superomedial calcaneonavicular ligament was provided by Barclay-Smith and a recent investigation is reported by Volkmann.[14,24]

The superomedial calcaneonavicular ligament is quadrilateral, inseparable from the inferior calcaneonavicular ligament. It originates from the medial and anterior borders of the sustentaculum tali. This band is directed upward, anteriorly, and laterally; twists upon itself; winds around the medial segment of the talar head; and inserts on the superomedial aspect of the navicular and, to a lesser degree, on the lateral aspect of the tuberosity of the navicular. The tibionavicular, tibioligamentous, and tibiocalcaneal components of the superficial deltoid ligament interlace with it. The segment of the ligament that does not connect with the deltoid ligament blends with the superior talonavicular ligament. The superficial aspect of the ligament is further hidden by a thick fascial or fibrocartilaginous layer forming the floor of the tunnel of the crossing tibialis posterior tendon. As mentioned by Barclay-Smith, "it requires great care to dissect away this fascial stratum, and to remove the deposited cartilage, in order to expose the proper calcaneonavicular fibers."[14]

The articular surface of this thick ligament is smooth and fibrocartilaginous, giving support to the medial aspect of the talar head, not to the inferior.

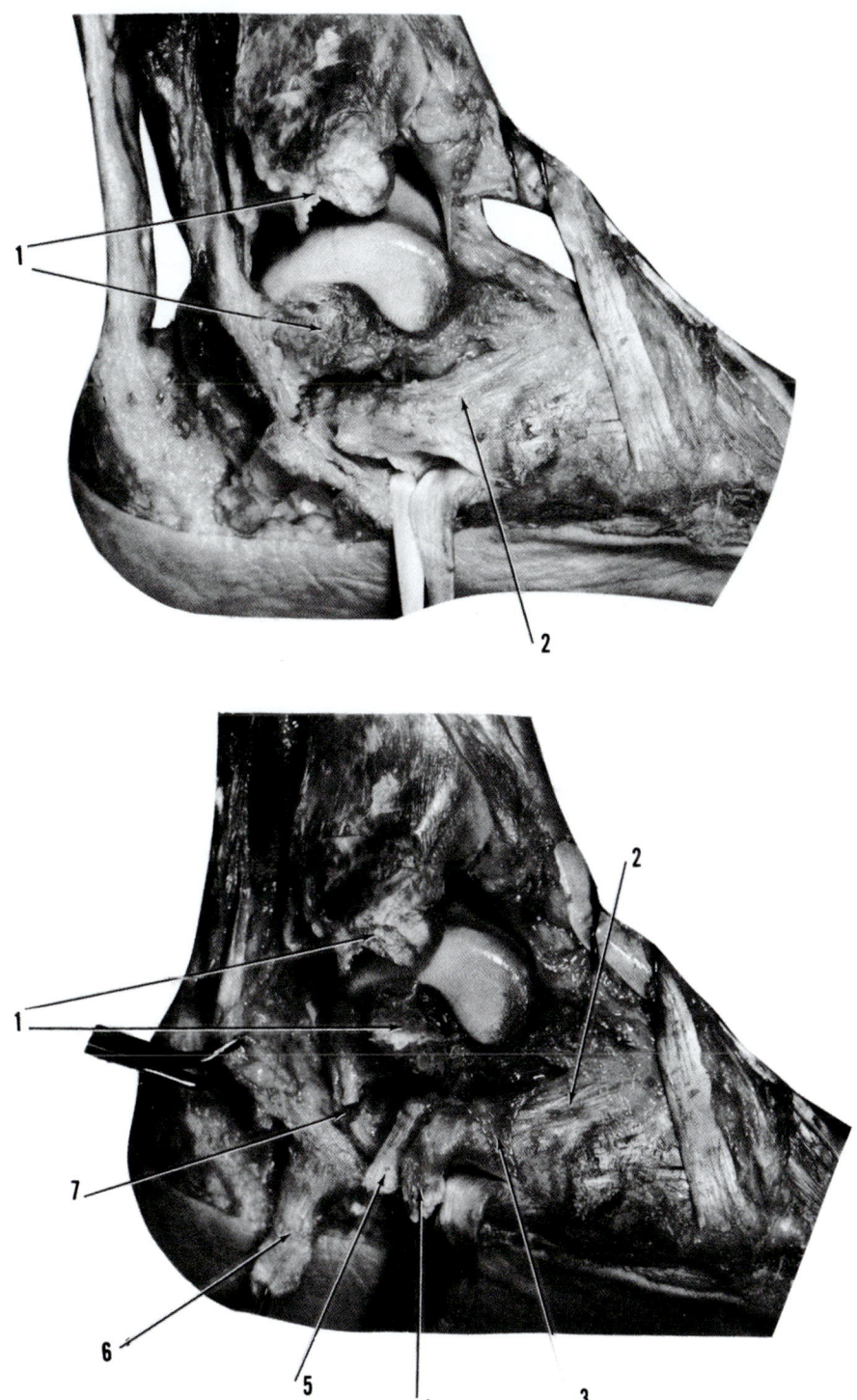

Figure 4.34 Medial aspect of ankle. (*1*, Origin and insertion areas of deep deltoid ligament; *2*, superomedial calcaneonavicular ligament; *3*, anterior border of sustentaculum tali; *4*, deltoid ligament, reflected tibioligamentous component; *5*, deltoid ligament, reflected tibiocalcaneal component; *6*, reflected flexor retinaculum; *7*, transected medial talocalcaneal ligament.)

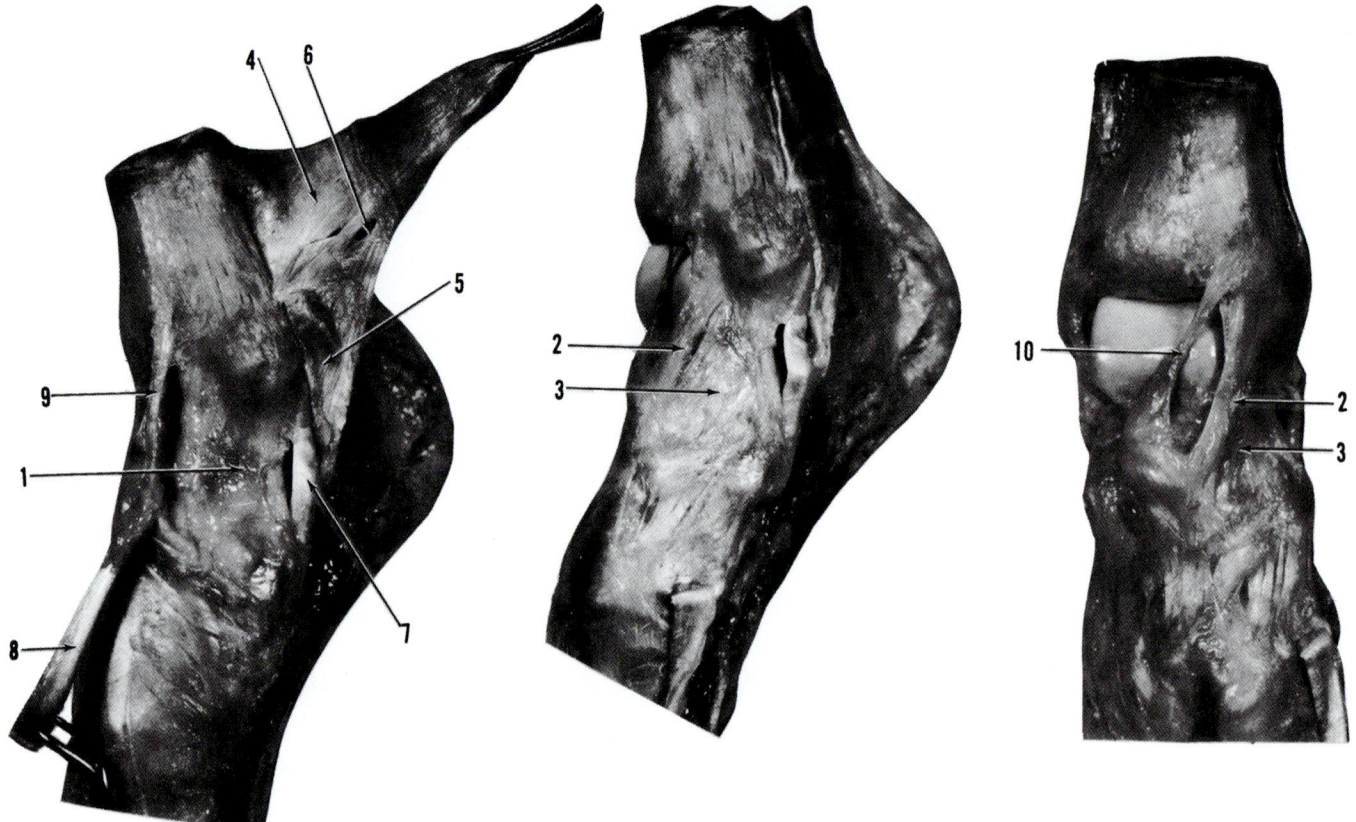

Figure 4.35 Medial aspect of ankle. (*1*, Deltoid ligament, superficial tibionavicular component covered by adipose tissue; *2*, deltoid ligament, superficial tibiotalar component; *3*, deltoid ligament, superficial tibionavicular ligament; *4*, superior extensor retinaculum; *5*, flexor retinaculum in continuity with 4; *6*, tunnel of tibialis anterior tendon; *7*, tibialis posterior tendon; *8*, reflected tibialis anterior tendon; *9*, deep attachment of oblique superomedial band of inferior extensor retinaculum; *10*, anterior talotibial ligament.)

▶ Inferior Calcaneonavicular Ligament

The inferior calcaneonavicular ligament (spring ligament; Figs. 4.42 and 4.43) is trapezoidal and fasciculated and corresponds to the inferior segment of the talar head unsupported by the articular surfaces. It originates from the upper part of a small excavation, the coronoid cavity, located on the inferior surface of the calcaneus between the anterior border of the sustentaculum tali and the cuboidal articular surface. The thick bundle of fibers extends forward, fans out, and inserts on the inferior surface of the navicular. This ligament is very fasciculated and the lateral bundle, the strongest, inserts on the beak of the navicular. Longitudinal intervals are set between the bundles and occasionally the ligament clearly has two components. A thick layer of adipose tissue covers the plantar aspect of the ligament and the fat extends through the longitudinal interligamentous intervals into the joint cavity and is covered by synovial tissue. The medial border of the ligament is in continuity with the superomedial calcaneonavicular ligament. Taniguchi et al,[25] based on the dissection of 48 feet, identified a specific calcaneonavicular on the plantar aspect in all of their specimens, named the third ligament. This ligamentous band originates from the notch between the calcaneal facets and inserts on the tuberosity of the navicular (Fig. 4.44).

▶ Lateral Calcaneonavicular Ligament and Bifurcate Ligament

The bifurcate ligament (ligament of Chopart; Fig. 4.45) is formed by the lateral calcaneonavicular ligament and the medial calcaneocuboid ligament. This ligament is disposed in a V and each component has a distinct origin on the os calcis.

The lateral calcaneonavicular ligament originates from the anteromedial corner of the sinus tarsi, immediately lateral to the facies articularis talaris anterior, and reaches the lateral aspect of a small tubercle (the intermediary tubercle).[26] The surface of origin measures approximately 1 cm.[26] The ligament extends anteriorly upward and medially and inserts on the posterosuperior segment of the lateral end of the navicular. The ligament measures an average of 2 to 2.5 cm in length and 1 cm in width.[27] Barclay-Smith considers two sets of fibers forming this ligament.[14] The inferior fibers are very short, fasciculated, and separated from the most lateral band of the inferior calcaneonavicular ligament by an interval filled with fat. The upper and the more superficial fibers are longer, stronger, and usually not fasciculated; they represent the main component of the ligament.

The medial calcaneocuboid ligament originates from the anterior aspect of the intermediary tubercle, lateral to the origin of the lateral calcaneonavicular ligament. It is directed

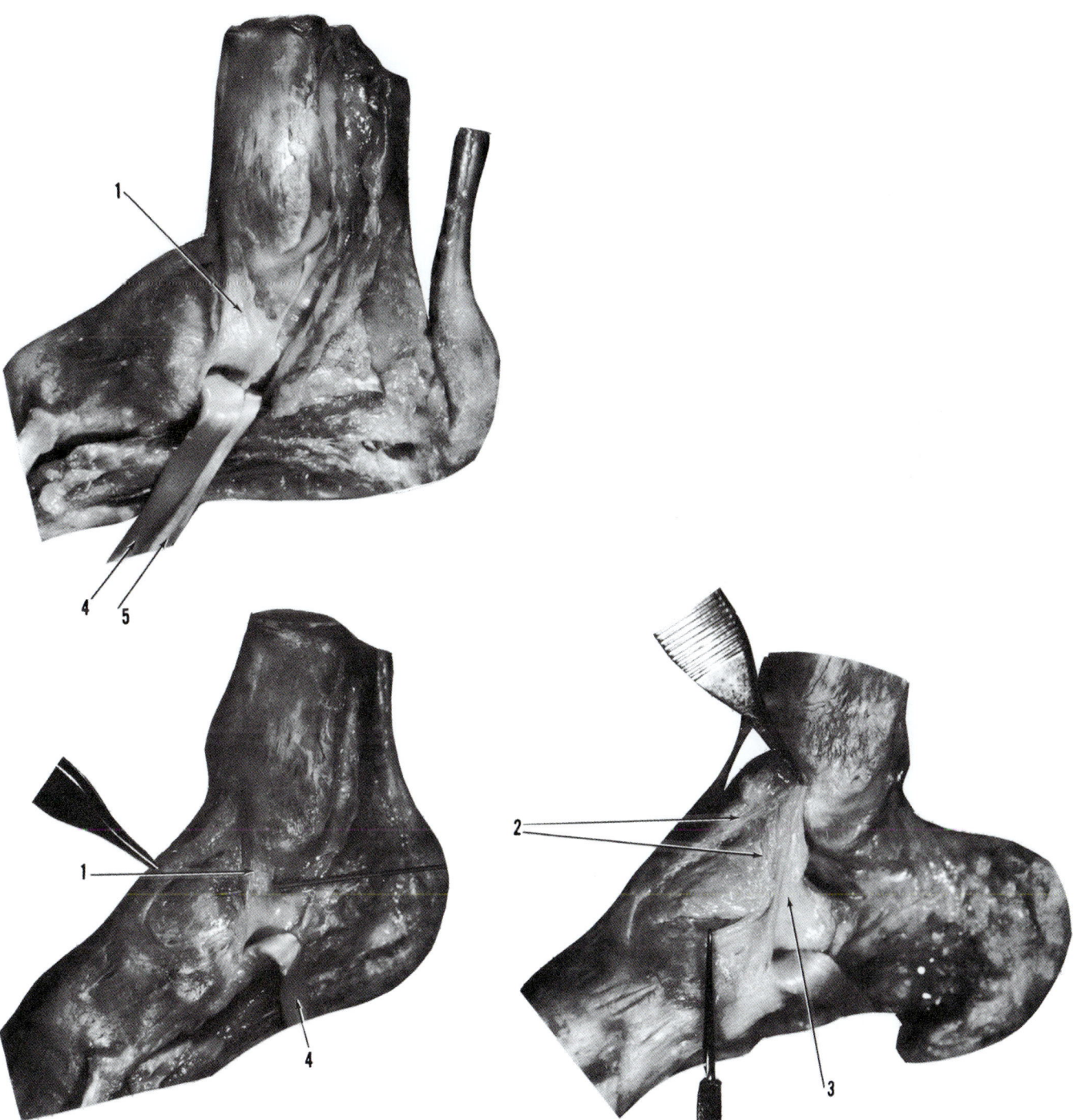

Figure 4.36 Medial aspect of ankle. (*1*, Deltoid ligament, tibioligamentous component; *2*, deltoid ligament, tibionavicular and superficial tibiotalar components; *3*, superomedial calcaneonavicular ligament covered by fibrocartilage; *4*, reflected tibialis posterior tendon; *5*, reflected flexor digitorum longus tendon.)

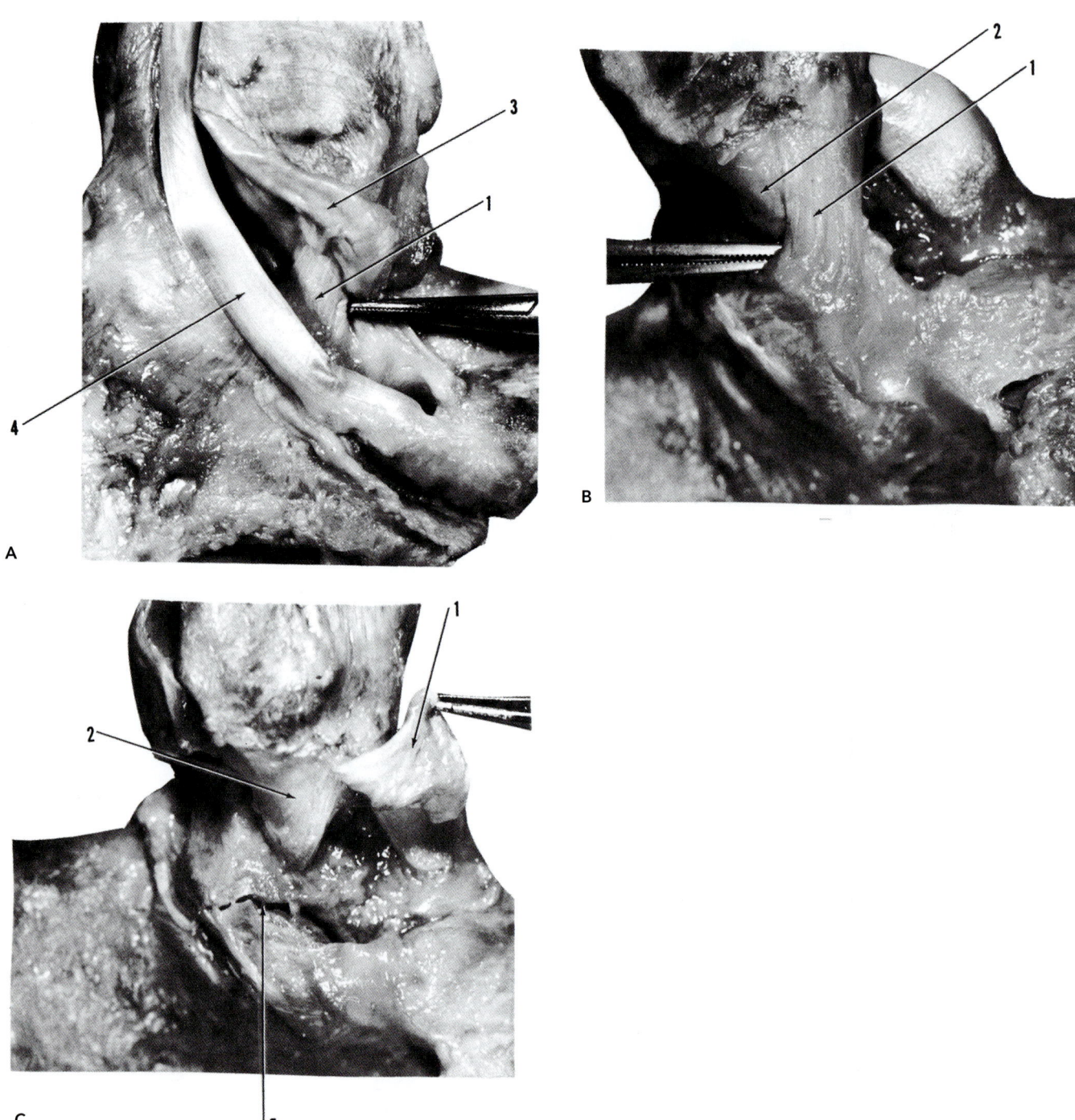

Figure 4.37 **Medial aspect of ankle. (A)** Deltoid ligament, tibiocalcaneal component (1), crossed by tibialis posterior tendon (4), exposed by reflecting its sheath and the aponeurosis cruris, superficial and deep, forming the flexor retinaculum (3). **(B)** Deltoid ligament, tibiocalcaneal component (1), covering deep tibiotalar component (2). **(C)** Reflected talocalcaneal component (1) of deltoid ligament exposing deep tibiotalar component (2) of deltoid ligament. (5, medial and posterior talocalcaneal articular interline.)

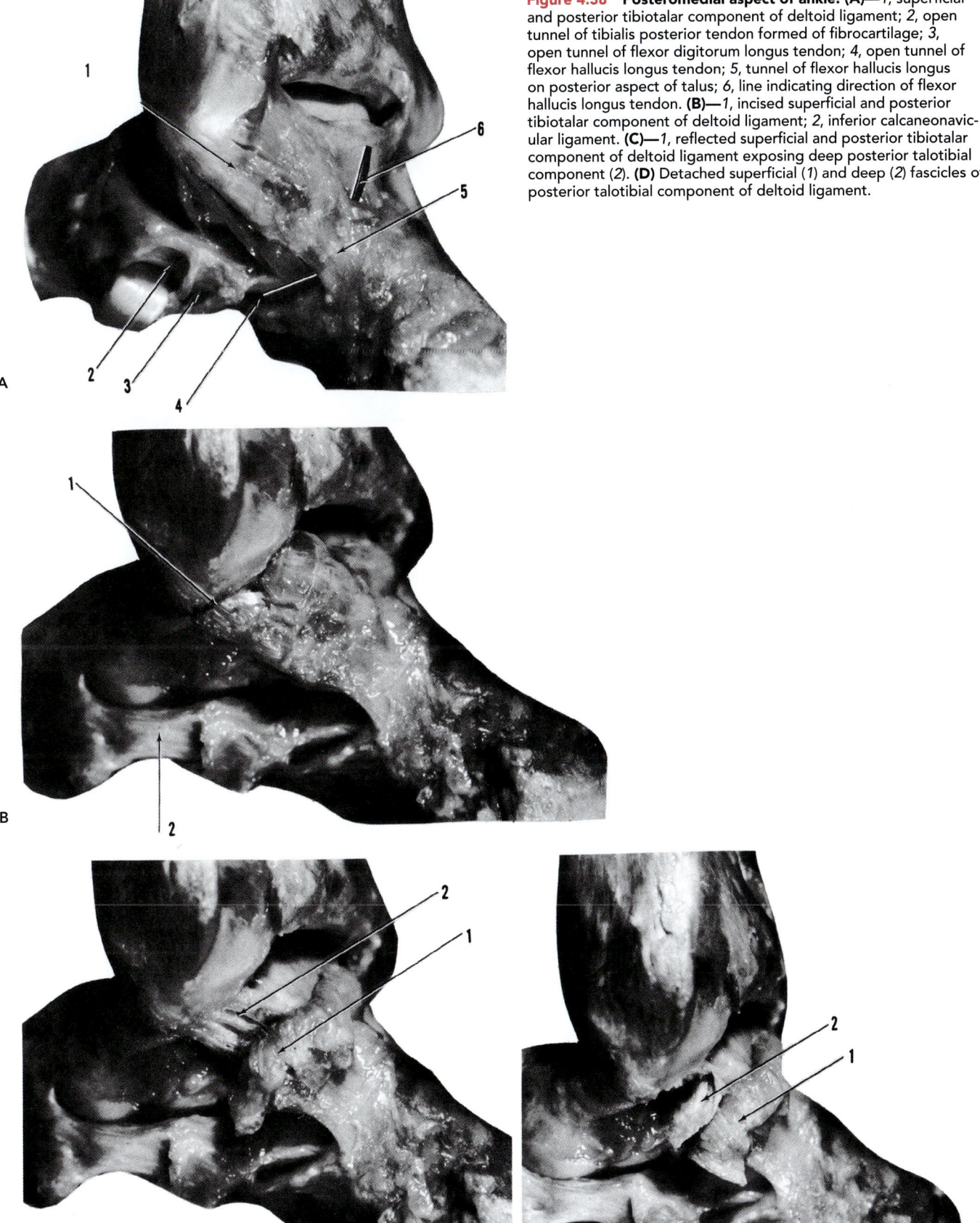

Figure 4.38 **Posteromedial aspect of ankle. (A)**—*1*, superficial and posterior tibiotalar component of deltoid ligament; *2*, open tunnel of tibialis posterior tendon formed of fibrocartilage; *3*, open tunnel of flexor digitorum longus tendon; *4*, open tunnel of flexor hallucis longus tendon; *5*, tunnel of flexor hallucis longus on posterior aspect of talus; *6*, line indicating direction of flexor hallucis longus tendon. **(B)**—*1*, incised superficial and posterior tibiotalar component of deltoid ligament; *2*, inferior calcaneonavicular ligament. **(C)**—*1*, reflected superficial and posterior tibiotalar component of deltoid ligament exposing deep posterior talotibial component (*2*). **(D)** Detached superficial (*1*) and deep (*2*) fascicles of posterior talotibial component of deltoid ligament.

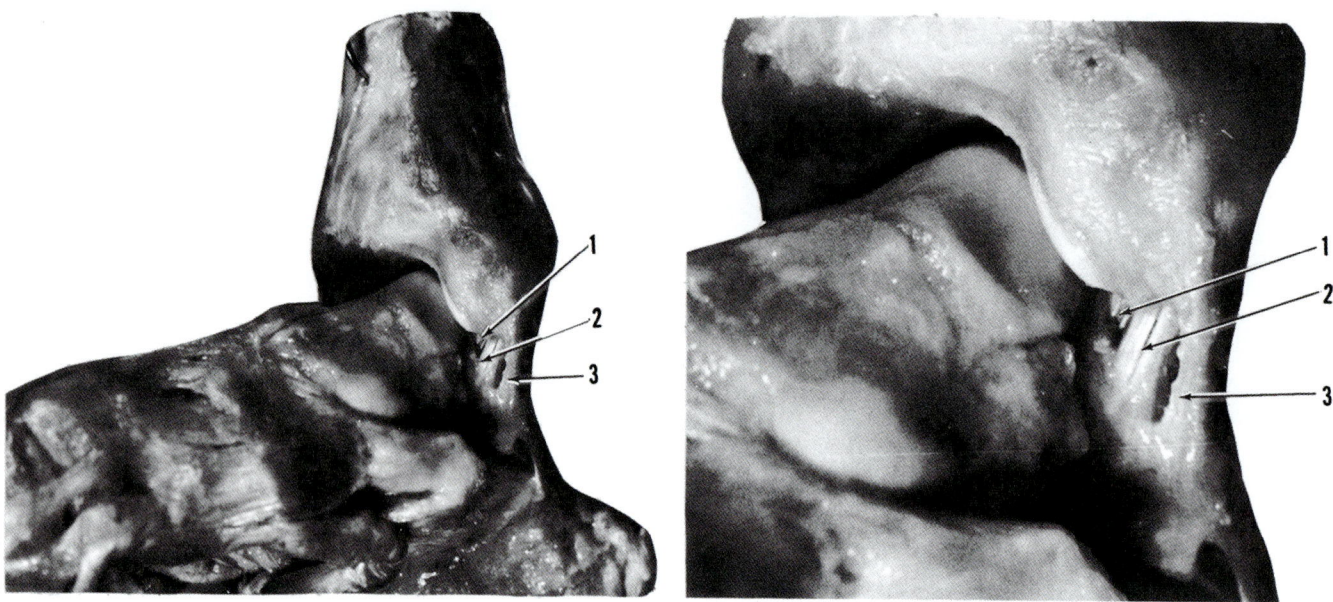

Figure 4.39 **Deltoid ligament.** (*1, 2,* Fasciculated deep component, talotibial; *3,* superficial tibiocalcaneal component.)

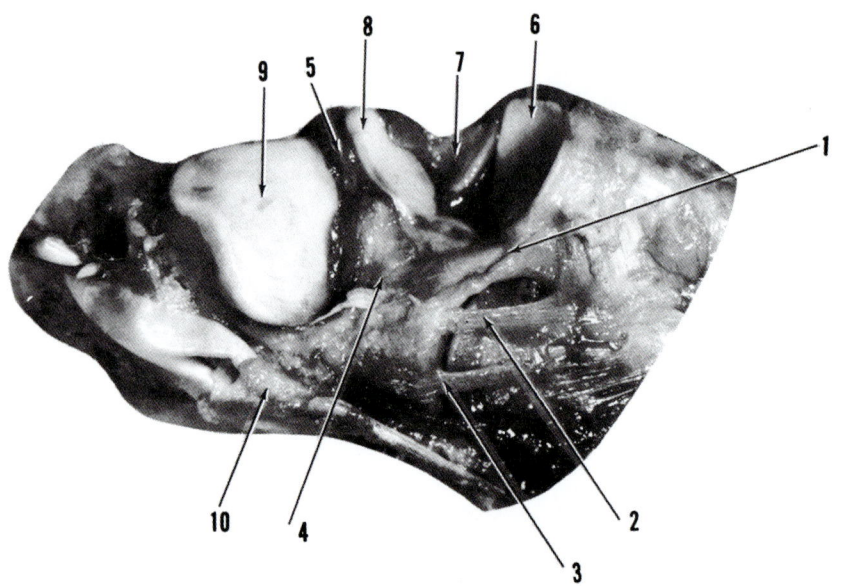

Figure 4.40 **Calcaneonavicularcuboid complex.** (*1,* Lateral calcaneonavicular ligament; *2,* medial calcaneocuboid ligament; *3,* dorsolateral calcaneocuboid ligament; *4,* sinus tarsi; *5,* canalis tarsi; *6,* navicular articular surface for talar head; *7,* inferior calcaneonavicular ligament; *8,* medial and anterior articular surfaces of os calcis; *9,* posterior articular surface of os calcis; *10,* inferior peroneal retinaculum.)

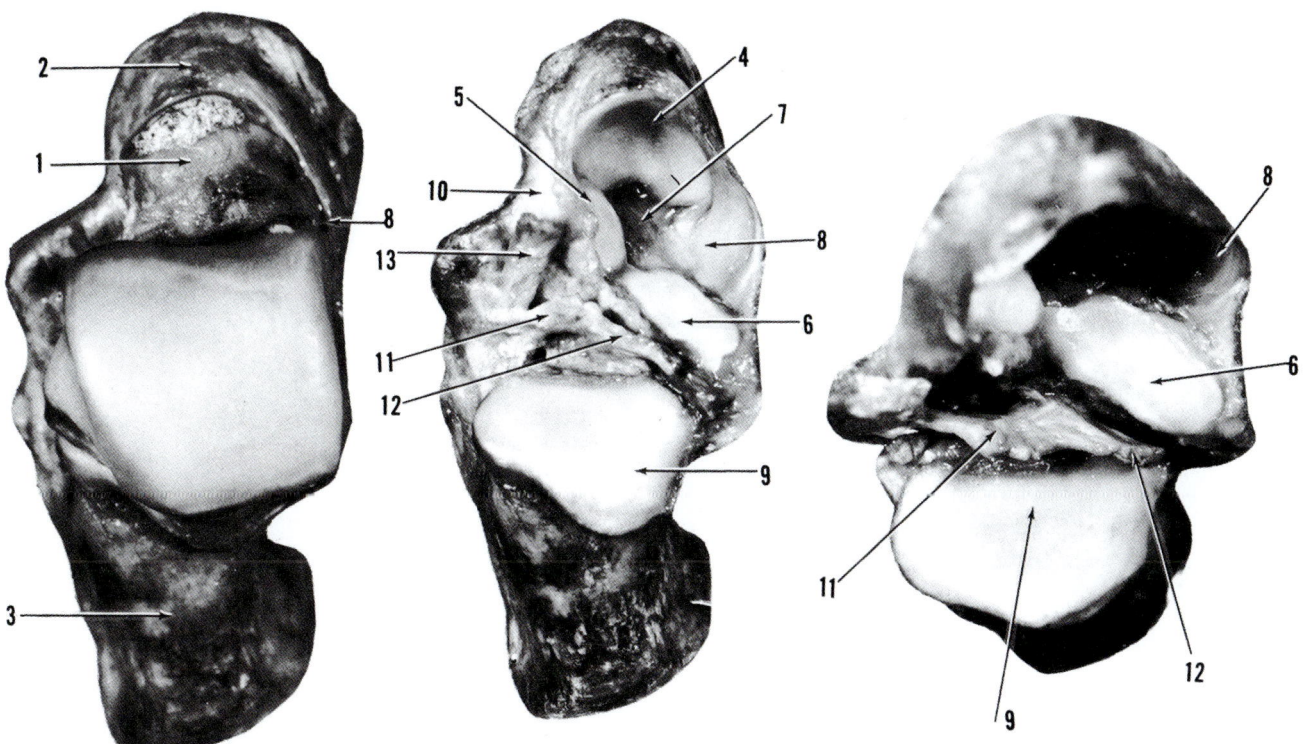

Figure 4.41 **Talocalcaneonavicular complex.** (*1,* Talus; *2,* navicular; *3,* os calcis; *4,* articular surface of navicular for talar head; *5,* anterior calcaneal surface; *6,* middle calcaneal surface; *7,* inferior calcaneonavicular ligament; *8,* superomedial calcaneonavicular ligament; *9,* posterior calcaneal surface; *10,* lateral calcaneonavicular ligament; *11,* medial root of inferior extensor retinaculum blending with interosseous talocalcaneal ligament [*12*] of canalis tarsi; *13,* cervical ligament.)

anteriorly and slightly inferiorly and inserts on the dorsum of the cuboid 1.5 cm anterior to the posterior border of the cuboid.[27] This ligament measures approximately 1 cm in length and 0.5 cm in width.[27]

The two arms of the bifurcate ligament form an average angle of 30° in the transverse plane and an average angle of 20° in the vertical or sagittal plane.[27]

The lateral calcaneonavicular ligament is usually stronger than the calcaneocuboid component. The latter may be absent and Köktürk provides the following information based on the dissection of 40 feet: both ligaments present in 57.5%, medial calcaneocuboid ligament absent in 40.0%, and lateral calcaneonavicular ligament absent in 2.5%.[26]

LIGAMENTS OF THE TALOCALCANEONAVICULAR JOINTS

The calcaneonavicular complex is a functional unit moving around the talus. The extracapsular ligaments of the sinus tarsi and tarsal canal are the major elements guiding the motion of the calcaneonavicular complex relative to the talus. Furthermore, any instantaneous motion between the calcaneus and the talus occurs simultaneously at the anterior and posterior talocalcaneal joints and at the talonavicular joint. In clinical and functional terms, the hindfoot carries the forefoot and vice versa.

The advantage of the functional rather than the conventional anatomic grouping of the ligaments is evident when one confronts the understanding and correction of clinical problems.

▶ Cervical Ligament

The cervical ligament (external talocalcaneal ligament, anterolateral talocalcaneal ligament, anterior talocalcaneal ligament, a portion of the interosseous ligament; Fig. 4.46) is the strongest ligament connecting the talus and the calcaneus.[14,28-30] It originates in the anteromedial segment of the sinus tarsi from the cervical tubercle located on the medial aspect of the bony eminence giving origin to the extensor digitorum brevis muscle. The prominence of the cervical tubercle is variable. The origin of the cervical ligament is posterolateral to the origin of the lateral calcaneonavicular ligament and anterior to the intermediate root of the inferior extensor retinaculum (Fig. 4.47). In the neutral position of the os calcis, the cervical ligament takes an oblique course and is directed upward, anteriorly, and medially and inserts on the inferior aspect of the talar neck, where a tubercle may be present. In our series of 100 tali, the tuberculum cervicis talus was recognized in 37%. The long axis of the ligament makes an angle of 45° to 50° with the long axis of the calcaneus in the sagittal plane and nearly parallels the average direction of the calcaneofibular ligament (Fig. 4.48). The position of the os calcis determines the orientation of the ligament. In valgus, the cervical ligament is more horizontal

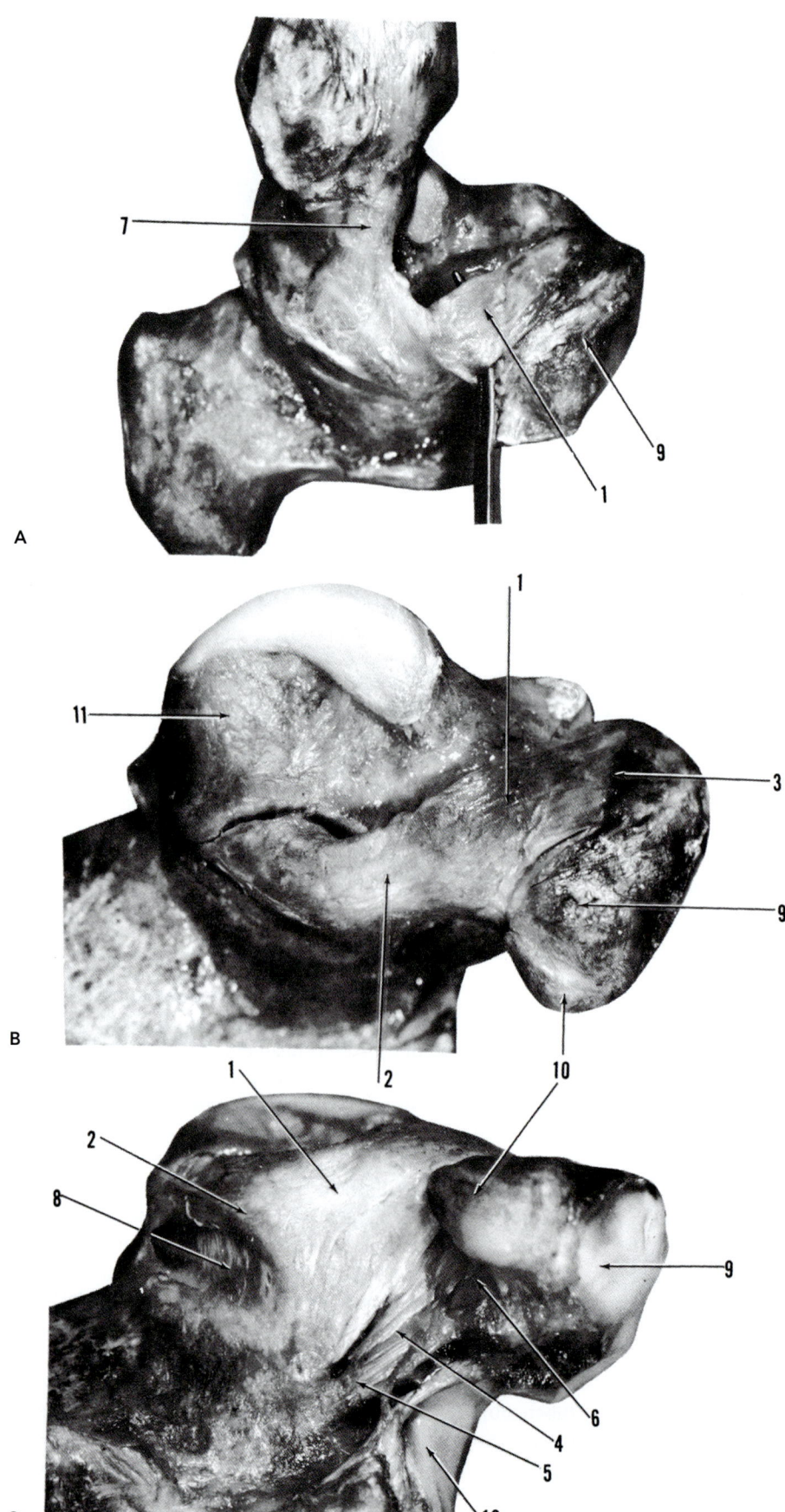

Figure 4.42 Superomedial calcaneonavicular ligament. (A) Medial view of ankle. (B) Medial view of talocalcaneonavicular complex. (C) Inferomedial view of talocalcaneonavicular complex. (1, Superomedial calcaneonavicular ligament; 2, origin of 7 from anterior border of sustentaculum tali; 3, insertion of 1 on superomedial aspect of navicular; 4, inferior calcaneonavicular ligament; 5, origin of 4 from coronoid fossa of os calcis; 6, insertion of 4 on inferior segment of navicular; 7, deltoid ligament, tibiocalcaneal component; 8, canal of flexor hallucis longus tendon on inferior surface of sustentaculum tali; 9, navicular; 10, tuberosity of navicular; 11, talus; 12, cuboidal surface of os calcis.)

Chapter 4: Syndesmology   197

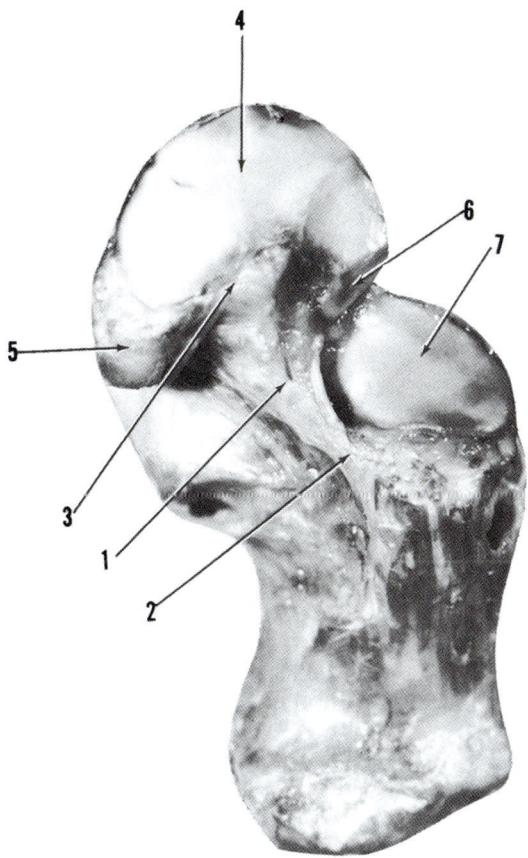

Figure 4.43 Inferior view of calcaneonavicular complex. (*1*, Inferior calcaneonavicular ligament; *2*, origin of 1 from coronoid fossa of os calcis; *3*, insertion of 1 on inferior surface of navicular [*4*]; *5*, tuberosity of navicular; *6*, articular surface of navicular for cuboid; *7*, articular surface of calcaneus for cuboid.)

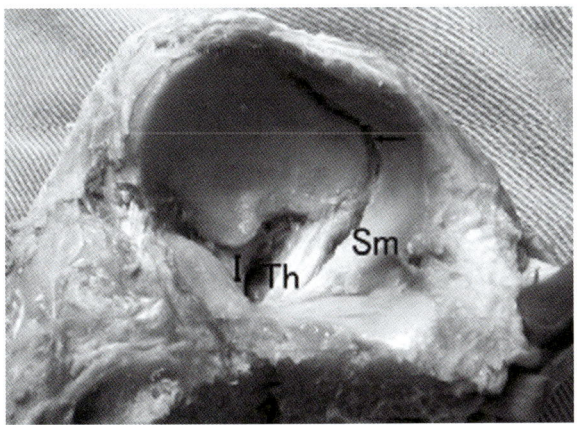

Figure 4.44 The fibers of the third ligament (*Th*) are distinct from both the superomedial calcaneonavicular ligament (*Sm*) and the inferior calcaneonavicular ligament (*I*). Note that the superomedial calcaneonavicular ligament runs along the medial margin of the talonavicular articular surface and does not attach to the tubercle of the navicular (*arrow*). (From Taniguchi A, Tanaka Y, Takakura Y, et al. Anatomy of the spring ligament. *J Bone Joint Surg Am*. 2003;85:2174-2178, Figure 2.)

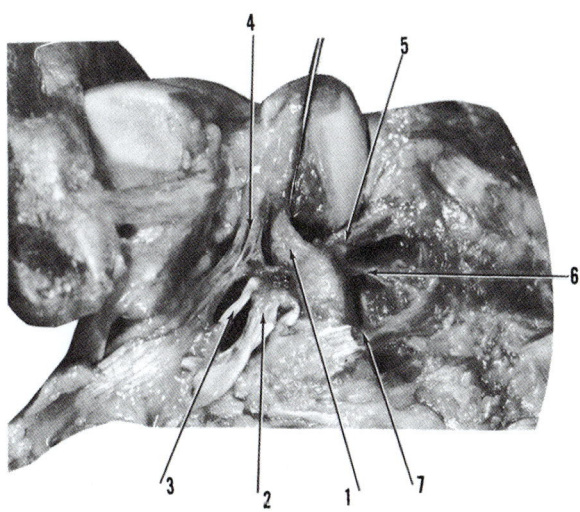

Figure 4.45 Dorsolateral view of sinus tarsi. (*1*, Cervical ligament; *2*, *3*, intermediate and medial roots of inferior extensor retinaculum; *4*, cervical attachment of medial root of inferior extensor retinaculum; *5*, lateral calcaneonavicular ligament; *6*, medial calcaneocuboid ligament; *7*, dorsolateral calcaneocuboid ligament.)

and it is more vertical in varus. The angle formed by the long axis of the ligament and the horizontal line in the frontal plane is 16° in valgus and 75° in varus as measured in the specimen shown in Figure 4.49. The cervical ligament is in the form of a rectangular band and its measurements are as follows: length, 20 mm; width, 10 mm; *or* length, 19.6 mm; width, 11.6 mm; thickness, 2.8 mm.[29] As mentioned by Smith, the cervical ligament is separate from the ligament of the canalis tarsi in the majority.[30] Of 22 feet, the two ligaments were continuous in one specimen and the ligaments were joined by an oblique band in another specimen.[30]

▶ **Ligament of the Tarsal Canal**

This ligament (interosseous talocalcaneal ligament; Figs. 4.50 and 4.51) of the tarsal canal is a flat, oblique band that originates from the sulcus calcanei of the tarsal canal close to the anterior capsule of the posterior talocalcaneal joint but independent of it.[14,29,30] The fibers are directed obliquely upward and medially, with an angle of inclination of 40° to 45° relative to the horizontal; they insert on the sulcus tali medially. Cahill provides the following average measurements of the ligament: length, 15 mm; width, 5.6 mm; thickness, 1.6 mm.[29] The inner fibers are shorter than the outer fibers.

The ligament of the tarsal canal may be distinguished from the thickened segment of the anterior capsule of the posterior talocalcaneal joint because the fibers of the latter are vertically oriented, whereas the former takes an oblique course. The ligament is crossed anteriorly in an X by the canalicular portion of the medial root of the inferior extensor retinaculum. The talar insertion of the ligament is joined by the talar portion of the medial root and by the "oblique talocalcaneal band."[29] The oblique talocalcaneal band extends from the calcaneal attachment of the intermediate extensor retinacular root to the talar portion of the

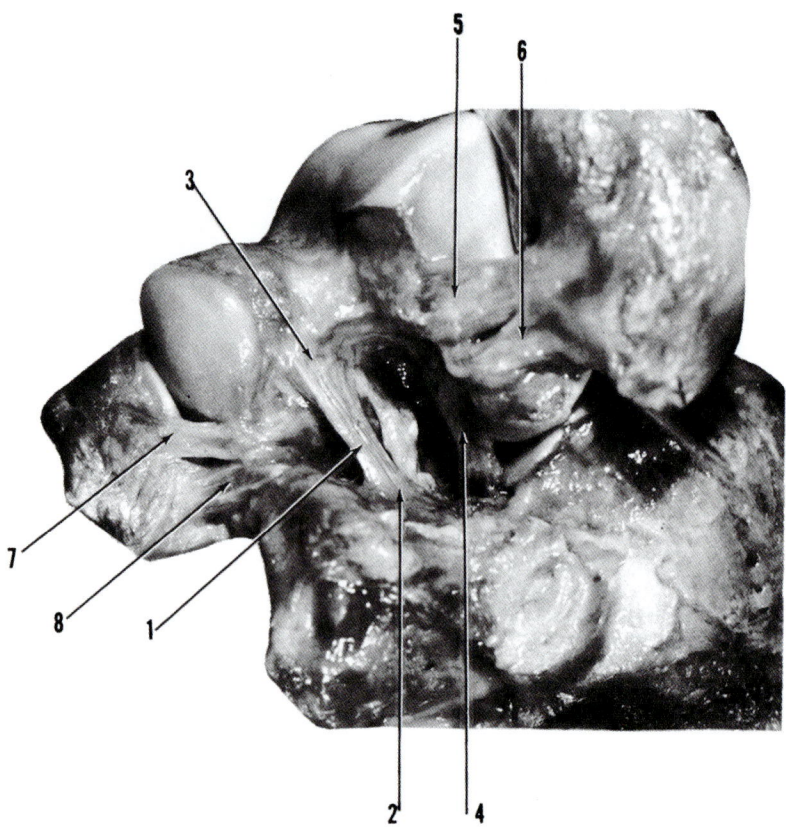

Figure 4.46 **Lateral view of sinus tarsi.** (*1*, Cervical ligament; *2*, origin of 1 from sinus tarsi; *3*, insertion of 1 on talar neck; *4*, capsule of posterior talocalcaneal joint; *5, 6*, anterior talofibular ligaments; *7, 8*, lateral calcaneonavicular ligaments.)

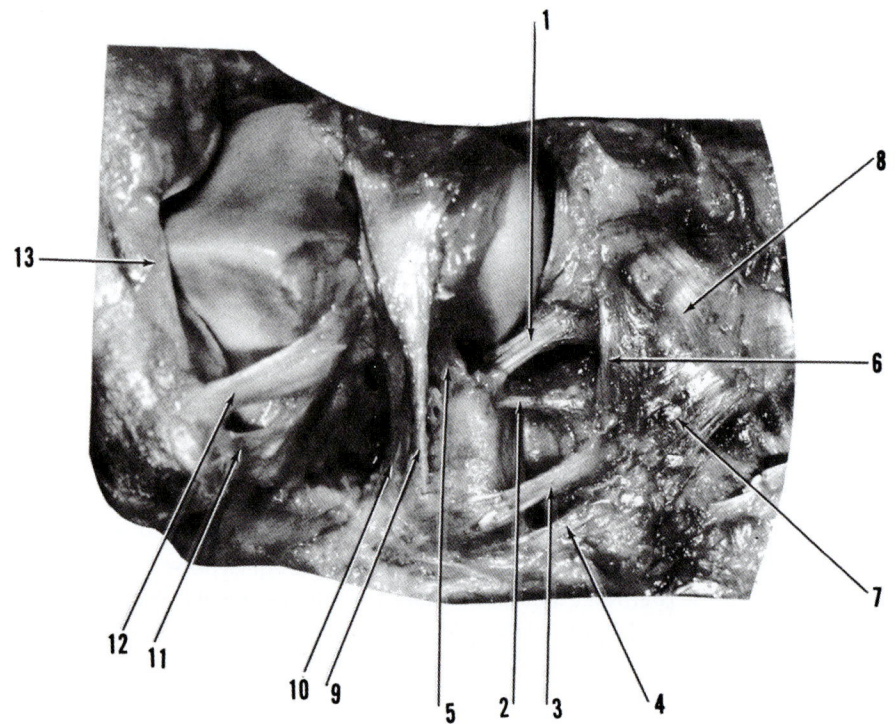

Figure 4.47 **Dorsal view of mid tarsus and ankle joint.** (*1*, Lateral calcaneonavicular ligament; *2*, medial calcaneocuboid ligament; *3*, dorsolateral calcaneocuboid ligament; *4*, lateral calcaneocuboid ligament; *5*, cervical ligament; *6*, dorsal cubonavicular ligament; *7*, dorsal cuneo$_3$ cuboid ligament; *8*, dorsal navicularcuneo$_3$ ligament; *9, 10*, intermediate and medial roots of inferior extensor retinaculum; *11, 12*, anterior talofibular ligaments; *13*, anterior tibiofibular ligament.)

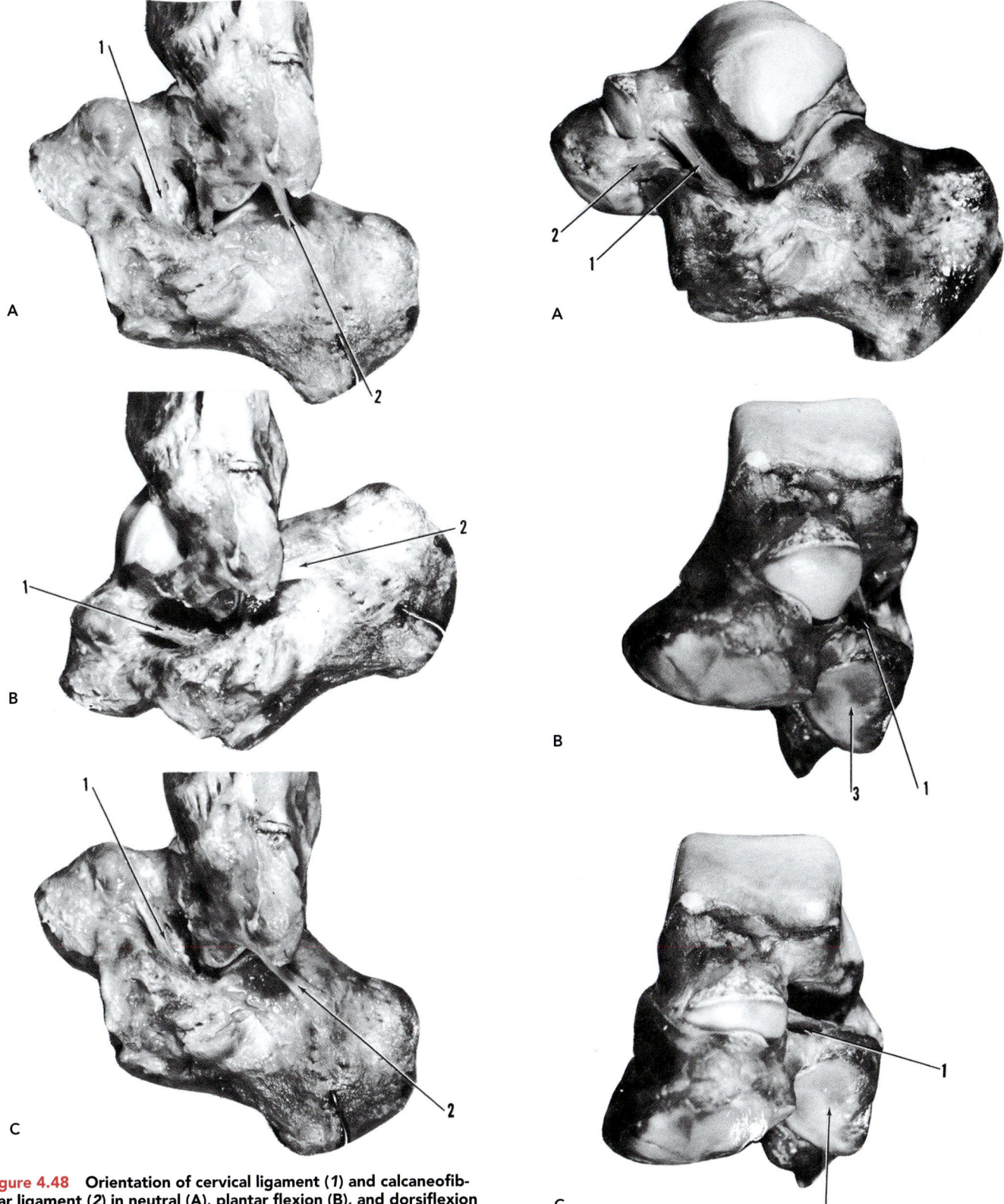

Figure 4.48 Orientation of cervical ligament (*1*) and calcaneofibular ligament (*2*) in neutral (**A**), plantar flexion (**B**), and dorsiflexion (**C**). In **A** and **C,** the ligaments are nearly parallel.

Figure 4.49 **Cervical ligament. (A)**—*1*, cervical ligament; *2*, lateral calcaneonavicular ligament. (**B**) Calcaneus (*3*) in varus. The cervical ligament (*1*) is nearly vertical. (**C**) Calcaneus (*3*) in valgus. The cervical ligament (*1*) is nearly horizontal.

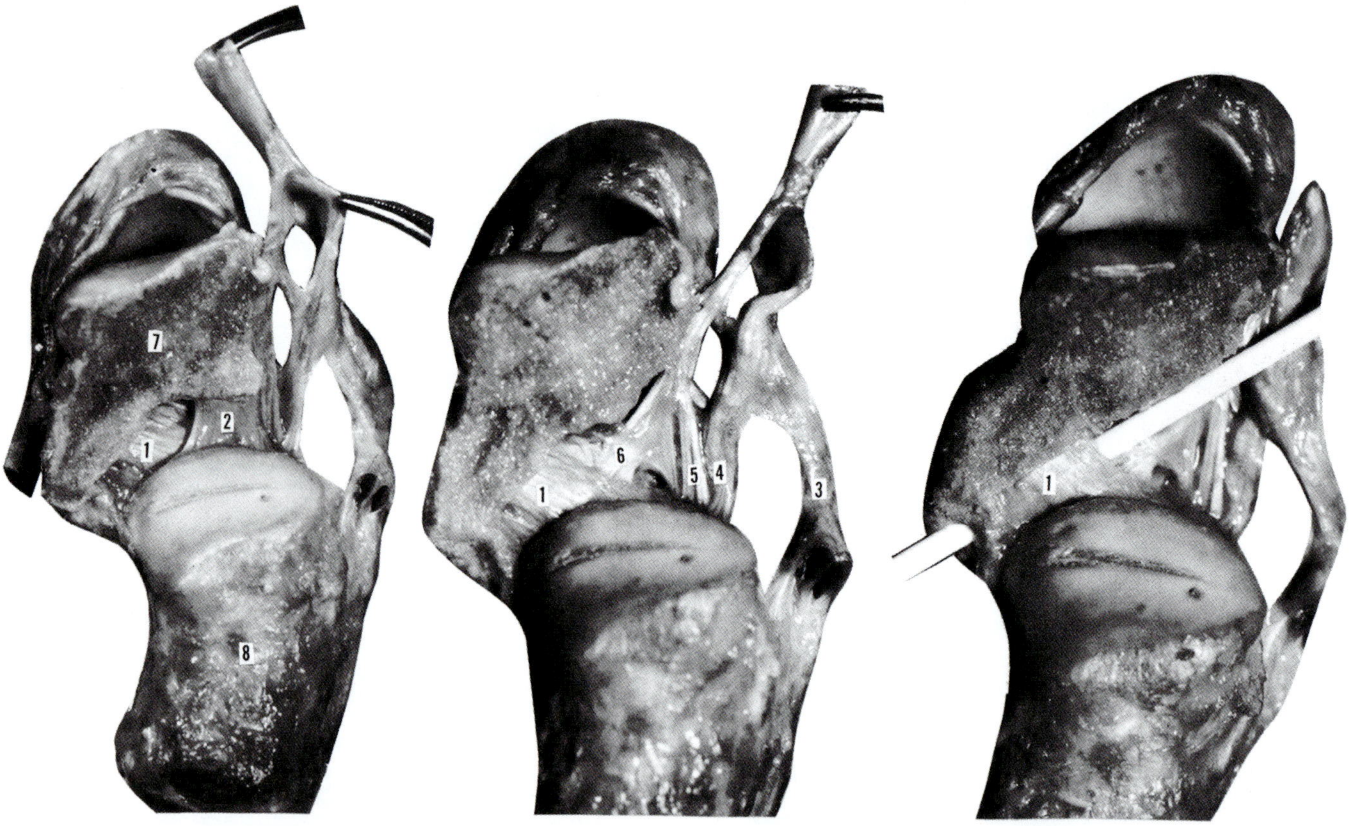

Figure 4.50 **Anatomic preparation of canalis tarsi.** Posterior half of talus is removed through an oblique osteotomy. (*1*, Talocalcaneal interosseous ligament of canalis tarsi; *2*, anterior capsular ligament of posterior talocalcaneal joint; *3*, insertion of lateral root of inferior extensor retinaculum on inferior peroneal retinaculum; *4*, intermediate root of inferior extensor retinaculum; *5, 6*, medial roots of inferior extensor retinaculum; *7*, talus; *8*, os calcis.)

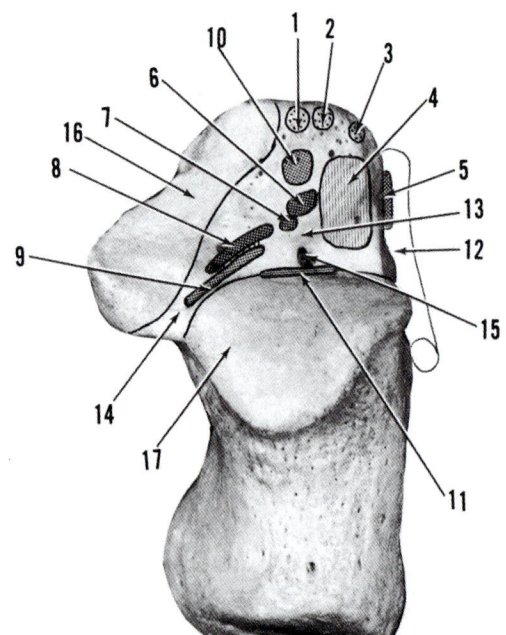

Figure 4.51 **Insertion sites in the sinus tarsi and canalis tarsi.** (*1*, Lateral calcaneonavicular ligament; *2*, medial calcaneocuboid ligament; *3*, dorsolateral calcaneocuboid ligament; *4*, extensor digitorum brevis muscle; *5*, lateral root of inferior extensor retinaculum; *6*, intermediate root of inferior extensor retinaculum; *7, 8*, medial roots of inferior extensor retinaculum; *9*, interosseous talocalcaneal ligament of canalis tarsi; *10*, cervical ligament; *11*, capsular ligament of anterior aspect of posterior talocalcaneal joint; *12*, tunnel of peronei; *13*, sinus tarsi; *14*, canalis tarsi; *15*, foramina of calcaneal antrum; *16*, anterior and middle calcaneal articular surfaces; *17*, posterior calcaneal articular surface.)

tarsal canal. These two talar extensions from the medial and intermediate roots of the extensor retinaculum were clearly recognized by Barclay-Smith in 1896.[14] In reference to the latter extension, Barclay-Smith describes "very closely associated with and lying on a plane anterior to that of the deep limb is a ligament which at its attachment to the os calcis is often blended with its outer band; passing upwards and inwards, it is attached to the groove on the astragalus, forming the roof of the canalis tarsi."[14]

▶ Lateral Talocalcaneal Ligament

The lateral talocalcaneal ligament (see Figs. 4.11 and 4.12) is a flat, short, rectangular ligament, parallel to the calcaneofibular ligament. It originates from the anteroinferior aspect of the lateral talar process, extends downward and posteriorly, and inserts on the os calcis just lateral to the posterior articular surface. This ligament is slightly anterior and medial to the calcaneofibular ligament. Occasionally it is difficult to separate these two ligaments because of their intimate adherence. The variation of this ligament and its relationship with the calcaneofibular ligament has been analyzed, as mentioned previously, by Trouilloud and colleagues.[9]

DiGiovanni et al[31] investigated the ligamentous attachments on the lateral talar process. Based on the dissection of 10 feet, they confirmed that "only the insertions of the ATFL and PTFL (posterior talofibular ligament), in addition to the origin of the LTCL (lateral talocalcaneal ligament), attached to the lateral process of the talus" and "these three ligaments formed a circumferential 'skirt' of ligamentous tissue."

Milner and Soames,[7] in a study based on the dissection of 40 feet, provided the following measurements in regard to the lateral talocalcaneal ligament: length, 15.5 ± 3.9 mm; width, 3.5 ± 2.5 mm. The ligament was observed in 55% (22 specimens) and was bilateral in 20% (8 specimens).

▶ Posterior Talocalcaneal Ligament

The posterior talocalcaneal ligament is a short, flat, quadrilateral ligament directed downward and laterally. It originates from the lateral surface and apex of the posterolateral talar tubercle and inserts on the superior and medial aspect of the os calcis. It may also give insertion to the fibrous roof of the flexor hallucis longus tunnel (see Fig. 4.18). At the talar origin, the posterior talocalcaneal ligament may interchange fibers with the posterior talofibular ligament. Occasionally, the posterior talocalcaneal ligament is formed by two fascicles. The lateral band originates from the posterolateral tubercle, extends downward and medially, and inserts on the dorsum of the os calcis. The medial band originates from the posteromedial talar tubercle, extends downward and laterally, and inserts on the superomedial aspect of the os calcis next to the insertion of the lateral band. The two fascicles form a V with a talar base and calcaneal apex.

When an os trigonum is present, the posterior talocalcaneal ligament originates from it and forms a trigonocalcaneal ligament.

▶ Medial Talocalcaneal Ligament

The medial talocalcaneal ligament (Fig. 4.52) is a short, strong ligament. It originates from the talar posteromedial tubercle, courses anteriorly and inferiorly, and inserts on the posterior border of the sustentaculum tali. It limits posteroinferiorly the medial opening of the tarsal canal. A second band may be present, originating from the same site but directed downward and posteriorly; this band inserts posterior to the sustentaculum tali and completes the groove lodging the flexor hallucis tendon.

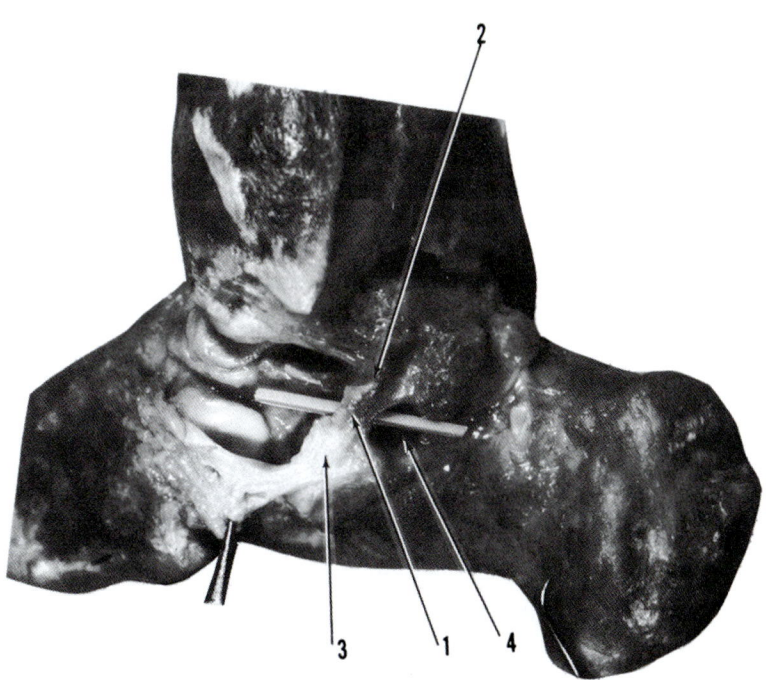

Figure 4.52 Medial aspect of hindfoot. (*1*, Medial talocalcaneal ligament; *2*, origin of 1 from talar posteromedial tubercle; *3*, insertion of 1 on posterior aspect of sustentaculum tali; *4*, medial opening of canalis tarsi.)

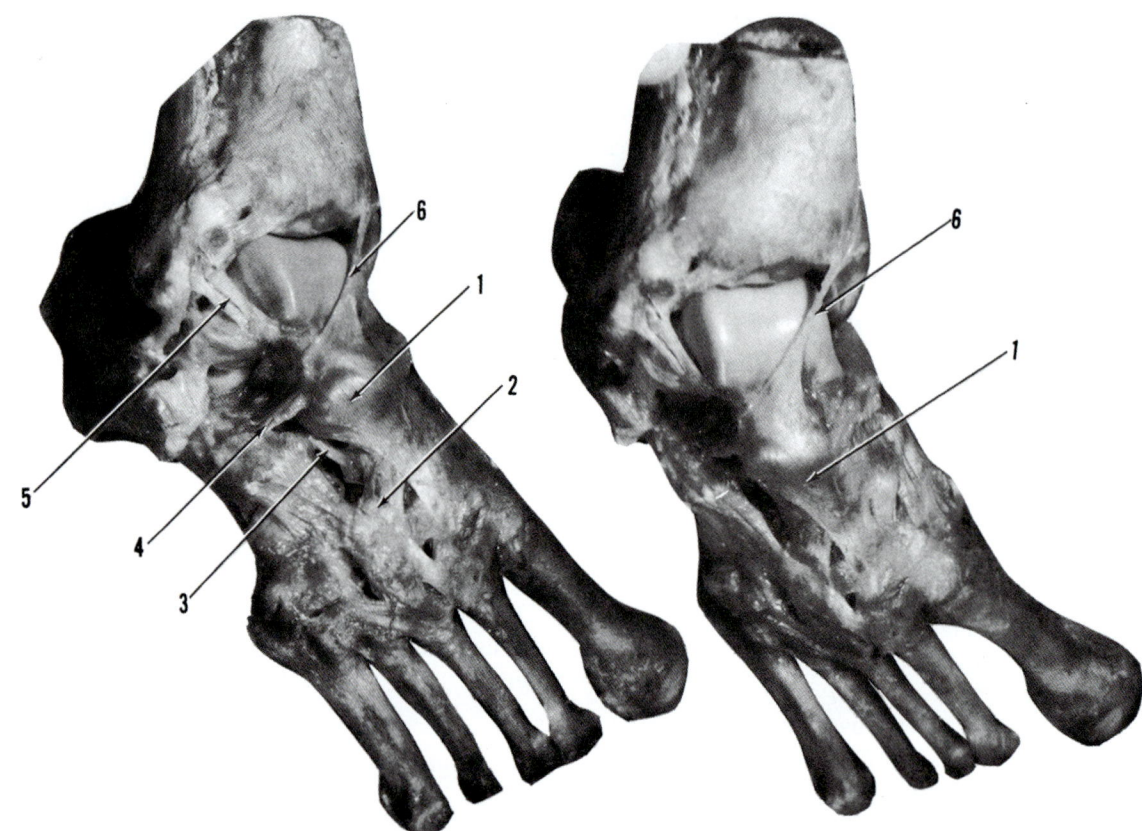

Figure 4.53 **Talonavicular ligament.** (*1*, Dorsal talonavicular ligament; *2*, dorsal cuneo[3] navicular ligament; *3*, lateral calcaneonavicular ligament; *4*, cervical ligament; *5*, anterior talofibular ligament; *6*, anterior tibiotalar ligament.)

▶ Talonavicular Ligament

The talonavicular ligament (Fig. 4.53) occupies the dorsal interval between the superomedial calcaneonavicular ligament and the lateral calcaneonavicular ligament. It is a capsular thickening. Barclay-Smith recognized two components: superficial and deep.[14] The superficial component originates from the dorsum of the talar neck and is a thin, long, broad band that courses anteromedially and inserts on the dorsum of the navicular. It crosses the superomedial calcaneonavicular ligament in an X and their fibers interlace. The deep component is shorter and deeper. It originates from the superomedial aspect of the talar neck, courses anterolaterally, passes under the superficial component, and inserts on the dorsum of the navicular.

LIGAMENTS OF THE CALCANEOCUBOID AND CUBONAVICULAR JOINTS

▶ Medial Calcaneocuboid Ligament

The medial calcaneocuboid ligament has already been described as the outer component of the bifurcate ligament (V ligament, ligament of Chopart) (see Fig. 4.45).

▶ Dorsolateral Calcaneocuboid Ligament

The dorsolateral calcaneocuboid ligament (see Fig. 4.45) originates from the dorsolateral corner of the anterior segment of the calcaneus close to the margin of the anterior articular surface of the calcaneus. It is directed, as a flat band, anteromedially and inserts on the dorsum of the cuboid at least 0.5 cm distal to the articular interline. Occasionally a smaller, more lateral band is present.

Dorn-Lange et al[32] investigated the morphology of the dorsal and lateral calcaneocuboid ligaments in 30 feet. They defined a dorsolateral ligament "when a wide band extended from the dorsal aspect to the lateral aspect of the foot."

In 56.6% (17 specimens), the dorsolateral ligament was a single tract; in 43.3 % (13 specimens), it was composed of two or more separate tracts; in 56.6% (17 specimens), there was an additional "lateral" ligament. The ligament was measured and defined as maximal ligament length along the medial fibers bundle and as minimum length at the lower edge of the ligament.

The measurements were as follows:

Dorsal calcaneocuboid ligament
Mean length, maximum: 23.4 ± 4.3 mm
Mean length, minimum: 19.3 ± 4.3 mm
Mean width, complete: 12.4 ± 5.4 mm

Chapter 4: Syndesmology

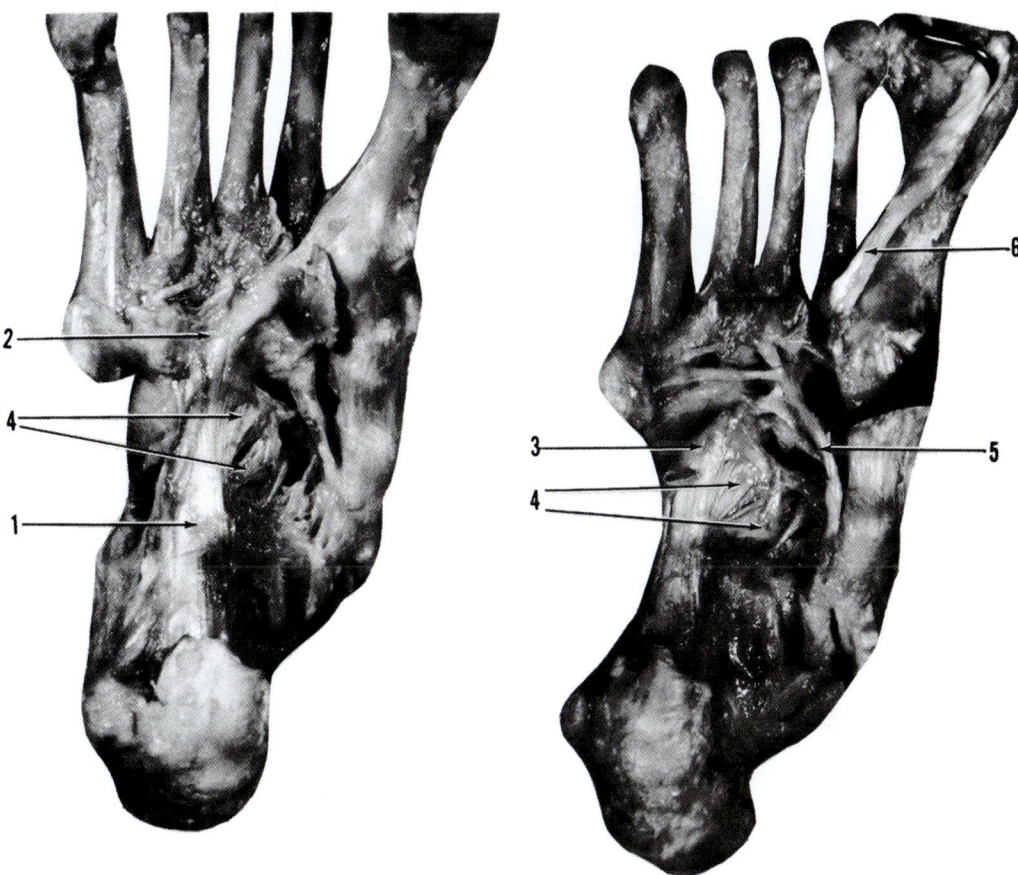

Figure 4.54 Plantar aspect of foot. (*1*, Long plantar ligament; *2*, superficial distal component of 1; *3*, deep insertion of 1 on cuboidal crest forming the long calcaneocuboid ligament; *4*, short plantar ligament or deep, short, calcaneocuboid ligament; *5*, plantar segment of tibialis posterior tendon; *6*, reflected peroneus longus tendon.)

Lateral calcaneocuboid ligament
   Length: 13.4 ± 3.9 mm
   Width: 5.9 ± 3.9 mm

Patil et al[33] investigated the morphology and the dimensions of the dorsal calcaneocuboid ligament (DCCL) in 30 preserved feet. The DCCL was a solitary structure in 66.6% and had two components in 33.3%.

The measurements of the ligaments were as follows:

Solitary DCCL
   Length
      Superior border: 18.6 ± 2.8 mm
      Inferior border: 17.3 ± 2.5 mm
   Width
      Calcaneal: 13.8 ± 2.2 mm
      Cuboid: 12.4 ± 2.1 mm
   Thickness: 2.6 ± 0.6 mm

Two components of DCCL
Superior component
   Length
      Superior border: 16.9 ± 2.1 mm
      Inferior border: 16.4 ± 2.8 mm
   Width
      Calcaneal: 9.3 ± 1.2 mm
      Cuboid: 10.6 ± 1.4 mm
   Thickness: 2.6 ± 0.4 mm

Lower component
   Length
      Superior border: 12.9 ± 2.9 mm
      Inferior border: 13.8 ± 3.0 mm
   Width
      Calcaneal side: 8.3 ± 1.4 mm
      Cuboid side: 7.2 ± 1.00 mm
   Thickness: 2.1 ± 0.4 mm

▶ Inferior Calcaneocuboid Ligament

The inferior calcaneocuboid ligament (long and short plantar ligaments) is a thick, powerful, longitudinally oriented ligament with two components: superficial or long and deep or short (Fig. 4.54). The superficial or long plantar ligament originates from the segment of the inferior surface of the os calcis extending from the anterior surface of the posterior tuberosities and their intertubercular segment to the anterior tuberosity. The strong longitudinal fibers pass over the calcaneocuboid joint and divide into two sets of fibers, deep and superficial. The deep fibers, representing the bulk of this component, insert on the oblique crest of the cuboid. The more superficial fibers form a thinner layer, cross the tunnel of the peroneus longus (contributing to its formation) and divide into four thinner slips inserting over the metatarsal bases 2 to 5. Paturet[10] describes the band directed to the base of the fifth metatarsal as a rectangular

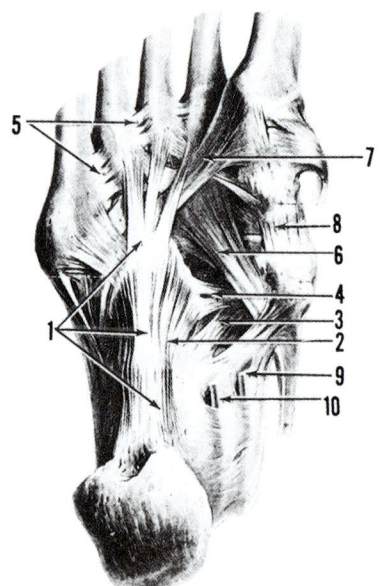

Figure 4.55 Plantar aspect of foot. (1, Longitudinal plantar ligament; 2, short plantar calcaneocuboid ligament; 3, plantar calcaneonavicular ligament; 4, plantar cubonavicular ligament; 5, intermetatarsal ligaments M5-M4, M4-M3; 6, tibialis posterior tendon; 7, peroneus longus tendon; 8, plantar cuneo1navicular ligament; 9, flexor digitorum longus tendon [cut through]; 10, flexor hallucis longus tendon [cut through].) (From Spalteholz W. *Hand Atlas of Human Anatomy*. Vol 1. JB Lippincott; 1903:219.)

ligament 20 to 25 mm in width, called the long cubo-fifth metatarsal ligament.[10] This band is also well illustrated by Spalteholz[34] (Fig. 4.55). The deep or short calcaneocuboid ligament (Fig. 4.56) originates from the anterior tuberosity of the os calcis. The strong, fasciculated fibers fan out, course anteromedially, and insert over the entire triangular surface located posterior to the crest of the cuboid. A strong band oriented almost transversely inserts on the nonarticulating surface of the beak of the cuboid. The deep component is covered by the longitudinal ligament only laterally and is in continuity medially with the inferior calcaneonavicular ligament.

Ward and Soames[35] studied the morphology and dimensions of the plantar calcaneocuboid ligaments in 59 feet specimens. In the long plantar ligament (LPL), structural variations were observed in 20.3% (12 specimens) in the form of medial twisting fibers in 11.8% (seven specimens), or lateral twisting fibers in 3.3% (two specimens), or additional bands in 5% (three specimens). On passing forward, the LPL split into either two or three bands and in 86% attached to the cuboid and the bases of M_2 to M_4. In 12% of the specimens, the attachment was to M_2-M_3, and in four specimens, it was from M_2 to M_5. In one specimen, the attachment was from M_1 to M_5, and in another specimen, the attachment of the LPL was only to the cuboid.

In the study of the short plantar ligament (SPL), some displayed superficial and deep bands, and in 39% of the specimens, the deep band had a distinct attachment to the calcaneus.

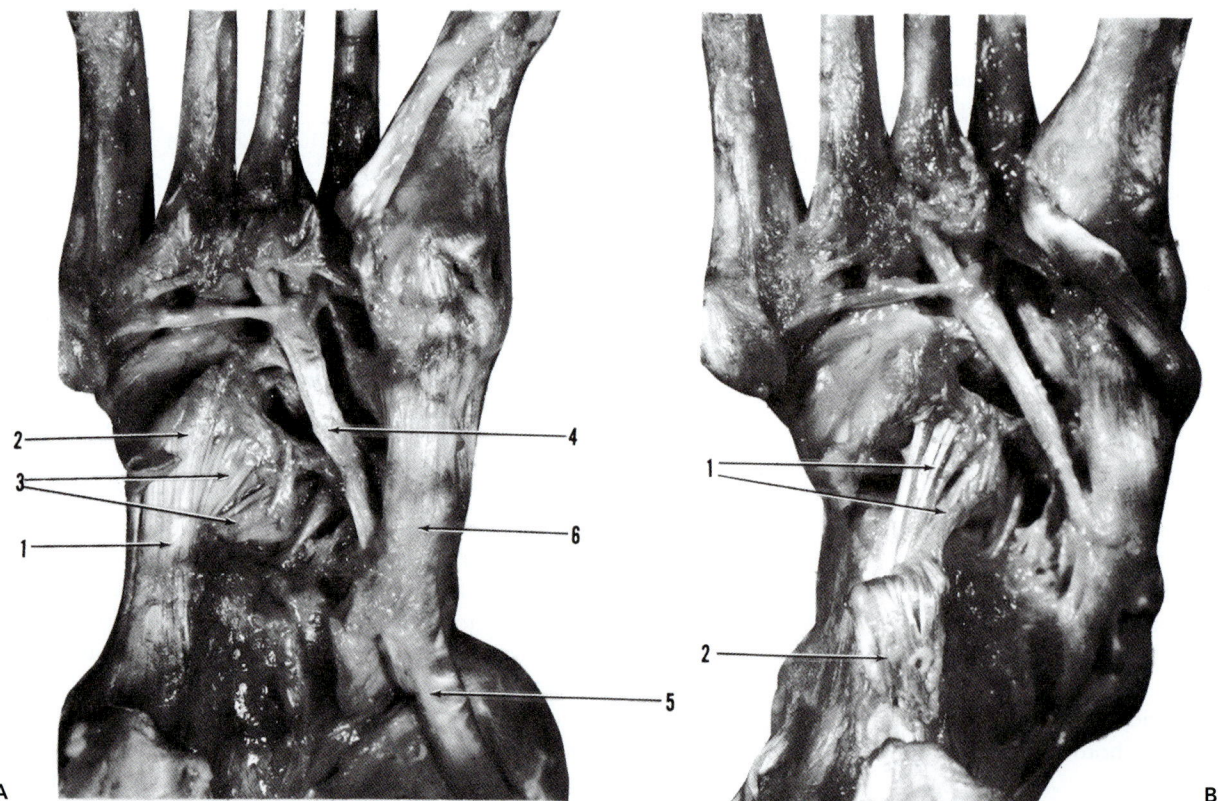

Figure 4.56 Plantar aspect of foot. (A)—1, long calcaneocuboid ligament; 2, insertion of 7 on cuboidal crest; 3, short, deep calcaneocuboid ligament; 4, 5, 6, tibialis posterior tendon and insertions. (B)—1, deep calcaneocuboid ligament; 2, reflected long calcaneocuboid ligament.

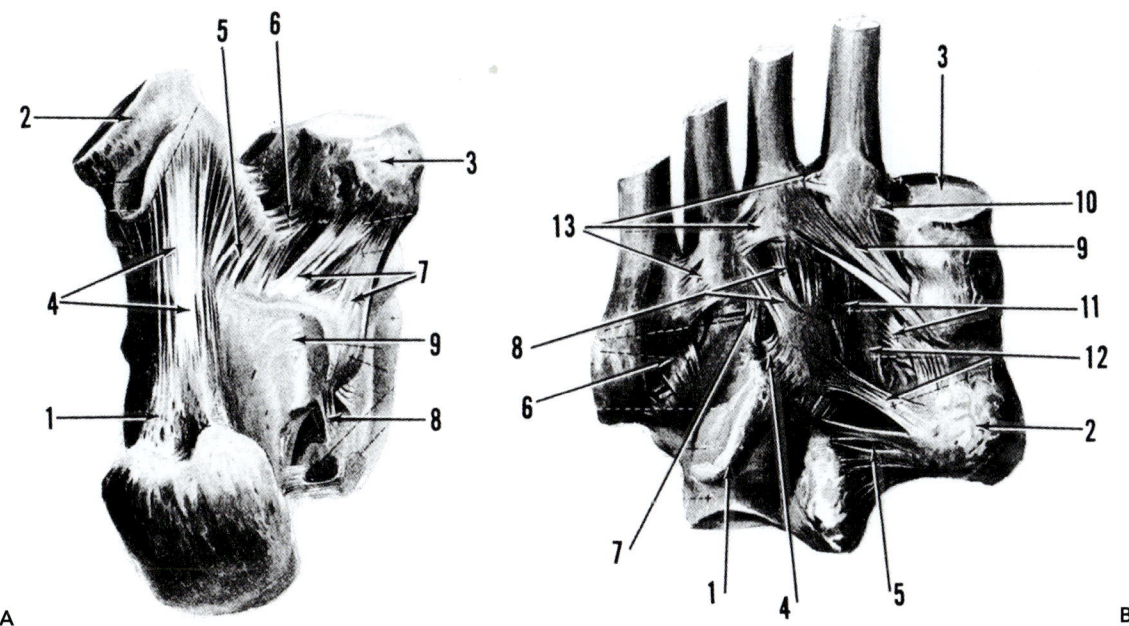

Figure 4.57 **(A)** Plantar view of hindfoot. (*1*, Os calcis; *2*, cuboid; *3*, navicular; *4*, long plantar or long calcaneocuboid ligament; *5*, short or deep calcaneocuboid ligament; *6*, plantar cubonavicular ligament; *7*, plantar calcaneonavicular ligament; *8*, medial talocalcaneal ligament; *9*, sulcus of flexor hallucis longus tendon.) **(B)** Plantar view of tarsus. (*1*, Cuboid; *2*, navicular; *3*, first cuneiform; *4*, plantar cuneo$_3$-cuboid ligament; *5*, plantar cubonavicular ligament; *6*, plantar cubo-M$_5$ ligament; *7*, plantar cubo-M$_4$ ligament; *8*, plantar cuneo$_3$-M$_3$, M$_4$ ligaments; *9*, long plantar cuneo$_1$-M$_3$, M$_2$ ligament; *10*, short plantar cuneo$_1$-M$_2$ ligament; *11*, plantar cuneo$_1$-cuneo$_2$, cuneo$_2$-cuneo$_3$ ligaments; *12*, plantar cuneo$_{2,3}$-navicular ligaments; *13*, intermetatarsal ligaments M$_5$-M$_4$, M$_4$-M$_3$, M$_3$-M$_2$.) (From Spalteholz W. *Hand Atlas of Human Anatomy.* Vol 1. JB Lippincott; 1903:219.)

The measurements of the ligaments were as follows:

Long plantar ligament
 Mid, mean length: 28.5 mm ± 10.5
 Mid, mean width: 10.7 mm ± 2.8

Short plantar ligament
 Mid, mean length: 18.2 mm ± 4.3
 Mid, mean width: 12.2 mm ± 3.3

▶ Cubonavicular Ligaments

There are three cubonavicular ligaments: dorsal, plantar, and interosseous.

The dorsal cubonavicular ligament (see Fig. 4.45) is a triangular ligament with a medial apex and a lateral base. It originates from the dorsal aspect of the navicular, anteromedial to the insertion of the lateral calcaneonavicular ligament. The fibers extend laterally and transversely, pass over the corner of the third cuneiform (wedged between the navicular and the cuboid), and insert on the dorsum of the cuboid in its distal half. Some fibers attach to the dorsum of the third cuneiform also.

The plantar cubonavicular ligament (see Figs. 4.55 and 4.57A) is a rectangular band that originates from the inferior surface of the cuboid along the medial border, posterior to the cuboid crest. It overlaps, in this segment, the insertional fibers of the deep calcaneocuboid ligament. The fibers course transversely and insert on the inferior surface of the navicular, distal to the insertion of the plantar calcaneonavicular fibers. Occasionally the plantar cubonavicular ligament is formed by two fascicles: these are more or less triangular, with the apex attached to the cuboid and the base to the navicular. These bands are directed medially and posteriorly.

The interosseous cubonavicular ligament is a very short, strong ligament that originates from a narrow, vertical segment of the medial surface of the cuboid, posterior to the third cuneiform articular surface. When a small articular surface is present for the navicular (45%-55%), the fibers originate above and below this articular surface. The fibers are transversely oriented and insert on the anteroinferior segment of the lateral end of the navicular.

LIGAMENTS OF THE CUNEONAVICULAR AND CUNEOCUBOID JOINTS

▶ Cuneonavicular Ligaments

Each cuneiform is united to the navicular by a dorsal and a plantar ligament. In addition, the first cuneiform is united to the navicular by the medial cuneonavicular ligament.

There are three dorsal cuneonavicular ligaments (Figs. 4.58 and 4.59). Each ligament, in the form of a flat fibrous band, arises from the distal segment of the dorsal surface of the navicular. The first cuneonavicular ligament extends straight anteriorly and inserts on the dorsum of the first cuneiform; it is the strongest of the three. The second and third ligaments are thinner and oblique and insert on the dorsum of the corresponding cuneiform. They are partially covered by an expansion from the talonavicular ligament. The

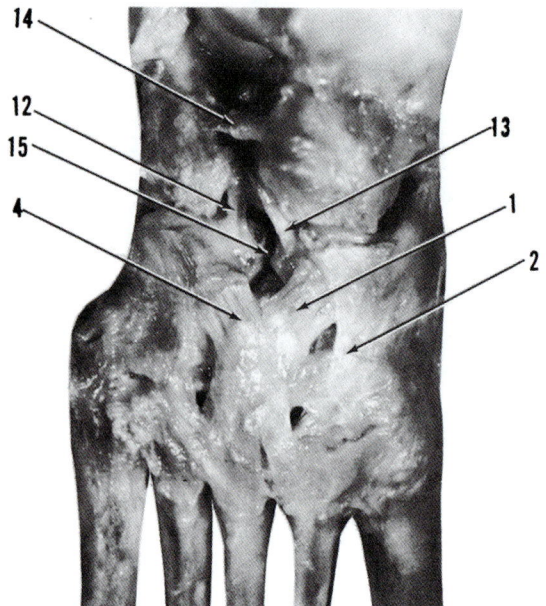
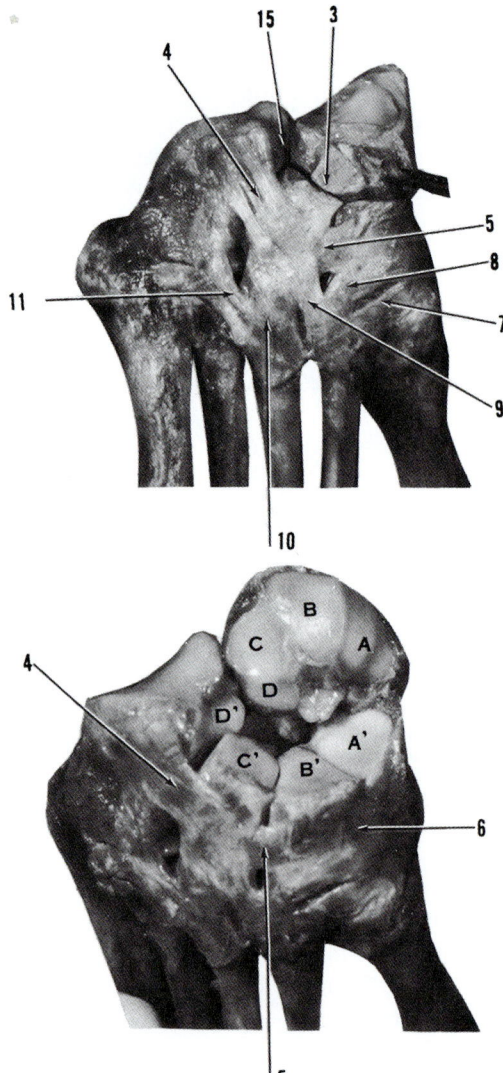

Figure 4.58 Dorsal aspect of tarsus. (1, Dorsal cuneo$_3$-navicular ligament; 2, dorsal cuneo$_2$-navicular ligament; 3, incised dorsal cuneo$_3$-navicular ligament; 4, dorsal cubocuneo$_3$ ligament; 5, dorsal intercuneiform C$_3$-C$_2$ ligament; 6, dorsal intercuneiform C$_2$-C$_1$ ligament; 7, dorsal cuneo$_1$-M$_2$ ligament; 8, dorsal cuneo$_2$-M$_2$ ligament; 9, dorsal cuneo$_3$-M$_2$ ligament; 10, dorsal cuneo$_3$-M$_3$ ligament; 11, dorsal cubo-M$_3$ ligament; 12, dorsal, medial calcaneocuboid ligament; 13, dorsal, lateral calcaneonavicular ligament; 14, cervical ligament; 15, cubonavicular articular interline; A, A', navicular and cuneiform$_1$ articular surfaces; B, B', navicular and cuneiform$_2$ articular surfaces; C, C', navicular and cuneiform$_3$ articular surfaces; D, D', navicular and cuboid articular surfaces.)

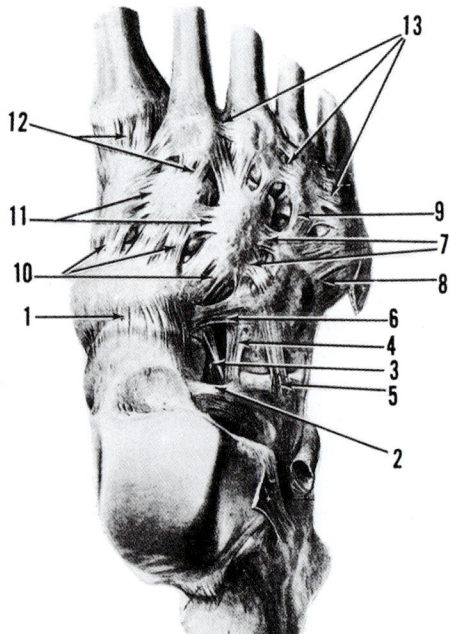

Figure 4.59 Dorsum of foot. (1, Dorsal talonavicular ligament; 2, cervical ligament; 3, calcaneonavicular component of bifurcate ligament; 4, calcaneocuboid component of bifurcate ligament; 5, dorsolateral calcaneocuboid ligament; 6, dorsal cubonavicular ligament; 7, dorsal cubo-cuneo$_3$ ligaments; 8, dorsal cubo-M$_5$ ligament; 9, dorsal cubo-M$_4$ ligament; 10, dorsal cuneo$_{1-2-3}$-navicular ligaments; 11, dorsal intercuneiform ligaments C$_1$-C$_2$, C$_2$-C$_3$; 12, dorsal cuneometatarsal ligaments C$_1$-M$_1$, C$_1$-M$_2$, C$_2$-M$_2$, C$_3$-M$_2$; 13, dorsal intermetatarsal ligaments M$_2$-M$_3$, M$_3$-M$_4$, M$_4$-M$_5$.) (From Spalteholz W. Hand Atlas of Human Anatomy. Vol 1. JB Lippincott; 1903:219.)

third dorsal cuneonavicular ligament forms a triangular complex in association with the dorsal cuneocuboid ligament and the dorsal cubonavicular ligament (see Fig. 4.45).

There also are three plantar cuneonavicular ligaments (see Figs. 4.56 and 4.57B). The first arises from the anterior and plantar aspect of the tuberosity of the navicular, extends anteriorly as a thick, rectangular, flat cuff, and inserts on the plantar tuberosity of the first cuneiform; this ligament is short and strong. The second and third ligaments arise from the inferior surface of the navicular, between the tuberosity and the beak. They are thin and deep and are masked by the expansions of the tibialis posterior tendon. Each ligament inserts on the posterior segment of the corresponding cuneiform crest. The third ligament is oriented anterolaterally and is the longest; the second ligament is the deepest.

The medial cuneonavicular ligament (Fig. 4.60) is a thick, strong ligament that extends from the medial aspect of the tuberosity of the navicular to the medial aspect of the first cuneiform and receives a few fibers from the tibialis posterior tendon.

The common synovial cavity of the naviculo-cuneiform$_{1-2-3}$ articulation extends expansions into the intercuneiform articulations C_1-C_2, C_2-C_3, the C_3-cuboid articulation, and the naviculocuboid articulation.

▶ **Cuneo$_3$-Cuboid Ligaments**

There are three cuneocuboid ligaments: dorsal, plantar, and interosseous.

The dorsal cuneo$_3$-cuboid ligament (see Figs. 4.58 and 4.59) is a broad, flat ligament extending obliquely anteromedially from the dorsum of the cuboid to the dorsal aspect of the third cuneiform. As mentioned previously, this ligament makes a triangular arrangement with the dorsal cubonavicular and the dorsal cuneo$_3$-navicular ligament. Occasionally this ligament is divided into two fascicles.

The plantar cuneo$_3$-cuboid ligament (see Figs. 4.56 and 4.57B) is a short ligament extending from the medial aspect of the cuboid crest and the segment of the medial border immediately behind it to the posterior segment of the third cuneiform crest.

The interosseous cuneo$_3$-cuboid ligament is a very short but thick ligament binding the two bones and located anterior to their articular surfaces.

INTERCUNEIFORM LIGAMENTS

There are two dorsal, two interosseous, and one plantar intercuneiform ligaments.

The dorsal intercuneiform ligaments (see Figs. 4.58 and 4.59) are small, rectangular bands transversely binding the cuneiforms, the first to the second and the second to the third.

There are two interosseous cuneiform ligaments. The medial interosseous (see Fig. 4.65) is a strong, thick, transverse ligament uniting the first cuneiform with the second. It is located in the angle of the intercuneiform articulating surfaces. Its origin on the first cuneiform is confined to the posterior half of the lateral surface, at least 8 mm posterior to the anterior border. The lateral interosseous ligament is also a short, strong band transversely uniting the second to the third cuneiform; it is located anterior to the intercuneiform articulating surfaces.

The plantar intercuneiform ligament (see Fig. 4.57B), a short ligament, originates on the posterolateral corner of the plantar surface of the first cuneiform. It is directed anterolaterally and inserts on the deeply located crest of the second cuneiform.

LIGAMENTS OF THE TARSOMETATARSAL JOINT

The tarsometatarsal joint (Lisfranc joint), connecting the cuneocuboid block to the bases of the metatarsals, has a complex joint interline configuration. The line is oblique, directed laterally and posteriorly, and presents a dorsolateral convexity corresponding to the transverse cubocuneiform arch (Fig. 4.61). A line drawn through the first metatarsal-cuneiform joint and extended laterally transects the shaft of the fifth metatarsal near the middle. A line drawn through the fifth metatarsal-cuboid joint and extended medially passes behind the head of the first metatarsal (Fig. 4.62).

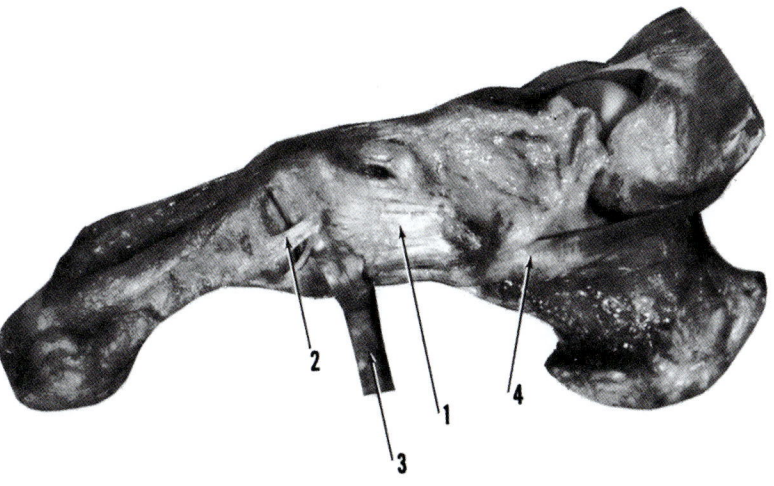

Figure 4.60 Medial aspect of foot. (*1*, Medial cuneo$_1$-navicular ligament; *2*, medial cuneo$_1$-ligament; *3*, reflected tibialis anterior tendon; *4*, tibialis posterior tendon.)

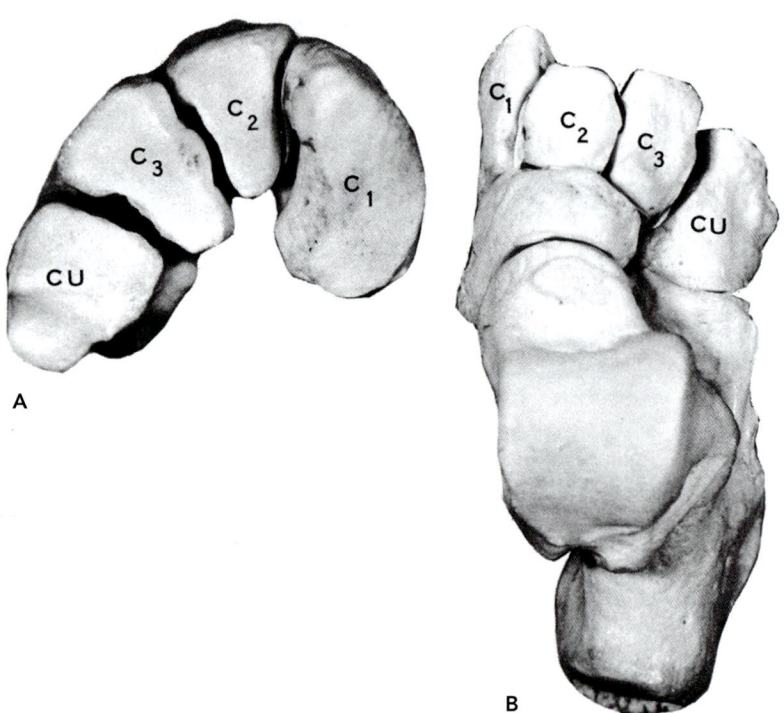

Figure 4.61 (A) Transverse arch formed by cuneiforms (C_1, C_2, C_3) and cuboid (*CU*). (B) Contour of distal cuneiform and cuboid interline with recess of C_2.

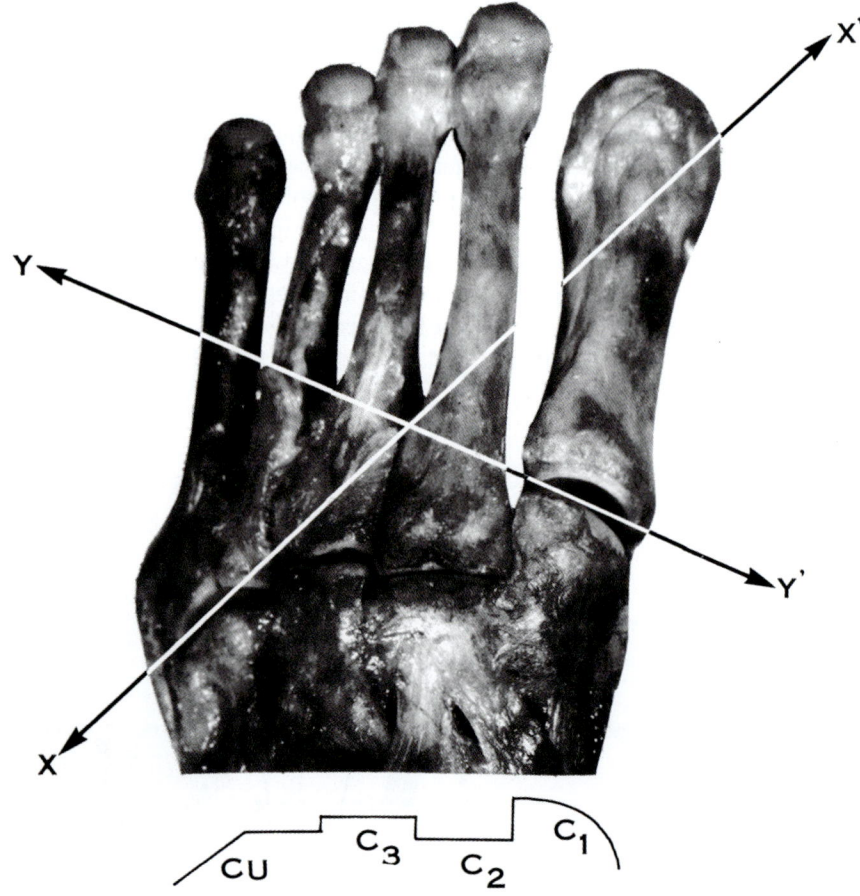

Figure 4.62 Lisfranc (tarsometatarsal) articular interline. Cuneiform$_2$ (C_2) is in recess relative to cuneiform$_1$ (C_1) and cuneiform$_3$ (C_3). A line *YY'* extended from the cuneiform$_1$-metatarsal$_1$ transects the shaft of metatarsal$_5$ in its midsegment. A line *XX'* extended from the cubo-metatarsal$_5$ interline passes behind the head of the first metatarsal. The base of M_2 is locked in the intercuneiform recess at the level of C_2. The cuneiform$_3$ is locked, to a lesser degree, in the intermetatarsal recess at the level of M_3. (*CU*, cuboid.)

The second cuneiform is in proximal recess of 8 mm relative to the first cuneiform and 4 mm relative to the third cuneiform; this creates the cuneiform mortise that will receive its tenon—the base of the second metatarsal. This arrangement enhances the stability of Lisfranc joint. The cuboid is in slight proximal recess of at least 2 mm relative to the third cuneiform; this creates a shallow metatarsal mortise receiving its tenon—the third cuneiform.

The ligaments connecting the cuboid and the cuneiforms to the metatarsal bases are the dorsal, plantar, and interosseous ligaments.

▶ Dorsal Ligaments

There are seven dorsal tarsometatarsal ligaments (see Figs. 4.58 and 4.59).

The base of the first metatarsal is united by a large, thick ligament to the first cuneiform (see Fig. 4.59). This ligament is in a dorsomedial location and is the strongest.

The base of the second metatarsal is secured by three ligaments to the dorsum of the first, second, and third cuneiforms. The first two have an anterolateral obliquity, whereas the third is directed anteromedially.

The base of the third metatarsal is connected by a dorsal ligament to the dorsum of the third cuneiform. An accessory cuboid-cuneiform$_3$-metatarsal$_3$ band may also be present, which is then in continuity with the ligament connecting the base of the fourth metatarsal to the cuboid.

The fifth metatarsal base is connected to the cuboid by a ligament that is in a dorsolateral location. Occasionally a transverse band extends from this ligament to the dorsum of the third cuneiform.

▶ Plantar Ligaments

The plantar cuneometatarsal ligaments (see Fig. 4.57B) are always present on the medial aspect of Lisfranc joint, but they are very variable in number and disposition on the lateral side.[36]

The cuneiform$_1$ is attached to the base of the metatarsal$_1$ by a broad, rectangular ligament. This ligament arises from the plantar aspect of the cuneiform$_1$ near the articular surface, extends slightly outward and distally, and inserts on the lateral half of the first metatarsal base.[36] Proximally, the fibers are seen to be in continuity with the fibers of the inferior cuneo$_1$-navicular ligament.

The cuneo$_1$-metatarsal$_{2,3}$ ligament is a very strong ligament, considered by Sappey to be the key of the tarsometatarsal arch.[15] The ligament originates from the inferolateral surface of the cuneiform$_1$ and soon divides into two bands.[36] The superficial band is the stronger and thicker; it courses obliquely outward and upward and makes a broad insertion on the base of metatarsal$_3$. The deep band is less developed and inserts on the base of metatarsal$_2$.

There is no ligament between cuneiform$_2$ and metatarsal$_2$ on the plantar aspect.

The plantar ligament cuneiform$_3$-metatarsal$_{3,4}$ is inconstant. It originates from the inferolateral surface of the third cuneiform and inserts on the bases of metatarsals 3 and 4. In a study of eight feet, Welti found this ligament absent in three and present with two bands in three (two, cuneo$_3$-metatarsal$_3$; one, cuneo$_3$-metatarsal$_4$).[36] The plantar ligaments between the cuboid and metatarsals 4 and 5 are often absent. Welti finds these ligaments absent in five feet of eight, present as two bands (cubometatarsal$_4$, cubometatarsal$_5$) in one, and present as only one band in two (cubometatarsal$_4$). The ligaments, when present, are small and rectangular. The long cubometatarsal$_5$ ligament, extending from the crest of the cuboid to the base of the fifth metatarsal as a quadrilateral ligament, is a component of the long plantar ligament.

▶ Interosseous Ligaments

There are three sets of interosseous ligaments (Fig. 4.63), corresponding to the first, second, and third cuneometatarsal spaces. There are none in the fourth interspace. An extensive study of the interosseous ligaments, based on the dissection of 50 adult feet, is provided by Thomas.[37]

The first interosseous cuneo$_1$-metatarsal$_2$ ligament (Lisfranc ligament, medial interosseous ligament) is the strongest ligament of the three (Figs. 4.64 and 4.65). It arises from the lateral surface of the first cuneiform in front of the intercuneiform ligament and under the articular surface corresponding to the second metatarsal. The ligament is directed obliquely outward and slightly downward and inserts on the lower half of the medial surface of the second metatarsal base. The ligament measures nearly 1 cm in height and approximately 0.5 cm in thickness. In 22%, this ligament is formed by two bands, each band being 3 to 4 mm thick. In 18%, one band is anterior and the other posterior and, in 4%, there is an inferior and a superior fascicle. The anterior band is nearly always the thinner.

Some secondary fibers may be seen in the interspace running from the first cuneiform near the attachment of Lisfranc ligament to the first metatarsal base. These fibers, seen in 30%, are less than 2 mm in size. In another 30%, small fibrous formations are present, 1 to 2 mm in thickness, extending from the metatarsal insertion of Lisfranc ligament to the base of the first metatarsal.[37]

Lisfranc ligament is separated by an interval of 1 to 2 mm from the dorsal surface of the peroneus longus tendon. Interosseous ligaments connect C_1-C_2, C_2-C_3, and C_3-cuboid.

The second interosseous cuneometatarsal ligament (middle interosseous ligament) has a complex ligamentous arrangement. It is located between the cuneiforms and metatarsals 2 and 3. The ligamentous arrangement in this interspace is very variable. Thomas[37] described the following possibilities, as seen on 50 feet (Fig. 4.66):

Type 1 (48%): The ligament forms a strong, obliquely placed triangular lamina extending from one cuneiform to the

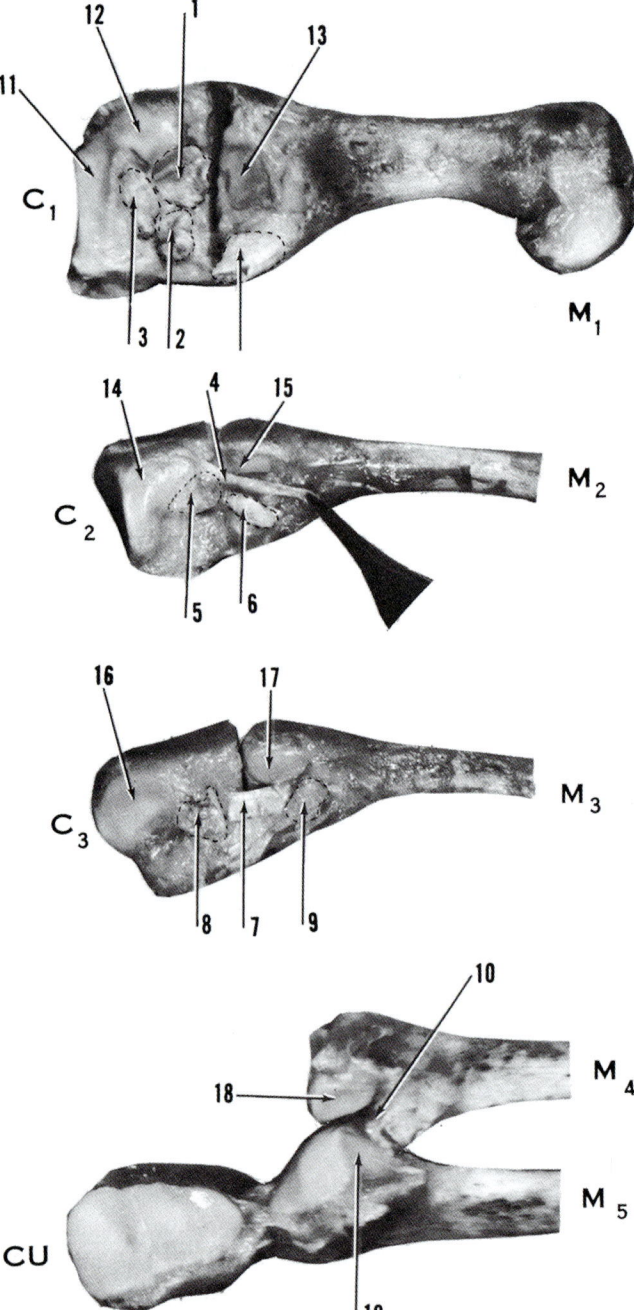

Figure 4.63 Lateral aspect of metatarsocuneiform joints (M_1-C_1, M_2-C_2, M_3-C_3) and intermetatarsal (M_4-M_5) joints. (*1*, Surface of origin of Lisfranc's ligament [cuneiform$_1$-metatarsal$_2$]; *2*, origin of accessory band of C_2-M_2 ligament; *3*, origin of intercuneiform C_1-C_2 ligament; *4*, cuneo$_2$-metatarsal$_3$ ligament; *5*, origin on intercuneiform C_2-C_3 ligament; *6*, origin of intermetatarsal M_2-M_3 ligament; *7*, cuneo$_3$-metatarsal$_3$ ligament; *8*, origin of cuneo$_3$-cuboid ligament; *9*, origin of intermetatarsal M_3-M_4 ligament; *10*, intermetatarsal ligament M_4-M_5; *11*, articular surface of C_1 corresponding to C_2; *12*, articular surface of C_1 corresponding to M_2; *13*, articular surface of M_1 corresponding to M_2; *14*, articular surface of C_2 corresponding to C_3; *15*, articular surface of M_2 corresponding to M_3; *16*, articular surface of C_3 corresponding to cuboid [CU]; *17*, articular surface of M_3 corresponding to M_4; *18*, *19*, articular surfaces of M_4-M_5; *arrowhead in C_2*, peroneus longus tendon.)

corresponding and opposite metatarsals. The origin on the cuneiform represents the apex of the triangle and is located anterior or inferior to the intercuneiform$_{2,3}$ ligament. The metatarsal insertion or base of the triangle is in close connection with the intermetatarsal ligament$_{2,3}$. The ligament divides the interspace into an upper and a lower segment. In 28%, the origin of the ligament is on the second cuneiform, and in 20% it is on the third cuneiform.

Type 2 (22%): A single ligamentous band is present, connecting the cuneiform and the metatarsal of the same ray. The connection of the third cuneiform and the third metatarsal occurs more frequently. The insertions are located under the intercuneiform and intermetatarsal ligaments.

Type 3 (8%): A longitudinal band is present simultaneously, corresponding to each cuneometatarsal ray.

Type 4 (4%): A quadrilateral lamina fills the entire second interspace, dividing it completely into an upper and a lower segment.

Type 5 (8%): This represents a complex arrangement. Longitudinal bands are present along with each cuneometatarsal ray and crossing fibers are present, forming an X. Fibers extend from the second cuneiform to the base of the third metatarsal. Other fibers unite the third cuneiform to the base of the second metatarsal.

Type 6 (10%): The ligament is absent.

The third interosseous cuneometatarsal ligament (lateral interosseous ligament) has a variable morphology. The following arrangements are described by Thomas[37] (Fig. 4.67):

Type 1 (32%; the most frequent arrangement): The ligament extends from the lateral aspect of the third cuneiform to the base of the third metatarsal. The origin is located anterior to the intercuneiform ligament. A similar unilateral arrangement may be present along the cubometatarsal$_4$ ray. This ligament is 2 to 3 mm in thickness.

Type 2 (14%): Two longitudinal bands are present, each corresponding to its cuneo$_3$-metatarsal$_3$ or cubometatarsal$_4$ ray.

Type 3 (20%): A V arrangement is present. The ligament originates from the lateral aspect of the third cuneiform (12%) or from the medial aspect of the cuboid (8%) and inserts on the third and fourth metatarsals. This ligament has very strong fibers.

Type 4 (16%): An oblique band extends from the lateral aspect of the third cuneiform to the base of the fourth metatarsal in 10%. In the remaining 6%, the oblique band originates on the cuboid and inserts on the base of the third metatarsal.

Type 5 (4%): This type is similar to type 4, but a second band is also present, ascending in an oblique manner from the anteroinferior corner of the third cuneiform to the dorsal aspect of the fourth metatarsal.

Type 6 (4%): This ligament, similar to the oblique ligament of type 5, is the only one filling the interspace; it arises from the intercuneiform ligament.

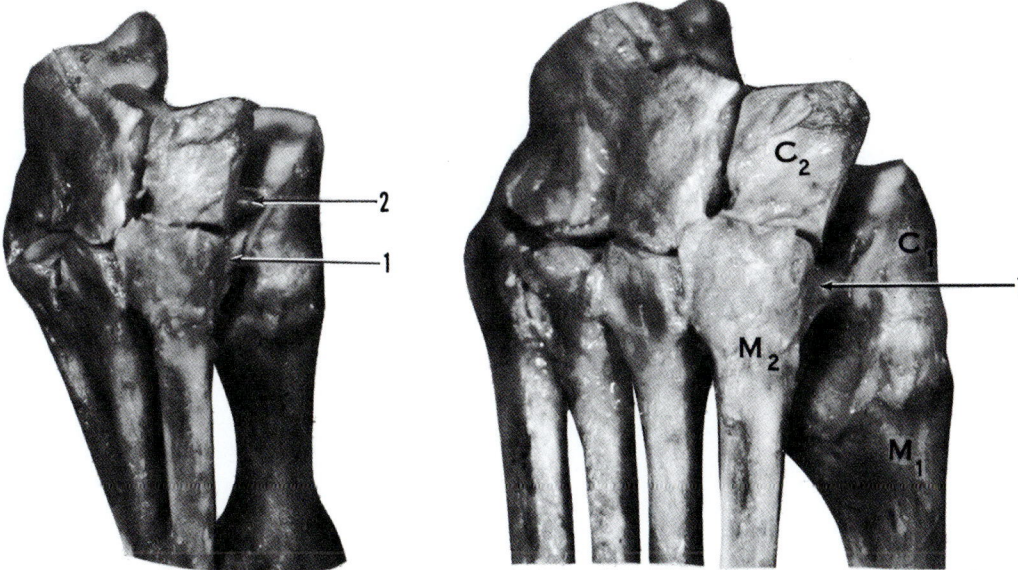

Figure 4.64 Lisfranc ligament. (1, Lisfranc ligament [cuneiform$_1$-metatarsal$_2$]; 2, intercuneiform [C$_1$-C$_2$] ligament.)

Type 7 (4%): There is a V disposition of the ligament (as in type 3) arising from cuneiform$_3$, supplemented by a strong ligament originating from the inferior surface of the intercuneiform ligament, coursing parallel to the fourth metatarsal band.

Type 8 (6%): Weak ligamentous fibers are arranged in an "X".

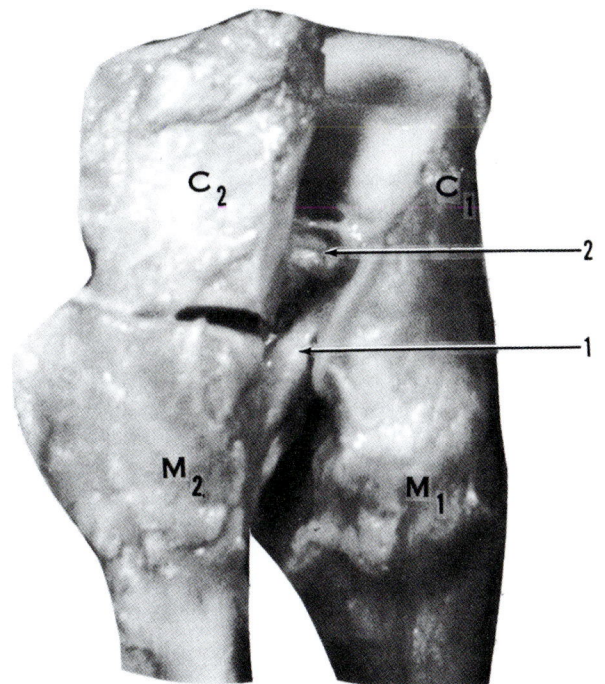

Figure 4.65 Lisfranc ligament. (1, Lisfranc ligament [cuneiform$_1$-metatarsal$_2$]; 2, intercuneiform [C$_1$-C$_2$] ligament.)

INTERMETATARSAL LIGAMENTS

The intermetatarsal ligaments are dorsal, plantar, and interosseous. There is no ligament between metatarsal$_1$ and metatarsal$_2$ on the dorsal or plantar aspect. The interosseous connection between metatarsals 1 and 2 is through poorly individualized weak fibers.

The dorsal intermetatarsal ligaments are three small, thin, flat bands located obliquely on the dorsum of the base of metatarsal$_{2,3}$, metatarsal$_{3,4}$, and metatarsal$_{4,5}$. The middle band is the strongest.

The plantar intermetatarsal ligaments also are three in number with a similar distribution. They are stronger than the dorsal ligaments. They are oriented obliquely, medially, and slightly anteriorly.

The three interosseous ligaments are very short and very strong, determining the intermetatarsal stability. They are located in the posterior aspect of the intermetatarsal space but anteroinferior to the articular surfaces. They are in close connection with the corresponding interosseous cuneometatarsal ligaments.

SYNOVIAL COMPARTMENTS OF THE LISFRANC JOINT

The Lisfranc joint is subdivided into three synovial compartments as described by Poirier et Charpy,[38] Testut,[39] Rouviere,[40] Pernkofp,[41] and recently by de Palma et al.[42] The first synovial compartment, internal, corresponds to the first cuneiform and the first metatarsal base (C$_1$-M$_1$). The second synovial compartment, middle, corresponds to the second and third cuneometatarsal joints (C$_2$-M$_2$ and C$_3$-M$_3$). The third synovial compartment, external, corresponds to the cuboid and the

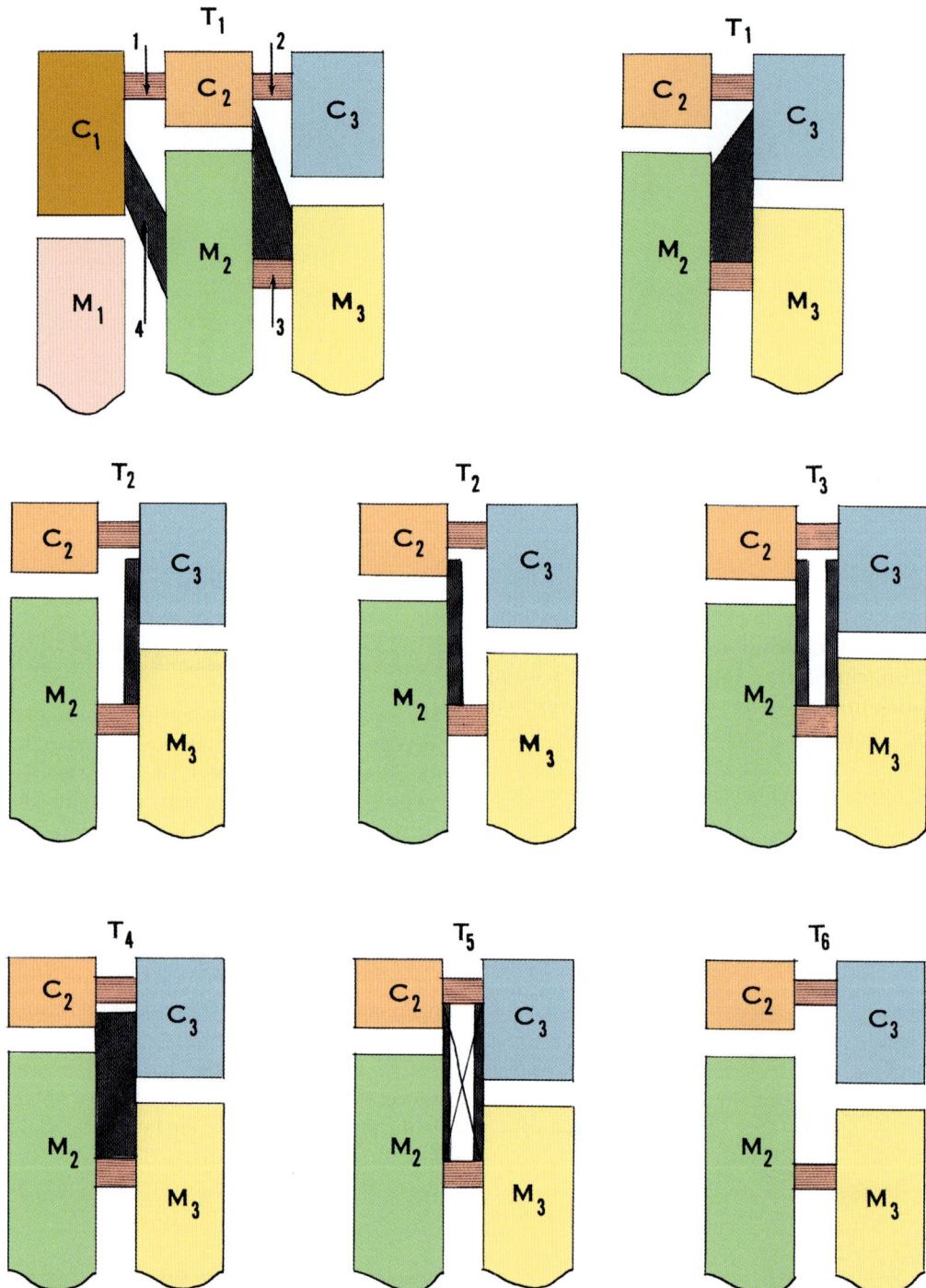

Figure 4.66 Variations of cuneometatarsal ligaments. *Type 1* (T_1), 48%: the second interosseous cuneometatarsal ligament forming a triangular lamina originating from C_2 or C_3 and attached to the metatarsals M_2, M_3. *Type 2* (T_2), 22%: a single ligament present C_3-M_3 (more frequently) or C_2-M_2. *Type 3* (T_3), 8%: two ligaments are present (C_3-M_3 and C_2-M_2). *Type 4* (T_4), 4%: a quadrilateral ligamentous lamina fills the interosseous interspace. *Type 5* (T_5), 8%: longitudinal ligamentous bands C_2-M_2, C_3-M_3 supplemented by crisscrossing fibers C_2 M_3, C_3-M_2. *Type 6* (T_6), 10%: absent ligament. (C_1, cuneiform$_1$; C_2, cuneiform$_2$, C_3, cuneiform$_3$; M_1, metatarsal$_1$; M_2, metatarsal$_2$; M_3, metatarsal$_3$, 1, intercuneiform C_1-C_2 ligament; 2, intercuneiform C_2-C_3 ligament; 3, intermetatarsal M_2-M_3 ligament; 4, Lisfranc ligament C_1-M_2.) (Adapted from Thomas L. Recherches sur les ligaments interosseux de l'articulation de Lisfranc: Etude anatomique et embryologique. *Arch Anat Histol Embryol.* 1926;5:110.)

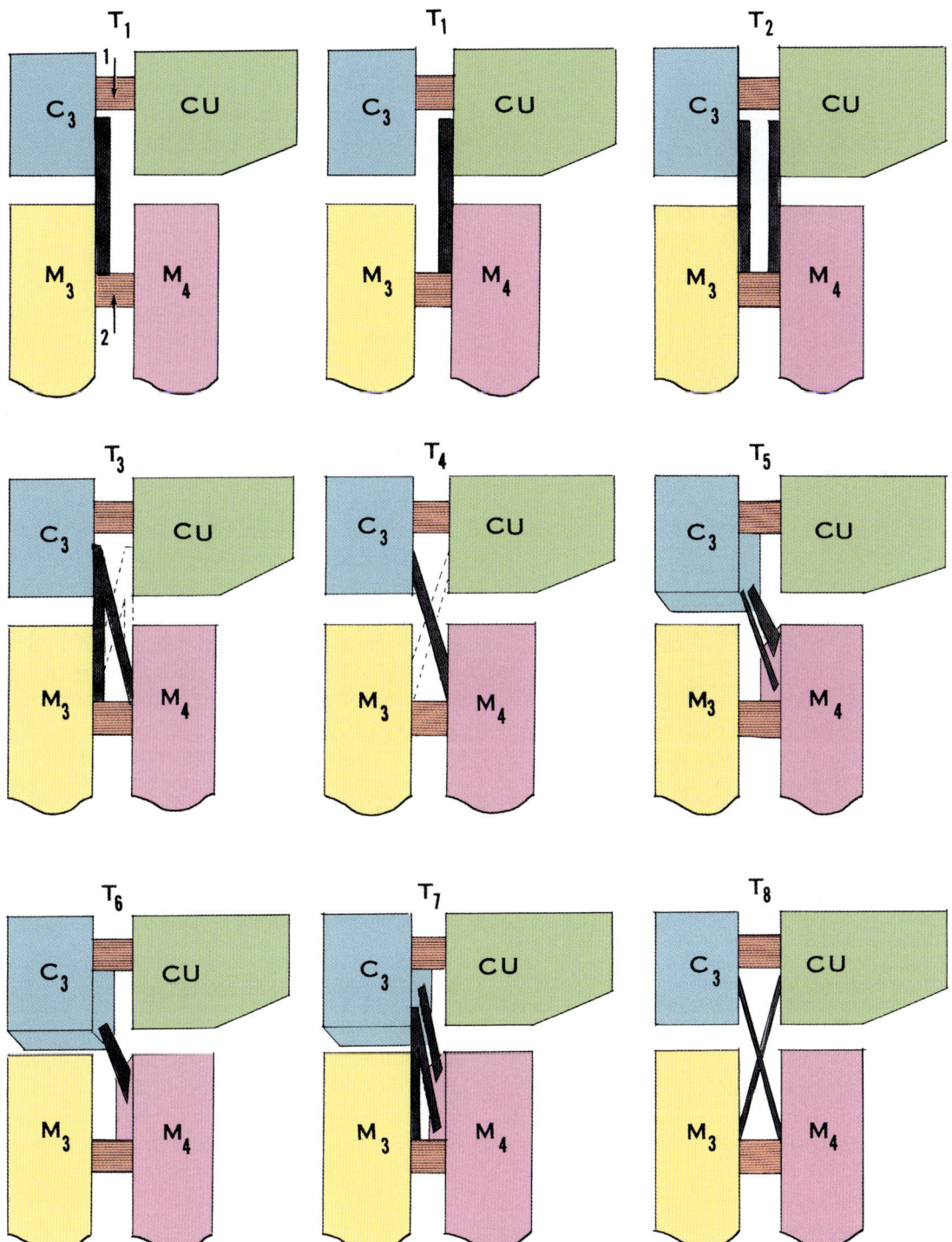

Figure 4.67 Variations of the ligaments of the third interosseous space. Type 1 (T_1), 32%: one ligament present (C_3-M_3 or CU-M_4). Type 2 (T_2), 14%: two ligaments present (C_3-M_3, CU-M_4). Type 3 (T_3), 20%: a V arrangement, the apex of the V being located on C_3 (12%) or on the CU (8%), the distal attachment being to M_3 and M_4. Type 4 (T_4), 16%: oblique ligament C_3-M_4 (10%) or CU-M_3 (6%). Type 5 (T_5), 4%: two oblique ligaments present (C_3-M_4). Type 6 (T_6), 4%: one short oblique band present, extending from the anteroinferior corner of C_3 to the dorsal aspect of M_4. Type 7 (T_7), 4%: a V disposition of the ligament with the apex attached to C_3 and the arms to M_3 and M_4, supplemented by an oblique C_3-M_4 ligament. Type 8 (T_8), 6%: weak ligamentous fibers arranged in X (C_3-M_4, Cu-M_3). (C_3, cuneiform$_3$, CU, cuboid; M_3, metatarsal$_3$, M_4, metatarsal$_4$, 1, C_3-CU ligament; 2, M_3-M_4 ligament.) (Adapted from Thomas L. Recherches sur les ligaments interosseux de l'articulation de Lisfranc: Etude anatomique et embryologique. *Arch Anat Histol Embryol.* 1926;5:110.)

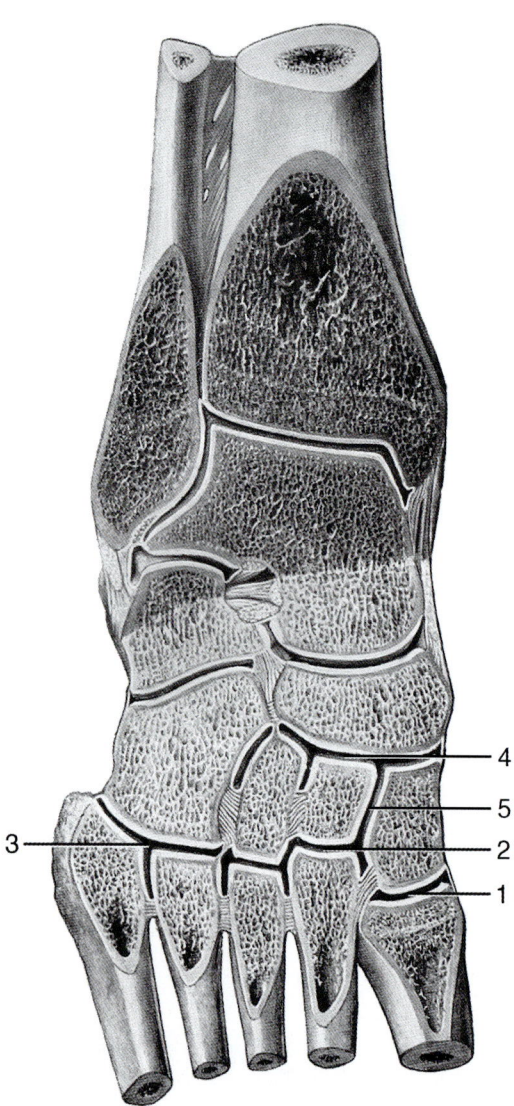

Figure 4.68 **Lisfranc synovial compartments.** Internal: C_1-M_1 (1); middle: C_2-M_2, C_3-M_3, (2) communicating through C_1-C_2 with the scaphocuneo joint (5); external: cubo-M_4-M_5 (3); naviculocuneiform C_1, C_2, C_3 joint (4). (Reprinted from Pernkopf E. *Atlas of Topographical and Applied Human Anatomy.* Urban and Schwarzenberg; 1963:402, Figure 376.)

bases of the fourth and fifth metatarsals (CU-M_4-M_5). The middle synovial compartment communicates posteriorly with the scapho-cuneosynovial cavity (Fig. 4.68).

LIGAMENTS OF METATARSOPHALANGEAL JOINTS AND PROXIMAL PHALANGEAL APPARATUS

At the level of the metatarsophalangeal joint of the lesser toes, the proximal phalanx and the fibrocartilaginous plantar plate form an anatomic and functional unit. They are both suspended from the sides of the metatarsal head through the collateral and the suspensory glenoid ligaments. Furthermore, the plantar plate is connected on each side by the deep transverse intermetatarsal ligament and gives insertion on the plantar side to the fibrous flexor tendon sheath, the two longitudinal septa of the plantar aponeurosis, the transverse head of the adductor hallucis, and vertical fibers extending to the superficial component of the plantar aponeurosis; some of these fibers are arciform and form a preflexor tendinous space retaining the premetatarsal adipose cushion (Figs. 4.69 to 4.71).[43] On the dorsal aspect, the plantar plate gives insertion to the accessory collateral ligament or the metatarsoglenoid suspensory ligament, the transverse lamina of the extensor aponeurosis, and the corresponding interossei muscles at the junction of the deep transverse intermetatarsal ligament with the plantar plate.[44]

The anatomical unit formed by the proximal phalanx, the plantar plate, and their insertional connections is called the phalangeal apparatus; this is the main articular unit of the ball of the foot.

▶ Metatarsophalangeal Ligaments of the Lesser Toes

The lateral ligaments of the metatarsophalangeal joints are divided into metatarsophalangeal collateral ligaments and metatarsoglenoid suspensory ligaments. The lateral ligaments on the peroneal side are thicker and stronger than those on the tibial side.

The metatarsophalangeal ligament originates on the lateral tubercle of the metatarsal heads. It is directed downward and anteriorly and inserts on the lateral tubercle of the base of the proximal phalanx.

The metatarsoglenoid ligament or suspensory ligament originates from the posteroinferior aspect of the lateral metatarsal tubercle of the head. It is triangular (fan shaped), and the fibers descend vertically in the posterior part and obliquely in the anterior part and insert on the lateral border of the plantar plate. The fibers are also in continuity with the lower borders of the metatarsophalangeal collateral ligament.

▶ Interphalangeal Joint Ligaments of the Lesser Toes

The collateral ligaments of the interphalangeal joints extend from the lateral aspect of the head of the corresponding phalanx to the base of the distally located phalanx. When sesamoid bones are present, as described in Chapter 2, they are then an integral part of the plantar plate and offer a small articular surface.

▶ Proximal Phalangeal Apparatus of the Big Toe

The two sesamoids, embedded in the thick fibrous plantar plate and united to the proximal phalanx of the big toe, form an anatomic and functional unit called (by Gillette) the sesamophalangeal apparatus (Fig. 4.72).[45] The sesamophalangeal apparatus moves backward or forward relative to the fixed metatarsal head; in hallux valgus or in traumatic displacements, the sesamoids always follow the proximal phalanx and are displaced with the latter, not with the metatarsal head.

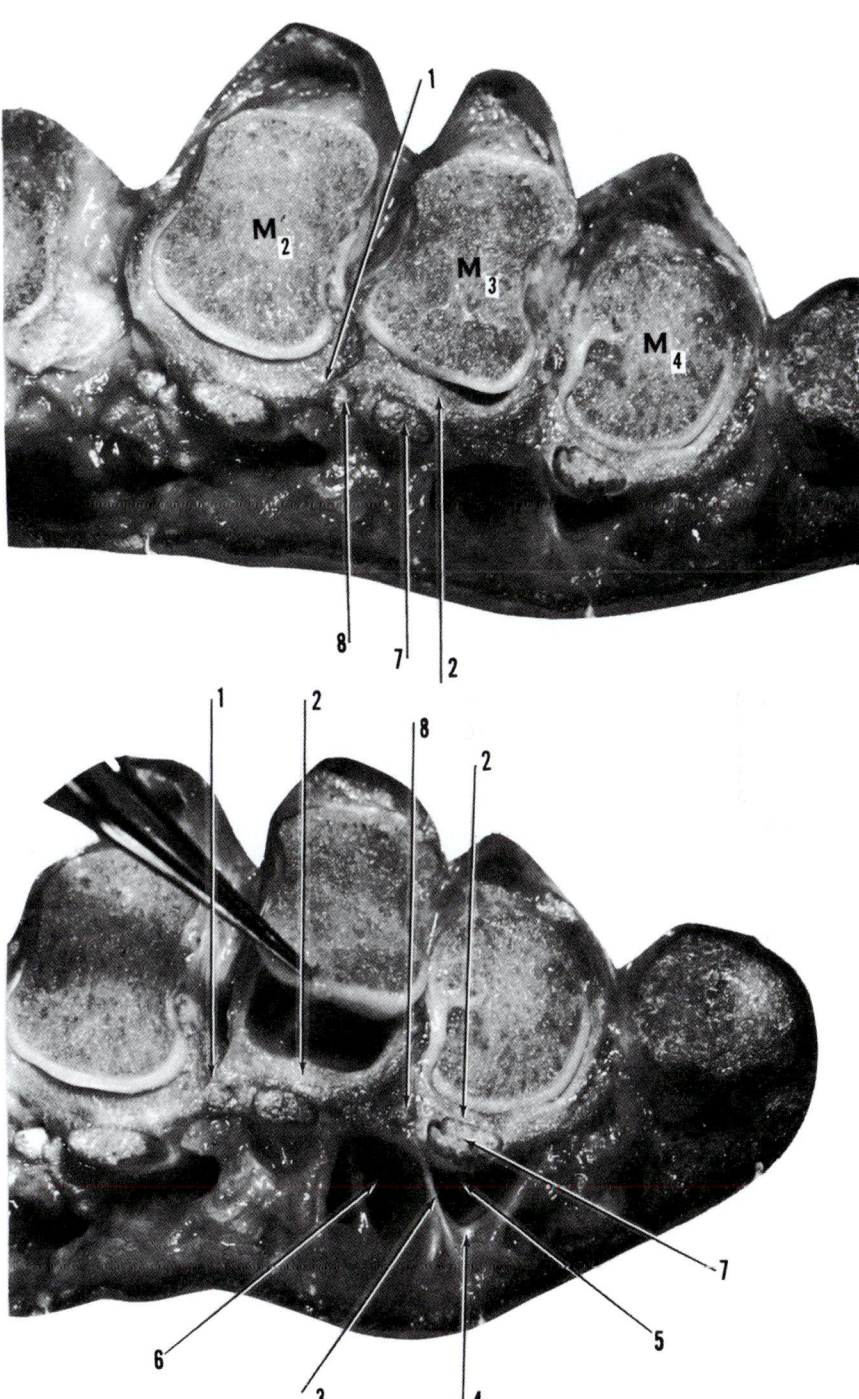

Figure 4.69 Cross-section through metatarsal heads 2, 3, and 4. (*1*, Deep transverse metatarsal ligaments; *2*, plantar plate, fibrocartilaginous; *3*, perpendicular fibers forming with the arciform fibers [*4*] a pretendinous space [*5*] lodging adipose cushion located on plantar aspect of long flexor tendons [*7*]; *6*, space located on plantar aspect of deep transverse metatarsal ligament, lodging the adipose body; *8*, lumbrical tendon in its canal.)

The smaller, upper portion of the metatarsal head is convex in the vertical and transverse direction and corresponds to the glenoid cavity of the proximal phalanx. The larger, inferior two-thirds of the metatarsal head has a median crest separating two small, obliquely oriented trochlear surfaces, each corresponding to a sesamoid. The medial sesamoid is slightly larger than the lateral and each sesamoid has an anteroposterior concavity that corresponds to the lateral contour of the metatarsal head and a slight transverse convexity. Occasionally, a definite smooth anteroposterior crest is recognizable, the mid axis of the sesamoid corresponding to the mid axis of the corresponding metatarsal trochlear surface.

The two sesamoids are united by a thick intersesamoid ligament (Figs. 4.72 and 4.73). Each sesamoid is united, by an ill-defined short sesamophalangeal ligament, to the base of the proximal phalanx, which makes the distal attachment to the plantar plate stronger on the sides and weaker centrally. On the intra-articular surface of the plantar plate, a transverse band

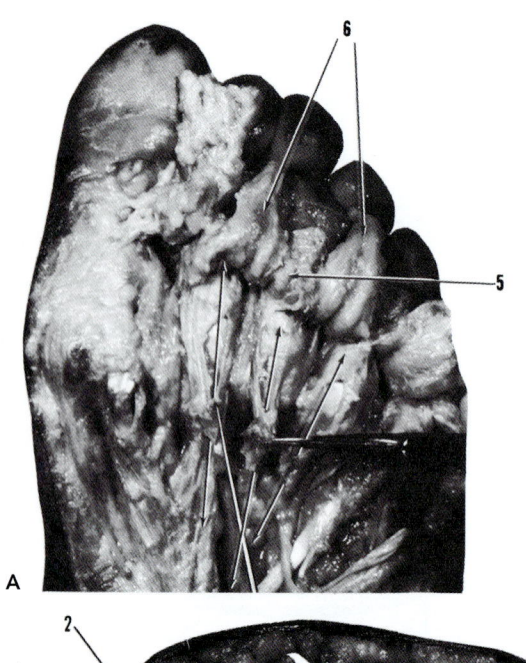

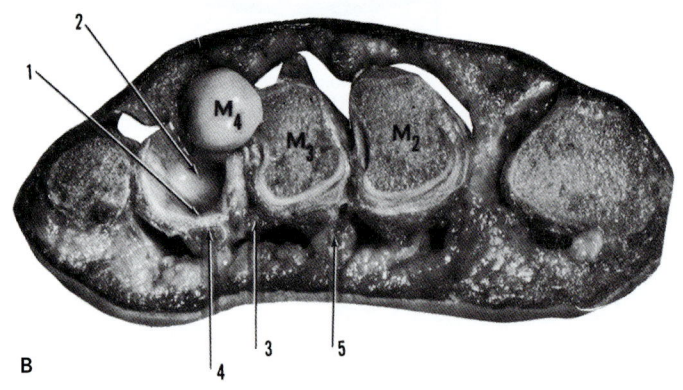

Figure 4.70 (**A**) *Arrows* indicate the direction of the long flexor tendons passing through the foramina delineated by the longitudinal septa of the plantar aponeurosis. (*5*, Adipose preflexor **tendon cushion, reflected;** *6*, **adipose body, reflected from the intermetatarsal head space.**) (**B**) **Cross-section through metatarsal heads M_{2-4}.** (*1*, Plantar plate; *2*, base of proximal phalanx; *3*, lumbrical tendon and canal; *4*, long flexor tendons and their fibrous tunnel; *5*, preflexor fat cushion retained within preflexor space [see Fig. 4.66].)

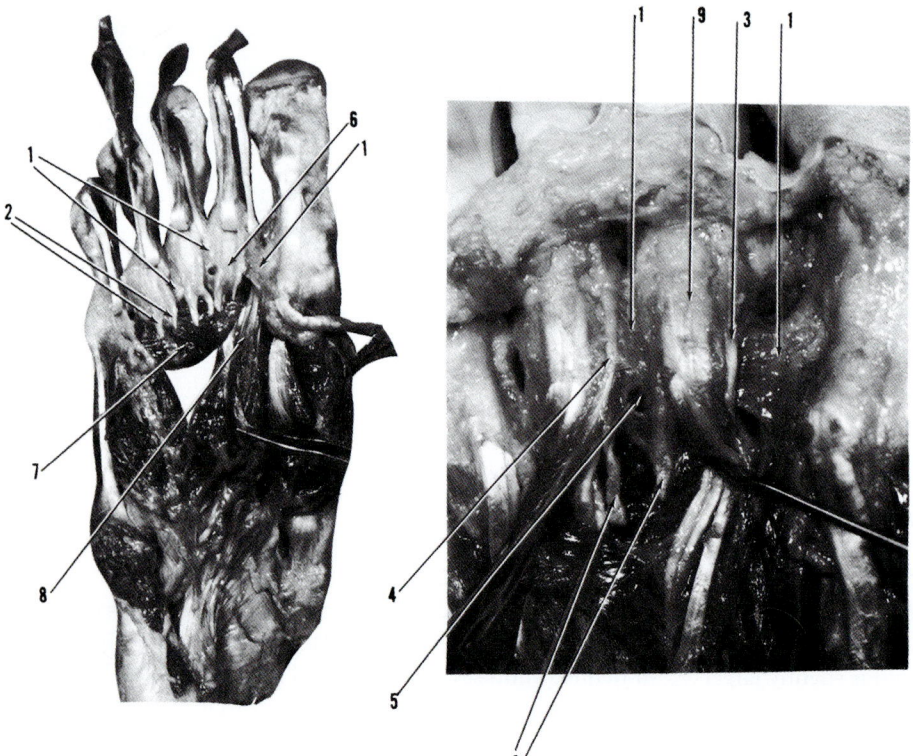

Figure 4.71 Deep transverse metatarsal ligament. (*1*, Deep transverse metatarsal ligament; *2*, insertion of longitudinal septa of plantar aponeurosis on plantar plate [*6*] and over aponeurosis covering transverse head of adductor hallucis muscle [*7*]; *3*, lumbrical tendon crossing plantar aspect of *1*; *4*, thin tunnel of lumbrical tendon; *5*, foramina for passage of common digital artery; *8*, oblique head of adductor hallucis muscle; *9*, flexor digitorum longus and brevis tendons.)

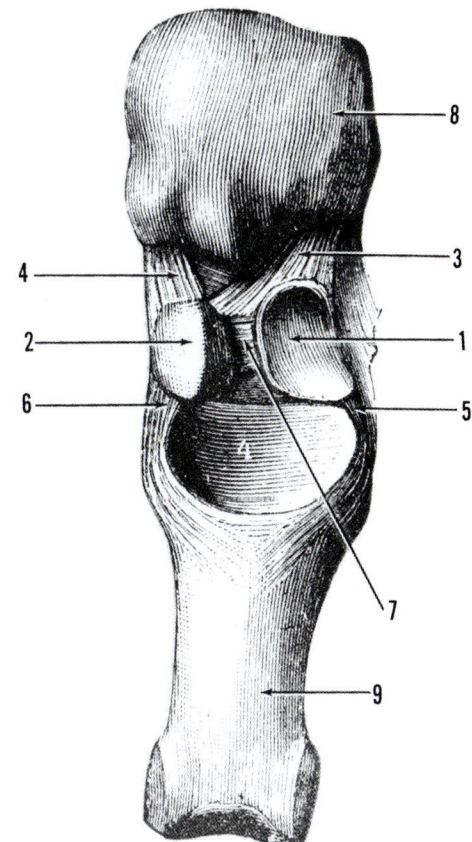

Figure 4.72 Phalangeosesamoid apparatus of the big toe. (*1*, Medial sesamoid; *2*, lateral sesamoid; *3*, medial metatarsosesamoid ligament; *4*, lateral metatarsosesamoid ligament; *5*, medial phalangeosesamoid ligament; *6*, lateral phalangeosesamoid ligament; *7*, intersesamoid ligament; *8*, head of first metatarsal; *9*, proximal phalanx of big toe.) (From Gillette. Des os sésamoides. *Anat Physiol Normal Pathol.* 1872;8:506.)

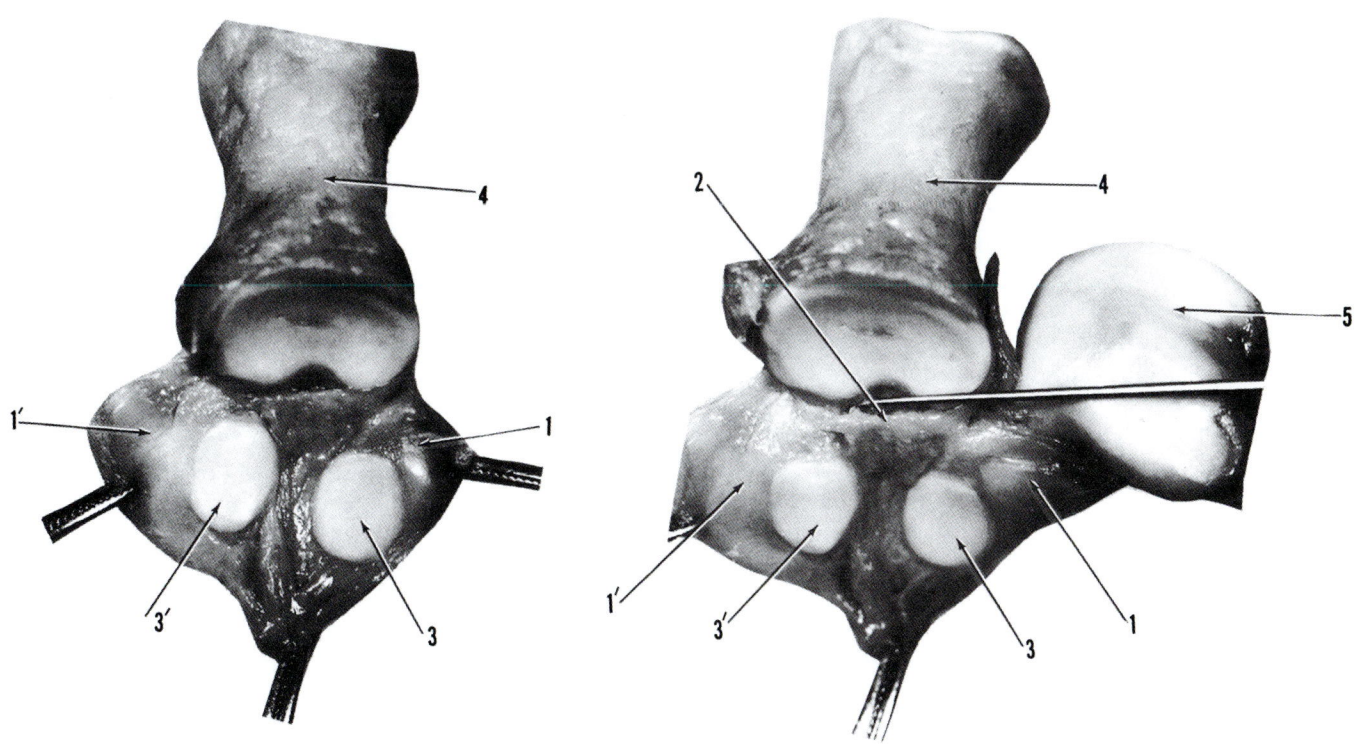

Figure 4.73 Phalangeosesamoid apparatus of the big toe. (Metatarsosesamoid ligaments, medial [*1'*] and lateral [*1*]; *2*, transverse band uniting the sesamophalangeal ligaments; sesamoids, medial [*3'*] and lateral [*3*]; *4*, proximal phalanx; *5*, metatarsal head.)

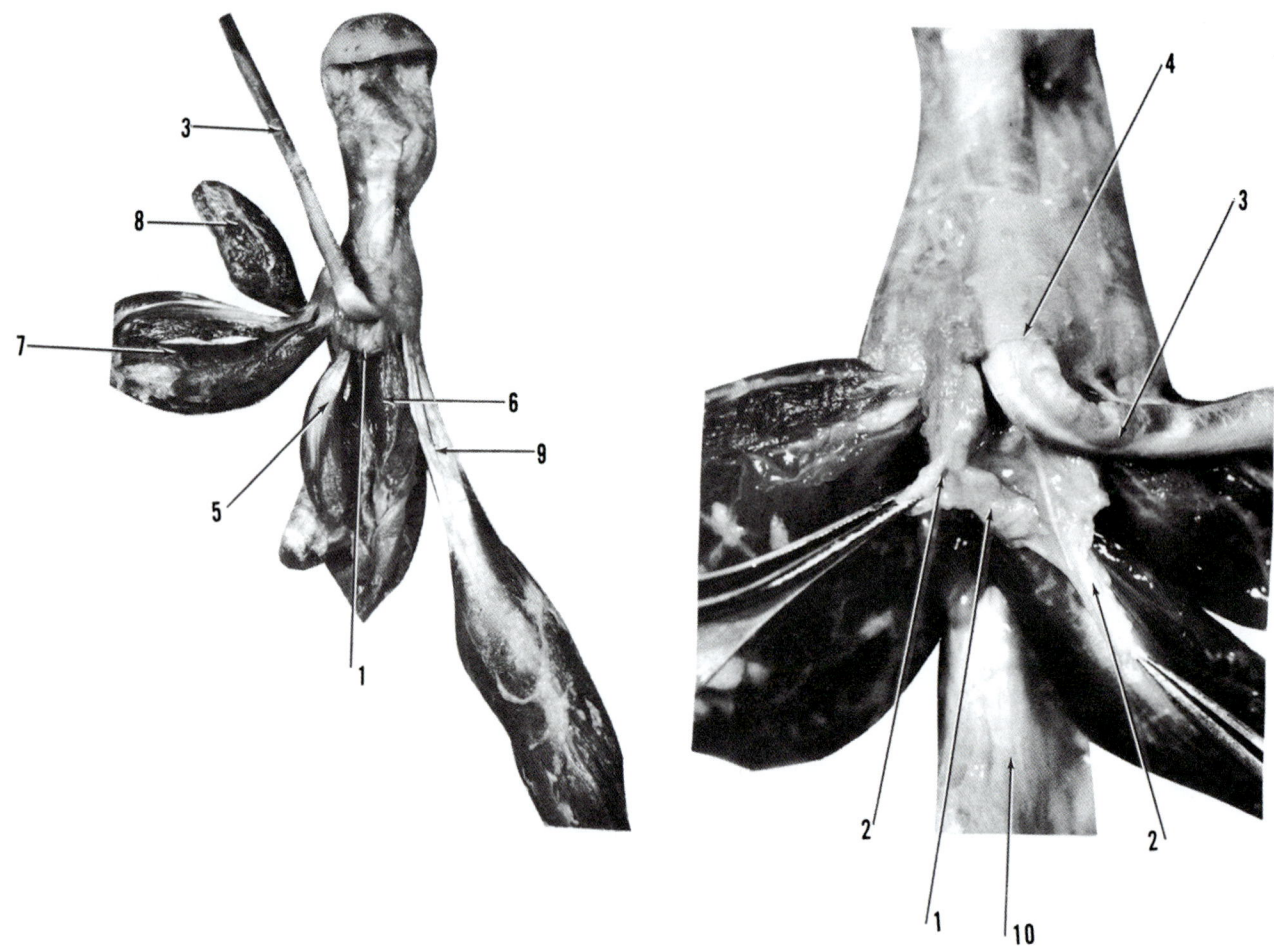

Figure 4.74 **Plantar aspect of the big toe.** (*1*, Proximal border of plantar plate; *2*, insertion of longitudinal septa on plantar plate; *3*, flexor hallucis longus tendon; *4*, flexor hallucis longus tunnel; *5*, flexor hallucis brevis muscle, lateral head; *6*, flexor hallucis brevis muscle, medial head; *7*, adductor hallucis muscle, oblique head; *8*, adductor hallucis muscle, transverse head; *9*, abductor hallucis muscle-tendon; *10*, first metatarsal.)

extends from one sesamophalangeal ligament to the other and the distal border of this band forms with the inferior concave border of the proximal phalanx a triangular small space lodging synovial tissue. The intersesamoid segment of the plantar plate corresponds to the crest of the metatarsal head and longitudinally running fibers cover the area and blend with the more distal transverse band. Obliquely oriented fibers may be seen crossing the most proximal segment of the plate in a medial-to-lateral direction. Each side of the plantar plate receives the insertion of the corresponding metatarsosesamoid suspensory ligament.

The proximal border of the plantar plate is complex (Fig. 4.74). The central segment is in continuity proximally with synovial-type tissue and anchors on the neck of the first metatarsal. This central segment provides attachment to the two vertical septa of the plantar aponeurosis of the first ray and also blends with the proximal segment of the fibrous tunnel of the flexor hallucis longus tendon. The lateral and medial segments of the proximal border of the plantar plate give partial insertion to the lateral and medial heads of the flexor hallucis brevis, respectively (Fig. 4.75).

The plantar surface of the plantar plate is raised on each side by the medial and lateral sesamoids. Between the two, a groove for the flexor hallucis longus tendon is formed, converted into a fibrous tunnel by arcuate fibers. These fibers receive contributions from the two vertical septa of the plantar aponeurosis. The floor of the long flexor tunnel is formed by a transverse fibrocartilaginous-like ligament. Occasionally a smaller transverse subband is seen proximally. A triangular tendon-like structure extends from the distal border of the transverse ligament and the apex fades away distally at the level of the proximal phalanx.

The sesamoids are foci of insertion. The proximal segment of each sesamoid gives insertion to the corresponding head of the flexor hallucis brevis. The lateral head of the flexor hallucis brevis enters into its own fibrous tunnel prior to the insertion on the sesamoid. The deep transverse metatarsal ligament attaches longitudinally along the lateral sesamoid. Dorsal to this ligament, the lateral sesamoid gives insertion to the oblique and transverse components of the adductor hallucis muscle. The medial sesamoid also receives insertional fibers from the abductor hallucis. Vertical fibrous bands extend from the sides

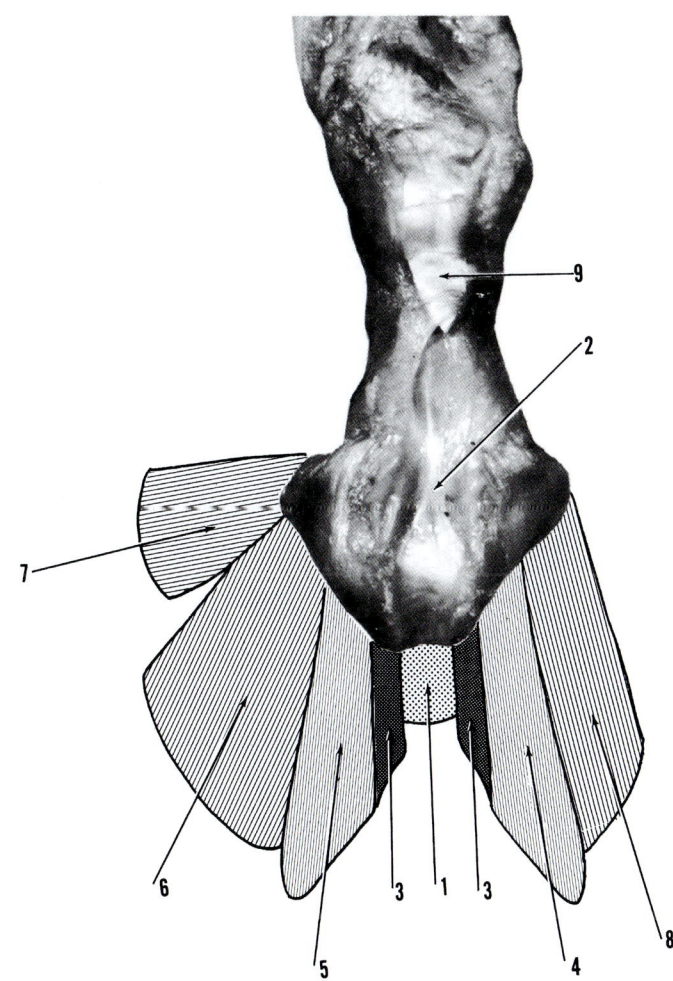

Figure 4.75 **Plantar aspect of plantar plate of the big toe and diagrammatic representation of the insertion sites.** (*1*, Plantar plate; *2*, triangular tendonlike structure extending from thick intersesamoid ligament to proximal phalanx; *3*, longitudinal septa; *4*, medial head of flexor hallucis brevis; *5*, lateral head of flexor hallucis brevis; *6*, oblique head of adductor hallucis; *7*, transverse head of adductor hallucis; *8*, abductor hallucis; *9*, flexor hallucis longus tendon.)

of the sesamoids and the flexor hallucis longus tendon sheath and connect with the superficial band of the plantar aponeurosis. Some of these fibers curve over the fibrous flexor tunnel and form a pre-flexor tendon compartment retaining an adipose cushion, which also covers both sesamoids. From the dorsal aspect, the transverse lamina of the extensor hallucis longus aponeurosis inserts along the lateral and medial borders of the plantar plate.

▶ Metatarsophalangeal Ligaments of the Big Toe

The metatarsal head is united to the proximal phalangeal apparatus by two sets of ligaments: the lateral collateral ligaments and the metatarsosesamoid suspensory ligaments (Figs. 4.76 to 4.78). These two sets originate from the lateral tubercle of the metatarsal head, the origin of the lateral collateral ligament slightly covering the origin of the suspensory ligament. From their origin, the ligaments fan out in a triangular manner. The lateral collateral ligament is directed downward anteriorly and inserts on the tubercle at the base of the proximal phalanx. The thick metatarsosesamoid or suspensory ligament descends vertically and inserts on the lateral and medial borders of the plantar plate. The posterior border of the lateral collateral ligament is in continuity with the suspensory ligament and the anatomic separation is nearly artificial. These two ligaments are identified mostly by their insertions.

▶ Interphalangeal Joint Ligaments of the Big Toe

The interphalangeal joint of the big toe may possess a sesamoid bone, median and transversely oriented, embedded in the plantar plate and located above the flexor hallucis longus tendon. The superior articular surface of the sesamoid is divided by a transverse crest into two facets—one anterior, articulating with the distal phalanx, and one posterior, corresponding to the head of the proximal phalanx. The sesamoid is connected to the sides of the distal phalanx with two small ligaments.[45] Two collateral ligaments extend from the lateral aspect of the proximal phalangeal head to the tubercle at the base of the distal phalanx.

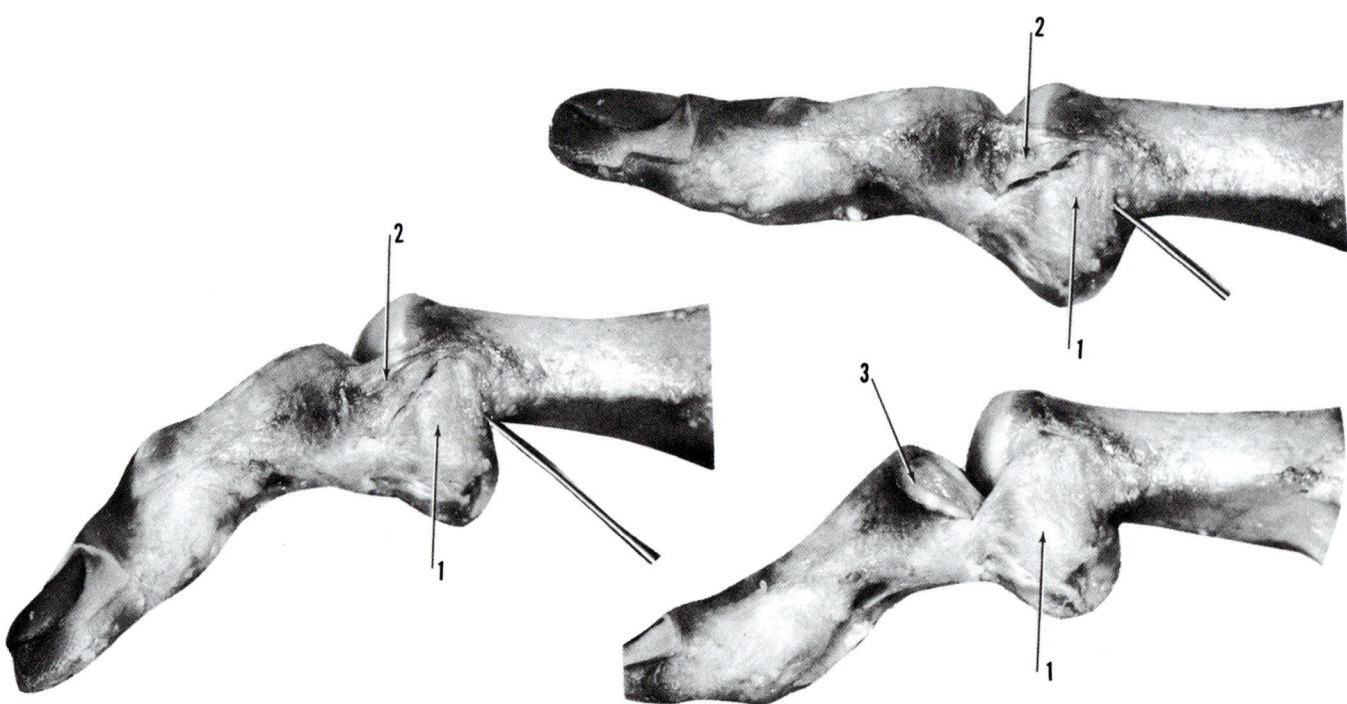

Figure 4.76 Metatarsophalangeal joint of the big toe; medial aspect. (*1*, Medial metatarsosesamoid or suspensory ligament; *2*, medial metatarsophalangeal ligament reflected as *3*.)

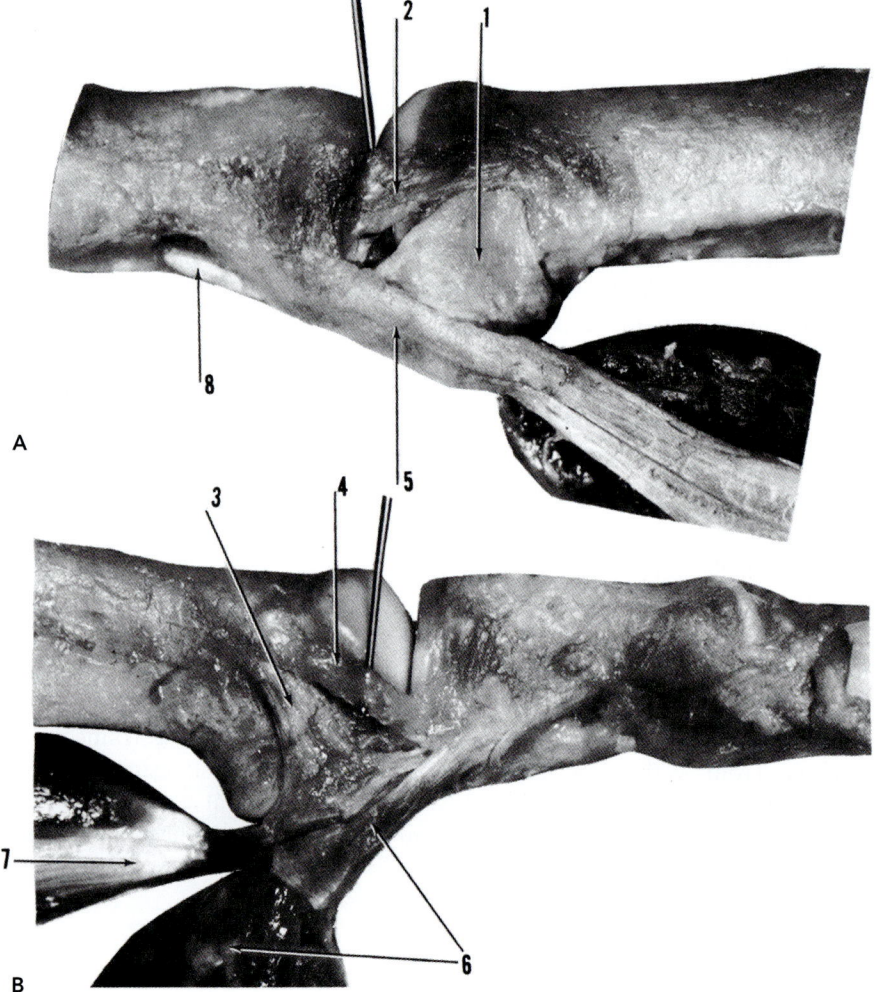

Figure 4.77 Metatarsophalangeal joint of the big toe. (A) Medial aspect. **(B)** Lateral aspect. (*1*, Medial metatarsosesamoid ligament; *2*, medial metatarsophalangeal ligament; *3*, lateral metatarsosesamoid ligament; *4*, lateral metatarsophalangeal ligament; *5*, tendon of abductor hallucis muscle; *6*, adductor hallucis muscle-tendon; *7*, flexor hallucis brevis, lateral head; *8*, flexor hallucis longus tendon.)

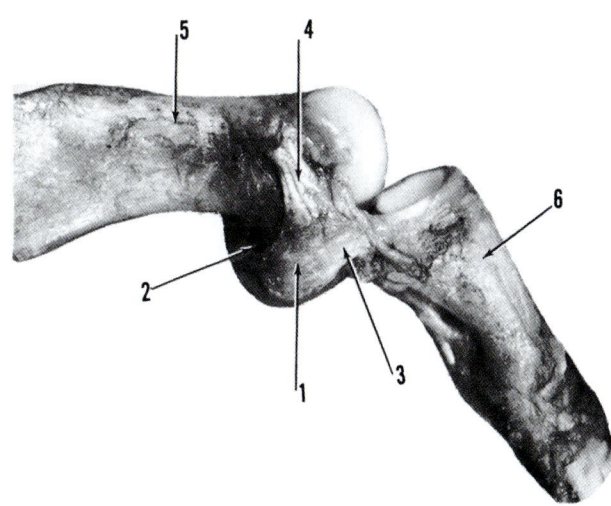

Figure 4.78 **Metatarsophalangeal joint of the big toe, lateral aspect.** (*1*, Sesamoid; *2*, proximal border of plantar plate; *3*, sesamophalangeal ligament; *4*, suspensory metatarsosesamoid ligament; *5*, metatarsal; *6*, proximal phalanx.)

REFERENCES

1. Morris HL. *The Anatomy of the Joints of Man*. Churchill; 1879:384.
2. Poirier P, Charpy A. *Traité d'Anatomie Humaine*. Vol 1. Masson; 1899:756-762.
3. Testut L. *Traité d'Anatomie Humaine*. Vol 1. Doin; 1921:630-638.
4. Prins JG. Diagnosis and treatment of injury to the lateral ligament of the ankle. *Acta Chir Scand Suppl*. 1978;486:23.
5. Ruth CJ. The surgical treatment of injuries of the fibular collateral ligaments of the ankle. *J Bone Joint Surg [Am]*. 1961;43:229.
6. Milner CE, Soames RW. Anatomical variations of the anterior talofibular ligament of the human ankle joint. *J Anat*. 1997;191:457-458.
7. Milner CE, Soames RW. Anatomy of the collateral ligaments of the human ankle joint. *Foot Ankle Int*. 1998;19(11):757-760.
8. Laidlaw PL. The varieties of the os calcis. *J Anat Physiol*. 1904;38:138.
9. Trouilloud A, Dia A, Grammont P, et al. Variations du ligament calcaneo-fibulaire (lig. calcane fibulare). Applications a la cinématique de la cheville. *Bull Assoc Anat*. 1988;72:31.
10. Paturet G. *Traité d'Anatomie Humaine*. Vol 2. Masson; 1951:704-727.
11. Dujarier CH. *Anatomie des Membres: Dissection—Anatomie Topographique*. 2nd ed. Masson; 1924:399-407.
12. Rouviére J, Canela Lazaro M. Le ligament péroneo-astragalocalcanéen. *Ann Anat Pathol Anat Normal*. 1932;9:745.
13. Beau A. Recherches sur le développement et la constitution morphologiques de l'articulation du cou-de-pied chez l'homme. *Arch Anat Histol Embryol*. 1939;26:238.
14. Barclay-Smith E. The astragalo-calcaneo navicular joint. *J Anat Physiol*. 1896;30:390.
15. Sappey PC. *Traité d'Anatomie Descriptive*. Vol 1. 4th ed. Delahaye, Lecrosnier; 1888:712-728.
16. Toldt C. *Anatomischer Atlas für Studirende und Ärzte*. 2nd ed. Urban und Schwarzenberg; 1900:242-243.
17. Warwick R, Williams PL, eds. *Gray's Anatomy*. 35th ed. WB Saunders; 1973:460-461.
18. Yashar J. Contribution à l'étude des ligaments des articulations tibiotarsienne et médio-tarsienne. *Arch Anat Histol Embryol Normal Exp*. 1961;44:25.
19. Pankovich AM, Shivaram MS. Anatomical basis of variability in injuries of the medial malleolus and the deltoid ligament. I. Anatomical studies. *Acta Orthop Scand*. 1979;50:217.
20. Fick R. *Handbuch der Anatomie und Mechanik der Glenke*. Vol 1. Fischer; 1904:410-414.
21. Bourgery J. *Traité Complet de l'Anatomie de l'Homme*. Vol 1. Hachette Livre-BnF; 1832.
22. Henle J. *Handbuch der Systematischen Anatomie des Menschen*. Vol 3. Braunschweig; 1856:160-163.
23. Lane AS. The causation, pathology and physiology of several of the deformities which develop during young life. *Guy's Hosp Rep*. 1887;44:254.
24. Volkmann R. Ein ligamentum "neglectum" pedis (lig. calcaneonaviculare mediodorsale seu sustentaculo-naviculare). *Verhandlungen Anat Ges*. 1970;64:483.
25. Taniguchi A, Tanaka Y, Takakura Y, et al. Anatomy of the spring ligament. *J Bone Joint Surg Am*. 2003;85:2174-2178.
26. Köktürk. Remarques sur le ligament de Chopart (lig. bifurcatum). *Comptes-Rendus Assoc Anat*. 1957;44:380.
27. Hovelacque A, Sourdin A. Note au sujet de quelques ligaments de l'articulation médio-tarsienne. *Ann Anat Pathol Anat Normal*. 1933;10:469.
28. Jones WF. *Structure and Function as Seen in the Foot*. 2nd ed. Baillière; 1949:120.
29. Cahill DR. The anatomy and function of the contents of the human tarsal sinus and canal. *Anat Rec*. 1965;153:1.
30. Smith JW. The ligamentous structures in the canalis and sinus tarsi. *J Anat*. 1958;92:616.
31. DiGiovanni CW, Langer PR, Nickish F, et al. Proximity of the lateral talar process to the lateral stabilizing ligaments of the ankle and subtalar joint. *Foot Ankle Int*. 2007;2:175-180.
32. Dorn-Lange NV, Nauck T, Lohrer H, et al. Morphology of the dorsal and lateral calcaneocuboid ligaments. *Foot Ankle Int*. 2008;29:942-949.
33. Patil V, Ebraheim N, Wagner R, et al. Morphometric dimensions of the dorsal calcaneocuboid ligament. *Foot Ankle Int*. 2008;5:508-512.
34. Spalteholz W. *Hand Atlas of Human Anatomy*. Vol 1. JB Lippincott; 1903:219, 223.
35. Ward KA, Soames RW. Morphology of the plantar valacaneocuboid ligaments. *Foot Ankle Int*. 1997;18:649-653.
36. Welti H. Contribution a l'étude du ligament I cuneiforme II/III metatarsiens—etude d'anatomie comparée. *Arch Histol Embryol*. 1966;48:373.
37. Thomas L. Recherches sur les ligaments interosseux de l'articulation de Lisfranc: Etude anatomique et embry. *Arch Anat Histol Embryol*. 1926;5:104.
38. Poirier P, Charpy P. *Traite d'"Anatomie Humaine*. Masson; 1899:784-785.
39. Testut L. *Traite d'Anatomie Humaine Livre II Arthrologie Tome*. Librairie Ovtave Doin; 1921:654.
40. Rouviere H. *Anatomie Humaine-Descriptive, topographique et fonctionelle*. Vol 3. 11th ed. Masson; 1979:336.
41. Pernkopf E. *Atlas of Topographical and Applied Human Anatomy*. Urban Schwarzenberg; 1963:402.
42. de Palma L, Santucci A, Sabetta SP, et al. Anatomy of Lisfranc joint complex. *Foot Ankle Int*. 1997;18(6):356-364.
43. Bojsen-Møller F, Flagstad KE. Plantar aponeurosis and internal architecture of the ball of the foot. *J Anat*. 1976;121:599.
44. Meyer P. Contribution à l'étude de la region métatarsophalangienne. *Comptes-Rendus Assoc Anat*. 1958;44:500.
45. Gillette. Des os sesamoides. *J Anat Physiol Normal Pathol*. 1872;8:506.

Myology

Shahan K. Sarrafian and Armen S. Kelikian

In the anatomic position, the foot is in a transverse plane relative to the leg; all the extrinsic tendons destined for the midfoot and forefoot make the necessary turn around the ankle and are retained by their corresponding retinacular systems acting as pulleys. The detailed anatomy of these retaining systems was discussed in Chapter 3.

ANTERIOR ASPECT OF THE ANKLE AND DORSUM OF THE FOOT

Four tendons are present on the anterior aspect of the ankle: the tibialis anterior, the extensor hallucis longus, the extensor digitorum longus, and the peroneus tertius.

▶ Tibialis Anterior

The flat tendon of the tibialis anterior acquires its first retaining tunnel under the superior extensor retinaculum (Fig. 5.1). From the anteromedial aspect of the ankle, the tendon courses toward the medial border of the foot. It makes a twist and inserts vertically over a tubercle on the inferomedial aspect of the first metatarsal base and on the medial aspect of the first cuneiform. Retaining tunnels are provided by the superomedial and inferomedial bands of the inferior extensor retinaculum. A terminal tunnel may be formed by the transverse retinacular band over the first metatarsal bone. The interretinacular segments of the tendon are covered by the thin dorsal aponeurosis of the foot.

Variations

The insertional variations of the tibialis anterior may be grouped under bifurcations, extensions of attachment, and loss of attachment.[1-3] Hallisy, in a comprehensive study of 290 ft, reported 90% with customary insertion of the tibialis anterior tendon on the base of the first metatarsal and first cuneiform and 10% with insertional variations (Fig. 5.2).[3]

Bifurcation

The tibialis anterior tendon may be bifid.[1-5] The anterior tendon inserts on the base of the first metatarsal and the posterior tendon on the first cuneiform. The division of the tendon may extend 1 to 2 cm above the cuneometatarsal joint or may, rarely, reach the muscular fibers or even separate the muscle fibers a length of 1.5 cm.[1] Between these two extremes, all the intermediaries may exist.

Extensions of Attachment

The tibialis anterior tendon may insert additionally on the navicular, forming a fan-shaped tendon; on the base of the proximal phalanx of the big toe; on the distal dorsal part of the first metatarsal; on the adjacent parts of the first metatarsal head and proximal phalanx[1]; on the inferior extensor retinaculum and dorsal aponeurosis of the foot; on the talus and calcaneus with another band reaching the navicular and the first cuneiform; on the neck of the talus and the capsule of the ankle joint; or on the plantar aponeurosis.[1-3,5-7]

Loss of Attachment

There may be loss of attachment with insertion on the first metatarsal base only.[3]

Additional Muscle Variants

Three additional muscles may be present as variants of the tibialis anterior muscle: musculus tibioastragalus anticus of Gruber, musculus tibiofascialis anticus of Macalister, or musculus tensor fasciae dorsalis pedis.[1-3,8,9]

Musculus Tibioastragalus Anticus of Gruber

Gruber describes three cases of a muscle located behind the tibialis anterior, originating from the tibia and the interosseous membrane and inserting on the lateral aspect of the talar

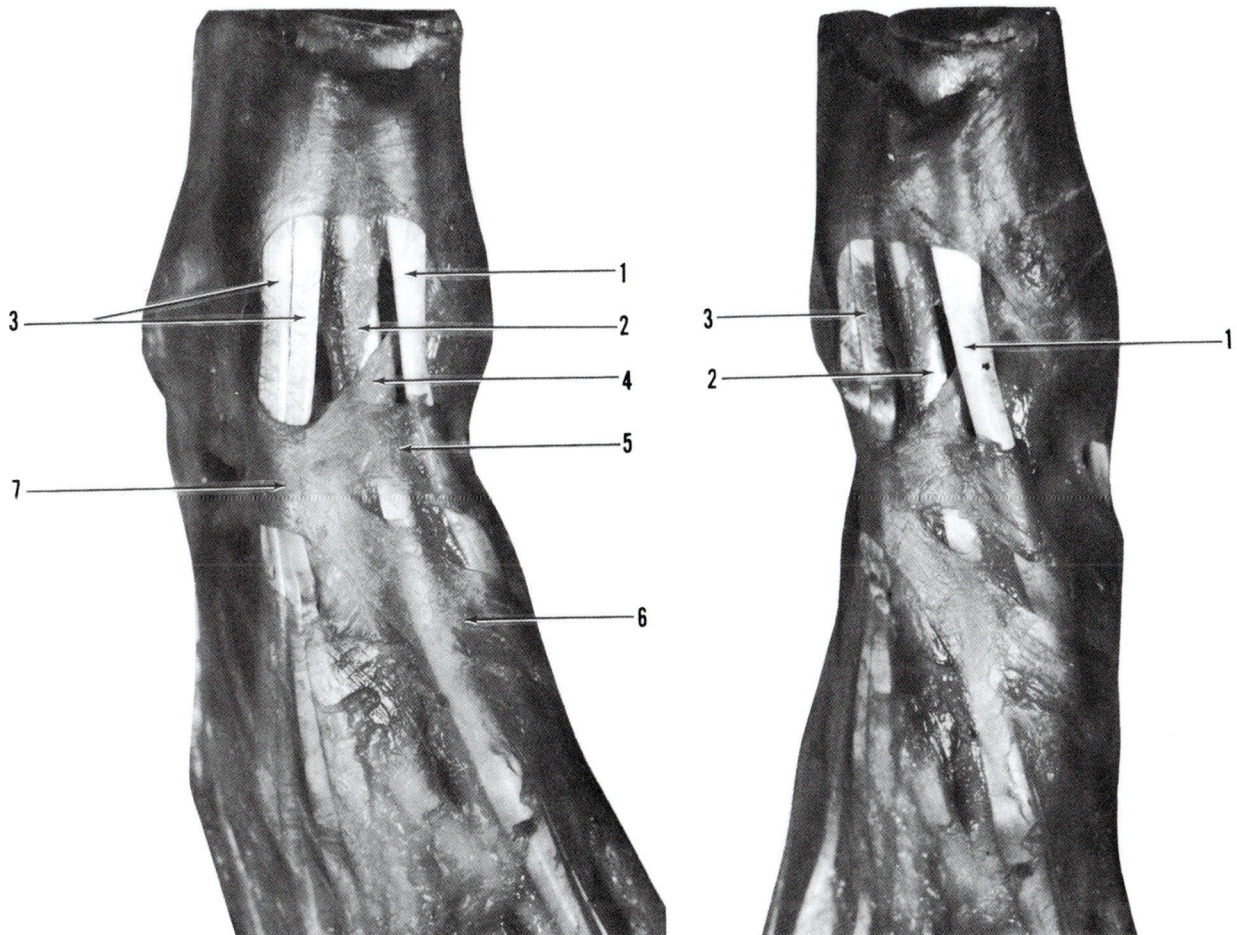

Figure 5.1 **Tibialis anterior tendon.** (*1*, Tibialis anterior tendon; *2*, extensor hallucis longus tendon; *3*, extensor digitorum longus tendons; *4, 5*, superior and inferior subdivisions of the superomedial band of the inferior extensor retinaculum, forming a tunnel for *1*; *6*, inferomedial band of inferior extensor retinaculum; *7*, stem of interior extensor retinaculum.)

neck.[8] Two of the three muscles had additional attachment to the medial malleolus, and one also had an attachment into the talonavicular joint and the navicular.[8]

Seelaus describes a similar muscle originating from the anterior surface of the lower third of the tibia, lateral to the anterior tibial crest, from the interosseous membrane, and from an intermuscular septum intervening between the muscle and the tibialis anterior (Fig. 5.3).[9] The tendon of the muscle is first medial to the tendon of the tibialis anterior and then is located behind it; it passes with the tendon of the tibialis anterior through the same inferior extensor retinacular compartment. The tendon of the tibioastragalus anticus pierces the capsule of the ankle joint and inserts in a fanlike manner into the anterosuperior aspect of the talar neck.

Musculus Tibiofascialis Anticus of Macalister and Musculus Tensor Fasciae Dorsalis Pedis

These muscles originate from the lower third of the anterior edge or the lateral side of the tibia.[1-3] The muscle is located over the tibialis anterior and inserts on the inferior extensor retinaculum over the extensor digitorum longus or on the dorsal aponeurosis of the foot.

▶ Extensor Hallucis Longus

At the level of the ankle, the extensor hallucis longus tendon is deep and lateral to the tibialis anterior tendon, and the muscle fibers descend very low on the lateral aspect of the tendon, reaching the level of the inferior extensor retinaculum (see Figs. 5.1 and 5.4). The tendon passes through its own fibrous tunnel and is directed anteriorly and slightly medially along the dorsum of the first metatarsal. It extends further distally, gradually enlarges, and inserts on the dorsum of the base of the distal hallucal phalanx.

At the level of the metatarsophalangeal joint, the extensor hallucis longus tendon is anchored by the extensor aponeurotic transverse lamina or sling, which extends from the sides of the tendon, wraps around the joint, and inserts on the base of the proximal phalanx and the sides of the plantar plate. Oblique

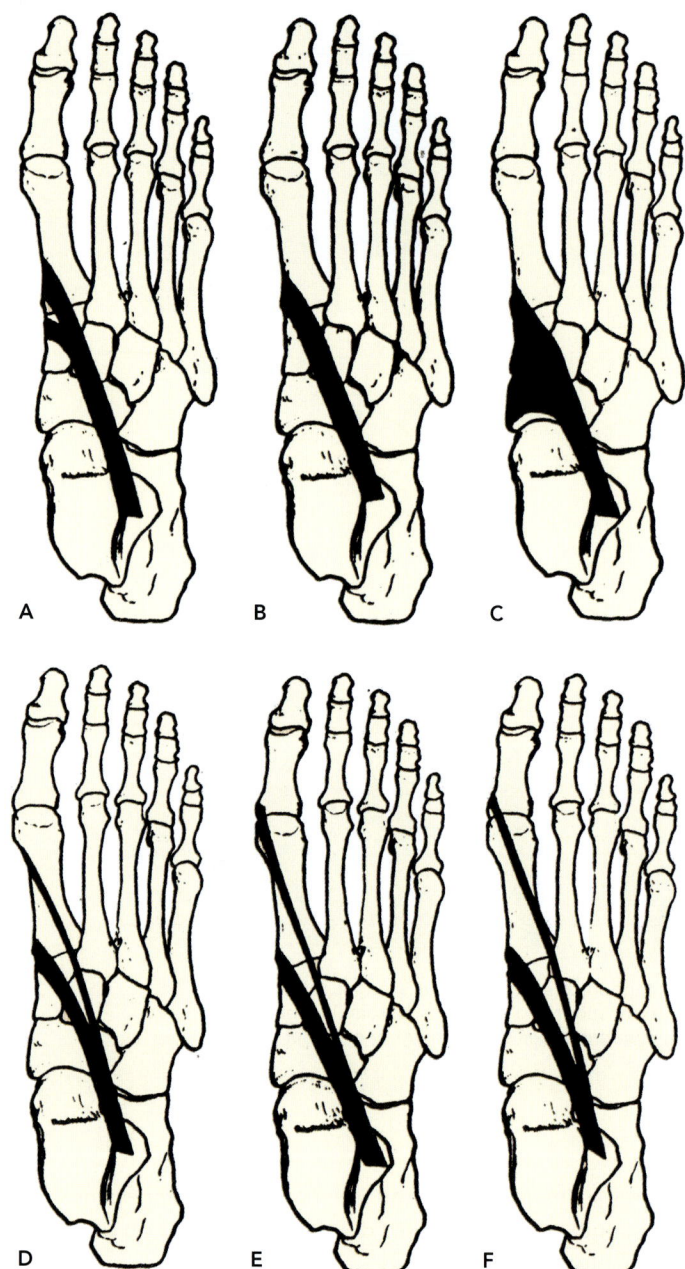

Figure 5.2 Insertional variations of the tibialis anterior tendon. The customary insertion on the adjacent areas of the first metatarsal and the medial cuneiform occurs in 90%. The variations occur in 10%. **(A)** Splitting of tibialis anterior tendon at or near insertion but not more than 25 mm from the latter (1%). **(B)** Insertion of tibialis anterior tendon into first metatarsal only (1.5%). **(C)** Fan-shaped insertion of tibialis anterior tendon into navicular, cuneiform$_1$, and metatarsal$_1$ (0.3%). **(D)** A slip of the tibialis anterior tendon inserting on the first metatarsal distally, representing in rudimentary form the musculus extensor ossis primi metatarsi (1%). **(E)** Accessory slip of tibialis anterior tendon inserting on the dorsum of the distal segment of the first metatarsal and the base of the proximal phalanx of the big toe (0.3%). **(F)** A slip of the tibialis anterior tendon inserting on the base of the proximal phalanx of the big toe, representing the musculus extensor primi internodii hallucis (2.3%). (From Hallisy JE. The muscular variations in the human foot: a quantitative study. *Am J Anat.* 1930;45[3]:411.)

aponeurotic fibers extend from the transverse lamina to the borders of the extensor tendon distally on each side, in a triangular shape. The insertional fibers of the transverse lamina are in close connection, medially with the abductor hallucis tendon and laterally with the adductor hallucis tendon (see Figs. 5.75, 5.76, and 5.83).

Variations

There are a number of variations involving the insertion of the extensor hallucis longus (Fig. 5.5).[1,2,10-12] A frequent variation is the tedious attachment to the proximal phalanx forming the musculus extensor primi internodii hallucis.[3] The percentage of occurrence of this variation, according to various sources, is as follows: in 290 ft, 23%; in 72 ft, 72%; and in 50 ft, 54% (approximate average, 50%).[3,10,12]

As described by Hallisy,[3] the variation with the extensor hallucis longus tendon giving an insertion to the distal segment of the first metatarsal representing the musculus extensor ossis primi metatarsi occurred in 1.5%. A proximal hallucal phalangeal slip may also be provided by the tibialis anterior tendon (in 8%) and by the extensor digitorum longus.[12]

Tate and Pachnik,[13] based on the dissection of 100 ft, described a tendinous slip originating from the extensor hallucis longus tendon, medially, just distal to the inferior extensor retinaculum and inserting into the capsule of the first metatarsophalangeal joint.

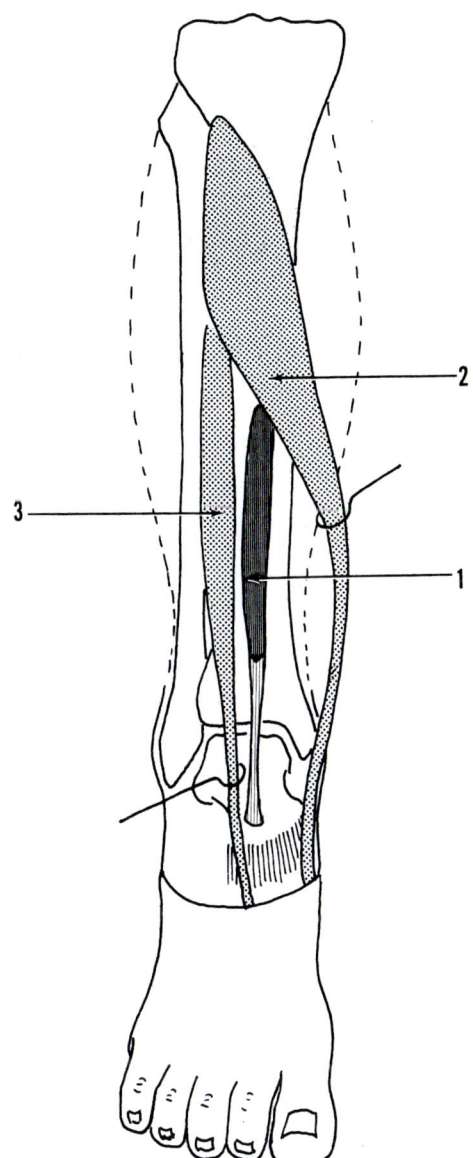

Figure 5.3 Musculus tibioastragalus anticus of Gruber. (*1*, Musculus tibioastragalus anticus of Gruber; *2*, tibialis anterior muscle; *3*, extensor hallucis longus muscle.) (From Seelaus HK. On certain muscle anomalies of the lower extremity. *Anat Rec.* 1927;35:187.)

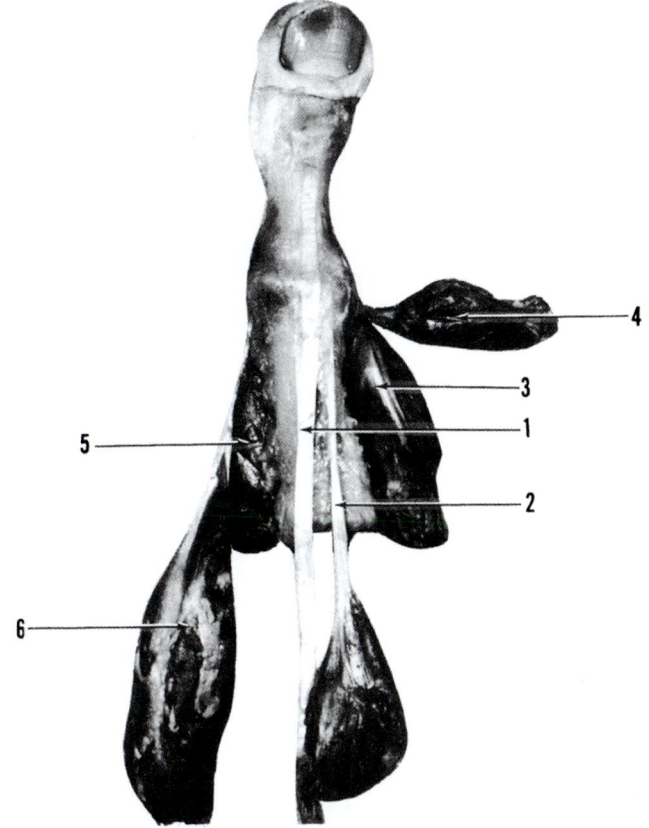

Figure 5.4 Dorsal aspect of big toe. (*1*, Extensor hallucis longus tendon; *2*, extensor hallucis brevis; *3*, adductor hallucis muscle, oblique head; *4*, adductor hallucis muscle, transverse head; *5*, flexor hallucis brevis, medial head; *6*, abductor hallucis muscle.)

They named this variation the extensor hallucis capsularis. It occurred in 86% of the dissections. In 2%, there was proximally a corresponding muscle. In 9%, the tendon originated from the tibialis anterior tendon. The average length of the tendon was 7.1 cm.

Lundeen et al[14] investigated the secondary tendinous slip of the extensor hallucis longus in 25 cadaver feet. The accessory tendon was present in 80% of the specimens. All the tendons originated from the medial aspect of the extensor hallucis longus tendon, "coursed anteriorly and slightly medially to their insertion. The length of these tendons ranged from 1.5 to 12.5 cm with an average of 4.2 cm."[14] In 19 of the 20 occurrences, the tendon in the distal 0.5 cm fanned out and inserted on the sling portion of the extensor apparatus at the level of the metacarpophalangeal joint. In one instance, the insertion was on the dorsum of the first metatarsal head.

Bibbo et al[15] dissected 32 ft to study the accessory extensor tendon of the first metatarsophalangeal joint originating from the extensor hallucis longus tendon or the tibialis anterior tendon and inserting "onto the dorsal/dorsomedial aspect of the 1st metatarsophalangeal joint capsule."

The accessory tendon was present in 81.25% and was originating from the extensor hallucis longus in 92.3% and from the tibialis anterior in 7.7%. The accessory tendon was found to be bilateral in 84.6%. The average free length of the accessory extensor tendon was 5.5 cm. The mean distance that the accessory and main tendons were able to be dissected from one another was 16.9 cm (range 12.4-27.5 cm). In 7.7%, a "small muscle belly, separate from extensor hallucis longus and tibialis anterior, provided origin to the accessory tendon." "The mean accessory tendon width was 2 mm (range <1 mm [thread-like] to 4 mm)"[15] (Fig. 5.6).

Boyd et al[16] investigated the extensor hallucis capsularis based on the dissection of 81 cadaver feet. The extensor hallucis capsularis was present in 88%. "In two instances, multiple accessory tendons were present in the same leg, one originating from the extensor hallucis longus and the other originating from the anterior tibial tendon."[16] "The origin of the extensor hallucis capsularis tendon was highly variable."[16]

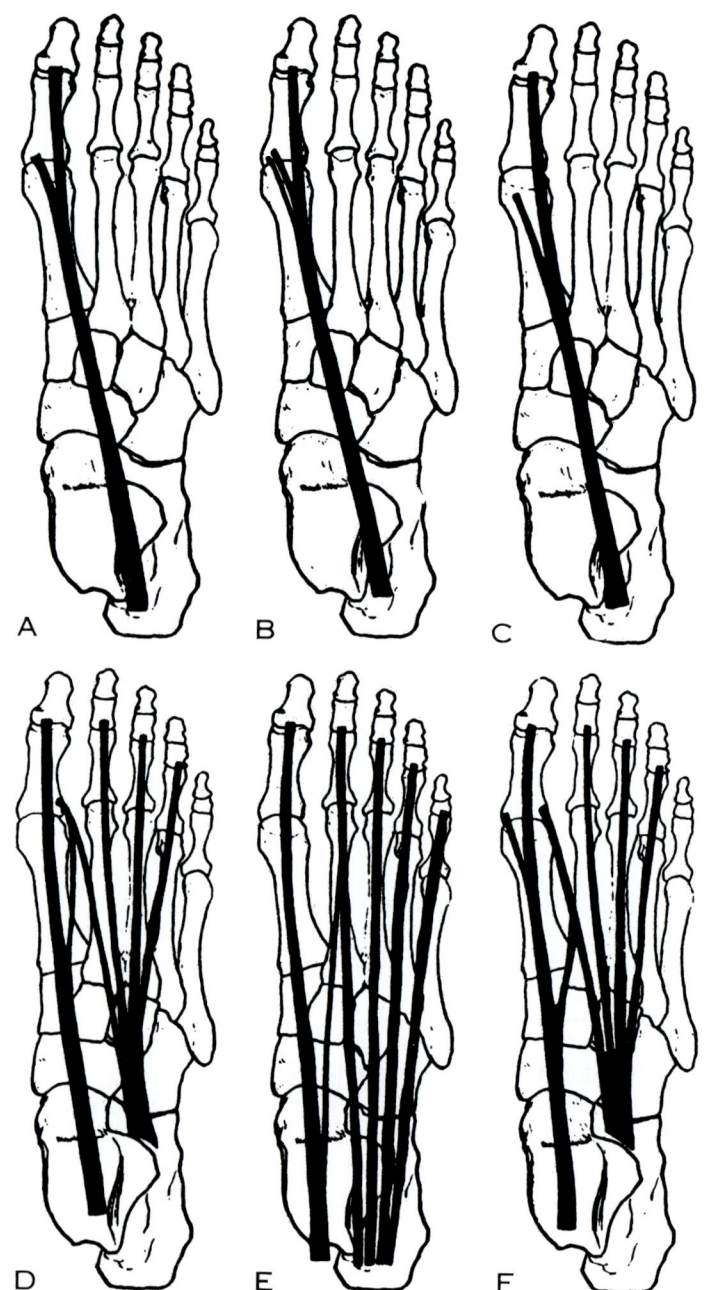

Figure 5.5 Insertional variations of the extensor hallucis longus tendon. (A) A slip from the extensor hallucis longus tendon to the base of the proximal phalanx of the big toe (23%), forming the musculus extensor primi internodii hallucis. (B) As in A but with two tendinous accessory insertional slips on the base of the proximal phalanx (1.5%). (C) A slip from the extensor hallucis longus tendon inserting on the distal segment of the first metatarsal (1.5%), representing the musculus extensor ossis primi metatarsi. (D) A slip from the extensor hallucis longus tendon joining the extensor hallucis brevis tendon (1%). (E) A slip from the extensor hallucis longus tendon joining the extensor digitorum longus tendon (0.3%). (F) Combined lateral expansion from the extensor hallucis longus tendon to a tendinous slip of the extensor digitorum longus inserting on the base of the proximal phalanx of the big toe and a second tendinous slip representing a musculus extensor primi internodii hallucis. (From Hallisy JE. The muscular variations in the human foot: a quantitative study. Am J Anat. 1930;45[3]:411.)

The extensor hallucis capsularis arose

- In 32%, from its own extensor hallucis longus muscle fascicle.
- In 62%, from a bifurcation point off the extensor hallucis longus itself.
- In 3%, from the tibialis anterior tendon.
- In 1%, from the extensor hallucis brevis (EHB) tendon.
- In 3%, it was undetermined.

In the group arising from the extensor hallucis longus, the point of divergence of the tendon from the extensor hallucis longus was at the level of the ankle in 24%, at the level of the navicular in 44%, and at the level of the proximal metatarsal in 31%.

In regard to the insertion, 99% of the extensor hallucis capsularis inserted into the first metacarpophalangeal joint capsule and 1% onto the base of the proximal phalanx. The average length of the extensor hallucis capsularis tendon was 10.8 cm ± 5 cm.

The width of the tendon was 1 mm or less in 36%, 1 to 2 mm in 48%, 2 to 3 mm in 15%, and more than 3 mm in 1% (see Fig. 5.6A). Other rare insertional variations may occur in combination with the insertion to the distal phalanx: two tendinous slips inserting on the proximal phalanx; one tendinous slip attached into the distal part of the dorsal aspect of the first metatarsal, a small slip extended to the most medial tendon of the extensor digitorum brevis; a tendinous extension to the extensor digitorum communis of the second toe; and a tendinous extension to the extensor digitorum brevis and to the base of the proximal phalanx (very rare).

▶ Extensor Digitorum Longus

The muscle fibers of the extensor digitorum longus extend distally on the lateral border of the common tendon to a level 8 to 10 mm proximal to the inferior extensor retinaculum (Figs. 5.7 and 5.8).[17] Initially unique, the extensor digitorum longus tendon divides into two tendons under the superior extensor retinaculum. Both tendons enter the common tunnel under the inferior extensor retinaculum; as they exit under the stem of the retinaculum, each divides into two tendons. The divided two lateral tendons reach the fifth and fourth toes, and the medial two tendons reach the third and the second toes, respectively. At the level of the metatarsophalangeal joint, the long extensor tendons of the second to the fourth toes are joined from the peroneal side by the corresponding extensor brevis tendons. This extensor tendinous ensemble forms a trifurcation system over the dorsum of the proximal phalanx and divides into a middle or central slip and two lateral slips. The central slip inserts on the dorsum of the middle phalanx and the capsule of the proximal interphalangeal joint. The two lateral slips, after receiving tendinous contribution mostly from the lumbrical on the tibial side, form two lateral tendons. These two tendons gradually converge on the dorsum of the middle phalanx and form a common terminal tendon that inserts on the dorsal capsule of the distal interphalangeal joint and on the base of the distal phalanx. The corresponding tendon of the extensor digitorum brevis inserts on the common extensor tendon laterally or forms the entire lateral slip on the peroneal side.[18,19]

The tendons of the extensor system are anchored at the level of the metatarsophalangeal joint and proximal phalanx by a fibroaponeurotic structure. The proximal segment of this aponeurosis has transversely oriented fibers originating from the lateral and medial borders of the flat aponeurotic tunnel surrounding the corresponding extensor tendons. The transverse aponeurotic fibers extend around the capsule of the metatarsophalangeal joint and blend on the plantar side with the plantar plate, the deep transverse metatarsal ligament, and the flexor tendon sheath. This firm insertion extends distally on the base of the proximal phalanx. The proximal segment of the extensor aponeurosis is termed the *transverse* or *quadrilateral lamina* or *extensor sling* (Figs. 5.9 to 5.11).[19]

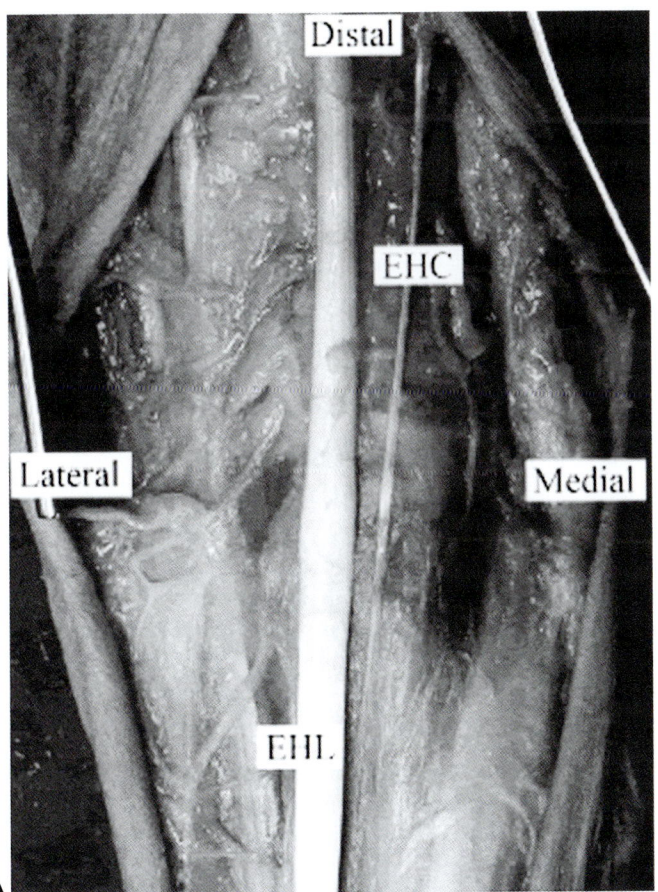
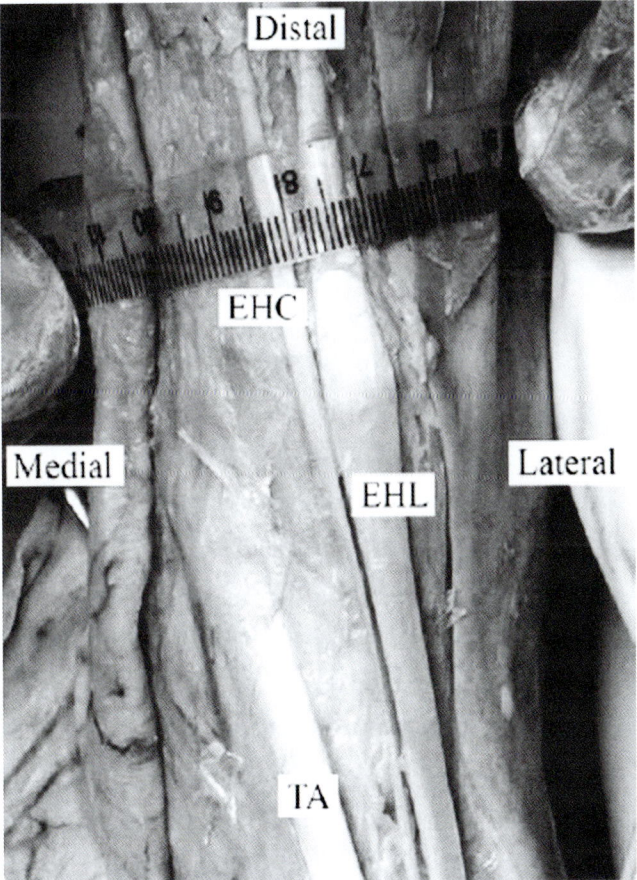

Figure 5.6 (A and B) Foot oriented vertically with the most distal segment at the top of the image. (*EHC*, extensor hallucis capsularis; *EHL*, extensor hallucis longus; *TA*, tibialis anterior.) (Boyd N, Brock H, Meier A, et al. Firoozbakhsh: extensor hallucis capsularis. Frequency and identification on MRI. *Foot Ankle Int.* 2006;3:181-184, Figure 1A and 1B. Copyright ©2006. Reprinted by Permission of SAGE Publications)

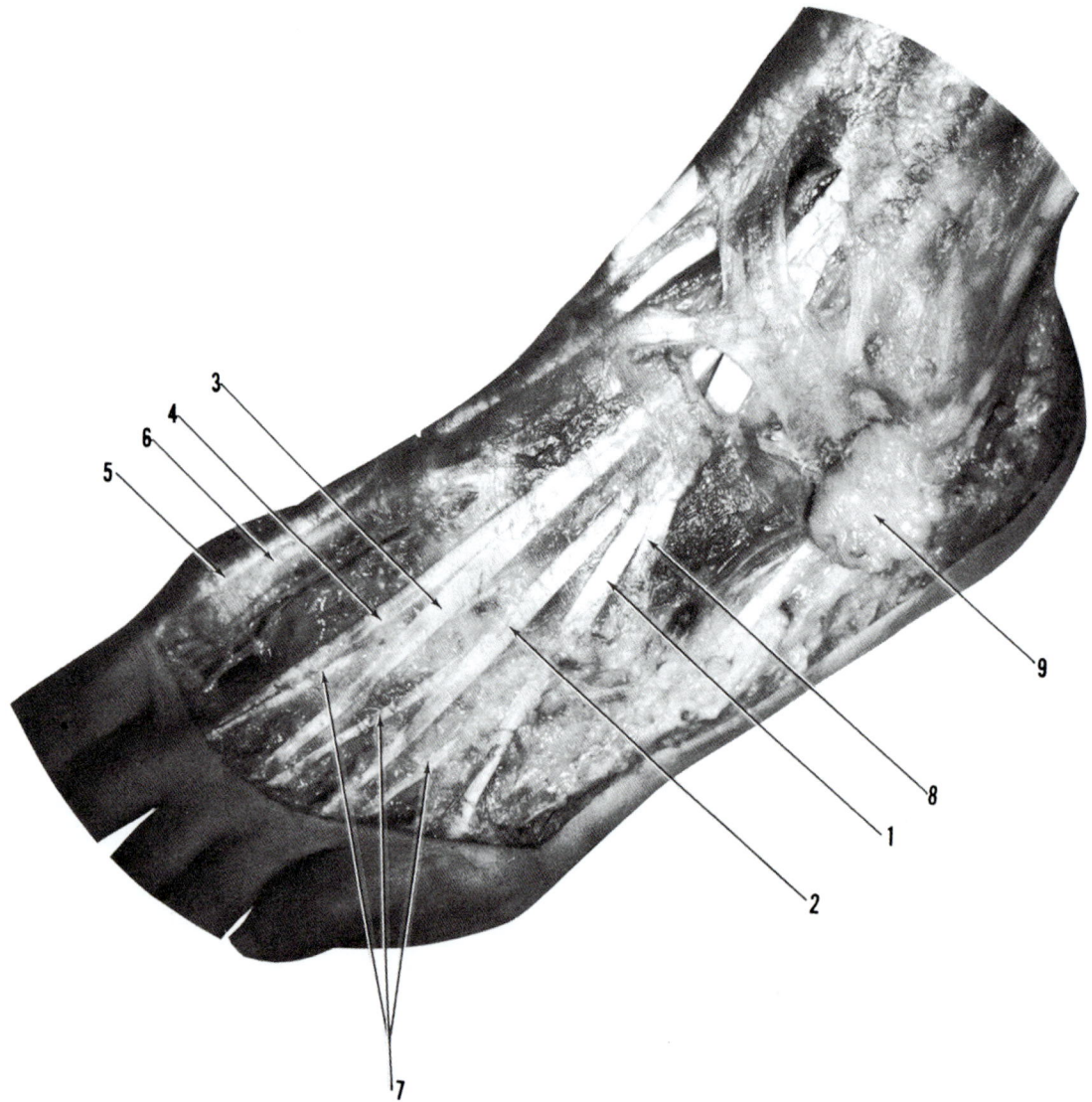

Figure 5.7 Extensor digitorum longus. (*1-4,* Extensor digitorum longus tendon to toes 5, 4, 3, 2; *5,* extensor hallucis longus tendon; *6,* extensor hallucis brevis tendon; *7,* extensor digitorum brevis tendons [none to the fifth toe]; *8,* peroneus tertius tendon; *9,* fat pad of prelateral malleolar fossa.)

Further distally, the extensor aponeurosis is formed by obliquely oriented fibers making up the extensor wing or extensor hood.[19] Tendinous expansions from the lumbrical or the minute expansion from the plantar interosseous to the middle slip forms the spiral fibers.[18,19] The triangular space located between the lateral tendons is filled by an aponeurotic structure called the *triangular lamina*.[18,19]

The fifth toe does not have a corresponding extensor brevis tendon; furthermore, beyond the base of the proximal phalanx, there is an atrophy of the fibrous apparatus, and usually the spiral fibers and the triangular lamina do not exist at this level (see Fig. 5.11).[18]

At the level of the proximal interphalangeal joint, transversely oriented fibers extend from the trifurcation tendons to the flexor tunnel.[18]

There are a number of variations involving the extensor digitorum longus.[1,2]

Individual Muscles

The level at which the common long extensor divides into the digital components proximally is very variable. The tendinous divisions may extend further proximally and divide the muscle mass into separate muscle units. The following variations are possible:

- Four muscle units followed by four tendons.
- One muscle unit corresponding to the lateral three long extensor tendons and one muscle corresponding to the tendon of the second toe, thus forming the extensor proper of the second toe.
- One muscle unit corresponding to the tendons of the second, third, and fourth toes and one muscle with a tendon to the fifth toe, the latter tendon combined with the peroneus tertius.

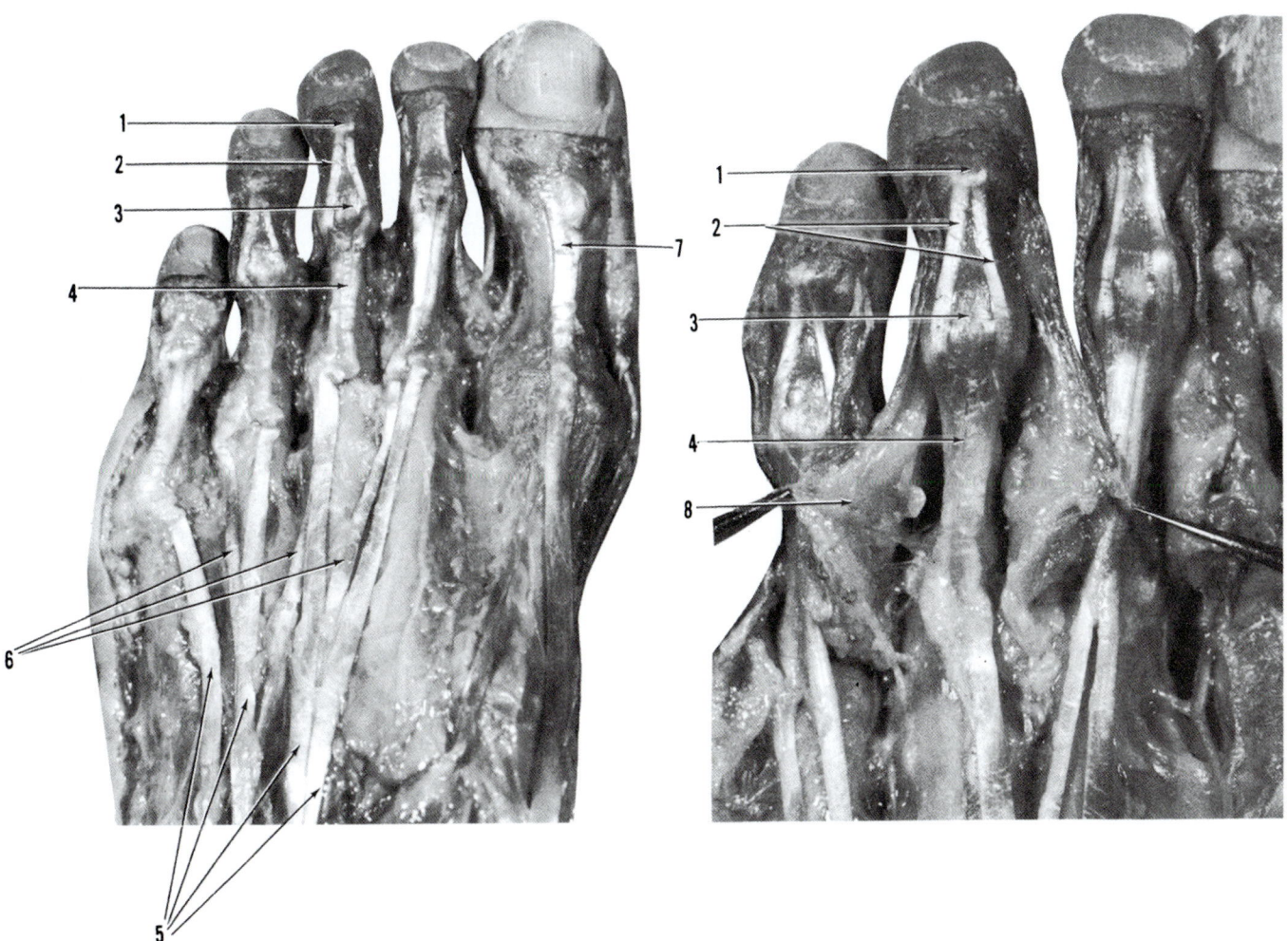

Figure 5.8 Extensor digitorum longus. (*1*, Extensor terminal tendon of third toe; *2*, lateral tendons of extensor tendon trifurcation; *3*, middle slip of extensor tendon trifurcation; *4*, extensor digitorum longus tendon joined by extensor digitorum brevis; *5*, extensor digitorum longus tendon; *6*, extensor digitorum brevis tendon; *7*, extensor hallucis longus tendon; *8*, adiporetinacular layer carrying superficial nerves and vessels.)

Bifid Tendons

Distally, the long extensor tendon of a lesser toe may be bifid, with the following distributions:

- Both tendons may insert on the same toe.
- The additional tendons of the third and fourth toes may insert laterally or medially on the adjacent toes.
- The additional tendon of the second toe may insert on the third toe, and that of the fifth toe may insert on the fourth toe.

Additional Slips

Additional tendinous slips from the extensor digitorum longus may insert on the metatarsal shaft, the extensor digitorum brevis tendon, the dorsal aponeurosis, or the big toe. Anastomotic fibrous bands, variable in number and location, may also unite the long extensor tendons of the adjacent toes.

▶ Extensor Digitorum Brevis

The extensor digitorum brevis muscle originates from the anterolateral aspect of the sinus tarsi (Fig. 5.12). The muscle is located between the lateral and intermediate roots of the inferior extensor retinaculum and is lateral to the cervical ligament and posterior to the origin of the dorsal calcaneocuboid ligament. Occasionally, a slip from the intermediary root divides the EHB from the extensor digitorum brevis of the lesser toes.

The muscle divides into four fascicles that terminate in four tendons located on the peroneal side of the first four toes. There is no extensor brevis tendon to the fifth toe. As mentioned previously, each extensor brevis tendon of the lesser toes joins the corresponding extensor digitorum longus tendon and may form the lateral slip of the trifurcation in its entirety. The extensor digitorum brevis to the first toe or EHB is located deep under the extensor hallucis longus

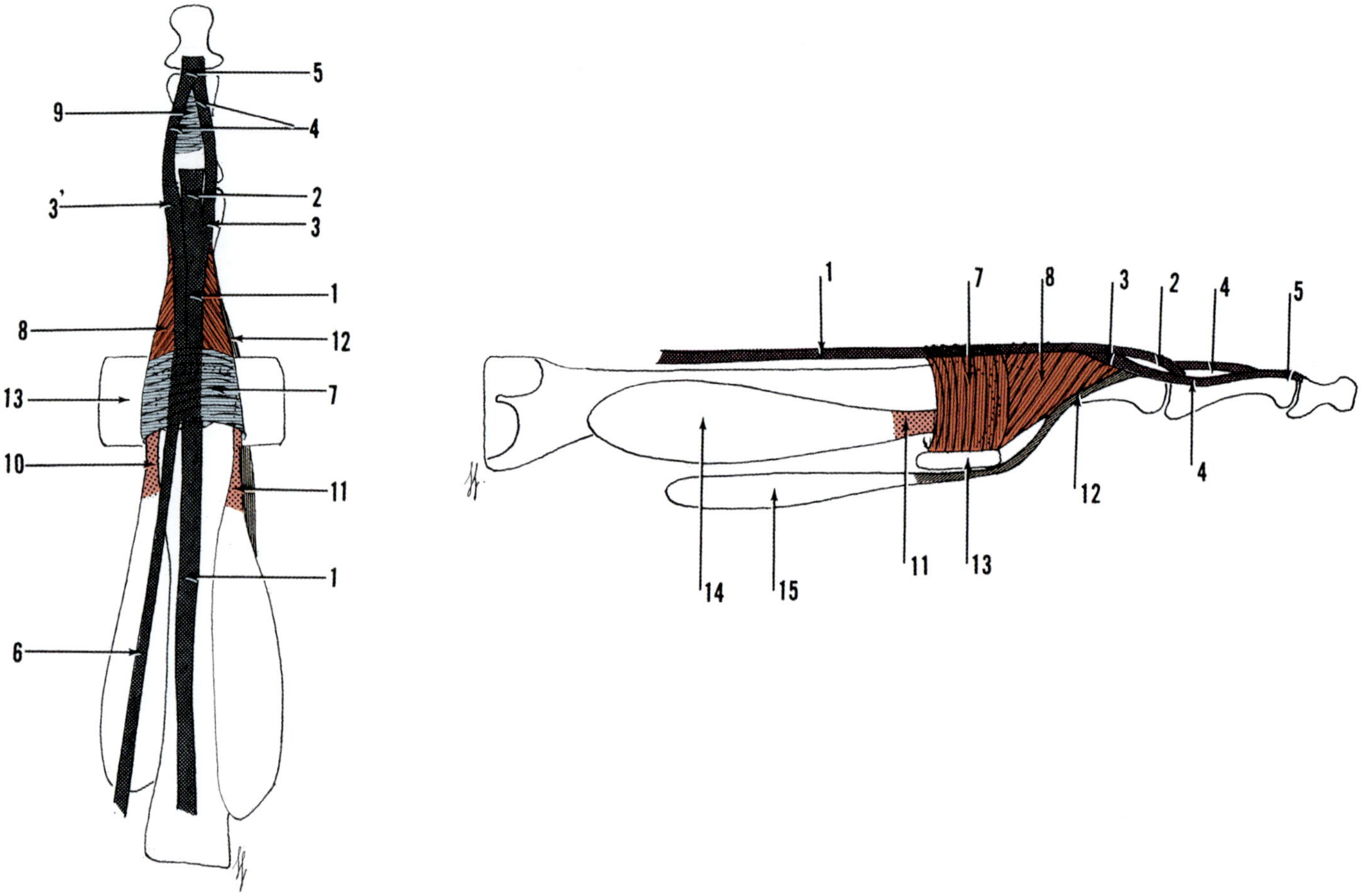

Figure 5.9 **Extensor complex of a lesser toe.** (*1*, Extensor digitorum longus tendon; *2*, middle slip of extensor tendon trifurcation; *3, 3'*, lateral slips of extensor tendon trifurcation; *4*, lateral tendons of extensor tendon trifurcation; *5*, terminal extensor tendon; *6*, extensor digitorum brevis tendon; *7*, transverse lamina of extensor aponeurosis or extensor sling; *8*, oblique component of extensor aponeurosis forming the extensor hood or wing; *9*, triangular ligament; *10, 11*, interossei tendons; *12*, lumbrical tendon; *13*, deep transverse metatarsal ligament; *14*, interosseous muscle; *15*, lumbrical tendon.)

and its aponeurosis; it enlarges distally and inserts on the dorsum of the proximal phalanx.

Lucien, in a study of 51 ft, reported that the normal division of the extensor digitorum brevis into four components occurs only in 26% and that in 72.5% an additional musculotendinous unit may be present.[20] The absence of a slip is rare.

Additional Musculotendinous Units

The additional musculotendinous units (Fig. 5.13) are of the following types: accessory medial head to the second, fourth, and third toes (in order of decreasing frequency); accessory digastric and trigastric muscles; extensions to the long extensor tendons; and extensions to the metatarsal and midtarsal bones.

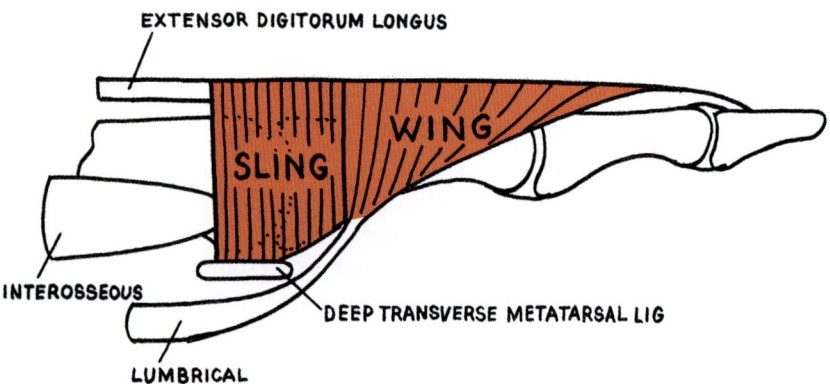

Figure 5.10 **Extensor aponeurosis of a lesser toe.**

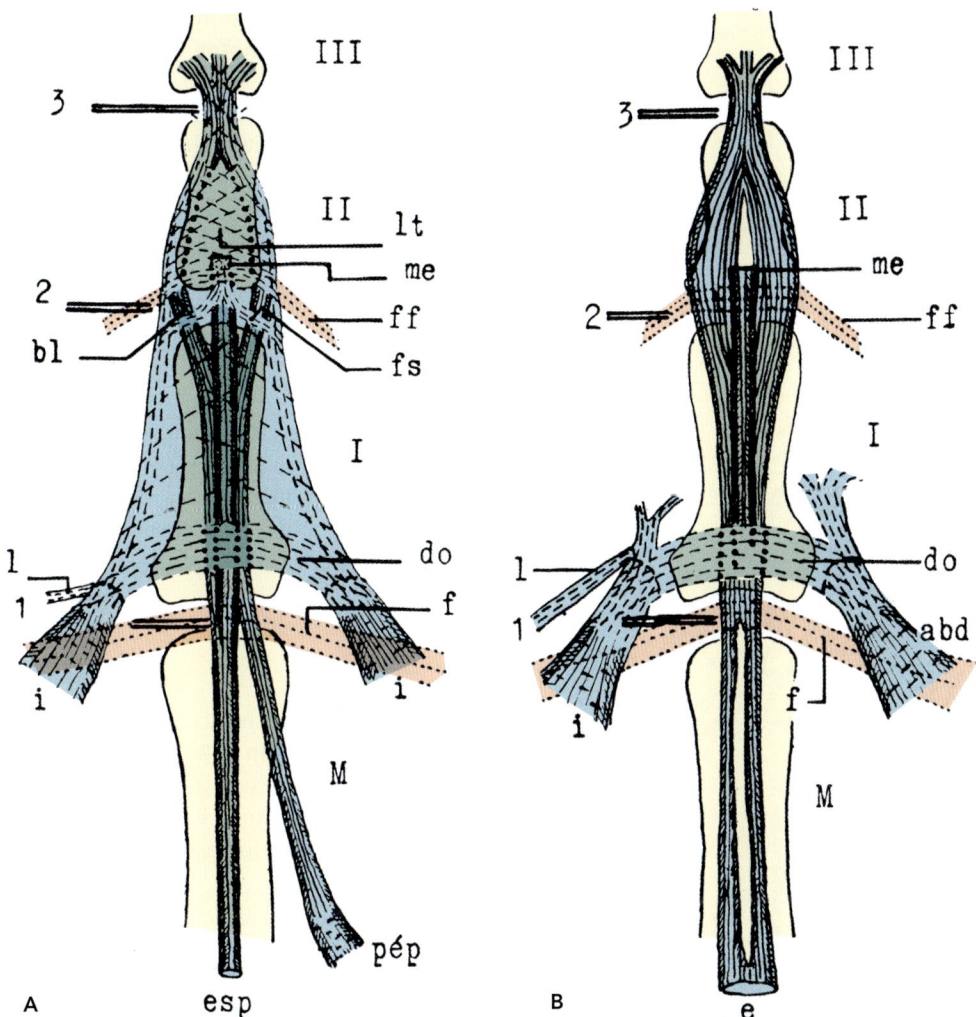

Figure 5.11 Internal structure of extensor mechanism of lesser toes. (A) Second toe, right foot. **(B)** Fifth toe, right foot. (*abd*, abductor of fifth toe; *bl*, lateral band of long extensor tendon; *do*, dorsal sling; *esp*, extensor digitorum longus tendon; *f*, perforating aponeurotic fibers arising from plantar aponeurosis; *ff*, fibers arising from sheath of long flexors; *fs*, spiral fibers; *i*, interossei; *l*, lumbrical; *lt*, triangular lamina; *M*, metatarsal; *me*, middle slip of long extensor tendon; *pep*, extensor digitorum brevis tendon; *I*, *II*, *III*, proximal, middle, and distal phalanges; *1*, *2*, *3*, level of metatarsophalangeal and interphalangeal joints.) (Adapted from Baumann JA. Valeur, variations et équivalences des muscles extenseurs, interosseux, adducteurs et abducteurs de la main et du pied chez l'homme. *Acta Anat.* 1948;4:10. By permission of S. Karger AG, Basel.)

The accessory medial head to the second toe occurs quite frequently (in 34%), and the well-developed muscle ends with a tendon that inserts on the medial aspect of the head of the proximal phalanx of the second toe.[20] Occasionally, this tendon terminates on the first dorsal interosseous aponeurosis. The origin of this muscle is variable. In the majority, it arises from the muscle fascicle to the second toe. It sometimes originates from the EHB, the EHB and the muscle fascicle to the second toe, or the middle cuneiform or cuboid.

The accessory medial head of the fourth toe originates from the corresponding muscle fascicle of the extensor digitorum brevis to the fourth toe. It is medial in location. Rarely, the unit is completely developed, and most frequently, the tendon terminates on the interosseous aponeurosis.

The accessory medial head of the third toe is very rare and originates from the fascicle to the second toe.

The digastric muscle is always formed by an accessory muscle arising from the second fascicle of the extensor digitorum brevis and is connected to an accessory muscle of the first or the second dorsal interosseous muscle. Two similar digastric muscles may be present, each connected separately to the accessory first and second dorsal interosseous muscles.

A trigastric muscle is formed when the accessory muscle arising from the second fascicle of the extensor brevis attaches simultaneously to the accessory first and second dorsal interosseous muscles.

Variations of Insertion and of Origin

The tendons of the extensor digitorum brevis of the lesser toes may insert on the corresponding base of the proximal phalanx, on the base of the metatarsal, or on the interosseous

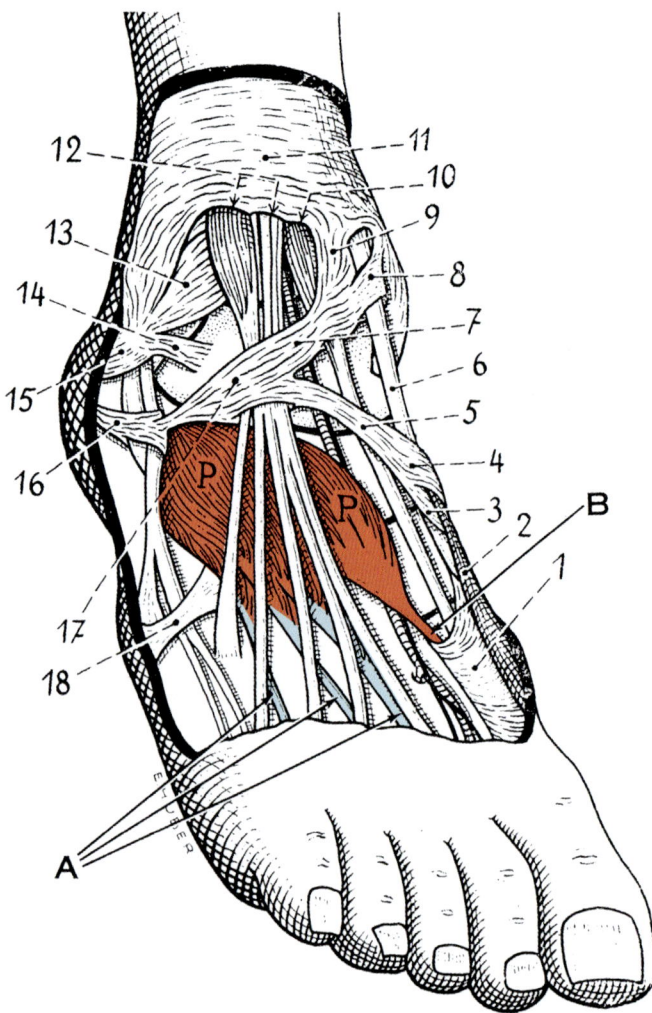

Figure 5.12 **Extensor digitorum brevis tendon to toes 2, 3, and 4 (A) and extensor hallucis brevis tendon (B).** (*1*, Medial transverse retinacular band of dorsum of foot; *2*, abductor hallucis muscle; *3, 4*, superficial and deep laminae of oblique inferomedial band of inferior extensor retinaculum; *5*, oblique inferomedial band of inferior extensor retinaculum; *6*, tibialis anterior tendon; *7*, oblique superomedial band of inferior extensor retinaculum; *8, 9*, superficial and deep components of oblique superomedial retinaculum forming tunnel of tibialis anterior tendon; *10*, extensor hallucis longus tendon; *11*, aponeurosis of leg; *12*, extensor digitorum longus and peroneus tertius tendons; *13*, anteroinferior tibiofibular ligament; *14*, anterior talofibular ligament; *15*, superior peroneal retinaculum; *16*, inferior peroneal retinaculum; *17*, stem of interior extensor retinaculum or frondiform ligament; *18*, lateral transverse band; *P*, extensor digitorum brevis muscle.) (Adapted from Meyer P. La morphologie du ligament annulair anterieur du coudepied chez l'homme. *Comptes-Rendus Assoc Anat.* 1955;84:281.)

aponeurosis. The EHB tendon may insert on the lateral aspect of the extensor hallucis longus tendon. The origin of the extensor digitorum brevis is also subject to variation, because this muscle may originate from the cuneiforms, the cuboid, or even the base of the metatarsals.[1,21]

Muscle Cuneo-Naviculo-Fascialis

Uzel et al[22] reported on an anomalous muscle on the dorsomedial aspect of the foot (m. cuneo-naviculo-fascialis) in a 7-year-old patient.

At surgery, "the anomalous muscle originated from the navicular and cuneiform bones and was composed of two distinct parts. The first part had a bipennate muscle belly, the proximal and distal portions of which originated from the dorsal aspects of the navicular and cuneiform bones. The tendon coursed medial to the first metatarsal bone and then plantarward toward the sole of the foot superficial to the abductor hallucis muscle and merged with the plantar fascia. The second part arose from the navicular… coursed medially and inserted in the plantar fascia."[22]

▸ Peroneus Tertius

The peroneus tertius tendon is lateral to the extensor digitorum longus tendon and passes in the same compartment or in a separate compartment under the inferior extensor retinaculum (see Figs. 5.12 and 5.14). The tendon is directed anteriorly and laterally, fans out, and inserts on the superior surface of the fifth metatarsal base.

Absence

The peroneus tertius muscle may be absent; LeDouble provides the following data: in 102 ft, absent in 10; in 537 ft, absent in 44; and in 120 ft, absent in 11 (759 ft total, absent in a total of 65 [8.5%]).[2] Reimann,[23] in a study of 200 cadaver feet, reports the peroneus tertius to be absent in 10%.

Insertional Variations

The following insertional variations of an additional tendinous slip of the peroneus tertius are possible:

- On the base of the fourth metatarsal. This additional slip is seen frequently and is usually smaller but occasionally equal to or even larger than the main tendon. It may also represent the sole insertion of the peroneus tertius tendon.
- On the fifth toe at the level of one of the phalanges or on the long extensor of the same toe.
- On the fifth metatarsal shaft or on the interosseous space.

LATERAL ASPECT OF THE ANKLE AND FOOT AND THE SOLE OF THE FOOT

▸ Peroneus Longus

The peroneus longus is shown in Figures 5.15 and 5.16.[2,24-26] The lateral surface of the fibula faces laterally in the middle third, becomes directed posteriorly in the distal fourth, and continues as the posterior surface of the lateral malleolus. The osseous twist is also followed by the peroneus longus tendon, which is lateral in the middle third, posterolateral in the distal fourth, and posterior to the peroneus brevis tendon behind the lateral malleolus.

The peroneus longus tendon is retained by three tunnels and makes three turns before reaching its destination. The first

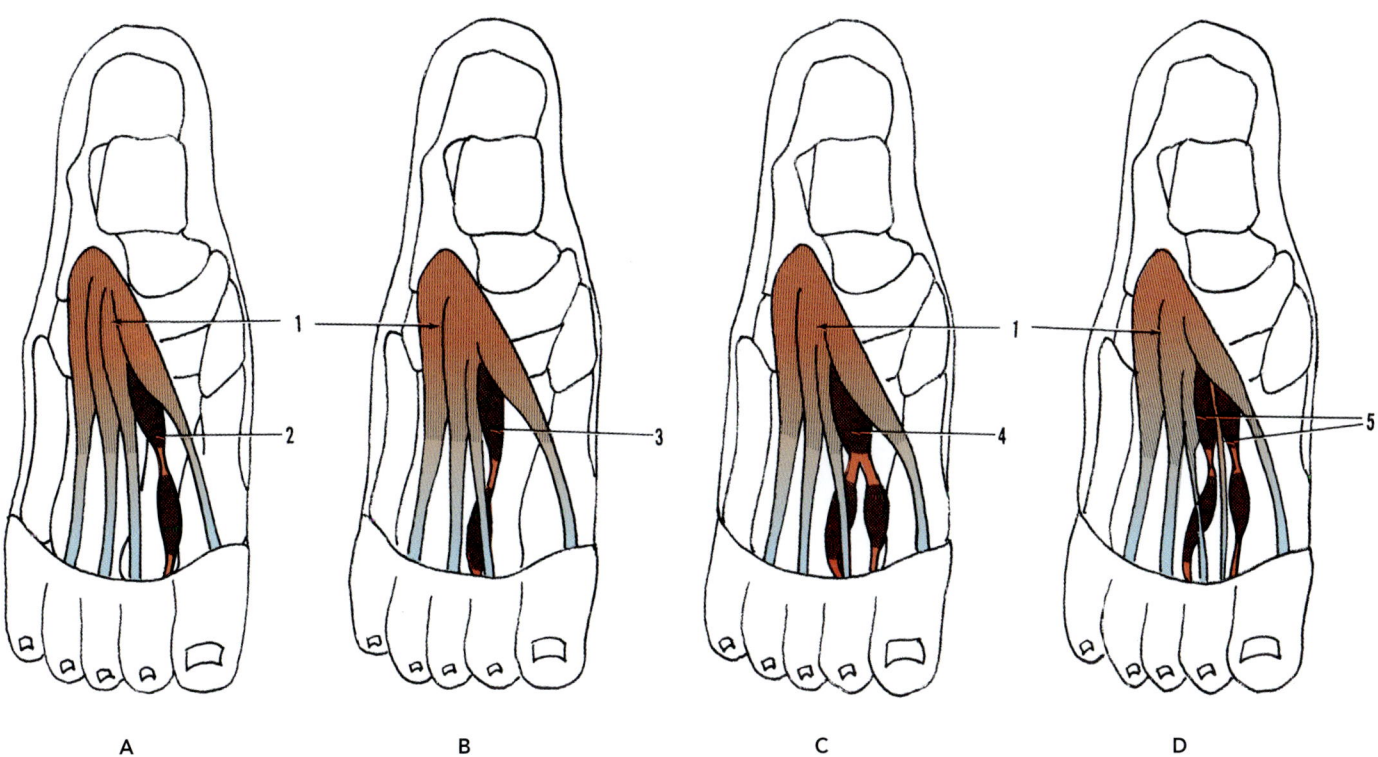

Figure 5.13 Variations of the extensor digitorum brevis—additional musculotendinous units. (*1*, Extensor digitorum brevis muscle; [**A**] *2*, digastric muscle formed proximally by additional portion derived from extensor digitorum brevis of second toe and connected to an accessory muscle of first dorsal interosseous; [**B**] *3*, digastric muscle derived proximally as in 2 but attached distally to an accessory muscle of second dorsal interosseous; [**C**] *4*, trigastric muscle formed proximally by an additional muscle derived from extensor digitorum brevis to second toe and attached distally to accessory muscles of first and second dorsal interossei; [**D**] *5*, two digastric muscles arising separately from extensor digitorum brevis and attached distally to accessory muscles of first and second dorsal interossei.) (Adapted from Lucien M. Sur les connexions entre le pédieux et les muscles interosseur dorsaux chez l'homme: Considérations sur le developpement du muscle pédieux. *Bibl Anat*. 1909;XIX:232.)

tunnel common to both peronei tendons is retromalleolar and is formed by the superior peroneal retinaculum. At the tip of the lateral malleolus, the tendon makes its first turn and is directed downward and anteriorly. It enters the inferior tunnel formed by the inferior peroneal retinaculum at the level of the processus trochlearis of the os calcis and makes its second turn; it is now directed inferiorly and medially. It makes its third turn around the lateral border of the foot between the cuboid and the base of the fifth metatarsal and enters the plantar tunnel. The tendon glides over the anterior convex slope of the cuboidal tuberosity (Fig. 5.17). It obliquely crosses the sole of the foot, oriented anteromedially, and inserts on the lateral tubercle of the base of the first metatarsal (Fig. 5.18). At times, it sends an extension to the plantar aspect of the first cuneiform, the base of the second metatarsal, and the first dorsal interosseous. The plantar peroneal tunnel is fibrous at the level of the cuboid and is formed by arciform fibers extended from the crest of the cuboid tuberosity to the anterior ledge of the cuboid. These fibers are deep to the long cuboideometatarsal ligament. This plantar segment of the tunnel is also reinforced by the extensions of the long plantar ligament to the base of the fourth and third metatarsals. The inner segment of the peroneal tunnel is roofed by a thinner layer of fibrous tissue.

A near-constant sesamoid, osseous or fibrocartilage, is present in the substance of the peroneus longus tendon at the level of the cuboid tubercle. Rarely, a sesamoid is found in the retromalleolar portion of the tendon and very exceptionally in the calcaneal portion of the tendon.

Picou describes the normal insertions of the peroneus longus tendon as taking place on the first metatarsal base; the first cuneiform, plantar aspect; and the first metatarsal, behind the head, on the superolateral border (Fig. 5.19).[25,26]

The slip to the first cuneiform is described by Picou as arising from the deep or dorsal surface of the peroneus longus tendon at the level of the sesamoid in the cuboid tunnel.[26] It is located near the posterior border and extends medially, and the fan-shaped end of the tendon terminates on the anterior aspect of the plantar surface of the first cuneiform (Fig. 5.20).

The slip to the anterior aspect of the first metatarsal arises from the anterior border of the tendon and is directed toward the base of the second metatarsal; it adheres very weakly to the second metatarsal but is braced against it by a transverse ligament acting as a fibrous bridge. The tendinous slip changes course and is directed toward the head of the first metatarsal. It passes through the first interosseous space and gives insertion from its two surfaces to the first dorsal interosseous muscle and

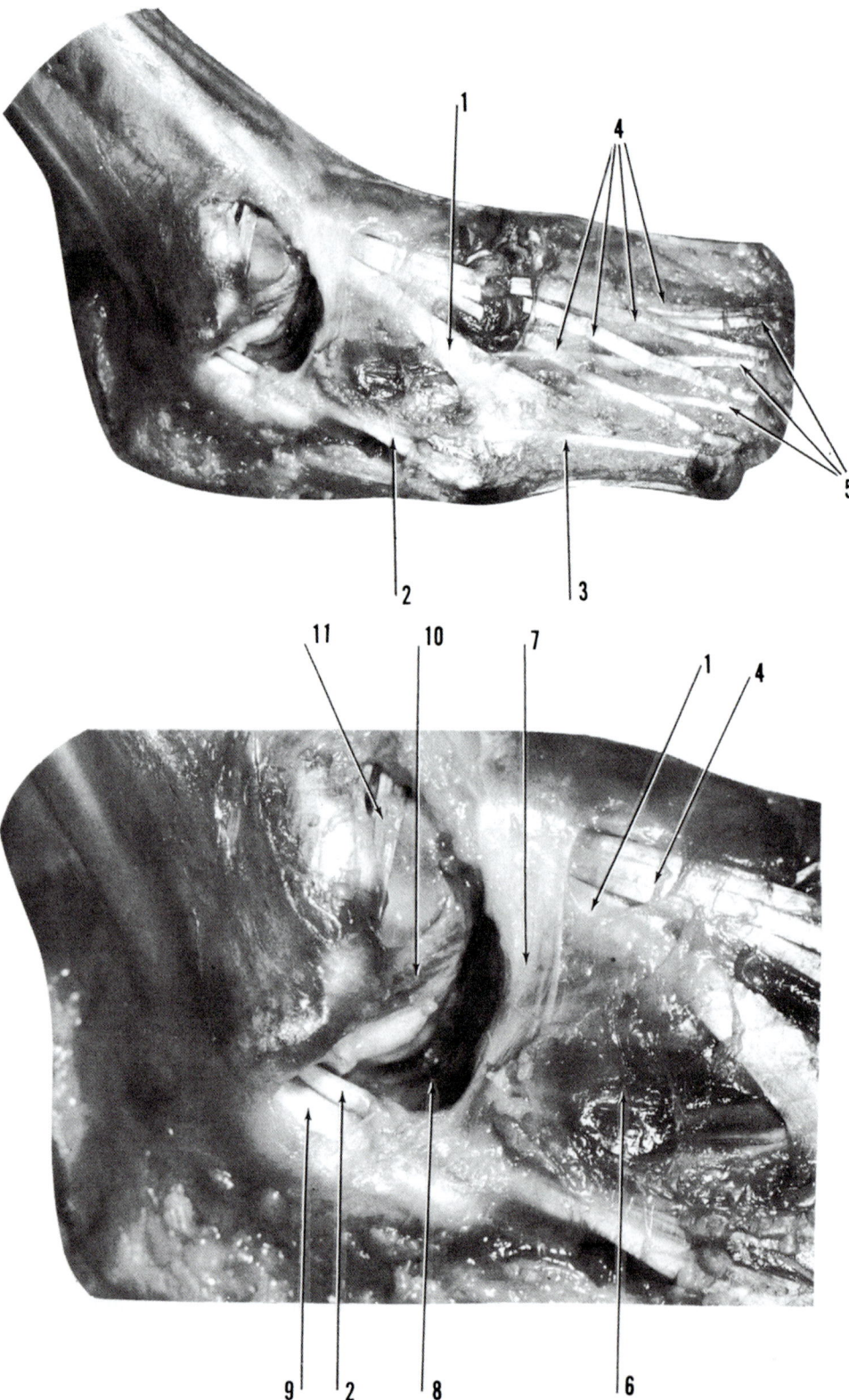

Figure 5.14 **Peroneus tertius tendon.** (*1*, Peroneus tertius tendon; *2*, peroneus brevis tendon; *3*, supplementary slip of *2*; *4*, extensor digitorum longus tendons; *5*, extensor digitorum brevis tendons 2, 3, 4; *6*, extensor digitorum brevis muscle origin; *7*, stem of inferior extensor retinaculum occupying middle and anterior segments of sinus tarsi [*8*]; *9*, peroneus longus tendon; *10*, anterior talofibular ligament; *11*, lower band of anterior tibiofibular ligament.)

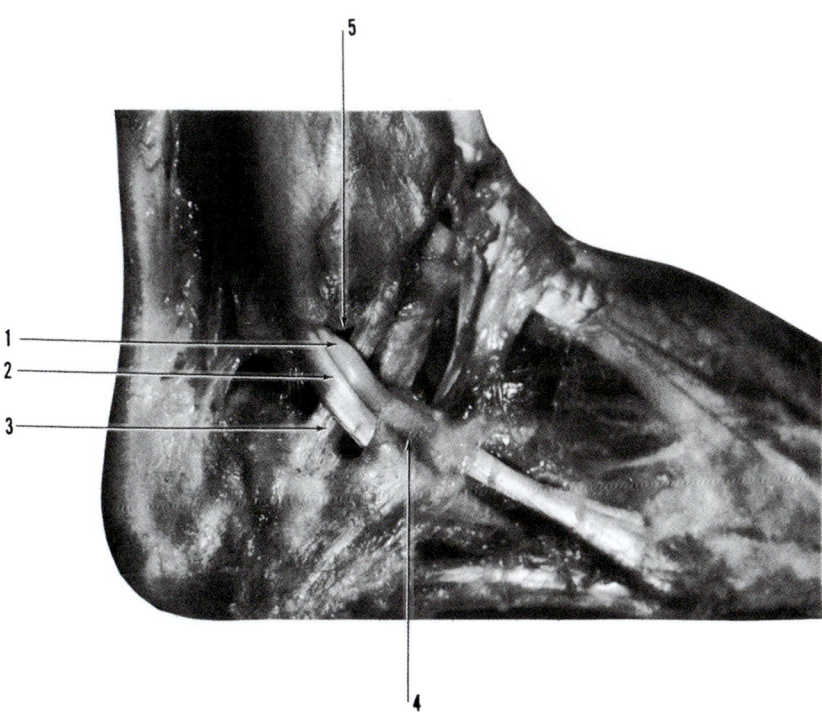

Figure 5.15 **Peroneus longus tendon.** (*1*, Peroneus brevis tendon; *2*, peroneus longus tendon; *3*, calcaneofibular ligament; *4*, inferior peroneal retinaculum; *5*, tip of lateral malleolus, free of insertion.)

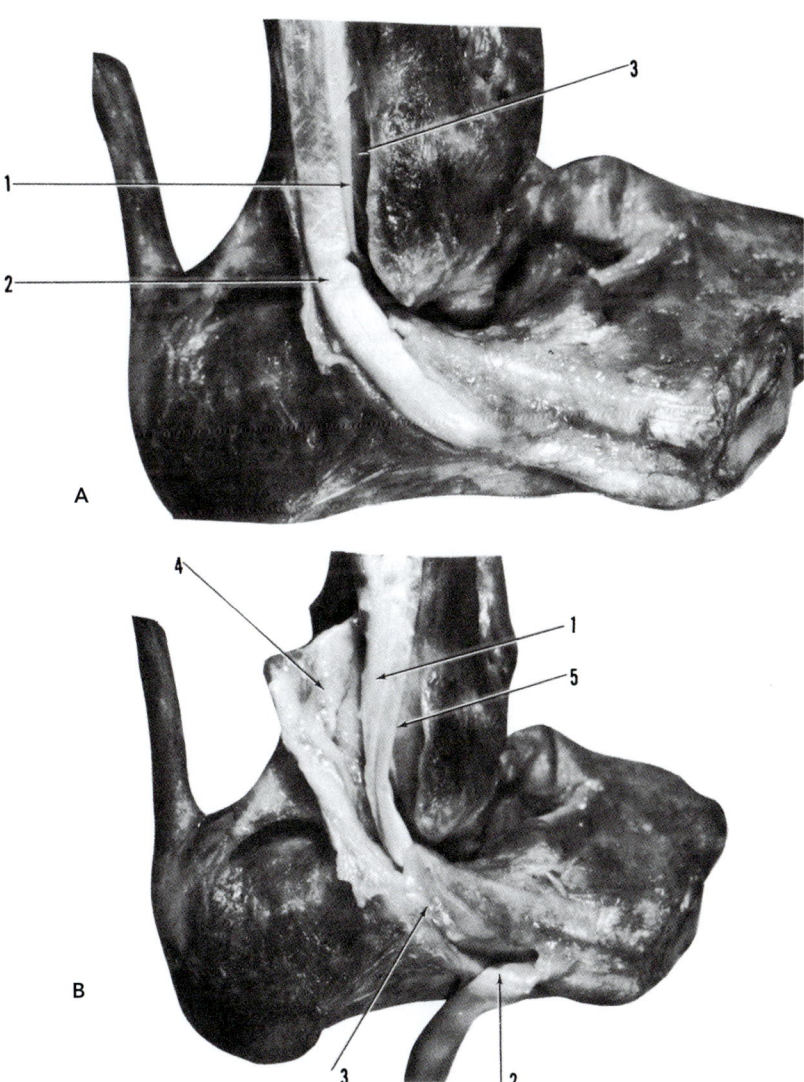

Figure 5.16 **Peroneus longus tendon. (A)** Superior peroneal retinaculum split. (*1*, Peroneus brevis tendon; *2*, peroneus longus tendon; *3*, sulcus of peronei.) **(B)** Peroneus longus tendon reflected. (*1*, Peroneus brevis tendon; *2*, reflected peroneus longus tendon; *3*, septum dividing inferior peroneal retinacular tunnel into two; *4*, deep surface of superior peroneal retinaculum; *5*, sulcus of peronei.)

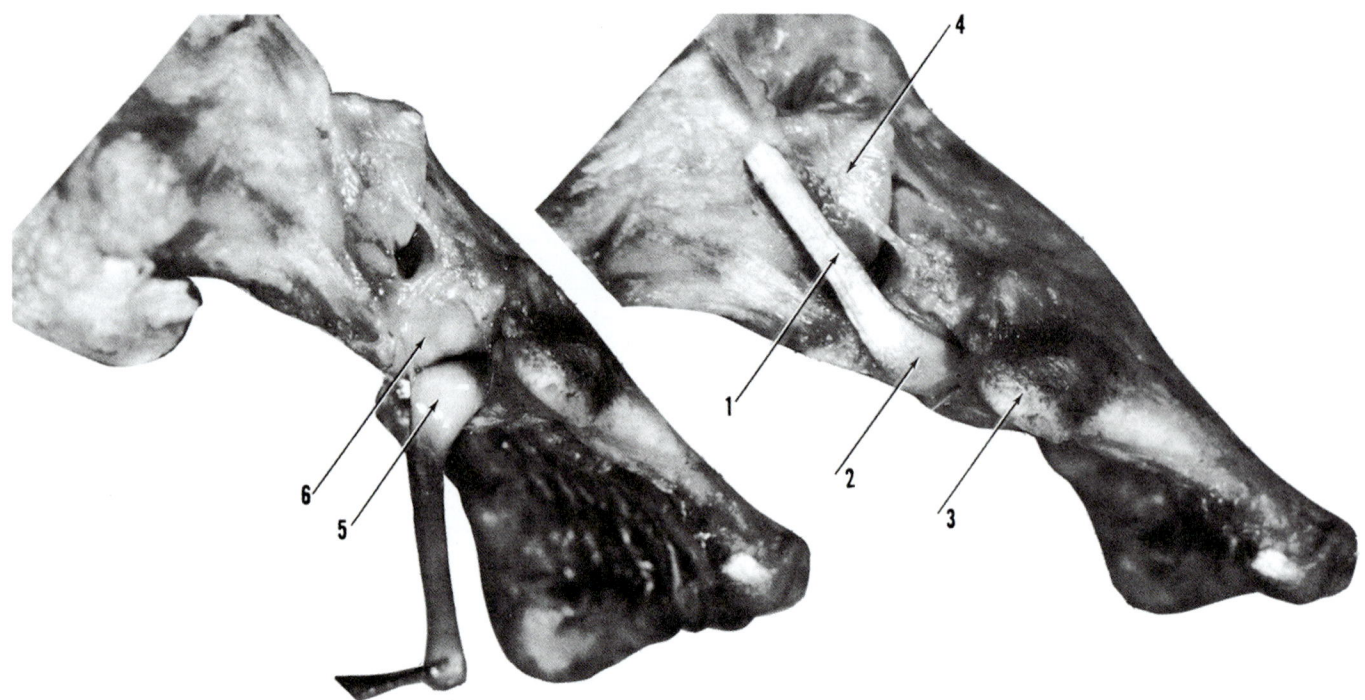

Figure 5.17 **Peroneus longus tendon.** (*1*, Peroneus longus tendon; *2*, portion of [*1*] reflected on tuberosity of cuboid and entering sole of foot; *3*, tuberosity of fifth metatarsal base; *4*, anterior segment or greater apophysis of os calcis; *5*, intra-articular sesamoid of peroneus longus tendon; *6*, cuboidal tuberosity for reflection of peroneus longus tendon.)

inserts 10 mm behind the first metatarsal head on its lateral aspect. This tendinous slip forms an arcade with medial concavity that forms, with the lateral surface of the first metatarsal, an oval aperture filled with adipose tissue giving passage to the dorsal vessels going to the sole of the foot.

In a study of 54 ft, Picou gives the following information concerning the occurrence of the insertional slips of the peroneus longus tendon: insertion on the cuneiform and metatarsal base, 95%; insertion on the metatarsal head, 89%; and insertion on the metatarsal base only, 5.5%.[24]

A fibrous expansion may connect the peroneus longus tendon at the level of the cuboidal sesamoid to the base of the fifth metatarsal and to the origin of the short flexor of the fifth toe and forms the anterior frenular ligament contained in the mesotenon. Occasionally, the anterior ligament may be large and represent an insertion of the principal tendon on the base of the fifth metatarsal. A posterior frenular ligament, which is sesamocuboid, may also exist. The rate of occurrence of these frenular ligaments, according to different sources, is as follows: anterior ligament, 80% in 30 ft, 63% in 30 ft; posterior ligament, 13% in 30 ft, and 10% in 30 ft.[2,25] The peroneus longus may receive a slip from the tibialis posterior tendon in 22%.[26]

Patil et al[27] investigated the insertion of the peroneus longus tendon in 30 preserved feet. The peroneus longus tendon inserted into the base of M_1 in all feet and there was an additional medial cuneiform insertion in 86.6% (23 ft).

An attachment band to the neck of M_1 was present in 10% (3 ft) and attachments to the bases of the lesser metatarsals were as follows: M_2 20% (6 ft), M_4 16.6 % (5 ft), M_5 23.3% (7 ft). An anterior frenular ligament was present in 83.3% (25 ft) and a posterior frenular ligament in 13.3% (4 ft). "An additional band and quite similar to the anterior frenular ligament was observed close to the first metatarsocuneiform joint in nine specimens (30%). This band gave the origins of the first and second dorsal interossei and first plantar interosseous muscles."[27]

▶ Peroneus Brevis

The peroneus brevis tendon is applied against the posterior surface of the lateral malleolus and glides in the retromalleolar canal (see Figs. 5.15 and 5.16). Just below the tip of the lateral malleolus, the tendon makes a turn anteriorly, following the contour of the bone. It is retained by the fibrous sheath of the peronei. The tendon is then directed downward, anteriorly, and slightly laterally, crossing the calcaneofibular ligament superficially. It passes above the calcaneal processus trochlearis through the tunnel formed by the inferior peroneal retinaculum. It fans out and inserts on the styloid apophysis of the fifth metatarsal.

Variations of the Lateral Peronei

The variations of the lateral peronei are multiple, and the descriptive terminology is even more variable, resulting in "a regrettable confusion."[1] To alleviate this, Testut has referred to the comparative anatomy and specifically to the peroneus digiti quinti in mammals (bears and cats).[1] He describes in the *Ursus americanus* three distinct peronei: long lateral peroneus,

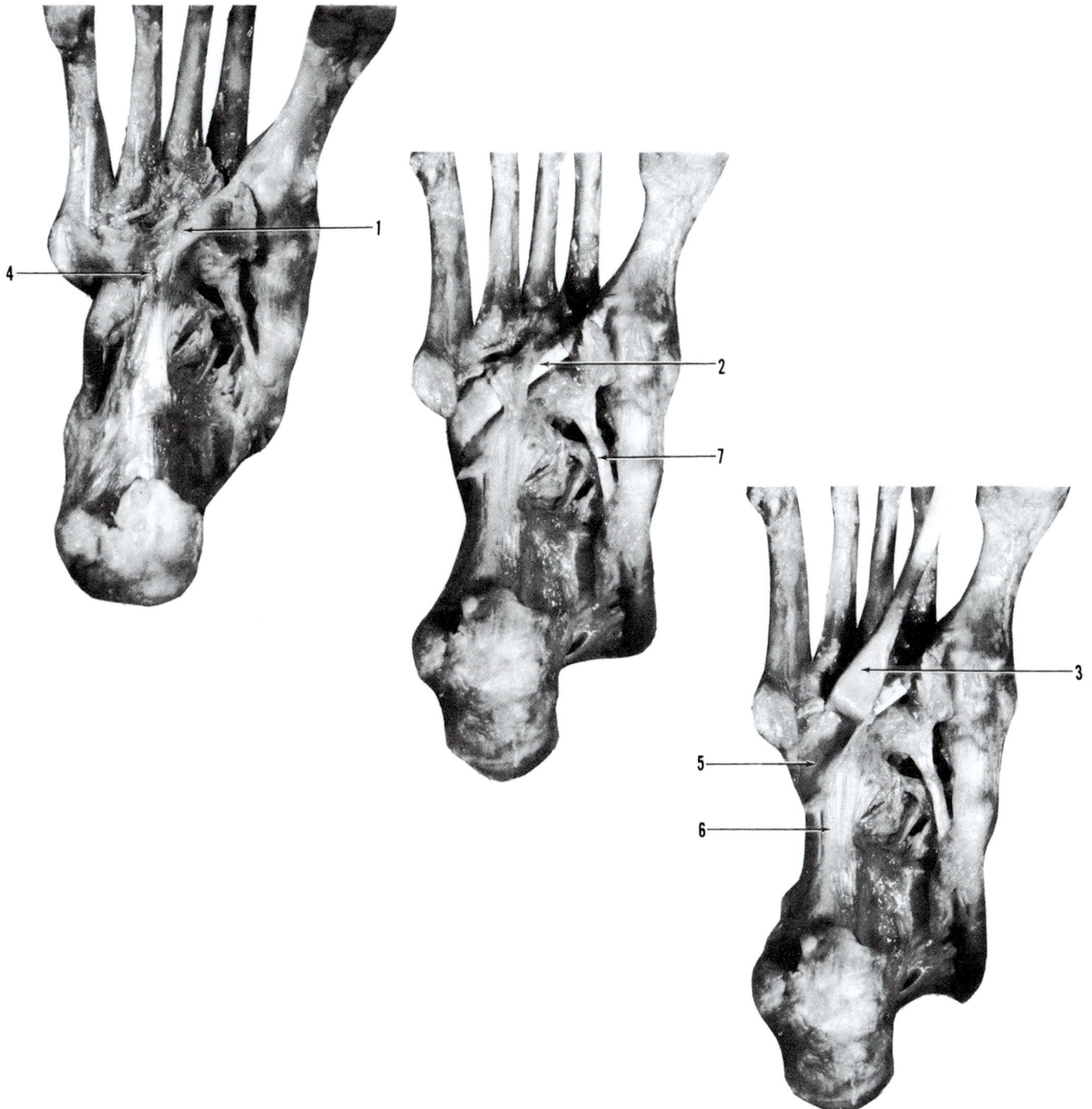

Figure 5.18 Peroneus longus tendon. (*1*, Sheath of peroneus longus tendon; *2*, peroneus longus tendon; *3*, reflected peroneus longus tendon with intratendinous sesamoid; *4*, distal segment of long plantar ligament contributing to formation of peroneus longus tunnel; *5*, peroneus longus sulcus; *6*, long calcaneocuboid ligament; *7*, plantar portion of tibialis posterior tendon.)

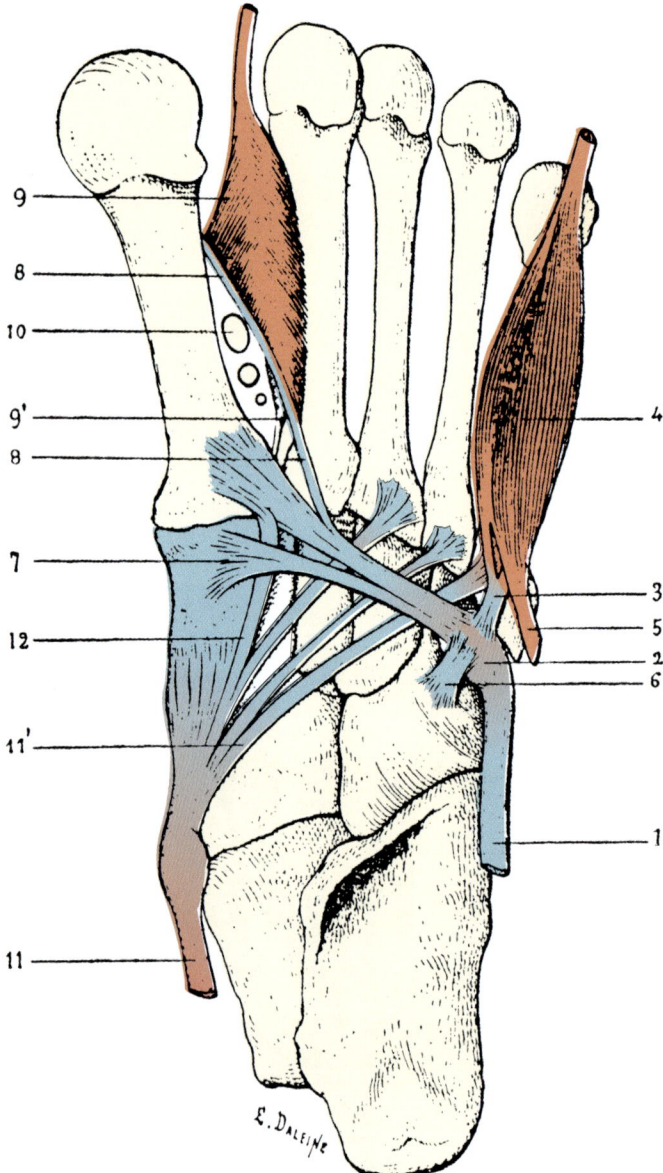

Figure 5.19 Normal insertions of peroneus longus tendon. (*1*, Peroneus longus tendon; *2*, sesamoid of *1*: *3*, anterior frenulum of sesamoid; *4*, short flexor muscle of fifth toe; *5*, expansion of *4* that inserts on fibrous tunnel of peroneus longus tendon; *6*, posterior frenulum of sesamoid [inconstant]; *7*, attachment of *1* on medial cuneiform; *8*, expansion of *1* forming an arcade of origin to the first dorsal interosseous muscle [*9*] and inserting on the superolateral corner of the first metatarsal neck; *9'*, origin of first dorsal interosseous from base of first metatarsal; *10*, dorsalis pedis vessels; *11*, tibialis posterior tendon; *11'*, expansion of *11* to base of fifth metatarsal [inconstant]; *12*, expansion of *11* to peroneus longus tendon [inconstant].) (Adapted from Picou R. Insertions inférieures du muscle long peronier lateral: anomalie de ce muscle. *Bull Soc Anat Paris.* 1894;8[7]:162.)

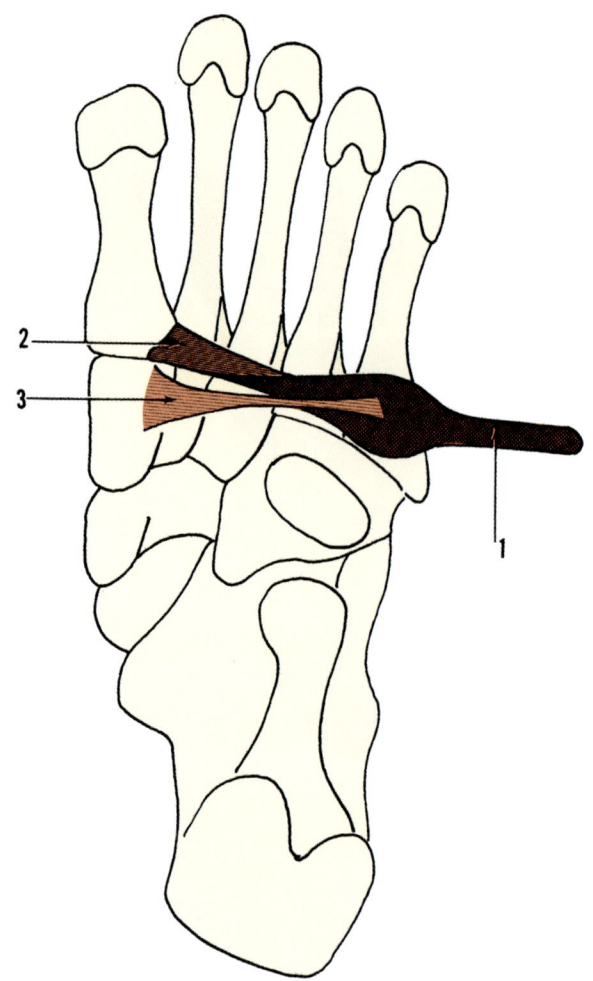

Figure 5.20 Slip of peroneus longus tendon to the first cuneiform. (*1*, Deep surface of peroneus longus tendon; *2*, superficial surface of *1* inserting on base of first metatarsal; *3*, deep slip arising from deep surface of *1* and inserting on first cuneiform.) (Adapted from Picou R. Insertions inférieures du muscle long peronier lateral: anomalie de ce muscle. *Bull Soc Anat Paris.* 1894;8[7]:162.)

short lateral peroneus, and peroneus digiti quinti. The latter is located between the previous two, is triangular in shape, and arises through its base from the fibula. The apex of the muscle is continued by a cylindrical tendon that turns around the lateral malleolus, glides over the dorsum of the fifth metatarsal, and inserts on the proximal phalanx of the fifth toe. In Testut's interpretation, the peroneus digiti quinti may be reproduced in man in a complete or incomplete form with the following classification:

A. —Complete
- Phalangeal insertion on the fifth toe with corresponding independent proximal muscle.
- Phalangeal insertion on the fifth toe with muscle fused to the peroneus brevis muscle.
- Phalangeal insertion on the fifth toe extending as a tendon slip from the peroneus brevis tendon. There is no corresponding muscle.

B. —Incomplete
- Type I: Peroneometatarsal muscle, the tendon terminating at the level of the fifth metatarsal head shaft or base.
- Type II: Peroneocuboidal muscle, the tendon inserting on the cuboid or peroneoperoneal longus muscle with the tendon inserting on the tendon of the latter. This corresponds then to the peroneus accessorius of Henle.

- Type III: External peroneocalcaneal muscle with the tendon inserting on the lateral surface of the calcaneus, thus corresponding to the peroneus quartus of Otto.
- Type IV: Peroneomalleolar muscle with the tendon terminating on the lateral malleolus.

The most common variation is the subvariety of the peroneus digiti quinti of Huxley, represented by a tendinous slip extending from the tendon of the peroneus brevis to the fifth ray. It pierces the tendon of the peroneus tertius and inserts on the base of the proximal phalanx of the fifth toe or on the extensor tendon or aponeurosis of the fifth toe, or on the fifth metatarsal head, shaft, or base (Fig. 5.21). The following data are given relative to the occurrence of the fifth digital tendinous extension from the peroneus brevis tendon: in 102 ft, the digital slip is well developed in 23% and vestigial in 13%, total 36% (Wood)[12]; in 100 ft, the slip is well developed in 21% and vestigial in 13%, total 34% (LeDouble)[2]; in 100 ft, the slip is present in 15.5% (Bhargava and colleagues).[28]

Reimann, in a study of 200 cadaver limbs, describes a tendinous extension slip from the peroneus brevis tendon in 79.5%.[23] This tendinous extension may insert on the following structures as follows:

- Extensor aponeurosis of the fifth toe
- Extensor aponeurosis of the fifth toe and fourth metatarsal shaft
- Fifth metatarsal shaft
- Fourth and fifth metatarsal shafts
- Fourth metatarsal shaft
- Peroneus tertius tendon
- Extensor aponeurosis of the fifth toe and peroneus tertius tendon
- Extensor aponeurosis of the fifth toe with loop formation around peroneus tertius tendon and insertion on fourth metatarsal shaft
- Fifth metatarsal shaft and peroneus tertius tendon
- Fourth and fifth metatarsal shafts and extensor aponeurosis of fifth toe

Bareither and coworkers, in a study of 298 cadaver limbs, found the extension of the tendinous slip from the peroneus brevis tendon to the extensor aponeurosis of the fifth toe in 59.7%.[29]

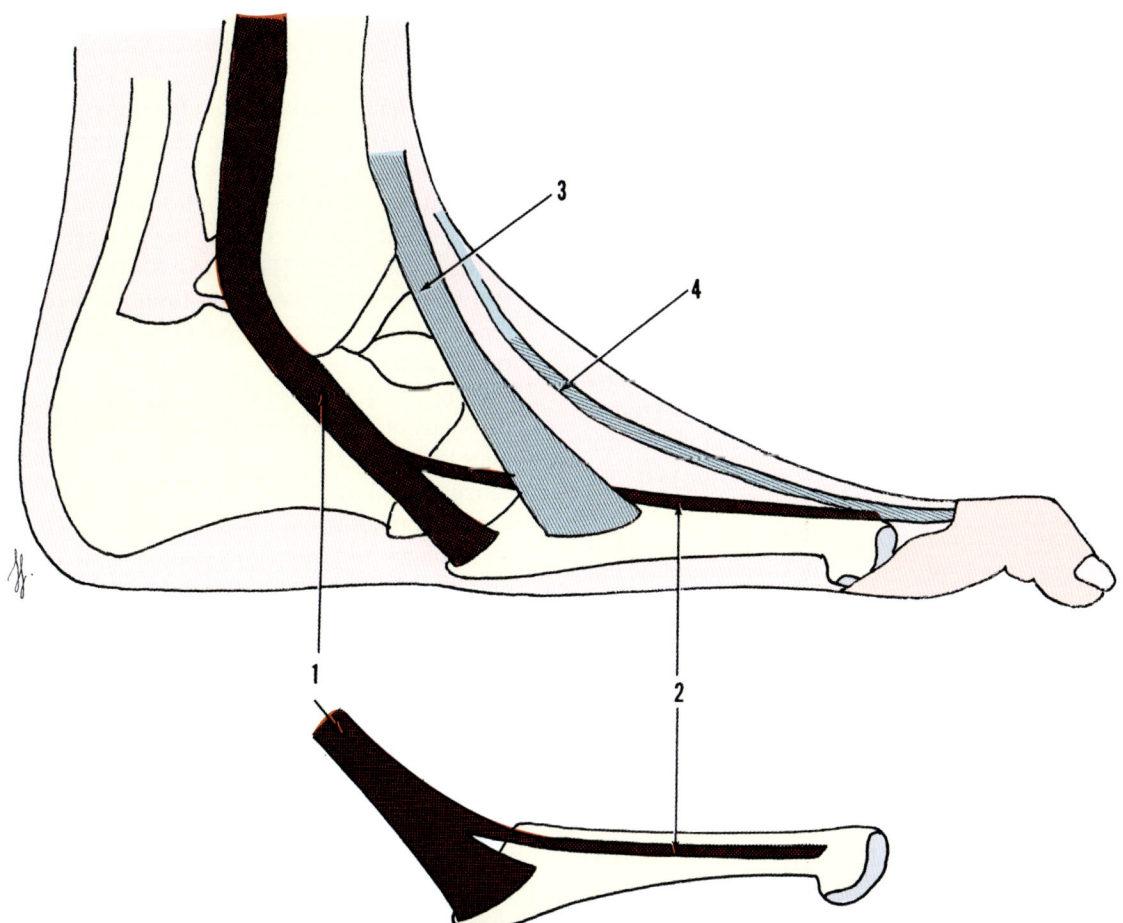

Figure 5.21 **Variation of lateral peronei.** (*1*, Peroneus brevis tendon; *2*, accessory slip passing through peroneus tertius [*3*] insertion and attaching to long extensor of fifth toe [*4*] or fifth metatarsal shaft.)

Of interest to the surgeon is the muscle peroneus quartus described by Otto in 1816: "This muscle originates from the external surface of the lower third of the fibula and continues as a very thin tendon up to the external surface of the calcaneus."[30] Gruber[31] has found the muscle peroneus quartus in 12% of 982 extremities, and Wood[12] in 3% of 70 extremities.

Hecker, in a comprehensive study of the variations of the lateral peronei, grouped (under the heading of the lateral peronei of the tarsus) the different forms of variations: lateral peroneocalcaneal muscle, peroneocuboid muscle, and peroneoperoneolongus muscle.[32] The frequency of occurrence of the lateral peronei of the tarsus has been stated as 13% in 47 adult feet and 20% in 16 embryonic feet.[32]

The majority of the variations are of the peroneocalcaneal type, forming the lateral peroneocalcaneus muscle. Hecker describes six types of variations (Fig. 5.22)[32]:

Type I: The muscle originates from the peroneus longus and the peroneus brevis muscle mass. The strong tendon (4 mm) glides through the retromalleolar tunnel and divides into two slips below the tip of the lateral malleolus. The thin anterior slip passes along the anterior border of the peroneus brevis tendon and inserts on the origin of the inferior extensor retinaculum and on the superolateral aspect of the os calcis. The thicker posterior slip diverges and inserts on the inferolateral aspect of the os calcis and on the septum separating the two compartments of the inferior peroneal retinaculum. With its diverging two slips, the lateral peroneocalcaneal tendon forms a buttonhole through which the tendon of the peroneus brevis passes.

Type II: The muscle derives from the peroneus brevis at the junction of the middle and lower thirds of the leg. The cylindrical tendon measures 2.5 mm in diameter and 5 cm in length and inserts on the lateral surface of the os calcis. The insertion is fan-shaped and located posterior to the inferior peroneal retinaculum and posterior to the peroneus longus tendon.

Type III: The muscle arises from the peroneus brevis muscle at the level of the inferior third of the leg. The thin tendon attaches on the lateral surface of the os calcis in close connection with the lower component of the inferior peroneal retinaculum.

Type IV: The muscle is similar to type III distally. Proximally, however, the muscle is larger and extends higher on the fibula and on the posterolateral intermuscular septum.

Type V: The muscle arises from the peroneus brevis in the lower third of the leg. At a level three fingerbreadths proximal to the tip of the lateral malleolus, a few musculotendinous fascicles separate from the muscular portion and spread in the fibrous tissue, forming the peroneocalcaneal ligament. The true tendinous formation appears further down and divides into three slips: anterior, middle, and posterior. The stronger middle slip inserts on a tubercle on the lateral surface of the os calcis, the thin anterior slip fans out and inserts anterior to the middle slip, and the vertical posterior slip inserts posterior and slightly more proximal to the middle slip.

Type VI: This muscle represents a lateral peroneal of the tarsus completely replacing the peroneus brevis. The muscle arises from the middle third of the lateral surface of the fibula, the anterior crest of the fibula, and the lateral intermuscular septum. The large muscle divides into three parts. The anterior tendon inserts on the os calcis, the dorsal calcaneocuboid ligament, and the lateral surface of the cuboid. The middle tendon has a broad, fan-shaped insertion on the lateral surface of the os calcis. The posterior tendon is thin and inserts posteriorly below the lateral malleolus. This type of variation is extremely rare.

Three other rare types of variation may also occur: peroneocuboid muscle, bifid peroneus longus tendon, and peroneoperoneolongus muscle. The peroneocuboid muscle originates from the lateral compartment in the inferior third, and the tendon inserts on the lateral surface of the cuboid. The bifid peroneus longus tendon forms a buttonhole through which the peroneus brevis tendon passes. The peroneoperoneolongus muscle originates from the inferior third of the lateral compartment, and the tendon inserts on the peroneus longus tendon.

Sobel and colleagues, in a recent anatomic investigation of the lateral peronei of 124 cadaveric legs, found the peroneus quartus in 21.7% with the following variations[33]:

- Peroneus quartus takes origin from the muscular portion of the peroneus brevis in the lower one-third of the leg and inserts on the peroneal tubercle of the calcaneus (Fig. 5.23): 63%.
- Peroneus quartus takes origin from the peroneus brevis and inserts into the peroneus longus just distal to the retromalleolar groove (Fig. 5.24): 3.7%.
- Peroneus quartus takes origin from the peroneus brevis muscular portion and inserts into the peroneus brevis just distal to the fibular groove (Fig. 5.25): 3.7%.
- Peroneus quartus takes origin from the peroneus brevis. The tendon divides into two tendinous slips that insert separately on the dorsum of the base and the head of the fifth metatarsal (Fig. 5.26): 7.4%.
- Peroneus quartus originates high in the leg from the peroneus longus and inserts into the peroneal tubercle of the calcaneus (Fig. 5.27): 7.4%.
- Peroneus quartus originates high in the leg from the peroneus longus and inserts back into the peroneus longus tendon just distal to the fibular groove (Fig. 5.28): 3.7%.
- Peroneus quartus originates from the peroneus brevis and inserts into the lateral retinaculum: 11.1%.
- Peroneus quartus originates from the peroneus longus and inserts into the peroneus brevis: 3.7%.

Interestingly, Sobel and coworkers found an attrition of 18% of the peroneus brevis tendon in the fibular groove when the peroneus quartus was present.[33]

Trono et al[34] reported on a case of peroneus quartus muscle and reviewed the literature. Sonmez et al[35] demonstrated the occurrence of bilateral peroneus quartus and peroneus digiti. Quinti muscles in both legs of a cadaver were associated with the presence of a bilateral tendinous slip extending from the

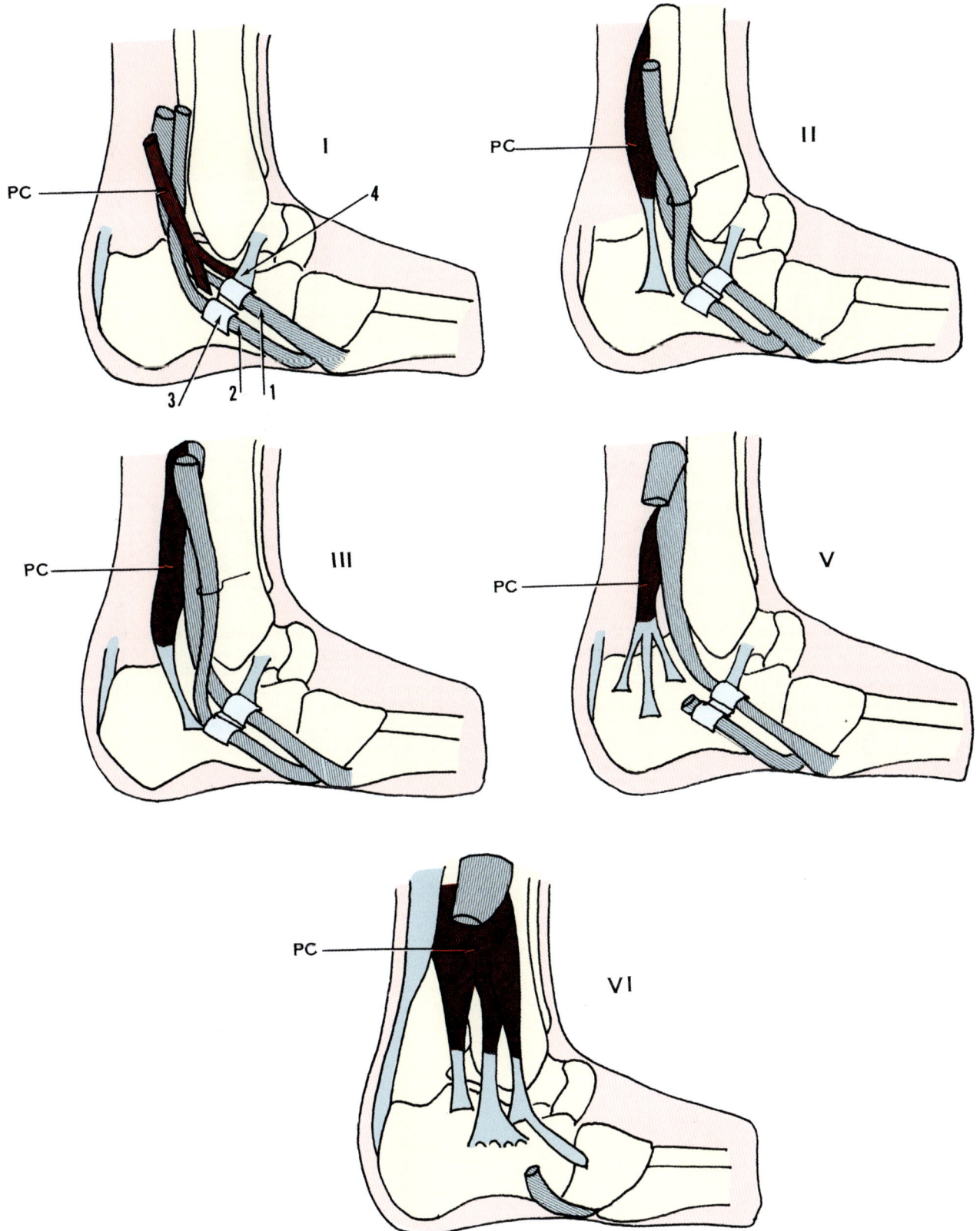

Figure 5.22 **Types of variation of lateral peronei.** (*PC*, peroneocalcaneal muscle; *1*, peroneus brevis tendon; *2*, peroneus longus tendon; *3*, inferior peroneal retinaculum; *4*, stem of inferior extensor retinaculum.) (Adapted from Hecker P. Etude sur le péronier du tarse: variations des péroniers latéraux. *Arch Anat Histol Embryol.* 1924;3:327.)

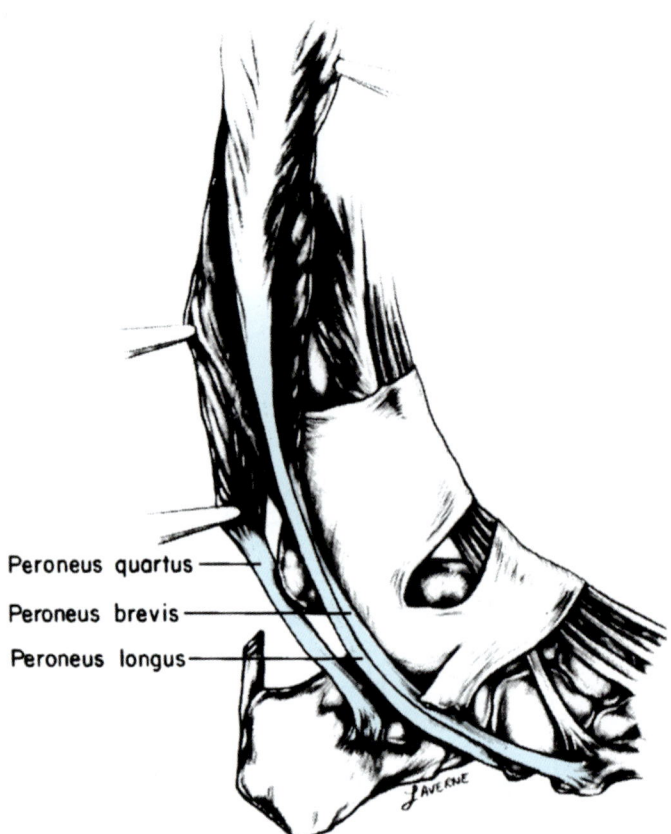

Figure 5.23 **The peroneus quartus takes origin from the lower one-third portion of the peroneus brevis and inserts into the peroneal tubercle of the calcaneus.** Hypertrophy of the peroneal tubercle is evident. (Adapted from Sobel M, Levy ME, Bohne WH. Congenital variations of the peroneus quartus muscle: an anatomic study. *Foot Ankle.* 1990;11[2]:81.)

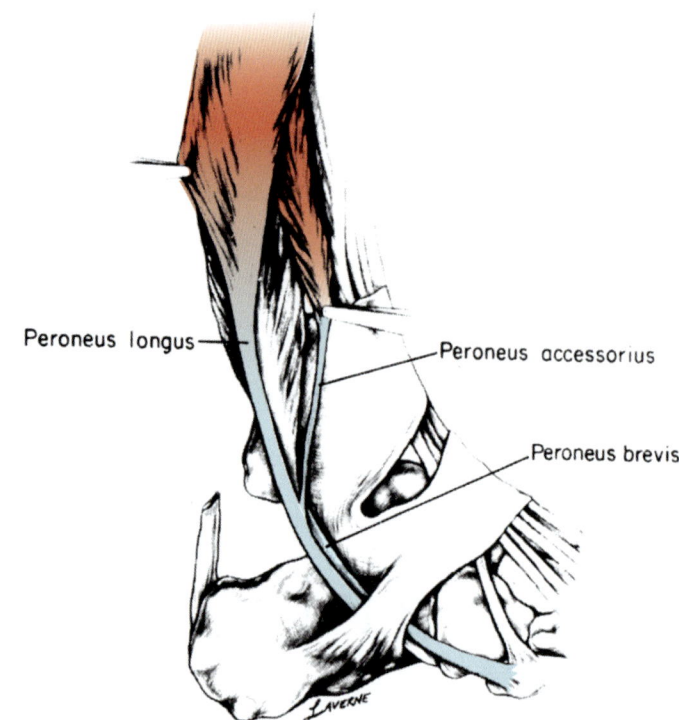

Figure 5.24 **The peroneus quartus takes origin from the peroneus brevis and inserts into the peroneus longus just distal to the fibular groove.** (Adapted from Sobel M, Levy ME, Bohne WH. Congenital variations of the peroneus quartus muscle: an anatomic study. *Foot Ankle.* 1990;11[2]:81.)

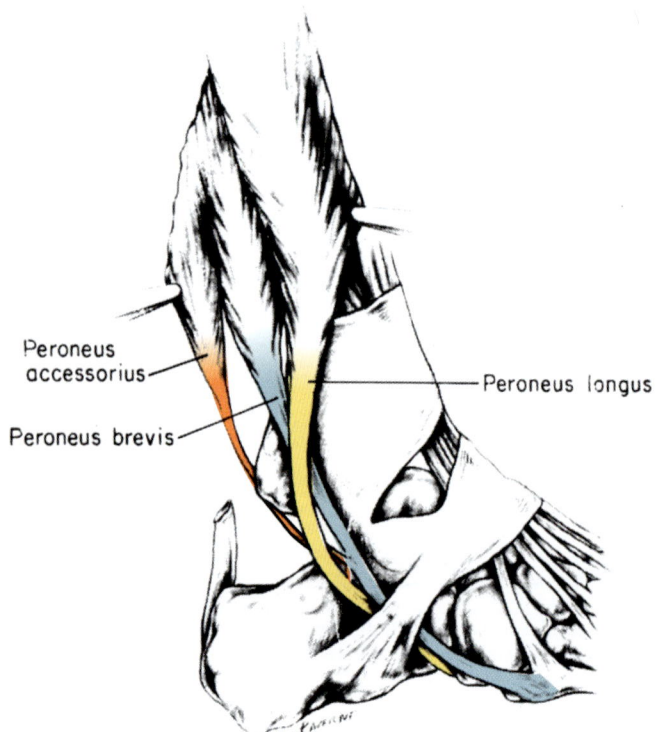

Figure 5.25 **The peroneus quartus takes origin from the peroneus brevis and inserts back into the peroneus brevis just distal to the fibular groove.** (Adapted from Sobel M, Levy ME, Bohne WH. Congenital variations of the peroneus quartus muscle: an anatomic study. *Foot Ankle.* 1990;11[2]:81.)

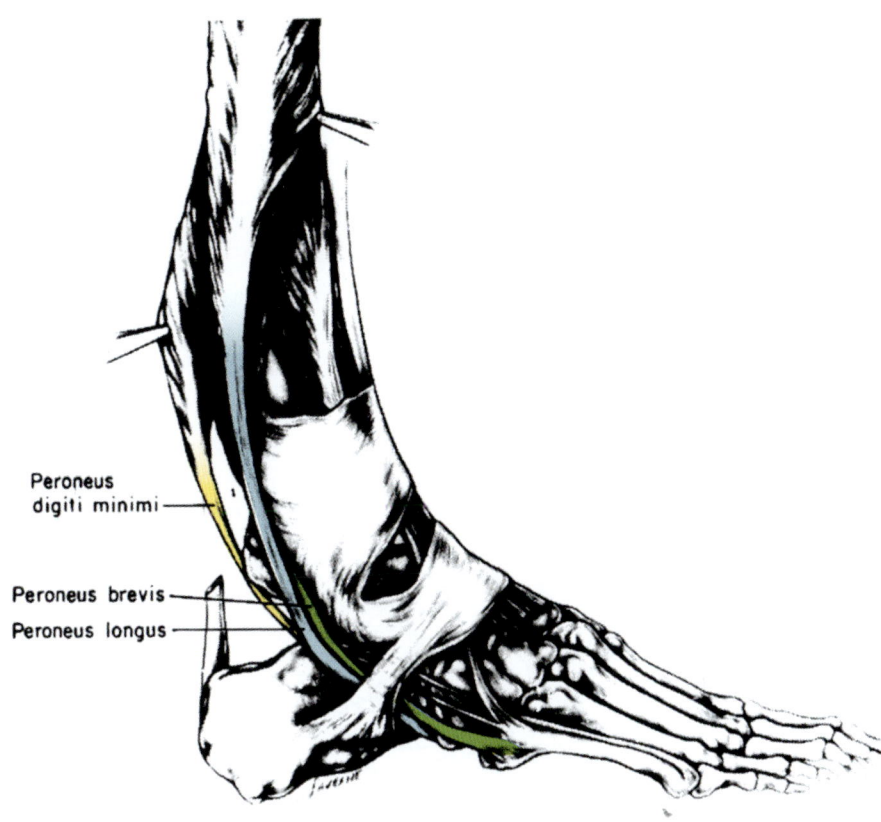

Figure 5.26 The peroneus digiti minimi quinti takes origin from the peroneus brevis and the tendinous portion splits into two tendons. One slip inserts dorsally at the base of the fifth metatarsal and the long slip inserts into the dorsum of the head of the fifth metatarsal. (Adapted from Sobel M, Levy ME, Bohne WH. Congenital variations of the peroneus quartus muscle: an anatomic study. *Foot Ankle*. 1990;11[2]:81.)

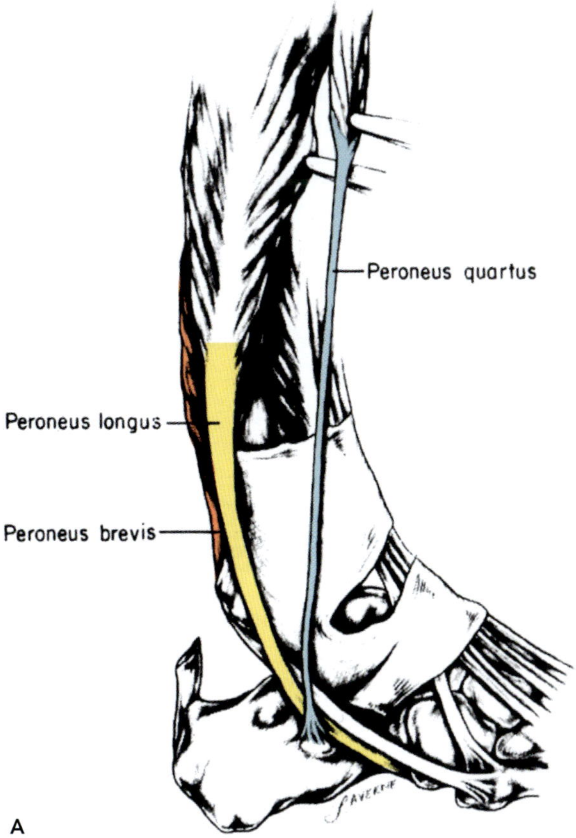

Figure 5.27 (A) The peroneus quartus takes origin high in the leg from the peroneus longus and inserts into the peroneal tubercle of the calcaneus. Hypertrophy of the peroneal tubercle is evident. **(B) The peroneus quartus takes origin high in the leg from the peroneus longus, courses under the tendon of the peroneus longus, and inserts into the peroneal tubercle of the calcaneus.** (Adapted from Sobel M, Levy ME, Bohne WH. Congenital variations of the peroneus quartus muscle: an anatomic study. *Foot Ankle*. 1990;11[2]:81.)

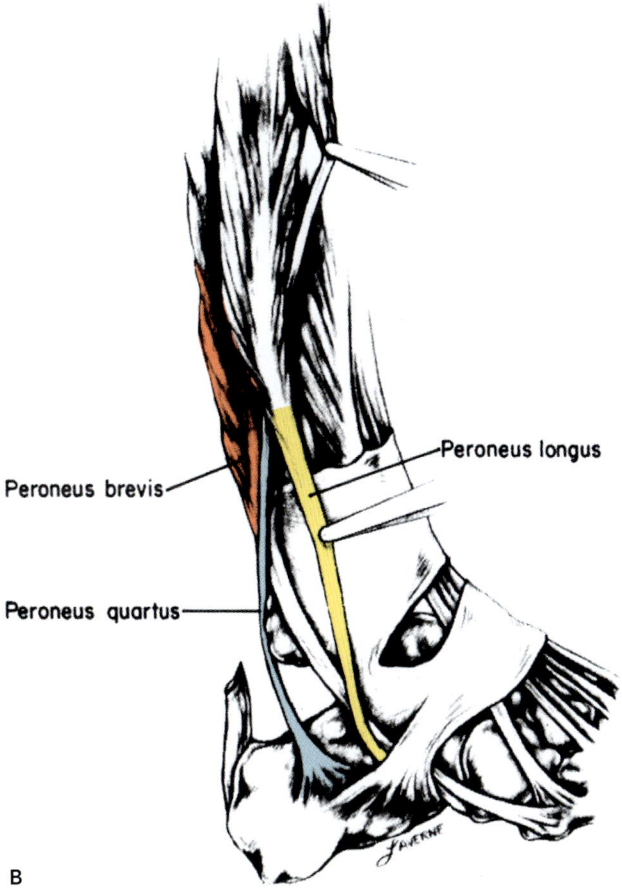

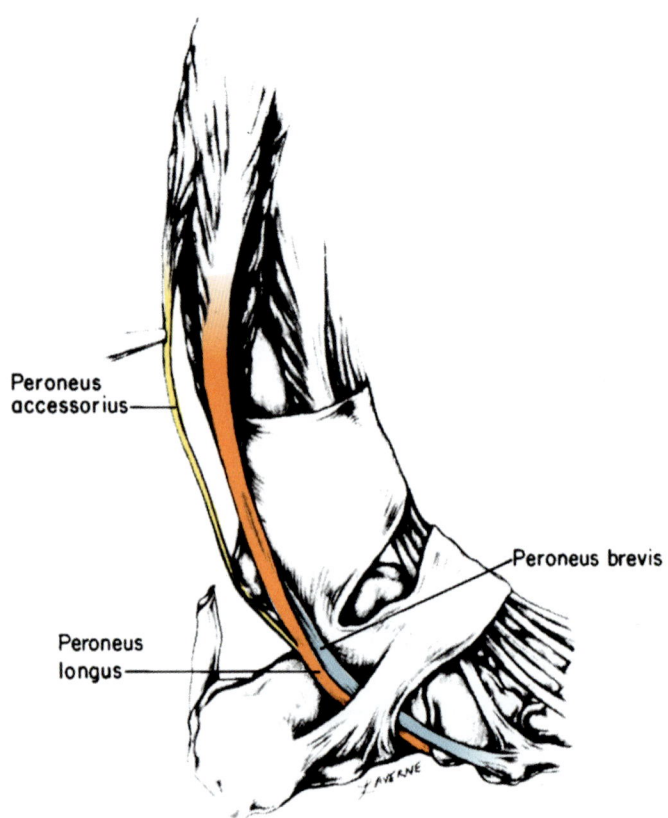

Figure 5.28 The peroneus quartus takes origin high in the leg from the peroneus longus and inserts back into the peroneus longus just distal to the fibular groove. (Adapted from Sobel M, Levy ME, Bohne WH. Congenital variations of the peroneus quartus muscle: an anatomic study. *Foot Ankle*. 1990;11[2]:81.)

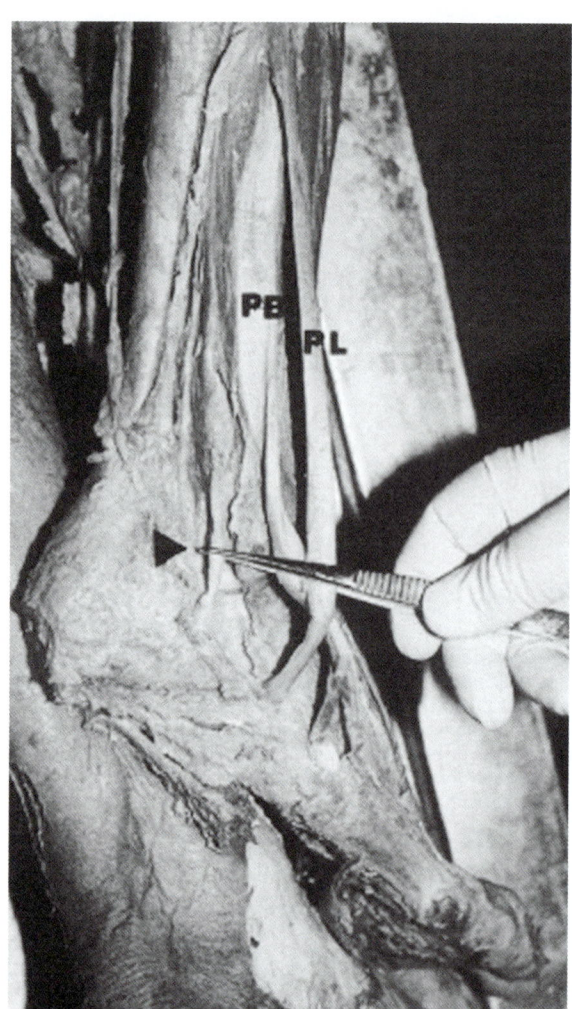

Figure 5.29 Lateral view of the right foot showing the tendon of the peroneus quartus inserting in the peroneal trochlea on the calcaneus (*arrowhead*). (*PB*, peroneus brevis tendon; *PL*, peroneus longus tendon.) (Reprinted from Sonmez M, Kosar I, Cimen M. The supernumerary peroneal muscles: case report and review of literature. *Foot Ankle Surg*. 2000;6:125-129, Figure 1, with permission from Elsevier.)

tibialis anterior tendon and inserting on the base of the proximal phalanx of the big toe (Figs. 5.29 to 5.31).

Zammit and Singh[36] reported the presence of the peroneus quartus muscle in 5.88% of dissected 102 cadaver legs and identified the peroneus quartus in 7.5% of 80 magnetic resonance imaging studies of symptomatic ankles. The overall incidence of occurrence of the peroneus quartus muscle was 6.69%. Moroney and Borton[37] reported in a surgical patient the occurrence of the peroneus quartus muscle in association with a second smaller muscle that "passed with the peroneus longus tendon toward the plantar aspect of the first metatarsal," but the final insertion of this muscle was not identified.

Gumusalan and Ozbag[38] reported in a dissected leg the presence of a peroneus quartus muscle originating "from the lateral surface of the fibula and posterior intermuscular septum almost 7.5 cm proximal to the distal tip of the fibula. The muscle belly was fusiform in shape and 4 cm long. Its width at the widest level was 7.7 cm, and the thickness was 3 mm. The muscle converged into a slender tendon, the length of which was 5.8 cm." The attachment was to the retrotrochlear eminence of the calcaneus.

Saupe et al[39] in a magnetic resonance imaging study of 65 asymptomatic ankles of volunteers reported evidence of the pronator quartus muscle in 17%. The attachment of the tendon was to the calcaneus (peroneocalcaneus externum), the cuboid bone (peroneocuboideus), or the peroneus longus tendon (peroneoperoneolongus).

MEDIAL ASPECT OF THE ANKLE AND FOOT AND THE SOLE OF THE FOOT

On the posteromedial aspect of the ankle-hindfoot, the tendon of the tibialis posterior crosses obliquely the medial aspect of the talus. The flexor digitorum longus crosses the very posteromedial aspect of the talus, then the medial border of the sustentaculum tali. The flexor hallucis longus passes through the posterior talar groove and crosses the inferior surface of the sustentaculum tali (Fig. 5.32). All three tendons make their turn with anterior concavity and pass through the tarsal tunnel and the porta pedis and penetrate the sole of the foot.

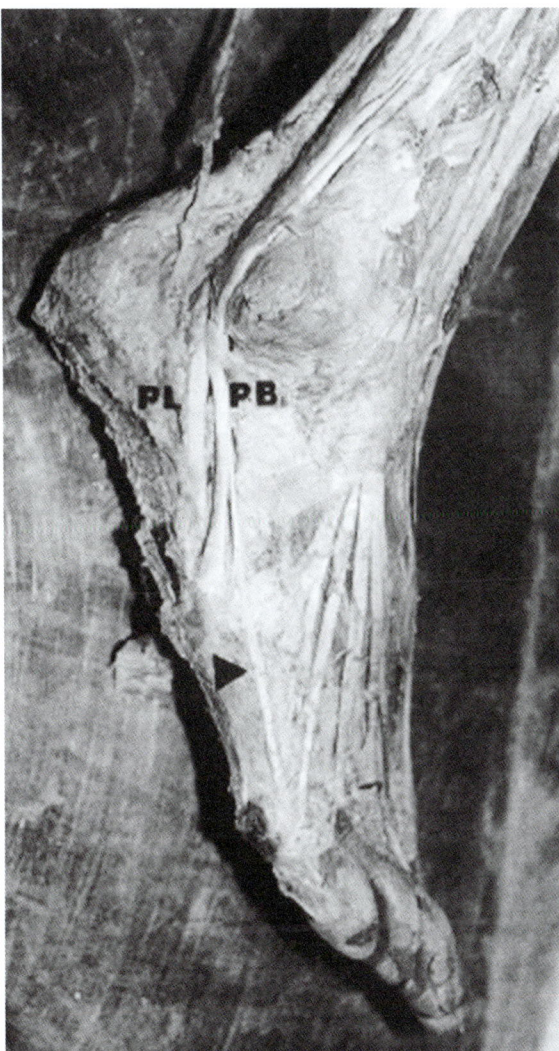

Figure 5.30 Lateral view of the foot showing the tendon of the peroneus digiti quinti inserting into the aponeurosis of the fifth toe (*arrowhead*). (*PB*, peroneus brevis tendon; *PL*, peroneus longus tendon.) (Reprinted from Sonmez M, Kosar I, Cimen M. The supernumerary peroneal muscles: case report and review of literature. Foot Ankle Surg. 2000;6:125-129, Figure 2, with permission from Elsevier.)

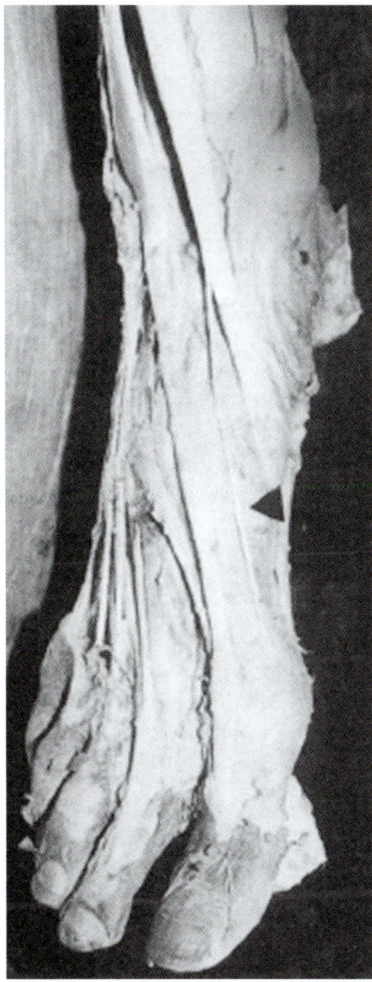

Figure 5.31 Superomedial view of the right foot showing the accessory tendon of tibialis anterior inserting into the base of the proximal phalanx of the big toe (*arrowhead*). (Reprinted from Sonmez M, Kosar I, Cimen M. The supernumerary peroneal muscles: case report and review of literature. Foot Ankle Surg. 2000;6:125-129, Figure 3, with permission from Elsevier.)

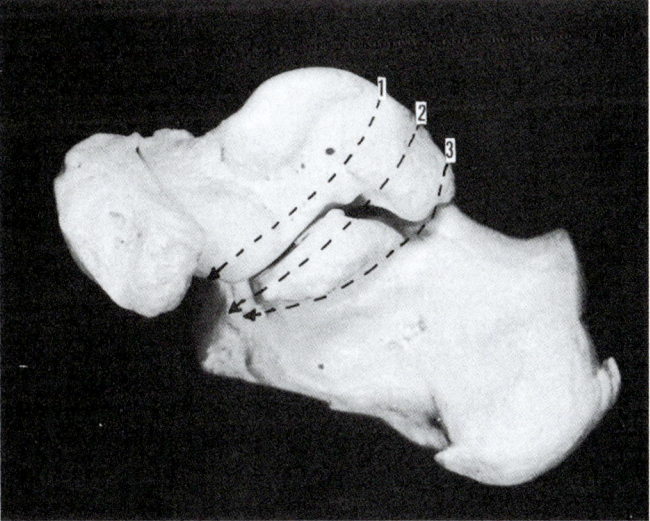

Figure 5.32 Medial aspect of the talocalcaneal joint. (*Dotted lines*, direction of 1, tibialis posterior tendon; 2, flexor digitorum longus tendon; 3, flexor hallucis longus tendon.)

On the posterior aspect of the medial malleolus and of the talus, each tendon is retained in a fibrous tunnel. The tunnel of the tibialis posterior crosses the medial aspect of the posterior talus, the medial aspect of the talar neck, and the inferior surface of the inferocalcaneonavicular ligament. The tibialis posterior tendon is thus transtalar during its course and crosses the tibiotalar and tibiocalcaneal components of the deltoid ligament. Further distally, it crosses the origin of the superomedial calcaneonavicular ligament and the inferior surface of the inferior calcaneonavicular ligament. The tibialis posterior tendon is located above the sustentaculum tali.

The tunnel of the flexor digitorum longus is adjacent to that of the tibialis posterior. The tendon of the flexor digitorum longus crosses the very posterior aspect of the medial talar surface, passes over the subtalar joint, and crosses the medial surface of the sustentaculum tali.

The tendon of the flexor hallucis longus passes through the fibrous retrotalar tunnel, which is at a distance from the fibrous tunnel of the flexor digitorum longus. Further down, the interval between the tendons narrows as the flexor hallucis longus converges medially. The tendon crosses the posterior talocalcaneal joint and passes under the inferior surface of the sustentaculum tali.

The superficial and deep layers of the flexor retinaculum are in close connection with the fibrous sheath of the tibialis posterior and flexor digitorum longus tendons. The interval between these two tunnels and that of the flexor hallucis longus is bridged by the deep aponeurosis that inserts laterally on the tunnel of the peronei; this creates a third compartment for the posterior tibial neurovascular bundle. The neurovascular compartment is superficial to the intertendinous interval and to the tunnel of the flexor hallucis longus.

▶ Tibialis Posterior Tendon

On the inferior aspect of the inferior calcaneonavicular ligament, the tibialis posterior tendon is flat and contains a fibrocartilaginous or bony sesamoid (Figs. 5.32 to 5.36). Just in front of the tuberosity of the scaphoid, the tendon divides into three components: anterior, middle, and posterior.

The anterior component is the largest of the three, in direct continuity with the main tendon, and inserts on the tuberosity of the navicular, the inferior capsule of the cuneo$_1$-navicular joint, and the inferior surface of the first cuneiform. This is a very broad insertion that engulfs the tuberosity of the navicular and reaches the first cuneiform, similar to a cuff.

The middle component is very deep and continues distally into the sole of the foot as a tarsometatarsal extension that inserts on the second cuneiform, the third cuneiform, and the cuboid, laterally and over the peroneal canal. Beyond this point, the metatarsal extension of the tendon passes deep or dorsal to the peroneus longus tendon, the two crossing in an "X." Three metatarsal tendinous slips are formed. The medial two slips make a twist, become sagittal in orientation, penetrate the narrow spaces between the bases of the corresponding metatarsals, and insert on the base of the second metatarsal laterally and the base of the third metatarsal medially, and on the base of the third metatarsal laterally and the base of the fourth metatarsal medially. The third tendinous slip is oriented transversely and inserts on the base of the fifth metatarsal; at times, this slip is absent.

The tarsometatarsal component of the tibialis posterior tendon also gives attachment to the Y-shaped origin of the flexor hallucis brevis. A detailed description of this Y-shaped or triangular component is provided by Lewis and by Martin.[40,41] The medial limb of the Y is in continuity with the tibialis posterior tendon. The lateral limb inserts on the cuboid and the lateral cuneiform. The stem of the Y provides attachment to the flexor hallucis brevis (Fig. 5.37).[40] The arms of the Y component may be united, forming a triangular fold that bends medially and gives attachment to the flexor hallucis brevis (Fig. 5.38).[41] This

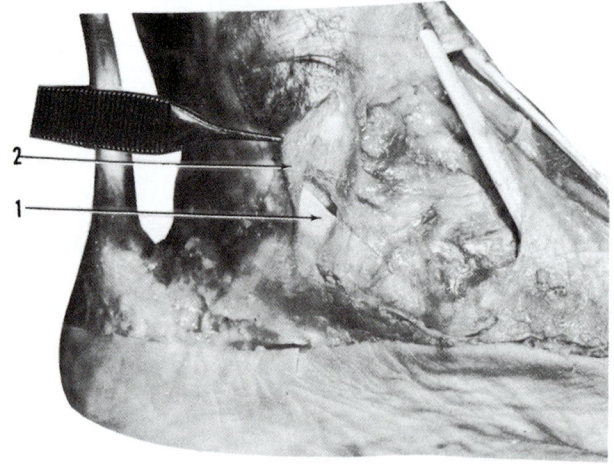

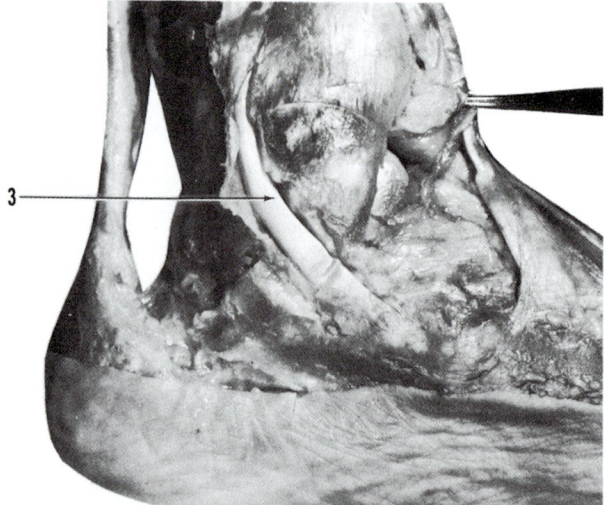

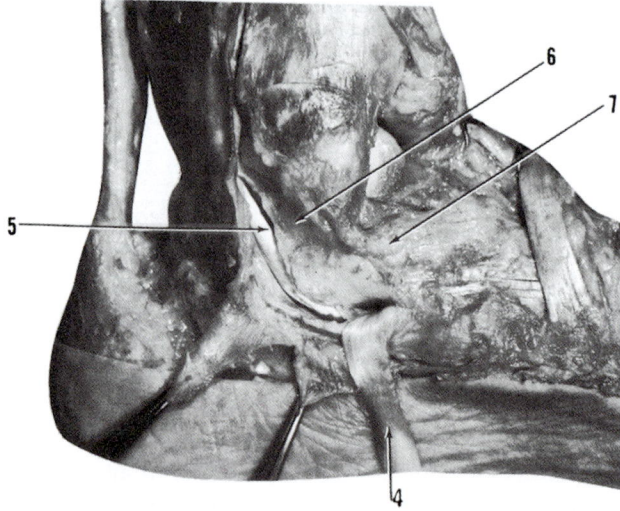

Figure 5.33 Medial aspect of the ankle and calcaneal canal. (*1*, Tibialis posterior tendon; *2*, reflected flexor retinaculum and fibrous sheath of *1*; *3*, retromedial malleolar position of tibialis posterior tendon; *4*, reflected tibialis posterior tendon; *5*, flexor digitorum longus tendon exposed through incised fibrous tunnel; *6*, sulcus of tibialis posterior tendon; *7*, origin of superomedial calcaneonavicular ligament.)

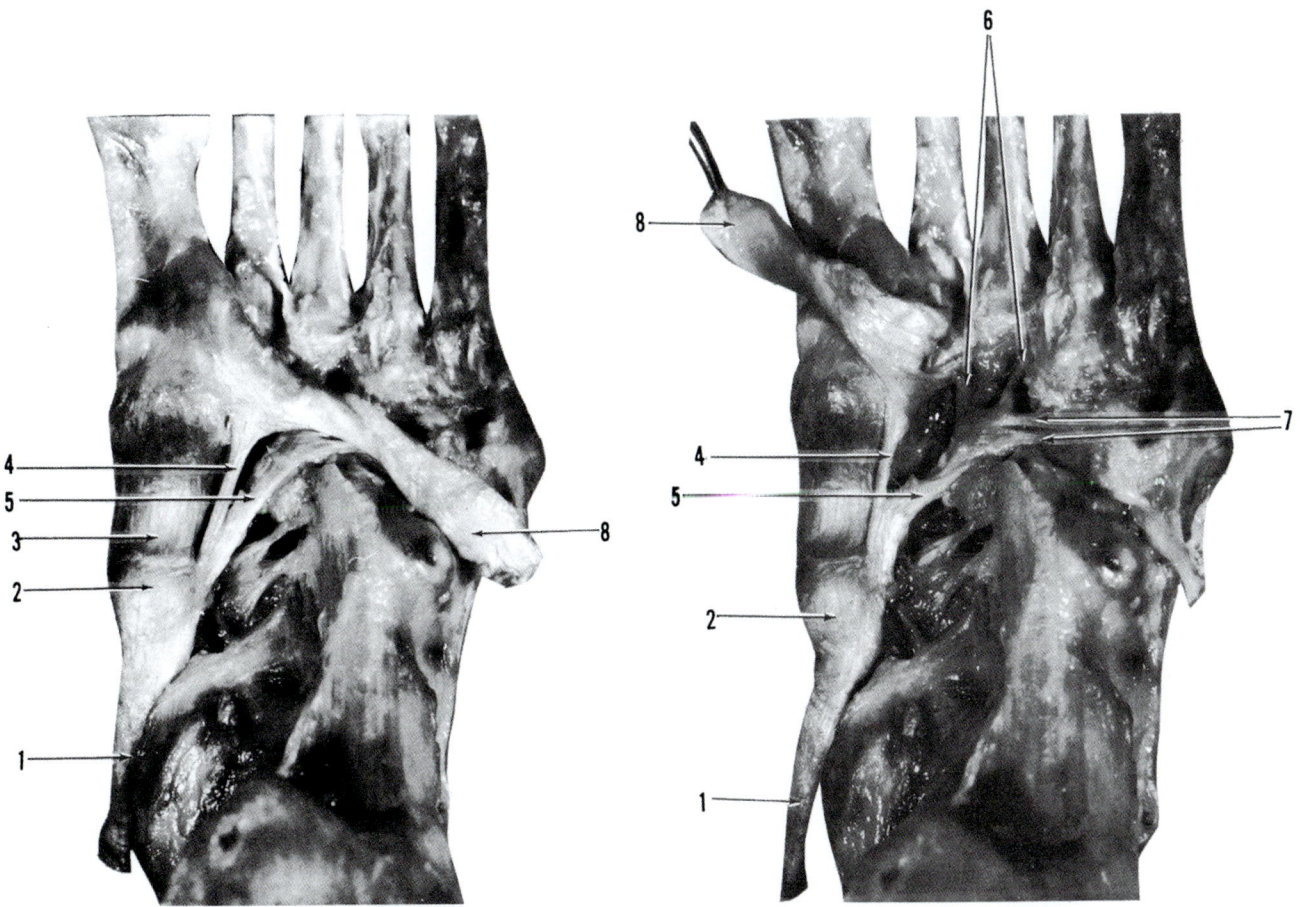

Figure 5.34 Tibialis posterior tendon. (*1*, Tibialis posterior tendon; *2*, insertion of *1* on tuberosity of navicular; *3*, insertion of *1* on medial cuneiform; *4*, insertion of *1* on peroneus longus tendon; *5*, plantar segment—cuneometatarsal—of *1*; *6*, insertional slips of *1* on metatarsal 2-3 and 3-4; *7*, insertional slips of *1* on metatarsals 4 and 5; *8*, peroneus longus tendon.)

brings forth the dynamic connection between the tibialis posterior tendon and the flexor hallucis brevis. Occasionally, the tarsometatarsal component of the tendon sends a sizable tendinous slip to the peroneus longus tendon close to its insertion on the base of the first metatarsal.

The posterior component of the tibialis posterior is recurrent and originates from the main tendon prior to its insertion on the tuberosity of the navicular. It is oriented laterally and posteriorly and inserts as a band on the anterior aspect of the sustentaculum tali. This complex insertion of the tibialis posterior tendon provides a firm grip on the planta pedis.

Bloome at al[42] investigated the insertion of the tibialis posterior tendon in 11 fresh frozen feet. The division of the tendon into three bands—anterior, middle, and posterior—was confirmed in all specimens. The approximate width of the tendinous bands in percentage of the total was anterior band 65%, middle band 15%, and posterior band 20%.

The insertion of the tendon on the navicular; the medial, middle, and lateral cuneiforms; the metatarsal bases of M_2, M_3, and M_4; and the sustentaculum tali was 100%. The additional insertion on the base of M_5 was 64%. An insertional band to the peroneus longus tendon was present in 36% and an attachment to the medial origin of the flexor hallucis brevis muscle in 82%. "A distinct slip from the anterior band to the abductor hallucis was seen in 5/11 (45%)."[42] An attachment to the spring ligament was present in 36%.

▶ Flexor Digitorum Longus and Flexor Hallucis Longus

In the upper compartment of the inferior segment of the calcaneal canal, above the interfascicular septum, the tendons of the flexor digitorum longus and the flexor hallucis longus converge (see Figs. 5.32, 5.33, 5.39, and 5.40). Both tendons pierce the medial intermuscular septum in a medial-to-lateral direction and enter the middle compartment of the sole of the foot. They cross in an X shape as the tendon of the flexor digitorum longus continues its oblique course—anteriorly and laterally— and passes superficial or plantar to the tendon of the flexor hallucis longus, which remains oriented anteriorly and slightly

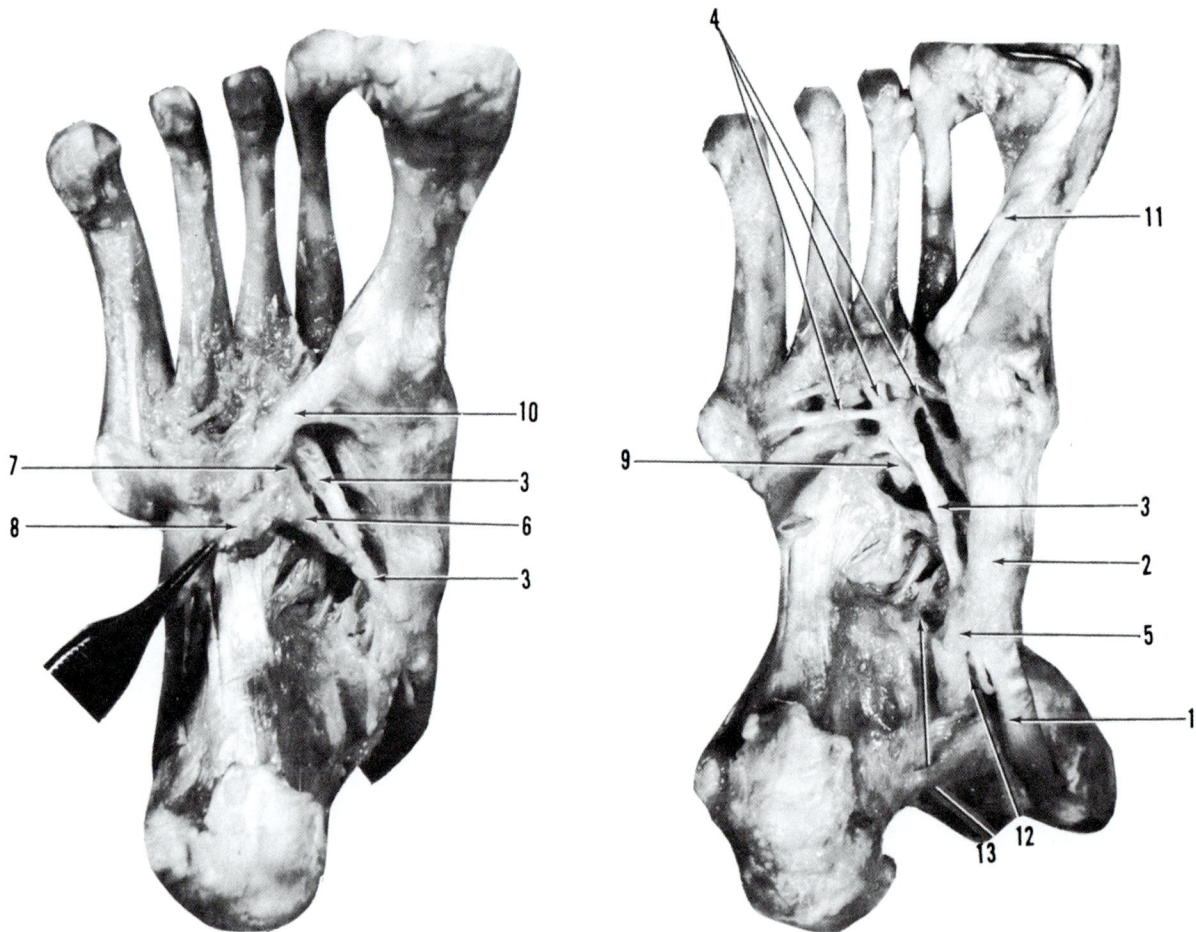

Figure 5.35 **Tibialis posterior tendon.** (*1*, Tibialis posterior tendon; *2*, insertion of *1* on tuberosity of navicular; *3*, plantar cuneometatarsal portion of *1*; *4*, metatarsal insertions of *1*; *5*, calcaneal, recurrent insertion band of *1*; *6*, band from tibialis posterior tendon forming medial arm of Y stem of origin of flexor hallucis brevis; *7*, lateral arm of Y stem of origin of flexor hallucis brevis muscle; *8*, stem of origin of flexor hallucis brevis muscle; *9*, lateral calcaneal insertion of *1*; *10*, peroneus longus tendon within its thin fibrous tunnel crossing superficially the metatarsal insertional bands of tibialis posterior tendon; *11*, reflected peroneus longus tendon; *12*, direction of flexor digitorum longus tendon; *13*, direction of flexor hallucis longus tendon.)

medially. A tendinous slip extends from the lateral border of the flexor hallucis longus and anastomoses with the flexor digitorum longus tendon after its segmentation (Fig. 5.41). The lateral border of the flexor digitorum longus tendon gives insertion to the quadratus plantae muscle.

The tendon of the flexor digitorum longus divides into four diverging tendons directed anteriorly and laterally; all four tendons give origin to the lumbrical muscles. Each long flexor tendon with its accompanying and more superficially placed flexor brevis tendon passes through an arch formed by the deep septa of the plantar aponeurosis at the level of the transverse head of the adductor hallucis. At the level of the plantar plate, both tendons enter the osteofibrous tunnel, the flexor brevis tendon still more superficial (plantar) to the long flexor tendon. The flexor brevis tendon bifurcates at the level of the proximal phalanx. The tendon of the flexor digitorum longus passes through the bifurcation and continues its distal course, now located more superficial to the tendon of the brevis. A slit appears in the midaxis of the flexor digitorum longus tendon. The latter gradually enlarges transversely at the distal end and inserts on the base of the distal phalanx.

The tendon of the flexor hallucis longus remains in the middle compartment, lateral to the medial intermuscular septum, for a short distance. Further distally, it passes through the medial septum into the medial compartment and obliquely crosses the lateral belly of the flexor hallucis brevis.[41] It passes through the fibrous arch formed by the two septa emanating from the deep surface of the plantar aponeurosis and reaches the intersesamoid interval. The tendon penetrates the osseofibrous flexor tunnel and courses distally. The terminal end gradually spreads in a transverse direction and inserts on the base of the distal phalanx.

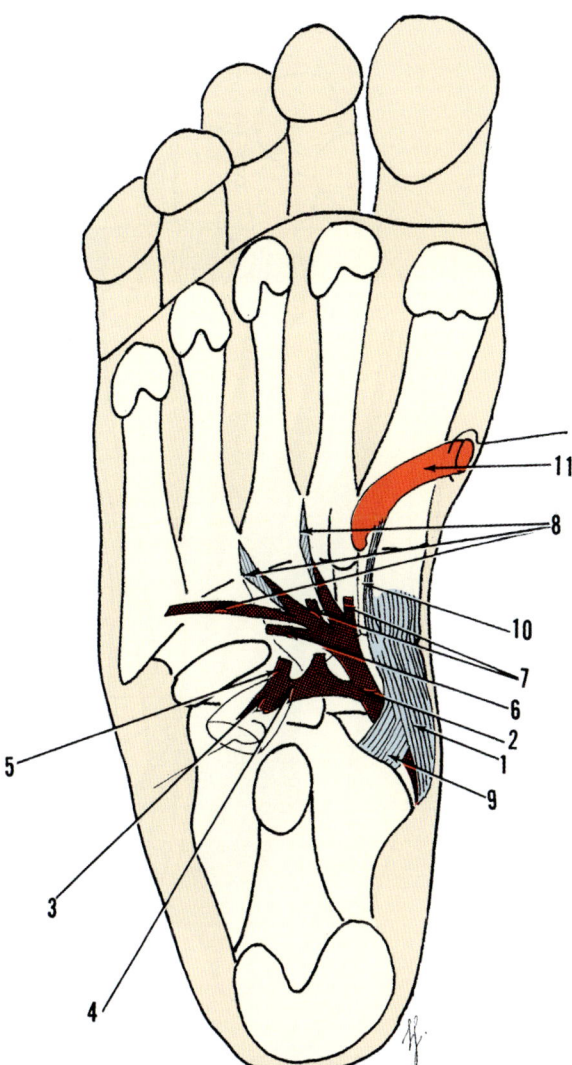

Figure 5.36 Insertion of tibialis posterior tendon. (1, Tibialis posterior tendon; 2, plantar cuneometatarsal component of 1; 3, Y stem of origin of flexor hallucis brevis muscle; 4, medial arm of 3; 5, lateral arm of 3; 6, cuboidal insertion of 1; 7, insertion of 1 on cuneiforms 3 and 2; 8, insertion of 1 between metatarsals 2-3 and 3-4 and on metatarsal 5; 9, recurrent calcaneal band of 1; 10, attachment slip of 1 to peroneus longus; 11, peroneus longus.)

Tendinous Connections

The variations basically involve the tendinous connection between the flexor hallucis longus and the flexor digitorum longus; the connection occurs after the segmentation of the latter. In the majority, the tendinous connection extends from the flexor hallucis longus to the flexor digitorum longus tendons with the following distribution: in 50 ft, 22% insert on the second tendon, 40% insert on the second and third tendons, 36% insert on the second through fourth tendons, and 2% insert on the second through fifth tendons; in 100 ft, 32% insert on the second tendon, 58% insert on the second and third tendons, and 10% insert on the second through fourth tendons.[1,2,40,41,43] The tendinous connection from the flexor digitorum longus to the flexor hallucis longus occurs less frequently: 12% in 50 ft, 29% in 100 ft, and 20.5% in 29

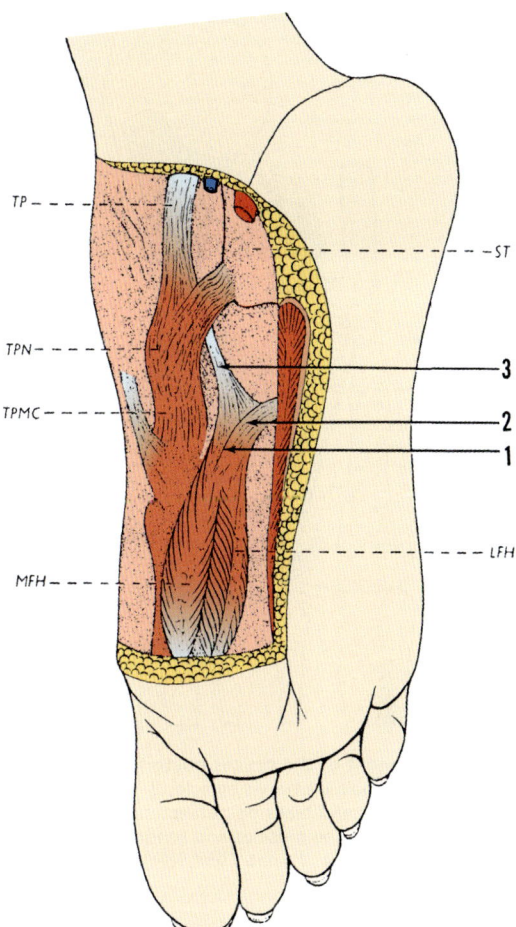

Figure 5.37 Y-shaped origin of the flexor hallucis brevis muscle. (1, Stem of origin of flexor hallucis brevis muscle; 2, lateral stem of origin; 3, medial stem of origin provided by tibialis posterior tendon; *LFH*, lateral head of flexor hallucis brevis; *MFH*, medial head of flexor hallucis brevis; *ST*, sustentaculum tali with attachment of recurrent band of *TP*; *TPMC*, medial cuneiform insertion, of tibialis posterior; *TPN*, navicular insertion of tibialis posterior; *TP*, tibialis posterior.) (Adapted from Lewis OJ. The tibialis posterior tendon in the primate foot. *J Anat.* 1964;98(2):209. By permission of Cambridge University Press.)

ft.[1,2,43] The absence of the connecting tendon is rare; Martin has observed two such cases.[41]

LaRue and Anctil[44] investigated the relationship of the flexor hallucis longus and the flexor digitorum longus in 24 ft. The tendons were "dissected through the knot of Henry and any attachments that existed between them were exposed." Three different configurations of the distal relationship of the flexor hallucis longus to the flexor digitorum longus were identified:

- Type 1: Attachment branching from the flexor hallucis longus tendon proximally to the flexor digitorum longus tendon in 41.6% (10 specimens).
- Type 2: Attachment branching from the flexor hallucis longus proximally to the flexor digitorum longus tendon and from the flexor digitorum longus proximally to the flexor hallucis longus tendon in 41.6% (10 specimens).
- Type 3: No attachment in 16.6% (4 specimens).

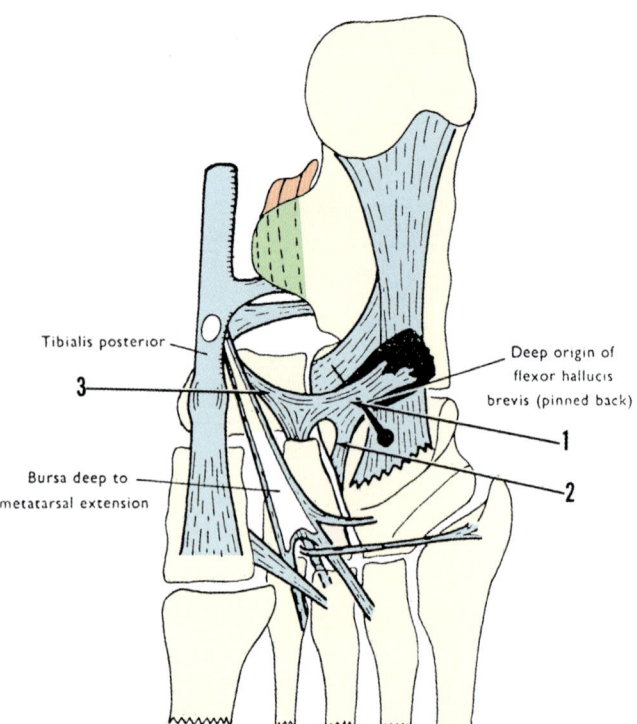

Figure 5.38 Attachment of the tibialis posterior tendon. (*1*, Y stem of origin of flexor hallucis brevis muscle; *2*, lateral arm of *1*; *3*, medial arm of *1* arising from tibialis posterior tendon.) (Adapted from Martin BF. Observation on the muscles and tendons of the medial aspect of the sole of the foot. *J Anat.* 1964;98(3):437. By permission of Cambridge University Press.)

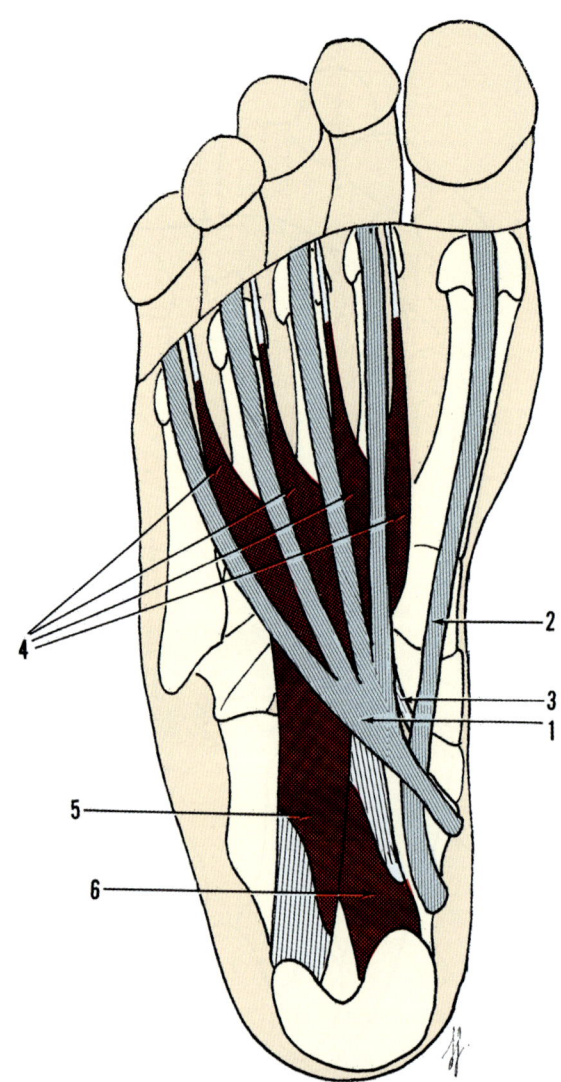

Figure 5.40 Flexor digitorum longus and flexor hallucis longus tendons. (*1*, Flexor digitorum longus tendon; *2*, flexor hallucis longus tendon; *3*, extension slip of *2-1*; *4*, lumbrical muscles; *5*, lateral head of quadratus plantae muscle; *6*, medial head of quadratus plantae muscle.)

There were no cases in with an attachment from the flexor digitorum longus to the flexor hallucis longus tendon alone[44] (Figs. 5.42 and 5.43).

Additional Muscles

Three additional muscles may be seen on the medial aspect of the ankle and tarsal tunnel: peroneocalcaneus internus, tibiocalcaneus internus and accessory soleus, and long accessory of the long flexors or of the quadratus plantae.

Peroneocalcaneus Internus Muscle

The peroneocalcaneus internus muscle was first described by Meckel.[45] It originates from the lower half of the medial surface of the fibula and partly by digitations from the flexor hallucis longus.[46-50] The tendon is directed downward and forward and enters

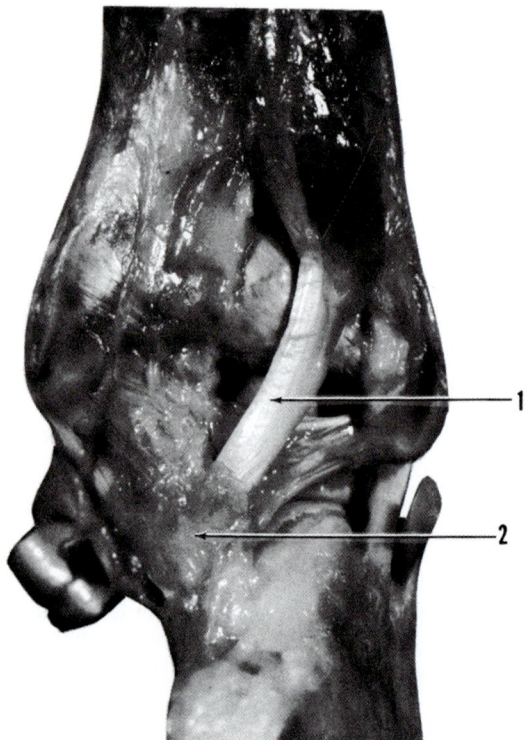

Figure 5.39 Posterior aspect of the ankle. (*1*, Flexor hallucis longus tendon; *2*, fibrous tunnel of *1* on posterior aspect of talus.)

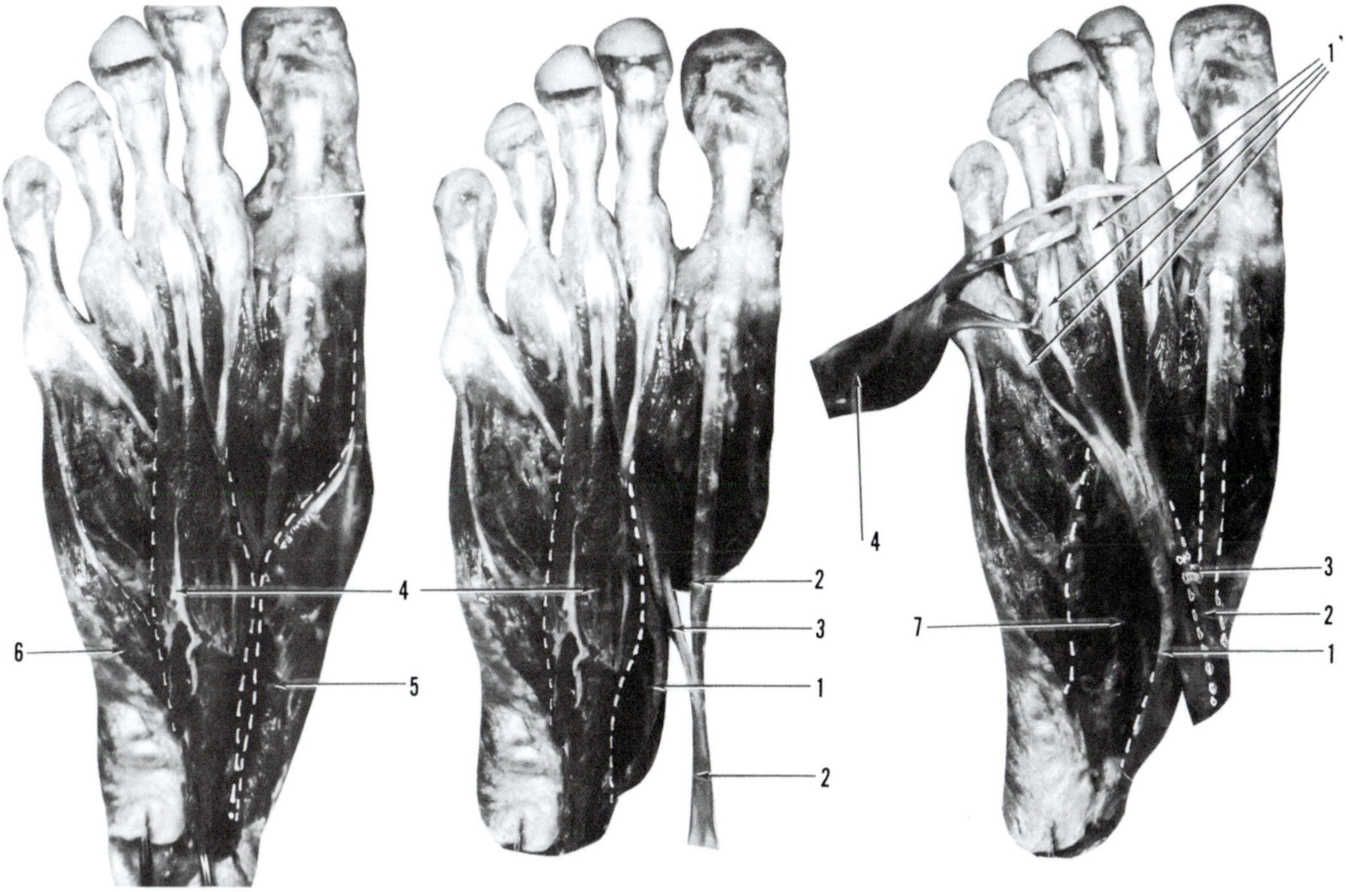

Figure 5.41 Plantar muscles, superficial layer. (*1, 1'*, Flexor digitorum longus tendons; *2*, flexor hallucis longus tendon; *3*, extension slip from *2* to *1*; *4*, flexor digitorum brevis muscle; *5*, abductor hallucis muscle; *6*, abductor of fifth toe; *7*, quadratus plantae muscle.) (LaRue BG, Anctil EP. Distal anatomical relationship of the flexor hallucis longus and the flexor digitorum longus tendons. *Foot Ankle Int*. 2006;7:528-532, Figure 1. Copyright ©2006. Reprinted by Permission of SAGE Publications.)

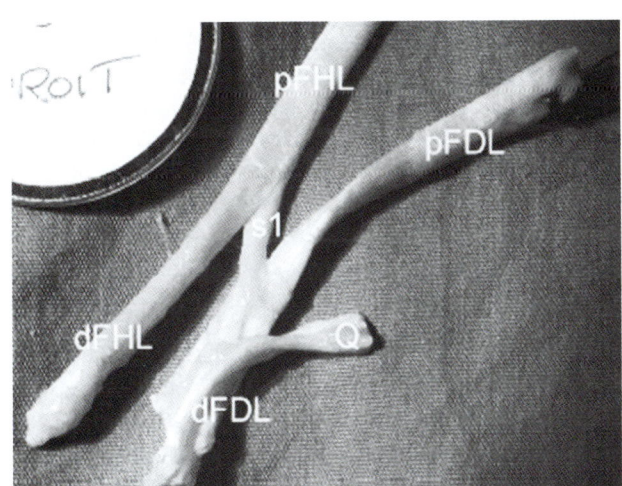

Figure 5.42 Type 2 configuration. (*dFDL*, distal flexor digitorum longus tendon; *dFHL*, distal flexor hallucis longus tendon; *pFDL*, proximal flexor digitorum longus tendon; *pFHL*, proximal flexor hallucis longus tendon; *s1*, tendinous slip from flexor hallucis longus to flexor digitorum longus; *s2*, tendinous slip from flexor digitorum longus to flexor hallucis longus.) (LaRue BG, Anctil EP. Distal anatomical relationship of the flexor hallucis longus and the flexor digitorum longus tendons. *Foot Ankle Int*. 2006;7:528-532, Figure 2. Copyright ©2006. Reprinted by Permission of SAGE Publications.)

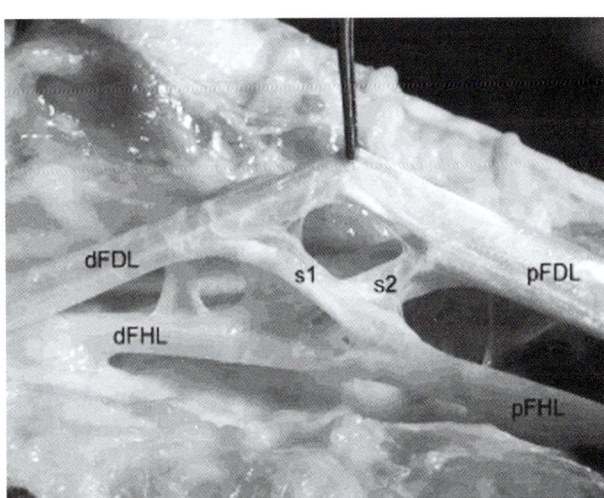

Figure 5.43 Type 1 configuration. (*dFDL*, distal flexor digitorum longus tendon; *dFHL*, distal flexor hallucis longus tendon; *pFDL*, proximal flexor digitorum longus tendon; *pFHL*, proximal flexor hallucis longus tendon; *Q*, quadratus plantae; *s1*, tendinous slip from flexor hallucis longus to flexor digitorum longus; *s2*, tendinous slip from flexor digitorum longus to flexor hallucis longus.) (LaRue BG, Anctil EP. Distal anatomical relationship of the flexor hallucis longus and the flexor digitorum longus tendons. *Foot Ankle Int*. 2006;7:528-532, Figure 2A. Copyright ©2006. Reprinted by Permission of SAGE Publications.)

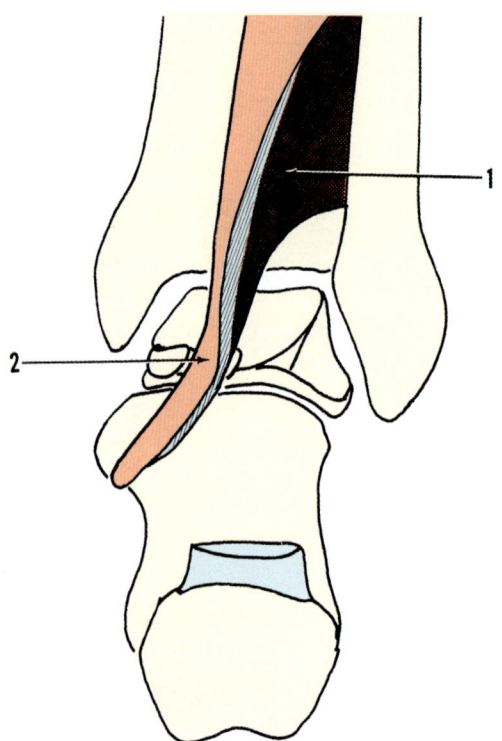

Figure 5.44 Peroneocalcaneus internus muscle. (*1*, Peroneocalcaneus internus muscle; *2*, flexor hallucis longus tendon.) (Adapted from Perkins JD Jr. An anomalous muscle of the leg: peroneo-calcaneous internus. *Anat Rec*. 1914;8:21.)

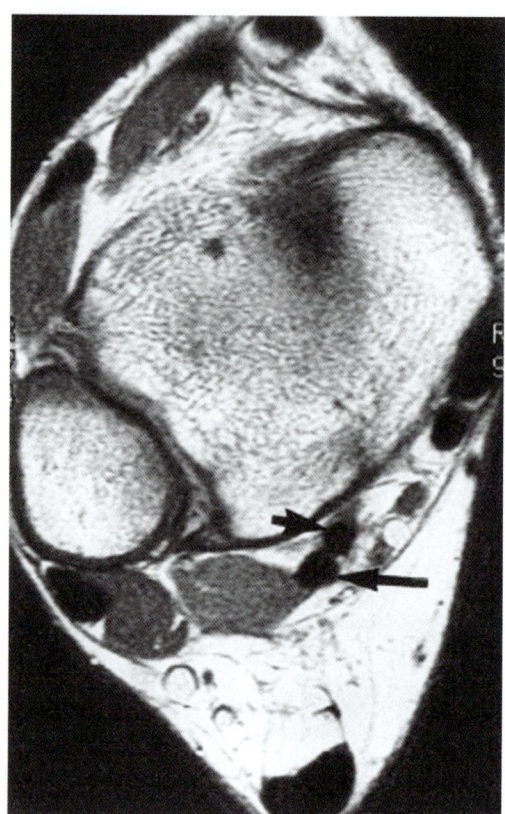

Figure 5.45 Axial proton density magnetic resonance image at the level of the distal tibiofibular syndesmosis demonstrating the peroneocalcaneus internus muscle (*long arrow*) and the flexor hallucis longus tendon (*short arrow*). (Seipel R, Linklater J, Pitsis G, et al. The peroneocalcaneus internus muscle: an unusual cause of posterior ankle impingement. *Foot Ankle Int*. 2005;10:890-893, Figure 2. Copyright ©2005. Reprinted by Permission of SAGE Publications.)

the same compartment as the flexor hallucis longus. It inserts on the distal segment of the medial calcaneal surface (Fig. 5.44).

Seipel et al[51] reported on the peroneocalcaneus internus muscle bilaterally in a 14-year-old boy complaining of posterior ankle pain with minimal activity. On preoperative magnetic resonance imaging, the peroneocalcaneus internus muscle was recognized at the level of the ankle, lateral to the flexor hallucis longus tendon muscle and the peroneocalcaneus internus tendon inserted into the base of the sustentaculum tali (Figs. 5.45 to 5.47). At surgery, the peroneocalcaneus internus muscle originated from the fibula—"its tendon coursing through the fibro-osseous tunnel lateral to the flexor hallucis longus tendon. There was no interdigitation with the normal flexor hallucis longus muscle."[51]

Tibiocalcaneus Internus and Accessory Soleus

Hecker describes the tibiocalcaneus internus originating from the medial crest of the tibia, the site of attachment measuring 7 to 8 cm (Fig. 5.48A,B).[32] The muscular portion measures 17 cm, followed by a tendinous portion of 4 cm, which inserts on the medial surface of the os calcis about 1 fingerbreadth anterior to the Achilles tendon. The posterior border of the muscle touches the soleus, and the separation is more or less artificial. This muscle is quite similar to the well-recognized variation of the accessory soleus muscle (Fig. 5.48C) that arises from the oblique line of the tibia, the deep fascia of the leg, or the deep surface of the soleus and inserts on the medial surface of the os calcis through a distinct tendon. This muscle is always located posterior to the neurovascular bundle.[52]

Romanus and colleagues found the accessory soleus muscle in 11 patients, 7 of whom had surgery.[53] They described the muscle as "enclosed by its own fascia and found to be completely separated from the ordinary soleus."[53] Dunn, in a case report, describes the soleus accessorius found surgically as follows: "The thick and fleshy muscle was enclosed in a complete fascial envelope and took origin from the ventral surface of the soleus muscle and from the crural fascia. It inserted by a short, thick tendon into the calcaneal tuberosity just anterior to the Achilles tendon."[54] Gordon and Matheson, in a case report, describe the accessory soleus as "emanating from the central surface of the soleus and deep fascia and inserting into the calcaneal tuberosity medial to the tendo-Achilles. This muscle was approximately 6 cm and entirely fleshy throughout its length."[55] Nichols and Kàlenak describe an accessory soleus with a "very narrow, distinct origin at the level of the flexor hallucis longus origin. It likewise had a very narrow insertion on the medial aspect of the calcaneus."[56] In the surgical setup, when the origin of the muscle is not specified, it is to be differentiated from the tibiocalcaneus internus muscle.

Brodie at al[57] reported on four cases of the accessory soleus muscle in symptomatic patients. Three cases were defined by

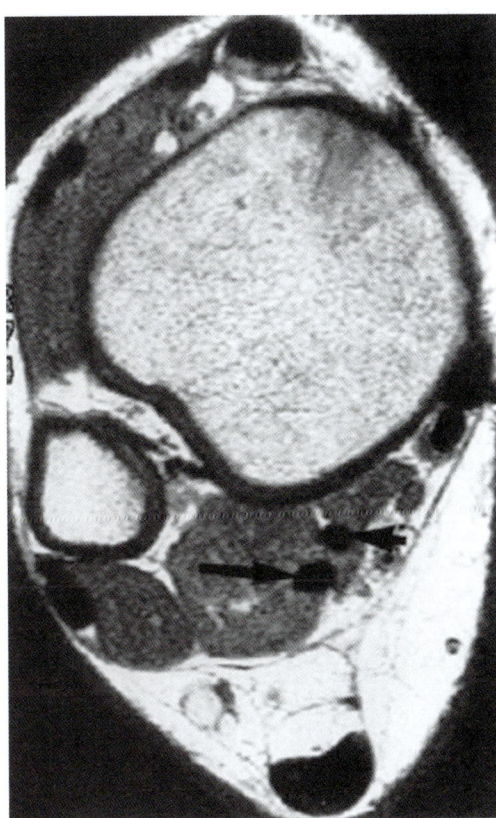

Figure 5.46 Axial proton density magnetic resonance image demonstrating the peroneocalcaneus internus tendon and muscle (*long arrow*) lateral to the flexor hallucis muscle tendon juncture (*short arrow*). (Seipel R, Linklater J, Pitsis G, et al. The peroneocalcaneus internus muscle: an unusual cause of posterior ankle impingement. Foot Ankle Int. 2005;10:890-893, Figure 3. Copyright ©2005. Reprinted by Permission of SAGE Publications.)

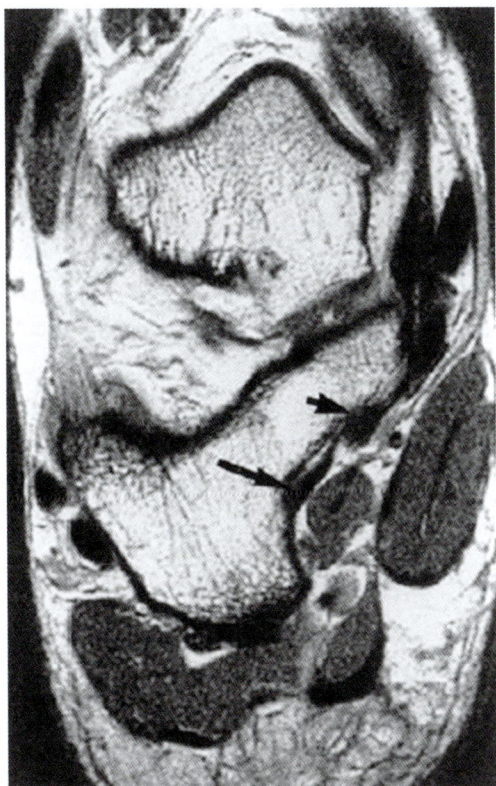

Figure 5.47 Coronal proton density magnetic resonance image demonstrating the calcaneal insertion of the peroneocalcaneus internus muscle on the base of the sustentaculum (*long arrow*). The flexor hallucis longus tendon is situated more medially and superiorly (*short broad arrow*). (Seipel R, Linklater J, Pitsis G, et al. The peroneocalcaneus internus muscle: an unusual cause of posterior ankle impingement. Foot Ankle Int. 2005;10:890-893, Figure 4. Copyright ©2005. Reprinted by Permission of SAGE Publications.)

magnetic resonance imaging. The accessory soleus muscle originated from the medial aspect of the soleus and inserted as muscle on the medial superior surface of the calcaneus, anteromedial to the Achilles tendon. The accessory soleus muscle in the surgical patient was defined as "a mass measuring 7 × 4 × 3 cm, enveloped in its own fascial sleeve, was excised from its origin off the Achilles tendon to its insertion, via a 1.5 cm tendon, anteromedial to the tendo-Achilles insertion on the calcaneus."[57]

Long Accessory of the Long Flexors or of the Quadratus Plantae

The long accessory of the long flexors or of the quadratus plantae (accessorius of the accessorius of Turner, second accessorius of Humphrey) extends from the lower third of the leg into the flexor digitorum longus or the quadratus plantae (Fig. 5.49). The variable origin may be from the fibula, tibia, deep aponeurosis of the leg, soleus, flexor hallucis longus, flexor digitorum longus in the leg, or peroneus brevis.[52] Nathan and coworkers confirmed the variable origin of this muscle and describe the following sites of origin: tibia, fibula, fasciae covering the deep compartment of the leg, transverse intermuscular septum, and calcaneus.[58] The attachment is fleshy, tendinous, or aponeurotic. The muscle may have a double head (long and short) or a single short head arising from the lower leg. The accessory muscle courses through the tarsal tunnel. It remains deep to the neurovascular bundle but occasionally may cross it superficially.[32] Frequently, it descends into the tarsal tunnel as a fleshy structure and may become tendinous in the planta or may remain fleshy until its insertion.[58]

The tendon courses in the planta and inserts on the undivided portion of the flexor digitorum longus tendon. The tendon passes deep or superficial to the latter or joins the lateral head of the quadratus plantae for a combined insertion.[32,52] The flexor digitorum accessorius longus occurs in 3.9% to 8% of legs.[12,58-60]

From a surgical point of view, as mentioned by Testut, the accessory soleus or the long accessory of the long flexors is over the deep crural aponeurosis at the level of the leg, and the posterior tibial neurovascular bundle is under the same aponeurosis.[52] To have access to the latter, the surgeon should retract or transect these muscles transversely and then incise the aponeurosis. In the inferior third of the leg, the tendon of the long accessory of the long flexors courses in the neurovascular tunnel. The tibiocalcaneus internus muscle-tendon unit is superficial and posterior to the tarsal tunnel.

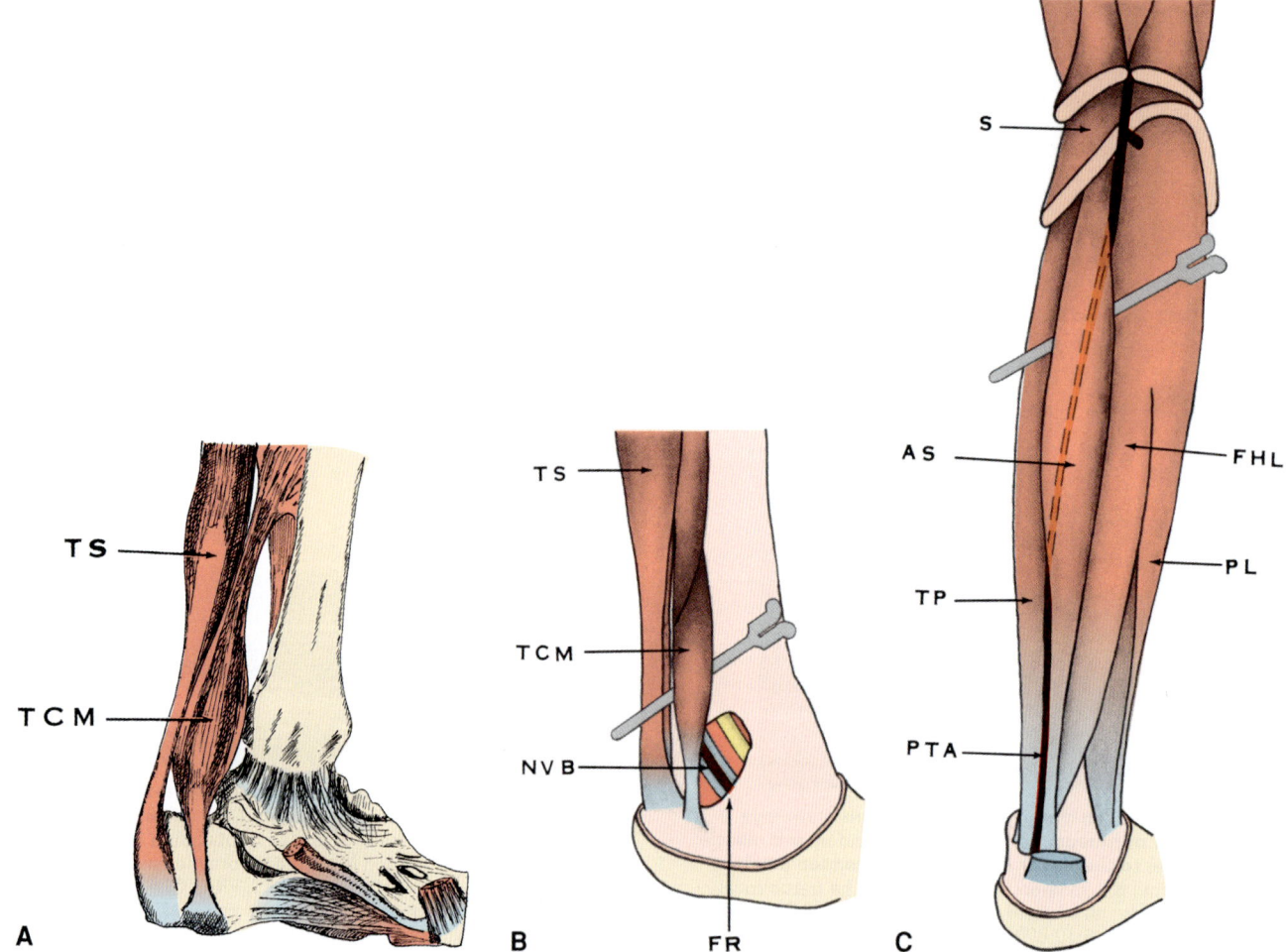

Figure 5.48 (A) Tibiocalcaneal muscle (*TCM*). (Adapted from Hecker P. Etude sur le péronier du tarse [Variations des péroniers latéraux]. *Arch Anat Hist Embr.* 1924;III:342.) (B) *TCM* superficial to neurovascular bundle (*NVB*), seen through a window in the flexor retinaculum (*FR*). Triceps surae (*TS*). (Adapted from Testut L. *Les anomalies musculaires considérées du point de vue de la ligature des artères*, P1. Paris, Doin; 1892.) (C) Accessory soleus (*AS*), soleus (*S*), flexor hallucis longus (*FHL*), peroneus longus (*PL*), tibialis posterior (*TP*), and posterior tibial artery (*PTA*). (Adapted from Testut L. *Les anomalies musculaires considérées du point de vue de la ligature des artères*. Doin; 1892:1.)

Páč and Malinovsky reported on the study of two flexor digitorum longus accessorius muscles.[61] The first muscle had two heads of origin: large and small. The large head originates from the posterior surface of the tibia in its middle third. The smaller medial head originates from the crural aponeurosis. The two fascicles unite and form a flat triangular unit, the medial component overlapping the lateral component. Above the medial aspect of the ankle, the muscle is continued by a narrow tendon that penetrates the tarsal tunnel and is within its own fibrous tunnel. The latter is located medial to the tunnel of the flexor hallucis longus and within the neurovascular tunnel (Fig. 5.50). The tendon of the flexor digitorum longus accessorius enters the planta pedis, along the tendon of the flexor hallucis longus, and expands into three slips that merge with the tendons of the long flexors of the toes. The most lateral slip of the long accessory tendon is joined by the tendinous connection band emanating from the flexor hallucis longus tendon (Fig. 5.51).

Of further interest was the fact that the quadratus plantae was absent in this specimen. The second flexor digitorum longus accessorius muscle originated from the posterior aspect of the tibia between the flexor digitorum longus and the tibialis posterior. The tendon courses distally under the tendon of the tibialis posterior and passes under the flexor retinaculum in its own tunnel and merges with the tendon of the long flexor of the toes at the level of the quadratus plantae.

Sammarco and Stephens described a flexor digitorum accessorium longus muscle located within the tarsal tunnel and compressing the posterior tibial nerve.[62] This muscle "originated from the medial aspect of the belly of the flexor hallucis longus and passed medially and posteriorly to loop around the posterior tibial nerve before entering the tarsal tunnel."[62]

Sammarco and Conti[63] reported on 104 patients with a diagnosis of tarsal tunnel syndrome with 37 (35.5%) patients within this group treated surgically. Among those treated surgically, the deep fascia of the leg in four feet and from the fibula and the deep fascia of the leg in two feet. The insertion of the accessory flexor digitorum longus was on the common tendon of the flexor digitorum longus deep in the sole of the foot in three feet and on the quadratus plantae in three feet. The average length of the accessory flexor digitorum longus was 12.3 cm. The tibiocalcaneus internus muscle originated from the tibia and the deep fascia of the leg and inserted on the calcaneus 4 cm anterior to the insertion of the Achilles tendon. The length of the muscle was 12 cm. Peterson et al[64] dissected 136 lower extremities to study the occurrence of the long accessory flexor muscle. The long accessory flexor muscle occurred in 8% (11 legs) out of 136 legs and was bilateral in 2. They found that five long accessory flexor muscles originated from the tibia and fascia of the deep posterior compartment and inserted on the quadratus plantae. Two of them had an additional insertion on the flexor digitorum longus. Six of the tendons began on the fibula just distal to the flexor hallucis longus origin; three inserted on the quadratus plantae and three inserted on the flexor digitorum. An additional head from the fibula was present on two of the six fibular origin muscles.[64]

Gumusalan and Kalaycioglu[65] reported on the flexor digitorum longus accessorius muscle in both legs of a cadaver. The muscle originated with two heads—medial and lateral—"from the median margin of the tibia, lateral margin of the fibula, posterior intermuscular septum, and the deep fascia at the distal part of the leg. Both heads came together just posterior and superficial to the tibial nerve and converged into a slender tendon which traversed the tarsal tunnel in the vicinity of the neurovascular bundle to reach the sole of the foot. It terminated by merging into the tendons of the quadratus plantae muscle."[65] The length of the flexor digitorum longus accessorius tendon

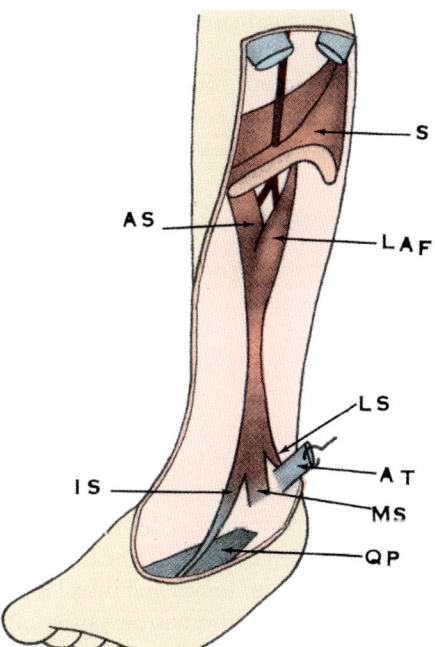

Figure 5.49 Long accessory of the flexors (*LAF*) and the accessory soleus (*AS*) fuse into one muscle that trifurcates distally into an inner slip (*IS*) inserting on the quadratus plantae; middle slip (*MS*) and lateral slip (*LS*) inserting on the calcaneus and in front of the Achilles tendon (*AT*). *S*, soleus. (Adapted from Testut L. *Les anomalies musculaires considérées du point de vue de la ligature des artéres.* Doin; 1892:1.)

causative factor of nerve compression in the tarsal tunnel was the accessory flexor digitorum longus muscle in six feet and the tibiocalcaneus internus muscle in one foot. The origin of the accessory flexor digitorum longus was from the tibia and the

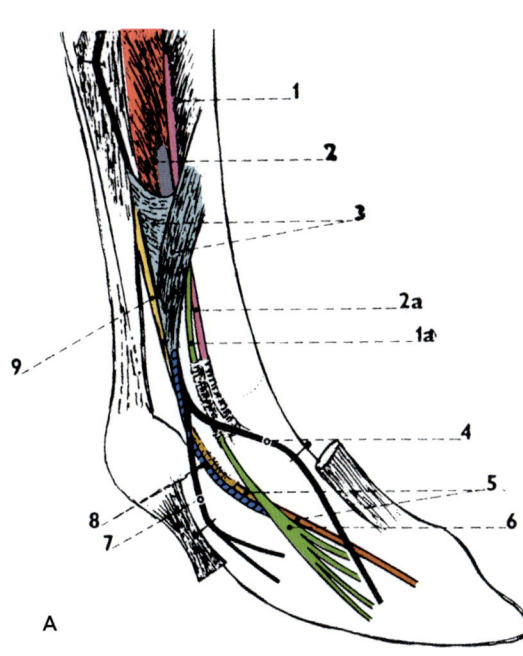
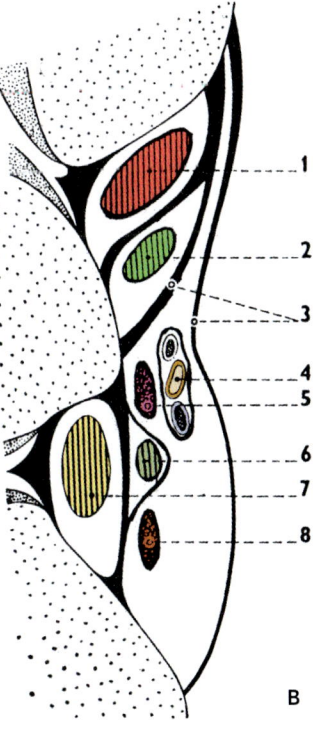

Figure 5.50 (A) Survey of muscle flexor digitorum longus. (*1*, muscle flexor digitorum longus; *1a*, tendon of the muscle flexor digitorum longus; *2*, muscle tibialis posterior; *2a*, tendon of the muscle tibialis posterior; *3*, medial and lateral heads of the muscle flexor digitorum longus accessorius; *4*, nerve plantaris medialis; *5*, tendon of the muscle flexor hallucis longus; *6*, distal part of the tendon muscle flexor digitorum longus; *7*, nerve plantaris lat; *8*, tendon of the muscle flexor digitorum longus accessorius; *9*, muscle flexor hallucis longus.) **(B) Diagram of osteofibrous canals in the region of the medial ankle.** (*1*, m tibialis posterior; *2*, muscle flexor digitorum longus; *3*, retinaculum flexorum; *4*, vasa tibialis posterior; *5*, n plantaris med; *6*, muscle flexor digitorum longus accessorius; *7*, muscle flexor hallucis longus; *8*, nerve plantaris lateral) (Adapted from Páč L, Malinovsky L Jr. M. flexor digitorum longus accessorius in the lower limb of man. *Anat Anz.* 1985;159:253.)

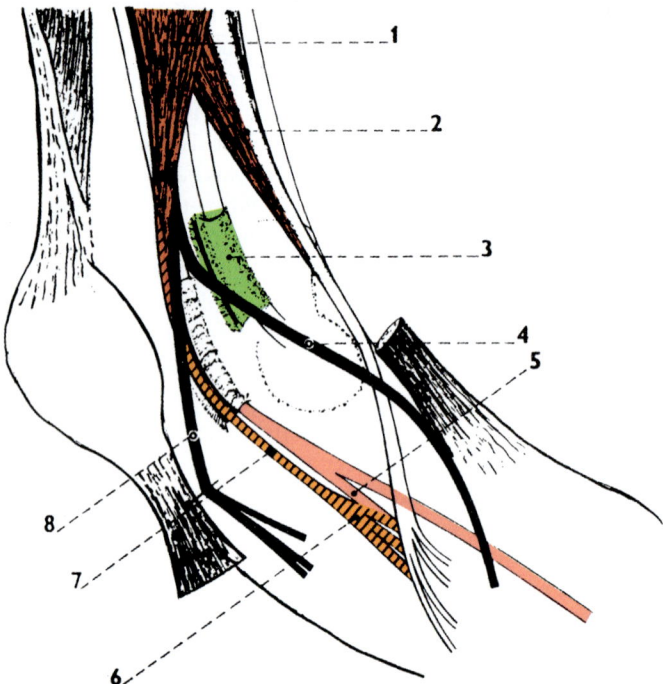

Figure 5.51 Mutual relation of the tendons of toe and big toe flexors in the planta pedis. (*1*, muscle flexor digitorum longus accessorius; *2*, muscle flexor digitorum longus [inclined medially]; *3*, tendon of the muscle tibialis posterior in the tendon sheath; *4*, nerve tibialis head; *5*, tendon link between the muscle flexor hallucis longus and muscle flexor digitorum longus accessorius; *6*, branching tendon of the muscle flexor digitorum longus accessorius; *7*, tendon of the muscle flexor digitorum longus accessorius; *8*, nerve plantaris lateral) (Adapted from Páč L, Malinovsky L Jr. M. flexor digitorum longus accessorius in the lower limb of man. *Anat Anz.* 1985;159:253.)

was 7.8 cm on the left and 6.8 cm on the right. The width of the tendon was 0.2 cm bilaterally (Figs. 5.52 to 5.54).

Kinoshita et al[66] reported on 41 patients (49 ft) with tarsal tunnel syndrome treated surgically. An accessory muscle was found in 16.3% of this group. The flexor digitorum longus accessorius was present in 12.2% and the accessory soleus in 4.1%. The flexor digitorum longus accessorius muscle "proximally attached to the intermuscular fascial septum in three feet, to the fascia of the flexor digitorum longus muscle in two, and to the fascia of the flexor hallucis longus muscle in one foot."[66] The accessory soleus was proximally attached to the deep fascia of the soleus. The distal connections to the toe flexors were assessed functionally.

▸ Flexor Digitorum Brevis

The flexor digitorum brevis arises from the posteromedial calcaneal tuberosity, the posterior third of the deep surface of the plantar aponeurosis, and the lateral and medial intermuscular septa (see Figs. 5.43 and 5.55). The calcaneal origin extends to the posterolateral tuberosity and is sandwiched between the origin of the plantar aponeurosis posteriorly, the abductor hallucis anteromedially, and the abductor digiti quinti anterolaterally. The muscular attachment to the deep surface of the plantar aponeurosis in the posterior third is dense, allowing separation only by sharp dissection. At this level, there is no potential space between the flexor digitorum brevis and the plantar aponeurosis. The muscle body is thick and narrow posteriorly and gradually spreads out transversely. In the midsegment of the foot, it divides into four muscular fascicles, each followed by a flat tendon centered on and superficial to the corresponding long flexor tendon. Both tendons pass through an arc formed by the vertical septa of the plantar aponeurosis and penetrate the osseofibrous tunnel. The flat tendon of the short flexor divides into two slips at the level of the base of the proximal phalanx.

The slips contour the long flexor tendon on each side, pass underneath, decussate fibers, and insert on the inferior aspect of the middle phalanx near the borders. They form a tendinous groove through which the long flexor tendon passes. The medial two tendons are usually larger than the lateral two.

Variations involving the flexor digitorum brevis are frequent. Nathan and Gloobe provide the following data on 100 ft: 37% had a normal flexor digitorum brevis and 63% had variations involving mostly the fifth toe and less frequently the fourth toe.[67] The variations involve the origin or the insertion of the muscle or both.

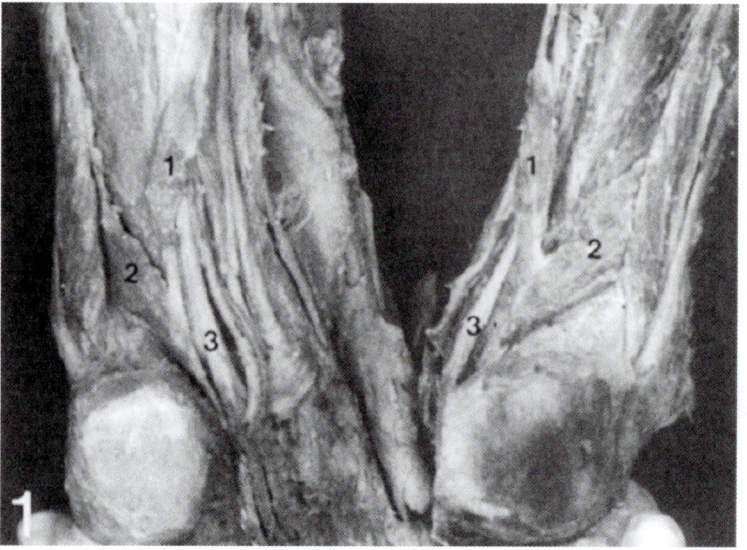

Figure 5.52 Bilateral double-headed flexor digitorum longus accessorius muscles in the distal one-third of the posterior deep compartment of both legs. (*1*, Medial head; *2*, lateral head; *3*, tibial nerve.) (Reprinted from Gumusalan Y, Kalaycioglu A. Bilateral accessory flexor digitorum longus muscle in man. *Ann Anat.* 2000;182:574, Figure 1, with permission from Elsevier.)

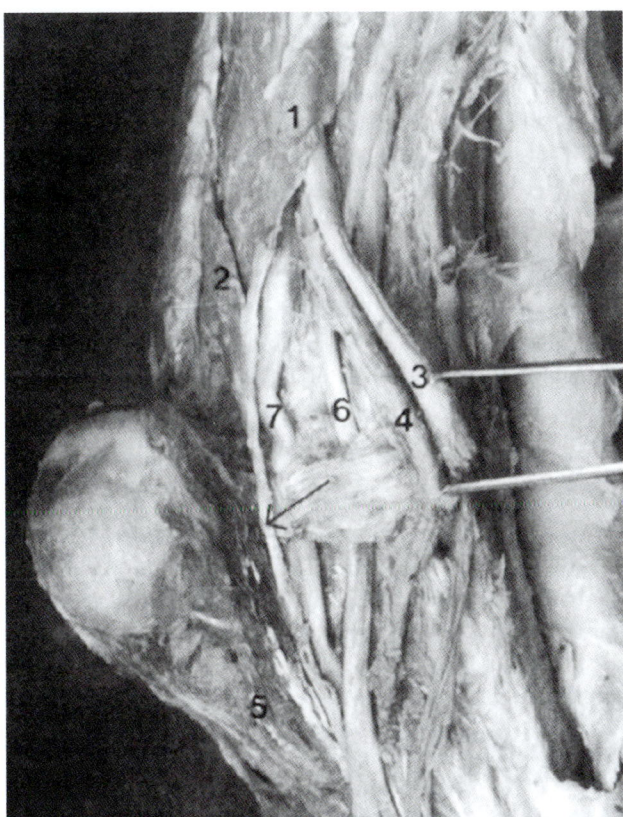

Figure 5.53 Flexor digitorum longus accessorius muscle with two heads. (*Arrow*, tendon of flexor digitorum longus accessorius; *1*, medial head; *2*, lateral head; *3*, tibial nerve; *4*, posterior tibial vessels; *5*, quadratus plantae; *6*, tendon flexor digitorum longus; *7*, tendon of flexor hallucis longus.) (Reprinted from Gumusalan Y, Kalaycioglu A. Bilateral accessory flexor digitorum longus muscle in man. *Ann Anat.* 2000;182:574, Figure 2, with permission from Elsevier.)

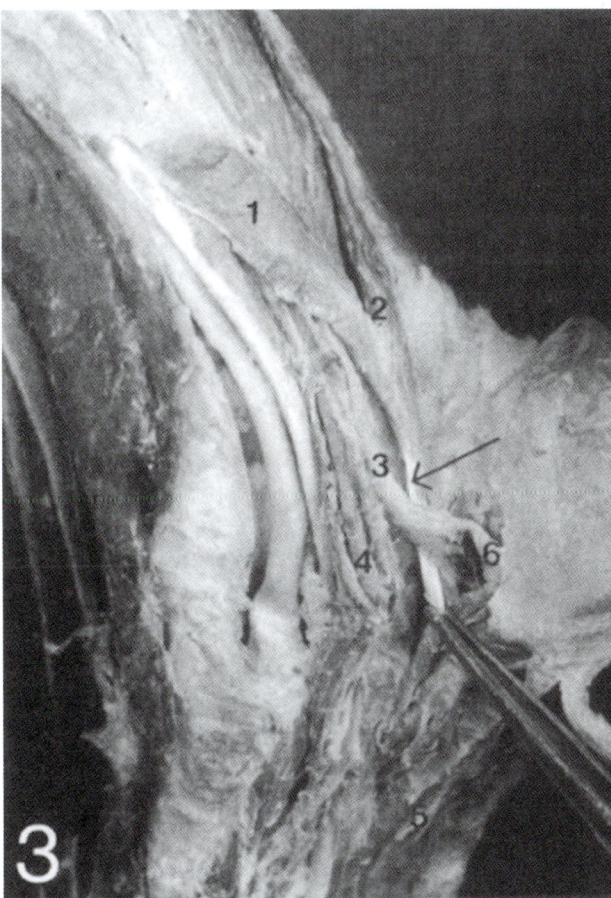

Figure 5.54 Flexor digitorum longus accessorius muscle to the right side. (*Arrow*, tendon of flexor digitorum longus accessorius; *1*, medial head; *2*, lateral head; *3*, tibial nerve; *4*, posterior tibial vessels; *5*, quadratus plantae; *6*, lateral plantar nerve.) (Reprinted from Gumusalan Y, Kalaycioglu A. Bilateral accessory flexor digitorum longus muscle in man. *Ann Anat.* 2000;182:574, Figure 3, with permission from Elsevier.)

Variations of Origin

In addition to the normal muscle, a second muscle may arise from the flexor digitorum longus and join the tendon of the brevis. Occasionally, this additional muscle arises from the tibialis posterior tendon. The flexor brevis to the fourth and fifth toe may arise from the long flexor or the lateral intermuscular septum. This muscle is then deeper than the rest of the flexor brevis.

The frequency of occurrence of these variations in 100 ft is as follows: an additional slip of the flexor digitorum brevis from the flexor digitorum longus to the fifth toe is present in 20% and from the flexor digitorum longus to the fourth and fifth toes in 3%; an additional slip from the tibialis posterior to the fifth toe occurs in 1%. A sole origin of the flexor digitorum brevis from the flexor digitorum longus to the fifth or fourth and fifth toes is present in 5%; a sole origin from the lateral intermuscular septum to the fifth toe occurs in 1%.[67]

Variations of Insertion

The variations of insertion of the flexor brevis are of these types: absence of tendon, unsplit tendon, or tendon fused to the long flexor. The absence of the flexor brevis tendon to the fifth toe occurs with the following frequency, according to various sources: in 5 of 50 ft (10%), in 22 of 136 ft (16.1%), in 135 of 540 ft (25%), in 14 of 100 ft (14%), and in 23 of 100 ft (25%) (total, 199 in 926 ft).[2,67] The average of absence of the flexor digitorum brevis to the fifth toe is 21.5%.

The brevis tendons of the fifth and fourth toes may be absent in 3%.[52] The unsplit tendon is seen in 5% (fifth or fourth toes) and runs parallel to the long flexor and inserts on the second phalanx.[1,52] The short flexor tendon of the fifth may fuse to the long flexor tendon in 2%.[1,52]

▶ Quadratus Plantae or Flexor Accessorius and Its Variations

The quadratus plantae (caro quadrata of Sylvius) is a flat, trapezoidal muscle formed by two heads: lateral and medial (see Figs. 5.40 and 5.43).

The lateral head is a tendinous origin and arises from the posterolateral calcaneal tuberosity and from the lateral segment of the calcaneocuboid ligament up to the cuboidal crest. The medial head has a fleshy origin from the lower segment of the medial surface of the os calcis in the calcaneal canal, from the

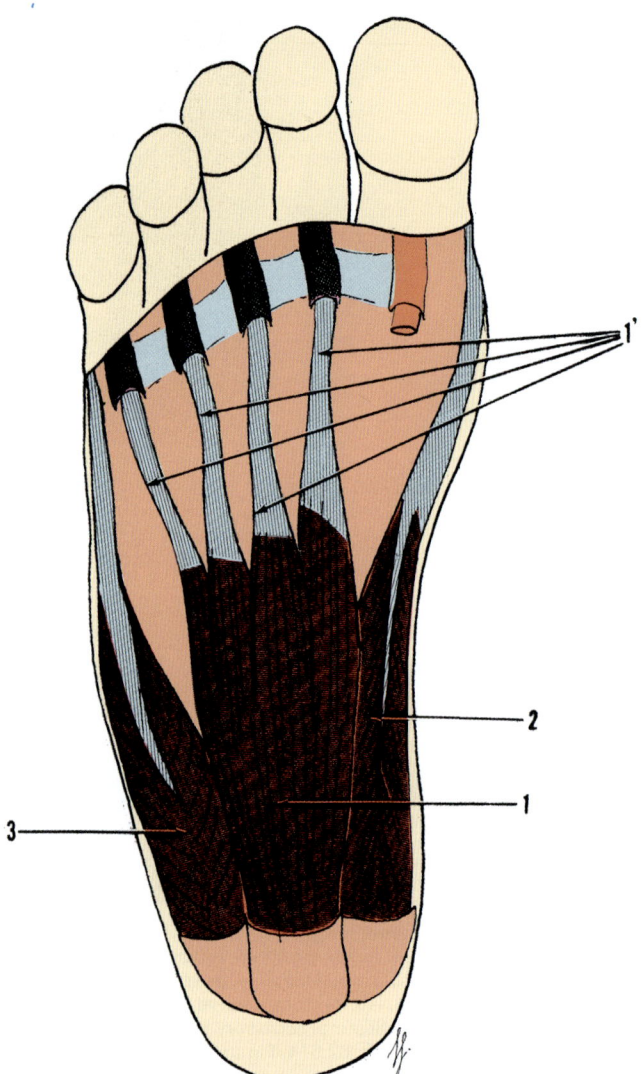

Figure 5.55 **Flexor digitorum brevis muscle.** (*1*, Flexor digitorum brevis; *1'*, tendons of flexor digitorum brevis; *2*, abductor hallucis muscle; *3*, abductor of fifth toe.)

anterior aspect of the posteromedial calcaneal tuberosity, and from the inferior surface of the interfascicular septum of the calcaneal canal. The medial head of the muscle forms the lateral wall of the lower segment of the calcaneal canal and is inferior to the interfascicular septum. Both heads, initially separated by a triangular space with an anterior apex, gradually unite. Most of the muscular fibers of the medial head terminate in a narrow tendon that inserts into the deep surface of the common long flexor tendon. The remaining fibers join the lateral head, and both heads insert with the fleshy fibers on the segmented tendons of the long flexor, mostly of the fifth toe, and on the anastomotic tendon between the flexor digitorum longus and the flexor hallucis longus. The flexor hallucis longus may occasionally receive some direct insertional fibers from the accessory flexor.

The quadratus plantae is sandwiched posteriorly between the short flexor and the osseoligamentous frame. A thin transverse fascia, occasionally thick, is interposed between the superficial surface of the accessory flexor and the deep surface of the flexor brevis; this transverse band extends from the medial to the lateral intermuscular septum (Fig. 5.56).

Lewis considers the medial head of the flexor accessorius or quadratus plantae "a uniquely human apomorphy, and the double-headed condition is unique to man" and mentions that "standard textbook accounts attributing the attachment of the flexor accessorius to the lateral border of the flexor digitorum longus are invalid, for only in some cases does this arrangement obtain."[68] He describes the tendinous arrangement of the quadratus plantae and the long flexor tendons in two layers: superficial and deep.[68] The flexor digitorum longus forms the superficial layer and passes laterally. It provides the long flexor tendon to the fifth toe and part of the long flexor tendons of the second, third, and fourth toes. A contribution may be given to the flexor hallucis longus tendon. The flexor hallucis longus, its digital extensions, and the medial head of the quadratus plantae with its digital extensions form the deep layer. Lewis considers the medial head of the quadratus plantae "a part of the flexor hallucis longus which has 'descended' to the sole."[68] The flexor accessorius longus muscle is considered as a part of the medial head having a partial origin in the leg, usually from the fibula in close association with the flexor hallucis longus (Fig. 5.57).[68] The lateral head of the quadratus plantae "frequently has no attachment to the lateral border of the flexor digitorum longus tendon... This head generally has a flat, narrow tendon of origin which passes between the long plantar ligament and abductor digiti minimi before expanding into a fleshy belly and contributes to the digital flexor tendon."[68]

The lateral head of the quadratus plantae "is not infrequently absent."[68] Winckler and Gianoli studied the quadratus plantae and its insertional variations in 15 ft.[69] It was their conclusion that the anatomy of the quadratus plantae is very variable. The lateral head may be absent. The larger medial head may have a more or less high origin in the calcaneal canal. An accessory head to the muscle may be present, originating from the fibula at a variable distance from the flexor hallucis longus origin or arising directly from the posterior surface of the latter. The quadratus plantae terminates in the majority of the cases on the tendinous expansions of the flexor hallucis longus tendon to the deep surface of the tendons of the flexor digitorum longus. "Rarely does the quadratus plantae insert on the lateral border of the flexor digitorum longus and when the latter occurs it is a partial insertion."[69] Only exceptionally does the quadratus plantae provide a tendinous slip to the flexor digitorum longus tendon of the fifth toe. The authors considered the quadratus plantae a dependent of the flexor hallucis longus muscle, a part of this muscle that has migrated toward the plantar region. The major insertional variations are as indicated in Figures 5.58 to 5.64.

Barlow reported a bilateral variation of the quadratus plantae.[70] The muscle was composed of three parts: superficial, intermediate, and deep. The superficial component "was a small muscle arising by two heads, a tendinous one from the medial tubercle of the calcaneum just medial to the long plantar ligament and a muscular one from the sheath of the flexor hallucis longus and flexor digitorum longus."[70] This component formed the long flexor of the fifth toe and provided an extension to the long flexor of the fourth toe (Fig. 5.65).

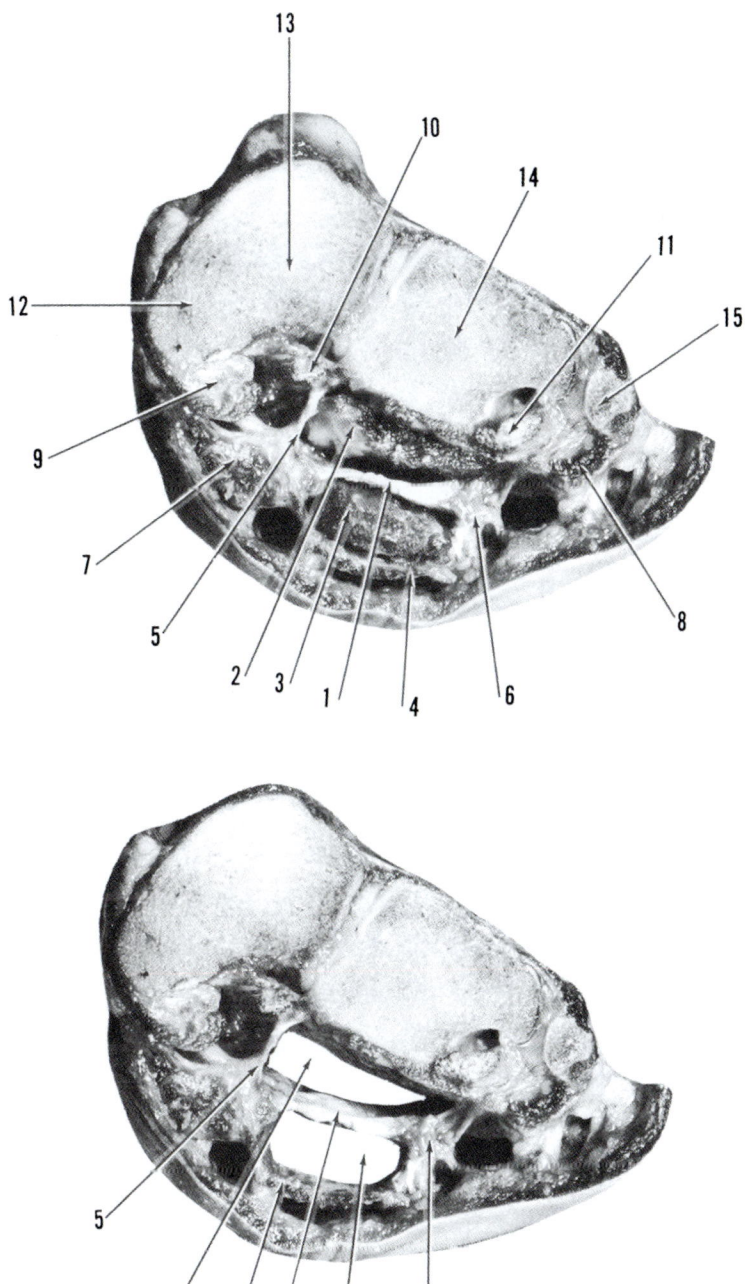

Figure 5.56 Cross-section of left foot passing through the cuboid and the navicular—anterior view. (*1*, Transverse septum extending from medial intermuscular septum to lateral intermuscular septum and dividing middle compartment of hindfoot into a deep compartment [*16*] for quadratus plantae muscle and a superficial compartment [*17*] for flexor digitorum brevis muscle; *2*, quadratus plantae muscle with tendon of flexor digitorum longus; *3*, flexor digitorum brevis muscle; *4*, middle segment of plantar aponeurosis; *5*, medial intermuscular septum; *6*, lateral intermuscular septum; *7*, abductor hallucis muscle; *8*, abductor of fifth toe; *9*, insertion of tibialis posterior tendon on navicular tuberosity; *10*, flexor hallucis longus tendon; *11*, peroneus longus tendon; *12*, tuberosity of navicular; *13*, navicular; *14*, cuboid; *15*, tuberosity of fifth metatarsal base.)

"The intermediate part of the muscle was the main source of the tendons to the fourth and fifth toes."[70] It originated by fleshy fibers from the medial surface of the calcaneum, behind the sustentaculum tali and as far as the medial calcaneal tubercle. The insertional tendon split to go to the fourth and fifth toes, the latter joined by the contribution of the superficial component. The deep part of the muscle originated "from the underside of the calcaneum in front and lateral to the sustentaculum tali and inserted into the tendons of the flexor digitorum longus."[70]

Barlow reported on three further variations of the quadratus plantae muscle.[71] In one specimen, a tendon sprang from the medial head of the muscle and provided approximately half of the fibers to the tendons of the third, fourth, and fifth toes and extended a tendinous band to the flexor hallucis longus (Fig. 5.66). In a second specimen, the flexor digitorum longus to the second toe had been replaced by a tendon from the medial head of the quadratus plantae. Furthermore, there was "a broad thin tendinous link with the flexor hallucis longus" (Fig. 5.67).[71]

In the third specimen, all the long flexors were arising from the quadratus plantae (Fig. 5.68). The tendons of the flexor digitorum longus and flexor hallucis longus were terminating in a "mass of fibrous tissue on the medial side of the foot situated in the hollow of the calcaneum, below the sustentaculum

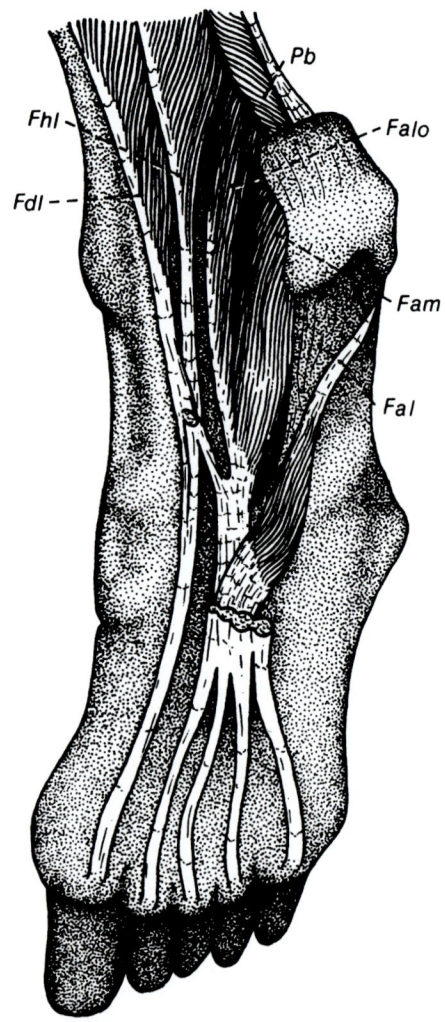

Figure 5.57 Sole of the right foot of *Homo sapien*. A flexor accessorius longus (*Falo*) is present, and the tendon of the flexor digitorum longus (*Fal*) gives a contribution to the tendon of flexor hallucis longus (*Fh 1*). Part of the flexor digitorum longus tendon has been removed to show the trilaminar arrangement of the tendons present in this foot. (*Fal*, lateral head of the flexor accessorius; *Fam*, medial head of the flexor accessorius; *Pb*, peroneus brevis.) (From Lewis OJ. *Functional Morphology of the Evolving Hand and Foot.* Clarendon Press; 1989:263.)

tali."[71] From the lateral side of this mass originated the quadratus plantae, giving origin to the four long flexor tendons. Furthermore, an entirely separate flexor hallucis longus tendon originated from the medial calcaneal tubercle.

Auvray reported on variations of the long flexors of the toes.[49] The flexor digitorum longus provided the long flexor tendons to the fourth and fifth toes. The lateral head of the quadratus plantae inserted on this component. The flexor hallucis longus tendon also provided the long flexor tendons to the second and third toes. The medial head of the quadratus plantae inserted on this component (Fig. 5.69).

The absence of the lateral head of the quadratus plantae is "far from being rare."[2] LeDouble mentions having observed 10 such cases.[2] The absence of the medial head is rare, and a bilateral case is reported by Morestin (Fig. 5.70).[72] The accessory flexor may be reduced in size or converted to a fibrous band.

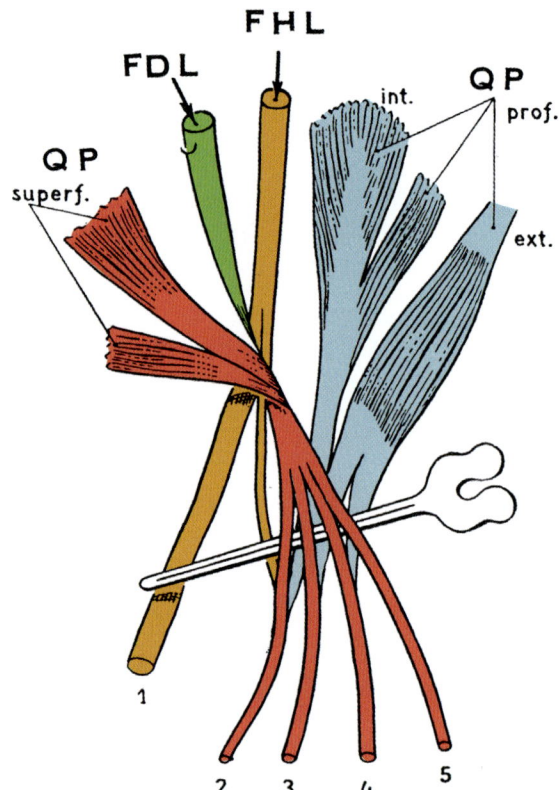

Figure 5.58 The medial head of the quadratus plantae is divisible into two parts: superficial and deep. The weak superficial component inserts on the two surfaces of the flexor digitorum longus (*FDL*) tendon and sparingly onto its lateral border. The deep component of the medial head and the lateral head insert onto the deep surface of the flexor digitorum longus tendons to the second, third, and fourth toes. A tendinous expansion from the flexor hallucis longus to the flexor digitorum longus tendon of the second toe is present. (*ext.*, external; *FDL*, flexor digitorum longus; *FHL*, flexor hallucis longus; *int.*, internal; *prof.*, deep; *QP*, quadratus plantae; *superf.*, superficial; *1-5*, tendons to toes 1-5.) (Adapted from Winckler G, Gianoli G. La véritable terminaison de la Chair Carrée de Sylvius [musc. quadratus, plantae]. *Arch Anat Histol Embryol [Strasb]*. 1955;38:47.)

▶ Intrinsic Muscles of the Big Toe

There are four intrinsic muscles of the big toe: extensor hallucis EHB (described previously); abductor hallucis; flexor hallucis brevis with two heads (medial and lateral); and adductor hallucis with two heads (oblique and transverse) (Fig. 5.71).

Abductor Hallucis

The abductor hallucis is a superficial, thick, flat elongated muscle extending from the tuberosity of the os calcis to the big toe (see Figs. 5.43, 5.55, and 5.71). It is the muscle of the medial border of the foot and originates from the inferior and medial aspect of the posteromedial calcaneal tuberosity through mostly tendinous fibers (the main origin), the deep surface of the plantar aponeurosis, the posterior end of the medial intermuscular septum, and the flexor retinaculum, which invests the muscle.[73]

The abductor hallucis muscle bridges the calcaneal canal and with the flexor retinaculum converts it into a tunnel (Fig. 5.72). The deep investing aponeurosis of the muscle is anchored

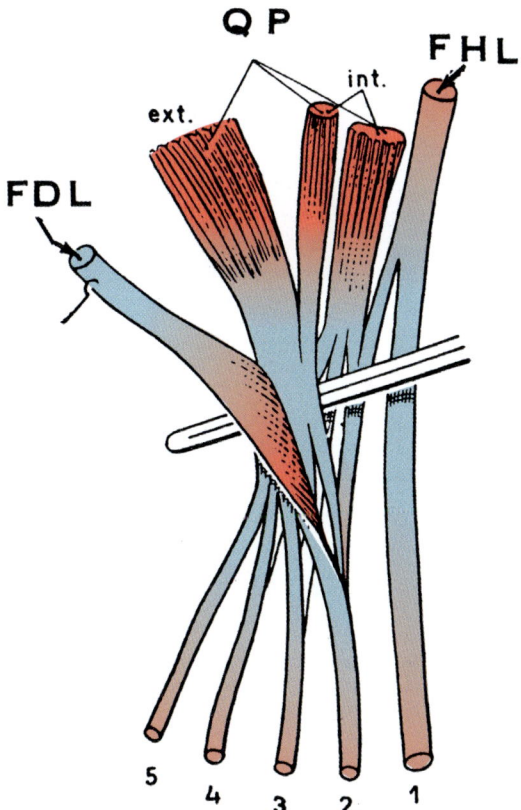

Figure 5.59 A trilaminar arrangement. The superficial layer is formed by the flexor digitorum longus (*FDL*) and the four lumbricals. The middle layer is formed by the tendons of the lateral head and, to a lesser degree, of the medial head of the quadratus plantae (*QP*) reaching the deep surfaces of the flexor digitorum longus tendons to the second, third, and fourth toes. The deep layer is formed by the tendinous expansion of the flexor hallucis longus (*FHL*) to the second toe flexor and the tendinous extensions of the quadratus plantae. The first extension of the latter joins the tendinous band of the flexor hallucis longus to the second toe, whereas the second and third tendinous extensions reach the deep surface of the flexor digitorum longus tendons to the third and fourth toes. (*ext.*, external; *int.*, internal; *1, 2, 3, 4, 5*, refer to the corresponding toes or digits 1st, 2nd, 3rd, 4th, and 5th.) (Adapted from Winckler G, Gianoli G. La véritable terminaison de la Chair Carrée de Sylvius [musc. quadratus, plantae]. Arch Anat Histol Embryol [Strasb]. 1955;38:47.)

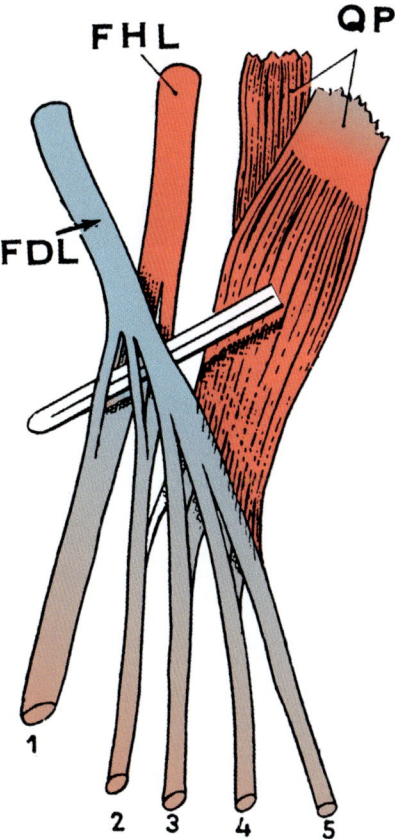

Figure 5.60 The flexor hallucis longus (*FHL*) tendon provides a strong expansion to the second toe. The flexor digitorum longus (*FDL*) provides tendinous bands to the flexor hallucis longus and to the tendinous contribution of the latter to the second toe. The quadratus plantae (*QP*) has only a medial head. The superficial layer of the quadratus plantae inserts on the lateral border of the flexor digitorum longus and its tendon to the fifth toe. The deep layer of the quadratus plantae inserts on the deep surface of the flexor digitorum longus tendons to the third, fourth, and fifth toes and minimally on the second toe. *1, 2, 3, 4, 5*, refer to the corresponding toes or digits 1st, 2nd, 3rd, 4th, and 5th. (Adapted from Winckler G, Gianoli G. La véritable terminaison de la Chair Carrée de Sylvius [musc. quadratus, plantae]. Arch Anat Histol Embryol [Strasb]. 1955;38:47.)

proximally to the medial surface of the os calcis through the attachment of the interfascicular septum (Figs. 5.73 and 5.74). Distally, the same investing aponeurosis makes fibrous connection with the common fibrous tunnel of the flexor digitorum longus and the flexor hallucis longus tendons. It also is adherent to the tunnel of the tibialis posterior tendon and to the tuberosity of the navicular. Poirier and Charpy described a frequently seen aponeurotic expansion detached from the superior border of the abductor muscle and in continuity with the inferior arm of the inferior extensor retinaculum.[74] The tendon of origin of the muscle is located on the deep or lateral aspect of the muscle. The tendon of insertion appears early on the superficial or medial aspect of the muscle. Distally, the tendon is flat, slightly twisted, fasciculated, and more plantar in location. Its inferolateral fibers insert on the medial sesamoid, in conjunction with the fibers of the medial head of the flexor hallucis brevis, and on the medial plantar tubercle of the proximal phalanx of the big toe. The superomedial fibers connect with the transverse lamina of the extensor aponeurosis (Figs. 5.75 and 5.76).

The variations of the abductor hallucis are limited. An extension from the anterior part of the abductor to the proximal phalanx of the second toe may be seen in 7%.[2] Occasionally, the entire muscle originates from the flexor hallucis longus.[2]

Flexor Hallucis Brevis

The flexor hallucis brevis has a Y-shaped fibrotendinous origin (see Figs. 5.37, 5.77, and 5.78).[40,41] The medial arm of the Y originates from the metatarsal component of the tibialis posterior tendon. The lateral arm originates from the lateral cuneiform and the cuboid, with some fibers inserting on the groove of the peroneus longus tendon and on the long and short plantar ligaments. The stem of the Y origin of the muscle resembles a triangular lamina or fold. The stem of the Y is considered by Martin as the deep origin of the muscle, whereas superficial fibers originate from the medial intermuscular septum, which

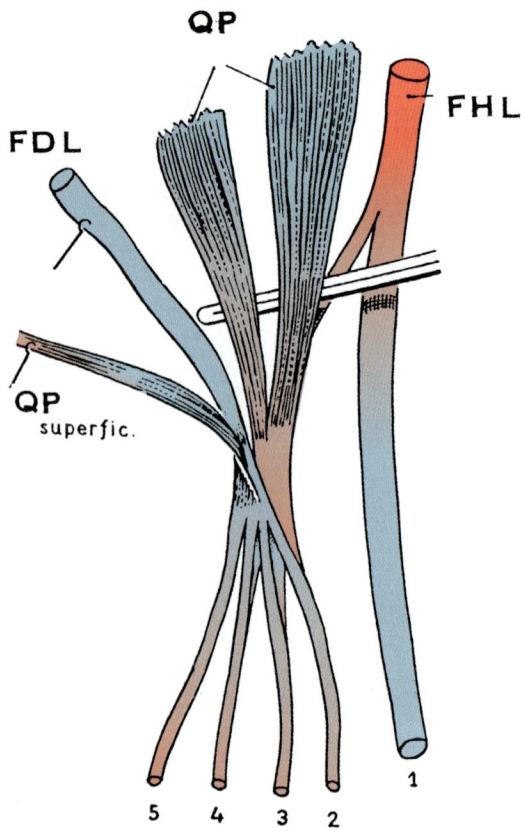

Figure 5.61 **The tendons are disposed in four layers.** First layer, superficial (plantar), formed by the small superficial layer of the medial head of the quadratus plantae (*QP*). Second layer formed by the tendons of the flexor digitorum longus (*FDL*). Third layer formed by the tendons of the deep layer of the medial head and the lateral head of the quadratus plantae. These tendons insert on the deep surface of the flexor digitorum longus tendons to the second, third, and fourth toes. The fourth layer is formed by the tendinous extensions of the flexor hallucis longus (*FHL*) to the flexor digitorum longus tendons of the second, third, and fourth toes. (*superfic.*, superficial; *1, 2, 3, 4, 5*, refer to the corresponding toes or digits 1st, 2nd, 3rd, 4th, and 5th.) (Adapted from Winckler G, Gianoli G. La véritable terminaison de la Chair Carrée de Sylvius [musc. quadratus, plantae]. *Arch Anat Histol Embryol [Strasb]*. 1955;38:47.)

Figure 5.62 **The flexor hallucis longus (*FHL*) provides an extension to the flexor digitorum longus (*FDL*) tendons to the second and third toes.** The flexor digitorum longus provides a tendinous band to the flexor hallucis longus. The quadratus plantae (*QP*) is large and has only the medial head, which divides into a superficial and a deep component. The superficial part inserts on the superficial surface and the lateral border of the common flexor digitorum longus tendon and the tendon to the fifth toe. The deep part of the quadratus plantae inserts on the tendinous expansions of the flexor hallucis longus and onto the tendon of the fourth toe. (*superf.* superficial; *prof.*, deep; *1, 2, 3, 4, 5*, refer to the corresponding toes or digits 1st, 2nd, 3rd, 4th, and 5th.) (Adapted from Winckler G, Gianoli G. La véritable terminaison de la Chair Carrée de Sylvius [musc. quadratus, plantae]. *Arch Anat Histol Embryol [Strasb]*. 1955;38:47.)

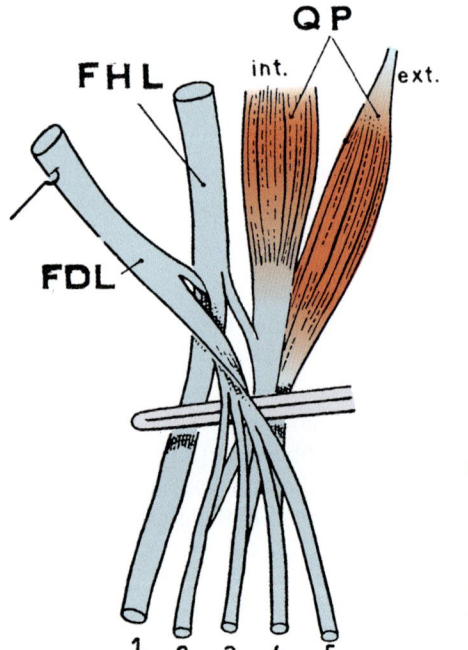

Figure 5.63 **The flexor hallucis longus (*FHL*) provides a weak expansion to the quadratus plantae (*QP*).** The flexor digitorum longus (*FDL*) provides a tendinous band to the flexor hallucis longus. The quadratus plantae has two heads. The inner head receives the extension from the flexor hallucis longus, and together they insert on the flexor digitorum longus tendons of the second, third, and fourth toes. The lateral head inserts on the lateral border of the medial head of the quadratus plantae. (*ext*, external; *int*, internal; *1, 2, 3, 4, 5*, refer to the corresponding toes or digits 1st, 2nd, 3rd, 4th, and 5th.) (Adapted from Winckler G, Gianoli G. La véritable terminaison de la Chair Carrée de Sylvius [musc. quadratus, plantae]. *Arch Anat Histol Embryol [Strasb]*. 1955;38:47.)

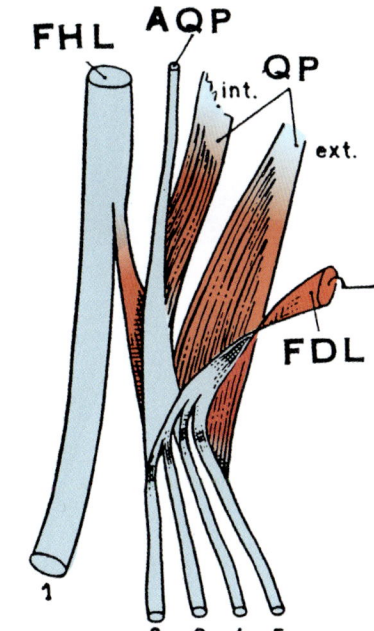

Figure 5.64 An accessory of the quadratus plantae (*AQP*) is associated with the medial head of the quadratus plantae (*QP*). Both join the strong tendinous expansion of the flexor hallucis longus (*FHL*) to the flexor digitorum longus (*FDL*) deep surface. (*int.* internal; *ext.* external; *1, 2, 3, 4, 5,* refer to the corresponding toes or digits 1st, 2nd, 3rd, 4th, and 5th.) (Adapted from Winckler G, Gianoli G. La véritable terminaison de la Chair Carrée de Sylvius [musc. quadratus, plantae]. *Arch Anat Histol Embryol [Strasb].* 1955;38:47.)

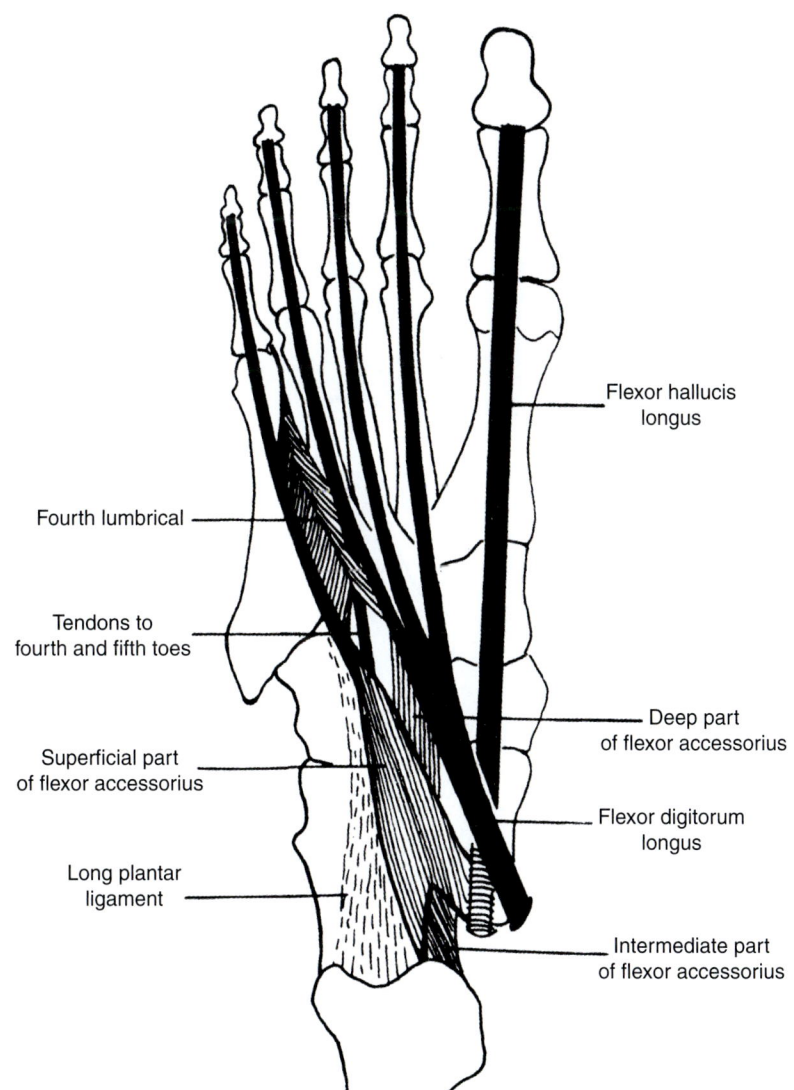

Figure 5.65 Flexor digitorum accessorius (quadratus plantae) composed of three parts: superficial, intermediate, and deep. The superficial originates with two heads from the medial calcaneal tubercle and the sheath of the flexor hallucis longus and flexor digitorum longus. It joins the lateral side of the tendon of the fifth toe and contributes to the tendon of the fourth. The intermediate head arises from the calcaneus medially, and its tendon splits into the tendons to both the fourth and fifth toes. The deep head arises from the medial surface of the calcaneus, in front of the sustentaculum tali, and inserts into the tendon of the flexor digitorum longus. (Republished with permission of John Wiley, from Barlow TE. An unusual anomaly of muscle flexor digitorum longus. *J Anat.* 1949;83:244; permission conveyed through Copyright Clearance Center, Inc.)

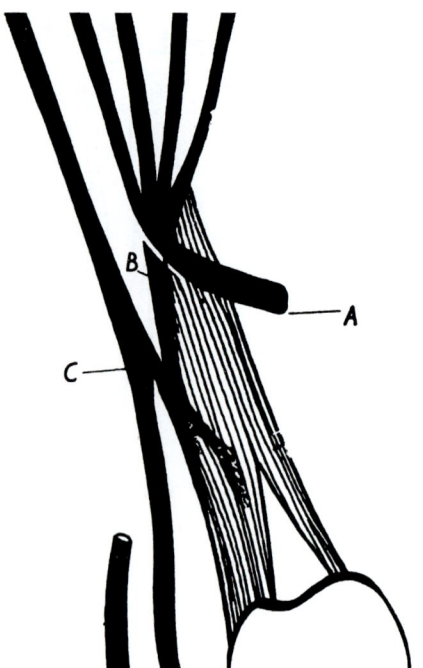

Figure 5.66 Left foot, left. (*A*, flexor digitorum longus turned laterally; *B*, tendon from accessorius to the lateral three toes; *C*, flexor hallucis longus with small tendinous attachment from accessorius.) (Republished with permission of John Wiley, from Barlow TE. The deep flexors of the foot. *J Anat.* 1983;87:308; permission conveyed through Copyright Clearance Center, Inc.)

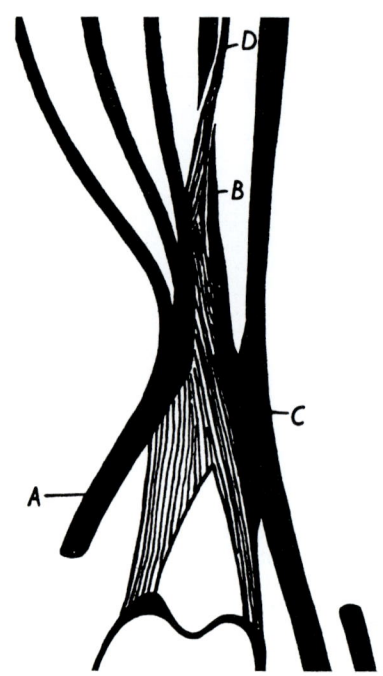

Figure 5.67 Right foot, right. (*A*, flexor digitorum longus turned laterally; *B*, tendon to second toe arising from accessorius; *C*, flexor hallucis longus with broad tendinous attachment to accessorius; *D*, first lumbrical.) (Republished with permission of John Wiley, from Barlow TE. The deep flexors of the foot. *J Anat.* 1983;87:308; permission conveyed through Copyright Clearance Center, Inc.)

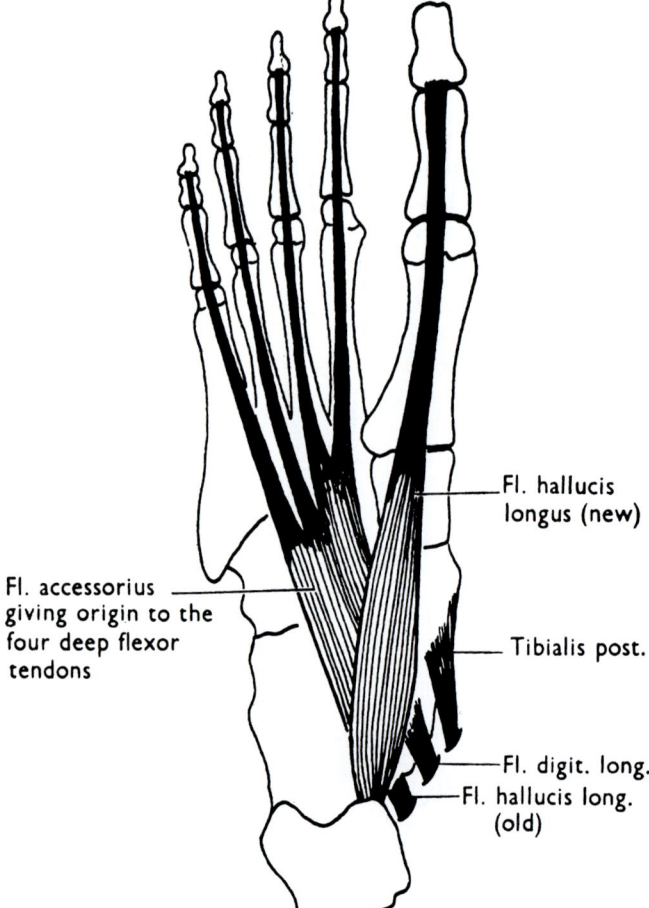

Figure 5.68 Complete divorcement of leg flexors from foot muscles showing flexor accessorius and the new plantar portion of flexor hallucis longus. (Republished with permission of John Wiley, from Barlow TE. The deep flexors of the foot. *J Anat.* 1983;87:308; permission conveyed through Copyright Clearance Center, Inc.)

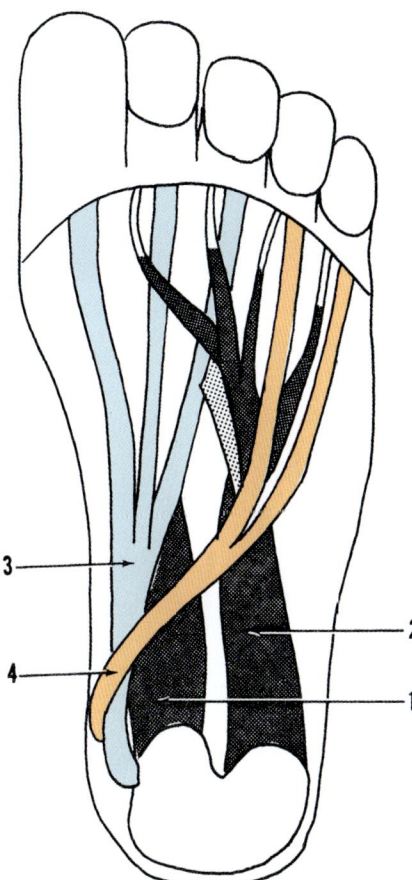

Figure 5.69 Insertional variation of the long flexors and of the quadratus plantae. (*1*, Medial head of quadratus plantae inserting on a common long flexor tendon [*3*] for toes 1, 2, and 3; *2*, lateral head of quadratus plantae inserting on a common long flexor tendon [*4*] for toes 4 and 5.) (Adapted from Auvray M. Anomalies musculaires et nerveuses. *Bull Soc Anat Paris.* 1896;10:223.)

creates an additional anchorage of the muscle to the medial calcaneal tubercle.[41] The Y-shaped origin of the muscle has been found in 46 of 50 ft (see Fig. 5.78).[41]

A large bursa is interposed between the proximal part of the muscle and the underlying medial cuneiform, first tarsometatarsal joint, and the terminal portion of the tunnel of the peroneus longus.[40] The flexor hallucis brevis muscle is oriented anteriorly and medially, crosses the first interosseous space and the first metatarsal, and divides into two parts, medial and lateral. The smaller lateral head is crossed obliquely by the tendon of the flexor hallucis longus, which imprints a groove. An insertional tendon appears on the plantar aspect of the lateral head and penetrates the plantar plate laterally through a flat tunnel at a distance from the adductor tendon (Fig. 5.79). The fibers insert on the plantar plate laterally; on the central, medial aspect of the lateral sesamoid; and on the base of the proximal phalanx laterally in conjunction with the corresponding fibers of the adductor hallucis. The medial head of the flexor hallucis brevis is larger and courses on the inner side of the flexor hallucis longus tendon. The fibers insert on the medial aspect of the plantar plate; on the lateral, central aspect of the medial sesamoid; and on the base

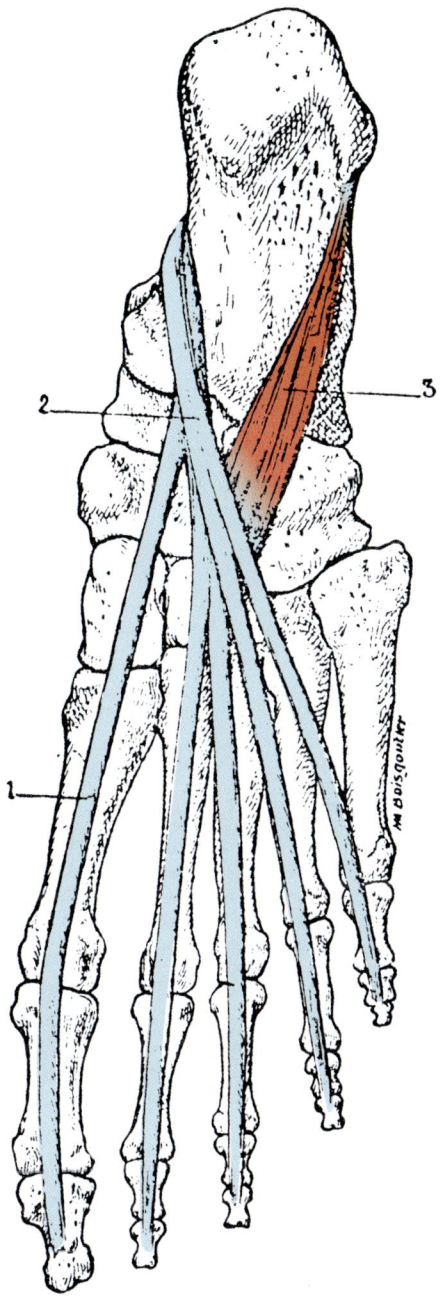

Figure 5.70 Absence of the medial head of the quadratus plantae muscle. (*1*, Flexor hallucis longus tendon; *2*, flexor digitorum longus tendon; *3*, lateral head of quadratus plantae.) (Adapted from Morestin H. Anomalie de l'accessoire du long fléchisseur commun des orteils. *Bull Soc Anat Paris.* 1895;11:46.)

of the proximal phalanx medially in conjunction with the corresponding fibers of the abductor hallucis. The parting of the two heads of the flexor hallucis brevis delineates a triangle at the level of the first metatarsal neck.

The following variations are mentioned by LeDouble[2]:

- Lateral head of the short flexor more or less united to the oblique adductor and occasionally inseparable from it
- Medial head inserting with the majority of its fibers on the tendon of the abductor hallucis

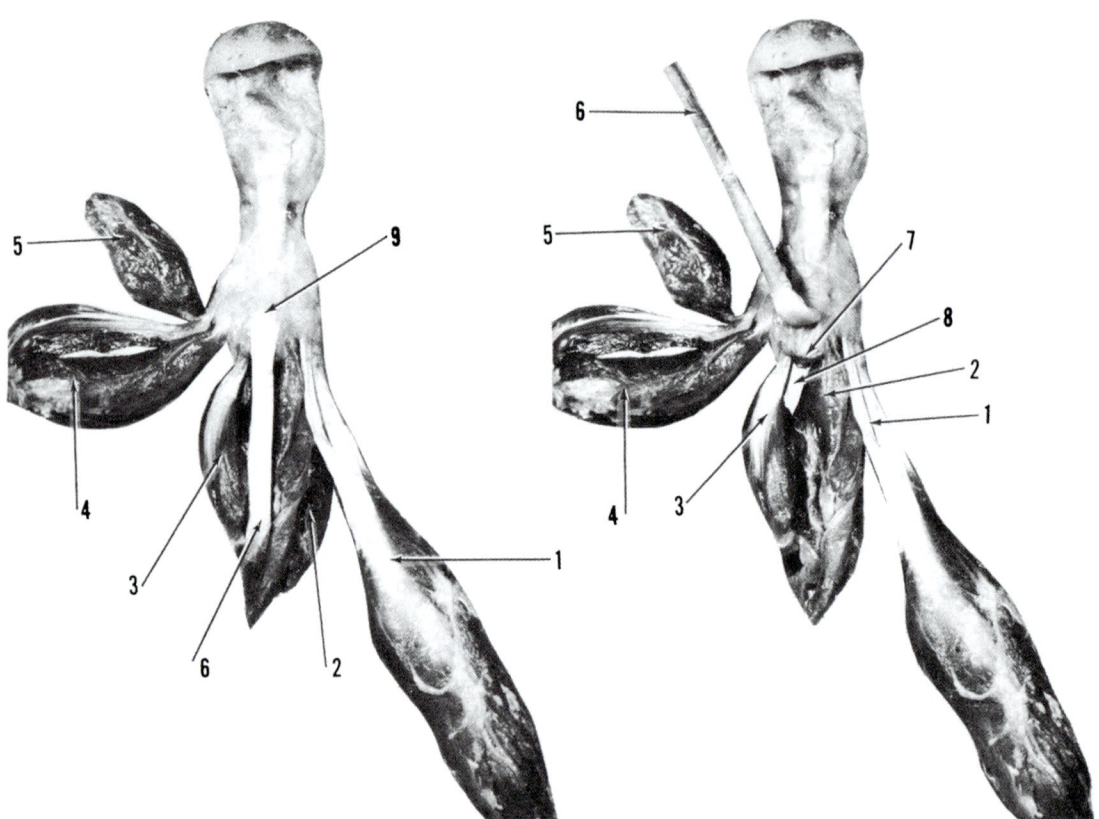

Figure 5.71 **Plantar aspect of the big toe.** (*1*, Abductor hallucis muscle; *2*, medial head of flexor hallucis brevis muscle; *3*, lateral head of flexor hallucis brevis muscle; *4*, oblique head of adductor hallucis muscle; *5*, transverse head of adductor hallucis muscle; *6*, flexor hallucis longus tendon; *7*, proximal border of plantar plate; *8*, triangular space between two heads of flexor hallucis brevis; *9*, fibrous tunnel of flexor hallucis longus tendon.)

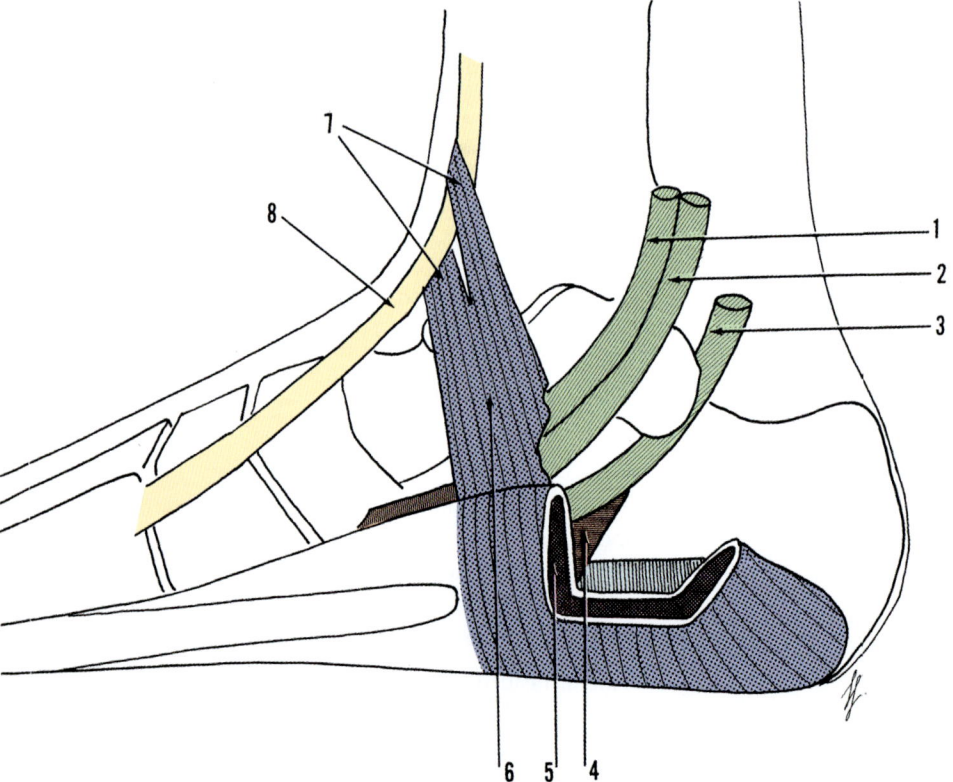

Figure 5.72 **Tarsal tunnel.** (*1*, Tibialis posterior tendon; *2*, flexor digitorum longus tendon; *3*, flexor hallucis longus tendon; *4*, interfascicular septum; *5*, abductor hallucis muscle; *6*, flexor retinaculum; *7*, apex of 6 forming tunnel disposition for tibialis anterior tendon [*8*].)

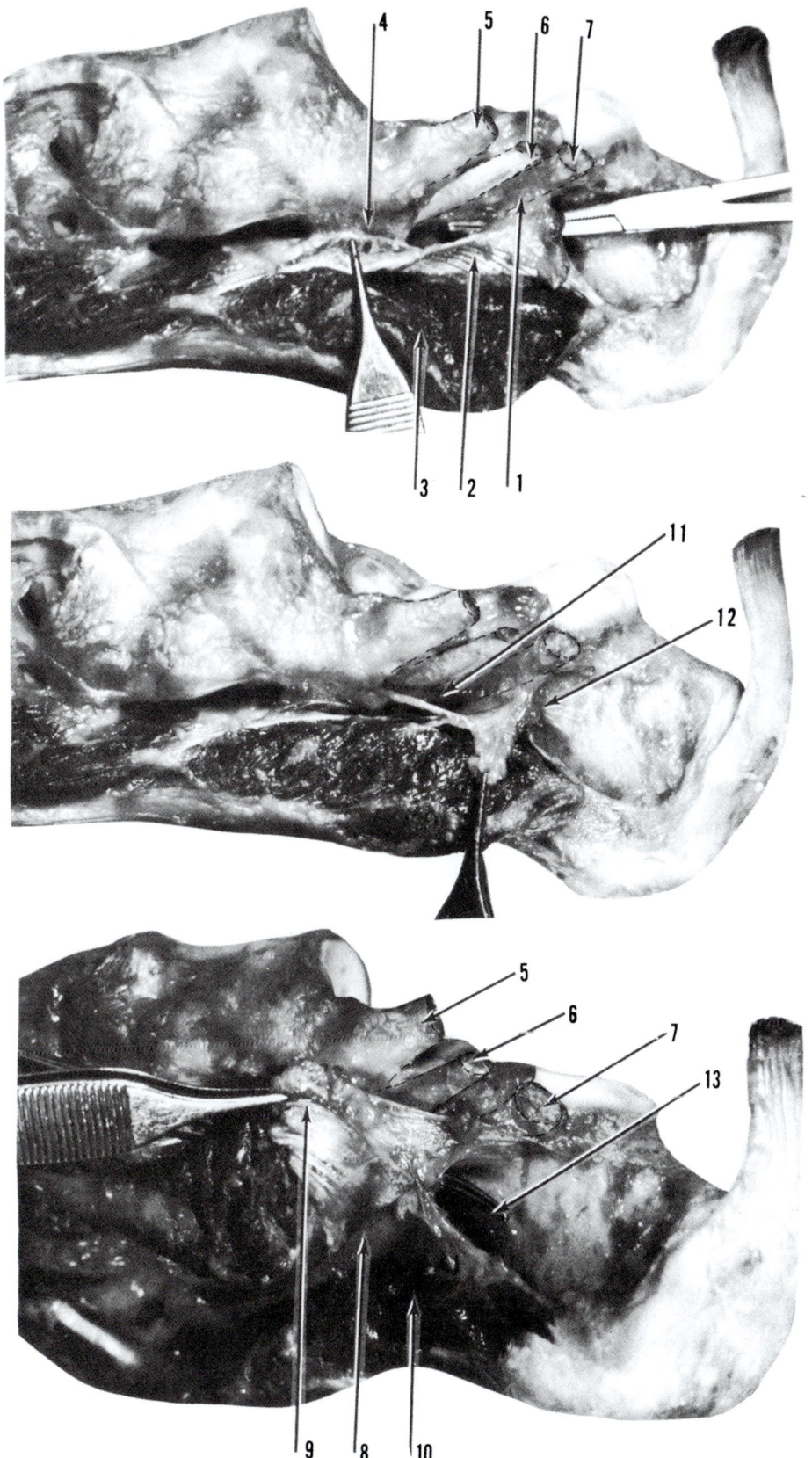

Figure 5.73 Upper and lower chambers of the calcaneal canal. (*1*, Interfascicular septum; *2*, deep investing aponeurosis of abductor hallucis muscle [*3*]; *4*, navicular attachment of investing fascia of abductor hallucis muscle; *5*, tendon of tibialis posterior; *6*, tendon of flexor digitorum longus; *7*, tendon of flexor hallucis longus; *8*, medial intermuscular septum; *9*, reflected calcaneal origin of abductor hallucis muscle; *10*, flexor digitorum brevis muscle; *11*, upper chamber of calcaneal canal; *12*, lower chamber of calcaneal canal with hemostat [*13*] passing through.)

268 Sarrafian's Anatomy of the Foot and Ankle

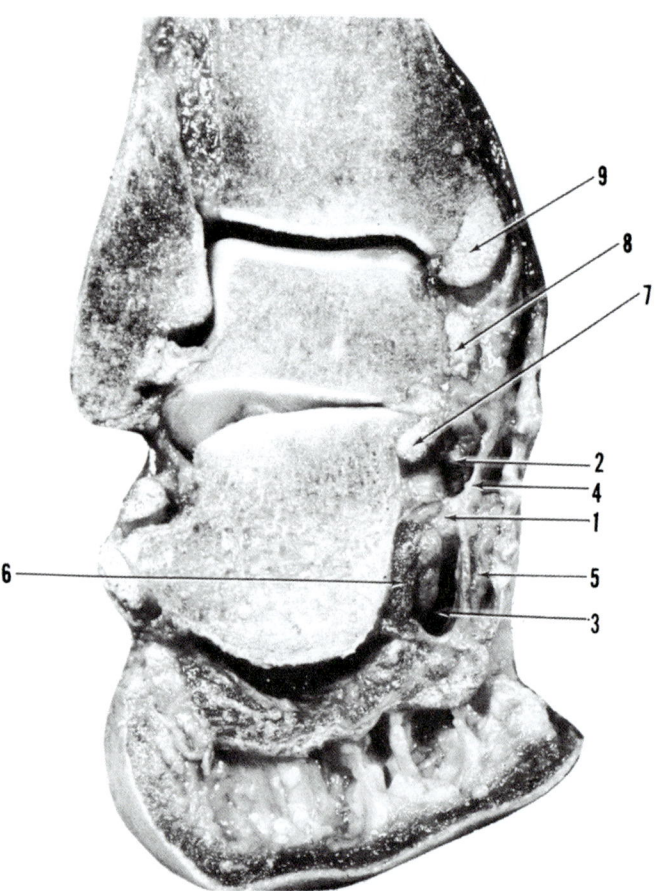

Figure 5.74 **Sagittal cross-section of ankle and hindfoot.** (*1*, Interfascicular septum; *2*, upper calcaneal chamber lodging medial plantar neurovascular bundle; *3*, lower calcaneal chamber lodging lateral plantar neurovascular bundle; *4*, deep investing fascia of abductor hallucis muscle [5]; *6*, quadratus plantae muscle; *7*, flexor hallucis longus tendon; *8*, flexor digitorum longus tendon; *9*, tibialis posterior tendon.)

- A small tendinous fascicle originating from the flexor hallucis and inserting on the first cuneiform (interosseous plantaris primus)
- A tendon extending from the short flexor to the proximal phalanx of the second toe
- Short flexor of the big toe reinforced by a tendinous extension from the flexor digitorum longus

Adductor Hallucis

The adductor hallucis is formed by two muscles, oblique and transverse (see Figs. 5.77, 5.80, and 5.81).

Oblique Head

The fibrous tunnel of the peroneus longus tendon inserts laterally on the crest of the cuboid and the base of the fourth and fifth metatarsals and medially on the lateral two cuneometatarsal joints. The oblique head of the adductor hallucis originates from the midsegment of the peroneus longus tunnel. It is through this simple relationship that the oblique head is said to arise from the anterior segment of the inferior calcaneocuboid ligament; the crest of the cuboid; the base of metatarsals 4, 3, and 2; and the cuneiforms. The origin of the muscle may form a fibrous arc extended from the base to the inferior border of the fourth metatarsal bone. This gives passage to the lateral plantar neurovascular bundle in the middle compartment of the planta pedis.

The oblique head of the adductor hallucis courses obliquely (anteromedially) toward the lateral aspect of the metatarsophalangeal joint of the big toe. Its lateral border crosses the underlying metatarsals 4, 3, and 2 and the corresponding interossei along an oblique line drawn from the base of the fourth metatarsal to the base of the proximal hallucal phalanx. The medial border is apposed to the flexor hallucis brevis muscle. Three components are recognizable in the distal segment of the adductor hallucis obliquum—medial, central, and lateral. All three components, prior to reaching their insertional destination, pass dorsal to the deep transverse metatarsal ligament (Figs. 5.82 and 5.83). The medial component with fleshy fibers inserts directly on the lateral sesamoid. The central component is the deepest and presents a tendinous band that takes a firm grip on the plantar aspect of the lateral sesamoid. The lateral component has a broad plantar tendon that inserts on the lateral sesamoid and the plantar lateral aspect of the proximal phalanx and gives minor contribution to the extensor aponeurosis (see Fig. 5.81). The phalangeal tendinous component may be traced as a definite band (Fig. 5.84).

Transverse Head

The transverse head of the adductor originates from the proximal border of the plantar plate of the fifth, fourth, and third metatarsophalangeal joints; the proximal border of the deep transverse metatarsal ligament between toes 5 and 4, 4 and 3, and 3 and 2; the longitudinal septa of the plantar aponeurosis to the fifth, fourth, and third toes; and the medial crux of the lateral component of the plantar aponeurosis (see Figs. 5.77, 5.80, and 5.85).[75]

Three transversely oriented muscular fascicles are formed. The most posterior is the longest and the most superficial. It arises from the fifth toe and the medial crux of the lateral plantar aponeurosis. It partially overlaps the second fascicle, which in turn overlaps the shortest, deepest, and most anterior component arising from the third toe. The three fascicles unite at the level of the second metatarsophalangeal joint, and a short tendon appears, which passes dorsal to the deep transverse metatarsal ligament of the first toe and reaches the tendons of the oblique head of the adductor. At this level, some fibers of the tendon of the transverse head insert on the extensor aponeurosis; the remaining fibers pass over the fibers of the oblique head at the level of the lateral sesamoid, share their insertion, and terminate on the fibrous sheath of the flexor hallucis longus.

Leboucq emphasized the independent insertion of the transverse head of the adductor hallucis and its connection with the sheath of the flexor hallucis longus.[76] Furthermore,

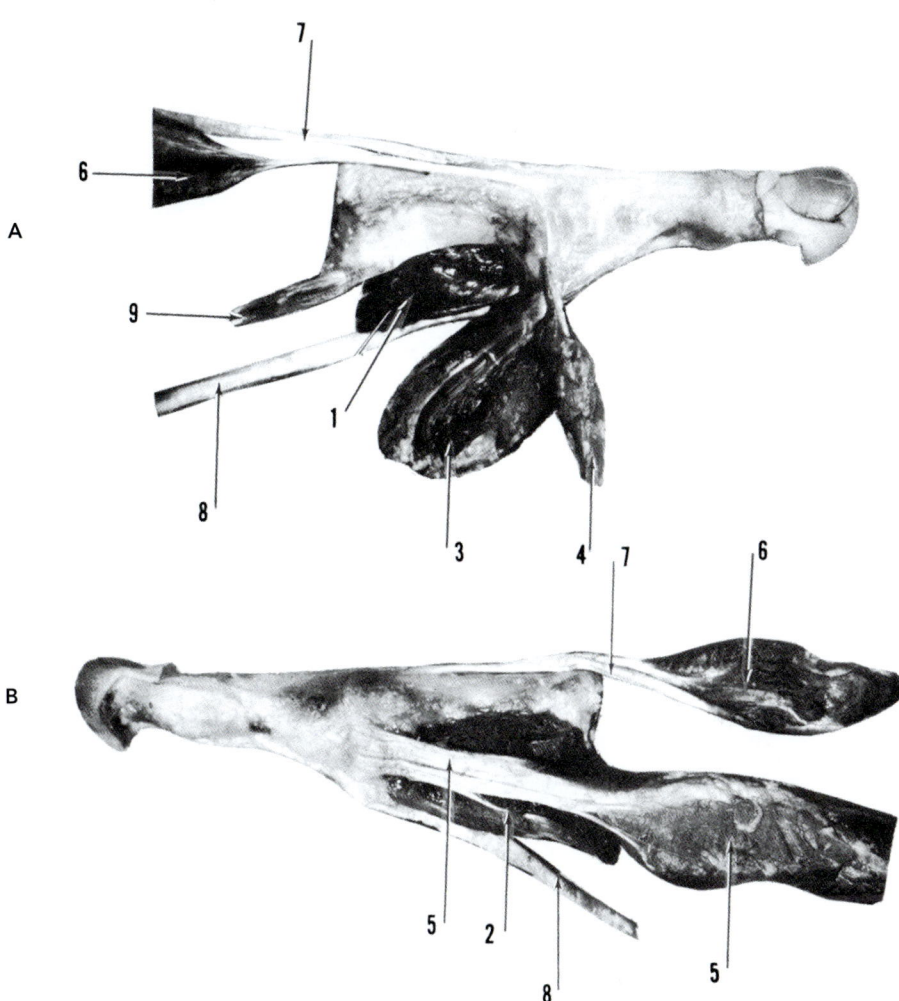

Figure 5.75 **(A) Lateral aspect of right big toe. (B) Medial aspect of right big toe.** (*1*, Lateral head of flexor hallucis brevis muscle; *2*, medial head of flexor hallucis brevis muscle; *3*, adductor hallucis, oblique head; *4*, adductor hallucis, transverse head; *5*, abductor hallucis muscle and tendon; *6*, extensor hallucis brevis muscle; *7*, extensor hallucis longus tendon; *8*, flexor hallucis longus tendon; *9*, insertion of peroneus longus tendon.)

he mentioned some fibers inserting on the deep surface of the flexor tendon sheath of the second, third, and fourth toes and a bifurcation of the insertion at the level of the distal end of the fifth metatarsal, some fibers passing dorsal to the long flexor of the little toe, and the remaining fibers passing plantar and uniting with the superficial plantar aponeurosis.

The transverse head of the adductor hallucis has no insertion on the metatarsals. Owens and Thordarson[77] investigated the insertion of the adductor hallucis tendon into the lateral sesamoid and the lateral aspect of the proximal phalanx of the great toe in 42 fresh frozen specimens. All specimens had conjoint insertional fibers of the adductor hallucis and of the flexor hallucis brevis, from the lateral sesamoid into the base of the proximal phalanx of the great toe. There was no separate phalangeal insertion of these tendons. An isolated surgical release of the adductor hallucis tendon is possible on the dorsal aspect of the deep transverse metatarsal ligament and the lateral surface of the lateral sesamoid. A distal lateral phalangeal release results in the combined release of the adductor hallucis and flexor hallucis brevis conjoint tendon.

The guideline for the safe surgical release of the adductor hallucis tendon is the deep transverse metatarsal ligament. At that level, the adductor tendon is dorsal to the ligament whereas the tendon of the flexor hallucis brevis is plantar to the ligament.

Variations

The following variations may be seen[2]: oblique adductor and transverse adductor.

Oblique Adductor
- Inseparable from the lateral head of the flexor hallucis brevis insertion on the tendon or the muscle of the lateral head of the short flexor
- A fascicle extending from the lateral border of the oblique adductor to the lateral aspect of the proximal phalanx of the second toe at the base

Transverse Adductor
- Origin only from the fifth-fourth or fourth-third plantar plate and corresponding deep transverse metatarsal ligaments
- Origin only from the joint of the fifth toe

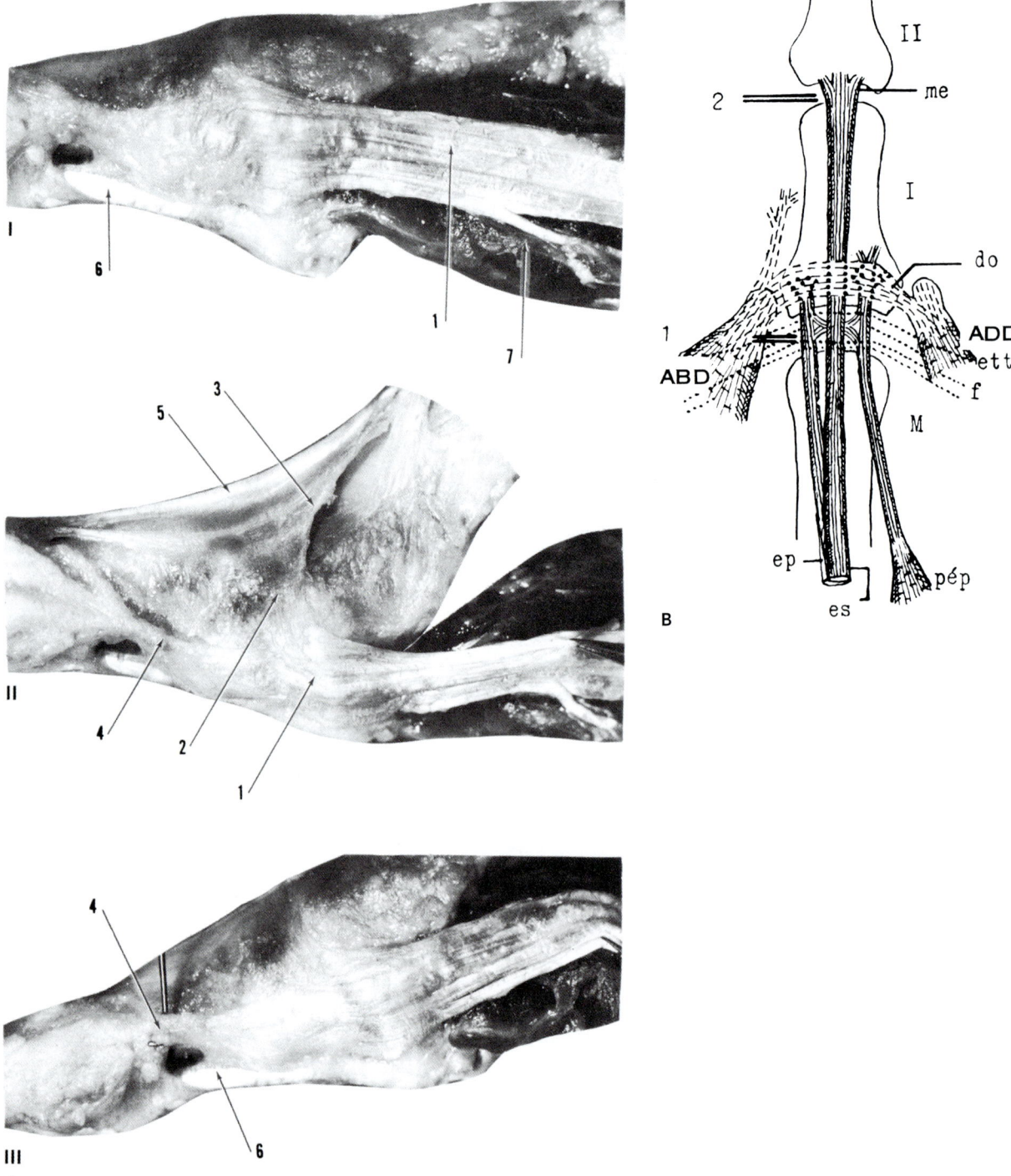

Figure 5.76 **(A) Medial aspect of the metatarsophalangeal level of the right big toe.** (*I*) In neutral. (*II*) In hyperextension. (*III*) In flexion. (*1*, Tendon of abductor hallucis muscle; *2*, transverse lamina of extensor aponeurosis; *3*, proximal border of [2]; *4*, phalangeal insertional band of [1]; *5*, extensor hallucis longus tendon; *6*, flexor hallucis longus tendon; *7*, medial head of flexor hallucis brevis muscle.) **(B) Internal structure of the extensor apparatus of the right big toe.** (*ABD*, tendon of abductor hallucis tendon and insertion fibers contributing to extensor sling; *ADD*, tendon of adductor hallucis contributing to dorsal sling; *do*, dorsal sling; *f*, perforating fibers arising from plantar aponeurosis; *ep*, deep fibers of extensor hallucis longus tendon; *es*, superficial fibers of extensor hallucis longus tendon; *M*, metatarsal; *me*, insertion of extensor hallucis longus tendon; *pép*, extensor hallucis brevis tendon; *I-II*, proximal and distal phalanges; *1-2*, level of metatarsophalangeal and interphalangeal joints.) (From Baumann JA. Valeur, variations et équivalences des muscles extenseurs, interosseux, adducteurs et abducteurs de la main et du pied chez l'homme. *Acta Anat.* 1948;4:10. By permission of S. Karger AG, Basel.)

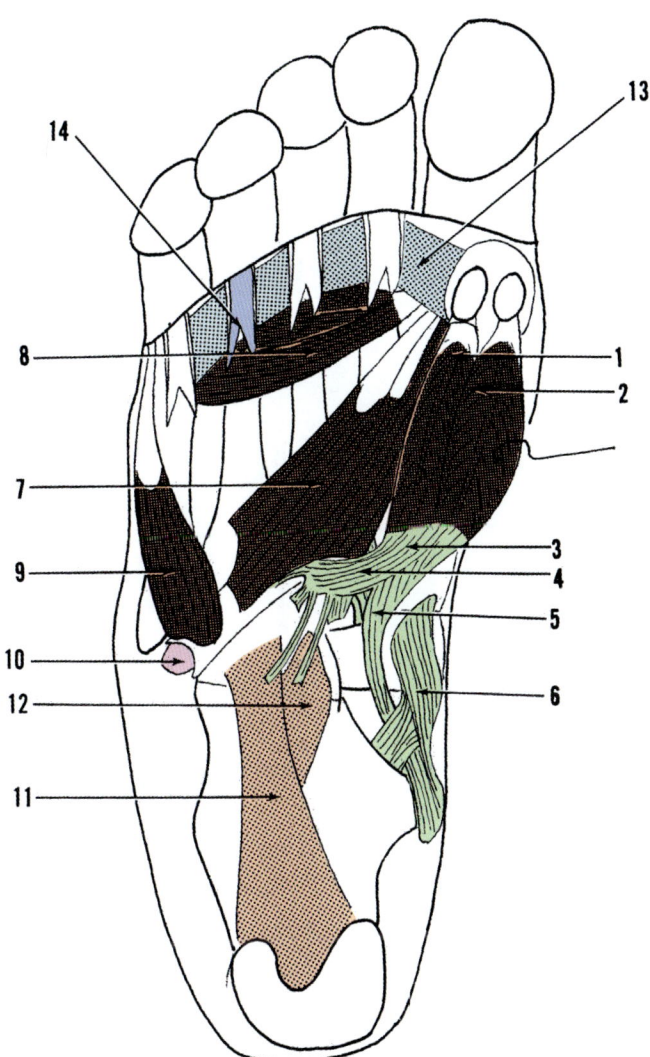
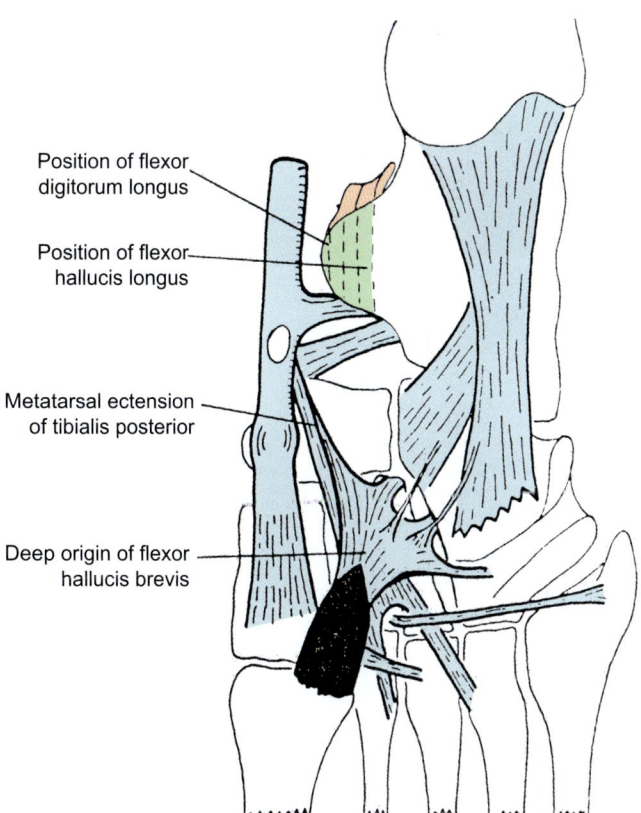

Figure 5.77 Flexor hallucis brevis. (*1*, Lateral head of flexor hallucis brevis; *2*, medial head of flexor hallucis brevis; *3*, stem of Y origin of flexor hallucis brevis; *4*, lateral arm of Y origin of flexor hallucis brevis; *5*, medial arm of Y origin of flexor hallucis brevis provided by tibialis posterior tendon [6]; *7*, oblique head of adductor hallucis muscle; *8*, transverse head of adductor hallucis muscle; *9*, short flexor of fifth toe; *10*, peroneus longus tendon; *11*, long calcaneocuboid ligament; *12*, short calcaneocuboid ligament; *13*, deep transverse metatarsal ligament; *14*, deep insertional septa of plantar aponeurosis.)

Figure 5.78 Origin of flexor hallucis brevis muscle. (Adapted from Martin BF. Observation on the muscles and tendons of the medial aspect of the sole of the foot. *J Anat.* 1964;98(3):437. By permission of Cambridge University Press.)

- Absent transverse component or replaced by an extremely thin contractile band
- Proximal extension of the muscle reaching the anterior border of the oblique adductor
- Additional muscle located in the first interosseous space. This is a small triangular muscle that measures about 1 cm and originates through its base from the distal third of the plantar border of the second metatarsal. It is located between the first dorsal interosseous and the oblique adductor, courses anteromedially, and inserts on the tendon of the transverse adductor

Cralley and Schuberth studied the transverse head of the adductor hallucis in 91 cadaver feet.[78] This muscle is absent in 6% and "is a highly variable muscle not only in origin and insertion but also in size."[78] The authors describe the insertion as "broad often without any discernible tendon." The insertion is into the lateral margin of the oblique head of the adductor hallucis and posterior to the lateral sesamoid bone. The origin is described as being from the deep transverse metatarsal ligament, the plantar ligament of the metatarsophalangeal joints of the lesser toes, "from the intermuscular septa of the third and fourth muscle layers and from the fibular syndesmosis of Henkel (1913), a portion of the plantar aponeurosis which extends to the plantar ligament (pad) of the fourth toe. This fleshy origin is often quite broad. Nowhere does this muscle originate from bony attachments."[78]

Arakawa et al[79] investigated the adductor hallucis muscle, oblique and transverse components, in respect to its origin and insertion, in 45 ft.

The oblique head of the adductor hallucis muscle was classified into types A, B, C, and D based on its origins.

- Type A, 47%, was subdivided into subtype 1, subtype 2, and subtype 3. In subtype 1, "muscle arose from the fibrous sheath of the tendon of the peroneus longus muscle, the long plantar ligament, the bases of the second, third, and fourth metatarsal bones, and lateral cuneiform bone."[79] This was designated as the common origin of the oblique head of the adductor hallucis muscle. In subtype 2, the muscle did not

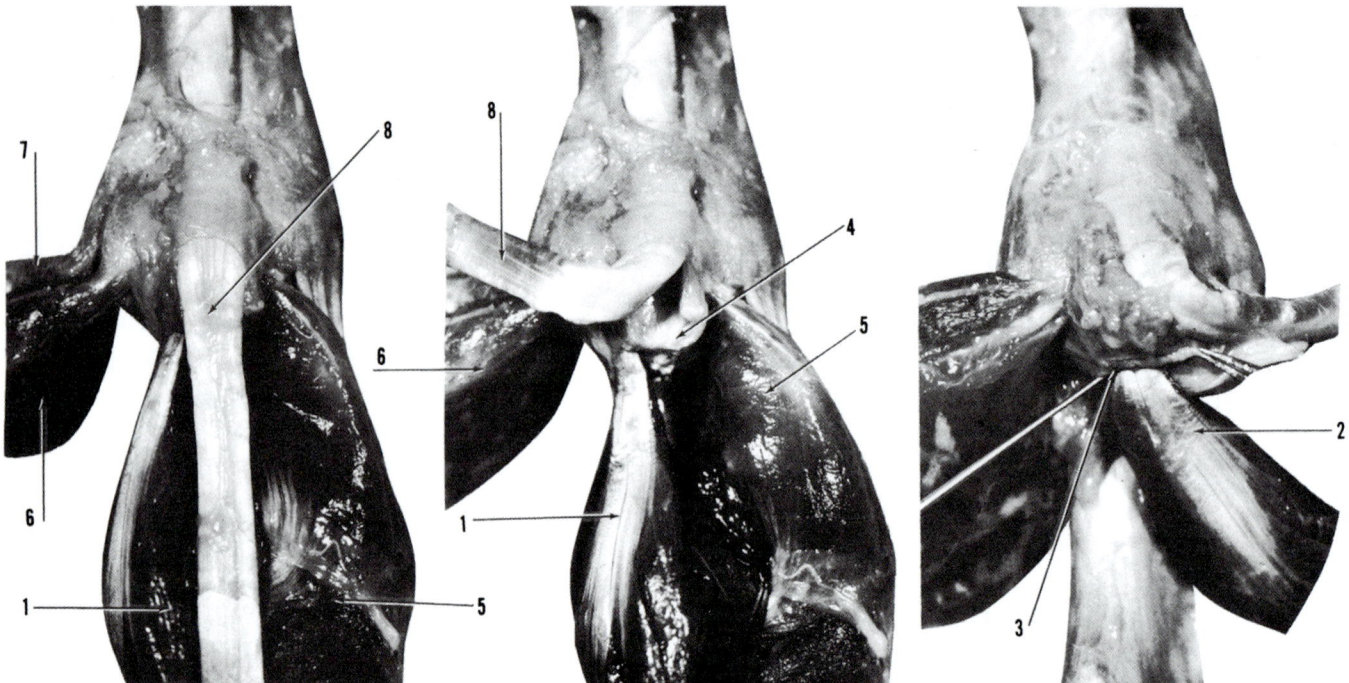

Figure 5.79 **Plantar aspect of the metatarsophalangeal joint of the big toe.** (*1*, Lateral head of flexor hallucis brevis; *2*, tendon of *1* entering its own tunnel [*3*] before inserting on lateral sesamoid; *4*, proximal border of plantar plate; *5*, medial head of flexor hallucis brevis; *6*, oblique head of adductor hallucis muscle; *7*, transverse head of adductor hallucis muscle; *8*, flexor hallucis longus tendon.)

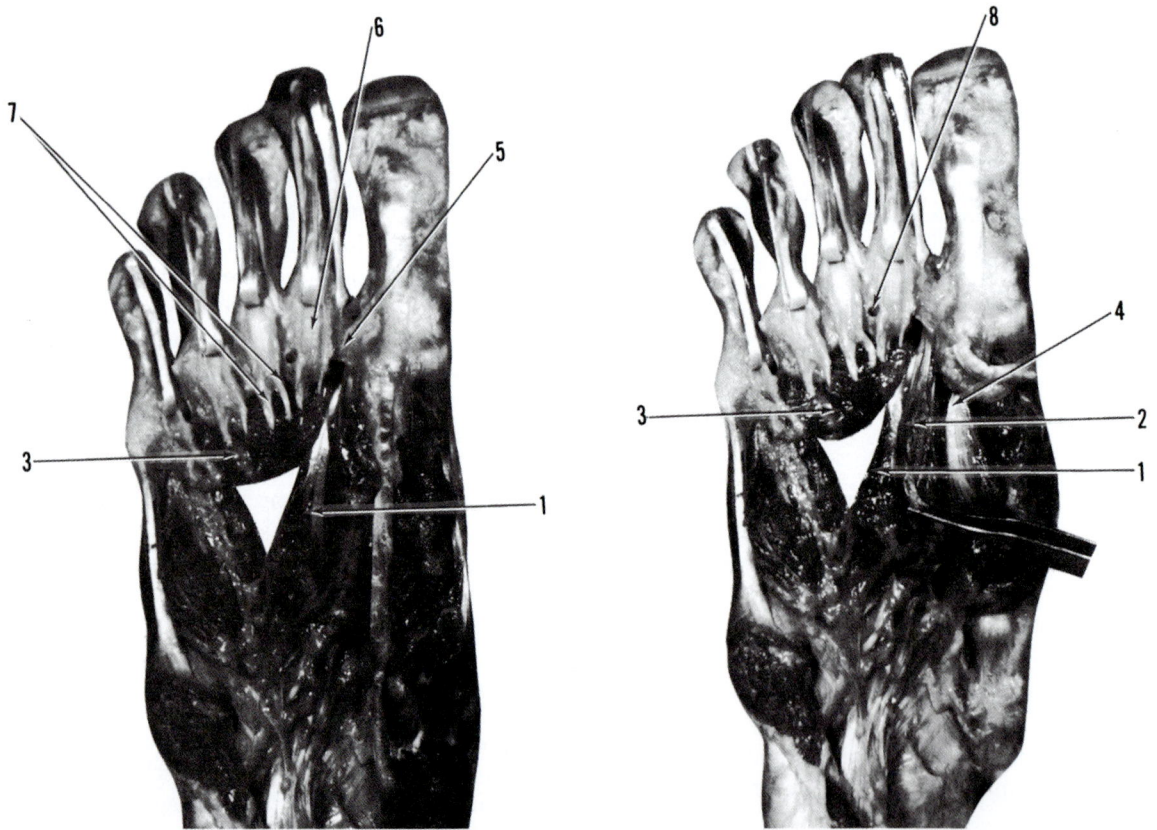

Figure 5.80 **Adductor hallucis.** (*1*, Oblique head of adductor hallucis muscle, lateral component; *2*, medial component of *1*; *3*, transverse head of adductor hallucis muscle; *4*, lateral head of flexor hallucis brevis muscle; *5*, deep transverse metatarsal ligament; *6*, plantar plate; *7*, deep insertional septa of plantar aponeurosis; *8*, foramen for common digital artery.)

Chapter 5: Myology 273

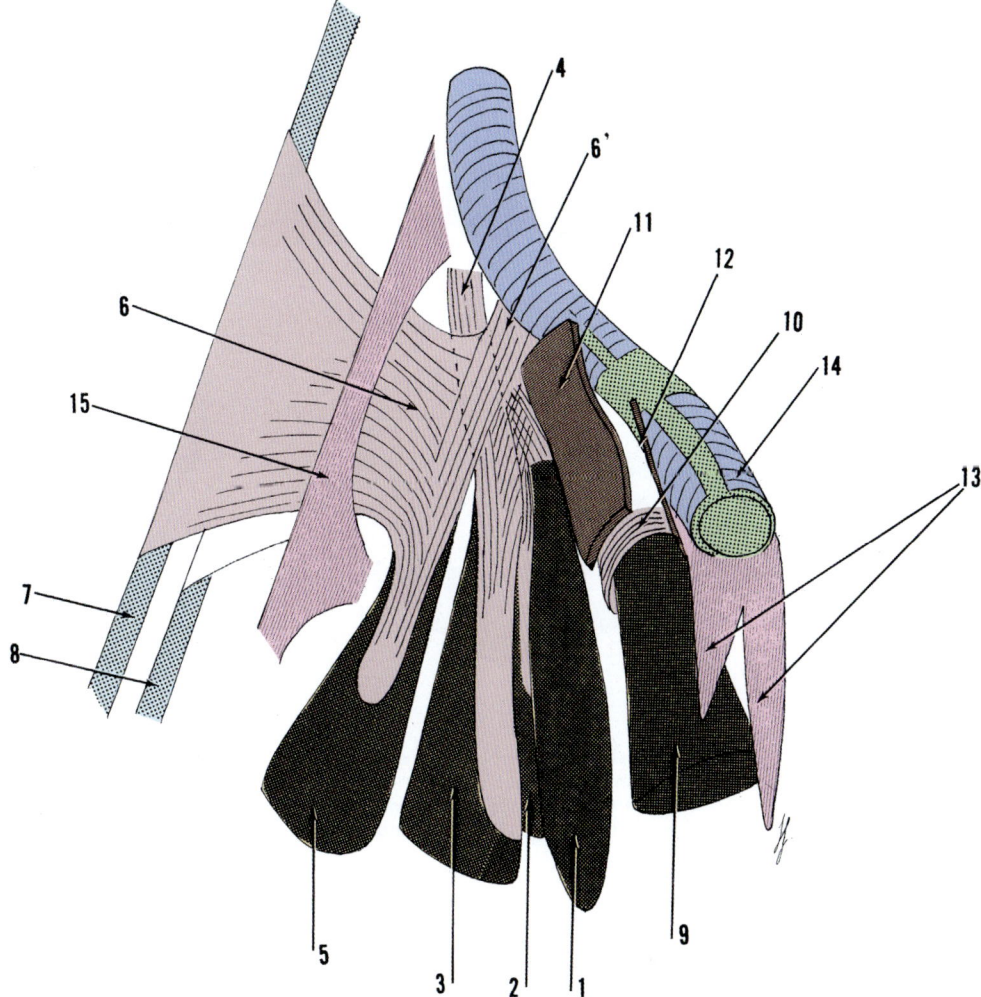

Figure 5.81 **Internal structure of plantar-lateral aspect of the right big toe.** The specimen is fanned out for display of anatomic details. (*1*, Medial component of oblique head of adductor hallucis muscle; *2*, central component of oblique head of adductor hallucis muscle; *3*, lateral component of oblique head of adductor hallucis muscle; *4*, phalangeal insertion of *3*; *5*, transverse head of adductor hallucis muscle with contribution to extensor aponeurosis [*6*] and insertion on flexor hallucis longus tendon tunnel [*6'*]; *7*, extensor hallucis longus tendon; *8*, extensor hallucis brevis tendon; *9*, lateral head of flexor hallucis brevis entering its own tunnel [*10*]; *11*, insertion of deep transverse metatarsal ligament; *12*, insertion of medial intermuscular septum; *13*, deep insertional septa of plantar aponeurosis; *14*, fibrous tunnel of flexor hallucis longus tendon; *15*, fibrous bridge extending from metatarsal to proximal phalanx; diagram after dissection under magnification ×8.)

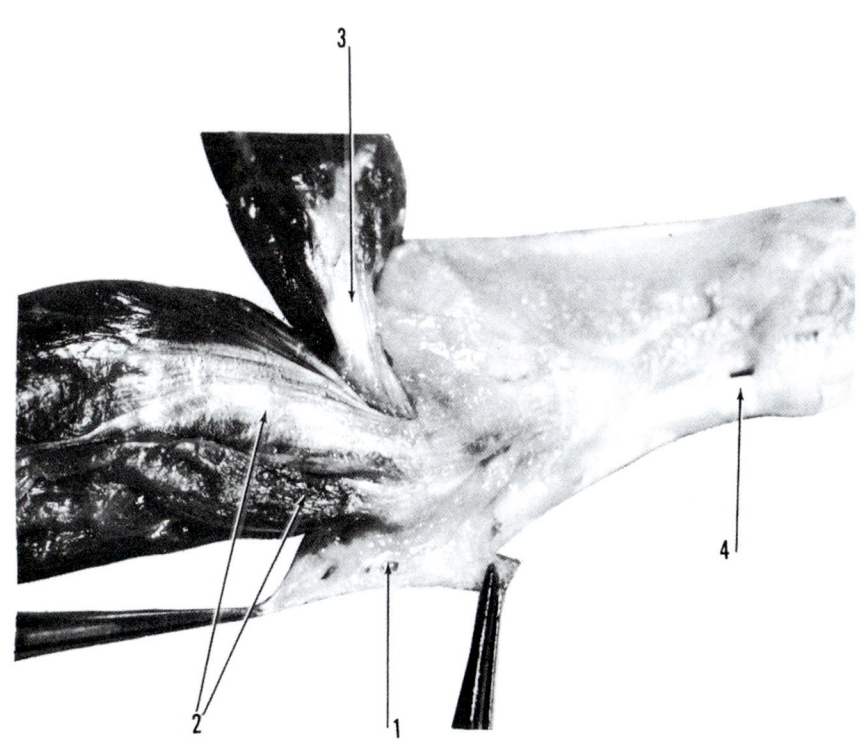

Figure 5.82 **Lateral aspect of metatarsophalangeal level of the right big toe.** (*1*, Deep transverse metatarsal ligament; *2*, components of oblique head of adductor hallucis muscle; *3*, transverse head of adductor hallucis muscle; both *2* and *3* pass dorsal to *1*; *4*, flexor hallucis longus tendon.)

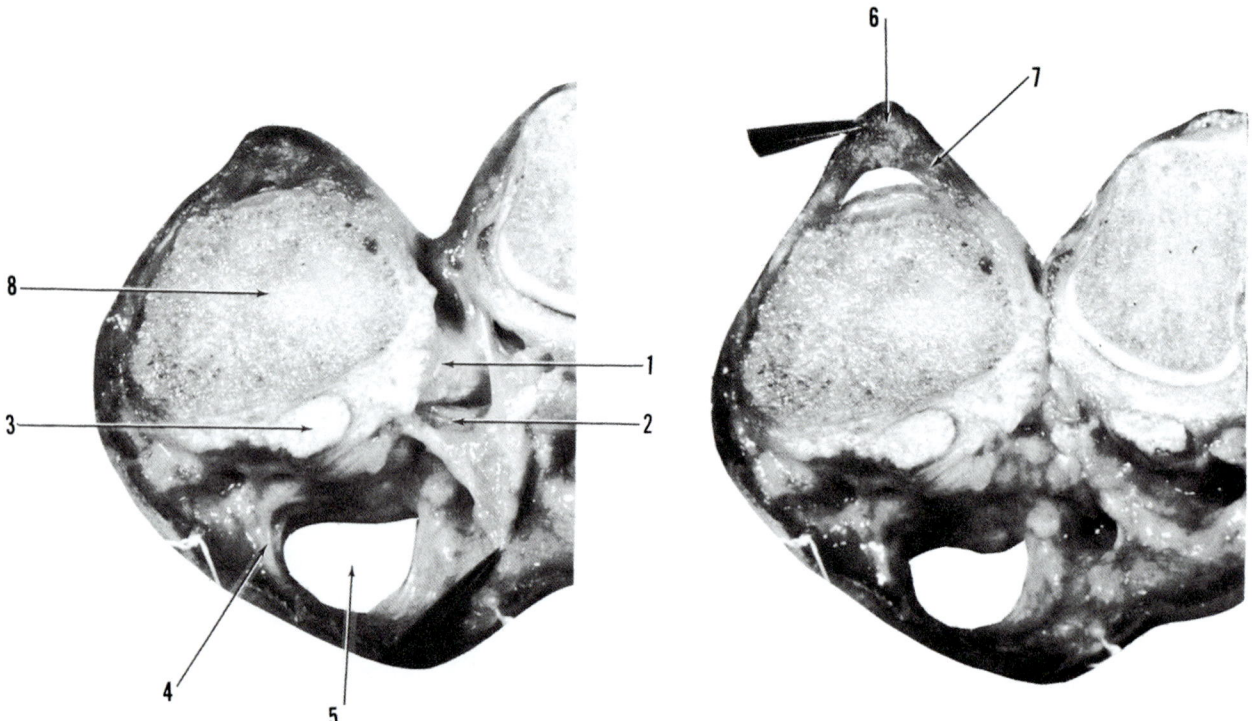

Figure 5.83 Cross-section through proximal phalanx of the big toe. (*1*, Adductor tendon passing dorsal to deep transverse metatarsal ligament [*2*]; *3*, flexor hallucis longus tendon and its fibrous sheath attached to *1*; *4*, arciform fibrous fibers forming a preflexor chamber [*5*] retaining preflexor adipose cushion; *6*, extensor hallucis longus tendon giving origin to transverse lamina [*7*].)

have an origin from the long plantar ligament. In subtype 3, the muscle did not arise from the lateral cuneiform bone (Fig. 5.86).

- Type B, 33%, is a "lateral type of the oblique head originated from the base of the fifth metatarsal bone by an aponeurotic slip in addition to the common origin site as in type A."[79]
- Type C, 9%, or wide type, arose laterally from the base of the fifth metatarsal bone as in type B. Medially, it originated "from the divided tendon of the tibialis posterior muscle, or the medial intermuscular septum, or the plantar tarsometatarsal ligaments extended between the medial cuneiform bone and the base of the second metatarsal bone or the divided tendon of the peroneus longus inserting into the first dorsal interosseous muscle, in addition to the common origin sites"[79] (Fig. 5.86).
- In type D (medial type), 11%, the muscle "originated from the divided tendon of the tibialis posterior muscle, or the medial intermuscular septum, or the plantar tarsometatarsal ligament spanned between the medial cuneiform bone and the base of the second metatarsal bone, or divided tendon of peroneus longus then inserting to the first dorsal interosseous muscle, in addition to the common origin sites"[79] (Fig. 5.86).

Muscle Bellies

The oblique head of the adductor hallucis had two muscle bellies: medial and lateral.

Insertion. The oblique head of the adductor hallucis inserted into the lateral sesamoid and the capsule of the metacarpophalangeal joint of the great toe in all except two feet. In one specimen, the insertion was an addition on the medial surface of the metacarpophalangeal joint and the base of the proximal phalanx of the second toe. In another specimen, the oblique head insertion extended to the medial sesamoid.

The Transverse Head of the Adductor Hallucis Muscle

This muscle was classified into types A, B, and C based on its origins.

- In type A, 40%, or narrow type, it originates "from the capsules of the third and fourth (metatarsophalangeal) joints and the deep transverse metatarsal ligaments spanning between the capsules."[79]
- In type B, 30% (lateral type), it originates "from the capsule of the third, fourth, and fifth (metatarsophalangeal) joints and the deep transverse metatarsal ligaments extending between the capsules."[79]
- In type C, 30% (wide type), the transverse head originates "from the aponeurosis spanning between the third plantar interosseous muscle and the fourth dorsal interosseous muscle" or from "deep band of fibular part of the plantar aponeurosis in addition to the capsules of the third, fourth, and

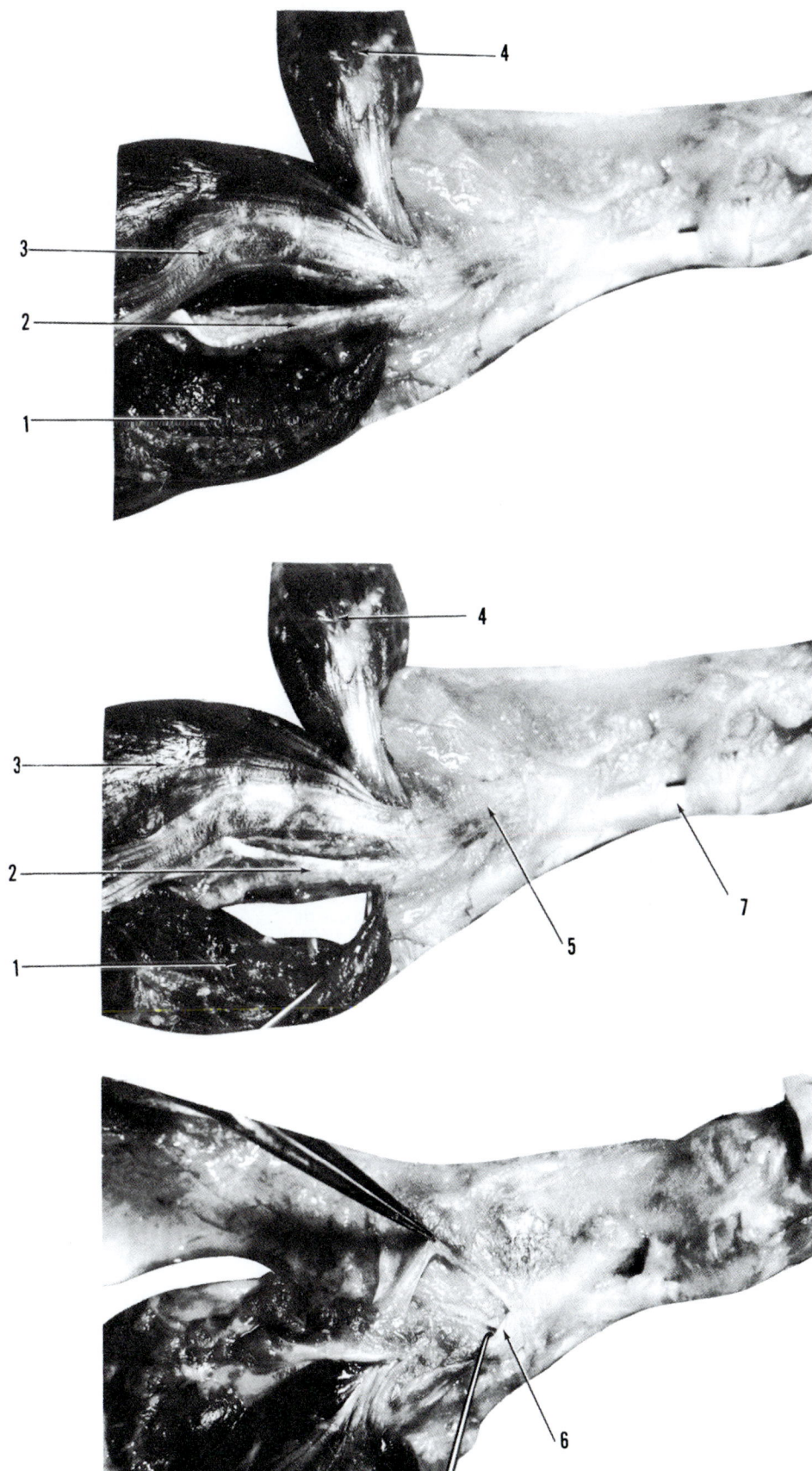

Figure 5.84 Insertion of adductor muscle of the big toe. (*1*, Medial component of oblique head of adductor hallucis; *2*, central component of oblique head of adductor hallucis; *3*, lateral component of oblique head of adductor hallucis; *4*, transverse head of adductor hallucis; *5*, phalangeal insertional band of 3, retracted with a hook [*6*]; *7*, flexor hallucis longus tendon.)

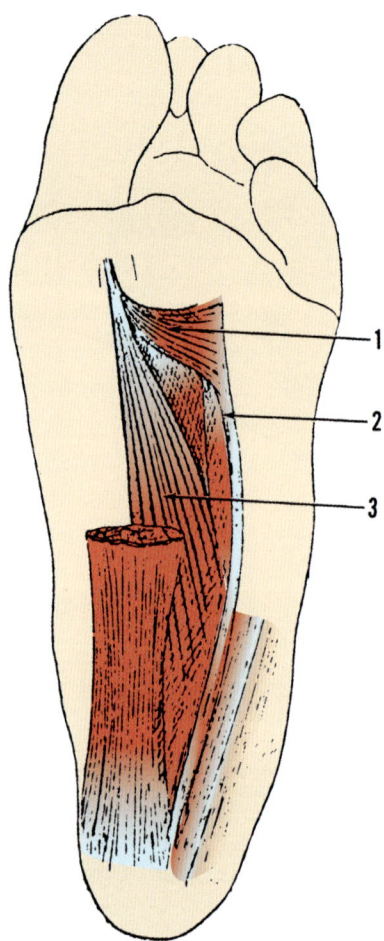

Figure 5.85 Origin of the transverse head of the adductor hallucis from the medial crux of the lateral component of the plantar aponeurosis. (*1*, Transverse head of adductor hallucis muscle; *2*, medial crux of lateral component of plantar aponeurosis; *3*, oblique head of adductor hallucis muscle.) (From Loth É. Etude anthropoligique de l'aponevrose plantaire. *Bull Mem Soc Anthropol Paris.* 1913:4:606.)

occasionally fifth (metacarpophalangeal) joints and the deep transverse metatarsal ligaments expanding between these capsules."[79]

Insertion. The transverse head of the adductor hallucis "inserted into the lateral sesamoid bone of the great toe, the capsule of the (metatarsophalangeal) joint and the lateral surface of the first proximal phalanx"[79] (Fig. 5.86).

▶ Intrinsic Muscles of the Fifth Toe

There are five intrinsic muscles of the fifth toe: abductor, short flexor, opponens, third plantar interosseous, and fourth lumbrical (see Intrinsic Muscles of the Lesser Toes, later) (see Figs. 5.43, 5.55, 5.77, and 5.80).

Abductor Digiti Minimi

The abductor digiti minimi is an elongated, fusiform muscle extending from the tuberosity of the os calcis to the base of the fifth toe. It is the muscle of the lateral border of the foot. It originates from the plantar aspect of the posterolateral tuberosity of the os calcis and extends to the adjacent posteromedial calcaneal tuberosity slightly anterior to the origin of the flexor digitorum brevis, from the deep surface of the fibular component of the plantar aponeurosis, and from the lateral intermuscular septum.

The fleshy fibers are directed forward and form an elongated muscle. The tendon appears in the substance of the muscle at the level of the calcaneocuboid joint and passes over the base of the fifth metatarsal. At this level, it may glide over the tuberosity of the metatarsal base, separated then by a bursa, or may (occasionally) receive fibers of attachment from it. From this point on, a substantial tendon appears, located in a lateral position. The tendon passes through the bifurcation arms or crux of the peroneal component of the plantar aponeurosis (Fig. 5.87). It still receives some fleshy fibers from its superior surface and extends distally, inserting on the plantar plate of the fifth metatarsophalangeal joint and the lateral aspect of the base of the proximal phalanx of the fifth toe. Frequently, the terminal tendon sends an extension into the extensor aponeurosis.

The variations occur in the form of additional muscle components:

- Muscle arising from the tuberosity of the fifth metatarsal and the overlying plantar aponeurosis, independent of the main component. It runs deep to the abductor (clear of its fibers) and inserts on the base of the proximal phalanx in conjunction with the abductor of the fifth toe, which may then be considered a "biventral muscle."[80]
- Abductor ossis metatarsi quinti. This is a fusiform long muscle that originates from the calcaneal posterolateral tuberosity and inserts on the apophysis of the fifth metatarsal. The muscle may be partially or totally adherent to the abductor of the fifth toe. LeDouble reported a frequency of 43% in 65 ft and 45% in 40 ft.[2]
- Accessory abductor of the fifth toe. LeDouble described an independent muscle that originates from the posterolateral tuberosity of the os calcis and the plantar aponeurosis about 1 cm from the origin of the abductor of the fifth toe and inserts separately on the base of the proximal phalanx of the fifth toe or joins the tendon of the abductor at the level of the fifth metatarsal base.[2] In another variety, the accessory abductor arises from the sheath of the peroneus longus and inserts separately on the basal phalanx of the fifth toe. Carmont et al[81] reported on an accessory abductor muscle of the fifth toe detected by a magnetic resonance imaging study of the right foot of a 6-year-old patient in which the muscle appeared to originate from the calcaneal tuberosity and to insert on the lateral aspect of the proximal phalanx of the fifth toe.

Flexor Digiti Minimi Brevis

The short flexor of the fifth toe originates from the fibrous sheath of the peroneus longus, the crest of the cuboid, the base of the fifth metatarsal, and the plantar aponeurosis.

A small fusiform muscle forms that courses lateral to the converging long flexor tendon and inserts on the plantar plate of the fifth metatarsophalangeal joint and the base of

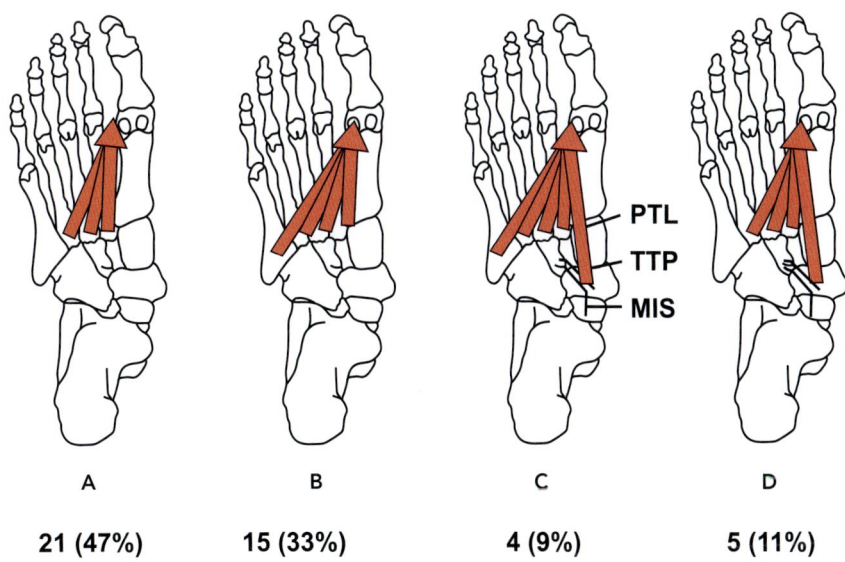

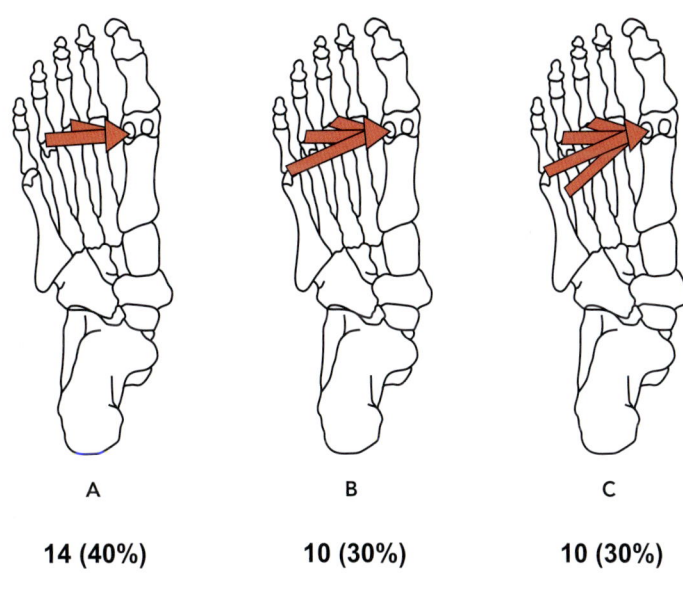

Figure 5.86 **Classification of adductor hallucis muscle, oblique head, and transverse head on the basis of their origins.** (* represents the origin of the transverse adductor from the broadly developed, deep band of the fibular part of the plantar aponeurosis. *MIS*, medial intermuscular septum; *PTL*, plantar tarsometatarsal ligament; *TTP*, tendon of tibialis posterior.) (Adapted from Arakawa T, Tokita K, Miki A, et al. Anatomical study of human adductor hallucis muscle with respect to its origin and insertion. *Ann Anat.* 2003;185:585-592.)

the proximal phalanx of the fifth toe. This insertion is located between the attachment of the abductor tendon and the flexor tendon sheath.

The short flexor may be more or less united to the abductor of the fifth toe and is always fused—completely or incompletely—to the opponens of the fifth toe.[1,74]

Opponens Digiti Quinti

The opponens digiti quinti is a flat, triangular muscle that originates from the sheath of the peroneus longus tendon and the crest of the cuboid. The tendon contours the base of the fifth metatarsal and gives origin to fleshy fibers that fan out and insert on the lateral border of the fifth metatarsal. The close connection of this muscle with the short flexor has been mentioned previously.

LeDouble recognized this muscle in more than 50% of his material.[2] Jones summarized the controversy surrounding this muscle very well: "The frequency of its occurrence as an independent muscle and the practically constant occurrence of fibers representing it, though partly incorporated in the short flexor, justifies its recognition as an entity entitled to its own name."[80]

The muscle is not listed in the *Nomina Anatomica* (PNA 1964).

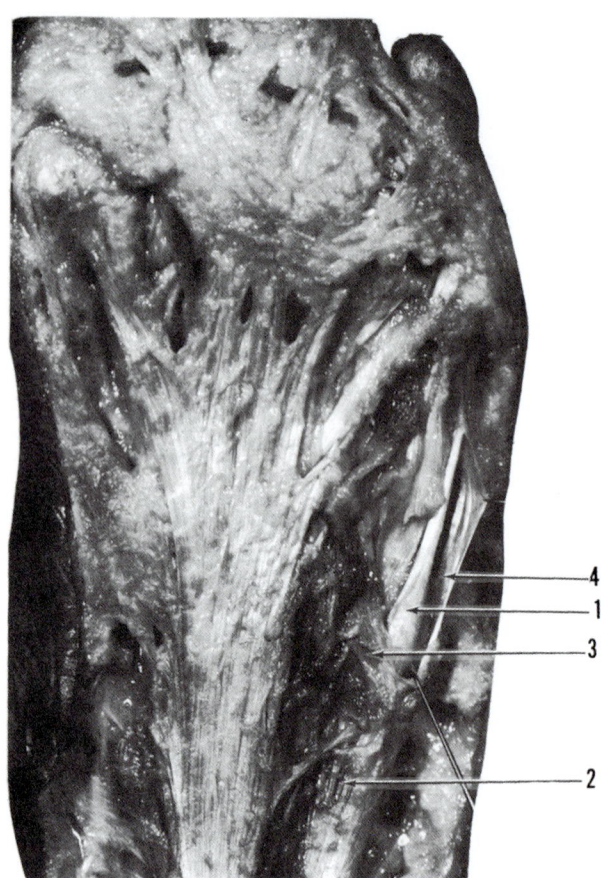

Figure 5.87 Tendon of the abductor digiti minimi. (*1*, Tendon of abductor muscle of fifth toe; *2*, lateral component of plantar aponeurosis; *3*, medial crux of *2*; *4*, lateral crux of *2*.)

▶ Intrinsic Muscles of the Lesser Toes

The intrinsic muscles of the lesser toes, excluding the muscles of the lateral compartment of the fifth toe, include four dorsal interossei, three plantar interossei, and four lumbricals (Figs. 5.88 to 5.90).

The functional axis of the foot passes through the second toe. The motions of abduction and adduction occur relative to this axis. The dorsal interossei are the abductors of the toes, the plantar interossei are the adductors, and the second toe possesses two dorsal interossei. The functional classification simplifies the location of the insertion of the interossei.

The first through the fourth dorsal interossei are inserted, respectively, on the tibial and the peroneal aspect of the second toe and the peroneal aspect of the third and fourth toes (acting as the abductors). The first through the third plantar interossei insert, respectively, on the tibial side of the third, fourth, and fifth toes (acting as adductors). The lumbricals are located on the tibial aspect of the corresponding toes.

Dorsal Interossei

The four dorsal interossei bipenniform muscles originate from the lateral surface of the metatarsals delineating the corresponding intermetatarsal space (Figs. 5.91 and 5.92).

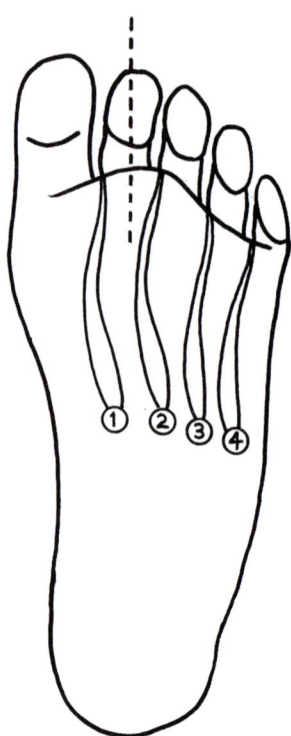

Figure 5.88 Insertion sites of lumbrical muscles. (*1, 2, 3, 4*, refer to the corresponding toes or digits 1st, 2nd, 3rd, and 4th.)

The first dorsal interosseous attaches to the entire tibial surface of the second metatarsal bone and to the inferior surface of its base. Dorsally, the attachment of the peroneal component extends to the anterolateral corner of the first cuneiform. The medial or tibial head arises from a tendinous arch that

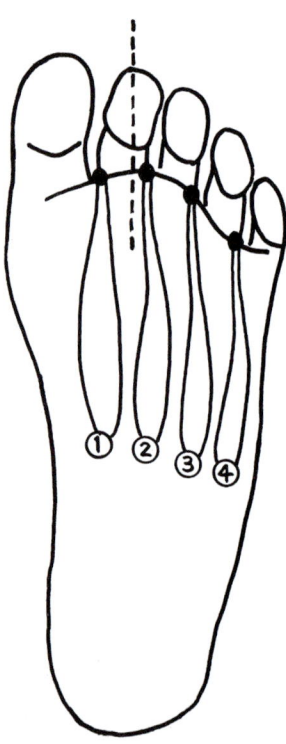

Figure 5.89 Insertion sites of dorsal interossei muscles. (*1, 2, 3, 4*, refer to the corresponding toes or digits 1st, 2nd, 3rd, and 4th.)

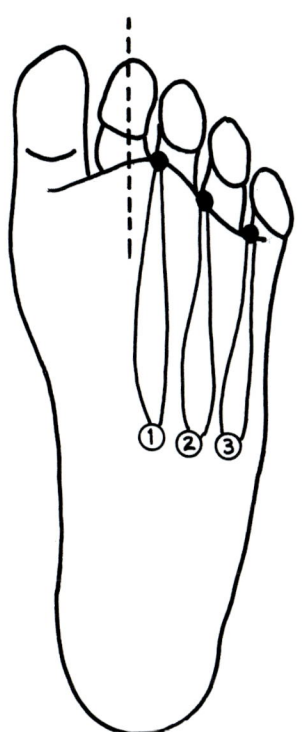

Figure 5.90 Insertion sites of plantar interossei muscles. (*1, 2, 3,* refer to the corresponding toes or digits 1st, 2nd, and 3rd.)

Plantar Interossei

The three plantar interossei are smaller than the corresponding dorsal interossei. They are single-headed and fusiform and arise from the inferior segment and border of the tibial surface of the third, fourth, and fifth metatarsals (see Figs. 5.91 and 5.92). Their origin extends to the base of the same metatarsals and to the metatarsal expansions of the inferior calcaneocuboid ligament.

Lumbricals

The lateral three lumbricals are bipenniform and arise from the intertendinous angle of the flexor digitorum longus tendons (see Figs. 5.92 and 5.93). The first lumbrical has a single origin from the tibial side of the long flexor to the second toe. Distally, the muscle-tendon units are located on the tibial side of the corresponding toe.

Insertion

Interossei

The tendons of the dorsal and plantar interossei, in their path to the toes, pass dorsal to the deep transverse metatarsal ligament (see Figs. 5.93 and 5.94), whereas the lumbrical tendons remain plantar (Fig. 5.95). Prior to their insertions, all the tendons of the toes are grouped and retained around the metatarsophalangeal joint by fibrous formations.

The long extensor tendon and the short extensor tendon are each located in a flat, independent tendon sheath and are centered over the corresponding metatarsal head. Within the tunnel, the deep surface of the tendon is connected to the sheath with fibrous bands, whereas on the dorsal aspect, a gliding or a bursal component is interposed between the tendon and the sheath.[84] The extensor tendon sheaths are formed by the distal segment of the common dorsal aponeurosis.

A fibrous annular formation originates from the sides of the extensor sheath, wraps around the metatarsophalangeal joint capsule (independent from it), and inserts on the plantar aspect along the sides of the plantar plate in conjunction with the deep transverse intermetatarsal ligament. This annular structure centralizes and stabilizes the extensor tendons. It represents the proximal segment of the digital extensor aponeurosis and is called the *transverse lamina* or *extensor sling* (Figs. 5.96 and 5.97). Meyer, in a cross-sectional study of 15 adult feet and 20 fetal feet supplemented by sagittal sections of 10 adult feet, provided a detailed account of the formation and arrangement of the retaining fibrous structures.[84] Proximal to the metatarsal heads, the extensor sheaths of two adjacent rays are united by the intertendinous segment of the dorsal common aponeurosis, which is superficial to the underlying dorsal interosseous aponeurosis covering the intermetatarsal space (Fig. 5.98). At this level, the quadrilateral intermetatarsal space is limited on each side by the corresponding lateral surfaces of the metatarsals. The dorsal aspect is limited by the dorsal interosseous aponeurosis and the plantar aspect by the proximal segment of the deep transverse

originates from the anterior border of the peroneus longus tendon near its insertion, crosses the base of the second metatarsal, and inserts on the anterior segment of the superolateral border of the first metatarsal (see Fig. 5.19).[24] This fibrous arcade with posteromedial concavity delineates, with the lateral surface of the first metatarsal, an elliptic space that gives passage to the pedal vessels. The frequency of occurrence of the arcade, according to various sources, is 89% in 54 ft, 74% in 27 ft, and 63.5% in 149 ft.[24,82,83]

The attachment of the medial head to the first metatarsal shaft may be by loose connective tissue only. If the fibrous arcade has a more proximal insertion on the base of the first metatarsal, the medial head of the interosseous may then attach to the lateral surface of the first metatarsal, not exceeding the proximal half of the surface or being limited to a few insertional fibers.[83]

The second dorsal interosseous originates from the entire peroneal surface of the second metatarsal and partially from the superior segment of the tibial surface of the third metatarsal. It may extend its origin to the dorsum of the lateral cuneiform.

The third dorsal interosseous originates from the entire peroneal surface of the third metatarsal and partially from the superior aspect of the tibial surface of the fourth metatarsal.

The fourth dorsal interosseous originates from the entire peroneal surface of the fourth metatarsal and partially from the superior aspect of the tibial surface of the fifth metatarsal.

The last two interossei receive some fibers from the plantar calcaneocuboid ligament.[80]

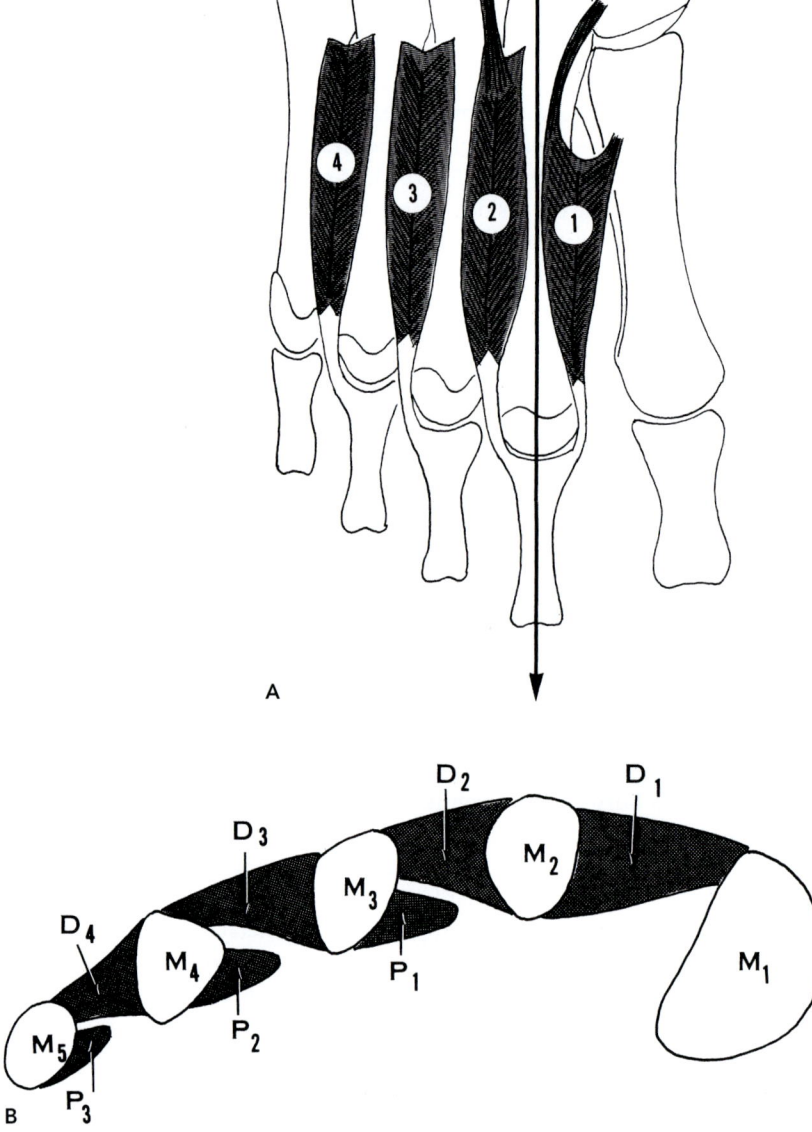

Figure 5.91 (A) Origin of dorsal interossei muscles 1 to 4. The first dorsal interosseous with an accessory origin from the first cuneiform. The second dorsal cuneiform with an accessory origin from the third cuneiform. The *arrow* indicates the axis of the foot passing through the second metatarsal. (B) Metatarsal origin of the dorsal and plantar interossei muscles. (D_1–D_4, dorsal interossei muscles 1-4; M_1–M_5, metatarsals 1-5; P_1–P_3, plantar interossei muscles 1-3.)

intermetatarsal ligament. An oblique fibrous expansion divides this chamber into two sections: large for the dorsal interosseous tendon and smaller for the plantar interosseous tendon. It is at this level that the dorsal interosseous makes its first insertion on the deep transverse intermetatarsal ligament.

Further distally, between the metatarsal heads, the extensor intertendinous aponeurosis advances plantarward as a wedge, carrying the dorsal adipose tissue and neurovascular structures, and unites with the dorsal interosseous aponeurosis (see Fig. 5.98). Multiple fascial septa now extend vertically plantarward from the apex of the united aponeurosis. A vertical lamina passes over each interosseous tendon and inserts on the deep transverse intermetatarsal ligament. This arrangement corresponds to the transverse lamina or extensor sling. Some septa pierce the transverse intermetatarsal ligament and connect with the deep longitudinal septa of the plantar aponeurosis. At this level, the dorsal interosseous is strongly attached to the lateral lower aspect of the capsule and glenoid ligament of the metatarsophalangeal joint and also to the lateral aspect of the plantar plate; it is also attached to the deep surface of the transverse lamina.

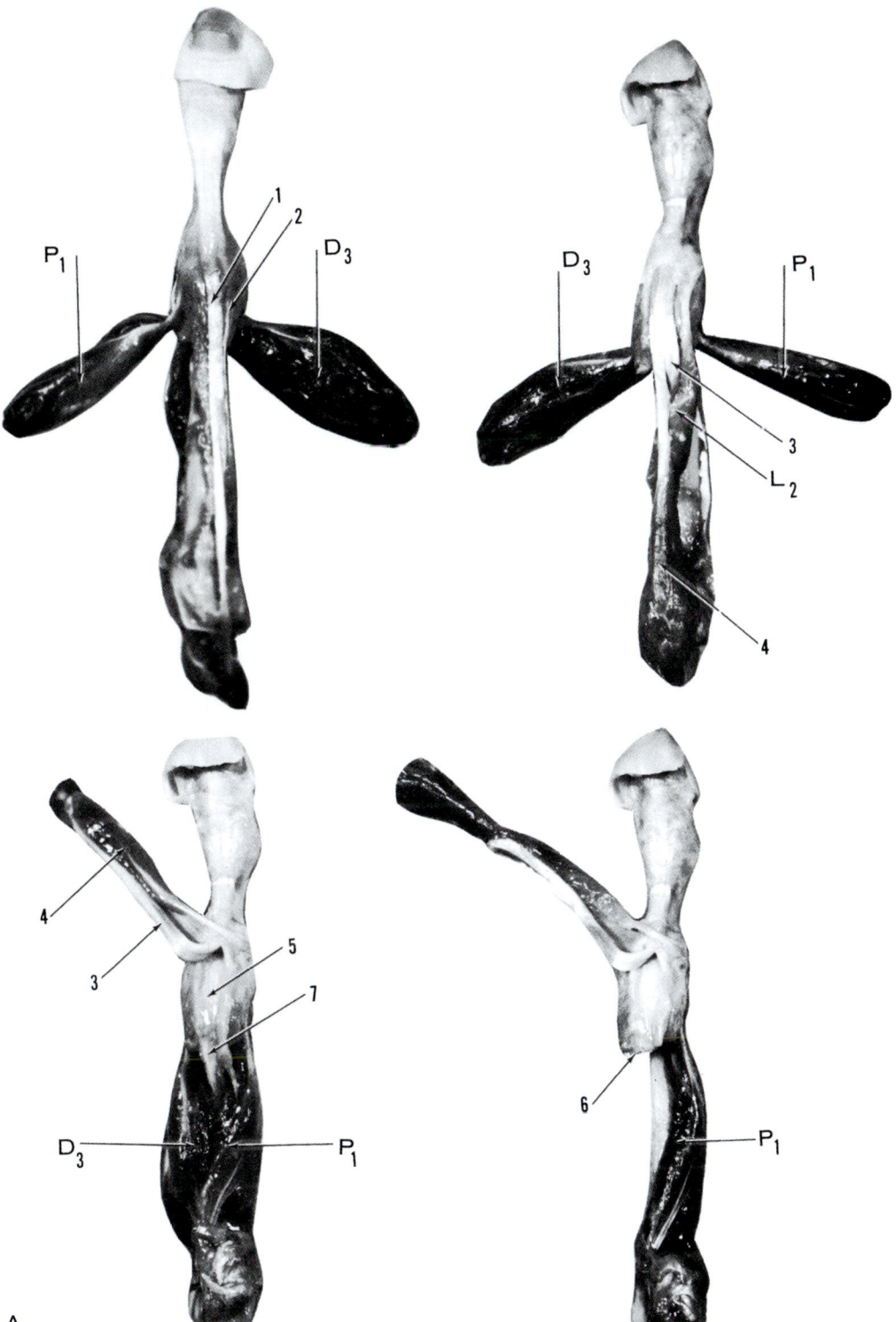

Figure 5.92 **(A) Right third toe.** (*Left*) Dorsal aspect. (*Right*) Plantar aspect. (*D3*, third dorsal interosseous muscle; *L2*, second lumbrical muscle; *P1*, first plantar interosseous muscle; *1*, long extensor tendon; *2*, extensor digitorum brevis tendon; *4*, flexor digitorum brevis muscle; *5*, plantar plate; *6*, proximal border of plantar plate; *7*, insertion of plantar aponeurosis septa.) **(B) Right third toe, peroneal aspect.** (*1*, Third dorsal interosseous muscle; *2*, superficial phalangeal tendon of *1*; *3*, deep phalangeal tendon of *1*; *4*, flexor digitorum brevis muscle and tendon; *5*, extensor aponeurotic lamina forming tunnel for tendon of *1*; *6*, split transverse lamina of extensor aponeurosis; *7*, flexor hallucis longus tendon; *8*, extensor digitorum longus tendon; *9*, extensor digitorum brevis tendon; *10*, capsule of metatarsophalangeal joint.)
(C) Right third toe, tibial side. (*1*, Lumbrical tendon and muscle; *2*, first plantar interosseous muscle and tendon; *3*, flexor digitorum brevis muscle and tendon; *4*, flexor hallucis longus tendon; *5*, extensor digitorum brevis tendon; *6*, proximal border of transverse lamina; *7*, proximal border of plantar plate; *8*, metatarsophalangeal collateral ligament; *9*, deep transverse metatarsal ligament.)

282 Sarrafian's Anatomy of the Foot and Ankle

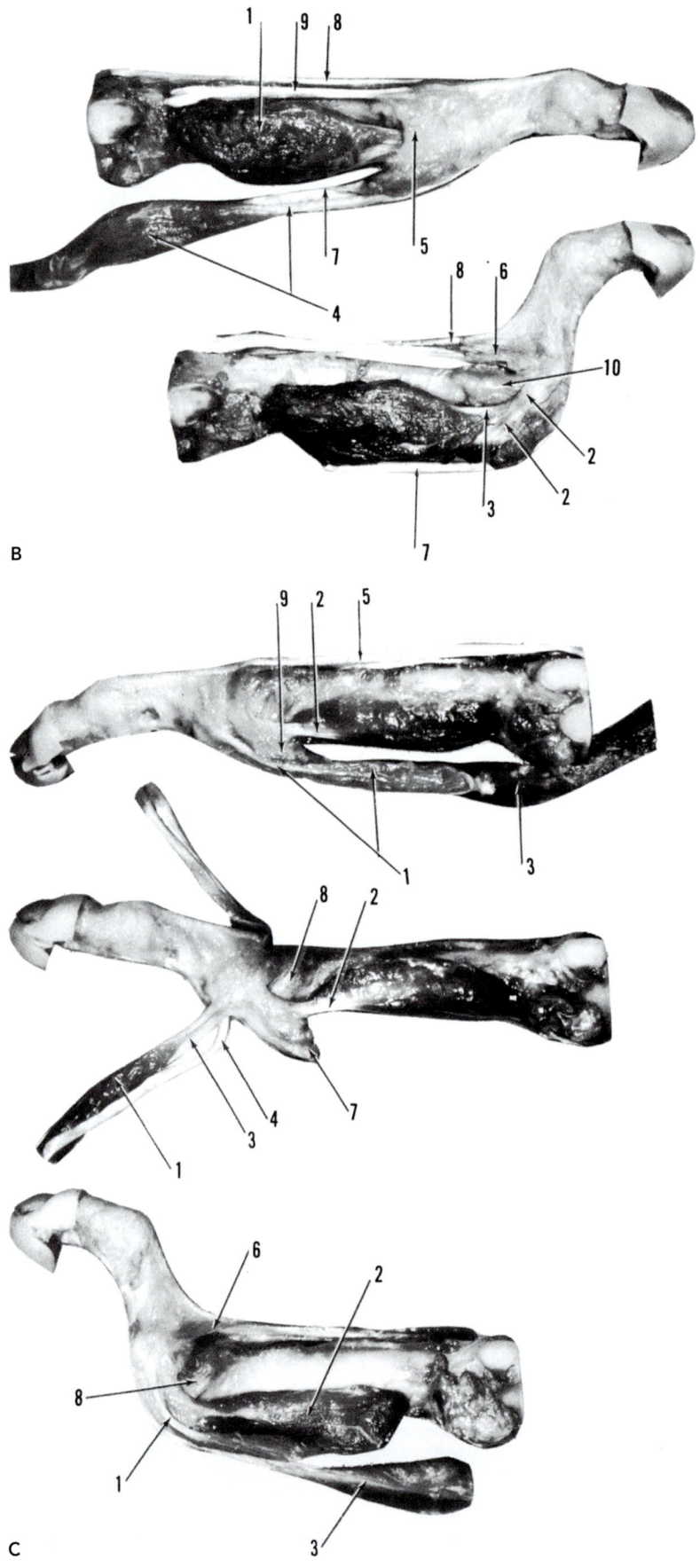

Figure 5.92 Cont'd

Chapter 5: Myology 283

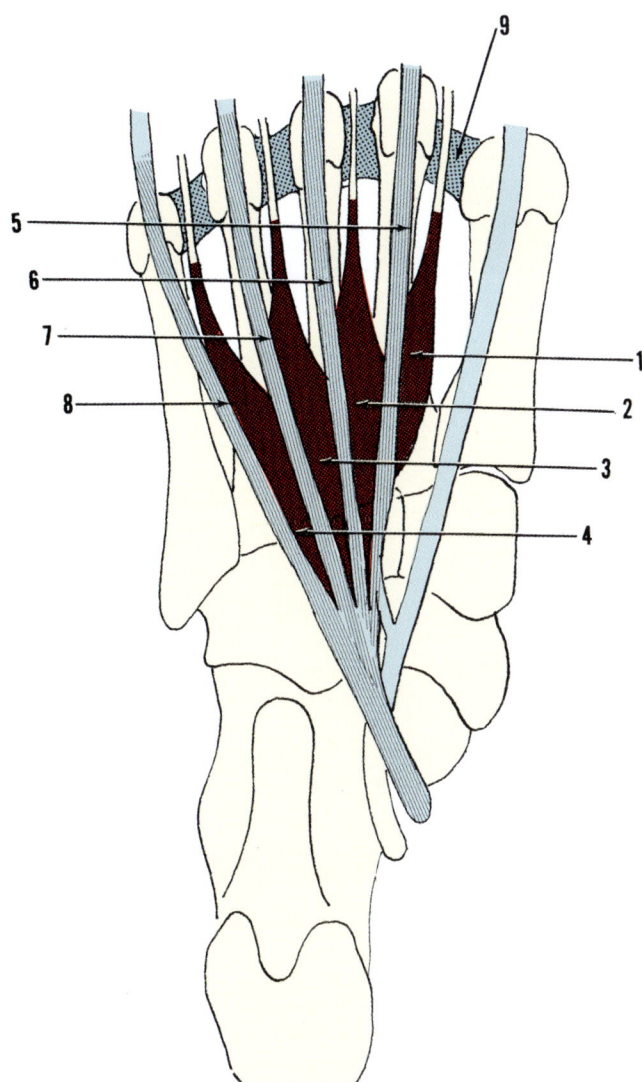

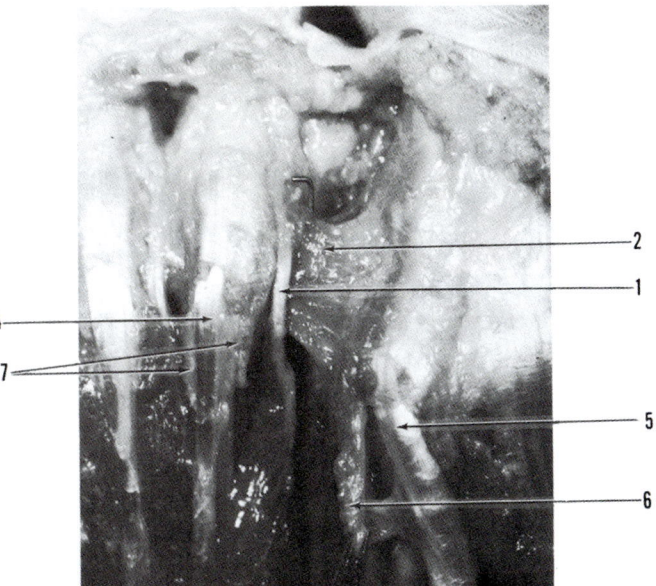

Figure 5.94 **Tendon of lumbrical.** (*1*, Tendon of lumbrical passing plantar to the deep transverse metatarsal ligament [*2*]; *3*, first dorsal interosseous tendon; *4*, flexor digitorum brevis tendon; *5*, flexor digitorum longus tendon with a central split; *6*, adductor hallucis tendon passing dorsal to the deep transverse metatarsal ligament [*2*].)

Figure 5.93 **Lumbricals.** (*1-4*, Lumbricals 1-4; *5-8*, flexor digitorum longus tendons 2-5; *9*, deep transverse metatarsal ligament.)

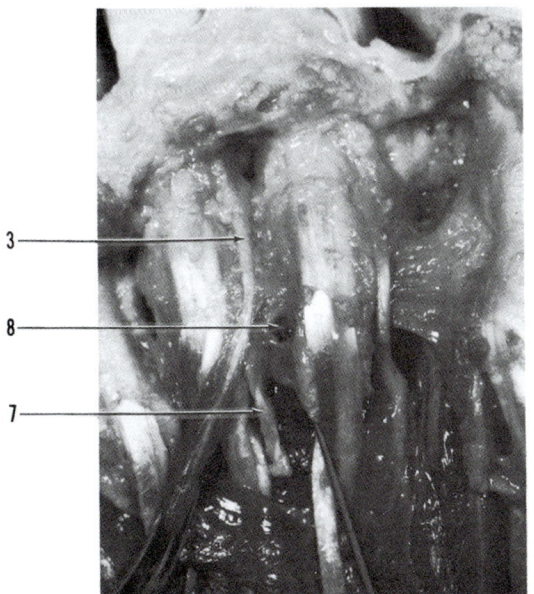

Figure 5.95 **Lumbrical tendons.** (*1*, Lumbrical tendon; *2*, deep transverse metatarsal ligament 1-2; *3*, lumbrical fascia forming thin tunnel to tendon; *4*, flexor digitorum brevis tendon; *5*, flexor hallucis longus tendon; *6*, *7*, deep insertional septa of plantar aponeurosis; *8*, foramen for common digital artery.)

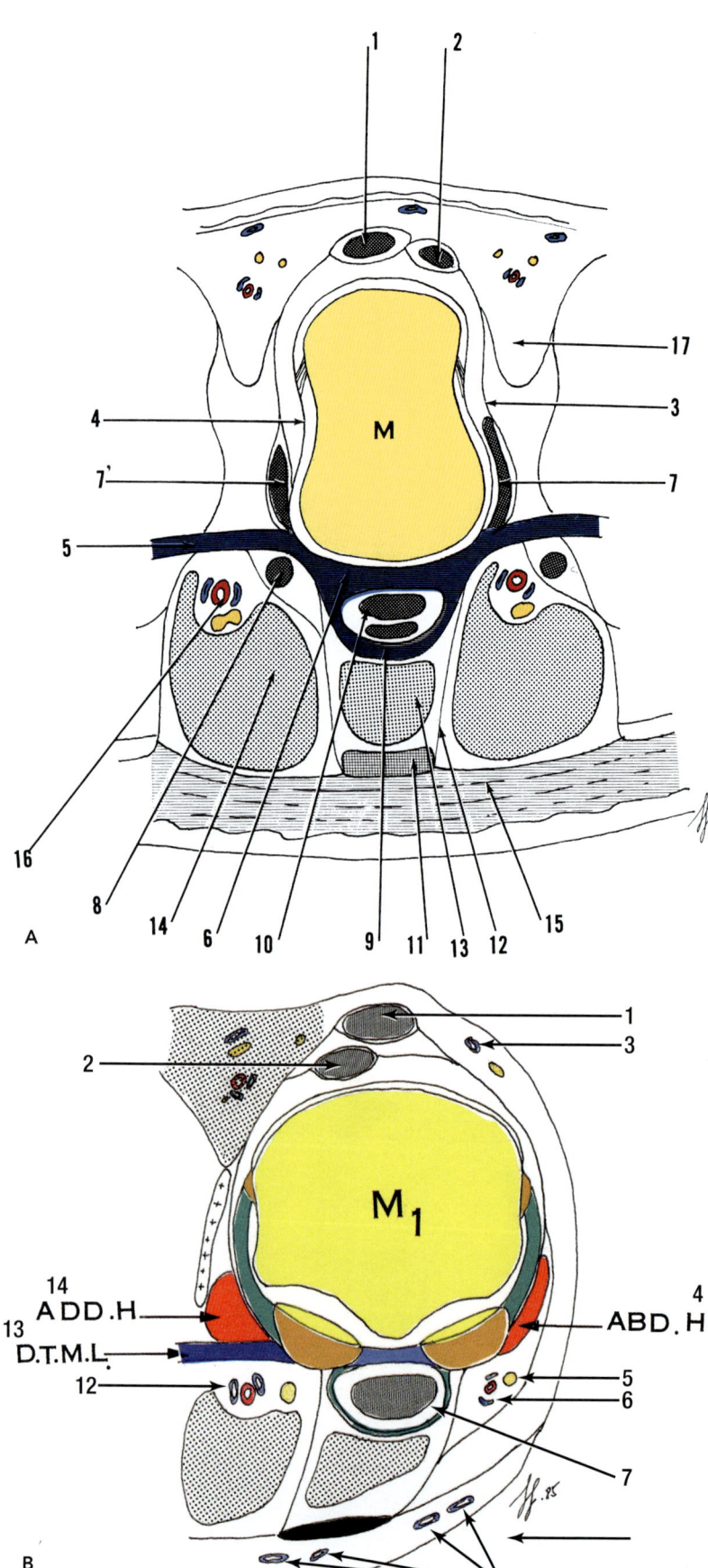

Figure 5.96 **(A) Cross-section of the ball of the left foot.** (*M*, lesser metatarsal head; *1*, extensor digitorum longus tendon; *2*, extensor digitorum brevis tendon; *3*, transverse lamina of extensor aponeurosis; *4*, capsule of metatarsophalangeal joint; *5*, deep transverse metatarsal ligament; *6*, plantar plate; *7, 7′*, interossei muscles located in narrow cleft formed by capsule and transverse lamina [*7*] or incorporated in split of transverse lamina [*7′*]; *8*, lumbrical tendon in its own tunnel on tibial side of joint; *9*, long flexor tunnel; *10*, long flexor tendons; *11*, longitudinal band of plantar aponeurosis; *12*, vertical thin fibrous band of plantar aponeurosis forming a preflexor tendon space lodging a preflexor adipose cushion [*13*]; *14*, fat body on plantar aspect of *5* covering neurovascular bundle [*16*]; *15*, transverse component of plantar aponeurosis; *17*, triangular adipofascial complex filling intermetatarsal capitular space and carrying superficial nerves and vessels.) **(B) Cross-section of the ball of the right foot.** (*M1*, first metatarsal head; *1*, extensor hallucis brevis; *2*, extensor hallucis longus; *3*, saphenous nerve; *4*, abductor hallucis; *5*, medial proper digital nerve; *6*, medial neurovascular bundle; *7*, flexor hallucis longus; *8*, veins; *9*, plantar aponeurosis; *10a*, pre-flexor adipose tissue; *10b*, triangular adipose complex filling intermetatarsal complex and carrying superficial nerves and vessel; fat pad covering the lateral neurovascular bundle; *11*, lateral digital nerve; *12*, lateral neurovascular bundle; *13*, deep transverse metatarsal ligament; *14*, adductor hallucis.)

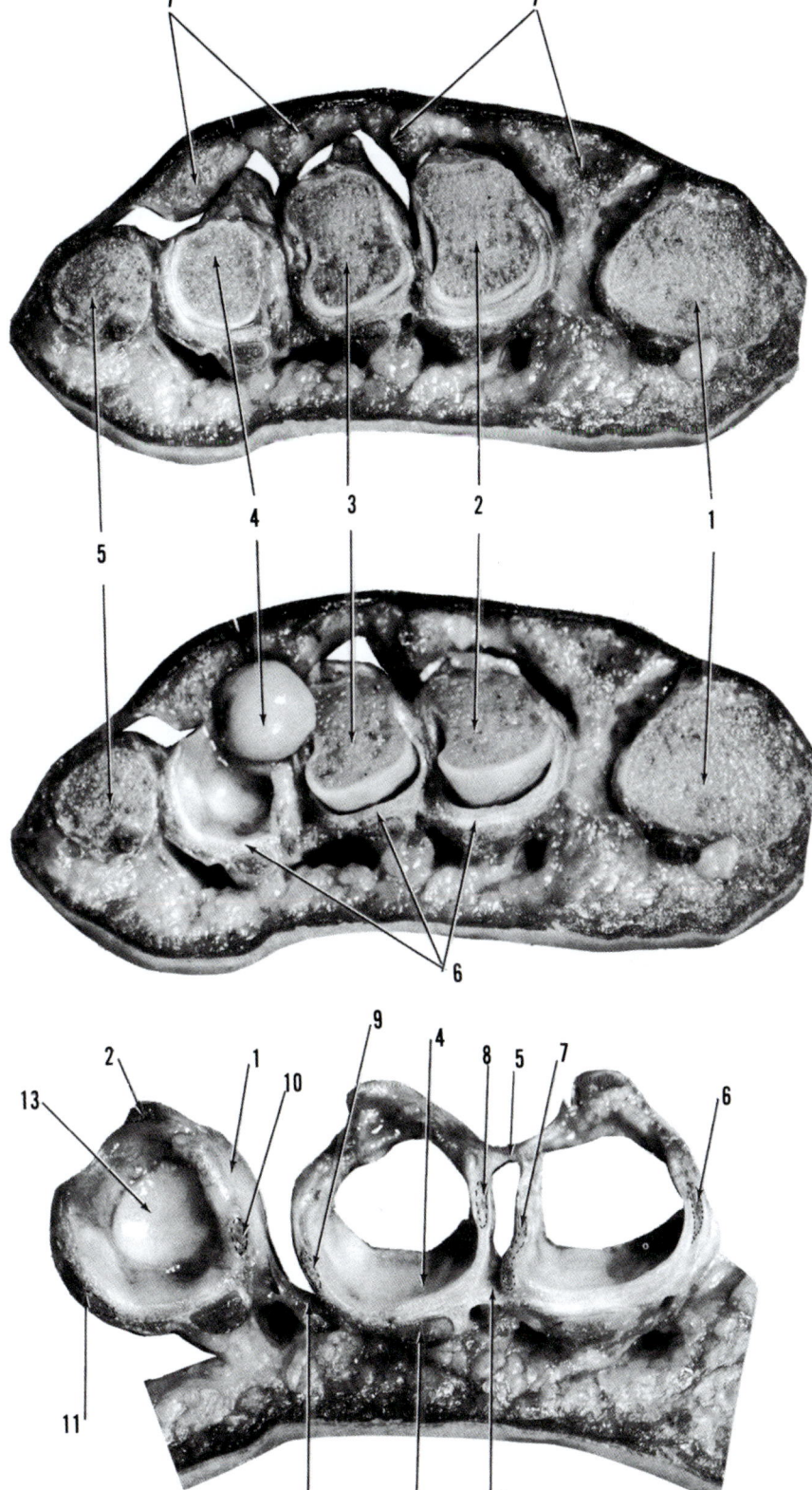

Figure 5.97 (A) (*Top* and *middle*) Cross-section passing through metatarsal heads 2, 3, and 4 and phalanges 1 and 5. (*6*, Plantar plates *2, 3, 4*; *7*, adipofascial triangular pads filling interspaces.) (*Bottom*) Extensor ring complex formed around the metatarsal heads. (*1*, Transverse lamina of extensor aponeurosis; *2*, extensor digitorum longus tendon of fourth toe; *3*, deep transverse metatarsal ligament; *4*, plantar plate; *5*, superficial transverse metatarsal ligament; *6*, insertional tendon of first dorsal interosseous; *7*, insertional tendon of second dorsal interosseous; *8*, insertional tendon of first plantar interosseous; *9*, insertional tendon of third dorsal interosseous; *10*, insertional tendon of second plantar interosseous; *11*, insertional tendon of fourth dorsal interosseous; *12*, long flexor tendons; *13*, base of proximal phalanx of fourth toe.) (B) Cross-section through metatarsal heads. (*Top*) (*1*, transverse lamina; *2*, capsule of metatarsophalangeal joint; *3*, plantar plate; *4*, fibrous tunnel for long flexors; *5*, insertional tendon of third dorsal interosseous muscle; *6*, second lumbrical; *7*, long flexor tendons.) (*Bottom*) (*1*, transverse lamina; *2*, capsule of metatarsophalangeal joint; *3*, point of junction of *1, 2*, plantar plate, and flexor tendon tunnel; *4*, insertional tendon of first plantar interosseous muscle; *5*, insertional tendon of third dorsal interosseous muscle; *6*, insertional tendon of second dorsal interosseous muscle; *7*, insertional tendon of first dorsal interosseous muscle.)

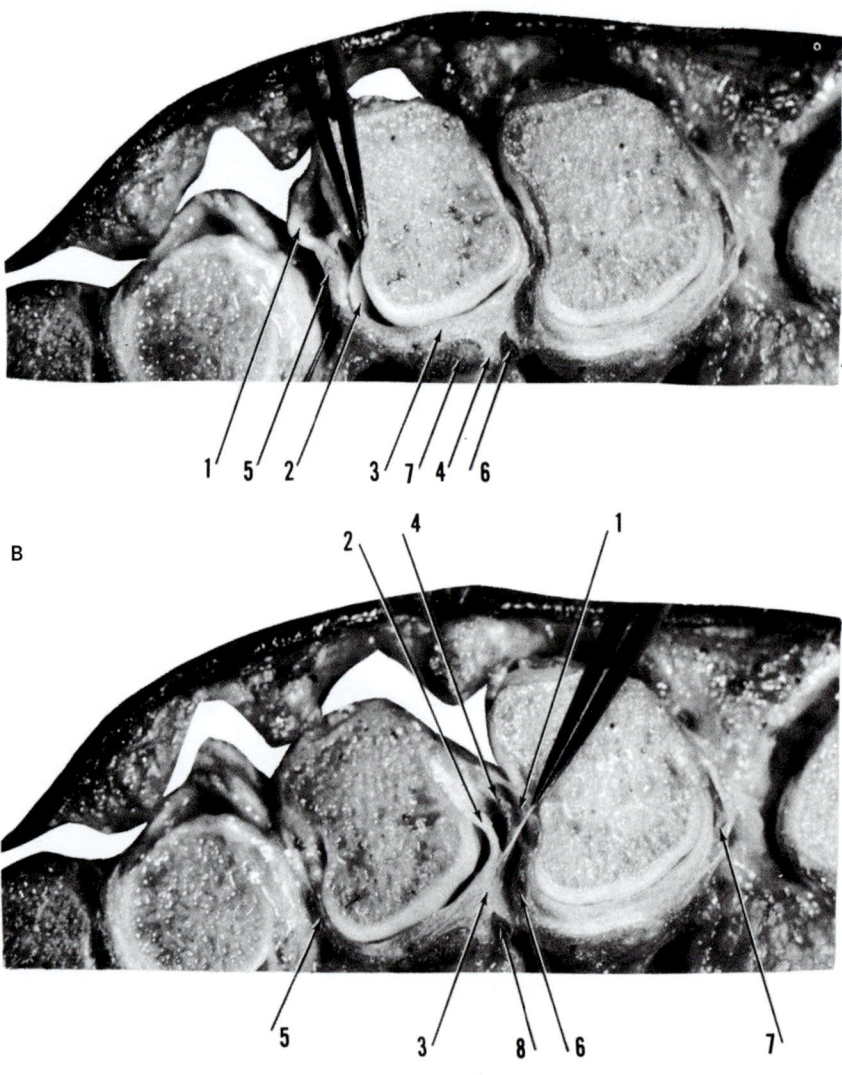

Figure 5.97 Cont'd

Occasionally, and especially with the second dorsal interosseous, two definite tendons are seen, corresponding proximally to a subdivision of the same muscle into two units. One tendon inserts on the plantar plate, the proximal phalanx, whereas the second tendon terminates on the deep surface of the transverse lamina.[19]

The plantar interossei have insertions similar to those of the dorsal interossei. At the level of the metatarsophalangeal joint, the tendons of the interossei are located in vertical clefts limited on one side by the capsule of the joint and on the other side by the transverse lamina (see Fig. 5.97B). At the level of the proximal phalanx, the interossei attach to the base of the corresponding phalanx and have no or very minimal contribution to the oblique component or extensor hood of the extensor mechanism (Fig. 5.99).

Baumann, analyzing the microanatomy of the extensor aponeurosis, brings forth the participation of the interossei muscles in the constitution of the transverse proximal component and the extensor hood.[18] In the fifth toe, however, the extensor hood is more or less atrophic, and the spiral contributory fibers from the intrinsics are absent.[19]

In summary, the interossei are inserted on the follwoing:

- The deep transverse intermetatarsal ligaments
- The lateral capsule and the glenoid ligament of the metatarsophalangeal joint
- The plantar plate of the metatarsophalangeal joint
- The deep surface of the transverse lamina
- The base of the proximal phalanx

Variations of the Interossei

A comprehensive study of the variations of the interossei muscles, based on 149 ft, has been reported by Manter.[83] These variations involve the origin, the insertion, and fusion or addition.

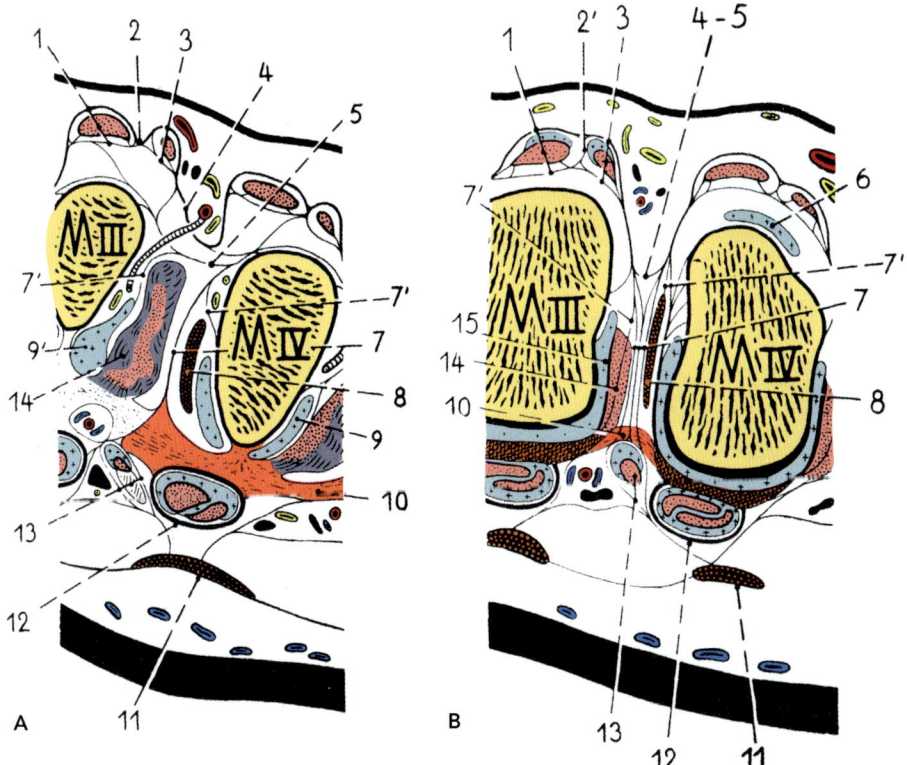

Figure 5.98 **Metatarsophalangeal region of the right foot. (A)** Anterior segment of a vertical and transverse section of the metatarsophalangeal region of the right foot, passing through the articular interlines at the level of the big toe and the fifth toe and through the intermetatarsal spaces between metatarsals 2, 3, and 4. Segment of the section passing through the third intermetatarsal space. **(B)** Anterior segment of a vertical and transverse cross-section of the metatarsophalangeal region of the right foot, passing through the metatarsal heads 3 and 4. (*1*, Tendinous portion of dorsal aponeurosis common to extensor tendons forming sheath to long extensor tendon; *2, 2′*, axial intertendinous portion of dorsal aponeurosis; *3*, tendinous portion of dorsal aponeurosis forming sheath to extensor digitorum brevis tendon; *4*, intertendinous interaxial portion of dorsal common aponeurosis; *5*, dorsal interosseous aponeurosis [*4* and *5* form dorsal transverse ligament]; *6*, superior articular cul-de-sac; *7*, interaxial lamina; *7′*, vertical laminae arising from *5* and inserting on metatarsals, articular capsules, and tendons of interossei; *8*, plantar interosseous tendon; *9, 9′*, lateral and inferior articular cul-de-sac; *10*, deep plantar transverse ligament; *11*, pretendinous band of superficial plantar aponeurosis; *12*, fibrous sheath of long flexor tendons; *13*, fibrous sheath of lumbrical tendon; *14*, dorsal interosseous tendon; *15*, articular capsule.) (Adapted from Meyer P. Contribution a l'étude de la region métatarso-phalangienne. *Bull Assoc Anat.* 1958;99:500.)

Variations of Origin

There are four variations of origin (Fig. 5.100).

Dorsal Interossei With Single Head. The dorsal interossei may have one head of origin only, and the frequency of occurrence is as follows: the fourth dorsal interosseous from the fifth metatarsal, 22.8%; the first dorsal interosseous from the second metatarsal, 11.4%; the second dorsal interosseous from the second metatarsal, 7.4%; the third dorsal interosseous from the fourth metatarsal, 3.4%; and the fourth dorsal interosseous from the fourth metatarsal, 1.3%.[83] The first two dorsal interossei remain grouped along the second metatarsal. The third and fourth dorsal interossei shift their origin laterally (except for a small percentage of the fourth dorsal interossei).

Dorsal Extension of Plantar Interossei. In the second intermetatarsal space, the second dorsal interosseous originates from the entire lateral surface of the second metatarsal and from the upper segment of the medial surface of the third metatarsal. In 15.5%, the "origin of the first plantar interosseous had extended dorsally on the third metatarsal at the expense of the second dorsal muscle which had lost, wholly or in part, its attachment to that bone."[83] In one case, only the third plantar interosseous extended dorsally on the fifth metatarsal.

Accessory Origins. The first and second plantar interossei and the second and third dorsal interossei may have plantar accessory origins.[83] The most frequently seen arrangement, occurring in 11.4%, is the presence of a plantar slip extending from the third dorsal interosseous to the first plantar interosseous. The second dorsal interosseous may extend plantarward, covering the first plantar interosseous without creating an attachment to it. The dorsal interossei may also receive tendinous slips from the extensor digitorum brevis, the peroneus brevis, and the peroneus tertius.

Fusion and Doubling of Muscle Bellies. The fusion may occur between the muscle bellies of the second plantar interosseous and the third dorsal interosseous (2.5%) or the first

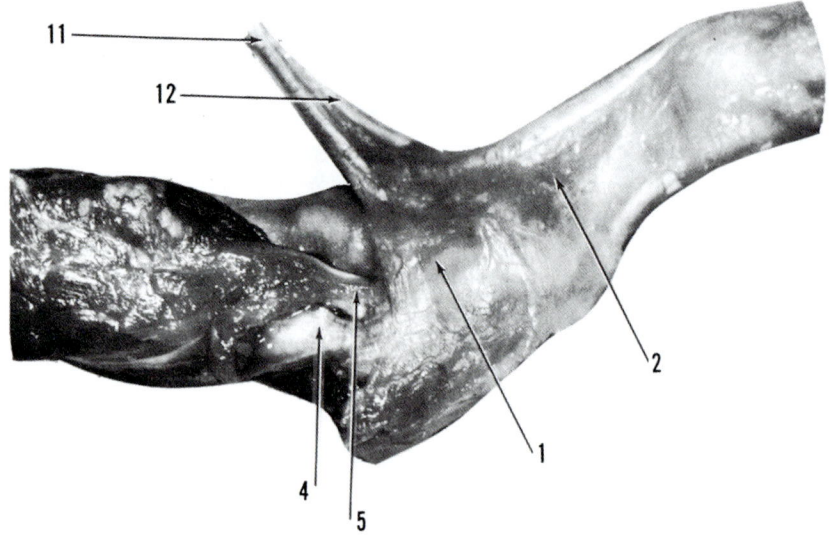
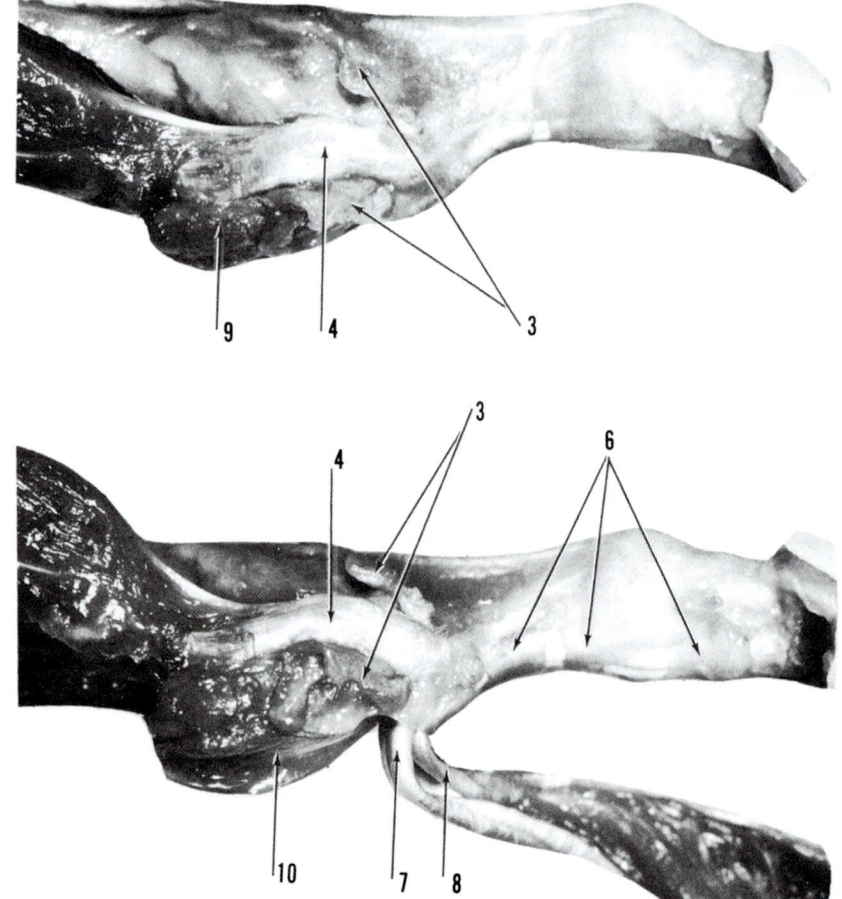

Figure 5.99 **Metatarsophalangeal region of the right third toe, peroneal side.** (*1*, Transverse lamina of extensor aponeurosis; *2*, oblique segment of extensor aponeurosis; *3*, split transverse lamina; *4, 5*, superficial and deep tendons of third dorsal interosseous tendon; *6*, pulleys of long flexor tendons; *7*, long flexor tendon; *8*, short flexor tendon; *9*, deep transverse metatarsal ligament; *10*, plantar plate; *11*, extensor digitorum brevis tendon; *12*, extensor digitorum longus tendon.)

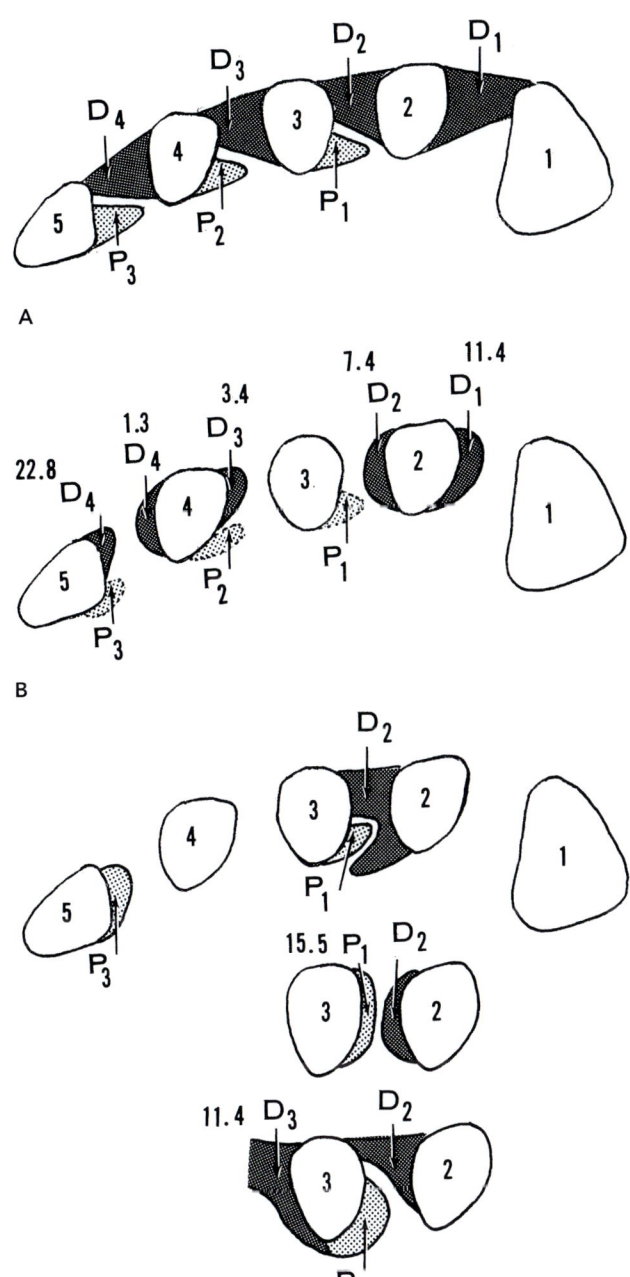

Figure 5.100 Variations of origin of the interossei muscles. **(A)** Normal pattern of origin. **(B)** Variation with origin of dorsal interossei from a single metatarsal. **(C)** Variation with extension of origin of D_2, D_3, P_1, and P_3. (D_1–D_4, dorsal interossei; P_1–P_3, plantar interossei; 1–4, metatarsals.) (From Manter JT. Variations of the interosseous muscles of the human foot. Anat Rec. 1945;93:117.)

Intermetatarsal Space	Muscle With Bifid Tendon	Insertion on Digits	Frequency
2	Second dorsal interosseous	Digits 2 and 3	3.4%
	First plantar interosseous	Digits 2 and 3	0.7%
3	Third dorsal interosseous	Digits 3 and 4	1.4%
	Second plantar interosseous	Digits 3 and 4	0.7%
4	Fourth dorsal interosseous	Digits 4 and 5	0.7%
	Third plantar interosseous	Digits 5 and 6	1.4

TABLE 5-1 Frequency of Occurrence of Bifid Tendons

plantar interosseous and the second dorsal interosseous (1.3%). Doubling of the muscle was observed only with the second dorsal interosseous (1.3%).[83]

Variation of Insertion

Bifid Tendons. Bifid tendons inserting each on the adjacent toe and involving mostly the second dorsal interosseous were observed with the frequency shown in Table 5.1.[83]

Additional Muscle. Leboucq described a small triangular muscle located between the first dorsal interosseous and the oblique head of the adductor hallucis. This muscle originates with a 1-cm base from the distal third of the plantar border of the third metatarsal, is directed obliquely and anteriorly, and terminates by a tendon inserting on the deep surface of the transverse head of the adductor. In certain cases, the muscle is replaced by an aponeurotic lamella having similar insertions and position. In a study of 60 ft, Leboucq observed such a muscle in 5%.[76]

Manter mentioned having observed "a tiny thread to a band about 4 mms wide" with similar position and insertion in 55.5% of 54 ft.[83]

LeDouble described an additional muscle originating from the midsegment of the inferior calcaneocuboid ligament or from the sheath of the peroneus longus.[2] It is separated from the plantar interossei by the deep branch of the lateral plantar nerve. It courses anteriorly and medially and inserts on the lateral aspect of the base of the proximal phalanx of the second toe.

Kalin and Hirsch studied the origins of the interossei in 10 ft.[85] They concluded that the interossei originate "not only from the metatarsal bones, but also from ligamentous tissue proximal to the tarsometatarsal joints,… from the fascia of adjacent muscles and the first dorsal interosseous muscle usually arises in part from a slip of the peroneus longus tendon."[85] More specifically, 88% of the dorsal interossei and 93% of the plantar interossei had a soft-tissue origin as well as a bony origin from the corresponding metatarsal shafts and bases.[85]

Lumbricals

The lumbrical tendons are located on the plantar and tibial aspects of the corresponding deep transverse intermetatarsal ligaments. They are retained within a tunnel formed by a septum extending from the sagittal band of the plantar aponeurosis and inserting between the lumbrical tendon and the digital neurovascular bundle. At the distal end of the deep transverse intermetatarsal ligament, the lumbrical tendon is directed anteriorly and dorsally. It joins the extensor hood, and most of the fibers remain concentrated on the tibial border distally, reaching the extensor middle and lateral slips. Few fibers insert on the base of the proximal phalanx.

Variations of the Lumbricals

Variation of Origin

The first lumbrical may originate from the tibialis posterior tendon or from this tendon and the tendon of the flexor hallucis longus. The second, third, and fourth lumbricals may originate from the flexor digitorum brevis.

Absence

The lumbrical may be absent. In a study of 100 ft (400 lumbricals), Schmidt and coworkers found 32 lumbricals absent (8%), with the following distribution: first lumbrical, 1 absent (0.25%); second lumbrical, 9 absent (2.25%); third lumbrical, 10 absent (2.5%); and fourth lumbrical, 12 absent (3%).[86]

Duplicity and Bifidity

The third and fourth lumbricals are sometimes double.[86] The fourth lumbrical may be bifid at the insertion.[86]

CALCANEAL (OF ACHILLES) AND PLANTARIS TENDONS

The calcaneal tendon is the conjoint tendon of the gastrocnemii and soleus. Large and strong, ovoid in contour, it measures 1.2 to 2.5 cm in width at the insertion and 5 to 6 mm in thickness at the level of the ankle.[87,88] Oriented nearly in the frontal plane, the tendon is invested by the superficial crural fascia. The tendon is larger at the insertion on the inferior half of the posterior calcaneal surface. Some of the insertional fibers are in continuity with the plantar aponeurosis.

Structurally, the fibers of the calcaneal tendon do not descend straight down but rotate to a variable degree in a spiral manner. This internal arrangement is analyzed by Cummins and coworkers and Jones.[80,87] At the onset, the tendinous fibers of the gastrocnemius are posterior to the fibers contributed by the soleus component. At 12 to 15 cm from the insertion, the fibers rotate from a medial to a lateral direction, as observed posteriorly. The gentle twist of the fibers is progressive, reaching a maximum at 2 to 5 cm from the insertion.[88]

During their descent, the medial fibers of the gastrocnemius component reach a lateral position posteriorly, whereas the middle fibers are straight laterally and the most lateral fibers are anterolateral in location. The fibers of the soleus component are subjected to the same rotation, bringing some of the anteriorly located fibers into a posterior position (Fig. 5.101).

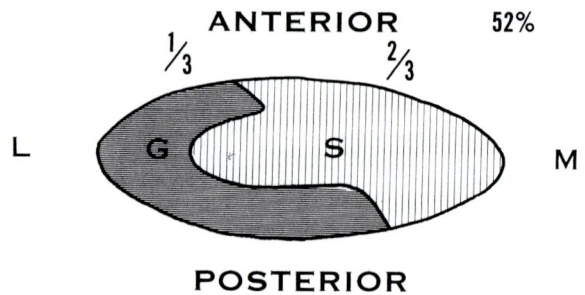
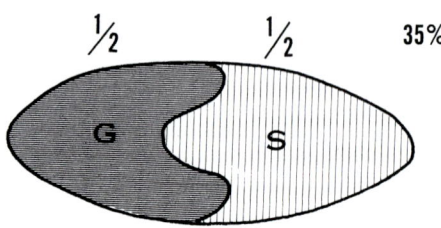
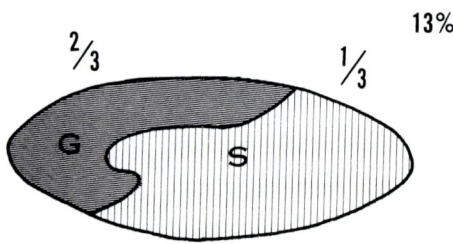

Figure 5.101 Degree of rotation of gastrocnemius-to-soleus portions of the calcaneal tendon (left extremity) at the level of insertion into the calcaneus. Occurrence in 100 specimens is indicated for each. (*G*, gastrocnemius; *L*, lateral; *M*, medial; *S*, soleus.) (Reprinted from Cummins JE, Anson JB, Carr WB, et al. The structure of the calcaneal tendon [of Achilles] in relation to orthopedic surgery with additional observations on the plantaris muscle. *Surg Gynecol Obstet*. 1946;83:107, with permission from Elsevier.)

The degree of rotation of the calcaneal tendon is variable, and the grouping and distribution shown in Table 5.2 are provided by Cummins and coworkers.[87]

The plantaris arises in close association with the lateral head of the gastrocnemius. The flat fusiform muscle is followed by a slender and long tendon that courses obliquely downward and medially between the soleus and the gastrocnemii. The tendon locates itself along the medial border of the calcaneal tendon and has a variable insertion, as reported by Cummins

TABLE 5-2 Posterior Contribution to Calcaneal Tendon[a]				
Group	Gastrocnemius	Soleus	%	Rotation
I	2/3	1/3	52	Minimum
II	1/2	1/2	35	
III	1/3	2/3	13	Maximum

[a]In 100 tendons.

Reprinted from Cummins JE, Anson JB, Carr WB, et al. The structure of the calcaneal tendon (for Achilles) in relation to orthopedic surgery with additional observations on the plantaris muscle. *Surg Gynecol Obstet*. 1946;83:107, with permission from Elsevier.

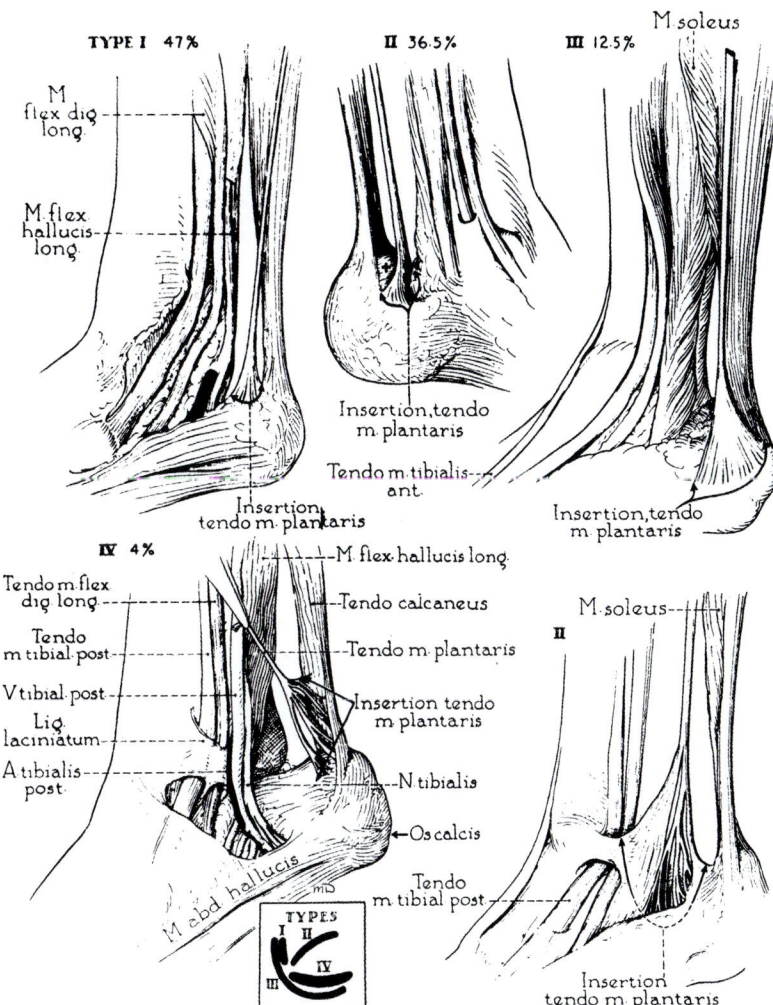

Figure 5.102 Types of tendinous insertion of plantaris muscle. (Adapted from Cummins EJ, Anson JB, Carr WB, et al. The structure of the calcaneal tendon [of Achilles] in relation to orthopedic surgery with additional observations on the plantaris muscle. *Surg Gynecol Obstet.* 1946;83:107.)

and coworkers, based on the analysis of 200 plantaris tendons (Fig. 5.102):

- Type I (47%): Fan-shaped expansion inserting into the medial aspect of the superior calcaneal tuberosity for the insertion of the calcaneal tendon.
- Type II (36.5%): Insertion on the os calcis, 0.5 to 2.5 cm anterior to the medial border of the calcaneal tendon. This insertion may radiate into the laciniate ligament and the fascia covering the medial aspect of the calcaneus.
- Type III (12.5%): Broad insertion investing the dorsal and medial surfaces of the adjacent terminal calcaneal tendon.
- Type IV (4%): Insertion on the medial border of the calcaneal tendon at a level 1 to 16 cm proximal to the insertion of the latter on the calcaneum. Occasionally a slip may reach the os calcis.[87]

The plantaris "is exceedingly variable in origin, structure and insertion" and is absent in 7.05%.[87]

REFERENCES

1. Testut L. *Les Anomalies Musculaires Chez l'Homme Expliquées par l'Anatomie Comparée: Leur Importance en Anthropologie.* Masson; 1884.
2. LeDouble AF. *Traité des Variations du Système Musculaire de l'Homme et de leur Signification au Point de Vue de l'Anthropologie et Zoologique.* Vol 2. Schleicher Frères; 1897.
3. Hallisy JE. The muscular variations in the human foot: a quantitative study. *Am J Anat.* 1930;45(3):411.
4. Chudzinski T. Contributions à l'étude des variations musculaires dans les races humaines. *Rev Anthropol.* 1882;5:613.
5. Macalister A. Additional observations on muscular anomalies in human anatomy (3rd series) with a catalogue of the principal muscular variations hitherto published. *Trans R Irish Acad.* 1875;25:1.
6. Knott JF. Muscular anomalies, including those of the diaphragm and subdiaphragmatic regions of the human body. *Proc R Irish Acad.* 1877-1883;3:627.
7. Macalister A. Further notes on muscular anomalies in human anatomy and their bearing upon homotypical myology. *Proc R Irish Acad.* 1866-1869:10.
8. Gruber W. Ueber einen musc. tibio-astragalus anticus des Menschen. *Arch Anat Physiol.* 1871:663.
9. Seelaus HK. On certain muscle anomalies of the lower extremity. *Anat Rec.* 1927;35:187.

10. Gruber W. Ueber die varietaeten des musc. extensor hallucis longus. *Reich und DuBoise—Reymond's Arch.* 1875:565.
11. Gruber W. Ein neuer fall von Musc. Extensor hallucis longus tricaudatus. *Reich und DuBoise—Reymond's Arch.* 1876:746.
12. Wood J. Variations in human myology observed during winter session of 1867-68 at King's College, London. *Proc R Soc Lond.* 1867-1868;16:438.
13. Tate R, Pachnik RL. The accessory tendon of extensor hallucis longus. Its occurrence and function. *J Am Podiatry Assoc.* 1976;66(12):899-907.
14. Lundeen RO, Latva D, Yant J. The secondary tendinous slip of the extensor hallucis longus (extensor ossis metatarsi hallucis). *J Foot Surg.* 1983;22:142-144.
15. Bibbo C, Arangio G, Patel DV. The accessory extensor tendon of the first metatarsophalangeal joint. *Foot Ankle Int.* 2004;6:387-390.
16. Boyd N, Brock H, Meier A, et al. Extensor hallucis capsularis: frequency and identification on MRI. *Foot Ankle Int.* 2006;3:181-184.
17. Paturet G. *Traité d'Anatomie Humaine, Vol II. Membres Superieur et Inferieur.* Masson et Cie; 1951:834.
18. Baumann JA. Valeur, variations et équivalences des muscles extenseurs, interosseux, adducteurs et abducteurs de la main et du pied chez l'homme. *Acta Anat.* 1947-1948;4:10.
19. Sarrafian SK, Topouzian LK. Anatomy and physiology of the extensor apparatus of the toes. *J Bone Joint Surg Am.* 1969;51(4):669.
20. Lucien M. Les chefs accessoires du muscle court extenseur des orteils chez l'homme. *Bibl Anat.* 1909;14:148.
21. Ruge G. Entwicklungsvorgänge an der Musculatur des Menschlichen Fusses. *Morphol Jahrbuch.* 1875;4:117.
22. Uzel M, Cetinus E, Gumusalan Y, et al. An anomalus muscle on the dorsomedial aspect of the foot (m. cuneo-naviculo-fascialis): case report. *Foot Ankle Int.* 2004;9:647-649.
23. Reimann R. Der variable streckapparat der kleinen zehe. *Gegenbaurs Morphol Jahrb.* 1981;127(2):188-209.
24. Picou R. Insertions inférieures du péronier lateral. *Bull Soc Anat Paris.* 1894;8(7):254-259.
25. Picou R. Quelques considérations sur les insertions du muscle long péronier lateral à la plante du pied. *Rev Orthop.* 1894:216-220.
26. Picou R. Insertions inférieures du muscle long péronier lateral: anomalie de ce muscle. *Bull Soc Anat Paris.* 1894;8(7):160-164.
27. Patil V, Frisch NC, Ebraheim NA. Anatomical variations in the insertion of the peroneus (fibularis) longus tendon. *Foot Ankle Int.* 2007;11:1179-1182.
28. Bhargava KN, Sanyal PK, Bhargava SN. Lateral musculature of the leg as seen in a hundred Indian cadavers. *Indian J Med Sci.* 1961;15:181-185.
29. Bareither DJ, Schuberth JM, Evoy PJ, et al. Peroneus digiti minimi. *Anat Anzeiger.* 1984;155:11-15.
30. Otto WA. Neve Seltene Beobachtungen, zur Anatomie, Physiologie und Pathologie. *Gehörig.* 1816:40.
31. Gruber W III. Monographie über den musculus peronaeus digiti V und sein reduktionen USW bei dem menschen, und über den homologen m. peronaeus digiti V USW bei den sängetieren. *Beobachtungen aus der Menschlichen und Vergleichenden Anatomie H.* 1879;7:35-80.
32. Hecker P. Etude sur le péronier du tarse: variations des péroniers latéraux. *Arch Anat Histol Embryol.* 1924;3:327.
33. Sobel M, Levy ME, Bohne WH. Congenital variations of the peroneus quartus muscle: an anatomic study. *Foot Ankle.* 1990;2(2):81-89.
34. Trono M, Tueche S, Quintart C, et al. Peroneus quartus muscle: a case report and review of the literature. *Foot Ankle Int.* 1999;20(10):659-662.
35. Sonmez M, Kosar I, Cimen M. The supernumerary peroneal muscles: case report and review of literature. *Foot Ankle Surg.* 2000;6:125-129.
36. Zammit J, Singh D. The peroneus quartus muscle, anatomy and clinical relevance. *J Bone Joint Surg Br.* 2003;85(8):1134-1137.
37. Moroney P, Borton D. Multiple accessory peroneal muscles: a cause of chronic lateral ankle pain. *Foot Ankle Int.* 2004;5:322-324.
38. Gumusalan Y, Ozbag D. A variation of fibularis quartus muscles: musculus fibulocalcaneus externum. *Clin Anat.* 2007;20:998-999.
39. Saupe N, Mengiardi B, Pfirrmann CWA, et al. Anatomic variants associated with peroneal tendon disorders: MR imaging findings in volunteers with asymptomatic ankles. *Radiology.* 2007;242(2):509-517.
40. Lewis OJ. The tibialis posterior tendon in the primate foot. *J Anat.* 1964;98(2):209.
41. Martin BF. Observations on the muscles and tendons of the medial aspect of the sole of the foot. *J Anat.* 1964;98(3):437.
42. Bloome DM, Marymont JV, Varner KE. Variations on the insertion of the posterior tibialis tendon: a cadaveric study. *Foot Ankle Int.* 2003;10:780-783.
43. Turner W. On variability in human structure with illustrations from the flexor muscles of the fingers and toes. *Trans R Soc Edinburgh.* 1865:24.
44. LaRue BG, Anctil EP. Distal anatomical relationship of the flexor hallucis longus and the flexor digitorum longus tendons. *Foot Ankle Int.* 2006;7:528-532.
45. Meckel JF. *Handbuch der Menschlichen Anatomie.* Halle und Berlin; 1815.
46. Macalister A. Additional observations on muscular anomalies in human anatomy. *Trans R Irish Acad.* 1872;25:125.
47. Curnow. Notes of some irregularities on muscles and nerves. *J Anat Physiol.* 1873;7:304.
48. Hartmann H. Anomalie du fléchisseur propre du gros orteil (muscle peroneo-calcanéen interne). *Bull Soc Anat Paris.* 1888;2:1044.
49. Auvray M. Anomalies musculaires et nerveuses. *Bull Soc Anat Paris.* 1896;10:223.
50. Perkins JD Jr. An anomalous muscle of the leg: peronaeo-calcaneus internus. *Anat Rec.* 1914;8:21.
51. Seipel R, Linklater J, Pitsis G, et al. The peroneocalcaneus internus muscle: an unusual cause of posterior ankle impingement. *Foot Ankle Int.* 2005;10:890-893.
52. Testut L. *Les Anomalies Musculaires Considérées du Point de Vue de la Ligature des Artères.* Doin; 1892:38-40.
53. Romanus B, Lindahl S, Stener B. Accessory soleus muscle: a clinical and radiographic presentation of eleven cases. *J Bone Joint Surg Am.* 1986;68(5):731.
54. Dunn AW. Anomalous muscles simulating soft-tissue tumors in the lower extremities. *J Bone Joint Surg Am.* 1965;47(7):1397.
55. Gordon SL, Matheson DW. The accessory soleus. *Clin Orthop.* 1976;97:129.
56. Nichols GW, Kàlenak A. The accessory soleus muscle. *Clin Orthop.* 1984;190:279.
57. Brodie JT, Dormans JP, Gregg JR, et al. Accessory soleus muscle: a report of 4 cases and review of literature. *Clin Orthop Relat Res.* 1997;337:180-186.
58. Nathan H, Gloobe H, Yosipovitch Z. Flexor digitorum accessorius longus. *Clin Orthop.* 1975;113:158.
59. Driver JR, Denison AB. The morphology of the long accessorius muscle. *Anat Rec.* 1914;8:341.
60. Lewis OJ. The comparative morphology of m. flexor accessorius and the associated long flexor tendons. *J Anat.* 1962;96(3):321.
61. Páč L, Malinovsky L Jr. M. flexor digitorum longus accessorius in the lower limb of man. *Anat Anz.* 1985;159:253-257.
62. Sammarco GJ, Stephens MM. Tarsal tunnel syndrome caused by the flexor digitorum accessorius longus. *J Bone Joint Surg Am.* 1990;72(3):453-454.
63. Sammarco GJ, Conti SF. Tarsal tunnel syndrome caused by anomalous muscle. *J Bone Joint Surg Am.* 1994;76-A(9):1308-1314.
64. Peterson DA, Stinson W, Lairmore JR. The long accessory flexor muscle: an anatomical study. *Foot Ankle Int.* 1995;16:637-640.
65. Gumusalan Y, Kalaycioglu A. Bilateral accessory flexor digitorum longus muscle in a man. *Ann Anat.* 2000;182:573-576.
66. Kinoshita M, Okuda R, Morikawa J, et al. Tarsal tunnel syndrome associated with an accessory muscle. *Foot Ankle Int.* 2003;2:132-136.
67. Nathan H, Gloobe H. Flexor digitorum brevis: anatomical variations. *Anat Anzeiger.* 1974;135:295.
68. Lewis OJ. *Functional Morphology of the Evolving Hand and Foot.* Clarendon Press; 1990:265, 266.
69. Winckler G, Gianoli G. La véritable terminaison de la chair carrée de Sylvius (musc. quadratus plantae). *Arch Anat Histol Embryol.* 1955;38:47.
70. Barlow TE. An unusual anomaly of m. flexor digitorum longus. *J Anat.* 1949;83:224.
71. Barlow TE. The deep flexors of the foot. *J Anat.* 1953;87:308.
72. Morestin H. Anomalie de l'accessoire du long fléchisseur commun des orteils. *Bull Soc Anat Paris.* 1895;11:46.
73. Baumann J. La région de passage de la loge posteriore de la jambe a la plante du pied. *Ann Anat Pathol Anat Normal Medico-Chirurg.* 1930;7(2):201.
74. Poirier P, Charpy A. *Traité d'Anatomie Humaine.* Vol 2. 2nd ed.. Masson et Cie; 1901:279, 284.
75. Loth E. Etude anthropologique de l'aponevrose plantaire. *Bull Mem Soc Anthropol Paris.* 1913;4:606.
76. Leboucq H. Les muscles adducteurs du pouce et du gros orteil. *Bull Acad R Med Belg.* 1893;7(1):26.
77. Owens S, Thordarson DB. The adductor hallucis revisited. *Foot Ankle Int.* 2001;3:186-191.

78. Cralley JC, Schuberth JM. The transverse head of adductor hallucis. *Anat Anzeiger*. 1979;146:400.
79. Arakawa T, Tokita K, Miki A, et al. Anatomical study of human adductor hallucis muscle with respect to its origin and insertion. *Ann Anat*. 2003;185:585-592.
80. Jones FW. *Structure and Function as Seen in the Foot*. 2nd ed. Baillière; 1949:134, 135, 176, 177, 181.
81. Carmont MR, Bruce C, Bass A, et al. An accessory abductor muscle of the fifth toe? An unusual cause of a lump in the foot. *Foot Ankle Surg*. 2002;8:125-128.
82. Harbeson AE. The origin of the first dorsal interosseous muscle of the foot. *J Anat*. 1934;68:116.
83. Manter JT. Variations of the interosseous muscles of the human foot. *Anat Rec*. 1945;93:117.
84. Meyer P. Contributions a l'étude de la region metatarsophalangienne. *Bull Assoc Anat*. 1958;99:500.
85. Kalin PJ, Hirsch BE. The origins and function of the interosseous muscles of the foot. *J Anat*. 1987;152:83.
86. Schmidt VR, Reissig D, Heinrichs HJ, Die MM. Lumbricales am fuss des menschen. *Anat Anzeiger*. 1963;113:450.
87. Cummins JE, Anson JB, Carr WB, et al. The structure of the calcaneal tendon (of Achilles) in relation to orthopedic surgery with additional observations on the plantaris muscle. *Surg Gynecol Obstet*. 1946;83:197.
88. Testut L. *Traité d'Anatomie Humaine*. Vol I. Doin; 1921:992.

Tendon Sheaths and Bursae

Shahan K. Sarrafian and Armen S. Kelikian

SYNOVIAL TENDON SHEATHS

The tendons of the leg at the level of the ankle and the plantar aspect of the foot engage in fibrous, fibro-osseous tunnels acting as pulleys or as retention systems. Within these tunnels, the tendons are surrounded by synovial sheaths to facilitate their gliding.

Structurally, a synovial tendon sheath has a parietal layer lining the deep surface of the fibrous or fibro-osseous canal, a visceral layer covering the tendon, and a mesotenon connecting the latter to the parietal lining. The synovial sheath forms a cavity closed at both ends, and proximally, synovial folds permit the play of the tendon through the sheath.

▶ Tibialis Anterior

The synovial tendon sheath of the tibialis anterior (Figs. 6.1 and 6.2) extends from above the proximal arm of the inferior extensor retinaculum to the level of the talonavicular interline. Hartman mentions that the synovial sac extends 5.75 cm proximal to a line joining the center of the malleoli.[1] The length of this synovial sheath is given as 6 to 8 cm or 8 to 10 cm.[2,3] Hartman reports that the distal end of the synovial sac reaches the talonavicular joint in 60%, is shorter in 22%, and is longer in 18%.[1] There is a complete mesotenon to the tibialis anterior tendon throughout the length of the sheath, located on the deep surface of the tendon.

▶ Extensor Hallucis Longus

The synovial tendon sheath of the extensor hallucis longus (see Figs. 6.1 and 6.2) starts lower than the synovial sac of the tibialis anterior tendon but extends more distally. It originates slightly above the upper arm of the inferior extensor retinaculum, at 1.75 cm proximal to the intermalleolar interline, just above the talotibial articular interline.[1,4] The lower limit of this synovial sac is more difficult to delineate; it usually reaches the level of the first cuneometatarsal joint. Less frequently, this distal end of the synovial sheath extends distal to the cuneometatarsal joint interline and advances more or less on the dorsum of the first metatarsal bone.[2] Hartman mentions that the synovial sac terminates at the level of the cuneometatarsal joint in 34%, proximal to it in 34%, and distal to it in 32% and that it may reach the lower third of the first metatarsal in 24%.

▶ Extensor Digitorum Longus

The synovial tendon sheath of the extensor digitorum longus (see Figs. 6.1 and 6.2) is a large but short synovial sac that enlarges as it extends distally and also covers the tendon of the peroneus tertius. It starts 2 to 3 cm above the ankle joint, about 1 cm above the upper limit of the extensor hallucis longus tendon sheath.[3] The synovial sac passes under the undivided segment of the inferior extensor retinaculum, enlarges to cover the diverging tendons, and ends at the level of the cuneonavicular joint in a large blind sac that is subdivided into small saclike projections that are 0.5 cm in length and are located on the superficial aspect of the tendons.[3] There is no prolongation over the tendon of the peroneus tertius.

▶ Extensor Digitorum Brevis

Lovell and Tanner describe synovial sheaths to the tendons of the extensor digitorum brevis (see Fig. 6.1) when the tendons are well developed.[3] The synovial sheath of the extensor digitorum brevis to the big toe is the longest, measuring 5.5 cm; it originates under the fascial band extending from metatarsal 1 to 2 and terminates at the proximal end of the proximal phalanx.

The synovial sheaths of toes 2, 3, and 4 are 3 to 4 cm in length; they start from close to where the tendons originate, pass under the digital extensor aponeurosis, and terminate at the level of the proximal phalanges.[3]

▶ Peroneus Longus and Peroneus Brevis

The synovial sheath of the peroneus longus and peroneus brevis is complex (Figs. 6.3 and 6.4). It is common to both tendons behind the lateral malleolus and bifurcates for a short distance

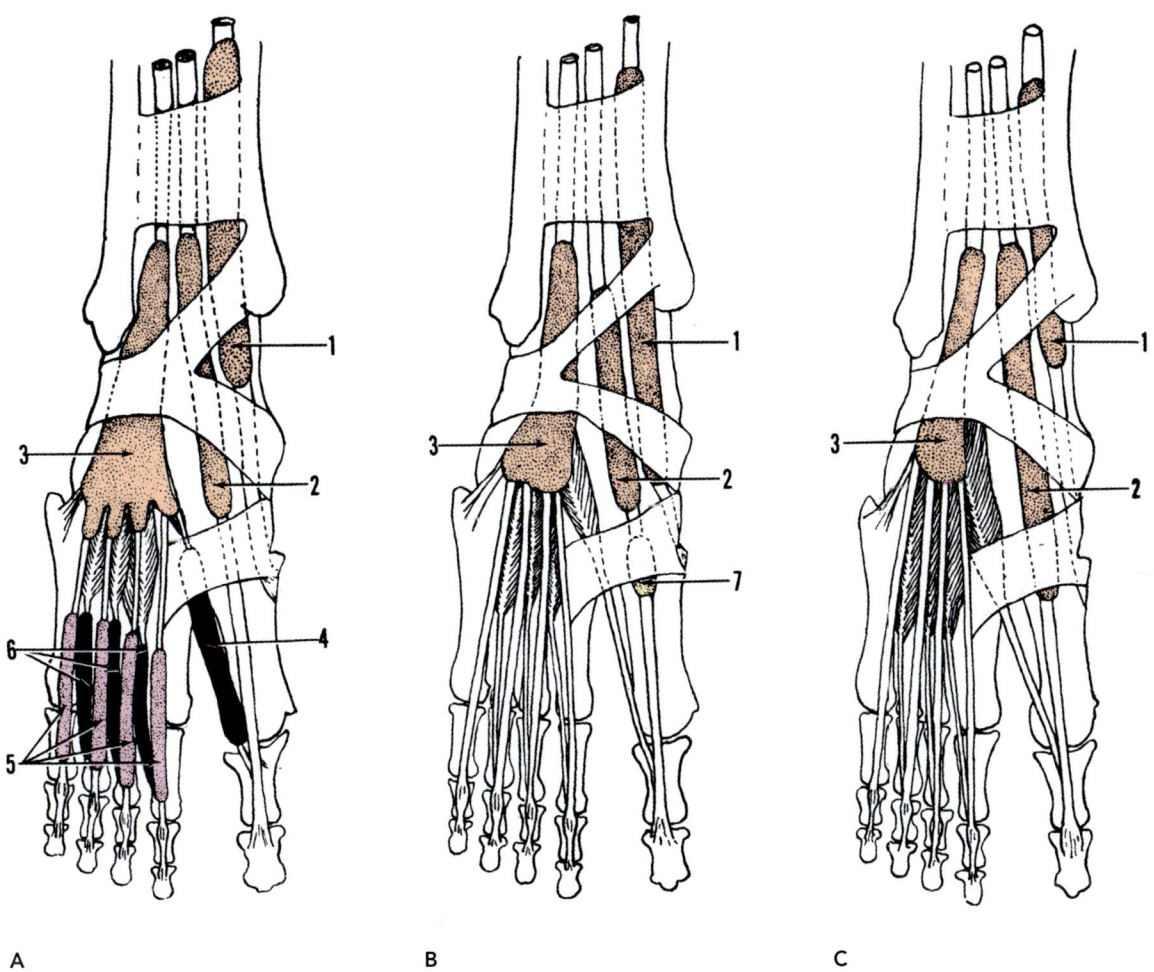

Figure 6.1 Extensor tendon sheaths. (A) According to Lovell and Tanner.[3] (B) According to most French anatomists. (C) According to most German anatomists. (1, tendon sheath of tibialis anterior; 2, tendon sheath of extensor hallucis longus; 3, tendon sheath of extensor digitorum longus; 4, tendon sheath of extensor hallucis brevis; 5, tendon sheath of extensor digitorum longus, digital portion; 6, tendon sheath of extensor digitorum brevis; 7, distal segment of extensor hallucis longus tendon sheath.) (Adapted from Jones FW. *Structure and Function as Seen in the Foot*. 2nd ed. Baillière Tindall & Cox; 1949:229-245.)

above and for a longer distance below the malleolus. The common synovial sheath extends 2.5 to 3.5 cm above the tip of the lateral malleolus.[3] The proximal bifurcation extends 2.5 cm on the peroneus longus and 1.5 cm on the peroneus brevis.[3] Inferiorly, the synovial sac bifurcates at the level of the peroneal tubercle of the calcaneus, which separates the two tendons. The bifurcation extension of the peroneus brevis is located above the tubercle and extends up to within 2 cm of the insertion of the tendon on the base of the fifth metatarsal or to the level of the calcaneocuboid joint.

The synovial sac of the peroneus longus terminates in the region of the groove of the cuboid. On the superficial surface of the tendon, the sac extends for about 1 cm distal to the peroneal tubercle, whereas on the osseous surface, it extends into the groove of the cuboid entering the planta pedis.[3]

In the sole of the foot, the peroneus longus tendon receives a second synovial sheath, which extends from the groove of the cuboid to the insertion of the tendon on the base of the first metatarsal. At the level of the cuboid, this synovial sac extends laterally less on the superficial surface of the tendon and more on the deep surface; this brings the two sacs close to one another on the osseous surface of the tendon. At this level, the two synovial sacs of the peroneus longus tendon are separated only by a thin, cellular, transparent lamella, or they may even communicate (about one-third of cases).[2]

Behind the lateral malleolus, the common synovial sheath of the peronei tendons is in close contact with the synovium of the ankle joint above and below the posterior talofibular ligament. The peronei tendon sheath and the calcaneofibular ligament cross each other in an "X" and are in intimate contact. The possible communication of the common synovial sheath of the peronei with the ankle joint is of importance in the arthrographic assessment of ligamentous injuries of the ankle joint.

According to Broström and Prins and based on their arthrographic assessment of injured ankles in healthy individuals, there is no communication between the synovial sheath of the peronei and the synovial cavity of the ankle joint.[5,6] The data provided by investigators is as follows: postmortem—in 18 ankles, 0 communication; in 40 ankles, 0 communication; in vivo—in 45 ankles, 0 communication; in 68 ankles, 0 communication; in 17 ankles, 14% communication; in 95 ankles, 26% communication.[5,7]

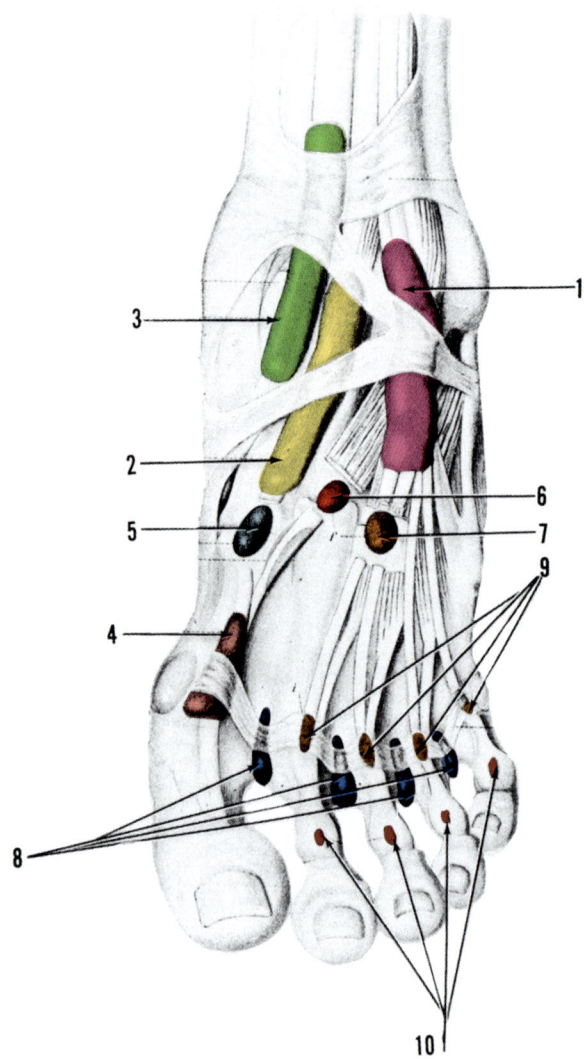

Figure 6.2 Tendon sheaths and bursae of the dorsum of the foot. (1, tendon sheath of extensor digitorum longus and peroneus tertius; 2, tendon sheath of extensor hallucis longus; 3, tendon sheath of tibialis anterior; 4, distal synovial space of extensor hallucis longus [may be tendon sheath or bursa]; 5, bursa between metatarso$_1$-cuneiform$_1$ joint and extensor hallucis longus tendon; 6, 7, bursae between tarsometatarsal joint and extensor digitorum brevis, extensor hallucis brevis; 8, intermetatarsophalangeal bursae seen in upper and anterior parts; 9, bursae between extensor digitorum longus tendons and dorsal extensor aponeurosis at level of metatarsophalangeal joint; 10, subcutaneous bursae over proximal interphalangeal joints.) (Adapted from Hartman H. Die sehnenscheiden und synovialsäcke des fusses. *Morphol Arbeit*. 1896;5:214.)

▶ **Tibialis Posterior**

The synovial sheath of the tibialis posterior tendon (Figs. 6.5-6.7) is 7 to 9 cm in length and starts 6 cm proximal to the tip of the medial malleolus. It descends along the tendon in the retromalleolar groove and terminates close to the tuberosity of the navicular, extending more on the osseous surface and less on the superficial surface. The tibialis posterior tendon has no mesotenon.

The synovial sheath sometimes communicates with that of the flexor digitorum longus or with the synovial cavity of the ankle joint (in 5.8% of cases).[3,6]

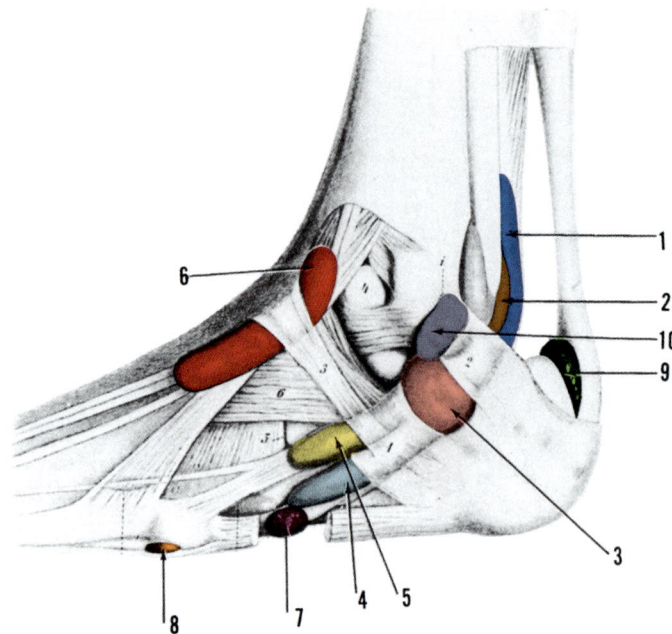

Figure 6.3 Tendon sheaths and bursae of the lateral aspect of the ankle and foot. The combined tendon sheath of the peronei tendons splits into two: peroneus longus and peroneus brevis above and peroneous longus and peroneus brevis below. (1, peroneus longus above; 2, peroneus brevis above; 3, peronei tendons; 4, peroneus longus below; 5, peroneus brevis below; 6, tendon sheath of extensor digitorum longus and peroneus tertius; 7, bursa between peroneus longus tendon and abductor digiti quinti; 8, bursa between metatarsal 5 and abductor digiti quinti; 9, pre-Achilles bursa; 10, lateral malleolar subcutaneous bursa.) (Adapted from Hartman H. Die sehnenscheiden und synovialsäcke des fusses. *Morphol Arbeit*. 1896;5:214.)

▶ **Flexor Digitorum Longus**

The synovial sheath of the flexor digitorum longus (see Figs. 6.5-6.7) has two components: malleolar and digital.

The malleolar synovial sac starts about 5 cm above the tip of the medial malleolus, slightly lower than the sac of the tibialis posterior. The synovial sac accompanies the tendon of the flexor digitorum longus in the calcaneal canal and terminates in the sole of the foot where the flexor digitorum longus tendon crosses that of the flexor hallucis longus. On the superficial aspect of the tendon, the sheath falls 1 cm short of this crossing point, and a mesotenon is present on its entire length.[3] The synovial sheath of the flexor digitorum longus may communicate with those of the tibialis posterior and flexor hallucis longus tendons.

The digital synovial sacs of the lesser toes envelop the tendons of the flexor digitorum longus and the flexor digitorum brevis. These synovial sheaths are independent and lie within the fibrous tunnels extending from the heads of the metatarsals to the bases of the distal phalanges. A comprehensive study of the vascular system within the tenosynovial tubes is provided by Hartman, Lovell and Tanner, and Ziegler.[1,3,8]

At the level of the proximal third of the proximal phalanx, the tendon of the flexor digitorum brevis is still superficial and it bifurcates. The slips of the divided tendon slide on each side of the long flexor tendon, decussate fibers under the tendon at the level of

Chapter 6: Tendon Sheaths and Bursae 297

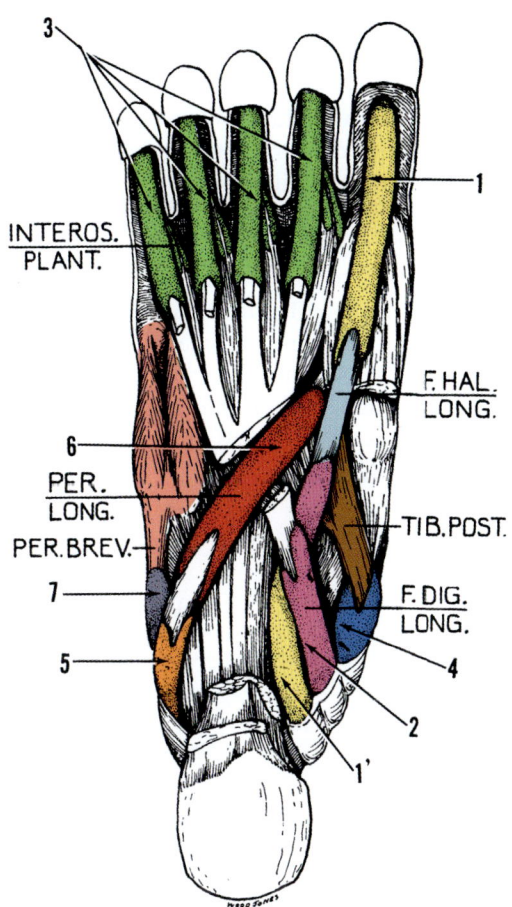

Figure 6.4 Tendon sheaths of the plantar aspect of the foot. (*1*, distal tendon sheath of flexor hallucis longus; *1′*, proximal tendon sheath of flexor hallucis longus; *2*, proximal tendon sheath of flexor digitorum longus; *3*, distal digital tendon sheath of flexor digitorum longus; *4*, tendon sheath of tibialis posterior; *5*, proximal tendon sheath of peroneus longus; *6*, distal tendon sheath of peroneus longus; *7*, tendon sheath of peroneus brevis.) (Adapted from Jones FW. *Structure and Function as Seen in the Foot*. 2nd ed. Baillière Tindall & Cox; 1949:229-245.)

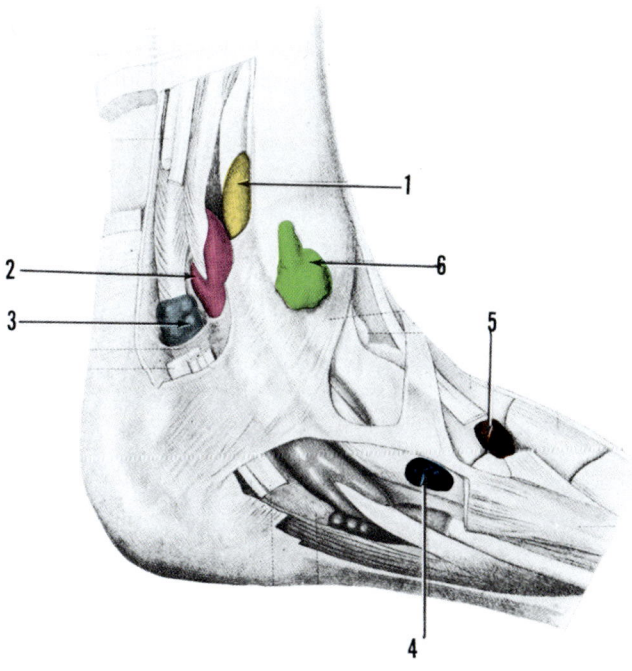

Figure 6.5 Tendon sheaths and bursae of the medial aspect of the ankle and foot. (*1*, tendon sheath of tibialis posterior; *2*, tendon sheath of flexor digitorum longus; *3*, tendon sheath of flexor hallucis longus; *4*, bursa between abductor hallucis and tibialis posterior tendon; *5*, bursa under tibialis anterior tendon near its insertion; *6*, subcutaneous medial malleolar bursa.) (Adapted from Hartman H. Die schnenscheiden und synovialsäcken des fusses. *Morphol Arbeit*. 1896;5:214.)

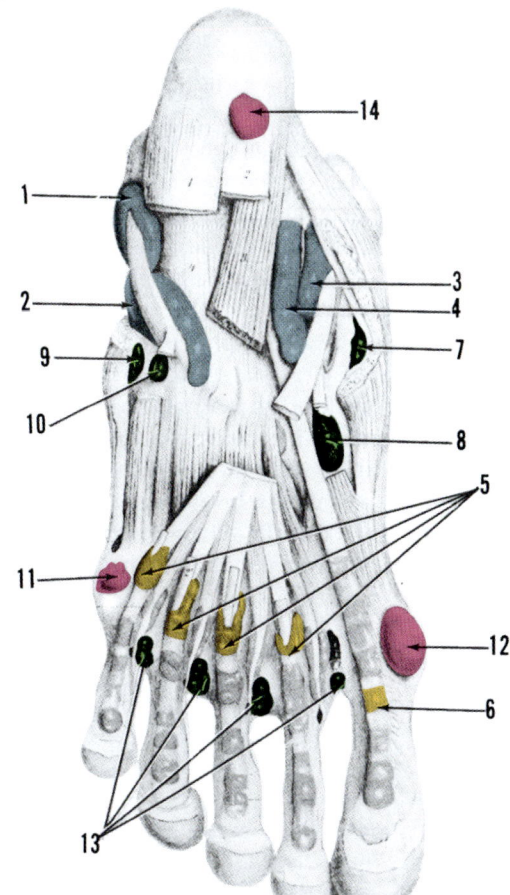

Figure 6.6 Tendon sheaths and bursae of the sole of the foot. (*1, 2*, proximal and distal segment of sheath of peroneus longus; *3*, tendon sheath of flexor digitorum longus, proximal segment; *4*, tendon sheath of flexor hallucis longus, proximal segment; *5*, digital segment of flexor digitorum longus tendon sheath; *6*, digital segment of flexor hallucis longus tendon sheath; *7*, bursa between abductor hallucis and tibialis posterior; *8*, bursa under origin of flexor hallucis brevis; *9*, bursa between metatarsal 5 and abductor of fifth toe; *10*, bursa under origin of flexor brevis and opponens of fifth toe; *11*, subcutaneous bursa under head of metatarsal 5; *12*, subcutaneous bursa under head of metatarsal 1; *13*, intermetatarsophalangeal bursae; *14*, plantar calcaneal subcutaneous bursa.) (Adapted from Hartman HO. Die schnenscheiden und synovialsäcke des fusses. *Morphol Arbeit*. 1896;5:214.)

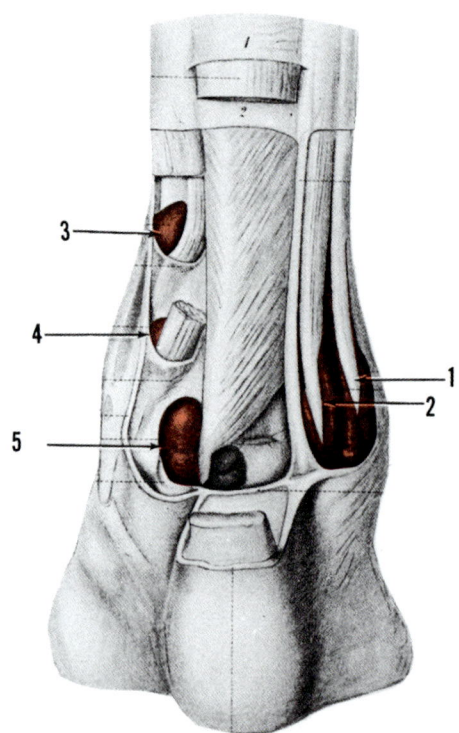

Figure 6.7 **Tendon sheath of the posterior aspect of the lower leg and the ankle.** (1, tendon sheath of peroneus longus; 2, tendon sheath of peroneus brevis; 3, tendon sheath of tibialis posterior; 4, tendon sheath of flexor digitorum longus; 5, tendon sheath of flexor hallucis longus.) (Adapted from Hartman H. Die schnenscheiden und synovialsäcke des fusses. *Morphol Arbeit.* 1896;5:214.)

the middle phalanx, and insert on the sides of the middle third of the middle phalanx. The flexor digitorum longus tendon courses through the bifurcation and inserts on the base of the distal phalanx. The distal segments of the flexor tendons are connected to the parietal layer of the tenosynovial membranes with short triangular mesomembranes, the vincula brevis. The vinculum brevis of each short flexor tendon slip has a free concave proximal border (Fig. 6.8) and has a variable location. Ziegler provides the following data on the location of the proximal border of the triangular vinculum of the flexor digitorum brevis in 300 toes: on the base of the shaft of the proximal phalanx, 52%; more proximal, 18%; distal to the middle of the proximal phalanx, 28.3%; more distal, 1.3%; on the base of the middle phalanx, 0.3%.[8]

The distal triangular vinculum brevis connecting the flexor digitorum longus tendon to the parietal tenosynovial sheaths extends from the middle or base of the middle phalanx to the distal phalanx. Proximal to the chiasma tedium, the flexor digitorum brevis tendinous slips are united by a horizontal synovial membrane that forms with the chiasma a bed for the flexor digitorum longus tendon. A transverse mesosynovial membrane connects the same tendons at the level of the proximal borders of the vincula brevis. This arrangement contributes to the formation of a closed space (see Fig. 6.8).

The vinculum longus connecting the previously described tenosynovial floor to the dorsal aspect of the flexor digitorum longus tendon has two parts: proximal and distal. The proximal vinculum longus originates on the midline of the long flexor tendon; it then splits into two sagittal plates, which gradually diverge, forming a tent, and insert along the horizontal tenosynovial membrane connecting the slips of the flexor digitorum brevis. This insertion is proximal to the chiasma tendinum. The form of this proximal vinculum longus is variable, and Ziegler provides the following data in 300 toes: tent form (see Fig. 6.8), 22.7%; one sagittal plate (Fig. 6.9), 16.7%; cordlike (see Fig. 6.9), 28%; one filament (see Fig. 6.9), 9.6%; multiple filament (see Fig. 6.9), 5.7%; meshlike, very narrow, 4%; absent vinculum longus, 10%; absent vinculum longus and horizontal connecting membrane, 3.3%.[8] The distal vinculum longus extends from the midline of the dorsal surface of the flexor digitorum longus to the level of or distal to the chiasma tendinum. It may be present as a sagittal plate, a filiform structure, or a multifilamentous complex (see Fig. 6.9). Accessory vincula may be present in toes 2 to 4.

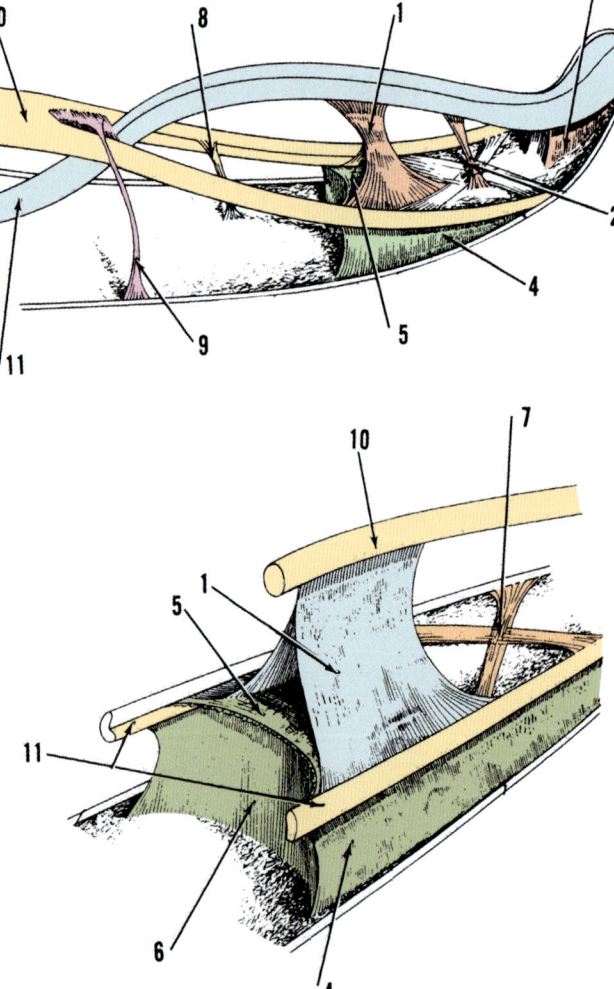

Figure 6.8 **Vincula of the flexor tendons of the lesser toes.** (1, proximal segment of long vinculum of flexor digitorum longus forming a tentlike arrangement; 2, distal segment of long vinculum of flexor digitorum longus; 3, short vinculum of flexor digitorum longus; 4, vinculum of flexor digitorum brevis; 5, horizontal mesomembrane; 6, transverse mesomembrane forming with 4 and 5 a closed space; 7, chiasma tendineum; 8, 9, accessory vincula; 10, flexor digitorum brevis tendon; 11, flexor digitorum longus tendon.) (Adapted from Ziegler EM. Zur morphologie der vincula tendinum menschlichen zehen erwachsener. *Anat Arz Bd.* 1972;130:404.)

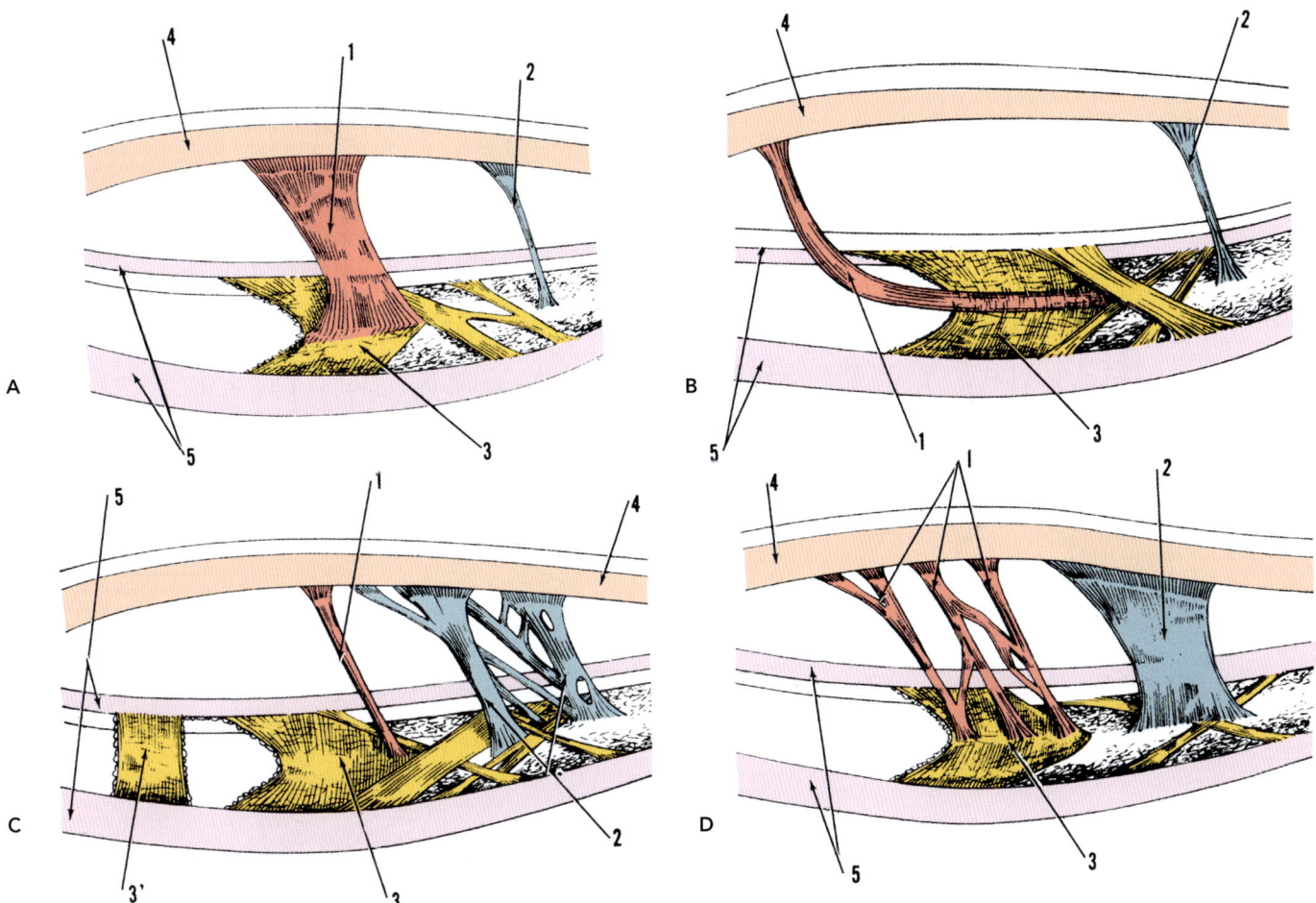

Figure 6.9 Varieties of the vinculum longus of the flexor digitorum longus of the lesser toe. (*Type A*) *1* is in sagittal plate configuration; *2* is filiform. (*Type B*) *1* is cordlike; *2* is filiform. (*Type C*) *1* is filiform; *2* is meshlike. (*Type D*) *1* is meshlike; *2* is in sagittal plate configuration. (*1*, proximal segment of vinculum longus of flexor digitorum longus; *2*, distal segment of vinculum longus of flexor digitorum longus; *3*, horizontal mesomembrane; *3'*, proximal horizontal membrane; *4*, flexor digitorum longus tendon; *5*, flexor digitorum brevis tendon.) (Adapted from Ziegler EM. Zur morphologie der vincula tendinum menschlichen zehen erwachsener. *Anat Arz Bd.* 1972;130:404.)

▶ Flexor Hallucis Longus

The synovial sheath of the flexor hallucis longus (see Figs. 6.4-6.7) has two components: proximal and distal. The proximal synovial sheath extends 1 cm proximal to the ankle joint and accompanies the tendon in the fibro-osseous tunnel of the talus, over the calcaneus, under the sustentaculum tali, and past the crossing of the flexor digitorum longus tendon, and it ends usually in the region of the cuneonavicular joint on the plantar aspect of the tibialis posterior tendon. This proximal synovial sheath measures 10 to 12 cm in length, has no mesotenon, and may communicate with the sheath of the flexor hallucis longus (in 20% of cases) and the sheath of the tibialis posterior tendon.[2,3,9] A communication may exist normally between the posterior aspect of the ankle joint and the synovial sheaths of the long flexor tendons and the tibialis posterior tendon; according to Prins, the posterior aspect of the ankle joint communicates with the sheath of the flexor hallucis longus in 13%, with the sheath of the flexor digitorum longus in 7%, and with the sheath of the tibialis posterior in 6% of normal cases.[6]

The distal or digital segment of the flexor hallucis longus sheath is longer than the sheath of the lesser toes and extends from near the base of the first metatarsal to the insertion of the tendon on the base of the distal phalanx. Communication between the proximal and the distal digital sheath is exceedingly rare; one case has been described by Chemin.[3,10]

In 34% of the big toes, the proximal vinculum is in the form of two quadrangular simple mesomembranes extending from the shaft of the proximal phalanx to the dorsal surface of the flexor hallucis tendon.[8] The proximal borders of these mesomembranes reach the level of the base of the proximal phalanx in 8% and the level of the head of the proximal phalanx or the interphalangeal joint in 25% of cases.[8] In 42%, a triangular mesomembrane extends from the parietal tendon sheath to the dorsal surface of the flexor hallucis longus tendon, up to its insertion.[8] The distal vinculum of the flexor hallucis longus tendon is a very weak structure but regularly present; an accessory vinculum to the same tendon is rarely present.

SYNOVIAL BURSAE

The synovial bursae are flat pouches present where there is excess pressure of friction (see Figs. 6.2, 6.3, 6.6, and 6.10). They are subject to considerable variation in both location and size.

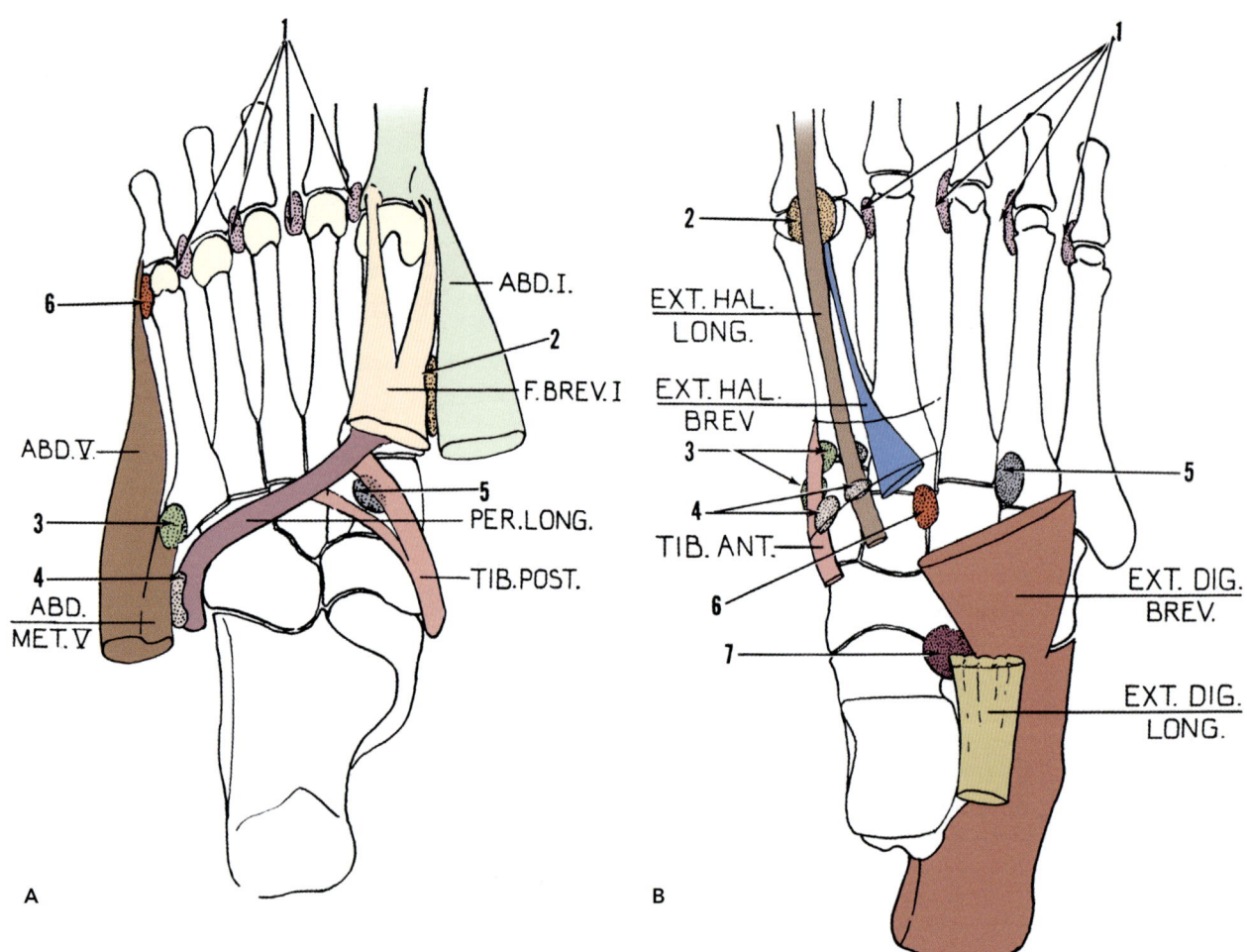

Figure 6.10 Bursae. (A) Plantar aspect of the foot. (*1*, intermetatarsophalangeal bursae; *2*, bursa between flexor hallucis brevis and abductor hallucis; *3*, bursa between abductor of fifth toe and base of metatarsal 5; *4*, bursa between abductor of fifth toe and peroneus longus tendon; *5*, bursa between tibialis posterior tendon and first cuneiform; *6*, bursa between abductor of fifth toe and fifth metatarsal head.) **(B)** Dorsal aspect of the foot. (*1*, lumbrical bursae; *2*, bursa under extensor hallucis longus tendon at metatarsophalangeal joint level; *3*, bursae under tibialis anterior tendon near its insertions; *4*, bursae superficial to tibialis anterior and extensor hallucis longus tendons; *5, 6*, bursae under extensor digitorum brevis and extensor hallucis brevis; *7*, bursa of sinus tarsi of "bursae mucosa Grüberi" inserting between deep surface of extensor digitorum longus and neck of talus.) (Adapted from Jones FW. *Structure and Function as Seen in the Foot*. 2nd ed. Baillière Tindall & Cox; 1949:229-245.)

▶ Subcutaneous

Subcutaneous bursae are found over the medial and the lateral malleoli of the ankle joint, the former being the larger. Subcutaneous retro-Achilles tendon bursae may be present, one or three in number, forming a superior, a middle, and a lower bursa.[11] A subcalcaneal bursa may be present between the tuberosity of the os calcis and the subcutaneous fat pad; this bursa occurs in 50% of the cases.[1] Gregoire refers to Lenoir's 1837 report attesting to the presence of a subcalcaneal bursa in all subjects.[12] Gregoire conducted his own anatomic investigation of the subcalcaneal bursa in 40 cadaver feet and could demonstrate the presence of such a bursa in one specimen only. He concluded that the serous subcalcaneal bursa of Lenoir was an exception. It is interesting to note that in 19 ft, he observed "under the greater tuberosity of the calcaneus a considerable rarefaction of the fibrous tracts extending from the plantar aponeurosis to the deep surface of the skin."[12]

At times, there was no trace of fibrous tracts, and the very loose cellular tissue would crumble under digital pressure. Subcutaneous bursae may be found over the dorsomedial aspect of the head of the first metatarsal and the dorsolateral aspect of the fifth metatarsal head. Plantar subcutaneous bursae may be located over the head of the first and fifth metatarsals.[1] Frequently, subcutaneous bursae are seen over the dorsum of the proximal interphalangeal joints.[1,13]

▶ Subfascial

Subfascial synovial bursae may be classified as follows:

- *Group I:* Bursae located between the origin or insertion of a tendon and the bone
- *Group II:* Bursae located
    - Under the tendon or the muscle crossing a bony prominence
    - Between tendons and ligaments
    - Between tendons and muscles gliding over each other or running close to each other[1]

Group I

The bursae of this group are as follows:

- Pre-Achilles tendon, retrocalcaneal bursa
- Bursae corresponding to the insertion of the tibialis anterior tendon
- Bursae corresponding to the insertion of the tibialis posterior tendon
- Bursae located between the tendons of the interossei and the metatarsophalangeal joint
- Bursae located between the common origin of the tendons of the short flexor and opponens of the fifth toe and the base of the fifth metatarsal
- Bursae located between the flexor hallucis brevis and the first cuneiform.

The retrocalcaneal tendon bursa is a large, constant bursa situated between the smooth upper part of the posterior end of the calcaneus and the deep surface of the Achilles tendon. The bursa is in the form of a triangle, with the apex inferior and the base superior. The upper border carries synovial fringes and extends 8 to 10 mm above the os calcis.[11]

The bursae in association with the terminal portion of the tibialis anterior tendon are often three in number.[9] A bursa is present between the tendon and the cuneometatarsal joint. A second bursa is located between the tendon and the first cuneiform bone. The third bursa is superficial, located between the tendon and the overlying extensor retinaculum.

The bursa corresponding to the insertion of the tibialis posterior tendon is found between the plantar component of the tibialis posterior tendon and the second cuneiform. This bursa is 2 cm long and may communicate with the second cuneometatarsal joint.[1]

The bursae of the interossei are located between the tendons of the interossei and the collateral ligaments of the metatarsophalangeal joints. Hartman provides the following data in regard to their occurrence in 38 ft: toe 2—dorsal interosseous 1, 4%; dorsal interosseous 2, 2%; toe 3—plantar interosseous 1, 38%; dorsal interosseous 3, 7%; toe 4—plantar interosseous 2, 55%; dorsal interosseous 4, 9%; toe 5—plantar interosseous 3, 16%.[1]

A pea-sized bursa may be present between the common origin of the tendons of the short flexor and opponent of the fifth toe and the base of the fifth metatarsal.[1] A bursa may also be seen between the tendon of the flexor hallucis brevis near its origin and the first cuneiform.

Group II

Bursae Under Tendon or Muscle Crossing Bony Prominence

The bursa of the sinus tarsi is located between the neck of the talus dorsolaterally and the inferior extensor retinaculum. This bursa is present in 56% of the cases and may extend anteriorly to the talonavicular joint and posteriorly to the ankle joint.[1] It may communicate with these joints or with the sheath of the extensor digitorum longus.[1]

The bursae of the extensor digitorum brevis are usually two in number. One bursa is located between the extensor hallucis brevis and the cuneometatarsal base. The second bursa is situated more laterally under the extensor digitorum brevis to the lesser toes.

The bursa of the extensor hallucis longus is found between the tendon and the cuneometatarsal joint. This bursa does not communicate with the joint but frequently opens, with a superficial bursa present on the dorsal aspect of the tendon at that level. Occasionally, the bursa may communicate with the sheath of the extensor hallucis longus, which then seems to extend up to the base of the first metatarsal.

A bursa is also found between the abductor of the fifth toe and the tuberosity of the fifth metatarsal.

Bursae Between Tendons and Aponeurosis

Bursae are described as being present between the long extensor tendons of the toes and the dorsal aponeurosis of the toes at the level of the metatarsophalangeal joints. When well developed, these could be considered as the distal sheaths of the long extensor tendons of the lesser toes. The bursa of the big toe is the largest and covers over one-third of the first metatarsal; at times, it is difficult to differentiate this bursa from a vaginal sheath.[1]

Bursae Between Close Tendons and Muscles

A bursa is present between the tendon of the peroneus longus and the abductor digiti minimi, where the former turns into the sole of the foot in the groove on the cuboid. Another bursa may be seen between the tibialis posterior tendon and the abductor hallucis at the level of the navicular and the first cuneiform.

▶ Intermetatarsophalangeal Bursae

Hartman provided a detailed description and a good illustration of the intermetatarsophalangeal bursae (see Figs. 6.2 and 6.3).[1] These bursae are located in the narrow intermetatarsal head space, between the tendons of the corresponding interossei. They cover the dorsal aspect, the distal border, and partially the plantar aspect of the deep transverse metatarsal ligament. Bursae 1 to 3 are constant, whereas bursa 4 is missing in 80% of cases. Communication between the joint and the adjacent bursa may occur. Bossley and Cairney studied the intermetatarsophalangeal bursae in cadaveric feet after injection of heated, dyed gelatin into the bursae.[14] In the second and third capitometatarsal interspace, "the bursa was flattened, oval, up to 3 cm long, lying in a vertical plane, applied to the metatarsal neck, the capsule of the joint and the proximal phalanx, and surrounded by a thin layer of loose connective tissue" (Fig. 6.11). The bursa was dorsal to the deep transverse metatarsal ligament, and at the distal margin of the latter, it was closely applied to the plantar digital neurovascular bundle coursing dorsally (Fig. 6.12). The bursa of the fourth interspace did not extend distally beyond the free border of the deep transverse metatarsal ligament, and thus was not in close contact with the corresponding plantar neurovascular bundle. Bossley and Cairney supplemented their anatomic study with a radiographic investigation of the bursa with angiographs in a group of patients (Fig. 6.13).[14]

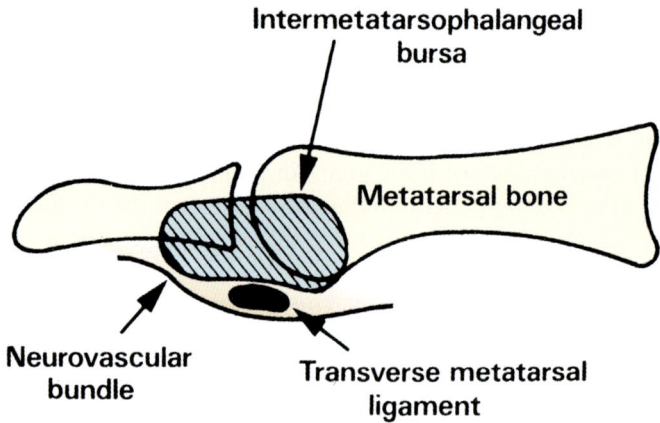

Figure 6.11 **Diagram of longitudinal section of the third–fourth web space.** Note relationship of bursa and neurovascular bundle. (Adapted from Bossley CJ, Cairney PC. The intermetatarsophalangeal bursa: Its significance in Morton's metatarsalgia. *J Bone Joint Surg Br.* 1980;62[2]:184.)

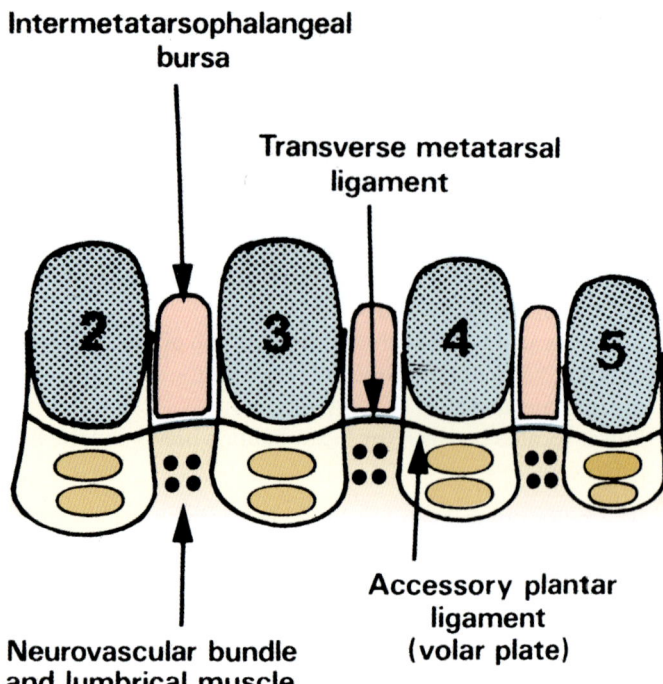

Figure 6.12 Diagram of transverse section across metatarsal necks. (Adapted from Bossley CJ, Cairney PC. The intermetatarsophalangeal bursa: Its significance in Morton's metatarsalgia. *J Bone Joint Surg Br.* 1980;62[2]:184.)

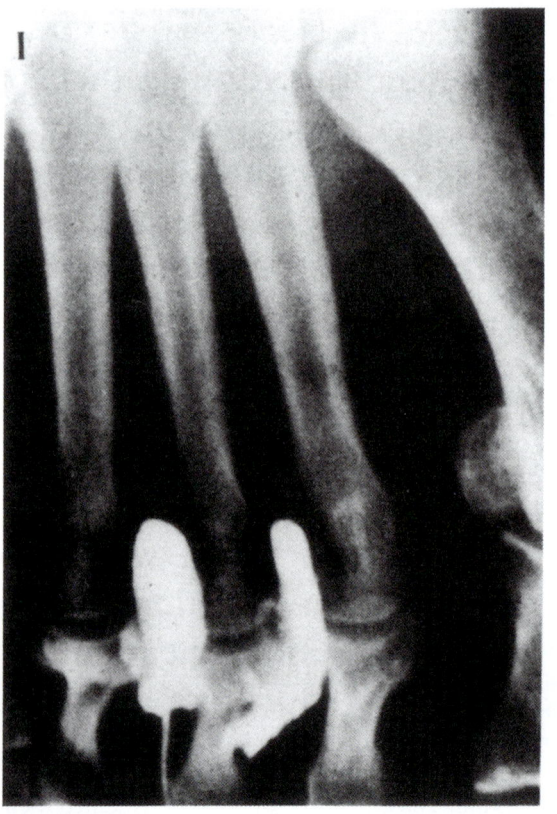
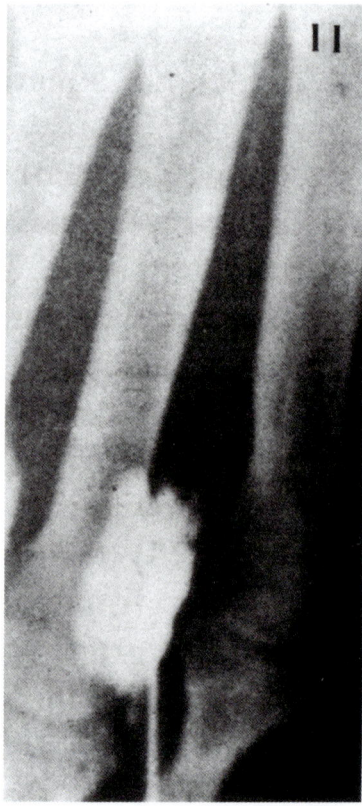

Figure 6.13 **(A)** Dye in intermetatarsophalangeal bursae in second–third and third–fourth web spaces. **(B)** Dye in bursa in fourth–fifth web space. Note that the distal end of the bursa is level with the joint. (Republished with permission of British Editorial Society of Bone and Joint Surgery, From Bossley CJ, Cairney PC. The intermetatarsophalangeal bursa: Its significance in Morton's metatarsalgia. *J Bone Joint Surg Br.* 1980;62[2]:184; permission conveyed through Copyright Clearance Center, Inc.)

Claustre and colleagues made an anatomic study of the intercapitometatarsal space in 25 ft and confirmed the existence of the intercapitometatarso bursa.[15] In the first and fourth interspaces, the bursa does not extend beyond the distal border of the deep transverse metatarsal ligament, whereas in the second and third interspaces, it extends 1 cm distal to the ligament. Midy and colleagues and Chauveaux and coworkers confirmed the presence of the supratransverse intermetatarsocapite bursa in an anatomic study of 25 ft.[16,17] In 14 ft suitable for dissection, the bursa was demonstrated in the second and third interspaces in 100%, whereas the bursa was present in the fourth interspace in 78.5% and in the first interspace in 71.4%. The bursa is dorsal to the deep transverse metatarsal ligament and is oval or elliptic with a greater anteroposterior sagittal axis. The length of the bursa is 2 to 3 cm for the second and third spaces and 2 cm for the first and fourth spaces. The height is 1 cm and the width is 0.5 to 1 cm in the coronal plane. The wall of the bursa is very fragile, almost soap bubble-like. In the second and third interspaces, the bursa extends beyond the distal border of the deep transverse metatarsal ligament and reaches the proximal phalanx, thus becoming an intermetatarsophalangeal bursa. In the fourth space, the bursa is located behind the posterior border of the ligament and is purely intermetatarsal in location. In the first space, it is in midposition, not extending beyond the anterior border of the ligament.

REFERENCES

1. Hartman H. Die Sehnenscheiden und synovialsäcke des fusses. *Morphol Arbeit.* 1896;5:214.
2. Poirier P, Charpy A. *Traité d'Anatomie humaine.* Vol 2. Masson; 1901:302-305.
3. Lovell AGH, Tanner HH. Synovial membranes with special reference to those related to the tendons of the foot and ankle. *J Anat.* 1908;42:414.
4. Testut L. *Traité d'Anatomie Humaine.* Vol 2. 7th ed. Doin; 1921: 1006-1007.
5. Broström L. Sprained ankles: II. Arthrographic diagnosis of recent ligament ruptures. *Acta Chir Scand.* 1965;129:485.
6. Prins JG. Diagnosis and treatment of injury to the lateral ligament of the ankle: a comparative clinical study. *Acta Chir Scand Suppl.* 1978;486:81.
7. Pascoet G. L'arthrografie tibio-tarsienne dans la traumatologie capsuloligamentaire du coup de pied. *Rev Chir Orthop [Suppl].* 1975;2:142.
8. Ziegler EM. Zur morphologie der vincula tendinum an menschlichen zehen erwachsener. *Anat Anz Bd.* 1972;130:404.
9. Jones FW. *Structure and Function as Seen in the Foot.* 2nd ed. Baillière, Tindall & Cox; 1949:229-245.
10. Chemin. Recherches sur les gaines synoviales tendineuses du pied. *Soc Biol Comptes Rendus.* 1896;3:237.
11. Testut L, Jacob O. *Traité d'Anatomie Topographique avec Applications Médico-Chirurgicales.* Vol. 2. Doin; 1909:1032-1033, 1036.
12. Gregoire R. Recherches sur la bourse sereuse sous-calcaneenne. *Bull Soc Anat Paris.* 1911;86:724.
13. Schreger. *De Bursis Mucosis Subcutaneis.* Erlangen; 1825.
14. Bossley CJ, Cairney PC. The intermetatarsophalangeal bursa: its significance in Morton's metatarsalgia. *J Bone Joint Surg Br.* 1980;62:184.
15. Claustre J, Bonnel F, Constans JP, et al. L'espace intercapito-metatarsien: aspects anatomiques et pathologiques. *Revue Rhumatologique.* 1983; 50:435.
16. Midy D, Chauveaux D, Le Huec JC. Etude des bourses sereuses intercapitometatarsiennes sus-transversaires. *Bull Assoc Anat (Nancy).* 1986;70(209):37.
17. Chauveaux D, Le Huec JC, Midy D. The supra-transverse intermetatarsocapital bursa: a description and its relation to painful syndromes of the forefoot. *Surg Radiol Anat.* 1987;9:13.

Angiology

Shahan K. Sarrafian and Armen S. Kelikian

ARTERIES

The arterial blood supply to the ankle and the foot (Fig. 7.1) is provided by three arteries: posterior tibial, anterior tibial, and peroneal.

The tibial arteries are the major suppliers of the foot, but the peroneal artery may predominate when the anterior and posterior tibial arteries are atrophic or absent in their distal segments. As described by Dubreuil-Chambardel, the anterior branch of the peroneal artery or perforating branch may supply the dorsalis pedis artery or the posterior branch of the peroneal artery may be the only supplier of the plantar arteries.[1] When the terminal segments of the posterior and anterior tibial arteries are absent simultaneously, the peroneal artery with its anterior and posterior branches is the sole supplier of the dorsal and plantar arterial network (Fig. 7.2).

The posterior tibial artery may be greatly attenuated or absent (Table 7.1). Adachi reports the absence of the posterior tibial artery as being nearly 2% (10 cases in 486 feet).[2] Dubreuil-Chambardel has never encountered a complete absence of the posterior tibial artery.[1]

The anterior tibial artery may be a very thin vessel distally or may terminate in the midleg, thus leaving the entire supply of the dorsum of the foot to the perforating branch of the peroneal artery. Such a variation occurs with the frequency shown in Table 7.2.

The peroneal artery is diminished in volume with the frequency shown in Table 7.3. Dubreuil-Chambardel has never seen this artery completely absent.[1] Edwards mentions that "either of its two terminal branches—the perforating or the posterior lateral malleolar—may be missing."[3]

▶ Dorsal Arterial Network of the Foot and Ankle

The dorsal arterial network of the foot is extremely variable, but these variations can be superimposed almost constantly on a general pattern termed "a very constant pattern," "a potential arterial pattern," or "a grundform."[1-4] As Huber points out, "any part of that network might be encountered as a vessel of significant size."[4]

The general pattern of this network is shown in Figure 7.3.[4] At the ankle joint interline, the anterior tibial artery is continued by the dorsalis pedis artery, which extends along an axis drawn from the middle of the transverse bimalleolar axis to the tip of the first intermetatarsal space. The dorsalis pedis artery gives origin at the level of the ankle to the anterior malleolar arteries, both medial and lateral. During its pedal course, the dorsalis pedis artery provides the following branches from its lateral side: artery to the sinus tarsi, lateral tarsal artery, artery to the proximal segment of the second intermetatarsal space, arcuate artery, and artery to the first intermetatarsal space.

The artery of the sinus tarsi may arise directly from the dorsalis pedis artery at the level of the talar neck. Directed transversely, it enters the sinus tarsi.

The lateral tarsal artery also originates at the level of the talar neck; it courses obliquely laterally and distally to the dorsum of the cuboid and divides into three longitudinal branches reaching the proximal segments of intermetatarsal spaces 2, 3, and 4.

The medial tarsal arteries, proximal and distal, as described by Huber (see Fig. 7.3) emanate from the medial aspect of the dorsalis pedis artery.[4] The proximal medial tarsal artery branches off from the dorsalis pedis artery at the level of the navicular and courses transversely. The distal medial tarsal artery originates from the dorsalis pedis artery at the level of C_2 and runs obliquely to the dorsum of C_1.

The artery to the proximal segment of the second intermetatarsal space takes off at the level of the middle cuneiform. It crosses the base of the second metatarsal and reaches the second intermetatarsal space. This longitudinal branch is connected to the first division branch of the lateral tarsal artery with a transverse branch on the dorsum of the lateral cuneiform.

The arcuate artery originates at the level of the first tarsometatarsal joint and transversely crosses the bases of the second, third, and fourth metatarsals. The arterial arcade is joined by the previously described longitudinal branches of the lateral tarsal artery. The arcuate artery gives origin to the proximal perforating arteries in intermetatarsal spaces 2, 3, and 4 and to the second, third, and fourth dorsal metatarsal arteries. The latter give a set of perforating branches proximal to the

Chapter 7: Angiology

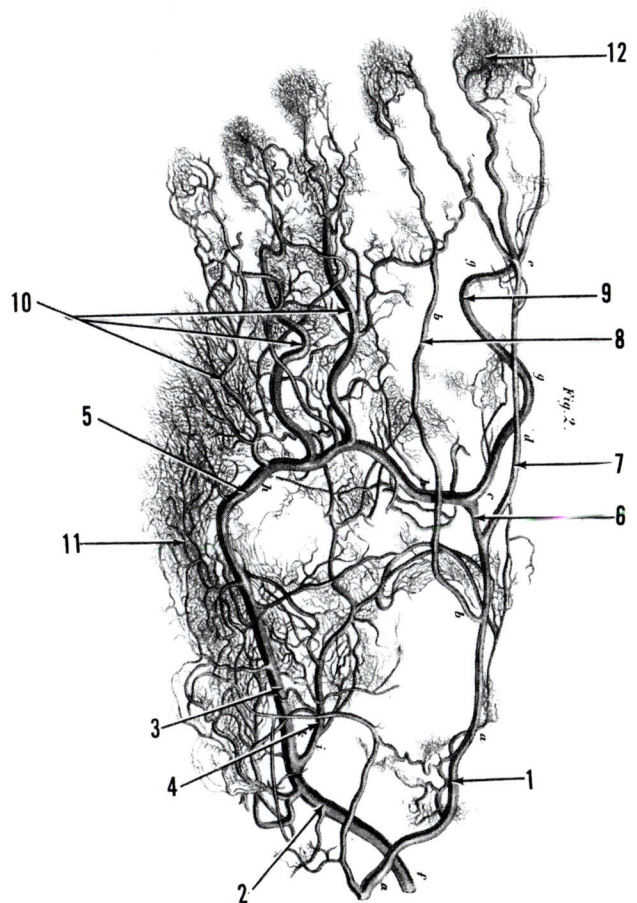

Figure 7.1 **Arterial tree of the foot, corrosion study.** (*1*, dorsalis pedis artery; *2*, posterior tibial artery; *3*, lateral plantar artery; *4*, medial plantar artery; *5*, plantar arc, deep; *6*, first proximal perforating artery; *7*, first dorsal interosseous artery; *8*, second dorsal interosseous artery; *9*, first plantar interosseous artery; *10*, plantar metatarsal arteries; *11*, dense arterial network of lateral border of foot; *12*, anastomotic network at level of pulp of big toe.) (From Hyrtl J. *Die Corrosions: Anatomie und Ihre Ergebnisse.* Braumüller; 1873:249.)

TABLE 7.2 Frequency of Absent or Very Thin Anterior Tibial Artery		
Author	Number of Feet	Frequency (%)
Dubreuil-Chambardel	165	2.4
Adachi	1239	7.1
Huber	200	3
Salvi	200	3
Schwalbe and Pfitzner	213	3.8
Quain	199	5.5
Total	2216	5.27

and forms the first proximal perforating artery. The first dorsal metatarsal artery provides two lateral branches to the first metatarsal and one anastomotic branch to the medial aspect of the second metatarsal neck. Farther distally, at the level of the web space, the artery divides into the dorsal digital artery of the big toe—providing both its dorsolateral and dorsomedial branches—and the dorsomedial artery of the second toe. The first dorsal metatarsal artery finally gives the first distal perforating artery. From its medial side, the dorsalis pedis artery provides two medial tarsal arteries taking off at the level of the navicular and the first cuneiform.

The perforating branch of the peroneal artery crosses the distal segment of the tibiofibular interspace, passes over the anterior aspect of the tibiofibular syndesmosis, contours the anterior border of the lateral malleolus, and establishes communication with the lateral malleolar and lateral tarsal arteries.

The previously described standard pattern of distribution of the branches of the dorsalis pedis artery occurs in 5.5%.[4] Huber, in a study of 200 feet, grouped the possible variations of pattern according to the level of origin of the arcuate artery and the number of dorsal metatarsal arteries provided by the latter. The individual arrangements are classified into the following four categories.

- *Group A* (35%) (Fig. 7.4): Arcuate artery arising at about the level of the first tarsometatarsal joint and giving rise to the following dorsal metatarsal arteries.
   - Group A_1 (16.5%): Dorsal metatarsal arteries 2, 3, and 4
   - Group A_2 (9%): Dorsal metatarsal arteries 2 and 3
   - Group A_3 (9.5%): Dorsal metatarsal artery 2
- *Group B* (19%) (see Fig. 7.4): Arcuate artery arising at about the level of the cuneonavicular joint, with the subgroups similar to those of group A.
   - Group B_1 (9%)
   - Group B_2 (6.5%)
   - Group B_3 (3.5%)

corresponding metatarsal heads, and farther distally, in the web space, they divide into the dorsal digital arteries. They give a perforating branch in the axis of the web space and a dorsoplantar anastomotic branch on the side of the corresponding proximal phalanx.

The first intermetatarsal artery or the first dorsal metatarsal artery continues the direction of the dorsalis pedis artery. At the base of the first intermetatarsal space, it plunges plantarward

TABLE 7.1 Frequency of Absent or Very Thin Posterior Tibial Artery		
Author	Number of Feet	Frequency (%)
Adachi	486	4.9 ± 0.98
Quain	211 ⎫	
Manno	66 ⎬ 380	8.4 ± 1.42
Dubreuil-Chambardel	103 ⎭	
Total	866	6.35

TABLE 7.3 Frequency of Very Thin Peroneal Artery		
Author	Number of Feet	Frequency (%)
Quain	208	2.8
Dubreuil-Chambardel	103	3.8

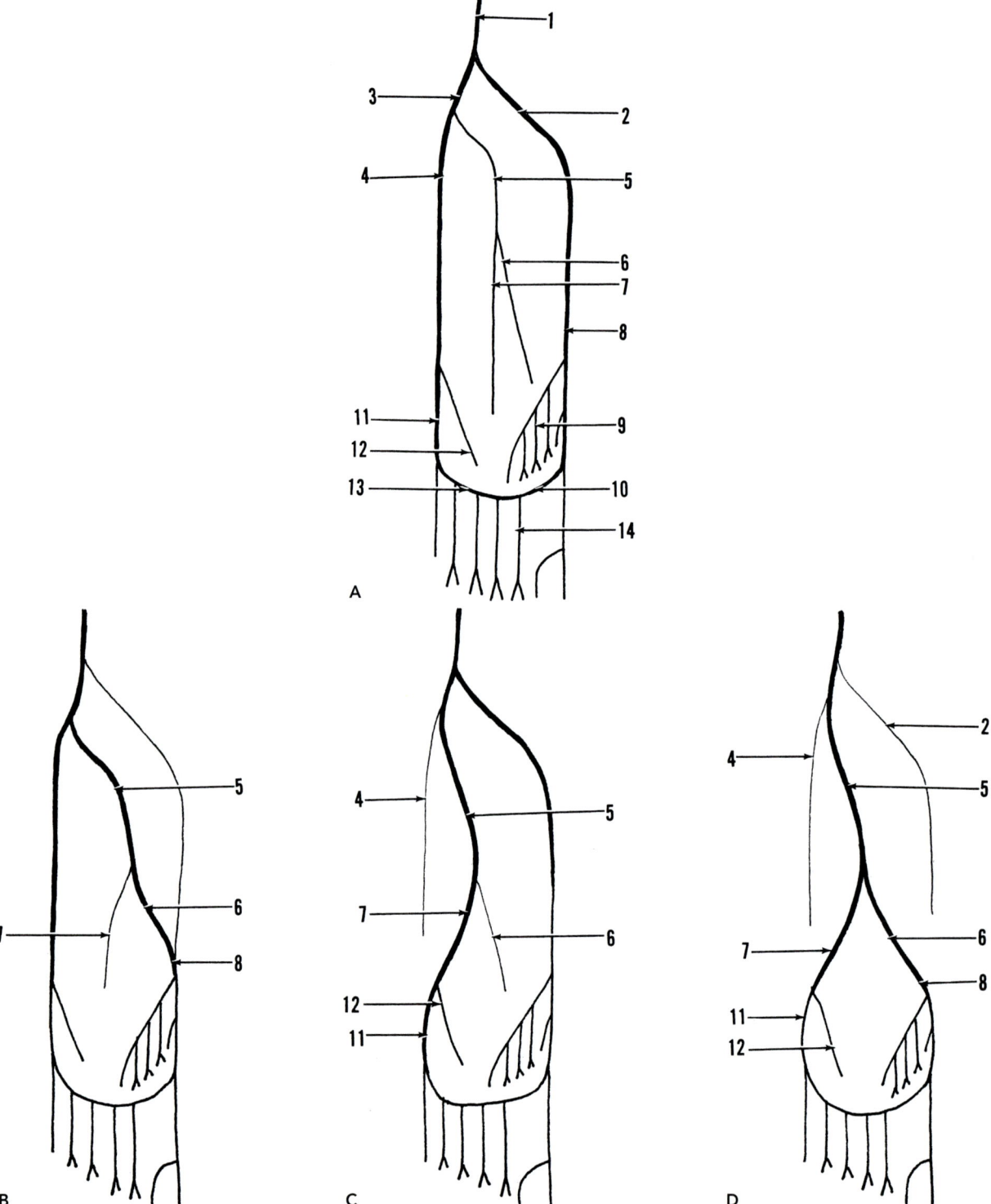

Figure 7.2 **Variations of the arteries of the leg and foot. (A)** Habitual pattern. (*1*, popliteal artery; *2*, anterior tibial artery; *3*, tibioperoneal arterial trunk; *4*, posterior tibial artery; *5*, peroneal artery; *6*, anterior peroneal artery; *7*, posterior peroneal artery; *8*, dorsalis pedis artery; *9*, dorsal metatarsal arteries; *10*, perforating artery of first interspace; *11*, lateral plantar artery; *12*, medial plantar artery; *13*, deep plantar arterial arc; *14*, first plantar metatarsal artery.) **(B)** The dorsalis pedis artery (*8*) is provided by the anterior peroneal artery (*6*). (*5*, peroneal artery; *7*, posterior peroneal artery.) **(C)** The posterior peroneal artery (*7*) supplies the lateral and medial plantar arteries (*11* and *12*). (*4*, posterior tibial artery, incomplete; *5*, peroneal artery, well developed; *6*, anterior peroneal artery.) **(D)** The peroneal artery (*5*) supplies the dorsalis pedis artery (*8*) through the anterior peroneal artery (*6*) and the plantar arteries (*11* and *12*) through the posterior peroneal artery (*7*). The anterior tibial artery (*2*) and the posterior tibial artery (*4*) are incomplete or absent. (From Dubreuil-Chambardel L. *Variations des Artères du Pelvis et du Membre Inférieur*. Maison; 1902:246.)

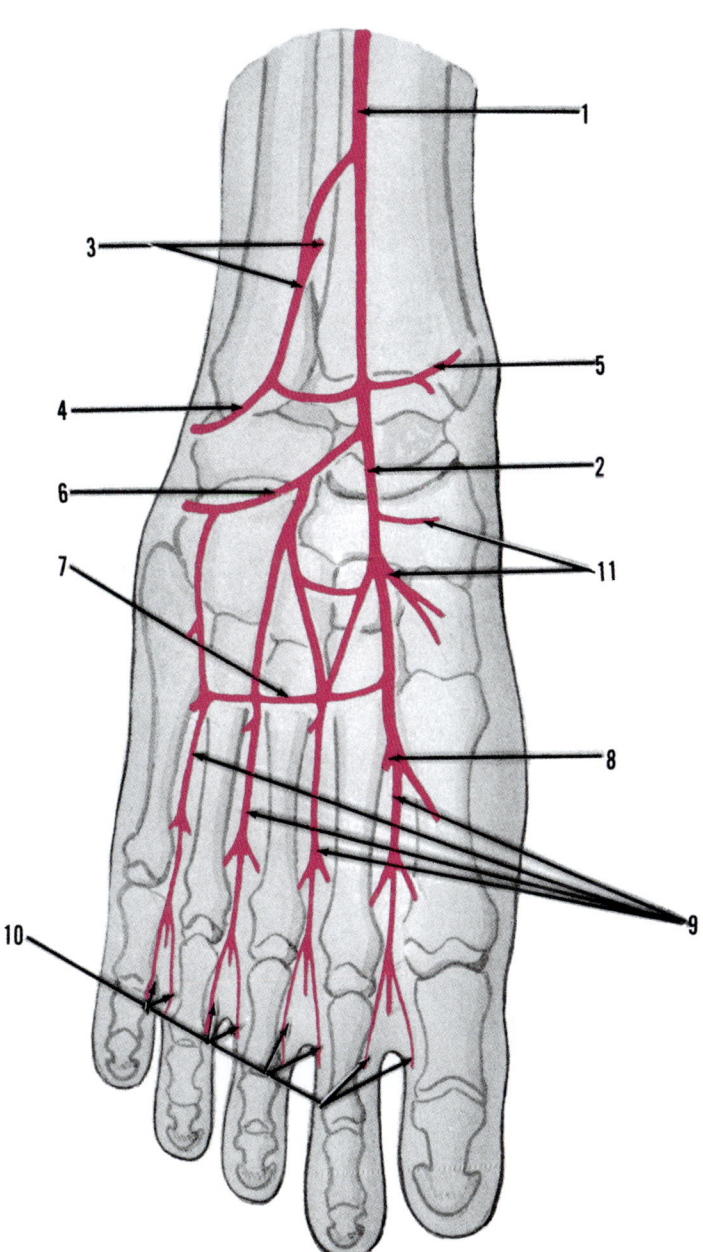

Figure 7.3 **The arterial network of the dorsum of the foot, general or potential pattern.** (*1*, anterior tibial artery; *2*, dorsalis pedis artery; *3*, anterior or perforating peroneal artery; *4*, anterior lateral malleolar artery; *5*, anterior medial malleolar artery; *6*, lateral tarsal artery; *7*, arcuate artery; *8*, first proximal perforating artery; *9*, dorsal metatarsal arteries; *10*, dorsal digital arteries; *11*, medial tarsal arteries.) (From Huber JF. The arterial network supplying the dorsum of the foot. *Anat Rec.* 1941;80:373. By permission of Alan R. Liss, Publisher.)

- *Group C* (34%) (Fig. 7.5): No arcuate artery present.
- *Group D* (12%) (see Fig. 7.5): Dorsalis pedis artery practically absent.

Adachi describes the "grundform" of the rete of the dorsalis pedis (Fig. 7.6) as formed transversely by the proximal lateral tarsal artery, the distal lateral tarsal artery, and the arcuate artery. These transverse or oblique components are anastomosed by three sagittal or longitudinal arteries, forming a complex network. The longitudinal arteries run parallel to the dorsalis pedis artery; they may be very thin, or one or two branches may be missing. These arteries continue as the dorsal metatarsal arteries and give off the proximal or posterior perforating arteries. The distal lateral tarsal artery is usually insignificant in size. When the sagittal arteries are thin, the supply to the dorsal metatarsal arteries is provided by the proximal perforating arteries. When the dorsal metatarsal arteries are thin, the proximal perforating arterial branches are also rudimentary.

Dorsalis Pedis Artery

At the level of the ankle joint interline, the anterior tibial artery is continued by the dorsalis pedis artery, which runs along a line extending from the middle of the transverse malleolar line to the proximal end of the first intermetatarsal space. During its course, the artery passes across the talus, the navicular, the second cuneiform, and the base of the second metatarsal. It penetrates the first intermetatarsal space limited anteriorly by the arch formed by the first dorsal

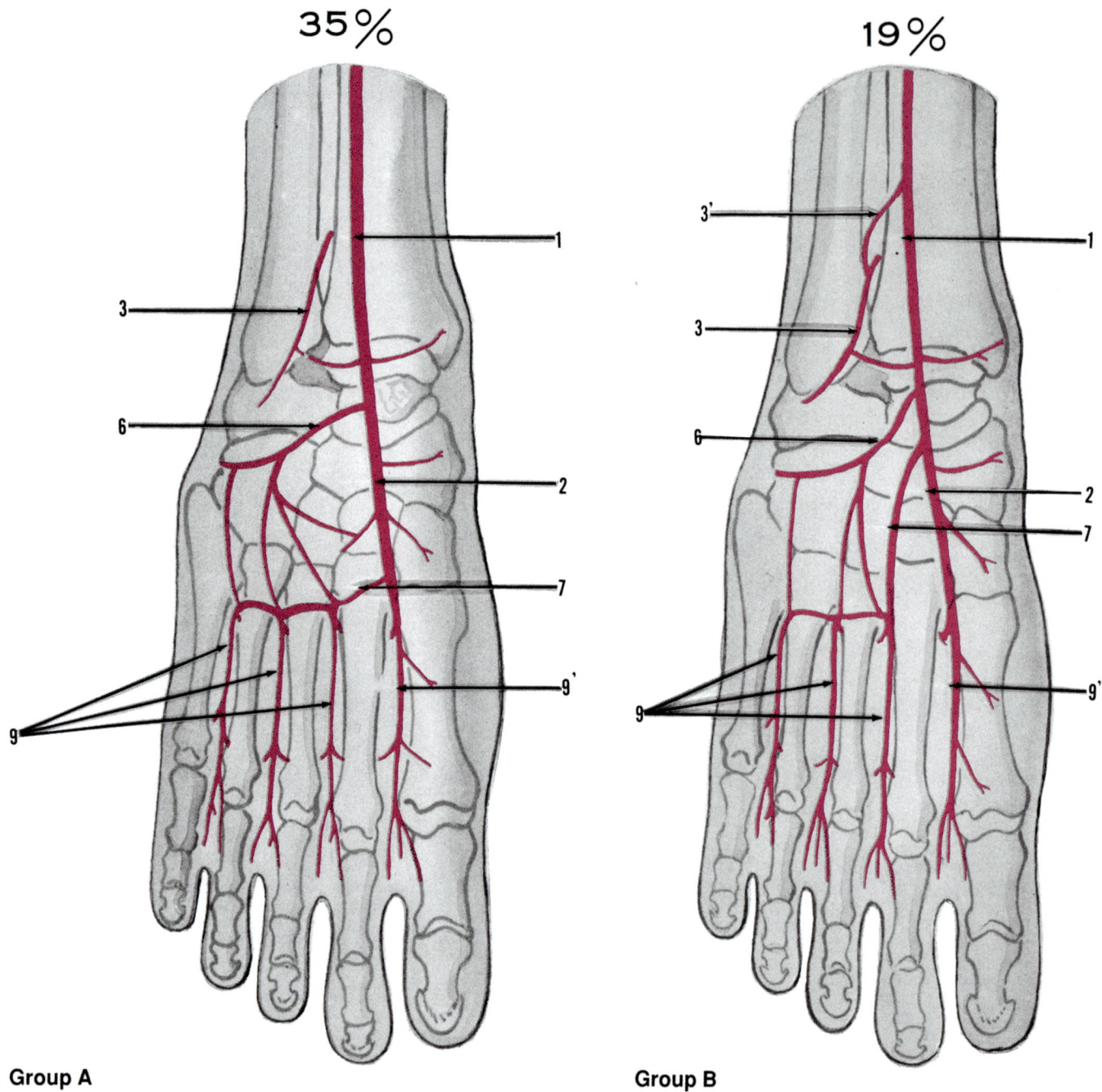

Figure 7.4 Variations of the arterial pattern on the dorsum of the foot. (*Group A*) Arcuate artery (7) arising at about the level of the first tarsometatarsal joint and giving rise to the dorsal metatarsal arteries 2, 3, and 4 (9). (*1*, anterior tibial artery; *2*, dorsalis pedis artery; *3*, anterior peroneal artery; *6*, lateral tarsal artery; *9'*, first dorsal metatarsal artery.) (*Group B*) Arcuate artery (7) arising at about the level of the cuneonavicular joint and providing the dorsal metatarsal arteries 2, 3, and 4 (9). (From Huber JF. The arterial network supplying the dorsum of the foot. *Anat Rec.* 1941;80:373. By permission of Alan R. Liss, Publisher.)

interosseous muscle and posteriorly by the base of the first and second metatarsals. It terminates by inosculation with the lateral plantar artery after making two 90° turns—one vertical and one horizontal-lateral. This standard course of the artery occurs in 73.5%.[4]

Variations

From a study of 200 feet, Huber reports the absence of the dorsalis pedis artery in 12% (see Fig. 7.5).[4] Adachi, from a group of 230 feet, reports a very thin dorsalis pedis artery in 3% (Fig. 7.7).[2]

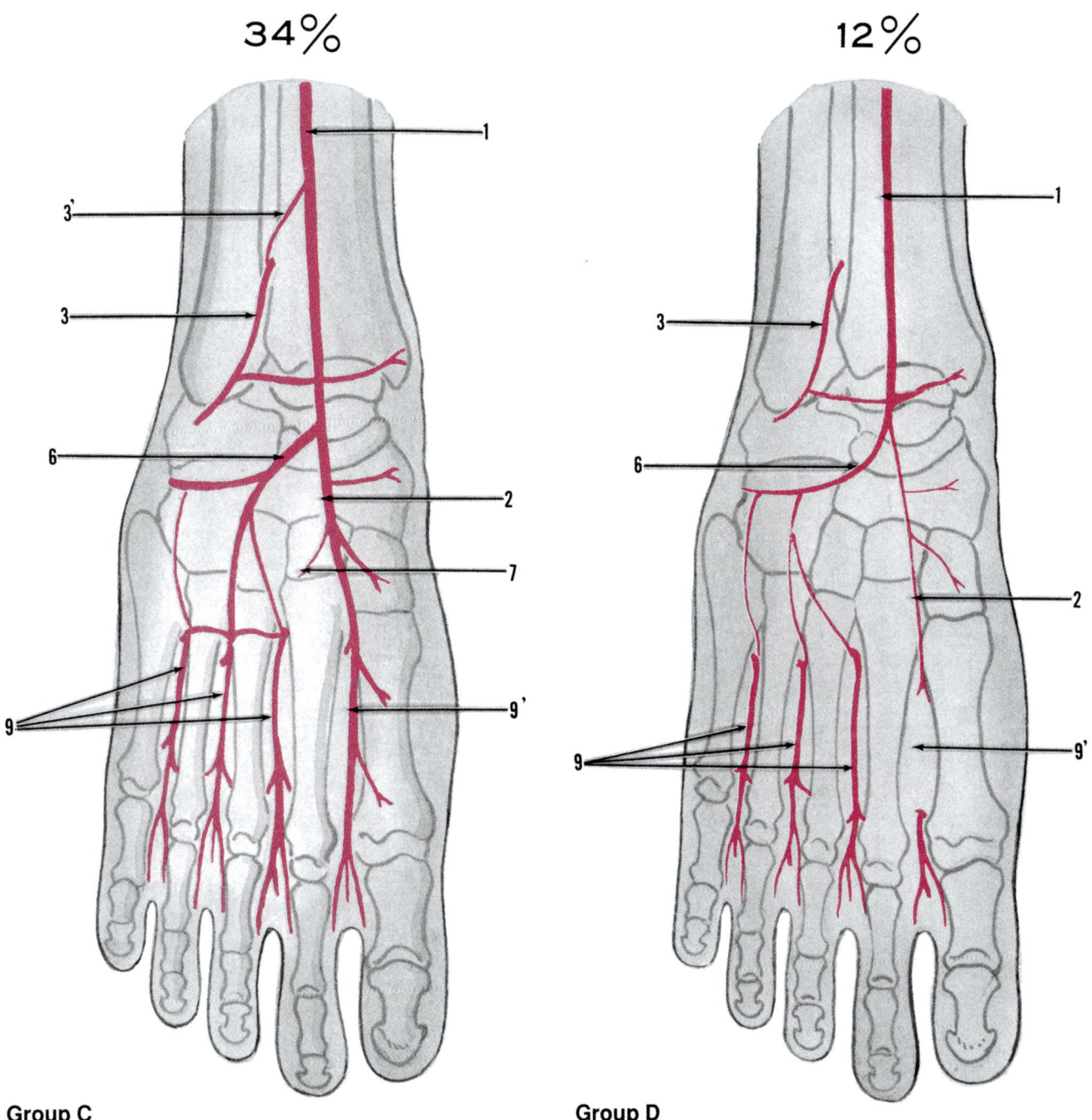

Figure 7.5 Variations of the arterial pattern on the dorsum of the foot. (*Group C*) Absent arcuate artery (*7*). (*1*, anterior tibial artery; *2*, dorsalis pedis artery; *3*, anterior peroneal artery; *3'*, anastomotic branch between anterior tibial artery and anterior peroneal artery; *6*, lateral tarsal artery providing dorsal metatarsal arteries 2, 3, and 4 (*9*); *9'*, first dorsal metatarsal artery.) (*Group D*) Practically absent dorsalis pedis artery (*2*). (*1*, anterior tibial artery; *3*, anterior peroneal artery; *6*, lateral tarsal artery; *9*, dorsal metatarsal arteries 2, 3, and 4; *9'*, absent first dorsal metatarsal artery.) (From Huber JF. The arterial network supplying the dorsum of the foot. *Anat Rec.* 1941;80:373. By permission of Alan R. Liss, Publisher.)

Lateral deviation of the artery occurs in 5.5%.[4] Such cases are also described by Dubreuil-Chambardel (1.8%) and Adachi (0.4%) (Fig. 7.8A).[1,2]

Medial deviation of the artery occurs in 3.5%.[4]

In about 5% (as mentioned previously), the tibialis anterior artery is absent or filiform in the distal segment, and the dorsalis pedis artery is supplied by the perforating branch of the peroneal artery (Fig. 7.9A).

The lower end of the anterior tibial artery is in the position of the perforating peroneal artery in 1.5% (Fig. 7.9B).[4]

The artery arises equally from the anterior tibial and the perforating peroneal artery in 0.5% (Fig. 7.10A).[4]

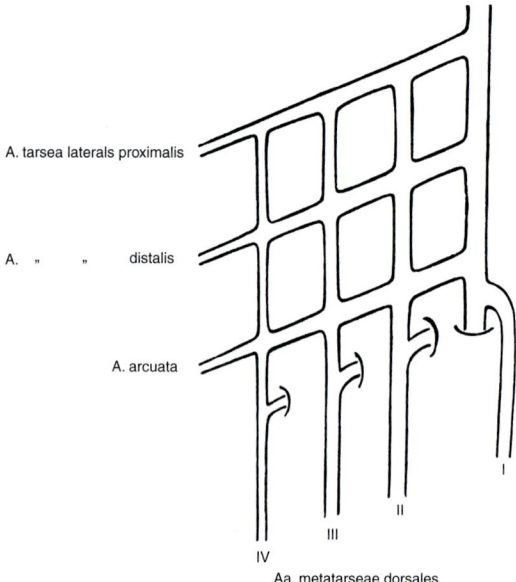

Figure 7.6 "Grundform" of the rete of the dorsalis pedis artery formed by the transversely oriented proximal, distal, and lateral tarsal arteries and the arcuate arteries connected by longitudinally oriented anastomotic branches and the dorsalis pedis artery. (From Adachi B. *Das Arteriensystem der Japaner*. Maruzen; 1928:251.)

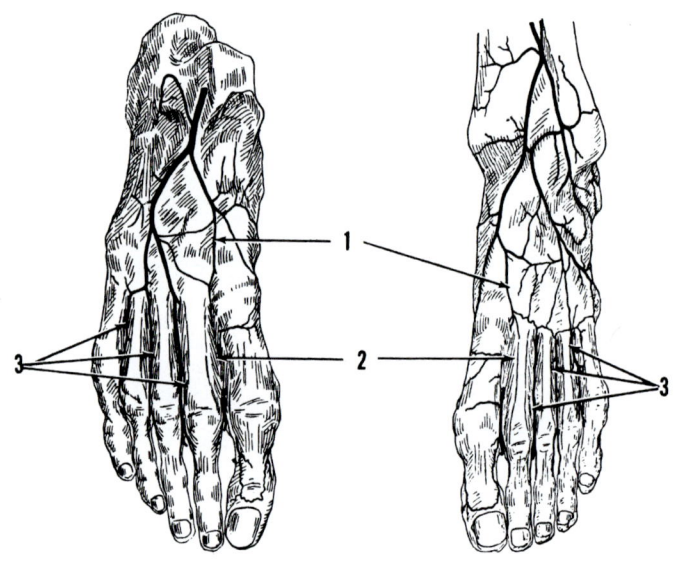

Figure 7.7 Very thin dorsalis pedis artery (*1*) and absent first dorsal metatarsal artery (*2*). (*3*, dorsal metatarsal arteries 2, 3, and 4.) (From Adachi B. *Das Arteriensystem der Japaner*. Maruzen; 1928:246-248.)

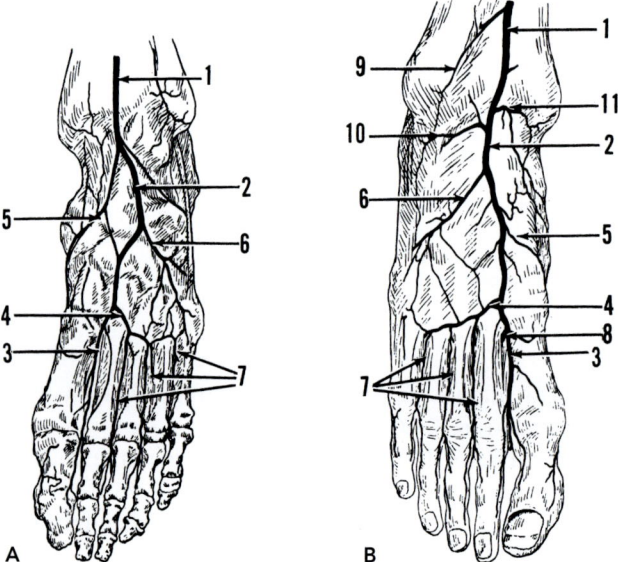

Figure 7.8 **(A) Lateral deviation of the dorsalis pedis artery. (B) General pattern of arterial distribution on the dorsum of the foot.** (*1*, anterior tibial artery; *2*, dorsalis pedis artery; *3*, first dorsal interosseous artery; *4*, arcuate artery; *5*, medial tarsal artery; *6*, lateral tarsal artery; *7*, dorsal metatarsal arteries 2, 3, and 4; *8*, first proximal perforating artery; *9*, anterior peroneal artery; *10*, anterior lateral malleolar artery; *11*, anterior medial malleolar artery.) (From Adachi B. *Das Arteriensystem der Japaner*. Maruzen; 1928:243.)

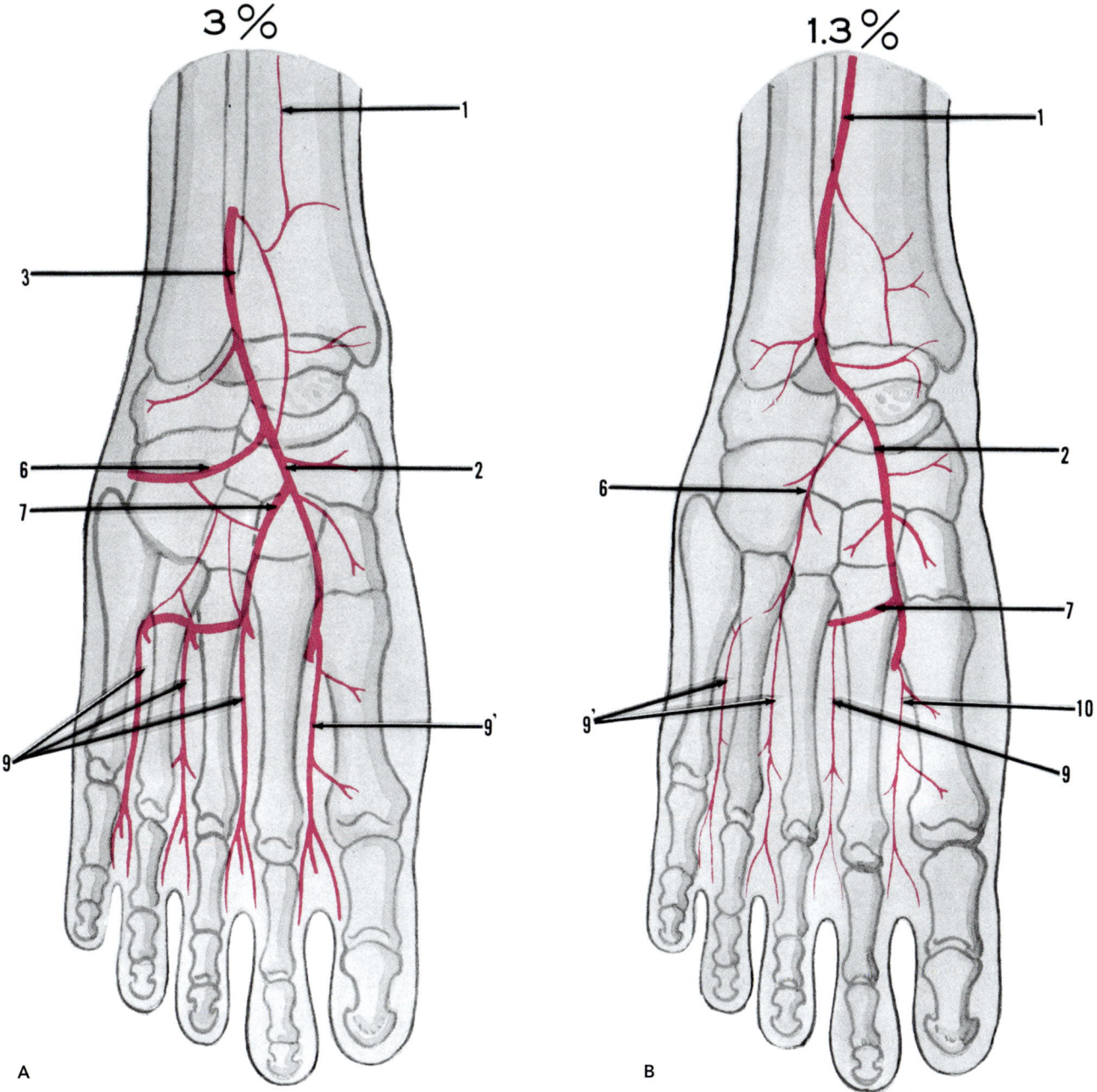

Figure 7.9 Variations of the arterial pattern on the dorsum of the foot. **(A)** Absent or filiform anterior tibial artery (*1*). The dorsalis pedis artery (*2*) is supplied by the anterior peroneal artery (*3*). (*6*, lateral tarsal artery; *7*, arcuate artery supplying the dorsal metatarsal arteries 2, 3, and 4 (*9*); *9'*, first dorsal metatarsal artery.) **(B)** The lower end of the anterior tibial artery (*1*) is in the position of the perforating peroneal artery. (*2*, dorsalis pedis artery; *6*, lateral tarsal artery supplying the dorsal metatarsal arteries 3 and 4; *7*, arcuate artery supplying second dorsal metatarsal artery [*9*]; *10*, first dorsal metatarsal artery.) (From Huber JF. The arterial network supplying the dorsum of the foot. *Anat Rec.* 1941;80:373. By permission of Alan R. Liss, Publisher.)

In very rare instances, the dorsalis pedis artery is formed by a branch of the posterior tibial artery passing around the medial malleolus and reaching the dorsum of the foot. This vessel is anastomosed by a transverse branch on the dorsum of the scaphoid, with the perforating branch of the peroneal artery supplying, in turn, the second, third, and fourth dorsal metatarsal arteries (Fig. 7.11).[1]

Caliber

The usual diameter of the dorsalis pedis artery is 2 to 3 mm, and in 6% of 50 feet, it was very small, not exceeding 1.5 mm.[5] The average diameter of the same artery at the upper limit of the extensor retinaculum is given as 2.79 mm.[6]

The continuation of the dorsalis pedis artery after giving off the lateral tarsal artery is reported by Adachi (230 feet) as being

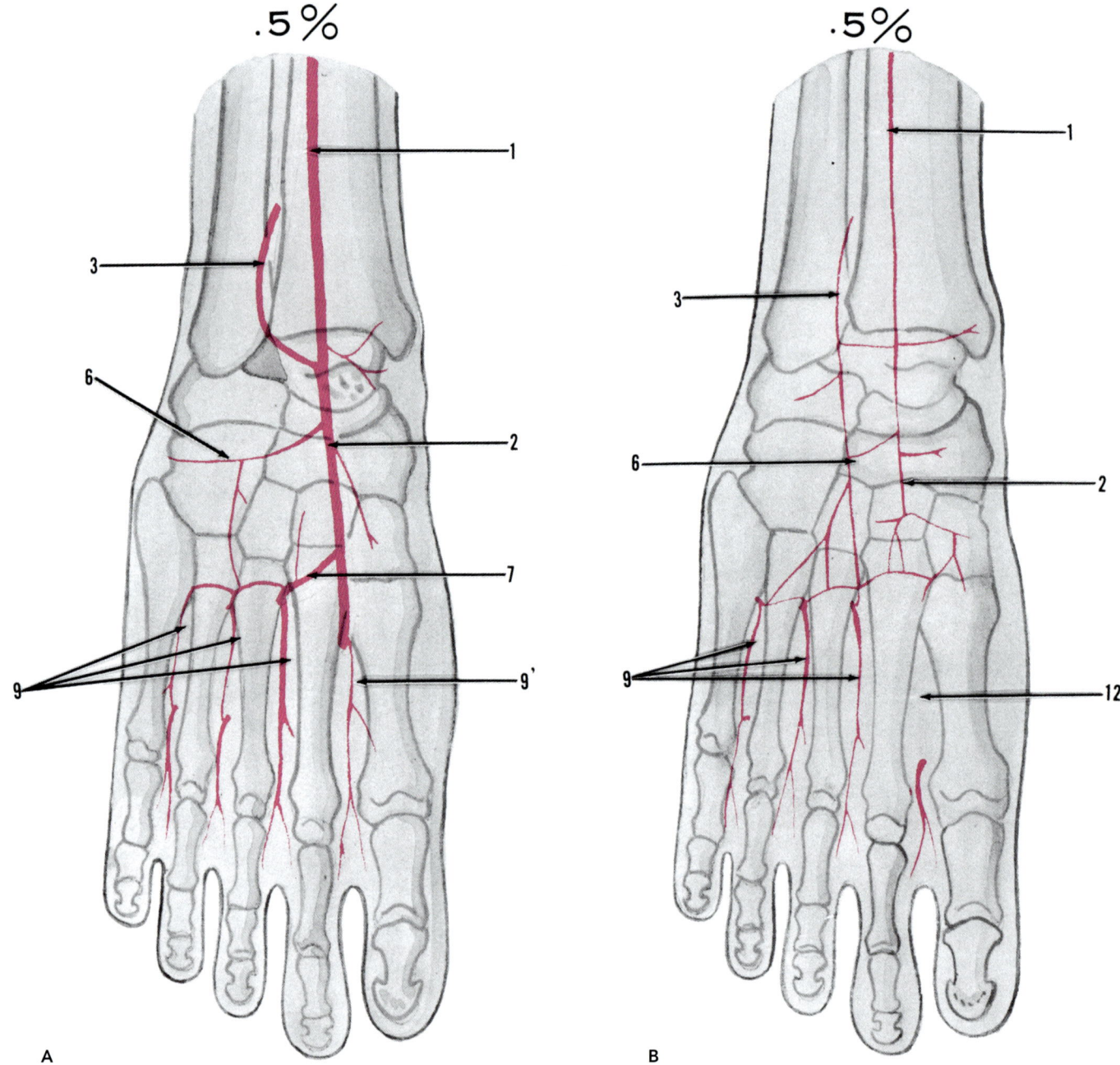

Figure 7.10 Variations of the arterial pattern on the dorsum of the foot. (A) The dorsalis pedis artery (*1*) arises equally from the anterior tibial artery (*1*) and the perforating peroneal artery (*3*). (*6*, lateral tarsal artery; *7*, arcuate artery; *9*, dorsal metatarsal arteries 2, 3, and 4; *9′*, first dorsal metatarsal artery.) **(B)** The lateral tarsal artery (*6*) is in continuity with the perforating peroneal artery (*3*). (*2*, incomplete dorsalis pedis artery; *9*, dorsal metatarsal arteries 2, 3, and 4 supplied by *6*; *12*, absent first dorsal metatarsal artery.) (From Huber JF. The arterial network supplying the dorsum of the foot. *Anat Rec.* 1941;80:373.)

larger than the latter in 86.5%, equal in 8.3%, and smaller in 5.2%.[2] Huber describes the lateral tarsal artery as being larger in 7% (200 feet).[4]

Lateral Tarsal Arteries

The lateral arteries are two, rarely three: it is the exception to have more than three.[2] The proximal lateral tarsal artery is the strongest. The second lateral tarsal artery is not significant and may be represented by only a connecting thin artery extending from the proximal lateral tarsal artery to the dorsalis pedis artery (Fig. 7.12).

Proximal

The proximal lateral tarsal artery originates from the dorsalis pedis at the level of the talar head, 0.5 cm proximal to this level (occasionally), or 0.5 cm distal (rarely).[2] This arterial branch

Chapter 7: Angiology 313

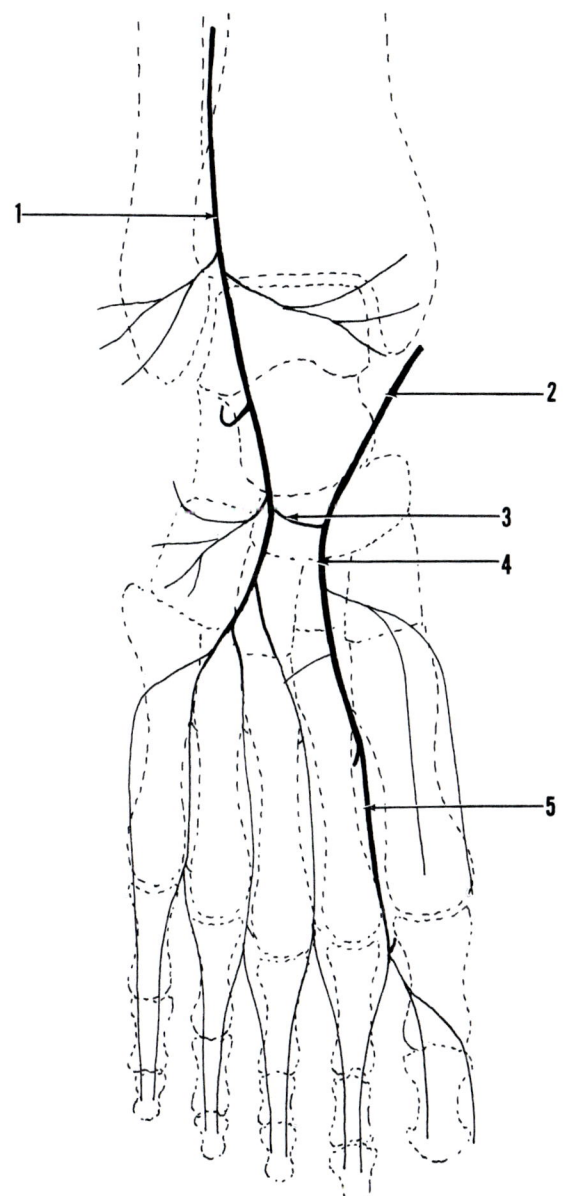

Figure 7.11 **Dorsalis pedis artery (4) formed by a branch of the posterior tibial artery (2) passing around the medial malleolus and reaching the dorsum of the foot.** (1, anterior peroneal artery; 3, anastomotic branch between 1 and 4; 5, first dorsal metatarsal artery.) (From Dubreuil-Chambardel L. *Variations des Artères du Pelvis et du Membre Inférieur*. 1902:225.)

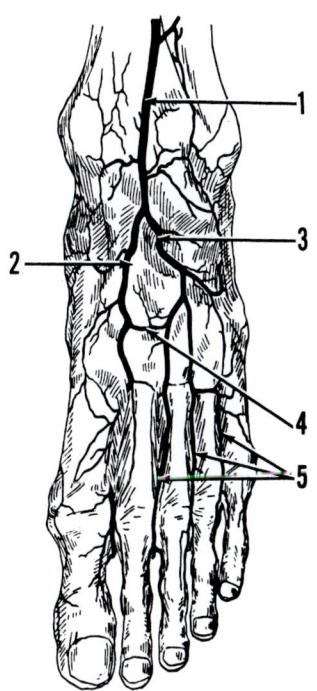

Figure 7.12 **Lateral tarsal arteries.** (1, anterior tibial artery; 2, dorsalis pedis artery; 3, proximal lateral tarsal artery; 4, distal lateral tarsal artery; 5, dorsal metatarsal arteries 2, 3, and 4.) (From Adachi B. *Das Arteriensystem der Japaner*. Maruzen; 1928:245.)

courses obliquely in a lateral and distal direction, crosses the calcaneonavicular junction and the dorsum of the cuboid, reaches the lateral border of the cuboid, passes under the peroneus brevis tendon, and anastomoses with the lateral plantar artery. At the level of the talar head, the proximal lateral tarsal artery provides arterial branches to the talar head and to the lateral anterior aspect of the talar body. In 21.7% to 32%, the artery provides direct origin to the artery of the sinus tarsi or forms with the perforating peroneal artery an arterial loop that gives origin to the artery of the sinus tarsi.[1,2,7] The artery forms an arterial anastomotic network in the tarsal sinus with contributions from the anterior lateral malleolar artery and the perforating peroneal artery. It also participates in the formation of the lateral malleolar arterial rete. At the level of the cuboid, the proximal lateral tarsal artery provides two, rarely three, longitudinal anastomotic branches with the arcuate artery; in some cases, these branches are large enough to continue distally as the fourth and third dorsal metatarsal arteries or, rarely, as the fourth, third, and second metatarsal arteries. The origin of the proximal lateral tarsal artery is variable and occurs at the following sites as reported by Huber in 200 feet: from the level of the junction of the talar head and neck, 58%; almost at the level of the ankle joint, 19.5%; from below the talonavicular joint, 19%; absent artery, 1.5%; extremely small artery, 1.5%; a continuation of the perforating peroneal artery, 0.5%.[4]

Gilbert et al,[8] in a comprehensive study, described the proximal lateral tarsal artery originating from the dorsalis pedis artery at the level of the talar neck in all 20 specimens. On the dorsum of the proximal-medial aspect of the cuboid, the proximal lateral tarsal divides into two branches—a longitudinal branch to the third intermetatarsal space and a transverse pedicle branch (unnamed previously).

The transverse pedicle branch courses the dorsum of the cuboid toward the groove for the peroneus longus tendon (Figs. 7.13 and 7.14). The artery provides an average of 15 nutrient vessels (range, 8-20 nutrient vessels) to the cuboid. It anastomoses at the lateral edge of the cuboid with the vertical descending segment of the anterior lateral malleolar artery and/or a branch of the lateral plantar artery. The division point of the longitudinal branch to the third intermetatarsal space and the transverse pedicle branch occurred, on average, 2 mm (range, 0-6 mm) lateral to the cuboid-third cuneiform joint.

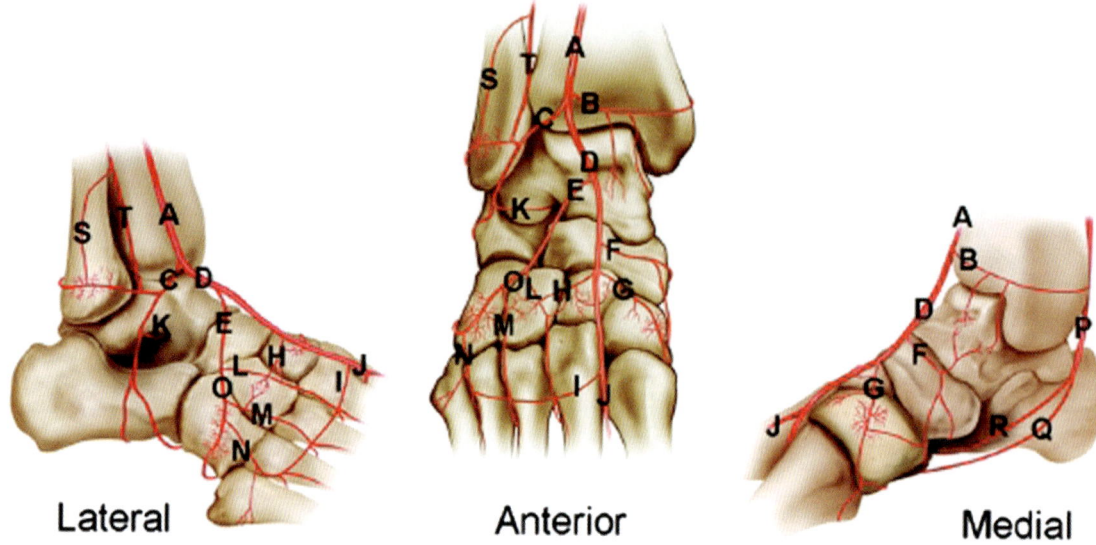

Figure 7.13 Overview of the extraosseous blood supply to the foot and ankle. (*A*, anterior tibial artery; *B*, anterior medial malleolar artery; *C*, anterior lateral malleolar artery; *D*, dorsalis pedis artery; *E*, proximal lateral tarsal artery; *F*, proximal medial tarsal artery; *G*, distal medial tarsal artery; *H*, distal lateral tarsal artery; *I*, arcuate artery; *J*, first dorsal metatarsal artery; *K*, artery of sinus tarsi; *L*, longitudinal branch to second intermetatarsal space; *M*, longitudinal branch to third intermetatarsal space; *N*, longitudinal branch to fourth intermetatarsal space; *O*, transverse pedicle branch; *P*, posterior tibial artery; *Q*, medial plantar artery; *R*, lateral plantar artery; *S*, fibular metaphyseal artery; *T*, perforating peroneal artery.) (From Gilbert BJ, Horst F, Nunley JA. Potential donor rotational bone graft using vascular territories in the foot and ankle. *J Bone Joint Surg Am.* 2004;86A[9]:1859, Figure 1.)

The average length of the proximal lateral tarsal artery from its origin from the dorsalis pedis to its division into the transverse pedicle branch and the longitudinal branch to the intermetatarsal space was 38 mm (range, 28-55 mm). The proximal lateral tarsal artery establishes communication with the second through fourth dorsal metatarsal arteries by way of three longitudinal branches to the second, third, and fourth intermetatarsal space. The longitudinal branch of the second intermetatarsal space anastomosed over the third cuneiform with the longitudinal branch to the second intermetatarsal space from the distal lateral tarsal artery (Fig. 7.15).

Distal

The origin of the distal lateral tarsal artery is very variable; it is often found on the dorsum of the second cuneiform or,

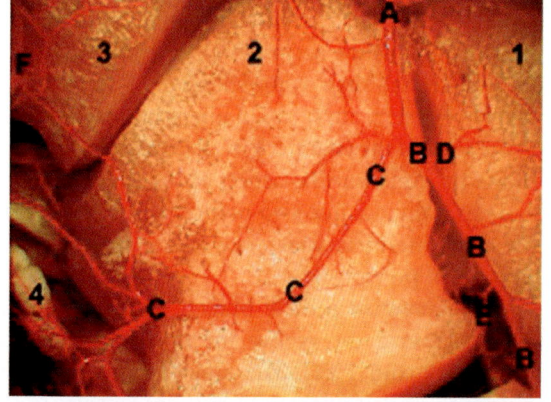
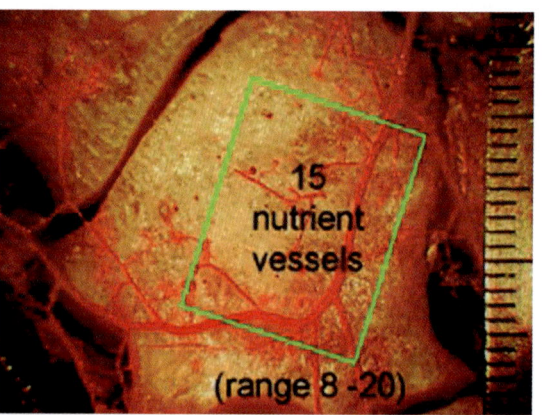

Figure 7.14 **(A) The dorsal extraosseous blood supply to the cuboid.** (*1*, third cuneiform; *2*, cuboid; *3*, calcaneus; *4*, os perineum; *A*, proximal lateral tarsal artery; *B*, longitudinal branch to the third intermetatarsal space; *C*, transverse pedicle branch; *D*, longitudinal branch to the second intermetatarsal space; *E*, longitudinal branch to the fourth intermetatarsal space; *F*, vertical descending branch of the anterior lateral malleolar artery.) **(B) The dorsal extraosseous supply to the cuboid in another specimen, with the vascular territory supplied by the transverse pedicle branch of the proximal lateral tarsal artery outlined in green.** (From Gilbert BJ, Horst F, Nunley JA. Potential donor rotational bone graft using vascular territories in the foot and ankle. *J Bone Joint Surg Am.* 2004;86A[9]:1861, Figure 3.)

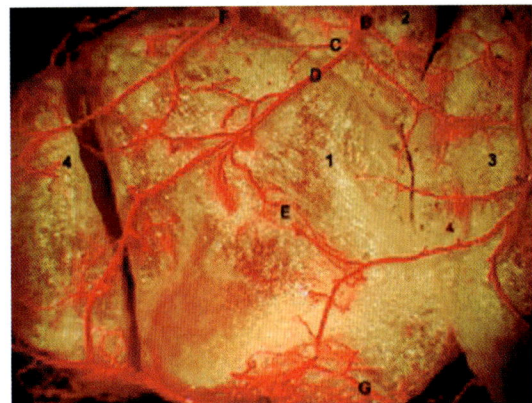
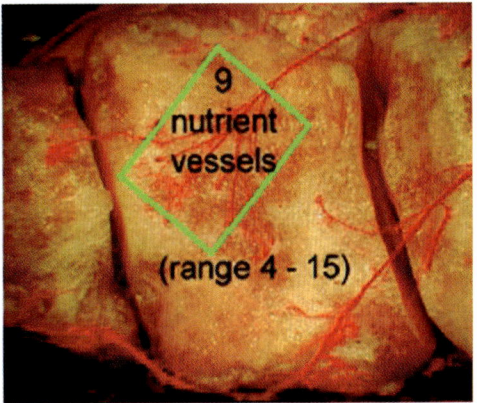

Figure 7.15 **(A) The extraosseous blood supply to the medial aspect of the first cuneiform.** (*1*, first cuneiform; *2*, second cuneiform; *3*, navicular; *4*, base of first metatarsal; *A*, proximal medial tarsal artery; *B*, distal medial tarsal artery; *C*, superomedial border branch of the distal medial tarsal artery; *D*, middle pedicle branch of the distal medial tarsal artery; *E*, inferior communicating branch of the distal medial tarsal artery; *F*, direct superomedial border branch of the dorsalis pedis artery; *G*, branch of the medial plantar artery.) **(B) The medial view of the extraosseous blood supplies the first cuneiform in another specimen, with the vascular territory supplied by the middle pedicle branch of the distal medial tarsal artery outlined in green.** (From Gilbert BJ, Horst F, Nunley JA. Potential donor rotational bone graft using vascular territories in the foot and ankle. *J Bone Joint Surg Am.* 2004;86A[9]:1862, Figure 4.)

occasionally, more proximal at the level of the $cuneo_2$-navicular joint.[2] The proximal lateral tarsal artery is usually larger than the distal, and Adachi provides the following information concerning their sizes in 230 feet: in 84%, the proximal lateral tarsal artery is larger; in 6%, the distal lateral tarsal artery is larger; in 10%, both are equal.[2]

The distal lateral artery as described by Gilbert et al[8] was present in all 20 specimens. It originates over the proximal half of the second cuneiform in 80% (16 specimens) and more proximally between the level of midnavicular and second cuneonavicular joint in 20% (4 specimens). From its origin, it courses across the dorsum of the second cuneiform (see Fig. 7.15) and provides its first branch medially, as the "lateral hook of the necklace to the second cuneiform," originating an average of 4 mm (range, 0-8 mm) medial to the articulation of the second and third cuneiforms. The distal lateral tarsal artery continues anterolaterally over the dorsomedial aspect of C_3 and divides into three branches—a plantar perforating branch, a transverse branch to C_3, and a longitudinal branch to the second intermetatarsal space.

The plantar perforating branch dives plantarward between C_2 and C_3 to anastomose with the plantar circulation and provide nutrient vessels to both of these bones. In 8 of 10 corrosion cast specimens, this branch originated directly from the distal lateral tarsal artery. In the other two specimens, it originated from the distal lateral longitudinal branch to the second intermetatarsal space.

The transverse branch crossed over the midsegment of C_3 and anastomosed with the longitudinal branch to the third intermetatarsal space (see Figs. 7.13 and 7.15A). This anastomosis was found in all specimens and occurred over the articulation of the cuboid and C_3 and provided an average of seven nutrient vessels (range, 2-11 nutrient vessels) to the dorsum of C_3. "In seven of the ten corrosion cast specimens, the transverse branch to the third cuneiform divided into two branches over the third cuneiform and then coalesced back into one branch before it united with the longitudinal branch to the third intermetatarsal space."[8]

The longitudinal branch to the second intermetatarsal space anastomoses over C_3 with the longitudinal branch to the second intermetatarsal space of the proximal lateral tarsal artery and forms the common longitudinal branch to the second intermetatarsal space. This arrangement was found in 8 of the 10 corrosion cast specimens. In the other two, either component was absent.

Medial Tarsal Arteries

Gilbert et al[8] provided a comprehensive study of the medial tarsal arteries, proximal and distal, and their findings were as follows.

Proximal Medial Tarsal Artery

This artery was present in all 20 specimens of their study. The artery originates from the dorsalis pedis artery at the level between the talonavicular and second cuneonavicular joint in 18 specimens. The artery travels nearly transversely along the dorsal aspect of the navicular, toward its inferomedial apex and bifurcates, uniting with the inferior communicating branch of the distal medial tarsal artery and continues inferomedially to anastomose with branches of the medial plantar artery (see Fig. 7.15). "Along its path, the proximal medial tarsal artery provided multiple nutrient vessels to the dorsum of the navicular, as well as a variable number of anastomotic branches to the distal medial tarsal artery."[8] It also sends a "medial recurrent tarsal artery to the talar neck and body."[8] In the remaining two specimens, "the proximal medial tarsal artery originated from the anterior tibial artery at the level of the tibiotalar joint. In one of these specimens, the proximal medial artery and the medial malleolar artery originated from a common trunk."[8] The artery "passed in a straight line from the tibiotalar joint to the medial posteroinferior corner of the first cuneiform" and "united with the inferior communicating branch of the distal medial tarsal artery and anastomosed with branches of the medial plantar artery. They sent a medial recurrent tarsal artery to the talar neck and body."[8]

Distal Medial Tarsal Artery

Gilbert et al[8] described this artery as present in all their 20 specimens. The distal medial tarsal artery originates from the dorsalis pedis artery at the level of the second cuneonavicular joint in 45% (9 of the 20 specimens). It originated more proximally at the level of the anterior half of the navicular in six specimens, and it originated more distally at the level of the posterior half of the second cuneiform in 5 specimens. The distal medial tarsal artery courses anteromedially. "The first main branch of the distal medial tarsal artery occurred over the medial half of the second cuneiform. This previously unnamed branch traveled in a U-shaped loop across the dorsum of the second cuneiform. The loop passed deep to the dorsalis pedis artery and supplied an average of 8 nutrient vessels (range, 3-14 nutrient vessels) to the dorsum of the second cuneiform. The lateral extent of this U-shaped loop anastomosed with the distal lateral tarsal artery."[8] "This U-shaped loop was an anastomotic necklace that draped down distally over the dorsal surface of the second cuneiform, connected the distal medial tarsal artery to the distal lateral tarsal artery, and provided multiple nutrient vessels to the dorsum of the second cuneiform along the way. This unnamed artery was evident in all specimens and is referred to here as the necklace of the second cuneiform" (see Fig. 7.15A).[8] Gilbert et al[8] referred to the "branch point of this artery off the distal medial tarsal artery as the medial hook of the necklace of the second cuneiform. The branch point of this artery off the distal lateral tarsal artery was referred to as the lateral hook to the 2nd cuneiform." The medial hook of the necklace to the second cuneiform branched off the distal medial tarsal artery an average 3 mm (range, 0-6 mm) lateral to the articulation of the first and second cuneiforms. The distal medial tarsal artery crossed the superior border of the first cuneiform and divided into two distinct and previously unnamed branches—a superomedial border branch and a middle pedicle branch.

The superomedial border branch was present in 18 of the 20 specimens. It supplied an average of three nutrient vessels (range, one to six nutrient vessels) to the first cuneiform. The middle pedicle branch was present in all specimens. It coursed across the medial aspect of C_1 and provided an average of nine nutrient vessels (range, 4-15 nutrient vessels) superior to the insertion of the tibialis anterior tendon. The middle pedicle branch anastomosed with a branch of the medial plantar artery. This occurred in 5 of the 10 corrosion cast specimens. In 3 of the 10 corrosion cast specimens, the middle pedicle branch supplied nutrient vessels to the medial aspect of the base of the first metatarsal. In the remaining two specimens, it anastomosed with the medial plantar artery and supplied nutrient vessels to the medial aspect of the base of M_1.

Another previously unnamed artery, termed by Gilbert et al[8] as the inferior communicating branch (see Fig. 7.16) originated from the middle pedicle branch about halfway between the navicular and the first metatarsal articular surface of the first cuneiform. This small vessel was oriented perpendicular to the middle pedicle branch. It coursed over the medial aspect of the first cuneiform, deep to the tibialis anterior tendon, and anastomosed with the proximal medial tarsal artery near the medial apex of the navicular. The inferior communicating branch provided an average of five nutrient vessels (range, 0-11 nutrient vessels) to the medial aspect of the first cuneiform.

Arcuate Artery

The arcuate artery originates from the dorsalis pedis usually at the level of the first tarsometatarsal joint; it crosses the base of the second, third, and fourth metatarsals almost transversely and provides the dorsal metatarsal arteries 2, 3, and 4 and, occasionally, the artery metatarsi dorsalis fibularis (see Figs. 7.3 and 7.8B).[2] The artery is present in only 54%, and the variable origin of the artery occurs at the following sites as reported by Huber in 200 feet: at the $cuneo_1$-$metatarsal_1$ level, 35% (group A); at the cuneonavicular level, 17% (group B); below the cuneonavicular level, 2%.[4] The dorsal metatarsal arteries provided by the arcuate artery occur with the following frequency in 200 feet: dorsal metatarsal arteries 2, 3, and 4—16.5% (group A),

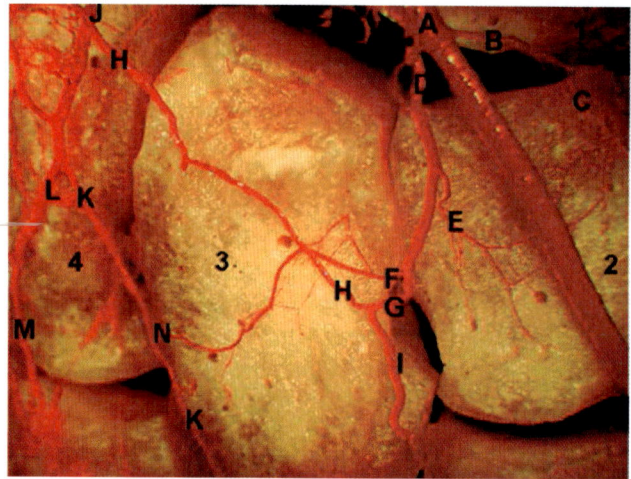

Figure 7.16 **The extraosseous blood supply to the dorsal surface of the second and third cuneiforms.** (*1*, navicular; *2*, second cuneiform; *3*, third cuneiform; *4*, cuboid; *A*, dorsalis pedis artery; *B*, distal medial tarsal artery; *C*, medial hook of the necklace to the second cuneiform; *D*, distal lateral tarsal artery; *E*, lateral hook of the necklace to the second cuneiform; *F*, transverse branch to the third cuneiform; *G*, distal lateral tarsal longitudinal branch to the second intermetatarsal space; *H*, proximal lateral tarsal longitudinal branch to the second intermetatarsal space; *I*, common longitudinal branch to the second intermetatarsal space; *J*, proximal lateral tarsal artery; *K*, longitudinal branch to the third intermetatarsal space; *L*, transverse pedicle branch of the proximal lateral tarsal artery; *M*, longitudinal branch to the fourth intermetatarsal space; *N*, site of anastomosis between the transverse branch of the distal medial tarsal artery to the third cuneiform and the longitudinal branch to the third intermetatarsal space. The ruler markings are in millimeters.) (From Gilbert BJ, Horst F, Nunley JA. Potential donor rotational bone graft using vascular territories in the foot and ankle. *J Bone Joint Surg Am.* 2004;86A[9]:1864, Figure 5A.)

9% (group B), 25.5% total; dorsal metatarsal arteries 2 and 3—9% (group A), 6.5% (group B), 15.5% total; dorsal metatarsal artery—9.5% (group A), 3.5% (group B), 13% total.[4]

First Dorsal Metatarsal Artery, First Plantar Metatarsal Artery, and Arterial Supply of the Big Toe

The first dorsal metatarsal artery originates from the dorsalis pedis artery, when the latter dives plantarward at the base of the first intermetatarsal space.

As described by Poirier and Charpy, the artery courses over the dorsum of the first dorsal interosseous muscle and divides into two branches—medial and lateral—at the level of the metatarsophalangeal joint of the big toe (Fig. 7.17).[9] The medial branch provides two dorsolateral collaterals to the big toe. The lateral branch terminates as the dorsomedial branch of the second toe.

Distally, in the web space, the first dorsal metatarsal artery plunges plantarward and bifurcates into its terminal branches, both medial and lateral. The medial plantar branch forms the plantar hallucal arteries, both fibular and tibial, whereas the lateral branch terminates as the medial plantar artery of the second toe. The lateral branch of the first plantar metatarsal artery joins the first dorsal metatarsal artery at the level of its plantar bifurcation. The plantar tibial hallucal artery crosses transversely between the midsegment of the proximal phalanx and the flexor hallucis longus tendon to reach the medial plantar aspect of the big toe, where it is joined by the medial bifurcation branch of the first plantar metatarsal artery (Fig. 7.18). Poirier and Charpy clearly state that, "it is the dorsal interosseous (metatarsal$_1$) and not the plantar interosseous (metatarsal$_1$) that provides the three inner plantar collaterals of the [first and second] toes" (Figs. 7.19 and 7.20).[9]

The first plantar metatarsal artery is considered a branch of the dorsalis pedis or a terminal branch of the lateral plantar artery. It arises at the level of the inferior border of the second metatarsal from the dorsalis pedis arterial area during its vertical course in the first intermetatarsal space.[5] It is directed medially and anteriorly, separated from the first dorsal metatarsal artery by the first dorsal interosseous muscle. It is located deep to the level of the oblique head of the adductor hallucis and the flexor hallucis brevis. Initially applied against the lateral surface of the first metatarsal, the artery passes between the bone and the flexor hallucis brevis muscle. At the level of the distal bifurcation triangle of this muscle, the first plantar metatarsal artery divides into two branches: lateral and medial. The lateral branch courses between the two heads of the flexor hallucis brevis and then passes plantar to the lateral head of the short flexor. It turns around the lateral sesamoid, pierces the deep lateral sagittal septum of the plantar aponeurosis for the big toe, courses on the plantar aspect of the deep transverse metatarsal ligament, and joins the first dorsal metatarsal artery at the point of bifurcation in the first web space. The medial branch of the first plantar metatarsal artery also emerges between the two heads of the short flexors of the big toe, passes around the medial sesamoid or between the two sesamoids, and terminates in the tibial plantar hallucal artery. This medial branch is joined by a thin branch from the medial plantar artery (see Figs. 7.17 and 7.18).

The description by Gilbert (see Fig. 7.18) of the arterial blood supply of the big toe and second toe is quite similar to that provided by Poirier and Charpy except for some further details and minor variations in interpretation.[5,9] The first dorsal metatarsal

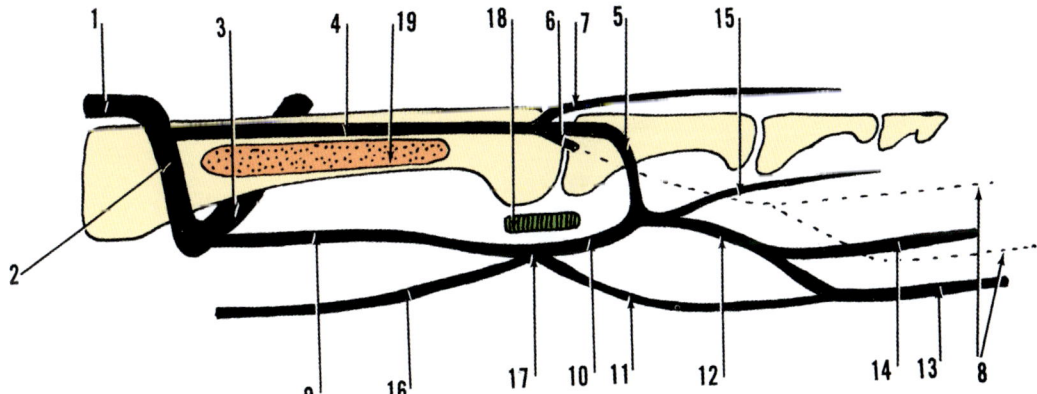

Figure 7.17 **Arterial supply of the big toe.** (*1*, dorsalis pedis artery; *2*, first proximal perforating artery or vertical descending portion of *1*; *3*, transverse segment or deep plantar arterial arc; *4*, first dorsal metatarsal artery; *5*, first distal perforating artery or vertical descending portion of *4*; *6*, medial division branch of first dorsal metatarsal artery, providing two dorsal collateral branches to big toe [*8*]; *7*, lateral division branch of first dorsal metatarsal artery, providing tibial dorsal collateral branch to second toe; *9*, first plantar metatarsal artery; *10*, lateral division branch of first plantar metatarsal artery; *11*, medial division branch of first plantar metatarsal artery; *12*, medial plantar division branch of vertical portion of first dorsal metatarsal artery, providing medial [*13*] and lateral [*14*] hallucal plantar arteries; *15*, lateral plantar division branch of vertical portion of first dorsal metatarsal artery, providing tibial plantar artery of second toe; *16*, arterial branch arising from medial plantar artery joins first plantar metatarsal artery; *17*, cruciate anastomosis formed by first plantar metatarsal artery and its two division branches joined by hallucal branch of medial plantar artery; *18*, deep transverse metatarsal ligament; *19*, first dorsal interosseous muscle arising from second metatarsal shaft.) (Diagram drawn in accordance with Poirier and Charpy's description.[9])

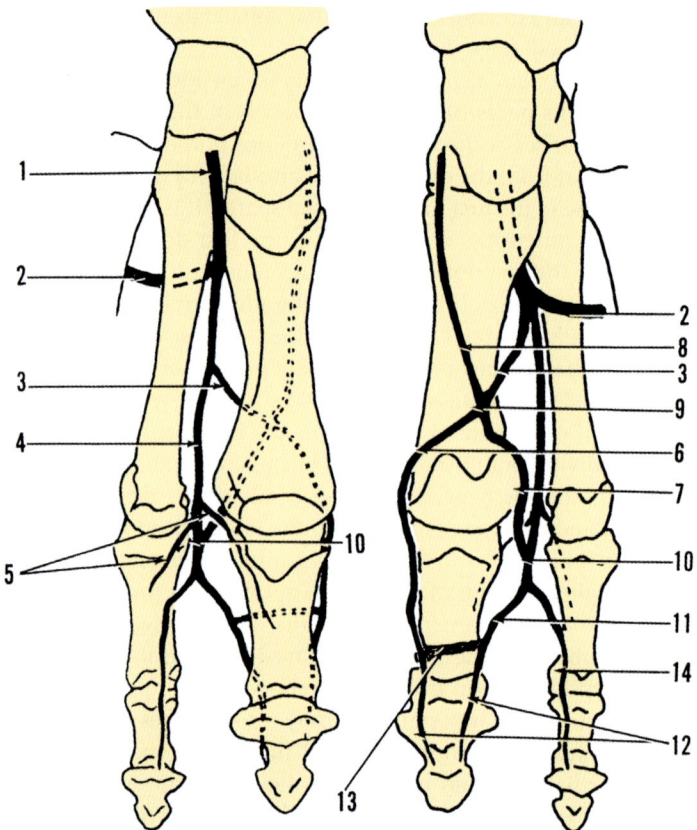

Figure 7.18 **Most common disposition of the first dorsal metatarsal artery.** (*1*, dorsalis pedis artery; *2*, transverse plantar arterial arc; *3*, first plantar metatarsal artery; *4*, first dorsal metatarsal artery; *5*, lateral and medial dorsal division branches of first dorsal metatarsal artery, forming dorsotibial collateral branch of second toe and dorsoperoneal collateral branch of big toe; *6*, medial division branch of first plantar metatarsal artery; *7*, lateral division branch of first plantar metatarsal artery; *8*, hallucal branch arising from medial plantar artery and forming cruciate anastomosis [*9*] with first plantar metatarsal artery and its division branches [*6, 7*]; *10*, descending vertical portion of first dorsal metatarsal artery joined by lateral division branch of first plantar metatarsal artery; *11*, common plantar hallucal artery; *12*, plantar hallucal arteries, medial and lateral, with their transverse anastomotic branch [*13*]; *14*, tibial and plantar collateral artery of second toe.) (From Gilbert A. In: Tubiana R, ed. *Chirurgie de la Main.* Masson et Cie; 1976.)

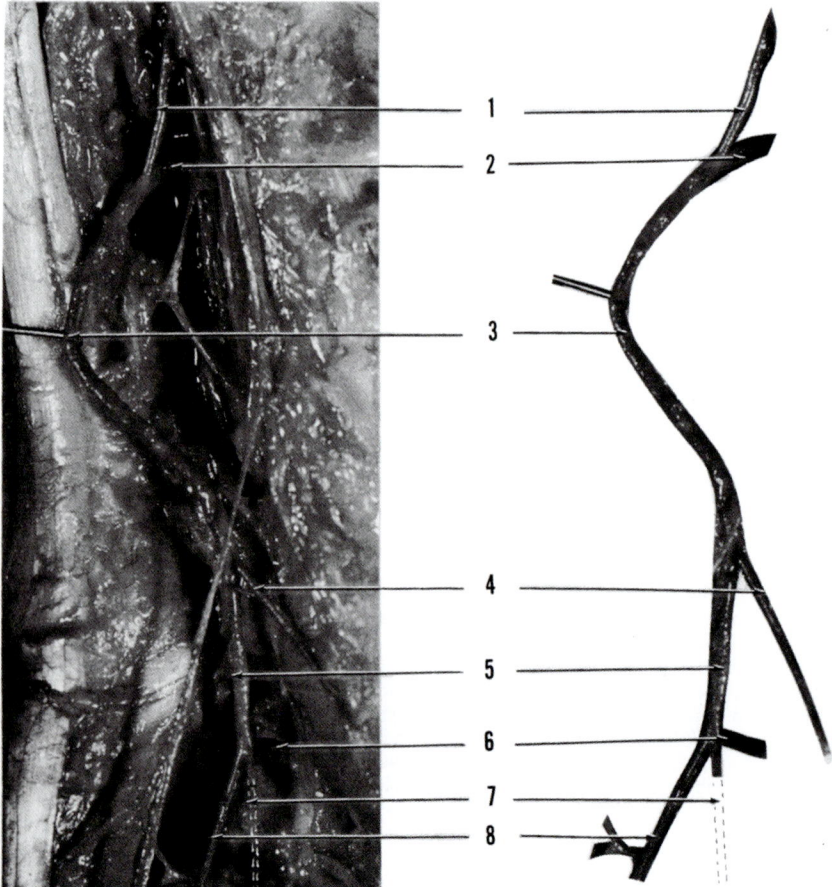

Figure 7.19 **Dorsal aspect of the first web space of the left foot.** Top is proximal. (*1*, thin dorsalis pedis artery; *2*, first proximal perforating artery provided from deep plantar arc and supplying first dorsal metatarsal artery [*3*]; *4*, dorsal collateral arterial branch to second toe; *5*, distal portion of first dorsal metatarsal artery; *6*, vertical descending portion of first dorsal metatarsal artery; *7, 3*, dorsal collateral branches of second and first toes.)

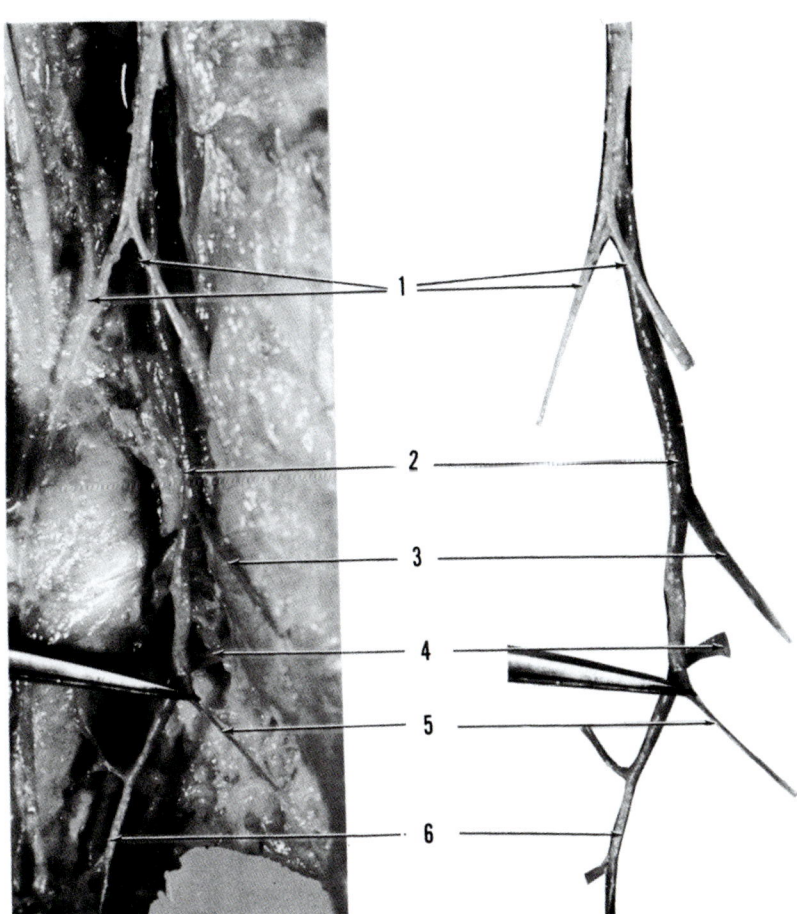

Figure 7.20 Relationship of the first dorsal metatarsal artery and the deep terminal branch of the deep peroneal nerve. Dorsal aspect of the first web space of the left foot; the big toe is on the left. (*1*, medial and lateral branches of deep peroneal nerve innervating first web space, crossing first dorsal metatarsal artery [*2*] superficially; *3*, proximal dorsal collateral arterial branch to second toe; *4*, vertical descending branch of first dorsal metatarsal artery; *5, 6*, dorsal collateral arterial branches to second and first toe supplied by first dorsal metatarsal artery; dorsal collateral artery to second toe is thin.)

artery arises from the dorsalis pedis artery as the latter enters the intermetatarsal space "limited anteriorly by the arch formed by the first dorsal interosseous muscle and posteriorly by the base of the two first metatarsals and their ligaments."[5] The first dorsal metatarsal artery passes under a muscular tunnel (about 15 mm long) formed by a belly of the first dorsal interosseous muscle and runs toward the web space in a subcutaneous position dorsal to the interosseous muscle.[5] In the web space, the artery provides a dorsal branch to the big toe and a dorsal branch to the second toe and dives plantarward. It branches into the larger lateral plantar digital artery of the big toe and the thinner medial plantar digital artery of the second toe. By means of a transverse anastomotic branch located between the proximal phalanx of the big toe and the flexor hallucis longus tendon, the lateral plantar artery of the big toe unites with the distal segment of the medial plantar artery and provides the major blood supply to the big toe. At the level of the first metatarsal neck, the first plantar metatarsal artery is joined by the thin medial plantar artery. Two arteries arise from this junction, and a "vascular cross" is formed. As described above, the lateral branch joins the first dorsal metatarsal artery in the web space. The distal medial branch forms the plantar tibial hallucal artery. Occasionally, the latter is formed solely by the medial plantar artery.

The plantar fibular hallucal artery and the dorsal tibial artery of the second toe are the predominating vessels.[3,5,10]

The dorsal hallucal arteries derive from the first dorsal metatarsal artery, and the medial branch is present only in the distal segment.[3,9] The medial branch may be supplied by the plantar medial hallucal artery through a vertical ascending branch.[3]

The first dorsal metatarsal artery provides muscular branches to the first dorsal interosseous muscle, articular branches to the metatarsophalangeal joints of the big toe and second toe, and cutaneous branches to the skin of the dorsum of the foot. The cutaneous branches arise from three main sites: proximal to the dorsal muscular arch of the first dorsal interosseous, distal to the same arch, and at the anterior aspect of the first web space.[5]

The caliber of the first dorsal metatarsal artery is 1 to 1.5 mm. The first plantar metatarsal artery is of similar size or smaller.[5]

Arterial Supply of the First Web Space

May and colleagues studied the neurovascular anatomy of the first web space in 50 fresh cadaver specimens.[11] The arterial anatomy was defined in regard to the variations of the first dorsal metatarsal artery and the distal communicating arterial anastomosis.

The first dorsal metatarsal artery was seen in two basic patterns (Fig. 7.21):

Type I (78%): The first dorsal metatarsal artery arises from the dorsalis pedis artery superficially at the base of metatarsals

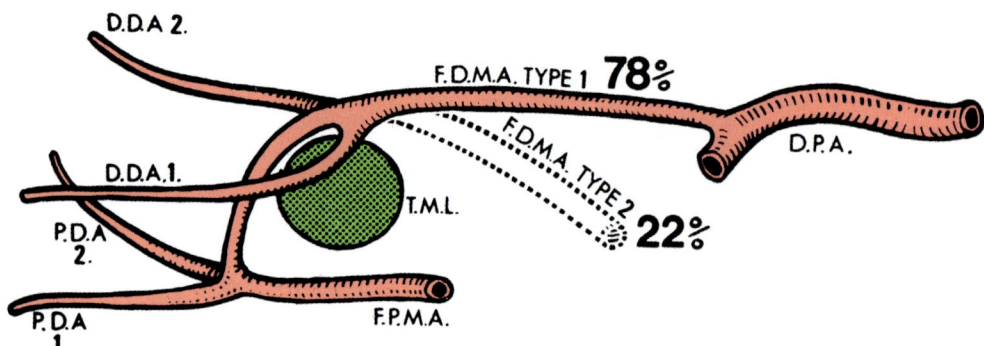

Figure 7.21 Diagram of arterial supply of the first web space showing two basic variations of the first dorsal metatarsal artery origin. (*DDA*, dorsal digital artery; *DPA*, dorsalis pedis artery; *FDMA*, first dorsal metatarsal artery; *FPMA*, first plantar metatarsal artery; *PDA*, plantar digital artery; *TML*, transverse metatarsal ligament.) (Adapted from May JW Jr, Chait LA, Cohen BE, O'Brien BM. Free neurovascular flap from the first web of the foot in hand reconstruction. *J Hand Surg*. 1977;2(5):387.)

1 and 2. It courses distally under the tendon of the extensor hallucis brevis, in the subcutaneous tissue. Proximally, it is covered by little or no first interosseous muscle.

Type II (22%): The first dorsal metatarsal artery arises deeply from the descending segment of the dorsalis pedis artery or from the plantar arterial tree. It ascends in the first metatarsal space and courses under or through the first dorsal interosseous muscle.

Both types of first dorsal metatarsal artery pass dorsal to the deep transverse metatarsal ligament and give small branches to the skin, muscle, and adjacent metatarsophalangeal joints. The artery courses distally, gives a small branch to the first and second toes, turns plantarward over the transverse metatarsal ligament, forms the distal communicating artery, and joins the first plantar metatarsal artery. Two large plantar digital arteries arise at the junction site and continue toward the tuft of the corresponding first and second toe. The variation of the anastomosis of the distal communicating artery is as follows (Fig. 7.22):

Type I (38%): The distal communicating artery anastomoses with the first plantar metatarsal artery.

Type II (26%): The distal communicating artery anastomoses with the plantar digital artery of the first toe.

Type III (28%): The distal communicating artery anastomoses with the plantar digital artery of the second toe.

In 8% of feet, minor variations to the three major patterns were noted.

The diameters of the arterial branches of the first web space and the distance of the origin from the edge of the web space are indicated in Table 7.4.

Variations of the First Dorsal Metatarsal Artery

The variations of the first dorsal metatarsal artery have been analyzed according to the origin and principal source of supply and the relationship with the first dorsal interosseous muscle.[2,4,5,12]

Variations Relative to the Source of Supply. With regard to the main source of the first dorsal metatarsal artery, in 230 feet, it is reported to be dorsal in 80.8% and plantar in 19.1%; in 200 feet, it is reported as dorsal in 76.5%, plantar in 8.5%, dorsal and plantar in 0.3%, and absent in 12%.[2,4]

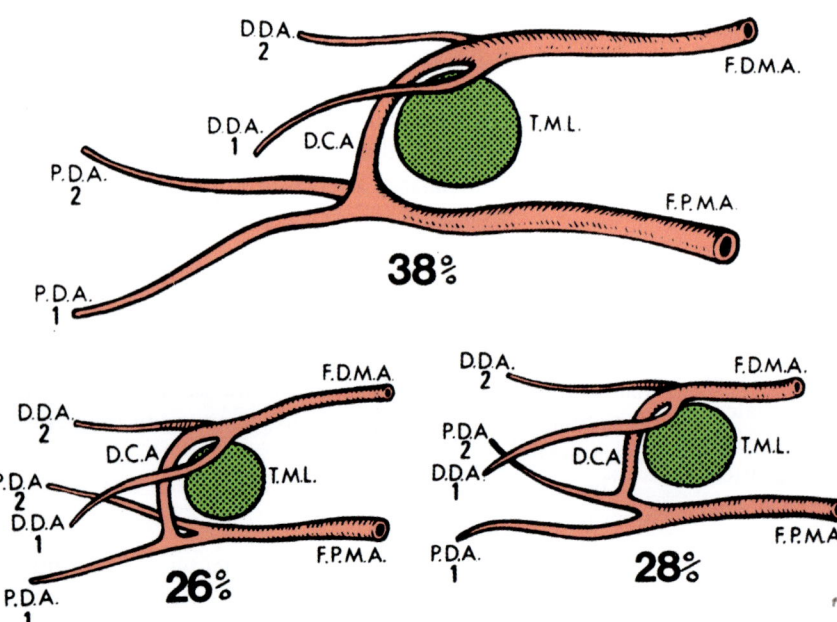

Figure 7.22 Patterns of distal communicating artery anastomosing. (*DCA*, distal communicating artery; *DDA*, dorsal digital artery; *DPA*, dorsal plantar artery; *FDMA*, first dorsal metatarsal artery; *FPMA*, first plantar metatarsal artery; *PDA*, plantar digital artery; *TML*, transverse metatarsal ligament.) (Adapted from May JW Jr, Chait LA, Cohen BE, O'Brien BM. Free neurovascular flap from the first web of the foot in hand reconstruction. *J Hand Surg*. 1977;2(5):387.)

TABLE 7.4 Size of Arteries Supplying the First Web Space of the Foot and Distance of Their Origins From the Web Edge in 50 Specimens				
	Diameter (mm)		Origin From Web Edge (cm)	
Vessel	Range	Average	Range	Average
First dorsal metatarsal artery	0.6-2.4	1.3	6.0-8.5	7.4
Dorsal digital arteries	0.3-1.5	0.7	1.6-3.8	2.4
Distal communicating artery	0.5-2.0	1.1	1.6-3.8	2.4
First plantar digital artery	0.4-2.0	1.1	1.5	2.3
Second plantar digital artery	0.4-2.0	0.9	1.5	2.3
First plantar metatarsal artery	0.6-3.0	1.5	Not dissected	Not dissected

Reprinted from May JW Jr, Chait LA, Cohen BE, et al. Free neurovascular flap from the first web of the foot in hand reconstruction. *J Hand Surg.* 1977;2(5):387, with permission from Elsevier.

Variations Relative to the First Dorsal Interosseous Muscle and to the Insertion of the Adductor of the Big Toe. Murakami, in a study of 40 feet, groups the variations of the first dorsal and first plantar metatarsal arteries into eight types (Fig. 7.23)[12]:

Type Ia (5%): The first dorsal and first plantar metatarsal arteries have a common trunk passing deep to the first dorsal interosseous muscle. The trunk reaches the plantar aspect of the first metatarsal bone and divides into the dorsal and plantar branches just proximal to the tendon of the adductor hallucis.

Type Ib (5%): The common trunk is more dorsal and passes close to the plantar aspect of the first dorsal interosseous muscle, and the division occurs just proximal to the adductor hallucis tendon.

Type Ic (12.5%): The common trunk is short, is located under the first dorsal interosseous muscle, and bifurcates, proximal to the distal border of the origin of the muscle, into the first dorsal and first plantar metatarsal arteries.

Type Id (25%): The common trunk bifurcates just distal to the origin of the first dorsal interosseous muscle.

Type II (25%): The dorsal and plantar arteries arise independently. The first dorsal metatarsal artery passes superficially to the first dorsal interosseous muscle, whereas the plantar artery passes deep to the same muscle.

Type III (17.5%): Both arteries arise independently. The dorsal artery passes just under the first dorsal interosseous muscle; the plantar artery descends on the plantar aspect of the first metatarsal bone.

Type IV (7.5%): The first dorsal metatarsal artery pierces the first dorsal interosseous muscle. The plantar artery is more plantar in location.

Type V (2.5%): The common trunk of both arteries passes dorsal to the first dorsal interosseous muscle and bifurcates just proximal to the adductor hallucis insertion.

Variations Relative to the First Dorsal Interosseous Muscle and to the Deep Transverse Metatarsal Ligament. Gilbert, in a study of 50 feet, groups the variations of the first dorsal metatarsal artery into five types (Fig. 7.24)[5]:

Types Ia and Ib (66%): Both metatarsal arteries arise independently. In type Ia, the first dorsal metatarsal artery passes under the small posterior belly of the first dorsal interosseous muscle but remains superficial to the main muscle and to the deep transverse metatarsal ligament. In type Ib, the dorsal artery passes through the first dorsal interosseous muscle.

Types IIa and IIb (22%): The dorsal and plantar metatarsal arteries have a common trunk located under the first dorsal interosseous muscle. The first dorsal metatarsal artery courses deep to the muscle and passes dorsal to the deep transverse metatarsal ligament.

Type IIa: A slender superficial branch is present passing superficially to the muscle and uniting at the anterior part of the web space with the dorsal metatarsal artery.

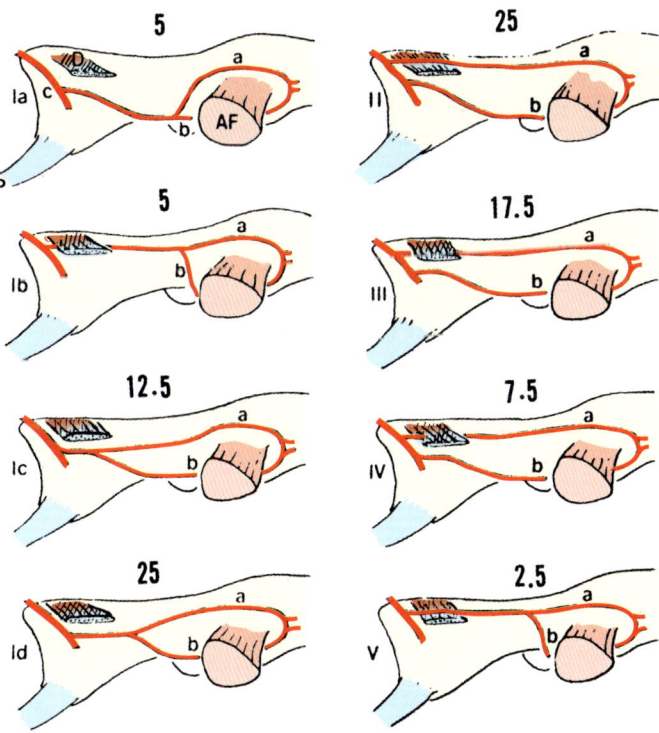

Figure 7.23 Variations in the origin and proximal course of the dorsal and plantar arteries in the first intermetatarsal space. (*a*, first dorsal metatarsal artery; *b*, first plantar metatarsal artery; *c*, deep plantar branch of dorsalis pedis artery; *D*, medial head of first dorsal interosseous muscle; *AF*, adductor hallucis and flexor hallucis brevis muscles; *P*, tendon of peroneus longus muscle.) (Adapted from Murakami T. On the position and course of the deep plantar arteries, with special reference to the so-called plantar metatarsal arteries. *Okajimas Folia Anat Jpn.* 1971;48:295.)

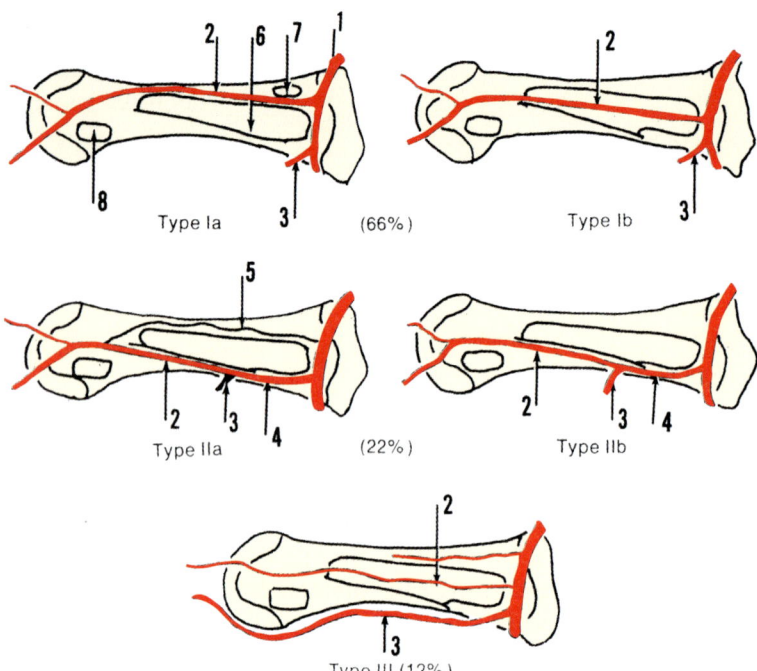

Figure 7.24 Anatomic variations of first dorsal metatarsal artery found in 50 specimens. (*1*, descending branch of dorsalis pedis artery; *2*, first dorsal metatarsal artery; *3*, first plantar metatarsal artery; *4*, common trunk to *2* and *3*; *5*, thin superficial first dorsal metatarsal artery; *6, 7*, origin of first dorsal interosseous muscle; *8*, deep transverse metatarsal ligament.) (Adapted from Gilbert A. In Tubiana R, ed. *La Main.* Masson et Cie; 1976.)

Type IIb: The superficial arterial branch is not present.

Type III (12%): The first dorsal interosseous artery is slender and passes through the first dorsal interosseous muscle. The first plantar metatarsal artery is well developed.

Leung and coworkers studied the arterial and venous supply of the first metatarsal web space in 70 feet.[13] Five dissections were done on fresh cadaver feet, and sixty-five dissections were carried out in surgery prior to toe transfer operations. The external diameter of the dorsalis pedis artery measured 1.3 mm in average, with a range of 1 to 1.9 mm. Seven types of arterial patterns were identified (Fig. 7.25):

Type I (28.6%): The superficial first dorsal metatarsal artery arises from the dorsalis pedis artery before the latter plunges into the first metatarsal space. The first dorsal metatarsal artery runs superficial to the first dorsal interosseous muscle, passes dorsal to the deep transverse metatarsal ligament, and divides into two branches, one for the big toe and one for the second toe. During the course, the artery gives off one to

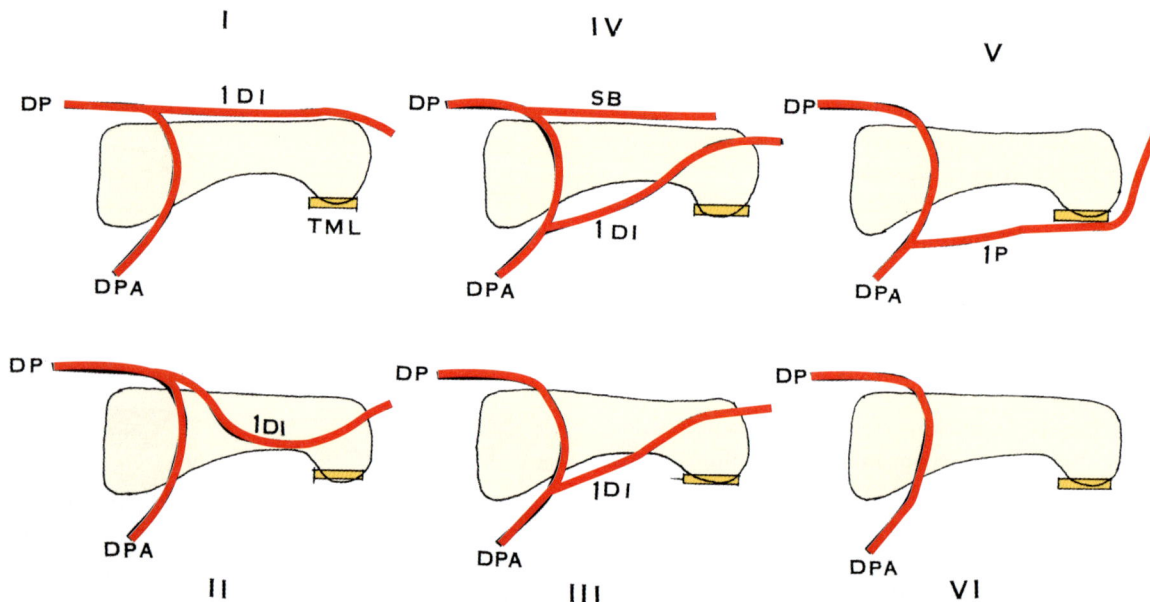

Figure 7.25 Six of the seven patterns of distribution of the dorsalis pedis artery of the first web space of the foot. (In type VII, this artery is absent.) (*1 DI*, first dorsal metatarsal artery [dorsal interosseous]; *1P*, first plantar metatarsal artery; *DP*, dorsalis pedis artery; *DPA*, deep plantar arch; *SB*, superficial branch; *TML*, transverse metatarsal ligament.) (Adapted from Leung PC, Wong WL. The vessels of the first metatarsal web space. *J Bone Joint Surg Am.* 1983;65A[2]:235.)

three small branches. The diameter of the first dorsal metatarsal artery ranges from 0.4 to 0.8 mm.

Type II (25.7%): The intramuscular first dorsal metatarsal artery passes through the first dorsal interosseous muscle and gives off three to five extremely small branches. The diameter of the artery ranges from 0.4 to 0.8 mm.

Type III (14%): The deep first dorsal metatarsal artery arises deep from the dorsalis pedis vertical portion. It runs along the plantar aspect of the first dorsal interosseous muscle, passes above or below the deep transverse metatarsal ligament, and divides into terminal branches to the big toe and second toe. The first dorsal metatarsal artery gives off 6 to 10 large branches to the bone, near the commencement of the artery and near the first metatarsal neck. The division into the terminal digital branches may occur more distally in the web space. The diameter of the artery ranges from 0.6 to 0.8 mm.

Type IV (5%): Deep and superficial first dorsal metatarsal arteries. A small superficial dorsal metatarsal artery branches off the dorsalis pedis artery superficially. This artery measures 0.1 to 0.3 mm in external diameter and terminates in fine branches in the web space without reaching the toes. The deep first dorsal metatarsal artery is similar to type III.

Type V (8%): The first plantar metatarsal artery. The first dorsal metatarsal artery is absent. The first plantar metatarsal artery has a large diameter (0.6-0.8 mm), runs plantar to the bone, and gives off 8 to 10 branches to the big toe. It passes plantar to the deep transverse metatarsal ligament and divides into multiple branches to the two toes. The adjacent plantar digital branches are smaller.

Type VI (1%): Absent first metatarsal artery, dorsal or plantar.

Type VII (4%): Absent dorsalis pedis artery.

Variations of the First Plantar Metatarsal Artery

The variations of the first plantar metatarsal artery, as described by Gilbert, involve mainly the origin.[5] The artery may branch off from the dorsalis pedis or the dorsal metatarsal artery. In one case in 50 feet, the artery branched from the plantar arterial arch, and in another, it branched from the terminal segment of the medial plantar artery.

The distal segment of the artery is fairly constant in its course and anatomic location at the level of the lateral sesamoid bone.

Variations of the Tibial Plantar Hallucal Artery

The tibial plantar hallucal artery has a variable origin. The artery may arise from the first dorsal metatarsal artery, the first plantar metatarsal artery, or the tibial superficial plantar artery.

In a study of 100 feet, Adachi found that the tibial plantar hallucal artery originates from the first dorsal metatarsal artery in 40%; from the first plantar metatarsal artery, fibular branch, in 35%, tibial branch, in 13%, both branches, in 5%; from the tibial superficial plantar artery in 1%; from the first dorsal metatarsal and first plantar metatarsal (tibial branch) arteries in 5%; and from the first dorsal metatarsal artery and the tibial superficial plantar artery in 1% (Fig. 7.26).[2]

Dorsomedial Hallucal Artery and Variations

The artery dorsalis hallucis tibialis or dorsal medial hallucal artery has a plantar or dorsal origin. As mentioned by Adachi, the artery originating from the first dorsal metatarsal artery and oriented toward the dorsotibial aspect of the big toe does not extend distally beyond the first metatarsophalangeal joint. The distal segment of the dorsomedial aspect of the big toe is supplied by a plantar branch arising from the plantar medial hallucal artery, turning around the proximal phalanx, and reaching the dorsotibial aspect of the big toe.[3] Poirier and Charpy describe the distal segment of the dorsotibial hallucal artery as being provided by the first dorsal metatarsal artery.[9] The principal source of the dorsomedial hallucal artery is described as plantar in 98.7% of 200 feet and 4.3% of 140 feet; as dorsal in 0.9% of 200 feet and 95.7% of 140 feet; and as plantar and dorsal in 0.4% of 200 feet and 0 of 140 feet.[1,2] The extreme differences are explained by the ethnic background (Japanese vs European).

Dorsal Metatarsal Arteries 2 to 4

The dorsal metatarsal arteries 2 to 4 have a double origin: dorsal and plantar (see Fig. 7.3). The dorsal source arises from the dorsal rete and the plantar source from the proximal or posterior perforating artery. According to the caliber of the supply vessel, one source may be considered to predominate or both sources may be of equal importance.

The respective sources of the dorsal metatarsal arteries 2 to 4 are as shown in Table 7.5. The dorsal source is provided predominantly by the arcuate artery, followed in frequency by the proximal lateral tarsal artery. The plantar source is provided by the proximal or posterior perforating artery.

Dorsal Digital Arteries

The dorsal digital arteries arise close to the metatarsophalangeal joints from the dorsal metatarsal artery, a branch of the plantar metatarsal artery passing dorsally through the distal part of the intermetatarsal space and forming the distal part of the dorsal metatarsal artery, or equally from the dorsal and plantar sources. The incidence of these sources of supply in 200 Western feet is shown in Table 7.6.

Posterior Perforating Arteries

The posterior perforating arteries (proximal perforating arteries, posterior communicating arteries) pass through the proximal end of the corresponding intermetatarsal spaces and join the dorsal metatarsal arteries.[4] They are important contributors to the latter, especially when the dorsal source is deficient. They may be absent in 3% to 5%.[4]

Anterior Perforating Arteries

The dorsal metatarsal artery gives origin to two dorsal digital arteries in the web space, plunges plantarward, forming the

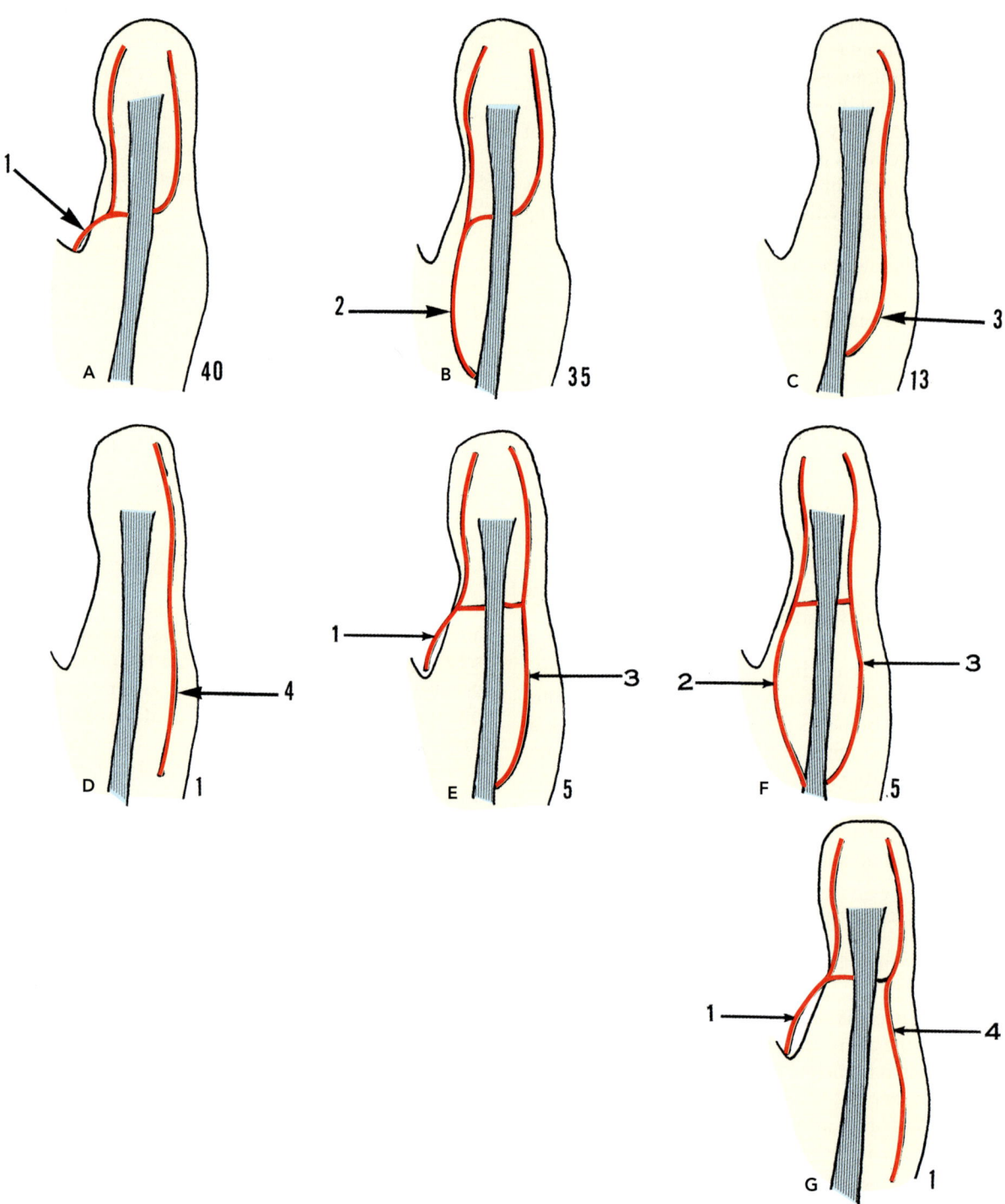

Figure 7.26 Variations of the origin of the tibial plantar hallucal artery. The tibial plantar hallucal artery is provided by **(A)** the first dorsal metatarsal artery (1); **(B)** the fibular branch of the first plantar metatarsal artery (2); **(C)** the tibial branch of the first plantar metatarsal artery (3); **(D)** the tibial superficial artery (4); **(E)** the first dorsal metatarsal artery (1) and the tibial branch of the first plantar metatarsal artery (3); **(F)** both branches of the first plantar metatarsal artery (2, 3); **(G)** the first dorsal metatarsal artery (1) and the tibial superficial metatarsal artery (4). (From Adachi B. *Das Arteriensystem der Japaner.* Maruzen; 1928:281.)

anterior perforating artery, supplies the plantar digital arteries, and is joined by the plantar metatarsal artery.[4] In the distal segment of the intermetatarsal space and in the web space, there are five communicating branches between the dorsal and plantar arteries: two arteries that arise from each side of the dorsal metatarsal artery at the metatarsal neck and course plantarward obliquely to unite with the corresponding plantar metatarsal arteries; one artery that is the continuation of the dorsal metatarsal artery and is usually called the *anterior perforating artery;* and two small arteries that connect on each side the dorsal and

TABLE 7.5 Source of Distal Metatarsal Arteries

	Dorsal Metatarsal Arteries (%)		
	II	III	IV
Adachi[2]			
Plantar	56.5	56.9	63.4
Dorsal	36	35.6	33.6
Plantar and dorsal	7.3	7.3	2.6
Huber[4] (200 Western feet)			
Dorsal	55	59	40.5
Plantar	33.5	23	37.5
Plantar and dorsal	6.5	10.5	0.5
Not present or classified	5	7.5	17

TABLE 7.6 Sources of Supply to Dorsal Digital Arteries[4]

	Dorsal Digital Arteries (%)			
Source	1 and 2	2 and 3	3 and 4	4 and 5
Dorsal	82.5	89	79	39
Plantar	10.5	8.5	10.5	53.5
Dorsal and plantar	0	2	3.5	2.5
Not classified	7	0.5	2	5

plantar digital arteries at the level of the side of the corresponding proximal phalanx.[4] Huber groups all five branches under the heading "anterior communicating branches."[4] The connections between the first dorsal metatarsal artery and the first plantar metatarsal artery are indicated in Figure 7.27.

Arteries of the Sinus Tarsi

The artery of the sinus tarsi (perforating vessel of the sinus tarsi, arteria anastomotica tarsi, ramus anastomicus tarsi) has a very variable origin (Figs. 7.28 and 7.29). Frequently, it arises from the lateral aspect of the dorsalis pedis artery at the level of the talar neck or from an anastomotic loop between the proximal lateral tarsal artery and the perforating peroneal artery.[7] The artery is always present. At the level of the talar neck, it gives off a few branches to the head, enters the sinus tarsi, supplies multiple branches to the talar body,

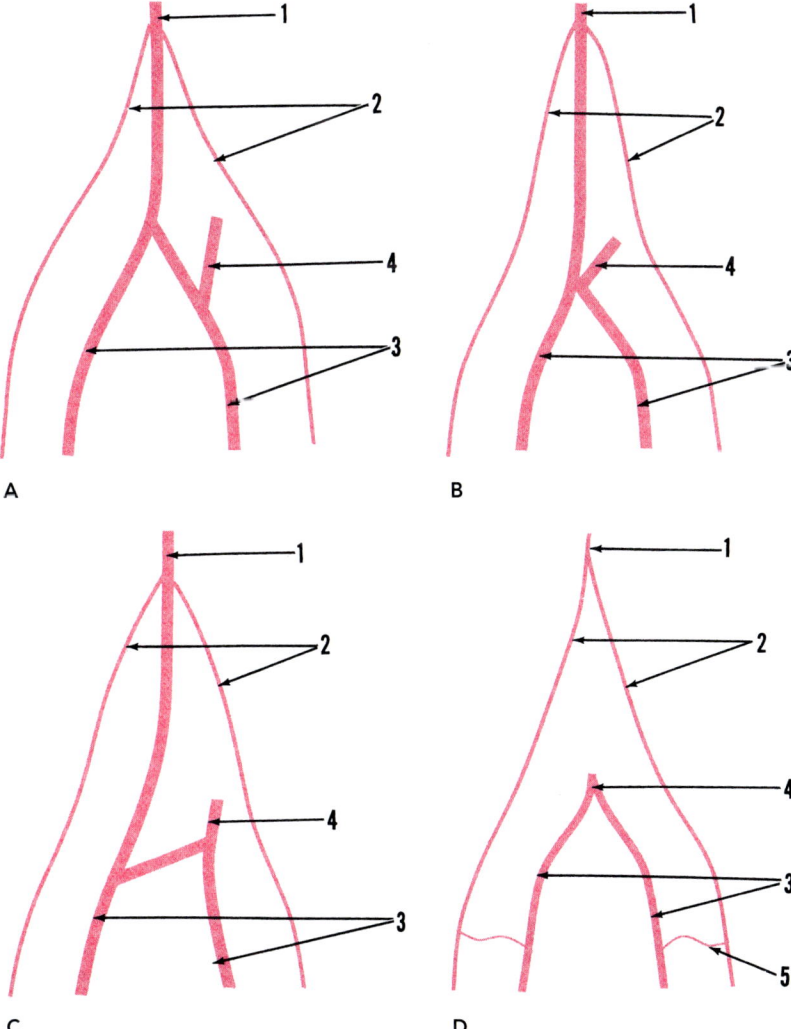

Figure 7.27 Anastomoses between the dorsal and plantar arteries in the interdigital spaces. (A–C) Examples of the ways in which the continuation of the dorsal metatarsal artery may contribute to the plantar digital arteries. **(D)** There is a connection between the dorsal and plantar digital arteries. (1, dorsal metatarsal artery; 2, dorsal digital arteries; 3, plantar digital arteries; 4, plantar metatarsal artery; 5, connection between dorsal and plantar digital arteries.) (From Huber JF. The arterial network supplying the dorsum of the foot. *Anat Rec*. 1941;80:373. By permission of Alan R. Liss, Publisher.)

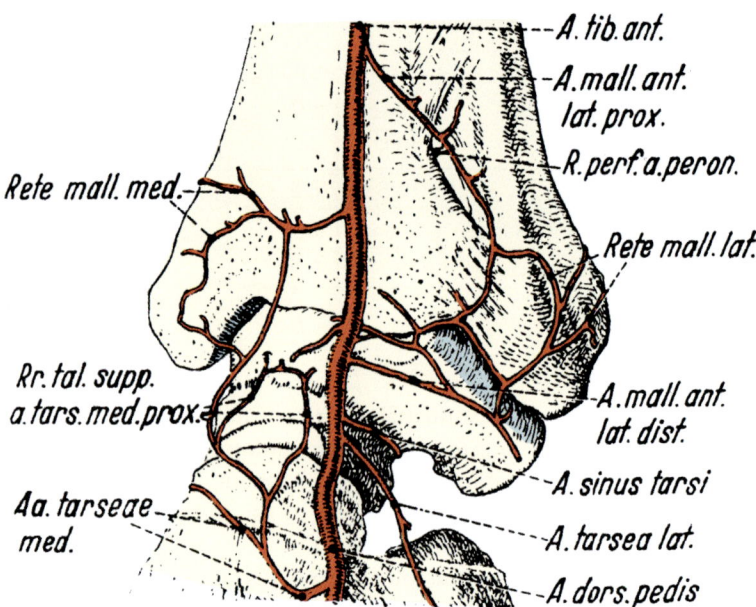

Figure 7.28 **Artery of the sinus tarsi arising from the dorsalis pedis artery.** The calcaneus has been removed. (Adapted from Wildenauer E. Die bluvesorgung des Talus. *Z Anat Entwicklungs*. 1950;115:32.)

and anastomoses with the artery of the tarsal canal emanating from the posterior tibial artery.

The caliber of the artery at the entrance of the sinus tarsi is reported by Adachi as being 1 to 1.5 mm and never more than 2 mm.[4] The origin of the artery of the sinus tarsi is reported to occur from the dorsalis pedis artery in 52% of 305 feet and 39.2% of 120 feet; from the lateral tarsal artery in 32% of 305 feet and 21.7% of 120 feet; from the anterior lateral malleolar artery in 9% of 305 feet and 11.7% of 120 feet; and from two equally strong arteries in 15.8% of 120 feet (proximal—dorsalis pedis, perforating branch of peroneal artery, 10%; distal—lateral tarsal artery, 5.8%).[1,2]

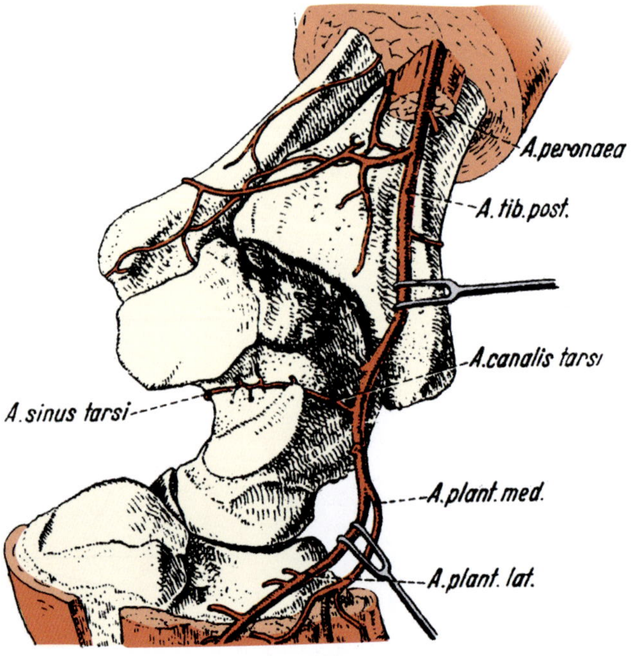

Medial Tarsal Arteries

The medial tarsal arteries are very variable in size and number (see Fig. 7.3). They might be two of equal size arising from the dorsalis pedis, one at the level of the middle of the navicular and the other just below the cuneonavicular articulation.[4] At times, there is only one proximal or one distal branch. Rarely are three branches present. These branches occur with the following frequency in 200 feet: two equal, 42%; one proximal, 13%; one distal, 13.5%; short common stem at the level of the proximal medial tarsus, divided into two branches (proximal and distal), 15%; minute branches, 16.5%.[4]

The medial tarsal arteries anastomose on the medial margin of the foot with the medial plantar artery. Adachi describes a significant anastomosis located on the medial margin of the foot between the first cuneiform and the muscles.[2]

Anterior Medial Malleolar Artery

The anterior medial malleolar artery originates from the dorsalis pedis artery just below the ankle joint (see Figs. 7.3 and 7.28). As mentioned by Huber, it is "not possible to decide in all cases on any one artery which should be called the anterior medial malleolar artery."[4]

The artery is directed transversely medially, passes under the tibialis anterior tendon, and at the level of the anterior border of the medial malleolus divides into two branches: superficial and deep. The superficial branch crowns the base of the medial malleolus and anastomoses with the terminal thin branch of

Figure 7.29 **Artery of the sinus tarsi and artery of the canalis tarsi arising from the posterior tibial artery.** (Adapted from Wildenauer E. Die bluvesorgung des Talus. *Z Anat Entwicklungs*. 1950;115:32.)

Anterior Lateral Malleolar Artery

The anterior lateral malleolar artery originates from the dorsalis pedis just below the ankle joint articular interline, usually 1 to 2 mm below the most common point of origin for the anterior medial malleolar artery (see Figs. 7.3 and 7.51).[4]

The artery is directed transversely laterally and passes under the tendons of the extensor digitorum longus and the peroneus tertius. At the level of the anterior border of the lateral malleolus, it descends vertically along the anterior border of the lateral malleolus and the lateral border of the tarsus and anastomoses with the proximal lateral tarsal artery and the lateral plantar artery.

The transverse segment of the anterior lateral malleolar artery anastomoses proximally with branches from the perforating peroneal artery and sends a transverse branch over the lateral malleolus. The latter anastomoses with a similar transverse branch emanating from the peroneal artery and contributes to the formation of the perimalleolar transverse arterial loop. The descending retromalleolar branch of the peroneal artery unites with the descending segment of the anterior lateral malleolar artery, forms a sagittal arterial loop, and contributes to the formation of the lateral malleolar arterial rete.

The variations occur relative to the origin, number, and size of the artery. The variations of origin are shown in Table 7.8. The anterior lateral malleolar artery is absent in 8%, may be double in 16%, and in 29% originates not from the dorsalis pedis but from the perforating branch of the peroneal artery.[1,2]

Gilbert et al[8] described the anterior lateral malleolar artery as present in all 20 specimens. This artery originated proximal to the tibiotalar joint in 30% (6 specimens), at the tibiotalar joint in 55% (11 specimens), and distal to the tibiotalar joint in 15% (3 specimens). On the average, the anterior lateral malleolar artery originated 2 mm (range, 6-7 mm) proximal to the tibiotalar joint. From its origin, the anterior lateral malleolar artery coursed transversely laterally across the anterior surface of the distal tibia, passing deep to the tendons of the extensor digitorum longus and peroneus tertius. It then divides into a vertical descending segment and a transverse segment just medial to the lateral malleolus articular surface in all specimens (see Fig. 7.51).

the posterior medial malleolar artery arising from the posterior tibial artery. The anastomotic network or medial malleolar rete provides small branches penetrating the medial malleolus near the base and coursing in a proximodistal direction. The deep branch of the anterior medial malleolar artery disappears in the deltoid ligamentous complex.

The variations occur relative to the origin, number, and size of the artery. The variations of origin are listed in Table 7.7. The anterior medial malleolar artery is absent in 16%, and occasionally, it is very insignificant.[1] It is usually smaller than the anterior lateral malleolar artery, and according to Adachi, the anterior lateral malleolar artery is larger in 69%, the anterior medial malleolar artery is larger in 7%, and both are equal in 24%.[2]

Gilbert et al.[8] described the anterior medial malleolar artery arising proximal to the tibiotalar joint in 45% (9 specimens) and at the tibiotalar joint in 55% (11 specimens). On the average, when the anterior medial malleolar artery originated from the anterior tibial artery, it arose 4 mm (range, 0-9 mm) proximal to the tibiotalar joint. The anterior medial malleolar artery traveled transversely medially, underneath the tibialis anterior tendon, and divided into a deep branch and a superficial branch. The deep branch of the anterior medial malleolar artery was present in all 10 corrosion cast specimens and supplied multiple nutrient vessels to the distal aspect of the tibia around the ankle mortise in 6 of the 10 specimens and provided direct nutrient branches to the neck of the talus in all 10 specimens. The superficial branch of the anterior medial malleolar artery was present in all 10 corrosion specimens. It bifurcated into a talar nutrient branch and a medial malleolar nutrient branch, and this bifurcation occurred also in all 10 corrosion cast specimens. In eight specimens, the superficial branch of the anterior medial malleolar artery sent a branch into the deltoid ligament from either the talar nutrient branch or from the medial malleolar nutrient branch. The talar nutrient branch anastomosed with the medial recurrent tarsal artery or another branch of the proximal medial tarsal artery to supply nutrient vessels to the talus. The medial malleolar nutrient branch provided the medial aspect of the medial malleolus with nutrient vessels.

TABLE 7.7 Variations of Origin of the Anterior Medial Malleolar Artery			
Origin	%		
	Adachi (59 Feet)	Dubreuil-Chambardel (235 Feet)	Huber (200 Feet)
At the level of the ankle joint articular interline	44		55-60 (or just below)
Below the interline	36	52	3-1 (about 1 cm)
Above the interline	20	32	8 (2-3 cm) 13-15 (just above)

TABLE 7.8 Variations of Origin of the Anterior Lateral Malleolar Artery			
Origin	%		
	Adachi (52 Feet)	Dubreuil-Chambardel (235 Feet)	Huber (200 Feet)
At the level of the ankle joint articular interline	31		60-65 (or 1-2 mm below)
Below the interline	61	52	
Above the interline	8	40	3 (just above)

The transverse segment anastomosed with the perforating peroneal artery and then continued laterally around the lateral malleolus. This transverse segment was present in all specimens and supplied an average of seven nutrient vessels (range, 2-15 nutrient vessels) to the anterior and lateral aspects of the lateral malleolus. Gilbert et al[8] also described, previously undescribed, a fibular metaphyseal artery originating from the perforating peroneal artery as the latter emerged over the tibiofibular syndesmosis. It traveled laterally over the distal fibular metaphysis and the anterolateral surface of the lateral malleolus to anastomose with the transverse branch of the anterior lateral malleolar artery near the anterolateral border of the lateral malleolus (see Figs. 7.13 and 7.15A). The fibular metaphyseal artery was identified in 90% (18 cases) and supplied multiple nutrient vessels to the anterolateral aspect of the distal fibular metaphysis. On the average, it provided 10 nutrient vessels (range, 4-15 own nutrient vessels) to this region. In two cases, the fibular metaphyseal artery supplied its usual nutrient vessels to the metaphysis of the fibula and ended without anastomosis with the transverse segment of the anterior lateral malleolar artery.

The anastomosis of the transverse segment of the anterior lateral malleolar artery with the peroneal artery was present in 60% (6 corrosion specimens out of 10). The anastomoses of the vertical descending segment of the anterior lateral malleolar artery with the lateral tarsal and lateral plantar arteries was present in 70% (7 corrosion specimens out of 10). In the other 30%, the vertical descending branch anastomosed only with the artery to the sinus tarsi. In 60% (6 corrosion specimens out of 10), the vertical descending branch was the primary origin of the artery of the sinus tarsi.

Perforating Branch of the Peroneal Artery

In the inferior segment of the leg, the peroneal artery divides into two branches: posterior and anterior. The anterior branch or perforating branch obliquely pierces the interosseous membrane, passes anteriorly, and courses over the anterior aspect of the distal tibiofibular syndesmosis behind the peroneus tertius tendon. It anastomoses with the transverse segment of the anterior lateral malleolar artery and contributes to the lateral malleolar sagittal and transverse perimalleolar arterial loops. Variations of termination are multiple, and according to Huber, the perforating peroneal artery may continue as the dorsalis pedis artery in 3% (see Fig. 7.9), contribute equally with the anterior tibial artery to the dorsalis pedis artery in 0.5% (see Fig. 7.10), or continue as the lateral tarsal artery in 0.5% (see Fig. 7.10).[4]

Huber also describes in 50% of the cases, an unrecognized artery branching from the anterior tibial artery about 5 cm above the ankle joint. This artery courses obliquely laterally and inferiorly and unites with the peroneal perforating branch as it pierces the interosseous membrane. This artery is a small branch in 13% or is equal to the perforating artery in about 20%; in 17%, it occupies the position of the latter.[4] When the distal segment of the anterior tibial artery is missing (1.5%), this oblique artery may be considered the link between the proximal segment of the anterior tibial artery and the perforating peroneal artery.

▶ Posterior and Plantar Arterial Network of the Foot and Ankle

Posterior Tibial Artery

On the posterior aspect of the ankle at the level of the tibial plafond, the tendons of the tibialis posterior, the flexor digitorum longus, and the flexor hallucis longus are applied against the posterior aspect of the tibia and are retained by their individual tunnels. The tunnels of the tibialis posterior and of the flexor digitorum longus are side by side and narrow and are separated from the larger tunnel of the flexor hallucis muscle–tendon unit by an interval. The neurovascular tunnel or fourth compartment is superficial to the intertendinous interval and to the tunnel of the flexor hallucis longus. At this level, the posterior tibial artery with its two accompanying veins is located in the tunnel, medial to the posterior tibial nerve (Figs. 7.30 and 7.31). As described previously, the neurovascular compartment is covered by the deep fascia cruris.

In the retromedial malleolar area, the passage zone curves anteriorly and the tendinous and neurovascular elements previously located in a frontal plane are in a nearly sagittal oblique plane. The neurovascular compartment is now posterior to the tunnel of the flexor digitorum longus and is superficial and medial to the intertendinous interval and to the tunnel of the flexor hallucis longus tendon. The posterior tibial artery follows the anterior concavity of its compartment and is accompanied by its two veins. The posterior tibial nerve is divided into the lateral and the medial plantar nerve. The lateral plantar nerve has already given the branch to the abductor digiti minimi muscle. The posterior tibial artery is not yet divided and is medial to the plane of the nerves.

The lower segment of the passage zone corresponds to the calcaneal canal and the porta pedis. The sustentaculum tali is the landmark. The tunnel of the tibialis posterior is located above the sustentaculum tali and is applied against the deltoid ligament. The tunnel of the flexor digitorum longus passes over the medial border of the sustentaculum tali, crossing the tibiocalcaneal portion of the deltoid ligament. The tunnel of the flexor hallucis longus is located over the inferior surface of the sustentaculum tali. The lateral wall of the calcaneal canal is further formed by the quadratus plantae applied against the medial concave surface of the os calcis, and the medial wall by the abductor hallucis muscle and its investing fascia. The interfascicular transverse septum (Fig. 7.32) originates from the fascia of the abductor hallucis, extends almost transversely laterally, and inserts along the inferior border of the flexor hallucis longus tunnel, just above the superior border of the quadratus plantae muscle. This transverse septum divides the lower part of the calcaneal canal into a superior and an inferior chamber. The posterior tibial artery bifurcates into the medial and lateral plantar arteries just proximal to the posterior border of the transverse septum. The medial plantar artery is the anterior branch and passes above the transverse septum. The lateral plantar artery is directed obliquely below the transverse septum. Relative to the sustentaculum tali, the bifurcation of the posterior tibial artery occurs at its posterior border, occasionally more proximal and rarely more distal.

According to various sources, the bifurcation level of the posterior tibial artery occurs with the following variations: under the posterior border of the sustentaculum tali, 67% and 61%; proximal to the posterior border of the sustentaculum tali (as far as 9-10 mm), 29% and 30%; distal to the posterior border of the sustentaculum tali (about 2-5 mm), 4% and 9%.[2,14] The level of arterial bifurcation may also vary relative to the level of bifurcation of the posterior tibial nerve. According to Adachi, in a study of 208 feet, the division of the posterior tibial artery occurs distal to the division of the posterior tibial nerve (usually 1-2 cm) in 86.5%, proximal to the division of the posterior tibial nerve (usually up to 0.5 cm) in 2%, and at the same level as the division of the posterior tibial nerve in 11.5%.[2]

The lateral plantar artery is usually larger than the medial plantar artery. The following frequencies of variations have been given: lateral plantar artery larger, 80.7% of 223 feet and 62.1% of 58 feet; medial plantar artery larger, 2.7% of 223 feet and 22.4% of 58 feet; both equal, 16.6% of 223 feet and 15.5% of 58 feet.[2,14]

In its distal segment, the posterior tibial artery provides the following four collateral branches:

- An anastomotic branch, which passes transversely under the flexor hallucis longus tendon, unites with a similar branch of the posterior peroneal artery and forms the posterior half of the perimalleolar arterial circle.
- The posteromedial malleolar artery, which courses transversely over the tendons of the flexor digitorum longus and the tibialis posterior. This branch anastomoses anteromedially with the anterior medial malleolar artery and contributes to the formation of the medial malleolar rete. It also

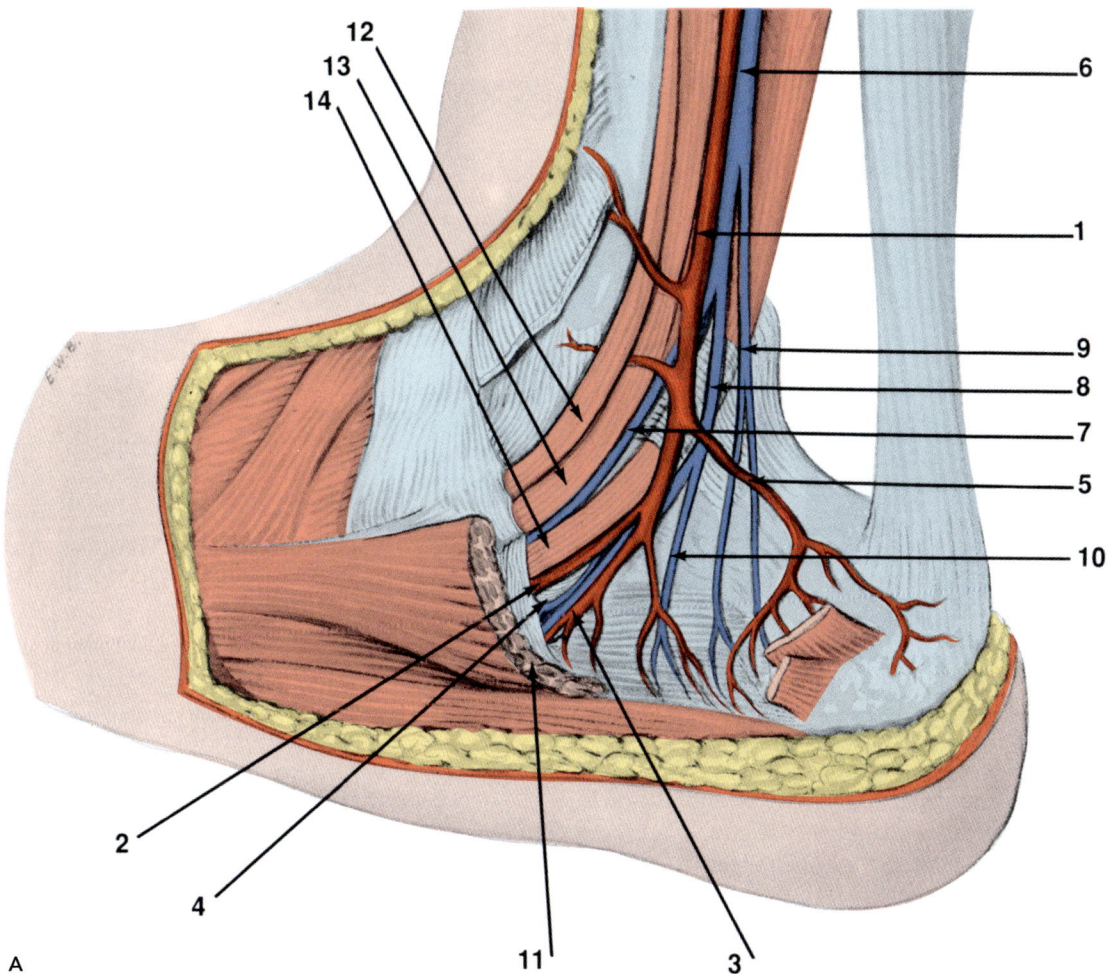

Figure 7.30 **(A) Medial tibiotalocalcaneal tunnel.** (*1*, posterior tibial artery; *2*, medial plantar artery passing above interfascicular ligament [*4*]; *3*, lateral plantar artery passing under interfascicular ligament [*4*]; *5*, posterior and medial arterial calcaneal branch; *6*, posterior tibial nerve; *7*, medial plantar nerve; *8*, lateral plantar nerve giving branch to abductor digiti quinti muscle; *9*, medial calcaneal nerve arising above bifurcation point of posterior tibial nerve; *10*, nerve to abductor digiti quinti; *11*, abductor hallucis muscle; *12*, tibialis posterior tendon; *13*, flexor digitorum longus tendon; *14*, flexor hallucis longus tendon.) **(B) Left foot, medial aspect.** The deltoid ligament is excised, exposing the talus, the medial malleolus, and the sustentaculum tali. (*1*, posterior tibial artery; *2*, lateral plantar artery; *3*, medial plantar artery; *4*, posteromedial calcaneal arterial branch; *5*, interfascicular septum; *6*, posterior tibial nerve; *7*, medial plantar nerve; *8*, lateral plantar nerve giving branch to abductor hallucis; *9*, medial calcaneal nerve; *10*, nerve to abductor digiti quinti; *11*, reflected flexor retinaculum; *12*, deep investing aponeurosis.)

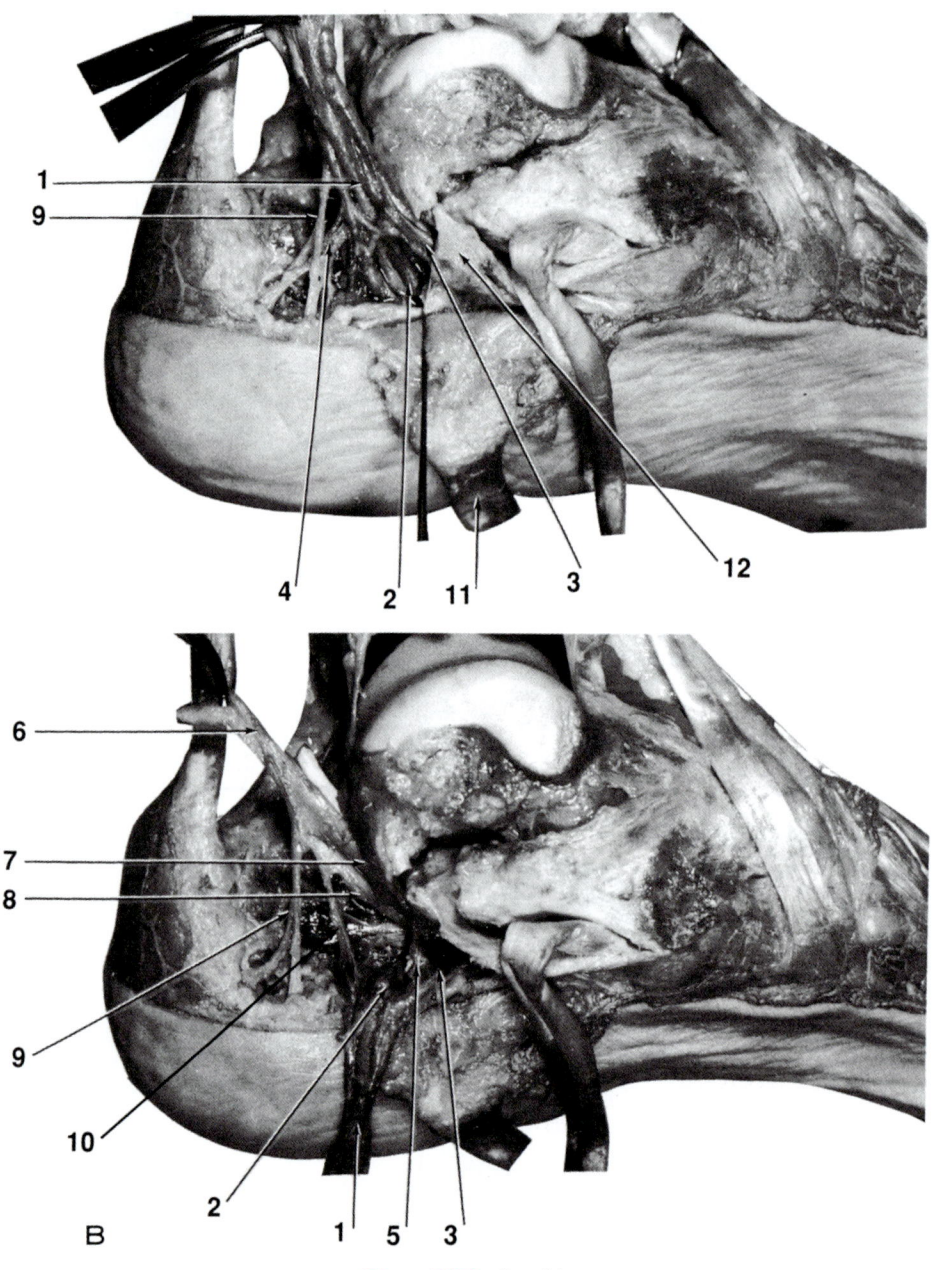

Figure 7.30 Cont'd

anastomoses with the medial tarsal arteries and provides cutaneous branches to the medial malleolar area.
- Calcaneal rami, which reach the calcaneus and the medial and posterior aspects of the heel.
- The artery of the tarsal canal (see Figs. 7.28 and 7.29).[7,15] This artery arises from the posterior tibial artery about 1 cm proximal to the bifurcation into the medial and lateral plantar arteries. It passes between the flexor digitorum longus and flexor hallucis longus tendon sheaths and enters the tarsal canal, where it anastomoses with the artery of the sinus tarsi. The size of the anastomosis varies, and the anastomosis may take place only in the talus.[7] In the sinus canal, the artery lies closer to the talus and provides larger branches to the talar body and smaller branches to the calcaneus. A deltoid branch takes off from the artery to the tarsal canal at 5 mm from its origin.[7] This artery passes between the calcaneotibial and talotibial components of the deltoid ligament, supplies the medial aspect of the talus, and anastomoses with the dorsalis pedis artery over the talar neck.[7] According to Mulfinger and Trueta, in 30 feet, the artery of the tarsal canal originates from the medial plantar artery in 16.6% and is duplicated in 3.3% and absent in 3.3%; in 30% the deltoid branch originates from the posterior tibial artery, and it is duplicated in 6.6%.[7]

Medial Plantar Artery

The medial plantar artery continues anteriorly and remains initially in the medial compartment of the sole of the foot on the inner side of the medial intermuscular septum (see Figs. 7.33, 7.34, 7.37, and 7.39). It is covered by the abductor hallucis

Chapter 7: Angiology   331

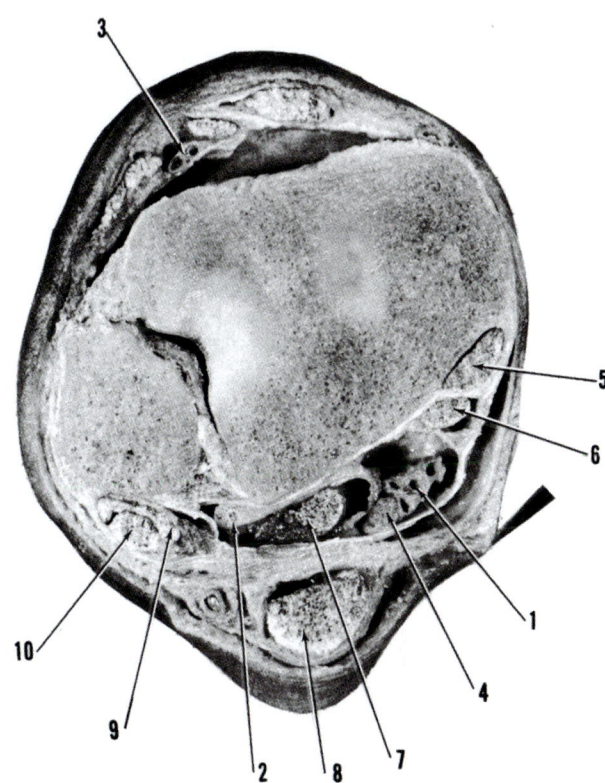

Figure 7.31 **Cross-section of the left ankle 2 cm proximal to the anterior colliculus of the medial malleolus.** (*1*, posterior tibial artery and accompanying veins; *2*, posterior peroneal artery and veins; *3*, anterior tibial artery and veins; *4*, posterior tibial nerve; *5*, tibialis posterior tendon; *6*, flexor digitorum longus tendon; *7*, flexor hallucis longus tendon and muscle; *8*, Achilles tendon; *9*, peroneus brevis tendon; *10*, peroneus longus tendon.)

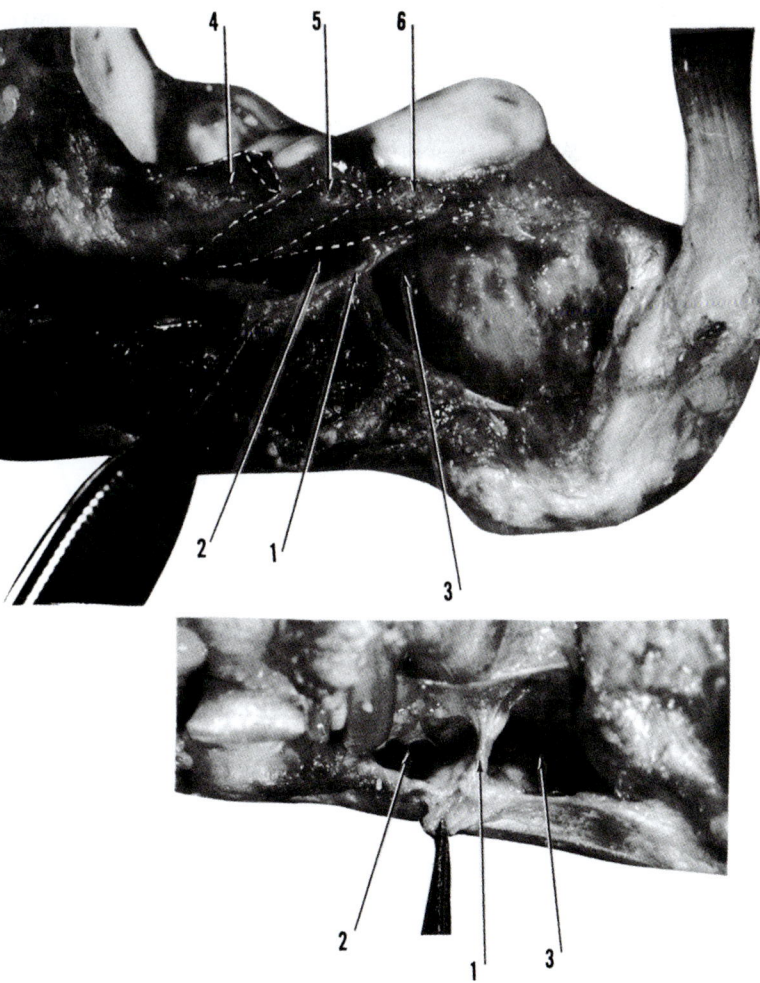

Figure 7.32 **Chambers of the calcaneal tunnel.** (*1*, interfascicular septum dividing calcaneal tunnel into upper [*2*] and lower [*3*] chambers; *4*, tibialis posterior tendon; *5*, flexor digitorum longus tendon; *6*, flexor hallucis longus tendon.)

muscle and crosses the tendon of the flexor digitorum longus at an acute angle; it runs parallel to the tibial side of the flexor hallucis longus tendon. It divides into two branches: superficial and deep. The stem may give origin to the deltoid arterial branches.[7]

Superficial Branch

The superficial branch emerges through the interval between the abductor hallucis and the flexor digitorum brevis and divides into two branches: the medial marginal plantar artery of the big toe (superficial tibial plantar artery) and the common plantar digital artery (see Fig. 7.34). The origin of the common plantar digital artery may be 1 to 1.5 cm or 5 to 6 cm from the origin of the medial plantar artery.[2]

The superficial tibial plantar artery runs constantly on the plantar aspect of the flexor hallucis brevis muscle, along the tibial side of the flexor hallucis longus. At the level of the first metatarsal neck, the artery passes between the bone and the flexor tendons and anastomoses with the first plantar metatarsal artery. The mode of termination of the superficial tibial plantar artery is variable. It may anastomose directly with the medial plantar hallucal artery or be the sole supplier of the latter(9); in these cases, the superficial tibial plantar artery courses on the plantar aspect of the medial head of the flexor hallucis brevis and remains on the tibial side of the flexor hallucis longus tendon until anastomosing with the medial plantar hallucal artery.

The superficial tibial plantar artery also may be very strong and replace the first plantar metatarsal artery.[2]

The stem of the common plantar digital arteries passes obliquely between the flexor digitorum brevis and the central plantar aponeurosis and provides the common superficial plantar digital arteries that unite with the first, second, and third plantar metatarsal arteries. The lateral terminal segment of the common superficial plantar digital artery may unite with the superficial branch of the lateral plantar artery and form the superficial plantar arch (see Fig. 7.34).

The superficial plantar arch formed by very slender arterial branches is present with the following frequency according to various sources: in 165 feet ("capillary caliber" arch), 28%; in 101 feet, 5%; in 66 feet, 30%; in 50 feet, 12% (well developed in 4%, frail in 8%).[1,2,14,16] A superficial branch—the medial superficial artery of the foot of Henle—is always quite large and arises from the medial plantar artery close to its origin. It crosses the deep surface of the abductor hallucis, emerges above the muscle, follows the superior border of the muscle, and terminates at the level of the metatarsophalangeal joint of the big toe.[9]

Deep Branch

The ramus profundus branches form the tibial side of the medial plantar artery near its origin, remains deep, and divides into two branches: tibial and lateral.[2]

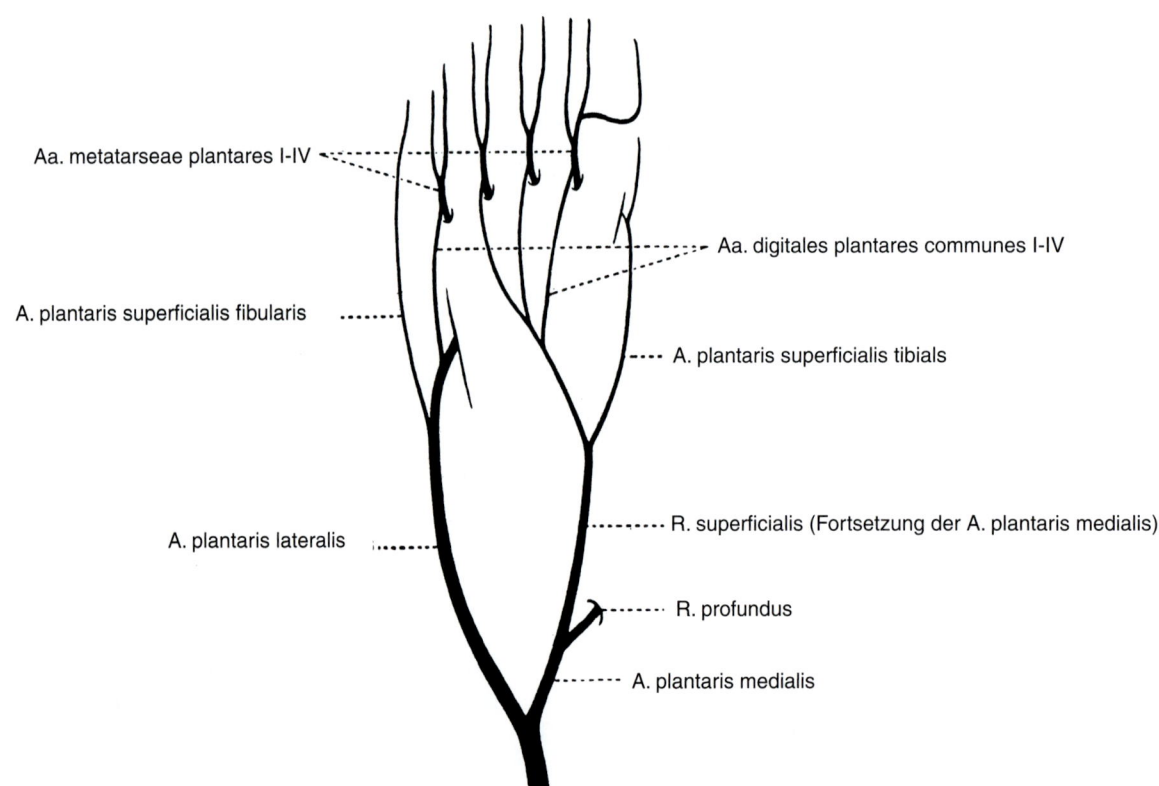

Figure 7.33 **The division branches of the medial plantar artery into the ramus superficialis and the ramus profundus.** The ramus superficialis provides the plantar-superficial tibial branch and the superficial common digital plantar arteries 1, 2, and 3. (From Adachi B. *Das Arteriensystem der Japaner*. Maruzen; 1928.)

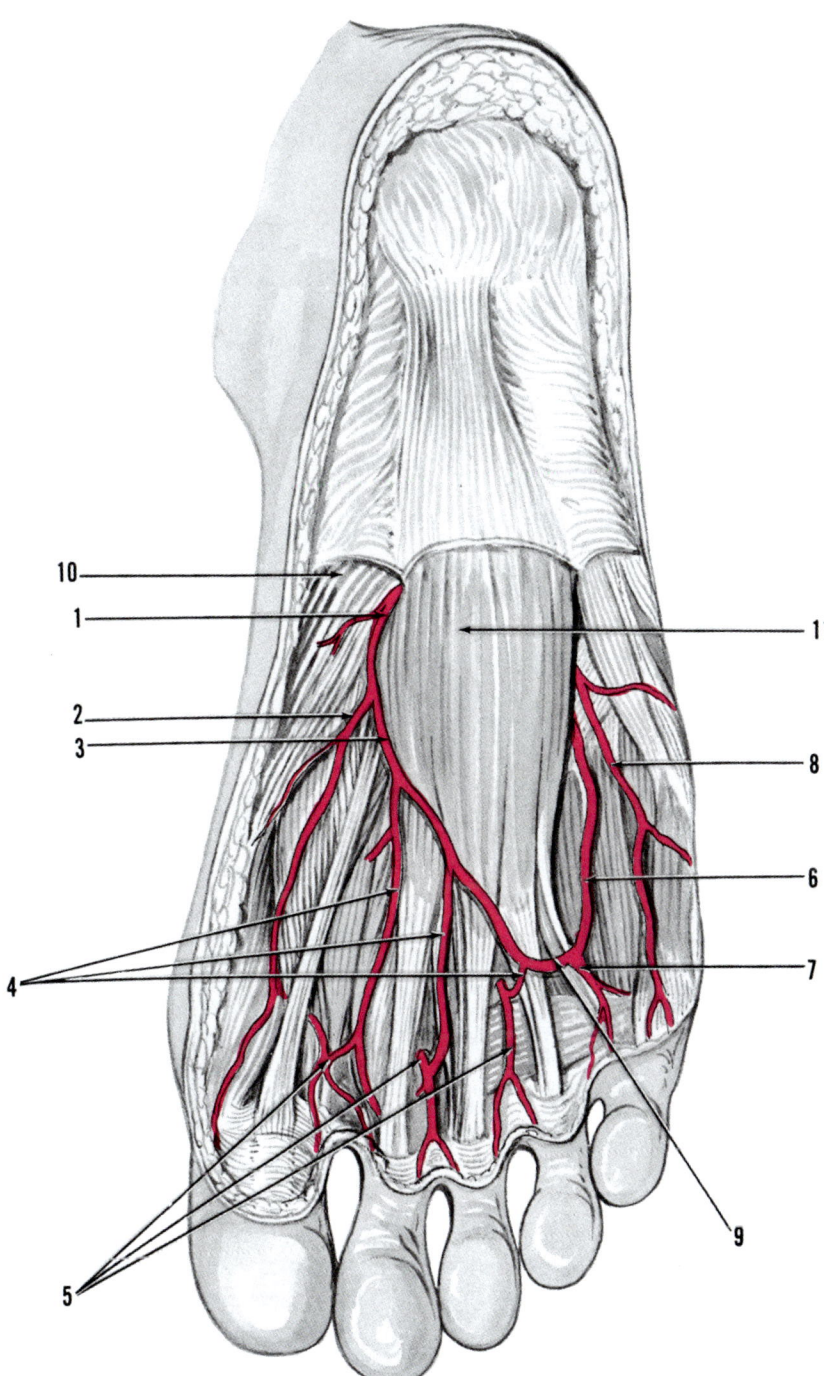

Figure 7.34 Superficial plantar arterial arc.
(*1*, superficial branch of medial plantar artery; *2*, tibial plantar superficial artery; *3*, common digital plantar superficial artery; *4*, superficial plantar digital arteries joining corresponding plantar metatarsal arteries [*5*]; *6*, superficial plantar digital artery to fourth web space joining plantar metatarsal artery to the same place [*7*]; *8*, fibular plantar superficial artery; *9*, superficial plantar arcade formed when *3* and *6* are anastomosed superficial to flexor digitorum brevis [*11*]; *10*, abductor hallucis muscle.) (From Aschner B. Zur Anatomie der Arterien der Fussohle. *Anat Hefte Beit Ref Anat Entwicklungs.* 1905;27:345.)

The tibial branch courses distally along the tibial skeletal margin of the foot, reaches the base of the first metatarsal, and anastomoses with the first plantar metatarsal artery (Figs. 7.35 and 7.36). In rare cases, it may even substitute for the latter. The same branch also occasionally continues into the dorsal tibial hallucal artery after emerging between the base of the first metatarsal bone and the abductor hallucis muscle. Further connections are established on the dorsomedial margin of the foot between branches of this artery and the dorsal arterial system.

The fibular branch penetrates even deeper into the planta pedis, passes dorsal to the peroneus longus tendon near its insertion on the base of the first metatarsal, and terminates on the tibial segment of the deep plantar arch (see Figs. 7.35 and 7.36). The fibular branch may arise directly from the medial plantar artery.

In a study of 100 feet, Adachi provides the following variations of the origin of the branches of the medial plantar artery: ramus profundus arising independently from the medial plantar artery, 63%; ramus profundus and superficial tibial plantar artery arising from the medial plantar artery through a short common trunk, 28%; medial plantar artery trifurcating into the superficial tibial plantar artery, ramus profundus, and common trunk of the plantar digital arteries, 9%.[2]

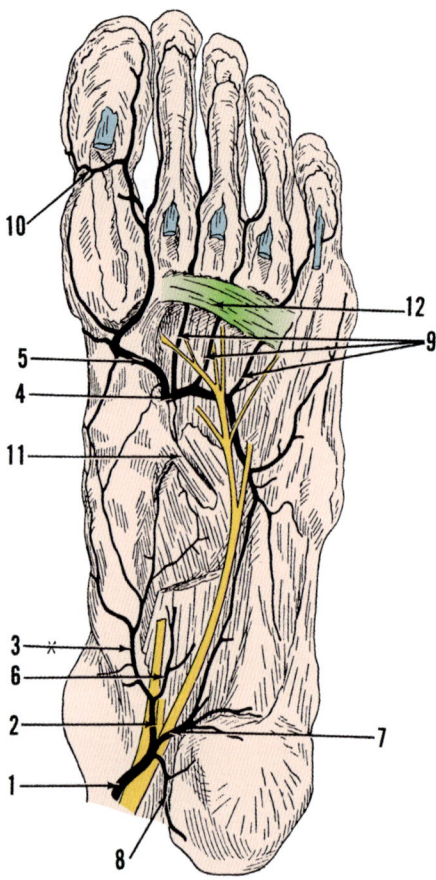

Figure 7.35 The deep branch of the medial plantar artery.
(*1*, posterior tibial artery; *2*, medial plantar artery; *3*, deep branch of medial plantar artery, which passes under peroneus longus tendon [*11*] and joins the deep plantar arc [*4*]; *5*, first plantar metatarsal artery; *6*, superficial branch of medial plantar artery; *7*, lateral plantar artery; *8*, medial calcaneal artery; *9*, plantar metatarsal arteries passing dorsal to transverse head of adductor hallucis muscle [*12*]; *10*, transverse plantar hallucal anastomotic branch passing on dorsal aspect of flexor hallucis longus tendon.) (Adapted from Adachi B. *Das Arteriensystem der Japaner*. Maruzen; 1928.)

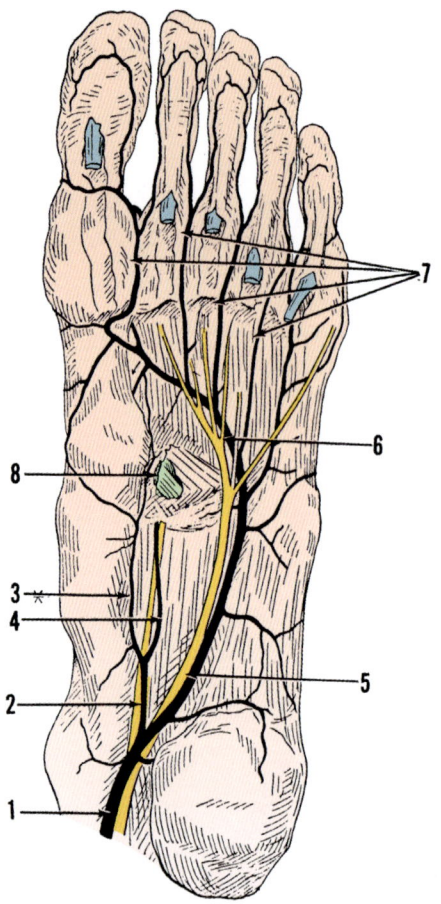

Figure 7.36 The deep branch of the medial plantar artery.
(*1*, posterior tibial artery; *2*, medial plantar artery; *3*, deep branch of medial plantar artery passing on dorsum of peroneus longus tendon [*8*; cut in this specimen]; *4*, superficial branch of medial plantar artery; *5*, lateral plantar artery; *6*, deep plantar arterial arc; *7*, plantar metatarsal arteries.) (Adapted from Adachi B. *Das Arteriensystem der Japaner*. Maruzen; 1928.)

Lateral Plantar Artery (Fig. 7.37)

The lateral plantar artery passes under the interfascicular septum of the calcaneal canal and enters the middle compartment of the foot. It courses obliquely and anterolaterally, under the fascia of the quadratus plantae muscle, and remains posterolateral to the lateral plantar nerve. It continues toward the base of the fifth metatarsal bone, pierces the lateral intermuscular septum, and extends forward between the lateral septum and the sheath of the abductor digiti quinti. On the medial aspect of the base of the fifth metatarsal and just distal to the latter, it gives off the superficial fibular plantar artery of the little toe. At about 2.5 cm distal to the fifth metatarsal base, the lateral plantar artery passes deep on the medial side of the flexor digiti quinti brevis, pierces again the lateral intermuscular septum, and enters the fascial space M_3 of the middle compartment. On the lateral border of the adductor hallucis obliquum, the artery penetrates the fascial space M_4 located between the adductor hallucis obliquum and the interossei muscles. The artery now has a nearly transverse course and crosses the base of metatarsals 4, 3, and 2 and terminates by inosculation with the perforating branch of the dorsalis pedis at the proximal end of the first intermetatarsal space. This deep arterial arch provides the proximal or posterior perforating arteries of the second to fourth intermetatarsal space communicating with the dorsal metatarsal arterial system and the second to fourth plantar metatarsal arteries. The first plantar metatarsal artery is considered a branch of the dorsalis pedis artery.

Deep Plantar Arch

The deep plantar arch is formed by inosculation of the deep plantar branch of the dorsalis pedis artery with the deep transverse component of the lateral plantar artery. The site of union of the two arteries is indicated by the thinnest portion of the arterial arch. This point of junction is not constant, indicating the variable contribution of each arterial component (Table 7.9, Fig. 7.38). Vann, in a study of 361 feet related to the formation of the deep plantar arch, reports the dorsalis pedis contribution to predominate in 80.8% and the lateral plantar artery in 15.23%.[17]

Chapter 7: Angiology   335

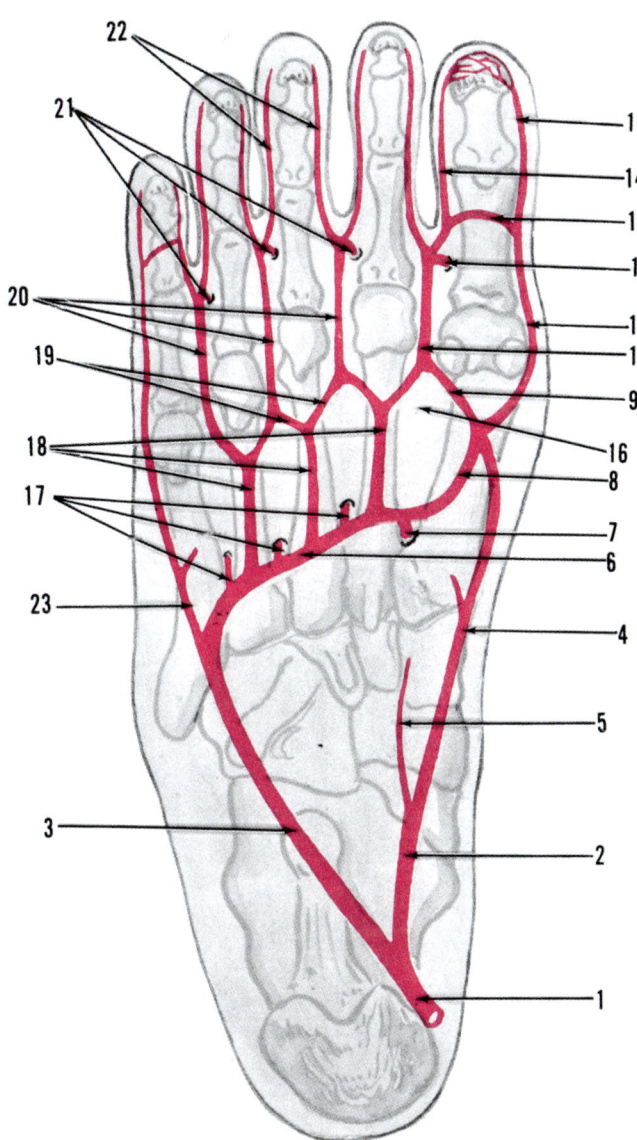

Figure 7.37 **Plantar arteries.** (*1*, posterior tibial artery; *2*, medial plantar artery; *3*, lateral plantar artery; *4*, superficial branch of medial plantar artery; *5*, deep branch of medial plantar artery; *6*, deep arterial plantar arc; *7*, first proximal perforating artery or vertical descending segment of dorsalis pedis artery, *8*, first plantar metatarsal artery; *9*, lateral division branch of first plantar metatarsal artery; *10*, medial division branch of first plantar metatarsal artery; *11*, common digital artery 1; *12*, first distal perforating artery or vertical descending segment of first dorsal interosseous artery; *13*, transverse plantar hallucal anastomotic branch passing dorsal to flexor hallucis longus tendon; *14*, lateral plantar hallucal artery; *15*, medial plantar hallucal artery; *16*, superficial common digital artery 1; *17*, proximal perforating arteries; *18*, plantar metatarsal arteries 2, 3, and 4; *19*, bifurcation of metatarsal arteries forming an arcade [in more usual form, medial limb of bifurcation is absent]; *20*, common digital arteries 2, 3, and 4; *21*, distal perforating arteries; *22*, plantar digital arteries; *23*, fibular plantar superficial artery.) (From Edwards EA. Anatomy of the small arteries of the foot and toes. *Acta Anat.* 1960;40:81. By permission of S. Karger AG, Basel.)

number of plantar metatarsal arteries supplied in each type of foot by these two arterial sources.

The plantar metatarsal arteries may be missing, as reported by Adachi, in the following percentages: 1, 2.3%; 2, 2.3%; 3, 0; 4, 6.1%, or they may be rudimentary and substituted for by the superficial plantar arterial system in the following frequency: 1, 16%; 2, 3%; 3, 0; 4, 19%.[2] The first plantar metatarsal artery may be substituted for by the tibial superficial plantar artery and the first common plantar digital artery. The second plantar metatarsal artery may be substituted for by the second common plantar digital artery and the fourth by the fibular superficial plantar artery or the fourth common plantar digital artery.

The four lateral plantar metatarsal arteries course "along the midline of the shafts of the medial four metatarsals not, as is usually stated, along the interosseous space."[3] These arteries course forward and remain superficial or plantar to the interossei muscles. The plantar metatarsal arteries 2 and 3 pass without exception deep or dorsal to the transverse head of the adductor hallucis muscle (Fig. 7.39). In 102 feet, Adachi reports only one case in which the second and third plantar metatarsal arteries divide into two branches at the proximal border of the muscle[2]; one branch passes plantar and the other dorsal to the muscle, forming an arterial loop, and they join again distally (Fig. 7.40). The plantar metatarsal artery 4 passes dorsal (75%) or plantar (25%) to the same muscle.[2] Distally, the plantar metatarsal artery bifurcates into two metatarsodigital branches. This division occurs at the level of a triangle centered on the head-neck of the metatarsal and is limited on each side by the corresponding interossei muscles (Fig. 7.41).[18] The base of the triangle is distal, corresponding to the entrance of the flexor

Plantar Metatarsal Arteries (See Fig. 7.37)

The four plantar metatarsal arteries arise from the deep plantar arch, and their blood supply is provided by the deep plantar branch of the dorsalis pedis or by the lateral plantar artery. The frequency of contribution of these two arterial sources to the individual plantar metatarsal artery is shown in Table 7.10. Figure 7.38 provides further information concerning the

TABLE 7.9 Frequency of Contributions of Arterial Components			
Deep Plantar Arterial Arch Formed by %	Dubreuil-Chambardel (203 Feet)	Manno (66 Feet)	Adachi (130 Feet)
Type I: Only deep plantar branch of dorsalis pedis artery	40.2	48.4	25.3 (type A)
Type II: Union of deep plantar branch of dorsalis pedis artery and lateral plantar arteries	55.8	51.6	67.6 (type B, 32.3; type C, 14.6; type D, 14.6; type E, 6.1)
Type III: Only lateral plantar artery	4		7 (type F)

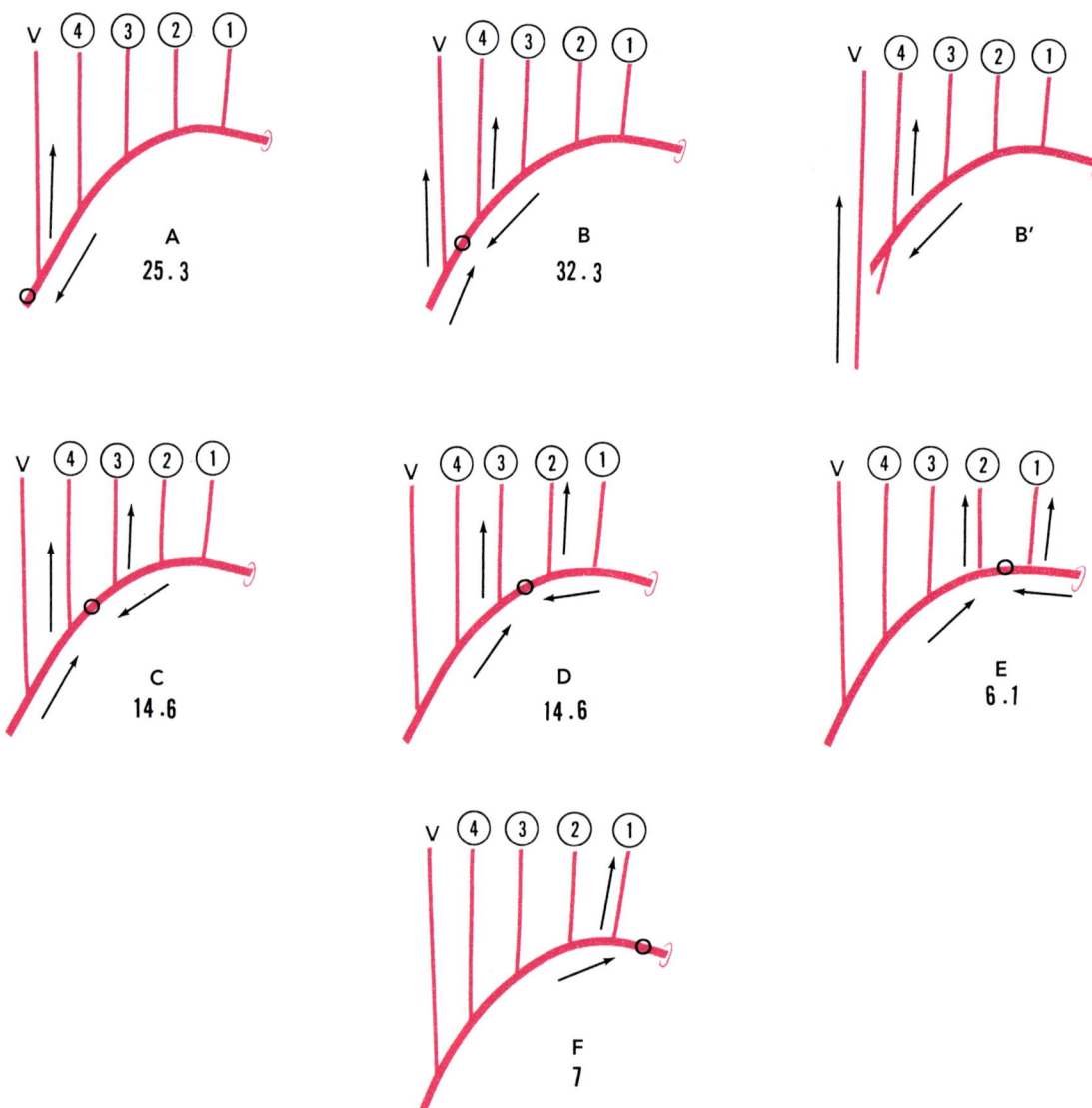

Figure 7.38 **Deep plantar arterial arch: variable contribution of the deep transverse component of the lateral plantar artery and of the deep plantar branch of the dorsalis pedis.** The site of union of the two arteries is indicated by a black circle representing the thinnest portion of the arterial arch. (*Type A*) The arch is formed only by the deep plantar branch of the dorsalis pedis and supplies the plantar meta-arteries 1 to 4 and the fibular plantar marginal artery V. (*Type B*) The point of junction is located between the plantar metatarsal artery 4 and the fibular plantar marginal artery V. The deep plantar branch of the dorsalis pedis supplies the plantar metatarsal arteries 1 to 4. (*Type B'*) The deep plantar arch is supplied only by the deep plantar branch of the dorsalis pedis artery. The fibular plantar marginal artery V is provided by the lateral plantar artery. (*Type C*) The point of junction is located between the plantar metatarsal arteries 3 and 4. The deep plantar branch of the dorsalis pedis artery provides the plantar metatarsal arteries 1 to 3. The lateral plantar artery provides the fibular plantar marginal artery V and the plantar metatarsal artery 4. (*Type D*) The point of junction shifts further medially and is located between the plantar metatarsal arteries 2 and 3. The deep plantar branch of the dorsalis pedis supplies the plantar metatarsal arteries 1 and 2. The lateral plantar artery supplies the fibular plantar marginal artery and the plantar metatarsal arteries 3 and 4. (*Type E*) The point of junction is located between the plantar metatarsal arteries 1 and 2. The deep plantar branch of the dorsalis pedis supplies only the first plantar metatarsal artery. The lateral plantar artery supplies the fibular plantar marginal artery V and the plantar metatarsal arteries 2, 3, and 4. (*Type F*) The deep plantar arterial arch is formed entirely by the lateral plantar artery. (The numbers indicate the percentage of occurrence of the indicated variations.) (From Adachi B. *Das Arteriensystem der Japaner.* Maruzen; 1928.)

TABLE 7.10 Contribution to Individual Plantar Metatarsal Arteries

Plantar Metatarsal Artery	Deep Plantar Branch of Dorsalis Pedis Artery (%)		Lateral Plantar Artery (%)	
	Adachi[a]	Manno[b]	Adachi[a]	Manno[b]
1	90.8	89.4	6.9	7.6
2	84.6	84.8	13.1	12.1
3	72.3	75.8	27.7	21.2
4	54.6	48.5	39.2	48.5

[a]130 feet.
[b]66 feet.

tunnel and the plantar plate. The apex is proximal. The bifurcation branches pass on each side of the corresponding flexor tunnel through an aperture located between the transverse head of the adductor hallucis muscle and the deep transverse metatarsal ligament. They course on the plantar aspect of the latter and join distally the corresponding plantar digital artery formed in the web space by the bifurcation of the distal perforating branch of the dorsal metatarsal artery. The medial limb of the lateral three bifurcations of the plantar metatarsal artery may be missing.[3] Also, the adjacent branches of the same bifurcation may unite and form an arterial arcade.[3]

Murakami describes two sets of plantar metatarsal arteries: superficial and deep (Fig. 7.42).[12] The superficial branches are located on the plantar aspect of the interossei muscles and are subdivided into two groups—the superficial metatarsal arteries (2-5) and the superficial intermetatarsal arteries (2-4). They all originate from the deep plantar arch, and almost all (38 of 40) are covered initially by the "accessory slips of the lateral two or three interosseous muscles arising from the lateral border of the plantar aponeurosis."[12]

The superficial metatarsal arteries course distally along the axis of the corresponding metatarsals and reach the triangular space described above. Except for the superficial metatarsal artery 2, they are separated from the bone by the interossei muscles.

The superficial intermetatarsal arteries course over the interossei in the intermetatarsal space in the direction of the web space and reach the proximal border of the deep transverse metatarsal ligament.

Any of the superficial arteries may take an oblique course when the deep plantar arch is formed entirely or almost completely by the deep plantar artery of the dorsalis pedis artery (see Fig. 7.38).

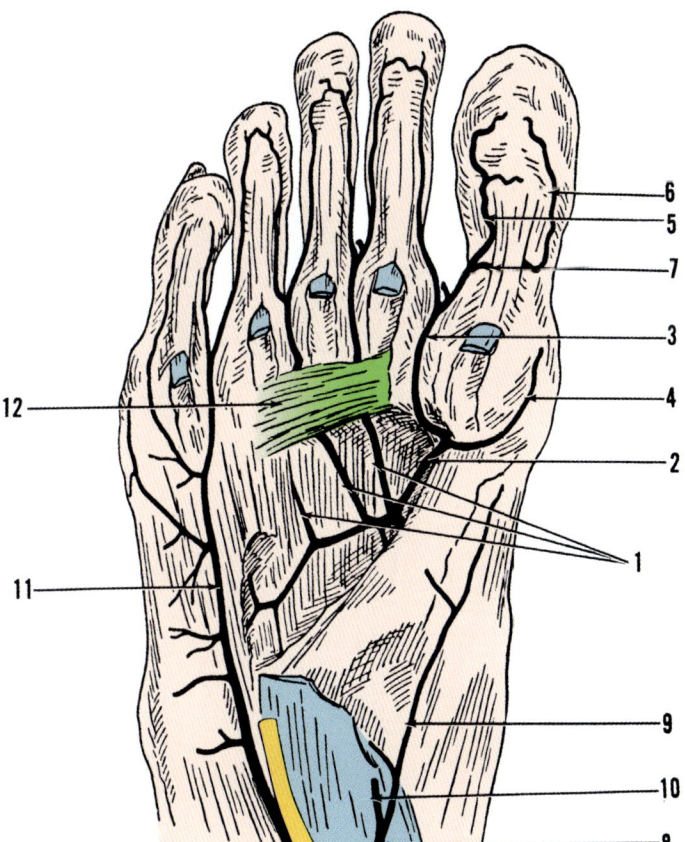

Figure 7.39 **The plantar metatarsal arteries 2, 3, and 4 pass dorsal to the transverse head of the adductor hallucis muscle.** (*1*, plantar metatarsal arteries 2, 3, and 4; *2*, first plantar metatarsal artery; *3*, lateral bifurcation branch of 2; *4*, medial bifurcation branch of 2; *5*, lateral plantar hallucal artery; *6*, medial plantar hallucal artery; *7*, transverse or anastomotic segment of plantar hallucal artery; *8*, medial plantar artery; *9*, tibial marginal plantar artery; *10*, deep branch of medial plantar artery; *11*, fibular marginal plantar artery; *12*, transverse head of adductor hallucis muscle.) (Adapted from Adachi B. *Das Arteriensystem der Japaner*. Maruzen; 1928:288.)

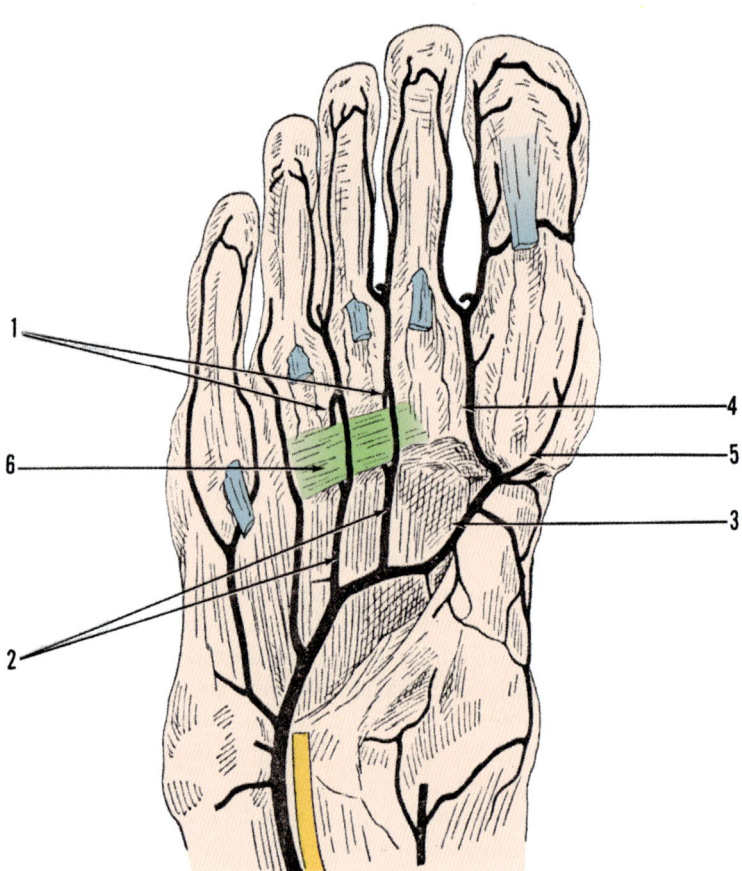

Figure 7.40 **The second and third plantar metatarsal arteries (2) form an arterial loop (1) around the transverse head of the adductor hallucis muscle (6).** (*3*, first plantar metatarsal artery; *4*, lateral division branch of *3*; *5*, medial division branch of *3*.) (Adapted from Adachi B. *Das Arteriensystem der Japaner*. Maruzen; 1928:289.)

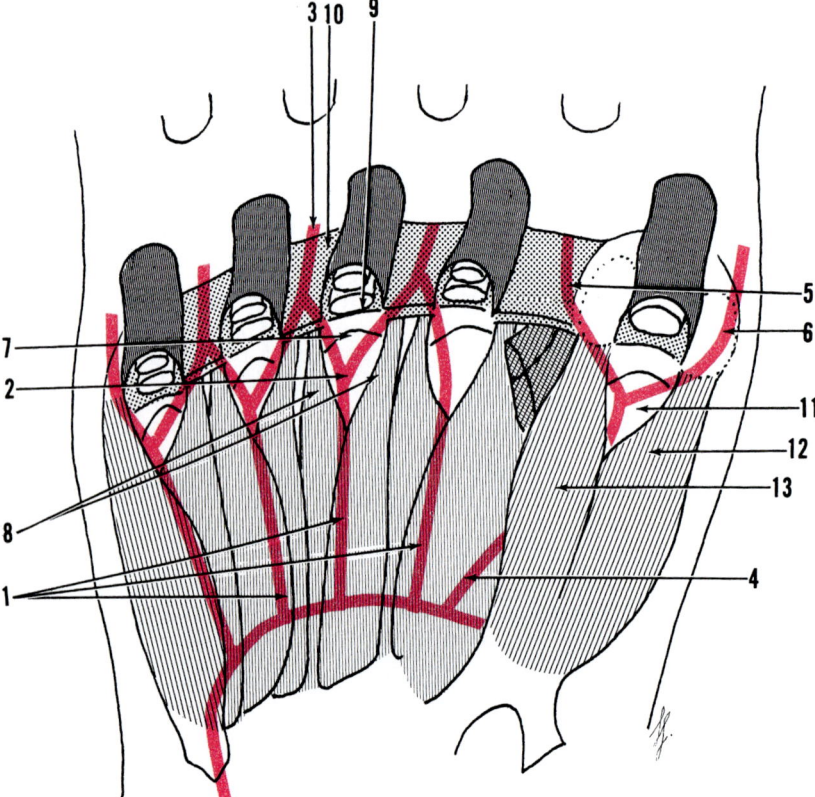

Figure 7.41 **The vascular triangle (7) overlies the plantar aspect of the metatarsal head.** The apex is proximal and the base distal, corresponding to the distal segment of the plantar plate (*9*). The sides are formed by the corresponding interossei muscle (*8*). Plantar metatarsal arteries (*1*) bifurcate at the level of the vascular triangle (*2*) and form at the level of the deep transverse metatarsal ligament (*10*) the common digital artery (*3*). The first plantar metatarsal artery (*4*) passes dorsal to the lateral head of the flexor hallucis brevis muscle (*13*) and reaches the vascular triangle (*11*) of the big toe, where it bifurcates into the lateral (*5*) and medial (*6*) branches. (*12*, medial head of flexor hallucis brevis muscle.)

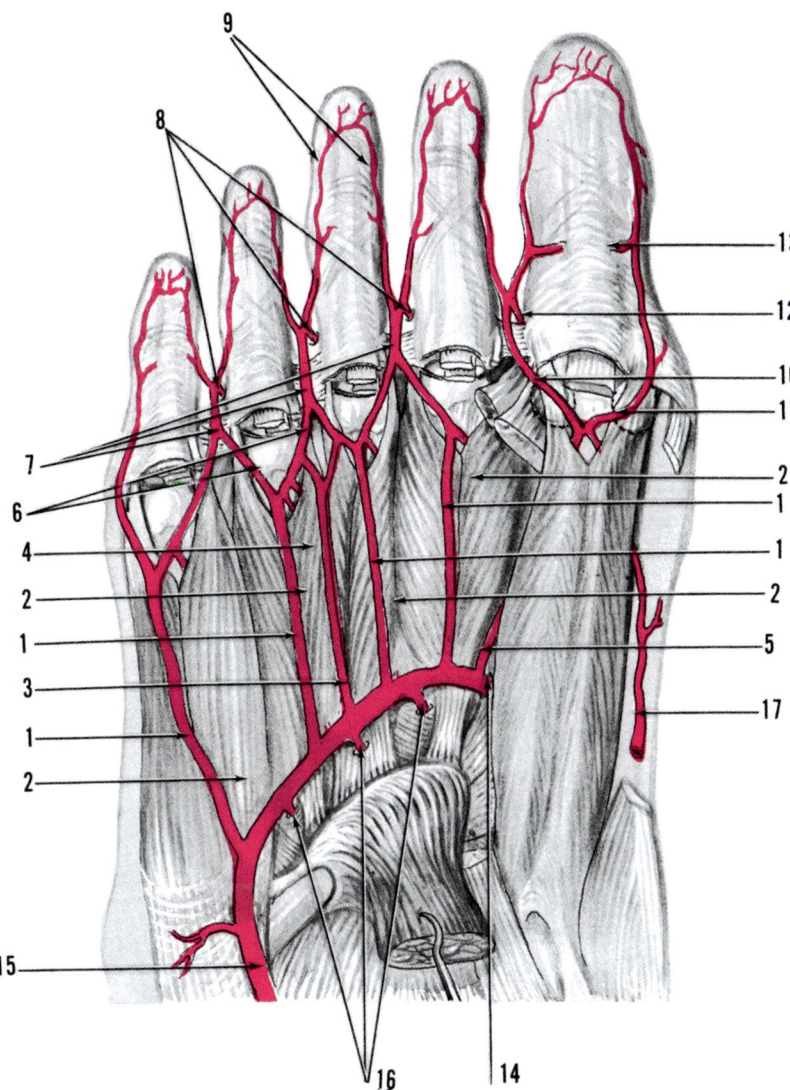

Figure 7.42 Potential pattern of the plantar metatarsal arteries. The first superficial plantar metatarsal artery, not represented in this diagram, passes plantar to the flexor hallucis brevis. It originates from the tibial plantar marginal artery and connects with the medial bifurcation branch of the first deep plantar metatarsal artery at the level of the vascular triangle of the big toe. In the first metatarsal interspace, Murakami considers the first dorsal interosseous artery as the first superficial plantar intermetatarsal artery and describes another slender branch, more plantar in position, as the first deep plantar intermetatarsal artery; the latter arises from the first deep plantar metatarsal artery. (*1*, superficial plantar metatarsal arteries, second to fifth; *2*, deep plantar metatarsal arteries, second to fifth; *3*, superficial plantar intermetatarsal artery; *4*, intermediary plantar metatarsal artery; *5*, first deep plantar metatarsal artery; *6*, lateral and medial bifurcation branches of plantar metatarsal artery; *7*, common plantar digital arteries; *8*, distal perforating arteries; *9*, plantar digital arteries, lateral and medial; *10*, lateral bifurcation branch of first deep plantar metatarsal artery; *11*, medial bifurcation branch of first deep plantar metatarsal artery; *12*, first distal perforating artery or descending segment of first dorsal interosseous artery; *13*, transverse anastomotic branch between plantar hallucal arteries; *14*, first proximal perforating artery or vertical descending segment of dorsalis pedis artery; *15*, lateral plantar artery; *16*, proximal perforating arteries; *17*, tibial plantar marginal artery, a superficial branch of medial plantar artery.) (From Murakami T. On the position and course of the deep plantar arteries, with special reference to the so-called plantar metatarsal arteries. *Okajimas Folia Anat Jpn.* 1971;48:295. https://www.jstage.jst.go.jp/article/ofaj1936/48/5/48_295/_article/-char/en)

The deep branches arise from the deep plantar arch or from the proximal perforating arteries. They penetrate the interossei muscles and are divided into two groups: deep metatarsal arteries (2-5) and deep intermetatarsal arteries (2-4).

The deep metatarsal arteries course distally on the plantar aspect of the metatarsal bones, between the plantar and dorsal interossei, and reach the triangular space at the neck of the corresponding metatarsal. The deep intermetatarsal arteries course distally between the plantar and dorsal interossei muscles in the intermetatarsal space. They descend on the medial surface of the lateral three metatarsal bones and enter the triangular space from the medial side. Any of the deep plantar arteries may also take an oblique course when the contribution of the dorsalis pedis to the deep plantar arch predominates.

Murakami's description, based on a study of 40 feet, provides the basis for the potential forms of the plantar metatarsal arteries, similar to the potential arterial system described on the dorsum of the foot.[4] Furthermore, it explains clearly that a "metatarsal" artery may be in a metatarsal or intermetatarsal position, the latter being the accepted location in most of the anatomy textbooks.

A fifth superficial plantar metatarsal artery is described by Murakami as the artery running distally between the third plantar interosseous muscle and the flexor digiti minimi brevis.[12] This artery may share a common trunk with the lateral marginal artery (Adachi's arteria plantaris superficialis lateralis). The lateral marginal artery, which may also arise independently from the lateral plantar artery, pierces the lateral intermuscular septum and courses distally between the flexor digiti minimi brevis and the abductor minimi muscles; it is present in 22.5%.[18]

The presence of the different components of the plantar "metatarsal" arteries is variable. The most commonly occurring arteries are the superficial plantar metatarsal arteries. Murakami provides data concerning these variations (Table 7.11).[12]

Plantar Digital Arteries of Lesser Toes

The plantar metatarsal arteries are the major source of blood supply to the lesser toes except the tibial aspect of the second toe. As described by Murakami, the superficial plantar metatarsal, the deep plantar metatarsal, and the deep plantar intermetatarsal arteries enter the triangular spaces located

TABLE 7.11 Frequency of Occurrence (%) of Plantar "Metatarsal" Arteries				
	Metatarsal Arteries		Intermetatarsal Arteries	
Plantar "Metatarsal" Arteries	Superficial	Deep	Superficial	Deep
Second	85[a]	22.5	32.5	32.5
Third	82.5	30	25	57.5
Fourth	62.5	57.5	22.5	67.5
Fifth	80	37.5	Mag[b] = 22.5	

[a]Includes the intermediate plantar metatarsal artery, which descends directly on the plantar surface of the second metatarsal bone.
[b]Mag, lateral marginal plantar artery.

on the plantar aspect of the second to fifth metatarsal necks (see Figs. 7.42 and 7.43).[12] The sides of the triangular space formed by the interossei muscles and the plantar aspect are crossed by the transverse head of the adductor hallucis muscle. In the triangular space, the superficial plantar metatarsal, deep plantar metatarsal, and deep plantar intermetatarsal arteries anastomose and form a common trunk. A pair of transversely directed anastomotic branches take off from the latter; these branches pass between the sides of the metatarsal neck and the interossei and form two dorsally directed perforating arteries that then anastomose with similar branches arising from the dorsal metatarsal artery.[4] The common plantar arterial trunk bifurcates into two terminal branches at the level of the triangular space. Each branch bends sharply and passes between the distal border of the transverse head of the adductor hallucis and the deep transverse metatarsal ligaments. The artery courses on the plantar aspect of the latter, along the flexor tendon sheath, and terminates as the corresponding proper plantar digital artery, which is joined by the bifurcation branch of the distal perforating branch of the corresponding dorsal metatarsal artery.

The superficial plantar intermetatarsal artery extends distally in the intermetatarsal space, passes dorsal to the deep transverse metatarsal ligament, and unites with the distal perforating branch of the dorsal metatarsal artery. The superficial plantar intermetatarsal artery may give two branches at the distal segment of the intermetatarsal space. These two branches are inconstant and, when present, join the terminal branches of the superficial plantar metatarsal, deep plantar metatarsal, and deep plantar intermetatarsal arteries to form an arterial arcade.

Adachi provides the following information with regard to the blood supplied by the plantar metatarsal artery to the toes in 100 feet: in web space 2 (toes 2 and 3), 84.8%; in web space 3 (toes 3 and 4), 96%; in web space 4 (toes 4 and 5), 76%.[2] The substitutions are provided by the dorsal metatarsal arteries, the common plantar digital arteries, and the superficial plantar fibular artery or lateral marginal artery.

The major blood supply to the lesser toes, except for the tibial side of the second toe, is provided by the proper plantar digital arteries. The dorsal digital arteries may be thin or short, ending in the proximal part of the dorsum of the proximal phalanx. In a lesser toe, one proper plantar digital artery may predominate.

Levame, in an arteriographic study of 11 feet (9 adult, 2 fetuses of 4 months), reports the tibial-sided proper plantar digital artery to predominate in toes 2 to 4.[10] The corresponding plantar digital artery on the fibular aspect of the toe is absent or always frail (Fig. 7.44).

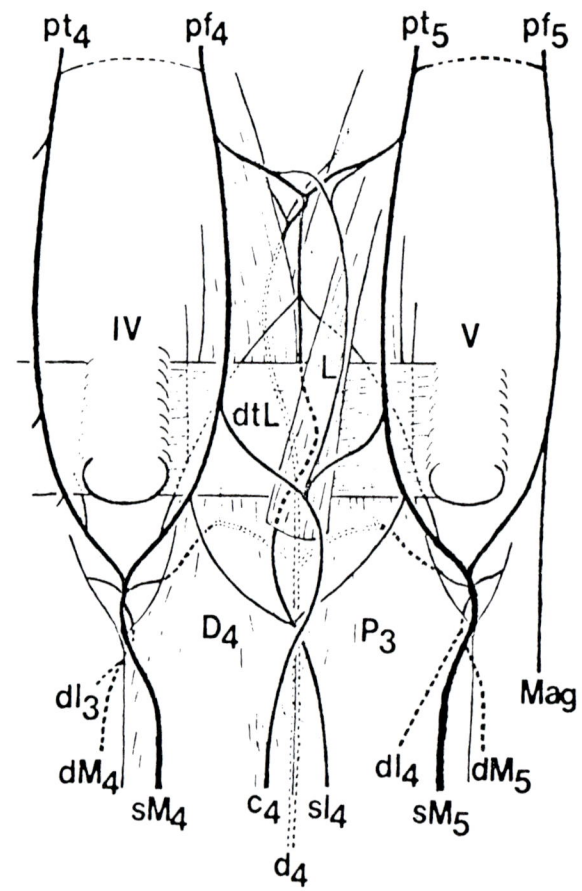

Figure 7.43 Ideal pattern of the branching and anastomosis of the deep metatarsal descending arteries. (*IV*, ray of fourth toe; *V*, ray of fifth toe; c_4, common superficial digital artery; d_4, dorsal interosseous artery; D_4, fourth dorsal interosseous muscle; dl_3, dl_4, deep plantar intermetatarsal arteries; dM_4, dM_5, deep plantar metatarsal arteries; *dtL*, deep transverse metatarsal ligament; *L*, lumbrical muscle; *Mag*, lateral marginal plantar artery; P_3, third plantar interosseous muscle; pt_4 and pf_4, tibial and fibular plantar arteries to the fourth toe; pt_5 and pf_5, tibial and fibular plantar arteries to the fifth toe; sl_4, superficial plantar intermetatarsal artery; sM_4, sM_5, superficial plantar metatarsal arteries.) (From Murakami T. On the position and course of the deep plantar arteries, with special reference to the so-called plantar metatarsal arteries. *Okajimas Folia Anat Jpn*. 1971;48:295. https://www.jstage.jst.go.jp/article/ofaj1936/48/5/48_295/_article/-char/en)

Chapter 7: Angiology

Posterior Peroneal Artery

The posterior peroneal artery is the posterior bifurcation branch of the peroneal artery. It descends vertically along the posterior tibiofibular ligament and is located in the compartment of the flexor hallucis longus muscle-tendon, which is covered by the deep crural aponeurosis. The artery is anterior in the narrow interval between the flexor hallucis longus and the peroneus brevis. Farther distally, the flexor hallucis longus tendon parts medially, thus enlarging the posterior intertendinous interval that would give access to the artery. During its downward course, the artery traces a curve with an anterior concavity behind the peronei tendons and terminates on the lateral surface of the os calcis. To reach its destination, the artery perforates the deep crural fascia but remains under the superficial fascia.

The posterior peroneal artery provides proximally two transverse anastomotic branches: medial and anterolateral. The medial transverse branch passes anterior to the tendon of the flexor hallucis longus and anastomoses with a similar branch emanating from the posterior tibial artery. The anterolateral branch is also transverse, passes between the peronei tendons and the lateral malleolus, and connects with the anterior lateral malleolar artery. These two transverse branches contribute to the formation of the transverse perimalleolar arterial circle. A third collateral branch takes off from the artery below the tip of the lateral malleolus, passes deep to the peronei tendons, and anastomoses anteriorly with the descending branch of the anterior lateral malleolar artery, forming a sagittal lateral malleolar arterial loop. Other small terminal branches anastomose with branches from the lateral tarsal artery and contribute to the formation of the lateral malleolar arterial rete.

Cutaneous branches are provided to the lateral aspect of the heel, and recurrent calcaneal branches ascend to the dorsal surface of the os calcis, anastomose with similar branches provided by the posterior tibial artery, and form an anastomotic arcade that contributes to the formation of the calcaneal arterial rete.

▶ Cutaneous Arterial Supply to the Foot and Ankle

To the Dorsum of the Foot and Ankle

The skin of the dorsum of the foot and ankle is supplied by the distal segment of the tibialis anterior artery, the dorsalis pedis artery, and the first dorsal metatarsal artery. Further contribution is given by the anterior peroneal artery, the dorsal arterial rete, and the marginal anastomotic branches along the medial and lateral borders of the foot. The dorsalis pedis artery and the first dorsal metatarsal artery form the arterial axis and are the major providers of the blood supply to the dorsal skin. The anterior peroneal artery furnishes most of the cutaneous vessels of the sinus tarsi, which are carried through the fat pad. The skin covering the extensor digitorum brevis has the poorest blood supply.[18] A quantitative study of the contribution of the dorsalis pedis and the first dorsal metatarsal arteries to the

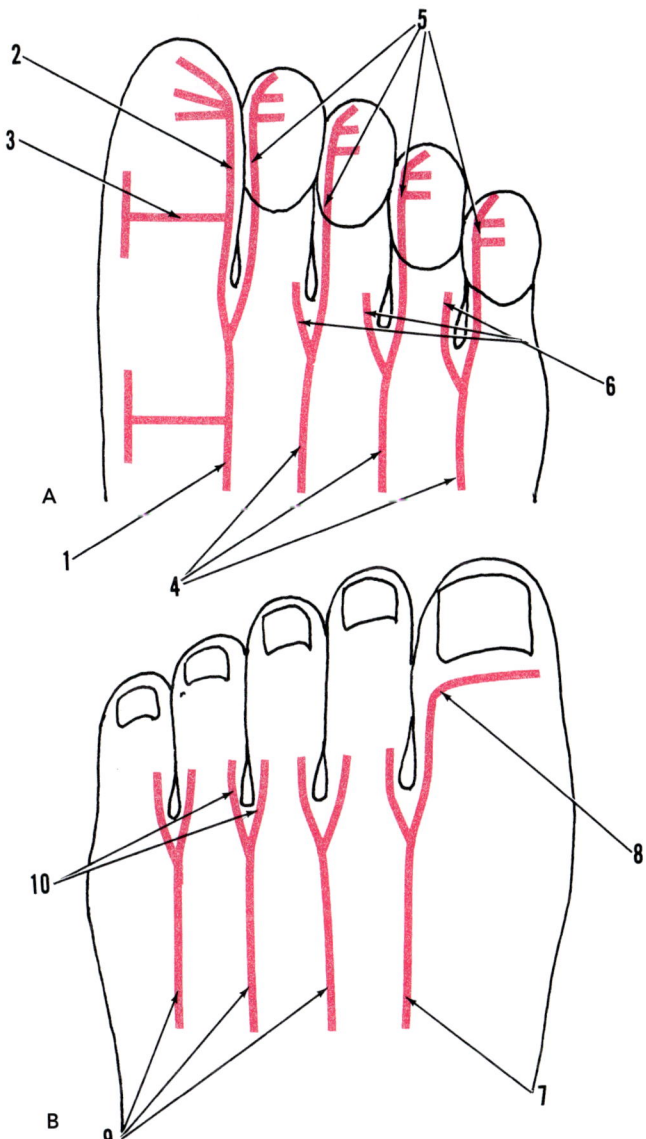

Figure 7.44 Arterial blood supply of the toes. (A) Plantar aspect. Five plantar digital collateral arteries are constant: the peroneal hallucal plantar artery (2) and the four tibial plantar digital arteries (5). The peroneal plantar digital arteries (6) are not well developed. (1, first plantar metatarsal artery; 3, anastomotic transverse plantar hallucal artery; 4, plantar metatarsal arteries.) **(B)** Dorsal aspect. One dorsal peroneal hallucal artery (8) is constant. The dorsal collateral arteries of the lesser toes (10) are not well developed. (7, first dorsal intermetatarsal artery; 9, dorsal metatarsal arteries of lesser toes.) (Reproduced from Levame JH. Les artères des orteils: etude anatomique et arteriographique: conclusions chirugicales. *J Chir.* 1963;86[6]:651. Copyright © 1963. Elsevier Masson SAS. All rights reserved.)

The proper plantar digital arteries terminate in a tuft, and this "terminal arborization is a major and constant site of communication between each pair of plantar digitals."[3] In the "adult" form of arborization, a proximal arcade is present at the level of the tuft.[3]

A transverse anastomotic branch may be seen passing between the plantar aspect of the proximal phalanx of the little toe and the flexor tendons.[3,12] Murakami cites the frequency of the occurrence of this anastomosis as 32.5% in 40 feet.[12]

blood supply of the skin of the dorsum of the foot and ankle in 23 feet is presented by Man and Acland.[6] The dorsal skin is divided into three zones (Fig. 7.45):

Zone 1: Extends from the superior border to the interior border of the inferior extensor retinaculum
Zone 2: Extends from zone 1 to the proximal border of the first dorsal interosseous muscle
Zone 3: Extends from zone 2 to the distal tip of the first web space.

In zone 1, the arterial branches pass between the arms of the extensor retinaculum. There are 5.4 arterial branches, with a diameter of 0.15 to 0.7 mm (average, 0.3 mm) and a mean total cross-sectional area of 0.53 mm.[2] Two-thirds of the branches pass between the tendons of the extensor digitorum longus and the extensor hallucis longus; one-third of the branches course more medially and then pass between the extensor hallucis longus tendon and the tibialis anterior tendon.

In zone 2, the dorsalis pedis artery is crossed obliquely by the extensor hallucis brevis. The purely cutaneous branches are 1.9 in number, with a mean total cross-sectional area of 0.16 mm.[2] If the arterial branches supplying the extensor hallucis brevis also are included with the assumption that they might reach the skin, the number of the arterial branches is 3.8, with a diameter of 0.15 to 0.7 mm (mean, 0.29 mm) and a mean total cross-sectional area of 0.30 mm.[2]

In zone 3, the provider is the first dorsal metatarsal artery. The cutaneous branches are 6.7 in number, with a diameter ranging from 0.15 to 0.33 mm (mean, 0.27 mm) and a mean total cross-sectional area of 0.45 mm.[2] When the first dorsal metatarsal artery is missing (14% in this study), the cutaneous branches are absent and "the cutaneous blood supply in such cases presumably comes from the subdermal plexus."[6]

To the Malleolar Skin

The blood supply of the malleolar skin is provided by the malleolar rete. The *lateral malleolar rete*, a fine-meshed subcutaneous network, is formed by arterial twigs emanating from the sagittal and the transverse perilateral malleolar arterial loops and the lateral tarsal artery. Small recurrent branches from the lateral plantar artery may reach the network. *The medial malleolar rete* over the medial malleolus has finer arterial branches, and the loose network is formed by the anterior and posterior medial malleolar branches and the medial tarsal artery.

To the Planta Pedis

The skin of the planta pedis is as well vascularized as the skin of the scalp.[18] In the midtarsal area, the small perforating vessels are numerous and are provided by the medial and, to a larger degree, the lateral plantar arteries. The medial vertical branches pass through the medial plantar sulcus between the abductor hallucis and the flexor digitorum brevis. The lateral perforating branches pass through the lateral plantar sulcus between the flexor digitorum brevis and the abductor digiti quinti.

At the anterior segment of the planta pedis, the skin is supplied by the cutaneous branches emanating from the common plantar digital arteries.

The skin of the medial aspect of the heel possesses more arteries than does that of the lateral aspect.[3] The medial calcaneal branches provided by the lateral plantar artery stem from two or three main branches, which then divide, pass through the flexor retinaculum, and reach the skin of the heel. Several other smaller branches originate farther distally. The first medial calcaneal branch may emanate from the end of the posterior tibial artery. The lateral calcaneal branches are provided by the posterior peroneal artery above and by the lateral tarsal artery below.

As mentioned by Edwards, the upper lateral calcaneal branch may stem from the posterior tibial artery and the lower calcaneal branches may arise from the lateral plantar artery or the anterior peroneal artery.[3]

Hidalgo and Shaw studied the plantar arterial blood supply in 15 fresh foot specimens.[19] Four zones of arterial skin anatomy were demonstrated[1]: the proximal plantar area,[2] the midplantar area,[3] the lateral foot, and[4] the distal foot (Fig. 7.46). In the proximal plantar area, there is an extensive subcutaneous arterial plexus that extends half the distance between the posterior border of the heel and the metatarsal heads. The vessels have a medial-lateral transverse orientation. This arterial plexus is supplied primarily by the dorsalis pedis and the lateral plantar arteries. The dorsalis pedis artery supplies the plexus by wraparound medial and lateral branches turning around

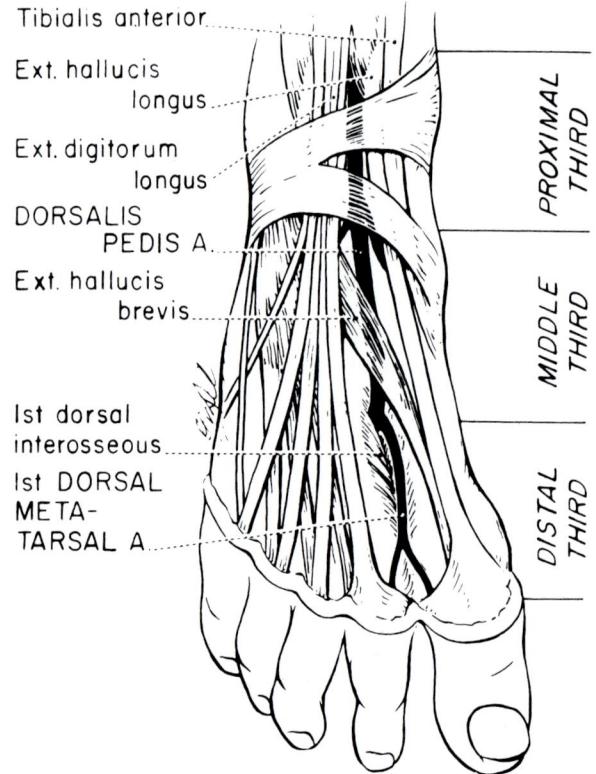

Figure 7.45 Zones of the skin of the dorsum of the foot.
(Adapted from Man D, Acland RD. The microarterial anatomy of the dorsalis pedis flap and its clinical applications. *Plast Reconstr Surg.* 1980;65(4):419.)

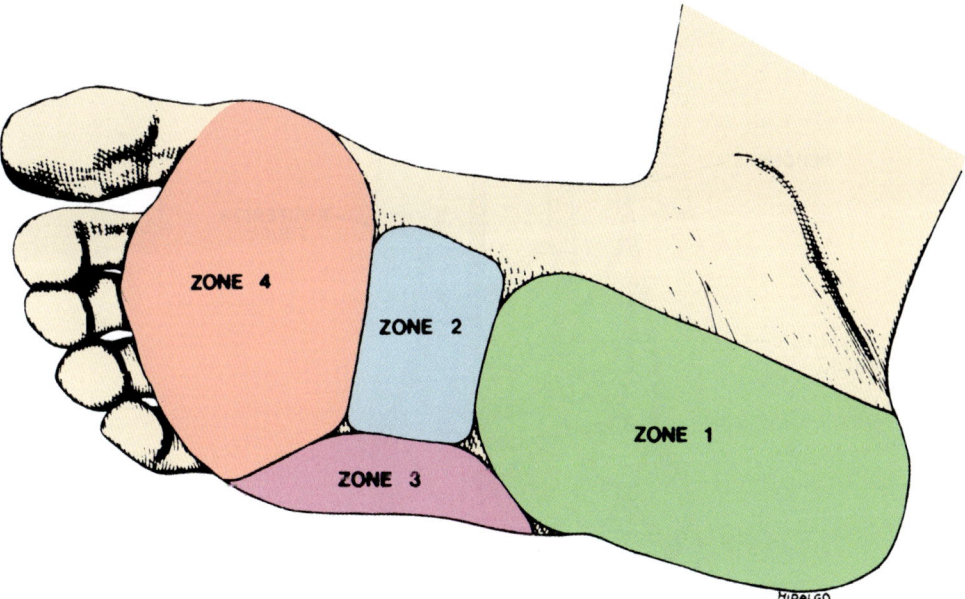

Figure 7.46 **Arterial anatomy.** (*Zone 1*, the proximal plantar area; *Zone 2*, the midplantar area; *Zone 3*, the lateral foot; *Zone 4*, the distal foot.) (From Hidalgo DA, Shaw WW. Anatomic basis of plantar flap design. *Plast Reconstr Surg.* 1986;78[5]:627.)

the medial and lateral sides of the foot (Fig. 7.47). The lateral plantar artery has multiple branches that descend vertically to reach the plexus. The medial plantar artery contributes far fewer branches, and in some specimens, the contribution appeared negligible. The peroneal artery contributed small lateral calcaneal branches to the plexus in the proximal heel area. The posterior tibial artery contributed small medial calcaneal branches to the medial aspect of the plexus in the proximal heel area. The midplantar area is a "watershed area, with blood supply reaching the skin from multiple sources."[19] Branches from the proximal plantar plexus supply the posterior segment, and branches from the deep plantar artery supply the anterior segment. Branches of the medial and plantar arteries supply the midplantar area from the sides (Fig. 7.48). No significant myocutaneous or fascia cutaneous vessels were demonstrated in this zone. The lateral plantar area is supplied with transverse branches from the dorsalis pedis wrapping around the lateral border of the foot and connecting with the corresponding branches from the lateral planter artery (Fig. 7.49). Proximally, the proximal plantar subcutaneous plexus provides arterial supply to this lateral zone. In the distal foot, vertical perforating branches arise from the plantar metatarsal and digital arteries, pass between the slips of the plantar fascia, and extend to the subdermal plexus. There is no subcutaneous plexus.[20] The subcutaneous vessels bifurcate in the web spaces into the plantar digital arteries.

▶ Arterial Blood Supply to the Superficial Muscles of the Sole and Dorsum of the Foot

The *extensor digitorum brevis* muscle receives two arterial branches from the proximal lateral tarsal artery.[21] The branches penetrate the muscle from the posteromedial aspect of the proximal segment. Small arterial branches arise from the dorsalis pedis artery and penetrate the extensor hallucis brevis component, at which level the latter crosses the artery distally.[18] Branches are also supplied to the muscle by the arcuate artery.

The *abductor hallucis* muscle is supplied by three to four arterial pedicles arising from the medial plantar artery as it crosses the interval between the abductor hallucis and the flexor digitorum brevis.[21] The arteries penetrate the muscle from the posterolateral aspect of the muscle.

The *flexor digitorum brevis* receives arterial branches proximally from the lateral plantar artery.[21] The branches penetrate the dorsal surface of the muscle. The middle segment of the muscle is supplied from the medial side by branches arising from the medial plantar artery.

The *abductor digiti minimi* receives two or three arterial branches from the lateral plantar artery.[21] The branches penetrate the posterior segment of the muscle.

▶ Osseous Arterial Blood Supply to the Foot and Ankle

Distal End of the Tibia and Fibula

The transverse perimalleolar arterial anastomotic circle, the medial and lateral malleolar rete, and the lateral malleolar sagittal arterial loop provide the blood to the distal tibia and fibula (Fig. 7.50). The anterior and posterior tibial and peroneal arteries are the providers of this arterial network. As described by Crock, "radiate epiphyseal arteries penetrate the distal tibial epiphysis" circumferentially and are located in a grid fashion near the epiphyseal plate or its remnant in the adult.[22] From this network, "branches drop vertically downward to end in the subchondral capillary bed," and a vertical branch penetrates the midsegment of the medial malleolus, which also receives radiate vessels from the nonarticular medial surface.[22] The lateral malleolus possesses a profuse arterial intraosseous network.

Gilbert et al[8] investigated the blood supply of the distal tibia, distal fibula, cuboid, and cuneiforms, thus defining vascular territories, enabling the surgeon to perform rotational vascularized pedicle bone-grafting procedures in the foot and ankle.

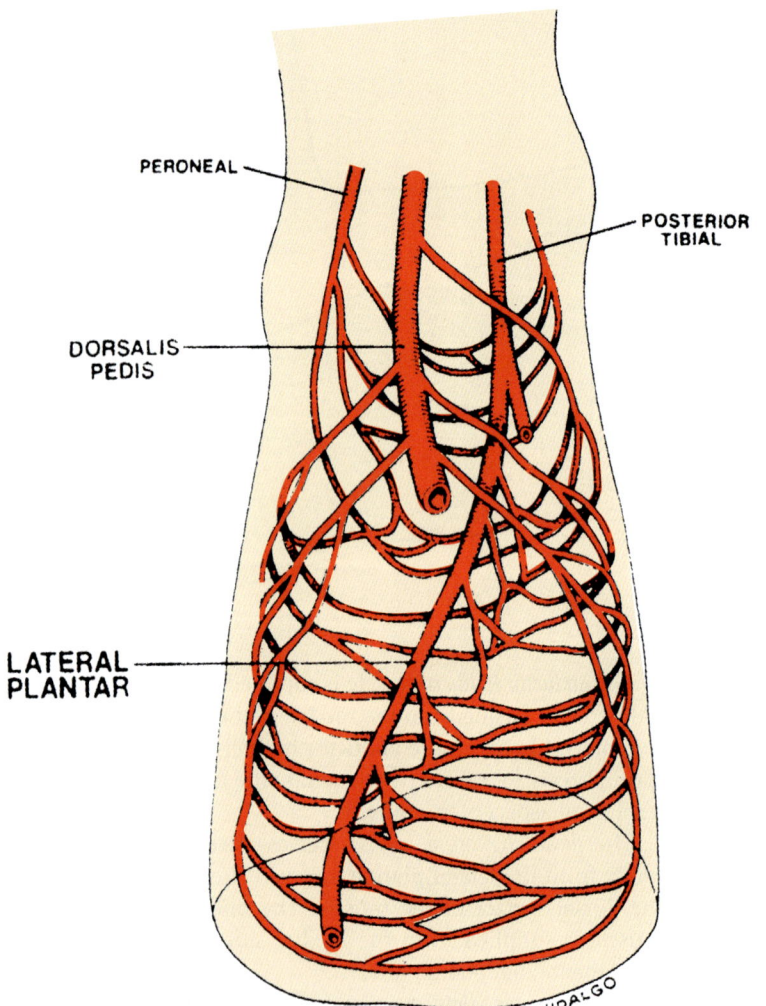

Figure 7.47 Zone 1 arterial supply. Proximal plantar subcutaneous arterial plexus seen through the dorsum of the foot. Extensive wraparound dorsal supply and multiple lateral plantar artery branches to the plexus are shown. (Adapted from Hidalgo DA, Shaw WW. Anatomic basis of plantar flap design. *Plast Reconstr Surg.* 1986;78[5]:267.)

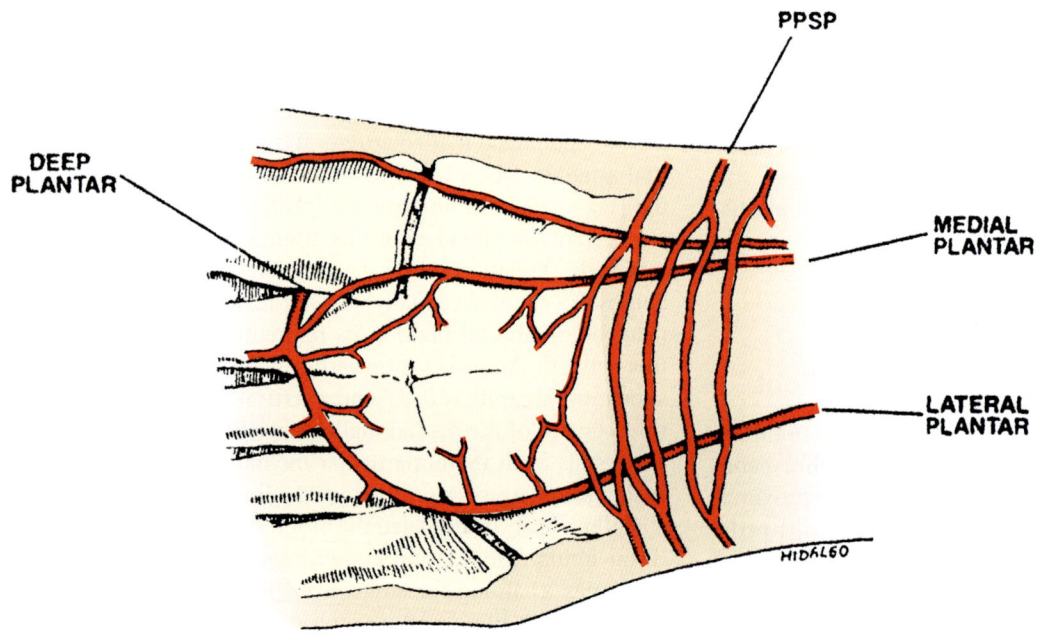

Figure 7.48 Zone 2 arterial supply. Plantar superficial plexus with large communicating branches from the lateral plantar artery. (*PPSP*, proximal plantar superficial plexus.) (Adapted from Hidalgo DA, Shaw WW. Anatomic basis of plantar flap design. *Plast Reconstr Surg.* 1986;78[5]:267.)

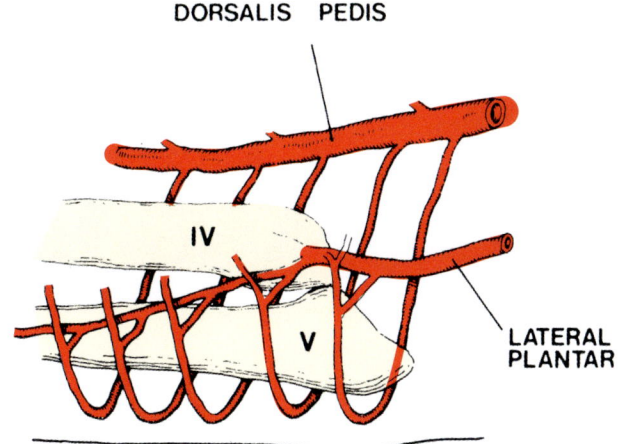

Figure 7.49 Zone 3 arterial supply: the lateral foot. The fourth and fifth metatarsals are seen within the wraparound dorsal and lateral plantar artery blood supply. (Adapted from Hidalgo DA, Shaw WW. Anatomic basis of plantar flap design. *Plast Reconstr Surg.* 1986;78[5]:267.)

They used two vascular injection techniques in 20 cadaver lower extremities. Ten specimens were subjected to injection with Batson's compound, soft-tissue digestion, and bone clearing utilizing a modified Spalteholz technique. Ten specimens were injected with latex and dissected. The anterior tibial artery was present in 95% (19 cases) of the specimens. In the remaining specimens, "the perforating peroneal artery was responsible for supplying the entire dorsal circulation of the foot."[8]

The authors defined in the distal tibia a new medial metaphyseal artery (Fig. 7.51).[1] Their findings were as follows.

Medial Metaphyseal Artery

The medial metaphyseal artery originates from the medial side of the anterior tibial artery at an average of 31 mm (range, 21-49 mm) proximal to the tibiotalar joint. It divides into the following three branches: branch to the medial malleolus, annular branch, and recurrent branch.

This arrangement occurred in only 6 of the 10 corrosion cast specimens. In the other four specimens, the annular and/or recurrent branch had a separate origin off the anterior tibial artery just proximal to the origin of the medial metaphyseal artery.

The branch to the medial malleolus always originated from the medial metaphyseal artery at an average of 32 mm (range, 21-43 mm) proximal to the tibiotalar joint. This branch coursed transversely medially from the anterior tibial artery for an average 8 mm (range, 3-12 mm) before it turned almost 90° to follow the long axis of the tibia down the ankle mortise and anastomosed with a branch of the anterior medial malleolar artery. Such an anastomosis occurred in 8 of the 10 corrosion specimens. In the other two specimens, the anterior medial malleolar artery originated exclusively from the medial metaphyseal branch to the medial malleolus as it reached the tibial plafond.

The annular branch was a derivative of the medial metaphyseal artery in 7 of 10 corrosion specimens. In the other three specimens, it came directly off the anterior tibial artery. The annular branch originated from the medial metaphyseal artery or the anterior tibial artery at an average of 40 mm (range, 26-51 mm) proximal to the tibiotalar joint. This annular branch wrapped transversely medially around the tibia, at about the level of the metaphysis to anastomose with the

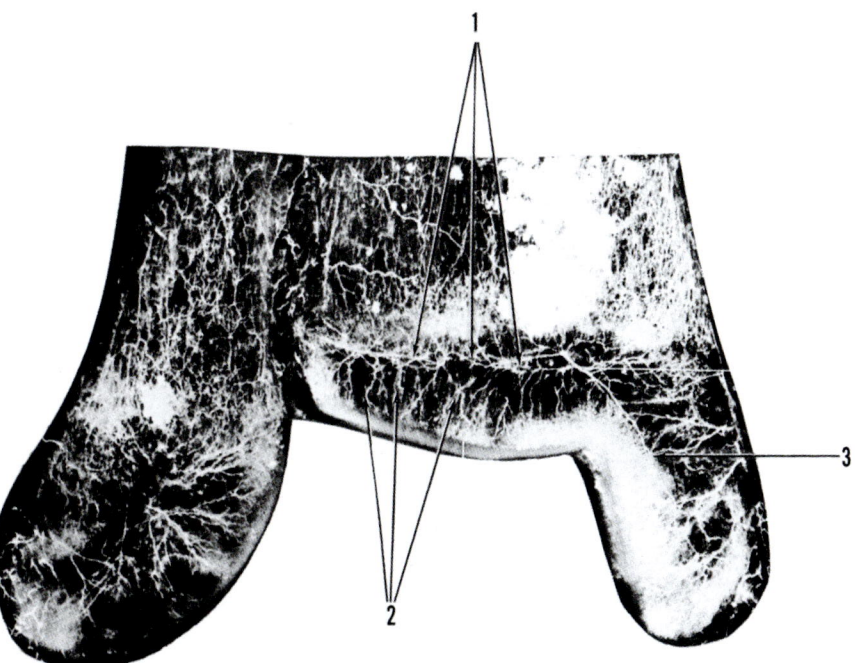

Figure 7.50 Osseous blood supply of the distal end of the tibia: a coronal section through the center of the lower ends of the tibia and fibula. The gridlike arrangement of the arterial network formed by the radiate arteries (*1*) is shown together with their vertically descending branches (*2*), which form the subchondral capillary bed. A medial malleolar descending artery (*3*) is indicated. (From Crock HV. *The Blood Supply of the Lower Limb Bones in Man: Descriptive and Applied.* Churchill Livingstone; 1967:74.)

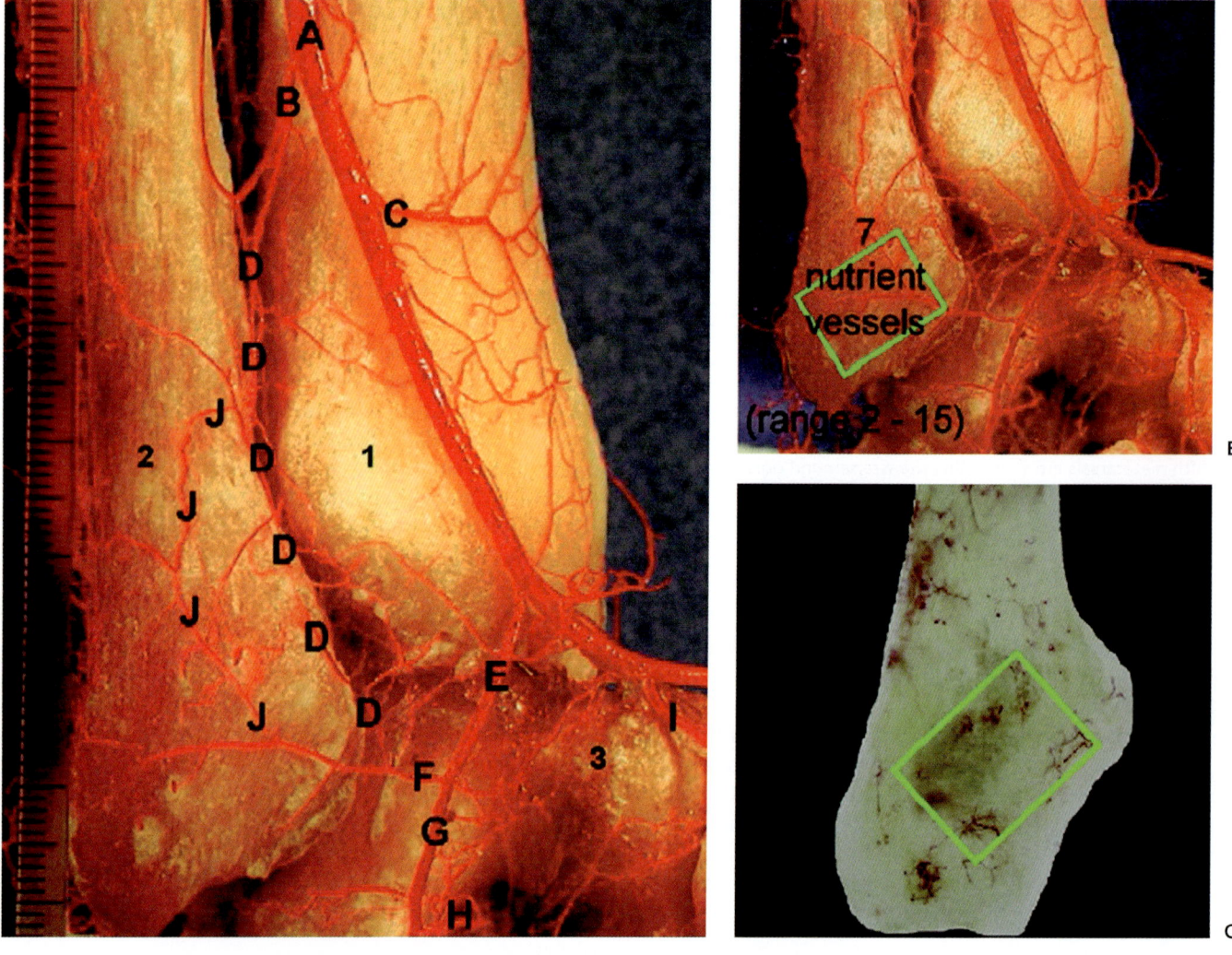

Figure 7.51 **(A)** Anterolateral view of the extraosseous blood supply to the foot and ankle. (*1*, tibia; *2*, fibula; *3*, talus; *A*, anterior tibial artery; *B*, lateral metaphyseal artery; *C*, medial metaphyseal artery; *D*, perforating peroneal artery; *E*, anterior lateral malleolar artery; *F*, transverse segment of the anterior lateral malleolar artery; *G*, vertical descending segment of the anterior lateral malleolar artery; *H*, artery to sinus tarsi; *I*, proximal lateral tarsal artery; *J*, fibular metaphyseal artery. Ruler markings are in millimeters.) **(B) The dorsal extraosseous blood supply to the distal aspect of the fibula, with the vascular territory supplied by the transverse segment of the anterior lateral malleolar artery outlined in green. (C) The dorsal intraosseous blood supply of the distal aspect of the fibula, with the vascular territory supplied by the transverse segment of the anterior lateral malleolar artery outlined in green.** (From Gilbert BJ, Horst F, Nunley JA. Potential donor rotational bone graft using vascular territories in the foot and ankle. *J Bone Joint Surg Am.* 2004;86A[9]:1860, Figure 2.)

posterior circulation (posterior tibial or peroneal artery). It sends numerous vessels to the superomedial aspect of the medial malleolus.

The recurrent branch arose from the medial metaphyseal artery in 6 of the 10 corrosion cast specimens, and it originated more proximally from the anterior tibial artery in four specimens. It originated from the medial metaphyseal artery or the anterior tibial artery at an average of 47 mm (range, 28-74 mm) proximal to the tibiotalar joint. This artery coursed in a proximal-medial direction, supplying multiple nutrient vessels to the anterior surface of the tibial diaphysis.

Lateral Metaphyseal Artery

This artery originates from the anterior tibial artery just proximal to the origin of the medial metaphyseal artery at an average of 37 mm (range, 24-63 mm) proximal to the tibiotalar joint. In 6 of the 10 corrosion cast specimens, the lateral metaphyseal artery originated directly from the anterior tibial artery. In the other four specimens, the lateral metaphyseal artery originated as a branch of the medial metaphyseal artery or one of its branches. In these cases, the lateral metaphyseal artery coursed laterally under the anterior tibial artery to return to its normal lateral position. The lateral metaphyseal artery supplies an average of six nutrient vessels (range, 1-15 nutrient vessels) to the distal dorsolateraltibial metaphysis.

Talus

The arterial blood supply to the talus is provided by the three major arteries: dorsalis pedis or anterior tibial, posterior tibial, and peroneal (Figs. 7.52 to 7.54).[7,15,23,24] More specifically, the providers are as follows:

- The artery of the sinus tarsi. As described previously, this artery arises more frequently from the dorsalis pedis artery or from any of the following: the proximal lateral tarsal artery, the anterior lateral malleolar artery, the perforating peroneal artery, or the anastomosis formed between the proximal lateral tarsal artery and the perforating peroneal artery.
- The artery of the tarsal canal, a branch of the posterior tibial artery or, less frequently, a branch of the medial plantar artery[7]
- The deltoid artery, a branch of the artery of the tarsal canal or, less frequently, a branch of the posterior tibial artery[7,15]
- Superomedial direct branches, provided by the dorsalis pedis artery
- Posterior direct branches, provided by the peroneal artery

The artery of the sinus tarsi and the artery of the tarsal canal anastomose in the canalis tarsi and form the major arterial axis of the talus. This arterial line is located posterior to the talar neck level. There is a large anastomosis between the deltoid branch of the artery of the tarsal canal and the arteries of the superior aspect of the neck, and this anastomotic periosteal network continues into the sinus tarsi and ends at the anterior edge of the talar articular surface of the lateral malleolus.[23]

Intraosseous Territory

The intraosseous territory of each artery is defined by Mulfinger and Trueta as follows[7]

Head. The superomedial half of the talar head is supplied by direct branches from the dorsalis pedis or anterior tibial artery that penetrate the upper surface of the neck. The inferolateral half of the talar head is supplied by branches from the artery of the sinus tarsi and its anastomosis or by direct branches from the lateral tarsal artery.

Body. The artery of the tarsal canal and its anastomosis provide four or five main branches, which are directed posterolaterally. They supply the lateral two-thirds of the talar body except for a small superior area in the middle third (supplied by the superior neck arteries), the lateral aspect of the posterior facet, and a variable amount of the lateral edge of the talar body.

The arteries from the anastomotic network in the tarsal sinus enter through the lateral anterior surface of the talar body and supply the lateral inferior segment and most of the posterior facet. The medial third or fourth of the talar body is supplied

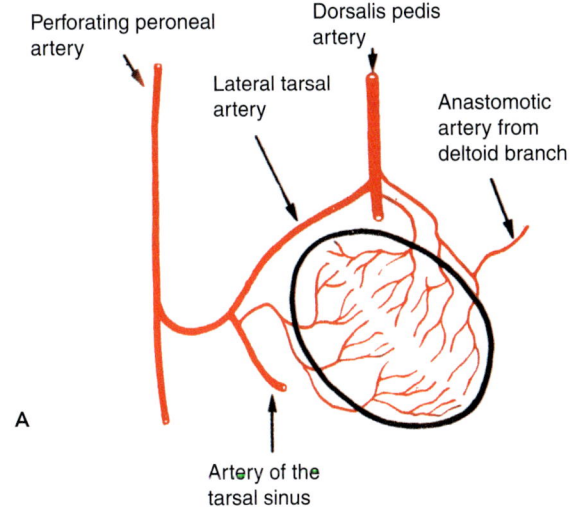

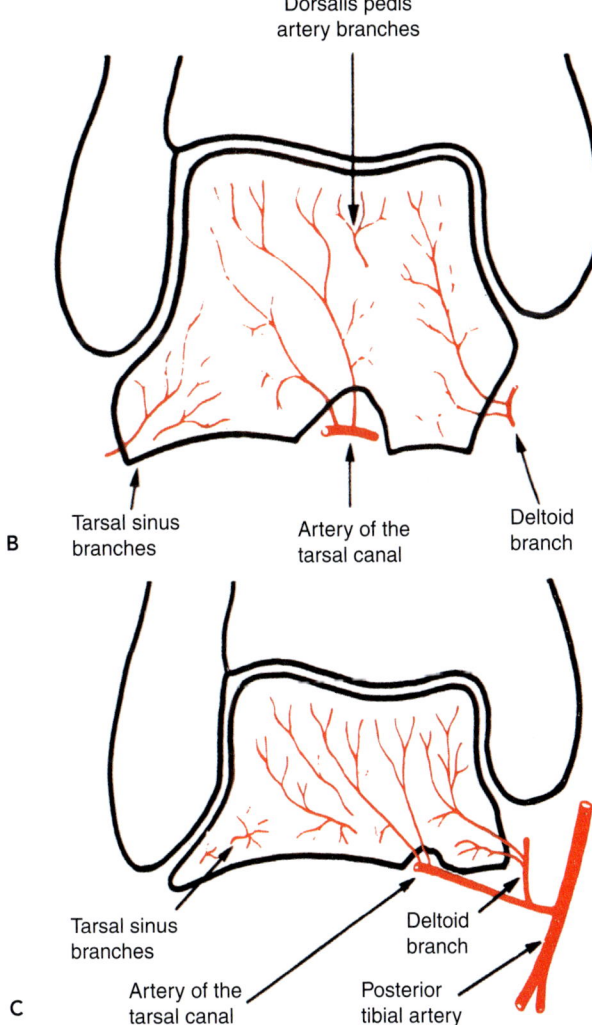

Figure 7.52 Blood supply to the talus in coronal sections. (A) Blood supply to the head of the talus. **(B)** Blood supply to the middle third of the talus. **(C)** Blood supply to the posterior third of the talus. (Adapted from Mulfinger GL, Trueta J. The blood supply of the talus. *J Bone Joint Surg Br.* 1970;52[1]:160.)

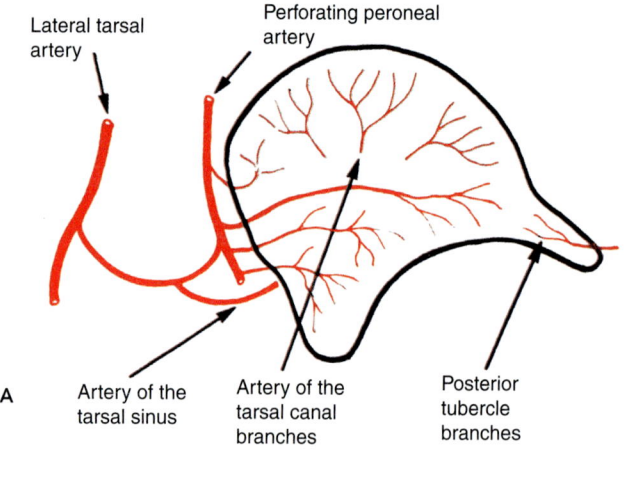

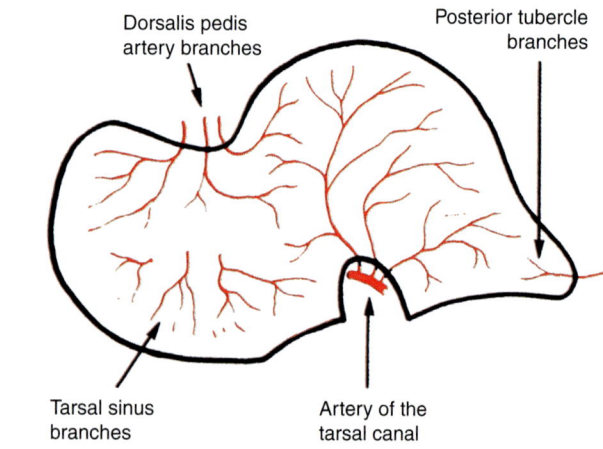

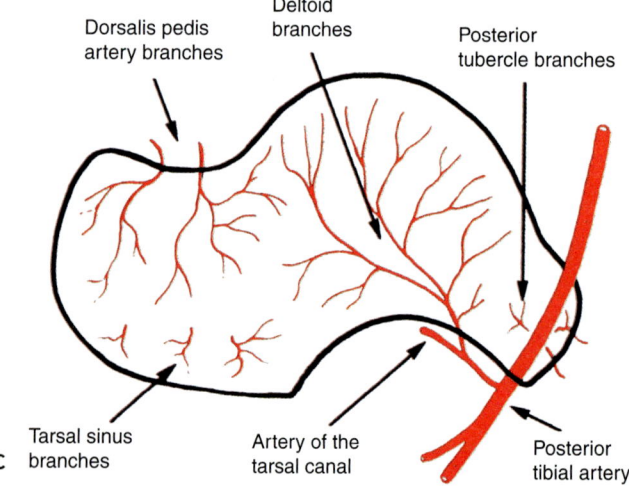

Figure 7.53 Blood supply to the talus in sagittal sections. (A) Blood supply to the lateral third of the talus. **(B)** Blood supply to the middle third of the talus. **(C)** Blood supply to the medial third of the talus. (Adapted from Mulfinger GL, Trueta J. The blood supply of the talus. *J Bone Joint Surg Br.* 1970;52[1]:160.)

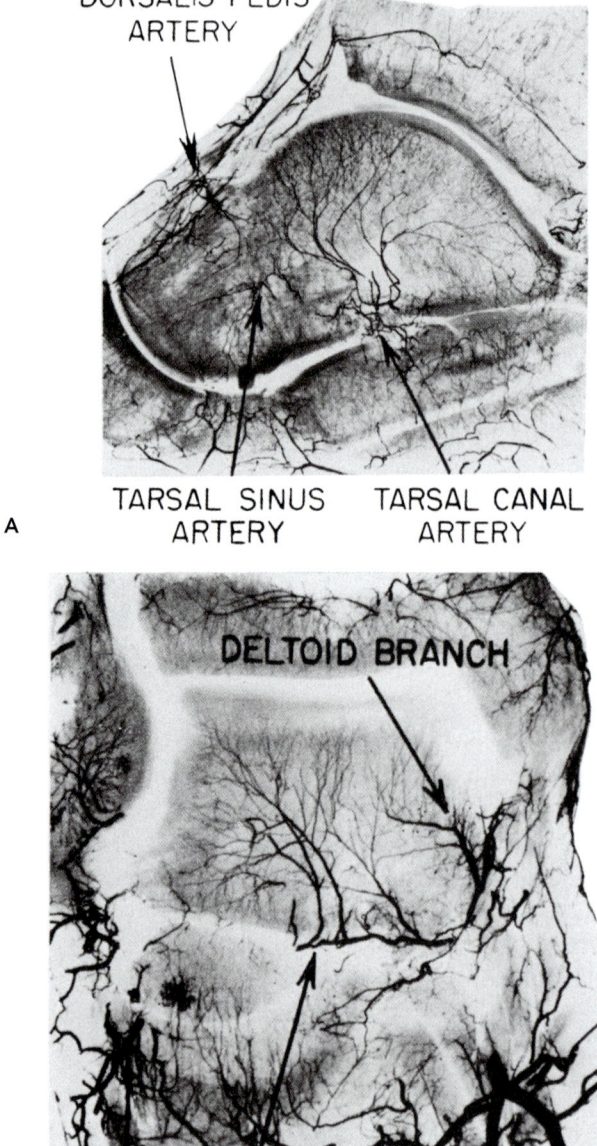

Figure 7.54 Blood supply to the talus. (A) Blood supply to the middle third of the talus through a sagittal section. **(B)** Blood supply to the middle third of the talus through a coronal section. (Republished with permission of British Editorial Society of Bone and Joint Surgery, From Mulfinger GL, Trueta J. The blood supply of the talus. *J Bone Joint Surg Br.* 1970;52[1]:160; permission conveyed through Copyright Clearance Center, Inc.)

Gelberman and Mortensen studied the extraosseous arterial blood supply of the talus in 23 specimens and the intraosseous supply in 14 specimens.[25]

The *extraosseous vascularity* is supplied by the anterior tibial, posterior tibial, tibial, and peroneal arteries (Figs. 7.55 and 7.56). The specific branches penetrate the talus through five nonarticulating surfaces: superior and inferior surfaces of the neck, medial surface of the body below the articular facet of the malleolus, sinus tarsi, and posterior tubercle. These surfaces are arterially penetrated as follows:

- Superior surface of the neck: By branches of anterior tibial artery; medial two-thirds: medial talar arteries of the medial

by the deltoid branches entering from the medial surface of the talus. The posterior tubercle is supplied by small branches from the posterior anastomotic network formed by the peroneal artery and the posterior tibial artery.

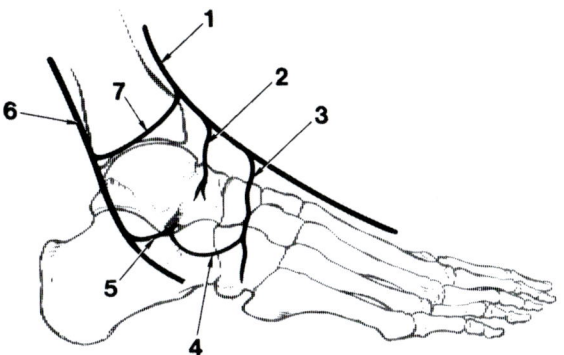

Figure 7.55 Schematic drawing of lateral ankle and foot with extraosseous arterial supply to the talus. (*1*, anterior tibial artery; *2*, lateral talar artery; *3*, lateral tarsal artery; *4*, posterior recurrent branch of lateral tarsal; *5*, artery of tarsal sinus; *6*, perforating peroneal; *7*, anterior lateral malleolar artery.) (Gelberman RH, Mortensen WW. The arterial anatomy of the talus. Foot Ankle. 1983;4[2]:64. Copyright ©1983. Reprinted by Permission of SAGE Publications.)

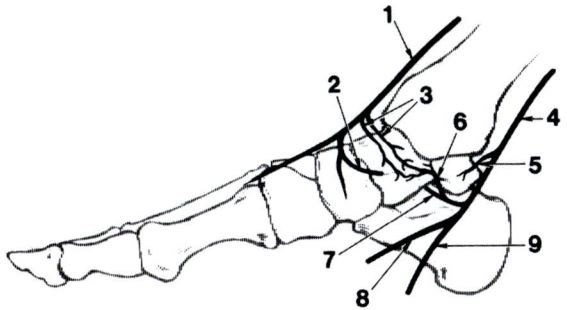

Figure 7.56 Schematic drawing of medial ankle and foot showing extraosseous arterial supply to the talus. (*1*, anterior tibial artery; *2*, medial recurrent tarsal artery; *3*, medial talar artery; *4*, posterior tibial artery; *5*, posterior tubercle artery; *6*, deltoid branches; *7*, artery of tarsal canal; *8*, medial plantar artery; *9*, lateral plantar artery.) (Gelberman RH, Mortensen WW. The arterial anatomy of the talus. Foot Ankle. 1983;4[2]:64. Copyright ©1983. Reprinted by Permission of SAGE Publications.)

recurrent tarsal arteries; lateral one-third: lateral talar arteries and lateral recurrent tarsal arteries.
- Inferior surface of the neck: Dual supply; artery of tarsal canal anastomosed with artery of sinus tarsi, forming an anastomotic artery in 83%.
- Medial surface of the body: Deltoid branch of posterior tibial artery in 91%. This branch anastomoses with branches from the medial talar artery and the medial recurrent tarsal artery. When absent, these last two arteries supply the talar body.
- Posterior talar tubercle: Direct branches from posterior tibial artery, which may anastomose with branches from peroneal artery.

The *intraosseous arterial supply* is as follows[25] (Fig. 7.57):

Head: The superior and medial two-thirds of the neck are supplied by superior neck vessels and the inferior and lateral one-third by branches from the sinus tarsi in 78.5%. In 21%, the superior neck vessels supply the entire head.

Body: The body receives branches from the anastomotic artery in the tarsal canal, the deltoid branches, and the sinus tarsi branch. Three to six branches from the artery of the tarsal canal penetrate the talar body and course posteriorly (Figs. 7.58 and 7.59). These branches supply the middle half of the body in 50% and the middle three-quarters of the body in 28.5%. In 14%, the deltoid branches are absent, and the artery of the tarsal canal supplies the medial half of the talar body. In 7%, the sinus tarsi branches

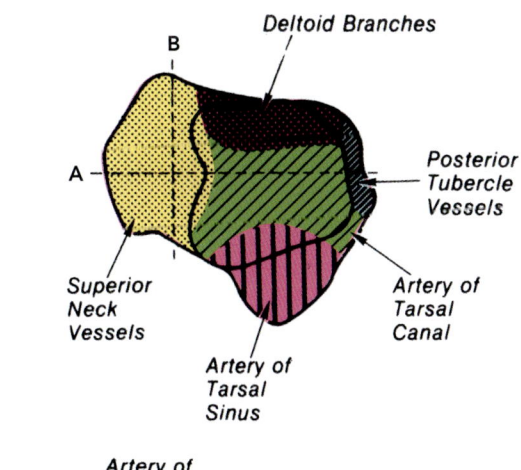

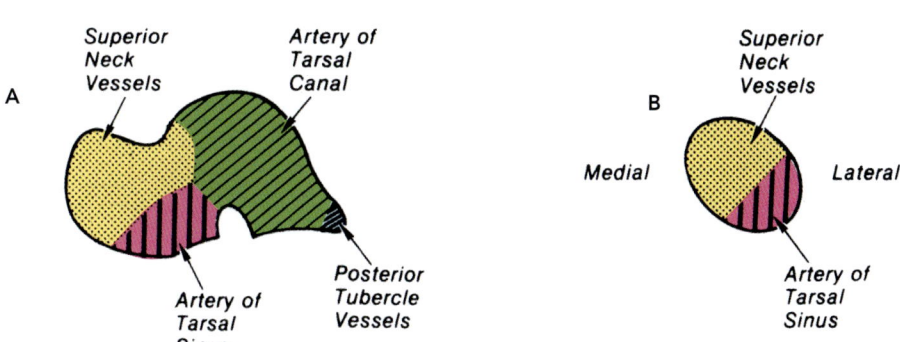

Figure 7.57 Internal vascularity of the talus: superior view. **(A)** Sagittal section through midtalus. **(B)** Coronal section through talar neck. (Adapted from Gelberman RH, Mortensen WW. The arterial anatomy of the talus. Foot Ankle. 1983;4[2]:64.)

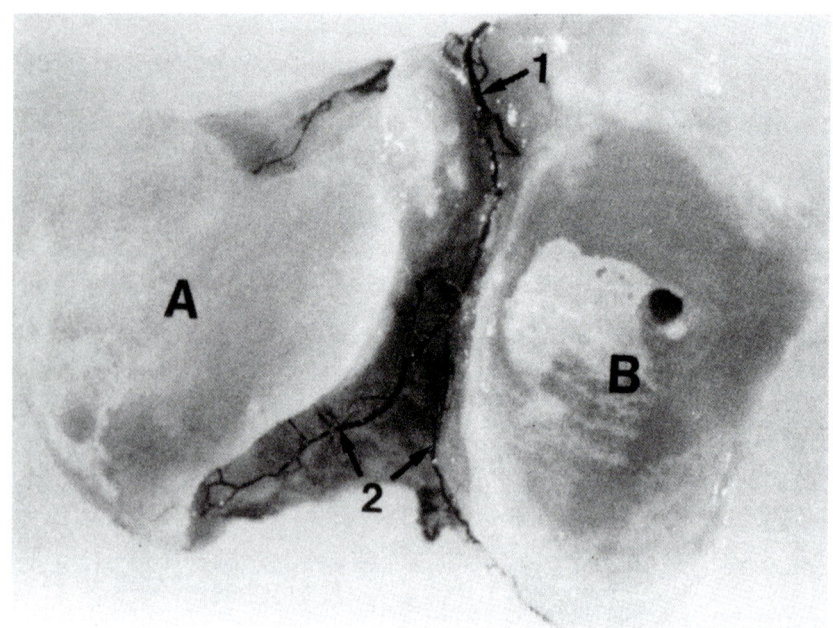

Figure 7.58 Inferior view of talus. (*1*, artery of tarsal canal; *2*, artery of tarsal sinus; *A*, head of talus; *B*, body of talus.) (Gelberman RH, Mortensen WW. The arterial anatomy of the talus. *Foot Ankle.* 1983;4[2]:64. Copyright ©1983. Reprinted by Permission of SAGE Publications.)

are absent, and the artery of the tarsal canal supplies the lateral half of the body. In 43%, branches of the superior neck supply a small area of the anterosuperior portion of the body.

The deltoid branches supply the medial one-quarter of the body in 64% and the medial half of the body in 21%. In 14%, the deltoid vessels are absent, and the artery of the tarsal canal supplies the medial segment of the body. Branches from the artery of the sinus tarsi supply the lateral one-quarter of the body in 57%, the lateral one-eighth in 28.5%, and the lateral half of the body in 7%. The artery to the sinus tarsi is absent in 7%, and the entire lateral aspect of the body is supplied by the artery of the tarsal canal.

The posterior talar tubercle receives direct branches in 57%.

It was the conclusion of the authors that "the single major arterial supply to the body of the talus was from the artery of the tarsal canal," and "the deltoid vessels constituted the most significant minor blood supply to the body."[25]

Variations

Mulfinger and Trueta report the following intraosseous territorial variations in 30 feet: lateral branches from the anastomotic network of the tarsal sinus supplying the lateral quarter of the body, 33.3%; superior neck vessels supplying approximately one-third of the body, 6.6%; superior neck vessels not penetrating the bone, 23.3%.[7]

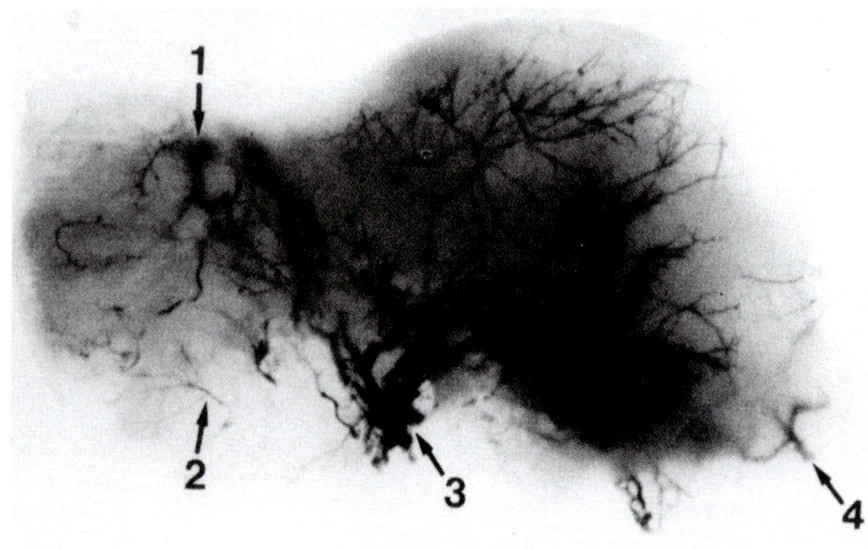

Figure 7.59 Photograph of cleared specimen, lateral view, showing the internal vascularity of the talus. (*1*, superior neck vessels; *2*, tarsal sinus branch; *3*, artery of tarsal canal; *4*, posterior tubercle branch.) (Gelberman RH, Mortensen WW. The arterial anatomy of the talus. *Foot Ankle.* 1983;4[2]:64. Copyright ©1983. Reprinted by Permission of SAGE Publications.)

Anastomosis

The intraosseous arteries may anastomose with each other. The anastomotic types and the frequency of their occurrence is reported by Mulfinger and Trueta in 30 feet as follows: between the superior neck arteries and the branches from the artery of the tarsal canal, 26.6%; between the inferior and superior branches in the head, 13.3%; between the branches from the artery of the sinus tarsi and the artery of the tarsal canal within the bone, 13.3%; between the posterior tubercle branches and the artery of the tarsal canal, 3.3%; between the deltoid branches and the artery of the tarsal canal, 3.3% (approximate total, 60%).[7] Gelberman and Mortensen found no significant intraosseous anastomoses in 43%.[25] In 28.5%, anastomoses were seen between the superior neck vessels and branches from the artery of the tarsal canal. In 43%, anastomoses were present between the deltoid branches and the artery of the tarsal canal. In 21%, anastomoses were seen between the latter and the posterior tubercle vessels.

Zchakaja, in a chronological study of the arterial blood supply in 68 feet, describes the following number of intraosseous talar arterial branches:

Newborn: Six to seven arterial branches penetrate the perichondrium from the lateral, inferior, superior, and medial surfaces and reach the ossification center, where they branch out.

Age group 13 to 14 years: Twenty-five to 26 arterial branches are present, of which 17 are constant and eight to nine are of the supplementary type.

The distribution of the branches is as follows:

- Upper surface: Six to seven branches with three permanent branches
- Lower surface: Four permanent branches and two to three supplementary
- Medial surface: Four to six branches, of which four are permanent
- Lateral surface: One to two branches entering through the anterior aspect of the lateral talar process
- Posterior surface: Two to four branches penetrating from each side of the posterior talar process

Age group 25 to 60 years: With aging, the supplementary arterial branches decrease in number (25-year-old age group) and disappear later (65-year-old age group) but the permanent arterial branches remain unchanged in number. However, the number of branches extending from the central anastomotic zone to the periphery decreases gradually with age, and only a few remain by the age of 65 years.[24]

Calcaneus

The calcaneus is supplied by a rich arterial network that yields branches penetrating from all the surfaces not covered by the articular surface (Fig. 7.60). The arteries providing the blood supply are the following:

- Medial calcaneal artery, branch of the posterior tibial artery
- Lateral calcaneal artery, branch of the peroneal artery
- Peroneal artery
- Posterior transverse calcaneal anastomotic arcade formed between the posterior tibial artery and the peroneal artery
- Lateral and medial plantar arteries
- Artery of the sinus tarsi and artery of the tarsal canal
- Direct branches from the proximal lateral tarsal artery and from the perforating peroneal artery

Zchakaja describes the blood supply to the os calcis (age group 13-14 years) as follows.[24]

Superior Surface

The *frontal part* of the superior surface is supplied by the arteries of the sinus tarsi and canalis tarsi and is supplemented by direct branches from the proximal lateral tarsal artery and the peroneal artery. These branches are small and six to nine in number, of which six branches are permanent and penetrate the bone at the following sites: two branches enter at 0.5 cm from the anterior articular surface for the cuboid, two branches enter at 0.5 cm anterior to the posterior calcaneal articular surface, and two branches enter at the base of the sustentaculum tali. The three supplementary arteries penetrate the bone in the inner half of the calcaneal canal.

The posterior part of the superior surface is supplied by the calcaneal anastomotic arcade between the tibialis posterior artery and the peroneal artery and by the peroneal artery proper. There are four to seven arterial branches, of which four branches are permanent and penetrate the bone at the following sites: two branches enter the bone at 0.5 to 1 cm posterior to the posterior calcaneal articular surface and two branches enter at 0.5 to 1 cm anterior to the posterior surface of the calcaneus.

Lateral Surface

The *anterior segment* of the lateral surface is supplied by a branch of the proximal lateral tarsal artery, and the *posterior segment* by the lateral calcaneal branches arising from the peroneal artery. Fifteen to 18 branches penetrate the bone almost at 90°, and 15 of these branches are permanent. Six of the permanent arteries are large and penetrate the bone at the following sites: one branch enters the bone at 0.5 to 1 cm posterior to the articular surface of the cuboid, one branch enters at the level of the posterior articular calcaneal surface, one branch penetrates at 0.5 to 1 cm posterior to the peronei tubercle, and three branches enter on the outer surface of the calcaneal tuberosity.

Medial Surface

The medial calcaneal surface is supplied anteriorly by the medial plantar artery and posteriorly by the medial calcaneal branches.

The medial surface is supplied by 12 to 16 arteries; of these, seven are of the permanent type. The five larger ones penetrate at the following sites: one penetrates the bone at 1 cm from the articular surface of the cuboid, one enters the bone at the base of the sustentaculum tali, two penetrate at the level of

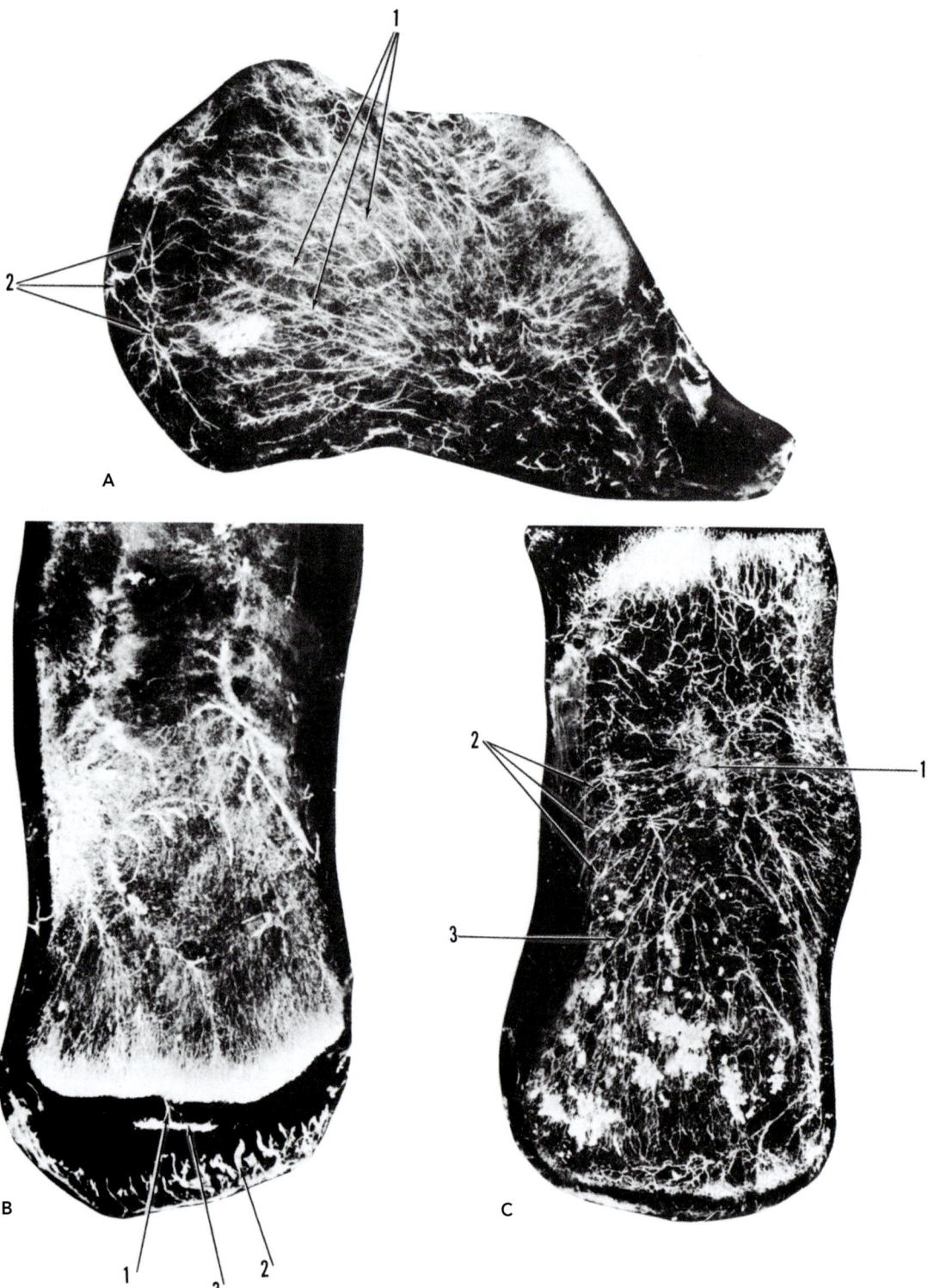

Figure 7.60 **Blood supply to the calcaneus. (A)** Sagittal section from the calcaneus viewed from the lateral side. Arteries penetrate the outer surface of the bone over a wide "waist area." Most of these give rise to recurrent branches (*1*), which pass backward to the epiphyseal zone of the heel, where they anastomose with epiphyseal arteries (*2*) across the site of the former growth plate. **(B)** Posterior half of a horizontal section through the middle of the calcaneus of a girl aged 11 years. The metaphyseal arteries (*1*) pass across the growth plate into the epiphysis (*3*). (*2*, vertical peripheral epiphyseal arteries.) **(C)** Horizontal section from the calcaneus of a woman aged 59 years. Peripheral penetrating arteries (*2*) converge to the center (*1*) and then sweep backward through recurrent branches (*3*) to the epiphyseal zone of the calcaneus. The periosteal network provides the radiate arteries that supply the facet areas and their subchondral capillary beds. (Reprinted from Crock HV. *The Blood Supply of the Lower Limb Bones in Man—Descriptive and Applied*. Churchill Livingstone; 1967.)

the posterior calcaneal tuberosity, and one enters the bone at 1 cm from the posterior rim. The foraminae of the remaining five to nine supplementary arteries are aligned parallel to the sulcus of the flexor hallucis longus tendon at 1 cm below the latter.

Plantar Surface

The plantar calcaneal surface is supplied by the lateral and medial plantar arteries. The surface is penetrated by five to six branches; of these, four branches are permanent and penetrate at the following sites: three branches enter the medial and lateral calcaneal tuberosities, and one branch enters the bone at 1 cm from the articular surface of the cuboid. The supplementary one to two branches penetrate the bone in the middle of the plantar surface.

Posterior Surface

The posterior calcaneal surface is supplied by the branches from the calcaneal anastomotic arcade between the posterior tibial artery and the peroneal artery, by the branches from the lateral and medial calcaneal arteries, and by the branches from the lateral and medial plantar arteries. This arterial network forms the calcaneal rete.

The arterial branches are five to eight in number (four permanent and one to three supplementary) and penetrate the posterior surface between the insertion of the Achilles tendon and the origin of the plantar aponeurosis. These branches are grouped in the middle of the posterior strip and represent the epiphyseal arteries.

The calcaneal intraosseous arteries, after penetrating the bone, turn anteriorly toward the center and anastomose. Many branches take a recurrent course posteriorly and reach the zone of the epiphysis.[16,22] The epiphyseal plate is perforated by five to six metaphyseal arterial branches.

In the newborn, Zchakaja describes arterial branches penetrating the perichondrium of the calcaneus from the medial surface (two to three branches), from the lateral surface (two branches), and from the superior surface (one to two branches).[24] These arteries converge on the ossification center and anastomose with each other. By 25 years of age, the supplementary arteries have decreased in number, and by 65 years of age, these arteries and the peripheral five arterial branches have disappeared.

Andermahr et al[26] investigated the extraosseous and intraosseous vascularization of the os calcaneum. The arteries of 13 lower leg and foot specimens of cadavers were injected with a polymer and subjected to maceration or were imbedded in plastic. The age group of the cadavers was 40 to 60 years, with no evidence of angiopathy. The examination revealed that 45% of the bone is vascularized via medial arteries and 45% via lateral arteries, whereas the remaining 10% is supplied by the sinus tarsi artery. The medial and lateral intraosseous arterial supply for the calcaneus is equal. Inside the bone, there is a watershed zone where the medial and lateral arterial supply meets in the midline (see Fig. 7.61).[1]

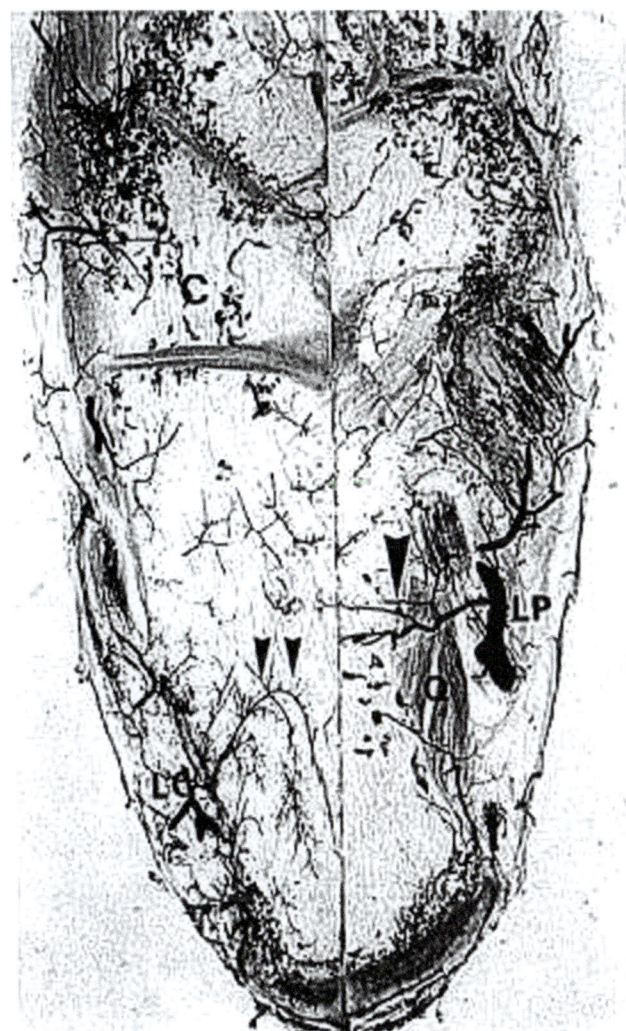

Figure 7.61 **Semicoronal sections of the cuboid (C) and calcaneus of human cadavers after injection of Biodur.** The lateral plantar artery (*LP*) delivers the medial calcaneal arteries (*single arrow*), which penetrate the bone through the quadrates plantae muscle (*Q*). On the lateral side of the calcaneus, the lateral calcaneal artery (*LC*) has one main intraosseous branch (*double arrow*) and smaller branches. The medial and lateral blood supply forms a watershed zone in the midline of the bone. (From Andermahr J, Helling HJ, Rehm KE, Koebke Z. The vascularization of the os calcaneum and the clinical consequences. *Clin Orthop Relat Res.* 1999;363:214, Figure 2.)

The medial half of the calcaneus receives the blood supply from the posterior tibial artery, which also provides the lateral calcaneal artery immediately proximal to the upper margin of the posterior calcaneus (see Fig. 7.62)[2] and separates into the medial and lateral plantar arteries. Two to four vessels, most commonly branches of the lateral plantar artery, penetrate the quadrates plantae at its origin and enter the bone immediately below the sustentaculum tali. The medial calcaneal arteries divide into four to six smaller vessels (0.5–1 mm in diameter) proceeding intraosseous to the midline of the anterior process, the posterior joint facet, tuber, and corpus (see Fig. 7.63).[1] The subperiosteal net delivers small arteries that penetrate the cortical bone on its entire surface. These smaller vessels do not penetrate into deep regions of the bone. They supply a subcortical zone of only 2 to 3 mm.

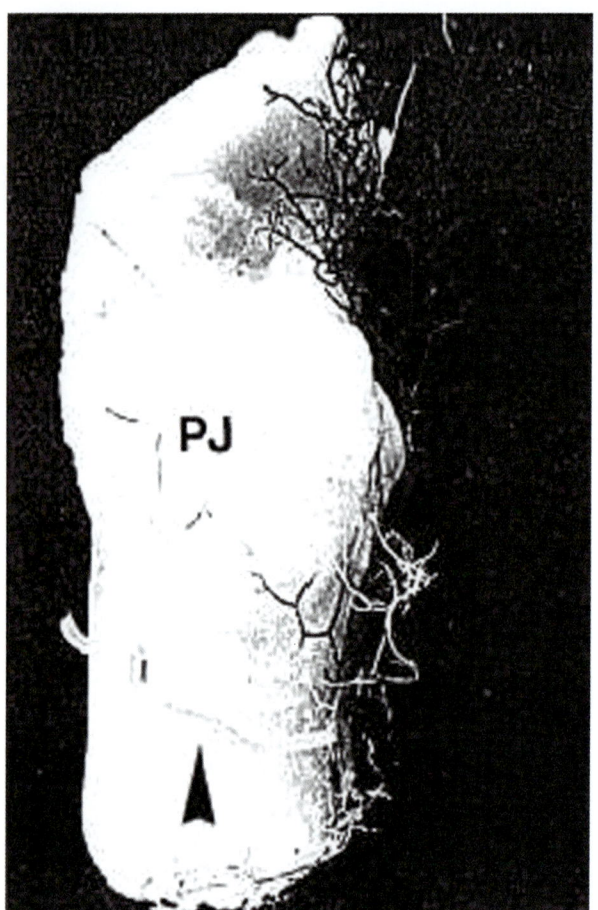

Figure 7.62 Upper view of a macerated human calcaneus bone after injection of Biodur. The lateral calcaneal artery (*arrow*) comes from the posterior tibial artery and crosses the tuber behind the posterior facet (*PJ*) on the lateral side, where it joins the large lateral anastomosis. (From Andermahr J, Helling HJ, Rehm KE, Koebke Z. The vascularization of the os calcaneum and the clinical consequences. *Clin Orthop Relat Res.* 1999;363:214, Figure 1.)

The lateral calcaneal artery is a branch of the posterior tibial artery, crossing over the tuber and penetrating the calcaneus immediately below the posterior joint surface and providing the lateral portion of the bone with circulation (see Fig. 7.64).[2,14,27] The lateral calcaneal artery forms a large extraosseous arcade with branches of the dorsalis pedis artery (see Fig. 7.65).[4]

There is a large artery through the tarsal sinus but the primary circulation enters the talus and not the anterior process of the calcaneus bone. Only small arterioles penetrate the calcaneal surface via the tarsal sinus and remain as short vessels immediately below the anteromedial and calcaneocuboid joint surfaces.

Navicular

The navicular receives its blood supply from the dorsal and plantar aspects and from the tuberosity. Velluda describes an artery on the dorsal side, a branch of the dorsalis pedis, that crosses the dorsum of the navicular and provides three to five branches.[28] Occasionally, there are direct branches to the dorsum from the dorsalis pedis. The plantar surface receives vessels from the medial plantar artery and the tuberosity from an anastomotic network formed by the union of these two source arteries.

Waugh, in a study of 21 injected navicular, describes at 8 weeks and 8 months a dense perichondral network of vessels that yields numerous arteries penetrating the cartilage and aiming toward the center (Figs. 7.66 to 7.68).[29] At 21 months, the ossification nucleus appears near the center and is fed by one nutrient artery. At 5 years of age, the ossification nucleus receives five to six arteries, but less commonly, it may be totally supplied by a single plantar or dorsal artery. With further growth, the multiple peripheral radial vessels are anastomosed and incorporated by the ossific nucleus. In the 4- to 5-year-old

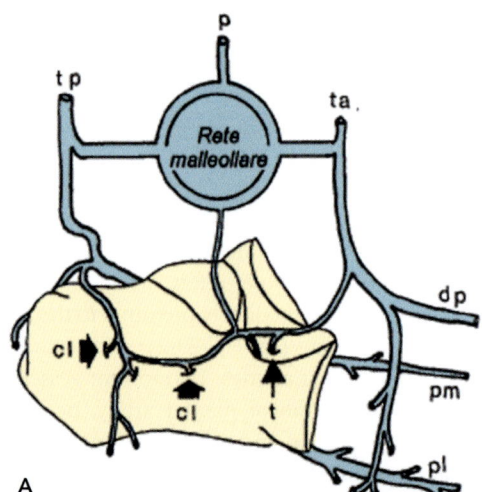
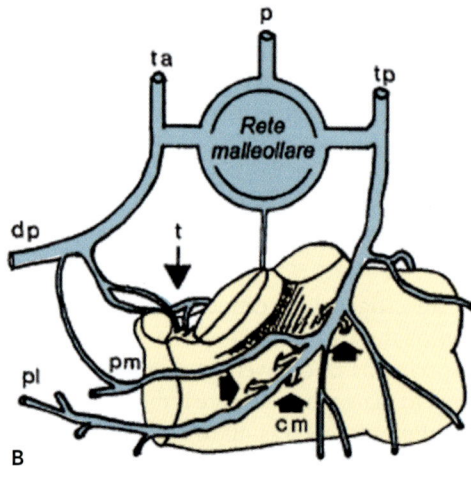

Figure 7.63 **(A) Diagram of the lateral calcaneal blood supply.** The main source is the tibialis posterior artery (*tp*) and the dorsalis pedis artery (*dp*). A smaller supply is delivered via the peroneal artery (*p*) which is lost amid the lateral malleolar net. (*Cl*, lateral calcaneal artery; *pl*, *pm*, lateral and medial plantar artery; *t*, sinus tarsi artery.) **(B) Diagram of the medial calcaneal blood supply.** The main supply is delivered via the tibialis posterior artery (*tp*). The medial calcaneal arteries (*cm*) are regular branches of the lateral plantar artery (*pl*). (*pm*, medial plantar artery; *t*, sinus tarsi artery; *ta*, anterior tibial artery.) (Adapted from Andermahr J, Helling HJ, Rehm KE, Koebke Z. The vascularization of the os calcaneum and the clinical consequences. *Clin Orthop Relat Res.* 1999;363:217.)

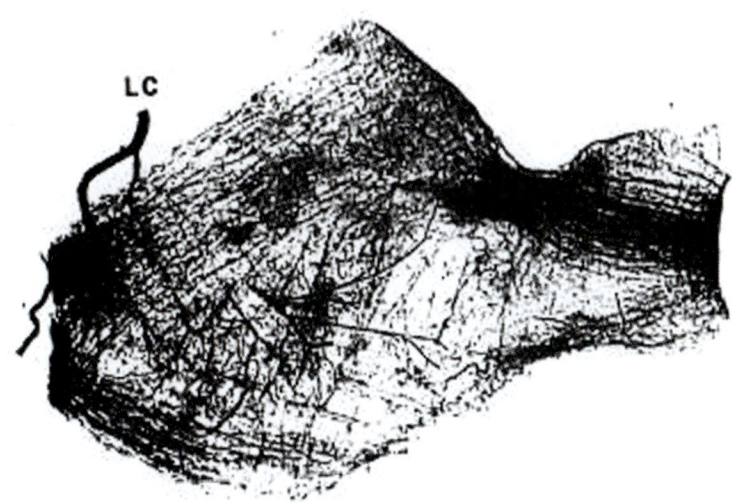

Figure 7.64 Sagittal section of a lateral macerated human calcaneus bone after injection of Biodur. The lateral calcaneal artery (*LC*) delivers 45% of the bone's blood supply. Smaller branches ultimately reach the posterior joint surface and neck. The neutral triangle serves as a conductive space for vessels supplying the anterior portion of the calcaneus. (From Andermahr J, Helling HJ, Rehm KE, et al. The vascularization of the os calcaneum and the clinical consequences. *Clin Orthop Relat Res.* 1999;363:216, Figure 4.)

age group, Zchakaja describes 8 to 10 vessels that penetrate the perichondrium and reach the ossification nucleus.[24] By 13 to 14 years of age, the navicular receives 15 to 21 arteries, of which 12 are permanent and three to nine are supplementary. They penetrate the bone at the following sites: dorsal surface—two to eight arteries, of which four are permanent, and one of these enters the tuberosity of the navicular; plantar surface—eight to nine arteries, of which five are permanent, and one of these enters the tuberosity of the navicular; medial margin—three to four arteries, of which three are permanent. Between 20 and 65 years of age, the supplementary arteries decrease in number.

Cuneiforms

The cuneiforms receive their blood supply from their dorsal, medial, and lateral surfaces.[24] These vessels are provided mostly by the dorsal arterial rete. According to Zchakaja, in the 13- to 14-year age group, the first cuneiform receives a total number of 21 to 24 arteries (17 permanent); the second cuneiform, 10 to 12 arteries (8 permanent); the third cuneiform, 14 to 16 arteries (11 permanent).[24] Between 21 and 65 years of age, the number of supplementary arteries decreases.

Cuboid

The cuboid receives its blood supply from the plantar arterial rete formed by the deep branches of the lateral and medial plantar arteries, with contribution from the dorsal arterial rete. The bone is penetrated by 25 to 27 arterial branches (12 permanent) from the dorsal, medial, lateral, and plantar surfaces. The plantar arterial branch predominates, and the larger vessel on the plantar aspect enters at the level of the cuboid tuberosity, and the remainder enters through the sulcus for the tendon of the peroneus longus.

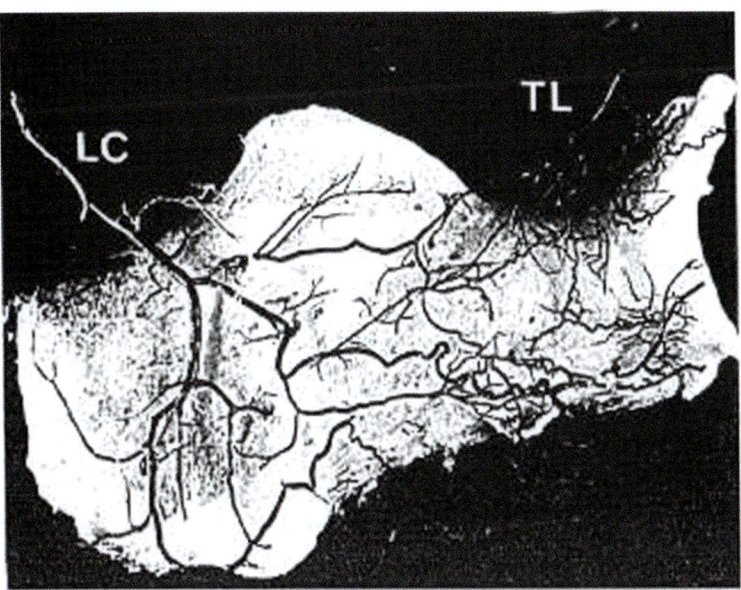

Figure 7.65 Lateral side of a macerated human calcaneus bone after injection of Biodur. The lateral calcaneal artery (*LC*) forms an anastomosis with the lateral tarsal artery (*TL*), a large branch from the dorsalis pedis artery. (From Andermahr J, Helling HJ, Rehm KE, et al. The vascularization of the os calcaneum and the clinical consequences. *Clin Orthop Relat Res.* 1999;363:215, Figure 3.)

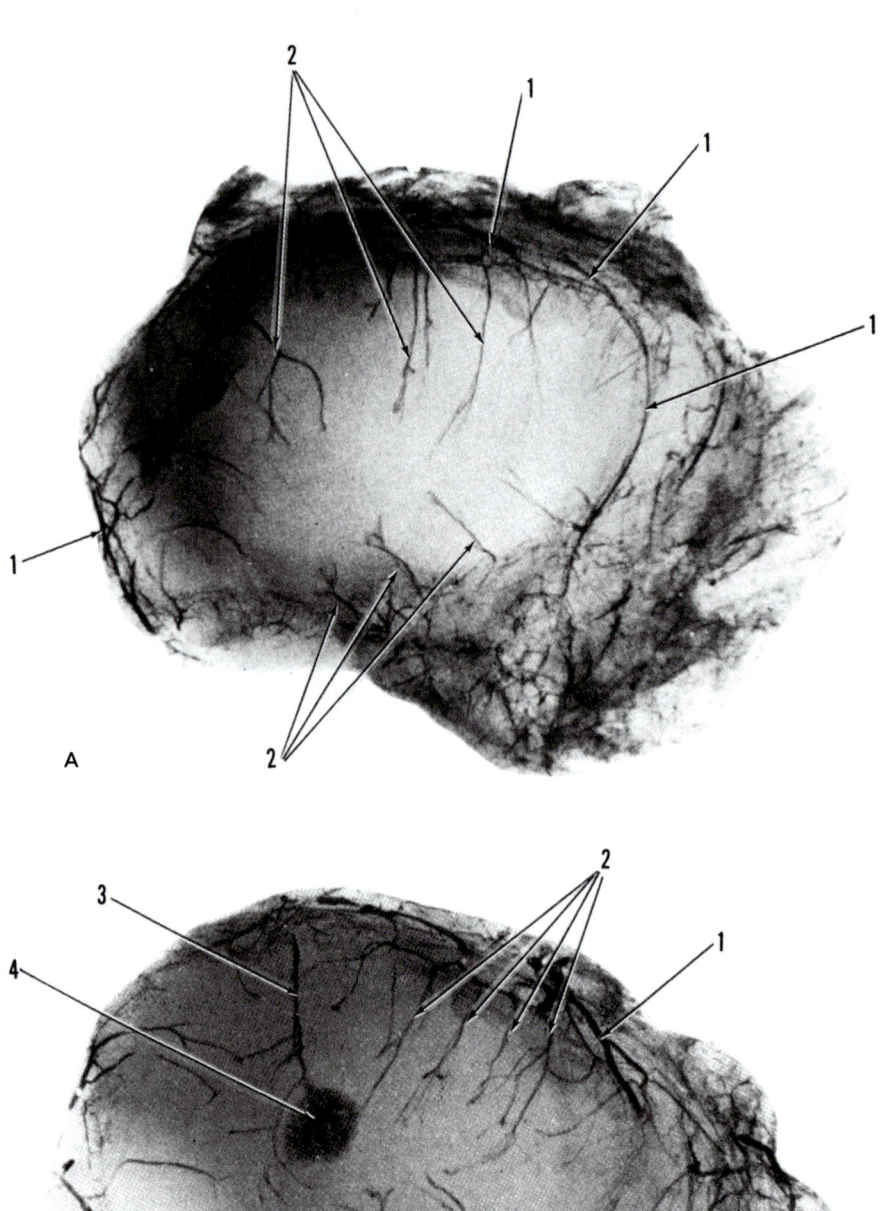

Figure 7.66 Blood supply to the navicular. (A) Fine-grain radiograph of an injected navicular from a girl aged 21 months. There is a rich perichondrial arterial network (*1*) with numerous radial penetrating arteries aiming to the center of the navicular (*2*). (B) Fine-grain radiograph of an injected navicular from a girl aged 21 months. The distribution is similar to (A) but a single artery–vein (*3*) reaches the ossifying nucleus (*4*). (Republished with permission of British Editorial Society of Bone and Joint Surgery, From Waugh W. The ossification and vascularisation of the tarsal navicular and their relation to Köhler's disease. *J Bone Joint Surg Br.* 1958;40[4]:765; permission conveyed through Copyright Clearance Center, Inc.)

Metatarsals

Lesser Metatarsals

Metatarsals 2, 3, and 4 have a similar pattern of arterial supply provided by the dorsal and plantar metatarsal arteries. As described by Zchakaja, in the age group of 13 to 14 years, the diaphysis is supplied by 13 to 14 arterial branches entering the bone from the dorsal (five or six branches), the medial (three or four branches), and the lateral (three or four branches) surfaces. The nutrient artery penetrates the lateral diaphyseal surface near the base and divides into two branches: distal and proximal. The distal branch is the strongest; it runs toward the epiphysis and divides into six to seven branches that anastomose with the metaphyseal vessels. The proximal branch is smaller, maintains the oblique direction of the mother stem, and reaches the base of the metatarsal. The metaphysis is supplied by seven arterial branches. Four to six arterial branches penetrate the epiphysis from the lateral and medial surfaces.

Metatarsal 5 receives its nutrient artery from the medial surface of the diaphysis and also receives arterial branches from the plantar aspect of the proximal diaphysis (three to five branches) in addition to the arterial supply from the dorsal (five to six branches) and medial (two to three branches) surfaces. Two arterial branches penetrate the lateral aspect of the tuberosity.

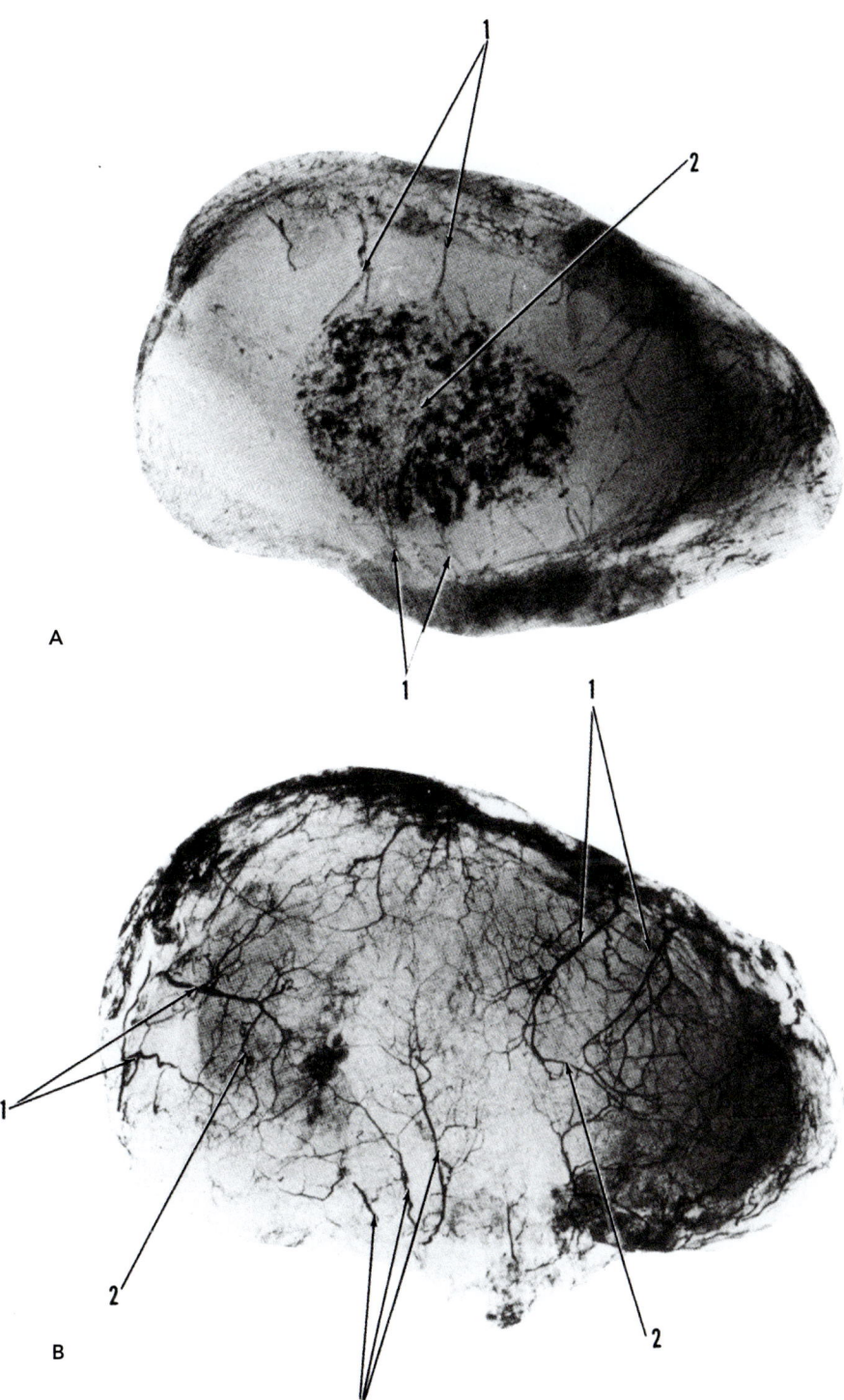

Figure 7.67 Blood supply to the navicular.
(A) Fine-grain radiograph of an injected and decalcified navicular from a girl aged 3.5 years. Radiate penetrating vessels (*1*) (six vessels counted from a study of the Spalteholz specimen) enter the central bony nucleus (*2*). **(B)** Fine-grain radiograph of an injected and decalcified navicular from a youth aged 19 years. Numerous radiate penetrating vessels (*1*) anastomose with each other (*2*) at the center and its periphery. (Republished with permission of British Editorial Society of Bone and Joint Surgery, From Waugh W. The ossification and vascularisation of the tarsal navicular and their relation to Köhler's disease. *J Bone Joint Surg Br.* 1958;40[4]:765; permission conveyed through Copyright Clearance Center, Inc.)

Distally, the metaphysis is supplied by three to four small arterial branches and the epiphysis by two to three branches entering from the medial and lateral aspects. At times, the lateral epiphyseal vessel is missing.

Shereff and colleagues studied the vascular anatomy of the fifth metatarsal in 15 fresh frozen feet by means of vascular injection techniques.[30] The extrinsic arterial circulation is provided by the dorsal and plantar metatarsal arteries and the inconsistent fibular marginal artery. The dorsal metatarsal artery of the fourth interspace originates from the arcuate artery, the lateral tarsal artery, or the proximal perforating artery of the fourth interspace. On the plantar aspect, the circulation is provided by the superficial plantar metatarsal artery running plantar to the intrinsic muscles along the midline of the fifth metatarsal shaft. Less often, a deep plantar intermetatarsal artery is present, coursing between the plantar and the dorsal interossei. In about 20%, the fibular plantar marginal artery, arising from the lateral plantar artery, contributes to the arterial

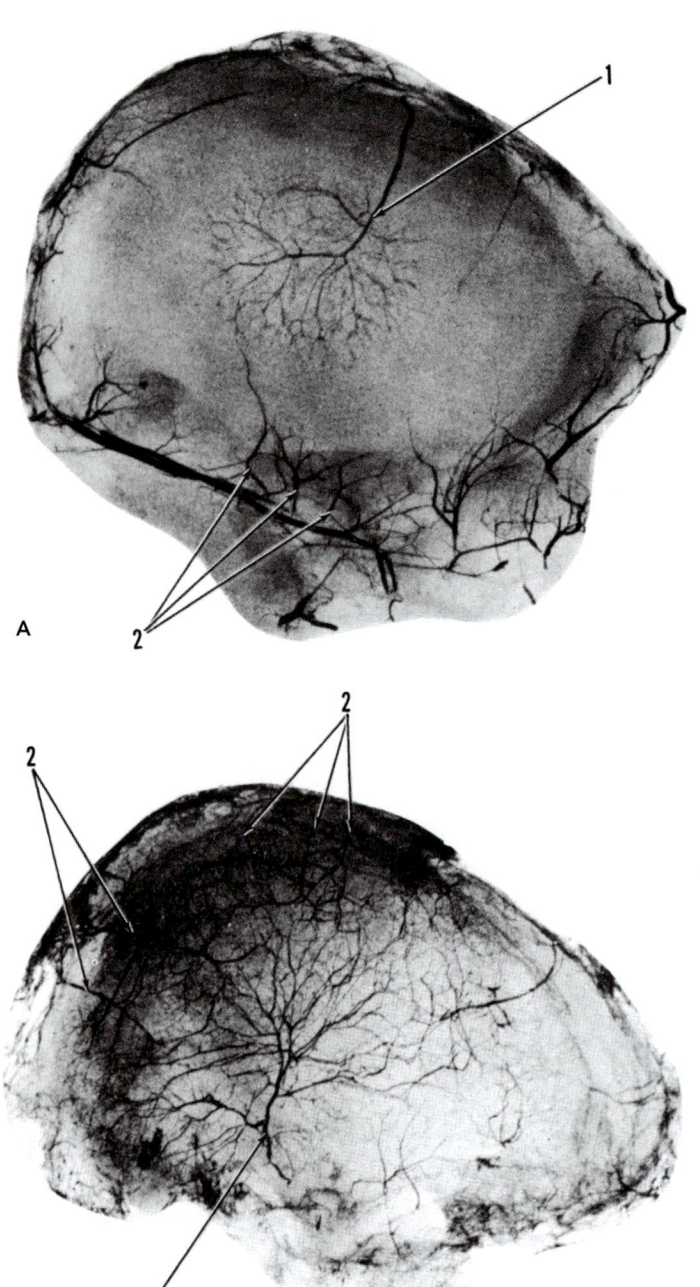

Figure 7.68 **Blood supply to the navicular. (A)** Fine-grain radiograph of an injected and decalcified navicular from a girl aged 4 years. A single main artery (*1*) from the dorsal surface branches and outlines the whole of the central bony nucleus. A few penetrating radiate vessels (*2*) are seen but take little part in the anastomotic network. **(B)** Fine-grain radiograph of a decalcified navicular from a boy aged 13 years. A large part of the bone is supplied by a single plantar artery (*1*). Other radial vessels (*2*) contribute to the blood supply of the bone. (Republished with permission of British Editorial Society of Bone and Joint Surgery, From Waugh W. The ossification and vascularisation of the tarsal navicular and their relation to Köhler's disease. *J Bone Joint Surg Br.* 1958;40[4]:765; permission conveyed through Copyright Clearance Center, Inc.)

blood supply coursing between the flexor digiti minimi brevis and the abductor minimi muscles. These source arteries course distally along the shaft of the fifth metatarsal and provide variable numbers of branches to the base, shaft, and head of the bone. They then participate in the intraosseous circulation, and "the greatest confluence of extraosseous vessels occurred at the medial side of the fifth metatarsal."[30] The intraosseous arterial supply is provided by a periosteal plexus, a nutrient artery, and metaphyseal and epiphyseal vessels. The periosteal plexus is formed by numerous branches arising from the dorsal and plantar sources. One single nutrient artery penetrates from the medial aspect at the junction of the proximal and middle third. Within the medullary canal, it divides into a shorter proximal branch supplying the metatarsal base and a longer distal branch supplying the metatarsal head. Metaphyseal and epiphyseal arterial branches arising from the source arteries to the base and head supply intracapsular branches to the tarsometatarsal and metatarsophalangeal joints, which penetrate the bone in nonarticular areas of the head and the base. The tuberosity of the fifth metatarsal is also supplied in a constant fashion by two arterial branches.

Leemrijse et al[31] studied the vascularization of the heads of the three central metatarsals of seven fresh cadaveric specimens in regard to the horizontal osteotomies of the metatarsal head. They used the latex injection method followed by dissection. The study of the first 12 metatarsals (in four specimens) was to define the normal vascularization without surgical interference. The dorsal metatarsal arteries terminate distally as well-defined

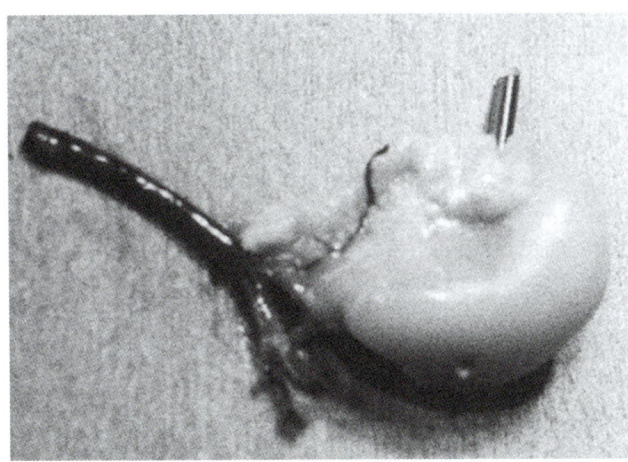

Figure 7.69 **The metatarsal head and its nutrient artery.** (Reprinted from Leemrijse T, Valti B, Oberlin C. Vascularization of the heads of the three central metatarsals: an anatomical study, its application and considerations with respect to horizontal osteotomies at the neck of the metatarsals. *Foot Ankle Surg.* 1998;4:57-62, Figure 7, with permission from Elsevier.)

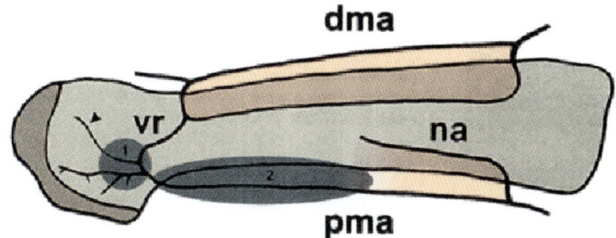

Figure 7.70 **The metatarsal heads have two arterial sources: (1) the dorsal metatarsal arteries (*dma*) and (2) the plantar metatarsal arteries (*pma*).** These two vessels typically anastomosed at two sites about the metatarsal heads forming a vascular ring (*vr*) and provided an extensive extraosseous arterial network around the metatarsal heads. Small arterial branches of this network run distally on the metatarsal cortex to enter the bone of the metatarsal head (*arrow*). The nutrient arteries traversed the cortex of the metaphysis close to the capsular and ligamentous insertions to provide multiple branches for the supply of the subchondral bone. (Adapted from Petersen WJ, Lankes JM, Paulsen F, Hassenpflug J. The arterial supply of the lesser metatarsal heads: a vascular injection study in human cadavers. *Foot Ankle Int.* 2002;23[6];491-495.)

dorsal capsular branches, which "anastomose with each other and with capsular branches of plantar origin to form a pericapsular network. At the level of the dorsal synovial fold, one or two fine vessels pass toward the head. They reach the bone in the extraarticular region. Subsequently, the dorsal metatarsal arteries divide to form the dorsal digital arteries. During their course along the intermetatarsal spaces, these dorsal metatarsal arteries give proximal and distal perforating branches to the plantar network"[31] and subsequently, the dorsal metatarsal arteries divide to form the dorsal digital arteries. The plantar metatarsal arteries give rise to plantar perforating arteries, which anastomose with their corresponding dorsal perforators. "Each of the plantar metatarsal arteries gives rise to 1 to 2 muscular branches. A branch to the head of the metatarsal and the capsule of the metatarsophalangeal joint arises from the medial side of each plantar metatarsal artery. It enters the articular cul-de-sac of the (metatarsophalangeal) joint under the plantar plate and divides into two clearly defined terminal branches—capsular and cephalic [Fig. 7.69]. The plantar vascular branch to the metatarsal head and capsule of the metatarsophalangeal joint is constant. The plantar metatarsal arteries subsequently divide into the proper plantar digital arteries."

Petersen et al[32] defined the vascularization of the lesser metatarsal heads of 20 cadaver feet using an epoxy resin injection method and a modified Spalteholz technique.

The metatarsal heads had two arterial sources—the dorsal metatarsal arteries, which arose from the dorsalis pedis artery, and the plantar metatarsal arteries, which are branches of the posterior tibial artery. These two vessels typically anastomosed at two sites about the metatarsal heads, forming a vascular ring and provided an extensive extraosseous arterial network around the metatarsal heads. Small arterial branches of this network run distally on the metatarsal cortex to enter the bone of the metatarsal head. The nutrient arteries traversed the cortex of the metaphysic close to the capsular and ligamentous insertions to provide multiple branches for the supply of the subchondral bone (Fig. 7.70).

First Metatarsal

Metatarsal 1 has an arterial supply pattern similar to that of the proximal phalanx of the lesser toes (Fig. 7.71). The nutrient artery penetrates the diaphysis in the middle of the lateral

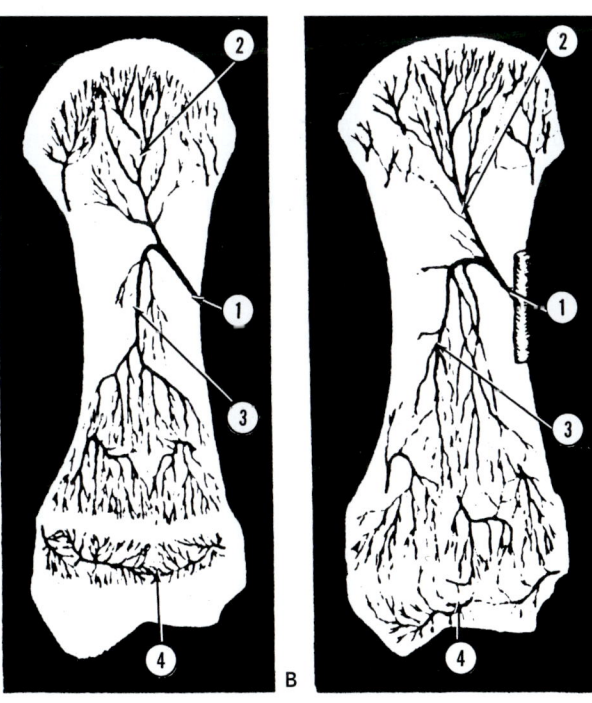

Figure 7.71 **Blood supply to the first metatarsal bone. (A)** In adolescent aged 12 to 13 years. The nutrient artery (*1*) divides into a short distal (*2*) and a long proximal (*3*) branch. The distal branch anastomoses with the distal metaphyseal and capital vessels. The proximal branch is stronger and is directed proximally toward the epiphysis, which in turn is supplied by arterial branches entering from its medial and lateral sides. (*4*, epiphyseal vessels.) **(B)** In the adult. (*1*, nutrient artery; *2*, distal division branch of *1*; *3*, proximal division branch of *1* anastomosing with the epiphyseal vessels [*4*].) (Reprinted by permission from Anseroff NJ. Die arterien des skelets der hand und des fusses des mensche. *Z Anat Entwicklungs.* 1937;106:204.)

surface at an angle of 90° and divides into two branches: proximal and distal. The distal branch is weaker; it runs distally and anastomoses with the arteries of the metaphysis and the head. The metaphysis receives four or five arterial branches, and the head receives 12 to 16 small arteries penetrating from its medial and lateral aspects. The proximal, stronger branch is directed proximally toward the epiphysis, which is supplied by four to eight arterial branches entering through the medial and lateral surfaces.

Shereff and colleagues studied the arterial supply to the first metatarsal and metatarsophalangeal joint in 32 feet specimens by means of vascular injection techniques.[33]

The first metatarsal and metatarsophalangeal joint are supplied by the first dorsal metatarsal artery, the first plantar metatarsal artery, and the superficial branch of the medial plantar artery. The three arteries form an abundant periosteal arterial system spreading out over the center of the diaphysis of the bone. These periosteal vessels penetrate the bone and anastomose with intraosseous branches deriving from the proximal branch of the nutrient artery. The first dorsal metatarsal artery provides one to two branches to the base of the first metatarsal, one or two branches to the shaft, and one to three branches to the metatarsal head. This artery supplies branches to the dorsal and lateral aspects of the first metatarsophalangeal joint and its capsule. The nutrient artery originates from the first dorsal metatarsal artery and perforates the lateral cortex in the distal third or at the junction of the middle third and distal third. The first plantar metatarsal artery provides one arterial branch to the base of the first metatarsal, one or two branches to the shaft, and one to three branches to the head from the plantar and the lateral aspect. No branches supply the dorsum of the metatarsophalangeal joint.

The superficial branch of the medial plantar artery was present in 75% and provides inconsistent branches to the first metatarsal throughout its course. It supplies one branch to the base of the bone, one to two branches to the shaft, and one to two capital branches to the medial side and, less frequently, to the plantar surface of the head.

The principal nutrient artery, after perforating the lateral cortex, courses obliquely through the nutrient foramen, enters the medullary canal, and divides into two branches—long proximal and short distal. The long proximal branch terminates and anastomoses with metaphyseal branches at the base. The distal arterial branch proceeds distally to the metatarsal head and gives terminal branches anastomosing with metaphyseal and capital vessels at the junction of the head and neck. During their course, both the proximal and distal arterial branches provide in a radiate manner numerous smaller endosteal branches. Metaphyseal arteries derived from the extracapsular branches penetrate the capsule, course along the neck, and penetrate at the junction of the head–neck of the metatarsal. Two to four metaphyseal arterial branches were identified for each metatarsal surface. The dorsal aspect of the head is penetrated by two large metaphyseal branches: dorsomedial and dorsolateral. They run distally and obliquely plantarward, supplying the dorsal two-thirds of the metatarsal head. Two smaller metaphyseal arteries penetrate the plantar aspect of the head and course dorsodistally, supplying the medial and lateral aspect of the plantar one-third of the head. In addition, four to six capital arteries penetrate the nonarticular surface of the head from the medial and lateral sides; extend toward the center of the head, anastomosing with the metaphyseal branches; and supply the medial and lateral one-fourth of the head (Fig. 7.72).

The position of the nutrient artery may be variable. Singh, in a study of 100 first metatarsals, gives the following distribution of the nutrient foramina (Fig. 7.73)[34]:

- Single lateral foramina: 62%
- Two foramina: 24%
    - Lateral and medial: 15%
    - Lateral and dorsal: 7%
    - Lateral and plantar: 2%
- Single plantar foramina: 11%
- Single medial foramina: 2%
- Single dorsal foramina: 1%

Jones et al[35] investigated the blood supply to the first metatarsal head in 22 fresh frozen specimens using latex injection and a modified Spalteholz technique. They correlated their findings with the Chevron osteotomy of the first metatarsal head. They described a first metatarsal "plantar arcade" "proximal to the first metatarsal head and sesamoids, providing two, three, or four pericapsular perforators"[35] (Fig. 7.74). The nutrient artery entered the metatarsal at or near the junction of the proximal and middle third of the shaft. Distally, several dorsolateral pericapsular perforators were supplied to the metatarsophalangeal joint.

Malal et al[36] mapped out the arrangement of the vascular supply to the first metatarsal and its relationship to the chevron osteotomy in 10 cadaveric specimens. They used the injection method with India ink-latex mixture followed by dissection.

"The nutrient artery to the first metatarsal shaft was found to arise from the first dorsal metatarsal artery in nine of the specimens. Whereas, it was found to branch directly from the dorsalis pedis artery in one specimen. The location of the nutrient artery was found to be very variable in the middle third of the metatarsal shaft laterally."[36]

"The first metatarsal received its extraosseous blood supply from the first dorsal metatarsal and first plantar metatarsal arteries (both branches of the dorsalis pedis artery) and from the superficial branch of the medial plantar artery (Fig. 7.75). A contribution from the medial plantar artery could not be identified in three of the specimens. All of the three vessels gave off branches to form a plexus on the plantar-lateral corner and the adjoining surfaces of the metatarsal neck. From the plantar-lateral plexus, a variable number of perforators entered the metatarsal head just proximal to the capsular attachment on its plantar-lateral aspect."[36] This study did not carry out the intraosseous topographic distribution of the vessels within the first metatarsal head–neck.

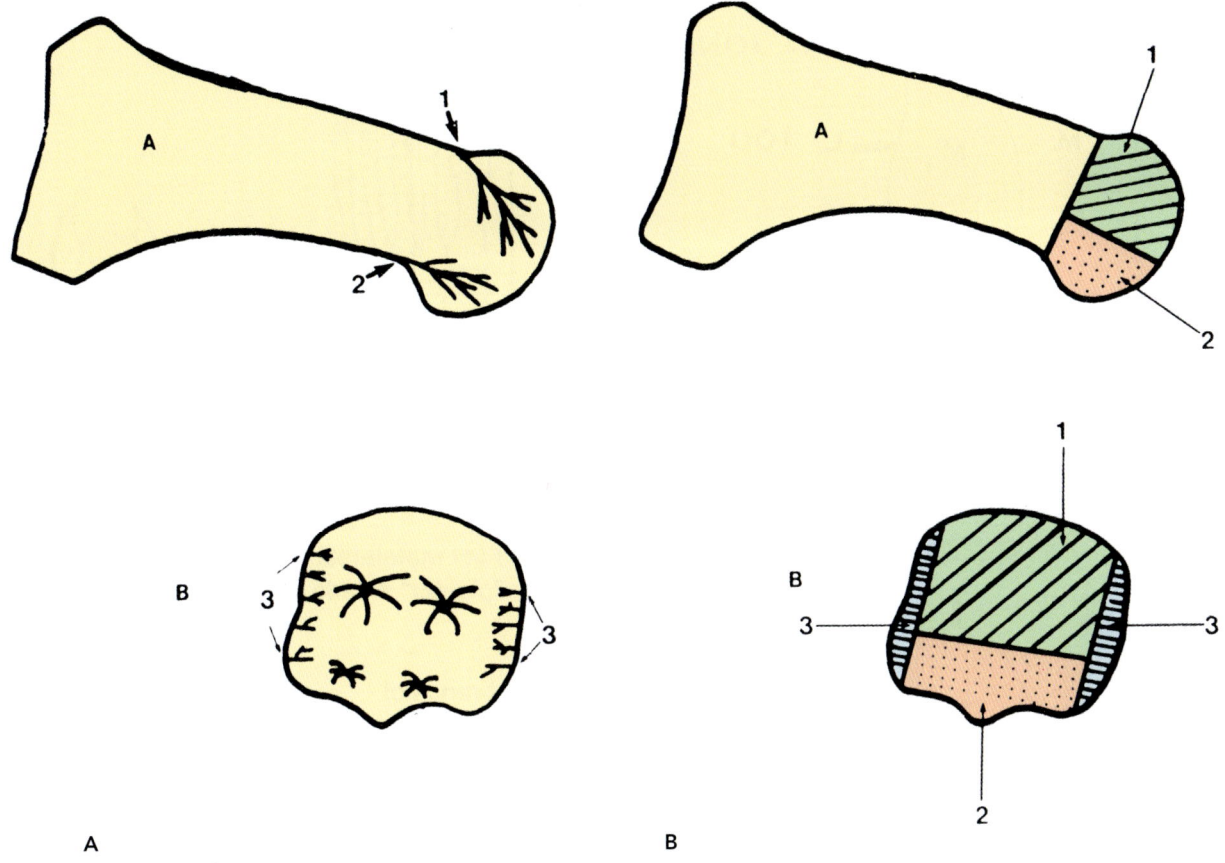

Figure 7.72 **Distribution of the intraosseous blood supply of the metatarsal head.** (A) Lateral view. (B) Axial view. The dorsal metaphyseal vessels (*1*) supply the dorsal two-thirds of the head, and the plantar metaphyseal vessels (*2*) supply the plantar one-third of the head. The capital arteries (*3*) supply the medial and lateral one-fourth of the head. (Adapted from Shereff MJ, Yang QM, Kummer FJ. Extraosseous and intraosseous arterial supply to the first metatarsal and metatarsophalangeal joint. *Foot Ankle.* 1987;5:81.)

Phalanges

The proximal phalanges receive their blood supply predominantly from the dorsal digital arteries; the middle phalanges are supplied by the plantar and dorsal digital arteries; and the distal phalanges have predominantly a plantar supply.[24]

In the age group of 13 to 14 years, the nutrient artery of the proximal phalanges penetrates the diaphysis from the lateral surface except for the artery of the fifth toe, which enters from the medial surface. In the bone, the nutrient artery divides into a distal, relatively weak branch and a proximal, stronger branch. The diaphysis receives 13 to 16 smaller branches entering mostly from the dorsal surface, to a lesser degree from the lateral and plantar surfaces, and minimally from the medial side. The epiphysis is supplied by four arterial branches.

The middle phalanges receive diaphyseal vessels from the periosteal network. These vessels penetrate the bone from the dorsal and plantar aspects. The epiphysis receives two arterial branches from the lateral and medial aspects.

The distal phalanx of the big toe has a large nutrient artery that penetrates the bone from the lateral rim of the middle diaphyseal segment; another large artery penetrates the bone from the plantar aspect. The metaphyseal area receives dorsal (six to eight) and plantar (four to six) branches. The epiphysis is penetrated by four to six branches from the dorsal and plantar aspects. As the nutrient artery enters the bone, it divides into a weak distal branch and a stronger proximal branch. The distal branch runs distally and anastomoses with the artery entering the tuft.

The distal phalanges of toes 2 through 5 have a similar pattern of blood supply. The diaphyseal vessel penetrates from the plantar surface in the middle third. The tuft is entered on each side by a branch, and the epiphysis receives two dorsal and two plantar arteries.

Vega and coworkers studied the arterial supply to the proximal phalanx of the hallux in six cadaver feet with injection-radiographic means.[37] The medial plantar hallucal artery rapidly attenuates and terminates in minute vessels supplying the medial aspect of the metatarsophalangeal joint and of the proximal phalanx. The prominent lateral plantar hallucal artery originates from the first plantar metatarsal artery and provides three major arterial branches (Fig. 7.76):

- Proximal: Smallest of the three, it supplies the capsule of the first metatarsophalangeal joint and terminates by supplying the base of the proximal phalanx.

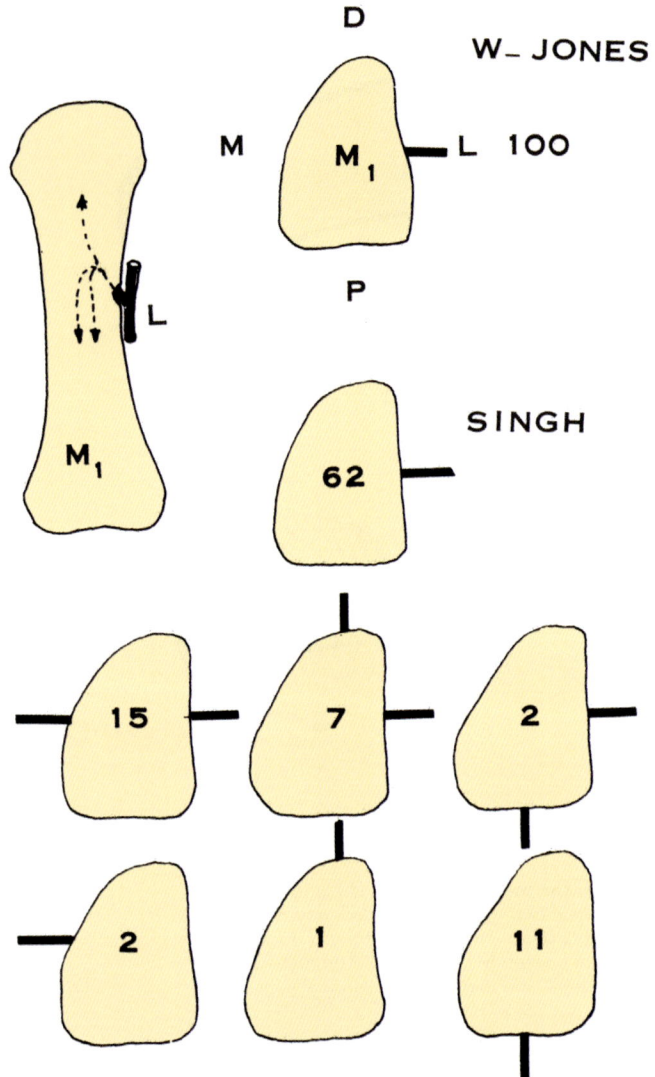

Figure 7.73 Distribution of the nutrient artery(ies) of the first metatarsal. (*D*, dorsal; *L*, lateral; *M*, medial; *P*, plantar.) Numbers indicate percentage of occurrence. (Adapted from Singh I. Variations in the metatarsal bones. *J Anat.* 1960;94:345.)

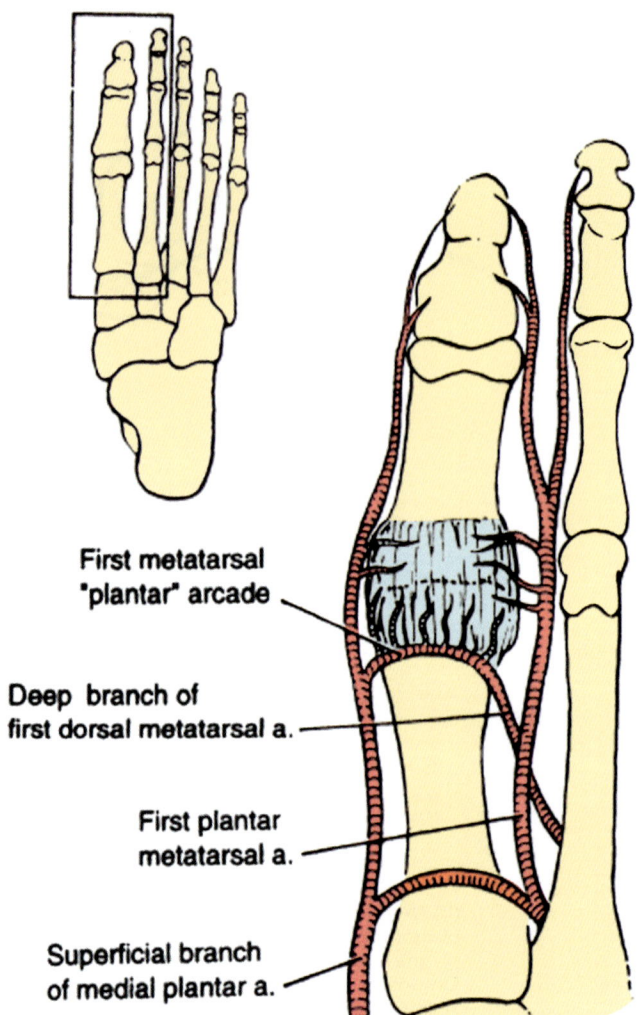

Figure 7.74 Plantar arterial network about the first metatarsophalangeal joint of the right foot. (Adapted from Jones KJ, Feiwell LA, Freedman EL, et al. The effect of chevron osteotomy with lateral capsular release on the blood supply to the first metatarsal head. *J Bone Joint Surg Am.* 1995;77:197-204.)

- Proximal transverse hallucal artery: Courses transversely from lateral to medial on the plantar aspect of the shaft of the proximal phalanx at about the level of the midshaft. The terminal branches anastomose with the medial plantar proper hallucal artery.
- Distal transverse hallucal artery: Courses transversely across the plantar aspect of the distal phalanx and supplies the distal phalanx, medial and lateral distal soft tissue of the hallux, and nail matrix.

The nutrient foramen was analyzed in 20 proximal phalanges with maceration technique. The foramen is located at the junction of the middle and distal third of the proximal phalanx. The artery bifurcates in the medullary canal and provides branches proximally and distally, supplying the head and base of the phalanx and anastomosing with corresponding metaphyseal arteries. Along its course, the nutrient artery provides small radial arteries supplying the cortical endosteum.

The dorsal hallucal arteries terminate in the proximal half of the hallux. The lateral dorsal hallucal artery provides a vertical communicating branch at 1 cm distal to the metatarsophalangeal joint communicating with the lateral plantar digital artery.

Sesamoids of the Big Toe

The two sesamoids of the metatarsophalangeal joint of the big toe receive their blood supply from the first plantar metatarsal artery. Two to three arteries penetrate the sesamoids from the sides, and one to two branches penetrate from the center. These multiple branches anastomose in the center of the sesamoid. Sobel and coworkers investigated the microvascular anatomy of the sesamoids in 15 cadaver specimens.[38] Each sesamoid has two major arterial sources (proximal and plantar) arising from the first plantar metatarsal artery and one minor arterial source (distal) entering through the capsular attachment. The proximal vessels enter

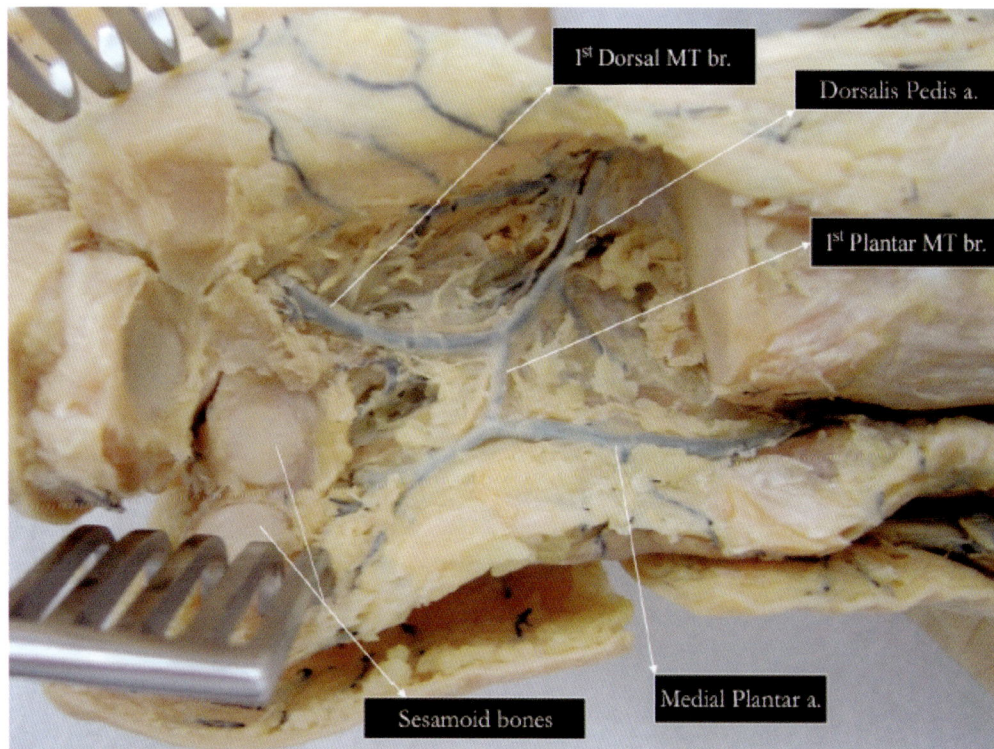

Figure 7.75 Photograph showing the main arteries supplying the first metatarsal (*MT*) head and the course of the dorsalis pedis. The first metatarsal has been removed for visualization. (From Malal JJ, Shaw-Dunn J, Kumar CS. Blood supply to the first metatarsal head and vessels at risk with a chevron osteotomy. *J Bone Joint Surg Am.* 2007;89A[9]: 2018-2022, Figure 1.)

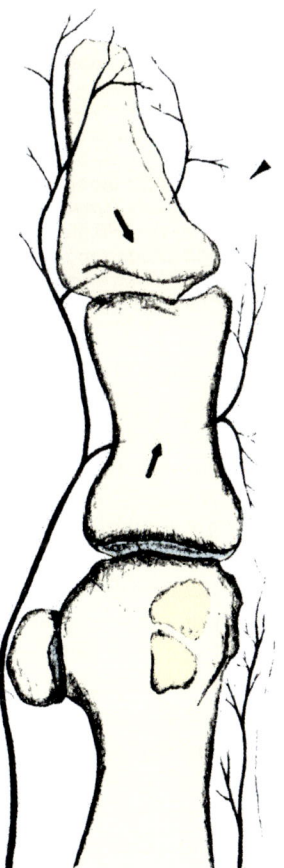

Figure 7.76 **Arterial blood supply of the big toe.** Proximal and distal transverse hallucal arteries (*arrows*) and their anastomosis (*arrowhead*). (Adapted from Vega M, Resnick D, Black JD, Haghighi P. The intrinsic and extrinsic arterial supply to the proximal phalanx of the hallux. *Foot Ankle.* 1985;5(5):257.)

the sesamoid at the attachment site of the flexor hallucis brevis. The plantar vessels penetrate the plantar surface near the midline and arborize throughout the bone, anastomosing with the proximal vessels. The contribution of the distal vessels is minimal. The lateral attachments of the sesamoids to the plantar plate and joint capsule are relatively avascular (see Fig. 7.77).

Chamberland et al[39] studied the vascularization of the hallucal sesamoids in 10 fresh frozen cadaver specimens. "The extraosseous blood supply to the sesamoids derives from branches of the medial plantar artery."[39] "Only one vessel constantly penetrates each sesamoid proximally and proceeds distally with variable amount of branching."[39] The intraosseous blood supply is abundant and appears to originate from vessels of the plantar, nonarticular surface of the sesamoids. The lateral and medial capsular attachments to the sesamoids also contain a small contribution to the sesamoid blood supply.

Vascular Anatomy of Tendons

Blood Supply of Achilles Tendon. Angiographic studies by Lagergren and Lindholm suggested that there is an avascular area in the calcaneal tendon between 2 and 6 cm from the insertion into the calcaneum.[40]

Carr and Norris[41] investigated the vascularity of the Achilles tendon based on the study of 16 fresh cadavers aged 56 to 79 years (average, 62.4 years) excluding any peripheral vascular disease or a history of diabetes. They injected barium sulfate and India ink to determine the blood supply of the tendon from the surrounding tissues and used a computer-assisted image analysis system to quantify the

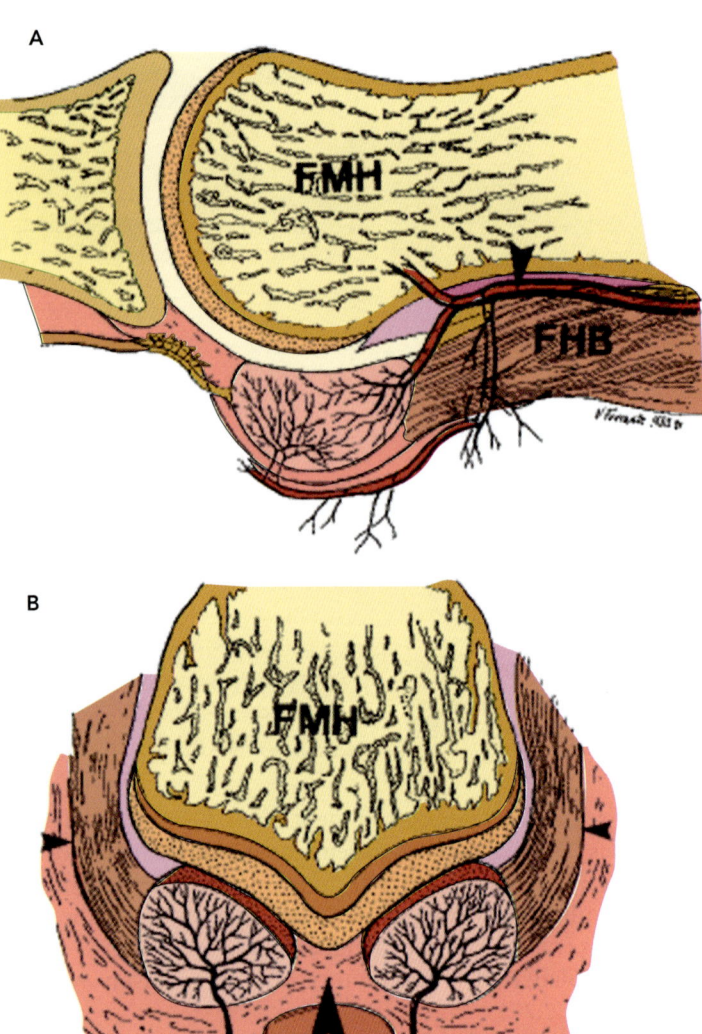

Figure 7.77 (A) Typical blood supply of the sesamoid complex. The proximal and plantar supply arises from branches of the first plantar metatarsal artery (*arrow*). The distal supply is minimal and enters through the capsular attachment. (B) Illustration of a coronal section through the sesamoid complex demonstrating the rich plantar blood supply and the absence of vascularity from the capsule (*small arrows*) and intersesamoid ligament (*large arrow*). (*FHB*, flexor hallucis brevis; *FMH*, first metatarsal head.) (Adapted from Sobel M, Hashimoto J, Arnoczky SP, Bohne WH. The microvasculature of the sesamoid complex: its clinical significance. *Foot Ankle*. 1992;13[6]:360.)

vascularity. "Numerous vessels were seen to be evenly distributed throughout the length of the paratenon and, on the anterior surface, vessels ran in the mesotenon toward the tendon"[41] (see Fig. 7.78).

"The number of vessels varied throughout the length of the tendon, most being at the insertion to the calcaneum and least at 4 cm above it" and "the mean of the relative cross-sectional area occupied by the intratendinous vessels was decreased in midsection of the tendon"[41] (Figs. 7.79 and 7.80).

Stein et al[42] determined the intravascular volume of the Achilles tendon segmentally using an injection of radioisotopes technetium-99. The Achilles tendon was divided into segments from 1 to 9 cm from the calcaneal insertion (see Fig. 7.81). The tendon segment at 4 cm had the lowest intravascular volume and the segment at 9 cm had the highest intravascular volume (Fig. 7.82).

Blood Supply of Tibialis Posterior Tendon. Frey et al[43] studied the vascularity of the posterior tibial tendon in 31 cadaveric limbs.

They injected three specimens with acrylic casting material and 28 specimens with an India ink-gelatin suspension mixture and then cleared with a modified Spalteholz technique. In all specimens, a zone of hypovascularity was present in the midportion of the posterior tibial tendon. This zone started approximately 4 cm from the medial tubercle of the navicular bone (approximately 1.5 cm distal to the medial malleolus) and runs proximally for an average of 1.4 cm (Fig. 7.83).[44]

Petersen et al[45] studied the vascularity pattern of the posterior tibial tendons by injection techniques and immunohistochemically using antibodies against laminin, a basic component of the basement membrane of blood vessels. The intravascular volume of the posterior tibial tendon was determined by injection of a solution of radioisotope technetium-99 and gelatinous ink into the lower legs of cadavers. "For analysis of the intravascular volume, the posterior tibial tendon was dissected into three segments (I, II, III) each 1 cm in length. For the immunohistochemical investigations, tissue was obtained from the same regions, but the length of each segment was 2 cms"[45] (Fig. 7.84).

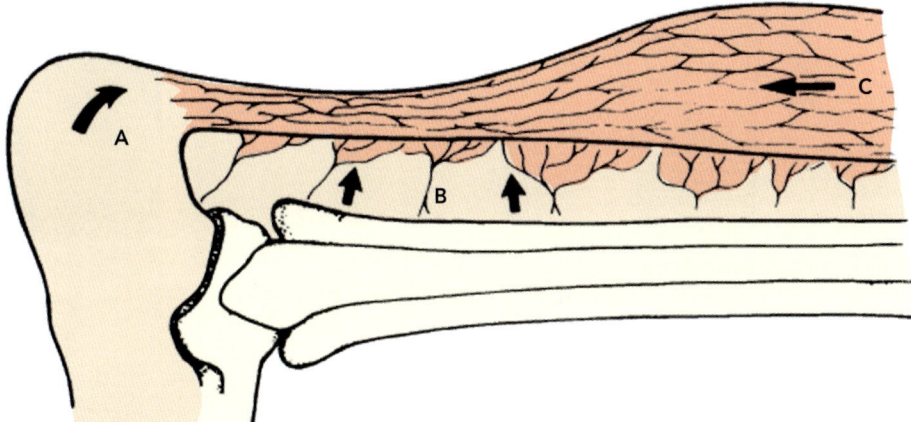

Figure 7.78 Diagram of the blood vessels of the paratenon, showing supply from the osseotendinous junction **(A)**, the mesotenon **(B)**, and the musculotendinous junction **(C)**. (Adapted from Carr AJ, Norris SH. The blood supply of the calcaneal tendon. *J Bone Joint Surg Br.* 1989;71B:100.)

The major blood supply of the posterior tibial tendon was from the posterior tibial artery. "Most of the tendon was covered by a paratenon in which blood vessels formed a web like network. From the paratenon, they penetrated the tendon tissue and anastomosed with intratendinous arterial network which was homogenous. In the region where the tendon passed around the medial malleolus, the longitudinally oriented intratendinous vascular network was interrupted and the tendon was avascular in the anterior part, directed toward the malleolus"[45] (Fig. 7.85).

The intravascular volume determined with radionucleoides indicated lowest intravascular volume in the middle segment (zone II retromalleolar) (Fig. 7.86).

Blood Supply of the Flexor Hallucis Longus Tendon

Petersen et al[46] investigated the blood supply of the flexor hallucis longus tendon. They utilized the previously described injection technique with India ink followed by Spalteholz clearing in 10 lower limbs and immunohistochemical proof of laminin in the wall of the vessels in 20 flexor hallucis longus tendons. Four zones of study—2 cm each—were defined as indicated in Figure 7.87 and, for the localization of laminin, a given tendon was divided into quarters, from anterior to posterior. "The injection specimens showed that the major blood supply for the flexor hallucis longus tendon proximally arose from the posterior tibial artery. The distal part was supplied by branches

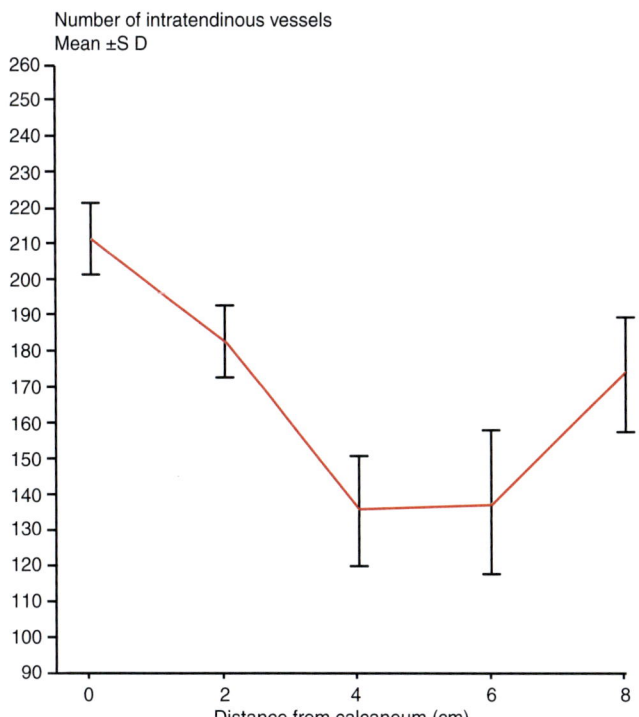

Figure 7.79 Graph of the number of intratendinous vessels at varying distances from the calcaneum. (Adapted from Carr AJ, Norris SH. The blood supply of the calcaneal tendon. *J Bone Joint Surg Br.* 1989;71B:100.)

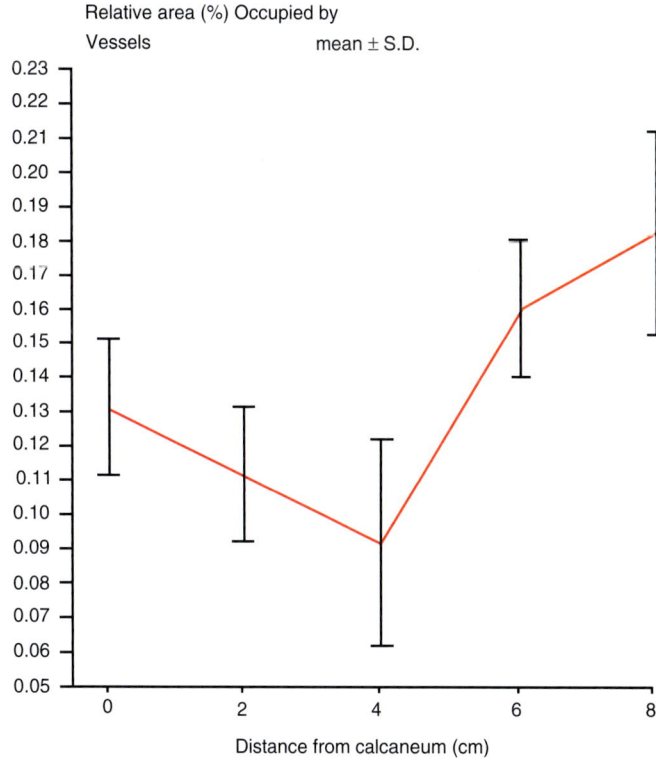

Figure 7.80 Graph showing the relative area of intratendinous vessels at various levels. (Adapted from Carr AJ, Norris SH. The blood supply of the calcaneal tendon. *J Bone Joint Surg Br.* 1989;71B:100.)

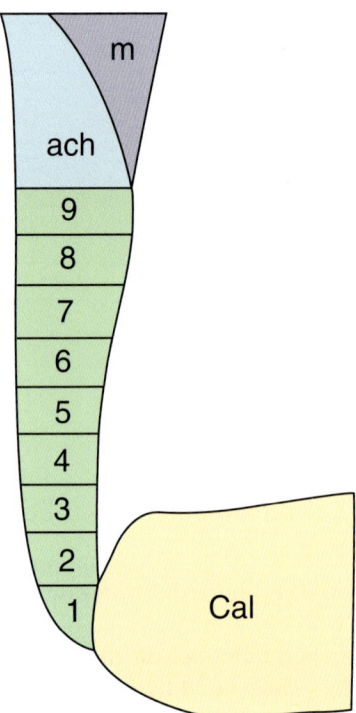

Figure 7.81 Schematic drawing of the Achilles tendon (*ach*), the musculus triceps surae (*m*), and the calcaneus (*cal*). The Achilles tendon was dissected into nine sections from 1 to 9 cm above the calcaneus. (Copyright © 2000. From Stein V, Laprell H, Tinnemeyer S, et al. Quantitative assessment of intravascular volume of the human Achilles tendon. *Acta Orthop Scand.* 2000;71[1]:61, Figure 1. Reproduced by permission of Taylor and Francis Group, LLC, a division of Informa plc.)

from the medial plantar artery. The tendon was widely covered by a peritenon where branches from both arteries formed a dense weblike network. From the peritenon, the blood vessels penetrated the tendon tissue and anastomosed with an intratendinous network. Within the tendon, the majority of the vessels were oriented longitudinally."[46]

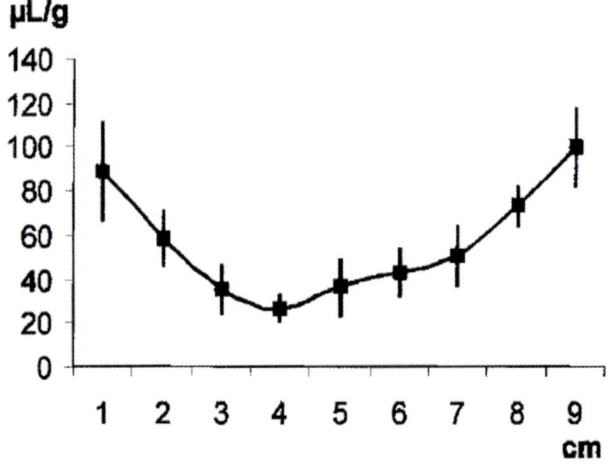

Figure 7.82 Diagram of intravascular volume per gram tendon of each cross-section from 1 to 9 cm above the calcaneal insertion of the Achilles tendon. The lower volume was found at 4 cm above the calcaneus. (Copyright © 2000. From Stein V, Laprell H, Tinnemeyer S, et al. Quantitative assessment of intravascular volume of the human Achilles tendon. *Acta Orthop Scand.* 2000;71[1]:61, Figure 3. Reproduced by permission of Taylor and Francis Group, LLC, a division of Informa plc.)

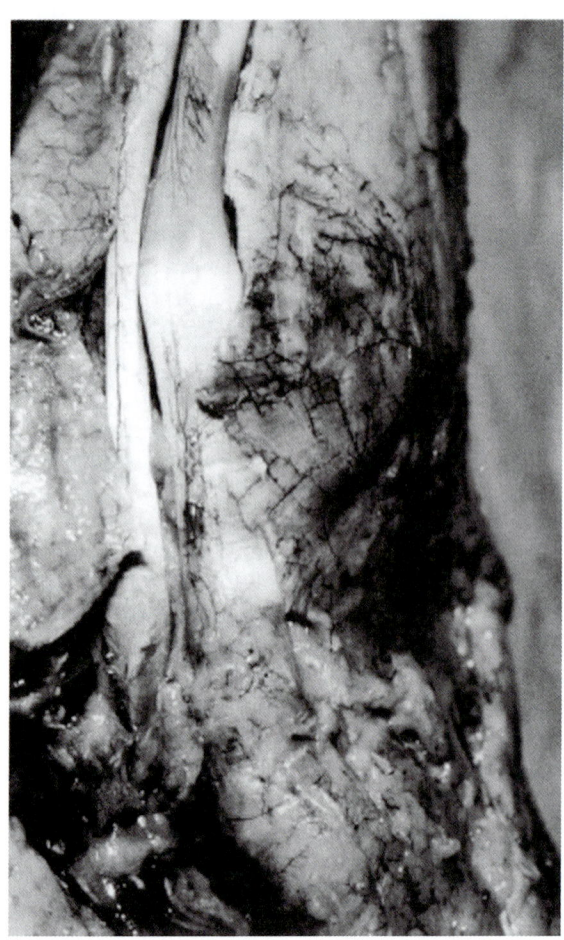

Figure 7.83 In the midportion of the posterior tibial tendon, a zone of hypovascularity can be seen. The zone starts approximately 40 mm from the medial tubercle of the navicular bone and runs proximally for an average of 14 mm. (From Frey C, Shereff M, Greenidge N. Vascularity of the posterior tibial tendon. *J Bone Joint Surg Am.* 1990;72:885, Figure 3.)

Avascular zones were defined in the flexor hallucis longus in the fibro-osseous tunnel posterior to the talus and in the segment of the tendon passing between the sesamoids at the level of the head of the first metatarsal.

The avascular zone posterior to the talus averaged 31.3 mm (range, 25-37 mm), and the average length of the avascular zone around the head of M_1 was 23.5 mm (range, 18-29 mm). Furthermore, "there was no immunochemical evidence proof of lamina in the anterior half of the segment which was located within the fibro-osseous tunnel posterior to the talus and positive immunoreactions could be found only in the posterior part of the gliding zone. A second zone negative for immunostaining for laminin was in the anterior part of the gliding zone where the tendon turned around the first metatarsal head" (Fig. 7.87).[46]

Blood Supply of Tibialis Anterior Tendon

Geppert et al[47] investigated the vascular supply to the tibialis anterior tendon in 12 fresh frozen cadaver specimens. They used the injection technique with India ink followed by clearing with modified Spalteholz technique.

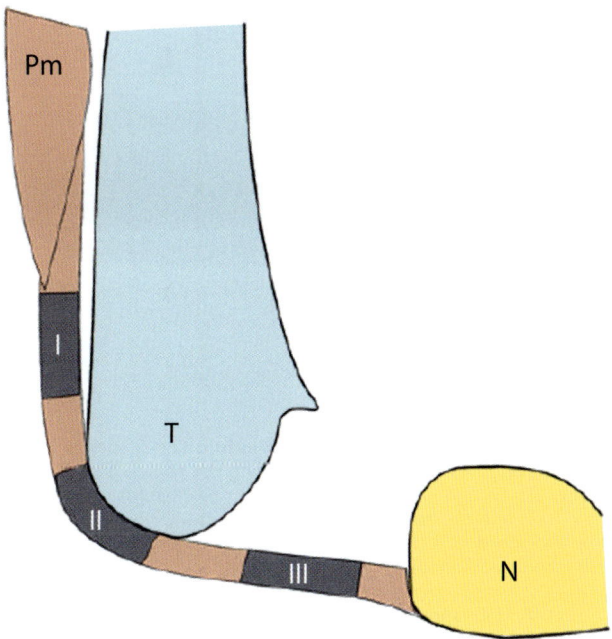

Figure 7.84 **Diagram of the posterior tibial tendon.** For analysis of the intravascular volume, the posterior tibial tendon was dissected into three segments (I, II, III)—each 1 cm in length from the same regions, but the length of each segment was 2 cm. (*N*, navicular; *Pm*, posterior tibial muscle; *T*, tibia). (Adapted from Petersen W, Hohmann G, Stein V, Tillmann B. The blood supply of the posterior tibial tendon. *J Bone Joint Surg Br*. 2002;84B[1]:141-144.)

On gross examination, the tibialis anterior tendon was supplied proximally by muscular branches from the anterior tibial artery. A rich vinculum was formed that supplied the undersurface of the tendon.

The tendon was well vascularized through its entire length including the region underlying the extensor retinaculum

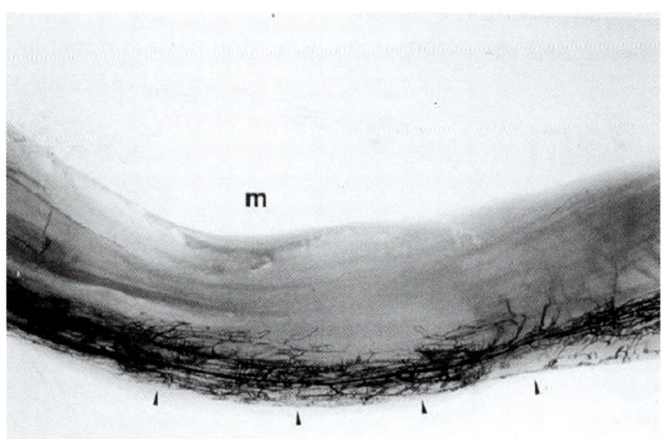

Figure 7.85 **Injection of India ink into a posterior tibial tendon shows that the terminal endings of the artery enter the tendon via a mesotenon (*arrowheads*) from the posterior aspect.** In the region where the tendon turns around the medial malleolus (*m*), the well-vascularized paratenon is absent and the distribution of vessels in the tendon is inhomogeneous. The posterior part of the tendon has a complete vascular network. The anterior part that is directed toward the medial malleolus is avascular. Detail is taken from the region where the tendon passes around the medial malleolus. (Republished with permission of British Editorial Society of Bone and Joint Surgery, From Petersen W, Hohmann G, Stein V, et al. The blood supply of the posterior tibial tendon. *J Bone Joint Surg Br*. 2002;84B[1]:141-144, Figure 2; permission conveyed through Copyright Clearance Center, Inc.)

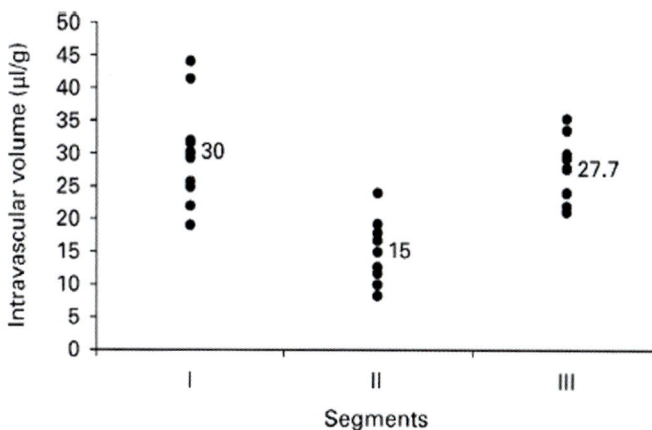

Figure 7.86 **Graphs showing the intravascular volume per gram of tendon.** The lowest volume was measured at segment II in the retromalleolar region. (Republished with permission of British Editorial Society of Bone and Joint Surgery, From Petersen W, Hohmann G, Stein V, et al. The blood supply of the posterior tibial tendon. *J Bone Joint Surg Br*. 2002;84B[1]:141-144, Figure 3; permission conveyed through Copyright Clearance Center, Inc.)

(Fig. 7.88). Near the tendon insertion, branches from the medial tarsal arteries and from the dorsalis pedis artery formed another rich vinculum. There was no evidence of a hypovascularity region in the tibialis anterior tendon.

Petersen et al[48] investigated the blood supply of the tibialis anterior tendon. They used the injection technique with India ink followed by preparation with the Spalteholz technique in 10 lower limbs.

They also used the immunohistochemical method (antibodies against laminin) in 20 tibialis anterior tendons obtained within 48 hours after death in patients aged 45 to 80 years old. The tendons were divided in six equal length segments from the musculotendinous junction to the insertion of the tendon (Fig. 7.89). "Within the tendon, the majority of the blood vessels are oriented in a longitudinal direction along the course of tendon fibers. The distribution of blood vessels within the tendon is not homogenous. The posterior half of the tendon has a complete vascular network extending from the musculotendinous juncture to the insertion zone at the medial cuneiform. In the middle part of the anterior half, the longitudinally oriented intratendinous vascular network is interrupted. In this zone, the tendon tissue is avascular and a well-vascularized peritenon is lacking" (Fig. 7.90).[48] The distance between the avascular zone and the tendon insertion is on average 10.1 mm (range, 5-16 mm). The avascular zone extends on average 56.6 mm (range, 45-67 mm). "In all specimens, the location of the avascular zone corresponded with the anatomical location of the inferior and superior extensor retinaculum."[48]

The immunohistochemical proof of laminin was positive in all investigated sections of the posterior half of the tendon. In the anterior half of both middle segments (three to four), there was no immunostaining for laminin.

Blood Supply of Peroneal Tendons

Sobel et al[49] investigated the microvascularity of the peroneal tendons in 12 fresh frozen cadaver limbs using the injection technique with India ink. The vascularity of the peroneal tendons was examined in situ and the harvested tendons, cleared

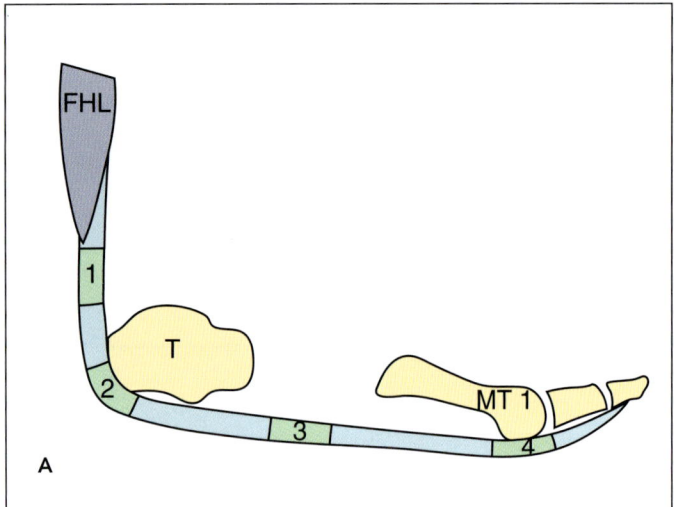

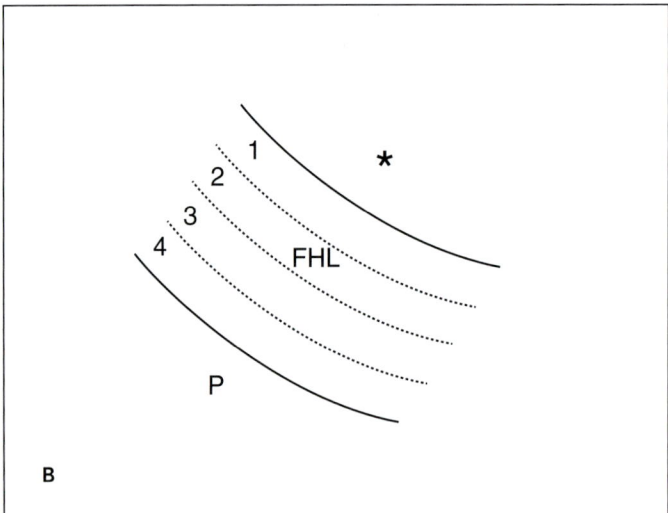

Figure 7.87 (A) Localization of segments 1-2-3-4 measuring each 1 cm for injection studies and 2 cm for immunohistochemical studies. (B) For the immunochemical analysis of the blood supply (proof of lamina in the wall of vessels), the presence of positive immunoreactions within different quarters of the tendon was noted. (1, anterior quarter adjacent to gliding surface; 2, 3, middle quarters; 4, peripheral quarter; *, localization of the bony pulley; FHL, flexor hallucis longus; P, peritendineum.) (Adapted from Petersen W, Pufe T, Zantop T, Paulsen F. Blood supply of the flexor hallucis longus tendon with regard to dancer's tendinitis: injection and immunohistochemical studies of cadaver tendons. Foot Ankle Int. 2003;8:592.)

using a modified Spalteholz technique, were evaluated under a dissecting microscope. Three zones (A, B, and C) were defined in a given tendon: zone A from the musculotendinous juncture to the proximal margin of the fibular groove, zone B behind the fibular groove, and zone C from the distal margin of the fibular groove to bony insertion. The tendons were supplied proximally by muscular branches from the posterior peroneal artery. "A rich vinculum supplied the entire length of the peroneus longus tendon from its periphery on the lateral side of the tendon. A separate vinculum supplied the peroneus brevis tendon along its periphery on the lateral side of the tendon and was more prominent in zones A and C and less prominent in zone B."[49] "A critical zone of hypovascularity was not demonstrated within either of the peroneus longus or peroneus brevis tendons in the 10 limbs with normal peroneus brevis tendon."[49]

Petersen et al[50] investigated the blood supply of the peroneal tendons with injection techniques and immunohistochemically by using antibodies for laminin. In the injection techniques, 10 lower limbs of fresh cadavers (aged 45-80 years) were used. In the immunohistochemical investigations, 20 peroneus longus and 20 peroneus brevis tendons together with their bony attachment sites were obtained at autopsies performed within 48 hours after death (age of subjects, 39-80 years). The tendons were divided into 2-cm segments[50] (Fig. 7.91).

The injection specimens indicated that the intratendinous distribution of blood vessels was not homogenous. "In the region where the peroneus brevis tendon passes through the

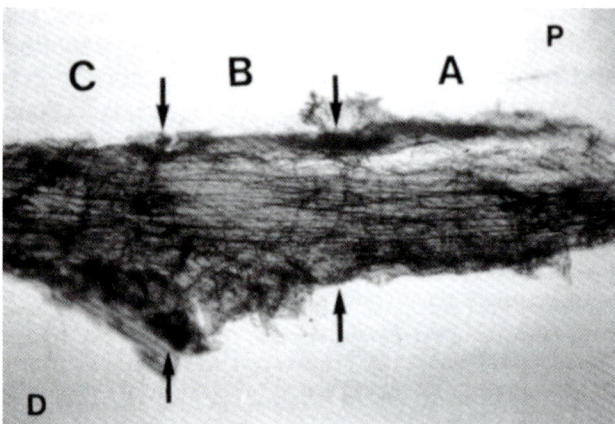

Figure 7.88 Cleared tibialis anterior tendon. The tendon is well vascularized through its entire length, including the region underlying the extensor retinaculum. (A, zone; D, distal; P, proximal.) A corresponding to the tibialis anterior tendon from its musculotendinous junction to the superior border of the inferior arm of the extensor retinaculum. (B, zone B, the region beneath the extensor retinaculum; C, zone C, the region of the tendon distal to the inferior retinaculum.) (From Geppert MJ, Sobel M, Hannafin JA. Microvasculature of the tibialis anterior tendon. Foot Ankle. 1993;14[5]:262, Figure 3. copyright ©1993. Reprinted by Permission of SAGE Publications.)

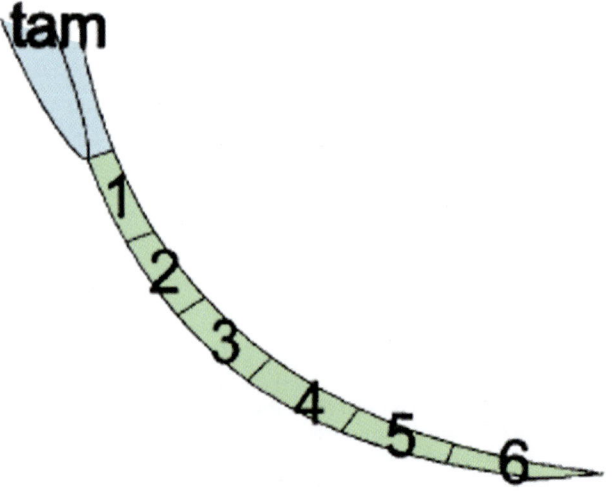

Figure 7.89 Schematic drawing showing the dissection of the tibialis anterior tendon for immunohistochemical investigations. The tendon was divided into six segments. (tam, tibialis anterior muscle.) (Adapted from Petersen W, Stein V, Tillmann B. Blood supply of the tibialis anterior tendon. Arch Orthop Trauma Surg. 1999;119:372.)

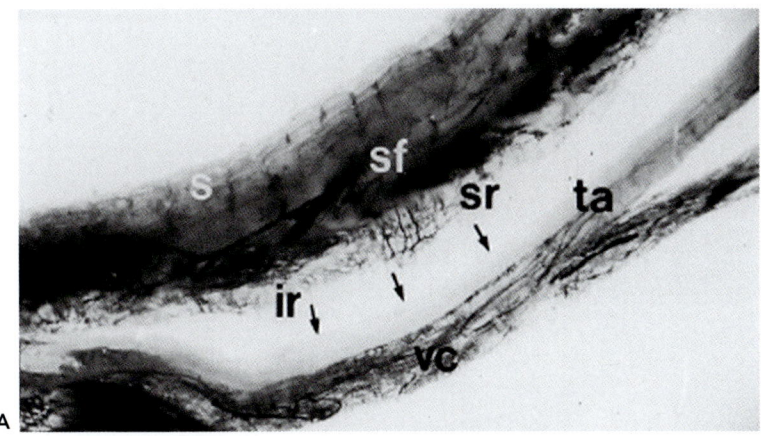

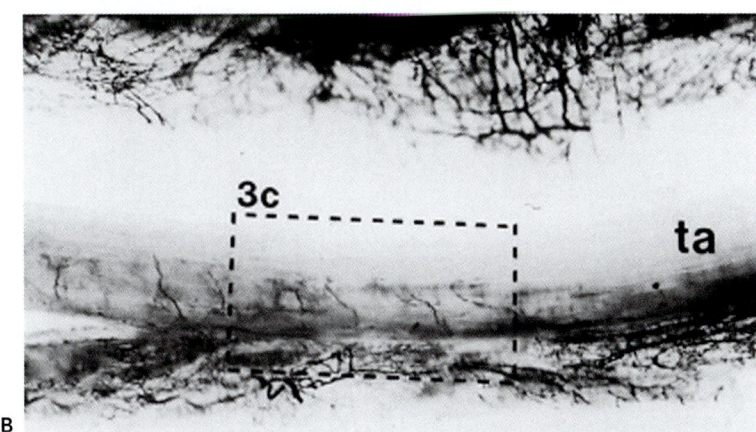

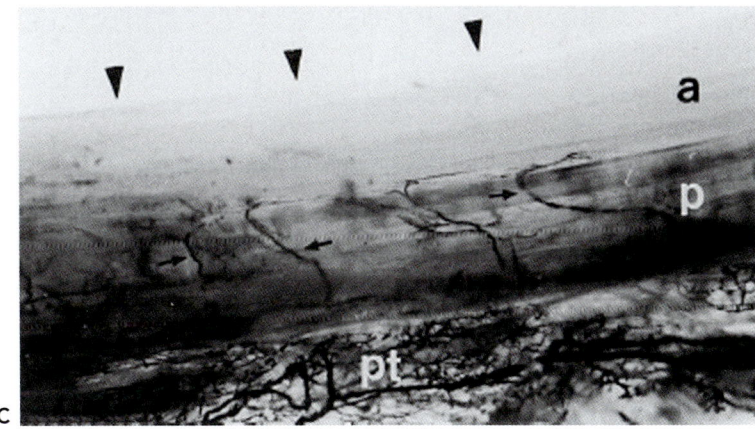

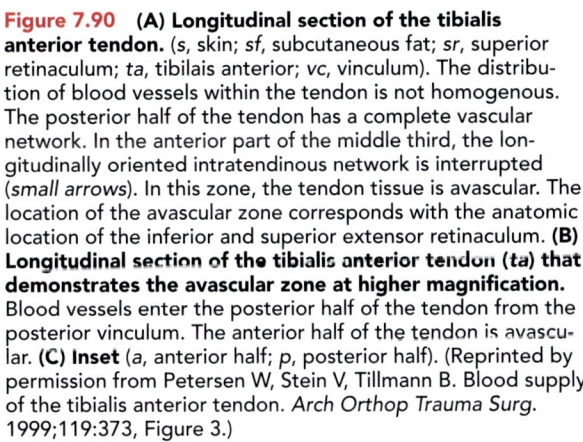

Figure 7.90 (A) Longitudinal section of the tibialis anterior tendon. (s, skin; sf, subcutaneous fat; sr, superior retinaculum; ta, tibilais anterior; vc, vinculum). The distribution of blood vessels within the tendon is not homogenous. The posterior half of the tendon has a complete vascular network. In the anterior part of the middle third, the longitudinally oriented intratendinous network is interrupted (*small arrows*). In this zone, the tendon tissue is avascular. The location of the avascular zone corresponds with the anatomic location of the inferior and superior extensor retinaculum. **(B) Longitudinal section of the tibialis anterior tendon (ta) that demonstrates the avascular zone at higher magnification.** Blood vessels enter the posterior half of the tendon from the posterior vinculum. The anterior half of the tendon is avascular. **(C) Inset** (a, anterior half; p, posterior half). (Reprinted by permission from Petersen W, Stein V, Tillmann B. Blood supply of the tibialis anterior tendon. *Arch Orthop Trauma Surg.* 1999;119:373, Figure 3.)

fibular groove, the longitudinally oriented intratendinous vascular network was interrupted and the tendon was nearly avascular."[50] The avascular zone of the peroneus brevis tendon had a variable longitudinal extension with an average length of 40 mm (range, 29-55 mm). The peroneus longus tendon had two avascular zones. In the region where the peroneus longus tendon curved around the lateral malleolus and the peroneal trochlea of the calcaneus, the anterior part of the tendon, which is directed toward the pulley, was avascular. This avascular zone had a variable length of an average 52 mm (range, 38-63 mm).

A second avascular zone was located more distally in the region where the tendon changes its direction and wraps around the cuboid. The length of the avascular zone was 25 mm in average length (range, 18-31 mm). The immunohistochemical investigation demonstrated for the peroneus brevis tendon no evidence of laminin in the segment of the peroneal groove of the fibula. Positive immunoreactions were found only in the posterior quarter of the retromalleolar gliding zone of six specimens.

"In the peroneus longus, there was no immunohistochemical evidence of laminin in the anterior part of the gliding zone where the tendon turns around the peroneal groove of the lateral malleolus and the calcaneus and in the region where the peroneus longus tendon turns around the cuboid."[50]

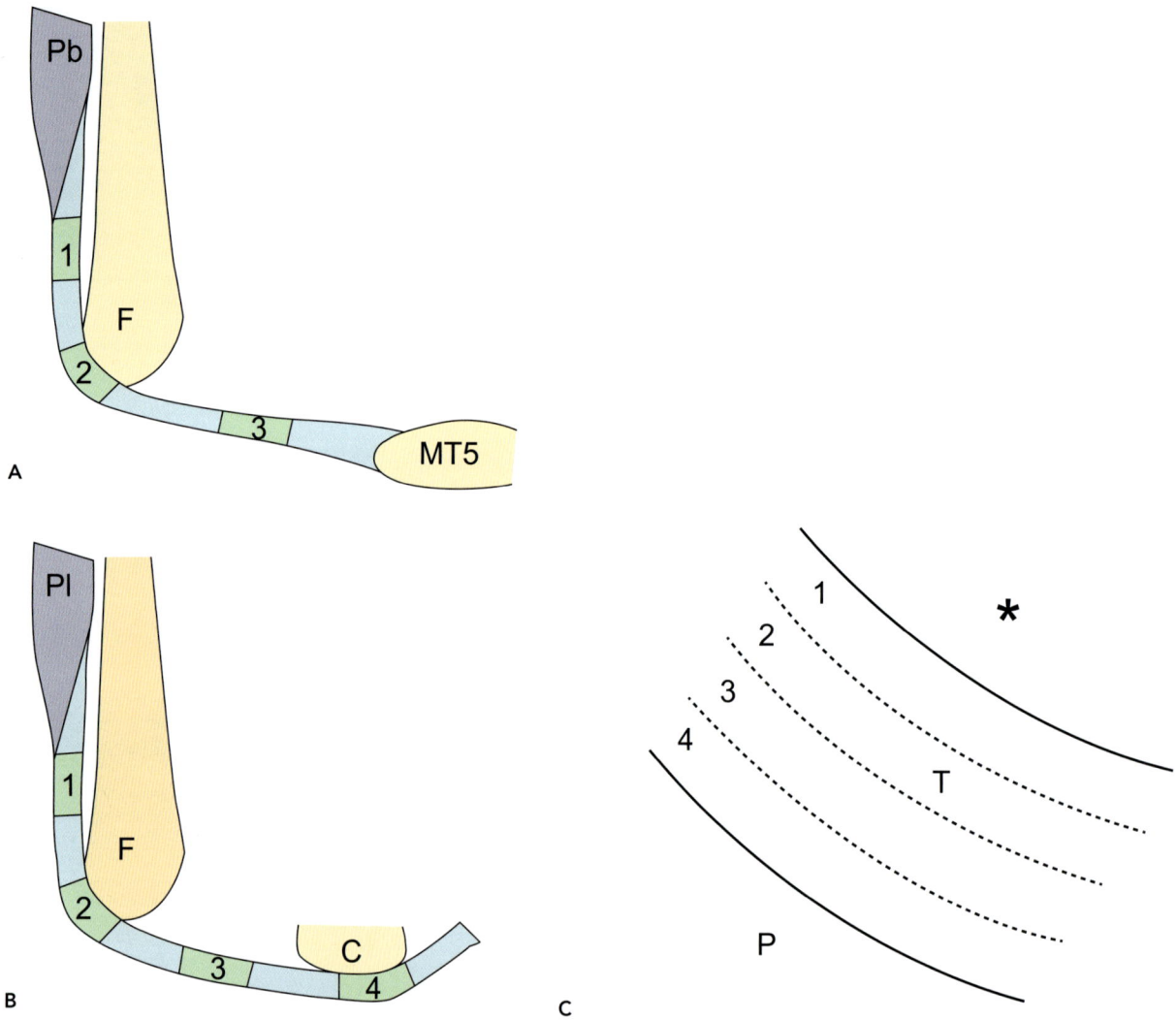

Figure 7.91 **(A) Location of three segments (dark marked) obtained from the peroneus brevis tendon for immunohistochemical proof of laminin.** (F, fibula; MT5, fifth metatarsal; PB, peroneus brevis muscle.) Segment 2 came from the region where the peroneus brevis wraps around the lateral malleolus. The segments measured 2 cm. **(B) Location of biopsies (dark marked) from the peroneus longus tendon for immunohistochemical investigations.** (PL, peroneus longus muscle.) From each tendon, four segments (length 2 cm) were obtained. (C, cuboid; F, fibula.) **(C) Presence of positive immunoreactions in different quarters of the tendon.** (1, anterior quarter adjacent to the gliding surface; 2, 3, middle quarters; 4, peripheral quarters; *, location of the bony pulley; P, peritendineum; T, tendon.) (Adapted from Petersen W, Bobka T, Stein V, et al. Blood supply of peroneal tendons. Injection and immunohistochemical studies of cadaver tendons. *Acta Orthop Scand.* 2000;71[2]:172.)

Vascular Anatomy of Nerves in Tarsal Tunnel

Flanigan et al[51] investigated the normal vascular supply of nerves in the tarsal tunnel with intra-arterial injection of latex in 20 lower extremities (aged 64-84 years). Detailed dissection was carried out using a dissecting microscope. Neurovascular segments were cleared with the Spalteholz method.

The blood supply of the posterior tibial nerve and its medial and lateral branches came directly from the corresponding arteries (Figure 7.92). The nutrient arteries were observed to be <1 mm in diameter, with the diameter decreasing distally within the terminal branches of the posterior tibial nerve. These vessels entered the posterior tibial nerve in the range of every 1 to 7 cm with intraspecimen means ranging from 3.0 to 3.8 cm (Fig. 7.93). One nutrient vessel from the posterior tibial artery was found to enter the nerve near the proximal border of the tarsal tunnel. Typically, the last nutrient artery from the posterior tibial artery (point zero) supplied the trifurcation point of the posterior tibial nerve about midway through the tarsal tunnel (Table 7.12). Distal to the trifurcation, the lateral and medial plantar nerves received most of the nutrient vessels from their corresponding arteries in shorter intervals ranging from 0.4 to 3.5 cm, with intraspecimen means ranging from 1.0 to 2.4 cm. In 65%, the lateral plantar nerve received nutrient vessels from the medial plantar artery (Fig. 7.94). The other nutrient vessels

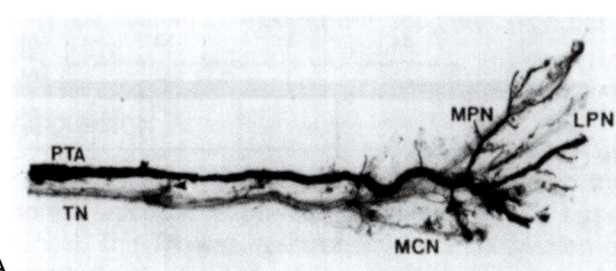
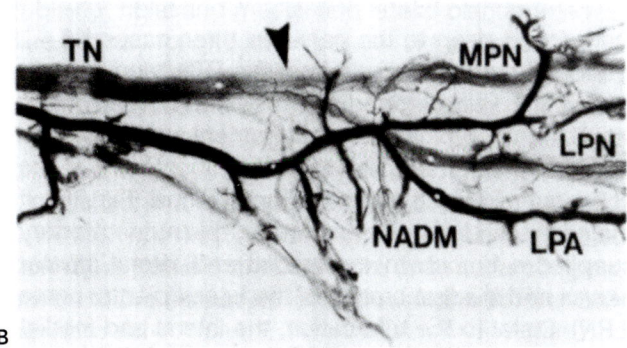

Figure 7.92 (A) Transilluminated view of posterior tibial neurovascular bundle and branches after clearing and microdissection. The nutrient vessels can be seen entering at regular intervals and form anastomosing arcades with proximal and distal nutrient vessels (*arrows*) via the intraneural longitudinal vessels. (B) **The nutrient vessels supplying the proximal border of the tarsal tunnel and the trifurcation point are illustrated.** The trifurcation point (*arrow*) is nourished by a vessel arising from a larger arterial branch of the posterior tibial artery; the vessel contributes a large branch to the lateral plantar nerve and a small branch to the medial plantar nerve. Also, this specimen contains the nutrient vessel from the medial plantar artery supplying the lateral plantar nerve (*). (*, vessel from medial plantar artery to lateral plantar nerve; *MCN*, medial calcaneal nerve; *MPN*, medial plantar nerve; *NADM*, nerve to abductor digiti minimi.) (Flanigan DC, Cassell M, Saltzman CL. Vascular supply of nerves in the tarsal tunnel. *Foot Ankle Int.* 1997;18[5]:288-292, Figure 1. Copyright ©1997. Reprinted by Permission of SAGE Publications.)

to the lateral plantar nerve came from the lateral plantar artery, with the most proximal of these nutrient arteries usually entering the corresponding plantar nerve at the distal border of the tarsal tunnel above the fascia of the abductor hallucis muscle (see Fig. 7.89).

The study of the microvasculature indicated that each nutrient artery bifurcated into a proximally and distally running longitudinal epineurial vessel that was associated with the lateral plantar fasciculus (Fig. 7.95). These longitudinal vessels usually anastomosed with other bifurcating nutrient vessels proximally and distally, forming an anastomotic arcade throughout the length of the nerve.

VEINS OF THE FOOT

The veins of the foot are divided into a dorsal and a plantar system. Contrary to the rest of the lower extremity, the flow in the foot is bidirectional, or when valves are present, the flow is from the depth of the planta to the superficial dorsal system.[52]

▶ Dorsal Veins of the Foot

There are two superficial venous networks and one deep venous network in the dorsum of the foot, separated by the superficial and the deep dorsal fasciae (Figs. 7.96 and 7.97).

Superficial Dorsal Venous Networks

The superficial dorsal veins and the greater and lesser saphenous veins with the dorsal venous arch constitute the superficial venous networks.

Superficial Dorsal Veins

The superficial dorsal veins are located immediately under the skin, superficial to the superficial dorsal aponeurosis of the foot.[53] They form a thin-meshed venous network with branches measuring up to 2 mm in diameter. The branches arise from the skin of the dorsum of the toes and from the superficial plantar veins. Other roots originate from the major dorsal venous arcade. The branches converge longitudinally to the anterior aspect of the ankle and join the saphenous venous system proximally. The superficial dorsal veins may take over the lesser saphenous vein when the latter does not reach the forefoot, or they may be connected to the deep venous system (dorsalis pedis or plantar) through a perforating vein.[52]

Greater and Lesser Saphenous Veins and the Dorsal Venous Arch

This superficial venous network starts with the dorsal veins of the toes, which represent the major drainage route of

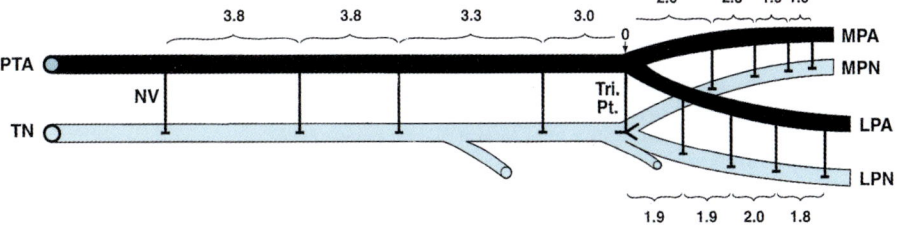

Figure 7.93 **Schematic diagram showing the mean distances between nutrient vessels starting from point zero.** The distances are greater in the tibial nerve as compared to its branches. (*LPA*, lateral plantar artery; *MPN*, medial plantar nerve; *NV*, nutrient vessel; *Tri. Pt*, trifurcation point.) (Adapted from Flanigan DC, Cassell M, Saltzman CL. Vascular supply of nerves in the tarsal tunnel. *Foot Ankle Int.* 1997;18[5]:288-292.)

TABLE 7.12 Positive Laminin Within the Gliding Zones of the Flexor Hallucis Longus Tendon, in Tendon Quarters 1 (Anterior), 2, 3, and 4 (Posterior)

Tendon Quarter	Posterior to Talus (n = 20)[a] (Segment 2)	Below First Metatarsal Head (n = 20)[a] (Segment 4)
1	0	0
2	0	0
3	7	14
4	20	20

[a]Total number of cases with a positive immunoreactivity within different quarters of the tendon diameter.
From Petersen W, Pufe T, Zantop T, Paulsen F. Blood supply of the flexor hallucis longus tendon with regards to dancer's tendinitis: injection and immunohistochemical studies of cadaver tendons. *Foot Ankle Int.* 2003;8:592, Table 2. Copyright ©2003. Reprinted by Permission of SAGE Publications.

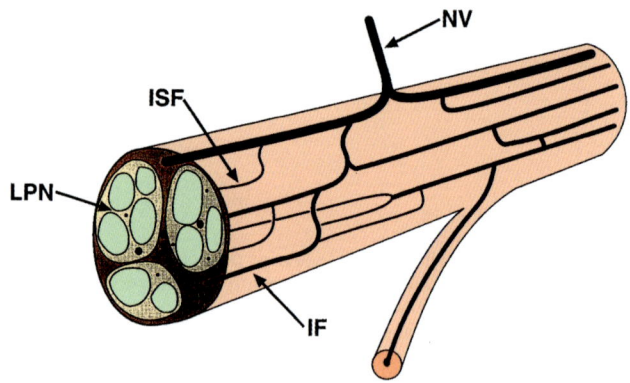

Figure 7.95 Schematic drawing illustrating the microvasculature of the posterior tibial nerve in the tarsal tunnel. (*IF*, interfascicular vessel; *ISF*, intrasubfascicular vessels; *LPN*, lateral plantar fasciculus; *NV*, nutrient vessel.) (Adapted from Flanigan DC, Cassell M, Saltzman CL. Vascular supply of nerves in the tarsal tunnel. *Foot Ankle Int.* 1997;18[5]:288-292.)

the toes. As described by Winckler, these veins are formed at the level of the distal and middle phalanges of the toe by a median vein draining the nail matrix and two collateral dorsal veins (Figs. 7.98 and 7.99).[53] The median vein bifurcates and joins the two dorsal veins in an "M"

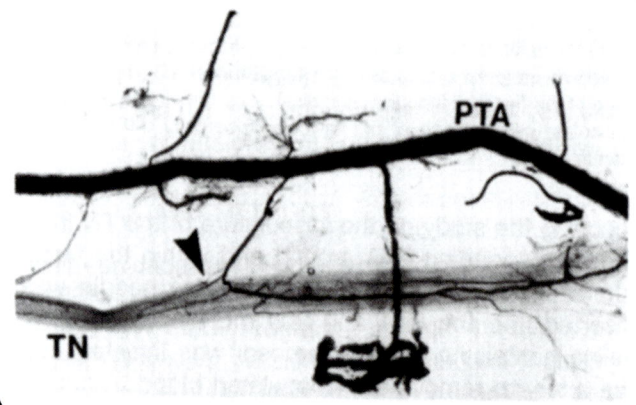

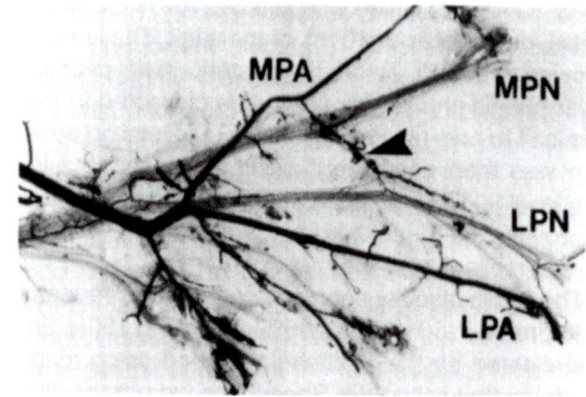

Figure 7.94 **(A) Tibial nerve specimen showing an asymmetrical splitting (*arrow*) of the nutrient vessel.** The larger branch from the split vessel supplied the distal aspect of the nerve consistently in all specimens with asymmetrical splitting. **(B) The nutrient vessel from the medial plantar artery supplying the lateral plantar nerve (*arrow*).** (*LPA*, lateral plantar artery; *LPN*, lateral plantar nerve; *MPA*, medial plantar artery; *MPN*, medial plantar nerve; *PTA*, posterior tibial artery; *TN*, posterior tibial nerve.) (Flanigan DC, Cassell M, Saltzman CL. Vascular supply of nerves in the tarsal tunnel. *Foot Ankle Int.* 1997;18[5]:288-292, Figure 4. Copyright ©1997. Reprinted by Permission of SAGE Publications.)

configuration. On the dorsum of the proximal phalanx, a transverse branch unites the two dorsal veins, and the network forms a vascular circle centered on the dorsum of the proximal interphalangeal joint. The adjacent dorsal veins of the toe unite in the web space and constitute the superficial dorsal metatarsal vein, which courses posteromedially to join the dorsal venous arch. Prior to the union in the web space, the medial dorsal digital vein receives the perforating interdigital vein that originates from the plantar superficial venous arch. The proximal end of the superficial dorsal metatarsal vein in turn is connected to the distal intermetatarsal perforating vein. The venous plexus on the plantar aspect of the pulp of the toe drains into two thin plantar digital veins, which end in either the interdigital vein or the plantar superficial venous arch.

The dorsomedial vein of the big toe and the dorsolateral vein of the fifth toe, after receiving the medial and lateral ends of the superficial plantar venous arch, join the dorsal venous arch on the medial and lateral sides, respectively, forming the greater saphenous vein on the anterior aspect of the medial malleolus and the lesser saphenous vein on the posterior aspect of the lateral malleolus. The dorsal venous arcade is convex anteriorly; it crosses the metatarsals at a variable level, 4 to 5 cm posterior to the web space, or may reach the level of the metatarsal heads.

On the dorsomedial aspect of the foot, the greater saphenous vein and the corresponding medial marginal vein of the dorsal venous arch receive the dorsal veins of the toes, plantar veins of the toes through the interdigital veins and the superficial plantar venous arch, superficial dorsal metatarsal veins, plantar metatarsal veins through the distal intermetatarsal perforating vein, and superficial plantar venous system through the superficial marginal connecting vein.

The greater saphenous vein and its root from the dorsal venous arch are also connected with the plantar system through perforating veins. These veins are mostly articular veins and course between the abductor hallucis and the tarsus. Winckler describes the following specific perforating veins

Chapter 7: Angiology 373

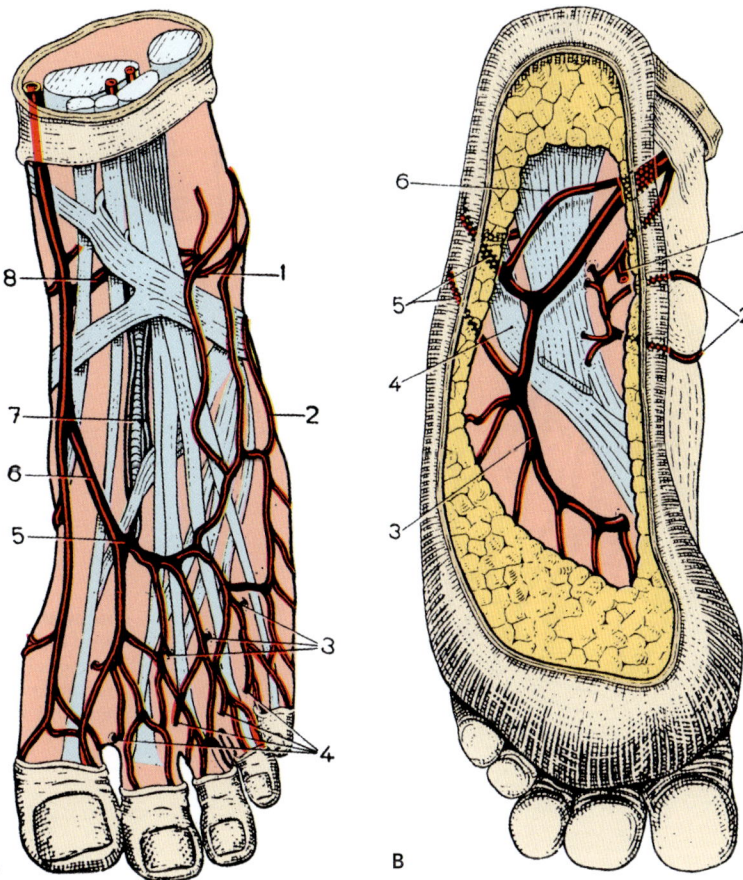

Figure 7.96 Dorsal and plantar veins of the foot. (A) Veins of the dorsal aspect of the foot. (*1*, anterolateral malleolar veins; *2*, lateral marginal vein; *3*, proximal interosseous perforating veins; *4*, distal perforating interdigital veins; *5*, communicating vein of first interosseous space; *6*, medial marginal vein; *7*, dorsalis pedis veins; *8*, anteromedial malleolar vein.) **(B)** Deep veins of the plantar aspect of the foot. (*1*, medial plantar vein; *2*, periscaphoid venous circle receiving articular veins; *3*, lateral plantar vein receiving plantar interosseous veins; *4*, peroneus longus tendon; *5*, peroneal communicating veins; *6*, calcaneocuboid ligament.) (Adapted from Winckler G. Les veines du pied. *Arch Anat Histol Embryol.* 1954-1955;37:175.)

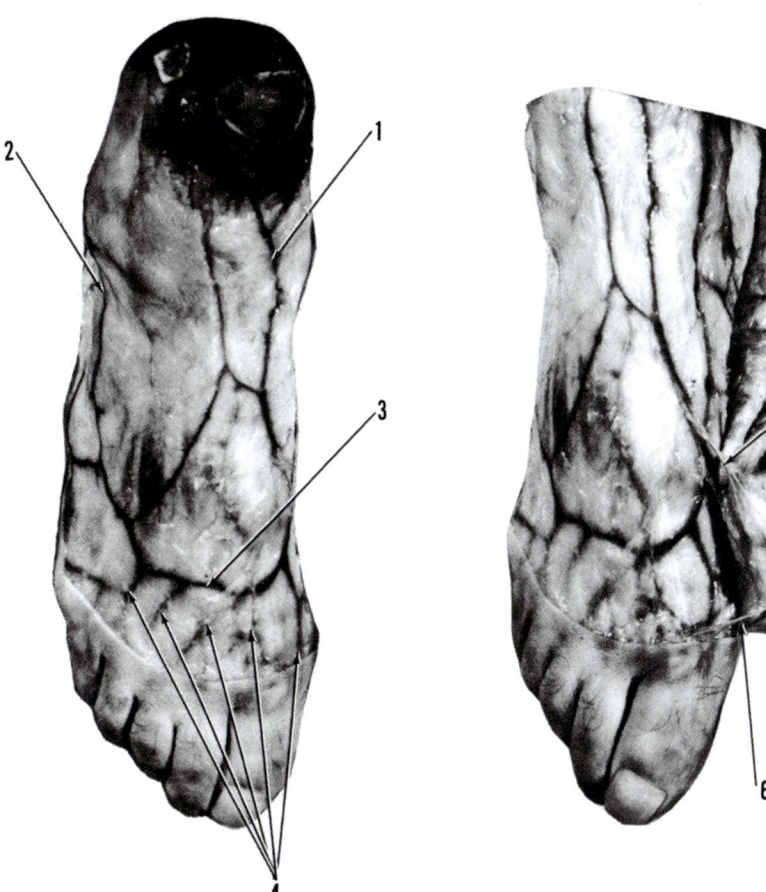

Figure 7.97 Veins of the dorsum of the foot. (*1*, greater saphenous vein; *2*, branch forming lesser saphenous veins; *3*, dorsal venous arc; *4*, dorsal superficial interosseous veins; *5*, *6*, superficial subcuticular venous branches.)

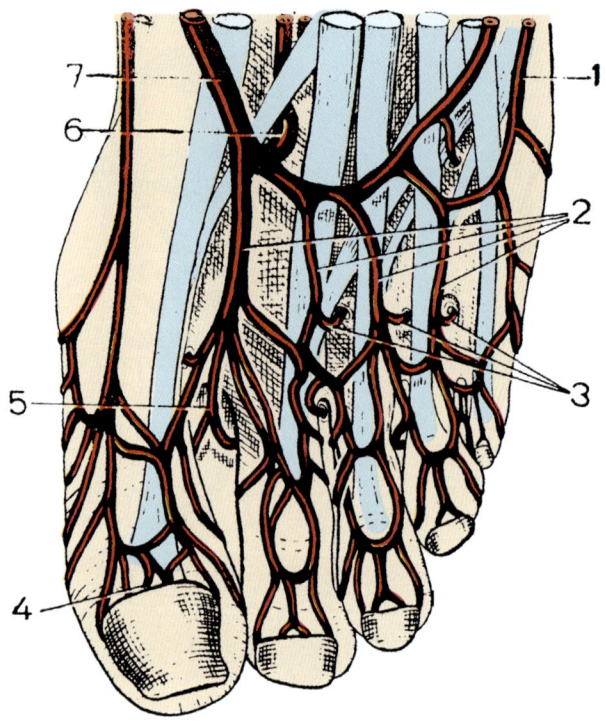

Figure 7.98 **Superficial venous system of the dorsal aspect of the web spaces and dorsal aspect of the toes.** (*1*, lateral marginal vein; *2*, superficial dorsal interosseous veins; *3*, perforating interosseous veins; *4*, ungual veins; *5*, interdigital vein of first web space; *6*, communicating vein of first interosseous interspace; *7*, medial marginal vein.) (Adapted from Winckler G. Les veines du pied. *Arch Anat Histol Embryol.* 1954-1955;37:175.)

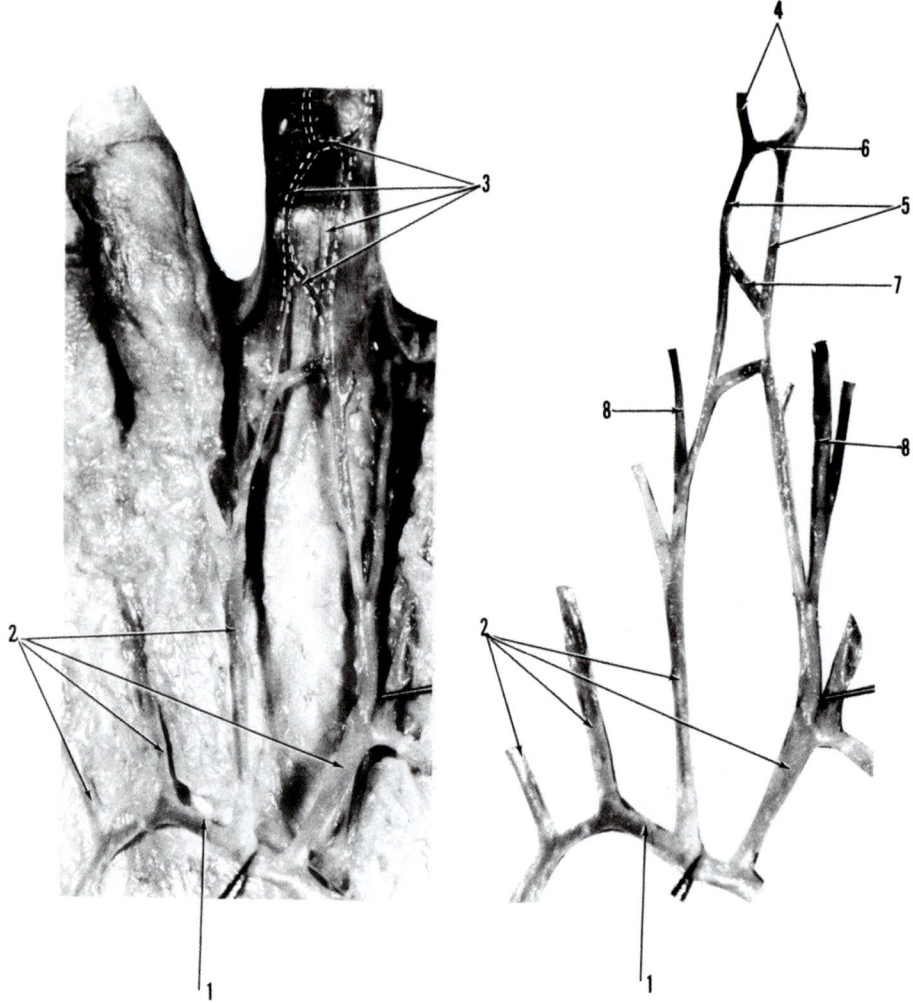

Figure 7.99 **Venous drainage system on the dorsum of the toe.** (*1*, dorsal venous arc; *2*, dorsal metatarsal [or interosseous] veins; *3*, venous circle centered on dorsum of proximal interphalangeal joint and formed by two dorsal collateral veins [*5*] anastomosed proximally [*7*] and distally [*6*] by transverse venous branches; dorsal ungual branches [*4*] continue with dorsal collateral veins; *8*, interdigital veins penetrating corresponding web space.)

draining into the greater saphenous vein or the medial marginal vein[53] (Figs. 7.100 and 7.101):

- A vein arising from the $cuneo_1$-$metatarsal_1$ joint level.
- Two periscaphoid veins arising from the scaphocuneiform and the calcaneocuboid joints. These veins form a periscaphoid venous circle.
- A vein uniting the medial plantar vein and the greater saphenous vein.
- A medial malleolar vein uniting the posterior tibial vein and the greater saphenous vein. This vein passes under the malleolus and receives superficial branches from the medial aspect of the heel and of the Achilles tendon.
- The communicating vein of the first interosseous space, a perforating vein connecting the dorsal venous arcade with the medial end of the deep plantar venous arch.

On the dorsal side, the greater saphenous vein and the dorsalis pedis or the anterior tibial veins are united by the anteromedial malleolar vein, which is located between the bifurcation arms of the inferior extensor retinaculum under the tendons of the extensor hallucis longus and the tibialis anterior.

On the dorsolateral aspect, the lateral marginal vein is of a smaller caliber and more variable than the corresponding medial marginal vein. It courses along the lateral border of the foot, crosses the peronei tendons, and passes behind the lateral malleolus, where it forms the lesser saphenous vein (see Fig. 7.100 and 7.102). It receives multiple (about 15) marginal, parallel veins arising from the superficial plantar venous system. These collaterals are distributed between the base of the fifth metatarsal and the heel. Two peroneal communicating veins, proximal and distal, are located on each side of the peroneus longus tendon as the latter makes its turn around the cuboid; these veins unite the lateral marginal vein with the lateral plantar veins. The distal communicating peroneal vein receives a branch that courses under the extensor digitorum brevis muscle and the tendon of the peroneus brevis and drains the dorsal calcaneocuboid joint. The proximal communicating peroneal vein receives a large vein from the plantar aspect of the calcaneocuboid joint.

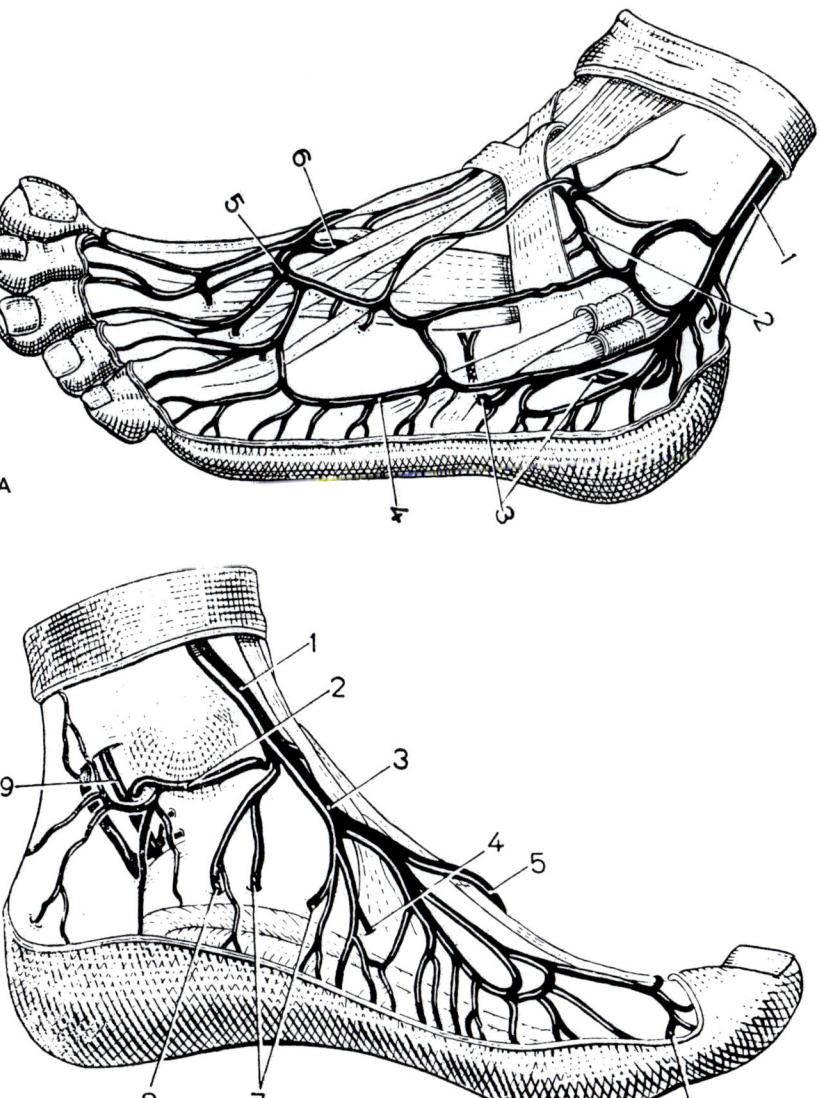

Figure 7.100 (A) Veins of the dorsolateral aspect of the foot. (1, lesser saphenous vein; 2, anterolateral malleolar vein; 3, communicating peroneal veins; 4, lateral marginal vein; 5, dorsal superficial venous arc; 6, communicating vein of first interosseous space.)
(B) Veins of the medial aspect of the foot. (1, major saphenous vein; 2, medial malleolar vein; 3, medial marginal vein; 4, articular vein arising from $cuneo_1$-$metatarsal_1$ joint; 5, superficial dorsal venous arc; 6, hallucal marginal communicating vein; 7, periscaphoid venous circle; 8, anastomosis between medial plantar vein and beginning of greater saphenous vein; 9, posterior tibial veins.) (Adapted from Winckler G. Les veines du pied. *Arch Anat Histol Embryol.* 1954-1955;37:175.)

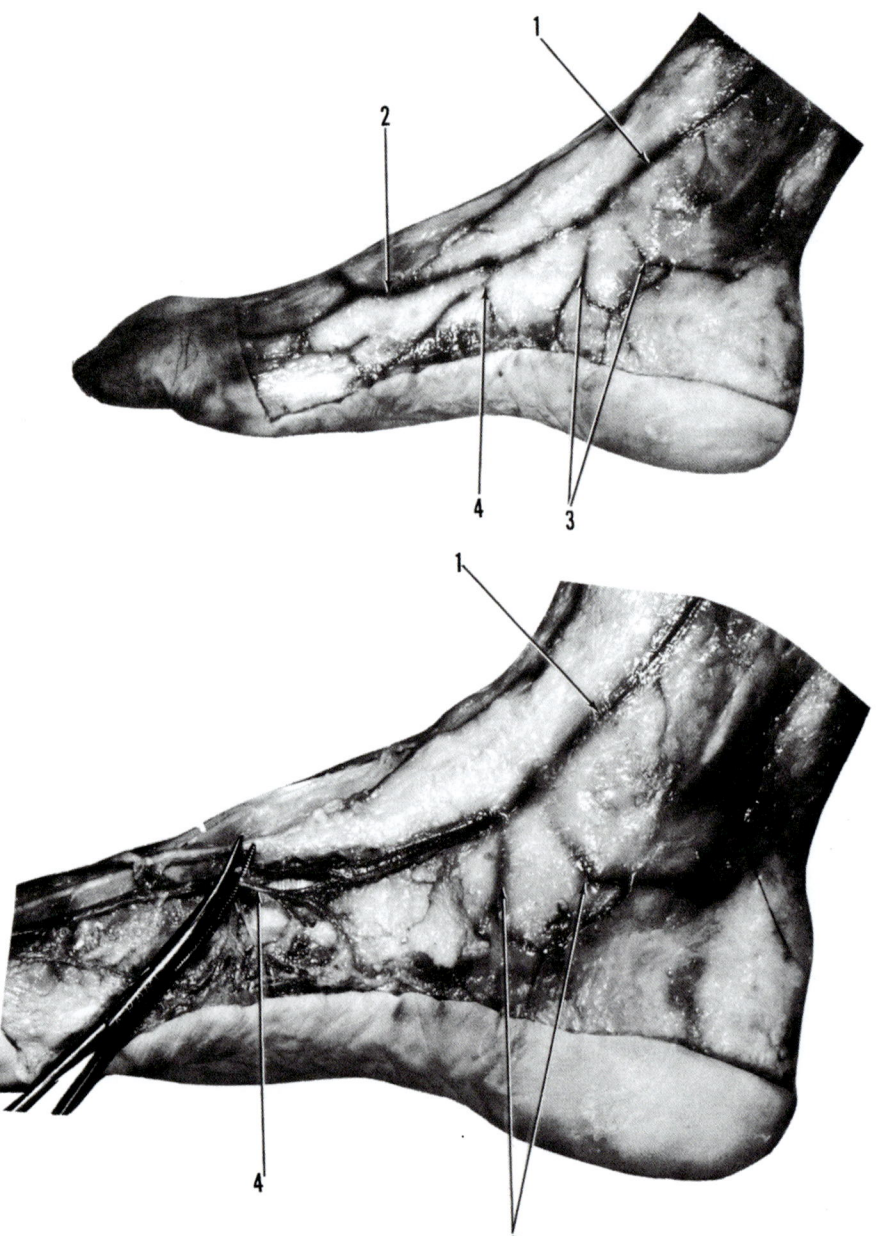

Figure 7.101 **Veins of the medial aspect of the foot.** (*1*, greater saphenous vein; *2*, superficial dorsal venous arc; *3*, periscaphoid venous circle; *4*, articular vein arising from cuneo$_1$-metatarsal$_1$ joint area.)

The medial aspect of the lateral marginal vein is connected to the dorsal venous system through an oblique venous network extending to the greater saphenous vein. These veins are variable in distribution. A set of anterolateral malleolar veins is almost constantly present, connecting the lesser saphenous vein and the anterior tibial vein and contributing to the formation of a lateral malleolar venous circle; they drain the ankle joint and the tibiofibular syndesmosis.

Kuster and coworkers, in a study of 10 feet, describe 6 to 12 perforating veins connecting the deep plantar venous systems with the dorsal venous system (Fig. 7.103).[52] In 53.8% of the 91 perforators, no valves were found; in 41.7%, one valve was present; in 4.3%, two valves were found. The valves, when present, face toward the superficial venous system, thus determining a plantar-to-dorsal venous flow. In the perforators with no valves and in the marginal superficial connecting veins uniting the superficial plantar venous system to the dorsal veins, the blood flow is bidirectional. The perforators have a diameter ranging from 0.9 to 1.8 mm.

Deep Dorsal Venous Network

The deep dorsal venous network is located under the deep fascia of the foot and consists of the veins accompanying the dorsalis pedis artery and its tributaries. There are two veins for one artery. This deep venous system communicates with the greater saphenous vein through the anteromedial malleolar vein, the lesser saphenous vein through the anterolateral malleolar vein, and the plantar metatarsal veins through the proximal and the distal perforating veins.

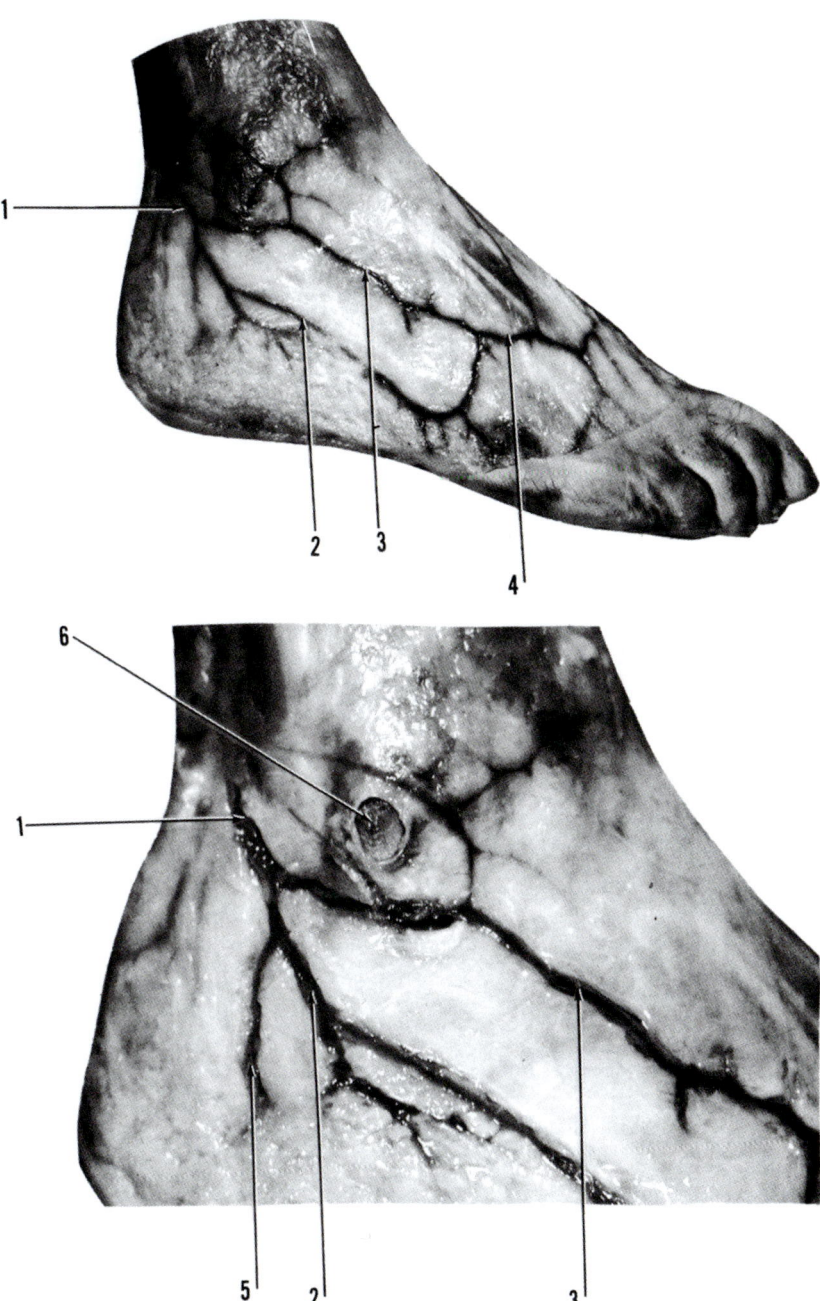

Figure 7.102 Veins of the lateral aspect of the foot. (*1*, lesser saphenous vein; *2*, lateral marginal vein; *3*, anastomotic branch between dorsal superficial venous arc [*4*] and *1*; *5*, lateral calcaneal vein; *6*, bursa of lateral malleolus.)

▶ Plantar Veins of the Foot

The plantar venous network is formed by a superficial and deep plantar system (see Fig. 7.96).

Superficial Plantar Venous Network

The superficial plantar venous network is formed by an extremely superficial, intradermal, and subdermal mesh (very thin) covering the sole of the foot; forming at the foot borders, the medial and lateral marginal veins end in the dorsal venous system, as described previously. These veins are valveless. The superficial midplantar region drains in a superficial venous arcade at the base of the toes. The medial and lateral ends of the venous arcade end dorsally by joining, respectively, the corresponding dorsal medial and lateral marginal veins of the first and fifth toes. The interdigital perforating veins originate from the superficial venous arcade, pass through the web space, and unite with the dorsal vein of the toe.

Deep Plantar Venous Network

The deep veins of the planta are represented by the veins accompanying the medial and lateral plantar arteries. The larger lateral plantar vein, single or double at the origin, forms distally the deep plantar venous arch.[53] It receives two communicating peroneal veins, the first proximal perforating interosseous or intermetatarsal vein, and the plantar metatarsal veins that connect with the dorsal metatarsal veins

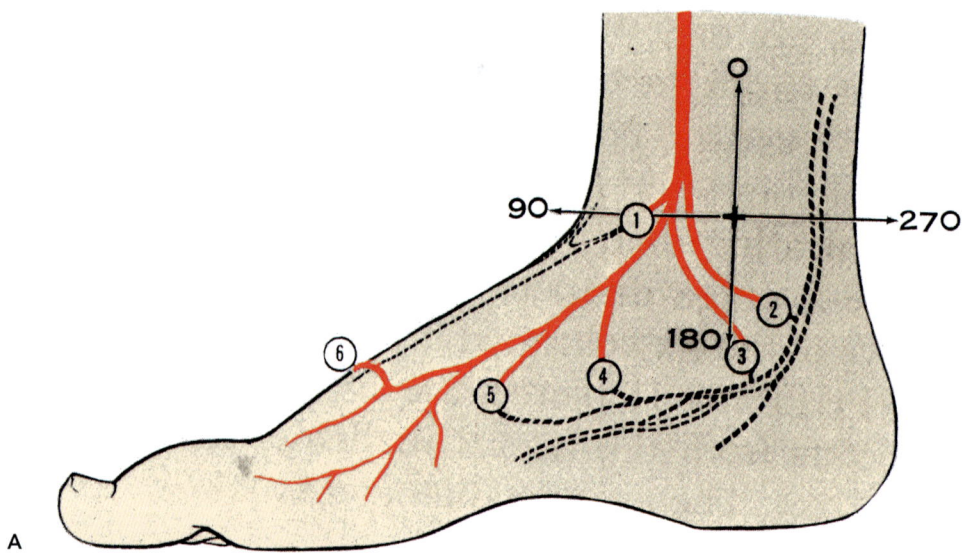

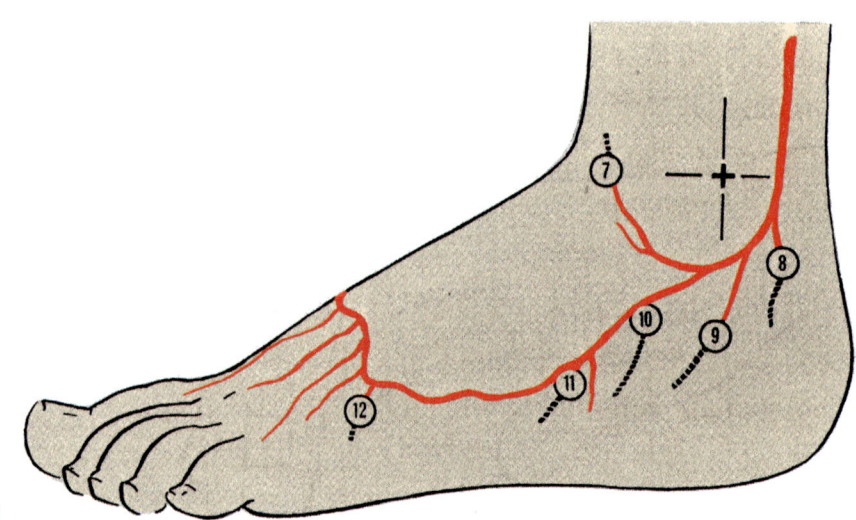

Figure 7.103 (A) Perforating veins that connect the deep veins with the greater saphenous vein. The circled numbers indicate the places at which the perforators pierce the fascia. Perforator 1 pierces the fascia 2.6 cm from the tip of the medial malleolus at 90°. It connects the greater saphenous vein with the dorsalis pedis vein and runs under the tendons of the extensor hallucis longus and tibialis anterior. Perforator 2 is inconstant. It appears 2.8 cm from the medial malleolus at 200° and communicates with the medial plantar veins. Perforator 3 pierces the fascia 3.4 cm from the medial malleolus at 180° and opens in the greater saphenous vein. It communicates with the deep plantar venous arch. Perforator 4 pierces the fascia 5.33 cm from the malleolus at 136°. Perforator 5 pierces the fascia 7.64 cm from the malleolus at 125°. Perforators 4 and 5 communicate with the medial plantar veins. Perforator 6 connects the dorsalis pedis vein with the dorsal venous arch and pierces the fascia between the first and second metatarsal bones at about 11 cm from the medial malleolus. **(B) Perforating veins that connect the deep veins with the lesser saphenous vein.** Perforator 7 perforates the fascia 2.64 cm from the lateral malleolus at 90°. It originates from the dorsalis pedis vein, passes deep to the extensor digitorum longus tendons, and connects with the lesser saphenous vein behind the lateral malleolus. Perforator 8 is inconstant. It pierces the fascia 2.8 cm from the tip of the lateral malleolus at 232°. Perforator 9 pierces the fascia 4.41 cm from the lateral malleolus at 180° and opens in the lesser saphenous vein. Perforator 10 pierces the fascia 3.42 cm from the lateral malleolus at 146°. Perforator 11 pierces the fascia at 6.1 cm from the lateral malleolus at 138.5° just behind the tuberosity of the fifth metatarsal. Perforator 12 is uncommon. It pierces the fascia 9.2 cm from the lateral malleolus at 116°. The cross-marks indicate the tips of the lateral and medial malleoli. (Adapted from Kuster G, Lofgren EP, Hollinshead WH. Anatomy of the veins of the foot. *Surg Gynecol Obstet.* 1968;127:817.)

through the proximal and distal perforating (interosseous) veins. The medial plantar vein is thinner and communicates on the medial margin of the foot with the periscaphoid veins and distally with the first perforating interosseous (intermetatarsal) vein.

▶ Direction of the Blood Flow in the Foot

In the leg and the thigh, the perforating veins have valves directing the flow from the superficial to the deep veins. "Because of the absence of valves in most of the perforating veins of the foot, the blood may indifferently pass from the foot to the leg through any deep or superficial vein and the saphenous system may be considered as an accessory drainage of the deep veins of the foot."[52] When valves are present in the perforating veins, they face the superficial veins.[52] Jacobson, in a venographic investigation, established that "part of the venous blood originating from the bones and muscles of the foot is drained by way of superficial veins. Thus, the supposition of Kuster about the function of superficial veins as an accessory drainage system for the deep veins of the feet is confirmed."[54] Askar and Aly further assessed the communicating venous system in the foot in 16 cadaveric feet using dissection and polyethylene casting.[55] Their findings indicated that on the dorsum of the foot, the digital, metatarsal, and communicating veins are equipped with valves that allow a venous flow only proximally toward the dorsal venous arch. Proximal to the dorsal arch, the venous blood may flow in a cephalad or in a plantar direction. The cephalad flow is along the saphenous veins and the venous plexus on the dorsum of the foot, which is continuous with the leg veins in front of the ankle. The plantar flow is through the distal saphenoplantar communicators to the deep plantar arch and then proximally through the posterior tibial veins. The deep dorsal veins may drain into the dorsalis pedis and tibialis anterior veins, the deep plantar arch through free valveless connections, or the subcutaneous veins through short dorsal communicators.

In the sole of the foot, the subcutaneous plantar venous network drains into the deep plantar arch via the plantar communicators and into the dorsal subcutaneous veins through the corresponding marginal veins. In the standing position, with the pressure exerted on the deep plantar veins, the tension in the plantar aponeurosis—impeding the circulation in the plantar communicators—favors the venous drainage through the marginal veins into the subcutaneous veins on the dorsum of the foot.

LYMPHATICS

The lymphatics of the foot are divided into superficial and deep channels.

▶ Superficial Lymphatics of the Foot

The superficial lymphatic vessels originate mainly from the skin of the toes, the skin of the sole of the foot, and the skin of the heel (Figs. 7.104 and 7.105).[56] The remaining segments of the skin of the foot contribute to the lymphatic channels through only very minuscule vessels.

Lymphatics of the Toes

The lymphatics of the toes form a true plexus and envelop the toes completely. The lymphatic network is less developed on the dorsum of the toe and better defined on the lateral, medial, and plantar aspects. Lymphatic rootlets converge on the sides of the toe and form dorsal and plantar digital channels that may be converted into two main lateral and medial lymphatic channels coursing parallel and dorsal to the digital arteries. At the level of the metatarsophalangeal joints, the lymphatic trunks of two adjacent toes may unite, or the four individual digital channels may form one common channel, which will then bifurcate and unite with the neighboring vessels. These multiple anastomoses result in a large lymphatic plexus covering the dorsum of the foot. At the level of the interdigital space, the lymphatic plexus is enriched by three to four lymphatic branches arising from the plantar aspect of the foot.[57] On the dorsum of the foot, Poirier and Charpy divide the superficial lymphatics into two collecting systems—medial and lateral.[57]

Medial System

The medial system is formed by the lymphatics of the big toe and the second toe and the skin of the inner third of the dorsum of the foot. This system is augmented by lymphatic branches arising from the sole of the foot. These medial marginal plantar branches, initially a total of 14 to 15, are reduced to 4 to 5 branches as they reach the dorsum of the foot. All the collectors converge and form longitudinal lymphatic channels coursing along the greater saphenous vein. They terminate in the inguinal nodes.

Lateral System

The lateral system is formed by the lymphatics of the third, fourth, and fifth toes of the lateral two thirds of the dorsal skin of the foot and of the anterior half of the lateral foot margin. The collectors are oriented posteromedially and join the channels along the greater saphenous vein. The superficial lymphatics of the posterior half of the lateral border of the foot and of the corresponding segment of the heel form two to three channels, pass behind the lateral malleolus, and course along the lesser saphenous vein. They terminate in the most superficial popliteal node.

Lymphatics of the Sole

As described by Sappey, the superficial lymphatics of the sole are divided into anterior, medial, and lateral groups[56]:

- The anterior group is formed by branches coursing toward the dorsum of the foot through the web space. There are two or three branches per web space.

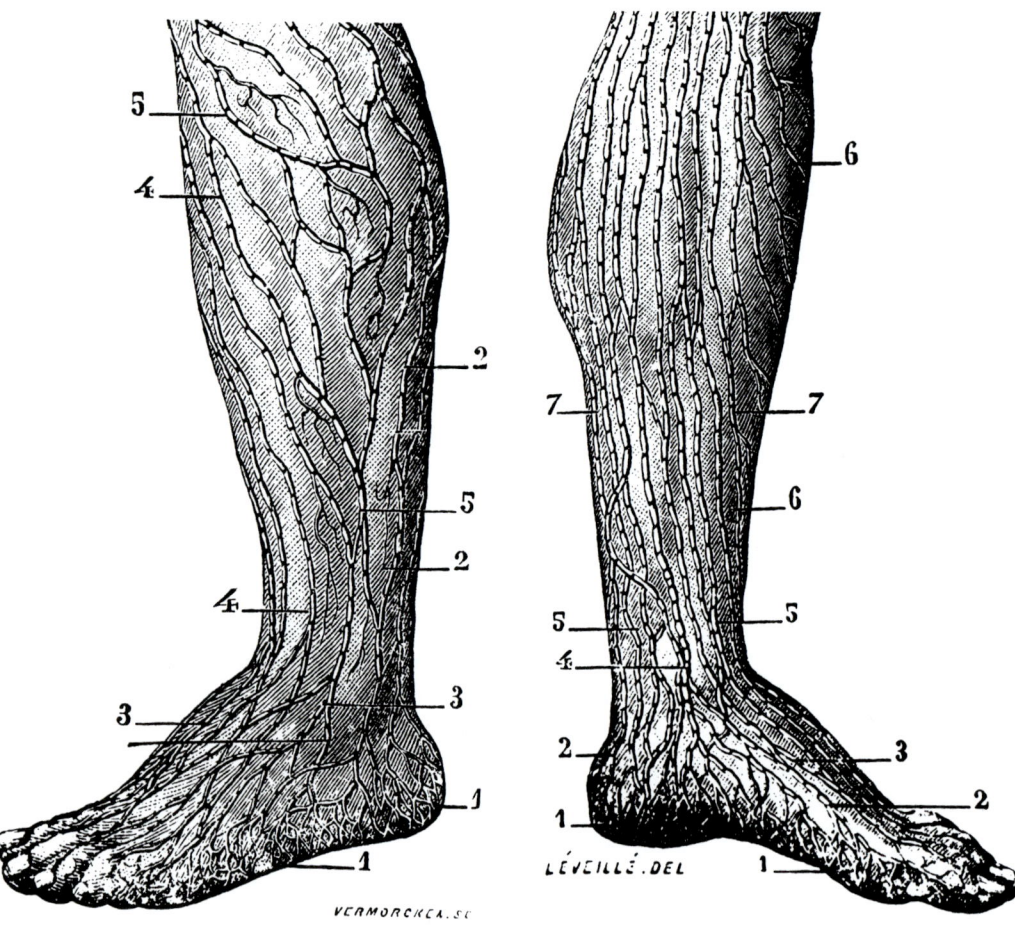

Figure 7.104 **Superficial lymphatics of the foot and leg.** **(A)** Lateral aspect. (*1*, lymphatic network of lateral borders of foot; *2*, lymphatic channels draining lateral border of foot and terminating in popliteal lymph nodes; *3*, lymphatic vessels of dorsum of foot draining toes and anterior segment of plantar region; *4*, lymphatic vessels crossing tibial crest.) **(B)** Medial aspect. (*1*, lymphatic network of inner aspect of sole of foot; *2*, lymphatic vessels that run from *1*; *3*, other lymphatic trunks of dorsal surface of foot; *4*, large lymphatic trunk passing in front of medial malleolus; *5*, lymphatic vessels located anterior and posterior to *4*; *6*, lymphatic vessels arising from lateral surface of leg; *7*, lymphatic vessels located on medial aspect of leg.) (From Sappey PC. *Traité d'Anatomie Descriptive*. Vol. 2: Angiologie. Lecrosnier; 1888:791.)

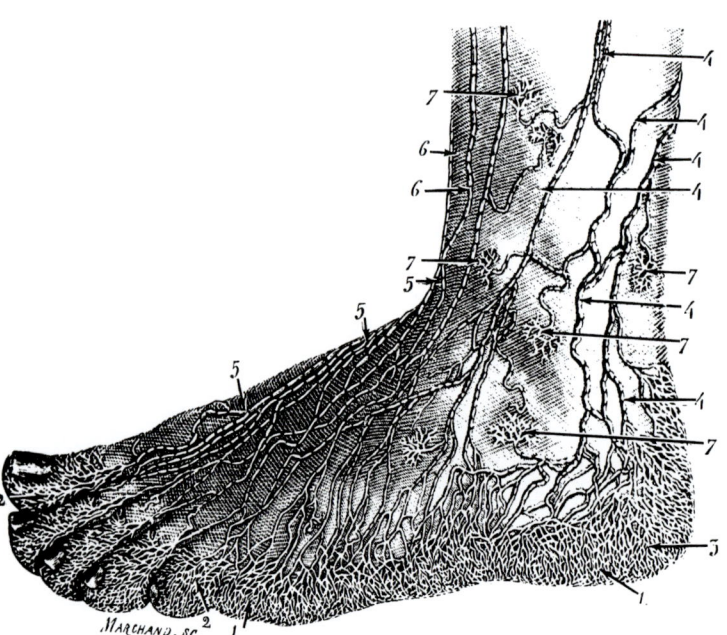

Figure 7.105 **Superficial lymphatics of the foot.** (*1*, lymphatic network of lateral border of foot; *2*, lymphatic network of toe; *3*, lymphatic network of skin of heel; *4*, lymphatic vessels that accompany lateral saphenous vein and terminate in popliteal lymph nodes; *5*, lymphatic trunks on dorsal surface of foot; *6*, lymphatic trunks that run from lateral to medial aspect of leg; *7*, lymphatic networks from which a single lymphatic vessel originates and connects with neighboring trunks.) (From Sappey PC. *Traité d'Anatomie Descriptive*. Vol. 2: Angiologie. Lecrosnier; 1888:789.)

- The medial group is formed by three or four lymphatic branches. Of these, three cross the medial border of the foot obliquely to reach the dorsal system and are located anterior to the medial malleolus; the fourth branch is posterior to the medial malleolus.
- The lateral group is formed by two to four vessels. Of these, one passes behind the lateral malleolus and the others pass in front to reach the dorsal system.

▶ **Deep Lymphatics of the Foot**

The deep lymphatics are satellites of the arterial trunks and are divided into three groups: dorsalis pedis and anterior tibial lymphatics, plantar and posterior tibial lymphatics, and peroneal lymphatics.

The dorsalis pedis and anterior tibial lymphatics originate in the planta pedis from the deep muscles. The lymphatic channels unite into one or two trunks, pass to the dorsum of the foot, and course along the dorsalis pedis and the tibialis anterior arteries. They also collect the deep lymphatics from the dorsum of the foot and terminate in the popliteal nodes.

The plantar and posterior tibial lymphatics originate in the sole and follow the plantar arteries and the posterior tibial artery. There are three or four collecting trunks around the latter: the trunks terminate in the popliteal nodes.[57]

The peroneal lymphatics have two collecting trunks accompanying the peroneal artery; they also terminate in the popliteal nodes.

▶ **Lymphatics of the Joints**

The lymphatics of the interphalangeal joints drain into the collecting channels of the dorsum of the foot.[58]

Lymphatics of the metatarsophalangeal joints are divided into plantar and dorsal lymphatics.[58] The lymphatic channels drain into the plantar metatarsal channels coursing along the plantar metatarsal arteries. The plantar lymphatics of the metatarsophalangeal joint of the big toe reach the dorsum of the foot and unite with the superficial saphenous system or the deep system accompanying the dorsalis pedis artery. The dorsal lymphatics empty into the superficial lymphatics of the dorsum of the foot and occasionally into the deep dorsal collecting channels.

The lymphatics of the ankle are divided into superficial and deep channels.[58] The superficial lymphatics are anterior and posterior; they course along the saphenous veins and reach the inguinal and the popliteal nodes. The deep lymphatics are divided into three groups: anterior, posteromedial, and posterolateral.

The deep anterior lymphatics start on the anteromedial and anterolateral aspects of the articular capsule and their corresponding ligaments. Their lymphatic channels are directed transversely toward the anterior tibial artery, where they join the longitudinal lymphatic channels along the artery. The deep posteromedial lymphatics emerge from the deltoid ligament and the posteromedial articular capsule and drain into the posterior tibial lymphatic channel. The deep posterolateral lymphatics originate from the posterolateral capsule and ligaments and merge with the peroneal lymphatic channels.

REFERENCES

1. Dubreuil-Chambardel L. *Variations des Artères du Pelvis et du Membre Inférieur*. Masson et Cie; 1925:191-271.
2. Adachi B. *Das Arteriensystem der Japaner*. Maruzen; 1928:215-291.
3. Edwards EA. Anatomy of the small arteries of the foot and toes. *Acta Anat*. 1960;40:81.
4. Huber JF. The arterial network supplying the dorsum of the foot. *Anat Rec*. 1941;80:373.
5. Gilbert A. Composite tissue transfers from the foot: anatomic basis and surgical technique. In: Daniller AI, Strauch B, eds. *Symposium on Microsurgery 14*. CV Mosby, 1976:230-241.
6. Man D, Acland RD. The microarterial anatomy of the dorsalis pedis flap and its clinical applications. *Plast Reconstr Surg*. 1980;65(4):419.
7. Mulfinger GL, Trueta J. The blood supply of the talus. *J Bone Joint Surg Br*. 1970;52(1):160.
8. Gilbert BJ, Horst F, Nunley JA. Potential donor rotational bone grafts using vascular territories in the foot and ankle. *J Bone Joint Surg*. 2004;86(9):1857-1874.
9. Poirier P, Charpy A. *Traité d'Anatomie Humaine. Vol 2: Angiologie*. Masson; 1902:839-847.
10. Levame JH. Les artères des orteils. Etude anatomique et artériographique: conclusions chirurgicales. *J Chir*. 1963;86(6):651.
11. May JW Jr, Chait LA, Cohen BE, et al. Free neurovascular flap from the first web of the foot in hand reconstruction. *J Hand Surg*. 1977;2(5):387.
12. Murakami T. On the position and course of the deep plantar arteries, with special reference to the so-called plantar metatarsal arteries. *Okajimas Folia Anat Jpn*. 1971;48:295.
13. Leung PC, Wong WL, Kok LC. The vessels of the first metatarsal web space. An operative and radiographic study. *J Bone Joint Surg Am*. 1983;65(2):235.
14. Manno A. Arteriae plantares pedis mammalium. *Int Monatsschr Anat Physiol*. 1905;22:293-359.
15. Wildenauer E. Die blutvesorgung des talus. *Z Anat Entwicklungsgeschichte*. 1950;115:32.
16. Aschner B. Zur Anatomie der Arterien der Fussohle. *Anat Hefte Beit Ref Anat Entwicklungs*. 1905;27:345.
17. Vann MH. A note on the formation of the plantar arterial arch of the human foot. *Anat Rec*. 1943;85:269.
18. Pyka RA, Coventry MB. Avascular necrosis of the skin after operations on the foot. *J Bone Joint Surg Am*. 1961;43:955.
19. Hidalgo DA, Shaw WW. Anatomic basis of plantar flap design. *Plast Reconstr Surg*. 1985;78[5]:627.
20. Kaplan IV, McCraw JB. *Plastic Surgery of the Foot and Ankle in Disorders of the Foot and Ankle*. 2nd ed. WB Saunders; 1991:1605.
21. Mathes SJ, Nahai F. *Clinical Atlas of Muscle and Musculocutaneous Flaps*. CV Mosby; 1979:263-307.
22. Crock HV. *The Blood Supply of the Lower Limb Bones in Man: Descriptive and Applied*. Livingstone; 1967:72-87.
23. Haliburton RA, Sullivan CR, Kelly PJ, et al. The extraosseous and intraosseous blood supply of the talus. *J Bone Joint Surg Am*. 1958;40(5):1115.
24. Zchakaja MJ. Blutversorgung der Knochen des Fusses (ossa pedis). *Fortschr Gebiete Röntgenol*. 1932;45:160.
25. Gelberman RH, Mortensen WW. The arterial anatomy of the talus. *Foot Ankle*. 1983;4(2):64.
26. Andermahr J, Hilling H-J, Rehm KE, et al. The vascularization of the os calcaneum and the clinical consequences. *Clin Orthop Relat Res*. 1999;363:212-218.
27. Quain R. *Anatomy of the Arteries of the Human Body*. Taylor and Walton; 1844.
28. Velluda C. Sur la vascularisation du scaphoid du tarse. *Ann Anat Pathol*. 1928;5:1016.
29. Waugh W. The ossification and vascularisation of the tarsal navicular and their relation to Köhler's Disease. *J Bone Joint Surg Br*. 1958;40(4):765.
30. Shereff MJ, Quing M, Kummer FJ, et al. Vascular anatomy of the fifth metatarsal. *Foot Ankle*. 1991;11(6):350.

31. Leemrijse T, Valti B, Oberlin C. Vascularization of the heads of the three central metatarsals: an anatomical study, its application and considerations with respect to horizontal osteotomies at the neck of the metatarsals. *Foot Ankle Surg.* 1998;4:57-62.
32. Petersen WJ, Lankes JM, Paulsen F, et al. The arterial supply of the lesser metatarsal heads: a vascular injection study in human cadaver. *Foot Ankle Int.* 2002;6:491-495.
33. Shereff M, Yang QM, Kummer FJ. Extraosseous and intraosseous arterial supply to the first metatarsal and metatarsophalangeal joint. *Foot Ankle.* 1987;8(2):81.
34. Singh I. Variations in the metatarsal bones. *J Anat.* 1960;94:345.
35. Jones KJ, Feiwell LA, Freedman EL, et al. The effect of chevron osteotomy with lateral capsular release on the blood supply of to the first metatarsal head. *J Bone Joint Surg Am.* 1995;77:197-204.
36. Malal JJ, Shaw-Dunn J, Kumar CS. Blood supply to the first metatarsal head and vessels at risk with chevron osteotomy. *J Bone Joint Surg Am.* 2007;89(9):2018-2021.
37. Vega M, Resnick D, Black JD, et al. The intrinsic and extrinsic arterial supply to the proximal phalanx of the hallux. *Foot Ankle.* 1985;5(5):257.
38. Sobel M, Hashimoto J, Arnoczky SP, et al. The microvasculature of the sesamoid complex: its clinical significance. *Foot Ankle.* 1992;13(16):359.
39. Chamberland PDC, Smith JW, Fleming L. The blood supply of the great toe sesamoids. *Foot Ankle.* 1993;14(8):435-442.
40. Lagergren C, Lindholm A. Vascular distribution in the Achilles tendon: an angiographic and macroangiographic study. *Acta Chir Scand.* 1958-1959;116:491-495.
41. Carr AJ, Norris SH. The blood supply of the calcaneal tendon. *J Bone Joint Surg Br.* 1989;71-B:100-101.
42. Stein V, Laprell H, Tinnemeyer S, et al. Quantitative assessment of intravascular volume of the human Achilles tendon. *Acta Orthop Scand.* 2000;71(1):60-63.
43. Frey C, Shereff M, Greenidje N. Vascularity of the posterior tibial tendon. *J Bone Joint Surg Am.* 1990;72:884-888.
44. Salvi G. Sull' arteria dorsale pedis. Atti della Societa Toscana di Scienze Naturalli, *Process Verbali.* 1898;12.
45. Petersen W, Hohmann G, Stein V, et al. The blood supply of the posterior tibial tendon. *J Bone Joint Surg Br.* 2002;84B:141-144.
46. Petersen W, Pufe T, Zantop T, et al. Blood supply of the flexor hallucis longus tendon with regards to dancer's tendinitis: injection and immunohistochemical studies of cadaver tendons. *Foot Ankle Int.* 2003;8:591-596.
47. Geppert MJ, Sobe M, Hannafin JA. Microvasculature of the tibialis anterior tendon. *Foot Ankle.* 1993;14(5):261-264.
48. Petersen W, Stein V, Tillman B. Blood supply of the tibialis anterior tendon. *Arch Orthop Trauma Surg.* 1999;119:371-375.
49. Sobel M, Geppert MJ, Hannafin JA, et al. Bohne microvascular anatomy of peroneal tendons. *Foot Ankle.* 1992;13(8):469-472.
50. Petersen W, Bobka T, Stein V, et al. Blood supply of peroneal tendons. Injection and immunohistochemical studies of cadaver tendons. *Acta Orthop Scand.* 2000;71(2):168-174.
51. Flannigan DC, Cassel M, Saltzman CL. Vascular supply of nerves in the tarsal tunnel. *Foot Ankle Int.* 1997;18(5):288-292.
52. Kuster G, Lofgren EP, Hollinshead WH. Anatomy of the veins of the foot. *Surg Gynecol Obstet.* 1968;127:817.
53. Winckler G. Les veines du pied. *Arch Anat Histol Embryol.* 1954-1955;37:175.
54. Jacobson BH. The venous drainage of the foot. *Surg Gynecol Obstet.* 1970;131:22.
55. Askar O, Aly SA. The veins of the foot: surgical anatomy and its relation to disorders of the venous return from the foot. *J Cardiovasc Surg.* 1975;16:53.
56. Sappey PC. *Traité d'Anatomie Descriptive. Vol 2: Angiologie.* Lecrosnier; 1888:790-795.
57. Poirier P, Charpy A. *Traité d'Anatomie Humaine: The Lymphatics.* Masson; 1902:1158-1170.
58. Rouvière H. *Anatomy of the Human Lymphatic System: A Compendium.* Edwards; 1938.

Nerves

Shahan K. Sarrafian, Armen S. Kelikian

The nerve supply to the foot and ankle is provided by the branches of the sciatic nerve. The saphenous nerve, a branch of the femoral nerve, gives limited contribution. The branches of the sciatic nerve innervating the foot and ankle are the sural nerve, the superficial peroneal nerve, the accessory deep peroneal nerve, the deep peroneal nerve, and the posterior tibial nerve with its medial and lateral plantar nerves.

SURAL NERVE

The sural nerve is formed by the union of the medial sural nerve—a branch of the tibial nerve—and the anastomotic peroneal communicating nerve arising from the lateral sural nerve or the common peroneal nerve (Figs. 8.1 to 8.3).

When the anastomotic branch is absent, the medial sural nerve usually predominates and covers the territory of the sural nerve. Occasionally the lateral sural nerve or the peroneal communicating nerve takes over the same territory of innervation. The frequency of occurrence of such variations is as indicated in Table 8.1.

The medial sural nerve (median sural nerve, external saphenous nerve, tibial saphenous nerve) arises from the tibial nerve in the popliteal space. It courses between the two heads of the gastrocnemius muscle covered by the deep aponeurosis. It pierces the latter in the middle of the leg, receives the anastomotic peroneal communicating nerve, and forms the sural nerve. The sural nerve courses along the lateral border of the Achilles tendon and is anterolateral to the short saphenous veins. It turns around the posterior border of the lateral malleolus and passes 1 to 1.5 cm from the tip of the lateral malleolus, from which it is separated by the tendons of the peronei and their sheaths (Figs. 8.4 and 8.5). At the level of the tuberosity of the fifth metatarsal, the nerve divides into two terminal branches, lateral and medial (Fig. 8.6). The lateral branch is a direct continuation of the main nerve and terminates as the dorsolateral cutaneous nerve of the fifth toe. The larger medial branch obliquely crosses the dorsolateral aspect of the foot; it passes over the tendon of the long extensor of the fifth toe and divides over the anterior aspect of the fourth interosseous space into the dorsomedial cutaneous nerve of the fifth toe and the dorsolateral cutaneous nerve of the fourth toe.

The sural nerve provides the lateral calcaneal branches (Fig. 8.7). One such branch originates 5 cm above the lateral malleolus and another 1.3 cm above and behind the tip of the lateral malleolus in 98% of the cases.[1] The sural nerve also supplies the lateral malleolar branch and an anastomotic branch that crosses the dorsum of the foot obliquely, passes under the dorsolateral vein, and unites with the lateral branch of the superficial peroneal nerve. Articular branches are provided by the sural nerve to the inferior tibiofibular joint, the ankle joint, and the talocalcaneal joint.

The anastomosis between the medial sural nerve and the peroneal communicating branch usually takes place at mid leg but may occur as low as in the lower quarter of the leg or as high as above the level of the knee joint.[2]

A very common location of the sural nerve is at "10 cm above the tip of the lateral malleolus just at the lateral border of the Achilles tendon."[1] The diameter of the sural nerve is 2 mm average (1.25-2.75 mm), according to Kosinski, or 3 mm average according to Horwitz.[1,2]

Ortigüela et al[3] investigated the anatomy of the sural nerve complex based on the dissection of 20 cadaveric limbs. All limbs had a medial sural cutaneous nerve and a sural nerve. A lateral sural cutaneous nerve was present in 19 of 20 limbs and, in 16 of 20 limbs, a peroneal communicating branch from the lateral sural cutaneous contributed to the sural nerve (Fig. 8.8).

The sural nerve was present in all specimens. In 80% of the specimens, it was formed by the union of the medial sural cutaneous nerve with the peroneal communicating branch at a point 11 to 20 cm proximal to the lateral malleolus (Fig. 8.8).[3] In the remaining 20%, the sural nerve was simply the continuation of the medial sural cutaneous nerve (Fig. 8.9).[3] The sural nerve coursed distally and laterally near the lesser saphenous nerve to pass 1.0 to 1.5 cm to the lateral malleolus. Two to 3 cm distal to the lateral malleolus, the nerve

384 Sarrafian's Anatomy of the Foot and Ankle

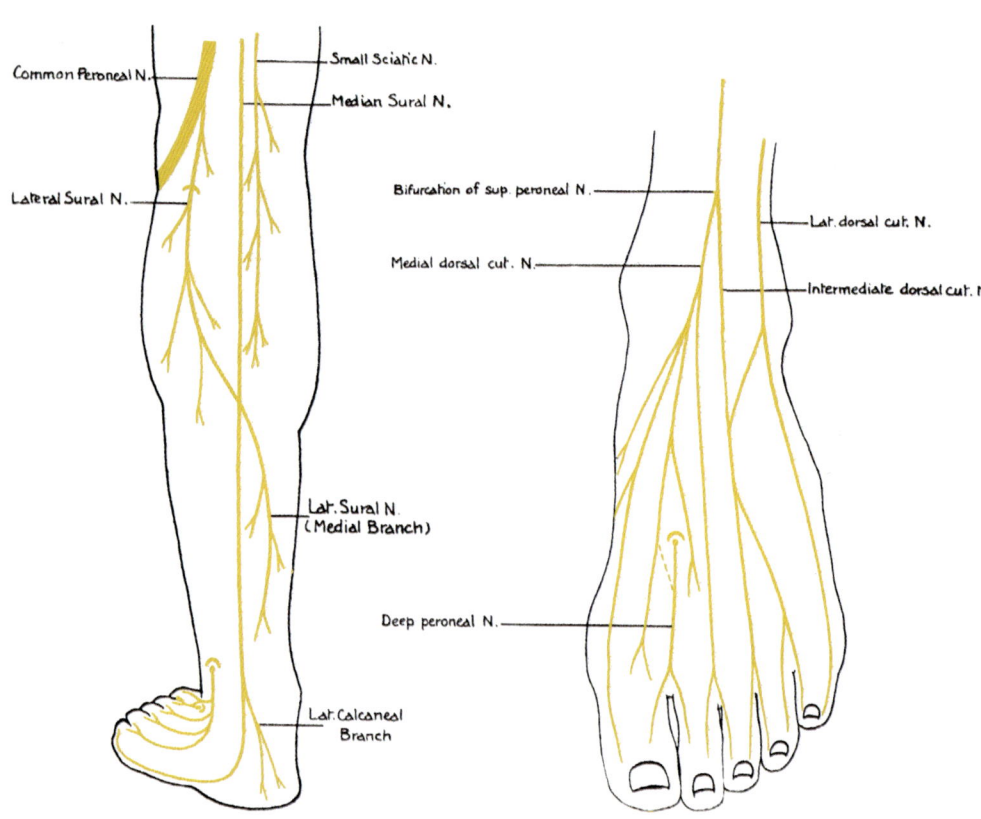

Figure 8.1 Sural nerve type A (53%) formed by the medial sural nerve only. The lateral sural nerve terminates in the posterior aspect of the leg. The sural nerve forms the lateral dorsal cutaneous nerve of the dorsum of the foot and provides an anastomotic branch to the intermediate dorsal cutaneous nerve—a branch of the superficial peroneal nerve, which is increased. (Republished with permission of John Wiley, from Kosinski C. The course, mutual relations and distribution of the cutaneous nerve of the metazonal region of the leg and foot. *J Anat.* 1926;60:274; permission conveyed through Copyright Clearance Center, Inc.)

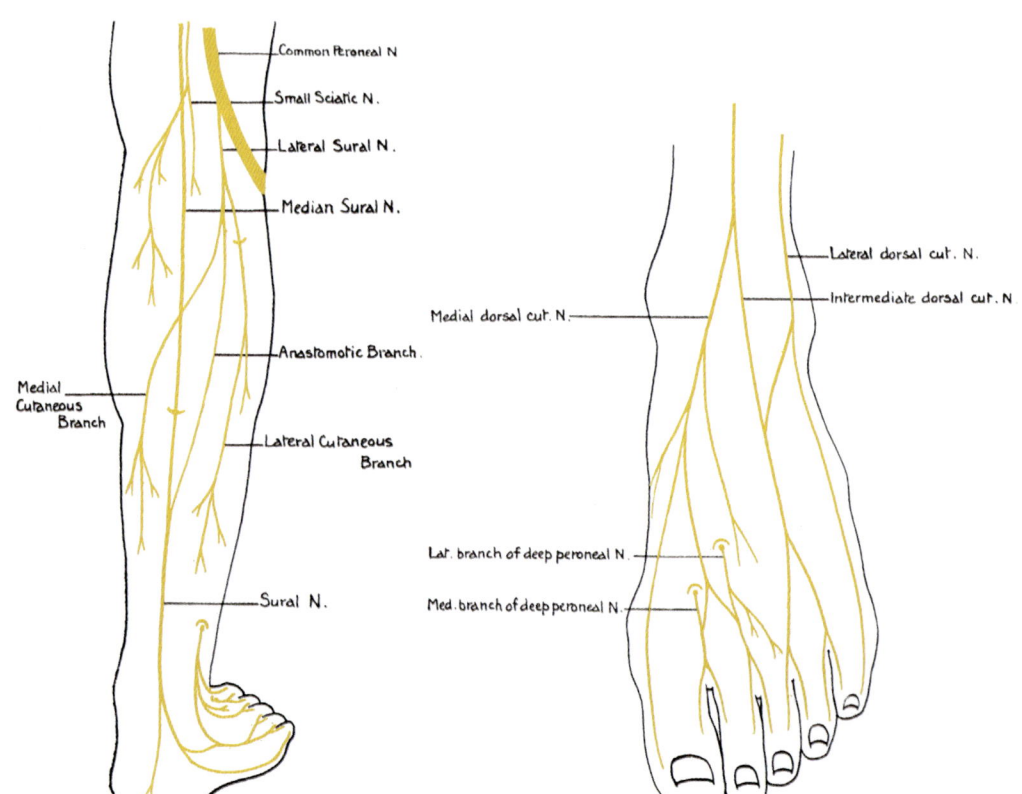

Figure 8.2 Sural nerve type B (40%) formed by two roots: the medial and lateral sural nerves, connected by an anastomotic branch. The sural nerve forms the lateral dorsal cutaneous nerve of the foot united to the intermediate dorsal cutaneous nerve by an anastomotic branch. The deep peroneal nerve is increased, with a medial branch innervating the first web space and a lateral branch innervating the second web space. (Republished with permission of John Wiley, from Kosinski C. The course, mutual relations and distribution of the cutaneous nerve of the metazonal region of the leg and foot. *J Anat.* 1926;60:274; permission conveyed through Copyright Clearance Center, Inc.)

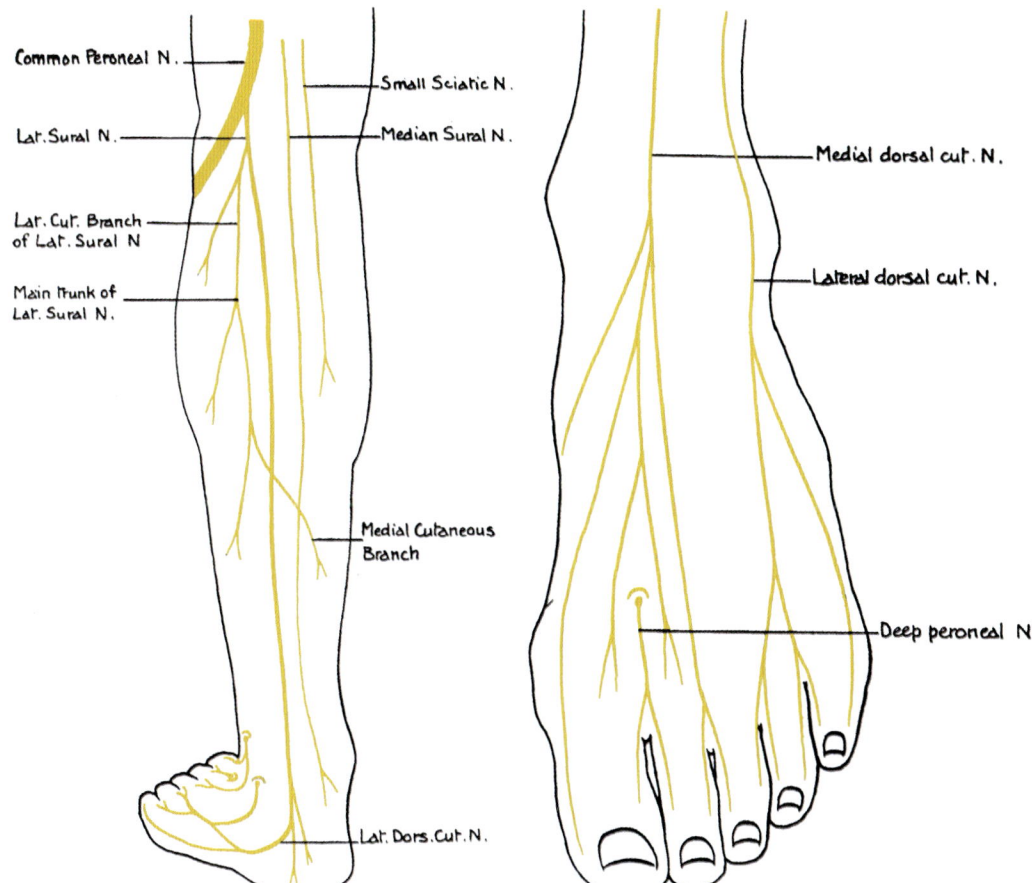

Figure 8.3 Sural nerve type C (6%) formed by the lateral sural nerve only arising from the common peroneal nerve. The sural nerve forms the lateral dorsal cutaneous nerve, which is increased. (Republished with permission of John Wiley, from Kosinski C. The course, mutual relations and distribution of the cutaneous nerve of the metazonal region of the leg and foot. J Anat. 1926;60:274; permission conveyed through Copyright Clearance Center, Inc.)

arborized into multiple cutaneous branches. The proximal diameter of the sural nerve ranged from 2.5 to 4 mm and distally from 2.0 to 3.0 mm.

Eastwood et al[4] conducted an anatomic-metric study of the sural nerve based on the dissection of 20 preserved cadaveric limbs. As illustrated in Figure 8.10, the parameters were determined and the position of the nerve trunk at reference points A–E was defined as indicated in Table 8.3. Furthermore, the branches of the sural nerve were described as major (>2 mm), smaller branches as minor, and their distribution was indicated in the defined reference zones of Table 8.2. This translates as 2 (1.9) major and 2 (2.15) minor branches posteriorly and as 3 (2.8) minor branches and 0.6 branches anteriorly.

The authors were able to describe 95% confidence limits for the course of the sural nerve trunk (Table 8.3). Thus, a longitudinal incision in the region of the fibula should be in front of the anterior limits for the course of the main trunk. Therefore, it should not be more than 1.7 cm posterior to the fibular crest at 10 cm proximal to the lateral malleolus (point A), 1.5 cm posterior at 5 cm proximal to the tip of the lateral malleolus (point B), and no more than 0.6 cm posterior to the tip of the malleolus itself (point C). With the foot in equines, it should

TABLE 8.1 Frequency of Occurrence of Sural Nerve or Other Nerve Functioning as Such				
			Functioning as Sural Nerve (%)	
Author	No. Legs	Sural Nerve with Two Roots (%)	Medial Sural Nerve	Lateral Sural Nerve or Peroneal Communicating Nerve
Catania	94	51	35	14
Kosinski	287	40.2 (type B)	53.8 (type A)	6 (type C)
Andreassi	144	63.9	34.7	1.4
Sockolow	500	52.2	43.8	3.6
Mogi	180	83.3	16.7	0
P'an	286	81.5	13.3	5.2
Williams	257	83.7	15.9	0.4

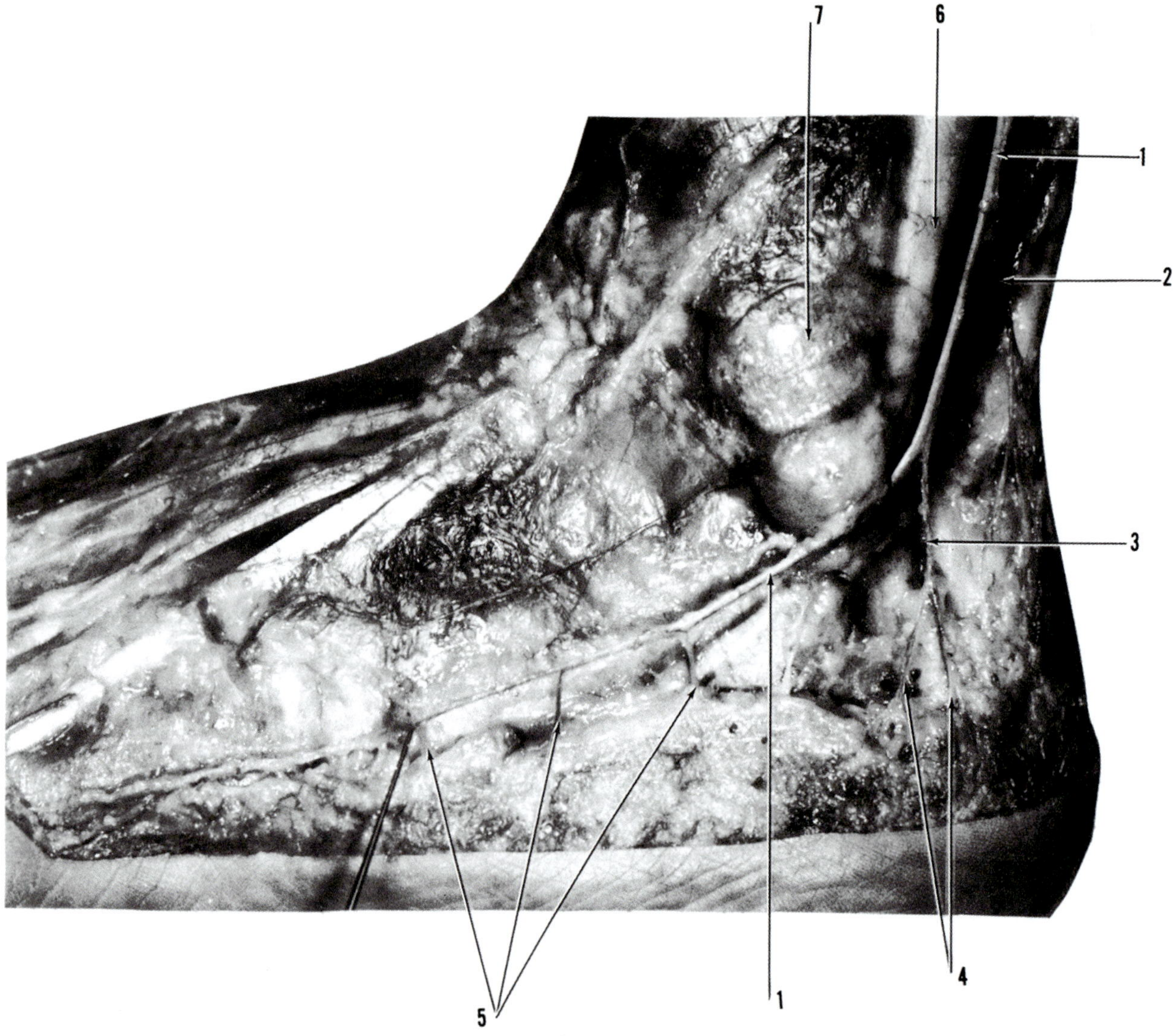

Figure 8.4 Sural nerve. (*1*, Sural nerve; *2*, branch of sural nerve to posterolateral aspect of Achilles tendon area and calcaneal region; *3*, lateral calcaneal branch of sural nerve with bifurcation branches [*4*]; *5*, branches of sural nerve to lateral border of foot; *6*, peronei tendons; *7*, lateral malleolus [sural nerve passes 1-1.5 cm below tip of lateral malleolus].)

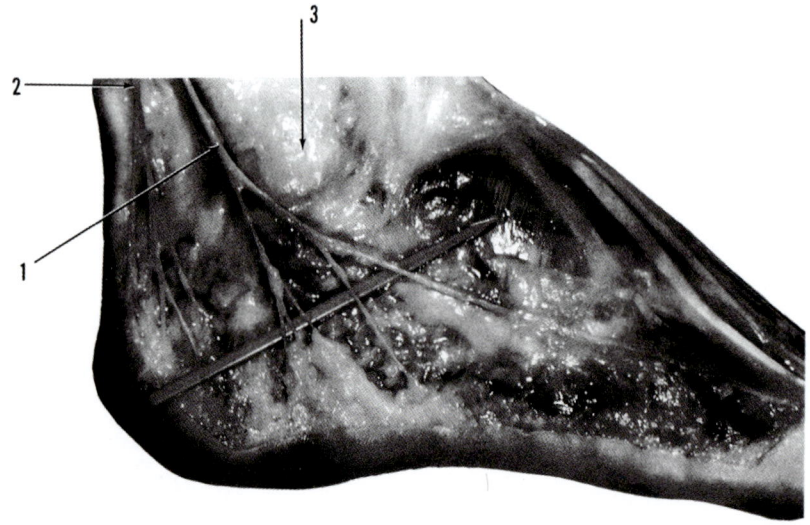

Figure 8.5 Sural nerve *(1)* dividing into lateral branches to the heel and the lateral border of the foot; lateral calcaneal nerve *(2)* dividing into multiple branches, lateral malleolar fat pad *(3)*.

Chapter 8: Nerves 387

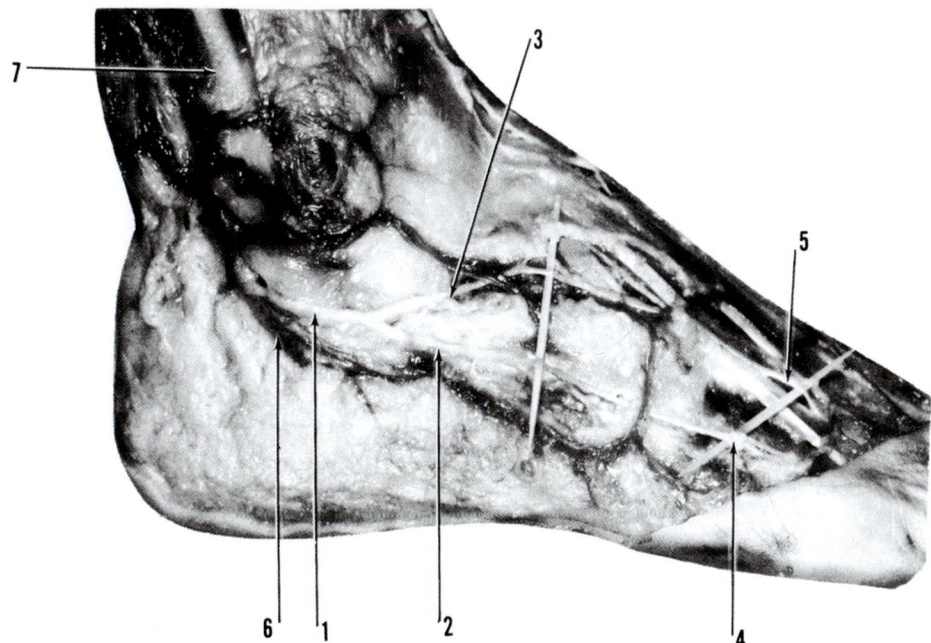

Figure 8.6 **Lateral aspect of the right foot and ankle.** (*1*, Sural nerve dividing into lateral branch [*2*] forming dorsolateral cutaneous nerve [*4*] and medial branch [*3*] uniting with intermediate dorsal cutaneous nerve [*5*] of superficial peroneal nerve; *6*, shorter saphenous vein; *7*, peronei tendons.)

not extend more than 0.7 cm distal to the tip of the lateral malleolus (point D) if the main trunk is to be avoided. Similarly, an incision designed to pass posterior to the sural nerve should be behind the posterior limits of the position of the main trunk (Table 8.3).

Lawrence and Botte[5] investigated the course and branching patterns of the sural nerve based on the dissection of 17 cadaver specimens. At 7 cm proximal to the lateral malleolus, the sural nerve was at a mean 26 mm (range, 16-36 mm) posterior to the edge of the fibula. The lesser saphenous vein was located superficial and lateral to the nerve. At the same level, the sural nerve was 2 mm lateral to the lateral order of the Achilles tendon. In the retromalleolar region, the sural nerve gave off an average of three branches (range, 1-5) that continued to the lateral aspect of the heel as lateral calcaneal branches (Figs. 8.11 to 8.13). In one case, there was a lateral malleolar branch (Fig. 8.12). In the hindfoot, the sural nerve was located at a mean distance of 14 mm (range, 3-22 mm) posterior and 14 mm (range, 1-26 mm) inferior to the tip of the lateral malleolus.

In the hindfoot, the sural nerve bifurcated and formed either terminal branches or a terminal branch and an anastomotic branch. A bifurcation or trifurcation occurred in 91%

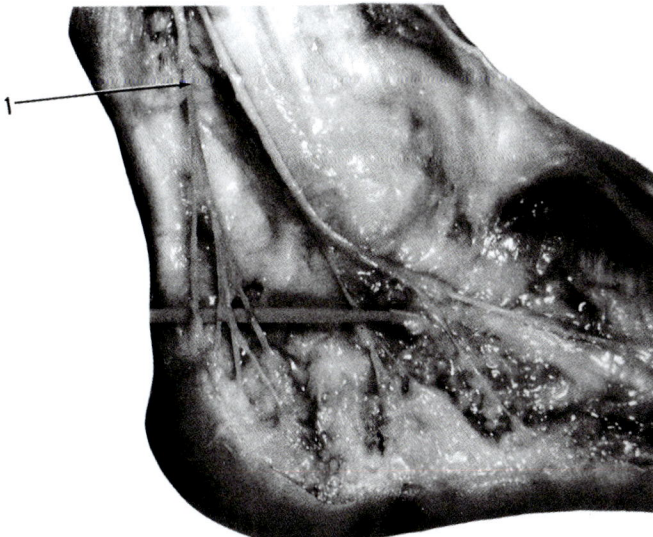

Figure 8.7 **Lateral calcaneal nerve (*1*) bifurcating into two branches: anterior and posterior.** The anterior branch subdivides into four branches supplying the lateral and posterior aspect of the heel. The posterior branch is just lateral to the insertion of the Achilles tendon and supplies the lateral posterior aspect of the heel.

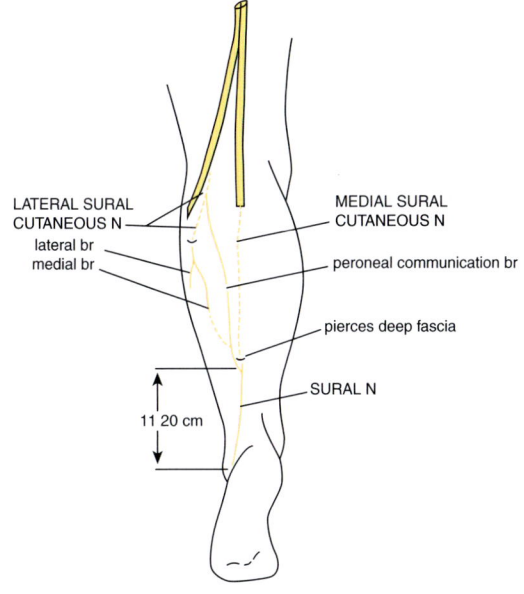

Figure 8.8 **Cutaneous nerves on the back of the leg that contribute to sural nerve.** In 3 of 10 cases, medial branch of lateral sural nerve was anastomosed to peroneal communicating branch.

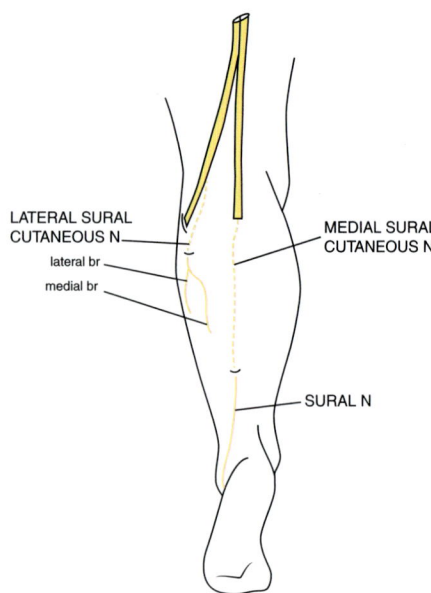

Figure 8.9 Formation of sural nerve as direct continuation of medial sural cutaneous nerve.

TABLE 8.2 Total Number of Posterior and Anterior Branches of the Sural Nerve in 20 Cases			
Site		Major	Minor
Posterior	X	7	9
	Y	20	13
	Z	11	21
	Total	38	43
Anterior	X	0	12
	Y	0	16
	Z	13	28
	Total	13	56

Eastwood DM, Irgau I, Atkins R. The distal course of the sural nerve and its significance for incisions around the lateral hindfoot. *Foot Ankle*. 1992;13(4):199-203, Table 1. Copyright ©1992. Reprinted by Permission of SAGE Publications.

(16 specimens). An anastomotic branch traversing medially toward the sinus tarsi was present in 24% (four cases) and remained superficial to the extensor digitorum brevis. This branch either formed an anastomosis with the intermediate dorsal cutaneous nerve or arborized in the region of the sinus tarsi (see Fig. 8.11). The lateral branch of the bifurcation continued toward the base of the dorsolateral branches of the fifth metatarsal.

Aktan Ikiz et al[6] conducted a comprehensive study of the sural nerve based on the dissection of 30 lower limbs. The sural nerve originated from the union of the medial and lateral cutaneous nerves of the leg which arise from the tibial nerve and the common peroneal nerve (see Fig. 8.19).

The lateral cutaneous nerve of the leg was present in 83.3% (25 specimens) and absent in 16.6% (five specimens) (Figs. 8.14 and 8.15). The origin of the lateral cutaneous nerve was an average 82.87 ± 74.52 mm below the bifurcation of the sciatic nerve.

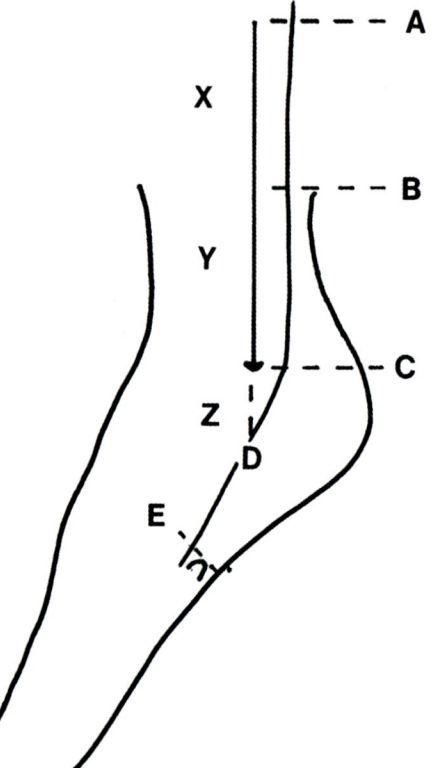

Position of the Main Nerve Trunk at Reference Points A–E	
Point	Position (mean ± SE cm)
A	2.5 ± 0.1
B	2.1 ± 0.1
C	1.4 ± 0.1
D	2.3 ± 0.2
E	1.3 ± 0.1

Figure 8.10 Landmarks to locate the sural nerve. Longitudinal arrow drawn along the fibular crest: the tip of the arrow is at tip of the lateral malleolus; curved black line represents the sural nerve; *A*, 10 cm proximal to tip of lateral malleolus; *B*, 5 cm proximal to tip of lateral malleolus; *C*, immediately posterior to tip of lateral malleolus; *D*, distance directly inferior to the tip of lateral malleolus, in line with the fibular crest; >, represents base of M_5; *E*, at level of base of M_5. (Eastwood DM, Irgau I, Atkins RM. The distal course of the sural nerve and its significance for incisions around the lateral hindfoot. *Foot Ankle*. 1992;13[4]:199-203, Figure 1. Copyright ©1992. Reprinted by Permission of SAGE Publications.)

TABLE 8.3 95% Confidence Limits for the Anterior and Posterior Extents of the Main Nerve Trunk Defined by the Mean ± 1.96 SD at Each of Points A–E

Point	Anterior (cm)	Posterior (cm)
A	1.7	3.2
B	1.5	2.7
D	0.6	2.2
C	0.7	3.9
E	2.1	0.5

Eastwood DM, Irgau I, Atkins R. The distal course of the sural nerve and its significance for incisions around the lateral hindfoot. *Foot Ankle.* 1992;13(4):199-203, Table 2. Copyright ©1992. Reprinted by Permission of SAGE Publications.

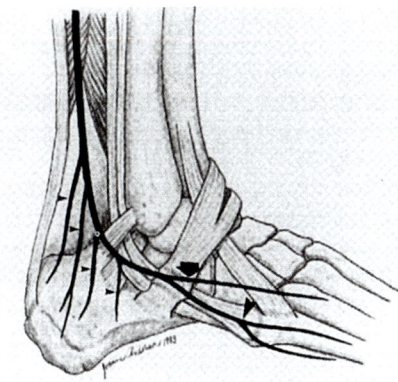

Figure 8.13 Sural nerve. Four lateral calcaneal branches (*small arrows*), an anastomotic branch (*large arrow*), distal bifurcation (*distal arrow*). (Lawrence SJ, Botte MJ. The sural nerve in the foot and ankle—an anatomic study with clinical and surgical implications. *Foot Ankle Int.* 1994;15[9]:490-494, Figure 4. Copyright ©1994. Reprinted by Permission of SAGE Publications.)

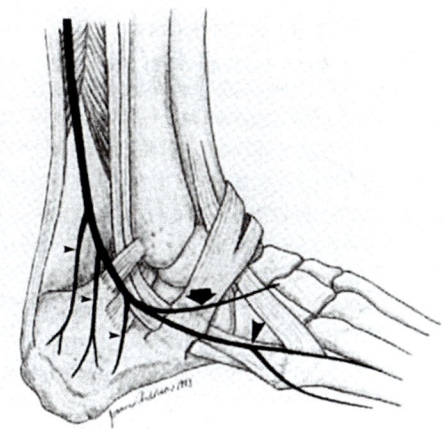

Figure 8.11 Sural nerve. Three lateral calcaneal branches (*small arrow*), anastomotic branch (*large arrow*). Division into dorsomedial and dorsolateral branches of M5 (*distal arrow*). (Lawrence SJ, Botte MJ. The sural nerve in the foot and ankle—an anatomic study with clinical and surgical implications. *Foot Ankle Int.* 1994;15[9]:490-494, Figure 2. Copyright ©1994. Reprinted by Permission of SAGE Publications.)

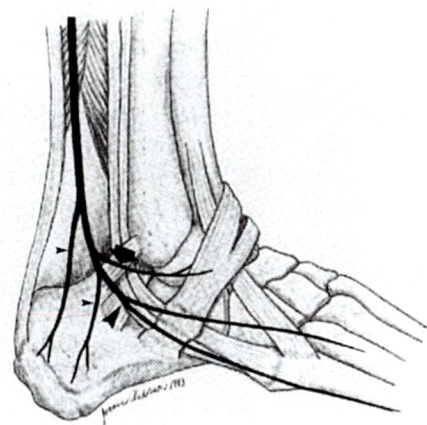

Figure 8.12 Sural nerve. Two lateral calcaneal branches (*small arrows*), a lateral malleolar branch (*large arrow*), proximal bifurcation (*distal arrow*). (Lawrence SJ, Botte MJ. The sural nerve in the foot and ankle—an anatomic study with clinical and surgical implications. *Foot Ankle Int.* 1994;15[9]:490-494, Figure 3. Copyright ©1994. Reprinted by Permission of SAGE Publications.)

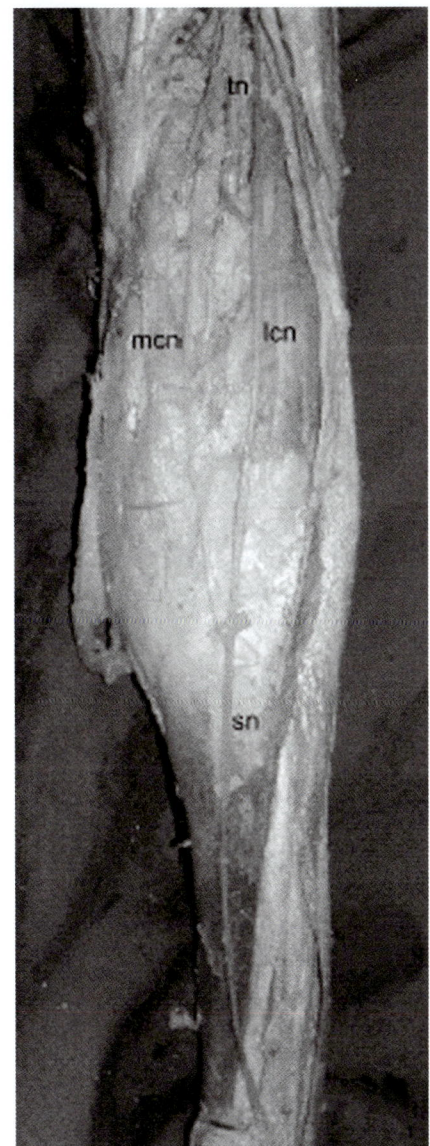

Figure 8.14 Sural nerve (*sn*), medial cutaneous nerve (*mcn*), and lateral cutaneous nerve (*lcn*). (Aktan Ikiz ZA, Ucerler H, Bilge O. The anatomic features of the sural nerve with emphasis on its clinical importance. *Foot Ankle Int.* 2005;7:942-946, Figure 1. Copyright ©2005. Reprinted by Permission of SAGE Publications.)

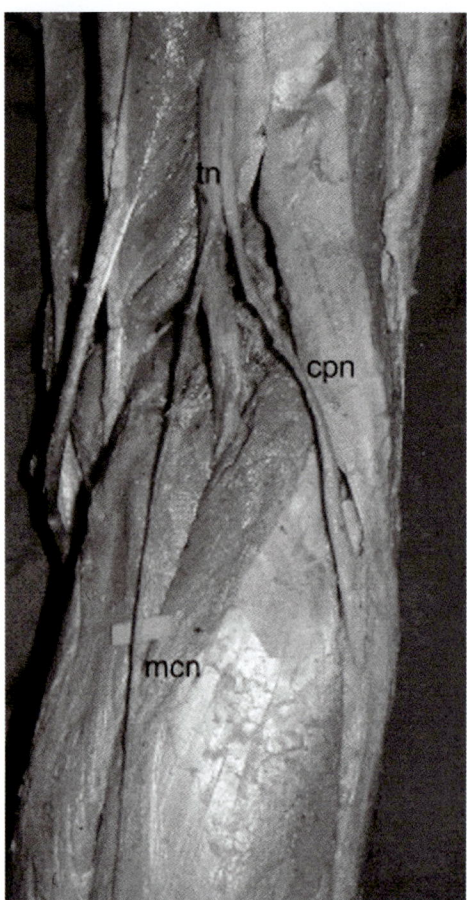

Figure 8.15 **Sural nerve.** Absence of lateral cutaneous nerve: medial cutaneous nerve (*mcn*) and common peroneal nerve (*cpn*). (Aktan Ikiz ZA, Ucerler H, Bilge O. The anatomic features of the sural nerve with emphasis on its clinical importance. *Foot Ankle Int.* 2005;7:942-946, Figure 2. Copyright ©2005. Reprinted by Permission of SAGE Publications.)

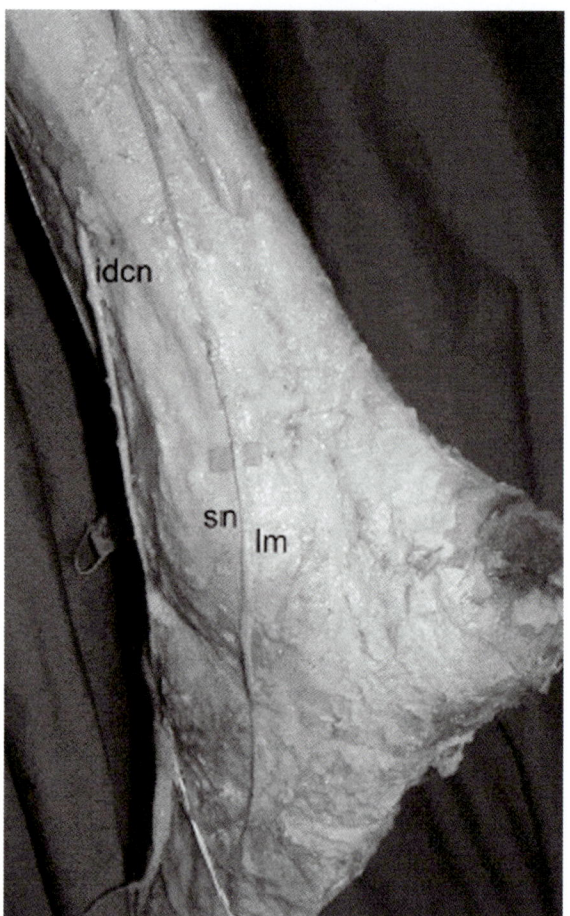

Figure 8.16 **Sural nerve passing over the lateral malleolus:** sural nerve (*sn*), intermediate dorsal cutaneous nerve (*idcn*), and lateral malleolus (*lm*). (Aktan Ikiz ZA, Ucerler H, Bilge O. The anatomic features of the sural nerve with emphasis on its clinical importance. *Foot Ankle Int.* 2005;7:942-946, Figure 11. Copyright ©2005. Reprinted by Permission of SAGE Publications.)

The medial cutaneous nerve of the leg derived from the tibial nerve in 93.3% (28 specimens) and was absent in 6.6% (two specimens). The origin of the medial cutaneous nerve was an average of 76.47 ± 67.42 mm below the bifurcation of the sciatic nerve.

An accessory communicating branch existed between the medial and lateral cutaneous nerves in 6.7% (two specimens).

The formation and course of the sural nerve was classified into five types:

Type 1: The sural nerve was formed by communication of the medial cutaneous nerve originating from the tibial nerve and the lateral cutaneous nerve originating from the common peroneal nerve in 60% (18 specimens).

Type 2: The lateral cutaneous nerve was absent in 16.7% (five cases) and the medial cutaneous nerve reproduced the normal course of the sural nerve.

Type 3: The medial cutaneous nerve became superficial and communicated with the lateral cutaneous nerve in the distal third of the leg in 10% (three specimens).

Type 4: The lateral cutaneous nerve and the medial cutaneous nerve passed down separately and did not form the sural nerve in 6.7% (two specimens).

Type 5: The medial cutaneous nerve was absent in 6.7% (two specimens). The lateral cutaneous nerve divided into three branches and the middle branch followed the standard course of the SN.

The median distance between the most prominent posterior aspect of the lateral malleolus and the sural nerve in all specimens was 12.76 ± 8.79 mm. The mean distance between the tip of the lateral malleolus and the sural nerve was 13.25 ± 6.88 mm. In 13.3% (4 specimens), the sural nerve was in contact with the tip of the lateral malleolus, and in 10% (3 cases), the sural nerve passed over the lateral malleolus (Fig. 8.16).

Webb et al,[7] based on the dissection of 30 preserved cadaveric lower limbs, analyzed and described the course of the sural nerve in relation to the Achilles tendon. The widths of Achilles tendon and horizontal distances of the sural nerve to the Achilles tendon lateral border were measured at 0, 4, 8, 12, and 16 cm from the Achilles tendon insertion into the calcaneum. The findings are presented in Table 8.4. At the level of insertion of the Achilles tendon into the calcaneum, the sural nerve was 17.5 mm lateral to the lateral border of the Achilles tendon and this is reduced to 7 mm lateral at 4 cm proximally.

TABLE 8.4 Widths of TA and Distances of Nerve From Muscle/Tendon

Distance from TA Insertion (cm)	TA Width (mm)	Horizontal Distance of Sural Nerve from TA Lateral Border (mm)
0	18.7 (11 to 28)	17.5 (3 to 40)
4	12.7 (8 to 16)	7.00 (3 to 14)
8	16.2 (13 to 31)	2.3 (−4 to 13)
12	28.2 (20 to 44)	−3.3 (0 to −16)
16	38.2 (25 to 58)	−10.4 (0 to −24)

TA, Tendoachilles.
Webb J, Moorjani N, Radfort M. Anatomy of the sural nerve and its relation to the Achilles tendon. *Foot Ankle Int.* 2000;21(6):475-477. Copyright ©2000. Reprinted by Permission of SAGE Publications.

The sural nerve curves medially as it courses proximally and crosses the lateral border of the Achilles tendon 9.83 cm (range, 6.55-16 cm) from the calcaneal insertion (Fig. 8.17).

Tashjian et al,[8] based on the dissection of 14 fresh frozen cadaver legs, investigated the distance from the distal tip of the fibula to the gastrocnemius-soleus juncture and then the distance of the sural nerve from the lateral border of the tendon at that level (Fig. 8.18).

The ratio of the distance of the gastrocnemius-soleus junction from the distal tip of the fibula divided by the length of the fibula was 0.5 (range, 0.5-0.6). The average width of the gastrocnemius-soleus complex at the junction was 58 mm (range, 44-69 mm) and the average distance of the sural nerve from the lateral border of the gastrocnemius-soleus complex at the level of the junction was 12 mm (range, 7-17 mm).

SUPERFICIAL PERONEAL NERVE

The superficial peroneal nerve (musculocutaneous nerve), a branch of the common peroneal nerve, after coursing in the anterolateral compartment of the leg, pierces the deep fascia cruris in the lower third of the leg and divides into the medial and the intermediate dorsal cutaneous nerves of the dorsum of the foot (Fig. 8.19). The piercing of the deep fascia of the leg by the superficial peroneal nerve occurs at different levels. In 100 legs, it occurred 12.5 cm above the tip of the lateral malleolus in 90%; 15 cm above the tip in 1%; 10 cm above the tip in 2%;

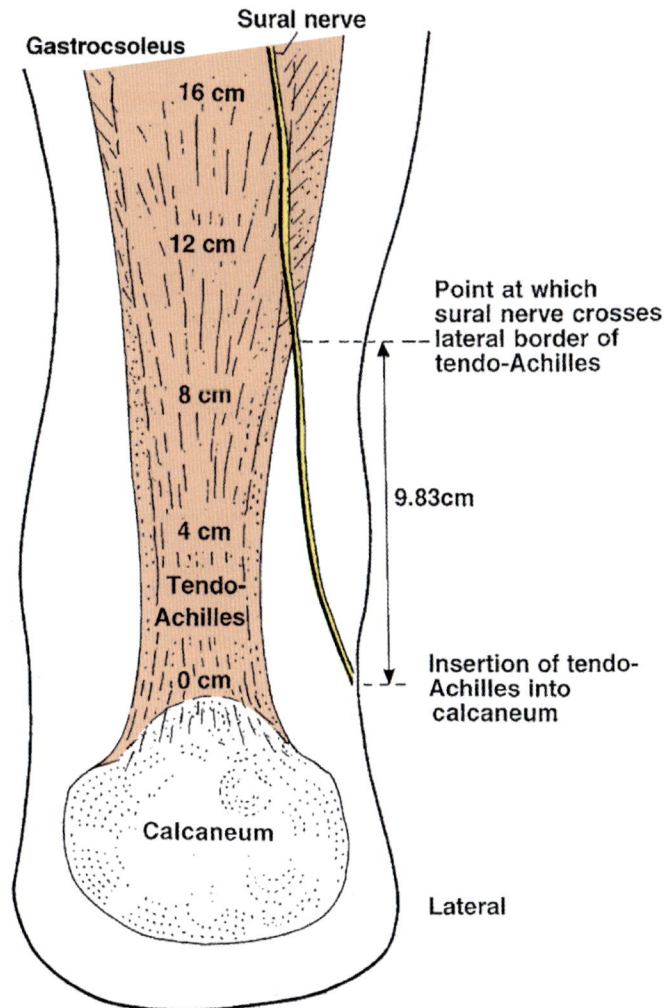

Figure 8.17 **Posterior view of the Achilles tendon and sural nerve.** (Adapted from Webb J, Moorjani N, Radfort M. Anatomy of the sural nerve and its relation to the Achilles tendon. *Foot Ankle Int.* 2000;21[6]:475-477.)

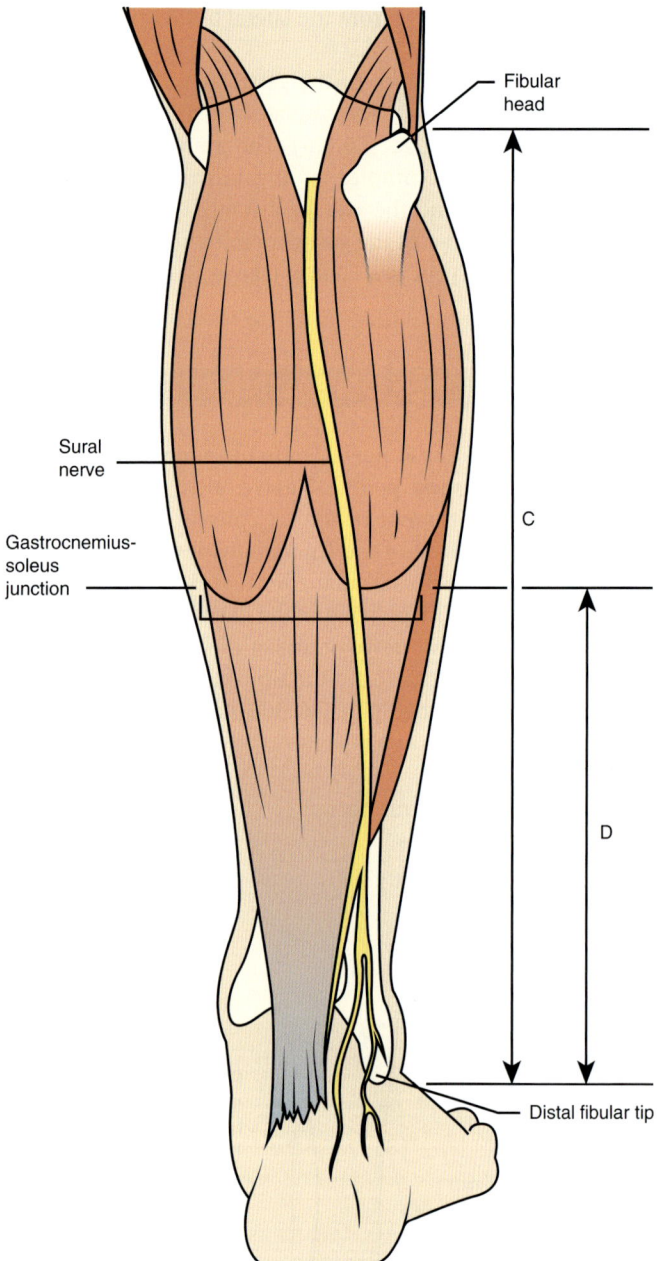

Figure 8.18 Posterior aspect of leg with gastrocnemius-soleus complex and sural nerve. **(A)** Width of gastrocnemius-soleus complex at the level of the musculotendinous junction. **(B)** Distance between the sural nerve and the lateral border of the gastrocnemius-soleus complex. **(C)** Length of fibula. **(D)** Distance from the distal fibula tip to the level of the musculotendinous junction. (Adapted from Tashjian RZ, Appel AJ, Banerjee R, et al. Anatomic study of the gastrocnemius-soleus junction and its relationship to the sural nerve. Foot Ankle Int. 2003;6:473-476.)

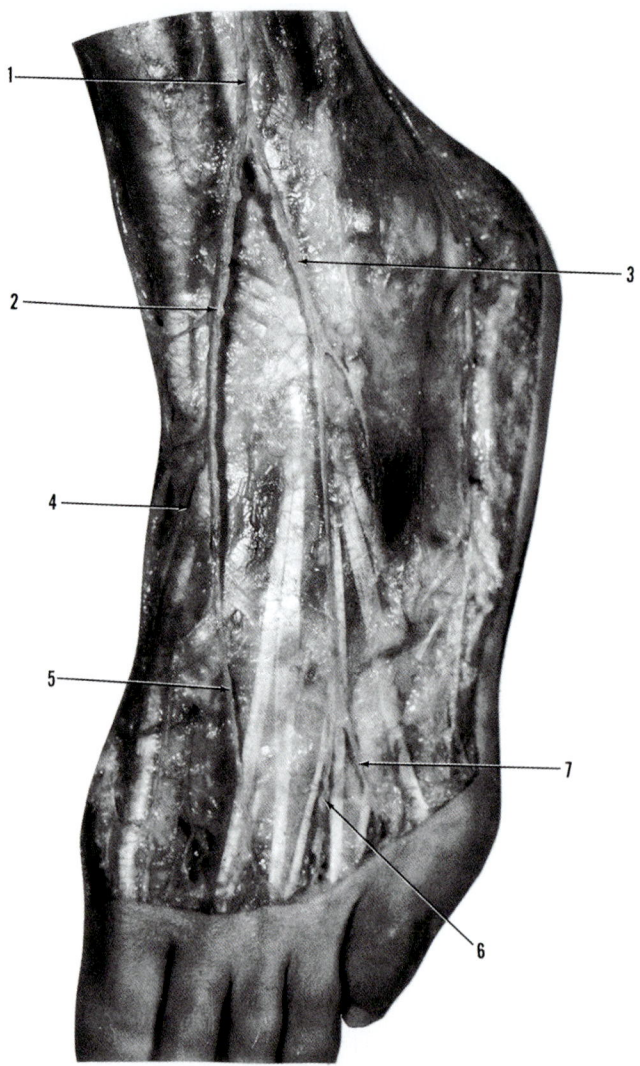

Figure 8.19 Superficial peroneal nerve (1) dividing into the intermediate dorsal cutaneous nerve (3) and the medial dorsal cutaneous nerve (2). The latter subdivides into the dorsomedial cutaneous nerve of the big toe (4) and the common digital nerve to the second web space (5). The intermediate dorsal nerve (3) supplies the dorsal cutaneous nerve of the third (6) and fourth (7) web spaces.

7.5 cm above the tip in 5%; and 5 cm above the tip in 2%.[1] In 118 legs, it occurred 10.5 cm above the tip of the lateral malleolus in 74.7% and at a higher level in 23.4%.[2]

When the division of the superficial peroneal nerve into its cutaneous branches occurs at a higher level, the medial dorsal cutaneous branch pierces the fascia cruris at 12.7 cm and the intermediate dorsal cutaneous branch at 4.7 cm above the tip of the lateral malleolus.[2] After becoming subcutaneous, the cutaneous common trunk of the superficial peroneal nerve divides into its terminal branches, usually 6.4 cm above the lateral malleolus; this division occurs below this level in 3% and above the same level in 5% (12.5 cm).[1] Cutaneous branches are provided by the common trunk, and the largest of these, the lateral malleolar branch, may anastomose with the lateral sural nerve or with an accessory branch of the sural nerve.[9]

The most common site of the superficial peroneal nerve is "10.5 cm above the tip of the external malleolus just within the anterior border of the fibula in the groove between the peroneal group of muscles and the extensor digitorum longus."[1] In this location, the nerve is subcutaneous in 91% and deep to the fascia in 9%.[1]

Adkinson and colleagues studied the anatomic variations in the course of the superficial peroneal nerve in 85 legs, with particular attention to the relationship between the nerve and the intermuscular septum between the lateral and anterior compartments of the leg.[10] In 73%, the superficial peroneal nerve was located in the lateral compartment and pierced the deep crural fascia an average of 13 cm (range, 3-18 cm) proximal to the lateral malleolus (Fig. 8.20). It divided into its terminal branches within 2 cm of its exit point.

In 14%, the superficial peroneal nerve passed into the anterior compartment of the leg, and in 13%, it pierced the crural fascia at 8 to 14 cm proximal to the lateral malleolus (Fig. 8.20). Within 1 to 3 cm of the exit site, the nerve divided into the terminal branches. In one specimen, the nerve divided in the lateral compartment and the two branches pierced the anterolateral intermuscular septum, passed into the anterior compartment, and surfaced through the crural fascia at 13 cm proximal to the lateral malleolus.

In 12%, the superficial peroneal nerve had branches in both the anterior and lateral compartments (Fig. 8.21). The anterior branch pierced the crural fascia at 10 to 17 cm from the lateral malleolus and the lateral branch at 4 to 10 cm. In one leg, the superficial peroneal nerve, located in the lateral compartment, coursed on the superficial surface of the peroneus longus muscle and passed through the crural fascia at 11 cm proximal to the lateral malleolus.

The intermediate dorsal cutaneous nerve (middle dorsal cutaneous nerve, external branch of the musculocutaneous nerve) is thinner than the medial branch and crosses the fifth and fourth extensor digitorum longus tendons obliquely and superficially. It courses over the third intermetatarsal space. At the anterior aspect of this space, the nerve provides the dorsolateral branch to the third toe and the dorsomedial branch to the fourth toe; it may also send an anastomotic branch to the sural nerve.

The medial dorsal cutaneous nerve is the largest bifurcation branch of the superficial peroneal nerve. It is directed medially toward the inner border of the foot. It crosses the inferior extensor retinaculum and takes a direction nearly parallel to the extensor hallucis longus tendon. The nerve divides into three branches: lateral, middle, and medial. The lateral branch takes off at the inferior border of the inferior extensor retinaculum, crosses the long extensor tendon of the second toe, and—in the anterior aspect of the second intermetatarsal space—divides into the dorsolateral branch of the second toe and the dorsomedial branch of the third toe. The middle branch courses in the interval corresponding to the first intermetatarsal space and, on the anterior aspect of the latter, divides into the dorsomedial branch of the second toe and the dorsolateral branch of the big toe. These two branches are very thin and receive reinforcement from the branches of the deep peroneal nerve. The medial branch is directed medially, crosses the extensor hallucis longus tendon superficially and obliquely, and then runs parallel to the tendon, forming the dorsomedial cutaneous nerve

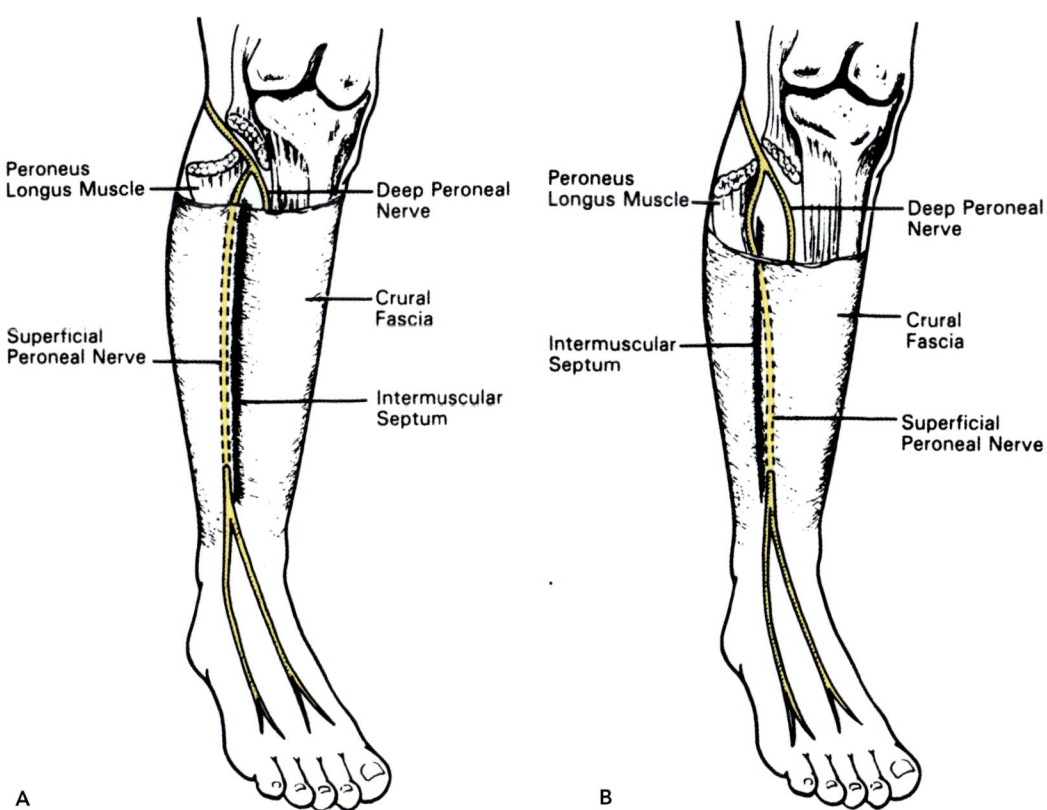

Figure 8.20 **Peroneal nerve. (A)** In 73%, the superficial peroneal nerve lies only in the lateral muscle compartment until, as it courses inferiorly, it pierces the crural fascia 3 to 18 cm proximal to the lateral malleolus. **(B)** In 14%, the superficial peroneal nerve passes through the crural fascia from the anterior muscle compartment. (Adapted from Adkinson DP, Bosse MJ, Gaccione DR, et al. Anatomical variations in the course of the superficial peroneal nerve. *J Bone Joint Surg Am.* 1991;73[1]:112.)

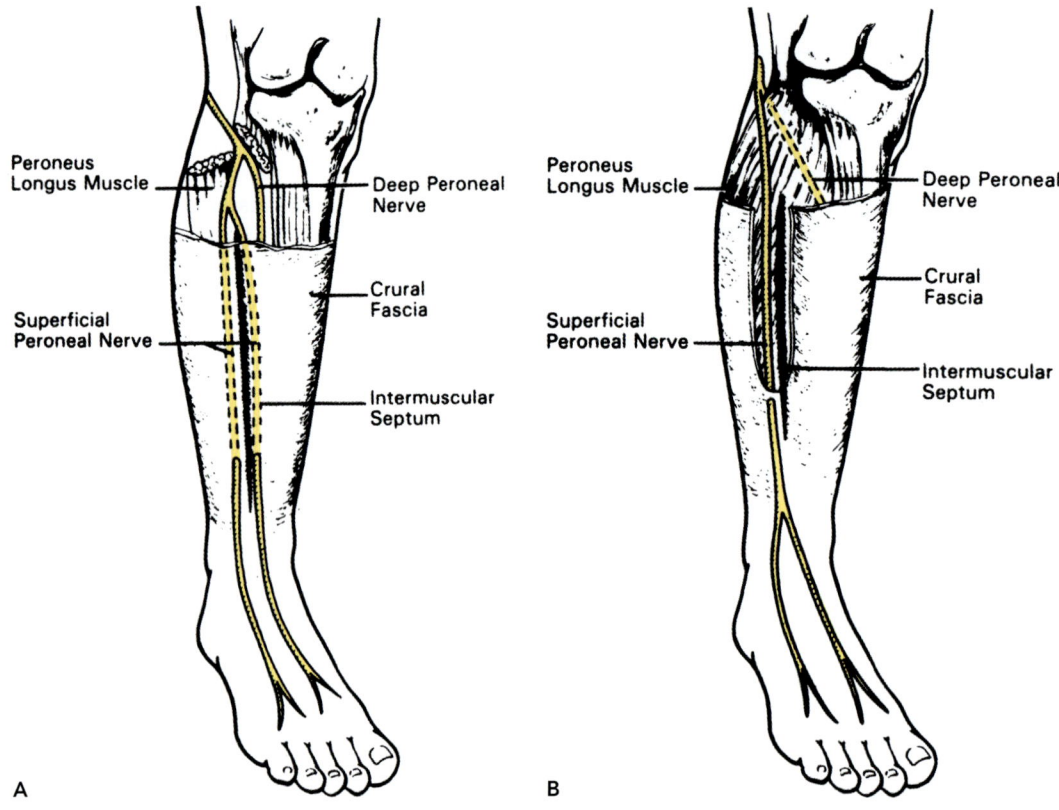

Figure 8.21 Peroneal nerve. (A) In 12%, the superficial nerve has branches in both the anterior and lateral compartments. (B) In 1%, the superficial peroneal nerve arises from the common peroneal nerve 1 cm from the posterior aspect of the fibular neck and never lies deep to the peroneus longus muscle. The nerve descends instead on the superficial surface of the peroneus longus muscle and pierces the crural fascia 11 cm proximal to the lateral malleolus. It then immediately divides into medial and intermediate dorsal cutaneous nerves of the foot. (Modified with permission from Adkinson DP, Bosse MJ, Gaccione DR, et al. Anatomical variations in the course of the superficial peroneal nerve. J Bone Joint Surg Am. 1991;73[1]:112.)

of the big toe. This nerve branch is subcutaneous but is located within or immediately under the superficial fascia of the foot and yet is superficial to the extensor hallucis longus tendon and its investing fascia. The medial cutaneous branch anastomoses at the level of the metatarsophalangeal joint of the big toe with a terminal branch of the saphenous nerve.

The accessory deep peroneal nerve, a branch of the superficial peroneal nerve, was first recognized by Bryce and described in three cases.[11-13] The thin branch passed through the substance of the peroneus brevis muscle and terminated once in the ligament of the ankle joint and twice in the extensor digitorum brevis.

A comprehensive study of the same nerve is provided by Winckler, who described it in seven cases (five adults and two newborns).[14] The branch of the superficial peroneal nerve to the peroneus brevis muscle, after providing the motor branches to the latter, courses along the posterior border of the peroneus brevis tendon, remains in the compartment of the peronei, and reaches the posterior aspect of the lateral malleolus. At this level, the nerve provides branches to the posterior talofibular ligament and to the calcaneofibular ligament and then turns around the lateral malleolus parallel to the tendon of the peroneus brevis, reaches the extensor digitorum brevis and innervates its two lateral heads (to the fourth and third toes), and terminates in the dorsal capsule of the calcaneocuboid joint. Prior to entering the extensor digitorum brevis, the accessory deep peroneal nerve provides branches to the anterior talofibular ligament and to the capsule of the ankle joint.

As described by Winckler, the accessory deep peroneal nerve is associated with a strong development of the peroneus brevis muscle and with the presence of an accessory tendon extending from the peroneus brevis muscle to the fifth toe as the peroneal extensor of the fifth toe.[14] The nerve may be purely sensory, innervating the ankle joint or certain articulations of the tarsal and tarsometatarsal joints; however, it is usually mixed, and it is never pure motor, innervating only the extensor digitorum brevis.

Lambert, in an electromyographic investigation of 50 healthy persons, found evidence of the presence of this accessory deep peroneal nerve in 22% of the examined limbs.[15]

DEEP PERONEAL NERVE

The deep peroneal nerve, after piercing the extensor digitorum longus muscle, joins the anterior tibial artery. In the upper third of the leg, the nerve is situated between the extensor digitorum longus and the tibialis anterior muscle. In the middle third, the nerve is located between the extensor hallucis longus and the tibialis anterior muscle. In the distal third of the leg, the deep peroneal nerve passes behind the obliquely directed extensor hallucis longus muscle-tendon, and at 2.5 to 5 cm above the ankle, the nerve is located between the latter tendon and the extensor digitorum longus tendon.[1]

The deep peroneal nerve is lateral to the anterior tibial artery proximally and distally, but some variations are possible. Horwitz, in a study of 100 legs, mentions that in 90% of the cases, the nerve is lateral to the artery in the upper and middle thirds of the leg, and then at 10 cm above the ankle joint, the nerve is anterolateral to the artery; at 5 cm above the joint, the nerve is again lateral to the artery.[1] In 4%, the nerve is lateral initially, crosses the artery posteriorly, and is medial farther down.[1] In 1%, the nerve is lateral initially, crosses the artery anteriorly, and is medial to the latter distally.[1]

The deep peroneal nerve divides into a medial and a lateral terminal branch at 1.3 cm above the ankle joint in 98% of the cases (Fig. 8.22).[1] In 2%, the branching occurs at 6.4 cm above the ankle joint or at the level of the ankle joint.[1] At the level of the ankle, the deep peroneal nerve is located under the reflected segment of the extensor pulley of the extensor hallucis longus tendon.

The medial branch usually is located medial to the dorsalis pedis artery. It is the larger branch and continues in the direction of the nerve. Initially it is located between the extensor hallucis longus tendon and the medial border of the extensor

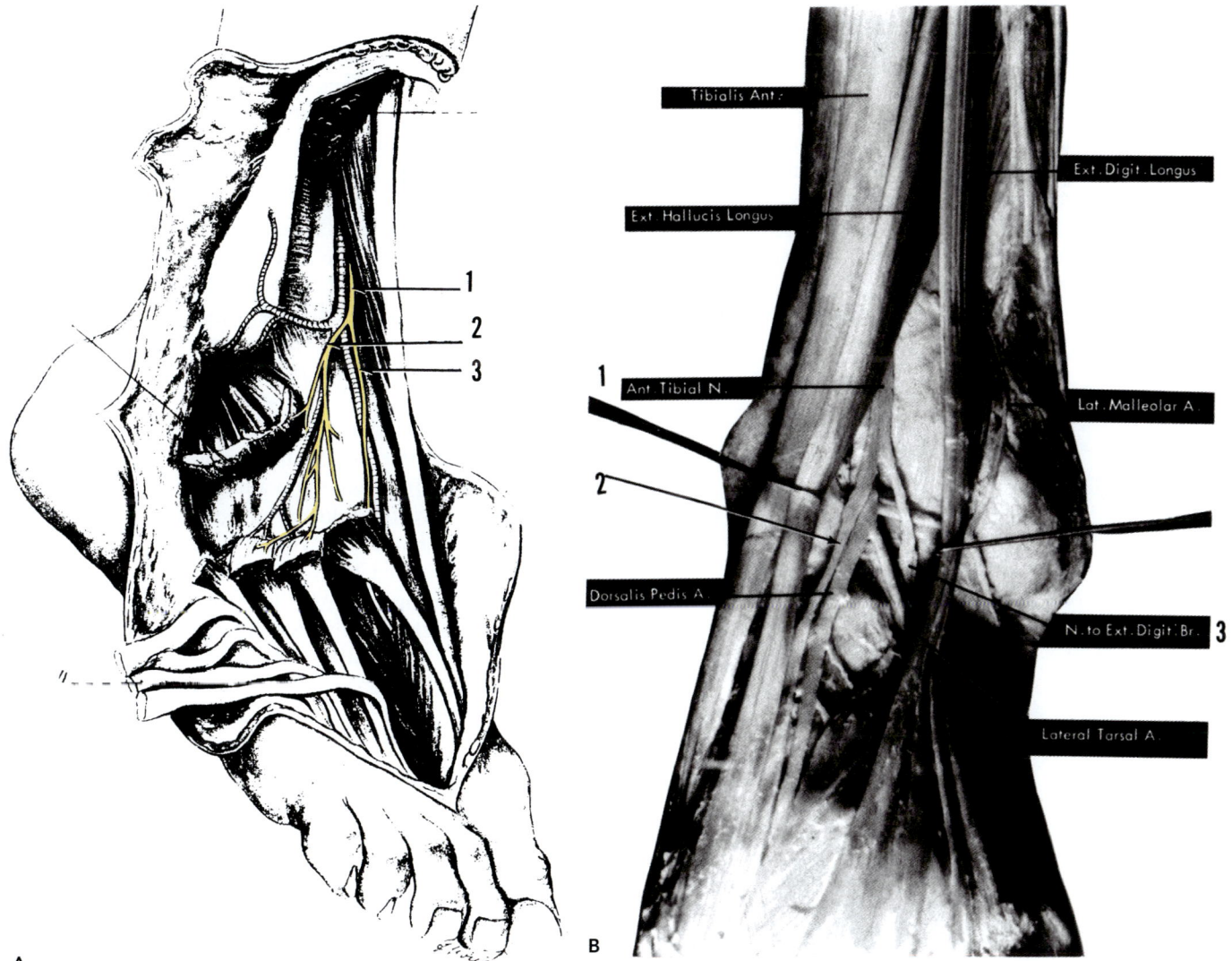

Figure 8.22 **(A) The deep peroneal nerve (*1*) divides into lateral (*2*) and medial (*3*) branches at the level of the ankle joint.** The lateral branch (*2*) supplies the extensor digitorum brevis muscle from the deep surface. It also provides articular branches. The medial division branch (*3*) courses under the extensor digitorum brevis of the hallux and reaches the dorsum of the first web space (the nerve has been sectioned at that level). **(B) The deep peroneal nerve (*1*) (or anterior tibial nerve) divides into a medial branch (*2*), which will reach the first web space and the lateral branch (*3*) or nerve to the extensor digiti brevis**. (A, Adapted from Hovelacque A. *Anatomie des Nerfs Craniens et Rachidiens et du Systeme Grand Sympathique*. Doin; 1927:612. B, From Cosentino R. *Atlas of Anatomy and Surgical Approaches in Orthopedic Surgery*. Vol 2. The Lower Extremity. Charles C Thomas; 1960.)

hallucis brevis muscle. It is crossed superficially and obliquely by the latter and reaches the first intermetatarsal space, where it pierces the deep dorsal aponeurosis of the foot. It is now located between the extensor hallucis brevis tendon medially and the long extensor of the second toe laterally. The nerve divides into two branches and supplies the dorsolateral cutaneous branch to the big toe and the dorsomedial cutaneous branch to the second toe (Fig. 8.23). Quite often the deep peroneal nerve joins the branches of the superficial peroneal nerve in going to the first web space.

The lateral branch of the deep peroneal nerve is directed anterolaterally, penetrates and innervates the extensor digitorum brevis muscle, and terminates into very thin branches that are applied against the tarsal skeleton and form the second, third, and fourth dorsal interosseous nerves. These branches provide the nerve supply to the tarsometatarsal, the metatarsophalangeal, and interphalangeal joints of the lesser toes.

The average diameter of the deep peroneal nerve is 1 to 3 mm, and the most constant site is 2.5 cm above the level of the ankle joint anteriorly, under the upper arm of the inferior extensor retinaculum between the extensor hallucis longus medially and the extensor digitorum longus laterally.[1]

The dorsal cutaneous nerve supply to the dorsum of the foot is very variable. Statistical information based on a collective study of 229 ft reported by the Anatomical Society of Great Britain and Ireland[16] is presented in Figures 8.24 to 8.27. When the territory of the sural nerve increases, that of the intermediate dorsal cutaneous branch decreases, and vice versa. In the same series, only in one case did the saphenous nerve supply the inner side of the big toe, and in another one, it reached the inner side of the head of the first metatarsal bone.[16]

Clarification is required at this time in regard to the data provided by this collective study as a misinformation has been initiated recently and is developing rapidly. In early October 1890, five questions were issued by the Committee of Collective Investigation of the Anatomical Society of Great Britain and Ireland. The fourth question concerned the distribution of the cutaneous nerves on the dorsum of the foot and toe.

At the Second Annual Report of this Committee for the year 1890 to 1891, the report was given by Arthur Thomson Lecturer on anatomy. Fifteen anatomists had participated and the report indicated that "a total of 229 feet have been examined and, in tabulating the results, the graphic method has been adopted in preference to the description. Twelve types are figured and lettered A, B, C, etc in order of their frequency." Their results were presented in a table depicting the 12 varieties. In our study, we have presented the 12 types with only improved graphics and due reference was given to the work of the Anatomical Society.

Kosinski[2] dissected 118 legs and reported on the cutaneous nerves on the dorsum of the foot. "For purposes of simplicity, the following three main types of distribution of cutaneous nerves on the dorsum of the foot may be considered" and he referred to types A (67%), B (17.1%), and C (13.7%). Each type was described in a complex manner with a digital formula followed by enlargement of distribution or absence. He also added a type D (0.85%) as "diminution of area supplied by deep peroneal nerve."

A "Kosinski affair" has been created because Canovas et al[17] are attributing the classification of the Anatomical Society in 12 types to Kosinski based on a nonexisting or erroneous reference and have reproduced our graphic presentation—without due reference—as "Figure 1, Distributions of the twelve types described by Kosinski and their reference."[14] Their corresponding reference is erroneous and does not exist. Unfortunately, the Kosinski classification K_1 to K_{12} has been adopted by Solomon et al[18] and subsequently by Aktan Ikiz and Ucerler.[19] The classification of the variation of the branches of the superficial peroneal nerve into 12 categories should be attributed to the Anatomical Society of Great Britain and Ireland and this error should be corrected by future investigators.

Blair and Botte[20] described the surgical anatomy of the superficial peroneal nerve in the ankle and foot based on the dissection and comprehensive study of 25 cadaver lower limbs. They classified their findings into types A, B, and C.

In type A (72%), the superficial peroneal nerve pierced the crural fascia to become subcutaneous at an average distance of 12.3 cm proximal to the ankle joint. At a mean distance of 4.4 cm proximal to the ankle joint, it divided into a large medial dorsal cutaneous nerve and a smaller laterally located intermediate dorsal cutaneous nerve (Fig. 8.28).

In type B (16%), the medial and intermediate dorsal cutaneous nerves arose independently from the superficial peroneal nerve. The intermediate dorsal cutaneous nerve pierced the

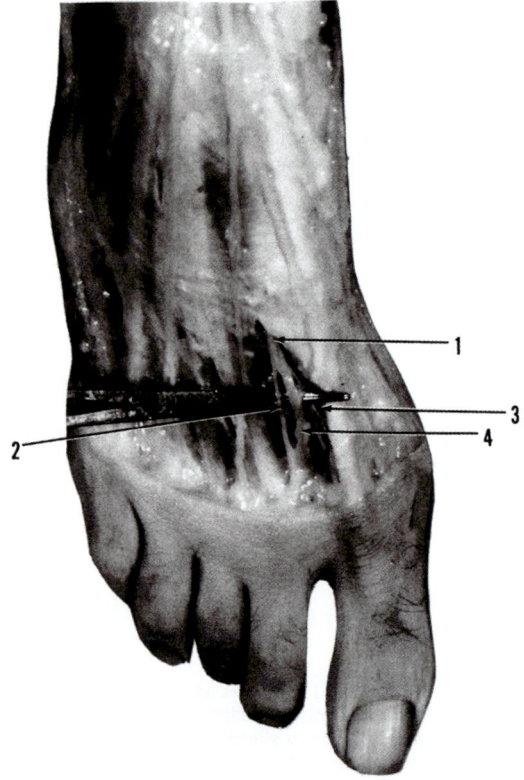

Figure 8.23 **Neurovascular bundle of the first web space.** Deep peroneal nerve (1) dividing into dorsomedial nerve (2) of the second toe and dorsolateral nerve (3) of the big toe; first dorsal metatarsal artery (4).

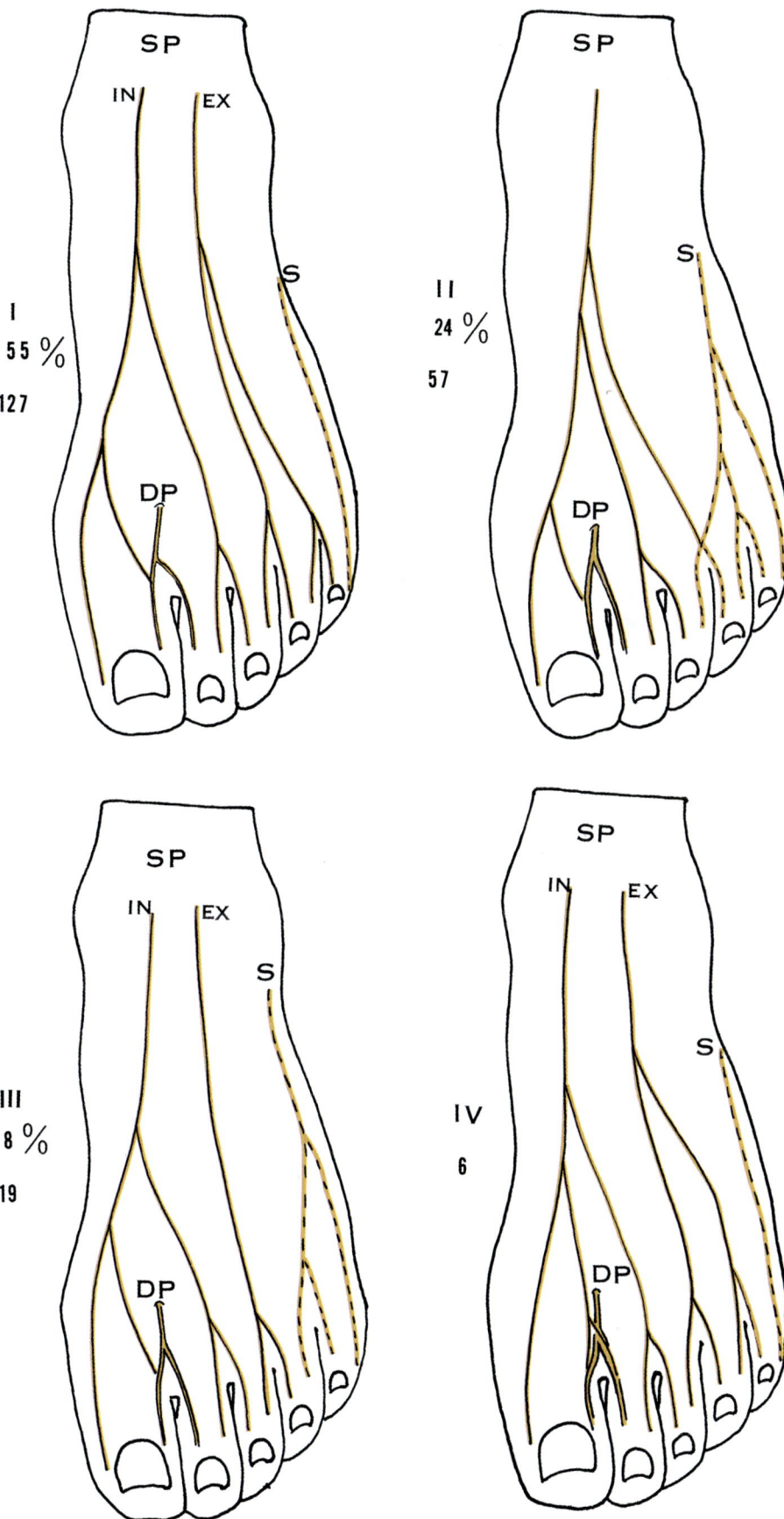

Figure 8.24 Variations in the distribution of the cutaneous nerves on the dorsum of the foot (229 ft examined). Roman numerals I to XII were used to classify the results in a decreasing frequency of occurrence pattern from maximum to minimum. The original classification was in capital letters, presented in a nonalphabetical manner (see Fig. 8.25). The correspondence of the Roman numbers to letters is as follows: I = A, II = B, III = C, IV = F, V = J, VI = D, VII = E, VIII = L, IX = G, X = H, XI = K, and XII = L. **Type I** (A) (55%): Most frequent distribution pattern, with the superficial peroneal nerve predominating. **Type II** (B) (24%): Sural nerve is increased. **Type III** (C) (8%): Sural nerve innervates the fourth web space and provides the lateral dorsal cutaneous branch of the little toe. **Type IV** (F) (6 of 229): Similar to type I but the superficial peroneal nerve provides two anastomotic branches to the deep peroneal nerve. (SP, superficial peroneal nerve; IN, internal division branch of SP, EX, external division branch of SP; DP, deep peroneal nerve; S, sural nerve.) (Adapted from Anatomical Society of Great Britain and Ireland. Report of Committee of Collective Investigation on the Distribution of Cutaneous Nerves on the Dorsum of the Foot. *J Anat Physiol.* 1891;26[pt I]:90.)

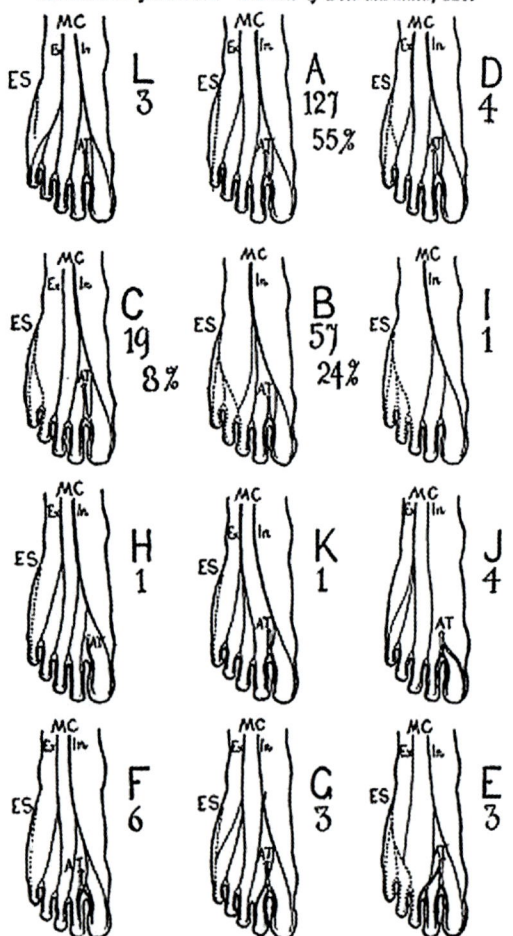

Figure 8.25 **Variations of the distribution of the cutaneous nerves on the dorsum of the foot** (229 ft examined). (From Report of Committee of Collective Investigation on the Distribution of Cutaneous Nerves on the Dorsum of the Foot. *J Anat Physiol.* 1891;26[pt I]:90, Table V.)

crural fascia posterior to the fibula 5.5 cm proximal to the ankle joint and coursed medially to cross the lateral aspect of the fibula at a mean distance 4.5 cm above the ankle joint (Fig. 8.29).

In type C (12%), the medial dorsal cutaneous nerve and the intermediate dorsal cutaneous nerve arose independently and the medial dorsal cutaneous nerve had a course similar to that in type A. The intermediate dorsal cutaneous nerve penetrated the crural fascia anterior to the fibula at an average of 4.9 cm above the ankle joint and continued in proximity to the anterior fibular border (Fig. 8.30).

From the topographic surgical point of view, "the medial dorsal cutaneous nerve was approximately one half the distance from the tip of the lateral malleolus to the medial malleolus. The intermediate dorsal cutaneous nerve was approximately one third the distance from the lateral malleolus to the medial malleolus."

Furthermore, "at the level of the ankle, the medial dorsal cutaneous nerve was usually found overlying the interval between the extensor digitorum longus and the extensor hallucis longus" and "the intermediate dorsal cutaneous nerve was usually located slightly lateral to the extensor digitorum longus."

Canovas et al[17] investigated the division of the superficial peroneal nerve in the leg and the distribution of the branches on the dorsum of the foot based on the dissection of 30 embalmed legs. The superficial peroneal nerve emerged through the crural fascia 11 cm on average from the distal tip of the lateral malleolus (range, 9-11.5 cm).

In 97% (29 cases), the superficial peroneal nerve divided above the extensor retinaculum into the medial dorsal cutaneous nerve and the intermediate dorsal cutaneous nerve. In 3% (one case), the two branches emerged from the crural fascia separately. An anastomosis between the medial dorsal cutaneous nerve and the intermediate dorsal cutaneous nerve was found in 47% (14 cases). Based on the 12 distribution patterns as defined by the Great Britain and Irish Anatomical Society,[16] their findings were as follows: type I, 80% (24 cases); type II, 10% (three cases); and type III, 10% (three cases).

Sayli et al[21] investigated the pattern of division of the superficial peroneal nerve in 30 fixed adult cadaver specimens. They adopted the classification of Blair and Botte.[20] Their findings were as follows: type A (73%), type B (13%), and type C (10%).

In type A, "the distance between the penetration point and the ankle joint was 10.41 ± 2.27 cm. The distance between the division point and the ankle joint was 3.70 ± 0.92 cm" (Fig. 8.31).

In type B, "the medial cutaneous branch pierced the fascia 11.2 ± 2.05 cm proximal to the ankle from the anterior compartment and had a similar course as in type A. The intermediate branch pierced the fascia posterior to the fibula 8.1 ± 1.93 cm proximal to the ankle joint and crossed anteriorly over the fibula 5.1 ± 1.01 cm proximal to the ankle" (Fig. 8.32).

In type C, "the medial dorsal cutaneous nerve pierced the crural fascia ~8.40 ± 0.42 cm proximal to the ankle joint and had a course similar to type A. The intermediate dorsal cutaneous nerve penetrated the fascia between the fibula and the tibia at about 6.43 ± 1.02 cm proximal to the ankle joint" (Fig. 8.33). In one case, "the deep peroneal nerve pierced the crural fascia more proximally and superficially and traveled parallel close to the superficial peroneal nerve at the ankle level" (Fig. 8.34).

The medial dorsal cutaneous nerve was almost located at the middle of the intermalleolar space with a mean perpendicular distance of 5.7 ± 0.9 cm from the tip of the medial malleolus and 5.3 ± 0.8 cm to the tip of the lateral malleolus. The intermediate dorsal cutaneous nerve was 6.91 ± 1.12 cm away from the medial malleolus and 3.9 ± 0.86 cm away from the lateral malleolus.

The findings of Sayli et al[21] were in agreement with the findings of Blair and Botte,[20] thus in an anatomic pool of 55 legs/ft.

Based on the dissection of 68 cadaver legs/ft, Solomon et al[18] reported on the variation in the distribution of the cutaneous nerves on the dorsum of the foot. In 35% (24 cases), the superficial peroneal nerve branched into the medial dorsal cutaneous nerve and the intermediate dorsal cutaneous nerve before piercing the crural fascia. The SPN or the IDCN pierced the crural fascia at 91 ± 23 mm to the tip of the lateral

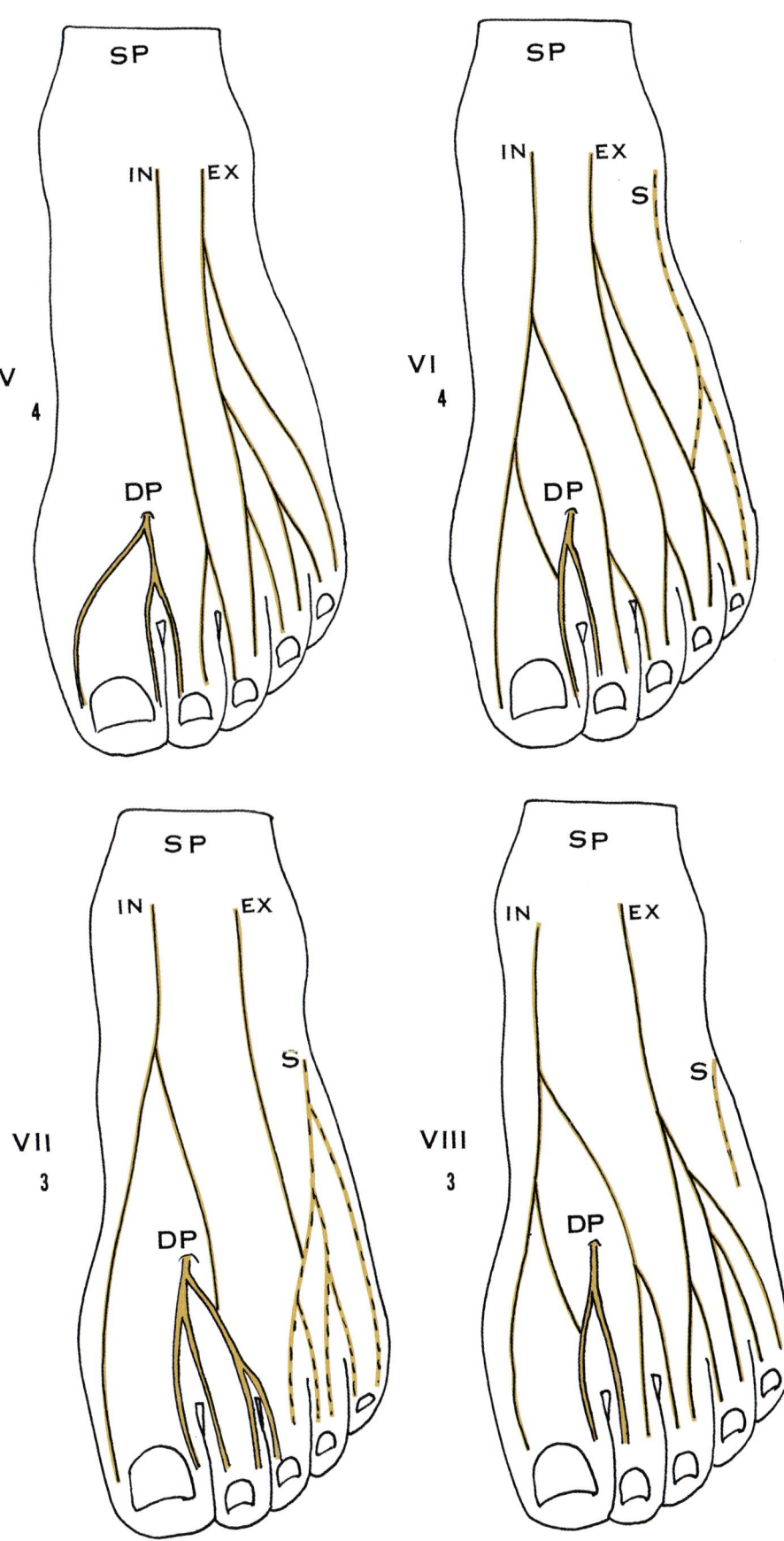

Figure 8.26 Variations in the distribution of the cutaneous nerves on the dorsum of the foot (229 ft examined). Type V (J) (4 of 229): The deep peroneal nerve predominates and the sural nerve is absent. **Type VI (D)** (4 of 229): Similar to type I except for anastomotic branch from the sural nerve to the external division branch (intermediate cutaneous branch) of the superficial peroneal nerve. **Type VII (E)** (3 of 229): The sural nerve and the deep peroneal nerve predominate. **Type VIII (L)** (3 of 229): The sural nerve is nearly absent. (*SP*, superficial peroneal nerve; *IN*, internal division branch of *SP*; *EX*, external division branch of *SP*; *DP*, deep peroneal nerve; *S*, sural nerve.) (Adapted from Anatomical Society of Great Britain and Ireland. Report of Committee of Collective Investigation on the Distribution of Cutaneous Nerves on the Dorsum of the Foot. *J Anat Physiol.* 1891;26[pt I]:90.)

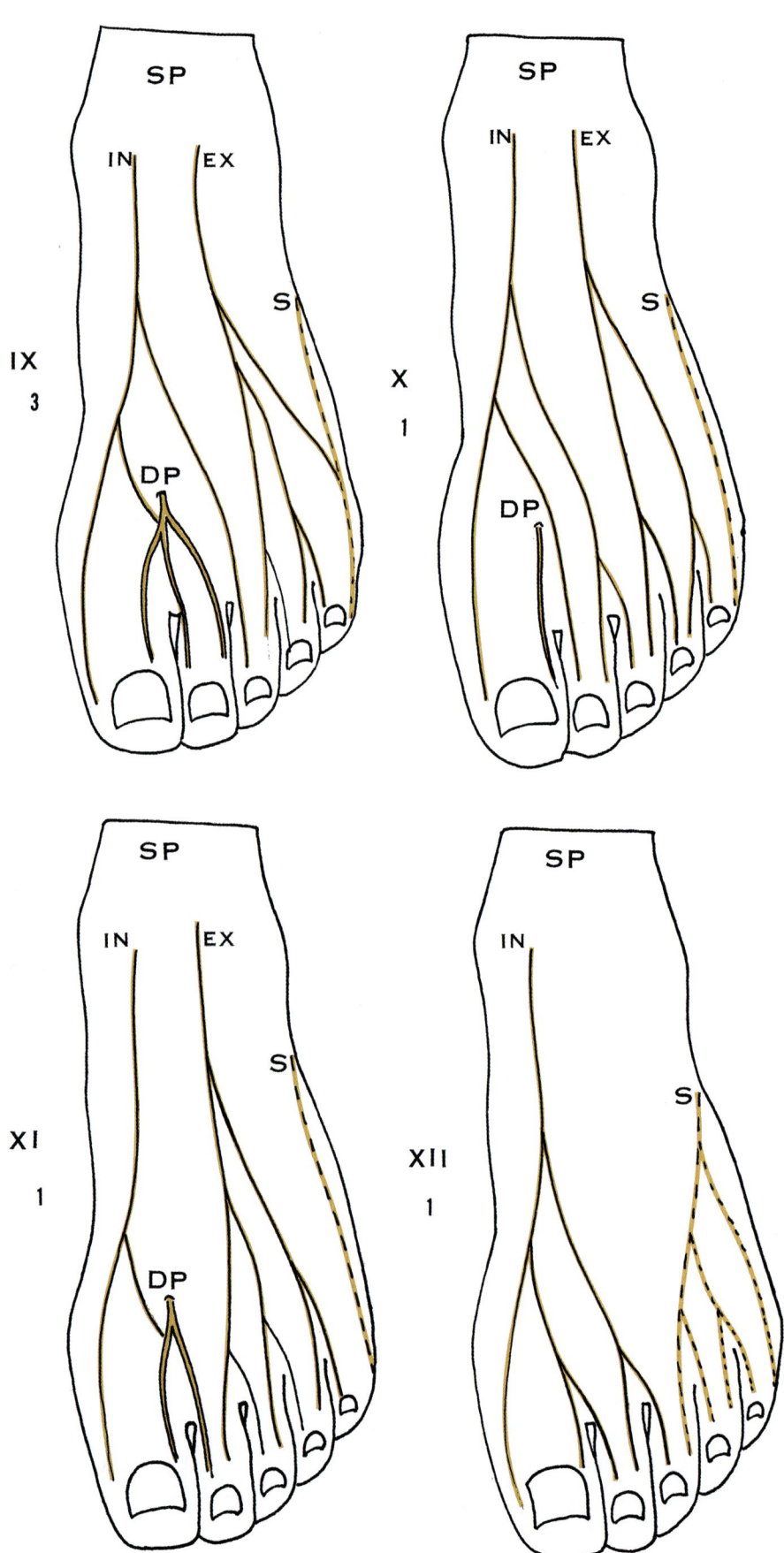

Figure 8.27 Variations in the distribution of the cutaneous nerves on the dorsum of the foot (229 ft examined). **Type IX (G)** (3 of 229): The deep peroneal predominates. The lateral peroneal nerve extends laterally. **Type X (H)** (1 of 229): The deep peroneal nerve has minimal contribution. **Type XI (K)** (1 of 229): The external division branch of the superficial peroneal nerve predominates. **Type XII (L)** (1 of 229): The deep peroneal nerve has no contribution. The sural nerve predominates. (*SP*, superficial peroneal nerve; *IN*, internal division branch of *SP*; *EX*, external division branch of *SP*; *DP*, deep peroneal nerve; *S*, sural nerve.) (Adapted from Anatomical Society of Great Britain and Ireland. Report of Committee of Collective Investigation on the Distribution of Cutaneous Nerves on the Dorsum of the Foot. *J Anat Physiol.* 1891;26[pt I]:90.)

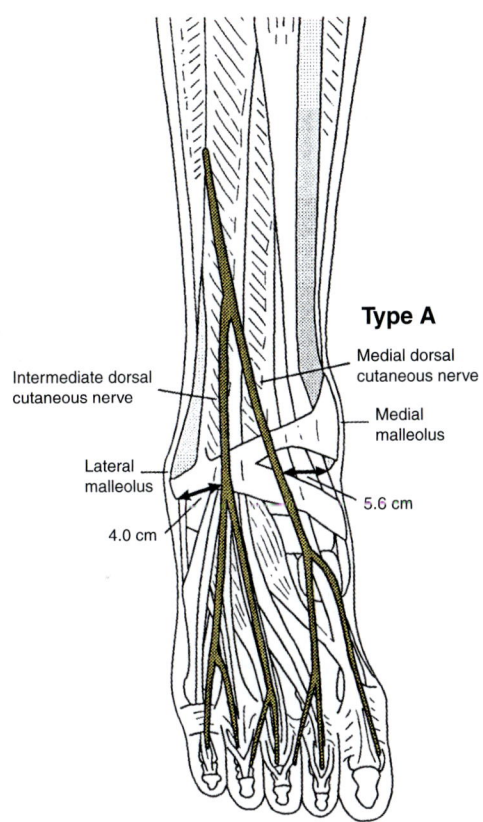

Figure 8.28 Course and branch pattern of superficial peroneal nerve in type A. (Adapted from Blair JM, Botte MJ. Surgical anatomy of the superficial peroneal nerve in the ankle and foot. *Clin Orthop Relat Res*. 1994;305:229-238, Figure 1.)

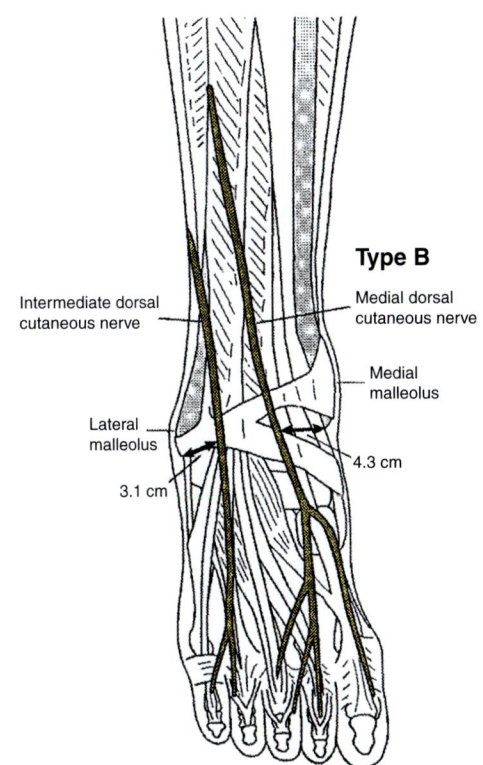

Figure 8.29 Course and branch pattern of superficial peroneal nerve in type B. (Adapted from Blair JM, Botte MJ. Surgical anatomy of the superficial peroneal nerve in the ankle and foot. *Clin Orthop Relat Res*. 1994;305:F229-F238, Figure 2.)

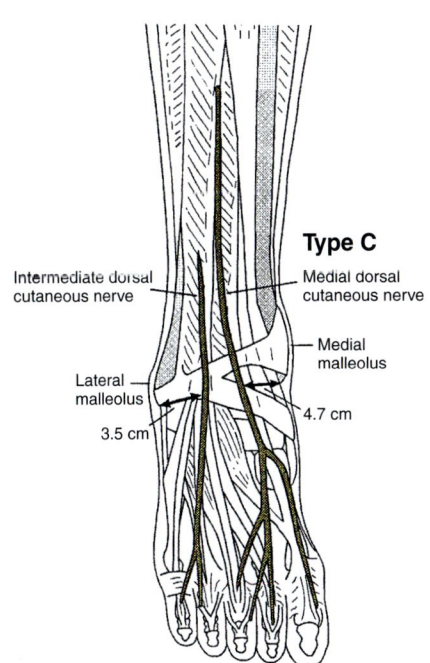

Figure 8.30 Course and branch pattern of superficial peroneal nerve in type C. (Adapted from Blair JM, Botte MJ. Surgical anatomy of the superficial peroneal nerve in the ankle and foot. *Clin Orthop Relat Res*. 1994;305:229-238. Figure 3.)

malleolus. The nerve was located at 3 ± 3 mm anterior to the anterior margin of the fibula at the level of the hiatus and at 23 ± 8 mm anterior to the margin of the malleolus at the level of the tip of the lateral malleolus. The sural nerve was located at an average of 7 ± 5 mm posterior to the lateral malleolus and an average 13 ± 7 mm distal to the tip of the lateral malleolus.

In 10% (seven cases), the sural nerve was tangent or crossed the distal tip of the lateral malleolus. In 6% (four cases), an anastomosis between the sural nerve and the intermediate dorsal cutaneous nerve was tangent to the tip of the lateral malleolus. In 59% (40 cases), the superficial peroneal nerve or the intermediate dorsal cutaneous nerve supplied branches to the lateral malleolar skin, and in 41% (28 cases), malleolar cutaneous branches were encountered.

The distribution pattern of innervations on the dorsum of the foot is presented in Figure 8.35.

Ucerler and Aktan Ikiz[22] investigated the variations of the branches of the superficial peroneal nerve based on the dissection of 30 cadaver lower limbs. They classified their findings into types 1, 2, and 3. In type 1 (63.3%), the nerve penetrated the crural fascia 80.15 ± 17.8 mm proximal to the intermalleolar line and then divided into the intermediate dorsal cutaneous and the medial dorsal cutaneous nerve. In type 2 (26.7%), the intermediate dorsal cutaneous nerve and the medial dorsal cutaneous nerve arose independently from the superficial

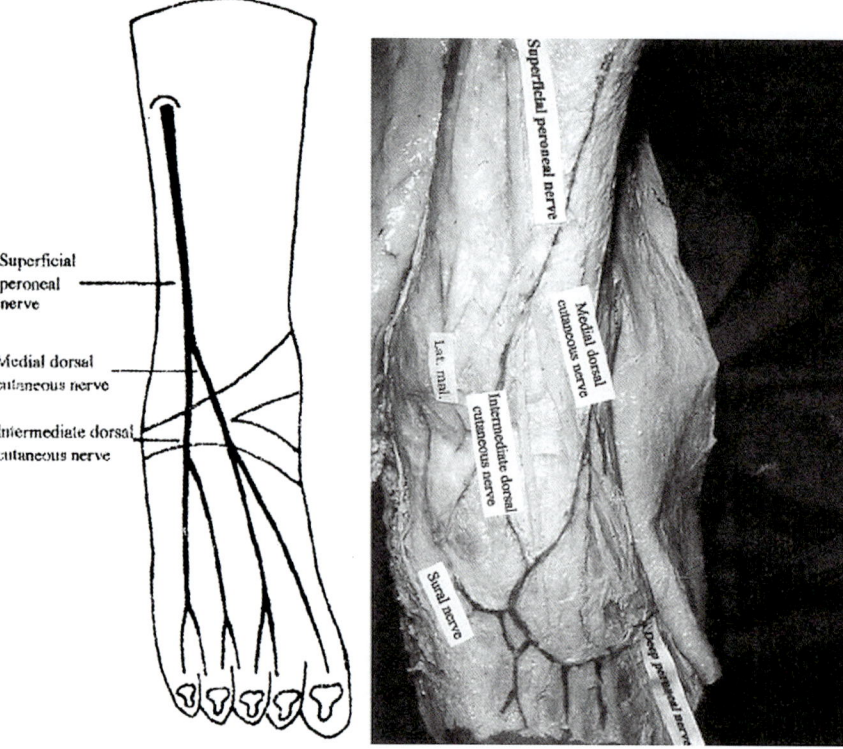

Figure 8.31 **Superficial peroneal nerve branching pattern type A.** (Reprinted from Sayli U, Tekdemyr Y, Cubuk HE, et al. The course of the superficial peroneal nerve: an anatomical cadaver study. *Foot Ankle Int*. 1998;4:63-69, Figure 1, with permission from Elsevier.)

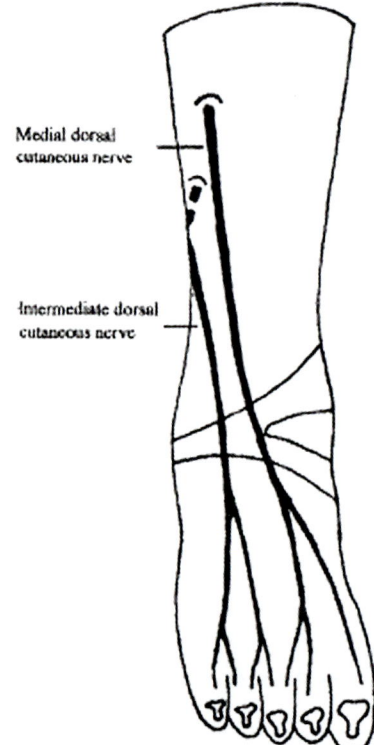
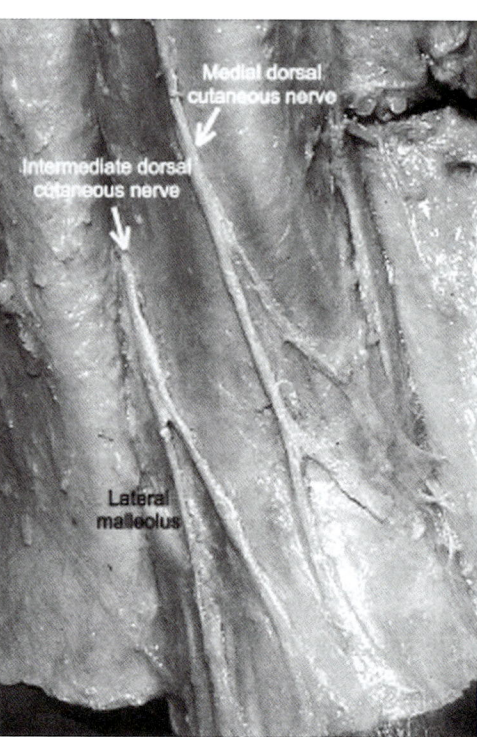

Figure 8.32 **Superficial peroneal nerve branching pattern type B.** (Reprinted from Sayli U, Tekdemyr Y, Cubuk HE, et al. The course of the superficial peroneal nerve: an anatomical cadaver study. *Foot Ankle Int*. 1998;4:63-69, Figure 2, with permission from Elsevier.)

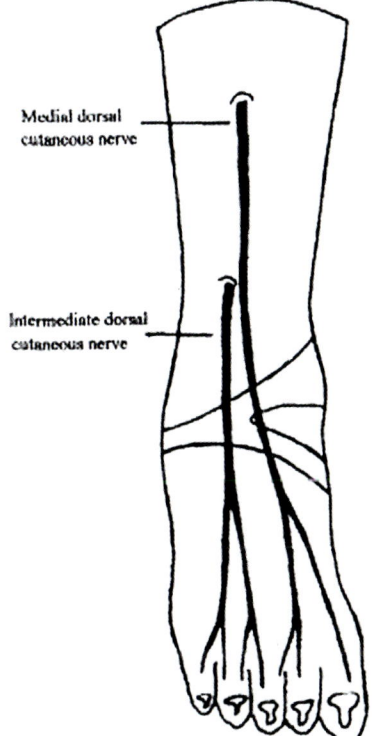
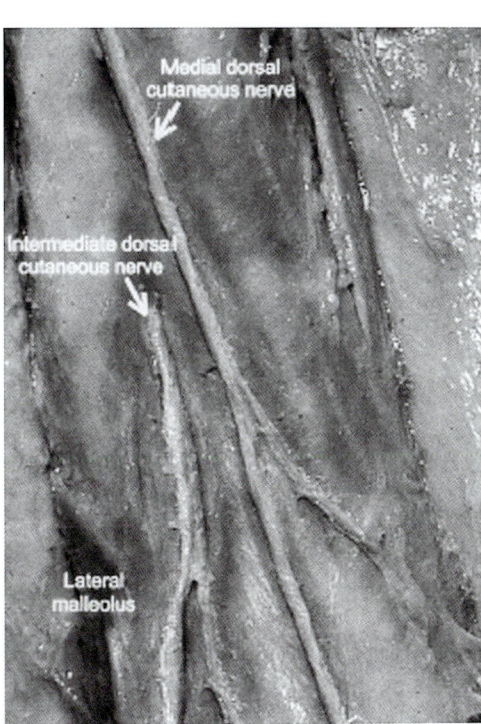

Figure 8.33 Superficial peroneal nerve branching pattern C. (Reprinted from Sayli U, Tekdemyr Y, Cubuk HE, et al. The course of the superficial peroneal nerve: an anatomical cadaver study. *Foot Ankle Int.* 1998;4:63-69, Figure 3, with permission from Elsevier.)

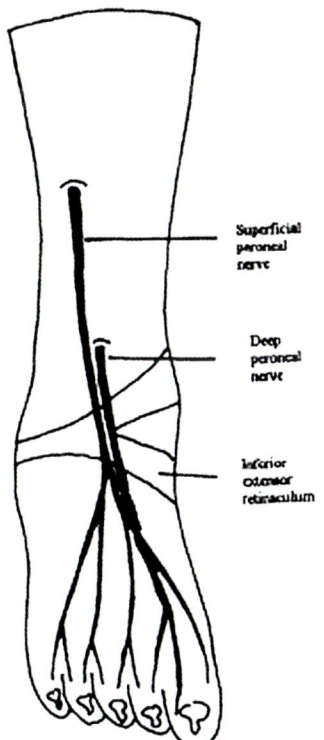
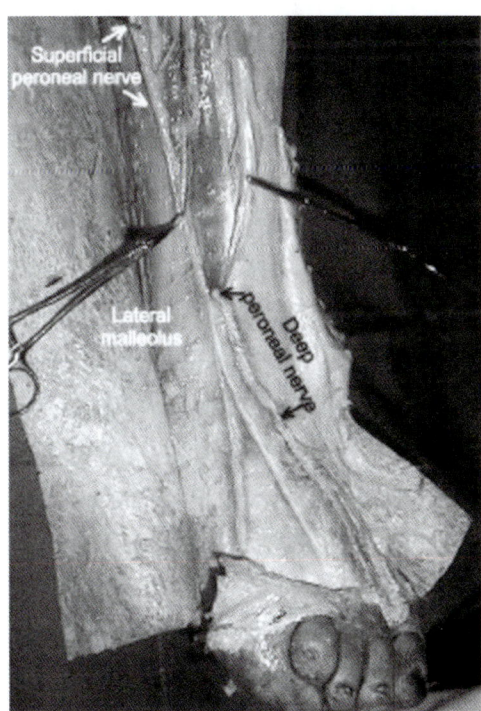

Figure 8.34 Deep peroneal nerve coursing close to the superficial peroneal nerve. (Reprinted from Sayli U, Tekdemyr Y, Cubuk HE, et al. The course of the superficial peroneal nerve: an anatomical cadaver study. *Foot Ankle Int.* 1998;4:63-69, Figure 4, with permission from Elsevier.)

peroneal nerve. In type 3 (10%), the superficial peroneal nerve penetrated the crural fascia 101.14 ± 70.27 mm proximal to the intermalleolar line as a single branch. This single branch had a course similar to the medial dorsal cutaneous nerve.

The intermalleolar distance, measured from the most prominent aspects of both malleoli, measured 98.70 ± 7.86 mm. The intermediate dorsal cutaneous nerve was 27.2 ± 7.8% of the intermalleolar distance and the medial dorsal cutaneous nerve was 53.4 ± 6.1% of the intermalleolar distance.

Aktan Ikiz and Ucerler[19] reported on the cutaneous nerve distribution of the sural nerve and of the superficial peroneal nerve, based on the same anatomic material of 30 cadaveric limbs. They classified their findings in seven types as indicated in Figure 8.36.

Miller and Hartman[23] investigated the origin and course of the dorsal medial cutaneous nerve of the first toe, based on the dissection of 12 ft. The dorsal medial cutaneous nerve of the first toe crosses dorsal to the extensor hallucis longus tendon proximal to the metatarso$_1$-cuneiform$_1$ joint (Fig. 8.37).

The average distance from the first metatarsocuneiform joint to the origin of the nerve was 40 mm (range, 8-61 mm). The average distance from the joint to where the nerve began to cross superficial to the extensor hallucis longus tendon was 32 mm (range, 8-50 mm). The nerve completed crossing

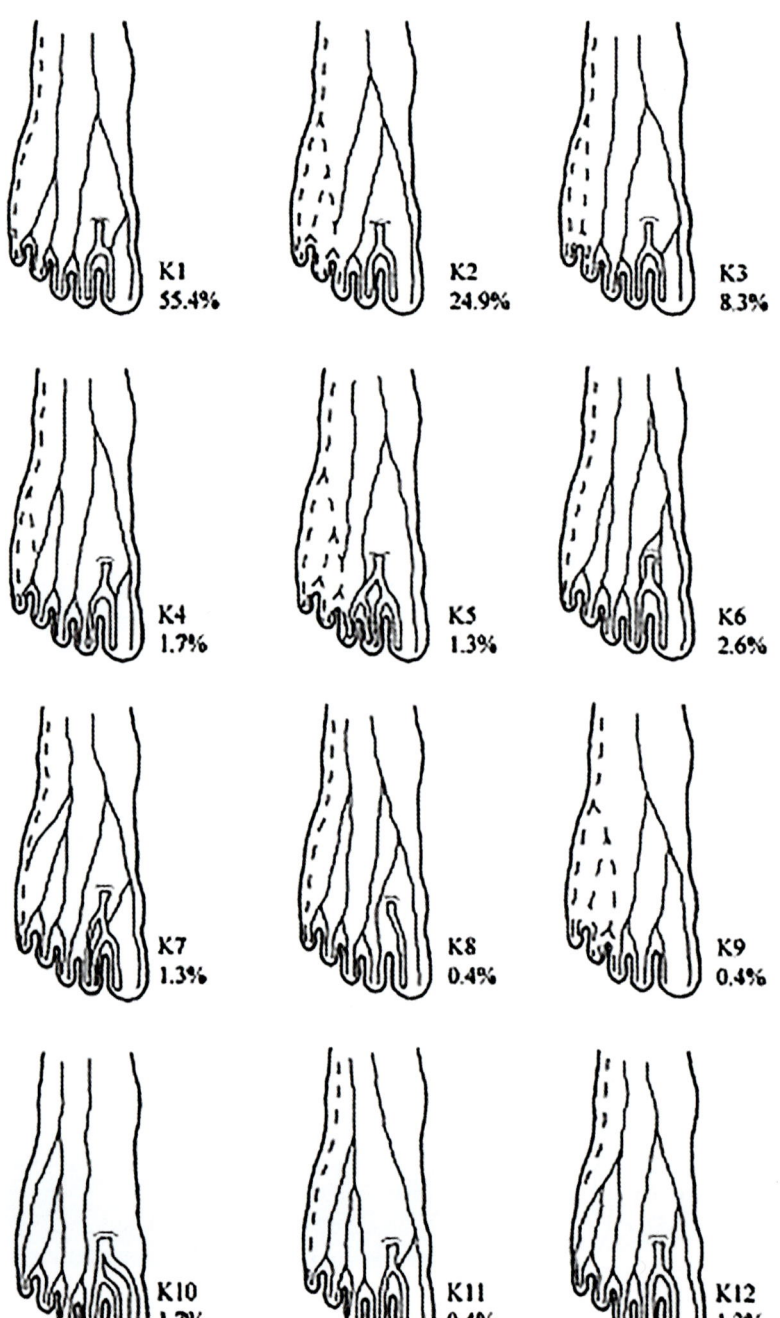

Figure 8.35 Innervation of the dorsum of the foot. Sural nerve (*dotted line*). Medial dorsal cutaneous nerve and intermediate dorsal cutaneous nerve (*continuous line*). Deep peroneal nerve (*double line*). (From Solomon LB, Ferris L, Tedman R, et al. Surgical anatomy of the sural and superficial fibular nerves with an emphasis on the approach to the lateral malleolus. *J Anat.* 2001;199:717-723, Figure 1.)

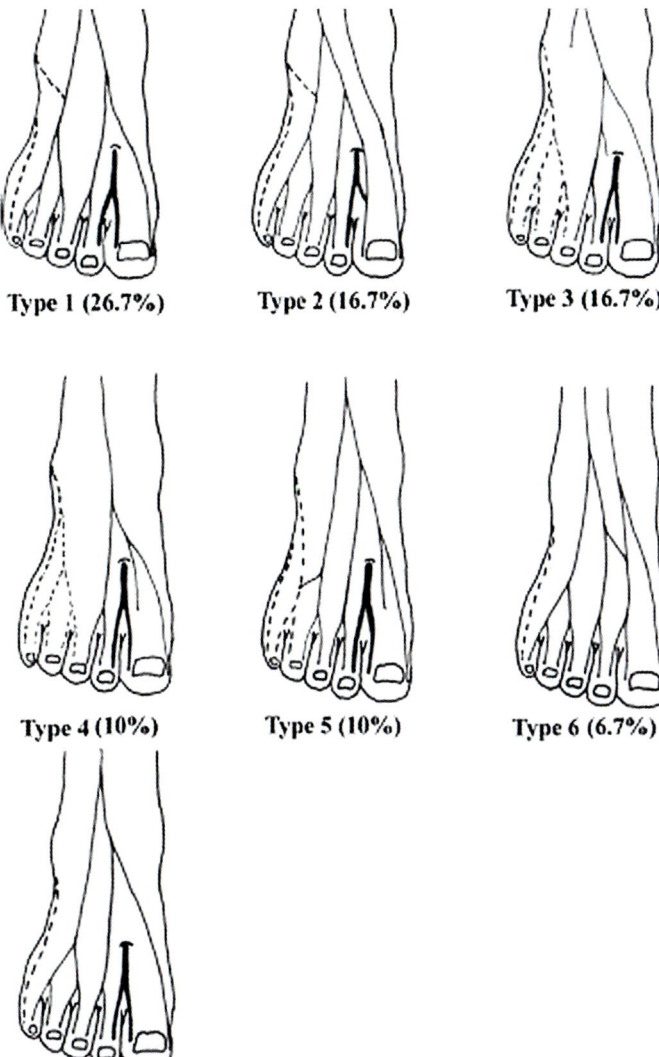

Figure 8.36 **Innervation of the dorsum of the foot and of the toes.** Sural nerve (*broken lines*); intermediate dorsal cutaneous nerve and medial dorsal cutaneous nerve (*continuous line*); deep peroneal nerve (*bold line*). (Aktan Ikiz ZA, Ucerler H. The distribution of the superficial peroneal nerve on the dorsum of the foot and its clinical importance. *Foot Ankle Int.* 2006;6:438-444, Figure 2. Copyright ©2006. Reprinted by Permission of SAGE Publications.)

the extensor hallucis longus tendon at an average distance of 16 mm proximal to the first metatarsocuneiform joint (range, 0-41 mm). The nerve did not overlie the tendon distal to the joint in any specimen. At the midpoint of the first metatarsal, the nerve was found at an average distance of 11 mm medial to the extensor hallucis longus tendon (range, 6-15 mm). At the metatarsophalangeal joint, the nerve was found at an average of 12 mm medial to the EHL tendon (range, 9-16 mm) (Fig. 8.38).

POSTERIOR TIBIAL NERVE

The posterior tibial nerve (tibial nerve) extends from the arcade of the soleus muscle to the calcaneal canal (Figs. 8.39 and 8.40). It is in direct vertical continuity with the sciatic nerve and shifts slightly to the medial side to reach the tibiotalocalcaneal canal; within this canal, the nerve divides into two terminal branches—medial and lateral plantar nerves.

In the upper two-thirds of its course, the posterior tibial nerve is located in the deep posterior compartment of the leg in the interval between the tibialis posterior muscle and the flexor digitorum longus anteriorly. Farther down, the nerve is located between the latter and the flexor hallucis longus.

In the interior third of the leg, the posterior tibial nerve is more superficial as the soleus and the gastrocnemii are converted to the Achilles tendon, thus exposing the nerve. The posterior tibial nerve now runs along the medial border of the Achilles tendon; the flexor hallucis longus tendon is lateral to the posterior tibial nerve and the flexor digitorum longus is anteromedial. Posteriorly and medially, the nerve is covered by the superficial and deep fasciae of the leg. The posterior tibial nerve remains lateral and slightly posterior to the posterior tibial artery.

The most common site of the posterior tibial nerve is 7.5 cm above the tip of the medial malleolus, in line with the medial border of the Achilles tendon.[1]

The terminal branches of the posterior tibial nerve are the medial and lateral plantar nerves (Figs. 8.41 and 8.42). The

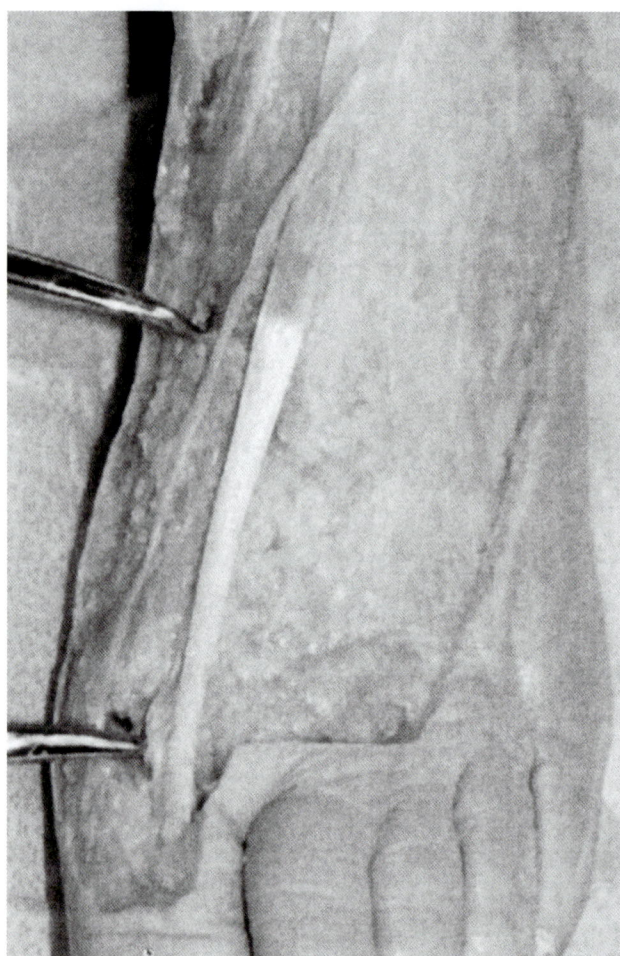

Figure 8.37 The medial dorsal cutaneous nerve to the great toe crosses dorsal to the extensor hallucis longus tendon proximal to the first metatarsocuneiform joint, which is indicated by the proximal hemostat. The second hemostat is at the level of the metacarpophalangeal joint. (Miller R, Hartman G. Origin and course of the dorsomedial cutaneous nerve to the great toe. *Foot Ankle Int*. 1996;17:620-622, Figure 3. Copyright ©1996. Reprinted by Permission of SAGE Publications.)

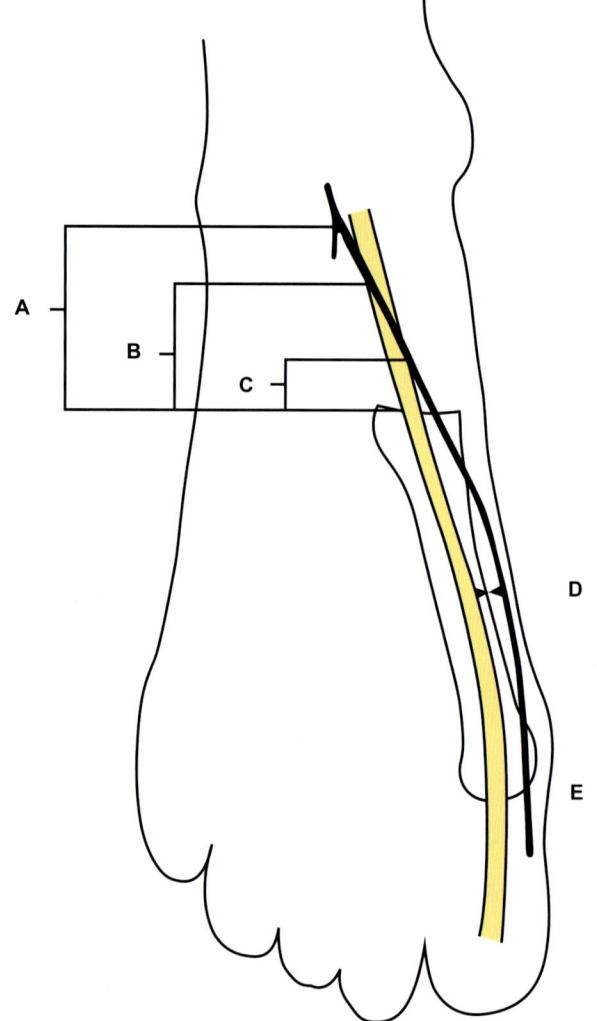

Figure 8.38 Medial dorsal cutaneous nerve. *(A)* Distance of origin of medial dorsal cutaneous nerve of first toe from the center of the first metatarsocuneiform joint. *(B)* Distance from the joint to where the nerve begins to cross the extensor hallucis longus tendon. *(C)* Distance to where the nerve finishes crossing over the tendon. *(D)* Distance of the nerve from the medial border of the extensor hallucis longus tendon at the midpoint of M1. *(E)* Distance of the nerve from the extensor hallucis longus tendon at the metacarpophalangeal joint. (Adapted from Miller R, Hartman G. Origin and course of the dorsomedial cutaneous nerve to the great toe. *Foot Ankle Int*. 1996;17:620-622.)

division occurs in the talocalcaneal tunnel, 1.3 to 2.5 cm proximal to the division of the posterior tibial artery.[1] The bifurcation of the posterior tibial nerve into its terminal branches occurs proximal to the medial malleolus; according to Horwitz, the bifurcation occurs 1.3 cm proximal to the tip of the medial malleolus and according to Macaggi, it occurs 1.5 cm proximal to the tip of the medial malleolus, with a higher bifurcation in 13.5%.[1,24] Hovelacque mentions having observed one bifurcation at 6 cm and another one at 10 cm above the tip of the medial malleolus.[25]

Dellon and Mackinnon studied the branching of the posterior tibial nerve in the tarsal tunnel in 31 cadaveric feet.[26] A reference line was determined extending "from the center of the medial malleolus to the center of the calcaneus, the malleolar-calcaneal axis" (Fig. 8.43). The bifurcation of the posterior tibial nerve was referred to this line, being at the level, proximal, or distal. In 90% of the feet, the bifurcation was within 1 cm of the malleolar-calcaneal axis, with 55% at the level, 16% at 1 cm distal, and 19% at 1 cm proximal to the reference line. In the remaining feet, the bifurcation was 2, 3, and 5 cm proximal to the axis and the authors concluded that in 95% the posterior tibial nerve bifurcates into its terminal branches within the tarsal tunnel. They defined the latter as extending 2 cm proximal and 2 cm distal to the malleolar-calcaneal axis. Havel and coworkers studied the branching of the posterior tibial nerve in the tarsal tunnel in 68 cadaveric feet.[27] They used the same malleolar-calcaneal axis as a reference line in their description. In 93%, the bifurcation occurred within the tarsal tunnel with the following distribution: at the axis, 38%; within ±1 cm of the axis, 76%; and within ±2 cm of the axis, 93%. Bifurcation proximal to the tunnel occurred in 7% (Fig. 8.44).

The posterior tibial nerve provides cutaneous, articular, and vascular branches.

The cutaneous branches are distributed to the skin of the medial malleolar area and to the inner aspect of the heel. The

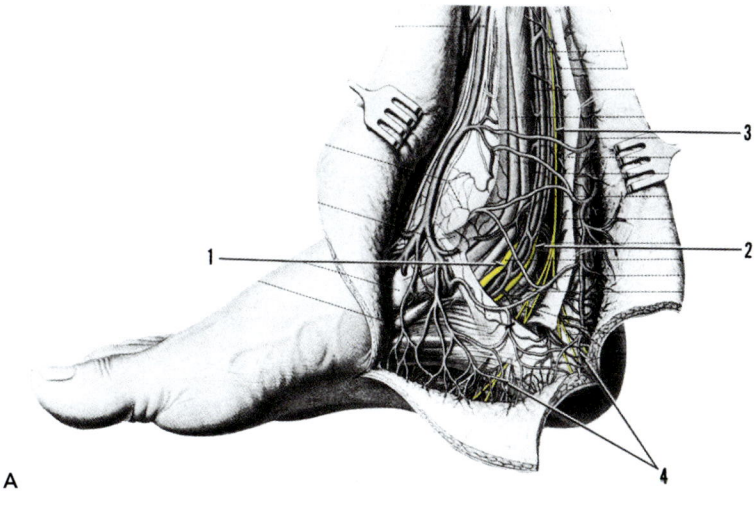

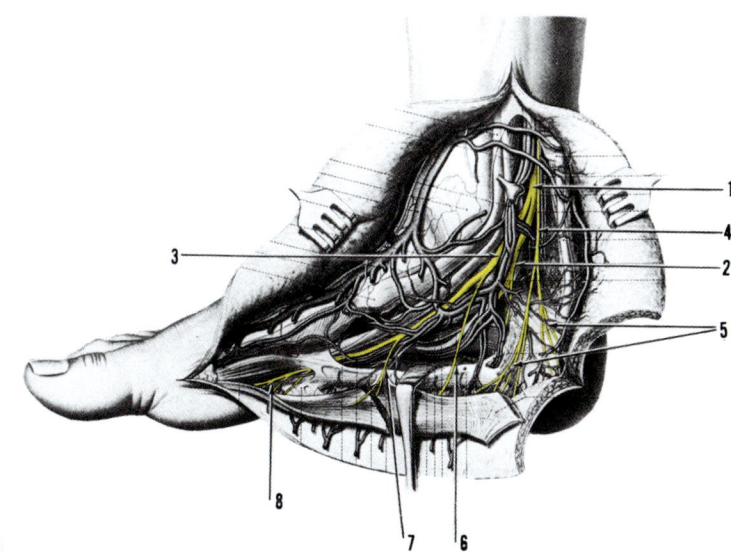

Figure 8.39 Medial aspect of the foot and ankle. (A) (1, Medial plantar nerve; 2, lateral plantar nerve; 3, calcaneal branch of posterior tibial nerve; 4, division branches of 3.) **(B)** Flexor retinaculum and abductor hallucis muscle reflected plantarward. (1, Posterior tibial nerve; 2, lateral plantar nerve; 3, medial plantar nerve; 4, calcaneal branch of posterior tibial nerve; 5, division branches of 4; 6, 7, branches to abductor hallucis muscle; 8, hallucal medial plantar nerve.) (Reprinted by permission from Lanz T, Wachsmuth W. *Praktische Anatomie Bein und Statik Erster Band.* 4th ed. Springer-Verlag; 1972:339-340.)

medial malleolar branch is very thin and perforates the aponeurosis of the ankle just proximal to the medial malleolus, supplies the skin covering the malleolus, and often anastomoses with a branch of the saphenous nerve.

The medial calcaneal nerve has a variable origin. Dellon and Mackinnon studied the origin of the nerve in 20 dissected feet and found posterior tibial nerve origin in 90% and lateral plantar nerve origin in 10%.[26]

In 40%, the medial calcaneal nerve origin was proximal to the tarsal tunnel and the nerve entered the heel from outside the tunnel (Fig. 8.45). In 25%, a single medial calcaneal nerve originated from the posterior tibial nerve within the tunnel, and in another 25%, two medial calcaneal nerve branches were found, both originating from the posterior tibial nerve—one proximal to and one within the tarsal tunnel. In 10% the origin was from the lateral plantar nerve within the tunnel.

Havel and colleagues studied the origin of the medial calcaneal nerve in 68 ft.[27] The origin was highly variable. A single medial calcaneal nerve was present in 79% and multiple branches in 21%. The most frequent pattern was a single medial calcaneal nerve arising from the posterior tibial nerve in 69%, with 34% within and 35% proximal to the tarsal tunnel. The medial calcaneal nerve originated also from the lateral plantar nerve as a single branch in 19% or as multiple branches from the posterior tibial nerve and lateral plantar nerve in 7%, and from the lateral plantar nerve and the medial plantar nerve in 3%. In 1%, the medial calcaneal nerve branched off from the medial plantar nerve as a single branch and, in 1%, it branched off from the posterior tibial nerve and medial plantar nerve as multiple branches.

The medial calcaneal branch pierces the aponeurosis at a variable point and immediately divides into two or three branches (Fig. 8.46), which at times could arise separately. The posterior branch or calcaneal branch proper is distributed to the skin covering the medial aspect of the Achilles tendon and the medial and posterior aspect of the heel. The two other anterior branches are plantar; they course along the inner border of the foot and pass through the very thick layer of adipose tissue, and the terminal branches are distributed to the skin of

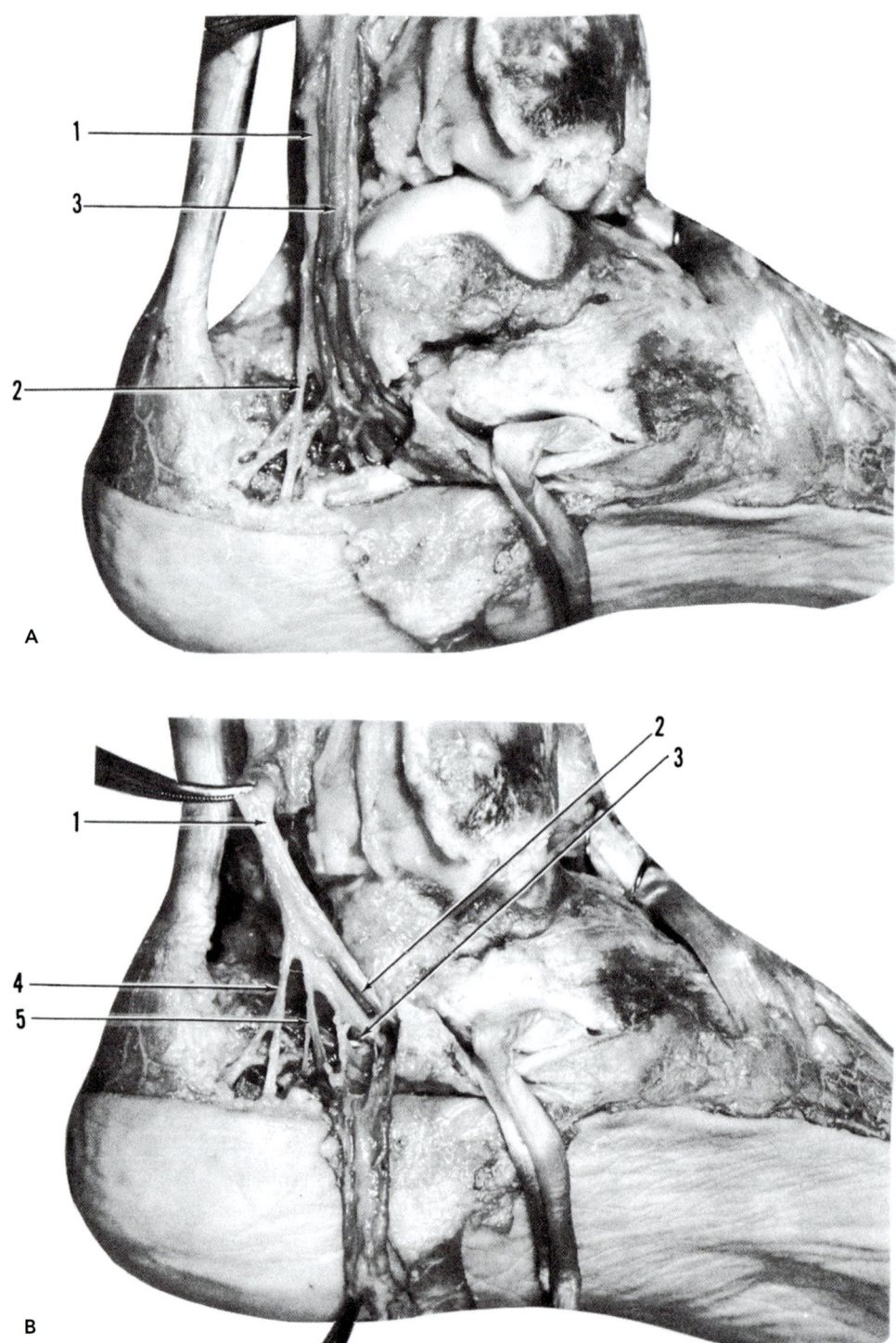

Figure 8.40 Medial aspect of the left ankle and foot. (A) (*1*, Posterior tibial nerve; *2*, calcaneal branch of *1*; *3*, posterior tibial vessels.) (B) Posterior tibial vessels reflected plantarward. (*1*, Posterior tibial nerve; *2*, medial plantar nerve; *3*, lateral plantar nerve; *4*, medial calcaneal cutaneous nerve branches; *5*, nerve to abductor digiti quinti.)

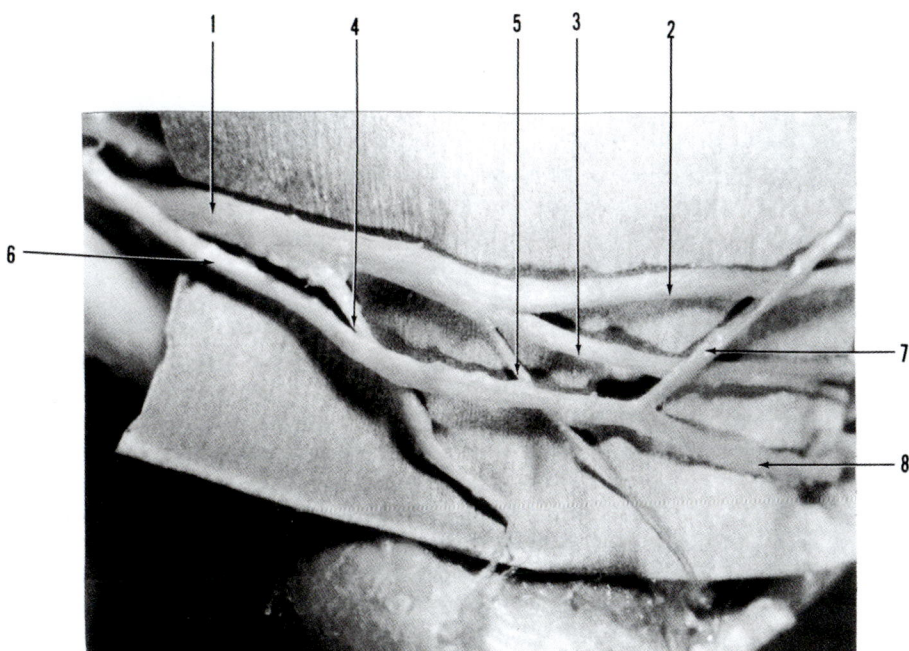

Figure 8.41 **Posterior tibial nerve (1) dividing into medial plantar nerve (2) and lateral plantar nerve (3).** Medial calcaneal nerve (4); branch to the abductor digiti quinti muscle (5) arising from the posterior tibial nerve just proximal to the lateral plantar nerve; posterior tibial artery (6) dividing into the medial (7) and lateral (8) plantar arteries. The arterial bifurcation is distal to the bifurcation of the posterior tibial nerve.

the posterior third of the sole (Fig. 8.47). Medially the terminal branches anastomose with the calcaneal branches of the saphenous nerve and the cutaneous branches of the medial plantar nerve. Laterally the terminal calcaneal branches anastomose with branches of the sural nerve, and anteriorly they anastomose with branches of the lateral plantar nerve.

The articular branches, one and occasionally two, arise from the posterior tibial nerve near its bifurcation. They are directed anteriorly, pass between the tibialis posterior tendon and the flexor digitorum longus tendon, and innervate the ankle joint. A few fibers penetrate between the deep and superficial layers of the deltoid ligament, whereas others remain on the surface of the superficial layer of the ligament.[28]

The vascular branches arise from the terminal portion of the posterior tibial nerve and form nerve loops around the posterior tibial artery; occasionally they form a plexus—the posterior tibial retromalleolar plexus of Lazorthe.[29] Among these vascular nerve branches there is usually one larger branch that bifurcates at the site of division of the posterior tibial artery, and each nerve branch accompanies the corresponding plantar medial and lateral arteries. This vascular branch anchors the bifurcation of the posterior tibial artery and nerve to each other.[30]

Davis and Schon[31] analyzed the branching of the posterior tibial nerve in 20 ankles, "starting 10 cm proximal to the medial malleolus to points 6 cm distal to the tibial nerve bifurcation." Measurements were made using the Dellon-Mackinnon medial-malleolar-calcaneal axis.

The posterior tibial nerve bifurcated into the medial plantar nerve and the LPN in the tarsal tunnel, within ±2 cm of the medial-malleolar-calcaneal axis in 90% and proximal to the tarsal tunnel in 10% (two cases) within, respectively, 5 and 9 cm proximal to the medial-malleolar-calcaneal axis.

The calcaneal nerves originated proximal to the tarsal tunnel in 70% and within only the tarsal tunnel in 30%. In 35%, "the sole origin of the calcaneal nerves was 7 cm or more proximal to the medial-malleolar-calcaneal axis." In 60% of the specimens, the calcaneal branches were multiple. The first branch or nerve to the abductor digiti minimi bifurcated from the lateral plantar nerve within 2 cm of the posterior tibial nerve bifurcation in 90%.

In 15% (three cases), branches of the first branch innervated the abductor hallucis in conjunction with branches from the medial plantar nerve (Figs. 8.48 and 8.49). In 5% (one case), the sole innervations of the abductor hallucis was from the posterior tibial nerve "originating 2 cm proximal to the tibial bifurcation" (Fig. 8.50).

In 90%, the innervations of the abductor hallucis were from branches of the medial plantar nerve "approximately 3 to 4 cm distal to the origin of the medial plantar nerve on the medial aspect of the abductor hallucis muscle."

Govsa et al[32] investigated the variations of the origin of the medial and inferior calcaneal nerves based on the dissection of 50 cadaveric feet. The medial calcaneal nerve originated from the following:

- Tibial nerve: 11 of 50 cases
- Lateral plantar nerve and tibial nerve: 9 of 50 cases
- Tibial nerve and medial plantar nerve: 6 of 50 cases
- Lateral plantar nerve: 7 of 50 cases
- Tibial nerve, medial plantar nerve, and lateral plantar nerve: 6 of 50 cases

The medial calcaneal nerve consisted of one major branch, two major branches, three major branches, and four major branches.

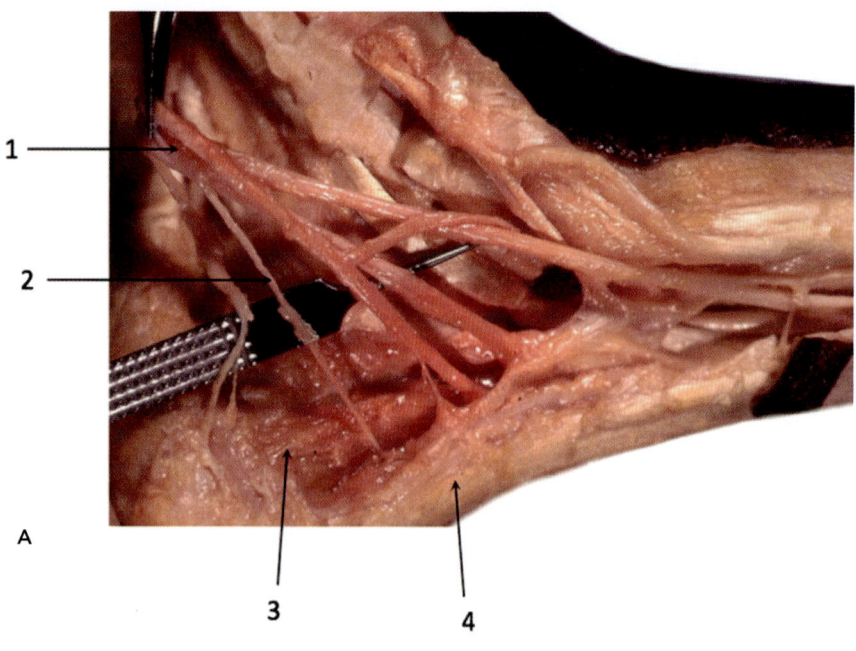

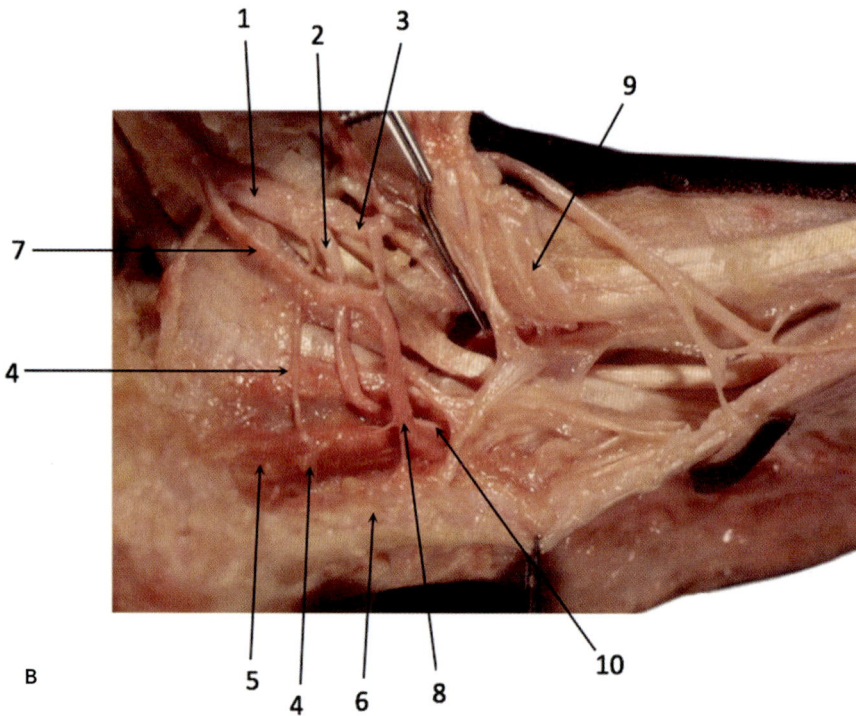

Figure 8.42 (A) Posterior tibial nerve (1); nerve branch to the abductor digiti quinti (2) passing between the quadratus plantae muscle (3) and the plantar aponeurosis overlying the origin of the flexor digitorum brevis (4). The abductor hallucis muscle has been reflected. (B) Posterior tibial nerve (1) dividing into lateral plantar nerve (2) and medial plantar nerve (3); nerve to abductor digiti quinti (4) arises just proximal to the lateral plantar nerve and passes between the abductor hallucis muscle (9) reflected in the present preparation and the quadratus plantae. Subsequently, the nerve to the abductor digiti quinti (4) passes between the quadratus plantae (5) and the common segment of the plantar aponeurosis and the flexor digitorum brevis (6); posterior tibial artery (7); lateral plantar artery (8); and the lateral plantar nerve enter the inferior calcaneal chamber (10).

The inferior calcaneal nerve originated from the tibial nerve or from the lateral plantar nerve shortly (9-11 mm) after the tibial nerve bifurcation. The patterns of origin of the inferior calcaneal nerve are as indicated in Figure 8.51.

▶ Medial Plantar Nerve

The medial plantar nerve (see Figs. 8.41, 8.42, and 8.52) is the anterior division branch of the posterior tibial nerve (Figs. 8.53 to 8.55). In general, it is larger than the lateral plantar nerve. Directed obliquely downward and anteriorly, it crosses the lateral surface of the posterior tibial artery and locates itself anterior to the medial plantar artery. Proximally the posterior tibial neurovascular bundle is contained in a neurovascular compartment limited posteriorly by the deep aponeurosis of the leg and located in the interval between the tunnels of the flexor hallucis longus laterally and the flexor digitorum longus anteromedially. In the lower segment, the calcaneal canal is subdivided into two chambers, upper and lower, by the semitransverse interfascicular septum extending from the deep investing fascia of the abductor hallucis to the upper border of the flexor accessorius immediately below the tunnel of the flexor hallucis

Chapter 8: Nerves 411

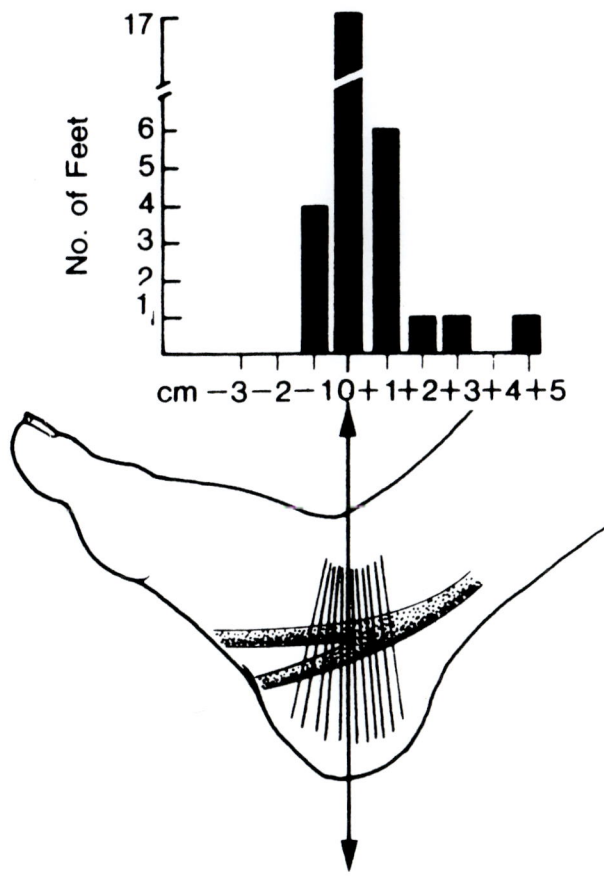

Figure 8.43 Distribution of location of bifurcation of tibial nerve with respect to malleolar-calcaneal axis. (Reproduced with permission from Dellon AL, Mackinnon SE. Tibial nerve branching in the tarsal tunnel. *Arch Neurol*. 1984;41:645. Copyright©1984.American Medical Association. All rights reserved.)

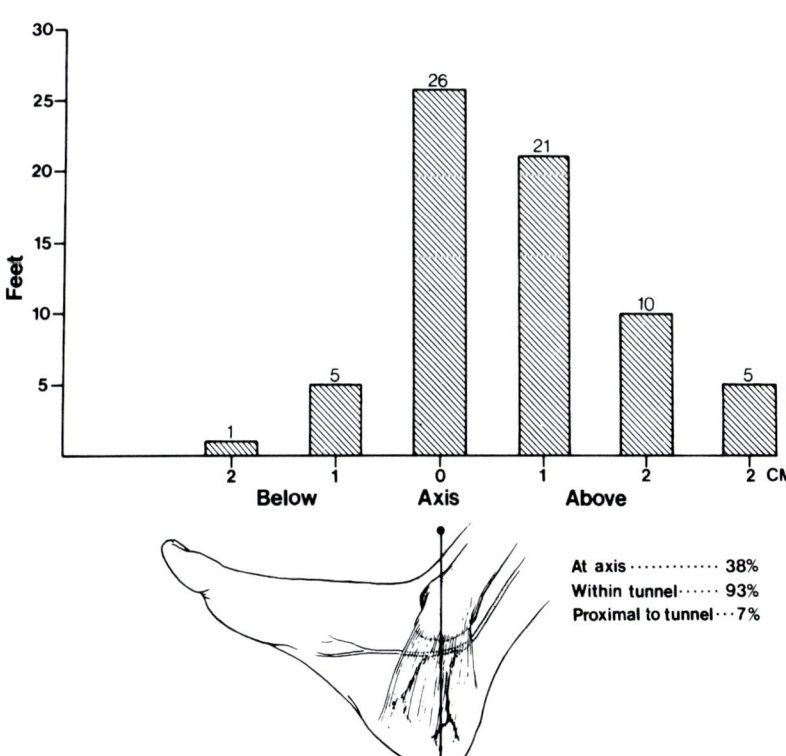

Figure 8.44 Distribution of posterior tibial nerve branching. (Havel PE, Ebraheim NA, Clark S, et al. Tibial nerve branching in the tarsal tunnel. *Foot Ankle*. 1988;9[3]:117. Copyright ©1988. Reprinted by Permission of SAGE Publications.)

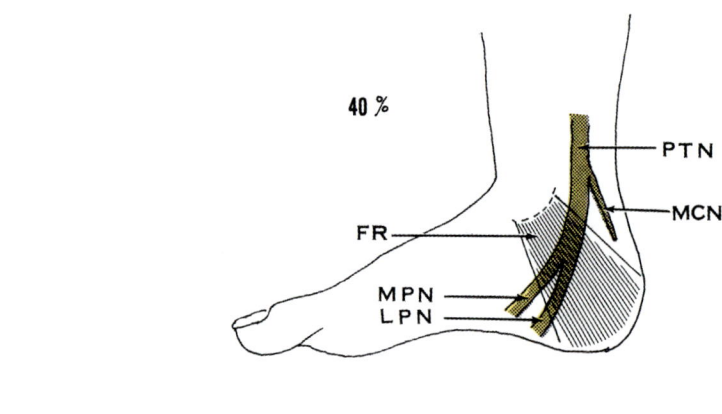
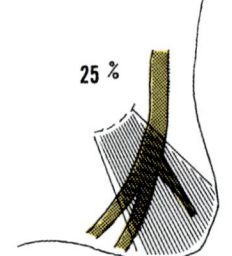
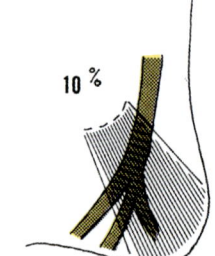
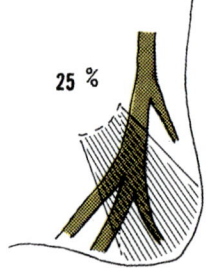

Figure 8.45 Pattern of origin of medial calcaneal nerve from posterior tibial nerve in 20 ft. (*PTN*, posterior tibial nerve; *MCN*, medial calcaneal nerve; *MPN*, medial plantar nerve; *FR*, flexor retinaculum.) (Adapted from Dellon AL, Mackinnon SE. Tibial nerve branching in the tarsal tunnel. *Arch Neurol*. 1984;41:645.)

longus. The medial plantar nerve and the medial plantar artery pass through the upper chamber, the nerve remaining anterior to the artery. They are covered medially by the superior segment of the abductor hallucis muscle and the laciniate ligament. At this level, the medial neurovascular bundle corresponds to the tunnel of the flexor hallucis longus tendon laterally. The medial plantar nerve leaves the calcaneal canal, penetrates the sole of the foot, and passes on the plantar aspect of intersection of the flexor hallucis longus and the flexor digitorum longus tendon. The nerve is located deep in the interval between the abductor hallucis and the flexor digitorum brevis and may be partially covered by the former. The medial plantar nerve now lies in the medial wall of the middle compartment of the sole of the foot, and at about the level of the base of the first metatarsal, the nerve divides into its terminal branches, medial and lateral.

During its course, the medial plantar nerve provides cutaneous, muscular, articular, and vascular branches. The cutaneous branches arise as soon as the nerve enters the sole of the foot. They are directed downward in the interval between the abductor of the big toe and the flexor digitorum brevis, perforate the aponeurosis, and supply branches to the skin of the inner aspect of the sole of the foot. They anastomose with terminal branches of the medial calcaneal nerve. The muscular branches to the abductor hallucis (two or, occasionally, three in number) branch off from the medial aspect of the medial plantar nerve as separate branches or as a common trunk. They are directed anteriorly and medially, pass through small fibrous tunnels, and enter the muscle from the lateral side into the deep surface.[30] The muscular branch to the flexor digitorum brevis is often double and arises from the lateral border of the nerve, usually at the same level as the nerve of the abductor hallucis; it is directed anteriorly and laterally and penetrates the muscle from its deep surface near the inner border at the junction of the posterior third and anterior two-thirds of the foot.[25] The articular branches arise from the medial border of the nerve, distal to the previous motor branches, and provide branches to the talonavicular and cuneonavicular joints. The vascular branches are very thin and variable in number (two or three) and reach the medial plantar artery and its branches.[30]

At the level of the base of the first metatarsal, the medial plantar nerve divides into its terminal branches, medial and lateral. The medial branch is the thinner of the two; it courses anteromedially over the medial head of the flexor hallucis brevis between the flexor hallucis longus laterally and the abductor hallucis tendon medially. It terminates as the medial plantar cutaneous nerve of the big toe, which also provides a sensory branch reaching the dorsomedial aspect of the distal phalanx of the big toe. During its course, the medial branch gives motor branches—one or two—to the medial head of the flexor hallucis brevis and often one branch to the lateral head of the same muscle. The lateral branch of the medial plantar nerve, the larger of the two, is located in the interval between the abductor hallucis brevis and the flexor digitorum brevis. This nerve now bulges into the middle compartment of the sole but still is separated from the latter by a layer of fascia.[33] It passes around the medial border of the flexor digitorum brevis, enters the superficial space (M_1) of the middle compartment of the sole, and divides into three common digital branches.[33]

The first common digital nerve is directed toward the first web space. It courses plantar to the lateral head of the short flexor of the big toe and is located between the flexor hallucis longus medially and the flexor digitorum longus to the second

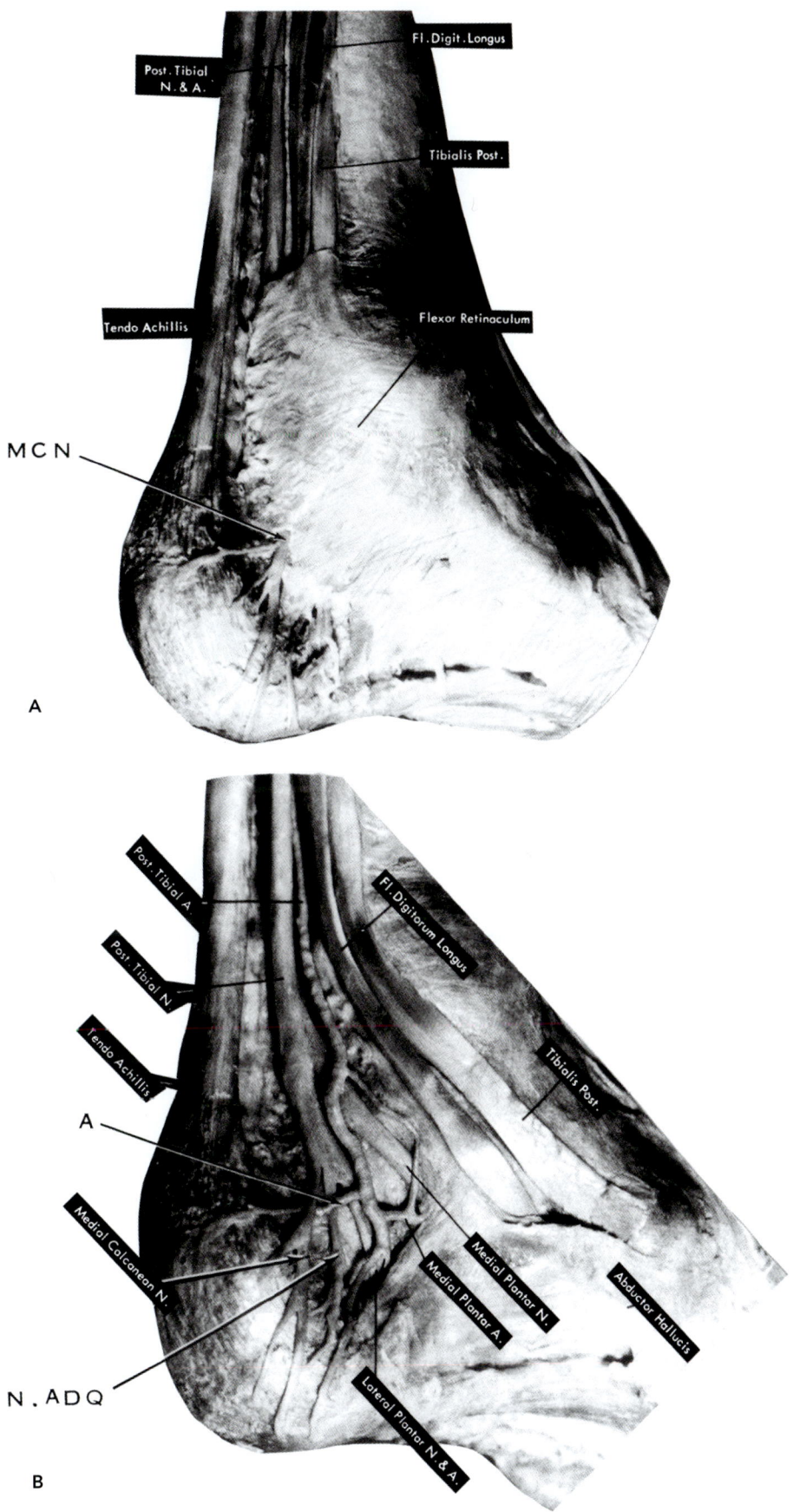

Figure 8.46 Medial calcaneal nerve (MCN). (A) Medial calcaneal nerve piercing the flexor retinaculum and dividing into multiple branches supplying the heel. **(B)** Medial calcaneal nerve arising low from the posterior tibial nerve and branching off at the heel. The nerve to the abductor digiti quinti (N.ADQ) arises just proximal to the lateral plantar nerve and is crossed near its origin by an arterial branch (A) of the posterior tibial artery. (From Cosentino R. *Atlas of Anatomy and Surgical Approaches in Orthopedic Surgery*. Vol 2. The Lower Extremity. Charles C Thomas; 1960:219.)

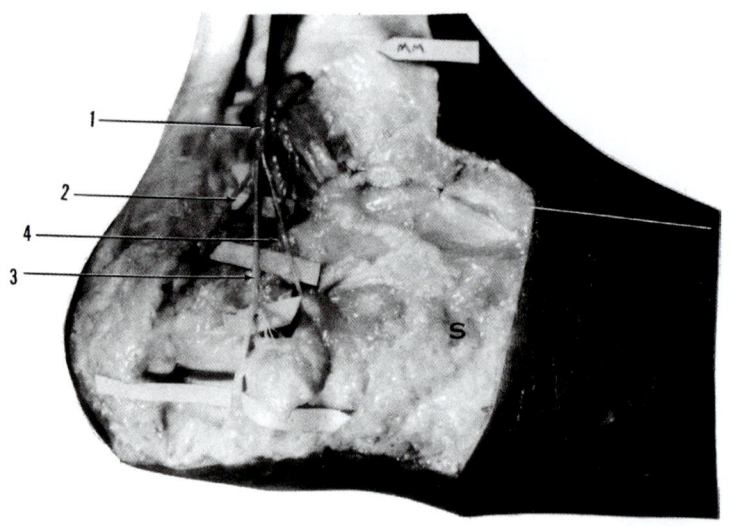
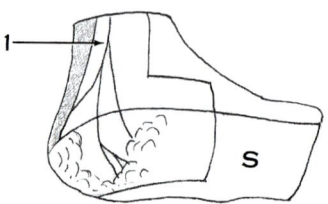

Figure 8.47 Medial calcaneal nerve (1) dividing into three branches: posterior (2), middle (3), and anterior (4). The posterior division branch (2) supplies the medial posterior heel; the middle branch (3) supplies the plantar aspect of the heel and reaches the lateral border of the heel; the anterior branch (4) supplies the plantar anterior aspect of the heel. (S, sole of the foot; MM, medial malleolus.)

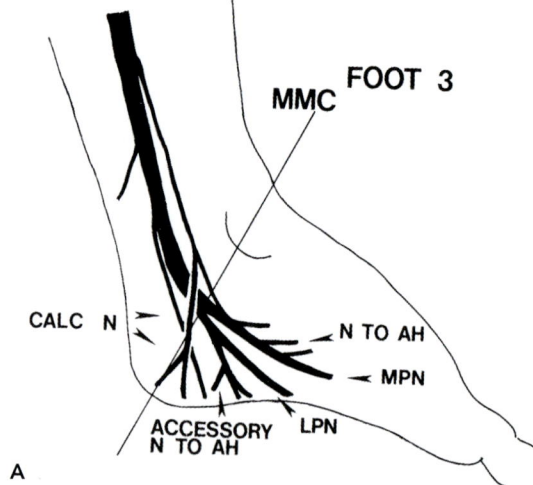
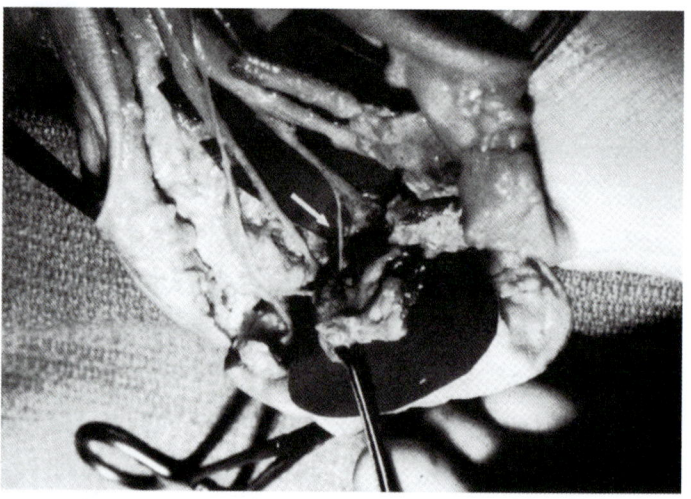

Figure 8.48 Plantar nerve. Diagram **(A)** and photograph **(B)** show a small branch of first branch of lateral plantar nerve coursing into the abductor hallucis muscle through its deep fascia (white arrow). Calc N, calcaneal nerve branch; LPN, lateral plantar nerve; MMC, medial malleolar calcaneal axis; MPN, medial plantar nerve; N TO AH, accessory nerve to the abductor hallucis muscle. (Davis TJ, Schon LC. Branches of the tibial nerve: anatomic variations. *Foot Ankle Int*. 1995;16[1]:23, Figure 4. Copyright ©1995. Reprinted by Permission of SAGE Publications.)

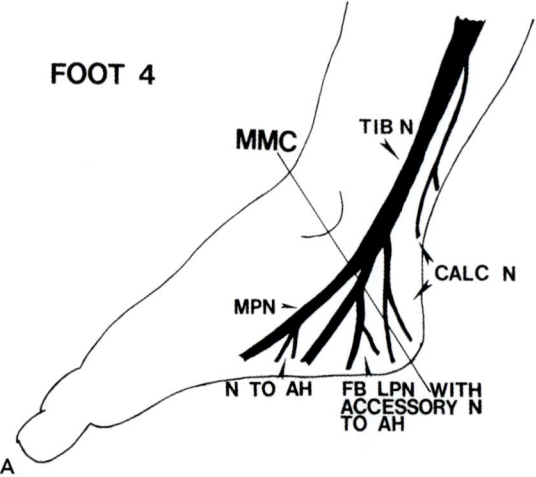
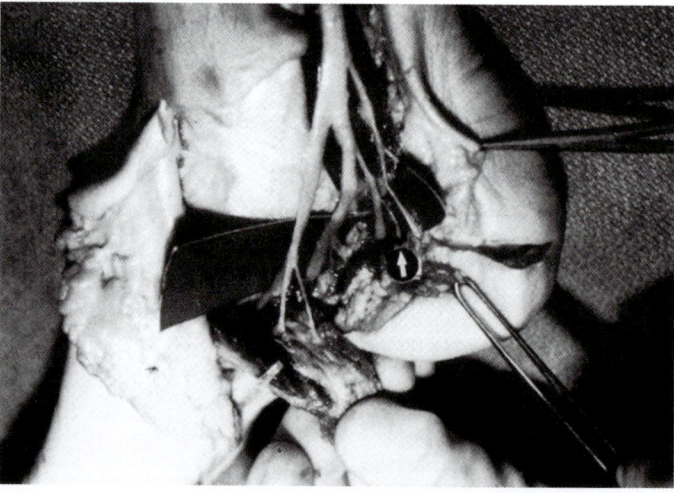

Figure 8.49 Medial plantar nerve. Diagram **(A)** and photograph **(B)** show both the branches of the medial plantar nerve innervating the abductor hallucis in their usual location and the accessory innervations of the abductor hallucis by a branch of the first branch of the lateral plantar nerve (white arrow). FB, flexor brevis; TIB N, tibial nerve. (Davis TJ, Schon LC. Branches of the tibial nerve: anatomic variations. *Foot Ankle Int*. 1995;16[1]:23, Figure 5. Copyright ©1995. Reprinted by Permission of SAGE Publications.)

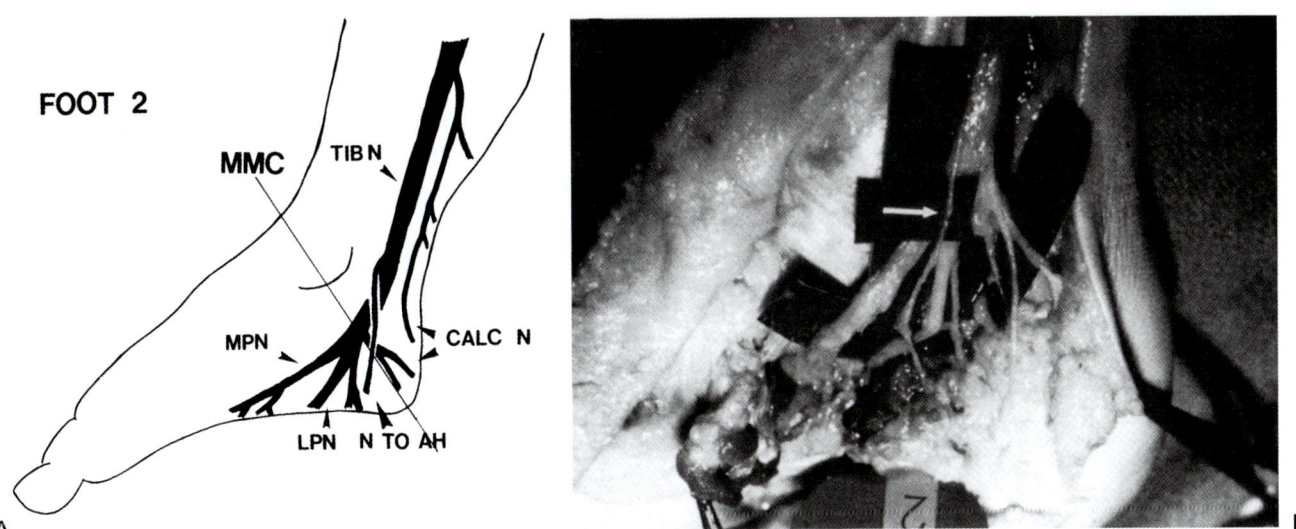

Figure 8.50 Tibial nerve. Diagram **(A)** and photograph **(B)** of foot show a branch of the tibial nerve running distally to innervate the abductor hallucis muscle (*white arrow*). No branches of medial plantar nerve were found innervating the abductor hallucis in this specimen. (Davis TJ, Schon LC. Branches of the tibial nerve: anatomic variations. *Foot Ankle Int.* 1995;16[1]:23, Figure 6. Copyright ©1995. Reprinted by Permission of SAGE Publications.)

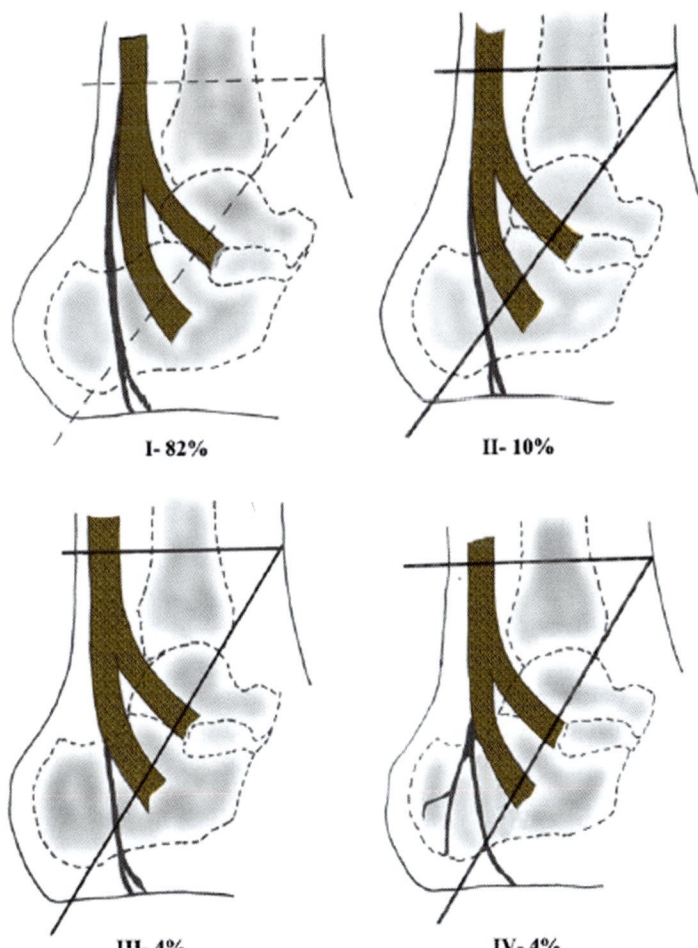

Figure 8.51 Patterns of origin of the inferior calcaneal nerve. The horizontal broken line represents the beginning of the tarsal tunnel, and the diagonal broken line represents the axis between the medial malleolus and the calcaneus. (Adapted from Govsa F, Bilge O, Ozer MA, et al. Variations in the origin of the medial and inferior calcaneal nerves. *Arch Orthop Trauma Surg.* 2006;126:6-14.)

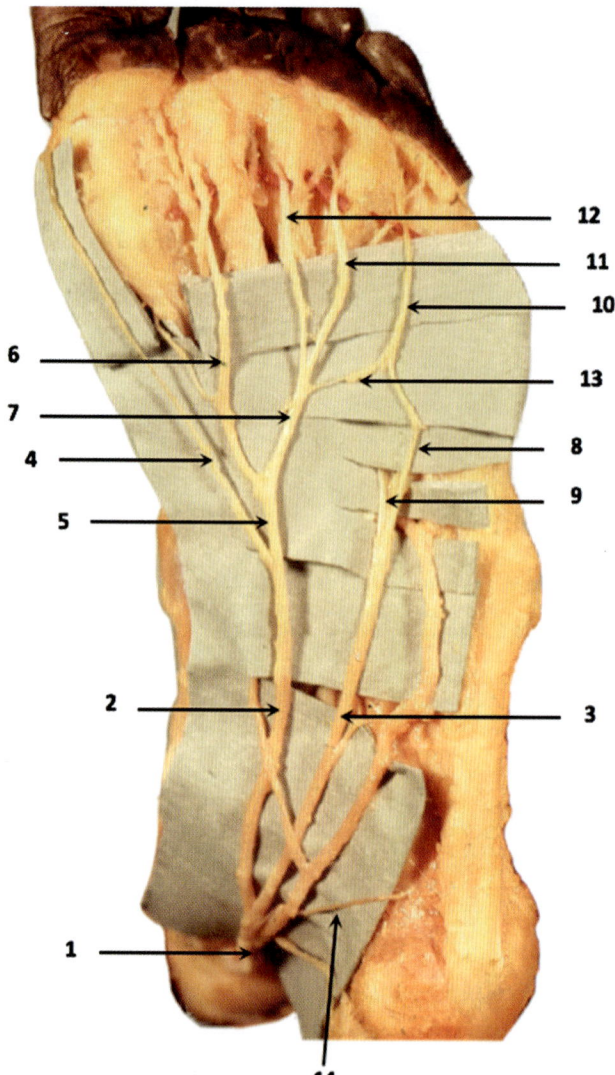

Figure 8.52 Nerves of the plantar aspect of the foot. Posterior tibial nerve (*1*); medial plantar nerve (*2*); lateral plantar nerve (*3*); medial division branch (*4*) of medial plantar nerve forming the medial plantar hallucal nerve; lateral division branch (*5*) of medial plantar nerve; first common plantar digital nerve (*6*); second and third common plantar digital nerve (*7*); fourth common digital nerve (*8*) or superficial branch of the lateral plantar nerve; deep branch (*9*) of the lateral plantar nerve; plantar digital nerve to third web space (*11*); plantar digital nerve to second web space (*12*); communicating branch (*13*) between the common digital nerve to the second and third web space (*7*) and the common digital nerve to the fourth web space (*10*); nerve to the abductor digiti quinti (*14*).

toe with its first lumbrical laterally. The nerve divides into the lateral plantar digital nerve of the big toe and the medial plantar digital nerve of the second toe. The bifurcation occurs proximal to or at the level of the deep transverse metatarsal ligament between the first and second toes. At this level, the nerve is joined by the lateral bifurcation branch of the first plantar metatarsal artery. The nerve is more plantar than the artery, and both are embedded in a protective fat body.[34] Farther distally, the nerves and the artery pass under the mooring ligament and the natatory ligament and reach the corresponding sides of the first and second toes. During its course, the first common digital nerve provides a branch to the first lumbrical and one to the lateral head of the short flexor of the big toe. It also provides a cutaneous branch and an anastomosis branch with the medial plantar hallucal nerve. The latter passes obliquely over the plantar aspect of the flexor hallucis longus tunnel.[25]

The second common digital nerve turns around the medial border of the flexor digitorum brevis and is directed anteriorly and laterally. It crosses superficially the short flexor tendon to the second toe and passes between this tendon and the longitudinal tract of the plantar aponeurosis. During its course, the nerve passes along the posterior border of the sagittal septa of the plantar aponeurosis to the second ray and divides into the lateral plantar nerve to the second toe and the medial plantar nerve to the third toe. Both are also embedded in a fat body at the level of the deep transverse metatarsal ligament and are joined by the digital artery merging from the space delineated by the proximal border of the same ligament and the transverse head of the adductor hallucis. The second common digital nerve provides, during its course, a branch to the second lumbrical muscle.

The third common digital nerve is directed anteriorly and laterally, crosses superficially the short flexor tendons corresponding to the second and third toes, and reaches the third interosseous space. The nerve courses under the plantar aponeurosis and makes a sharp turn against the free posterior border of the lateral sagittal septum of the aponeurosis of the third digit. The nerve divides into the lateral digital branch of the third toe and the medial digital branch of the fourth toe. Very often the third common digital nerve receives an anastomotic branch from the superficial branch of the lateral plantar nerve; the location and type of this anastomosis are very variable. As described by Hovelacque (see Fig. 8.53), most frequently the anastomotic branch arises from the lateral plantar nerve and is directed anteriorly and medially, coursing between the plantar aponeurosis and the short flexor of the toes and joining the third common digital nerve near its bifurcation. Sometimes the anastomotic branch passes deep to the short flexor tendons of the fifth and fourth toes and emerges between the tendons of the third and fourth toes. Rarely the anastomosis is double or Y-shaped, or it may extend obliquely outward and anteriorly from the medial plantar nerve to the lateral plantar nerve. Jones and Klenerman studied the communicating branches between the medial and lateral plantar nerves in 25 dissected feet.[35] The anastomotic branch was present in all feet, extending obliquely forward and medially from the common plantar digital nerve of the fourth web space to the common plantar digital nerve of the third web space. The anastomotic branch was usually applied to the deep surface of the plantar aponeurosis, "often with a branch penetrating its substance." In 90% of the specimens, the communicating branch was thinner than the corresponding common plantar digital nerve, and in 10% it was of similar size (Fig. 8.56).

▶ **Lateral Plantar Nerve**

In the proximal segment of the talocalcaneal canal, the lateral plantar nerve (see Figs. 8.41, 8.42, and 8.52) is located initially behind the posterior tibial artery, crosses the latter near its

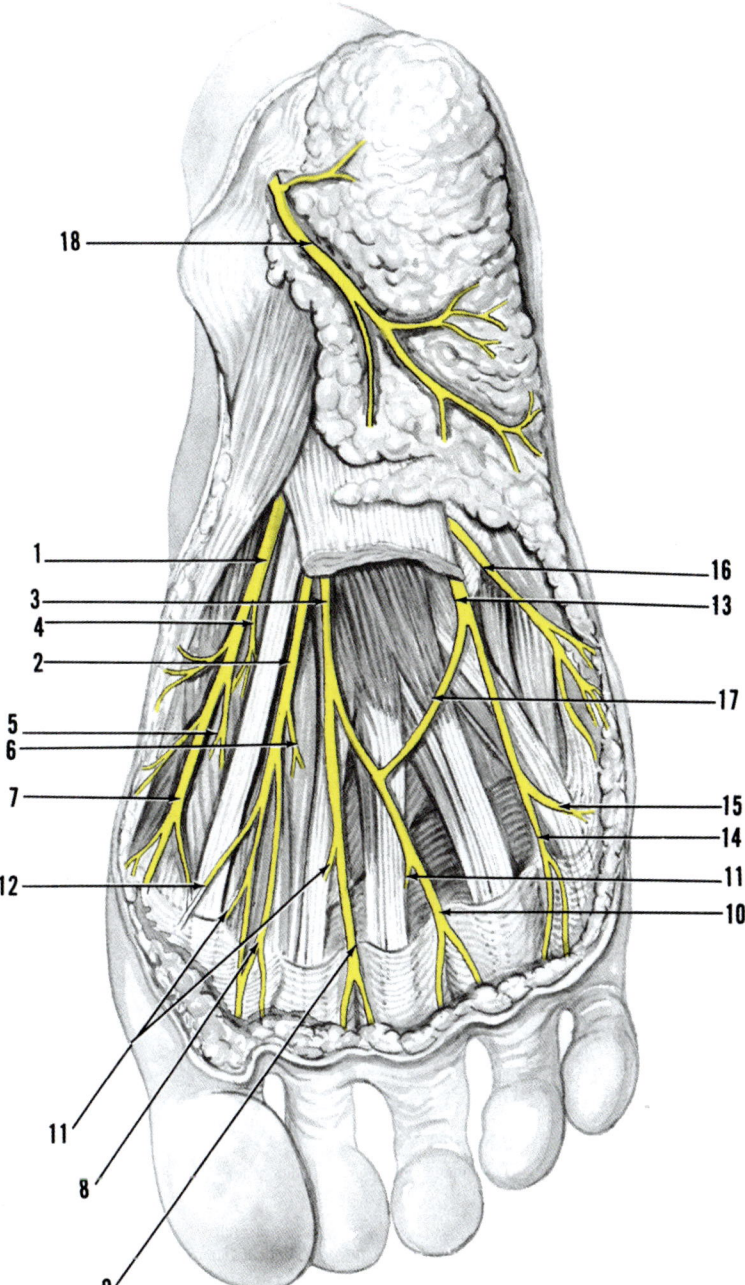

Figure 8.53 Plantar aspect of the right foot—superficial layer. (*1*, Medial division branch of medial plantar nerve; *2*, first common digital nerve, branch of lateral division branch of medial plantar nerve; *3*, second and third common digital nerve trunk, branch of lateral division branch of medial plantar nerve; *4, 5*, motor branches to flexor hallucis brevis arising from medial division branch of medial plantar nerve; *6*, motor branch to first lumbrical muscle; *7*, medial plantar hallucal nerve, a continuation branch of medial division branch of medial plantar nerve; *8*, plantar digital nerve to first web space; *9*, plantar digital nerve to second web space; *10*, plantar digital nerve to third web space; *11*, cutaneous branches; *12*, anastomotic branch between first common digital nerve and medial plantar hallucal nerve; *13*, fourth common digital nerve, a division branch of superficial branch of lateral plantar nerve; *14*, plantar digital nerves to fourth web space; *15*, lateral plantar cutaneous nerve of little toe; *16*, lateral plantar cutaneous nerve, a division branch of superficial branch of lateral plantar nerve; *17*, anastomotic branch between common digital nerve to third web space and common digital nerve to fourth web space; *18*, medial calcaneal nerve, branch of posterior tibial nerve.) (Adapted from Hovelacque A. *Anatomie des Nerfs Craniens et Rachidiens et du Système Grand Sympathique Chez l'Homme.* Doin; 1927.)

bifurcation, and courses between the more anteriorly located medial plantar artery and the more posteriorly located lateral plantar artery (see Figs. 8.53 to 8.55).

In the lower segment of the tarsal tunnel, the lateral plantar nerve penetrates the lower calcaneal chamber limited anteriorly by the free border of the interfascicular ligament, medially by the abductor hallucis with its investing fascia, and laterally by the medial head of the quadratus plantae. Subsequently, the lateral plantar nerve enters the middle plantar space located between the quadratus plantae and the flexor digitorum brevis. It runs obliquely, anteriorly and laterally, passing plantar to the quadratus plantae and anterior to the lateral plantar vessels. It now pierces the lateral intermuscular septum and extends forward. Opposite the base of the fifth metatarsal bone, the nerve divides into terminal branches.

At the level of the tarsal tunnel, the first branch taking off from the lateral plantar nerve is the nerve to the abductor digiti quinti. The origin of this nerve is from the lateral plantar nerve near the bifurcation of the posterior tibial nerve or slightly more proximal, arising then from the posterior tibial nerve (see Figs. 8.41 and 8.42). It penetrates the narrowed posterior segment of the lower calcaneal chamber. At this level, the investing fascia of the abductor hallucis muscle is thicker laterally because of the reinforcement from the interfascicular ligament in continuity

418 Sarrafian's Anatomy of the Foot and Ankle

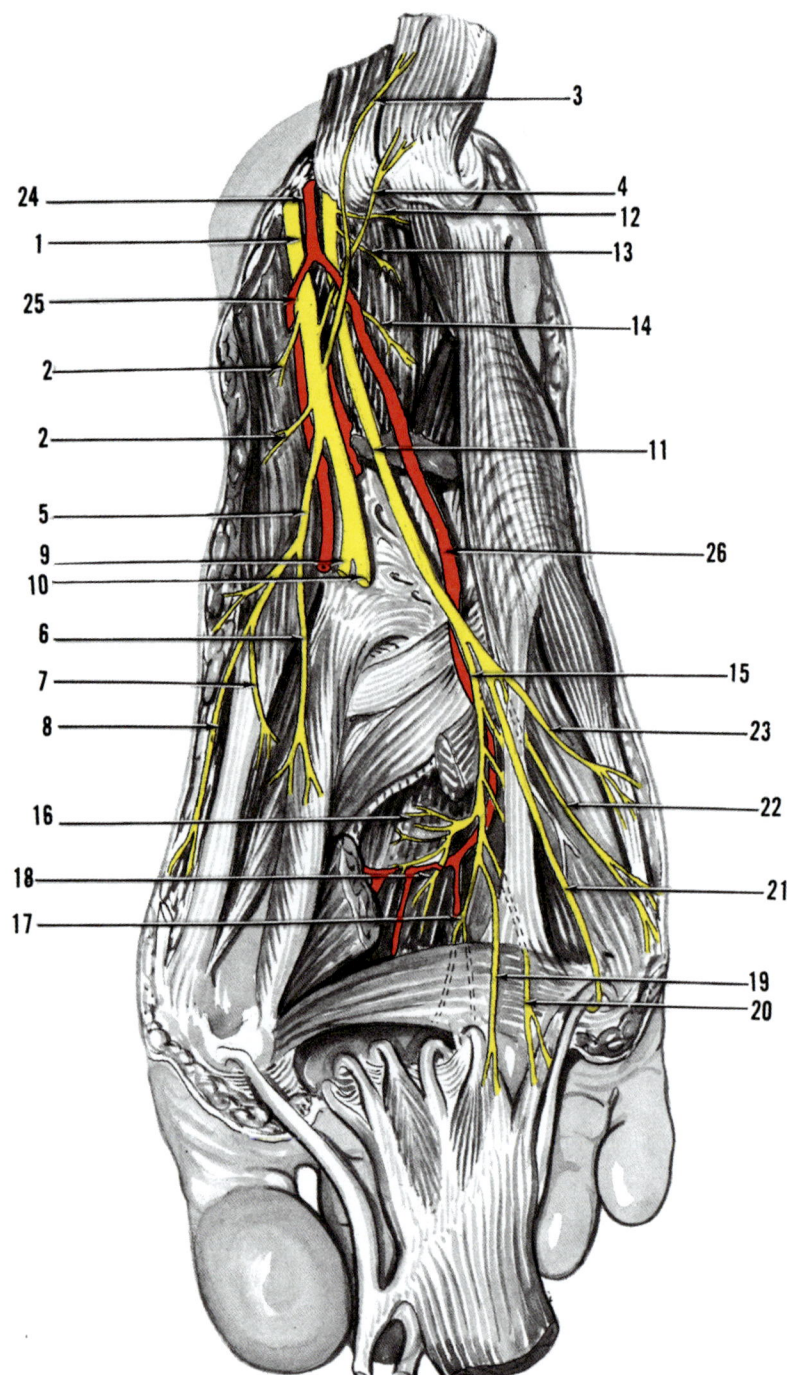

Figure 8.54 Plantar aspect of the right foot—deep layer. (*1*, Medial plantar nerve; *2*, anterior and posterior motor nerves to abductor hallucis muscle; *3, 4*, motor branches to flexor digitorum brevis muscle; *5*, medial division branch of medial plantar nerve; *6*, motor branch to lateral head of flexor hallucis brevis, providing also a branch to medial head of same muscle; *7*, motor branch to medial head of flexor hallucis brevis muscle; *8*, medial plantar hallucal nerve; *9, 10*, division branches of lateral division branch of medial plantar nerve; *11*, lateral plantar nerve; *12*, motor branch to abductor digiti quinti muscle; *13*, posterior motor branch to quadratus plantae muscle; *14*, anterior motor branch to quadratus plantae muscle; *15*, deep branch of lateral plantar nerve; *16*, motor branches to oblique head of adductor hallucis muscle; *17*, motor branch to transverse head of adductor hallucis muscle, providing also an articular branch; *18*, motor branch to interossei muscles of third interspace; *19*, motor branch to third lumbrical muscle; *20*, motor branch to fourth lumbrical muscle; *21*, common digital nerve to fourth web space; *22*, lateral collateral nerve to fifth toe; *23*, lateral plantar cutaneous nerve; *24*, posterior tibial artery; *25*, medial plantar artery; *26*, lateral plantar artery.) (Adapted from Hovelacque A. *Anatomie des Nerfs Craniens et Rachidiens et du Système Grand Sympathique Chez l'Homme.* Doin; 1927.)

with the medial intermuscular septum. At the lower border of the abductor hallucis, the nerve to the abductor digiti quinti makes a turn and courses almost transversely laterally, passing anterior to the medial calcaneal tuberosity located between the quadratus plantae and the underlying flexor digitorum brevis–plantar aponeurosis complex, and penetrates the abductor digiti quinti on its deep surface near its origin.

Roegholt dissected 20 ft and found this motor branch to be present in all his preparations and he termed it the *inferior calcaneal nerve*.[36] He correlated the clinical entity of heel pain with a possible compression of this nerve by a calcaneal spur. Clinical correlation between heel pain and a medial calcaneal nerve branch arising from the posterior aspect of the lateral plantar nerve was made by Tanz.[37] This nerve branch lies deep to the abductor hallucis, the plantar aponeurosis, and the short flexor, runs inferiorly and then laterally, coursing in front of the tuber-calcanei, and "it obviously would be vulnerable to pressure of a calcaneal spur, to local irritation, trauma, or other inflammation, edema or to venous engorgement."[37]

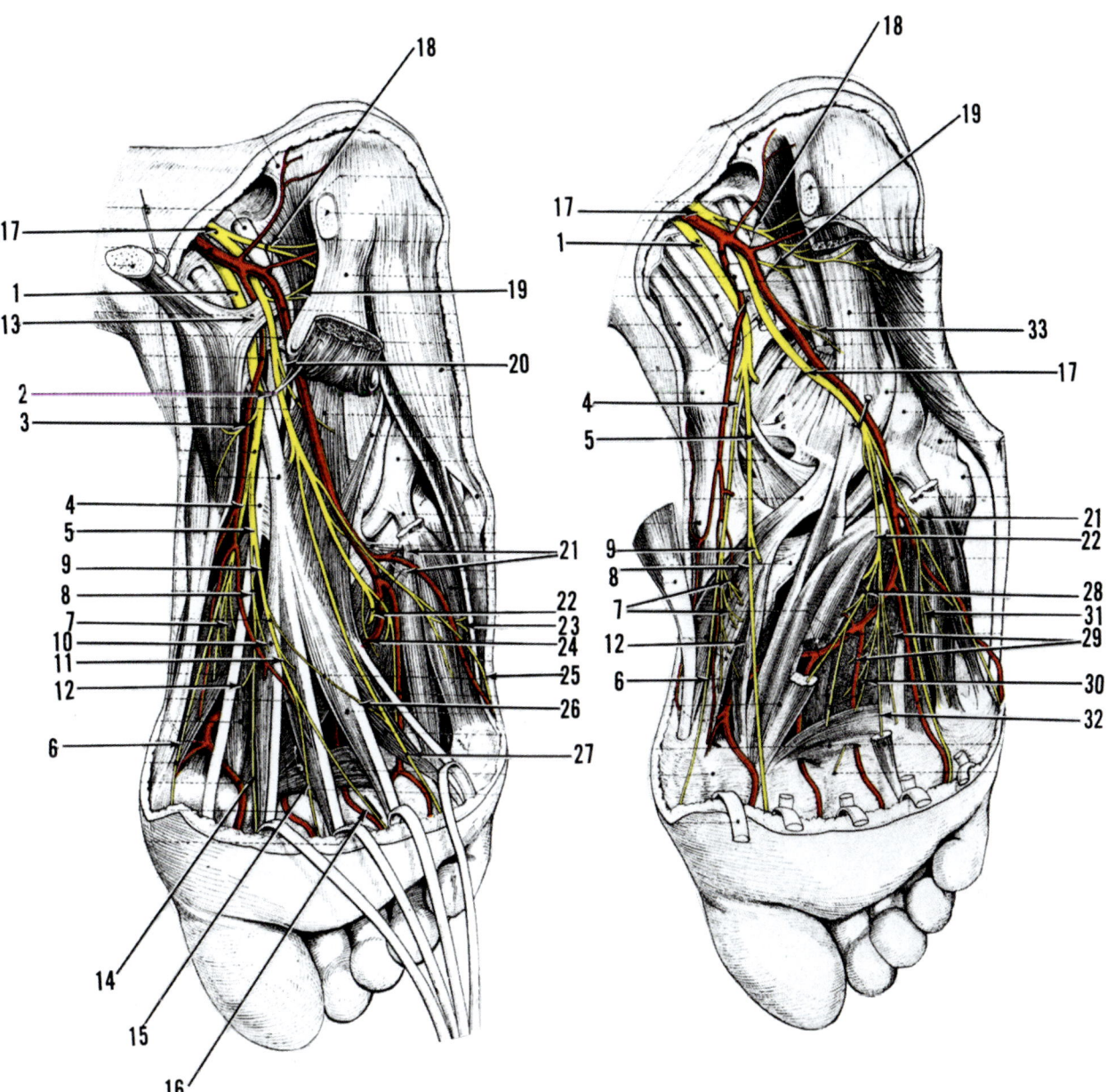

Figure 8.55 Plantar aspect of the right foot—superficial and deep layers. (*1*, Medial plantar nerve; *2*, motor branch to flexor digitorum brevis muscle; *3*, motor branch to abductor hallucis; *4*, medial division branch of medial plantar nerve; *5*, lateral division branch of medial plantar nerve; *6*, medial plantar hallucal nerve; *7*, motor branches to medial head of flexor hallucis muscle; *8*, first common digital nerve; *9*, common trunk of second and third common digital nerves; *10*, motor branch to first lumbrical muscle; *11*, motor branch to second lumbrical muscle; *12*, motor branch to lateral head of flexor hallucis brevis muscle; *13*, interfascicular septum; *14*, plantar digital nerve to first web space; *15*, plantar digital nerve to second web space; *16*, plantar digital nerve to third web space; *17*, lateral plantar nerve; *18*, motor branch to abductor digiti quinti muscle; *19*, posterior motor branch to quadratus plantae muscle; *20*, anterior motor branch to quadratus plantae muscle; *21*, motor branch to opponens of fifth toe; *22*, deep branch of lateral plantar nerve; *23*, motor branch to short flexor of fifth toe; *24*, motor branch to interossei of third interspace; *25*, lateral plantar cutaneous nerve of fifth toe; *26*, anastomotic branch between trunk of second-third common digital nerve and fourth common digital nerve; *27*, fourth common digital nerve; *28*, motor branches to adductor hallucis oblique head, interossei of second space, and transverse head of adductor hallucis; *29*, motor branches to interossei muscles of second and third interspaces; *30*, motor branch to transverse head of adductor hallucis muscle; *31*, motor branch to opponens of fifth toe; *32*, motor branch to third lumbrical muscle; *33*, motor branch to calcaneocuboid ligament.) (Adapted from Dujarier CH. *Anatomie des Membres: Dissection-Anatomie Topographique*. 2nd ed. Masson; 1924.)

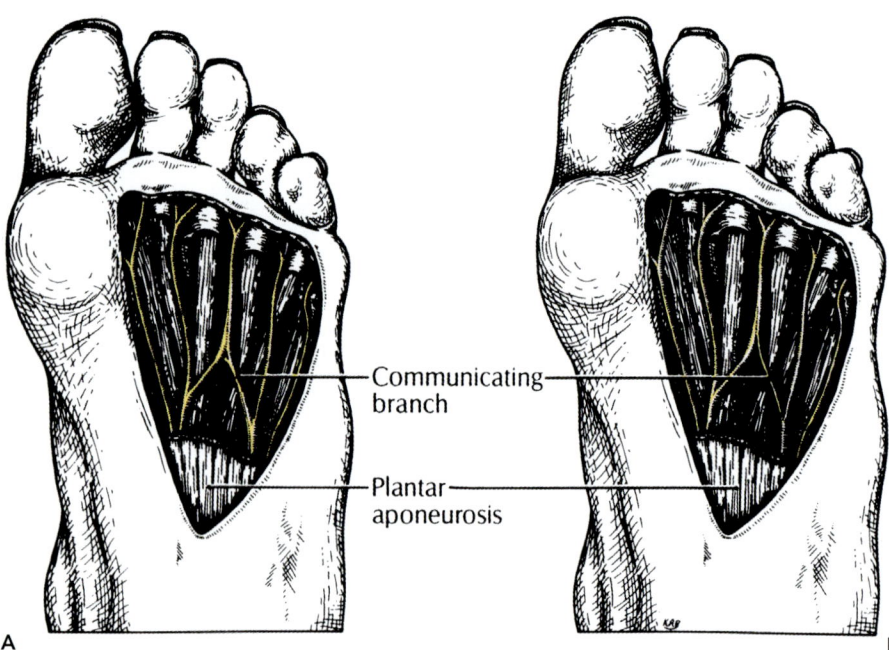

Figure 8.56 **Communicating branch.** The common pattern of communicating branch in **(B)** (thin) and the variation observed in **(A)** (thick). (Adapted from Iones JR, Klenerman L. A study of the communicating branch between the medial and the lateral plantar nerves. *Foot Ankle*. 1984;4[6]:313.)

Arenson and colleagues studied the inferior calcaneal nerve, a branch of the lateral plantar nerve, in 30 ft.[38] In all 30 feet, the inferior calcaneal nerve originated from the lateral plantar nerve, passed between the abductor hallucis muscle and the medial head of the quadratus plantae muscle, and coursed laterally 5.5 mm (in average) anterior to the medial process of the calcaneal tuberosity, passing between the flexor digitorum brevis muscle and the long plantar ligament. It crossed over the lateral head of the quadratus plantae muscle and terminated in the proximal portion of the abductor digiti quinti muscle. "In certain instances, branches were found to innervate the calcaneal periosteum, the flexor digitorum brevis muscle, and the lateral head of the quadratus plantae muscle."[38]

Przylucki and Jones dissected four feet to study a nerve branch that courses laterally just anterior to the medial tuberosity of the calcaneus.[39] It originates 2 cm below the tip of the medial malleolus from the lateral plantar nerve, courses downward and slightly anteriorly, and passes between the abductor hallucis muscle and the medial head of the quadratus plantae muscle. "It then takes an almost direct lateral course across the plantar aspect of the feet. It rests on the proximal most portion of the long plantar ligament… 0.5 to 1.0 cm anterior to the distal border of the medial calcaneal tuberosity. In the area of the lateral head of the quadratus plantae muscle, it divides into anterior and posterior branches, both of which enter the abductor digiti quinti muscle at its musculotendinous junction. Along its plantar course, a branch is also given off, entering the flexor digitorum brevis muscle."[39]

Baxter and Thigpen, using cadaver dissections and surgical observations, describe the mixed nerve of the abductor digiti quinti as follows: "as either a separate branch, as the authors have sometimes found it, or as a branch off the lateral plantar nerve. It enters underneath the fascia of the abductor hallucis muscle, passes through its fascial leash and exits distally beneath the abductor hallucis thick unyielding inferior fascial edge; then it immediately turns lateral to pass beneath the calcaneus. The plantar fascia and flexor digitorum brevis muscle both originate plantar to the nerve from the medial tuberosity of the calcaneus or 'heel spur,' if present. The thin, fibrous origin of the quadratus plantae muscle and the long plantar ligament lie dorsal to the nerve and barely separate the nerve from the bony inferior medial ridge of the calcaneus. The ridge is prominent and provides good fulcrum over which the nerve can be stretched. The nerve then terminates in a fan of three or four branches into the proximal portion of the abductor digiti quinti muscle"[40] (Figs. 8.57 and 8.58).

Rondhuis and Huson dissected the first branch of the lateral plantar nerve in 34 adult feet and traced the course of the nerve in serial sections of 4 fetal feet.[41] In all 34 ft, the first branch branched off from the lateral plantar nerve. The first branch passes through a separate canal bordered medially by the abductor hallucis and laterally by the medial head of the quadratus plantae muscle. It courses plantarward and "gives a nerve branch running sometimes to the insertion of the quadratus plantae muscle and always running to the periosteum covering the medial process of the calcaneal tuberosity. A branch of the latter runs just in front of the medial process of the calcaneal tuberosity in lateral direction giving branches to the long plantar ligament and mostly accompanying vas nutria into the latero-plantar part of the calcaneus. At first, the first branch crosses the quadratus plantae muscle obliquely in a plantar direction, turning then into a horizontal plane running now lateralward."[41] It gives a nerve branch to the proximal part of the flexor digitorum brevis muscle and terminates in the proximal part of the abductor digiti minimi muscle, dividing into a branch running proximalward and distalward (Figs. 8.59 and 8.60).

Hamm and Sanders studied the anatomic variations of the nerve to the abductor digiti quinti muscle in 39 cadaveric feet.[42] The nerve was present in 100% of the specimens. It originated as the posterior branch of a trifurcation of the posterior tibial nerve in 46%. It was a branch of the lateral plantar nerve in 49% and was a direct branch from the posterior tibial nerve in 5%.

The lateral plantar nerve also provides motor branches to the quadratus plantae. Generally two in number, these are more anterior than the preceding motor branch. They penetrate each head of the muscle from the plantar aspect. Quite often the nerve enters between the two muscular heads and then divides into muscular branches for each and also provides a branch to the calcaneocuboid ligament.[25,29]

There are two terminal branches of the lateral plantar nerve, superficial and deep.

▶ Superficial Branch

The superficial branch is located in the interval between the flexor digitorum brevis and the abductor digiti quinti; from its inferior surface, it provides for the outer aspect of the sole

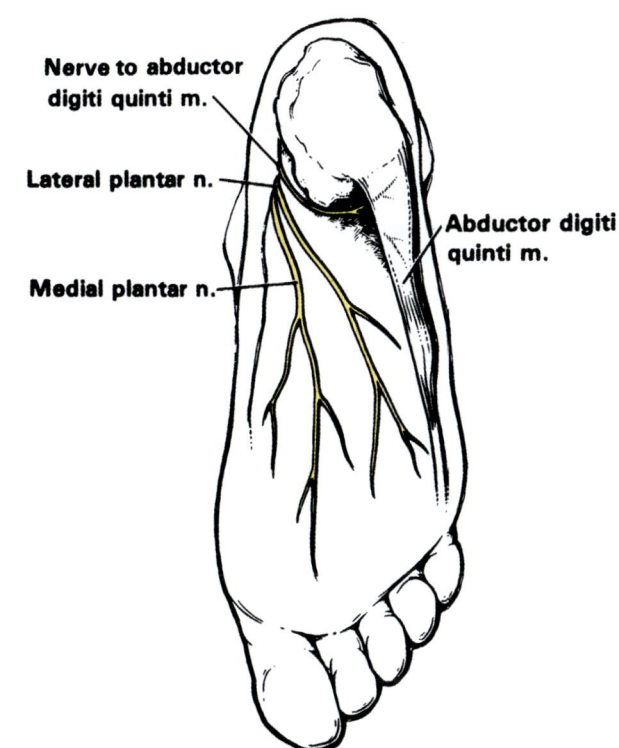

Figure 8.57 Nerve to abductor digiti quinti muscle as seen in cadaver dissection. (Adapted from Baxter DE, Thigpen CM. Heel pain: operative results. *Foot Ankle.* 1984;5[1]:16.)

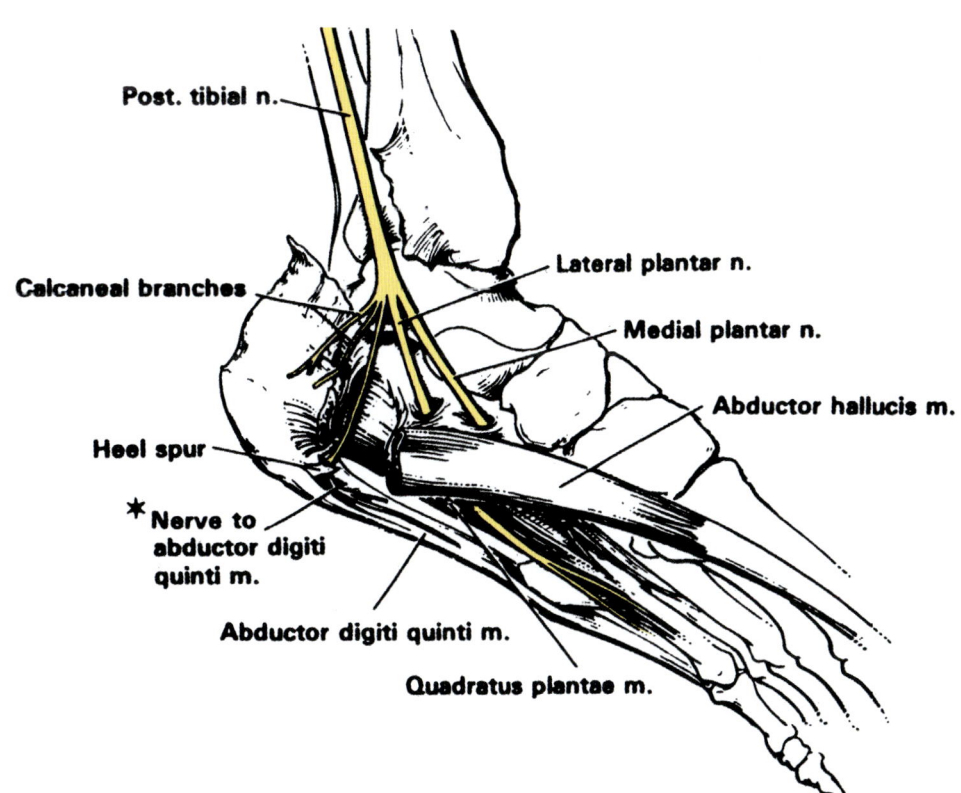

Figure 8.58 The abductor hallucis muscle with its deep fascia has been transected, exposing the nerve to the abductor digiti quinti muscle. (Adapted from Baxter DE, Thigpen CM. Heel pain: operative results. *Foot Ankle.* 1984;5[1]:16.)

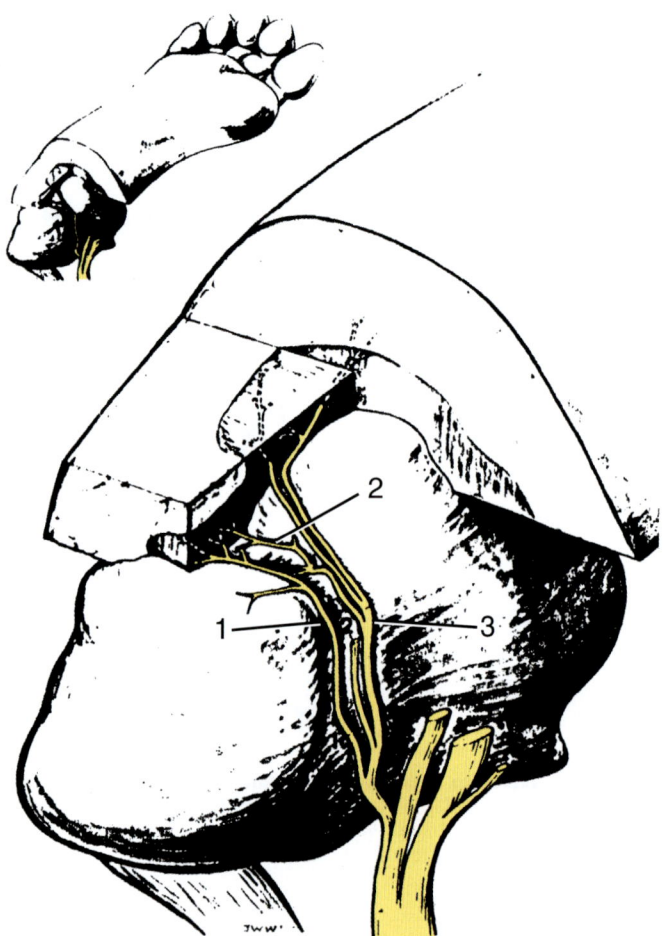

Figure 8.59 Graphic three-dimensional reconstruction of the ramification pattern of the first branch made from horizontal sections. (*1*, Branch running to the medial process of the calcaneal tuberosity, bifurcating into a branch covering the perichondrium of the medial process and into another one running to a more lateral part of the calcaneal perichondrium; *2*, branch to the flexor digitorum muscle; *3*, branches to the abductor digiti minimi muscle.) (Adapted from Rondhuis JJ, Huson A. The first branch of the lateral plantar nerve and heel pain. *Acta Morphol Neerl Scand.* 1986;24:269.)

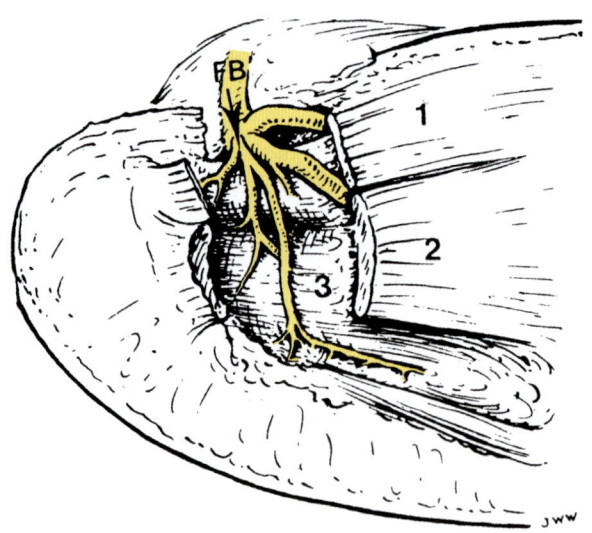

Figure 8.60 **The first branch and its ramification pattern as dissected in an adult foot.** Parts of the abductor hallucis (*1*) and flexor digitorum (*2*) muscles have been removed in order to show the first branch running across the quadratus plantae muscle (*3*) in a plantar direction, then turning into a horizontal plane to proceed laterally. (Adapted from Rondhuis JJ, Huson A. The first branch of the lateral plantar nerve and heel pain. *Acta Morphol Neerl Scand.* 1986;24:269.)

several cutaneous branches, which pass through the plantar aponeurosis. It also provides from its lateral border a branch for the short flexor and another branch for the opponens of the fifth toe. These motor branches may arise more anteriorly from the lateral plantar cutaneous branch of the fifth toe or even from the deep branch.[25] The superficial branch now divides into the fourth common digital nerve and the lateral plantar cutaneous nerve to the fifth toe. The lateral plantar cutaneous nerve to the fifth toe is directed obliquely anteriorly and laterally, crosses the short muscles of the fifth toe, and runs along its lateral border. The fourth common digital nerve turns around the lateral border of the flexor digitorum brevis, enters the middle plantar space M_1, and divides into the lateral plantar nerve of the fourth toe and the medial plantar nerve of the fifth toe. As described above, it is this nerve to the fourth space that provides the anastomotic branch with the third common digital nerve.

▶ Deep Branch

The deep branch of the lateral plantar nerve follows the direction of the lateral plantar artery, perforates the lateral intermuscular septum 2.5 cm distal to the tuberosity of the fifth metatarsal, and enters the middle plantar space M_3 and subsequently M_4 dorsal to the oblique head of the adductor hallucis. The nerve, posterior to the artery, now courses between the adductor hallucis muscle and the plantar interossei. It passes across the metatarsals 4, 3, and 2 near their base and traces a curve with a posteromedial concavity.

During its course, the deep branch of the lateral plantar nerve provides, from its concavity, articular branches to the tarsal and the tarsometatarsal joints. From its convexity, the nerve gives off motor branches to the lateral two or three lumbricals, to the interossei of the second, third, and fourth space, and to the transverse head of the adductor hallucis; the branches of the latter penetrate the muscle from the posterior border of the dorsal surface.

The deep branch of the lateral plantar nerve terminates by providing branches to the oblique head of the adductor hallucis and the muscles of the first interosseous space. One of the most posterior branches to the adductor hallucis perforates the muscle from the depth to the surface and, before reaching the lateral head of the flexor hallucis, anastomoses with a similar branch provided by the medial plantar nerve. This motor anastomosis, described by Hallopeau, is the equivalent of the Riche and Cannieu motor anastomosis seen in the hand.[25,43] The very thin anastomosis occurs in the substance of the flexor hallucis brevis or on the plantar aspect of the latter, dorsal to the flexor hallucis longus tendon.[43]

Chou et al[44] dissected 26 fresh cadaver feet and found Hallopeau anastomotic nerve in four specimens (15%) (Fig. 8.61).

SAPHENOUS NERVE

The saphenous nerve is the terminal branch of the femoral nerve. It courses with the femoral artery, and at the tendinous arch of the adductor magnus, it perforates the fascial covering of the adductor canal. It passes to the medial aspect of the knee deep to the sartorius, pierces the fascia lata between the sartorius and the gracilis, and becomes subcutaneous. It now runs distally in the leg behind the medial border of the tibia, just posterior to the greater saphenous vein. It divides into two branches: one branch, smaller, terminates at the level of the ankle, whereas the second branch passes in front of the medial malleolus and provides branches to the medial side of the foot, extending up to the medial side of the big toe. This branch anastomoses with the medial branch of the superficial peroneal nerve.

Horwitz provides the following data concerning the level of the terminal division of the saphenous nerve: 15 cm from the medial malleolus in 89%, 12.5 cm from the medial malleolus in 5%, 7.5 cm from the medial malleolus in 3%, and 5 cm from the medial malleolus in 3%.[1]

The most constant site of the saphenous nerve is 18 cm above the medial malleolus at the medial border of the tibia, superficial to the deep fascia and posterior or posteromedial to the saphenous vein.[1] The average diameter of the nerve is 3 mm.[1]

CUTANEOUS INNERVATION OF THE FOOT

A schematic representation of the cutaneous innervation of the foot is shown in Figure 8.62. On the dorsum of the foot, the superficial peroneal nerve innervates most of the central dorsal aspect of the foot. The intermediate dorsal cutaneous branch provides the dorsolateral branch to the third toe and the dorsomedial branch to the fourth toe. The lateral branch of the medial dorsal cutaneous nerve provides the dorsomedial branch to the third toe and the dorsolateral branch to the second toe. The middle branch of the medial dorsal cutaneous nerve provides the dorsomedial branch to the second toe and the dorsolateral branch to the big toe in conjunction with the deep peroneal nerve. The medial branch of the medial dorsal cutaneous nerve provides the dorsomedial branch to the big toe. The innervation by the dorsal digital nerve extends to the proximal two thirds of the toes. The distal dorsal segments of toes 1 to 3 and the tibial half of the fourth toe are innervated by the medial plantar nerve. The dorsolateral aspect of the foot, the proximal two-thirds segment of the dorsum of the fifth toe, and the lateral two-thirds segment of the fourth toe are innervated by the sural nerve. The distal segments of the dorsum of the fifth toe and lateral fourth toe are supplied by the lateral plantar nerve. The saphenous nerve innervates the dorsomedial segment of the foot and may extend to the dorsomedial aspect of the big toe. On the plantar aspect, the medial and central segment of the heel is supplied by the medial calcaneal nerve, and the lateral half of the heel is supplied by the lateral calcaneal nerve. The major central and medial aspect of the sole, the plantar aspect of toes 1 to 3, and the medial aspect of the fourth toe are supplied by the medial plantar nerve, and the lateral aspect of the sole, the plantar aspect of the fifth toe, and the lateral half of the fourth toe are innervated by the lateral plantar nerve.

Variations of the innervation of the dorsum of the foot and toes are multiple, as described in Figures 8.6, 8.7, and 8.19. Ziólkowski and colleagues studied the skin innervation of the foot in 160 lower limbs of human fetuses aged 4 to 8 months.[45]

The superficial peroneal nerve was present in 96.88% and absent in 3.12%. In the latter group, the innervation is provided in the medial half by the saphenous nerve and the deep peroneal nerve and in the lateral half by the sural nerve. In 8.13%, the superficial peroneal nerve reaches the lateral side of the fifth toe. The deep peroneal nerve innervates alone the adjacent sides of the first and second toes in 45.63%, and in combination with superficial and saphenous nerves, it innervates the remaining group. In 10%, the superficial peroneal nerve supplies the first interspace alone. The deep peroneal nerve may extend its innervation to the medial side of the third toe (7.5%) and may reach the medial side of the fourth toe and, rarely, the medial side of the big toe. The sural nerve innervates only the lateral margin

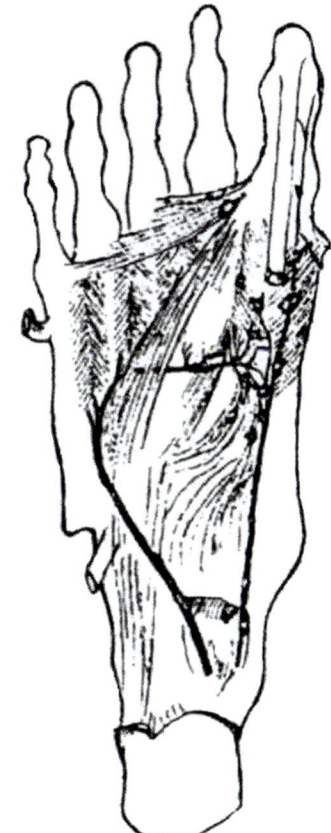

Figure 8.61 Original illustration by Hallopeau of the anastomotic branch. (Chou LB, Choi LE, Ramachandra T, et al. Variation of nerve to flexor hallucis brevis. *Foot Ankle Int.* 2008;29[10]:1042-1044, Figure 1. Copyright ©2008. Reprinted by Permission of SAGE Publications.)

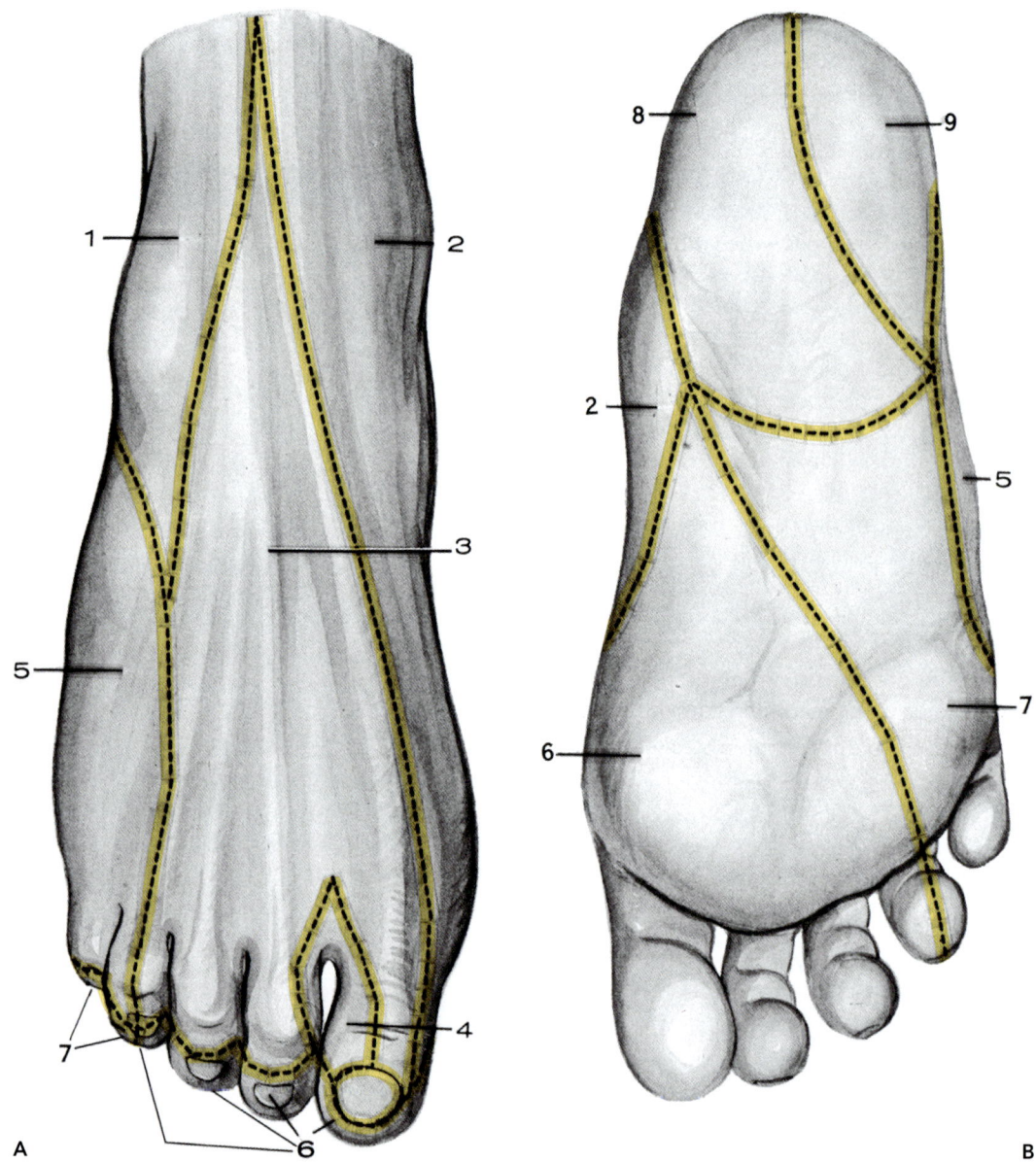

Figure 8.62 Cutaneous innervation of the foot. (A) Dorsum of the foot. (B) Sole of the foot. (1, Peroneal cutaneous nerve; 2, saphenous nerve; 3, superficial peroneal nerve; 4, deep peroneal nerve; 5, sural nerve; 6, medial plantar nerve; 7, lateral plantar nerve; 8, medial calcaneal nerve; 9, lateral calcaneal nerve.)

of the fifth toe in 38.75%. It supplies the fifth toe and the lateral margin of the fourth, third, and second toe in 54.38%. In 6.88%, the sural nerve does not contribute to the cutaneous digital innervation. The saphenous nerve reaches the dorsum of the feet in 9.38%.

The medial aspect of the hallux is supplied in 90% by the superficial peroneal nerve, in 6.88% by the saphenous nerve, and in 3.12% by the combination of the two or by the former and the deep peroneal nerve. The detailed information in regard to the dorsal innervation of the toes is as presented in Table 8.2. The plantar innervation of the toes is as presented in Table 8.3. In 1.25%, the posterior tibial nerve remained undivided and provided all the plantar digital nerves.

NERVES OF THE JOINTS OF THE FOOT AND ANKLE

The first comprehensive study of the innervation of the joints of the foot and ankle was provided by Rudinger.[28] The more recent studies include those of Morin and Roasenda, Lippert, Gardner and Gray, and Champetier.[46-49] The contribution to the innervation of the joints by the accessory deep peroneal nerve has been described by Bryce and Winckler, as presented previously.[11-14]

The ankle joint is innervated by all the nerves crossing the joint, but the more important contribution is from the deep nerves (Fig. 8.63). This innervation is extremely variable.[49]

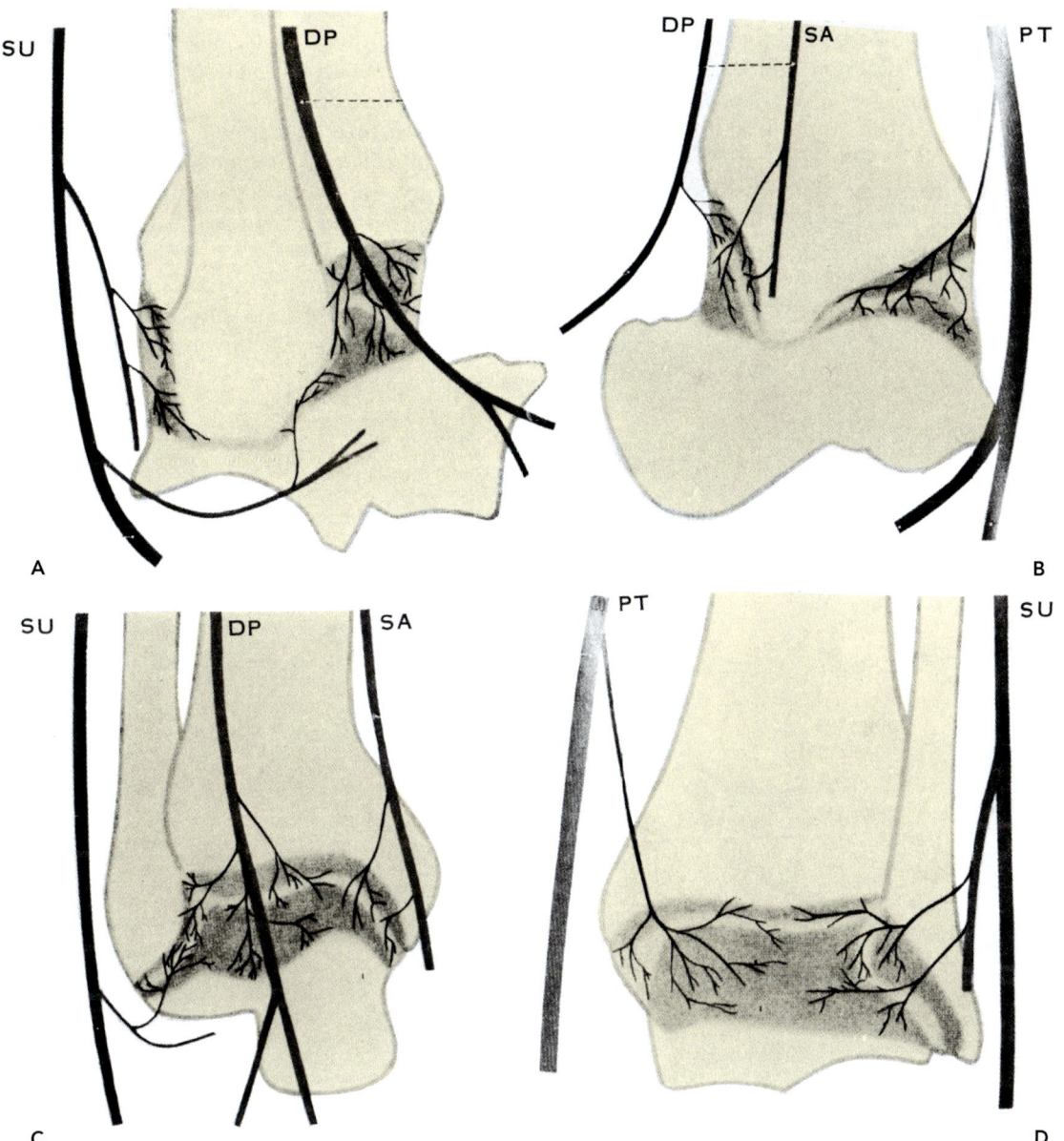

Figure 8.63 Innervation of the ankle joint. (A) Lateral aspect. (B) Medial aspect. (C) Anterior aspect. (D) Posterior aspect. (*SU*, sural nerve; *DP*, deep peroneal nerve; *PT*, posterior tibial nerve; *SA*, saphenous nerve.) (Adapted from Lippert J. Zur Innervation der menschlichen Fussgelenke. *Anat Entwgesh*. 1962;123:229.)

The articular branches from the deep peroneal nerve, three to five in number, arise at the level of the articular interline.[47,49] A branch may arise proximally in the distal third of the leg, covered by the tibialis anterior tendon. Some branches may have a low origin below the ankle joint interline, and they have then a recurrent course to reach the joint. The articular branches from the deep peroneal nerve are located behind the tendons and may pass anterior or posterior to the anterior tibial artery. They innervate the anterior aspect of the capsule of the ankle joint, the anterior and inferior tibiofibular ligament, and the anterior talofibular ligament. The posterior tibial nerve provides three to five articular branches and innervates the entire medial aspect of the articulation and the posterior and anterior aspect of the medial malleolus.[47,49] It extends its innervation to the anterior and posterior aspects of the ankle joint. The articular branches originate from the posterior tibial nerve when the latter divides below the medial malleolus; they may, however, originate from the medial plantar nerve or even the lateral plantar nerve when the division of the posterior tibial nerve is proximal to the level of the medial malleolus. There are also quite often articular branches arising proximally at the junction of the middle third and the distal third of the leg.[49] The nerve to the abductor hallucis from the medial plantar nerve may give articular branches to the ankle joint.

To reach the joint, the articular branches pass lateral or medial to the flexor digitorum longus and always lateral to the tibialis posterior tendon between the deep surface of the sheath and the capsuloligamentous plane.[49]

The saphenous nerve has a modest contribution, with two short branches to the anterior aspect of the medial malleolus and the corresponding capsuloligamentous plane at the same location. These articular branches originate at the level of the medial malleolus and pass behind the tendon of the tibialis anterior before entering the capsule of the joint.

The sural nerve provides articular branches to the perilateral malleolar capsule and ligament. Anterior branches arise sometimes from a long premalleolar branch at the level of the distal third of the leg. Inferior branches take off from the submalleolar arcade of the nerve; these branches pass over the peronei tendons and reach the joint. Posterior branches take off directly from the trunk of the sural nerve and pass deep to the peronei tendons or may originate from a long posterior branch of the sural nerve. The articular branches cross the adipose tissue between the Achilles tendon and the flexors and reach the ankle joint posteriorly.

Champetier describes an inconstant contribution to the innervation of the ankle joint from the superficial peroneal nerve; anterolateral and anteromedial branches may be provided by the superficial peroneal nerve to the ankle joint.[49] This nerve may also supply an articular branch through the accessory deep peroneal nerve.

The talotarsal joint receives its nerve supply from the posterior tibial nerve, the medial plantar nerve, the deep peroneal nerve, the sural nerve, and, when present, the accessory deep peroneal nerve (Fig. 8.64).[47,48] The posterior talocalcaneal joint

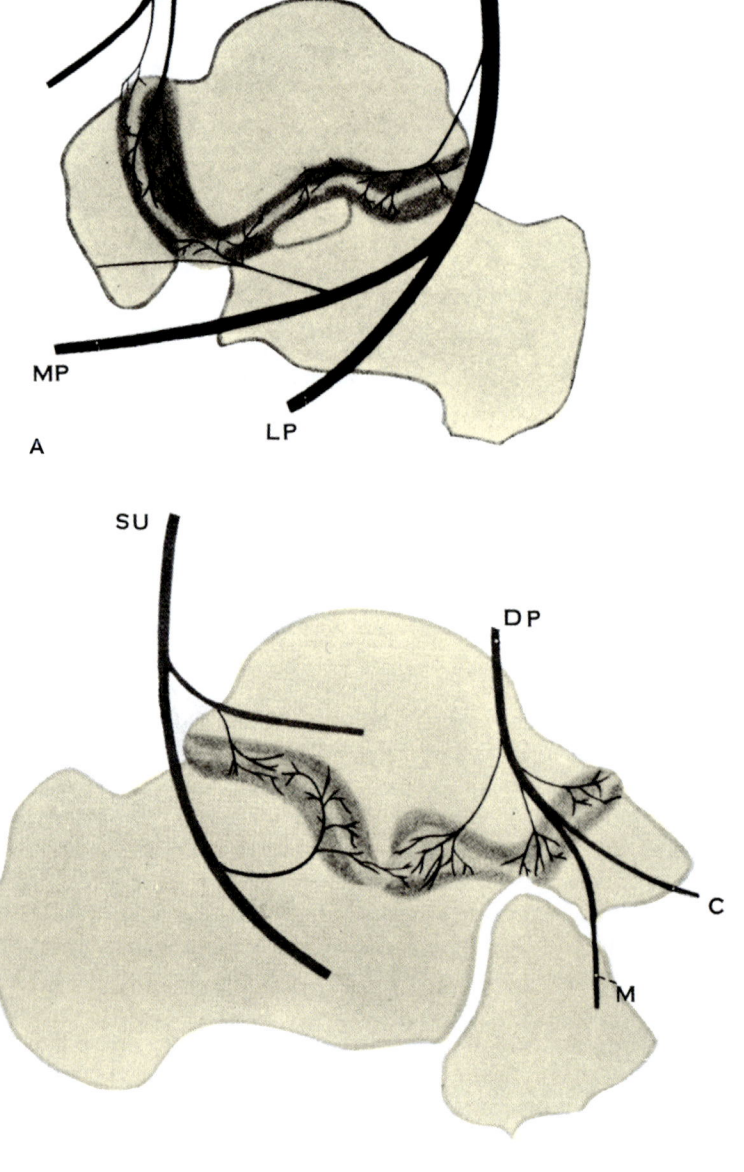

Figure 8.64 Innervation of the talocalcaneonavicular joint. (A) Medial aspect. (B) Lateral aspect. (PT, posterior tibial nerve; DP, deep peroneal nerve; SU, sural nerve; MP, medial plantar nerve; LP, lateral plantar nerve; M, muscular branch of deep peroneal nerve; C, cutaneous branch of deep peroneal nerve.) (Adapted from Lippert J. Zur Innervation der menschlichen Fussgelenke. Anat Entwgesh. 1962;123:229.)

is innervated medially by a branch from the posterior tibial nerve and laterally by two branches from the sural nerve. The sinus tarsi receives nerve twigs from a branch of the deep peroneal nerve, and the canalis tarsi receives nerve twigs from the posterior tibial nerve. The talocalcaneonavicular joint is supplied on the inferomedial aspect by the medial plantar nerve and on the dorsomedial, dorsal, and lateral aspects by the branches from the deep peroneal nerve; the lateral aspect of the joint may receive a branch from the accessory deep peroneal nerve.

On the plantar aspect, all the articular connections of the cuboid with the surrounding bones are innervated by the lateral plantar nerve before it gives off its deep branch (Fig. 8.65).[47,48] On the dorsal aspect, the calcaneocuboid joint is supplied by branches from the sural nerve, the deep peroneal nerve, and the accessory deep peroneal nerve. Dorsally, the cuboid-lateral cuneiform joint is supplied by the deep peroneal nerve, and the cuboid-metatarsals 4 and 5 are innervated by branches from the sural nerve and the lateral branch of the superficial peroneal nerve.

The cuneonavicular joints, the intercuneiform joints, and the cuneometatarsal 1–3 joints are all innervated on the dorsum by the deep peroneal nerve. On the plantar side the medial plantar nerve innervates the same joints except for the joints of the lateral cuneiform, which are supplied by the lateral plantar nerve.[47,48]

The intermetatarsal joints between metatarsal bases 1, 2, 3, and 4 are innervated on the dorsum by the deep peroneal nerve.[47,48] On the plantar aspect, the intermetatarsal joint 1 to 2 is supplied by the medial plantar nerve and the intermetatarsal joints 2 to 3, 3 to 4 by the deep branch of the lateral plantar nerve. The intermetatarsal joint 4 to 5 is supplied on the plantar side by the lateral plantar nerve before giving off its deep branch, and on the dorsal aspect by branches from the sural nerve and the lateral branch of the superficial peroneal nerve.

The metatarsophalangeal joints and the interphalangeal joints of the toes receive their main supply from the plantar interdigital nerves (Fig. 8.66).[47,48]

The digital branches of the medial plantar nerve give articular branches to the plantar aspects of the metatarsophalangeal joints of the first, second, and third toes and the medial aspect of the fourth toe. The digital branches of the lateral plantar nerve provide articular branches to the plantar aspect of the metatarsophalangeal joint of the fifth toe and the lateral aspect of the fourth toe. The plantar aspects of the metatarsophalangeal joints of the second, third, and fourth toes also receive long filaments arising from the deep branch of the lateral plantar nerve.

The medial dorsal cutaneous branch of the superficial peroneal nerve supplies sensory branches to the dorsomedial aspect of the metatarsophalangeal joint and to the interphalangeal joint of the big toe, whereas the deep peroneal nerve supplies the same joints on the dorsolateral aspect and the digital joints of the second toe medially. The digital branches of the intermediate dorsal cutaneous nerve can be traced up to the tip of the third toe, the lateral aspect of the second toe, and the

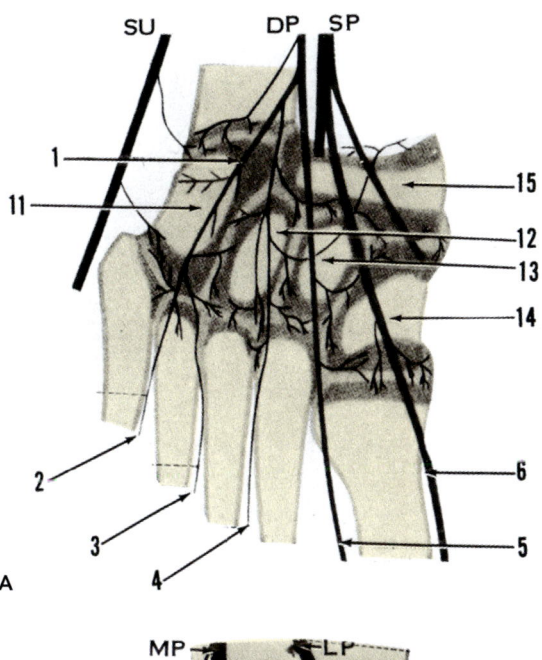

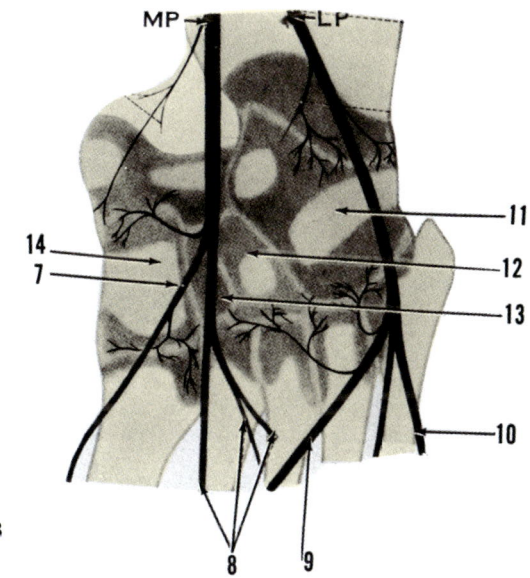

Figure 8.65 Innervation of the tarsus and the tarsometatarsal joint. (A) Dorsal aspect. (B) Plantar aspect. (*SU*, sural nerve; *DP*, deep peroneal nerve; *SP*, superficial peroneal nerve; *MP*, medial plantar nerve; *LP*, lateral plantar nerve; *1*, muscular branch of deep peroneal nerve; *2*, nerve to dorsal interosseous space 4; *3*, nerve to dorsal interosseous space 3; *4*, nerve to dorsal interosseous space 2; *5*, cutaneous branch of deep peroneal nerve; *6*, dorsotibial cutaneous hallucal nerve; *7*, plantar tibial cutaneous hallucal nerve; *8*, common digital plantar nerves; *9*, deep branch of lateral plantar nerve; *10*, plantar lateral cutaneous branch to fifth toe; *11*, cuboid; *12*, third cuneiform; *13*, second cuneiform; *14*, first cuneiform; *15*, navicular.) (Adapted from Lippert J. Zur Innervation der menschlichen Fussgelenke. *Anat Entwgesh*. 1962;123:229.)

medial aspect of the fourth toe, but "in most cases branches of these nerves could not be traced to the metatarsophalangeal and interphalangeal joints."[48] The lateral dorsal cutaneous nerve, a branch of the sural nerve, provides articular filaments to the metatarsophalangeal joint of the fifth and the fourth toe, "but branches to the interphalangeal joints of these toes were inconstant."[48]

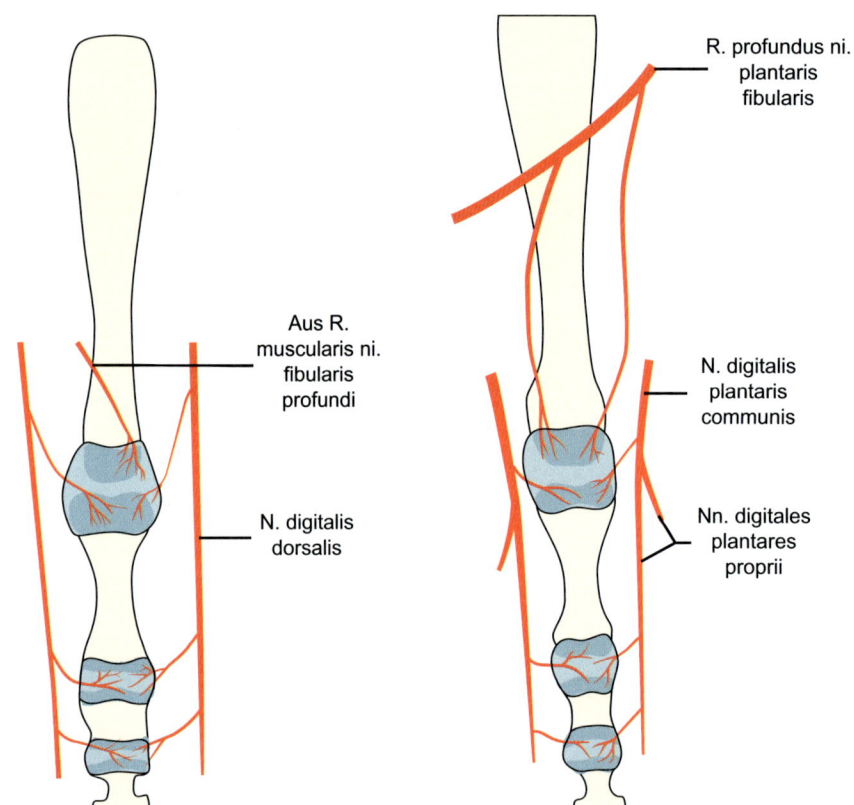

Figure 8.66 Innervation of the lesser toes.
(A) Dorsal aspect. **(B)** Plantar aspect. (Reprinted by permission from Lippert J. Zur Innervation der menschlichen Fussgelenke. *Anat Entwgesh*. 1962;123:229.)

REFERENCES

1. Horwitz MT. Normal anatomy and variations of the peripheral nerves of the leg and foot. *Arch Surg*. 1938;36:626.
2. Kosinski C. The course, mutual relations and distribution of the cutaneous nerve of the metazonal region of the leg and foot. *J Anat*. 1926;60:274.
3. Ortigüela ME, Wood MB, Cahill DR. Anatomy of the sural nerve complex. *J Hand Surg Am*. 1987;12(6):1119-1123.
4. Eastwood DM, Irgau I, Atkins R. The distal course of the sural nerve and its significance for incisions around the lateral hindfoot. *Foot Ankle*. 1992;13(4):199-203.
5. Lawrence SJ, Botte MJ. The sural nerve in the foot and ankle: an anatomic study with clinical and surgical implications. *Foot Ankle Int*. 1994;15(9):490-494.
6. Aktan Ikiz ZA, Ucerler H, Bilge O. The anatomic features of the sural nerve with emphasis on its clinical importance. *Foot Ankle Int*. 2005;7:560-567.
7. Webb J, Moorjani N, Radfort M. Anatomy of the sural nerve and its relation to the Achilles tendon. *Foot Ankle Int*. 2000;21(6):475-477.
8. Tashjian RZ, Appel AJ, Banerjee R, et al. Anatomic study of the gastrocnemius-soleus junction and its relationship to the sural nerve. *Foot Ankle Int*. 2003;6:473-476.
9. Cruveilhier J. *Anatomie Descriptive*. Vol 4. Bechet Jeune; 1836:868.
10. Adkinson DP, Bosse MJ, Gaccione DR, et al. Anatomical variations in the course of the superficial peroneal nerve. *J Bone Joint Surg Am*. 1991;73(1):112.
11. Bryce TH. Note of a case in which the deep accessory peroneal nerve supplied the extensor brevis digitorum pedis on both sides in the same subject. *J Anat Physiol*. 1903-1904;38:79.
12. Bryce TH. Long muscular branch of the musculocutaneous nerve of the leg. *J Anat*. 1896-1897;31:5.
13. Bryce TH. Deep accessory peroneal nerve. *J Anat*. 1900-1901;35:69.
14. Winckler G. Le nerf péronier accessoire profond: Etude d'anatomie comparée. *Arch Anat Histol Embryol*. 1934;18:186.
15. Lambert EH. The accessory deep peroneal nerve: a common variation in innervation of extensor digitorum brevis. *Neurology*. 1969;19:1169.
16. Thomas A. The distribution of the cutaneous nerves on the dorsum of foot. Second Annual Report of the Committee of Collective Investigation of the Anatomical Society of Great Britain and Ireland for the year 1890-1891. *J Anat Physiol*. 1891;26(76):89-90.
17. Canovas F, Bonnel F, Kouloumdjian P. The superficial peroneal nerve at the foot: organization, surgical applications. *Surg Radiol Anat*. 1996;18:241-244.
18. Solomon LB, Ferris L, Tedman R, et al. Surgical anatomy of the sural and superficial fibular nerve with an emphasis on the approach to the lateral malleolus. *J Anat*. 2001;199:717-723.
19. Aktan Ikiz ZA, Ucerler H. The distribution of the superficial peroneal nerve on the dorsum of the foot and its clinical importance in flap surgery. *Foot Ankle Int*. 2006;6:438-444.
20. Blair LM, Botte MJ. Surgical anatomy of the superficial peroneal nerve in the ankle and foot. *Clin Orthop Relat Res*. 1994;305:229-238.
21. Sayli U, Tekdemyr Y, Cubuk HE, et al. The course of the superficial peroneal nerve: an anatomical cadaver study. *Foot Ankle Int*. 1998;4:63-69.
22. Ucerler H, Aktan Ikiz ZA. The variations of the sensory branches of the superficial peroneal nerve course and clinical importance. *Foot Ankle Int*. 2005;11:942-946.
23. Miller R, Hartman G. Origin and course of the dorsomedial cutaneous nerve of the great toe. *Foot Ankle Int*. 1996;17:620-622.
24. Macaggi NA. Sul livetto di biforcazione del nervo tibiale posteriore. *Arch Ital Chirurg*. 1921;3:507.
25. Hovelacque A. *Anatomie des Nerfs Craniens et Rachidiens et du Système Grand Sympathique Chez l'Homme*. Doin; 1927:627-635.
26. Dellon AL, Mackinnon SE. Tibial nerve branching in the tarsal tunnel. *Arch Neurol*. 1984;41:645.
27. Havel PE, Ebraheun NA, Clark SE, et al. Tibial nerve branching in the tarsal tunnel. *Foot Ankle*. 1988;9(3):117.
28. Rudinger N. *Die Gelenknerven des Menschlichen Körpers*. Enke Erlangen; 1857.
29. Paturet G. *Traité d'Anatomie Humaine*. Vol 2. Masson; 1951:1067-1069.
30. Dujarier CH. *Anatomie de Membres: Dissection-Anatomie Topographique*. 2nd ed. Masson; 1924:323.
31. Davis TJ, Schon LC. Branches of the tibial nerve: anatomic variations. *Foot Ankle Int*. 1995;16(1):22-29.

32. Govsa F, Bilge O, Ozer MA. Variations in the origin of the medial and inferior calcaneal nerves. *Arch Orthop Trauma Surg*. 2006;126:6-14.
33. Grodinsky M. A study of the fascial spaces of the foot and their bearing on infections. *Surg Obstet Gynecol*. 1929;49(6):737.
34. Bosjen-Møller F, Flagstad KE. Plantar aponeurosis and internal architecture of the ball of the foot. *J Anat*. 1976;121:599.
35. Jones JR, Klenerman L. A study of the communicating branch between the medial and lateral plantar nerves. *Foot Ankle*. 1984;4(6):318.
36. Roegholt MN. Een nervus calcaneus inferior als overbrenger van de pijn bij calcaneodynie of calcanensspoor en de daaruit volgende therapie. *Ned Tijdschr v Geneeskd*. 1940;84:1898.
37. Tanz SS. Heel pain. *Clin Orthop*. 1963;28:169.
38. Arenson DJ, Cosentina GL, Suran SM. The inferior calcaneal nerve: an anatomical study. *J Am Podiatry Assoc*. 1980;70:552.
39. Przylucki H, Jones CL. Entrapment neuropathy of muscle branch of lateral plantar nerve. *J Am Podiatry Assoc*. 1981;71:119.
40. Baxter DE, Thigpen CM. Heel pain: operative results. *Foot Ankle*. 1984;5(1):16.
41. Rondhuis JJ, Huson A. The first branch of the lateral plantar nerve and heel pain. *Acta Morphol Neerl-Scand*. 1986;24:269.
42. Hamm JT, Sanders M. Anatomic variations of the nerve to the abductor digiti quinti muscle. Proceedings of the Third Annual Summer Meeting of the American Foot and Ankle Society, July 1987. *Foot Ankle*. 1987;8(2):123.
43. Hallopeau P. Note sur le nerf de l'adducteur oblique du gros orteil. *Bull Mem Soc Anat Paris*. 1900;2:1078.
44. Chou LB, Choi LE, Ramachandra T, et al. Variation of nerve to flexor hallucis brevis. *Foot Ankle Int*. 2008;10:1042-1044.
45. Ziólkowski M, Sudev E, Porwolik K, et al. Skin innervation of the foot in human fetuses. *Folia Morphol (Warsz.)*. 1987;46(1-2):57.
46. Morin F, Roasenda F. *Le Enervazioni Articolari*. Minerva Medica Torino; 1948.
47. Lippert J. Zur Innervation der menschlichen Fussgelenke. *Z Anat Entwgesh*. 1962;123:299.
48. Gardner E, Gray DJ. The innervation of the joints of the foot. *Anat Rec*. 1968;161:141.
49. Champetier J. Innervation de l'articulation tibio-tarsienne (articulatio talo-cruralis). *Acta Anat*. 1970;77:398.

Cross-Sectional and Topographic Anatomy

Shahan K. Sarrafian and Armen S. Kelikian

I. CROSS-SECTIONAL ANATOMY

The cross-sectional anatomy provides the foundation for the topographical, surgical anatomy.

The compartmental anatomy of the tibiotalocalcaneal tunnel is best understood when considered in continuity with the posterior compartment of the leg.

A cross-sectional study was conducted in the transverse, oblique, and coronal planes in two fresh frozen lower legs and feet. In the major first specimen, the sections were made as indicated in Figure 9.1. This provided transverse sections of the distal leg-ankle 1 cm apart, followed by oblique section blocks of the hindfoot, tarsus, and coronal sections up to the base of the proximal phalanx of the big toe. The second specimen provided coronal sections of the hindfoot and tarsus. Previous cross-sectional materials were incorporated for further clarification or demonstration of the anatomy.

TRANSVERSE CROSS-SECTIONS OF THE DISTAL LEG AND ANKLE

As shown in Figure 9.2, Section 8 is 8 cm proximal to the level of the medial malleolus (distal surface of section). The tibia and fibula are united by the interosseous membrane and the leg is enveloped by the superficial aponeurosis cruris. Four compartments are delineated: anterior, lateral, posterior superficial, and posterior deep. The posterior compartment has been divided into a superficial and deep compartment by the deep aponeurosis cruris. The latter originates from the posteromedial border of the tibia, adheres initially to the superficial aponeurosis cruris, and then diverges transversely to insert on the posterior wall of the lateral compartment.

The anterior compartment contains the extensor digitorum muscle, the extensor hallucis muscle, the tibialis anterior, which is becoming tendinous, and the anterior tibial neurovascular bundle. The vessels are against the bone, with the nerve anterior.

The neurovascular bundle is located between the tibialis anterior and the extensor hallucis longus muscle.

The lateral compartment lodges the peroneus longus and brevis muscles. The superficial posterior compartment contains the gastrocnemius-soleus muscle. Located in the deep posterior compartment are the musculotendinous flexor hallucis longus and the tibialis posterior tendon anterior to the musculotendinous flexor digitorum longus. The posterior tibial neurovascular bundle is also located in this deep compartment against the deep crural aponeurosis. The peroneal artery is just posterior to the interosseous membrane.

Section 7 is 7 cm proximal to the level of the medial malleolus (distal surface of section; Fig. 9.3). The partition of the compartments and the contents are similar to those in Section 8 except for the slight decrease in size of the posterior superficial compartment.

Section 6 is 6 cm proximal to the level of the medial malleolus (distal surface of section; Fig. 9.4). The partition of the compartments is unchanged. The lateral compartment is shifting posteriorly. The superficial posterior compartment is decreasing in size.

Section 5 is 5 cm proximal to the level of the medial malleolus (distal surface of section; Fig. 9.5).

A major change occurs: a *fifth compartment* appears. A new aponeurotic structure appears in the deep posterior compartment. It originates at the posteromedial border of the tibia, courses posteriorly, remaining adherent to the deep aponeurosis cruris, curves back anteriorly, and attaches to the posterior aspect of the tibia. It delineates a deep posteromedial fifth compartment, which lodges the tendons of the tibialis posterior and the flexor digitorum longus. The remaining larger segment, deep posterolateral, contains the posterior tibial neurovascular bundle and the musculotendinous flexor hallucis longus. The lateral compartment has shifted into a posterior position relative to the fibula. In the anterior compartment, a tunnel has formed for the tibialis anterior tendon.

Section 4 is 4 cm proximal to the level of the medial malleolus (distal surface of section; Fig. 9.6). The interosseous membrane has disappeared. The tibial metaphysis is united to the

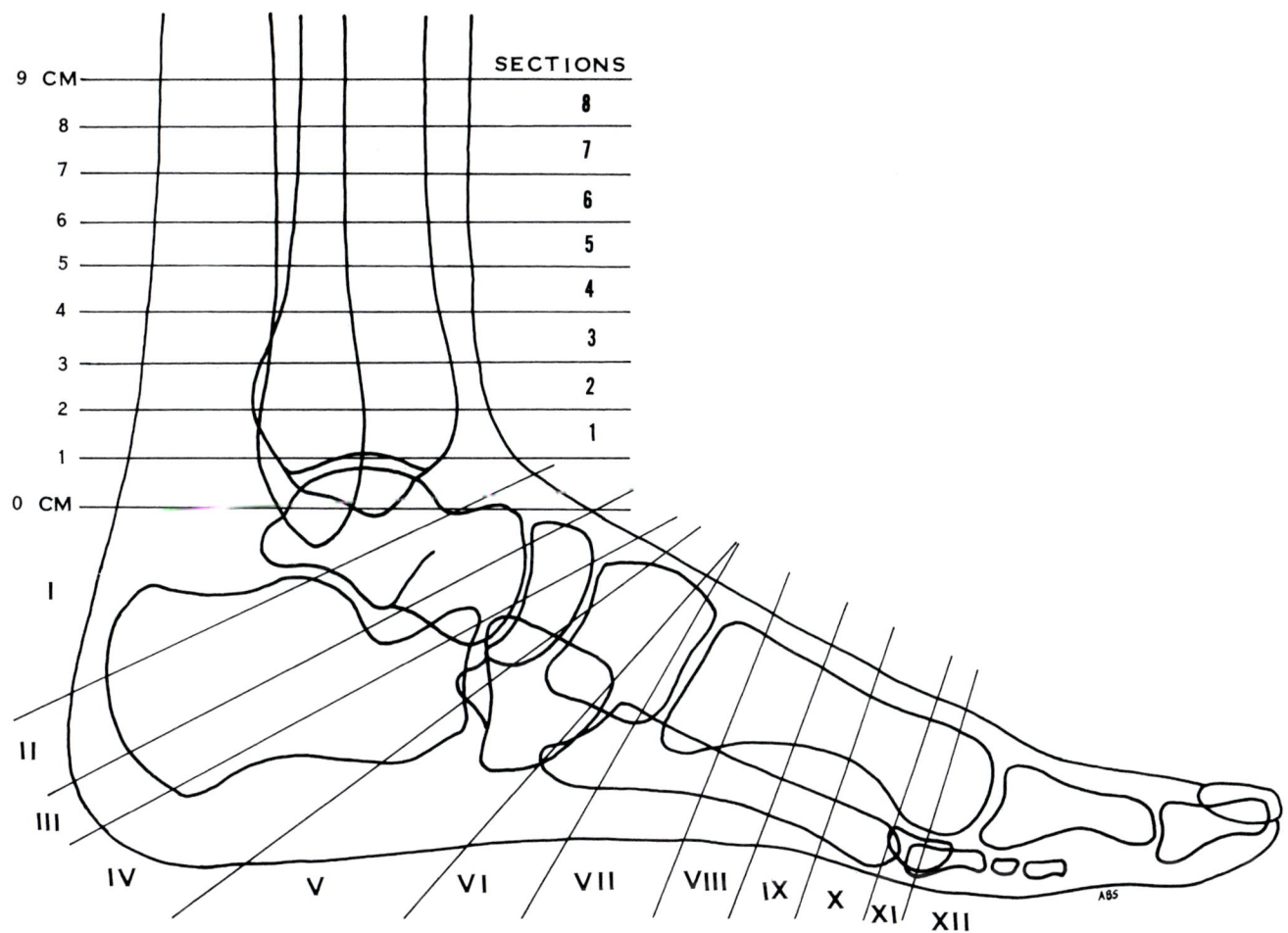

Figure 9.1 **Cross-sections (transverse, oblique, and coronal) of a left foot.** This is the key figure for all sections to locate the level of the cut. The distal leg has been sectioned transversely starting at 9 cm proximal to the tip of the medial malleolus. Eight sections were made, 1 cm apart, numbered 8 to 1. The remaining foot was sectioned obliquely, in the coronal plane, into 12 sections numbered I to XII. The exact levels of the cuts are indicated by the lines drawn relative to the skeletal frame. The sections are identified by their number and the specification of the surface viewed: proximal or distal.

distal fibula through the syndesmosis. Five compartments are present, as in the previous section. The tibialis posterior tendon is medial to the flexor digitorum longus tendon; the crossing of the two tendons has occurred and this level is considered the beginning of the tibiotalocalcaneal tunnel. A triangular aponeurotic space is present, superficial to the deep posterior compartment. It lodges a medial calcaneal neurovascular bundle. The anterior peroneal artery is now seen anterior to the tibiofibular syndesmosis.

Section 3 is 3 cm proximal to the level of the medial malleolus (distal surface of section; Figs. 9.7 and 9.8).

The tibial distal metaphysis is quadrilateral with concave-convex fit at the tibiofibular syndesmosis. The deep posterior compartment is now reduced in size and four tunnels are formed corresponding to the posterior aspect of the tibia. The common deep compartment previously lodging the tibialis posterior tendon and the flexor digitorum tendon is divided into two tunnels, the most medial corresponding to the tibialis posterior tendon and the lateral to the flexor digitorum longus tendon. Similarly, the deep posterolateral compartment is divided by a septum into two tunnels, the medial for the posterior neurovascular bundle and the larger lateral for the flexor hallucis tendon-muscle. The peroneal tunnel is posterior to the fibula.

The superficial posterior compartment has decreased in size. One clearly sees how the superficial aponeurosis cruris splits to enclose the Achilles tendon and remains adherent at this level to the deep aponeurosis cruris. Both unite laterally with the peroneal compartment.

This level represents the tibial section of the tibiotalocalcaneal tunnel.

Section 2 is 2 cm proximal to the level of the medial malleolus (distal surface of section; Fig. 9.9). The disposition of the compartments is similar to that in Section 3.

Section 1 is 1 cm proximal to the top of the medial malleolus. This section passes through the malleoli and the talu (distal surface of section; Figs. 9.10 and 9.11).

The tunnel of the tibialis posterior is posterior to the medial malleolus. The tunnels of the flexor digitorum longus, the posterior tibial neurovascular bundle, and the flexor hallucis

432 Sarrafian's Anatomy of the Foot and Ankle

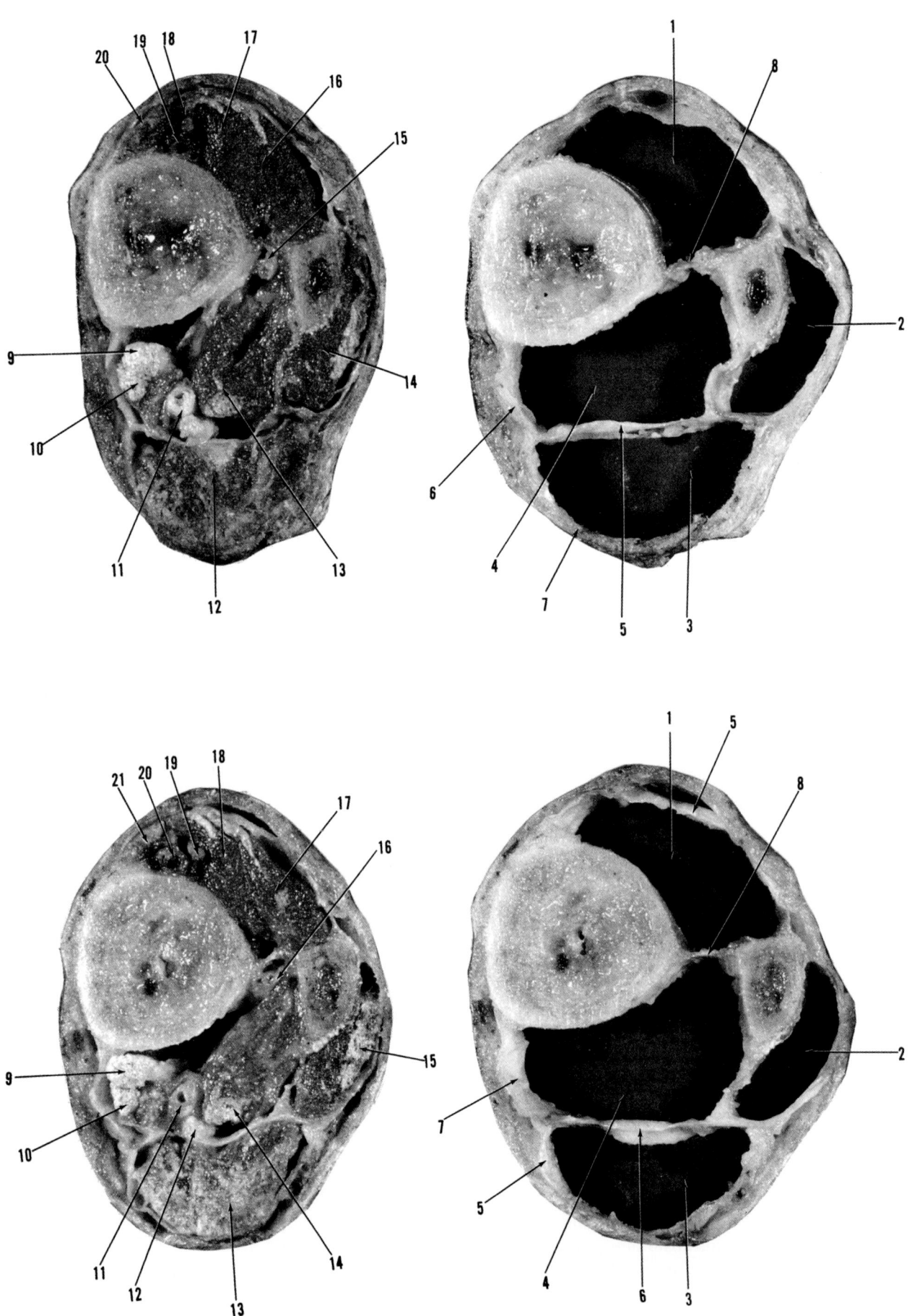

Figure 9.2 **Section 8.** Cross-section of leg at 8 cm proximal to tip of medial malleolus. Distal surface of section. (*1*, anterior compartment; *2*, lateral compartment; *3*, posterior superficial compartment; *4*, posterior deep compartment; *5*, deep aponeurosis cruris; *6*, adherent portion of superficial and deep aponeurosis cruris; *7*, superficial aponeurosis cruris; *8*, interosseous membrane; *9*, tibialis posterior tendon; *10*, flexor digitorum longus tendon; *11*, posterior tibial neurovascular bundle located within deep posterior compartment; *12*, triceps surae; *13*, flexor hallucis longus; *14*, peronei; *15*, peroneal vessels; *16*, extensor digitorum longus; *17*, extensor hallucis longus; *18*, anterior tibial nerve; *19*, anterior tibial vessels; *20*, tibialis anterior.)

Figure 9.3 **Section 7.** Cross-section of leg at 7 cm proximal to tip of medial malleolus. Distal surface of section. (*1*, anterior compartment; *2*, lateral compartment; *3*, posterior superficial compartment; *4*, posterior deep compartment; *5*, superficial aponeurosis cruris; *6*, deep aponeurosis cruris; *7*, adherent portion of superficial and deep aponeurosis cruris; *8*, interosseous membrane; *9*, tibialis posterior tendon; *10*, flexor digitorum longus tendon; *11*, posterior tibial vessels; *12*, posterior tibial nerve; *13*, triceps surae; *14*, flexor hallucis longus; *15*, peronei; *16*, peronei vessels; *17*, extensor digitorum longus; *18*, extensor hallucis longus; *19*, anterior tibial nerve; *20*, anterior tibial vessels; *21*, tibialis anterior tendon.)

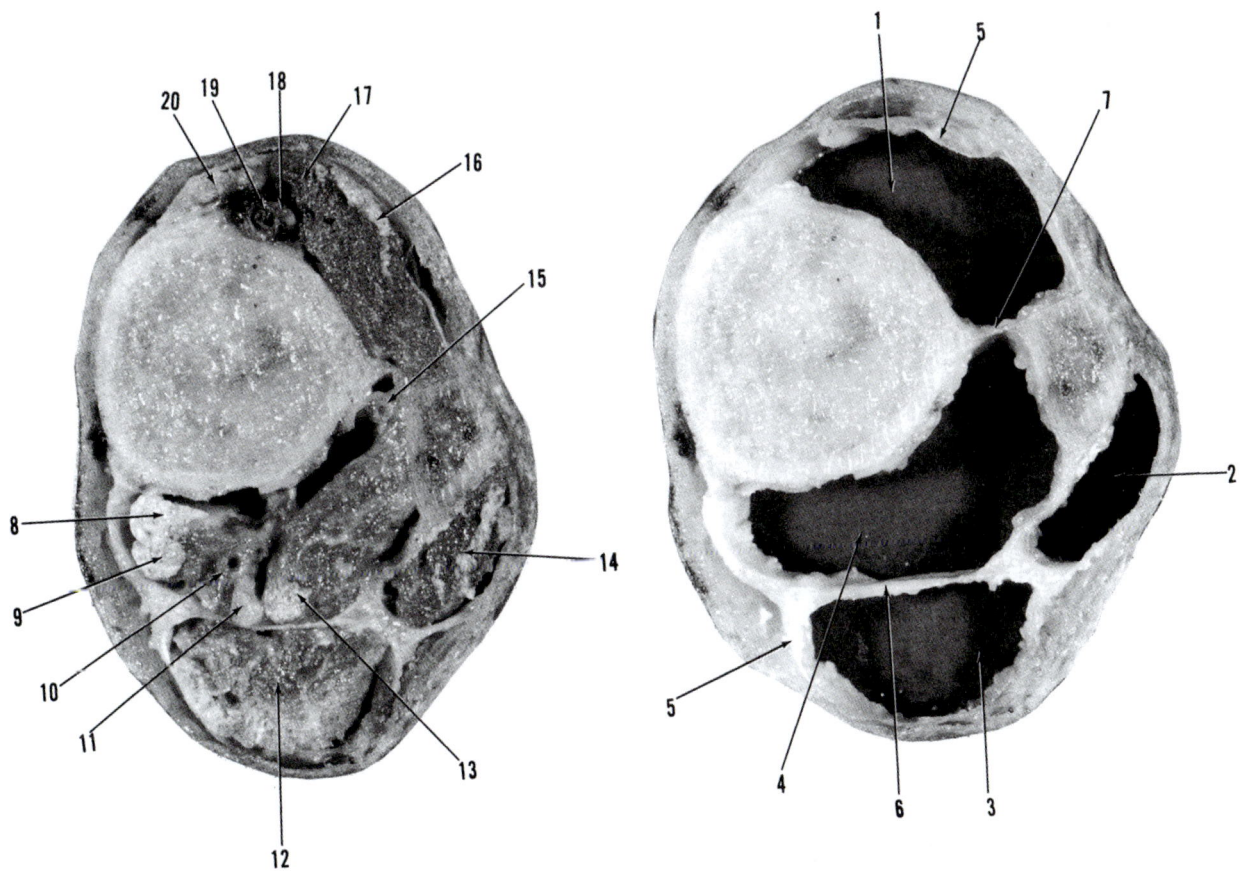

Figure 9.4 **Section 6.** Cross-section of leg at 6 cm proximal to tip of medial malleolus. Distal surface of section. (*1*, anterior compartment; *2*, lateral compartment; *3*, posterior superficial compartment; *4*, posterior deep compartment; *5*, superficial aponeurosis cruris; *6*, deep aponeurosis cruris; *7*, intermuscular septum; *8*, tibialis posterior tendon; *9*, flexor digitorum longus tendon; *10*, posterior tibial vessels; *11*, posterior tibial nerve; *12*, triceps surae; *13*, flexor hallucis longus; *14*, peronei; *15*, peroneal vessels; *16*, extensor digitorum longus; *17*, extensor hallucis longus; *18*, anterior tibial nerve; *19*, anterior tibial vessels; *20*, tibialis anterior tendon.)

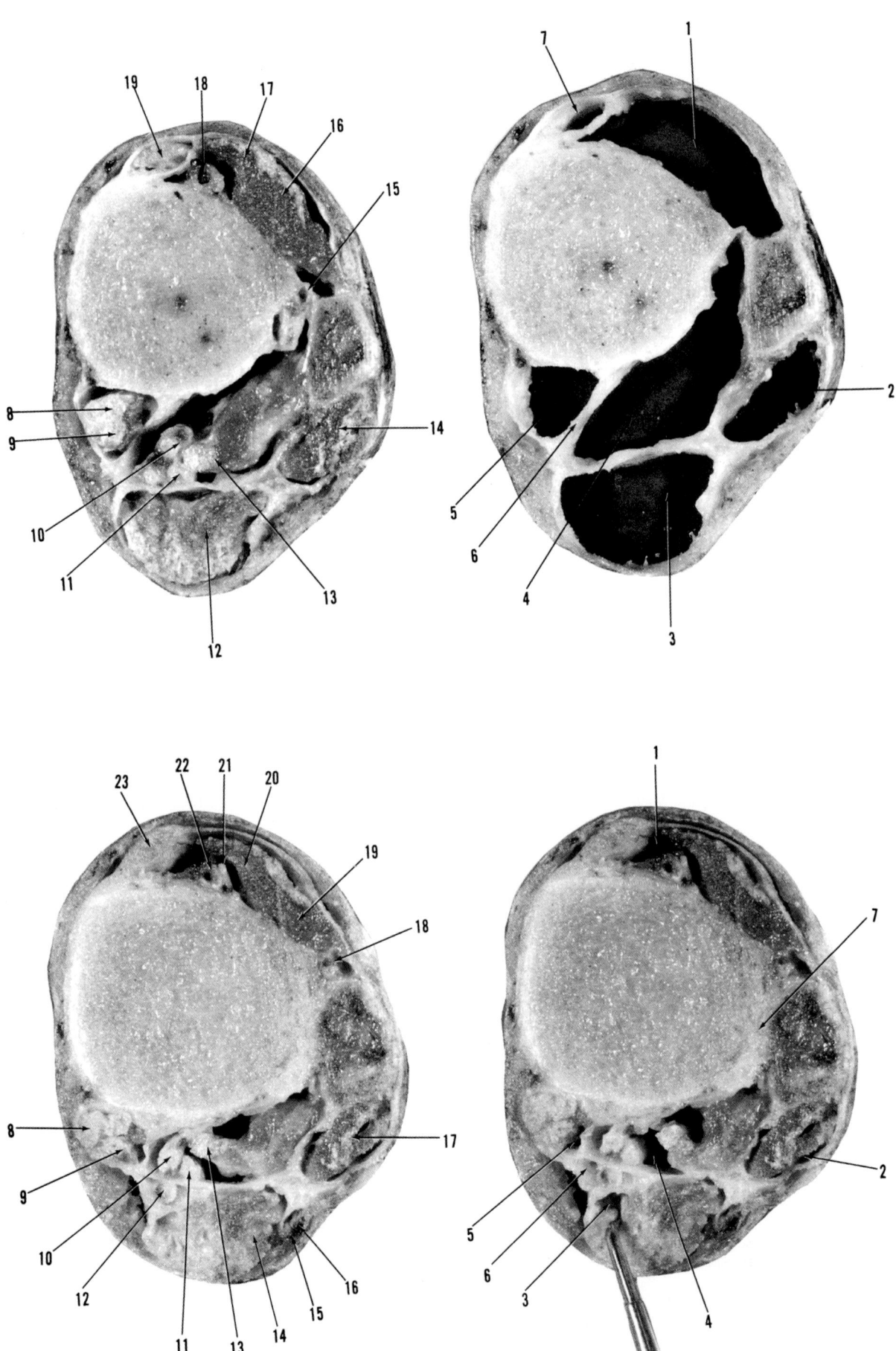

◀ **Figure 9.5** **Section 5.** Cross-section of leg at 5 cm proximal to tip of medial malleolus. Distal surface of section. (*1*, anterior compartment; *2*, lateral compartment; *3*, posterior superficial compartment; *4*, posterior deep compartment; *5*, fifth posterior compartment; *6*, aponeurosis of fifth compartment; *7*, tunnel of tibialis anterior tendon; *8*, tibialis posterior tendon; *9*, flexor digitorum longus tendon; *10*, posterior tibial vessels; *11*, posterior tibial nerve; *12*, triceps surae; *13*, flexor hallucis longus tendon muscle unit; *14*, peronei; *15*, peroneal vessels; *16*, extensor digitorum longus; *17*, extensor hallucis longus; *18*, anterior tibial neurovascular bundle; *19*, tibialis anterior tendon.)

◀ **Figure 9.6** **Section 4.** Cross-section of leg at 4 cm proximal to tip of medial malleolus. Distal surface of section. (*1*, anterior compartment; *2*, lateral compartment; *3*, posterior superficial compartment; *4*, posterior deep compartment; *5*, fifth posterior compartment; *6*, tunnel for medial calcaneal neurovascular bundle; *7*, tibiofibular syndesmosis; *8*, tibialis posterior tendon; *9*, flexor digitorum longus tendon; *10*, posterior tibial vessels; *11*, posterior tibial nerve; *12*, medial calcaneal neurovascular bundle; *13*, flexor hallucis longus tendon-muscle unit; *14*, triceps surae; *15*, sural nerve; *16*, short saphenous vein; *17*, peronei; *18*, anterior peroneal vessels; *19*, extensor digitorum longus; *20*, extensor hallucis longus; *21*, anterior tibial nerve; *22*, anterior tibial vessels; *23*, tibialis anterior tendon.)

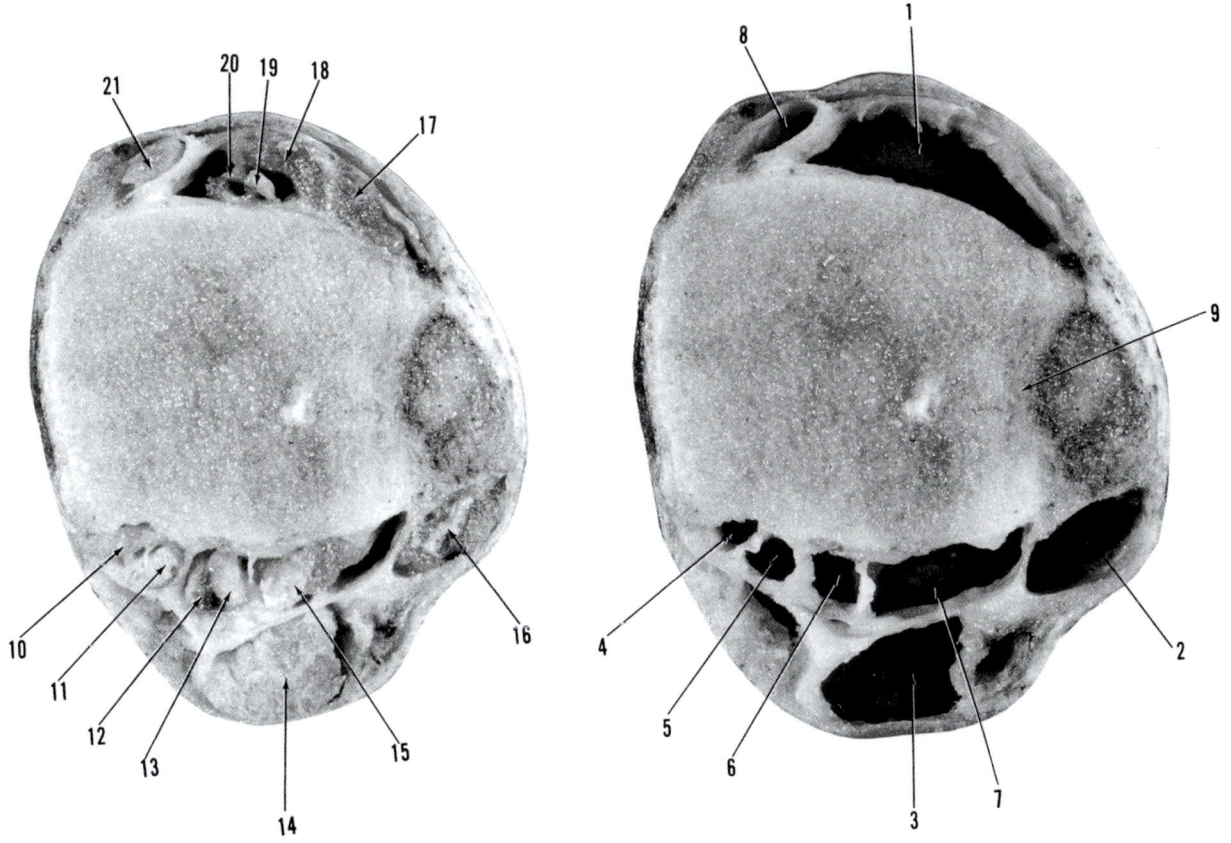

Figure 9.7 **Section 3.** Cross-section of ankle at 3 cm proximal to tip of medial malleolus. Distal surface of section. (*1*, anterior compartment; *2*, lateral compartment; *3*, posterior superficial compartment; *4*, tunnel of tibialis posterior tendon; *5*, tunnel of flexor digitorum longus tendon; *6*, tunnel of posterior tibial neurovascular bundle; *7*, tunnel of flexor hallucis longus tendon-muscle unit; *8*, tunnel of tibialis anterior tendon; *9*, tibiofibular syndesmosis; *10*, tendon of tibialis posterior; *11*, tendon of flexor digitorum longus; *12*, posterior tibial vessels; *13*, posterior tibial nerve; *14*, Achilles tendon [musculotendinous]; *15*, flexor hallucis longus tendon-muscle unit; *16*, peronei; *17*, extensor digitorum longus; *18*, extensor hallucis longus; *19*, anterior tibial nerve; *20*, anterior tibial vessels; *21*, tendon of tibialis anterior.)

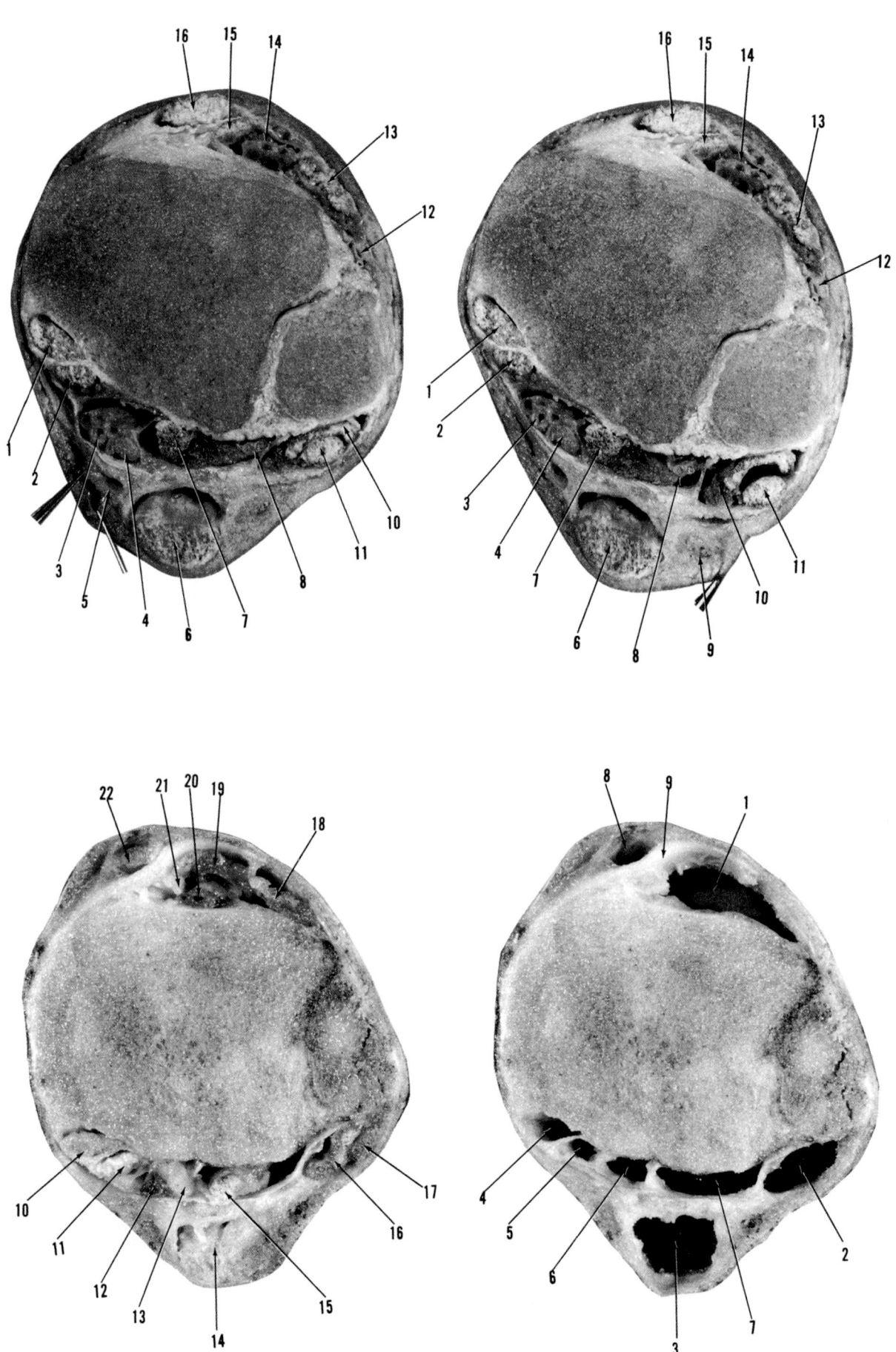

◀ **Figure 9.8** **Section 3.** Cross-section of ankle at 3 cm proximal to tip of medial malleolus. Distal surface of section from nonsequential specimen. (*1*, tibialis posterior tendon and tunnel; *2*, flexor digitorum longus tendon and tunnel; *3*, posterior tibial vessels and tunnel; *4*, posterior tibial nerve and tunnel; *5*, medial calcaneal neurovascular bundle and tunnel; *6*, Achilles tendon and tunnel; *7*, flexor hallucis longus tendon-muscle and tunnel; *8*, posterior peroneal vessels; *9*, sural nerve and short saphenous vein; *10*, frayed peroneus brevis tendon; *11*, peroneus longus tendon; *12*, anterior peroneal vessels; *13*, extensor digitorum longus tendon within tunnel; *14*, anterior tibial neurovascular bundle; *15*, extensor hallucis longus tendon under frondiform ligament; *16*, tibialis anterior tendon and tunnel.)

◀ **Figure 9.9** **Section 2.** Cross-section of ankle at 2 cm proximal to tip of medial malleolus. Distal surface of section. (*1*, anterior compartment; *2*, peronei compartment; *3*, tunnel of Achilles tendon; *4*, tunnel of tibialis posterior tendon; *5*, tunnel of flexor digitorum longus tendon; *6*, posterior tibial neurovascular tunnel; *7*, tunnel of flexor hallucis longus muscle-tendon unit; *8*, tunnel of tibialis anterior tendon; *9*, inferior extensor retinaculum superomedial arm; *10*, tibialis posterior tendon; *11*, flexor digitorum longus tendon; *12*, posterior tibial vessels; *13*, posterior tibial nerve; *14*, Achilles tendon; *15*, flexor hallucis longus tendon-muscle unit; *16*, peroneus brevis tendon; *17*, peroneus longus tendon; *18*, extensor digitorum longus; *19*, extensor hallucis longus; *20*, anterior tibial vessels; *21*, anterior tibial nerve; *22*, tibialis anterior tendon.)

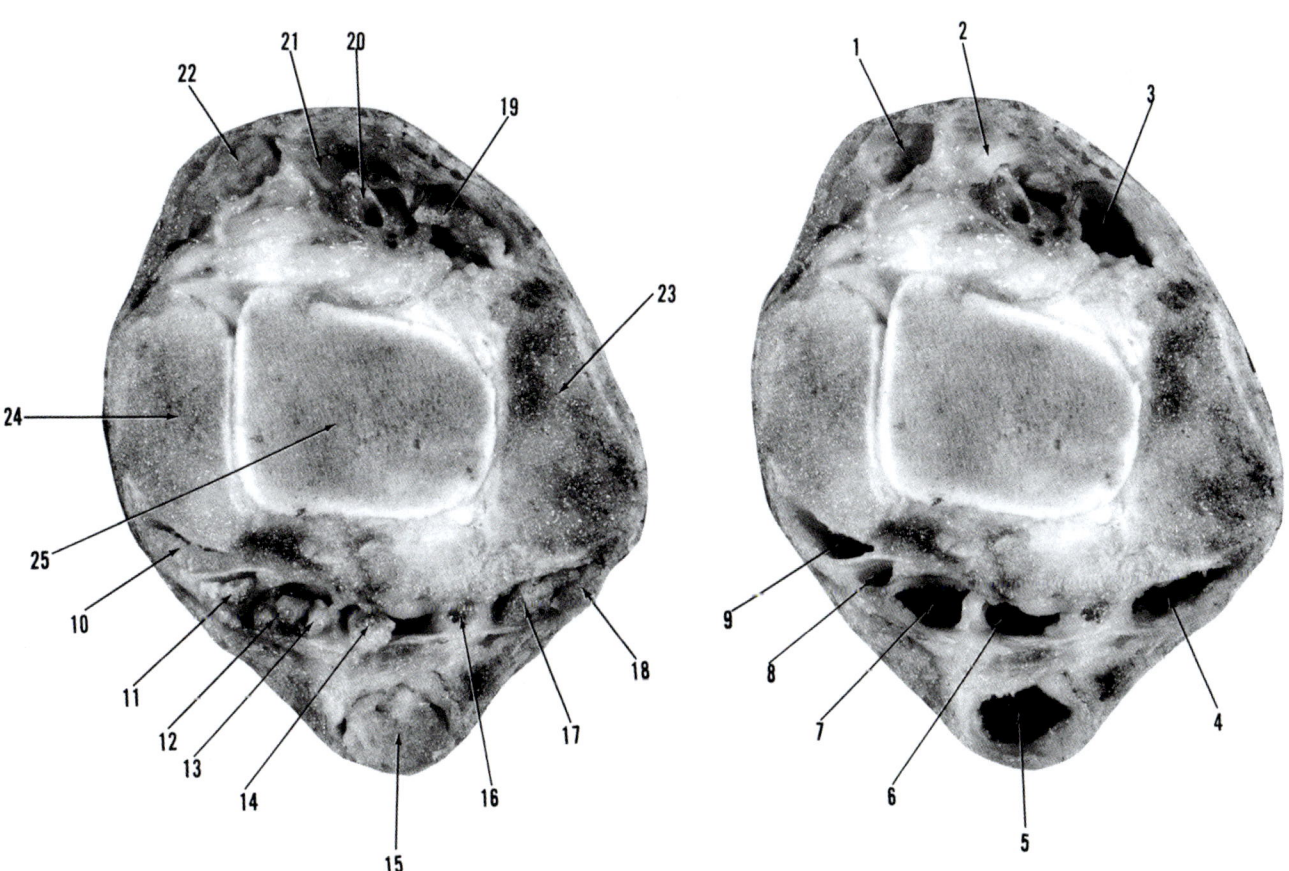

Figure 9.10 **Section 1.** Cross-section of ankle at 1 cm proximal to tip of medial malleolus. Distal surface of section. (*1*, tunnel of tibialis anterior tendon; *2*, superomedial band of inferior extensor retinaculum determining tunnel of extensor hallucis longus tendon and anterior tibial neurovascular bundle; *3*, tunnel of extensor digitorum longus; *4*, tunnel of peronei; *5*, tunnel of Achilles tendon; *6*, tunnel of flexor hallucis longus tendon; *7*, tunnel of posterior tibial neurovascular bundle; *8*, tunnel of flexor digitorum longus tendon; *9*, tunnel of tibialis posterior tendon; *10*, tibialis posterior tendon; *11*, flexor digitorum longus tendon; *12*, posterior tibial vessels; *13*, posterior tibial nerve; *14*, flexor hallucis longus tendon; *15*, Achilles tendon; *16*, posterior peroneal vessels; *17*, peroneus brevis tendon; *18*, peroneus longus tendon; *19*, extensor digitorum longus; *20*, anterior tibial neurovascular bundle; *21*, extensor hallucis longus tendon; *22*, tibialis anterior tendon; *23*, lateral malleolus; *24*, medial malleolus; *25*, talus.)

longus correspond to the posterior aspect of the tibiotalar joint. The peroneal tunnel is located on the posterior surface of the lateral malleolus. The posterior peroneal artery is located in the tunnel of the flexor hallucis longus. The Achilles tendon tunnel has further decreased in size, corresponding to the size of the tendon. Anteriorly, the inferior extensor retinaculum has formed the tunnels of the tibialis anterior, the anterior tibial neurovascular bundles, the extensor hallucis longus, and the extensor digitorum longus.

OBLIQUE SECTIONS OF THE HINDFOOT-TARSUS FOLLOWED BY TRANSVERSE SECTIONS OF THE TARSUS AND FOREFOOT IN THE CORONAL PLANE (SEE FIG. 9.1)

Section I is an oblique section passing through the posterior talocalcaneal joint. The distal surface of section is shown in Figure 9.12.

The tunnels of the tibialis posterior tendon, the flexor digitorum longus, the posterior tibial neurovascular bundle, and the flexor hallucis longus tendons are oriented in a near sagittal plane rather than in a coronal plane as seen in the previous sections.

Section II is an oblique section of the calcaneotalonavicular. The distal surface of this section is shown in Figure 9.13.

The tibialis posterior tendon and its tunnel are applied on the superomedial calcaneonavicular ligament. The flexor digitorum longus and tunnel are located on the medial surface of the sustentaculum tali and the flexor hallucis longus tendon and tunnel occupy the lower surface of the sustentaculum tali. The posterior tibial neurovascular bundle is located in a large sagittally oriented tunnel limited medially by the flexor retinaculum, laterally by the tunnel of the flexor hallucis longus, further posteriorly by the quadratus plantae and its investing fascia, and anteriorly by the tunnel of the flexor digitorum longus.

Section III is an oblique section of the calcaneotalonavicular. The dorsal surface of the section is shown in Figure 9.14. This section clearly depicts the calcaneal tunnel. The medial wall of the tunnel is formed by the abductor hallucis muscle and its investing fascia, the lateral thicker than the medial. The lateral wall is formed by the concave surface of the calcaneus buttressed by the quadratus plantae and its aponeurosis. The interfascicular lamina extends from the fascia of the quadratus plantae to the lateral investing aponeurosis of the abductor hallucis. It divides the calcaneal canal into two chambers: anterosuperior for the medial plantar neurovascular bundle and posteroinferior for the lateral plantar neurovascular bundle. The common tunnel of the flexor digitorum longus and flexor hallucis longus forms the roof of the superior calcaneal chamber. The tibialis posterior tendon has inserted on the tuberosity of the navicular.

Section IV is an oblique section of the calcaneocubonavicular cuneiforms. The distal surface of section is shown in Figure 9.15.

Figure 9.11 Section 1. Cross-section of ankle at 1 cm proximal to tip of medial malleolus. Talar dome removed. Distal surface of section of nonsequential specimen. (*1*, tibialis posterior tendon and tunnel; *2*, flexor digitorum longus tendon and tunnel; *3*, posterior tibial vessels and tunnel; *4*, posterior tibial nerve and tunnel; *5*, flexor hallucis longus tendon and tunnel; *6*, Achilles tendon and tunnel; *7*, sural nerve; *8*, short saphenous vein; *9*, peroneus brevis tendon, frayed, and tunnel; *10*, peroneus longus tendon and tunnel; *11*, posterior peroneal vessels; *12, 13*, posterior tibiofibular ligaments; *14*, lateral malleolus; *15*, synovial fringe of tibiofibular syndesmosis; *16*, extensor digitorum longus tendons and tunnel; *17*, anterior tibial vessels; *18*, anterior tibial nerve; *19*, extensor hallucis tendon and tunnel; *20*, tibialis anterior tendon and tunnel; *21*, greater saphenous vein; *22*, medial malleolus.)

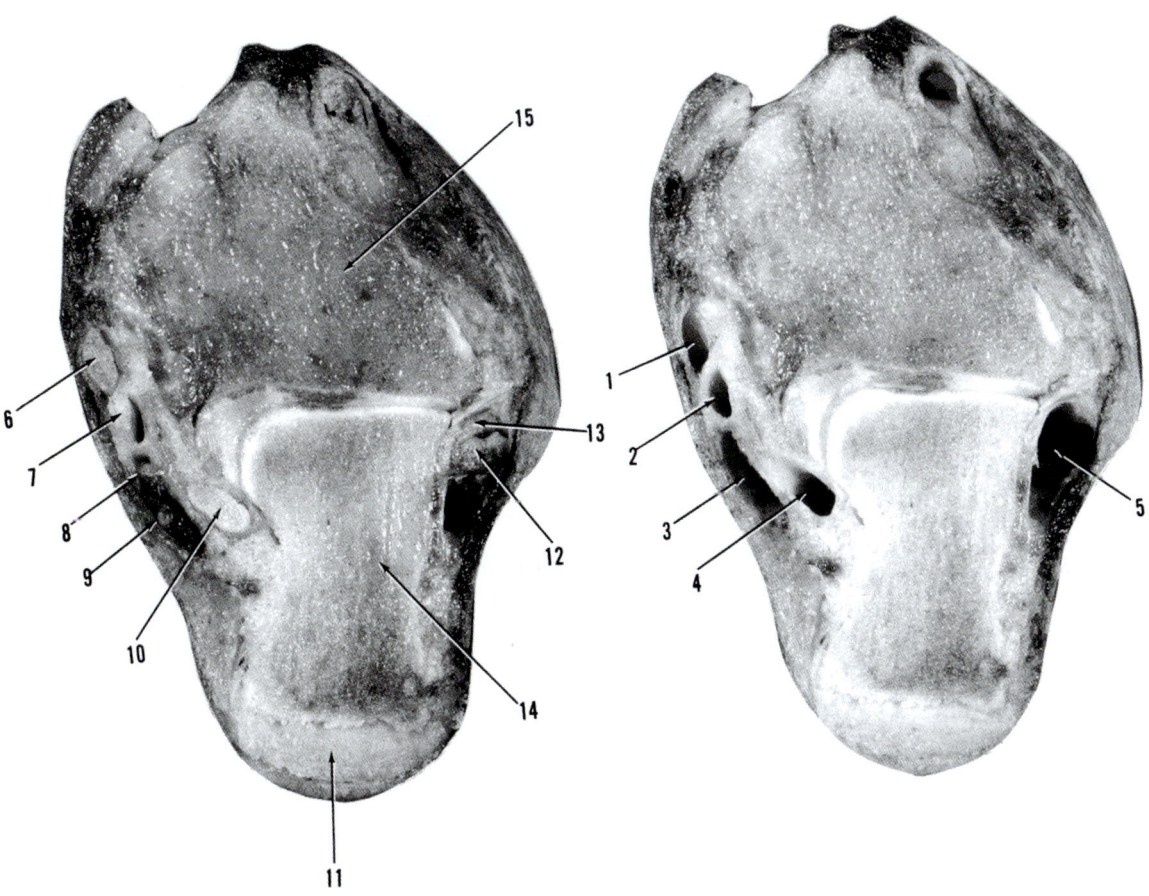

Figure 9.12 Section I. Oblique section talocalcaneal passing through the posterior talocalcaneal joint. Distal surface of section. (*1*, tunnel of tibialis posterior tendon; *2*, tunnel of flexor digitorum longus; *3*, tunnel of posterior tibial neurovascular bundle; *4*, tunnel of flexor hallucis longus; *5*, tunnel of peronei tendons; *6*, tibialis posterior tendon; *7*, flexor digitorum longus tendon; *8*, medial plantar neurovascular bundle; *9*, lateral plantar neurovascular bundle; *10*, flexor hallucis longus tendon; *11*, Achilles tendon; *12*, peroneus longus tendon; *13*, peroneus brevis tendon; *14*, calcaneus; *15*, talus.)

The long flexor tendons have crossed, and the flexor digitorum longus is inferior or plantar to the tendon of the flexor hallucis longus. The medial plantar neurovascular bundle now courses within the medial intermuscular septum. The latter forms the lateral investing layer of the larger abductor hallucis muscle and continues as a septum interposed between the abductor hallucis muscle and the flexor digitorum brevis muscle.

Section V is an oblique section of the calcaneocubonavicular cuneiforms. The proximal surface of the section, distal to section IV, is shown in Figure 9.16.

The flexor hallucis longus is separated from the flexor digitorum longus-quadratus plantae by a septum. The tibialis posterior is insertional. The three compartments of the sole are clearly identified: lateral, central, medial. The lateral compartment lodges the abductor digiti quinti and the medial compartment lodges the abductor hallucis muscle. The central compartment is subdivided into a superficial compartment for the flexor digitorum brevis and an intermediary compartment for the quadratus plantae and the flexor digitorum longus. The medial plantar neurovascular bundle is carried within the medial intermuscular septum. The lateral plantar neurovascular bundle is located between the transverse aponeurosis of the quadratus plantae and a thin aponeurosis that is more superficial.

A different view of Section V is provided in Figure 9.17. This figure shows the distal surface of a coronal section through cuboid, cuneiforms 1 to 3, and the base of metatarsal 5.

The peroneus longus tendon and its tunnel are under the cuboid and covered by the lateral compartment lodging the abductor digiti quinti. The middle or central compartment is divided by a transverse septum into the superficial compartment for the flexor digitorum brevis and the intermediary compartment lodging the flexor digitorum longus and the quadratus plantae. The flexor hallucis longus is medial to the flexor digitorum longus. The medial compartment lodging the abductor hallucis muscle is under the first cuneiform. The medial and lateral intermuscular septa are clearly identified. At both insertional sites of the transverse septum of the central compartment are the medial plantar neurovascular bundle on the medial side and the lateral plantar neurovascular bundle on the lateral side. On the most dorsal aspect of the central compartment, a short, sturdy transverse septum is present uniting the apices of the first and third cuneiforms.

Section VI is a coronal section through cuneiforms$_{1\text{-}2\text{-}3}$, the cuboid, and the base of metatarsal 5 (Fig. 9.18). The proximal surface of the section is shown. The disposition of the compartments is similar to that of the previous section. The fifth metatarsocuboid joint is apparent.

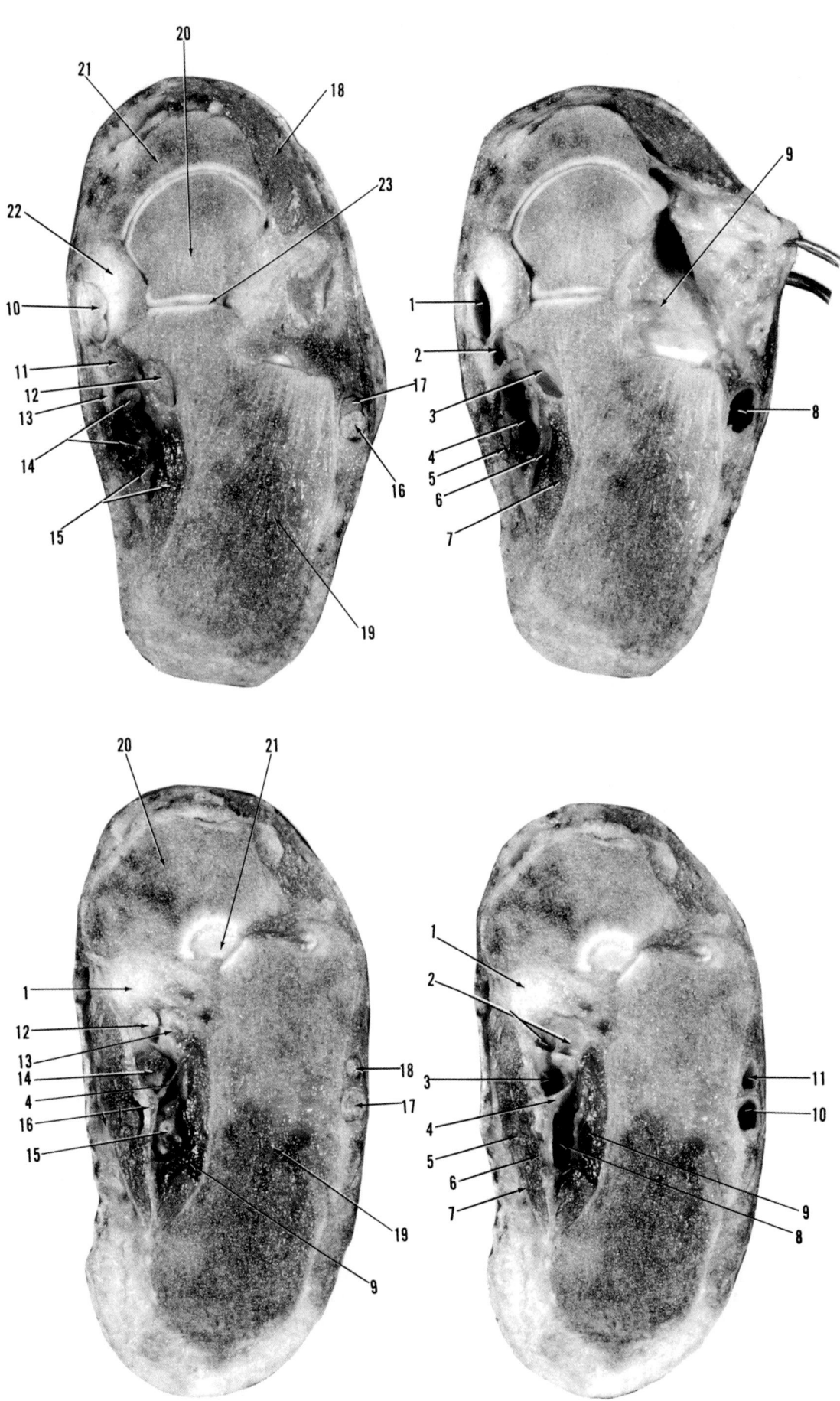

◀ **Figure 9.13** **Section II.** Oblique section calcaneotalonavicular. Distal surface of section. (*1*, tunnel of tibialis posterior tendon; *2*, tunnel of flexor digitorum longus tendon; *3*, tunnel of flexor hallucis longus tendon; *4*, tunnel of posterior tibial neurovascular bundle; *5*, flexor retinaculum; *6*, investing fascia of quadratus plantae medial head; *7*, quadratus plantae medial head; *8*, tunnel of peronei tendons; *9*, talar body; *10*, tibialis posterior tendon; *11*, flexor digitorum longus tendon; *12*, flexor hallucis longus tendon; *13*, flexor retinaculum; *14*, posterior tibial neurovascular bundle; *15*, quadratus plantae with investing fascia; *16*, peroneus longus tendon; *17*, peroneus brevis tendon; *18*, extensor digitorum brevis muscle; *19*, calcaneus; *20*, talar head; *21*, navicular; *22*, superomedial calcaneonavicular ligament; *23*, talocalcaneal joint.)

◀ **Figure 9.14** **Section III.** Oblique section calcaneotalonavicular. Distal surface of section. (*1*, insertion of tibialis posterior tendon on navicular; *2*, tunnel of flexor digitorum longus tendon and of flexor hallucis longus tendon; *3*, tunnel of medial plantar neurovascular tunnel; *4*, interfascicular ligament; *5*, abductor hallucis muscle; *6*, lateral investing fascia of abductor hallucis muscle; *7*, medial investing fascia of abductor hallucis muscle; *8*, tunnel of lateral plantar neurovascular bundle; *9*, quadratus plantae medial head; *10*, tunnel of peroneus longus tendon; *11*, tunnel of peroneus brevis tendon; *12*, flexor digitorum longus tendon; *13*, flexor hallucis longus tendon; *14*, medial plantar neurovascular bundle; *15*, lateral plantar neurovascular bundle; *16*, insertion of interfascicular ligament on lateral investing fascia of abductor hallucis bundle; *17*, peroneus longus tendon; *18*, peroneus brevis tendon; *19*, calcaneus; *20*, navicular; *21*, small segment of talar head.)

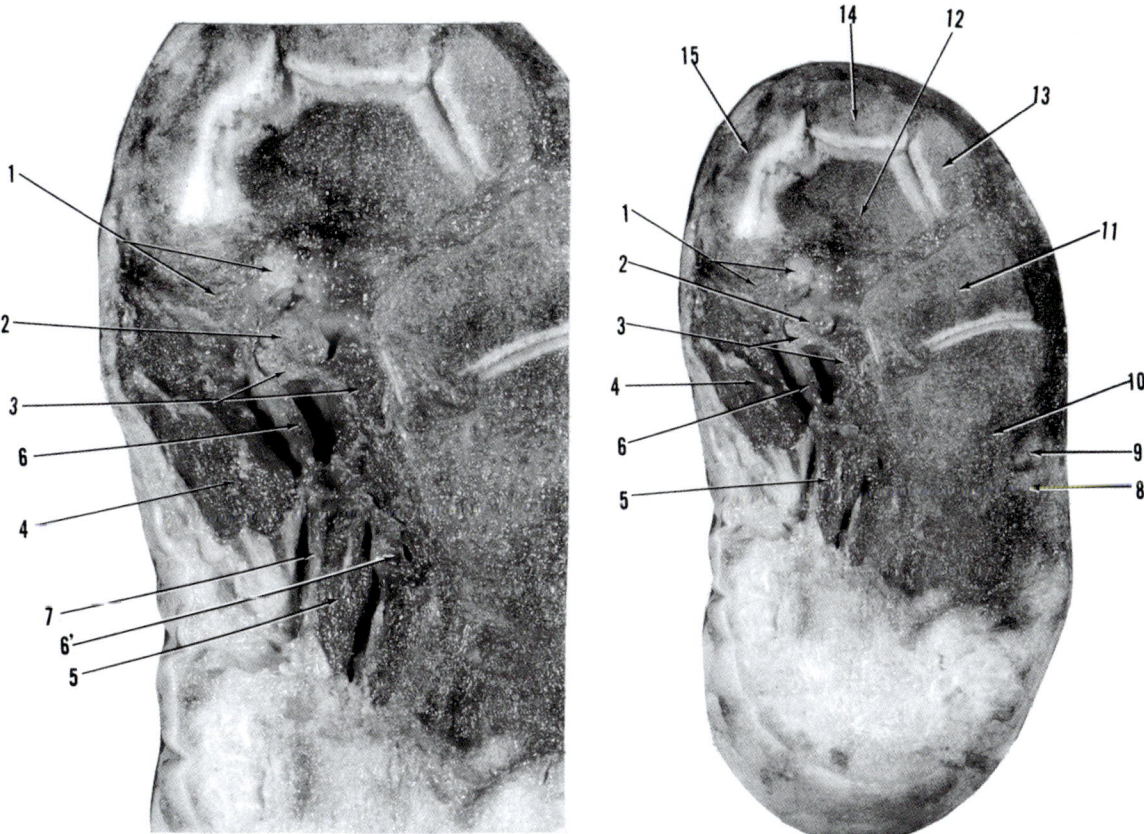

Figure 9.15 **Section IV.** Oblique section calcaneocubonavicular-cuneiforms. Distal surface of section. (*1*, insertional and deep plantar component of tibialis posterior tendon; *2*, flexor hallucis longus tendon; *3*, flexor digitorum longus tendon and contribution from the quadratus plantae muscle; *4*, abductor hallucis muscle; *5*, flexor digitorum brevis muscle; *6*, medial plantar neurovascular bundle within substance of medial intermuscular septum; *6′*, lateral plantar neurovascular bundle; *7*, medial intermuscular septum; *8*, peroneus brevis tendon; *9*, peroneus longus tendon; *10*, calcaneus; *11*, cuboid; *12*, navicular; *13*, lateral cuneiform; *14*, middle cuneiform; *15*, medial cuneiform.)

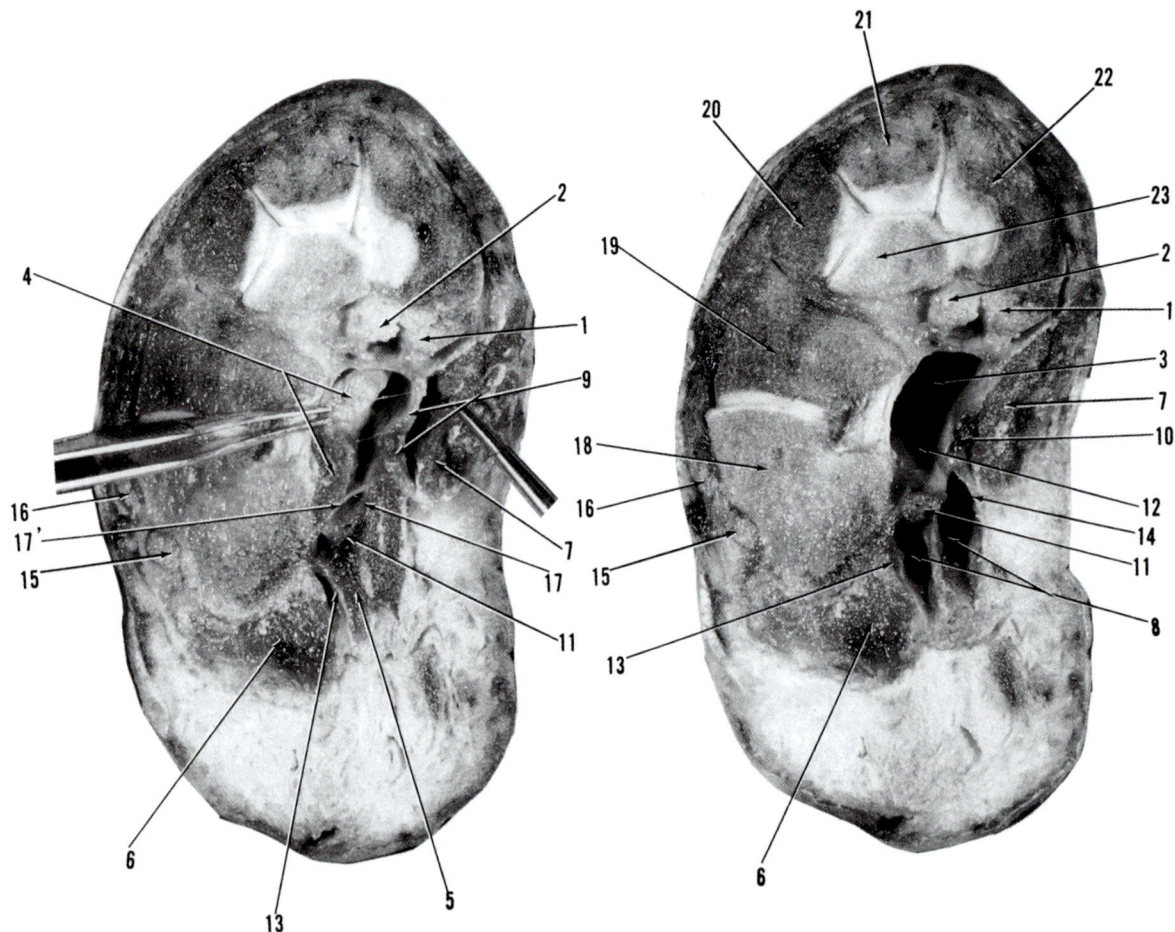

Figure 9.16 Section V. Oblique section calcaneocubonaviculo-cuneiforms. Proximal surface of section. (*1*, tibialis posterior tendon; *2*, flexor hallucis longus tendon; *3*, tunnel of flexor digitorum longus and quadratus plantae; *4*, flexor digitorum longus tendon and quadratus plantae; *5*, flexor digitorum brevis; *6*, abductor digiti quinti muscle; *7*, abductor hallucis muscle; *8*, compartment of flexor digitorum brevis; *9*, medial plantar neurovascular bundle carried within the medial intermuscular septum; *10*, medial plantar neurovascular bundle; *11*, lateral plantar neurovascular bundle; *12*, intermediary component of central compartment; *13*, lateral intermuscular septum; *14*, medial intermuscular septum; *15*, peroneus longus tendon; *16*, peroneus brevis tendon; *17*, superficial investing thin fascia of lateral plantar neurovascular bundle; *17′*, transverse aponeurosis, thick, dividing the central compartment into superficial and intermediary compartments; *18*, calcaneus; *19*, cuboid; *20*, lateral cuneiform; *21*, middle cuneiform; *22*, medial cuneiform; *23*, navicular.)

The distal surface of Section VI is shown in Figure 9.19. This is a coronal section through cuneiform 1 and metatarsal bases 2 to 5.

The peroneus longus tendon is well represented, crossing obliquely the bases of metatarsals 5-4-3. The flexor hallucis longus has its own tunnel located between the lateral wall of the medial compartment and the medial aspect of the intermediary deep segment of the central compartment. The dividing transverse septum of the latter is now very thin, membranous like. The medial plantar neurovascular bundle is in its own triangular channel within the medial intermuscular septum. The lateral plantar neurovascular tunnel is seen at the lateral end of the transverse membrane, within the lateral intermuscular septum.

Section VII is a coronal section through cuneiform$_1$ and metatarsal bases 2 to 5. The proximal surface of the section is shown (Fig. 9.20).

The oblique peroneus longus tunnel and tendon are seen at the base of metatarsals 2-3-4 and at the base of cuneiform 1.

The central intermediary compartment is triangular, lodging the flexor digitorum longus. This compartment is barely separated from the superficial central compartment by the thin transverse aponeurosis. The tunnel of the flexor hallucis longus is clearly delineated, adjacent to the central intermediary compartment and to the tunnel of the medial plantar neurovascular channel on its plantar aspect. The lateral plantar neurovascular bundle is located within the lateral intermuscular septum.

A different view of Section VII is provided by Figure 9.21. The figure shows the distal surface of a coronal section through the base of metatarsals 1 to 5.

The peroneus longus has inserted on the base of the first metatarsal. The origin of the oblique head of the adductor hallucis is seen. The central superficial and intermediary compartments are about to coalesce because the separating membrane is extremely thin. The tunnel of the flexor hallucis longus is again well delineated and located under the first metatarsal. The lateral plantar artery is seen under the fourth metatarsal

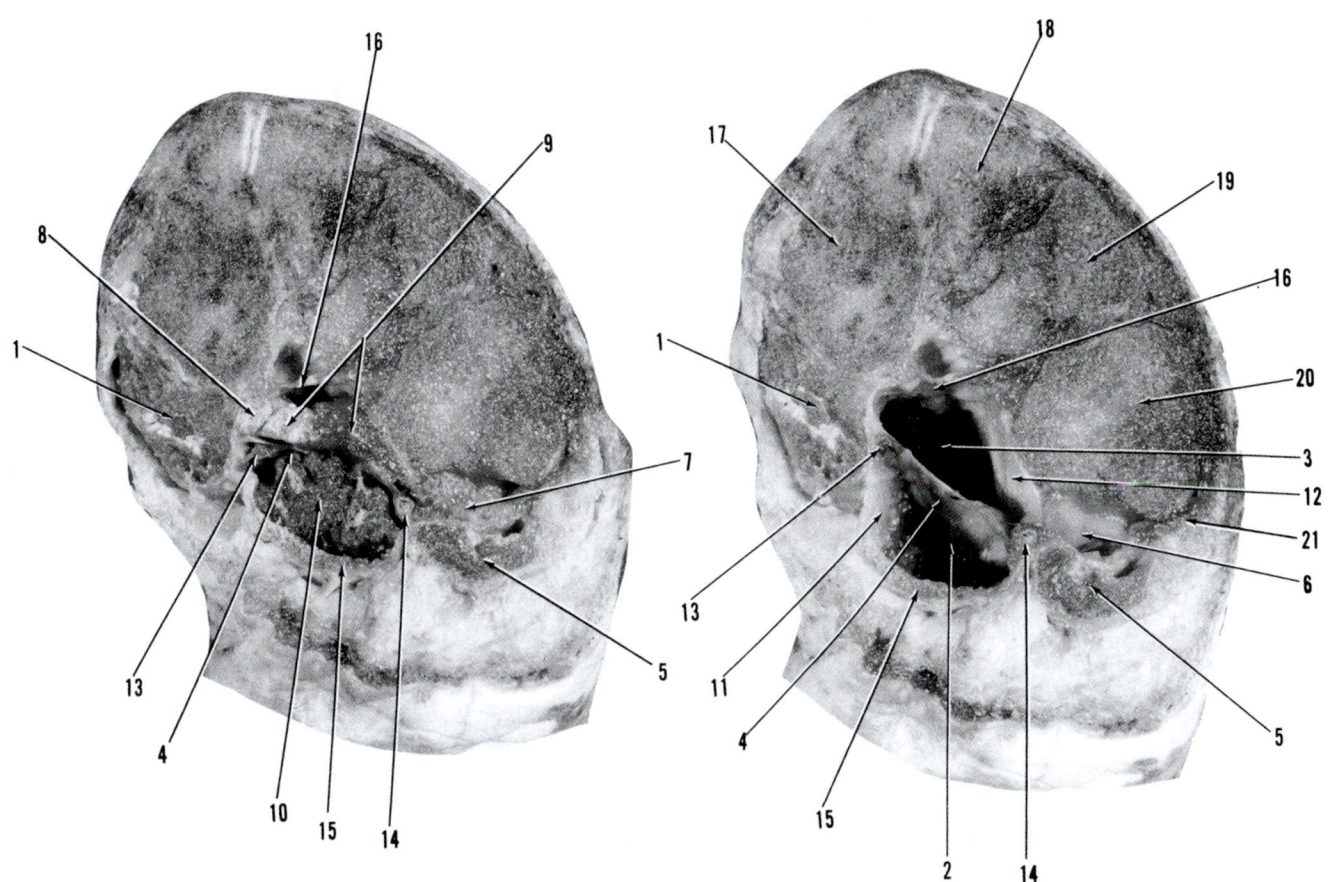

Figure 9.17 Section V. Coronal section through cuboid, cuneiforms 1, 2, 3, and base of metatarsal 5. Distal surface of section. (*1*, abductor hallucis muscle; *2*, superficial component of the central compartment; *3*, intermediary component of the central compartment; *4*, transverse septum dividing the central compartments into superficial and intermediary compartments; *5*, lateral compartment with abductor digiti quinti; *6*, tunnel of peroneus longus tendon; *7*, peroneus longus tendon; *8*, flexor hallucis longus tendon; *9*, flexor digitorum longus tendon and quadratus plantae located in the central intermediary compartment; *10*, flexor digitorum brevis located in the central superficial compartment; *11*, medial intermuscular septum; *12*, lateral intermuscular septum; *13*, medial plantar neurovascular bundle; *14*, lateral plantar neurovascular bundle; *15*, central segment of plantar aponeurosis; *16*, transverse intercuneiform ligament; *17*, medial cuneiform; *18*, middle cuneiform; *19*, lateral cuneiform; *20*, cuboid; *21*, segment of the metatarsal 5 base.)

and deep to the adductor hallucis. The dorsalis pedis artery is between the first and second metatarsal bases dorsally.

Section VIII is a coronal section through the metatarsal shafts 1 to 5. The distal surface of the section is shown in Figure 9.22.

The oblique head of the adductor is well developed, delineating the beginning of the adductor compartment and space. The superficial and intermediary central spaces have united. The tunnel of the flexor hallucis longus is located between the adductor hallucis and the flexor hallucis brevis lateral head. The metatarsal arteries are seen. The interossei spaces are defined.

Section IX is a coronal section through the mid segment of metatarsal shafts 1 to 5. The proximal surface of the section is shown in Figure 9.23.

The oblique head of the adductor is well delineated, determining the adductor compartment and dorsally the adductor space. The thin investing fascia of the adductor inserts laterally on the interossei fascia and separates the adductor space from the central intermediary space. The flexor hallucis brevis, lateral head, is in intimate contact with both the adductor hallucis and the medial head of the flexor hallucis brevis. The intermediary central compartment lodges the flexor digitorum longus, the corresponding lumbricals, and the tendons of the flexor digitorum brevis. The flexor hallucis longus is lodged in a tunnel delineated by the adductor hallucis and the flexor hallucis brevis. The interosseous spaces with the corresponding interossei and intermetatarsal arteries are clearly seen. The lateral compartment is limited to the undersurface of the fifth metatarsal. On the dorsal surface, the superficial dorsal aponeurosis, the extensor digitorum longus-brevis (tendinous with the intertendinous fascia), and the dorsal interossei fascia are demonstrated.

A different view of section IX is provided in Figure 9.24. The figure shows the distal surface of a coronal section through the mid metatarsal shafts 1 to 5.

The disposition of the spaces and compartments is similar to that in the previous section.

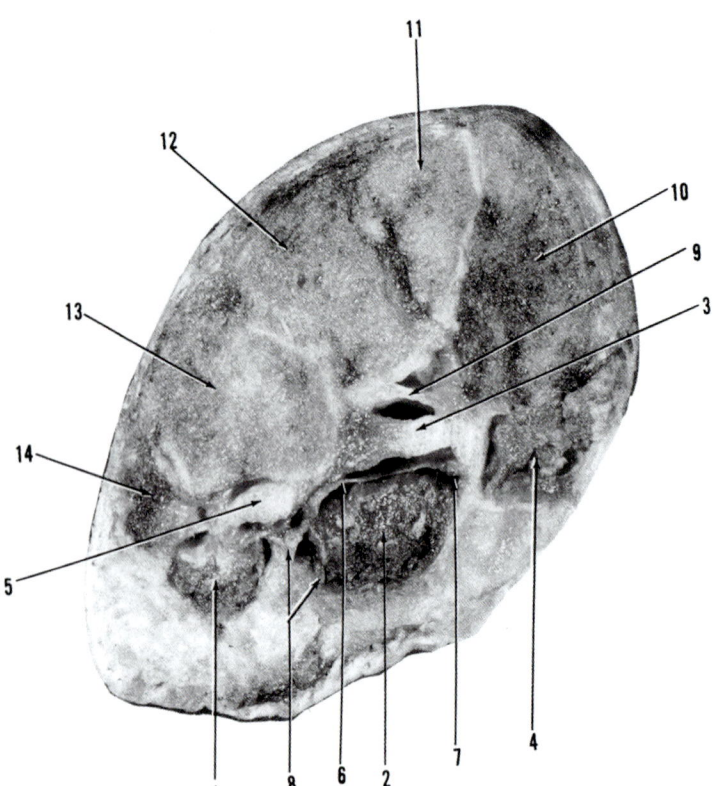

Figure 9.18 Section VI. Coronal section through cuneiforms 1, 2, 3, cuboid, and metatarsal$_5$ base. Proximal surface of section. (*1*, lateral compartment with abductor digiti quinti; *2*, central superficial compartment with flexor digitorum brevis; *3*, central intermediary compartment with flexor digitorum longus and quadratus plantae; *4*, medial compartment with abductor hallucis muscle; *5*, peroneus longus tendon; *6*, transverse septum dividing the central compartment into superficial and intermediary; *7*, medial plantar neurovascular bundle; *8*, lateral plantar neurovascular bundle; *9*, transverse intercuneiform ligament; *10*, medial cuneiform; *11*, middle cuneiform; *12*, lateral cuneiform; *13*, cuboid; *14*, base metatarsal$_5$.)

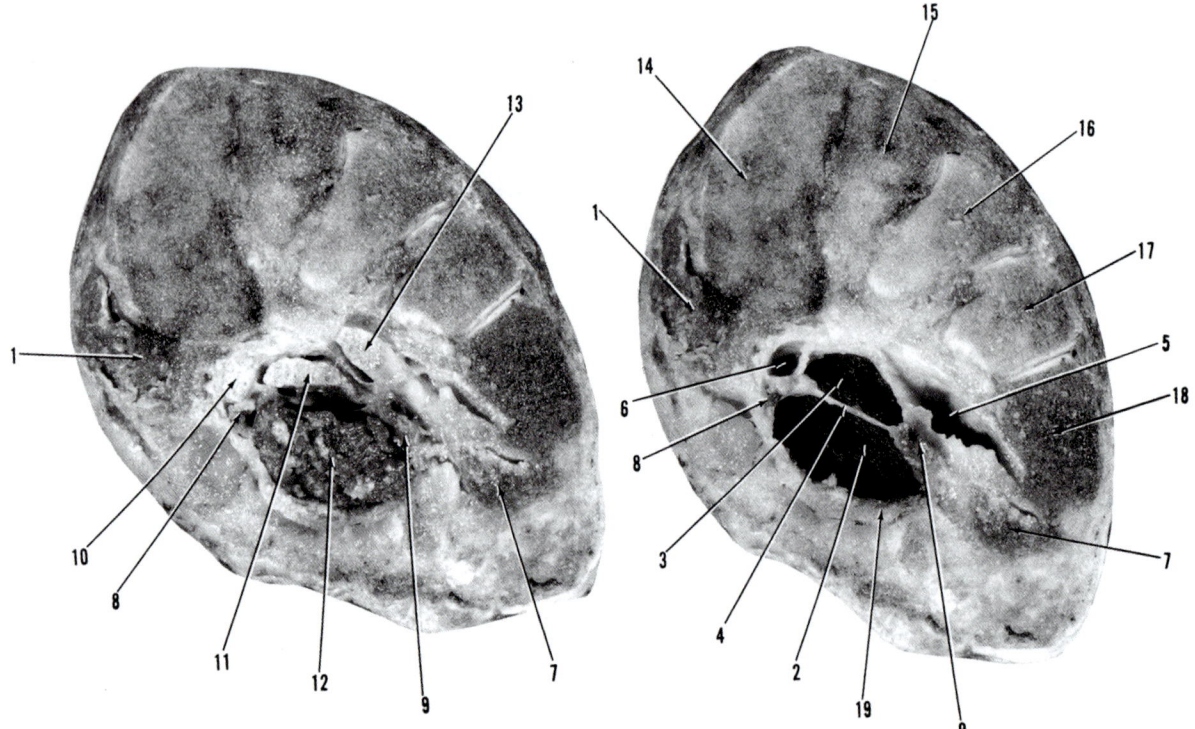

Figure 9.19 Section VI. Coronal section through first cuneiform and metatarsal bases 2, 3, 4, 5. Distal surface of section. (*1*, medial compartment with abductor hallucis muscle; *2*, central compartment, superficial component; *3*, central compartment, intermediary component; *4*, transverse septum dividing the central compartment into superficial and intermediary; *5*, tunnel of peroneus longus tendon; *6*, tunnel of flexor hallucis longus tendon; *7*, lateral compartment for the abductor digiti quinti; *8*, medial plantar neurovascular bundle; *9*, lateral plantar neurovascular bundle; *10*, flexor hallucis longus tendon; *11*, flexor digitorum longus tendon and quadratus plantae in central intermediary compartment; *12*, flexor digitorum brevis in central superficial compartment; *13*, peroneus longus tendon; *14*, medial cuneiform; *15*, metatarsal base 2; *16*, metatarsal base 3; *17*, metatarsal base 4; *18*, metatarsal base 5.)

Chapter 9: Cross-Sectional and Topographic Anatomy 445

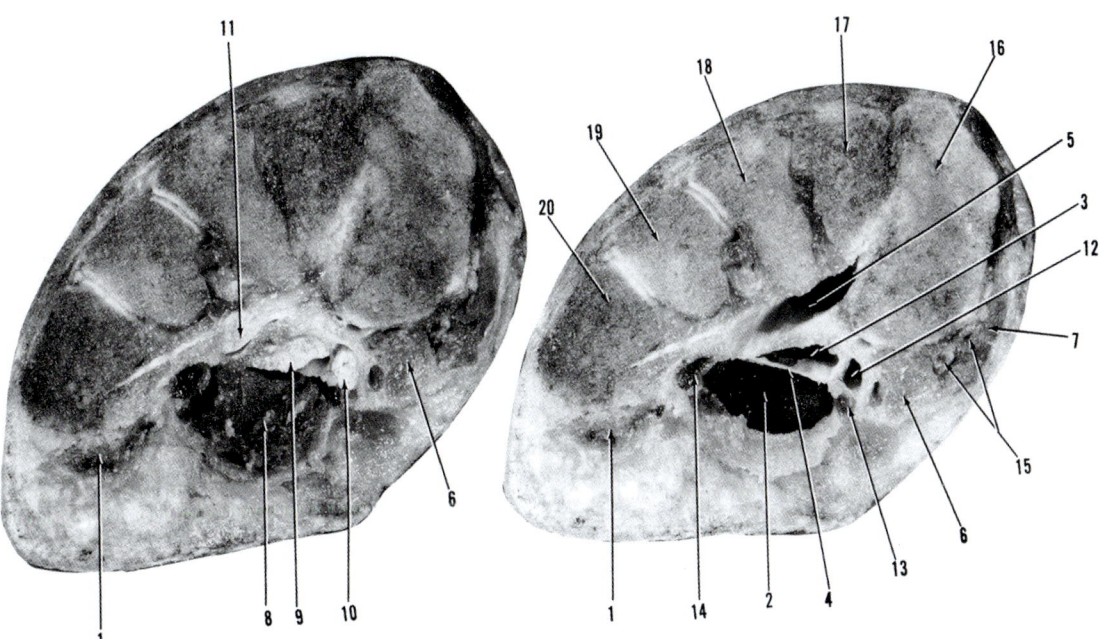

Figure 9.20 **Section VII.** Coronal section through cuneiform$_1$ and bases of metatarsals 2 to 5. Proximal surface of section. (*1*, lateral compartment with abductor digiti quinti; *2*, central superficial compartment; *3*, central intermediary compartment; *4*, transverse septum, thin at this level, between the superficial and intermediary components of the central compartment; *5*, tunnel of peroneus longus tendon; *6*, medial compartment with flexor hallucis brevis; *7*, medial compartment with tendon of abductor hallucis; *8*, flexor digitorum brevis in central superficial compartment; *9*, flexor digitorum longus with small portion of quadratus plantae in central intermediary compartment; *10*, flexor hallucis longus tendon; *11*, peroneus longus tendon; *12*, tunnel of flexor hallucis longus; *13*, medial plantar neurovascular tunnel; *14*, lateral plantar neurovascular tunnel; *15*, medial branches of medial plantar artery and vein; *16*, medial cuneiform; *17*, metatarsal base 2; *18*, metatarsal base 3; *19*, metatarsal base 4; *20*, metatarsal base 5.)

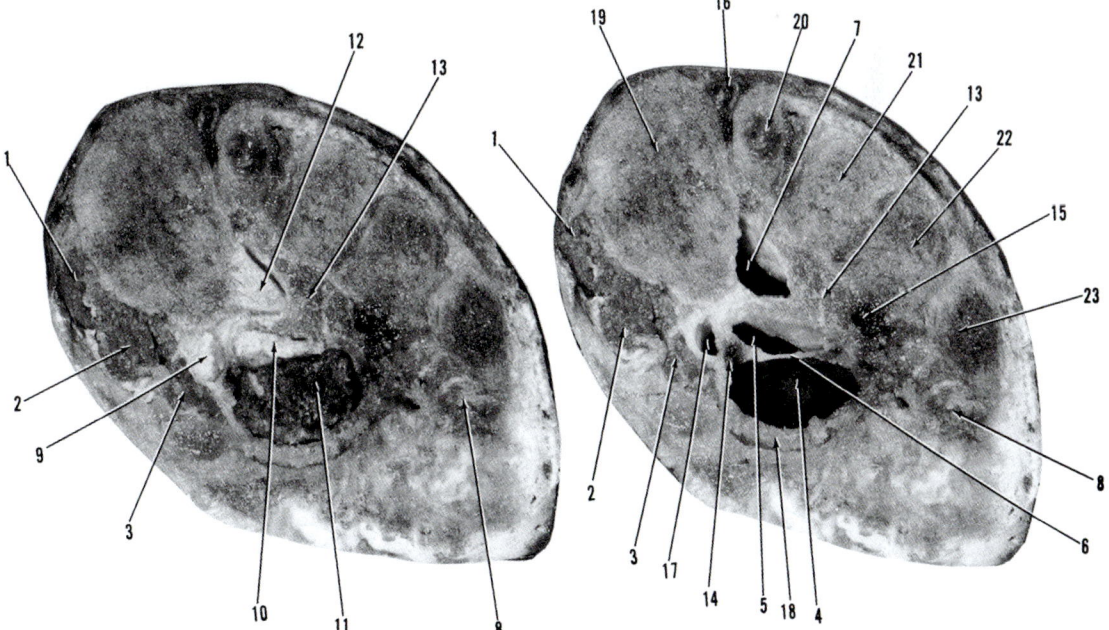

Figure 9.21 **Section VII.** Coronal section through bases of metatarsals 1 to 5. Distal surface of section. (*1*, abductor hallucis muscle; *2*, flexor hallucis brevis, medial head; *3*, flexor hallucis brevis, lateral head; *4*, central superficial compartment; *5*, central intermediary compartment; *6*, very thin end portion of the transverse septum dividing the central compartment into superficial and intermediary; *7*, tunnel for terminal portion of peroneus longus tendon; *8*, lateral compartment with abductor digit quinti; *9*, flexor hallucis longus tendon; *10*, flexor digitorum longus tendon in central intermediary compartment; *11*, flexor digitorum brevis in central superficial compartment; *12*, terminal portion of peroneus longus tendon; *13*, adductor hallucis muscle, oblique head; *14*, medial plantar neurovascular bundle; *15*, lateral plantar vessels; *16*, first dorsal metatarsal vessels; *17*, tunnel of flexor hallucis longus; *18*, central segment of plantar aponeurosis; *19*, metatarsal, base; *20*, metatarsal base 2; *21*, metatarsal base 3; *22*, metatarsal base 4; *23*, metatarsal base 5.)

The adductor compartment and space, the central intermediary compartment, and the interossei compartments are well delineated. The lateral and medial compartments are in very close contact with the adjacent muscles. The tunnel of the flexor hallucis is most superficial.

Section X is a coronal section through the distal segment of the metatarsal shafts 1 to 5. The proximal surface of the section is shown in Figure 9.25.

The adductor compartment space and the central intermediary compartments are smaller. The sagittal septa of the plantar aponeurosis projecting into the central intermediary compartment are already seen. The adductor compartment is separate from the medial compartment lodging the flexor hallucis brevis, the flexor hallucis longus, and the adductor hallucis.

The vertical fibers of the plantar aponeurosis projecting into the dermis are seen with abundant plantar veins.

A different view of section X is provided in Figure 9.26. The figure shows the distal surface of a coronal section through the distal segment of the metatarsals 2 to 4 and the heads of metatarsals 1 and 5.

The transverse head of the adductor hallucis is seen. The vertical septa of the plantar aponeurosis have formed near-tunnels to the long flexor tendons of toes 2 to 4. The fibrous tunnels of the flexor hallucis longus and of the long flexor of the fifth toe

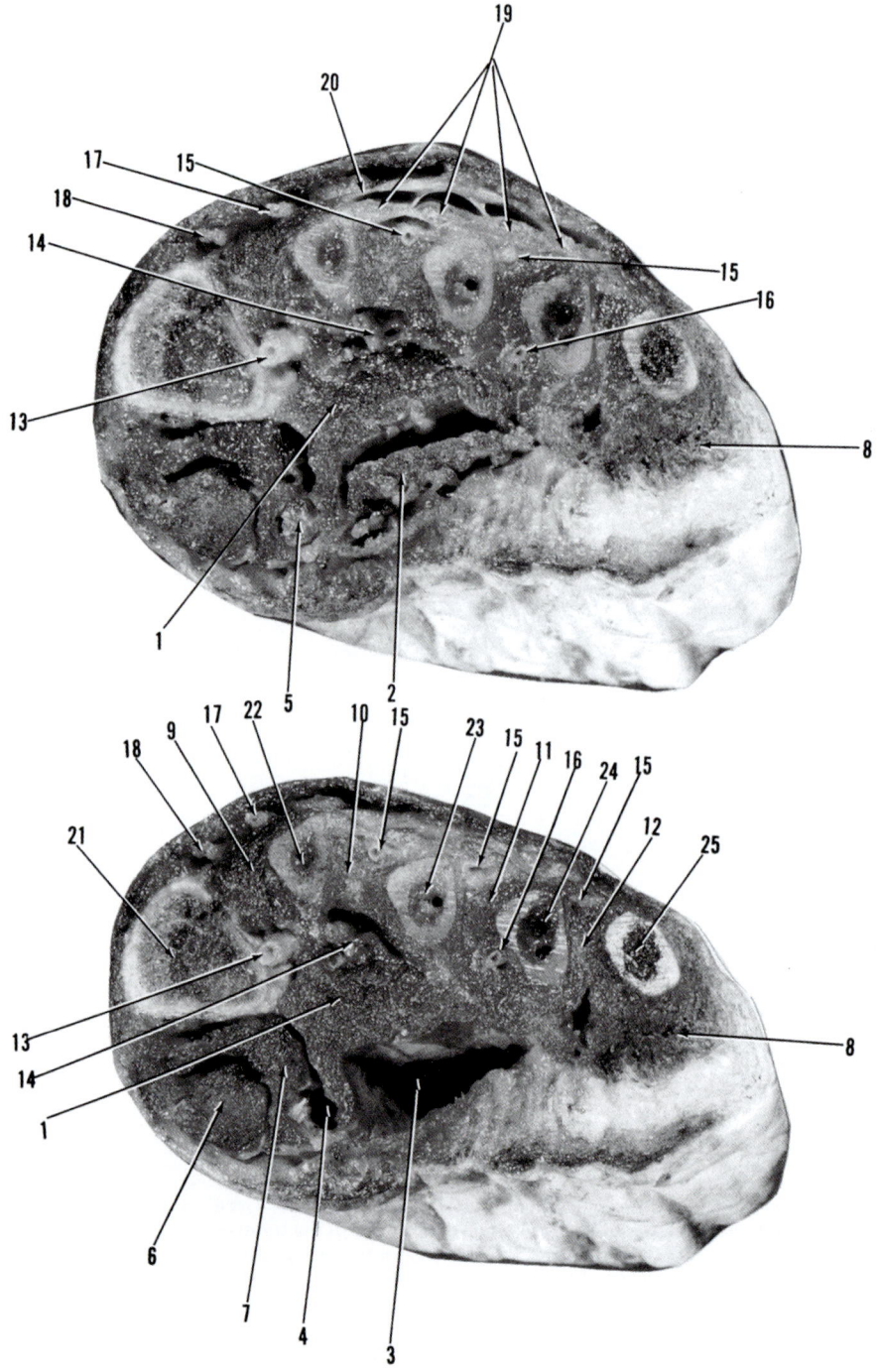

Figure 9.22 Section VIII. Coronal section through metatarsal shafts 1 to 5. Distal surface of section. (1, adductor hallucis muscle, oblique head, in adductor compartment; 2, flexor digitorum longus and brevis tendons and lumbricals in central intermediary compartment; 3, central intermediary compartment. The central superficial compartment has ended; 4, tunnel of flexor hallucis longus tendon located between the adductor hallucis and the lateral head of the flexor hallucis brevis; 5, flexor hallucis longus tendon; 6, flexor hallucis brevis medial head and abductor hallucis; 7, lateral head of flexor hallucis brevis; 8, lateral compartment and intrinsic muscles of fifth toe; 9, first dorsal interosseous muscle; 10, second interosseous space and interossei muscles: second dorsal interosseous and first plantar interosseous; 11, third interosseous space and interossei muscles: third dorsal interosseous and second plantar interosseous; 12, fourth interosseous space and interossei muscles: fourth dorsal interosseous and third plantar interosseous; 13, first plantar metatarsal artery; 14, lateral plantar artery and second plantar metatarsal artery; 15, dorsal second, third, fourth metatarsal arteries; 16, third plantar metatarsal artery; 17, first dorsal metatarsal artery; 18, branch of deep peroneal nerve; 19, extensor digitorum longus, brevis tendons with their investing aponeurosis; 20, dorsal aponeurosis of the foot; 21, first metatarsal shaft; 22, second metatarsal shaft; 23, third metatarsal shaft; 24, fourth metatarsal shaft; 25, fifth metatarsal shaft.)

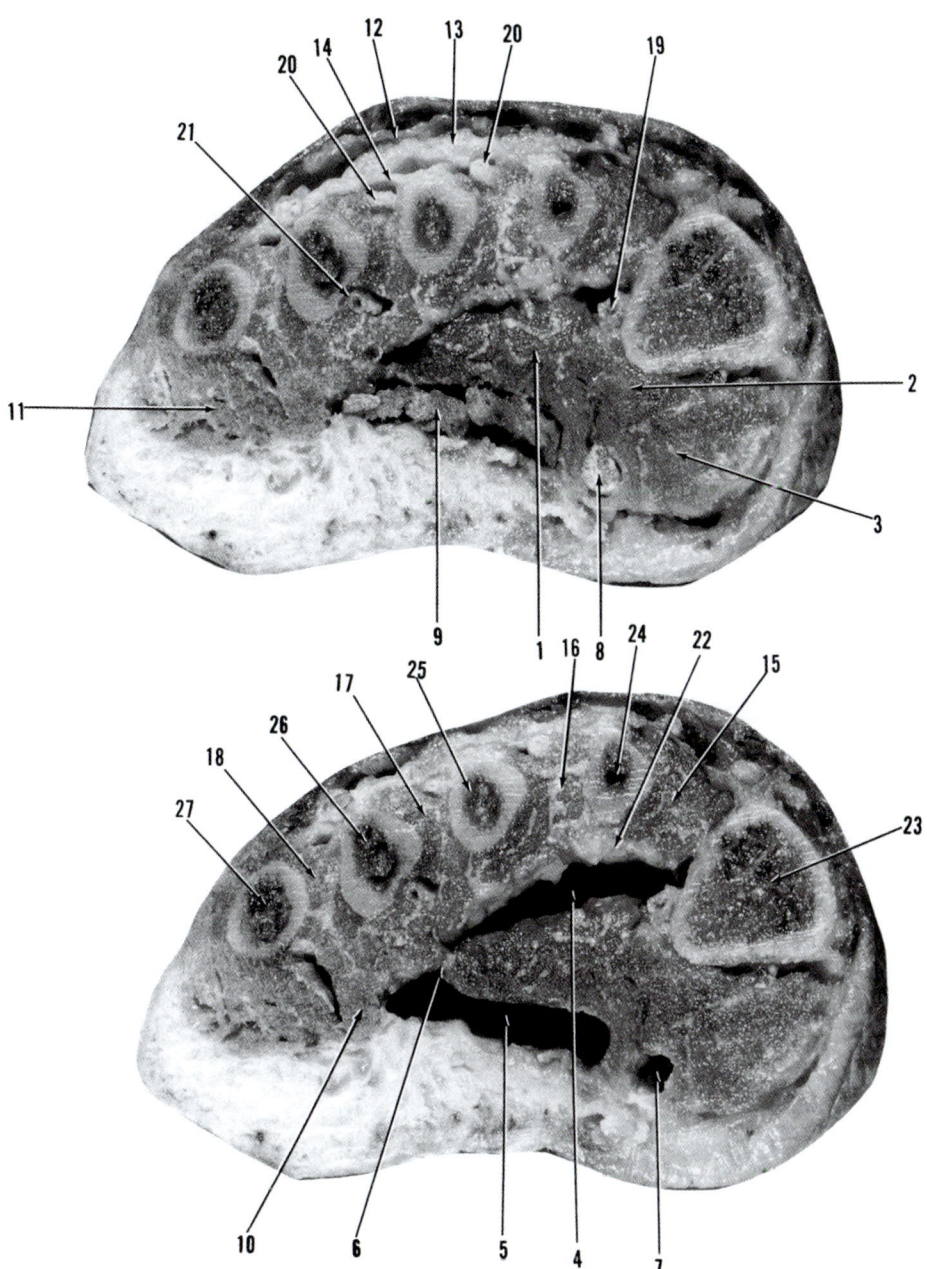

Figure 9.23 Section IX. Coronal section through metatarsal shafts 1 to 5. Proximal surface of section. (*1*, adductor hallucis muscle oblique head and adductor compartment; *2*, flexor hallucis brevis lateral head; *3*, flexor hallucis brevis medial head and abductor hallucis; *4*, adductor space or deep central space between interossei and adductor compartment; *5*, central intermediary compartment. The central superficial compartment has ended; *6*, attachment of the investing fascia of the oblique head of the adductor hallucis muscle to the interossei fascia separating the deep central space (adductor space) from the central intermediary compartment; *7*, tunnel of flexor hallucis longus tendon; *8*, tendon of flexor hallucis longus; *9*, flexor digitorum longus, brevis tendons, and lumbricals; *10*, attachment of third plantar interosseous muscle; *11*, lateral compartment with intrinsic muscles of the fifth toe; *12*, dorsal superficial extensor aponeurosis of the foot; *13*, extensor digitorum longus and brevis tendons and investing fascia; *14*, dorsal interosseous aponeurosis; *15*, first interosseous space and first dorsal interosseous muscle; *16*, second interosseous space and interossei: second dorsal interosseous and first plantar interosseous; *17*, third interosseous space and interossei: third dorsal interosseous and second plantar interosseous; *18*, fourth interosseous space and interossei: fourth dorsal interosseous and third plantar interosseous; *19*, first plantar metatarsal artery; *20*, dorsal metatarsal arteries; *21*, third plantar metatarsal artery; *22*, interossei fascia; *23*, first metatarsal shaft; *24*, second metatarsal shaft; *25*, third metatarsal shaft; *26*, fourth metatarsal shaft; *27*, fifth metatarsal shaft.)

are demonstrated. The interosseous spaces are well delineated. The adductor space between the interossei and the transverse head of the adductor hallucis is present.

Section XI is a coronal section through the head of the first metatarsal and its sesamoids, the head of the fifth metatarsal, and the necks of metatarsals 2 to 4. The proximal surface of this section is seen in Figure 9.27.

The transverse head of the adductor hallucis is very thin. The flexor hallucis longus, the flexor digitorum longus, and the corresponding tendons of the flexor digitorum brevis have their own fibrous tunnels. The flexor hallucis longus tunnel is located between the medial and lateral sesamoids. The interossei spaces are present.

The distal surface of the coronal section through metatarsophalangeal joints 1 to 4 and the base of the proximal phalanx of the fifth toe illustrates Section XI (Fig. 9.28).

The fibrous flexor tunnels are located on the plantar aspect of the corresponding plantar plates. The interossei spaces have disappeared. The interossei tendons are seen in their insertional positions on each side of the corresponding lesser metatarsal head. The dorsal aponeurosis of the first interspace is substantial. The first transverse deep intermetatarsal ligament is well delineated. The plantar neurovascular bundles are seen on the plantar aspect of the plantar metatarsal ligament and are located between the corresponding fibrous flexor tunnels.

Section XI is shown in Figure 9.29. Part I of Figure 9.29 is a close-up view of the coronal section through the sesamoid ring of the big toe (proximal surface of section). Part II of Figure 9.29 is a close-up view of the coronal section through the metatarsal head of the big toe (distal surface of section).

The sesamoid articular surfaces are oriented obliquely and articulate with the corresponding concave metatarsal articular

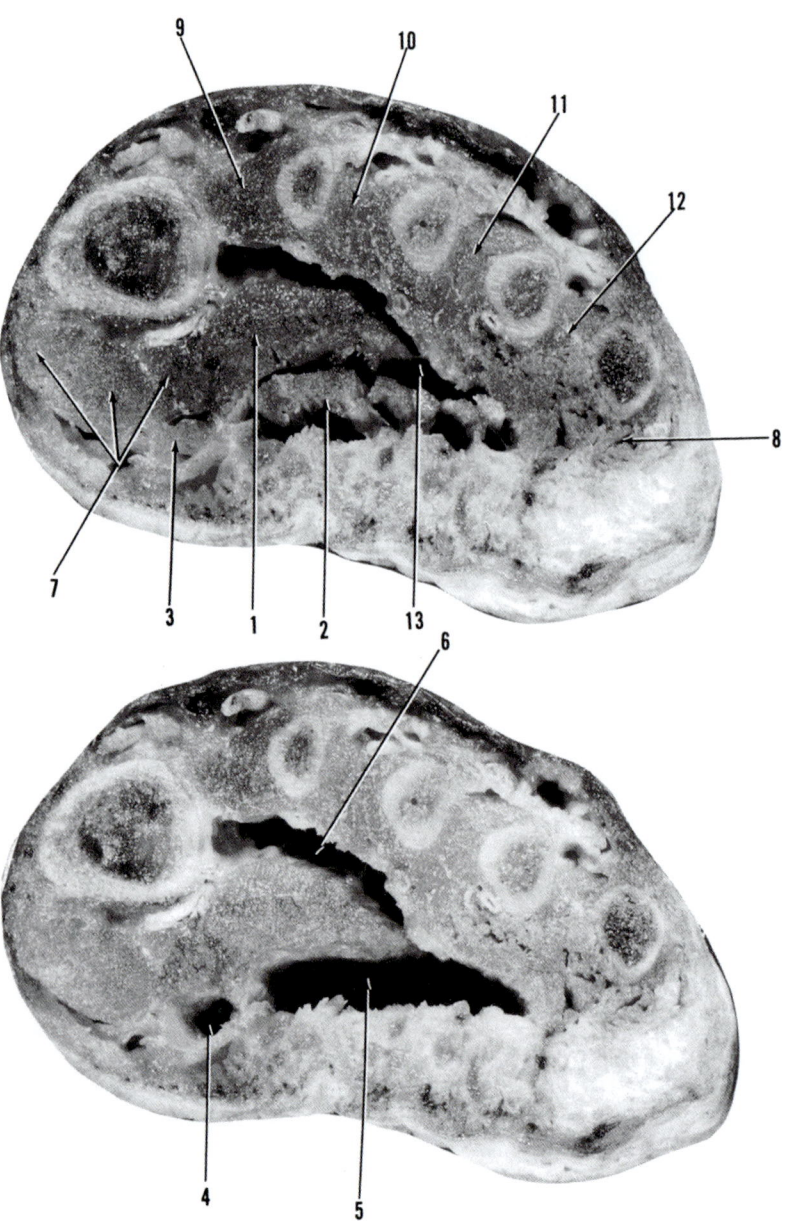

Figure 9.24 Section IX. Coronal section through metatarsal shafts 1 to 5. Distal surface of section. (1, adductor hallucis oblique head and adductor compartment; 2, flexor digitorum longus-brevis tendons and lumbricals; 3, flexor hallucis longus tendon; 4, flexor hallucis longus tunnel; 5, central intermediary compartment; 6, adductor space; 7, flexor hallucis brevis and abductor hallucis; 8, lateral compartment and intrinsic muscles of fifth toe; 9, first interosseous space and first dorsal interosseous muscle; 10, second interosseous space and interossei: second dorsal interosseous and first plantar interosseous; 11, third interosseous space and interossei: third dorsal interosseous and second plantar interosseous; 12, fourth interosseous space and interossei: fourth dorsal interosseous and third plantar interosseous; 13, investing fascia of adductor hallucis inserting on the interosseous fascia.)

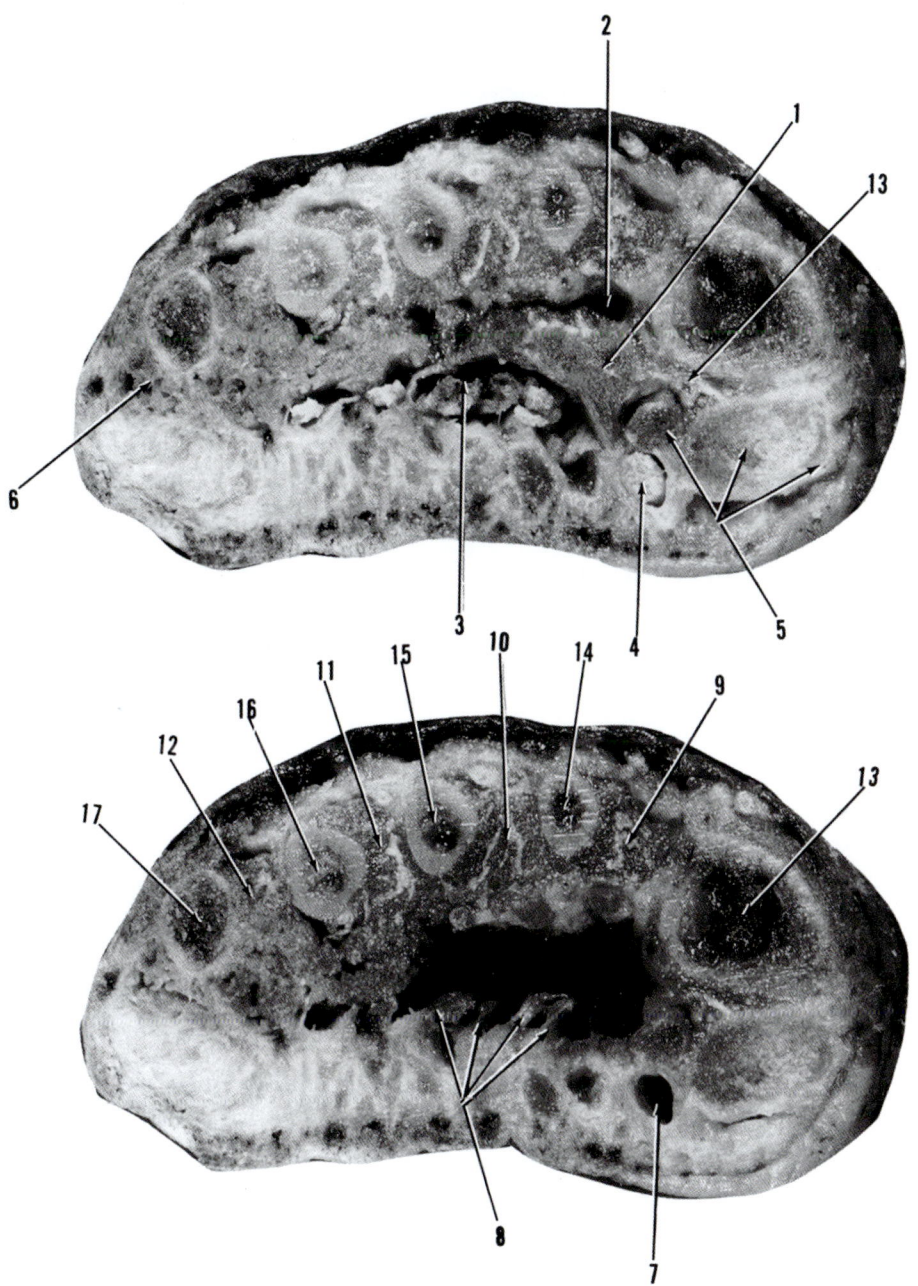

Figure 9.25 Section X. Coronal section through metatarsal shafts 1 to 5. Proximal surface of section. (*1*, adductor hallucis, oblique head, and adductor compartment; *2*, adductor space between adductor compartment and interossei fascia; *3*, flexor digitorum longus, brevis tendons, and lumbricals; *4*, flexor hallucis longus tendon; *5*, flexor hallucis brevis, lateral medial heads, and abductor hallucis; *6*, lateral compartment; *7*, tunnel of flexor hallucis longus tendon; *8*, longitudinal septa from central division bands of plantar aponeurosis; *9*, first dorsal interosseous space and muscle; *10*, second dorsal interosseous space and muscle; *11*, third dorsal interosseous space and muscle; *12*, fourth dorsal interosseous space and muscle; *13*, first metatarsal shaft; *14*, second metatarsal shaft; *15*, third metatarsal shaft; *16*, fourth metatarsal shaft; *17*, fifth metatarsal shaft.)

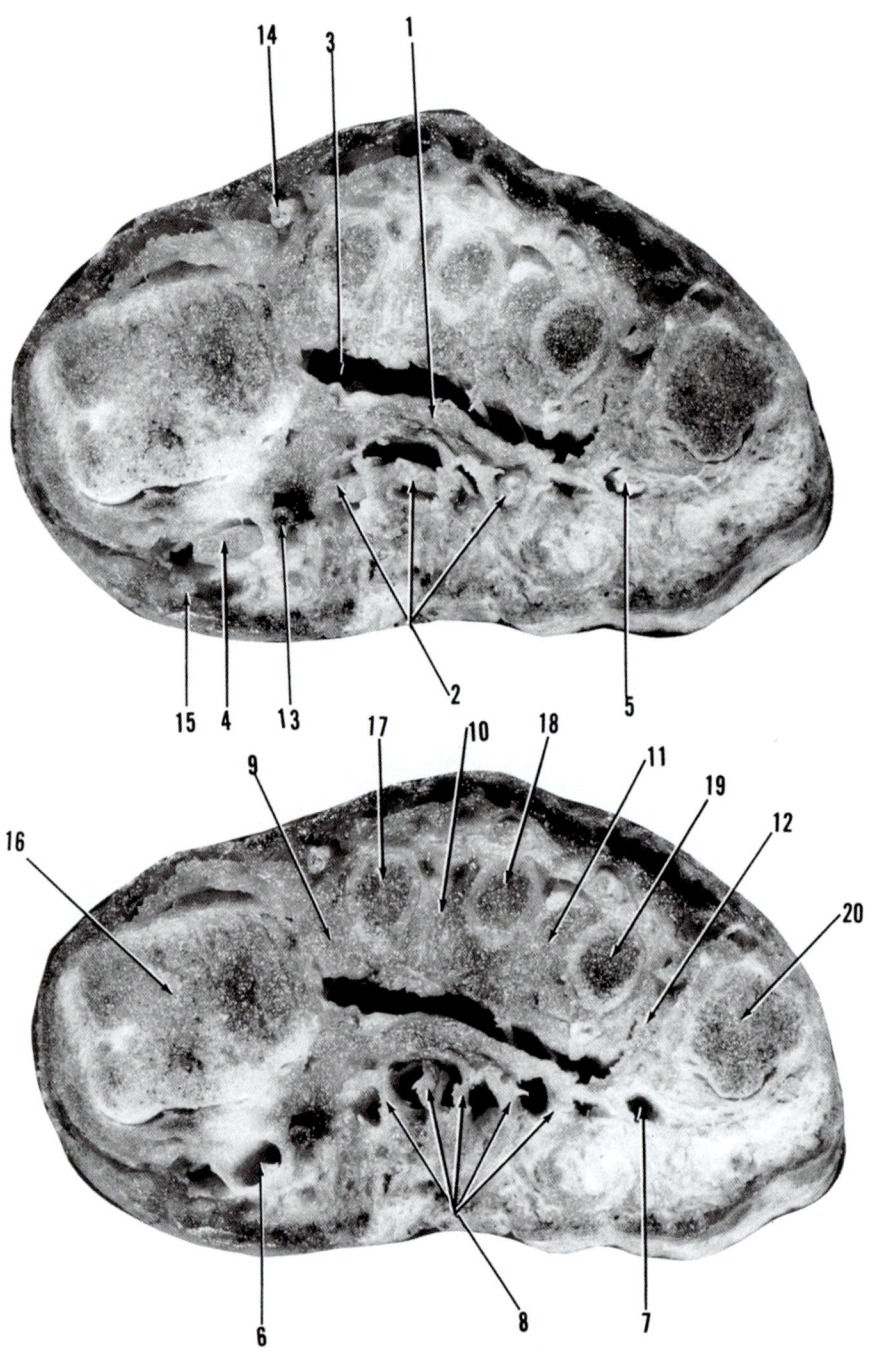

Figure 9.26 Section X. Coronal section through first and fifth metatarsal heads, and the shafts of metatarsals 2, 3, 4. Distal surface of section. (*1*, adductor hallucis transverse head; *2*, flexor digitorum longus and brevis tendons 2, 3, 4; *3*, adductor space; *4*, flexor hallucis longus tendon; *5*, flexor digitorum longus and brevis, tendon 5; *6*, tunnel of flexor hallucis longus tendon; *7*, tunnel of flexor digitorum longus, brevis of tendon 5; *8*, vertical septa from longitudinal bands of plantar aponeurosis forming a tunnel to the flexor tendons; *9*, first interosseous space and muscle; *10*, second interosseous space and muscles; *11*, third interosseous space and muscles; *12*, fourth interosseous space and muscles; *13*, plantar lateral hallucal artery; *14*, first dorsal metatarsal artery; *15*, plantar medial hallucal nerve; *16*, proximal phalanx, hallux; *17*, metatarsal shaft 2; *18*, metatarsal shaft 3; *19*, metatarsal shaft 4; *20*, proximal phalanx fifth toe.)

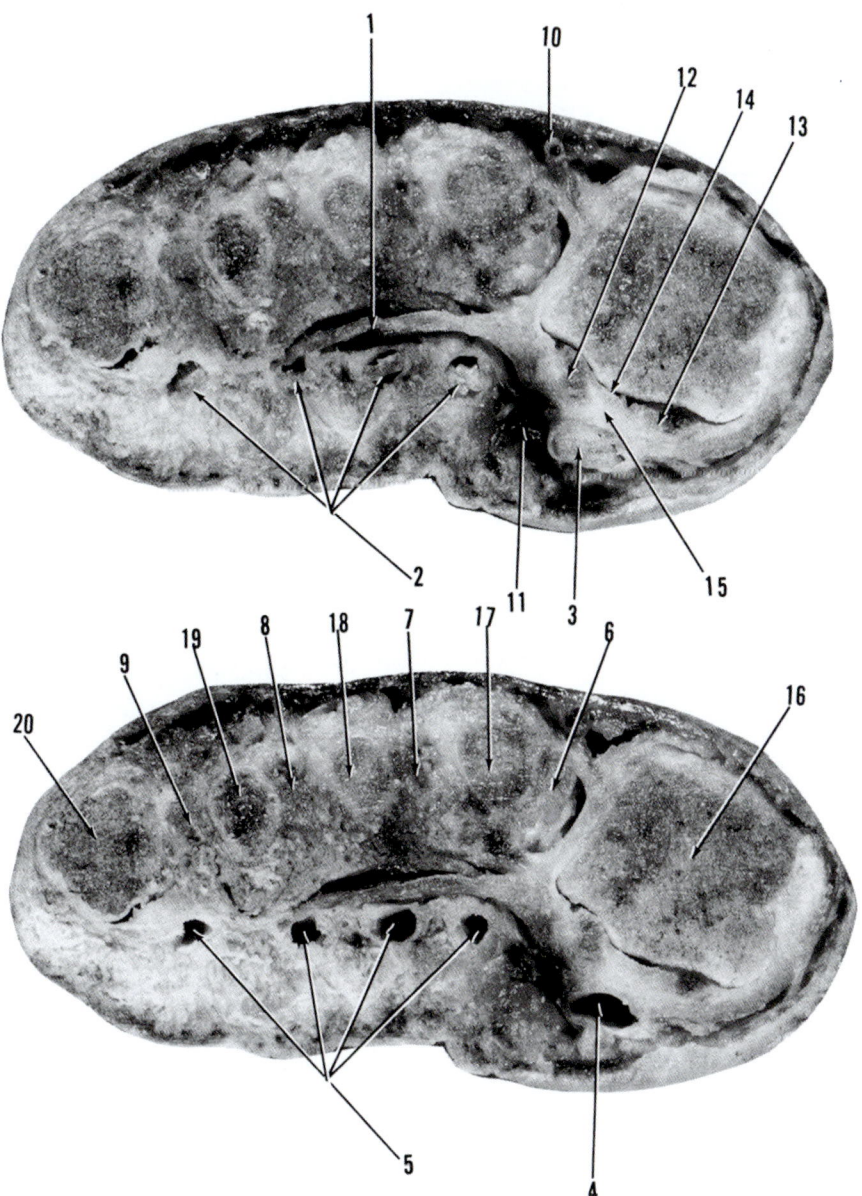

Figure 9.27 Section XI. Coronal section through the heads of the first and fifth metatarsals and the necks of metatarsals 2 to 4. Proximal surface of section. (*1*, adductor hallucis, transverse head; *2*, flexor digitorum longus, brevis tendons; *3*, flexor hallucis longus tendon; *4*, flexor hallucis longus tunnel; *5*, flexor digitorum longus, brevis tunnels; *6*, first interosseous space and muscle; *7*, second interosseous space and muscles; *8*, third interosseous space and muscles; *9*, fourth interosseous space and muscles; *10*, first dorsal metatarsal artery; *11*, lateral plantar hallucal vessels; *12*, lateral hallucal sesamoids; *13*, medial hallucal sesamoid; *14*, crista metatarsal, head; *15*, hallucal plantar plate and intersesamoid ligament; *16*, metatarsal head$_1$; *17*, metatarsal shaft 2; *18*, metatarsal shaft 3; *19*, metatarsal shaft 4; *20*, metatarsal head 5.)

surfaces separated by a crest. The soft-tissue ring with the incorporated sesamoids, the intersesamoid ligament, and the fibrous tunnel of the flexor hallucis longus form a unit. The first deep transverse metatarsal ligament is clearly seen extending from the lateral sesamoid to the fibrous tunnel and the plantar plate of the second toe. The neurovascular tunnel is plantar to the ligaments and the adductor is dorsal to the same.

Section XII is a coronal section through metatarsophalangeal joints 1 to 4 and the proximal phalanx of the fifth toe. The proximal surface of the section is shown in Figure 9.30.

Three niches for the metatarsal heads are demonstrated. Each niche is formed by the base of the proximal phalanx, the attached capsuloligamentous cuff, and the plantar plate. In the big toe, the sesamoids are embedded in the plantar plate.

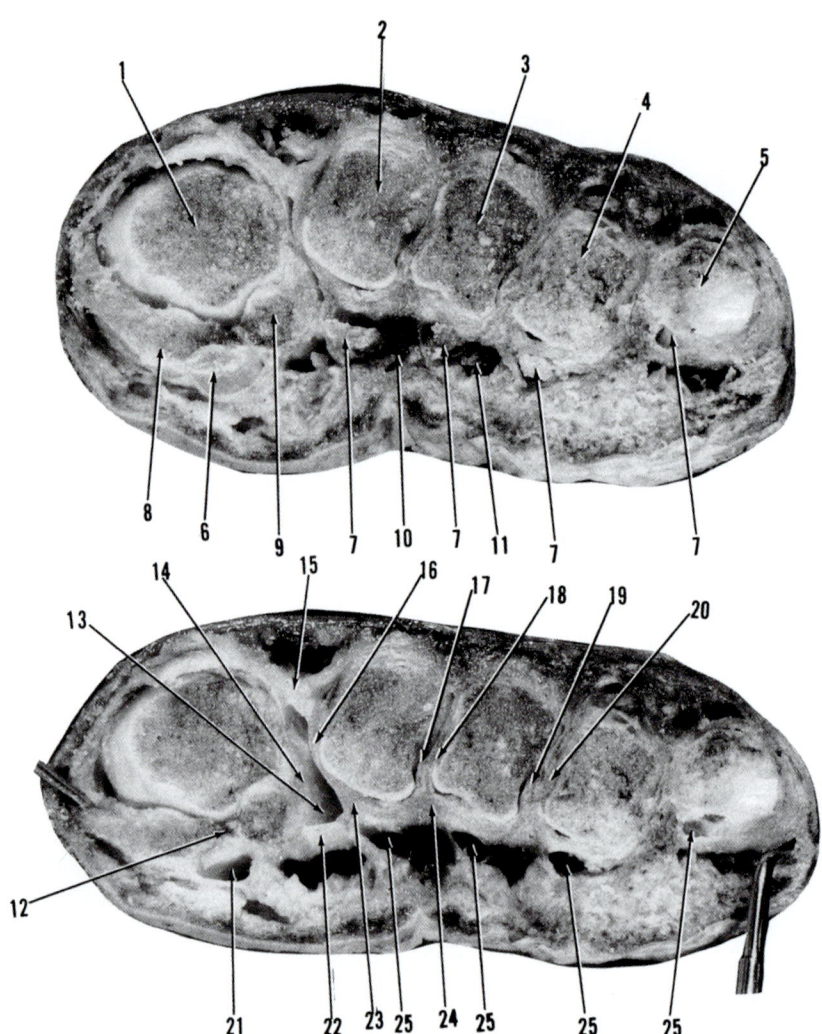

Figure 9.28 Section XI. Coronal section through metatarsophalangeal joints 1 to 4 and proximal phalanx of fifth toe. Distal surface of section. (*1*, metatarsal head 1; *2*, metatarsal head 2; *3*, metatarsal head 3; *4*, metatarsal head 4; *5*, proximal phalanx fifth toe; *6*, flexor hallucis longus tendon; *7*, flexor digitorum longus, brevis tendons; *8*, medial hallucal sesamoid; *9*, lateral hallucal sesamoid; *10*, second plantar intermetatarsal vessels; *11*, third plantar intermetatarsal vessels; *12*, intersesamoid ligament; *13*, first dorsal intermetatarsal space; *14*, adductor hallucis tendon; *15*, dorsal interosseous aponeurosis; *16*, tendon of first dorsal interosseous muscle; *17*, tendon of second dorsal interosseous muscle; *18*, tendon of first plantar interosseous muscle; *19*, tendon of third dorsal interosseous muscle; *20*, tendon of second plantar interosseous muscle; *21*, tunnel of flexor hallucis longus; *22*, first deep intermetatarsal transverse ligament; *23*, plantar plate; *24*, second deep intermetatarsal transverse ligament; *25*, tunnels of flexor digitorum longus, brevis tendons.)

II. TOPOGRAPHIC ANATOMY

ANTERIOR ASPECT OF THE ANKLE AND DORSUM OF THE FOOT

The anterior aspect of the ankle is a passage zone from the anterior compartment of the leg to the dorsum of the foot. Morphologically, the distal narrow leg gradually enlarges at the bimalleolar level and is in continuity with the foot plate. The latter is convex dorsally in the proximal and mid segments. Distally, at the level of the metatarsal heads, the foot plate is larger and horizontal.

▶ Surface Anatomy

The lateral and medial malleoli are easily palpated. The lateral malleolus is more distal—about 1 cm—and more posterior than the medial malleolus. The bimalleolar axis is thus turned posterolaterally, with an average angle of rotation of 20° to 30°. A line, nearly horizontal, drawn 2 cm proximal to the tip of the lateral malleolus and 1 cm proximal to the tip of the medial malleolus closely delineates the talotibial joint anterior interline (Fig. 9.31).

On the anterior aspect of the ankle, the tendons of the tibialis anterior medially and of the extensor digitorum longus laterally are easily palpated. Lateral to the latter and medial to the former are the medial and lateral premalleolar depressions

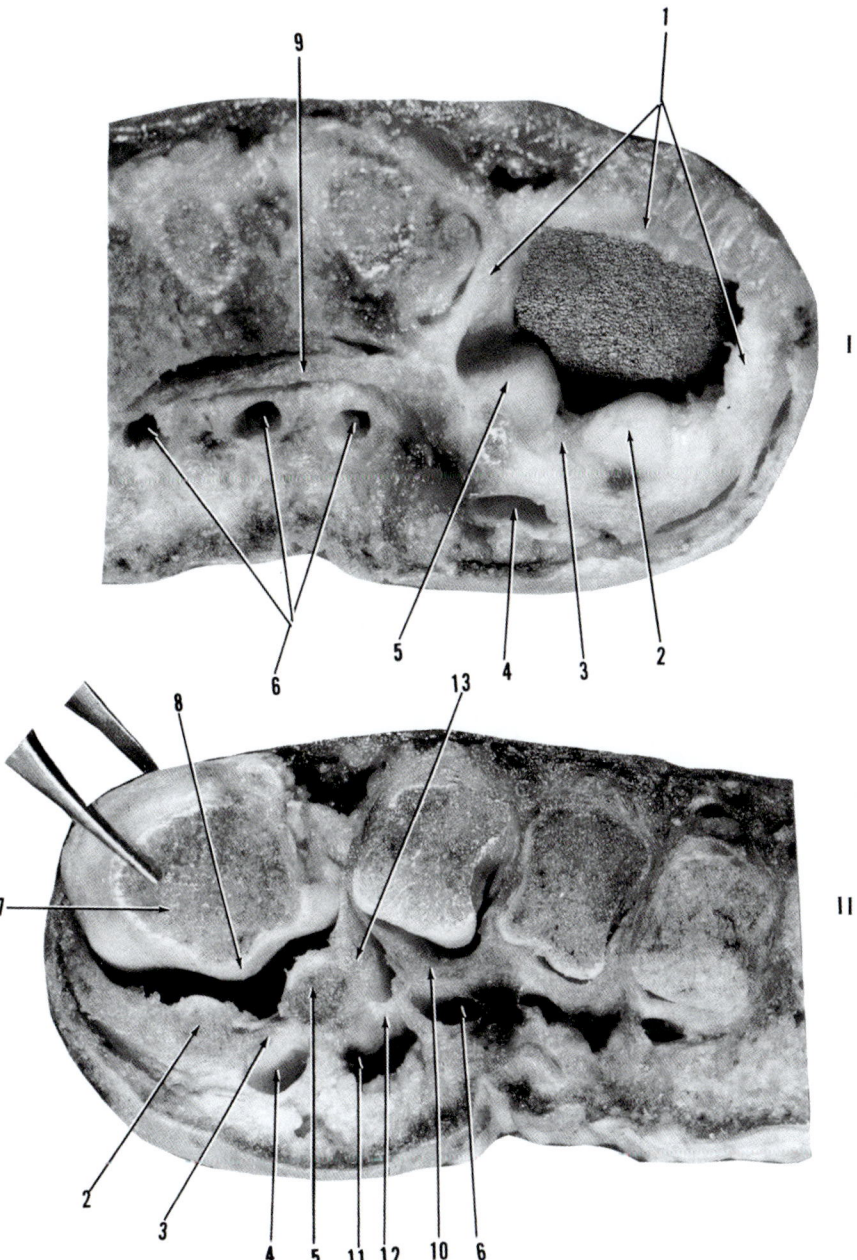

Figure 9.29 Section XI. **(I)** Close-up of coronal section through sesamoid ring of big toe. Proximal surface of section. Left foot **(II)**. Close-up of coronal section through metatarsal head of big toe. Distal surface of section. (*1*, capsuloligamentous "ring" of first metatarsal head; *2*, medial hallucal sesamoid; *3*, intersesamoid ligament; *4*, tunnel of flexor hallucis longus tendon; *5*, lateral hallucal sesamoid; *6*, tunnels of flexor digitorum longus brevis; *7*, head first metatarsal; *8*, crista hallucal head; *9*, transverse head adductor hallucis; *10*, plantar plate; *11*, interspace for "fat body" and plantar neurovascular bundle; *12*, first deep transverse intermetatarsal ligament; *13*, adductor hallucis tendon.)

where the synovium of the ankle joint may bulge in the presence of effusion. Between these two tendons (although deeper) is the tendon of the extensor hallucis longus; the tibialis anterior pulse may be taken just lateral to this tendon. A line drawn from the midpoint of the bimalleolar axis to the tip of the first intermetatarsal space traces the direction of the dorsalis pedis artery when the latter is present in its typical location (see Fig. 9.31). The dorsalis pedis pulse is felt for along this line, lateral to the extensor hallucis longus tendon and distal to the inferior extensor retinaculum. In young individuals, the pulse of the first dorsal metatarsal artery may be found in the first intermetatarsal space and felt up to the level of the head of the first metatarsal. A lateral premalleolar fat pad may be seen and palpated. At the level of the sinus tarsi, a second soft tissue bulge is frequently found, representing the well-developed origin of the extensor digitorum brevis muscle.

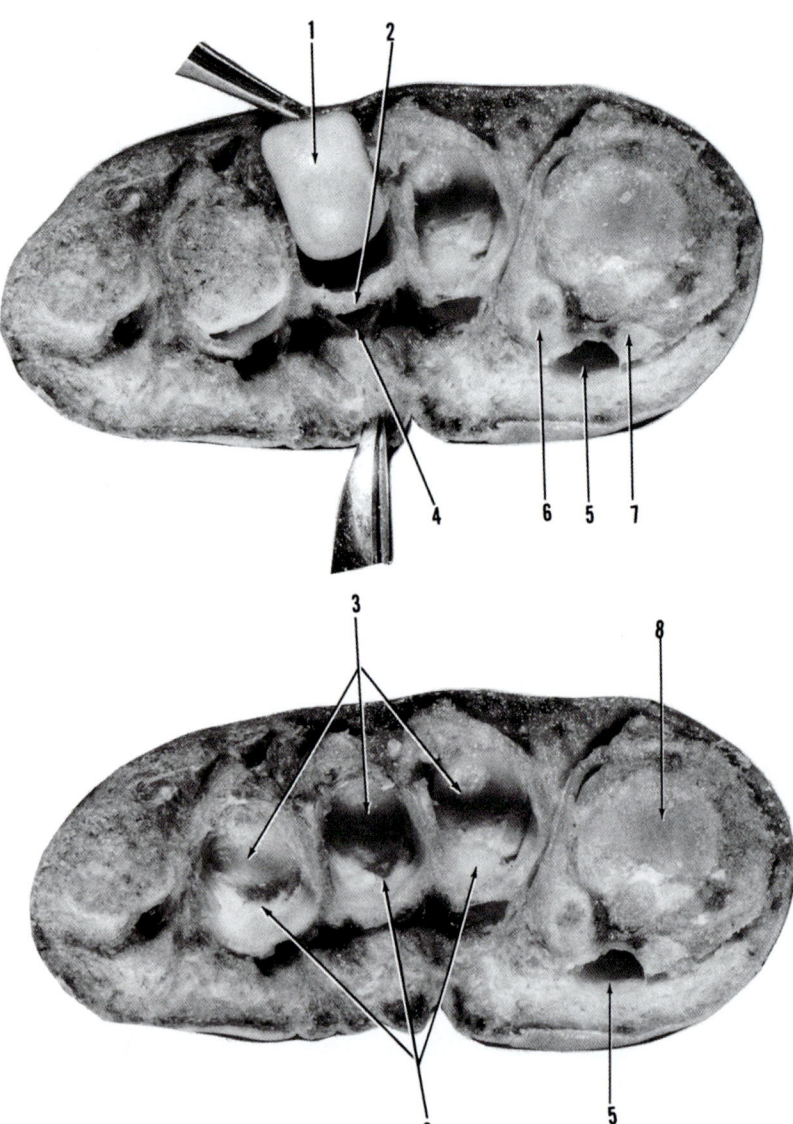

Figure 9.30 Section XII. Coronal section through metatarsophalangeal joints 1 to 4 and proximal phalanx of fifth toe. Proximal surface of section. (*1*, metatarsal head 3; *2*, plantar plate; *3*, proximal articular surfaces of proximal phalanges toes 2, 3, 4; *4*, flexor digitorum longus, brevis tunnel; *5*, flexor hallucis longus tunnel; *6*, lateral hallucal sesamoid; *7*, medial hallucal sesamoids; *8*, proximal articular surface of proximal phalanx big toe.)

On the lateral borders of the foot, the tuberosity of the fifth metatarsal is easily found. The calcaneocuboid joint line is one fingerbreadth proximal to this tuberosity. On the medial border of the foot, the tuberosity of the navicular is palpated and, farther distally, the tubercle of the first metatarsal base; the latter is located at the midpoint of the medial border of the foot. The talar head is located medially at the midpoint of a line joining the tuberosity of the navicular to the tip of the medial malleolus. A line drawn across the foot from the calcaneocuboid interline to the middle of a line connecting the head of the talus with the tuberosity of the navicular closely locates Chopart's joint line.[1] A line, slightly convex anteriorly, drawn across the foot from the tuberosity of the fifth metatarsal to the tubercle of the first metatarsal base closely corresponds to Lisfranc's joint interline.[1]

On the dorsum of the foot, in addition to the digital extensor tendons and the tibialis anterior tendon, the examining hand may palpate the intermediate cutaneous branch of the superficial peroneal nerve, which in certain individuals stands up like a thin, tense cable when the foot is inverted and plantar flexed. This nerve courses in the direction of the third web space.

▶ Skin and Subcutaneous Layer and Superficial Veins and Nerves

Skin and Subcutaneous Layer

The skin on the anterior aspect of the ankle and the dorsum of the foot is thin and supple and may be easily moved over the underlying structures. At the level of the lateral border of the foot, it is more intimately connected to the subcutaneous tissue and appreciably loses its mobility.

The cleavage lines of the dorsal skin are shown in Figure 9.32. Along the tibial aspect of the leg and across the anterior aspect of the ankle and the dorsum of the big toe, the lines run parallel

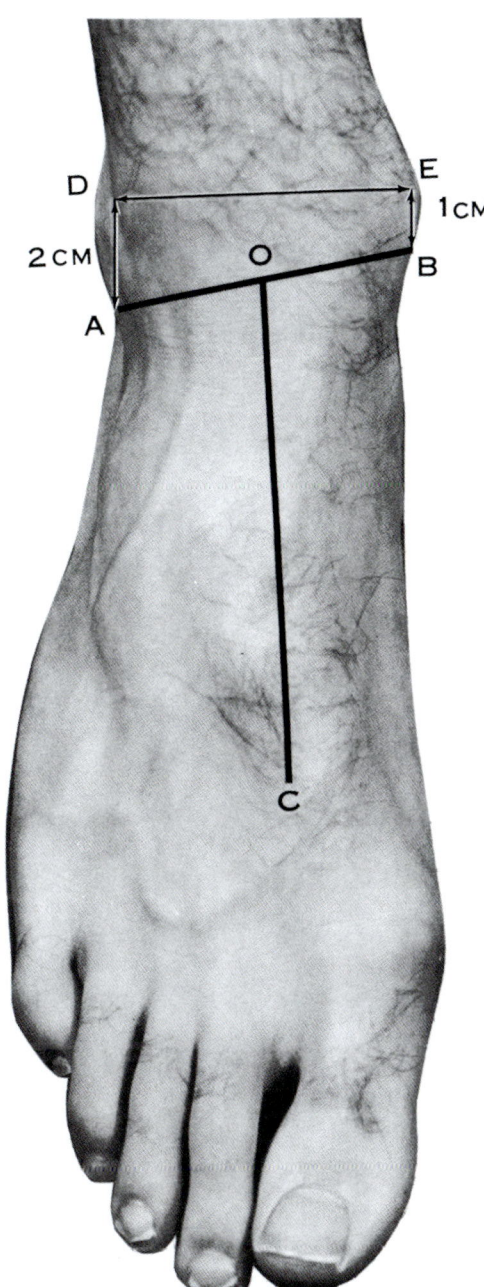

Figure 9.31 **The dorsal vascular axis.** The bimalleolar axis of the ankle is indicated by the line AB. Point O is the middle of line AB. Point C is the proximal end of the first intermetatarsal space. Line OC indicates the direction and location of the dorsalis pedis artery. Line DE indicates the location of the talotibial articular interline. It is 2 cm proximal to the tip of the lateral malleolus and 1 cm proximal to the tip of the medial malleolus.

to the long axis of the foot. In the remaining segment of the dorsum of the foot, the cleavage lines veer laterally, and at the level of the fifth ray, the obliquity of the lines may reach 45°. Around the lateral aspect of the ankle, the cleavage lines follow more or less the contour of the lateral malleolus. Over the lateral and the medial borders of the foot, the lines are longitudinally oriented. Surgical incisions parallel to the cleavage lines leave finer linear scars, whereas incisions at right angles to these lines are subjected to increased tension and may leave wider scars.

The subcutaneous tissue is formed by a loose-meshed connective tissue, lamellar in structure, and mobile relative to the underlying structures. It contains a variable amount of adipose tissue. This layer may form a thin transparent fascia covering or carrying the superficial nerves and veins and may be reflected with ease, exposing the superficial dorsal aponeurosis.

Superficial Veins

The superficial veins of the dorsum of the foot and the anterior ankle are usually superficial to the sensory nerves (Figs. 9.33 and 9.34).[2] The venous network is formed centrally by longitudinally and obliquely oriented veins and distally by the dorsal venous arcade, which receives the superficial dorsal metatarsal veins.

The dorsomedial vein of the big toe, a set of parallel superficial veins crossing the medial border of the foot, and the medial deep perforating veins join the proximal medial extension of the dorsal venous arcade to form the greater saphenous vein. The greater saphenous vein courses anterior to the medial malleolus and receives most of the longitudinally oriented dorsal veins from its lateral border. A medial malleolar vein crosses the medial malleolus inferiorly and transversely and unites the greater saphenous vein with the posterior tibial vein.

The medial perforating veins surface between the superior border of the abductor hallucis and the tarsus. They are usually four in number, one located at the level of the cuneo$_1$-metatarsal$_1$ joint, two periscaphoid, and one more proximal, arising from the medial plantar vein.

On the dorsum of the first web space, a perforating vein connects the dorsal venous arcade with the medial end of the deep plantar venous arch. The proximal lateral extension of the dorsal venous arcade receives a set of parallel veins (average number, 15) crossing the lateral border of the foot; this forms the lesser saphenous vein, which courses along the posterior aspect of the lateral malleolus.

The lateral perforating veins join the lesser saphenous vein. They are the peroneal perforating veins, distal and proximal. The distal peroneal perforating vein emerges on the lateral border of the peroneus brevis tendon near its insertion and arises from the dorsal aspect of the calcaneocuboid joint. The proximal peroneal perforating vein originates from the plantar aspect of the calcaneocuboid joint, emerges deep to the peroneus longus tendon, and unites with the lesser saphenous vein. The lesser saphenous vein also receives, from its medial border, the deep lateral malleolar veins that pass under the extensor digitorum longus tendons and unite with the dorsalis pedis vein.

The venous flow in the foot is bidirectional but, when valves are present, the flow is from the depth of the planta pedis to the superficial dorsal system.

Superficial Nerves

The superficial nerves of the dorsum of the foot are provided by the superficial peroneal nerve, the terminal branch of the deep peroneal nerve, the lateral sural nerve, and the saphenous nerve (see Figs. 9.33, 9.35, and 9.36).

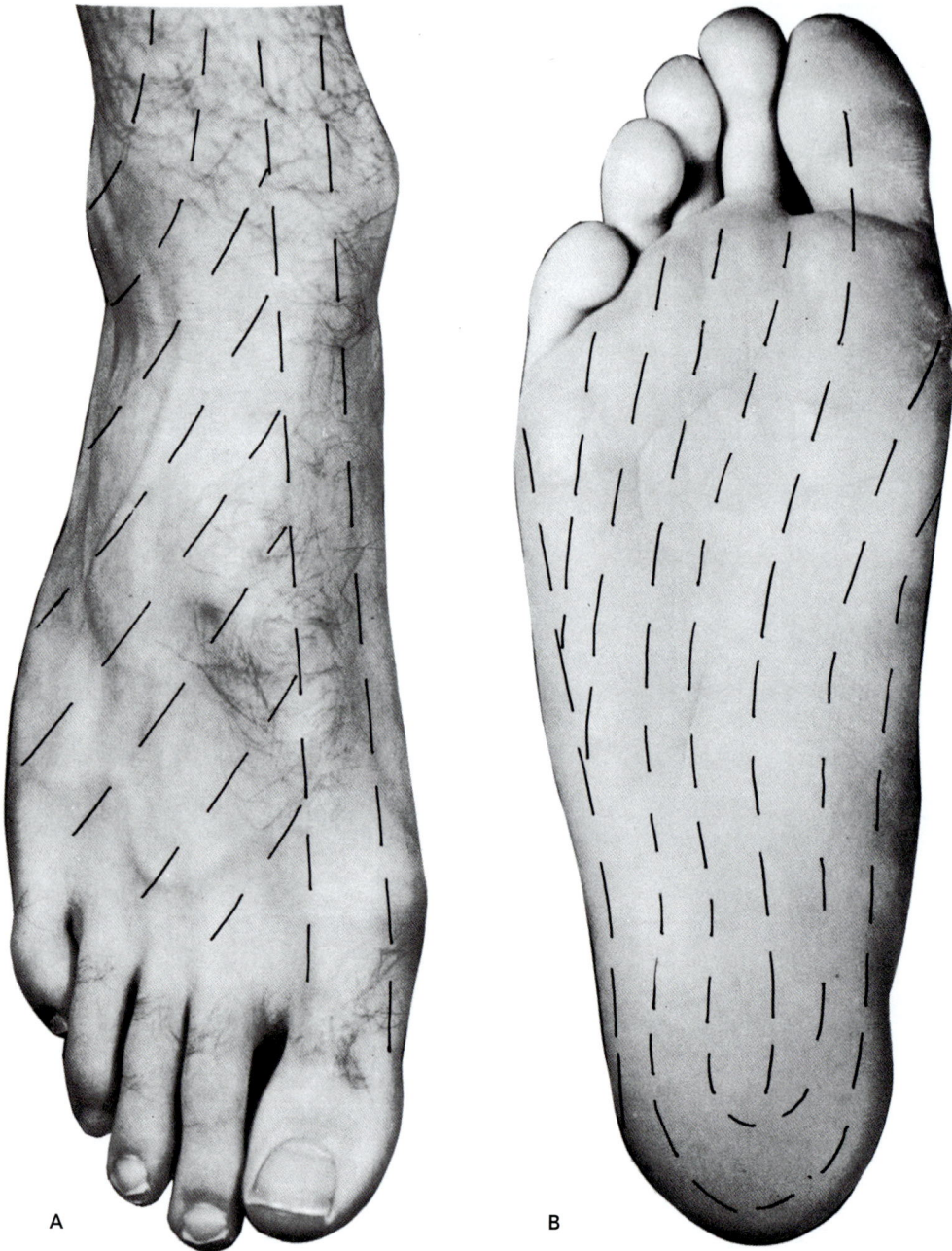

Figure 9.32 **The cleavage lines of the dorsal and plantar skin of the foot.**[20] **(A)** On the dorsal and medial aspect, the cleavage lines are parallel to the medial border of the foot. In the remaining surface, the lines are oblique, making about a 45-degree angle with the long axis of the foot. **(B)** On the plantar aspect, the lines are longitudinally oriented with a slight curvature, convex to the fibular side. At the level of the heel, the lines are arciform and parallel to the plantar border of the heel. Incisions placed in the cleavage lines leave fine linear scars, whereas incisions at right angles to these lines may leave wide scars.

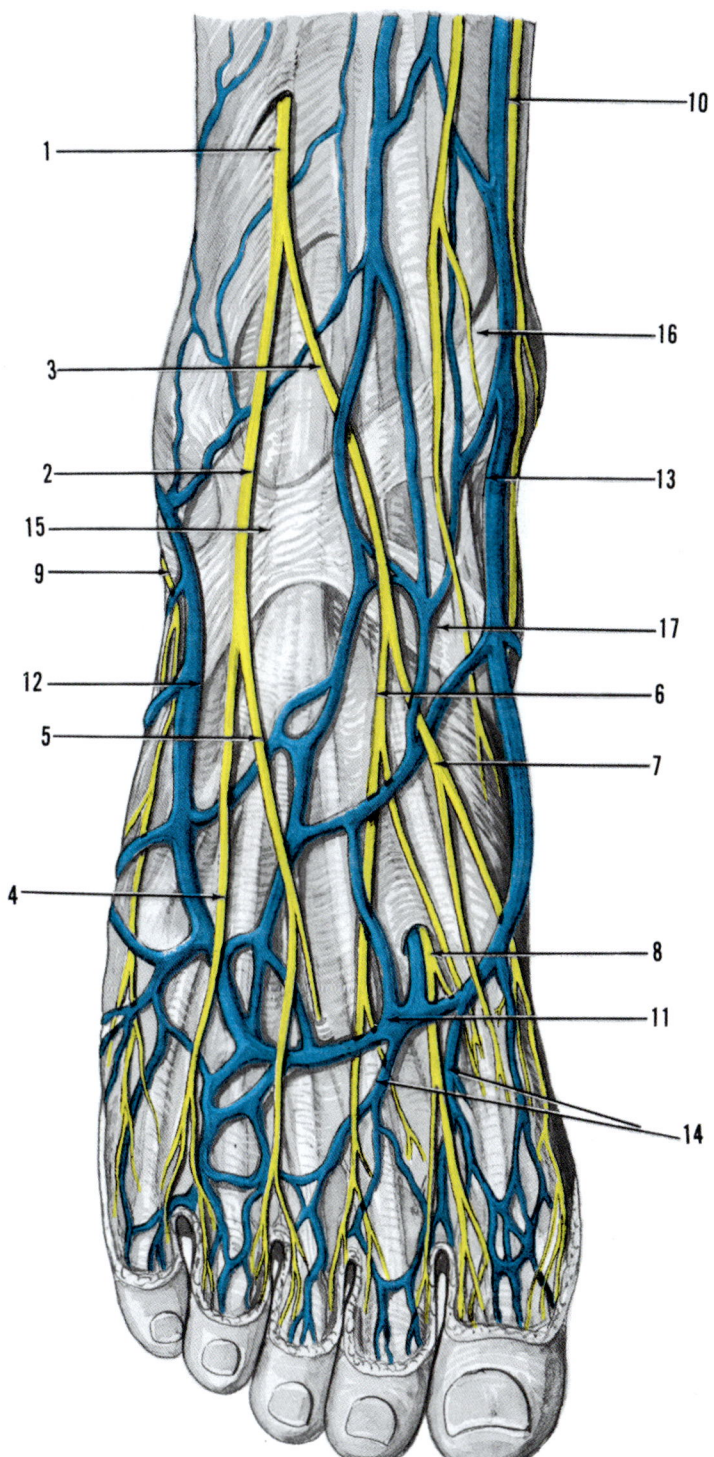

Figure 9.33 Superficial layer of the dorsum of the foot and ankle. (*1*, superficial peroneal nerve; *2*, intermediate dorsal cutaneous nerve; *3*, medial dorsal cutaneous nerve; *4*, dorsal cutaneous nerve to fourth web space; *5*, dorsal cutaneous nerve to third web space; *6*, dorsal cutaneous nerve to second web space with branch to dorsum of big toe; *7*, dorsomedial cutaneous nerve to big toe; *8*, nerve branch from deep peroneal nerve to first interspace; *9*, sural nerve; *10*, saphenous nerve; *11*, dorsal venous arcade; *12*, lesser saphenous vein; *13*, greater saphenous vein; *14*, dorsal metatarsal veins; *15*, stem of inferior extensor retinaculum; *16*, superomedial band of inferior extensor retinaculum; *17*, inferomedial band of inferior extensor retinaculum.)

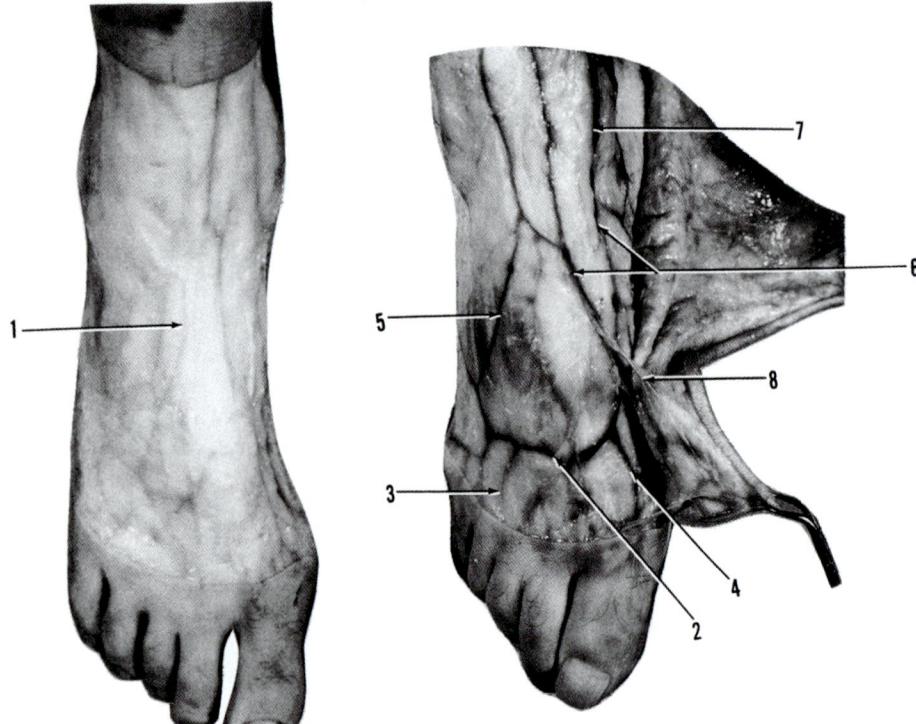

Figure 9.34 **The superficial veins are under the dorsal aponeurosis (1).** (*2,* dorsal venous arcade; *3,* dorsal metatarsal vein; *4,* dorsomedial hallucal vein; *5,* lateral dorsal longitudinal vein; *6,* medial dorsal longitudinal veins; *7,* greater saphenous vein; *8,* terminal nerve branch to the skin.)

The superficial peroneal nerve trunk is usually found subcutaneously along the anterior border of the fibula, 10.5 cm above the tip of the lateral malleolus, in the groove between the peroneal group of muscles and the extensor digitorum longus.[3] The nerve divides into its terminal branches—intermediate and medial dorsal cutaneous nerves—at an average of 6.5 cm proximal to the tip of the lateral malleolus.[3] The intermediate dorsal cutaneous nerve courses along the tibiofibular syndesmosis, passes over the root of the inferior extensor retinaculum, crosses obliquely the fifth and fourth extensor digitorum longus tendons, and courses over the third intermetatarsal space. This nerve can be palpated through the skin. Distally, the nerve divides into the dorsolateral branch of the third toe and the dorsomedial branch of the fourth toe. An anastomotic branch to the sural nerve may be present. The variations of distribution of the sensory nerves are dealt with in Chapter 8.

The medial dorsal cutaneous branch is located laterally over the anterior aspect of the ankle and overlies the extensor digitorum longus tendons. It runs parallel to the extensor hallucis longus tendon, crosses the inferior extensor retinaculum, and, distal to the latter, divides into three branches: lateral, middle, and medial.

The lateral branch obliquely crosses the long extensor tendon of the second toe and bifurcates in the anterior segment of the second intermetatarsal space into the dorsomedial branch of the third toe and the dorsolateral branch of the second toe.

The middle branch courses superficially over the first intermetatarsal space and divides into two thin branches supplying the dorsomedial aspect of the second toe and the dorsolateral aspect of the big toe. These two branches are reinforced by the deep peroneal nerve.

The medial branch is directed medially; it crosses the extensor hallucis longus tendon and forms the dorsomedial cutaneous nerve of the big toe. This is the superficial nerve branch that is to be looked for and reflected laterally during the bunionectomy of the big toe through a medial approach.

The intermediate and medial dorsal cutaneous nerves are to be dealt with in the anterolateral approach to the lateral malleolus and the ankle joint, in the anterolateral portal of ankle arthroscopy, in the lateral approach for a triple arthrodesis, in the transverse or longitudinal approach for a tarsometatarsal mobilization, in the midtarsal osteotomy, or in the central metatarsal osteotomies. The longitudinally oriented superficial nerves are most vulnerable in the transverse dorsal incisions.

The saphenous nerve is located on the anterior aspect of the medial malleolus, posteromedial to the greater saphenous vein, and may extend along the medial border of the foot and reach the medial aspect of the big toe.

The sural nerve, after turning around the lateral malleolus, divides into two branches—lateral and medial—at the base of the fifth metatarsal bone. The lateral branch terminates as the dorsolateral nerve of the fifth toe. The medial branch obliquely crosses the long extensor tendon of the fifth toe and forms the dorsomedial branch to the fifth toe. As mentioned previously, an anastomotic branch may be present between the sural nerve and the lateral division branch of the intermediate dorsal cutaneous nerve.

accompanying deep veins. It is attached to the dorsal skeletal frame medially and laterally and creates a true osteofascial space: spatium dorsalis pedis.[4] Laterally, the aponeurosis attaches on the os calcis, the cuboid, and the tuberosity and the lateral border of the fifth metatarsal bone. The medial marginal insertion extends from the sustentaculum tali to the tuberosity of the scaphoid and the medial border of the first metatarsal bone.

The superficial dorsal aponeurosis extends vertical fibers to the skin and closes the dorsal subcutaneous space along its margins. Distally, the thin aponeurosis attaches to the fibrous sheath of the extensor tendons, and proximally, it is in continuity with the inferior extensor retinaculum.

The inferior extensor retinaculum is a retention system acting as multiple pulleys for the tendons crossing the anterior aspect of the ankle and of the foot, preventing their bowstringing (Figs. 9.37 and 9.38). Their surgical preservation or reconstruction is essential.

At first sight, the delineation of the borders of this retinaculum might not be very clear, because distally, it is in continuity with the dorsal aponeurosis and proximally with the distal segment of the aponeurosis cruris and the superior extensor retinaculum. The inferior extensor retinaculum originates from the sinus tarsi and sinus canal with three roots: lateral, intermediate, and medial (Fig. 9.39). The lateral root inserts on the lateral border of the sinus tarsi and over the inferior peroneal retinaculum; it is lateral to the origin of the extensor digitorum brevis muscle. The intermediate root originates in the center of the sinus tarsi, medial to the extensor digitorum brevis muscle and posterior to the cervical ligament. The medial root originates in the sinus tarsi, next to the intermediate root; in the canalis tarsi, it is anterior to the interosseous ligament and sends an arm to the talar roof of the tarsal canal. The lateral and intermediate roots envelop the origin of the extensor digitorum brevis, unite, and form the stem of the inferior extensor retinaculum. The medial root courses superomedially and attaches to the deep surface of the stem immediately medial to the extensor digitorum longus tendons, contributing to the formation of the powerful lateral retention sling for these tendons. Anteriorly, the retinacular stem divides into two arms, superomedial and inferomedial. The superomedial arm passes over the tendon of the extensor hallucis longus, covers the tendon of the tibialis anterior, and inserts on the anterior aspect of the medial malleolus. On the medial border of the extensor hallucis longus tendon, deep retinacular fibers loop around the tendon posteriorly and insert on either the talar neck or the deep surface of the lateral sling. These recurrent fibers form a retention tunnel for the extensor hallucis longus tendon. Farther medially, the superomedial arm of the retinaculum reaches the tibialis anterior tendon and forms two retention systems: superior and inferior. The superior tunnel has a very thin or absent superficial cover, whereas the deep layer is thick and inserts on the medial malleolus. The inferior tunnel is well structured. The anterior and posterior walls of the tunnel unite on the medial border of the tendon and insert on the anterior aspect of the medial malleolus.

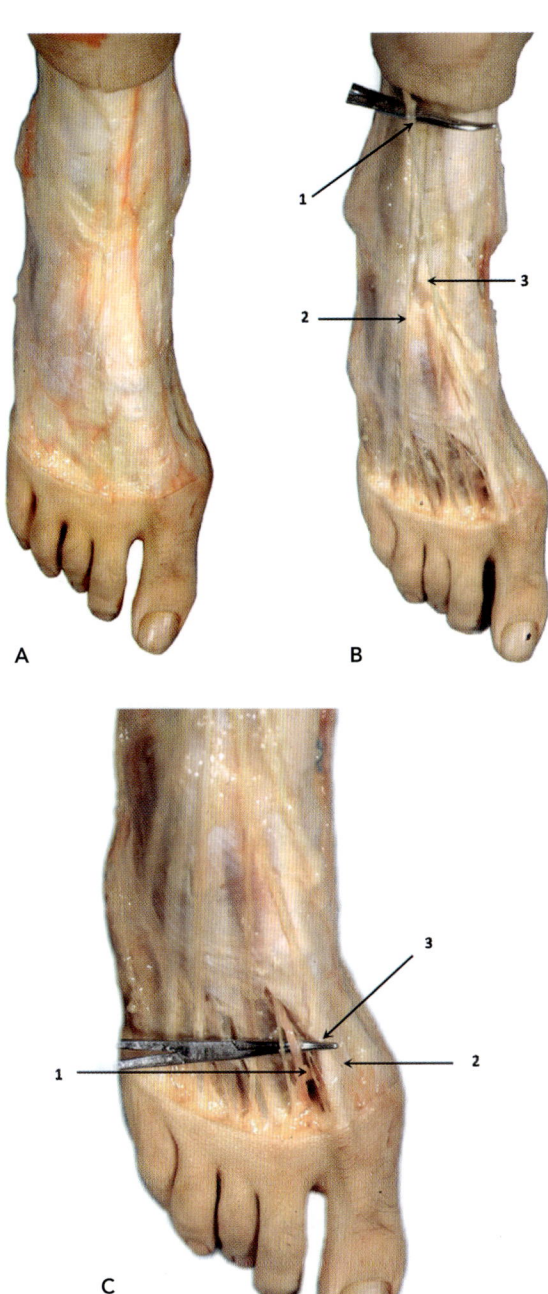

Figure 9.35 Superficial nerves of the dorsum of the foot. (A) The superficial nerves are under the superficial dorsal aponeurosis. **(B)** (*1*, trunk of superficial peroneal nerve; *2*, intermediate division branch of superficial peroneal nerve; *3*, medial division branch of superficial peroneal nerve.) **(C)** (*1*, lateral branch of deep peroneal nerve; *2*, medial branch of deep peroneal nerve; *3*, first dorsal metatarsal artery.)

▶ Dorsal Aponeurosis and Dorsal Fascial Spaces and Contents

Dorsal Aponeurosis

The superficial dorsal aponeurosis of the foot is encountered after reflection of the skin and the subcutaneous layer carrying the fascia superficialis and the incorporated superficial veins and nerves. This thin, semitransparent layer invests the musculotendinous units, the arteries, and their

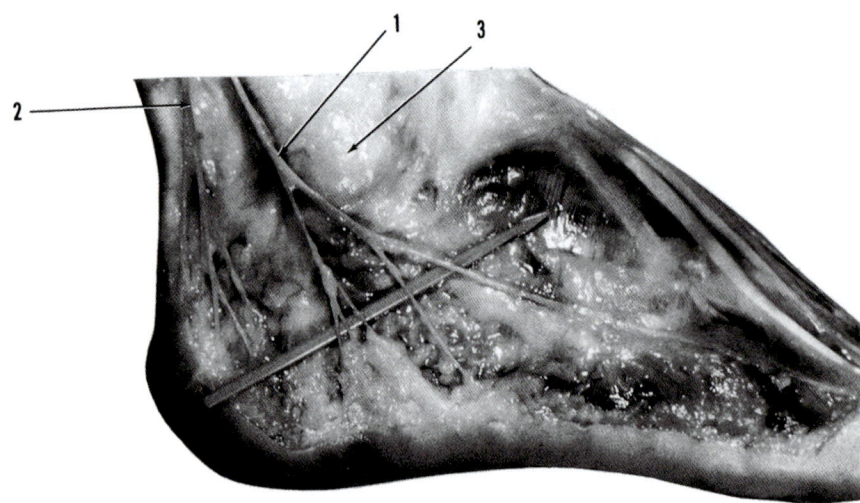

Figure 9.36 **Sural nerve.** (*1*, sural nerve trunk; *2*, lateral calcaneal nerve, branch of sural nerve; *3*, premalleolar fat pad).

The inferomedial arm of the retinaculum courses anteromedially and reaches the medial border of the foot at the level of the cuneonavicular joint. The fibers pass over the dorsalis pedis vessels, the deep peroneal nerve, and the extensor hallucis longus tendon—and, as they reach the tibialis anterior tendon, they form a terminal tunnel for the latter. This segment of the retinaculum splits into deep fibers, which insert on the navicular and medial cuneiform, and superficial fibers, which are in continuity with the investing fascia of the abductor hallucis muscle.

In 25% of the cases, the inferior extensor retinaculum has an oblique superolateral extension band that gives to the retinaculum a cruciate configuration. This band originates from the lateral sling, from the superomedial band, or from both. It courses upward and laterally and inserts on the lateral surface of the lateral malleolus and the lateral crest of the lower segment of the fibula.

Dorsal Fascial Spaces and Contents

The dorsal osteoaponeurotic space of the foot is subdivided into four fascial gliding spaces by three layers of tissue (see Fig. 9.42).[4]

The first layer is formed by the tendons of the tibialis anterior, extensor hallucis longus, extensor digitorum longus, and peroneus tertius, surrounded by their synovial sheaths or peritenon. The tendons are united to each other with loose connective tissue. Laterally and medially, this loose connective tissue blends with the superficial dorsal aponeurosis.

The second layer is muscular and is formed by the extensor digitorum brevis and its investing fascia. This fascia, attached to the deep surface of the extensor hallucis longus synovial sheath, passes over the dorsalis pedis vessels and the deep peroneal nerve. It encounters the medial border of the extensor digitorum brevis, where it splits into two investing layers, superficial and deep. On the lateral margin of the muscle, the two layers unite and the aponeurosis inserts on the deep surface of the superficial dorsal aponeurosis and on the tarsal skeleton.

The third layer, neurovascular, is formed by an adipoconnective lamina carrying the dorsalis pedis vessels with their tributaries and the deep peroneal nerve with its branches. At the level of the metatarsals, the dorsal interosseous aponeurosis is the last investing layer. The four gliding fascial spaces are the potential spaces located between the dorsal aponeurosis, the three soft tissue layers, and the dorsal osteoligamentous frame.

First Layer

On the anterior aspect of the ankle, the crossing tendons are grouped over the distal tibia and do not cover the anterior aspect of the malleoli (see Fig. 9.37). The tibialis anterior tendon on the medial side and the extensor digitorum longus tendon with the peroneus tertius tendon laterally are more superficial than the centrally located extensor hallucis longus tendon.

The reflection of the superficial dorsal aponeurosis reveals the same tendons on the dorsum of the foot but in a diverging pattern. On the medial aspect, the tendon of the tibialis anterior is directed obliquely anteromedially and plantarward, winds around the medial border of the foot, and inserts on the base of the first metatarsal inferomedially and on the medial aspect of the first cuneiform. The synovial tendon sheath of the tibialis anterior tendon extends from above the superior arm of the inferior extensor retinaculum to the level of the talonavicular joint.

The extensor hallucis longus tendon is located lateral to the tibialis anterior tendon. It is directed anteromedially, diverging slightly from the tibialis anterior tendon. The tendon approaches the first metatarsal bone at an acute angle; it courses on the dorsolateral aspect of the bone and remains centralized on the dorsum of the metatarsophalangeal joint of the big toe. The lateral border of the extensor hallucis longus is an important guideline because it parallels the direction of the vascular axis of the dorsum of the foot. The synovial sheath of the extensor hallucis tendon extends from just above the upper arm of the inferior extensor retinaculum to the level of the $cuneo_1$-$metatarsal_1$ joint.

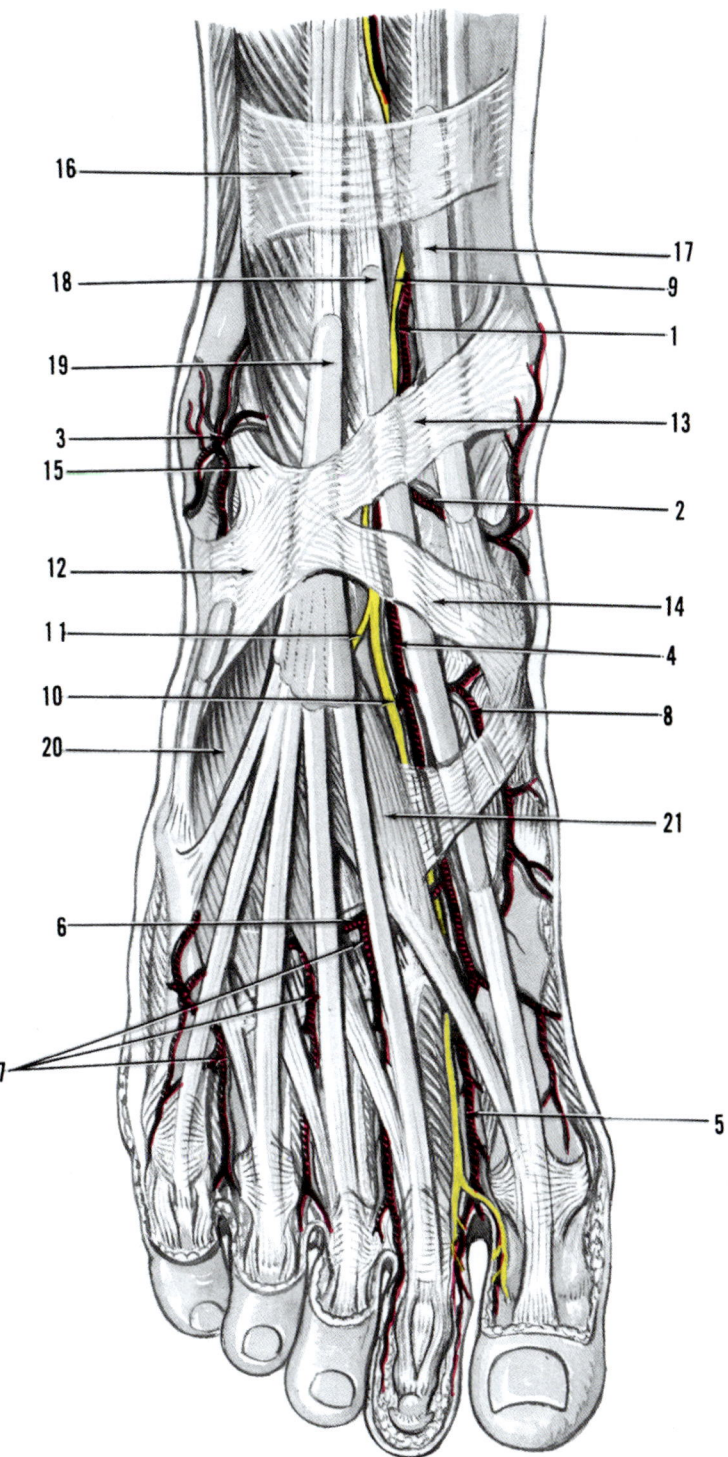

Figure 9.37 First layer of the dorsum of the foot and ankle. (*1*, anterior tibial artery; *2*, anterior medial malleolar artery; *3*, anterior lateral malleolar artery; *4*, dorsalis pedis artery; *5*, first dorsal metatarsal artery; *6*, arcuate artery; *7*, dorsal metatarsal arteries 2, 3, 4; *8*, medial tarsal artery; *9, 10*, deep peroneal nerve; *11*, motor nerve branch to extensor digitorum brevis; *12*, inferior extensor retinaculum; *13*, superomedial band of inferior extensor retinaculum; *14*, inferomedial band of inferior extensor retinaculum; *15*, superolateral band of inferior extensor retinaculum; *16*, superior extensor retinaculum; *17*, tibialis anterior tendon; *18*, extensor hallucis longus tendon; *19*, extensor digitorum longus tendon; *20*, extensor digitorum brevis muscle to toes 2, 3, 4; *21*, extensor hallucis brevis muscle.)

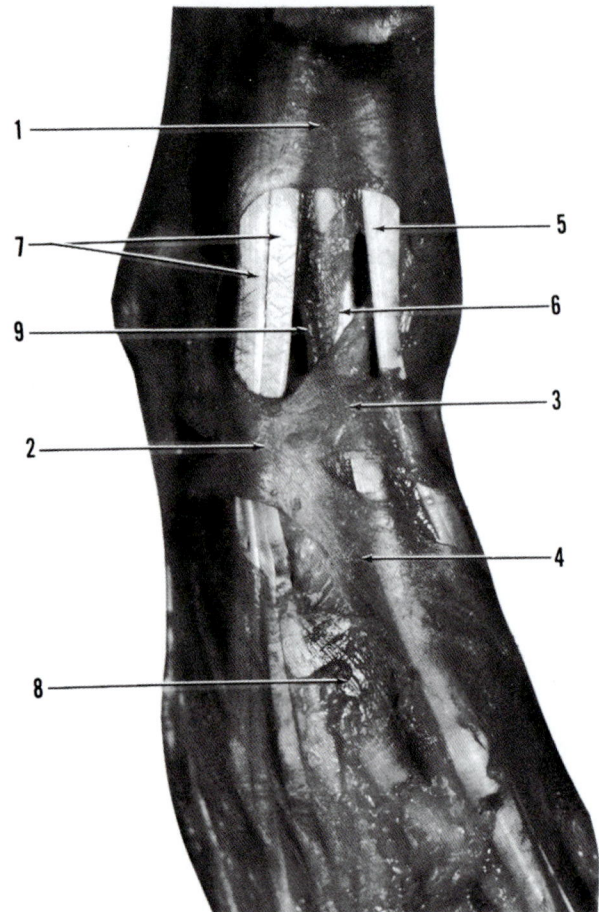
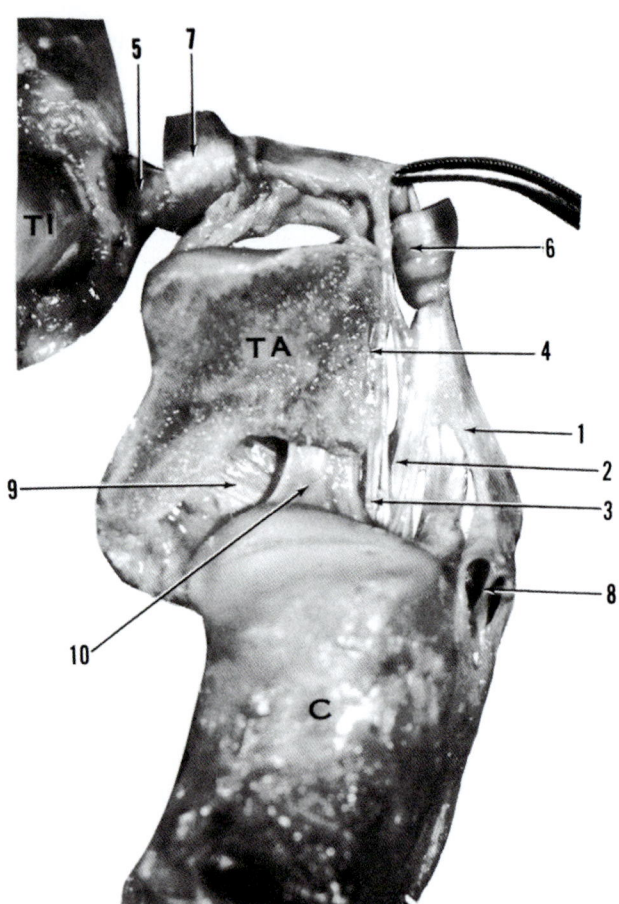

Figure 9.38 **Dorsum of the ankle and foot.** (*1*, superior extensor retinaculum; *2*, stem of inferior extensor retinaculum; *3*, superomedial band of inferior extensor retinaculum; *4*, inferomedial band of inferior extensor retinaculum; *5*, tibialis anterior tendon; *6*, extensor hallucis longus tendon; *7*, extensor digitorum longus tendons; *8*, extensor digitorum brevis muscle; *9*, neurovascular bundle—deep peroneal nerve and dorsalis pedis artery.)

Figure 9.39 **The roots of the inferior extensor retinaculum on the right foot.** The posterior aspect of the talus is removed, exposing the canalis tarsi. (*C*, calcaneum; *TA*, talus; *TI*, tibia; *1*, lateral root of inferior extensor retinaculum; *2*, intermediary root of inferior extensor retinaculum; *3*, medial root of inferior extensor retinaculum; *4*, talar attachment of 3; *5*, superomedial attachment of inferior extensor retinaculum on tibia; *6*, tendon of extensor digitorum longus; *7*, tibialis anterior tendon; *8*, inferior peroneal retinaculum; *9*, interosseous ligament of canalis tarsi; *10*, anterior capsular ligament of posterior talocalcaneal joint.)

The extensor digitorum longus tendons, usually two in number, are located under the stem of the inferior extensor retinaculum and divide into four tendons as they exit from their retinacular tunnel. On the dorsum of the foot, these tendons fan out, cross the extensor digitorum brevis muscle, may exchange thin connecting fibers, and reach their respective toes 2 to 5. The long extensor tendons to the fourth and fifth toes are oriented anterolaterally.

The peroneus tertius tendon is lateral to the tendons of the extensor digitorum longus. The tendon diverges anterolaterally, obliquely crosses the underlying extensor digitorum brevis muscle, fans out, and inserts on the superior surface of the fifth metatarsal base; this tendon is absent in 8.5% of the cases.

The common synovial tendon sheath of the extensor digitorum longus and the peroneus tertius starts about 1 cm proximal to the tendon sheath of the extensor hallucis longus. It enlarges distally and forms a triangular sac that terminates at the level of the cuneonavicular joint. Four small synovial projections may extend farther distally over the four toe extensors. The tenosynovial compartments described previously are normally flat, unimpressive structures, but they have great relevance when involved by an inflammatory or infectious process.

Second Layer

The extensor digitorum brevis muscle originates in the sinus tarsi between the superficial and intermediate roots of the inferior extensor retinaculum. Initially, the muscle covers the lateral half of the tarsus, is directed anteromedially, and divides into four small muscles followed by their corresponding tendons. The extensor hallucis brevis component is the largest of the four, and it obliquely crosses the distal segment of the dorsalis pedis artery. When the muscle is well developed, the medial border covers the mid segment of the same artery. The tendon of the extensor hallucis brevis joins the extensor hallucis longus from the peroneal side and is deep to the latter and its extensor lamina.

The extensor digitorum brevis tendons to the second, third, and fourth toes join the long extensor tendinous complex from the peroneal side. Proximally, they are deeper relative to the long extensor tendon. The fifth toe does not have an extensor brevis muscle and cannot be a donor of long extensor tendon as a graft.

Reflection of the extensor digitorum brevis and its aponeurosis reveals the connective tissue layer carrying the dorsal pedis vessels and the deep peroneal nerve, with their divisions (Figs. 9.40 and 9.41).

Third Layer

As mentioned previously, the dorsalis pedis vascular axis is delineated by a line joining the midpoint of the bimalleolar axis to the proximal end of the first interosseous space.

At the level of the ankle joint interline, the tibialis anterior artery becomes the dorsalis pedis artery. Above the ankle joint, the artery is covered by the extensor hallucis longus tendon. At the ankle, the extensor hallucis longus tendon crosses the dorsalis pedis artery and is then medial to the artery. Under the inferior extensor retinaculum, the artery is

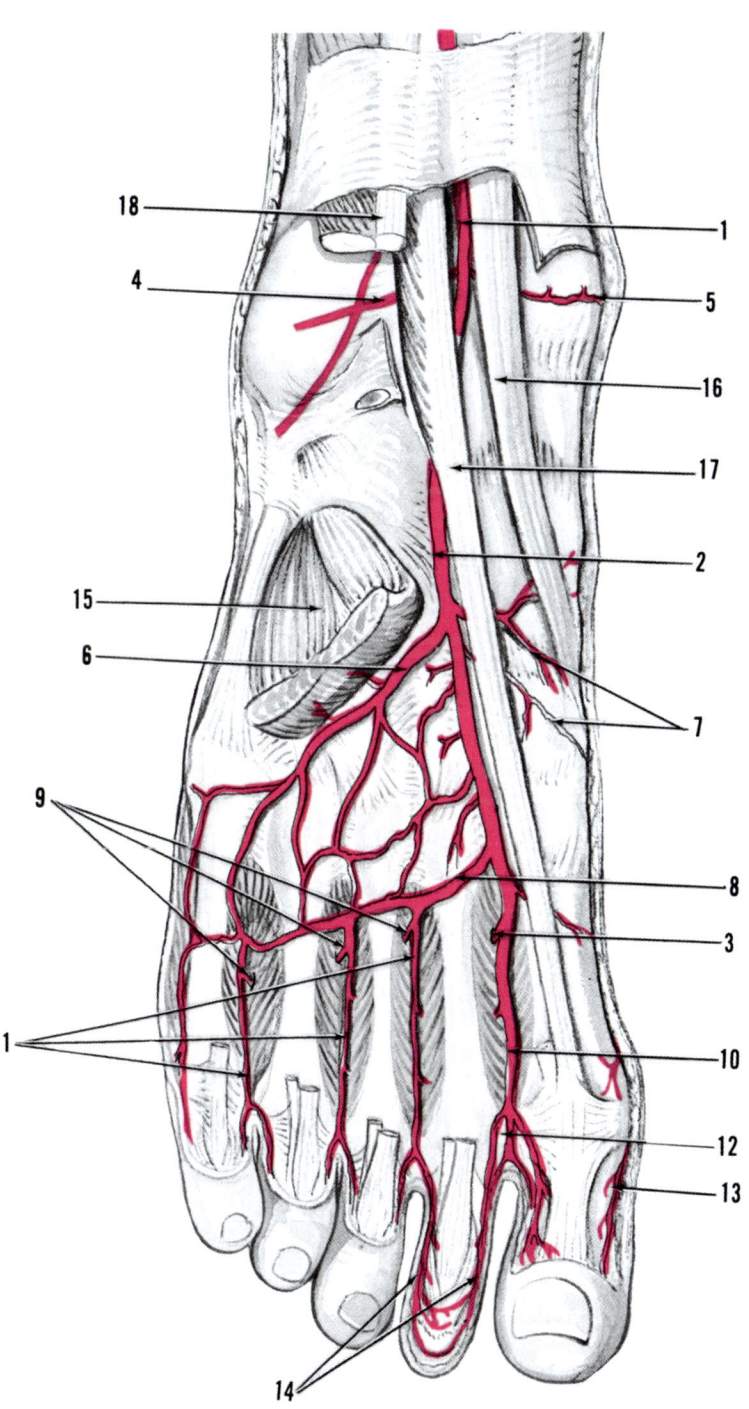

Figure 9.40 Deep layer of the dorsal aspect of the foot and ankle. (*1*, anterior tibial artery; *2*, dorsalis pedis artery; *3*, first proximal perforating artery; *4*, anterior lateral malleolar artery; *5*, anterior medial malleolar artery; *6*, lateral tarsal artery; *7*, medial tarsal arteries; *8*, arcuate artery; *9*, proximal perforating arteries 2, 3, 4; *10*, first dorsal metatarsal artery; *11*, dorsal metatarsal arteries 2, 3, 4; *12*, first distal perforating artery; *13*, dorsomedial hallucal artery; *14*, dorsal digital collateral arteries; *15*, extensor digitorum brevis muscle; *16*, tibialis anterior tendon; *17*, extensor hallucis longus tendon; *18*, extensor digitorum longus tendon.)

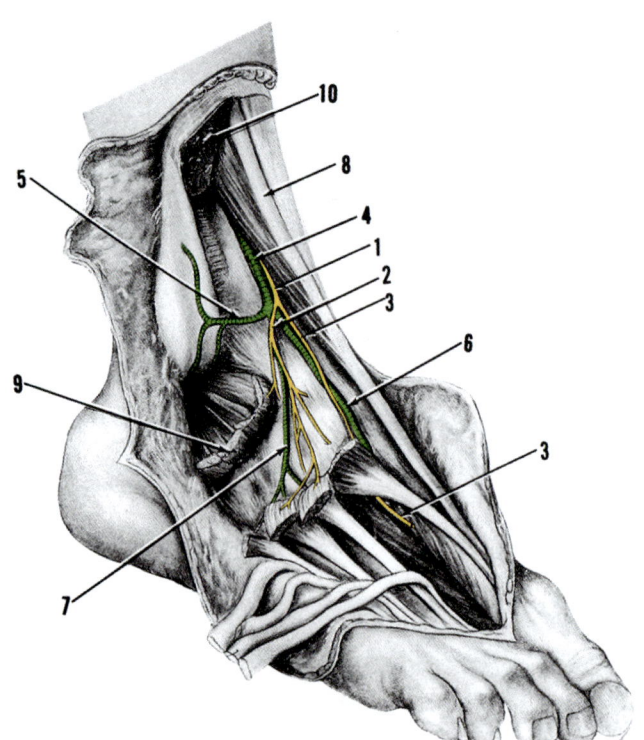

Figure 9.41 Terminal branch of anterior tibial nerve or deep peroneal nerve. (*1*, anterior tibial nerve or deep peroneal nerve; *2*, lateral division branch of [*1*], motor branch to extensor digitorum brevis [*9*]; *3*, medial division branch of [*1*], sensory deep peroneal branch to first web space; *4*, anterior tibial artery; *5*, lateral malleolar artery; *6*, dorsalis pedis artery; *7*, lateral tarsal artery; *8*, extensor hallucis longus; *9*, transected extensor digitorum brevis; *10*, transected extensor digitorum communis.) (Adapted from Hovelacque H. *Anatomie des Nerfs Craniens et Rachidiens et du Système Grand Sympathique.* Doin; 1927.)

deep and located posterolateral to the tunnel of the extensor hallucis longus tendon.

The two accompanying veins and the deep branch of the peroneal nerve located on the lateral side of the vessels are all applied against the osteoarticular layer (Fig. 9.42). Lateral detachment of the roots of the inferior extensor retinaculum and of the origin of the extensor digitorum brevis followed by medial reflection of this entire unit will carry all the tendons but leave the neurovascular structures against the joint.

For the anesthetic block of the deep peroneal nerve, the needle is introduced between the extensor hallucis longus tendon and the long extensor tendon to the second toe, as indicated by the vertical arrow in Figure 9.42. The needle passes medial to the extensor digitorum brevis, down onto the osseoligamentous frame, and is drawn slightly dorsally; thus, it remains under or within the third layer of the dorsum of the foot.

Distal to the inferior extensor retinaculum, the dorsalis pedis artery is located lateral to the extensor hallucis longus tendon and medial to the medial border of the extensor hallucis brevis muscle. In the mid segment of the foot, the artery is covered by the medial border of the same muscle, and distally, it is lateral to the tendon of the same muscle.

To expose the dorsalis pedis artery, a skin incision is made on the dorsum of the foot along a line extending from the midpoint of the bimalleolar axis to the base of the first interosseous space. The superficial aponeurosis is incised, followed by incision of the second aponeurosis along the medial border of the extensor digitorum brevis, which is retracted laterally, providing access to the artery.

The previous description of the dorsalis pedis artery applies to the majority of the cases. However, the artery may be absent in 12% of the cases or may have a lateral deviation in 5.5% and a medial deviation in 3.5%.[5]

The dorsalis pedis artery plunges plantarward at a 90-degree angle through the space limited by the arch of the first dorsal interosseous muscle and the bases of the first and second metatarsals. After making another 90-degree lateral turn, it inosculates with the deep branch of the lateral plantar artery. This 90 to 90-degree vascular corner located between the first and second metatarsal bases must be taken into serious consideration during basal corrective osteotomy of the first metatarsal (Fig. 9.43). At the level of the ankle, the dorsalis pedis artery provides the transversely oriented anterior lateral and medial malleolar arteries; these two arteries are deep to the tendons crossing the ankle. The transverse malleolar arteries are to be considered during arthroscopy of the ankle, using the anterolateral and anteromedial portals.

At the level of the talar neck, a few talar branches take off, including the artery of the sinus tarsi. The lateral tarsal artery originates at the level of the talar head and courses obliquely over the dorsum of the cuboid under the extensor digitorum brevis. It provides the arterial branches to the extensor digitorum brevis, contributes to the vascularization of the talus, and divides over the cuboid into two or three longitudinal arterial branches, which join the arcuate artery. The latter originates from the dorsalis pedis artery at the level of the cuneo$_1$-metatarsal$_1$ joint, crosses transversely the bases of the second, third, and fourth metatarsals, and provides the dorsal metatarsal arteries 2 to 4.

The first dorsal metatarsal artery takes off from the terminal segment of the dorsalis pedis artery and courses over the first dorsal interosseous muscle. It provides the dorsal arteries to the big toe and the dorsotibial artery to the second toe. It plunges plantarward at the first web space and becomes the first distal perforating artery.

The dorsal metatarsal arteries 2 to 4 course in their respective intermetatarsal spaces. Each provides the proximal perforating artery in the proximal segment of the interspace, supplies the dorsal arteries to the adjacent toes, and terminates as the distal perforating artery in the web space. At the level of the metatarsal necks, the dorsal metatarsal artery also provides two transverse plantar anastomotic branches. The medial tarsal arteries take off from the medial aspect of the dorsalis pedis artery at the level of the navicular and the cuneonavicular joint and course transversely under the tibialis anterior tendon. The transversely crossing arcuate artery and the longitudinal tributaries of the lateral tarsal artery are dealt with during tarsometatarsal surgical mobilization.

The deep branch of the peroneal nerve is lateral to the anterior tibial vessels (see Fig. 9.41). Just proximal to the ankle joint interline, the nerve divides into medial and lateral branches. Under the inferior extensor retinaculum, the nerves remain lateral to the dorsalis pedis vessels. The larger medial branch

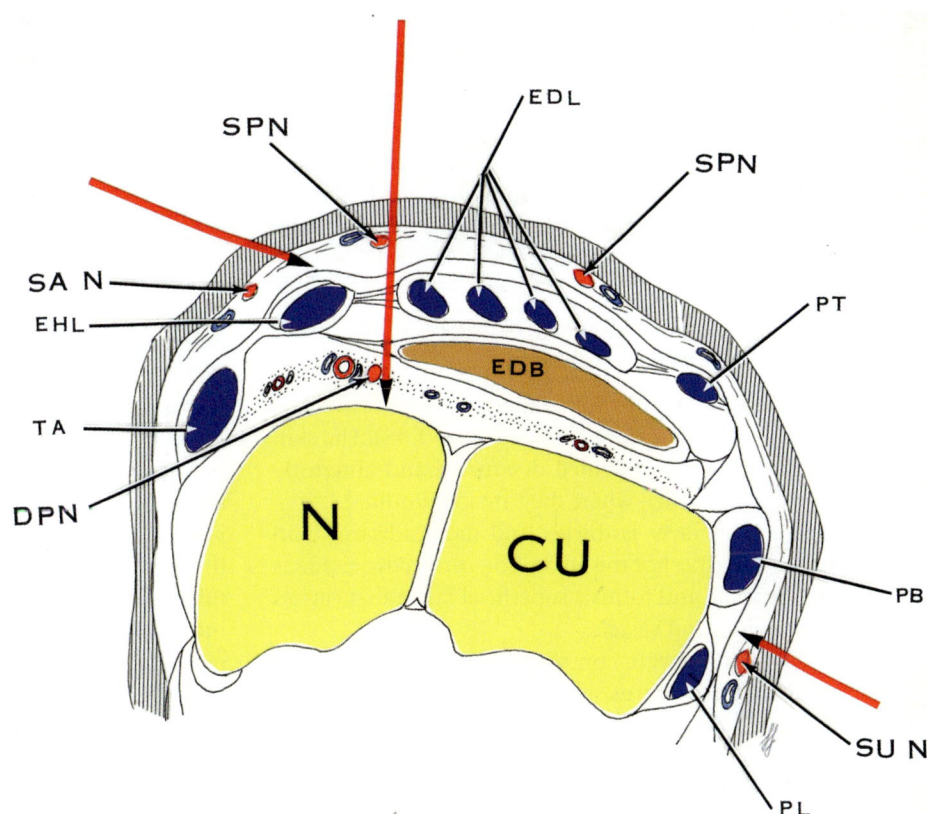

Figure 9.42 Coronal cross-section of the (right) foot passing through the anterior tarsus—view of anterior segment. (*CU*, cuboid; *DPN*, deep peroneal nerve lateral to dorsalis pedis vessel; *EDB*, extensor digitorum brevis; *EDL*, extensor digitorum longus tendons; *EHL*, extensor hallucis longus tendon; *N*, navicular; *PB*, peroneus brevis tendon; *PL*, peroneus longus tendon; *PT*, pronator teres tendon; *SAN*, saphenous nerve; *SPN*, superficial peroneal nerve; *SUN*, sural nerve; *TA*, tibialis anterior tendon.) *Vertical arrow* indicates site of injection to block the deep peroneal nerve. The *lateral side arrow* indicates the injection site for the sural nerve. The *medial side arrow* indicates the plane of injection to block the superficial peroneal nerve. (Adapted from Bellocq P, Meyer P. Contribution à l'étude de l'aponevrose dorsale du pied [fascia dorsalis pedis, P.N.A.]. *Acta Anat.* 1957;30:67.)

continues the direction of the nerve trunk and courses along the medial side of the dorsalis pedis artery. At the base of the first intermetatarsal space, the nerve divides into two branches: the dorsolateral branch of the big toe and the dorsomedial branch of the second toe.

The lateral branch of the deep peroneal nerve is directed anterolaterally and innervates the extensor digitorum brevis muscle. Both medial and lateral branches provide articular filaments to the tarsal skeleton, the tarsometatarsal joints, and the digital joints.

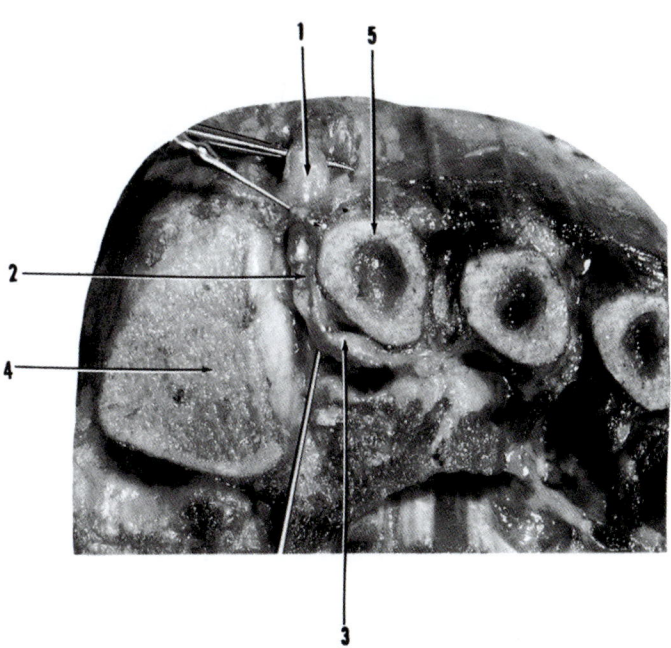

Figure 9.43 The 90-degree to 90-degree vascular corner in the proximal segment of the first intermetatarsal space. (*1*, dorsalis pedis artery; *2*, descending vertical branch of dorsalis pedis artery making a 90-degree angle; *3*, horizontal branch of dorsalis pedis artery joining the lateral plantar artery under the second metatarsal at 90-degree angle; *4*, base of first metatarsal; *5*, shaft of second metatarsal.)

POSTEROLATERAL ASPECT OF THE ANKLE AND FOOT

The posterolateral aspect of the ankle and foot comprises the concave region located between the lateral border of the Achilles tendon and the peronei tendons. It extends distally over the convex lateral aspect of the heel and the lateral border of the foot up to the tuberosity of the fifth metatarsal.

▶ Skin, Subcutaneous Layer, and Superficial Veins and Nerves

The skin is mobile proximally but relatively fixed over the heel and the lateral border of the foot (Figs. 9.44 and 9.45). The skin cleavage lines are oblique, oriented downward and anteriorly except on the lateral border, where they are longitudinal.

The subcutaneous layer is thicker and more adipose than that of the anterior aspect of the ankle. The connective tissue is organized in lamellae and forms a superficial fascia that carries the superficial nerves and vessels.

The short saphenous vein courses along the lateral border of the Achilles tendon, turns around the lateral malleolus, and reaches the lateral aspect of the foot. It receives from its inferior border an average of three lateral calcaneal veins, and from its anterior border, it receives the anterolateral malleolar vein arising from the dorsalis pedis vein. Farther distally, two peroneal communicating veins—proximal and distal—are tributaries of the short saphenous vein. The proximal peroneal vein arises from the plantar aspect of the calcaneocuboid joint and passes deep to the peroneus longus tendon. The distal peroneal vein arises from the dorsum of the calcaneocuboid joint and passes between the peroneus brevis and the peroneus longus tendon to join the lesser saphenous vein.

The retromalleolar branch of the posterior peroneal artery, after piercing the deep and superficial aponeurosis, accompanies the short saphenous vein and provides the lateral arterial calcaneal branches.

Proximal to the ankle joint, the sural nerve is lateral to the lesser saphenous vein. With the latter, the nerve courses behind the posterior border of the lateral malleolus and the retained peronei tendons (see Fig. 9.36). The nerve passes 1 to 1.5 cm distal to the tip of the lateral malleolus. It is anterior to the vein and remains posterior to the peronei tendons. At times, the peronei tendons are crossed by the nerve. At the level of the tuberosity of the fifth metatarsal base, the sural nerve divides into its two terminal branches. From its posterior border, the nerve provides two lateral calcaneal branches originating about three fingerbreadths and one fingerbreadth proximal to the tip of the lateral malleolus. Farther distally, the nerve provides from its lower border a set of three to four vertical or slightly oblique lateral marginal branches. In a transverse surgical incision across the sheath of the peronei tendons, the sural nerve is to be dealt with.

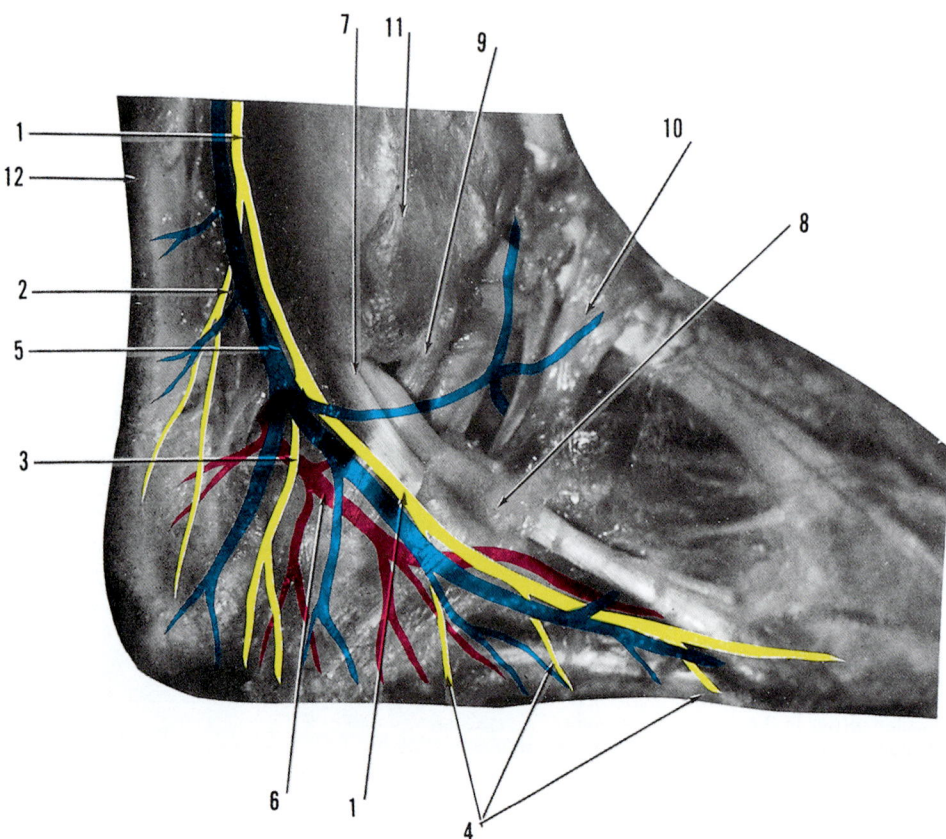

Figure 9.44 Lateral aspect of the ankle and hindfoot. (*1*, sural nerve; *2*, lateral calcaneal nerve, posterior branch; *3*, lateral calcaneal nerve, anterior branch; *4*, plantar lateral branches of sural nerve; *5*, shorter saphenous vein; *6*, lateral calcaneal artery; *7*, peronei tendons; *8*, inferior peroneal retinaculum; *9*, origin of calcaneofibular ligament; *10*, stem of inferior extensor retinaculum; *11*, lateral malleolus; *12*, Achilles tendon.)

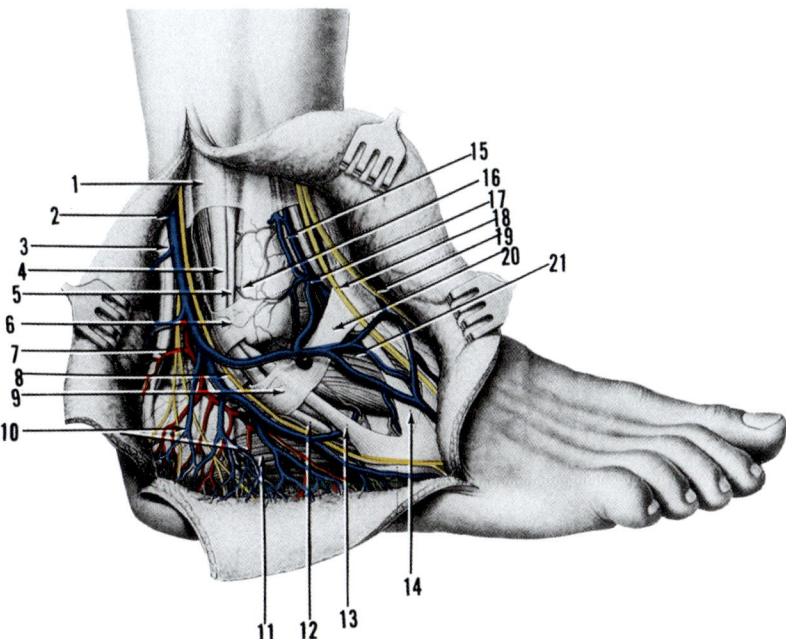

Figure 9.45 Lateral aspect of ankle and hindfoot. (*1*, superficial fascia cruris; *2*, short saphenous vein; *3*, Achilles tendon; *4*, peroneus longus tendon; *5*, peroneus brevis tendon; *6*, superior peroneal retinaculum; *7*, lateral calcaneal nerve, branch of sural nerve; *8*, sural nerve; *9*, inferior peroneal retinaculum; *10*, lateral calcaneal vascular rami; *11*, abductor digiti minimi muscle; *12*, peroneus longus tendon; *13*, peroneus brevis tendon; *14*, peroneus tertius tendon; *15*, anterior peroneal artery; *16*, communicating branch of peroneal arteries; *17*, lateral malleolar artery; *18*, superficial peroneal nerve, lateral branch; *19*, superficial peroneal nerve, medial branch; *20*, inferior extensor retinaculum; *21*, extensor digitorum brevis muscle.) (Adapted from Lang J, Wachsmuth W. *Praktische Anatomie Bein und Statik.* Springer-Verlag; 1972:345.)

Superficial Aponeurosis and Superficial Posterolateral Compartment

The superficial aponeurosis, after investing the Achilles tendon, covers the space between the latter and the fibrous proximal tunnel of the peronei tendons formed by the lateral expansion of the deep crural aponeurosis. Inferiorly, the superficial aponeurosis is reinforced and forms the superior peroneal retinaculum or lateral annular ligament, a quadrilateral lamina that originates from the tip and posterior border of the lateral malleolus. This lamina is oriented posteroinferiorly and inserts over the lateral aspect of the os calcis. The short saphenous vein and the sural nerve cross this lamina superficially and obliquely.

Farther distally, a second reinforcement of the superficial aponeurosis contributes to the formation of the inferior peroneal retinaculum. The latter originates from the posterior segment of the lateral rim of the sinus tarsi in common with the lateral root of the inferior extensor retinaculum. It is directed posteroinferiorly, crosses the trochlear process (to which it provides fibers of attachment), and terminates on the lateral tuberosity of the os calcis. The inferior peroneal retinaculum forms two tunnels at the level of the trochlear process. The upper tunnel lodges the peroneus brevis tendon, and the lower tunnel, the peroneus longus tendon.

The common synovial sheath of the peronei tendons extends proximally about two fingerbreadths from the tip of the lateral malleolus. Distally, the synovial sheath bifurcates at the level of the trochlear process. The sheath of the peroneus brevis tendon terminates about one fingerbreadth short of the insertion of the tendon. The synovial sheath of the peroneus longus reaches the plantar groove of the cuboid.

Below the free tip of the lateral malleolus, the peronei tendons cross the calcaneofibular ligament in an "X" (Fig. 9.46).

An incision of the superficial aponeurosis along the lateral border of the Achilles tendon provides safe entrance to the pre-Achilles space (filled centrally by the pre-Achilles fat pad) and leads to the deep aponeurosis.

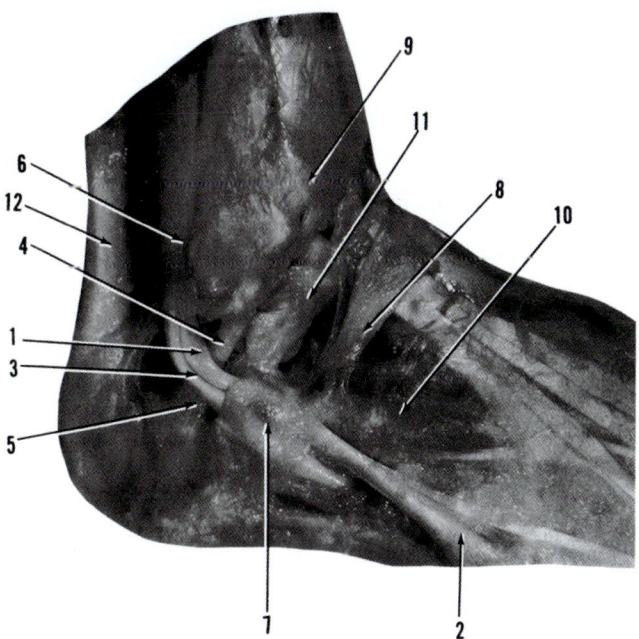

Figure 9.46 Lateral aspect of ankle. (*1*, peroneus brevis tendon; *2*, insertion of peroneus brevis tendon; *3*, peroneus longus tendon; *4*, calcaneofibular ligament passing under the peronei tendons; *5*, insertion site of calcaneofibular ligament; *6*, superior peroneal retinaculum; *7*, inferior peroneal retinaculum; *8*, inferior extensor retinaculum; *9*, anterior tibiofibular ligament; *10*, extensor digitorum brevis muscle; *11*, prelateral malleolar fat pad; *12*, Achilles tendon.)

Deep Aponeurosis, Superior Peroneal Tunnel

The deep aponeurosis cruris adheres to the retromalleolar superior peroneal tunnel (Fig. 9.47).

The distal extension of the deep aponeurosis toward the dorsum of the os calcis and the talus may acquire thick fibers and forms the fibulotalocalcaneal ligament of Rouvière and Canela Lazaro.[6] This ligament originates from the medial lip of the fibular canal for the peroneal tendons and from the lower segment of the posterior tibiofibular ligament. It is flat anteroposteriorly, enlarges as it courses inferomedially, and divides into two bands—inferolateral or fibulocalcaneal and superomedial or talofibular. The fibulocalcaneal component is the larger and inserts transversely over the dorsum of the os calcis. The talofibular component is oriented transversely and terminates over the posterolateral tubercle of the talus and the fibrous tunnel of the flexor hallucis longus tendon.

The fibulotalocalcaneal ligament is present in 60% of the cases; it covers the posterior talofibular ligament and is separated from the latter by adipose tissue.[6] This ligament is tight with dorsiflexion of the foot, and it contributes to the equinus deformity in clubfeet.

Incision of the deep aponeurosis in the posterolateral compartment above the ankle joint line gives access to a triangular interval with a proximal apex and a distal base. The lateral border of the space is formed by the peroneus brevis muscle, the medial border by the flexor hallucis. Enlargement of the triangular space provides access to the posterolateral end of the tibia and to the posterior tibiofibular joint.[7] The posterior peroneal vessels longitudinally cross the space and are to be dealt with in the surgical exposure (Fig. 9.48).

POSTEROMEDIAL ASPECT OF THE ANKLE AND THE TIBIOTALOCALCANEAL TUNNEL

The posteromedial aspect of the ankle and the tarsal tunnel or calcaneal canal constitute the major passageway from the posterior compartment of the leg to the sole of the foot.

▶ Surface Anatomy

The medial malleolus is felt with ease. The sustentaculum talus is found about 2.5 cm below the tip of the medial malleolus. At the midpoint of the line uniting the tuberosity of the scaphoid to the tip of the medial malleolus is located the head of the talus. The tendon of the tibialis posterior may be palpated prior to its scaphoid insertion. The posterior tibial pulse is found one fingerbreadth behind the medial malleolus.

▶ Skin, Subcutaneous Layer, and Superficial Veins and Nerves

The skin is mobile over the medial malleolus but semifixed over the medial aspect of the heel. The skin cleavage lines are oriented as indicated in Figure 9.49. The subcutaneous tissue has a lamellar constitution and may form a thin fascia superficialis carrying the superficial veins and nerves. Longitudinally, oriented veins course over the superficial fascia, which bridges the interval between the posterior tibia and the medial border of the Achilles tendon. The superficial veins collect the medial calcaneal veins. A transverse vein crosses the lower border of the medial malleolus, unites the greater saphenous vein to the posterior tibial vein, and contributes to the formation of the medial malleolar venous rete.

Two perforating veins are located around the scaphoid and surface at the upper border of the abductor hallucis muscle. These veins arrive from the plantar aspect of the scaphocuneiform and calcaneocuboid joints. A third perforating vein unites the greater saphenous vein with the medial plantar vein.

Sensory, longitudinally oriented nerve filaments are provided by the saphenous nerve. A medial calcaneal sensory nerve trunk, a branch of the posterior tibial nerve, perforates

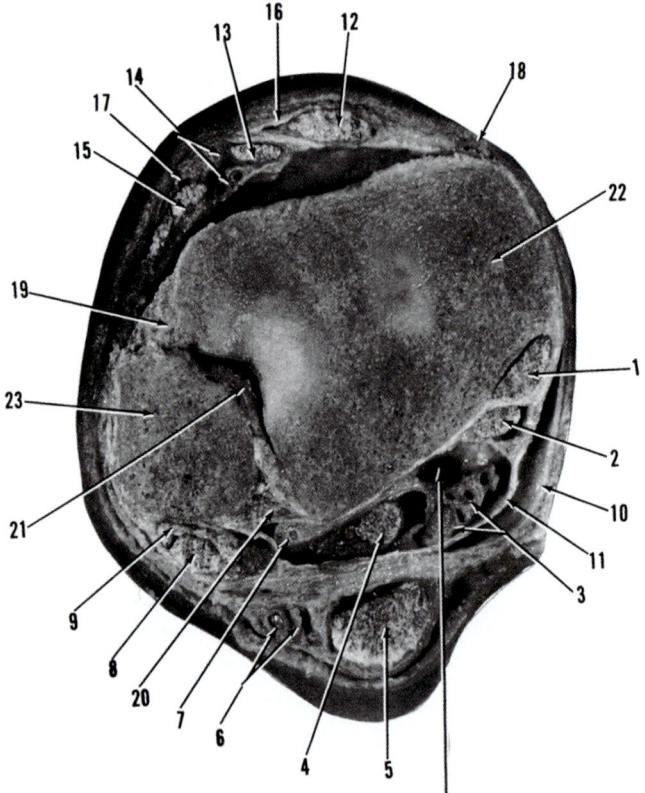

Figure 9.47 **Cross-section of the ankle 2 cm proximal to tip of medial malleolus.** (*1*, tibialis posterior tendon and tunnel; *2*, flexor digitorum longus tendon and tunnel; *3*, posterior tibial neurovascular bundle and tunnel; *4*, flexor hallucis longus tendon-muscle and tunnel; *5*, Achilles tendon and tunnel; *6*, sural nerve and short saphenous vein; *7*, posterior peroneal vessels; *8*, peroneus longus tendon and tunnel; *9*, peroneus brevis tendon, frayed; *10*, superficial aponeurosis cruris; *11*, deep aponeurosis cruris; *12*, tibialis anterior tendon and tunnel; *13*, extensor hallucis longus tendon; *14*, deep peroneal nerve and dorsalis pedis vessels; *15*, extensor digitorum longus tendons; *16*, *17*, inferior extensor retinaculum; *18*, greater saphenous vein; *19*, anterior tibiofibular ligament; *20*, posterior tibiofibular ligament; *21*, synovial fringe in tibiofibular syndesmosis; *22*, tibia; *23*, lateral malleolus.) *Vertical arrow* indicates the injection site to block the posterior tibial nerve.

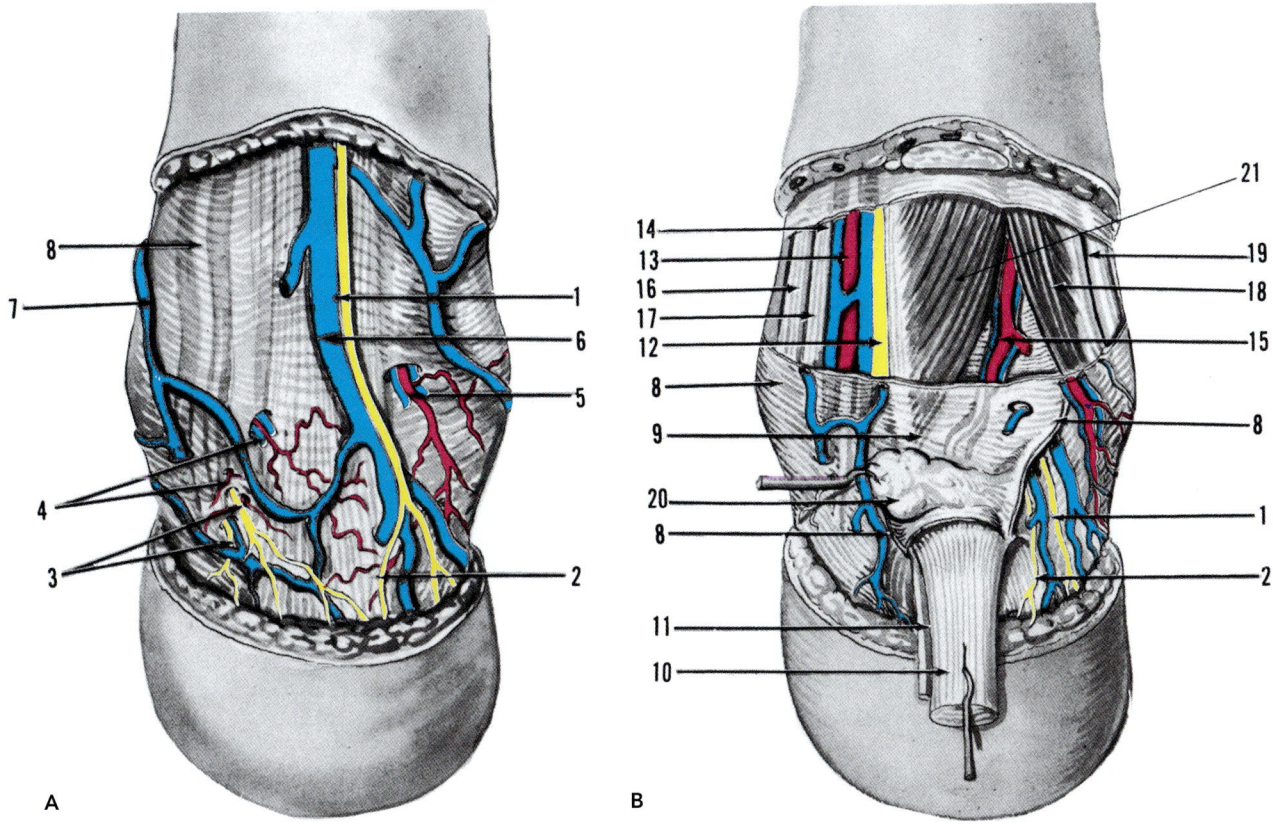

Figure 9.48 Posterior aspect of the ankle. (A) Superficial aspect. (B), Deep aspect. (1, sural nerve; 2, lateral calcaneal nerve, posterior branch; 3, medial calcaneal and posteromedial nerve branches of posterior tibial nerve; 4, posteromedial and medial calcaneal arteries, branch of posterior tibial artery; 5, lateral calcaneal artery, branch of posterior peroneal artery; 6, lesser saphenous vein; 7, posterior medial malleolar vein; 8, superficial aponeurosis cruris, which splits and invests Achilles tendon [10] and plantaris tendon [11]; 9, deep aponeurosis cruris; 12, posterior tibial nerve; 13, posterior tibial artery; 14, posterior tibial vein; 15, posterior peroneal artery and veins; 16, tibialis posterior tendon; 17, flexor digitorum longus tendon; 18, peroneus brevis muscle-tendon; 19, peroneus longus tendon; 20, pre-Achilles tendon fat pad located in "safe zone" between superficial and deep aponeuroses cruris; 21, flexor hallucis longus.) (Adapted from Testut L, Jacob O. *Traité d'Anatomie Topographique avec Applications Médico-Chirurgicales.* Vol 2. 2nd ed. Doin; 1909:1036, 1045.)

the superficial aponeurosis just proximal to the superior border of the abductor hallucis muscle. It courses superficially and divides into two branches, posterior and anterior.

The posterior branch subdivides into two terminal branches supplying the posterior and medial aspects of the heel. The anterior branch subdivides also into two branches coursing obliquely across the heel and the proximal sole. These branches reach the lateral border of the foot. They provide the sensory branches to the plantar aspect of the heel and proximal sole (Fig. 9.50).

Superficial and Deep Aponeurosis and Tibiotalocalcaneal Tunnel

At the level of the distal leg posteriorly, the superficial aponeurosis splits and incorporates the triceps surae. The deep aponeurosis covers the tibialis posterior, the flexor digitorum longus, the flexor hallucis longus muscles, and the posterior tibial neurovascular bundle. It forms the deep compartment of the leg separated from the triceps surae and its investing superficial aponeurosis. Distally, a new fascial layer covers the tibialis posterior and the flexor digitorum longus muscles. Beyond the point where the two muscles cross, the corresponding tendons pass through individual fibrous tunnels covered by the deep aponeurosis. The flexor hallucis longus muscle and the posterior tibial neurovascular bundle are in a common compartment under the deep aponeurosis. At the level of the talotibial joint line or just proximal to it, a fascial plane appears, forming a tunnel to the flexor hallucis longus muscle–tendon unit and separating the latter from the posterior tibial neurovascular bundle. This fascial plane covers the free interval between the flexor hallucis longus tunnel and the tunnel of the flexor digitorum longus. All four tunnels, three tendinous and one neurovascular, are covered by the deep aponeuroses and are retained in the deep compartment. The superficial compartment is now reduced to the Achilles tendon and the plantaris tendon. The space between these two compartments has enlarged and is filled with the pre-Achilles adipose tissue; it is considered a

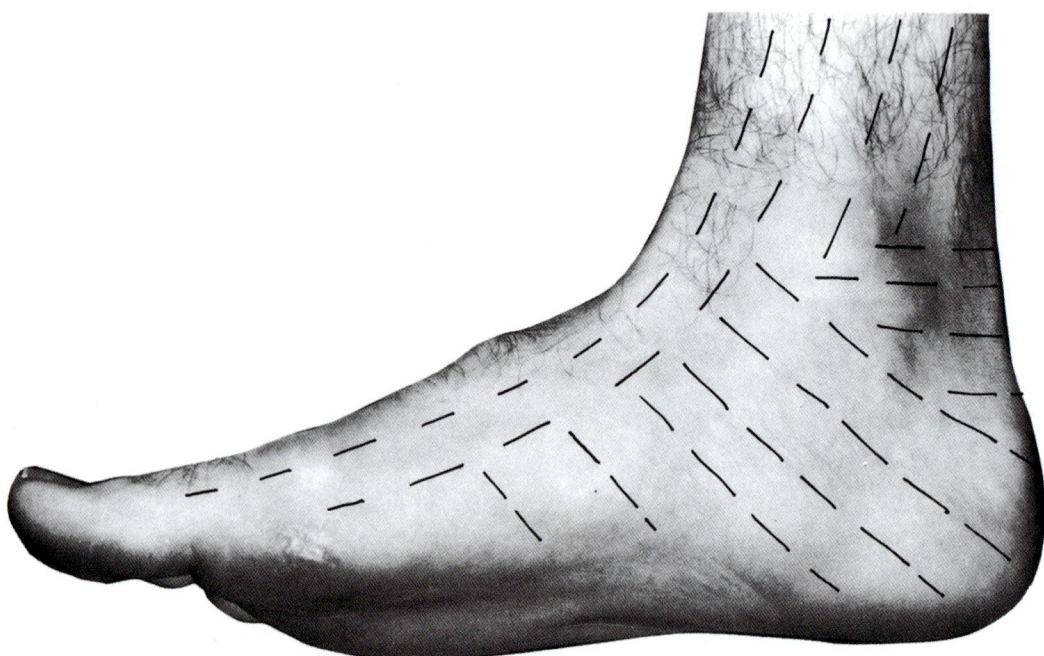

Figure 9.49 **The cleavage lines of the skin on the medial aspect of the ankle and foot.**[20] The cleavage lines are longitudinally oriented on the dorsomedial aspect. The lines are transverse and parallel on the posterior aspect of the ankle and are oblique in the remaining segment of the foot.

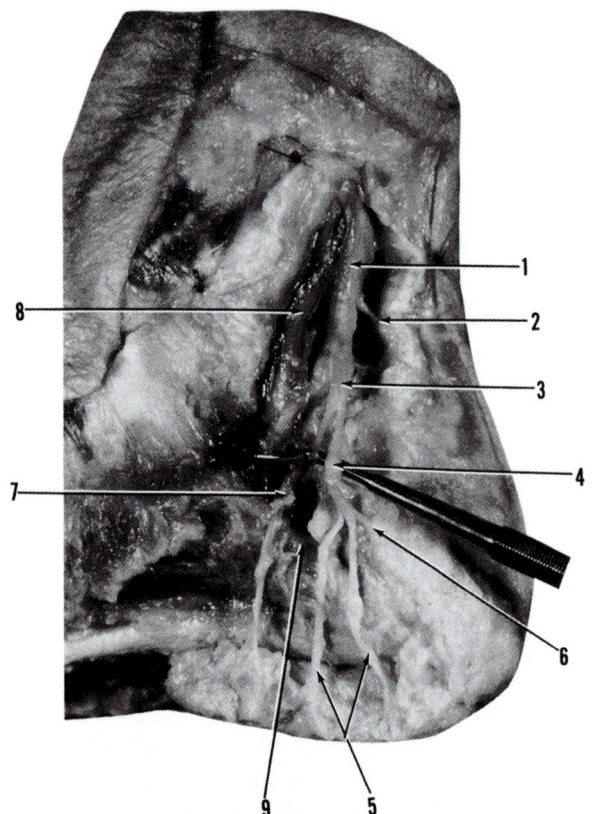

Figure 9.50 **Posteromedial aspect of ankle and hindfoot.** (*1*, posterior tibial nerve; *2*, nerve branch to Achilles tendon; *3*, medial calcaneal nerve [MCN]; *4*, posterior division branch of MCN; *5*, cutaneous subdivision branches of (*4*); *6*, posterior calcaneal division branch; *7*, anterior division branch of MCN; *8*, posterior tibial artery; *9*, abductor hallucis muscle.)

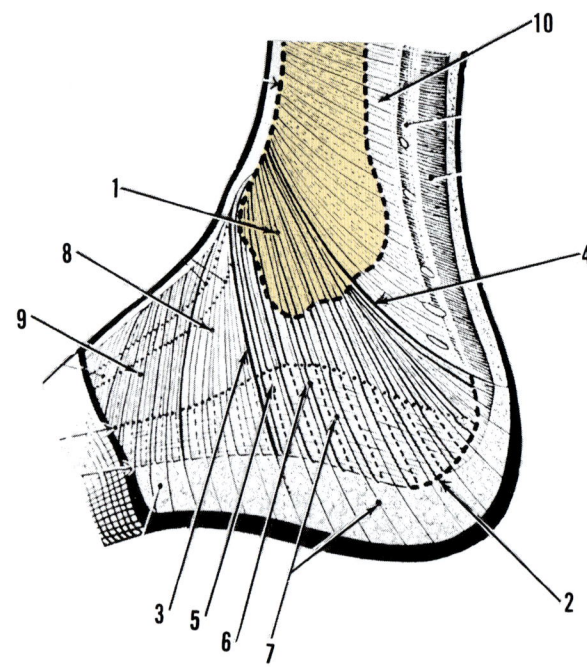

Figure 9.51 **Flexor retinaculum.** (*1*, apex of flexor retinaculum; *2*, posteromedial border of calcaneum; *3*, anterior border of flexor retinaculum; *4*, posterosuperior border of flexor retinaculum; *5*, deep layer of flexor retinaculum investing abductor hallucis muscle; *6*, superficial layer of flexor retinaculum investing abductor hallucis muscle; *7*, superficial fibers of flexor retinaculum continued by retinaculum cutis; *8*, superficial dorsal aponeurosis of foot; *9*, inferomedial band of inferior extensor retinaculum; *10*, adherent superficial and deep aponeuroses of leg.) (Adapted from Bellocq P, Meyer P. Le ligament annulaire interne du cou-de-pied. *Arch Anat Histol Embryol.* 1954;37:23.)

posteromedial "safe" zone. The superficial and the deep fasciae are adherent at the level of the fibrous sheath of the tibialis posterior and the flexor digitorum longus tendon in the retromedial malleolar position, and farther down, they form the flexor retinaculum. The segment of the deep investing fascia that formed the tunnel of the flexor hallucis longus and separated the latter from the neurovascular bundle continues distally as the investing fascia of the quadratus plantae muscle.

Flexor Retinaculum

The flexor retinaculum or laciniate ligament formed by the fusion of the superficial and deep aponeuroses of the leg is triangular in shape with malleolar apex, inferior base, and anterior and posterior borders (Fig. 9.51).[8] The delineation of the last two borders is difficult because they are in continuity: the posterior with the superficial aponeurosis of the leg and the anterior with the dorsal aponeurosis of the foot. A vertical line extended from the anterior border of the medial malleolus to the medial border of the foot marks approximately the anterior border of the flexor retinaculum. The posterior border follows more or less an oblique line drawn from the anterior border of the medial malleolus to the posterosuperior corner of the os calcis. The descending fibers of the retinaculum reach the superior border of the abductor hallucis muscle, split, and incorporate the muscle; they are in continuity with the plantar fascia. The superficial apical fibers of the flexor retinaculum insert on the subcutaneous anterior and medial surfaces of the medial malleolus. The deep apical fibers contribute to the formation of the tibialis anterior tunnel, insert on the deep surface of the superior extensor retinaculum, and exchange fibers with the superomedial band of the inferior extensor retinaculum.

Tibiotalocalcaneal Tunnel

The tibiotalocalcaneal tunnel extends from the posteromedial aspect of the ankle to the plantar aspect of the navicular to the crossing point of the flexor digitorum longus and flexor hallucis longus tendons (Figs. 9.52 and 9.53).[9,10] This passageway is concave anteriorly and may be divided into two compartments: upper or tibiotalar and lower or talocalcaneal.

Tibiotalar Compartment

The osseous canal of the tibiotalar compartment is formed by the posterior aspect of the distal tibia, the retromedial malleolar surface, the posterior border of the talus with its central sulcus flanked by the posterior talar tubercles, and the posterior

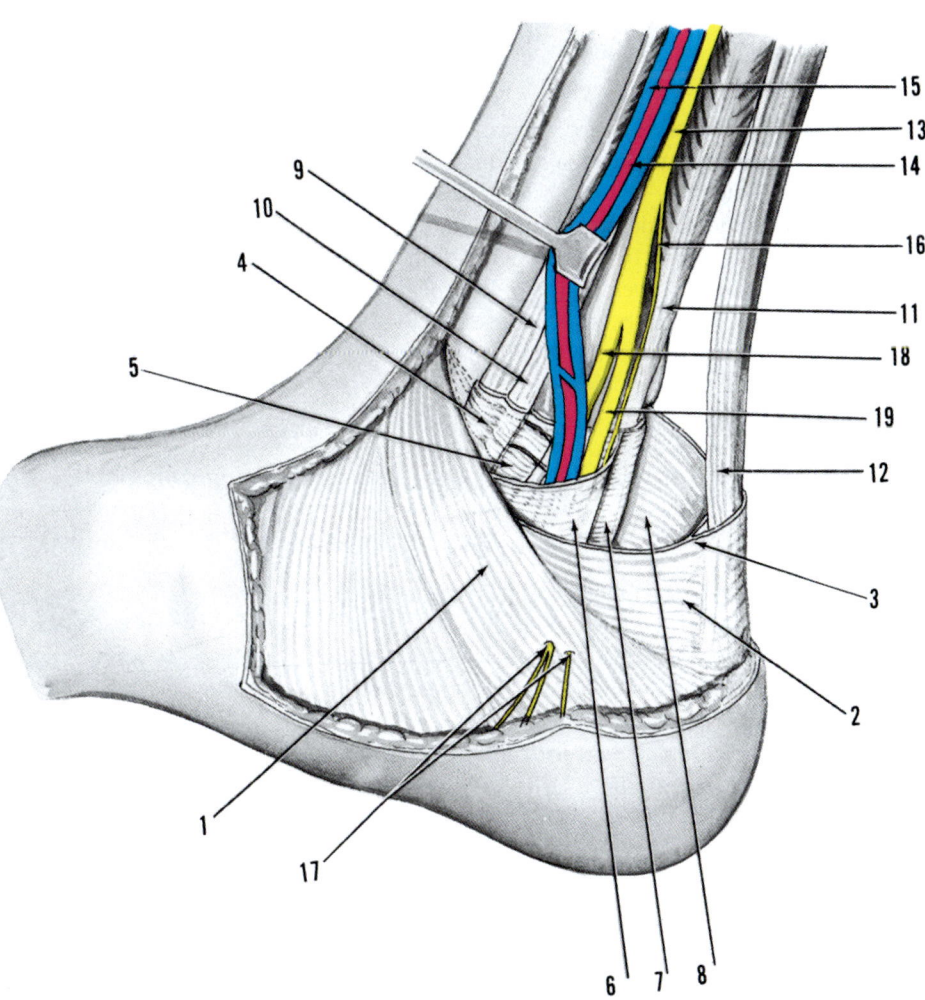

Figure 9.52 Proximal aspect of the tibiotalocalcaneal canal. The posterior tibial arteriovenous bundle is retracted anteriorly to expose the posterior tibial nerve and its division branches. (*1*, flexor retinaculum; *2*, superficial aponeurosis splitting [*3*] to incorporate Achilles tendon [*12*]; *4*, deep aponeurosis covering fibrous tunnels to tibialis posterior tendon [*9*] and flexor digitorum longus tendon [*10*]; *5*, intermediary intertendinous aponeurosis forming floor of neurovascular compartment; *6*, deep aponeurosis forming roof of neurovascular compartment and continuing over tunnel of flexor hallucis longus tendon [*7*]; *8*, "safe zone," in front of Achilles tendon and behind neurovascular tunnel; *11*, flexor hallucis longus tendon; *13*, posterior tibial nerve; *14*, posterior tibial artery; *15*, posterior tibial vein; *16*, posteromedial calcaneal nerve piercing aponeurosis at *17*; *18*, medial plantar nerve; *19*, lateral plantar nerve.)

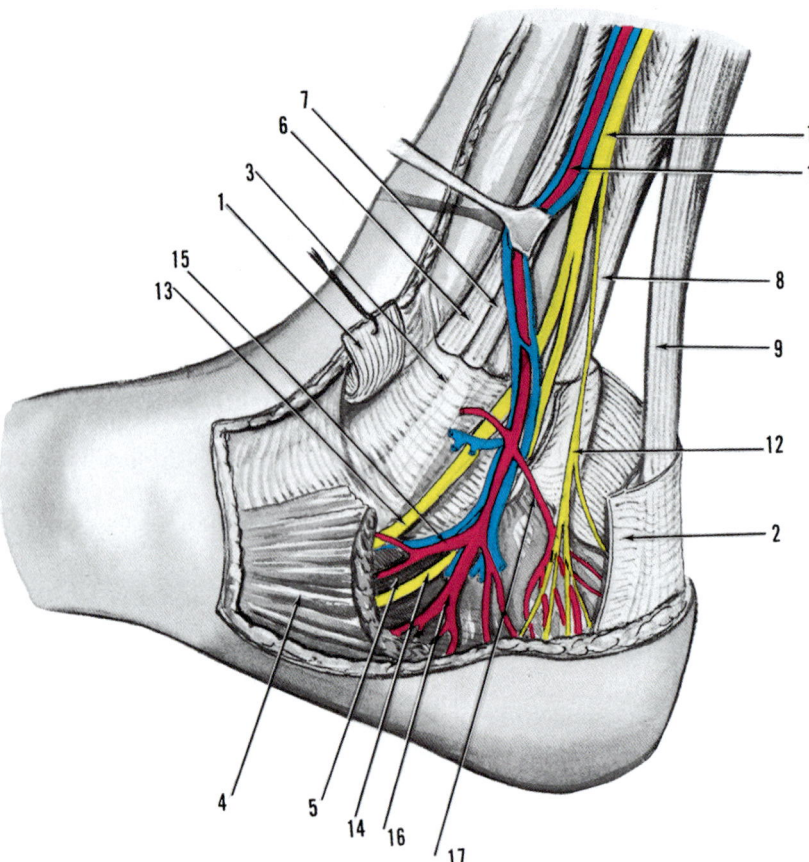

Figure 9.53 Deep aspect of the tibiotalocalcaneal canal. (1, reflected apex of flexor retinaculum; 2, superficial aponeurosis investing Achilles tendon [9]; 3, deep aponeurosis contributing to formation of fibrous tunnel of tibialis posterior tendon [6] and flexor digitorum longus tendon [7]; 4, abductor hallucis muscle; 5, interfascicular septum dividing calcaneal canal into upper and lower chambers; 8, flexor hallucis longus tendon; 10, posterior tibial nerve; 11, posterior tibial artery and veins; 12, posteromedial calcaneal nerve; 13, medial plantar nerve passing through upper chamber of calcaneal canal; 14, lateral plantar nerve passing through lower chamber of calcaneal canal; 15, medial plantar artery; 16, lateral plantar artery; 17, medial calcaneal artery.) (Adapted from Dujarier C. *Anatomie des Membres Dissection—Anatomie Topographique*. 2nd ed. Masson; 1924.)

segment of the medial talar surface. The canal is converted into a large compartment by the deep aponeurosis of the leg. The latter is attached medially to the posteromedial border of the tibia and the posterior border of the medial malleolus and laterally to the fibrous sheath of the peronei tendons. Anteriorly, the deep aponeurosis is covered by or adherent to the superficial aponeurosis. Posteriorly, the two aponeuroses part; the superficial aponeurosis courses toward the medial border of the Achilles tendon and the deep aponeurosis is directed laterally toward the fibrous tunnel of the peronei tendons. Distally, the deep aponeurosis is attached to the superomedial surface of the os calcis (Fig. 9.54). In the proximal tibial segment of the tunnel are located, from a medial to a lateral direction, the following structures:

- The fibrous tunnel of the tibialis posterior tendon
- The fibrous tunnel of the flexor digitorum longus adherent to the former
- The superficial compartment for the posterior tibial neurovascular bundle
- The large, loose compartment for the flexor hallucis longus muscle-tendon unit and the peroneal vessels laterally (Fig. 9.55)

In the distal malleolar-talar segment of the tunnel, the same relationship is present with some modifications. The flexor hallucis longus is all tendinous and passes through a strong fibrous tunnel on the posterior border of the talus. The peronei vessels have parted. The posterior tibial neurovascular compartment

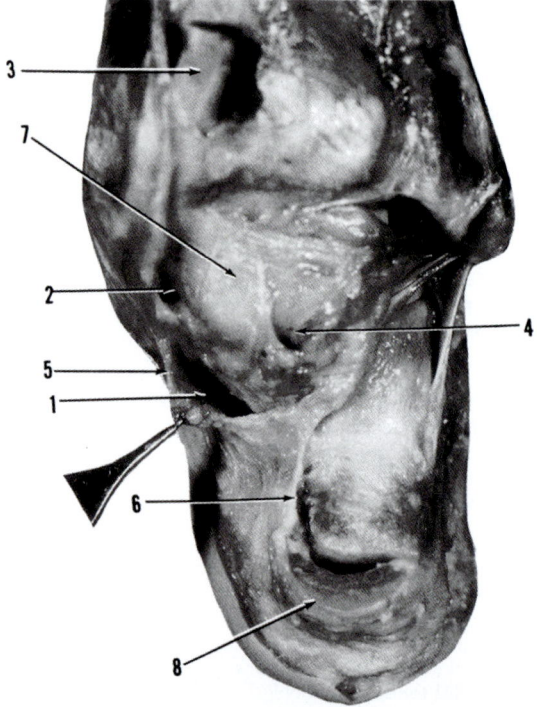

Figure 9.54 Posterior aspect ankle-hindfoot. (1, tunnel of posterior tibial neurovascular bundle; 2, tunnel of flexor digitorum longus tendon; 3, tibialis posterior tendon; 4, tunnel of flexor hallucis longus tendon; 5, adherent superficial and deep aponeurosis cruris; 6, superficial aponeurosis cruris; 7, intermedial aponeurosis cruris of Baumann; 8, Achilles tendon.)

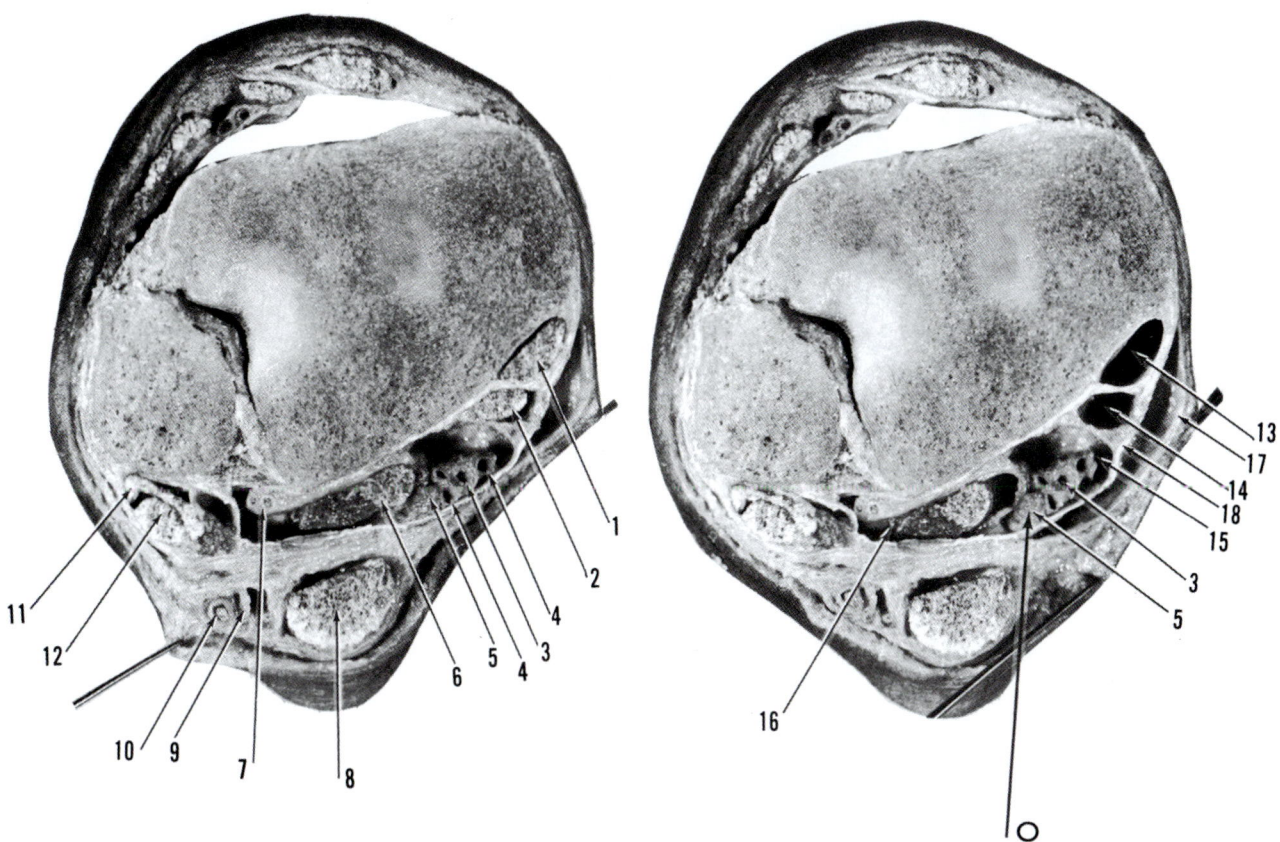

Figure 9.55 **Cross-section of the left ankle 2 cm proximal to the tip of the medial malleolus.** A needle inserted tangentially along the medial border of the Achilles tendon reaches the posterior tibial nerve, avoiding the vascular bundle (direction indicated by the *arrow* O). This is a safe guide for anesthetic block of the posterior tibial nerve. (*1*, tibialis posterior tendon; *2*, flexor digitorum longus tendon; *3*, posterior tibial artery; *4*, posterior tibial veins; *5*, posterior tibial nerve; *6*, flexor hallucis longus tendon and muscle; *7*, posterior peroneal vessels; *8*, Achilles tendon; *9*, sural nerve; *10*, saphenous vein; *11*, peroneus brevis tendon; *12*, peroneus longus tendon; *13*, tunnel of tibialis posterior tendon; *14*, tunnel of flexor digitorum longus tendon; *15*, tunnel of posterior tibial neurovascular bundle; *16*, tunnel of flexor hallucis longus tendon and muscle; *17*, superficial aponeurosis; *18*, deep aponeurosis.)

is superficial and overlies the tunnel of the flexor hallucis longus and the intertendinous interval between the latter and the flexor digitorum longus tunnel.

Within the tibiotalar compartment, the tunnel of the tibialis posterior tendon attaches to the posterior tibia, the medial and lateral crests of the retromalleolar canal, and the posterior talotibial fibers of the deltoid ligament. The tunnel of the flexor digitorum longus is usually lateral and occasionally posterolateral to the tunnel of the tibialis posterior tendon and attaches to the posterior tibia, the posterior capsule of the talotibial joint and the posterior bimalleolar ligament, and the posteromedial talar tubercle with the reaching posterior talotibial fibers of the deltoid ligament.

The neurovascular tunnel is more superficial, covering the tunnel of the flexor hallucis longus and the interval between the latter and the flexor digitorum longus tunnel. Within this compartment are located, medially to laterally, the posterior tibial veins (three), artery, and nerve (see Figs. 9.55 and 9.56). Proximal to the tip of the medial malleolus (1.3-1.5 cm), the posterior tibial nerve divides into its terminal medial and lateral plantar branches.[3] The posterior tibial artery is still undivided.

The tunnel of the flexor hallucis longus tendon is the most lateral in the deep compartment and attaches medially to the posterior tibia, the posterior tibiotalar capsule, and laterally to the fibrous sheath of the peronei tendons, the posterior talofibular ligament, and the talar component of the fibulotalocalcaneal ligament of Rouvière and Canela Lazaro. Further distally, the lateral insertion of the flexor hallucis longus tunnel continues along the posterior talar sulcus and lateral and medial posterior talar tubercles, and the posteromedial corner of the posterior talocalcaneal joint capsule.[6]

Talocalcaneal Tunnel

The osseous canal of the talocalcaneal or tarsal tunnel is formed from above downward by the medial surface of the talus and the inferomedial segment of the navicular, the sustentaculum tali, and the curved, excavated medial surface of the os calcis. The surface is buttressed above by the superficial deltoid ligament and below by the quadratus plantae muscle. The talocalcaneal canal is converted to a tunnel by the covering flexor retinaculum above and the abductor hallucis muscle with its

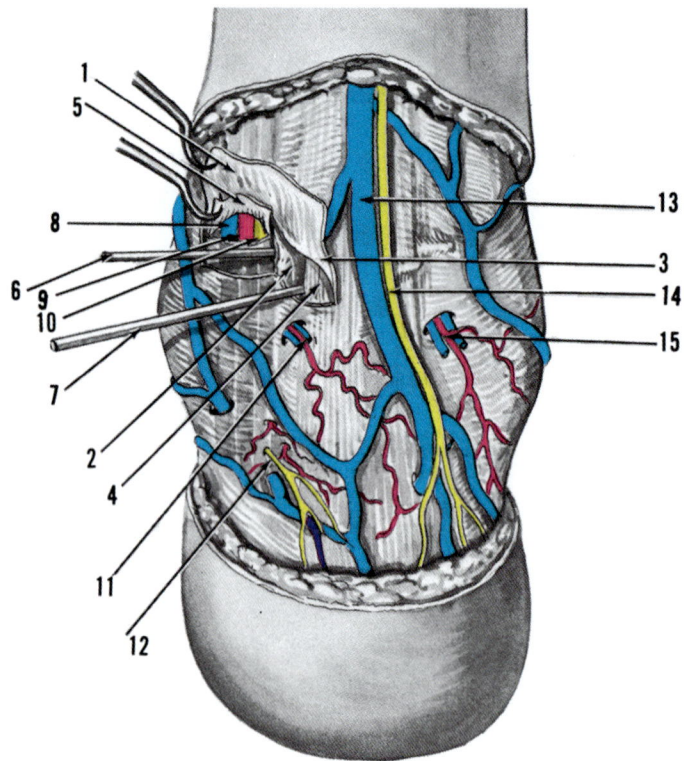

Figure 9.56 **Posterior aspect of the ankle.** (*1*, superficial aponeurosis, reflected upward; *2*, anterior split layer of one investing Achilles tendon [*4*]; *3*, posterior split layer of one investing Achilles tendon; *5*, deep aponeurosis reflected upward exposing posterior tibial neurovascular bundle in VAN sequence [*8*, posterior tibial vein; *9*, posterior tibial artery; *10*, posterior tibial nerve]; *6*, probe passing between deep and superficial aponeuroses; *7*, probe passing on anterior aspect of Achilles tendon but deep to anterior split layer of superficial aponeurosis; *11*, posterior calcaneal artery; *12*, posteromedial cutaneous nerve; *13*, lesser saphenous vein; *14*, sural nerve; *15*, lateral calcaneal artery, branch of posterior peroneal artery.) (Adapted from Testut L, Jacob O. *Traité d'Anatomie Topographique avec Applications Médico-Chirurgicales*. Vol 2. 2nd ed. Doin; 1909:1036.)

investing fascia below. Anterior to the flexor retinaculum, the aponeurotic coverage is provided by the superficial dorsal aponeurosis of the foot and the inferomedial band of the inferior extensor retinaculum. Within the talocalcaneal compartment, the tunnel of the tibialis posterior tendon attaches to the posterior talotibial segment of the deltoid ligament, the calcaneotibial component of the deltoid ligament, the superomedial calcaneonavicular ligament crossing the anterior talocalcaneal joint, and the inferior calcaneonavicular ligament.

Subsequently, the tibialis posterior tendon divides into three parts: navicular, plantar, and recurrent. The recurrent part inserts on the sustentaculum tali and contributes to the roof of the distal segment of the tunnel.

The tunnel of the flexor digitorum longus attaches to the posteromedial talar tubercle, the posterior talotibial fibers of the deltoid ligament, and the medial border of the sustentaculum tali and the tibiocalcaneal component of the deltoid ligament. It shares distally a common tunnel with the flexor hallucis longus tendon.

The tunnel of the flexor digitorum longus crosses the medial opening of the tarsal canal. It is a useful guideline for the surgical location of the mid segment of the medial talocalcaneal joint interline. Occasionally, the tunnel may shift downward and partially cover the tunnel of the flexor hallucis longus, which is attached to the lateral and medial borders of the osseous canal formed on the inferior surface of the sustentaculum tali. The bony canal disappears at the anterior border of the os calcis, and the tunnels of the flexor hallucis longus and the flexor digitorum longus lose their intermediary septum and share a common tunnel.[10] This segment of the tunnel corresponds to the master knot of Henry.[7] It is located on the inner aspect of the anterior segment of the os calcis, "a thumb's width lateral to the navicular tubercle."[7] The roof of the tunnel corresponds to the inferior calcaneonavicular ligament reinforced by a thick fibrous plate and by the recurrent segment of the tibialis posterior tendon. Medially, the tunnel is attached to the deep aponeurosis of the abductor hallucis muscle, and laterally, it is attached to the os calcis. The floor of the common tunnel is thin and corresponds to the compartment of the medial plantar neurovascular bundle.

The neurovascular tunnel is initially superficial and corresponds to the interval between the tunnel of the flexor digitorum longus and the tunnel of the flexor hallucis longus (Fig. 9.57). Gradually, as the latter approaches the former, the intertendinous space disappears and the neurovascular tunnel is located on the medial aspect of the os calcis, posterior to the flexor hallucis longus tunnel.

In the lower segment of the calcaneal tunnel, the neurovascular compartment is divided into an upper and a lower chamber by the transversely oriented interfascicular septum (see Figs. 9.57 and 9.58). The lower neurovascular chamber is limited laterally by the quadratus plantae muscle covering the medial calcaneal surface, medially by the abductor hallucis muscle covered by the deep aponeurosis, above by the interfascicular septum, and below by the interspace between the inferior borders of the abductor hallucis and of the quadratus plantae. The upper neurovascular chamber is limited laterally by the tunnel of the flexor hallucis longus, medially by the flexor retinaculum, above by the tunnel of the flexor digitorum longus, and below by the interfascicular septum.

The posterior tibial artery divides into the medial and lateral plantar arteries proximal to the free concave border of the interfascicular septum. The medial plantar nerve and vessels penetrate the upper chamber of the calcaneal canal, whereas the lateral

Chapter 9: Cross-Sectional and Topographic Anatomy 475

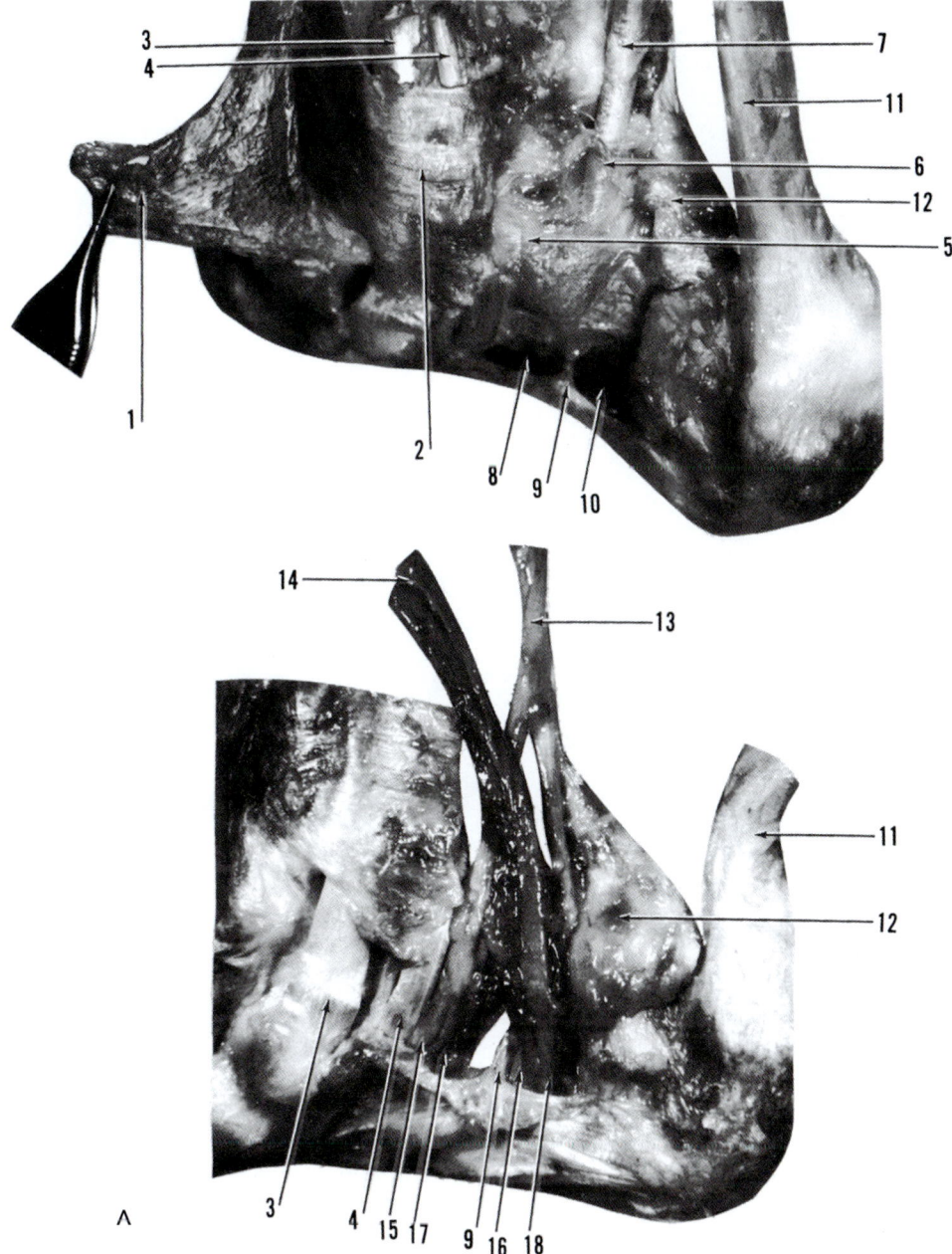

Figure 9.57 (A) Talocalcaneal canal. The medial plantar nerve and artery pass in the upper calcaneal chamber; the lateral plantar nerve and artery pass in the lower calcaneal chamber. (1, reflected flexor retinaculum, superficial aponeurosis; 2, deep aponeurosis covering tunnel of tibialis posterior [3] and flexor digitorum longus tendons [4]; 5, intermediary aponeurosis interposed between tunnels of the flexor digitorum longus [4] and flexor hallucis longus [6] tendons; 7, flexor hallucis longus muscle-tendon; 8, upper chamber of calcaneal canal; 9, interfascicular septum; 10, lower chamber of calcaneal canal; 11, Achilles tendon; 12, pre-Achilles fat pad; 13, posterior tibial nerve with proximal division; 14, posterior tibial artery and veins reflected anteriorly; 15, medial plantar nerve; 16, lateral plantar nerve; 17, medial plantar artery; 18, lateral plantar artery.) (B) Sagittal cross-section of the ankle and foot. (I) Cross-section passing through the posterior talocalcaneal joint. (1, tibialis posterior tendon; 2, flexor digitorum longus tendon; 3, flexor hallucis longus tendon; 4, deep investing layer of flexor retinaculum; 5, superficial investing layer of flexor retinaculum; 6, abductor hallucis muscle being invested by 4 and 5; 7, interfascicular septum; 8, upper calcaneal chamber; 9, lower calcaneal chamber; 10, quadratus plantae muscle; 11, peroneus brevis tendon; 12, peroneus longus tendon; 13, peroneal trochlea.) (II) Cross-section passing at the level of the sustentaculum tali (ST). (1, tibialis posterior tendon applied against tibiocalcaneal component of deltoid ligament; 2, flexor digitorum longus tendon applied against medial border of sustentaculum tali; 3, flexor hallucis longus tendon applied against inferior surface of sustentaculum tali; 4, flexor retinaculum with its deep [5] and superficial [6] layers investing abductor hallucis muscle [7]; 8, flexor digitorum brevis muscle; 9, interfascicular septum; 10, upper calcaneal chamber; 11, lower calcaneal chamber; 12, quadratus plantae muscle.)

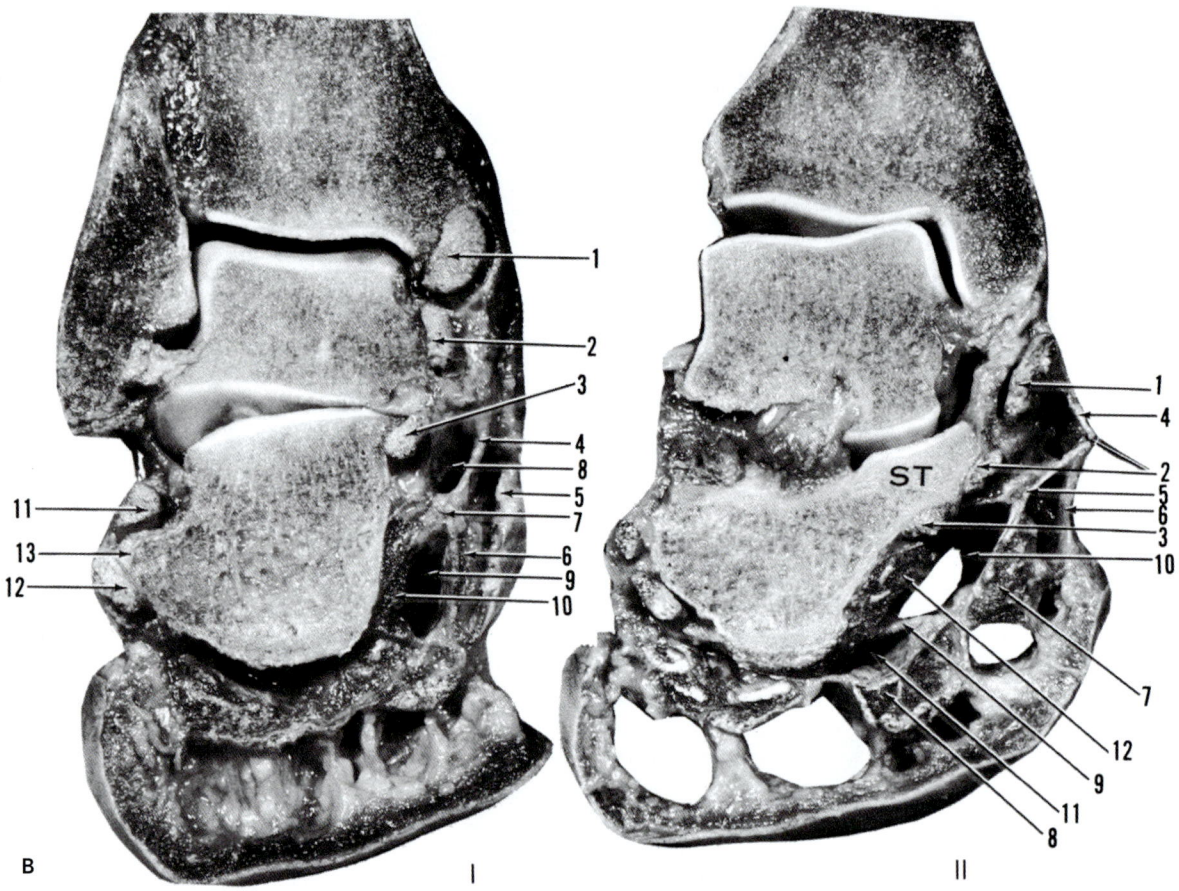

Figure 9.57 Cont'd

plantar nerve and vessels penetrate the lower chamber and reach the middle plantar compartment of the planta pedis. In both chambers, the nerve is anterior to the corresponding artery.

The posterior tibial nerve bifurcates into the medial and lateral plantar nerves at 1.3 to 1.5 cm proximal to the tip of the medial malleolus.[3] Higher bifurcation occurs in 13.5%.[3] Hovelacque has observed one bifurcation at 6 cm and another at 10 cm proximal to the tip of the medial malleolus.[11] The bifurcation of the posterior tibial artery into the medial and the lateral plantar artery occurs 1.3 to 2.5 cm distal to the bifurcation of the posterior tibial nerve; this occurs in the majority of cases (86.5%).[3,12] Occasionally, the bifurcation of both is at the same level (11.5%) or, rarely, that of the artery is proximal to that of the nerve (2%).[12] The posterior tibial nerve has the most common site of location at 7.5 cm proximal to the tip of the medial malleolus, in line with the medial border of the Achilles tendon but located in the neurovascular compartment.[3] The medial calcaneal nerve branches from the posterotibial nerve proximal to the bifurcation or may originate from the medial plantar nerve. It pierces the aponeurosis at a variable level, and as described previously, it divides into two main calcaneal branches. The long motor branch of the abductor digiti minimi takes off from the lateral plantar nerve in the canal.

The posterior tibial artery provides proximally two transverse anastomotic branches—lateral and medial. The lateral branch passes under the flexor hallucis longus tendon and unites with a similar branch of the posterior peroneal artery. The medial branch courses over the tunnels of the flexor digitorum longus and tibialis posterior tendons and anastomoses with the anterior medial malleolar artery. This branch supplies the skin overlying the medial malleolus. At about 1 cm proximal to the bifurcation of the posterior tibial artery originates the artery of the tarsal canal.[13] It passes between the tunnels of the flexor digitorum longus and flexor hallucis longus tendons and enters the tarsal canal. The artery of the tarsal canal occasionally originates from the medial plantar artery (16.6%) or may be double (3.3%) or absent (3.3%).[13]

A deltoid arterial branch takes off from the artery of the tarsal canal at 5 mm from its origin. It passes between the tibiocalcaneal and the talotibial components of the deltoid ligament. Occasionally, the deltoid branch originates from the posterior tibial artery (30%), or it may be double (6.6%).[13]

SURGICAL ANATOMY OF THE TIBIOTALOCALCANEAL NEUROVASCULAR TUNNEL AND MEDIAL CALCANEAL NERVES

The surgical anatomic knowledge of the tibiotalocalcaneal neurovascular tunnel and of the location of the medial calcaneal nerves is of importance to the surgeon dealing with the clinical problems of tarsal tunnel syndrome, compression of the nerve

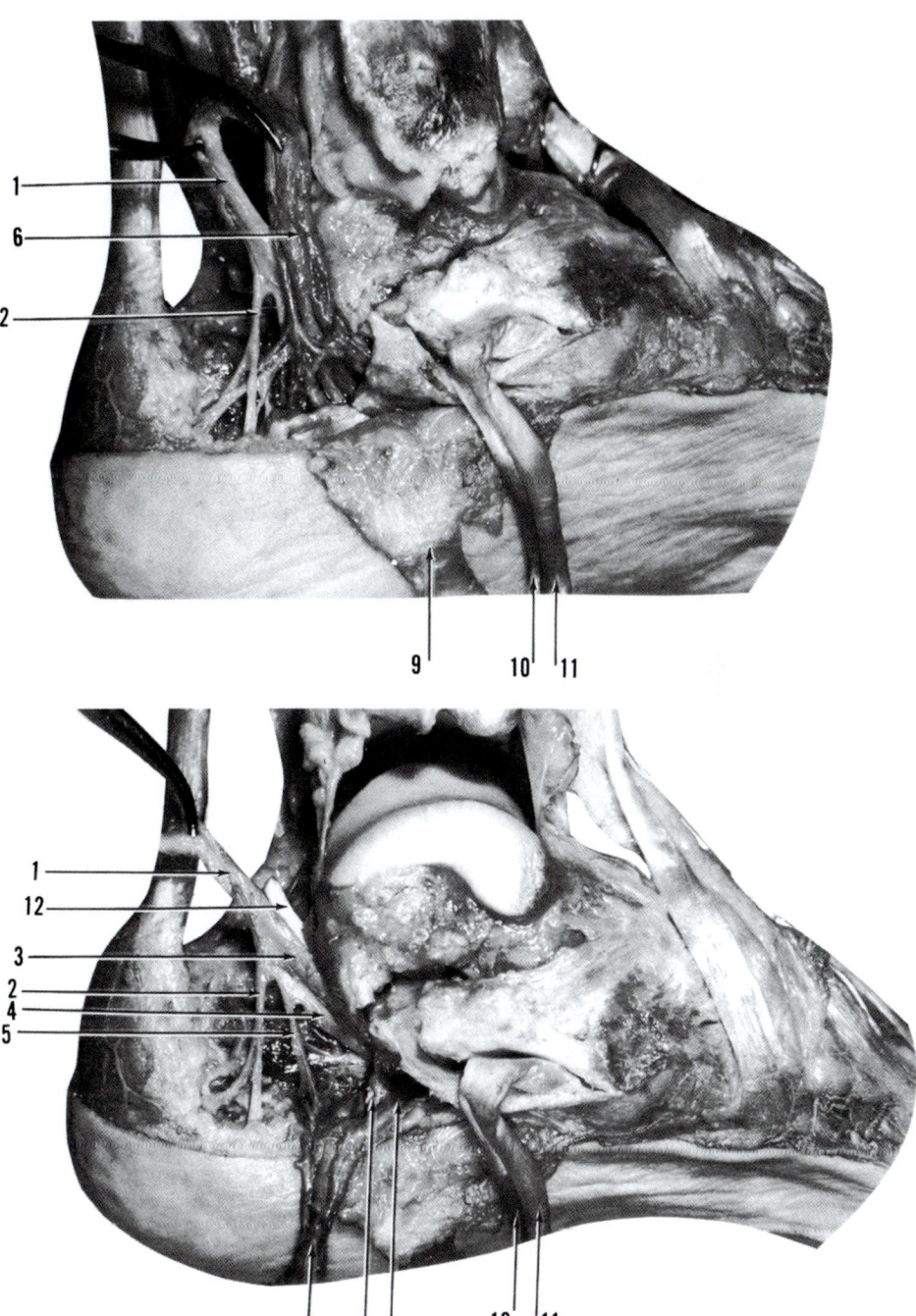

Figure 9.58 **Neurovascular bundle in the tibiotalocalcaneal canal.** (*1*, posterior tibial nerve; *2*, posteromedial calcaneal nerve; *3*, medial plantar nerve; *4*, lateral plantar nerve; *5*, motor branch abductor digiti quinti; *6*, posterior tibial artery veins covering posterior tibial nerve in top figure and reflected downward in bottom figure; *7*, upper calcaneal chamber; *8*, interfascicular septum; *9*, reflected flexor retinaculum; *10*, reflected flexor digitorum longus tendon; *11*, reflected tibialis posterior tendon; *12*, flexor hallucis longus tendon.)

to the abductor digiti quinti, exposure of the medial surface of the fractured calcaneus, and compression of the lateral plantar neurovascular bundle in the lower calcaneal tunnel.

For this purpose, a foot specimen was dissected in a sequential "revealing" manner to highlight some of the practical anatomic points.

After the removal of the skin (Fig. 9.59), the medial aspect of the region appears "homogenous," with complete continuity of the aponeurosis cruris, the flexor retinaculum, and the aponeurosis pedis. There are no anatomic landmarks to "differentiate" the flexor retinaculum. The heel adipose pad-cup has extended its coverage from the heel-sole to over the proximal segment of the abductor hallucis. The medial calcaneal nerves are not visible yet to the surgeon and are hidden in the substance of the thick adipose tissue.

A curved incision is made just posterior to the convex digitally felt posterior border of the tibialis posterior and flexor digitorum longus tendons and stops short of reaching the proximal border of the abductor hallucis. This incision passes through the adherent superficial and deep aponeurosis cruris and reveals the posterior tibial neurovascular bundle superficially located.

The posterior tibial veins are most superficial and medial. The posterior tibial artery is more lateral. The posterior tibial nerve is further lateral and "deep." The nerve is brought into the field and the common trunk of the medial calcaneal nerve

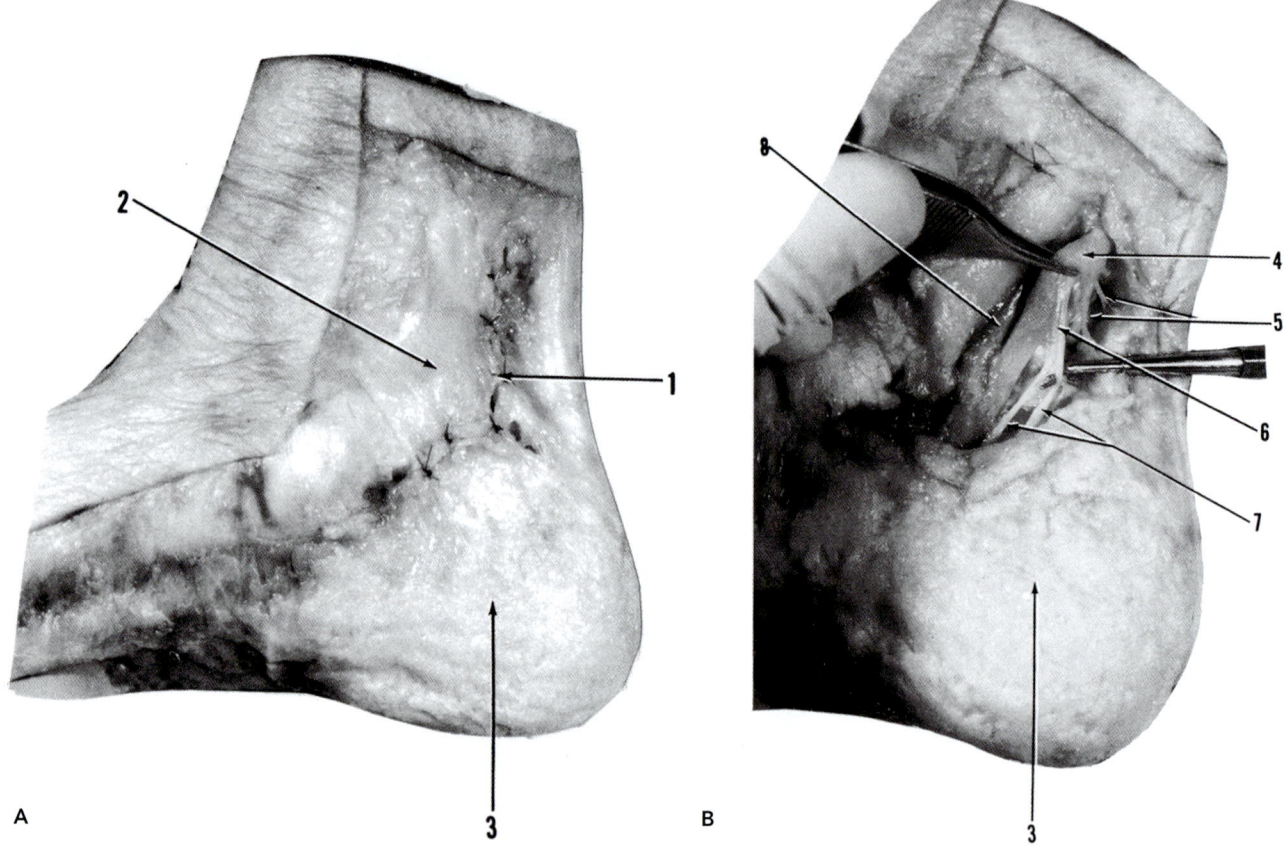

Figure 9.59 **Tibiotalocalcaneal tunnel. (A)** Skin removed. (*1*, an incision made along the posterior tibial neurovascular tunnel and closed with sutures; *2*, tunnel and tendons of tibialis posterior and flexor digitorum longus; *3*, adipose heel cup.) **(B)** The branches of the medial calcaneal nerve are not seen. They are embedded in the adipose heel cup. (*4*, posterior tibial nerve; *5*, nerve branches to the Achilles tendon; *6*, medial calcaneal nerve [MCN]; *7*, division branches of MCN; *8*, posterior tibial artery.)

is identified subdividing into two branches. A few short sensory branches are seen coursing toward the posterior aspect of the deep aponeurosis. Retraction of the posterior tibial nerve posteriorly reveals the flexor hallucis longus tendon covered by the intermediary fascia (of Baumann) (Fig. 9.60). This tendon is thus the most lateral structure within the tibiotalar tunnel.

Retraction of the posterior vascular bundle posteriorly reveals the multiple transversely running tethering vessels that limit the posterior mobilization. Short of sacrificing these important branches, the mobilization of the posterior tibial vessels is easier when carried anteriorly. By passing the probe under the common trunk of the medial calcaneal nerve (Fig. 9.61) and applying proximal rhythmic traction, the direction of and the "projected" location of the division branches within the thick heel adipose cup could be determined. This leads to the dissection of the branches, each into an initial subdivision of two and then off into multiple filaments. At this point, the proximal border of the abductor hallucis is identified. The vulnerability of the medial calcaneal nerve branches is thus evident during a transverse approach to the calcaneus or during the oblique exposure of the nerve to the abductor digiti quinti. Further dissection of the medial calcaneal branches reveals their transverse and oblique course within the substance of the adipose pad and superficial to the abductor hallucis, the short flexor, and the plantar aponeurosis (Fig. 9.62). These sensory branches are thus truly in a weight-bearing position. In this anatomic preparation, one appreciates the oblique proximal border of the abductor hallucis muscle that is attached to the fibrous tunnel of the tibialis posterior tendon anteriorly and to the medial aspect of the calcaneal tuberosity posteriorly. These close attachments limit the mobilization of the muscle.

In the next step, the medial calcaneal nerve and its branches, including the adipose fat pad, have been removed (Fig. 9.63). The subdivision of the posterior tibial nerve into the medial (anterior) and the lateral (posterior) plantar nerves are seen. The nerve to the abductor digiti quinti is in the field taking off from the origin of the lateral plantar nerve and passing between the medial head of the quadratus plantae laterally and the deep surface of the abductor hallucis medially.

Distal retraction of the proximal border of the abductor hallucis reveals the lower calcaneal chamber (Fig. 9.64) limited above by the transverse interfascicular ligament, laterally by the medial head of the quadratus plantae, and medially by the abductor hallucis muscle. The lateral plantar neurovascular

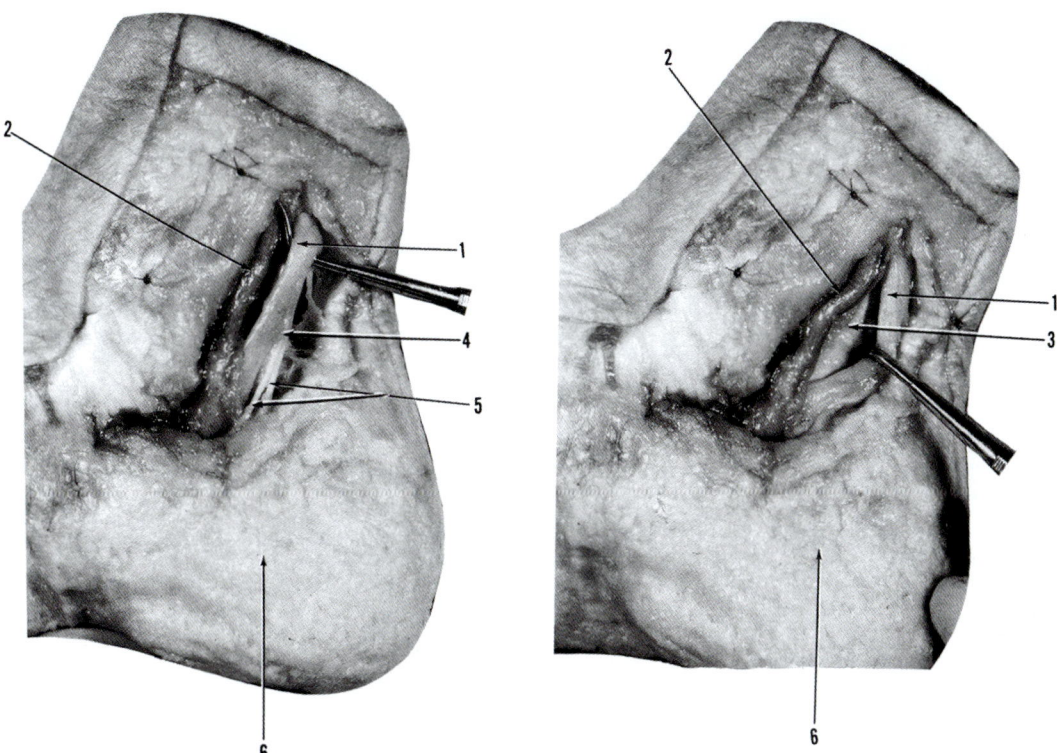

Figure 9.60 Tibiotalocalcaneal tunnel. The aponeurosis of the posterior tibial neurovascular tunnel is incised, opened, and tagged with sutures. (*1*, posterior tibial nerve; *2*, posterior tibial artery; *3*, flexor hallucis longus tendon covered by the intermediate fascia. The tendon is exposed by retracting the nerve; *4*, medial calcaneal nerve [MCN]; *5*, division branches of MCN; *6*, adipose heel cup.)

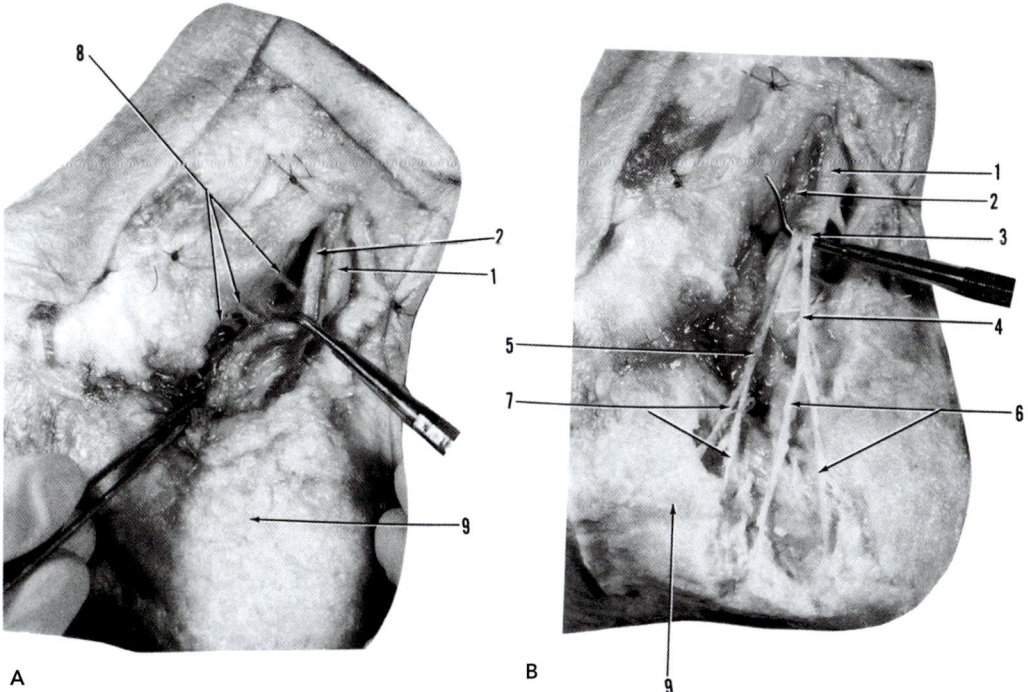

Figure 9.61 Tibiotalocalcaneal tunnel. (A) The posterior retraction of the posterior tibial artery (*2*) is limited by the anterior short-anchoring vessels (*8*). **(B)** The elevation of the medial calcaneal nerve trunk (*3*) with a probe may indicate the course of the division branches (*4*, *5*, *6*, and *7*) through the adipose mantle (*9*).

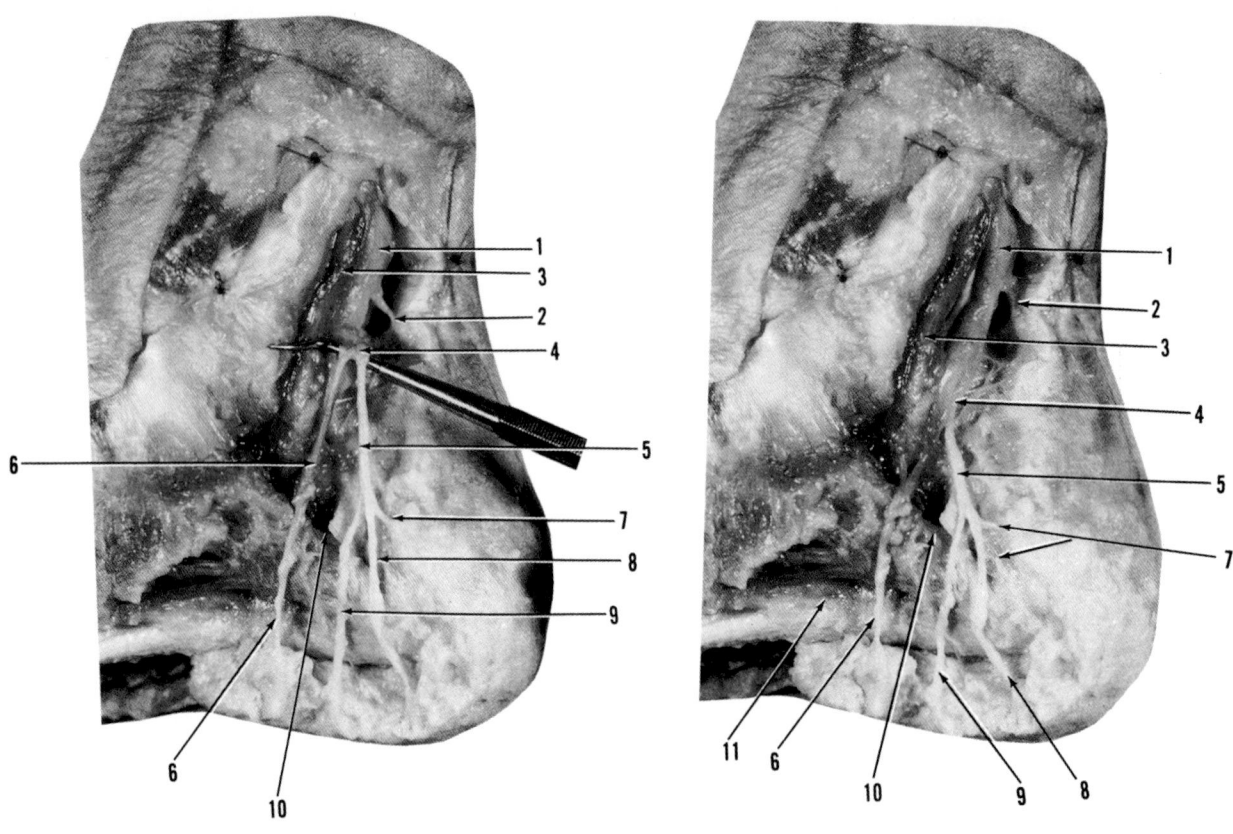

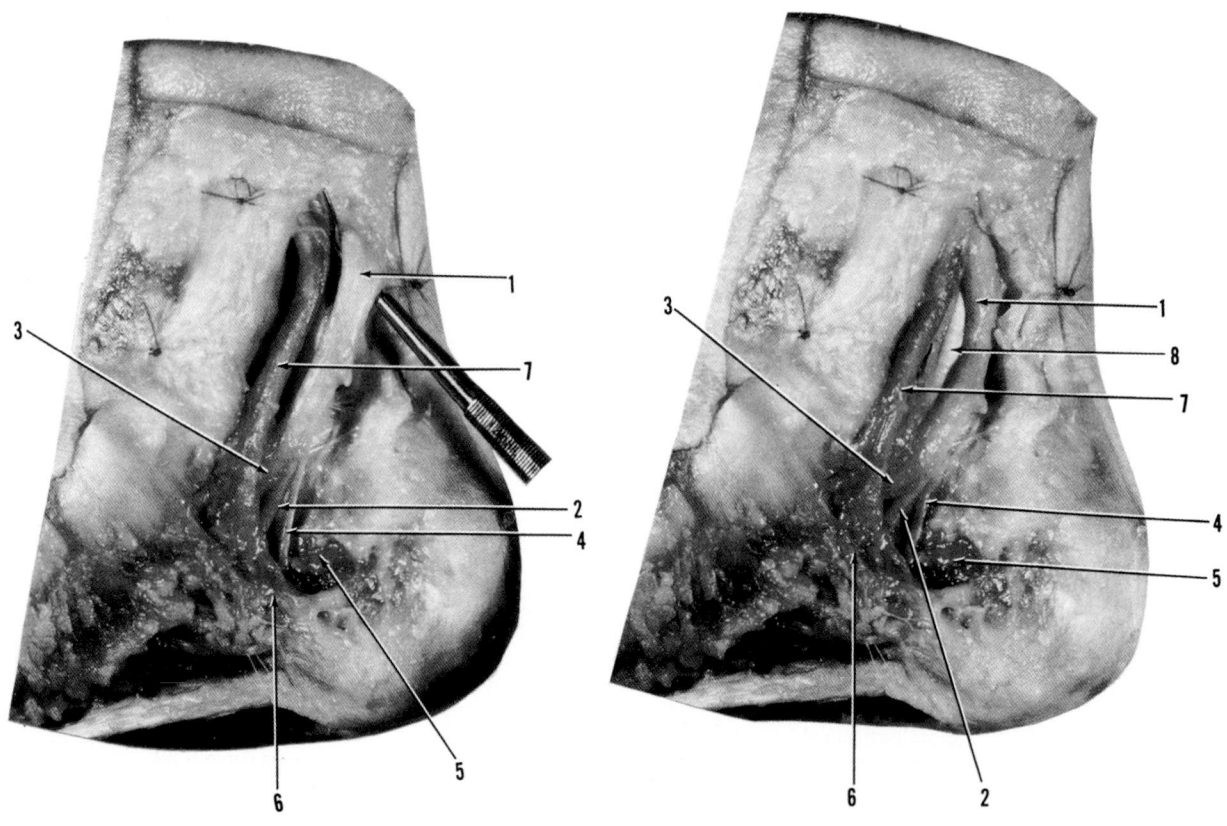

Chapter 9: Cross-Sectional and Topographic Anatomy   481

◀ Figure 9.62 **Tibiotalocalcaneal tunnel.** The adipose tissue has been removed to expose the abductor hallucis and the central compartment. The branches of the medial calcaneal nerve (4) exit from the tarsal tunnel above the superior border of the abductor hallucis muscle (10) and course superficial to the central compartment (11). (1, posterior tibial nerve; 2, nerve branch to Achilles tendon; 3, posterior tibial artery; 4, medial calcaneal nerve [MCN]; 5, posterior division branch of MCN; 6, anterior division branch of MCN; 7, posterior calcaneal nerve branches; 8, 9, terminal branches of posterior division branch of MCN; 10, abductor hallucis muscle; 11, central compartment.)

◀ Figure 9.63 **Tibiotalocalcaneal tunnel.** The medial calcaneal nerve has been excised. The division of the posterior tibial nerve (1) into the lateral plantar nerve (2) and the medial plantar nerve (3) has occurred. The nerve to the abductor digiti quinti (4) takes off from the origin of the lateral plantar nerve (2) and courses between the quadratus plantae (5) and the abductor hallucis muscle (6). The posterior tibial artery (7) has not divided yet. The tendon of the flexor hallucis longus and the covering fascia (8) are exposed by retracting the posterior tibial nerve (1) posteriorly.

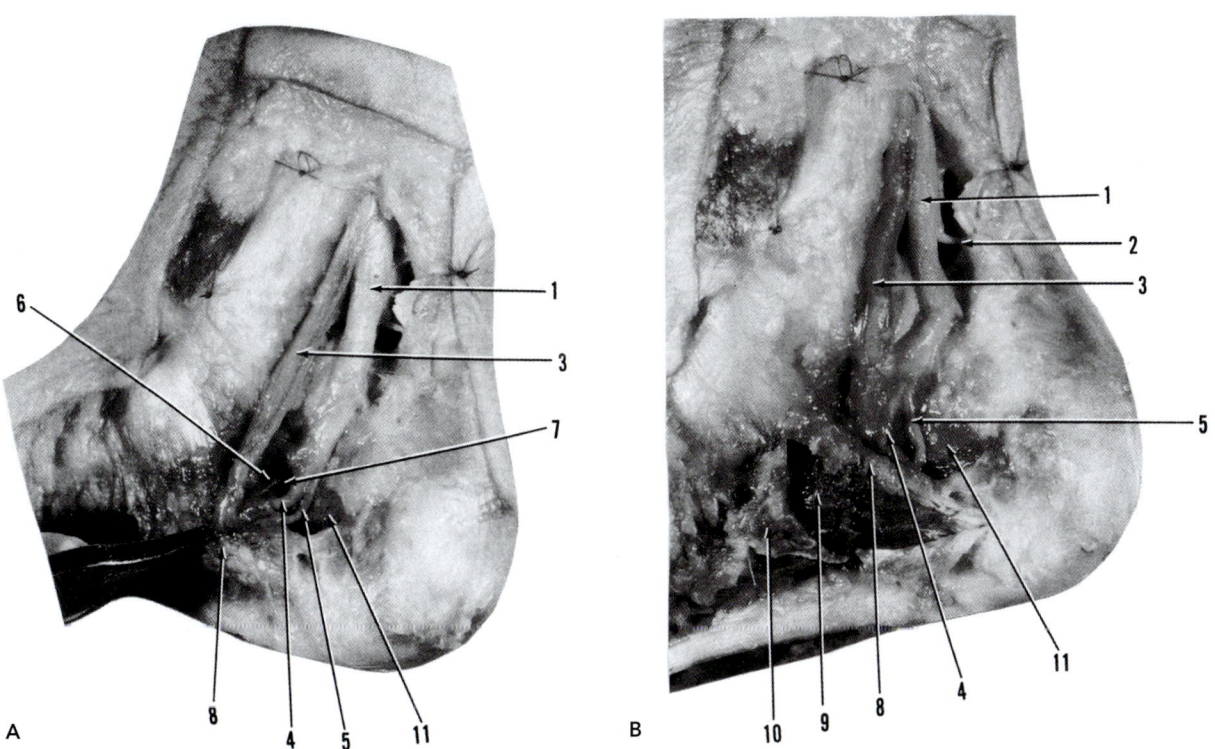

Figure 9.64 **Tibiotalocalcaneal tunnel: neurovascular compartment.** (A) Distal retraction of the dorsal border of the abductor hallucis muscle (8) brings into view the interfascicular ligament (6) and the lower calcaneal chamber (7) through which are passing the lateral plantar nerve (4) and the nerve to the abductor digiti quinti (5). (B) The superficial investing fascia (1) of the abductor hallucis muscle (9) has been incised and reflected. It is a thin layer. (1, posterior tibial nerve; 2, posterior nerve branch to Achilles tendon; 3, posterior tibial artery; 4, lateral plantar nerve; 5, nerve to abductor digiti quinti; 6, interfascicular ligament; 7, lower calcaneal chamber; 8, proximal border of abductor hallucis muscle; 9, abductor hallucis muscle; 10, superficial investing fascia of abductor hallucis; 11, quadratus plantae, medial head.)

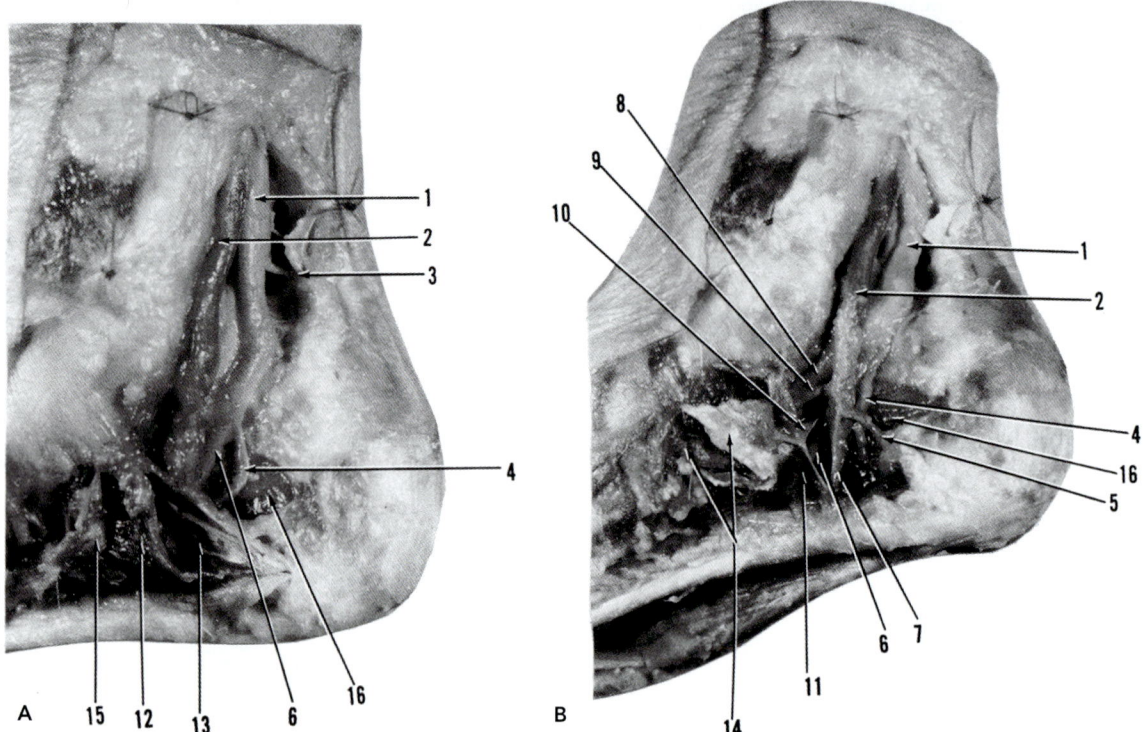

Figure 9.65 Tibiotalocalcaneal tunnel: neurovascular compartment. (A) After reflection of the superficial investing fascia (15) of the abductor hallucis followed by the reflection of the muscle (12), the lateral or deep investing aponeurosis (13) of the same muscle is exposed. It is thick and reinforced by the adherent medial intermuscular septum. (B) As a final step, the lateral investing fascia of the abductor hallucis and the adherent medial intermuscular septum are detached from the calcaneus and reflected forward (14) to bring into full view the interfascicular ligament (10) and its vertical component (11). Below the interfascicular ligament is the lower calcaneal chamber providing passage to the lateral plantar nerve (6) and artery (7). Above the same ligament is the upper calcaneal chamber giving passage to the medial plantar nerve (8) and artery (9). In both chambers, the nerve is anterior to the corresponding artery. The nerve to the abductor digiti quinti (4) is in full view, coursing across the medial head of the quadratus plantae (16) and passing deep to the compartment of the flexor digitorum brevis. This nerve is crossed by a medial calcaneal arterial branch (5). (1, posterior tibial nerve; 2, posterior tibial artery; 3, posterior nerve branch for the Achilles tendon; 4, nerve to the abductor digiti quinti; 5, medial calcaneal arterial branch; 6, lateral plantar nerve; 7, lateral plantar artery; 8, medial plantar nerve; 9, medial plantar artery; 10, interfascicular ligament, transverse component; 11, interfascicular ligament, vertical arm; 12, detached abductor hallucis bundle; 13, deep investing thick fascia of abductor hallucis muscle, reinforced by the adherent medial intermuscular septum; 14, detached and reflected lateral investing fascia of abductor hallucis and adherent medial intermuscular septum; 15, reflected superficial aponeurosis of abductor hallucis muscle; 16, quadratus plantae, medial head.)

bundle and the nerve to the abductor digiti quinti are located in this chamber.

The next step consists of analyzing the proximal segment of the abductor hallucis. Its superficial investing fascia has been incised and reflected: it is relatively thin. This is followed (Fig. 9.65) by the reflection of the muscle from its origin to reveal its medial investing layer, which is thick, aponeurotic, and formed by the adherent medial investing fascia of the muscle and the medial intermuscular septum. During a surgical decompression of the nerve to the abductor digiti quinti, the observation of a thick medial wall is thus normal.

As a final step, the medial aponeurosis is detached from its insertion and reflected. This now reveals all the components of the tibiotalocalcaneal tunnel. The interfascicular ligament is clearly seen with its transverse and vertical components. The former divides the calcaneal tunnel into the upper and lower calcaneal chambers and inserts on the medial surface of the abductor hallucis aponeurosis and on the proximal border of the quadratus plantae. The vertical component of the ligament inserts on the medial intermuscular septum.

The upper calcaneal chamber gives passage to the medial plantar neurovascular bundle (nerve anterior to artery), and the lower calcaneal chamber gives passage to the lateral plantar neurovascular bundle (nerve anterior to the artery) and to the nerve to the abductor digiti quinti. It should be noticed also that a medial calcaneal arterial branch crosses transversely the latter nerve.

The bifurcation of the posterior tibial artery occurs just proximal to the free border of the interfascicular ligament. The posterior tibial nerve has divided more proximally.

The lower calcaneal chamber leads to the plantar central intermediary compartment. It is the passageway between the sole of the foot, the tibiotalar tunnel, and the posterior compartment of the leg.

SOLE OF THE FOOT

▶ Surface Anatomy

The sustentaculum tali located 2.5 cm below the medial malleolus, the tubercle of the navicular, and the tuberosity of the base of the fifth metatarsal are important points of reference. Delorme has provided guidelines for the location of the plantar neurovascular bundles and the intermuscular septa.[14]

A vertical line is drawn along the posterior border of the medial malleolus and continues transversely across the heel. A line is drawn from the tubercle of the navicular to the sustentaculum tali. With the foot held at 90°, the intersection of these two lines indicates the point of division of the posterior tibial artery (Fig. 9.66).

A line is drawn from the tuberosity of the fifth metatarsal to the bifurcation point of the posterior tibial artery and to the medial end of the plantar fold of the big toe. These lines determine, with the medial border of the foot, a triangle that encompasses the plantar arteries.

A line drawn from the midpoint of the transverse heel line to the third web space indicates the direction of the lateral intermuscular septum. The portion of this line located within the above-traced triangle represents the direction of the posteroanterior portion of the lateral plantar artery.

A line drawn transversely from the tubercle of the first metatarsal intersects the anterior border of the previously traced triangle and indicates the position of the deep lateral plantar arch.

The midpoint of the inner half of the transverse heel line is marked and connected to the first web space; this line indicates the medial intermuscular septum. The portion of this line located within the previously described triangle locates the posteroanterior portion of the medial plantar artery.

▶ Skin

The skin of the sole of the foot is tight and fixed. It is thick at the level of the heel and the lateral margin and the ball of the foot; it is thinner along the medial longitudinal arch. The cleavage lines run longitudinally and have a lateral convexity. These lines are arcuate at the heel (see Fig. 9.32).

▶ Subcutaneous Tissue and Superficial Vessels and Nerves

The subcutaneous tissue is fit to bear weight and to act as a cushion (Fig. 9.67).

At the level of the heel, the thickness is close to 2 cm. Fibrous lamellae are arranged in a complex spiral fashion around the os calcis and form multiple chambers retaining the adipose tissue (Figs. 9.68 and 9.69). Similarly, farther anteriorly, especially in the ball of the foot, vertical fibers connect the dermis to the plantar aponeurosis. These connections fix the skin and retain the adipose tissue.

A very superficial intradermal and subdermal venous network covers the sole of the foot and forms, at the foot margins, the medial and lateral marginal veins that drain into

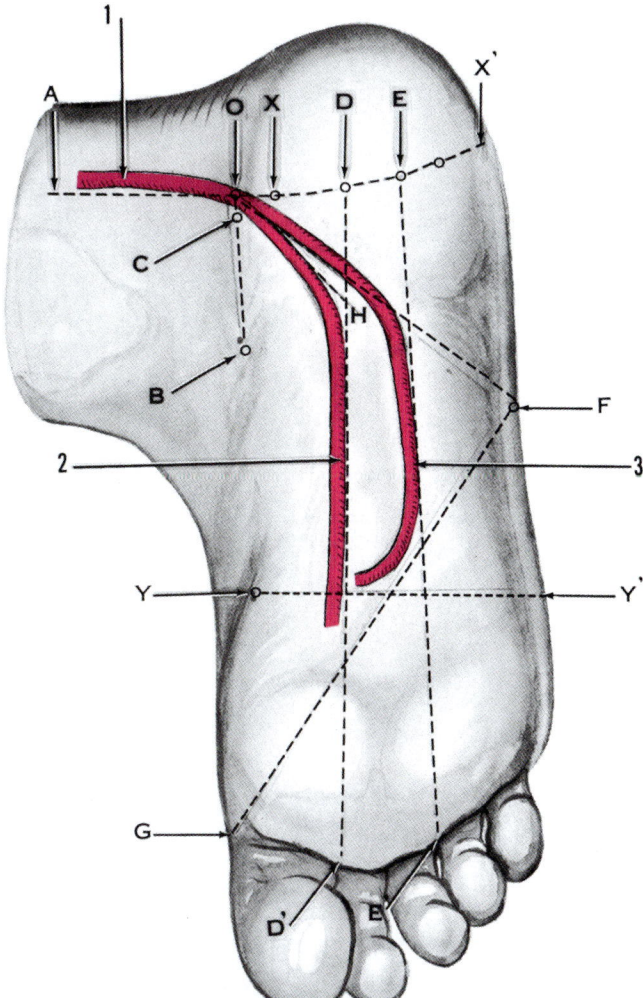

Figure 9.66 **Guidelines to the posterior tibial artery and the plantar arteries.** (*1*, posterior tibial artery; *2*, medial plantar artery; *3*, lateral plantar artery; *AX*, line tangential to posterior border of tibia; *B*, tuberosity of navicular; *C*, sustentaculum tali; *BC*, line that extended posteriorly intersects line *AX* at *O*, which represents bifurcation point of posterior tibial artery into medial and lateral plantar arteries; *AX*, line extends transversely across heel and forms line *XX'*; *E*, midpoint of *XX'*; *D*, midpoint of *XE*; *D'*, first web space; *E'*, third web space; *F* tuberosity of fifth metatarsal; *G*, medial border of flexion crease of big toe; *Y*, tuberosity of first metatarsal; *DD'*, line indicating direction of medial intermuscular septum; *EE'*, line indicating direction of lateral intermuscular septum.) Both plantar arteries are incorporated in the V formed by the line *OFG*. Each plantar artery has an oblique and a posteroanterior longitudinal portion. The oblique portion of the medial plantar artery is situated along with line *OH*. *H* is located on the line *DD'* at a point equidistant from points *B* and *C*. The longitudinal section of the medial plantar artery is along the medial intermuscular septum line, within the previously determined V. The oblique portion of the lateral plantar artery is along the line *OF*, extending from *O* up to its intersection with *EE'*. The longitudinal portion of the lateral plantar artery is located along the *EE'* line within the vascular V. The transverse portion of the lateral plantar artery is located along a transverse line *YY'* drawn across the sole. (After Delorme E. Ligature des artères de la pause de la main ET de la planet du pied. *Mem Accad Med.* 1882. Cited in Testut L, Jacob O. *Traité d'Anatomie Topographique avec Applications Médico-Chirurgicales.* Vol 2. 2nd ed. Doin; 1909:1084.)

the dorsal veins. The superficial mid plantar region drains into a distal superficial venous arcade joining at each end of the dorsomedial and dorsolateral marginal veins of the first and fifth toes.

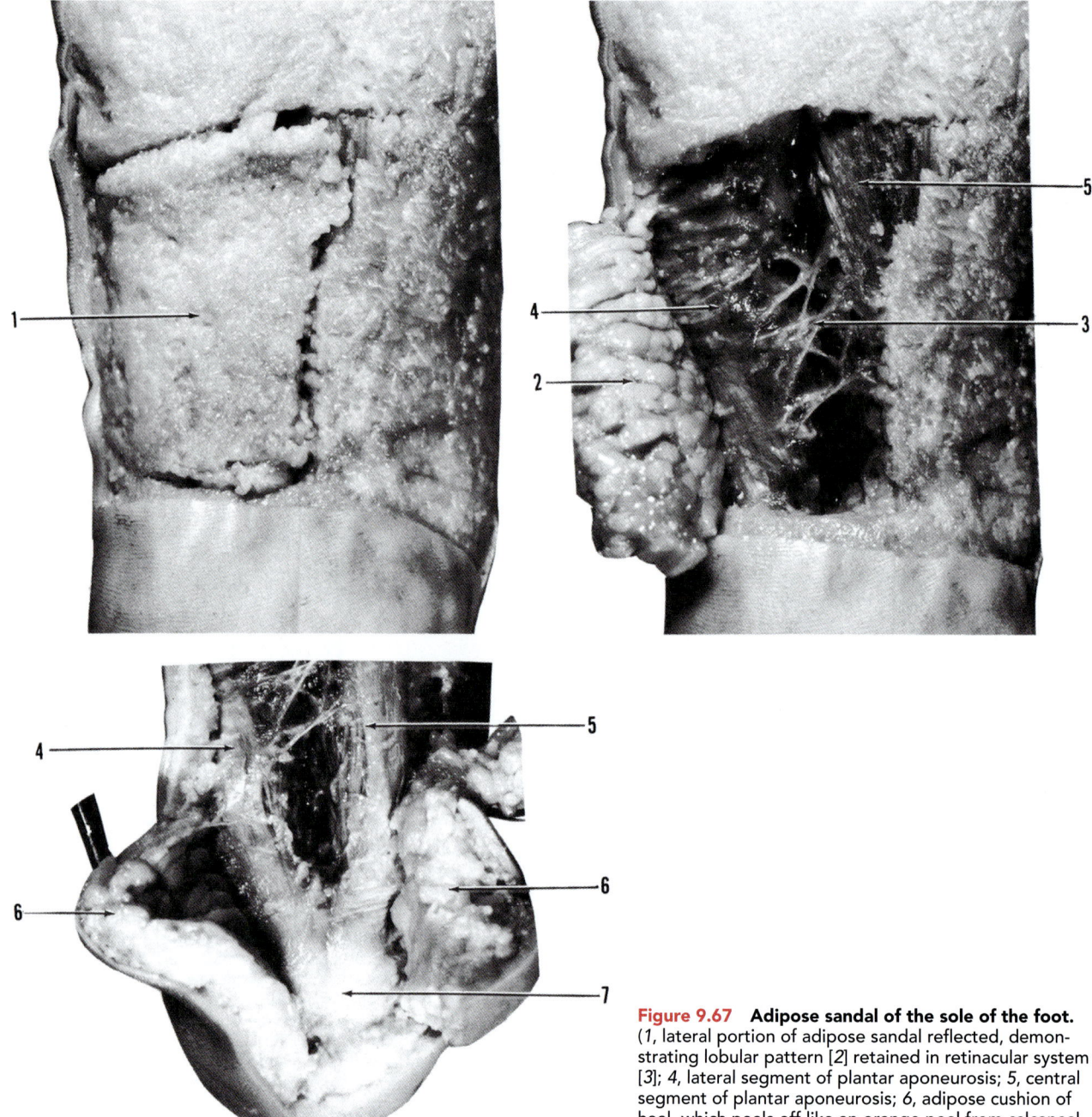

Figure 9.67 Adipose sandal of the sole of the foot. (*1*, lateral portion of adipose sandal reflected, demonstrating lobular pattern [*2*] retained in retinacular system [*3*]; *4*, lateral segment of plantar aponeurosis; *5*, central segment of plantar aponeurosis; *6*, adipose cushion of heel, which peels off like an orange peel from calcaneal tuberosity, where a large bursa is present [*7*].

The arterial blood supply of the sole of the foot is rich. In the mid segment, multiple small perforating vessels pass through the medial and lateral sulci of the sole and supply the skin. They are provided by the lateral and medial plantar arteries. The ball of the foot is vascularized by perforating cutaneous branches arising from the common plantar digital arteries. The medial aspect of the heel is supplied by the medial calcaneal arteries provided by the lateral plantar artery. The first medial calcaneal branch may emanate from the end of the posterior tibial artery. The lateral aspect of the heel is supplied by the posterior peroneal or the posterior tibial artery. The anterior calcaneal branches may be supplemented by the lateral plantar artery, the anterior peroneal artery, or the lateral tarsal artery.

The sural nerve provides two calcaneal branches to the lateral aspect of the heel. The medial calcaneal nerves are branches of the posterior tibial nerve. The most posterior branch supplies the medial aspect of the heel. The anterior medial calcaneal nerve courses anterolaterally through the thick adipose tissue accompanying the medial calcaneal artery and supplies the skin to the posterior third of the sole. The remaining segment of the sole is innervated by the medial plantar nerve in its inner two-thirds and by the lateral plantar nerve in its outer one-third.

Chapter 9: Cross-Sectional and Topographic Anatomy 485

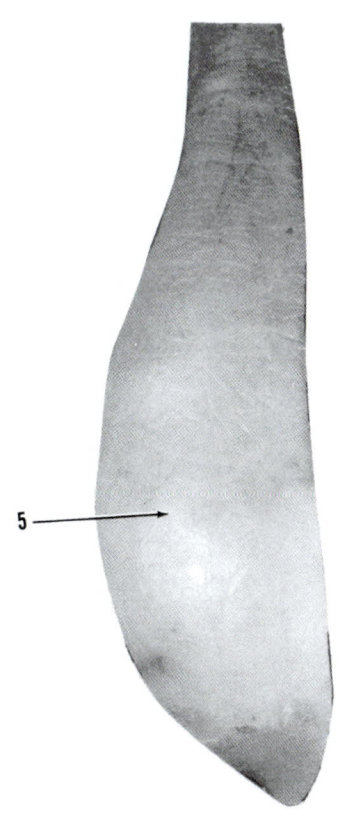
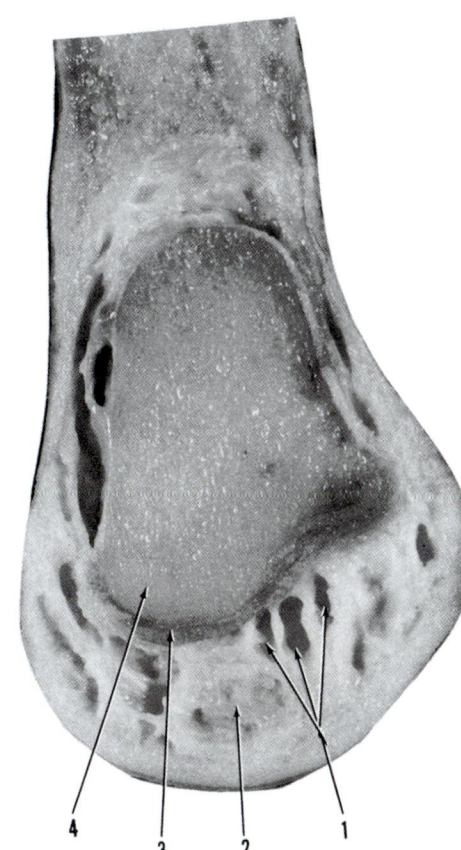

Figure 9.68 **Coronal section of the posterior aspect of the heel (5).** (*1*, vertical fibrous septa forming macro chambers for the retention of the adipose tissue; *2*, in this specimen, a localized degeneration and collapse of the retaining fibrous septa has occurred. The lesion is filled with very friable tissue and is retained by a fibrous wall. This may be considered an early stage of pressure necrosis with the skin still intact; *3*, insertion of the plantar aponeurosis; *4*, medial plantar calcaneal tuberosity.)

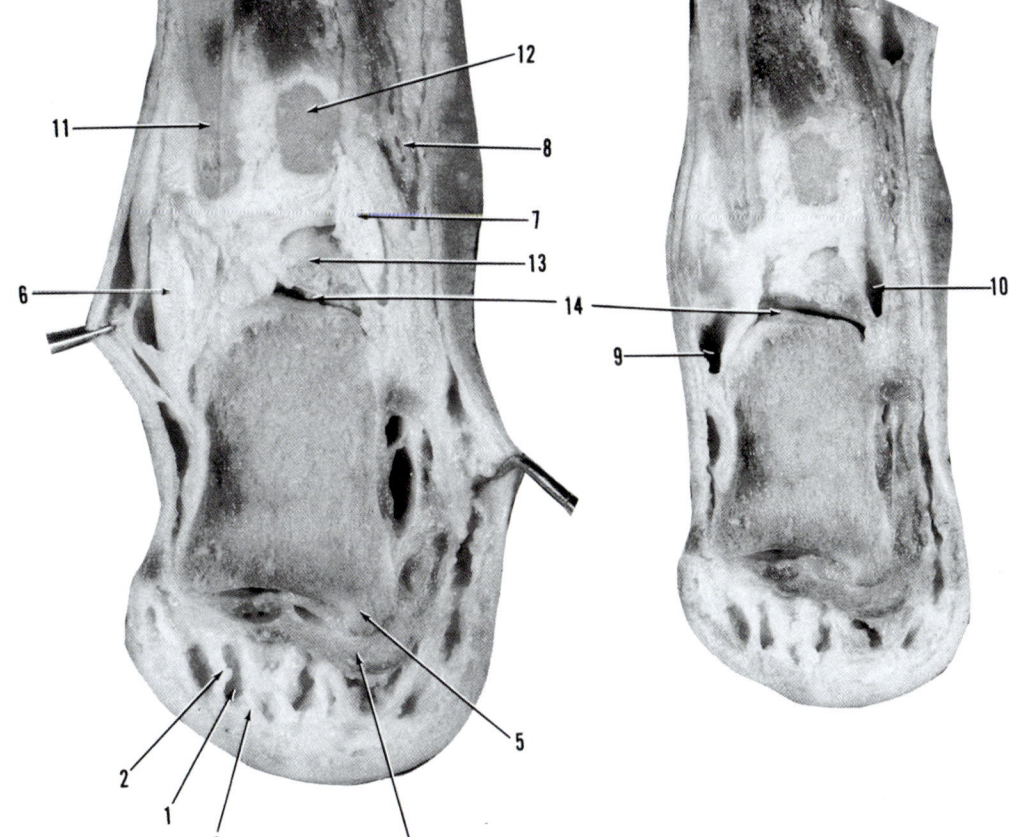

Figure 9.69 **Coronal section passing through posterior talocalcaneal joint, the fibula, and the tibia of the left foot.** Proximal segment of section. (*1*, macro chamber for retention of adipose tissue; *2*, vertical fibrous septum; *3*, fibrous heel cup providing insertion to the vertical septa; *4*, insertional site of plantar aponeurosis and origin of flexor digitorum brevis; *5*, plantar medial calcaneal tuberosity; *6*, peronei tendons; *7*, flexor hallucis longus tendon; *8*, posterior tibial vessels within tunnel; *9*, tunnel of peronei tendons; *10*, tunnel of flexor hallucis longus tendon; *11*, posterior aspect of lateral malleolus; *12*, distal tibia; *13*, posterior aspect of talus; *14*, posterior talocalcaneal joint.)

Hidalgo and Shaw, in a comprehensive study of the cutaneous and subcutaneous nerve and arterial anatomy of the plantar skin, provided guidelines for safe plantar incision and flaps.[15,16]

Four zones of arterial anatomy were demonstrated: proximal plantar, mid plantar, lateral foot, and distal foot (Fig. 9.70).

In zone 1 of the proximal plantar skin, the arterial branches are oriented transversely and are the largest ones found in the subcutaneous tissues of the plantar surface. The subcutaneous plexus is extensive and extends half the distance between the base of the heel and the metatarsal heads. This plexus is supplied primarily by the dorsalis pedis and the lateral plantar arteries. The dorsalis pedis artery supplies the plexus by branches that reach it from both medial and lateral directions around the sides of the forefoot. The lateral plantar artery has multiple vertical descending branches that reach the plexus, the largest being in the calcaneal area. The medial plantar artery contributes far fewer branches, much smaller in diameter, to the plexus. The peroneal artery contributes small lateral calcaneal

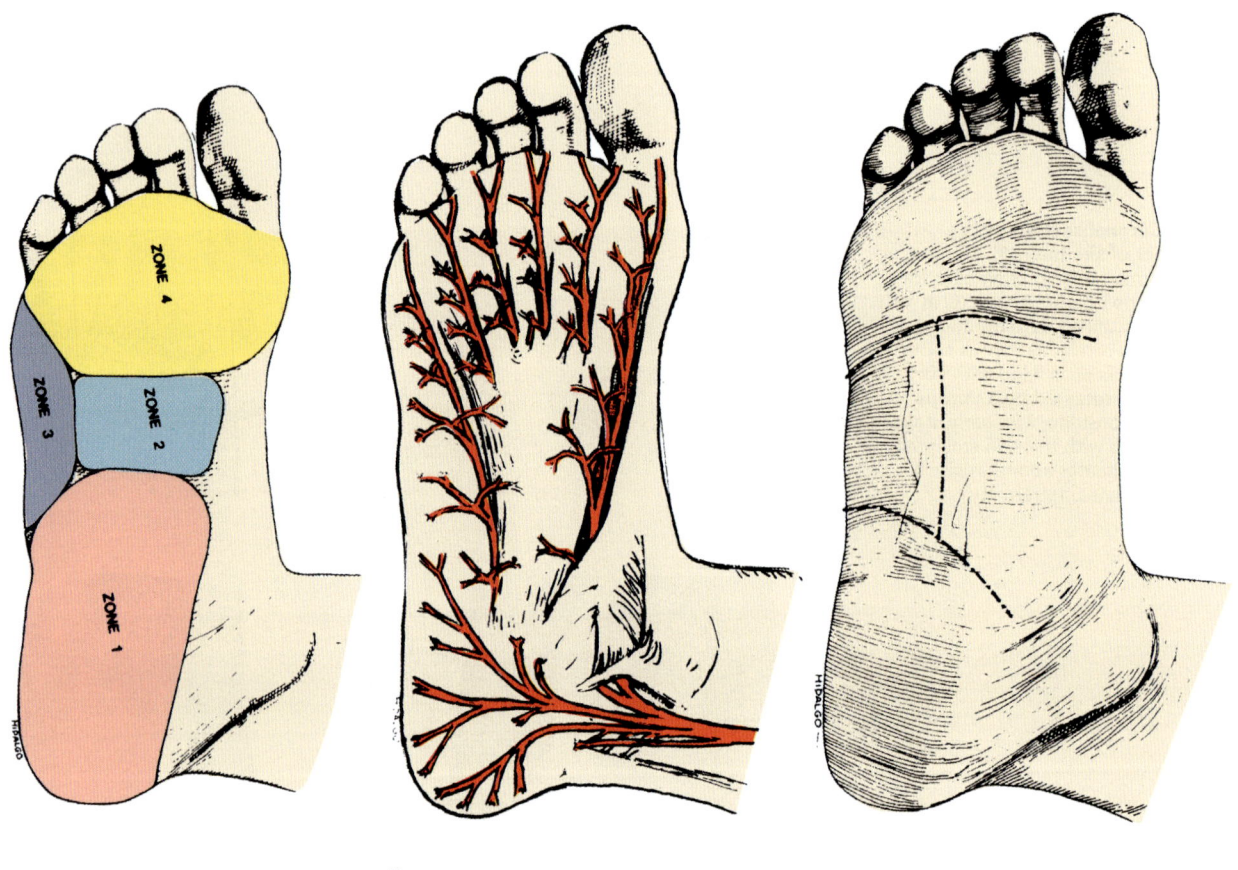

Figure 9.70 **(A) Arterial anatomy of the sole of the foot.** (*Zone 1*, proximal plantar skin.) The arterial branches are oriented transversely. The subcutaneous plexus is extensive and extends half the distance between the base of the heel and the metatarsal heads. This plexus is supplied primarily by the dorsalis pedis providing branches from the lateral and medial borders of the foot and the lateral plantar arteries providing vertical descending branches. *Zone 2* is a watershed area, receiving blood supply from many sources: proximally from the plantar subcutaneous plexus, on the sides by branches from the lateral and medial plantar arteries, and distally from the deep plantar artery. Minimal branches perforate the plantar aponeurosis to reach the skin. *Zone 3* is supplied by lateral branches from the dorsalis pedis artery connecting with branches from the lateral plantar artery. *Zone 4:* The ball of the foot is supplied by cutaneous branches from the deep arterial plantar arcade and the plantar metatarsal arteries. These branches descend vertically to the subdermal plexus without forming a subcutaneous plexus. The vessels are numerous. **(B)** Nerve supply of the sole of the foot. The heel and proximal sole are supplied by transversely and obliquely coursing branches of the medial calcaneal nerve. These branches lie approximately 4 mm deep to the skin surface. The lateral and medial plantar nerves are located in the intermuscular troughs—lateral and medial—and provide side branches to the mid plantar segment. No nerve branches pierce vertically the central aponeurotic segment. The sensory branches of the medial and lateral plantar nerves become subcutaneous at 3 cm proximal to the metatarsal heads and then course longitudinally. **(C)** Safe plantar incisions. The first line is oblique and lies anterior to the heel. Incisions proximal to this line should be oriented in a medial-lateral direction and should not be designed perpendicular to the course of the branches of the medial calcaneal nerve. The second safe incision is midline in mid segment. The third safe incision is transverse, 3 cm proximal to the metatarsal heads. Longitudinal plantar incisions in the distal skin have a better chance of preserving the skin innervation. (Adapted from Hidalgo DA, Shaw WW. Anatomic basis of plantar flap design. *Plast Reconstr Surg.* 1986;78(5):632.)

branches to the lateral aspect of the plexus in the proximal heel area and the posterior tibial artery contributes small medial calcaneal branches to the medial aspect of the plexus in the proximal heel area.

Zone 2 of the mid plantar skin is a watershed area, with blood supply reaching the skin from multiple sources. Posteriorly, branches of the proximal plantar subcutaneous plexus supply this area, which also receives branches from the sides of the lateral and medial plantar arteries and from the deep plantar artery distally. The contributions to the blood supply of the skin by the flexor digitorum brevis or the plantar aponeurosis are minor.

Zone 3 of the lateral foot is the middle third of the plantar skin, lateral to the plantar fascia. The arterial supply is from branches of the dorsalis pedis artery curving around the lateral border of the foot and connecting with branches from the lateral plantar artery.

In zone 4 of the distal foot, the cutaneous branches arise from the deep arterial plantar arcade and the plantar metatarsal arteries. The branches pass between the division slip of the plantar aponeurosis and "perforate vertically to the subdermal plexus without forming a subcutaneous plexus as in the proximal plantar area. These vessels are numerous and evenly distributed throughout the distal forefoot."[17]

Hidalgo and Shaw defined the nerve supply to the plantar skin by the branches of the medial calcaneal nerve and the lateral and medial plantar nerves.[15,16] The medial calcaneal nerve fans out over the heel into parallel branches that run in a mediolateral direction approximately 4 mm deep to the skin surface. The medial and lateral plantar nerves have sensory branches that run to the plantar skin distal to the heel and that reach the subcutaneous tissue from the deeper planes via clefts between the plantar fascia and the muscles that flank it, but they do not traverse the thick plantar fascia. Sensory branches to the distal foot course under the plantar fascia and become subcutaneous about 3 cm proximal to the metatarsal heads. The nerves then course obliquely to the skin over the metatarsal heads.[16]

On the basis of the innervation pattern of the skin, Hidalgo and Shaw delineated safe plantar incision (see Fig. 9.70).[15,16] The first incision line is oblique and lies anterior to the heel. Incisions proximal to this line should be oriented in a medial lateral direction and should not be designed perpendicular to the course of the branches of the medial calcaneal nerve. The incision should be perpendicular only at the most lateral aspect of the heel, near the terminal portion of the nerve branches. The plane of dissection is on the surface of the calcaneus and the plantar fascia distally so that the nerve branches are preserved superficially.

The second safe incision line (see Fig. 9.70) is in the midfoot segment, distal to the heel region. This incision is midline over the plantar aponeurosis and lies between the medial and lateral plantar nerve territories that do course around the medial and lateral borders of the plantar aponeurosis and supply the corresponding half of the skin. There are no nerve fibers piercing the plantar fascia.

A third safe incision line is transverse, 3 cm proximal to the metatarsal heads (see Fig. 9.70). This line marks the emergence of the web space subcutaneous branches. Transverse incisions distal to this line may leave anesthetic distal skin. Longitudinal plantar incisions in this distal skin segment have better chances of preserving the skin innervation. From the arterial point of view, in the proximal plantar area (zone 1; see Fig. 9.70), skin flaps may be based either medially or laterally on the dorsal arterial supply. However, a medially based flap simultaneously preserves the skin innervation. In the mid plantar area (zone 2; see Fig. 9.70), the arterial dorsal supply pattern allows the raising of medially or laterally based flaps in the subcutaneous plane, superficial to the plantar aponeurosis. This area is well supplied by regional subcutaneous sources, ucho that dissection superficial to the fascia is both practical and reliable.[15]

The skin innervation is preserved in these laterally or medially based flaps, but the degree of mobilization may require proximal intraneural dissection of the medial or lateral plantar nerve.

In the lateral foot (zone 3; see Fig. 9.70), a laterally based flap may be raised based on the dorsal supply from the dorsalis pedis arterial branches curving around the lateral border of the foot. The innervation is provided from branches of the lateral plantar nerve that are to be preserved.

In the distal foot or forefoot (zone 4), cutaneous arterial branches arise between the longitudinal slips of the plantar fascia and perforate vertically to the subdermal plexus without forming a subcutaneous plexus, as in the proximal plantar area. In this area, because of the vertical arterial supply, a V-Y skin transposition may be possible to cover defects of 2 to 4 cm.[17]

As defined by Shaw and Hidalgo, a medially based large plantar flap is delineated for design of a large flap for the coverage of a heel ulcer.[16] The flap is incised laterally and the subcutaneous tissue is raised off the abductor digiti minimi muscle. At the lateral intermuscular cleft, the subcutaneous branches of the lateral plantar nerve are identified. The portion of the flap that crosses the plantar aponeurosis distally is incised and the subcutaneous tissue of the flap is elevated directly off the fascia. At the level of the medial intermuscular cleft, branches of the medial plantar nerve are identified. As the flap is elevated in a proximal direction, the nerve branches from the medial and the lateral plantar nerves are separated from the main nerve trunks for a short distance, thus providing the rotational mobility of the flap. All of the lateral plantar arterial branches to the flap are divided with the medially based design. A laterally based flap is used less commonly.

▶ Adipose Mantle

The entire sole of the foot is invested by an adipose mantle that forbids exposure of the branches of the medial calcaneal nerve in the surgical setting and distally hides the more exposable digital nerves (Fig. 9.71).

Plantar Aponeurosis, Intermuscular Septa, and Compartments

Plantar Aponeurosis

The plantar aponeurosis is a strong fibrous structure with three components: central, lateral, and tibial (Figs. 9.72 and 9.73).

The central component is the strongest and the thickest and has a glistening appearance. It is triangular in contour with a proximal apex originating from the posteromedial calcaneal tubercle and a distal base. At the origin, the aponeurosis measures 1.5 to 2 cm in width; it narrows slightly and then gradually enlarges as it progresses anteriorly. At mid metatarsal level, the fibers group into five longitudinally oriented bands that diverge. Just proximal to the level of the metatarsal heads, each band divides into three components, one superficial and two deep.

The superficial fibers insert subcutaneously in the distal segment of the ball of the foot. The deep fibers reach the depth in the form of two sagittal septa around each flexor tendon.

The lateral component of the plantar aponeurosis is thick posteriorly and thin anteriorly. It originates from the lateral margin of the medial calcaneal tubercle, extends in the direction of the cuboid, and divides into a lateral component (which inserts on the base of the fifth metatarsal) and a medial deep component (which extends to the plantar plate of the fourth toe). Through the bifurcation of this, aponeurosis passes the tendon of the abductor digiti quinti.

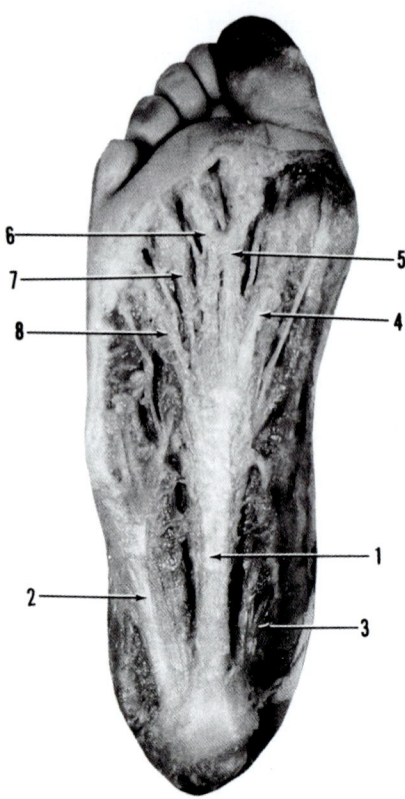

Figure 9.72 Plantar aponeurosis. (*1*, central component; *2*, lateral component; *3*, medial component; *4-8*, longitudinal superficial bands.)

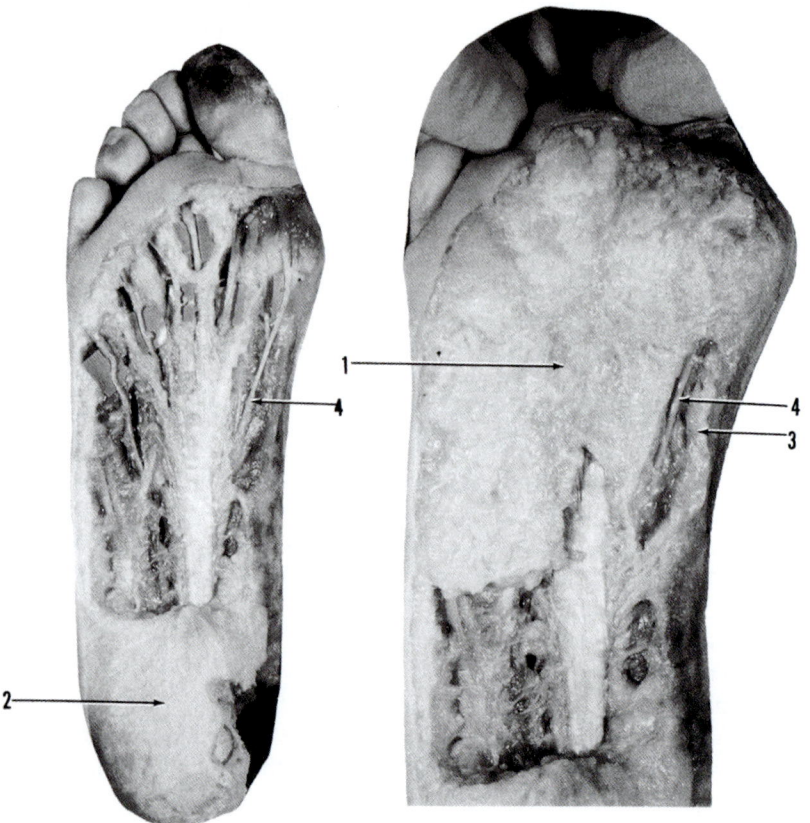

Figure 9.71 The adipose mantle of the sole (*1*) and heel (*2*). The medial plantar hallucal nerve (*4*) is embedded under the adipose tissue, which is to be reflected (*3*) to expose the nerve.

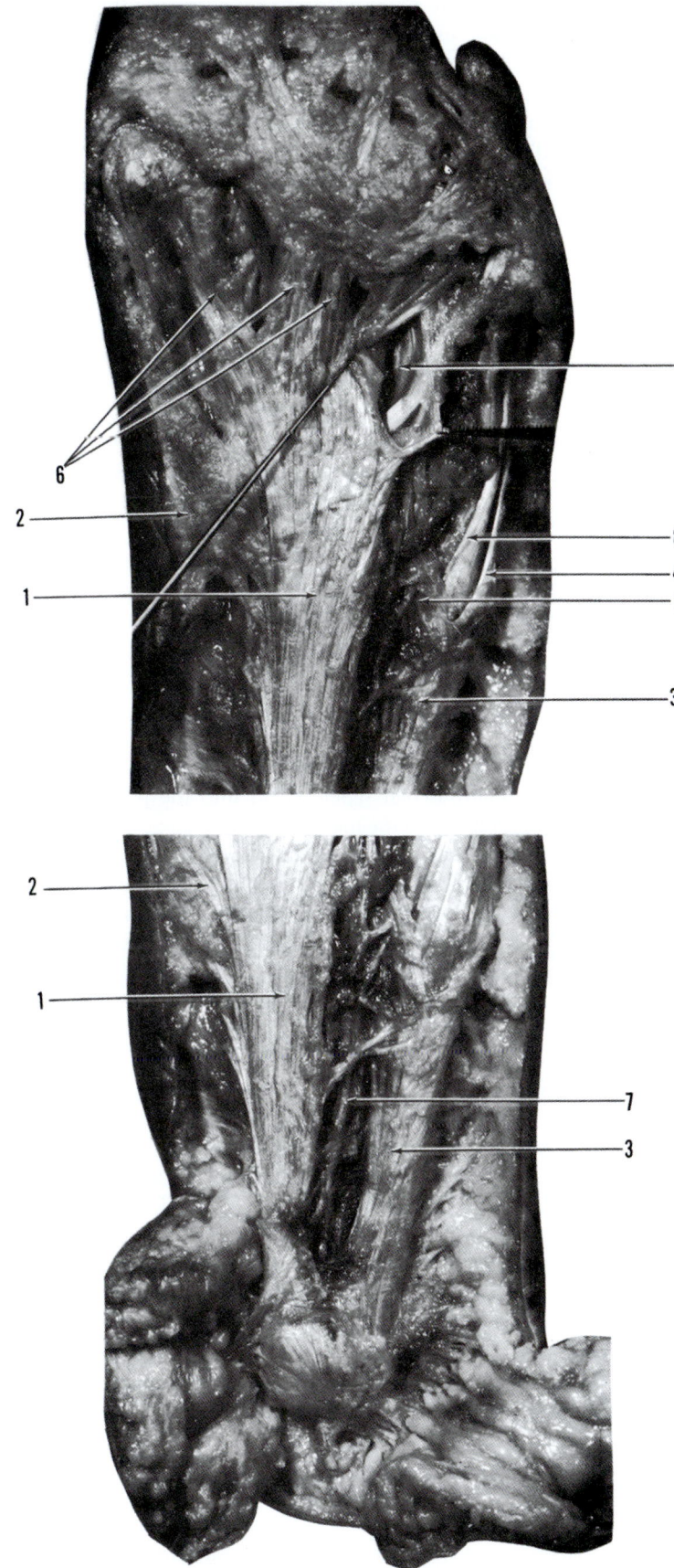

Figure 9.73 **Plantar aponeurosis.** (*1*, central segment; *2*, medial segment; *3*, lateral segment; *4*, lateral crus of lateral segment; *5*, medial crus of lateral segment; *6*, longitudinal bands of central segment; *7*, lateral intermuscular septum; *8*, tendon of abductor digiti quinti passing through crura of lateral component; *9*, lateral intermuscular septum pierced by long flexor tendon of fifth toe.)

The medial component of the plantar aponeurosis is thin posteriorly and thicker anteriorly. It forms the covering fascia of the abductor hallucis and is in continuity medially with the dorsal aponeurosis of the foot, the inferior arm of the inferior extensor retinaculum, and the flexor retinaculum.

Two longitudinal grooves, lateral and medial, are present on each side of the central component of the plantar aponeurosis. The lateral groove is better defined and larger than the medial and extends from the level of the calcaneal tubercle to the level of the fifth metatarsal tuberosity. This interval is bridged by a complex retinacular network uniting the central and the lateral components of the plantar aponeurosis. The retinacular fibers form a retaining system for the adipose lobules. Through this interval emerge the cutaneous branches arising from the lateral neurovascular bundle.

The medial groove located between the central and medial components is better defined in its proximal half and gives passage to the cutaneous branches arising from the medial plantar neurovascular bundle.

From the mid segment of the sulci surfaces, on the medial side, the medial plantar neurovascular bundle of the big toe and, on the lateral side, the lateral plantar neurovascular bundle of the fifth toe.

Intermuscular Septa

From the borders of the central component of the plantar aponeurosis, two intermuscular septa extend into the planta pedis—the lateral septum and the medial septum.

The lateral intermuscular septum is attached to the medial calcaneal tubercle, the calcaneocuboid ligament, and the sheath of the peroneus longus. Distally, the septum splits, encloses the third plantar interosseous muscle, and inserts on the medial border of the fifth metatarsal shaft and the medial aspect of the base of the proximal phalanx of the little toe.

The medial intermuscular septum originates from the medial plantar calcaneal tuberosity. In the proximal segment, it is thick and adheres to the lateral investing aponeurotic layer of the abductor hallucis muscle. It bridges the calcaneal canal. At the level of the sustentaculum tali, it provides insertion to the transverse interfascicular ligament and to the vertical arm of the latter. It is perforated in the proximal third by the lateral plantar neurovascular bundle and farther distally by the flexor digitorum longus tendon. Dorsally or in the depth, it is attached to the navicular, the medial cuneiform, and the lateral aspect of the first metatarsal shaft after passing between the adductor hallucis and the flexor hallucis brevis, and it contributes to the formation of their investing sheaths.

Compartments

The sole of the foot in its proximal two-thirds is divided into three compartments: central, medial, and lateral. The distal third is the ball of the foot, which extends from the distal segments of the metatarsals to the proximal segments of the toes.

Central Compartment

The central compartment is formed superficially by the central segment of the plantar aponeurosis, laterally by the lateral intermuscular septum, and medially by the medial intermuscular septum. The floor or deep surface corresponds proximally to the tarsal bones, their plantar ligamentous structures, the tendon of the tibialis posterior with its ramifications, and the covering peroneus longus tendon with its sheath. Distally, the floor is formed by the central metatarsals 2 to 4 and the interossei muscles covered by the interossei fascia.

The intermuscular septa are considered as "carriers" of the corresponding medial and lateral plantar neurovascular bundles. On cross-sectional studies, the neurovascular bundles have their own fascial tunnels in the proximal segments. The central compartment is divided into a superficial, an intermediary, and a deep compartment. The superficial central compartment is an enclosed compartment lodging the flexor hallucis brevis (Fig. 9.74). It does not communicate with the deep compartments or the calcaneal tunnel. It is important for the surgeon to know the anatomic relationship of the medial and plantar neurovascular structures (Figs. 9.75 and 9.76). There are no nerve branches on the superficial proximal two-thirds of the central segment of the plantar aponeurosis. The "midline" is the safe zone. The medial plantar nerve in the proximal two-thirds is located within the medial intermuscular septum and can be seen through this

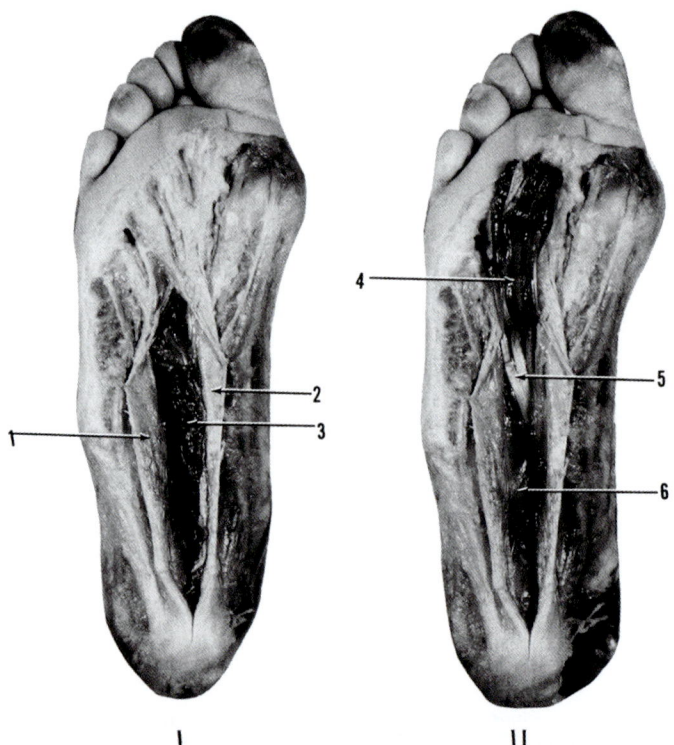

Figure 9.74 **Central superficial compartment. (I)** The central segment of the plantar aponeurosis is incised on midline and reflected (*1, 2*) to expose the flexor digitorum brevis muscle (*3*). **(II)** The flexor digitorum brevis muscle is detached from its origin and retracted distally (*4*), bringing into full view the central superficial compartment. The latter is limited dorsally by an investing fascia covering the quadratus plantae (*6*) and the proximal segment of the flexor digitorum longus tendons (*5*).

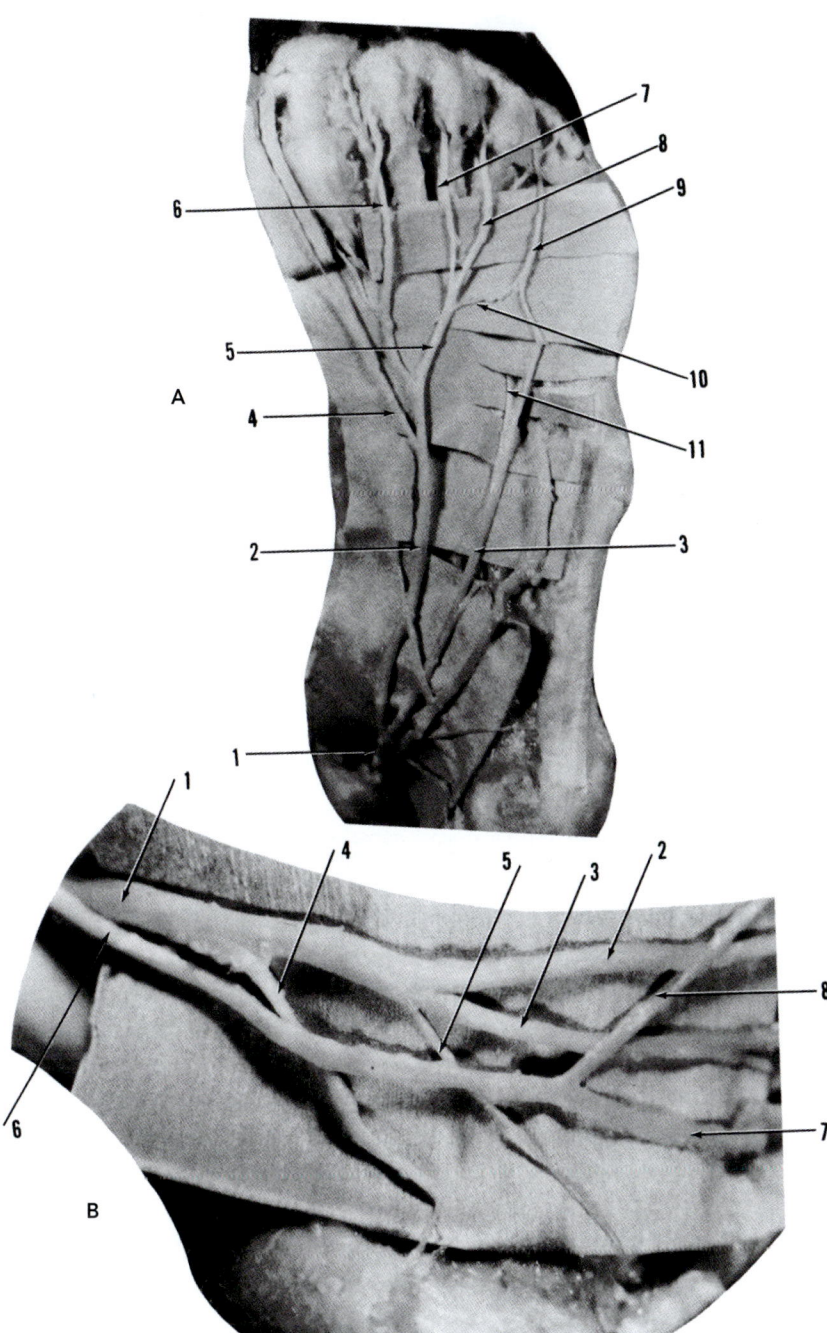

Figure 9.75 **The nerve supply to the sole of the foot.** (A) (*1*, posterior tibial nerve; *2*, medial plantar nerve; *3*, lateral plantar nerve; *4*, plantar medial hallucal nerve; *5*, common digital nerve for the second and third web space; *6*, digital branch for the first web space; *7*, digital branch for the second web space; *8*, digital branch for the third web space; *9*, digital branch for the fourth web space; *10*, communicating branch between the branches to the third and fourth web spaces; *11*, deep branch of lateral plantar nerve.) (B) (*1*, posterior tibial nerve; *2*, medial plantar nerve; *3*, lateral plantar nerve; *4*, trunk of medial calcaneal nerve; *5*, nerve to abductor digiti quinti; *6*, posterior tibial artery; *7*, lateral plantar artery; *8*, medial plantar artery.)

septum in the depth and within the medial wall of the superficial central compartment (Fig. 9.77).

The medial plantar nerve to the hallux surfaces from the medial intermuscular cleft at about the level of the first metatarsocuneiform joint (Figs. 9.72 and 9.78). It courses superficially across the medial compartment but is "embedded" in the adipose mantle. The lateral distal branches of the medial plantar nerve pierce the medial intermuscular septum laterally, turn around the medial border of the flexor digitorum brevis, and course for a short distance obliquely between the deep surface of the plantar aponeurosis and the flexor digitorum brevis.

They are surgically vulnerable at that level. This same superficial space is penetrated from the lateral side by the anastomotic branch between the third common digital nerve and the fourth common digital nerve, a branch of the lateral plantar nerve. This anastomotic branch may, however, be absent. The superficial common plantar digital arteries arising from the lateral superficial branch of the medial plantar artery join, in this space, the corresponding common digital branches of the medial plantar nerve. Occasionally, a superficial arterial branch is given off by the lateral plantar artery and joins the medial superficial group to form the superficial arterial arcade. The superficial common

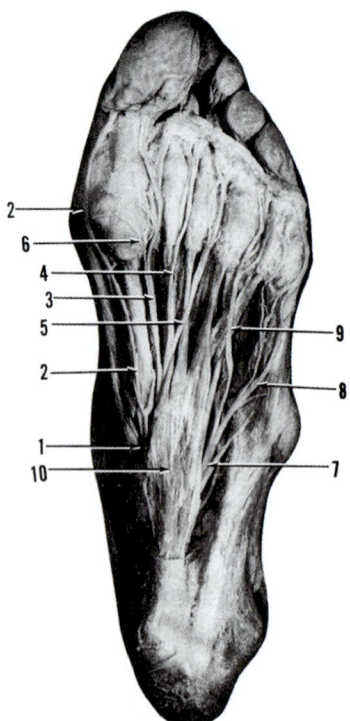

Figure 9.76 **Innervation of the sole of the foot: nerves in situ.** (*1*, medial plantar nerve; *2*, medial plantar hallucal nerve; *3*, digital branch to the first web space; *4*, digital branch to the second web space; *5*, digital branch to the third web space; *6*, small nerve branches to the metatarsophalangeal joint of the hallux; *7*, lateral plantar nerve; *8*, lateral plantar nerve to the fifth toe; *9*, digital branch to the fourth web space; *10*, flexor digitorum brevis.) The superficial branches of the medial and lateral plantar nerves merge from the side of the central compartment. (From Cosentino R. *The lower extremity.* In: *Atlas of Anatomy and Surgical Approaches in Orthopedic Surgery*. Charles C Thomas; 1960:Figure 112.)

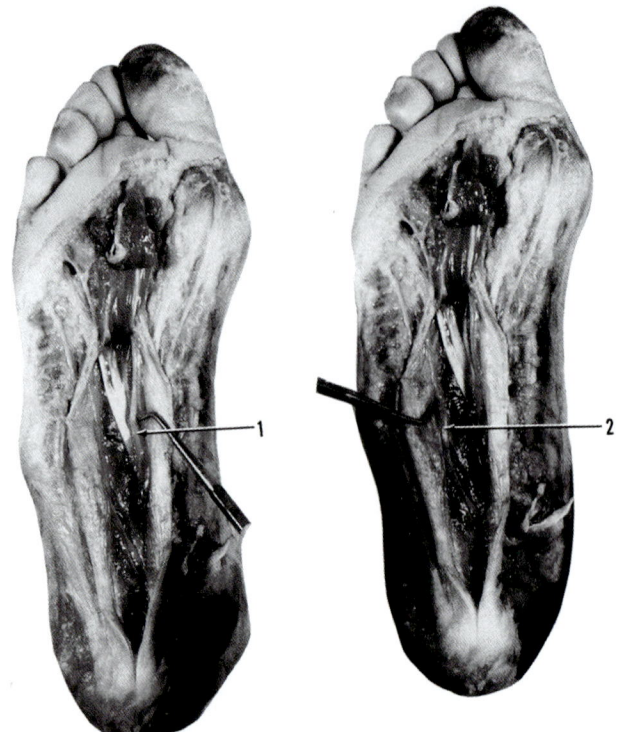

Figure 9.77 **Central superficial compartment.** The medial plantar nerve (*1*) is seen through transparency within the medial intermuscular septum. The lateral plantar nerve (*2*) is seen within the lateral intermuscular septum.

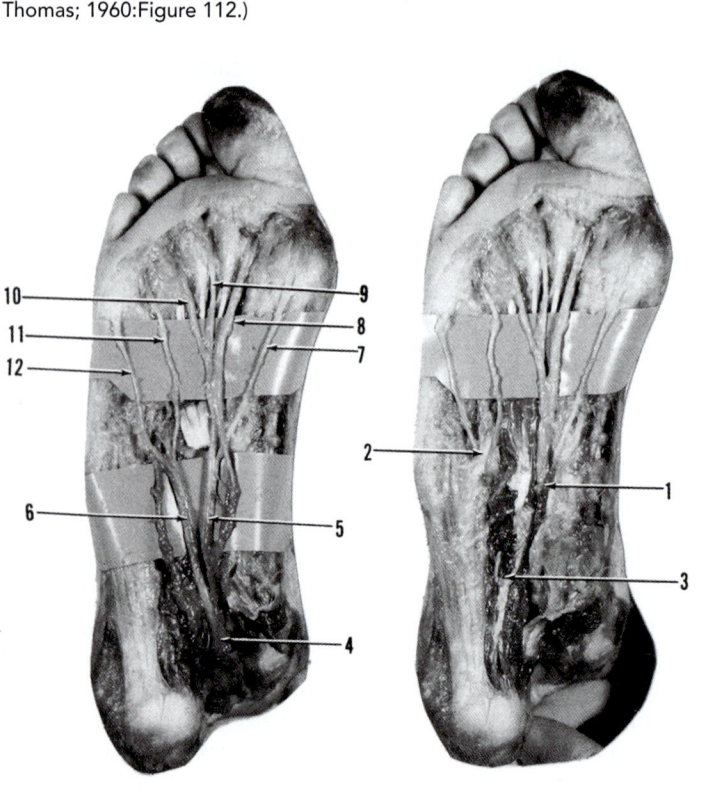

Figure 9.78 **The plantar nerves of the sole of the foot. (I)** The nerves exposed. **(II)** The nerves in situ. (*1*, medial intermuscular trough; *2*, lateral intermuscular trough; *3*, flexor digitorum brevis muscle; *4*, posterior tibial nerve; *5*, medial plantar nerve; *6*, lateral plantar nerve; *7*, medial plantar hallucal nerve; *8*, plantar digital nerve to the first web space; *9*, plantar digital nerve to the second web space; *10*, plantar digital nerve to the third web space; *11*, plantar digital nerve to the fourth web space; *12*, plantar lateral digital nerve to the fifth toe.) In this specimen, no anastomotic branch is present between the nerves to the third and fourth web spaces.

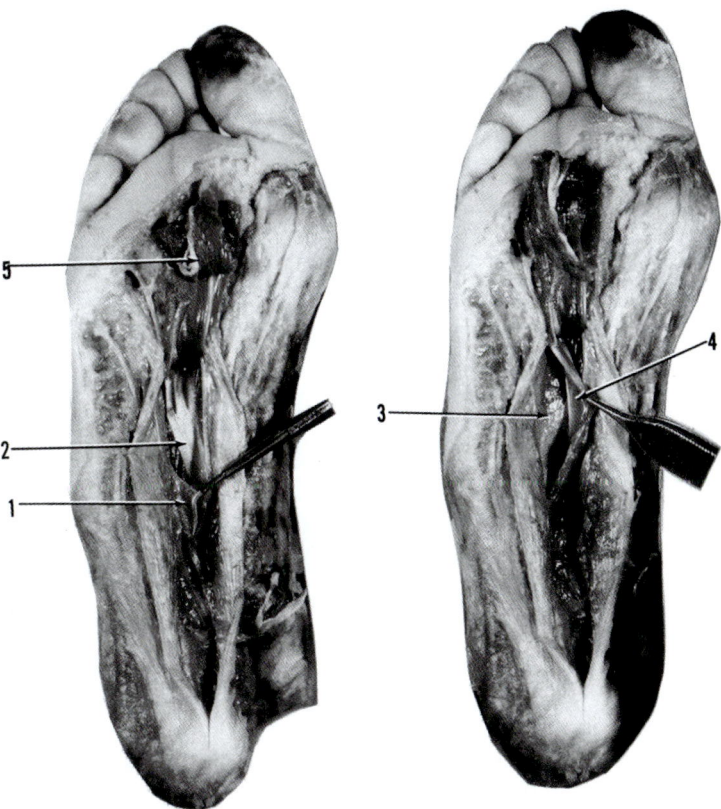

Figure 9.79 **The central intermediary compartment.** The probe is raising the distal border (*1*) of the thin fascia investing the quadratus plantae muscle. The flexor digitorum longus (*2*) is seen distally. The reflection of the quadratus plantae and flexor digitorum longus tendon (*4*) brings into view the ceiling (*3*) of the central intermediary compartment. The flexor digitorum brevis has been reflected (*5*) to expose the floor of the central intermediary compartment.

digital neurovascular bundles become relatively superficial between the superficial bands of the plantar aponeurosis. They course toward the corresponding intermetatarsal head interval and are covered by fat bodies.

The superficial central compartment is separated from the intermediary central compartment by a fascial layer that is thick proximally (Fig. 9.79). The intermediary compartment lodges the quadratus plantae and the proximal segment of the flexor digitorum longus (Fig. 9.80). The floor of the compartment is formed by the tarsal bones with their plantar ligamentous structures, the peroneus longus tendon sheath, and the fascia covering the oblique head of the adductor and a segment of metatarsals 4, 3, 2 with their interossei muscles. The lateral plantar neurovascular bundles enter the intermediary central compartment through the medial intermuscular septum, course over the proximal segment of the quadratus plantae (Figs. 9.81 to 9.83), and can be seen through transparency within the substance of the lateral intermuscular septum (see Fig. 9.77). The lateral plantar nerve remains anterior to the lateral plantar artery and its accompanying two veins. The nerve to the abductor of the fifth toe, which has taken off near the origin of the lateral plantar nerve, crosses the space in its most posterior aspect and penetrates the abductor of the fifth toe from its deep surface. Two small branches of the lateral plantar nerve pass under the lateral plantar vessels and supply the quadratus plantae and the calcaneocuboid ligament (Fig. 9.84). The lateral plantar artery provides muscular branches to the flexor digitorum brevis and the abductor digiti minimi. The flexor digitorum longus tendon passes through the medial intermuscular septum, anterior to the lateral neurovascular bundle. The margins of the septum are closely adherent to the tendon; however, the seal may yield to pressure. The long flexor of the fifth toe passes through the distal end of the lateral intermuscular septum to reach its destination. The lumbricals are located on the tibial aspect of the long flexor tendons. The first lumbrical originates from the tibial border of the tendon to the second toe; the other three lumbricals take off from the corresponding intertendinous spaces 2 to 4.

The adductor hallucis muscle is invested by a Y-shaped fascia that determines the deep central adductor compartment and the adductor space located between the interossei fascia and the fascia covering the dorsal surface of the adductor hallucis (Fig. 9.85).

The lateral plantar artery and nerve, after emerging from the mid plantar space, extend forward and are located between the lateral intermuscular septum and the deep sheath of the abductor digiti quinti muscle. About 2.5 cm distal to the base of the fifth metatarsal bone, the artery passes deep to the medial aspect of the short flexor of the fifth toe, pierces again the lateral intermuscular septum, and enters the adductor space (Fig. 9.86). Just distal to the fifth metatarsal base, the lateral plantar artery gives off the superficial fibular plantar artery of the little toe and may provide the fourth superficial common digital plantar artery, which contributes to the formation of the superficial plantar arterial arcade.

The lateral plantar nerve is initially anterior and then medial to the artery. Opposite the base of the fifth metatarsal, the nerve divides into one deep and two superficial branches (lateral and

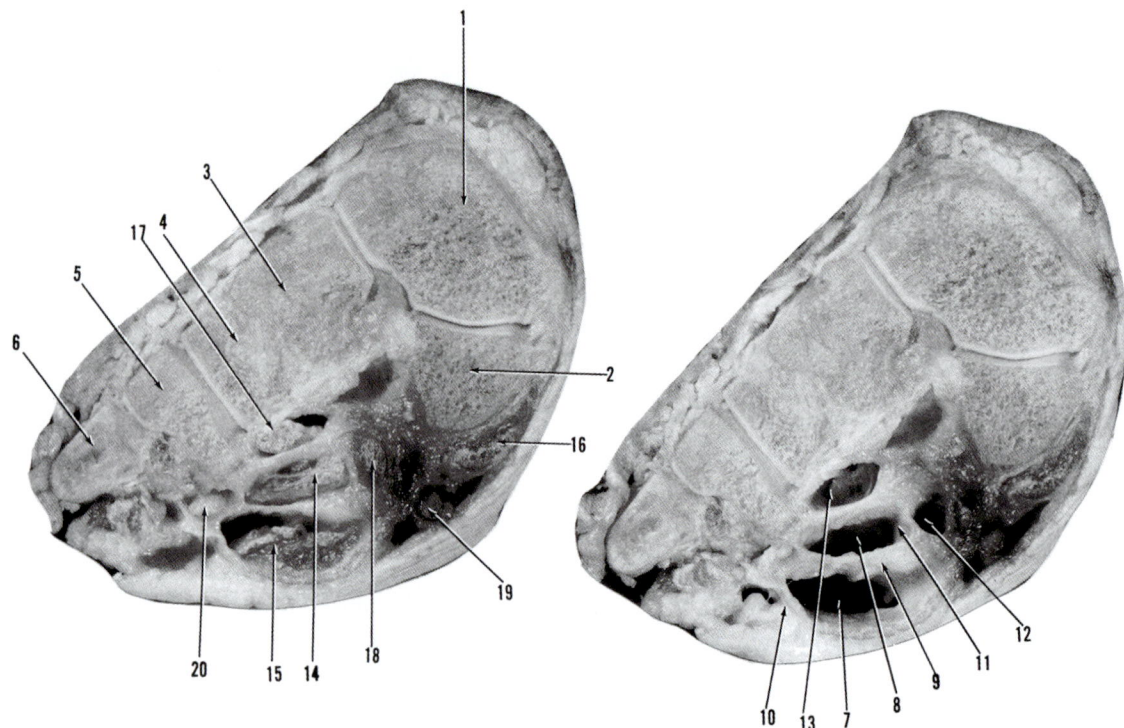

Figure 9.80 Cross-section passing through the navicular, cuneiforms 1 and 3, cuboid, and metatarsal bases 4 to 5 of left foot. Proximal surface of section. (*1*, navicular; *2*, first cuneiform, lower segment; *3*, third cuneiform, lower segment; *4*, cuboid; *5*, base metatarsal 4; *6*, base metatarsal 5; *7*, central superficial compartment; *8*, central intermediary compartment; *9*, transverse septum dividing the central compartment into superficial and intermediary; *10*, lateral intermuscular septum; *11*, medial intermuscular septum; *12*, tunnel of flexor hallucis longus tendon; *13*, tunnel of peroneus longus tendon; *14*, flexor digitorum longus with quadratus plantae; *15*, flexor digitorum brevis; *16*, abductor hallucis; *17*, peroneus longus tendon; *18*, flexor hallucis longus tendon; *19*, medial plantar neurovascular bundle; *20*, lateral plantar neurovascular bundle.)

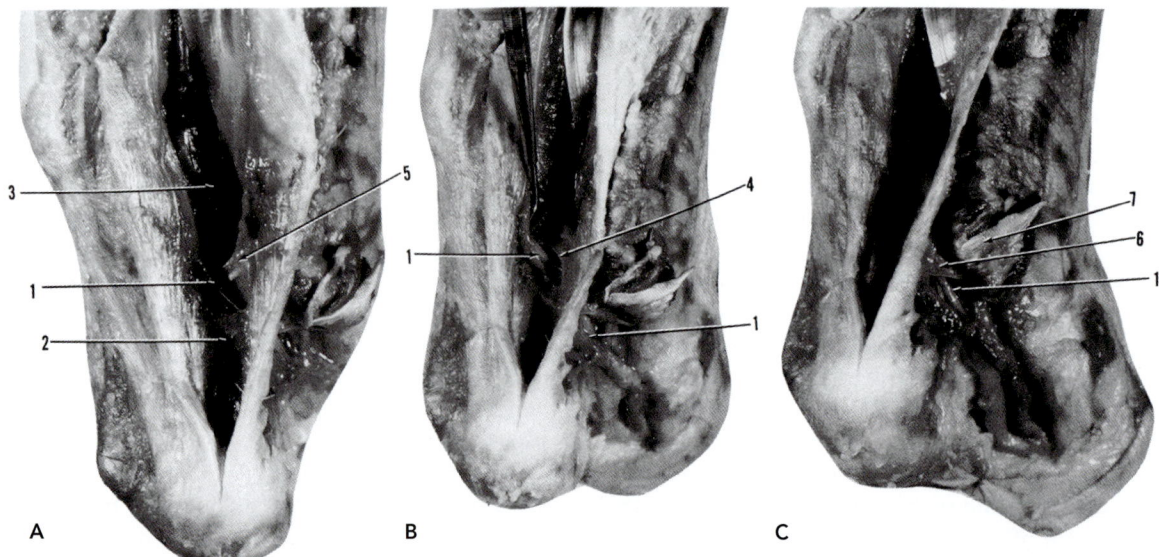

Figure 9.81 Communication between lower calcaneal chamber and central intermediary compartment of the sole of the foot. (A) In the central intermediary compartment, the lateral plantar neurovascular bundle (*1*) is "sandwiched" between a thick overlying fascia (*2*) and the transverse aponeurotic ligament (*5*) separating the proximal segment of the quadratus plantae from the neurovascular bundle and the superficial central compartment. The thin aponeurotic layer covering distally the lateral plantar bundle and the quadratus plantae has been removed. **(B)** The entrance of the lateral plantar neurovascular bundle (*1*) from the lower calcaneal chamber into the intermediary central compartment through foramina (*4*) in the medial intermuscular septum. **(C)** The lateral plantar neurovascular bundle passing through the lower calcaneal chamber, under the transverse interfascicular ligament (*6*) well exposed by reflecting the abductor hallucis muscle and its fascia (*7*).

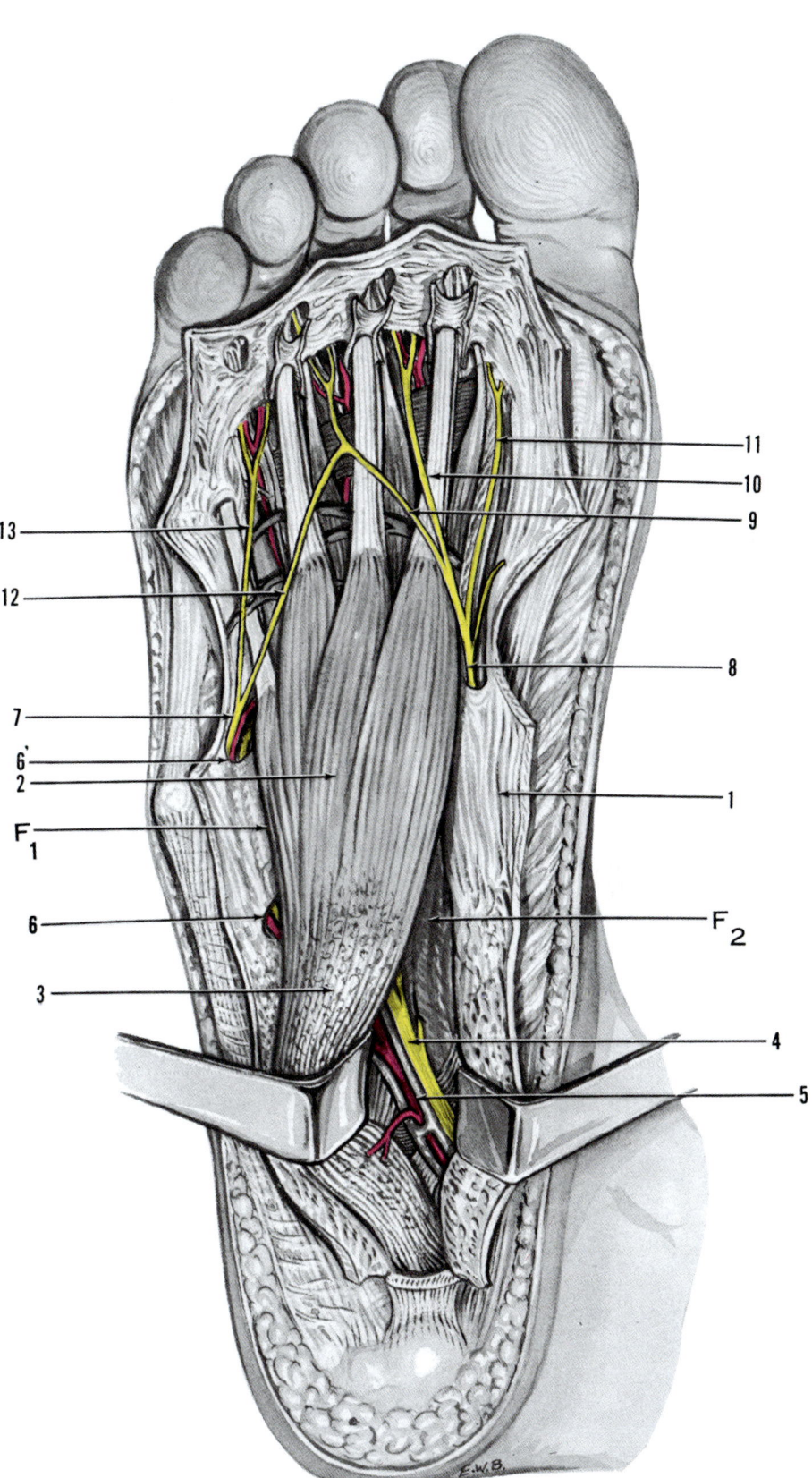

Figure 9.82 **Central compartment of the sole of the foot.** (F_1, fascial space 1 between central segment of plantar aponeurosis [*1*] and flexor digitorum brevis [*2*], which is adherent to *1* in the posterior third [*3*], where the space obliterates; F_2, fascial space 2 between flexor digitorum brevis and quadratus plantae-flexor digitorum longus [this space is crossed posteriorly by lateral plantar nerve (*4*) passing anterior to lateral plantar artery (*5*) and veins; lateral neurovascular bundle pierces lateral intermuscular septum twice—to leave the central compartment (*6*) and to reenter the latter (*6′*)]; *7*, superficial branch of lateral plantar nerve; *8*, superficial division branch of medial plantar nerve passing around medial border of flexor digitorum brevis and dividing into common digital plantar nerve to the third web space [*9*], the second web space [*10*], and the first web space [*11*]; *12*, anastomotic branch between third [*9*] and fourth [*13*] common digital plantar nerves.) (Adapted from Testut L, Jacob O. *Traité d'Anatomie Topographique avec Applications Médico-Chirurgicales.* Vol 2, 2nd ed. Doin; 1909:1081.)

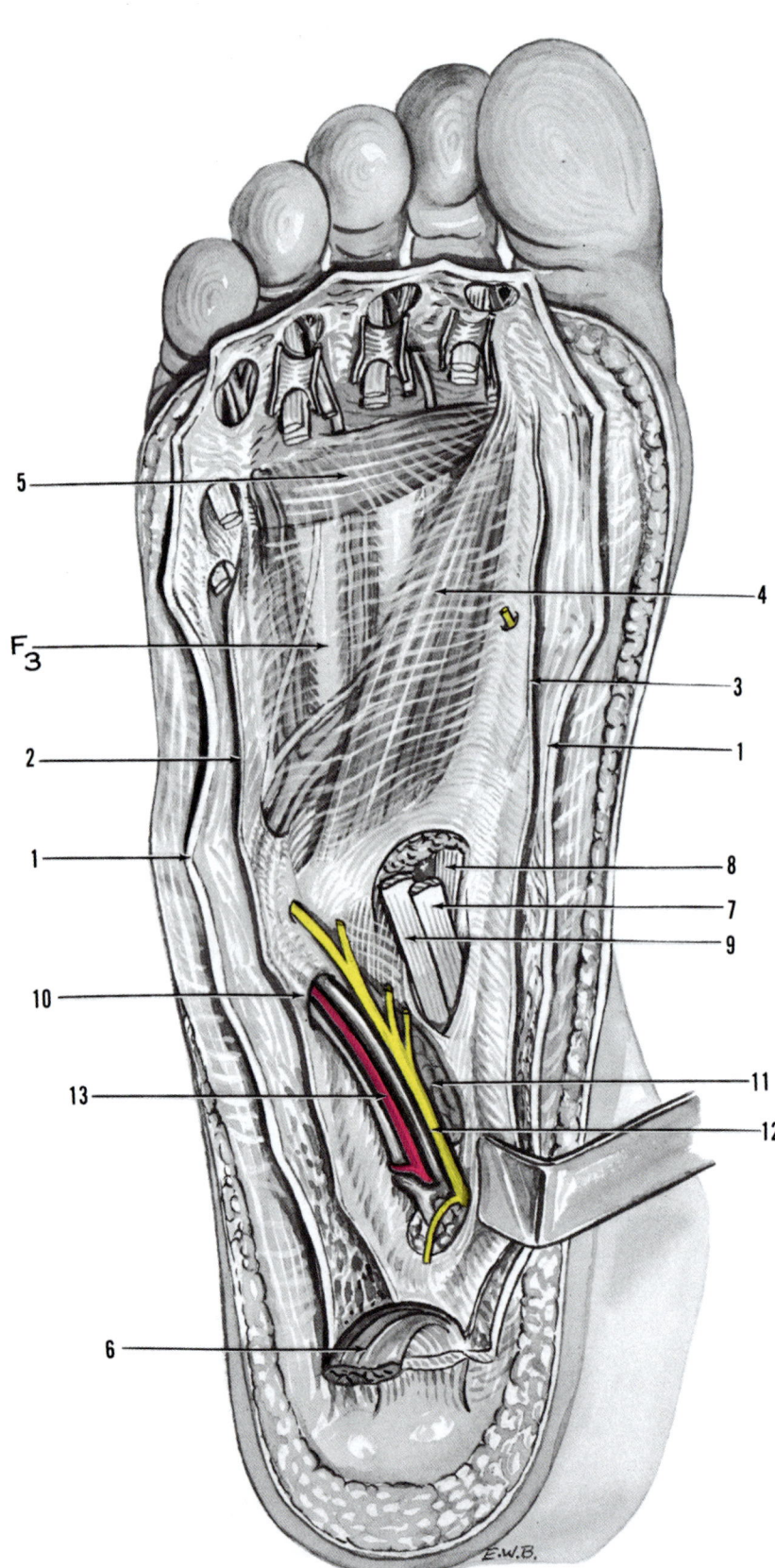

Figure 9.83 Central compartment of the sole of the foot. (F_3, fascial space 3, proximally between the flexor digitorum longus-quadratus plantae and the tarsus, distally between flexor digitorum longus and adductor hallucis oblique head, including a segment of plane of the interossei muscles; *1*, plantar aponeurosis; *2*, lateral intermuscular septum; *3*, medial intermuscular septum; *4*, adductor hallucis muscle, oblique head; *5*, adductor hallucis muscle, transverse head; *6*, flexor digitorum brevis reflected posteriorly; *7*, flexor digitorum longus tendon; *8*, flexor hallucis longus tendon; *9*, expansion band of flexor hallucis longus; *10*, foramen of exit of lateral plantar vessels; *11*, quadratus plantae muscle; *12*, lateral plantar nerve; *13*, lateral plantar artery and veins.) (Adapted from Testut L, Jacob O. *Traité d'Anatomie Topographique avec Applications Médico-Chirurgicales.* Vol 2. 2nd ed. Doin; 1909:1078.)

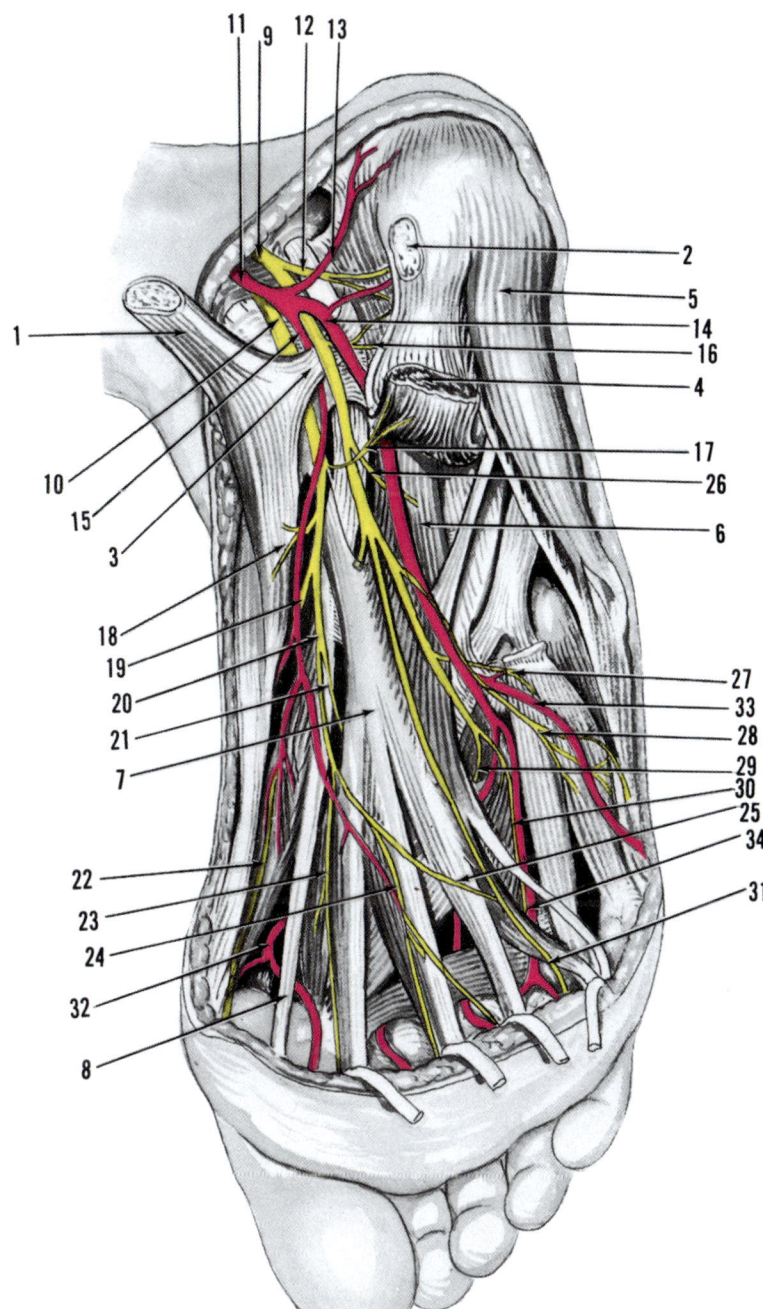

Figure 9.84 Plantar aspect of the foot. (*1*, abductor hallucis muscle detached from its origin [*2*]; *3*, interfascicular septum; *4*, flexor digitorum brevis; *5*, abductor digiti quinti; *6*, quadratus plantae; *7*, flexor digitorum longus; *8*, flexor hallucis longus; *9*, lateral plantar nerve; *10*, medial plantar nerve; *11*, posterior tibial artery; *12*, motor nerve branch to abductor digiti quinti; *13*, medial calcaneal artery; *14*, lateral plantar artery; *15*, medial plantar artery; *16*, posterior motor nerve branch to quadratus plantae; *17*, motor nerve branch to flexor digitorum brevis; *18*, motor nerve branch to abductor hallucis muscle; *19*, medial division branch of medial plantar nerve providing motor branches to medial head of flexor hallucis brevis and forming medial plantar hallucal nerve [*22*]; *20*, lateral division branch of medial plantar nerve providing motor branch to first lumbrical muscle [*21*] and then branch to lateral head of flexor hallucis brevis and forming first common superficial digital nerve [*23*]; the nerve courses laterally and provides second and third common superficial digital nerves [*24*] and anastomotic branch [*25*] to fourth common superficial nerve [*31*]; *26*, anterior motor nerve branch to quadratus plantae muscle; *27*, motor nerve branch to opponens digiti quinti; *28*, motor nerve branches to flexor digiti quinti; *29*, deep motor branch of lateral plantar nerve; *30*, motor nerve branch to adductor hallucis, transverse head; *32*, first plantar metatarsal artery; *33*, superficial plantar lateral artery to fifth toe; *34*, fourth plantar metatarsal artery.) (Adapted from Dujarier C. *Anatomie des Membres Dissection: Anatomie Topographique.* 2nd ed. Masson; 1924:322.)

medial). The deep lateral neurovascular bundle makes a medial turn, perforates the lateral intermuscular septum, and penetrates the adductor space. The lateral superficial nerve is located in the interval between the flexor digitorum brevis and the abductor digiti quinti. It provides motor branches to the short flexor, opponens, and abductor of the fifth toe and continues as the lateral plantar cutaneous nerve of the latter. The medial superficial nerve branch obliquely and superficially crosses the short flexor tendon to the fifth toe. It provides the common digital nerve to the fourth interosseous space and an anastomotic branch to the nerve of the third web space (see Fig. 9.82).

Variations of the pattern of division of the lateral plantar nerve are possible and the superficial branch may initially have a common stem that subsequently bifurcates.

The deep lateral neurovascular bundle advances transversely under the interossei fascia and then into the adductor space deep to the oblique head of the adductor hallucis. The artery is anterior to the nerve (see Fig. 9.86). Motor branches are provided to the oblique and transverse heads of the adductor hallucis, the two lateral lumbricals, and the interossei of the third, second, and first intermetatarsal spaces; a branch may extend into the lateral head of the short flexor of the hallux. This last

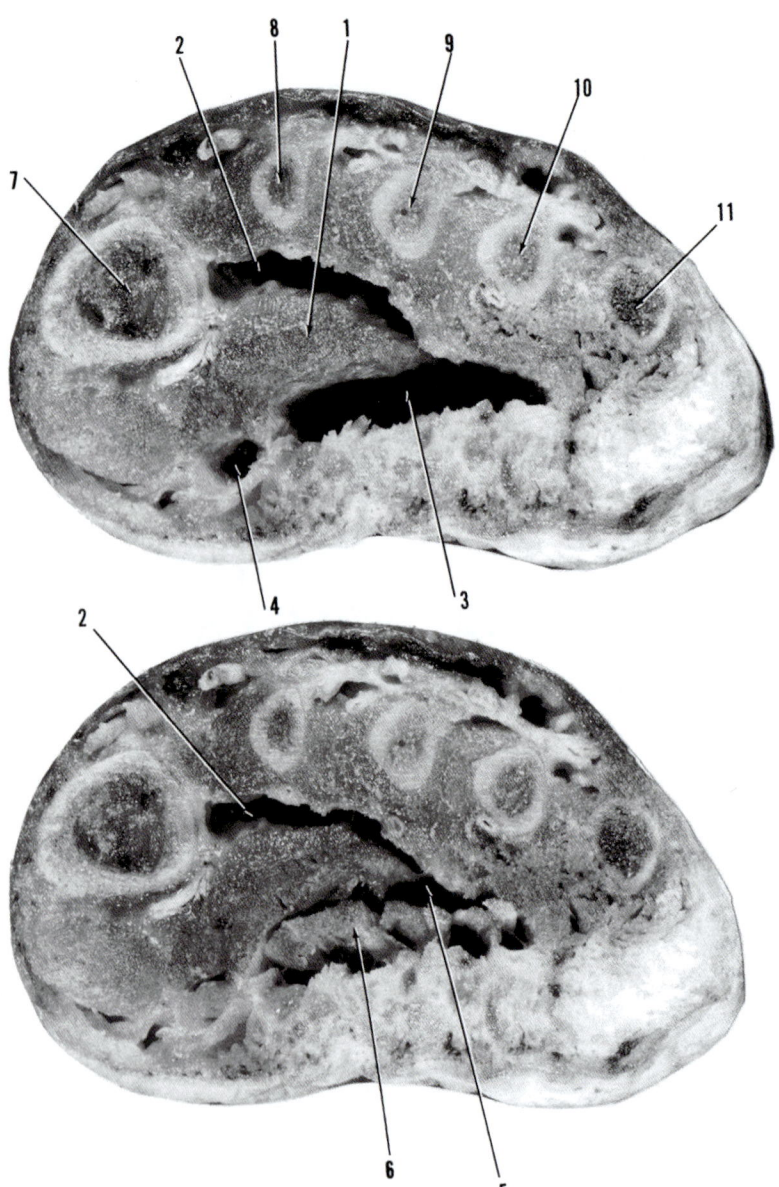

Figure 9.85 Coronal section through the metatarsal shafts of left foot distal surface of section. (*1*, adductor hallucis oblique head and adductor compartment; *2*, adductor space between adductor compartment and interossei fascia; *3*, central intermediary compartment; *4*, tunnel of flexor hallucis longus tendon; *5*, investing fascia of adductor muscle attached to the interosseous fascia and separating the adductor space (*2*) or deep space of the central compartment from the intermediary central compartment (*3*); *6*, flexor digitorum longus, brevis tendons, and lumbricals; *7-11*, metatarsals 1-5.).

branch may send an anastomotic branch to a similar motor branch arising from the medial plantar nerve and may form the anastomotic motor branch of Hallopeau, the equivalent of the Riche and Cannieu motor anastomosis as seen in the hand.[18] The lateral plantar artery crosses the bases of metatarsals 4, 3, and 2 and terminates by inosculation in the perforating deep branch of the dorsalis pedis at the base of the second metatarsal. It forms the plantar arterial arcade that provides the metatarsal arteries 1 to 4 and the proximal intermetatarsal perforating arteries 2, 3, and 4. The potential division of the metatarsal arteries into deep and superficial metatarsal and intermetatarsal arteries is presented in Chapter 7.

A pyogenic collection of the adductor space may invade the central intermediary compartment and from there extend into the lower calcaneal chamber and reach the posterior compartment of the leg.

Lateral Compartment

The lateral compartment is formed by the lateral intermuscular septum medially and the lateral component of the plantar aponeurosis on the plantar and lateral aspects. The lateral aponeurosis provides dorsolateral fibers that insert over the os calcis, the sheath of the peronei, and subsequently, the base and shaft of the fifth metatarsal. Three muscles are present in this compartment: the abductor digiti quinti, the short flexor, and the opponens of the fifth toe.

The abductor digiti quinti originates from the posterolateral and posteromedial tuberosities of the os calcis, the deep surface of the plantar aponeurosis, and the lateral intermuscular septum. The muscle is directed anterolaterally, and at the level of the base of the fifth metatarsal, it may glide over a bursa or receive supplementary fibers of attachment. The shiny, flat tendon passes through the bifurcation of the lateral plantar

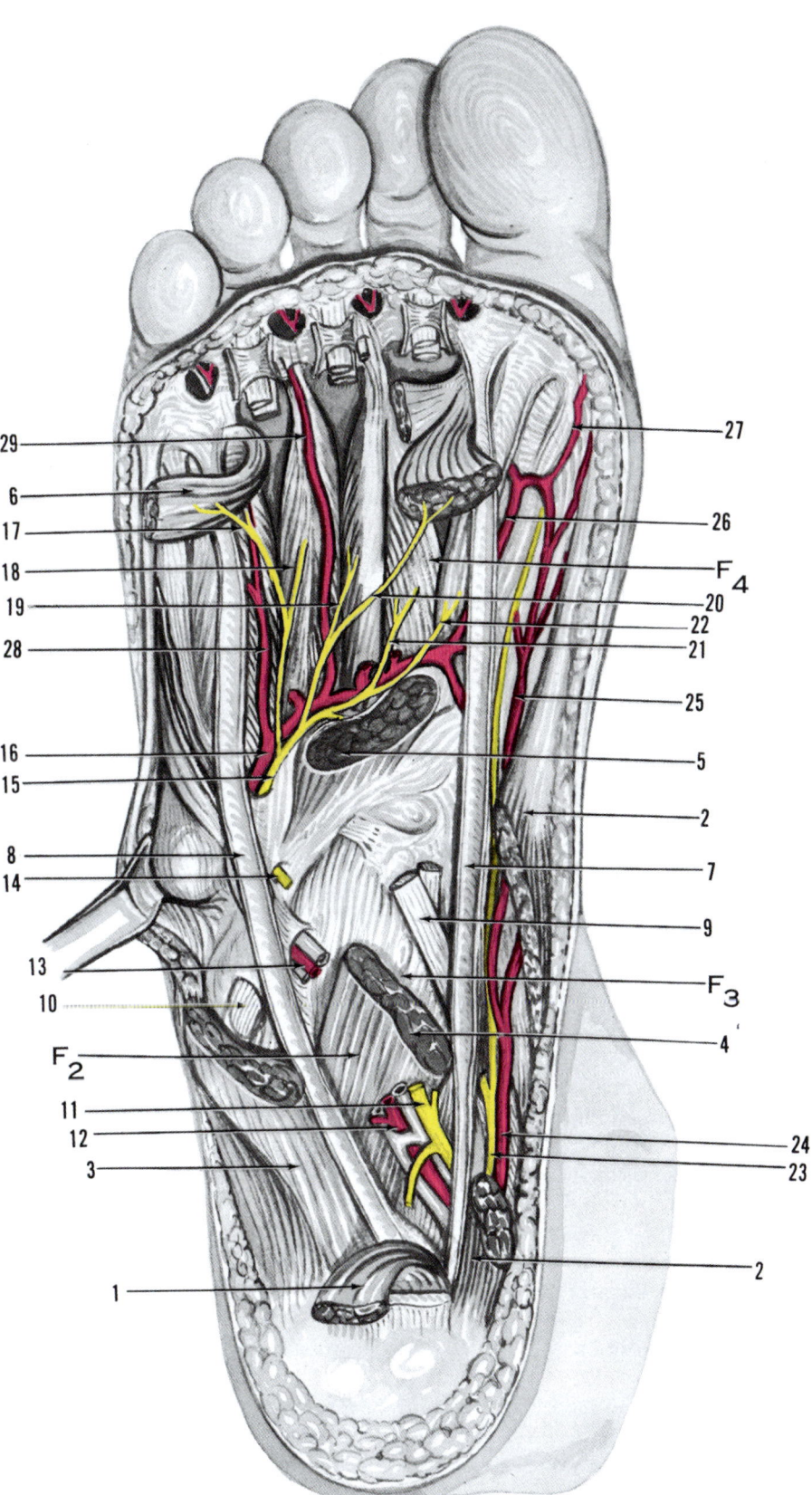

Figure 9.86 Central compartment of the sole of the foot. (F_4, fascial space 4 between oblique head of adductor hallucis muscle and plane of interossei; F_3, fascial space 3, posterior segment, between quadratus plantae muscle and osteoligamentous plane of tarsus; F_2, fascial space 2 between quadratus plantar muscle and reflected flexor digitorum brevis; *1*, flexor digitorum brevis muscle, reflected posteriorly; *2*, abductor hallucis muscle; *3*, abductor digiti quinti muscle; *4*, quadratus plantae muscle; *5*, adductor hallucis muscle, oblique head; *6*, adductor hallucis muscle, transverse head; *7*, medial intermuscular septum; *8*, lateral intermuscular septum; *9*, flexor digitorum longus tendon; *10*, peroneus longus tendon; *11*, lateral plantar nerve, exiting at *14*; *12*, lateral plantar artery, exiting at *13*; *15*, lateral plantar nerve, deep branch, passing posterior to deep branch of lateral plantar artery [*16*]; *17*, motor nerve branch to transverse head of adductor hallucis; *18*, motor nerve branch to second plantar interosseous muscle; *19*, motor nerve branch to first plantar interosseous muscle; *20*, motor branch to oblique head of adductor hallucis; *21*, motor branch to second dorsal interosseous muscle; *22*, motor branch to lateral head of flexor hallucis brevis; *23*, medial plantar nerve; *24*, medial plantar artery; *25*, superficial tibial plantar artery; *26*, first plantar metatarsal artery; *27*, medial plantar hallucal artery; *28*, *29*, plantar metatarsal arteries.)

aponeurosis and inserts on the lateral aspect of the proximal phalanx of the fifth toe and in the plantar plate of the metatarsophalangeal joint of the same toe. The deep covering fascia of the muscle is attached to the long calcaneocuboid ligament, the peroneus longus tendon sheath, and, more anteriorly, the flexor digiti quinti brevis fascia. A space is present between the deep investing fascia and the muscle. With increased pressure, the space yields into the peroneus longus tunnel or into the mid compartment.

The short flexor of the fifth toe is covered almost completely by the abductor muscle of the same toe. This small and thin muscle originates from the sheath of the peroneus longus tendon and the base of the fifth metatarsal. It inserts through a flat tendon on the base of the proximal phalanx of the toe laterally.

The opponens of the fifth toe is located on the inner aspect of the short flexor of the toe and has a common origin with the latter. The muscle inserts on the anterior two-thirds of the fifth metatarsal shaft. Quite often, this muscle is absent or fused to the short flexor.

Medial Compartment

The medial compartment of the foot is limited laterally by the medial intermuscular septum and on the plantar and medial sides by the medial component of the plantar aponeurosis. The latter inserts along the first metatarsal shaft, medial cuneiform, and navicular. Within the compartment are located the abductor hallucis muscle, the flexor hallucis brevis muscle, and the flexor hallucis longus tendon.

The abductor hallucis muscle originates from the medial calcaneal tuberosity, the deep surface of the plantar aponeurosis, the posterior end of the medial intermuscular septum, and the flexor retinaculum. It establishes fascial connections with the medial surface of the os calcis through the interfascicular septum of the calcaneal canal and with the common sheath of the flexor digitorum longus and the flexor hallucis longus tendon. Further connections are established at the level of the tuberosity of the navicular. The lateral border of the muscle is quite adherent to the plantar aponeurosis. The tendon of insertion appears on the medial aspect of the muscle; it is flat and slightly plantar in location. The inferolateral fibers insert on the medial sesamoid of the big toe in conjunction with the medial head of the flexor hallucis brevis. The superomedial fibers contribute to the transverse lamina of the extensor aponeurosis.

The flexor hallucis brevis muscle has a Y-shaped tendinous origin. The medial limb of the Y is in continuity with the tibialis posterior tendon and the lateral limb is anchored to the cuboid and the lateral cuneiform.

The muscle is oriented anteromedially, crosses obliquely the first interosseous space, and, before reaching the metatarsophalangeal joint of the big toe, divides into two heads—lateral and medial. The lateral head, which is crossed by the flexor hallucis longus tendon, has a spiral twist to its fibers and inserts on the lateral aspect of the plantar plate, the lateral sesamoid, and the base of the proximal phalanx of the big toe in conjunction with the tendon of the adductor hallucis. As mentioned previously, the medial head of the short flexor has a common insertion with the tendon of the abductor hallucis.

The tendon of the flexor hallucis longus, after being crossed on its plantar aspect by the flexor digitorum longus tendon, provides a tendinous slip to the latter but remains in the medial compartment and courses initially between the medial intermuscular septum and the abductor hallucis. It obliquely crosses the lateral head of the flexor hallucis brevis and enters the fibrous tunnel at the level of the plantar plate of the big toe.

The medial plantar neurovascular bundle reaches the medial compartment through the upper chamber of the calcaneal canal (see Fig. 9.84). The nerve is anterior to the artery. As the flexor digitorum longus tendon becomes oblique to enter the middle compartment, the neurovascular bundle passes over the same tendon superficially. The artery crosses the nerve superficially and locates on the medial side of the nerve. Until their branching, the medial plantar nerve and artery remain on the medial side of the flexor hallucis longus tendon and nearly within the substance of the medial intermuscular septum. The nerve provides two motor branches to the abductor hallucis muscle; they are located two and three fingerbreadths behind the tuberosity of the navicular and enter the muscle from the deep lateral border.[7] These branches pass through fibrous tunnels and superficially cross the vessels. A third motor branch is provided by the medial plantar nerve to the flexor hallucis brevis and penetrates the muscle from the medial border. Slightly distal to the level of the tuberosity of the fifth metatarsal, the medial plantar nerve divides into two branches: medial and lateral. The medial branch courses along the lateral side of the abductor hallucis tendon, provides multiple motor branches to the medial head of the flexor hallucis brevis, and terminates as the medial plantar digital nerve of the big toe. The lateral branch bifurcates and its medial branch innervates the lateral head of the flexor hallucis brevis and the first lumbrical and terminates as the common plantar digital nerve to the first web space. The lateral branch of the bifurcation turns around the medial border of the flexor digitorum brevis and divides into the motor branches to the second lumbrical and the sensory common plantar digital nerves to the second and third web spaces. The nerve to the last space may receive an anastomotic branch from the common digital nerve of the fourth space.

The medial plantar artery, located on the medial side of the nerve, has variable divisions. In general, the artery divides into two branches, superficial and deep. The superficial branch emerges between the abductor hallucis and the flexor digitorum brevis and divides into the superficial tibial plantar artery of the big toe and the common plantar digital artery. The former courses over the flexor hallucis brevis muscle on the tibial side of the flexor hallucis longus tendon. On the medial border of the first metatarsal neck, the superficial tibial plantar artery passes between the medial head of the flexor hallucis brevis and the bone and anastomoses with the first plantar metatarsal artery.

The common plantar digital artery crosses obliquely the flexor hallucis longus tendon, passes between the plantar aponeurosis and the flexor digitorum brevis, and provides the common digital plantar arteries 1 to 3, which will join the corresponding plantar metatarsal arteries. As mentioned previously, a superficial plantar arterial arcade is formed when the third common digital plantar artery receives a similar superficial branch from the lateral plantar artery.

The deep branch of the medial plantar artery is divided into a tibial and a peroneal branch. The deep tibial branch courses along the skeletal margin of the foot and may anastomose with the first plantar metatarsal artery or continue into the dorsal tibial hallucal artery. The deep peroneal branch passes dorsal to the peroneus longus tendon near its insertion and terminates in the deep plantar arterial arch.

A fascial space is present between the deep surface of the abductor hallucis muscle and its investing fascia. This is a closed space and may yield only into the subcutaneous space.

BALL OF THE FOOT AND BIG TOE

▶ Surface Anatomy

The ball of the foot extends from the level of the metatarsal necks to the distal plantar digital flexion crease. The skin is convex in the sagittal plane as it curves dorsally. The flexion crease is convex distally, with the apex centered on the second toe. It crosses the toes at the level of the proximal phalanges, and in the little toe, it may reach the proximal interphalangeal joint. The five metatarsal heads and the medial and the lateral sesamoids of the big toe are easily felt through the skin.

▶ Skin

The skin of the ball of the foot is thick and semimobile. It tenses and acquires fixation with the extension of the toes. The subcutaneous adipose layer is thin at the level of the dermal insertion of the longitudinal bands of the plantar aponeurosis. The cushioning of the ball of the foot is provided by the pretendinous submetatarsal adipose cushions and the intermetatarsal fat bodies.[19]

Subcutaneous bursae may be present under the heads of the first and fifth metatarsals. Venous longitudinal branches arising from the distal venous arcade course distally toward the corresponding web spaces to drain in the dorsal venous system.

▶ Plantar Aponeurosis and Subcompartments and Contents

The plantar aponeurosis, proximal to the metatarsal heads, is structured into five bands—one medial, three central, and one lateral. The medial and the lateral bands course obliquely over the metatarsophalangeal joint area of the big and little toes. The central bands diverge and proceed individually toward the first interdigital space, the third toe, and the fourth interdigital space. They insert into the dermis distal to the metatarsophalangeal joint and segmentally close the subcutaneous space. The distal fibers pass over the natatory ligaments and contribute to their formation. No fibers reach or insert on the skin at the level of the plantar digital crease, where a transverse band of adipose tissue is interposed between the skin and the most frontal part of the natatory ligament.

Proximal to the metatarsal heads, transversely oriented aponeurotic thin bands cross the plantar aponeurosis and extend into the dermis. Adipose tissue is retained between the layers. The medial and lateral ends of these transverse bands turn anteriorly and contribute to the formation of the natatory ligaments.

The longitudinally oriented aponeurotic bands, the transverse fasciculi proximally and the transversely oriented natatory ligaments distally, delineate spaces that are oval to quadrilateral in shape. Adipose tissue corresponding to the fat bodies protrudes in these spaces and forms the monticule of the skin. Within these windows course superficially the superficial common plantar digital arteries 1 to 4 and the common digital plantar nerves to spaces 1 to 4. The common plantar digital arteries are deeper and well covered with the fat body.

The medial plantar nerve of the big toe courses under the medial prong of the plantar aponeurosis. The lateral plantar nerve of the fifth toe and the accompanying plantar arterial branch pass under the lateral prong of the plantar aponeurosis.

Proximal to the metatarsal heads, each longitudinal band of the plantar aponeurosis extends, on each side of the corresponding long flexor tendon, two aponeurotic septa (Fig. 9.87). These septa insert on the interosseous fascia, the fascia of the transverse head of the adductor hallucis, the deep transverse metatarsal ligament, and the plantar plate and its junction with the accessory collateral ligament of the metatarsophalangeal joint. The two septa of a given band may interchange fibers proximally and form a foramina through which the long flexor tendons pass and may also extend insertional fibers to the adjacent septa.

The longitudinal septa separate the long flexor tendon from the lumbrical muscle and the origin of the latter limits the proximal extension of the sagittal septum.

At the level of the metatarsal heads, the septa are in continuity distally with vertical fibers (Figs. 9.88 and 9.89). These fibers arise from the sides of the fibrous flexor tendon sheath and from the plantar plate. They course plantarward, connect with the longitudinal aponeurotic band, and insert with the latter on the skin. Some of the vertical fibers arch over the flexor tendon sheath and form a compartment filled with adipose tissue, called the "submetatarsal cushion."[19] Both sesamoids of the big toe are covered by such a common cushion.

At the level of the metatarsophalangeal joint on the tibial side, a fascia splits off the longitudinal septum and forms a compartment for the lumbrical tendon. The intermetatarsal capitular space, over the plantar aspect of the transverse metatarsal ligament, is occupied by an encapsulated fat body that covers the common plantar digital neurovascular bundle.[19]

Distal to the level of the metatarsal heads, the fibrous sheaths of the flexor hallucis longus and of the flexor digitorum longus-brevis are joined by a transversely directed retinacular ligament, arching from sheath to sheath, called the "mooring ligament."

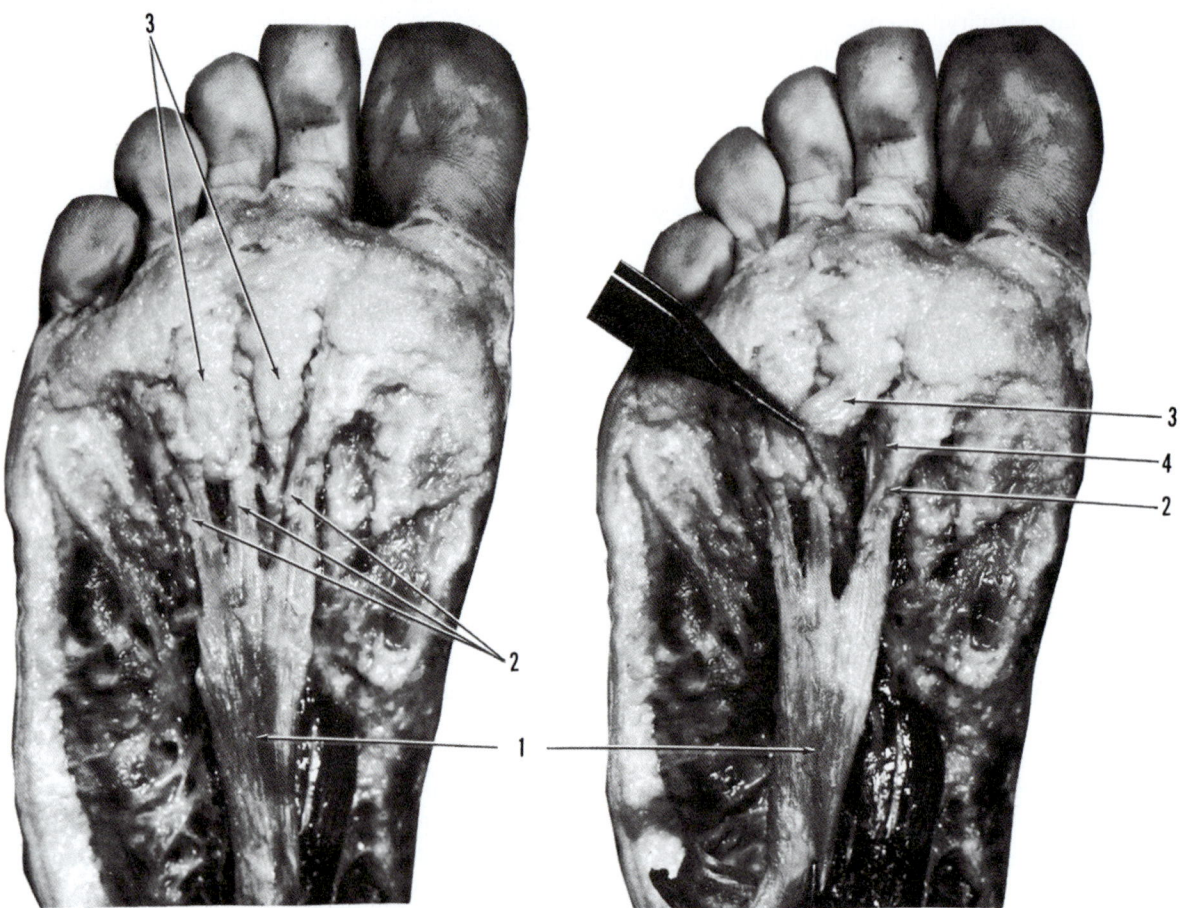

Figure 9.87 **Longitudinal bands of the plantar aponeurosis.** (*1*, plantar aponeurosis; *2*, longitudinal superficial tracts 2, 3, and 4 of plantar aponeurosis; *3*, fat bodies; *4*, septum of deep component of longitudinal tract of plantar aponeurosis.)

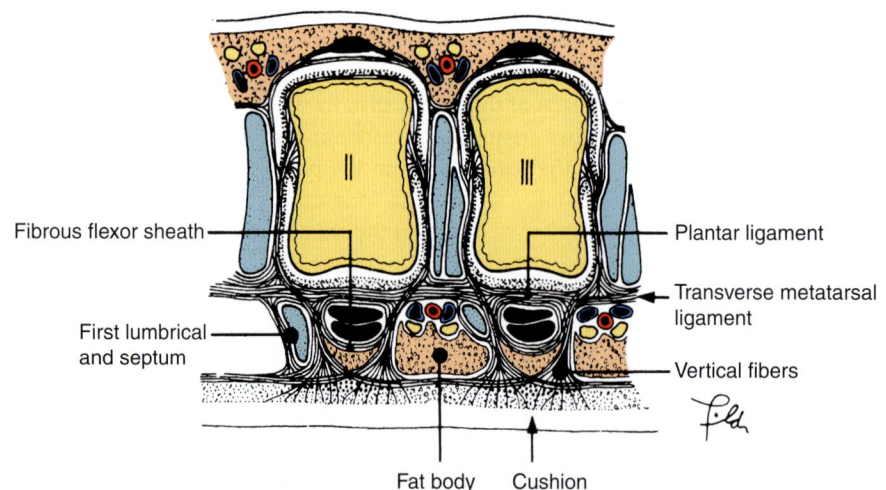

Figure 9.88 **Cross-section through metatarsal heads 2 and 3.** (From Bojsen-Møller F. Anatomy of the forefoot, normal and pathologic. *Clin Orthop.* 1979;142:17.)

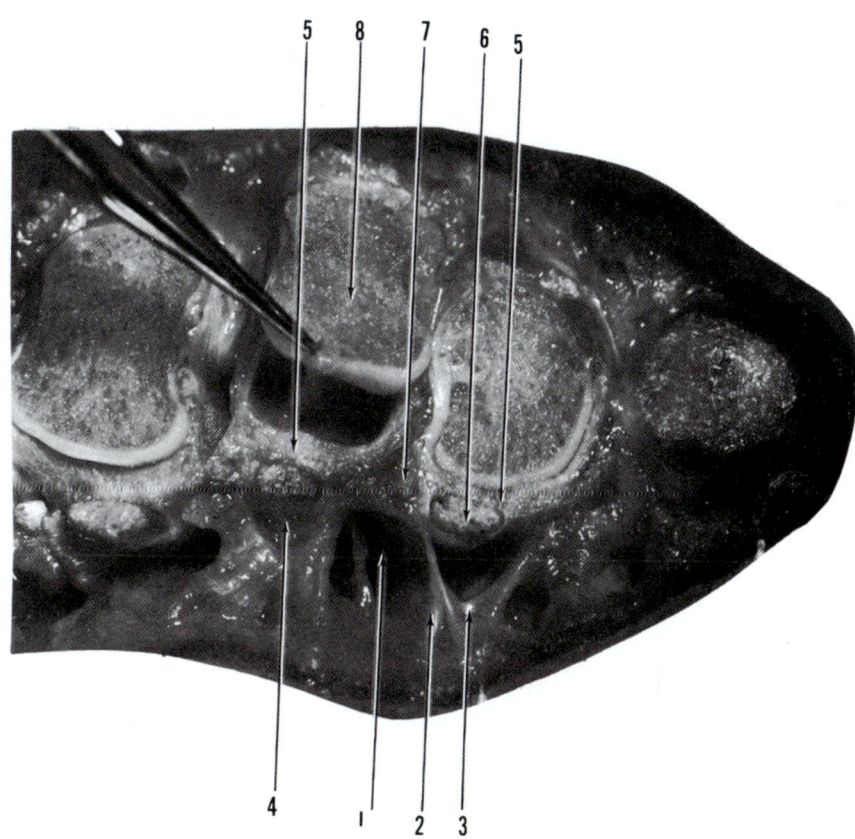

Figure 9.89 **Cross-section passing through metatarsal heads 2, 3, and 4.** (*1*, chamber retaining fat body; *2*, vertical fibers arising from flexor tendon sheath; *3*, arciform fibers forming chamber of fatty, preflexor cushion [*4*]; *5*, plantae plate; *6*, flexors digitorum longus and brevis in their fibrous tunnel; *7*, lumbrical tendon; *8*, metatarsal head.)

The distal segment of the ball of the foot and web space is crossed transversely by the natatory or interdigital ligament. This ligament has a multilamellar (six to eight transverse layers) or retinacular weblike structure.[19] It is deep to the insertional fibers of the longitudinal bands of the plantar aponeurosis. It attaches to the flexor tendon sheath and the mooring ligament and covers the intertendinous space on the plantar aspect of the web space. The plantar digital neurovascular bundle passes dorsal to this ligament. Superficially, the natatory ligament attaches to the dermis and retains within its layer a substantial amount of adipose tissue.

Proximal transection of the plantar aponeurosis and detachment of the longitudinal septa allows reflection of the aponeurosis. The superficial common plantar digital nerves and arteries now are crossing the plantar aspect of the flexor digitorum brevis tendons. These structures with the flexor digitorum longus are retracted to bring into view the transverse head of the adductor hallucis and a segment of the interossei covered by their fascia.

The transverse head of the adductor hallucis arises from the proximal border of the plantar plate of the third, fourth, and fifth metatarsophalangeal joints; the proximal border of the deep transverse metatarsal ligament of the second, third, and fourth spaces; and the lateral crux of the lateral segment of the plantar aponeurosis.

The covering fascia gives attachment to the longitudinal septa of the plantar aponeurosis. The transversely oriented muscle fibers overlap and the longest fibers are the most posterior and have a lateral origin. The transverse head of the adductor hallucis joins the oblique head for a common insertion on the lateral aspect of the proximal phalanx of the big toe and the lateral sesamoid.

Opposite the proximal border of the second, third, and fourth deep transverse metatarsal ligaments and the transverse head of the adductor hallucis, small apertures for the passage of the common plantar digital arteries are present. These openings are seen at times as a foramina through the substance of the deep transverse metatarsal ligament. Reflection of the transverse head of the adductor hallucis brings into view the origins of the common plantar digital arteries and of the premetatarsal vascular triangle.

Over the central metatarsals 2 to 4, the vascular triangle is located on the plantar aspect of the corresponding metatarsal neck (Fig. 9.90). The base is distal and formed by the proximal border of the plantar plate, the apex is proximal, and the sides are formed by the parting interossei muscles. The plantar metatarsal artery bifurcates in this space into lateral and medial branches. Each branch passes between the distal border of the transverse head of the adductor of the big toe and the proximal border of the deep transverse metatarsal ligament and courses on the plantar aspect of the latter as the common digital plantar artery. Quite often only the lateral limb of the bifurcation is substantial or present, and this continues as the common digital plantar artery and joins distally, in the web space, the distal perforating branch of the corresponding dorsal metatarsal artery, which in turn divides into the plantar digital arteries of the adjacent toes.

the lateral sesamoid, the lateral border of the plantar plate, the lateral head of the flexor hallucis brevis, and the distal end of the medial intermuscular septum.

Anterior to the aponeurotic septa, the metatarsophalangeal joint is covered by the pretendinous, premetatarsal fat or cushion. The cushion is retained in the compartment by vertical fibers extending from each side of the joint and arching at a distance over the fibrous tunnel of the flexor hallucis longus tendon. This adipose cushion covers both sesamoids.

Distally, the medial ends of the anchoring arms of the natatory ligaments insert on the long flexor tunnel. Proximally, the lateral septum may send a strong connecting band to the medial septum of the second toe, and it is also a termination point for the medial intermuscular septum.

The deep transverse metatarsal ligament joins the lateral border of the plantar plate of the big toe to the medial border of the plantar plate of the second toe. The adductor tendons reach the big toe dorsal to the deep transverse metatarsal ligament. The tendon of the transverse head of the adductor inserts on the extensor aponeurosis and the remaining fibers pass over the insertional fibers of the oblique head of the adductor hallucis, share their insertion on the lateral sesamoid, and terminate on the fibrous sheath of the flexor hallucis longus.

The oblique head of the adductor hallucis has three components: medial, central, and lateral. The medial component, with fleshy fibers, inserts directly on the lateral sesamoid. The central deep component is tendinous and takes a firm grip on the plantar aspect of the lateral sesamoid. The lateral component has a broader tendon that inserts on the lateral sesamoid and the plantar lateral aspect of the proximal phalanx, with minor contribution to the extensor aponeurosis (Fig. 9.92).

The lateral head of the flexor hallucis penetrates the plantar plate through a flat tunnel laterally at a distance from the tendons of the adductor hallucis. The fibers insert on the lateral aspect of the plantar plate, the central and medial aspects of the lateral sesamoid, and the lateral aspect of the proximal phalanx. The tendons of the adductor hallucis and of the lateral head of the short flexor of the big toe are conjoint only at the distal insertional point.

The medial head of the flexor hallucis brevis inserts on the medial aspect of the plantar plate, the lateral and central aspect of the medial sesamoid, and the medial aspect of the base of the proximal phalanx in conjunction with the abductor hallucis tendon (Fig. 9.93). The inferolateral tendinous fibers of the latter insert on the medial sesamoid and on the medial plantar tubercle of the proximal phalanx of the big toe. The superomedial tendinous fibers connect with the medial aspect of the transverse lamina of the hallucal extensor aponeurosis. A triangle is formed on the plantar aspect of the first metatarsal neck and is similar to the ones found in the lesser toes (see Fig. 9.90). This triangle has a distal base that corresponds to the proximal border of the plantar plate. The apex and the sides are formed by the parting of the two heads of the flexor hallucis brevis muscle. The first plantar metatarsal artery, after coursing proximally on the plantar aspect of the first dorsal interosseous muscle, passes from the lateral side between the flexor hallucis brevis muscle and the first metatarsal shaft. It appears in the depths

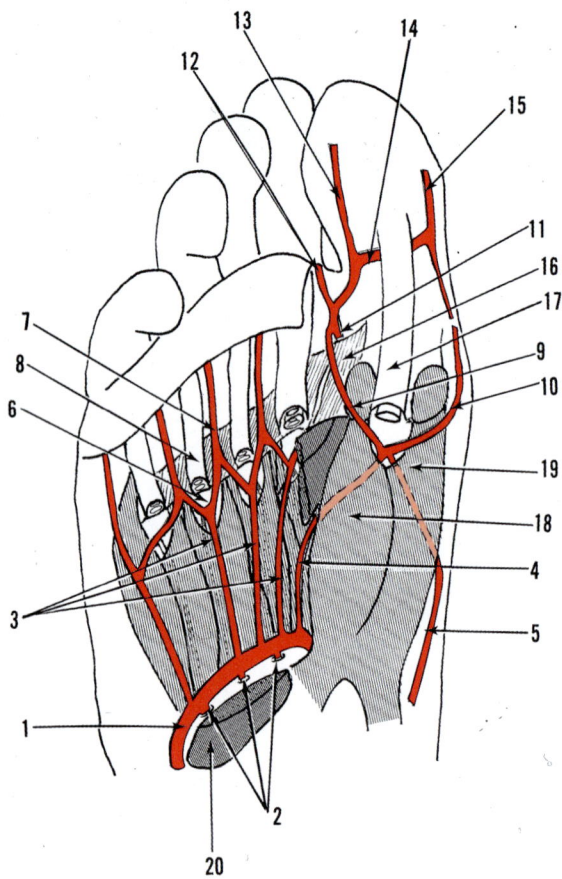

Figure 9.90 Disposition of the plantar arteries in the forefoot. (*1*, plantar arterial arcade; *2*, proximal perforating arteries; *3*, metatarsal arteries 2, 3, 4; *4*, first plantar metatarsal artery; *5*, medial branch of medial plantar artery; *6*, vascular triangle formed by interossei and proximal border of plantar plate; *7*, common plantar digital artery; *8*, flexor tunnel; *9*, lateral division branch of first plantar metatarsal artery; *10*, medial division branch of first plantar metatarsal artery; *11*, vertical segment of first dorsal metatarsal artery; *12*, medial plantar artery of second toe; *13*, lateral plantar hallucal artery; *14*, transverse anastomotic branch of plantar hallucal arteries; *15*, medial plantar hallucal artery; *16*, deep transverse metatarsal ligament; *17*, flexor hallucis longus tunnel; *18*, flexor hallucis brevis, lateral head; *19*, flexor hallucis brevis, medial head; *20*, adductor hallucis muscle, oblique head.)

Further details concerning the contribution of the metatarsal arteries to the digital arteries are provided in Chapter 7.

▶ Big Toe

The prominent head of the first metatarsal is covered on the plantar and the dorsomedial aspect by two subcutaneous bursae.

On the plantar aspect, a thin layer of subcutaneous fat is present, which covers the oblique superficial aponeurotic tract of the plantar fascia. Two deep aponeurotic septa extend from the superficial tract on each side of the flexor hallucis longus tendon (Fig. 9.91). The medial septum inserts on the medial sesamoid, the medial border of the plantar plate, and the medial head of the flexor hallucis brevis. The lateral septum inserts on

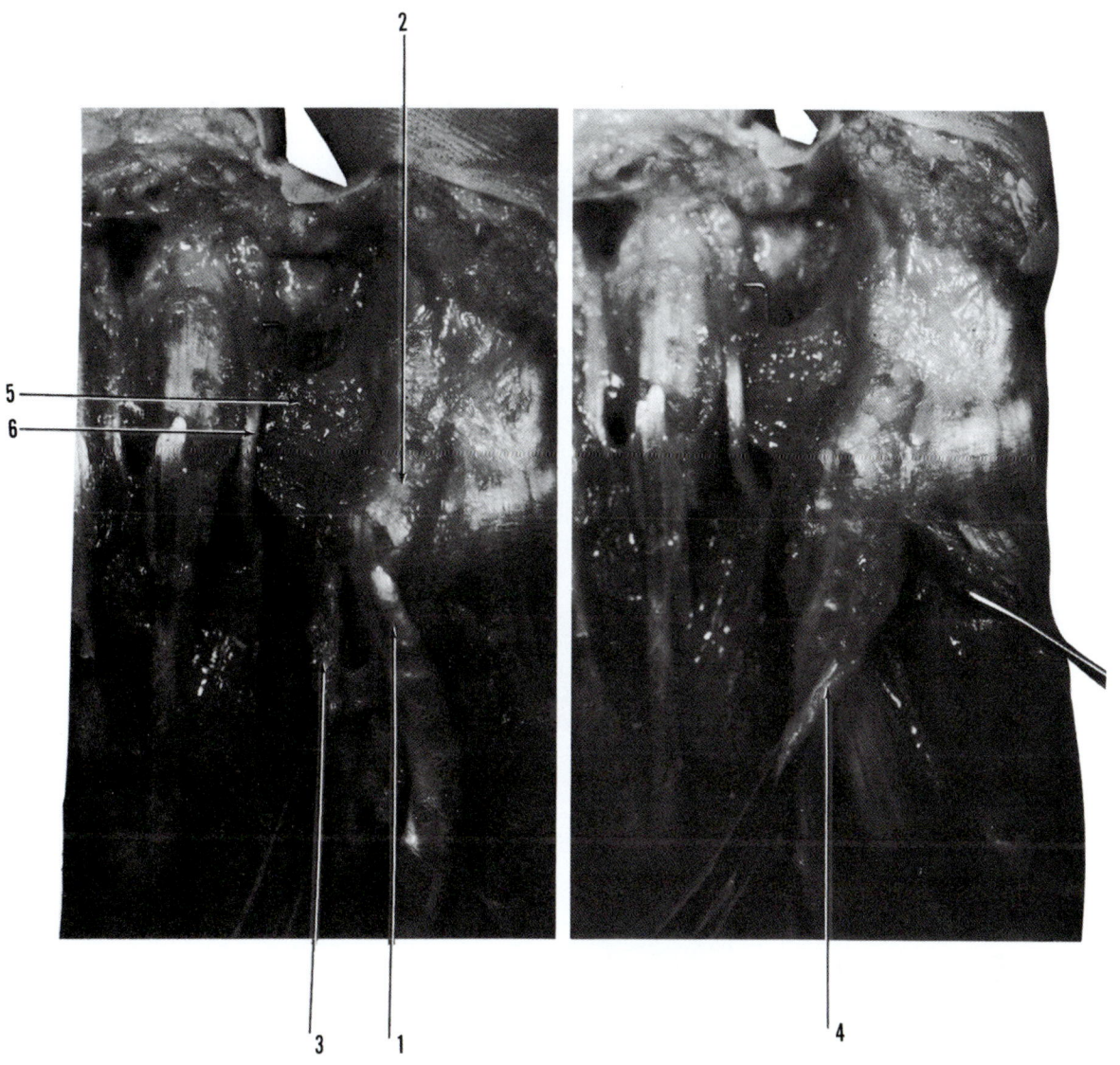

Figure 9.91 **Plantar aspect of the first intercapitular space.** (*1*, flexor hallucis longus; *2*, tunnel of 1; *3*, lateral vertical septum of first longitudinal band of plantar aponeurosis; *4*, medial vertical septum of first longitudinal band of plantar aponeurosis; *5*, intermetatarsal ligament; *6*, lumbrical tendon.)

of the described triangle and bifurcates into lateral and medial branches. The deep medial branch of the medial plantar artery passes between the medial head of the flexor hallucis brevis and the first metatarsal shaft from the medial side and joins the bifurcation point of the first plantar metatarsal artery (see Fig. 9.90). The anastomosis and the branching form a cruciform arterial pattern. The medial division branch of the first plantar metatarsal artery passes plantar to the flexor hallucis longus tendon, turns over or around the medial sesamoid, and joins the tibial plantar hallucal artery, which is a branch of the perforating branch of the first dorsal metatarsal artery. The medial division branch of the first plantar metatarsal artery is joined on the medial aspect of the big toe by the medial or tibial marginal artery, which is a lateral division of the superficial branch of the medial plantar artery. The lateral division branch of the first plantar metatarsal artery exits from the vascular triangle and crosses the plantar aspect of the lateral head of the flexor hallucis brevis and the adductor hallucis. It passes around the lateral sesamoid on the plantar aspect of the deep transverse metatarsal ligament and joins the perforating branch of the first dorsal metatarsal artery in the first web space. Subsequent to this anastomosis, the first dorsal metatarsal artery divides into the plantar lateral artery of the big toe and the medial plantar artery of the second toe.

The lateral plantar hallucal artery sends a transverse branch across the mid segment of the proximal phalanx between the bone and the flexor hallucis longus tendon and forms the medial plantar hallucal artery, which is joined by the medial division branch of the first plantar metatarsal artery. The lateral plantar hallucal artery is the major artery of the big toe and the variations of the arterial supply are presented in Chapter 7.

The first common plantar digital nerve provides the lateral plantar nerve to the big toe, which passes plantar to the deep transverse metatarsal ligament. The medial plantar digital nerve

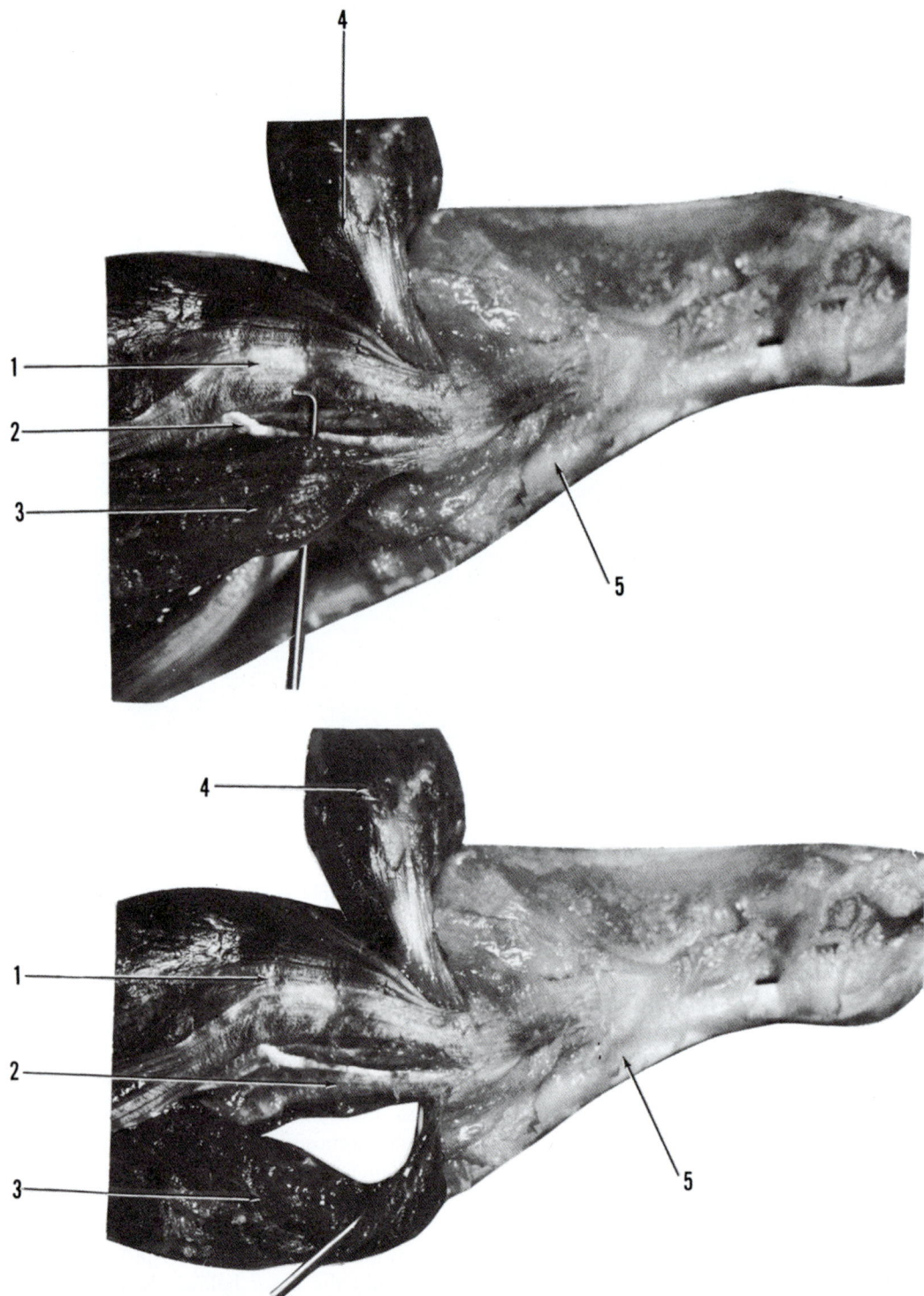

Figure 9.92 **Lateral aspect of the big toe.** The first metatarsal is removed, and the proximal phalanx is preserved. (*1-3*, three components of adductor hallucis oblique head—lateral [*1*], central [*2*], medial [*3*]; *4*, transverse component of adductor hallucis; *5*, flexor hallucis longus tendon within its tunnel.)

Chapter 9: Cross-Sectional and Topographic Anatomy   507

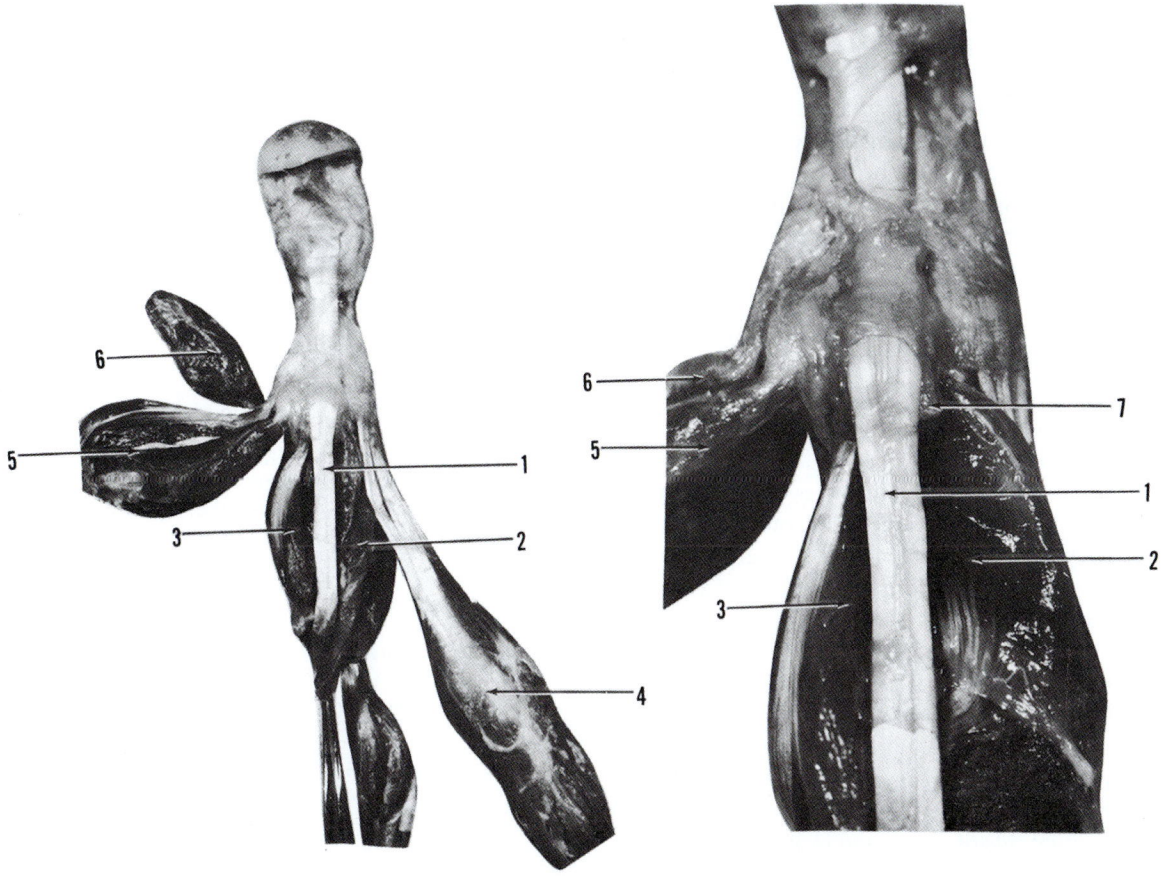

Figure 9.93 **Plantar aspect of the big toe.** (*1*, flexor hallucis longus tendon; *2*, flexor hallucis brevis muscle, medial head; *3*, flexor hallucis brevis muscle, lateral head; *4*, abductor hallucis muscle; *5*, adductor hallucis muscle, oblique head; *6*, adductor hallucis muscle, transverse head; *7*, proximal border of plantar plate.)

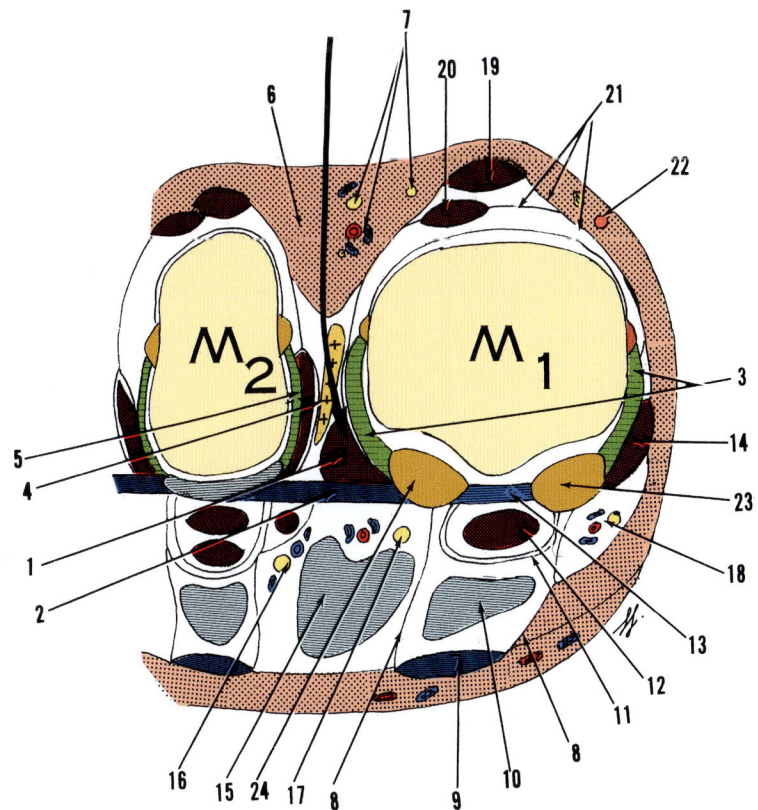

Figure 9.94 **Surgical approach to the first web space and to the adductor hallucis tendon is indicated by the vertical arrow.** (*1*, adductor hallucis tendon wedged between the deep transverse metatarsal ligament (*2*) and capsule (*3*) of the metatarsophalangeal joint of the hallux; *2*, deep transverse metatarsal ligament; *3*, capsule-collateral ligaments of metatarsophalangeal joint of the hallux; *4*, bursa interposed between metatarsal heads 1-2; *5*, tendon of first dorsal interosseous muscle; *6*, adipose wedge; *7*, branches of deep peroneal nerve and first dorsal metatarsal vessels; *8*, vertical septum extended from plantar aponeurosis; *9*, longitudinal band of plantar aponeurosis; *10*, preflexor tendon-tunnel fat pad; *11*, tunnel of flexor hallucis longus; *12*, flexor hallucis longus tendon; *13*, intersesamoid ligament; *14*, abductor hallucis tendon; *15*, fat body covering the plantar digital neurovascular bundle; *16*, plantar tibial digital neurovascular bundle to the second toe; *17*, plantar lateral digital neurovascular bundle to the first toe; *18*, plantar medial digital neurovascular bundle to the first toe; *19*, extensor hallucis longus tendon and extensor hallucis brevis tendon [*20*] with the transverse lamina [*21*]; *22*, dorsomedial hallucal nerve; *23*, medial hallucal sesamoid; *24*, lateral hallucal sesamoid.)

of the big toe courses along the medial side of the flexor hallucis longus tunnel. It is superficial to the corresponding tibial plantar hallucal artery.

On the dorsal aspect of the big toe, the dorsal veins and superficial nerve branches are located within or under a superficial fascia. The dorsomedial vein of the big toe joins the medial arm of the dorsal venous arcade and contributes to the formation of the greater saphenous vein.

The distal dorsal arterial supply of the big toe is provided by a branch of the first dorsal metatarsal artery or, predominantly, by a branch from the plantar medial hallucal artery. Details of variations are presented in Chapter 7.

In the first web space, the first dorsal metatarsal artery dives plantarward and is accompanied by the perforating veins leading to the dorsal venous arcade.

The dorsomedial nerve of the big toe is provided by the medial branch of the medial dorsal cutaneous nerve of the foot. The dorsolateral aspect of the big toe is innervated by the medial division branch of the deep peroneal nerve and may receive contribution from the medial dorsal cutaneous branch of the superficial peroneal nerve.

Reflection of the superficial fascia and of the neurovascular structures exposes the extensor aponeurosis anchoring the extensor hallucis longus tendon to the lateral and medial aspects of the plantar plate and to the sides of the proximal phalanx. A supplementary slip of the extensor hallucis longus is found on the medial side of the tendon in an average of 50%; this slip inserts on the proximal phalanx. The extensor hallucis brevis tendon is located on the peroneal side of the extensor hallucis longus tendon, under the extensor aponeurosis. The possible variations concerning the supplementary tendinous slip to the dorsum of the big toe are presented in Chapter 5.

The surgical access to the adductor hallucis insertional tendon is as indicated by the large vertical arrow in Figure 9.94. The dissection is to pass through the adipose wedge between metatarsals 1 and 2. The dorsal metatarsal artery and the division branches of the deep and superficial peroneal nerves are dissected "bluntly" and retracted sideways. Quite often, the dorsal aponeurosis may form a superficial transverse ligament that is incised, giving access to the depth of the interspace. The adductor tendon is "in the depth" wedged between the lateral capsule and sesamoid of the big toe and the attached deep transverse metatarsal ligament. It is covered by a fascia. The plantar digital neurovascular bundles—medial of the second toe and lateral of the big toe—are located under the deep transverse metatarsal ligament.

REFERENCES

1. Testut L, Jacob O. *Traité d'Anatomie Topographique Avec Applications Médico-Chirurgicales.* Vol 2. 2nd ed. Doin; 1909:1022-1114.
2. Winckler G. Les veines du pied. *Arch Anat Histol Embryol.* 1954-1955;37:175.
3. Horwitz MT. Normal anatomy and variations of the peripheral nerves of the leg and foot. *Arch Surg.* 1938;36:626.
4. Bellocq P, Meyer P. Contribution a l'étude de l'aponevrose dorsale du pied (Fascia dorsalis pedis, P.N.A.). *Acta Anat.* 1957;30:67.
5. Huber JF. The arterial network supplying the dorsum of the foot. *Anat Rec.* 1941;80:737.
6. Rouvière J, Canela Lazaro M. Le ligament péronéo-astragalocalcanéen. *Ann Anat Pathol Anat Normal.* 1932;9:745.
7. Henry AK. *Extensile Exposure.* 2nd ed. Williams & Wilkins; 1957:268-308.
8. Belloc P, Meyer P. Le ligament annulaire interne du cou-de-pied. *Arch Anat Histol Embryol.* 1954;37:23.
9. Baumann J. La région de passage de la loge postérieure de la jambe à la plante du pied. *Ann Anat Pathol Anat Normal.* 1930;7:201.
10. Bellocq P, Meyer P. Contribution a l'étude du canal calcanéen. *Comptes Rendus Assoc Anat.* 1956;89:292.
11. Hovelacque A. *Anatomie des Nerfs Craniens et Rachidiens et du Système Grand Sympathique Chez l'Homme.* 2nd ed. Doin; 1927: 627-635.
12. Adachi B. *Das Arteriensystem der Japaner.* Maruzen; 1928:215-291.
13. Mulfinger GL, Trueta J. The blood supply of the talus. *J Bone Joint Surg Br.* 1970;52(1):160.
14. Delorme E. Ligature des artères de la paume de la main et de la plante du pied. *Mem Acad Med.* 1882. Cited in Testut L, Jacob O. *Traité d'Anatomie Topographique Avec Applications Médico-Chirurgicales.* Vol 2. 2nd ed. Doin; 1909:1084.
15. Hidalgo DA, Shaw WW. Anatomic basis of plantar flap design. *Plast Reconstr Surg.* 1986;78(5):627.
16. Shaw WW, Hidalgo DA. Anatomic basis of plantar flap design: clinical applications. *Plast Reconstr Surg.* 1986;78(5):637.
17. Kaplan IB, McGraw JB. Plastic surgery of the foot and ankle. In Jahss M, ed. *Disorders of the Foot and Ankle: Medical and Surgical Management.* Vol 2. 2nd ed. WB Saunders; 1991:1595.
18. Hallopeau P. Note sur le nerf de l'adducteur oblique du gros orteil. *Bull Mem Soc Anat Paris.* 1900;75:1078.
19. Bojsen-Møller F, Flagstad KE. Plantar aponeurosis and internal architecture of the ball of the foot. *J Anat.* 1976;121(3):599.
20. Cox HT. The cleavage lines of the skin. *Br J Surg.* 1941;29:234.

Functional Anatomy of the Foot and Ankle

Shahan K. Sarrafian and Armen S. Kelikian

TERMINOLOGY OF MOTION

Until a consensus is reached, we will use the triaxial orthogonal coordinate system X-Y-Z of the human body and of the leg and its transposition into the foot to provide the basis for a sound definition of the movements occurring at the foot-ankle complex. The clinical terminology is well entrenched and will be preserved as long as we refer also to the coordinate system understood by all. Some undeniable difficulties still persist at the level of the foot when function is defined relative to the long axis of the foot passing from the heel through the second metatarsal and second toe. For example, the terms *metatarsus primus varus* and *hallux valgus* describe correctly the position of the segments relative to the sagittal mid plane of the body, whereas the contradiction is apparent when one labels, for example, the *abductor hallucis* and the *adductor hallucis* muscles. Factually, the abductor hallucis muscle is an adductor and the adductor muscle is an abductor of the hallux. Such contradiction, however, does not exist in the French anatomic studies.

The rationale of the transposition of the leg-ankle coordinate of motion to the foot axes is seen when one considers the embryologic evolution of the foot.[1] Initially, the foot is axially aligned with the leg and the three orthogonal coordinates of the leg-foot are the same with a transverse, vertical, and longitudinal axis of motion. As the embryo foot makes its first 90° of rotation relative to the leg, the transverse axis of the foot remains unchanged, whereas the longitudinal axis of the foot generates the same type of motion as the vertical axis of the leg-ankle; the vertical axis of the foot generates the same type of motion as the longitudinal axis of the leg-ankle (Fig. 10.1). This concept of Huson's facilitates the integration of the terminology of motion. However, on a habitual and clinical basis, we will still use some commonly accepted terms such as *supination* and *pronation* (in parallel with intracarpal supination-pronation between the first and second carpal rows of the wrist) and *valgus* and *varus* (because these may well be present in a dynamic fashion in clinical entities and correspond well to the standard axis references of the body-leg). We have some difficulty accepting as a functional component of inversion a motion of inversion (adduction-inversion, plantar flexion) or eversion as a component of eversion (abduction-eversion, dorsal flexion), as expressed by Huson.[1]

The use of supination-pronation (adduction-supination-plantar flexion; abduction-pronation-dorsal flexion) obviates this terminologic difficulty. Furthermore, we will also preserve the terminology of hindfoot and forefoot, which presents descriptive facility from the clinical point of view.

Each axis of the orthogonal coordinate system generates a rotary motion occurring in a plane perpendicular to the axis as follows:

- Transverse axis X generates motion in the sagittal plane.
- Vertical axis Y generates motion in the transverse or horizontal plane.
- Longitudinal axis Z generates motion in the frontal or coronal plane.

The types of motion occurring around the X, Y, and Z axes are as follows:

Tibiotalar (Fig. 10.2)
  Transverse axis X: dorsiflexion or extension and plantar flexion or flexion in the sagittal plane
  Vertical axis Y: internal rotation, external rotation in the transverse plane
  Longitudinal axis Z: adduction-abduction of the talus or supination-pronation of the talus or lateral-medial talar tilt
  The motions around the Y and Z axes are secondary.
Motion of the foot plate (talocalcaneonavicular, midtarsal, tarsometatarsal) around the talus (see Fig. 10.2). These motions occur around the obliquely oriented and movable axes, but they can be converted into their vectorial orthogonal components X, Y, and Z.
  Transverse axis X: dorsiflexion, plantar flexion in the sagittal plane.
  Vertical axis Y: abduction-adduction in the transverse or horizontal plane
  Longitudinal axis Z: supination in the frontal plane or counterclockwise rotation on the right and clockwise rotation on the left when facing the foot in an anteroposterior direction. The medial border of the foot is elevated. Pronation in the frontal plane or clockwise rotation on the right and

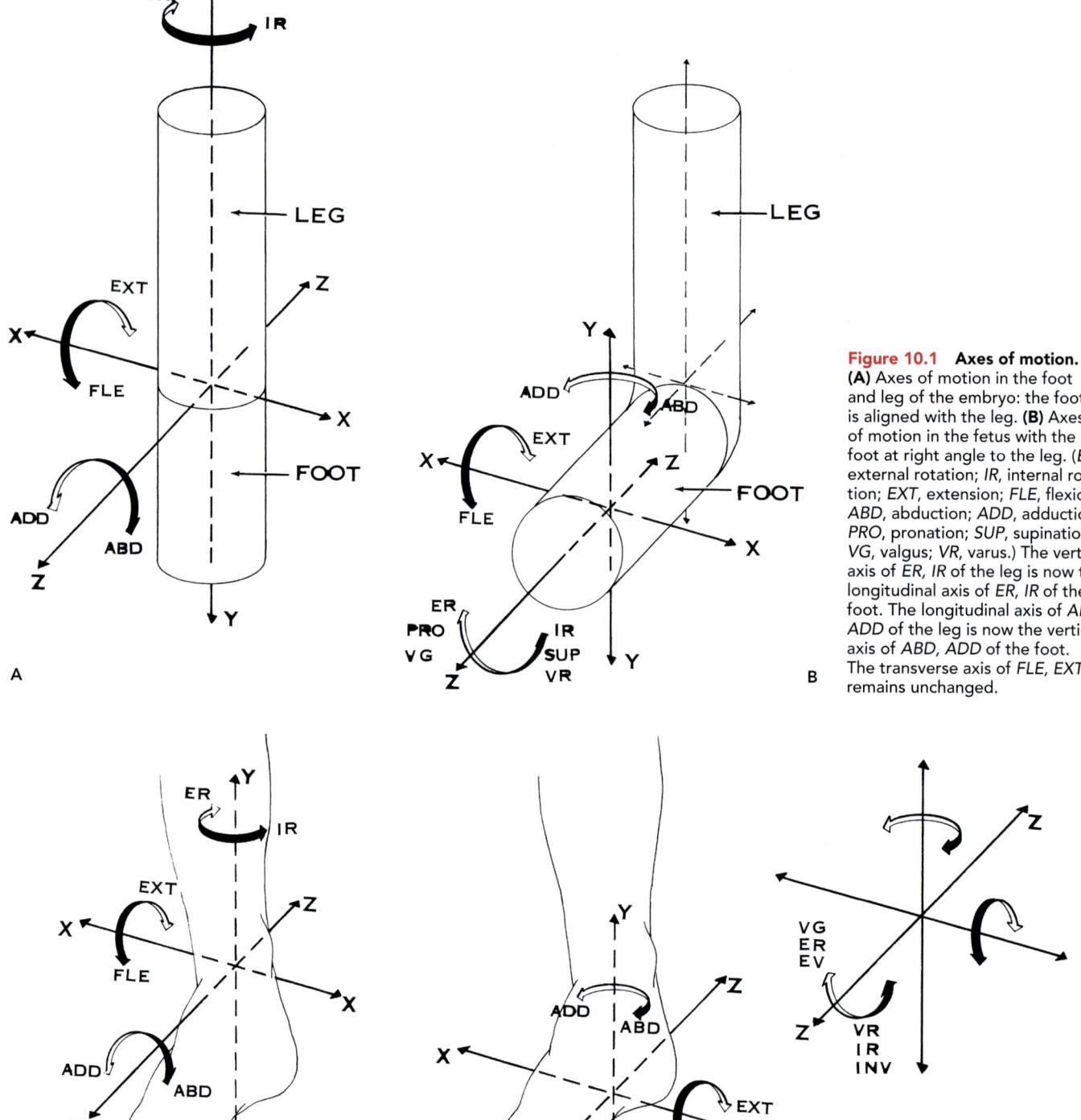

Figure 10.1 Axes of motion. **(A)** Axes of motion in the foot and leg of the embryo: the foot is aligned with the leg. **(B)** Axes of motion in the fetus with the foot at right angle to the leg. (*ER*, external rotation; *IR*, internal rotation; *EXT*, extension; *FLE*, flexion; *ABD*, abduction; *ADD*, adduction; *PRO*, pronation; *SUP*, supination; *VG*, valgus; *VR*, varus.) The vertical axis of *ER, IR* of the leg is now the longitudinal axis of *ER, IR* of the foot. The longitudinal axis of *ABD, ADD* of the leg is now the vertical axis of *ABD, ADD* of the foot. The transverse axis of *FLE, EXT* remains unchanged.

Figure 10.2 **(A)** Axes of motion of the ankle and leg. YY axis of *ER, IR* of the leg-talus. XX' axis of *FLE, EXT* of the talus. ZZ axis of *ASD, ADD* of the talus. **(B)** Axes of motion of the foot plate. YY axis of *ADD, ABD*, XX axis of *FLE, EXT*. ZZ axis of *SUP, PRO*. **(C)** Different terminology used for the motion around the longitudinal axis ZZ, VG, ER, EV and VR, IR, INV. (*ER*, external rotation; *IR*, internal rotation; *FLE*, flexion; *EXT*, extension; *ASD*, abduction; *ADD*, adduction; *VG*, valgus; *VR*, varus; *EV*, eversion; *INV*, inversion.)

counterclockwise rotation on the left when facing the foot in an anteroposterior direction. The lateral border of the foot is in elevation. The motion around this axis may also be termed internal-external rotation, endorotation-exorotation, or, by some, inversion-eversion.

AXIS OF MOTION: FIXED VERSUS MOBILE, SINGLE VERSUS MULTIPLE

The axis of motion is the imaginary line around which the motion occurs. An inclined axis is reduced vectorially to its three components in the orthogonal coordinate system, thus generating motion in three planes, with predominance of the planes of motion in function of the magnitude of the corresponding vectorial component.

The concept of triplane motion is now firmly established with the recent biomechanical investigations of Ambagtsheer,[2] Van Langelaan,[3] Benink,[4] and Lundberg and colleagues.[5-7] Furthermore, the concept of a fixed axis of motion has evolved toward the instantly moving axis of motion with accompanying helical motion, introducing the concept of rotation combined with translation around the axis.[1] Huson, in the early 1960s, challenged the concept of a fixed axis functioning like hinges,[8] and Van Langelaan concluded that "movements are found to take place around an axis which moves continuously and the position of which could be approximated with the aid of a bundle of discrete helical axes."[2]

FIELD OF MOTION

The functional capacity of the foot and ankle is expressed by the contour and dimensions of its field of motion (Fig. 10.3).[9] The dimensions of the field of motion include all possible spatial displacements of the forefoot, with the distal leg remaining stationary. The field of motion of the foot and ankle is oval

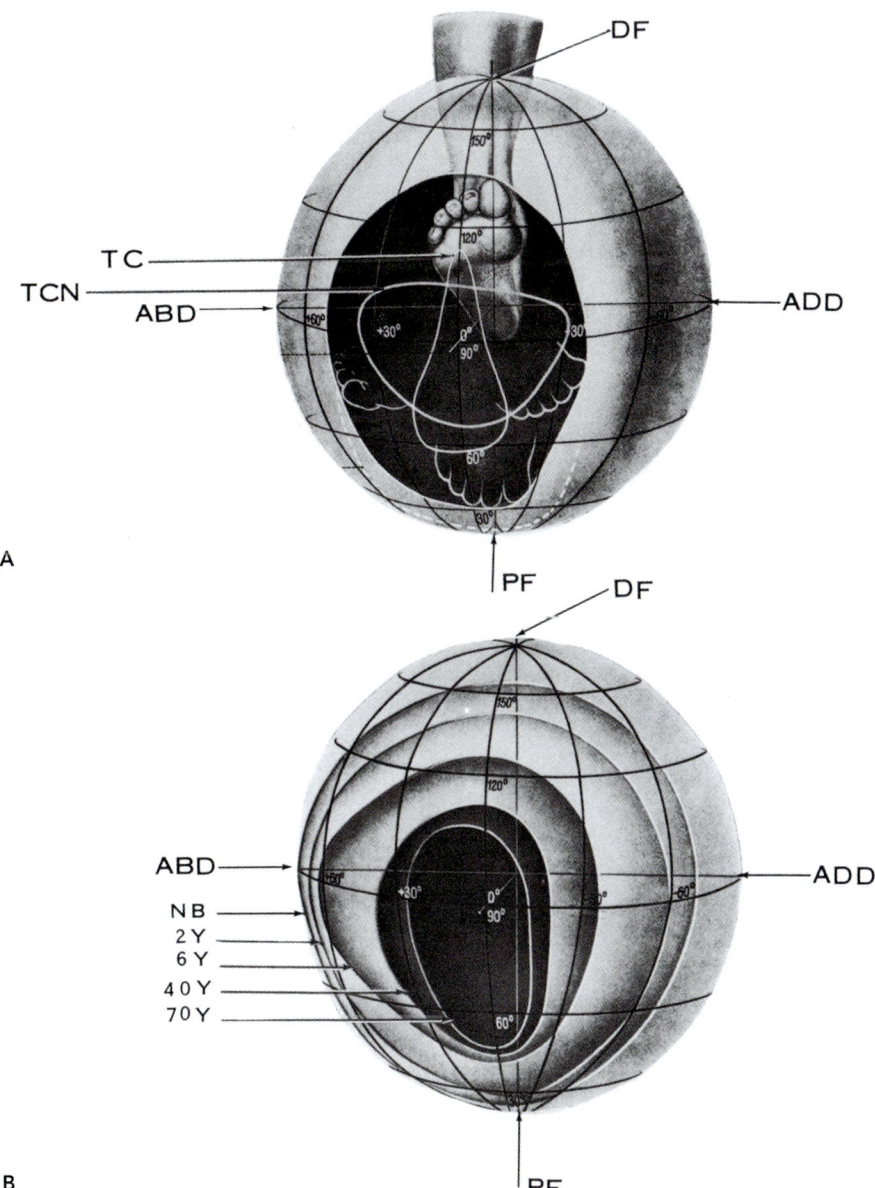

Figure 10.3 Field of motion of the foot-ankle complex. With aging, there is transverse constriction of the field of motion. (A) Oval contour of the field of motion. (B) Field of motion in different age groups. (TC, field contribution of talocrural joint; TCN, field contribution of talocalcaneonavicular joint; DF, dorsiflexion; PF, plantar flexion; ABD, abduction; ADD, adduction; NB, newborn; 2Y, 2 years old; 6Y, 6 years old; 40Y, 40 years old; 70Y, 70 years old.) (Adapted by permission from Lang J, Wachsmuth W. Praktische Anatomie: Ein Lehr-und Hilfsbuch der anatomischen Grundlagen ärztlichen Handelns. Vol 1, Part 4. Springer-Verlag; 1972:370.)

in contour. The vertical segment of the field is determined mainly by the talocrural joint and the transverse segment by the foot plate. The functional capacity of the foot and ankle is age dependent. The functional field is the largest in the newborn and it gradually constricts with aging, more in the transverse segment than in the vertical. At the age of 2 to 6 years, the field is transversely oval; at the age of 40 years, it is converted into a high oval; and, by the age of 70 years, it is narrow, limited mainly to the vertical segment.[8] In terms of functional capacity, the foot at the age of 70 years can dorsiflex and plantarflex but has a limited capacity to adapt to walking on uneven ground.

ANKLE JOINT

▶ Axis of Motion

Single Axis of Motion

According to Inman, the empirical axis of the ankle joint passes slightly distal to the tips of the malleoli at 5 ± 3 mm (range, 0-11 mm) distal to the tip of the medial malleolus and 3 ± 2 mm (range, 0-12 mm) distal to and 8 ± 5 mm anterior to the tip of the lateral malleolus.[10] The axis is inclined downward and laterally in the frontal plane (Fig. 10.4) and is rotated posterolaterally in the horizontal or transverse plane (Fig. 10.5).

In the frontal plane, the angle between the empirical axis of the ankle and the midline of the tibia is 82.7° ± 3.7°, with a range of 74° to 94° (Fig. 10.6).[10] In the transverse plane, the angle of the ankle axis with the transverse axis of the knee is 20° to 30°.[10]

Multiple Axes of Motion

Barnett and Napier[11] and Hicks[12] recognize two axes to the ankle joint: a dorsiflexion axis inclined downward and laterally and a plantar flexion axis inclined downward and medially (Fig. 10.7). The changeover occurs within a few degrees of the neutral

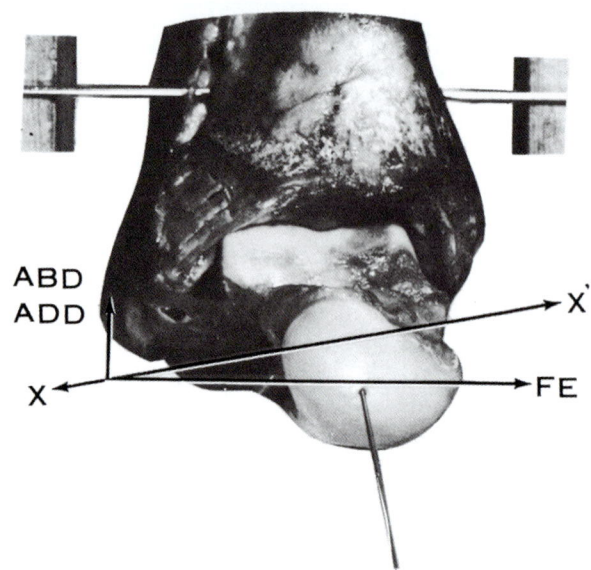

Figure 10.4 Axis of the ankle joint. The axis of the ankle joint XX' is inclined as indicated and has two vectorial components: the major transverse component, which generates the motion of flexion-extension (*FE*), and the lesser vertical component, which generates the motion of the abduction-adduction (*ABD-ADD*).

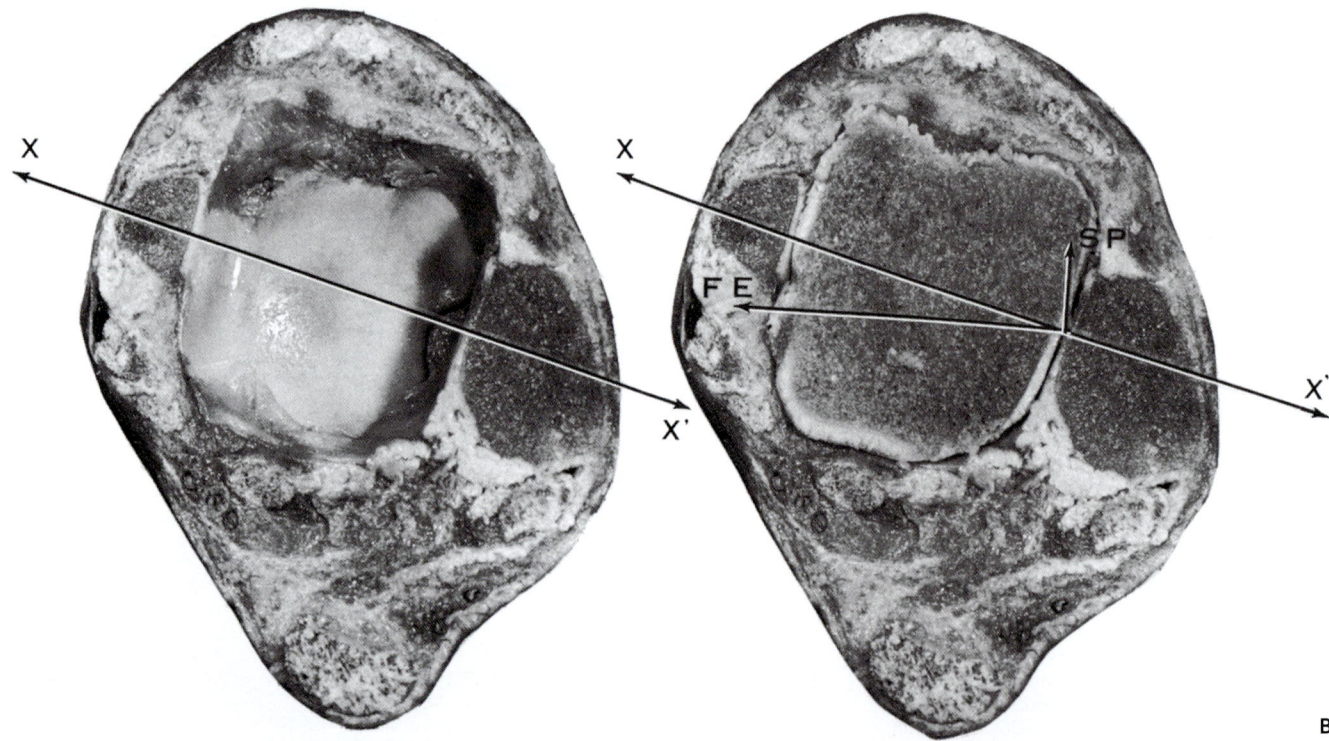

Figure 10.5 Cross section of the ankle 2 cm above the tip of the medial malleolus, indicating the oblique orientation of the axis of motion of XX' of the ankle in the transverse plane. The axis XX' has a major transverse component for flexion-extension (*FE*) and a minor longitudinal component for supination-pronation (*SP*). **(A)** Cross section demonstrating the two malleoli and the tibial plafond. **(B)** Cross section with the dome of the talus lodged in the ankle mortise.

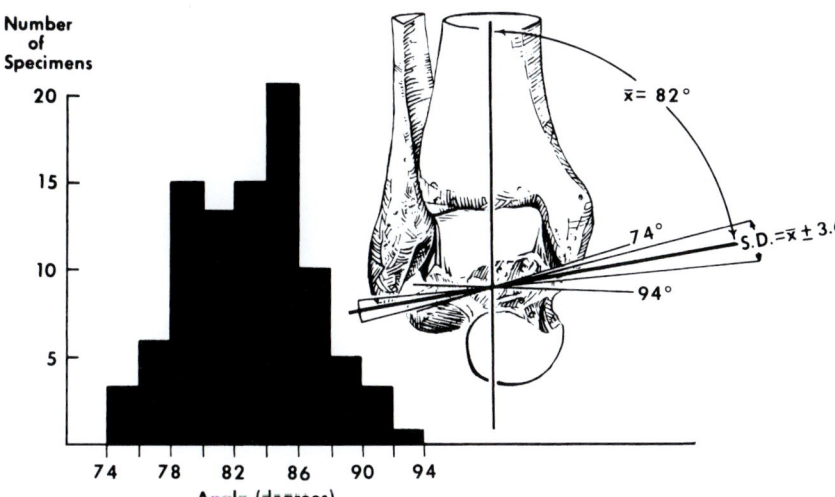

Figure 10.6 **Variations in the angle between the midline of the tibia and the empirical axis of the ankle.** This histogram reveals a considerable spread of individual values. (From Inman TV. *The Joints of the Ankle*. Williams & Wilkins; 1976:27.)

position of the talus (Figs. 10.8 and 10.9). Barnett and Napier[11] based their conclusions on the determination of the curvatures of the lateral and medial marginal profiles of the talar trochlea. The center of the curvature being the axis of motion, the lateral profile is "almost always an arc of a true circle and in all positions of the talus the axis of rotation must pass through the center of this circle."[11] The medial profile is formed by the arcs of two circles with different radii. The arc of a small circle, occupying the anterior one third of the medial profile, corresponds to the dorsiflexion arc; the center of the circle is high in location. The arc of a large circle, occupying the posterior two-thirds of the medial profile, corresponds to the plantar flexion arc; the center of the circle is low in location.

Lundberg and colleagues analyzed the axis of the talocrural joint by roentgen stereophotogrammetry in eight healthy human volunteers.[13] Tantalum beads, 0.8 mm in size, were inserted in their corresponding bones as markers. Under full weight-bearing, for each individual, the foot was carried by the supportive platform from 30° of plantar flexion to 30° of dorsiflexion in increments of 10°. The helical axis for each pair of consecutive positions was determined. Their investigation "fully supports the findings of Barnett and Napier and Hicks that the talocrural joint uses different axes for plantar flexion and dorsiflexion."[13] Based on their data, the mean inclinations of the axes in the eight subjects were as follows, with 0° corresponding to a horizontal axis: negative (−) corresponding to an axis inclined downward in a medial direction and positive (+) corresponding to an axis inclined downward laterally (Fig. 10.10).

Plantar Flexion	Inclination of Axis
30°-20°	−12°
20°-10°	−8.25°
10°-0°	+8.25°
Dorsiflexion	
0°-10°	+15.5°
10°-20°	+18.87°
20°-30°	+22.5°

When projected onto a horizontal plane, the axes passed through the malleoli (Fig. 10.11).

Sammarco and coworkers studied the instant centers of rotation and surface velocities at the point of contact in 24 normal weight-bearing ankles and six non–weight-bearing ankles.[14] In the weight-bearing group, the locations of the instant centers of rotation were as follows: 12 ankles, within the body of the talus; 8 ankles, one or two centers below the body of the talus; 2 ankles, above the joint surface; and 2 ankles, on the joint surface. In the six non–weight-bearing ankles, there was also scattered distribution of the centers of rotation. The motion pattern from plantar flexion to dorsiflexion was distraction of the joint surfaces at the beginning, sliding throughout the arc of motion, and jamming of the joint surfaces at the end of the motion (Fig. 10.12).

▶ Range of Motion

Dorsiflexion and plantar flexion are the major components of the motion at the talocrural joint. The minor components are the rotations around the vertical and the longitudinal axes.

The range of ankle flexion-extension is variable. The methodology used—clinical, roentgenographic, anatomic (cadaveric)—accounts for some of the reported discrepancies.

The reported normal ranges of motion at the ankle joint are shown in Table 10.1. During the stance phase of the gait, the ankle motion, as reported by Stauffer and colleagues, is 24.4° in average (range, 20°-31°), with 10.2° dorsiflexion (range, 6°-16°) and 14.2° plantar flexion (range, 13°-17°).[15] Motion around the vertical axis, external-internal rotation of the talus, occurs at the ankle joint. Close[16] and Close and Inman[17] report a range of 5° to 6° of external rotation of the talus (relative to the tibia) as active or passive dorsiflexion takes place at the ankle and "this rotation is reversed as the ankle is plantar flexed." Close also mentions 5° to 6° of horizontal rotation occurring at the ankle joint during the stance phase of walking.

McCullough and Burge, in an experimental setup, applied a rotary torque of 3 N · m on the talus about a vertical axis and measured the horizontal talar rotation under variable degrees

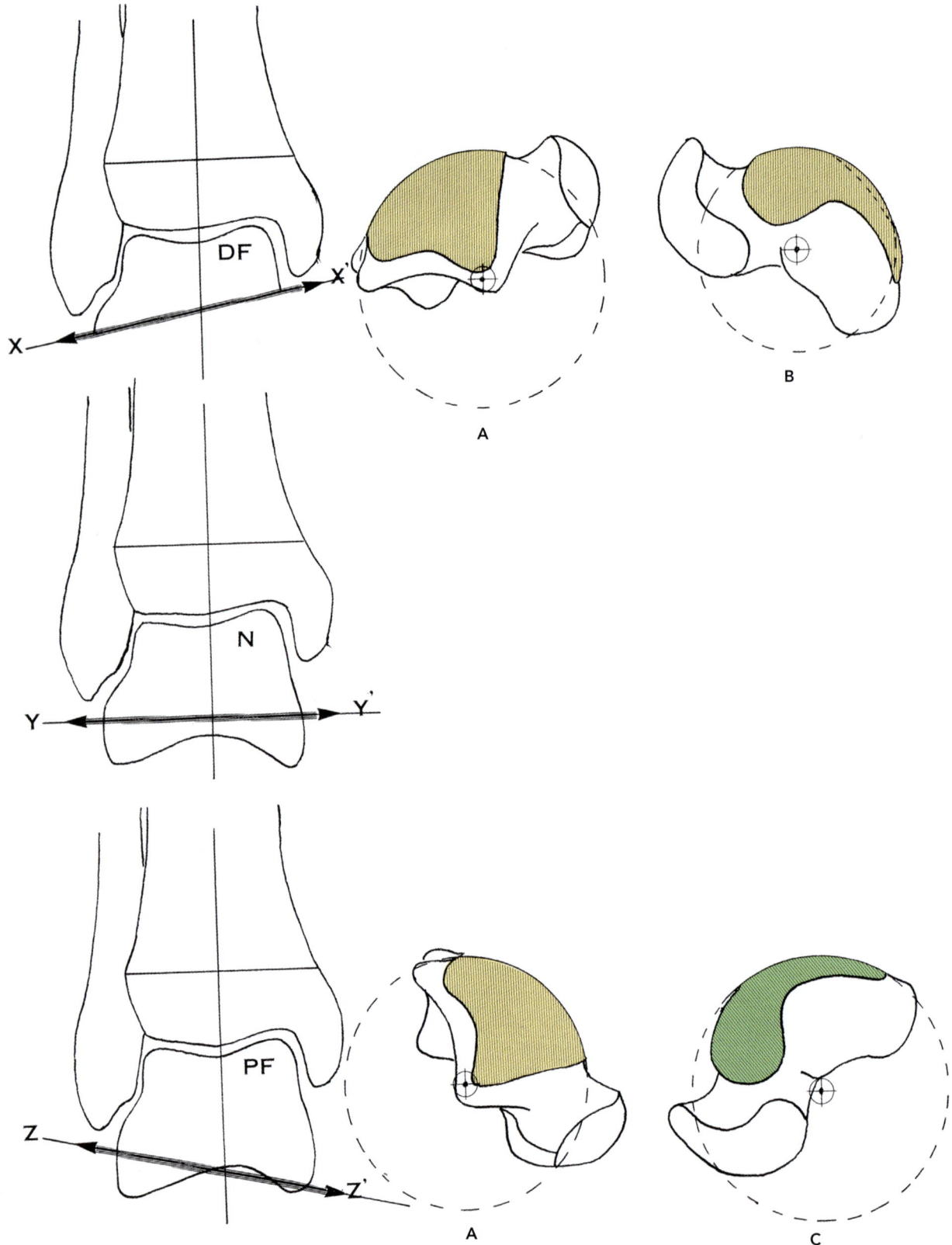

Figure 10.7 Ankle joint axis variation. In dorsiflexion (*DF*), the axis of motion *XX'* is inclined downward and laterally. In plantar flexion (*PF*), the axis of motion *ZZ'* is inclined downward and medially. Near neutral (*N*), the axis of motion *YY'* is almost horizontal. The lateral trochlear contour (*A*) is an arc of a true circle. The medial trochlear contour is more complex. Its anterior third or dorsiflexion arc (*B*) belongs to a smaller circle as compared with the posterior two-thirds or plantar flexion arc (*C*), which belongs to a large circle. (Adapted from Barnett CJ, Napier JR. The axis of rotation at the ankle joint in man: its influence upon the form of the talus and the mobility of the fibula. *J Anat.* 1952;86:1.)

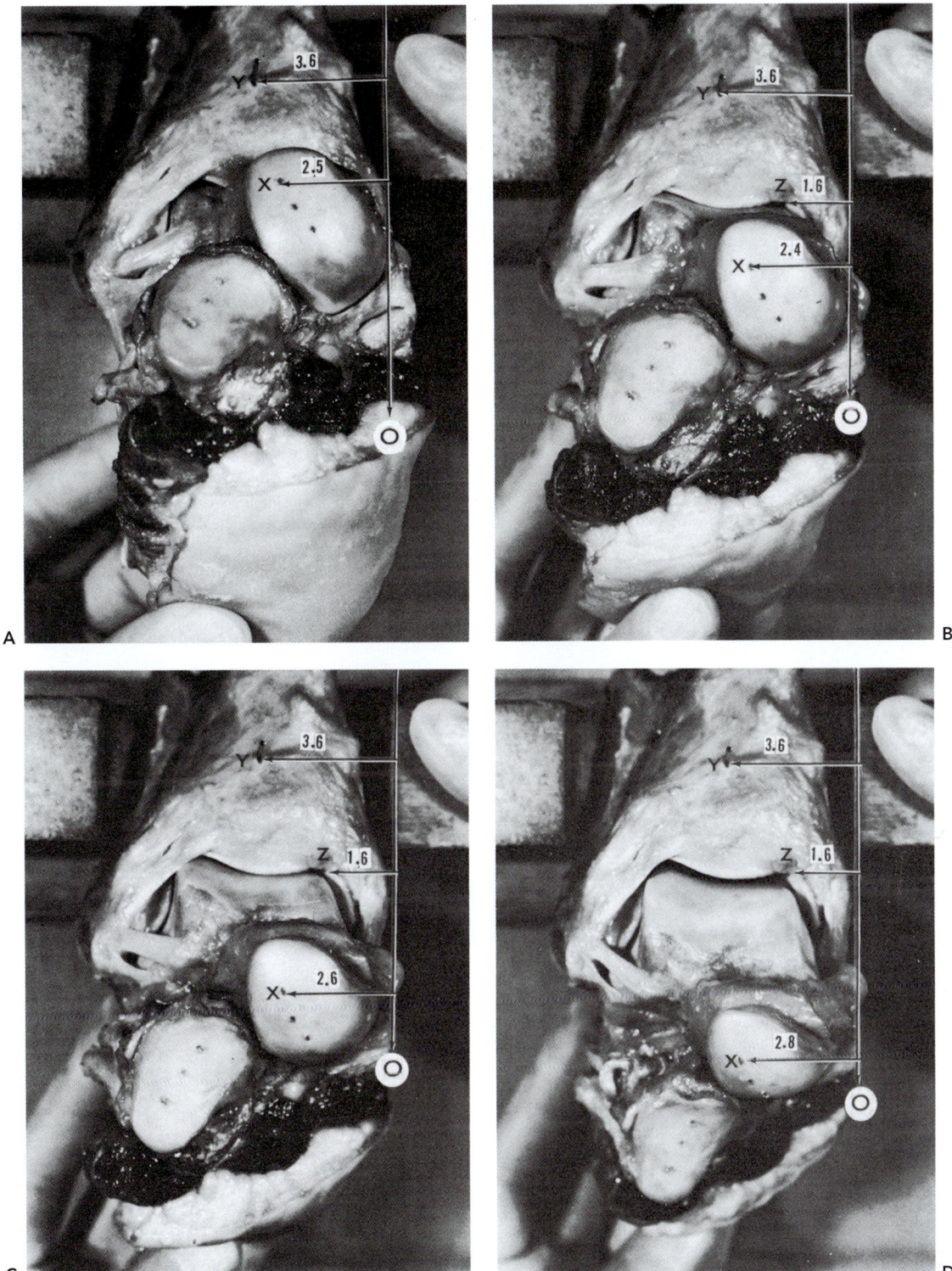

Figure 10.8 Ankle and hindfoot specimen. Tibia and fibula are stabilized. The talus is carried from dorsiflexion **(A)** to neutral **(B)** and plantar flexion **(C and D)**. A vertical reference line *O* is traced. The distance of the tibial reference points *Y* and *Z* from the line *O* remains constant (3.6 and 1.6 cm). A drill point *X* is taken as a reference point on the talar head. The distance from point *X* to the vertical reference line *O* is measured in all four positions: dorsiflexion distance, 2.5 cm; neutral distance, 2.4 cm; plantar flexion distance, 2.6 cm; maximum plantar flexion distance, 2.8 cm. The data indicate that, in this specimen, during dorsiflexion the talus is displaced upward and laterally around an oblique axis inclined downward and laterally. In neutral, the axis is transverse, whereas in plantar flexion the axis is inclined downward and medially as the talar reference point is displaced downward and laterally.

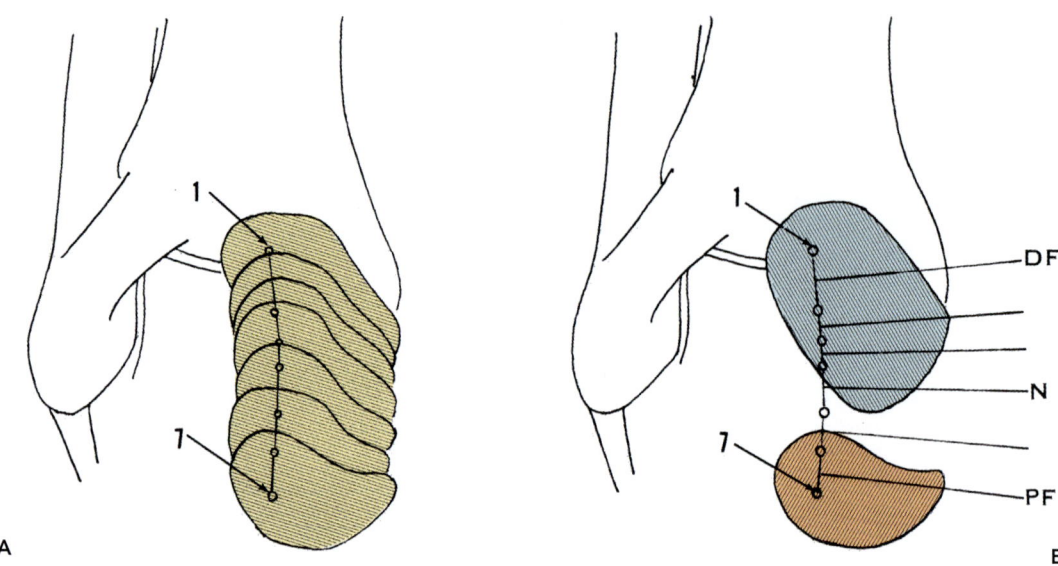

Figure 10.9 **(A)** Tracings of the displacements of the talar head reference point from dorsiflexion (*1*) to plantar flexion (*7*). **(B)** Motion axes drawn, perpendicular to the displacement lines. The axis is inclined laterally and downward in dorsiflexion and medially and downward in plantar flexion. The changeover in direction occurs very close to the neutral position of the ankle. (*DF*, dorsiflexion; *N*, neutral; *PF*, plantar flexion.)

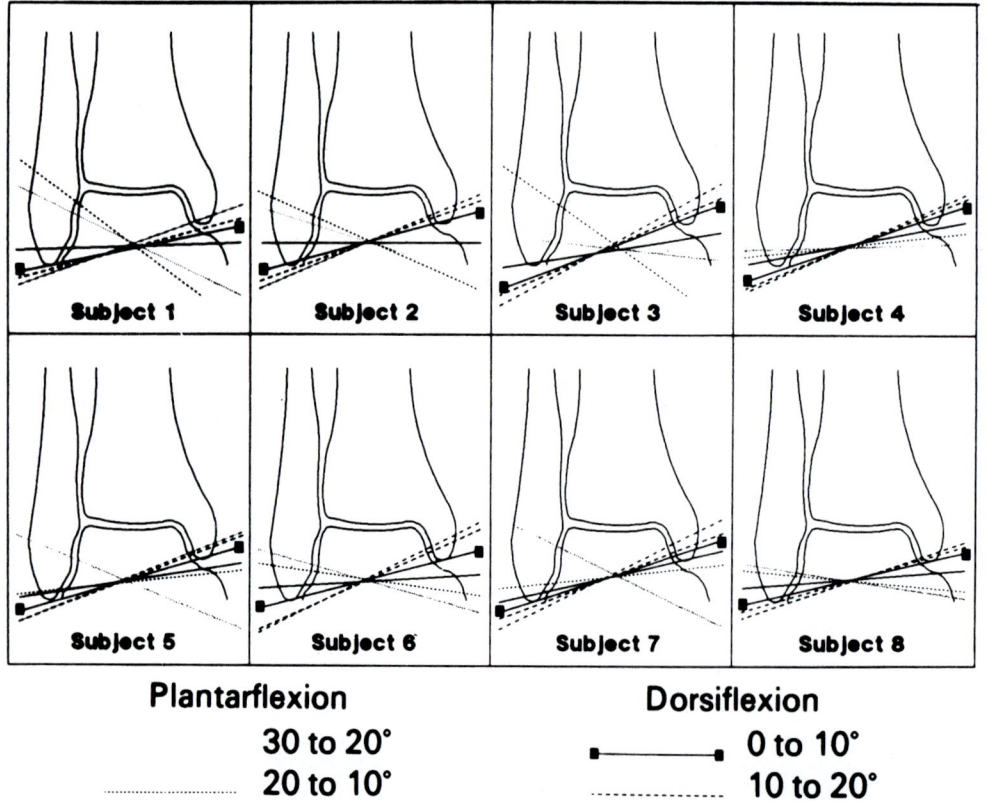

Figure 10.10 Discrete helical axes of the talocrural joint of each subject from each 10° interval from 30° of plantar flexion to 30° of dorsiflexion projected onto a coronal plane. All plantar flexion axes are more horizontal, or inclining downward and medially, than are the dorsiflexion axes. (Republished with permission of British Editorial Society of Bone and Joint Surgery, from Lundberg A, Svensson OK, Nemeth G, et al. The axis of rotation of the ankle joint. *J Bone Joint Surg Br.* 1989;71[1]:94; permission conveyed through Copyright Clearance Center, Inc.)

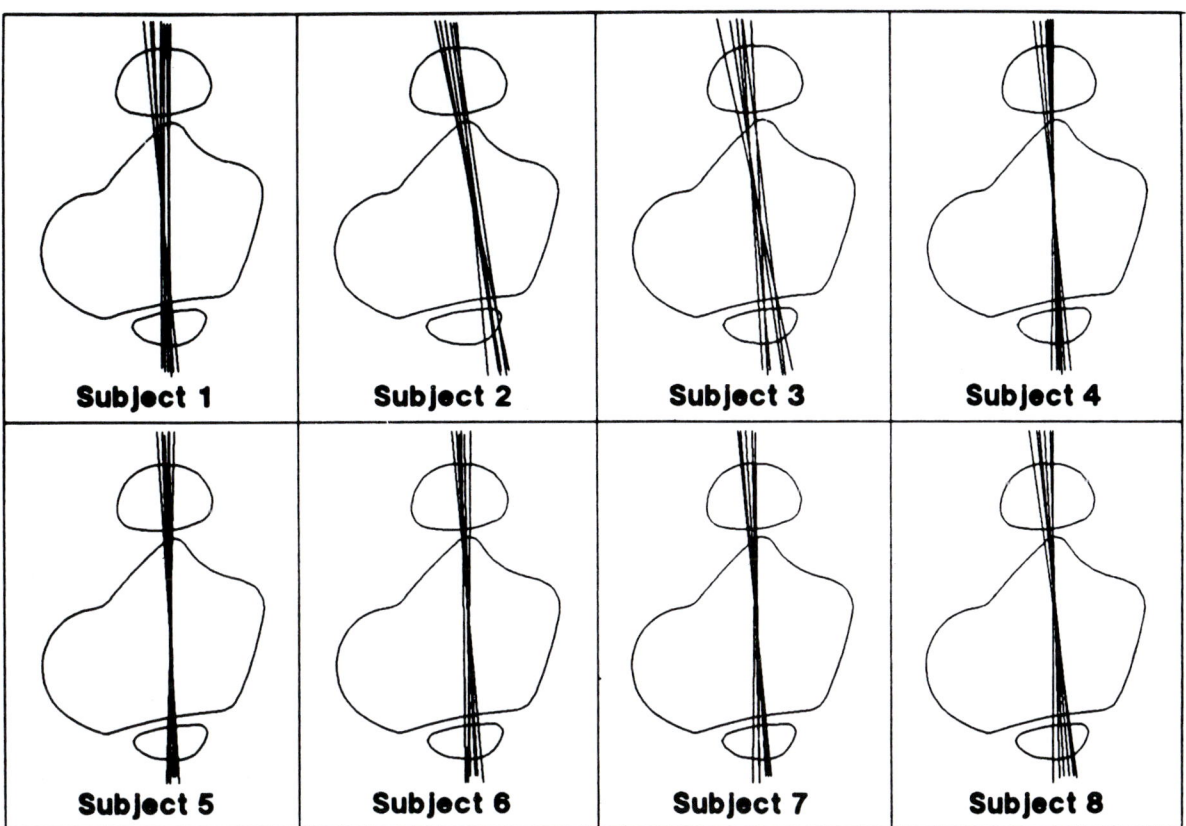

Figure 10.11 **Discrete helical axes of the talocrural joint projected onto a horizontal plane.** Axes tend to fall parallel to a transverse plane through the malleoli. (Republished with permission of British Editorial Society of Bone and Joint Surgery, from Lundberg A, Svensson OK, Nemeth G, et al. The axis of rotation of the ankle joint. *J Bone Joint Surg Br*. 1989;71[1]:94; permission conveyed through Copyright Clearance Center, Inc.)

of vertical load.[18] At a minimum load of 9.8 N (1 kg), the mean range of horizontal talar rotation was 24.1°. With increasing load from 9.8 N (1 kg) to 490 N (50 kg), the horizontal rotation decreased in a linear fashion for a total value of 7.5° ± 1.5° (Fig. 10.13). The range of rotation was nearly the same in plantar flexion and dorsiflexion.

Lundberg and colleagues, using the roentgen stereophotogrammetric technique described previously, analyzed the horizontal rotation of the talus in eight healthy volunteers.[5] From 0° to 30° of dorsiflexion, there was a consistent pattern of increasing external rotation, which reached 8.9°. From 0° to 10° of plantar flexion, there was a minimal amount of internal rotation (1.4° ± 0.9°) followed by a minimal amount of external rotation (0.6° ± 3°) at 30° of plantar flexion (Fig. 10.14).

A small amount of consistent supinatory rotation of the talus around the longitudinal axis was also recorded as the foot moved from 30° of plantar flexion to 30° of dorsiflexion.

Lundberg and colleagues, using the same methodology, studied the talar motion during rotation of the leg under weight-bearing conditions.[7] With external rotation of the leg from 0 to 10°, the talus moved triaxially, with dorsiflexion of 4.3° ± 3.5°, minimal supination of 1.5° ± 1.6°, and external rotation of 0.7° ± 2.5°. When the leg turned internally 20°, the talus rotated externally 5.0° ± 2.0°, with associated minimal pronation of 0.7° ± 0.5° and a trace of plantar flexion of 0.1° ± 1.9°.

From dorsiflexion to plantar flexion at the ankle joint, the articular surfaces of the talus and the malleoli remain in contact. Considering that the superior talar surface is larger anteriorly than posteriorly, with an average difference of 4.2 mm (2-6 mm), the question of potential "play" of the talus in the ankle mortise at full plantar flexion is raised. This, however, does not occur. In full plantar flexion, the posterior two-thirds of the talar dome remains in the ankle mortise (Fig. 10.15), thus minimizing the potential difference between the transverse diameter of the talus and the bimalleolar transverse distance. Furthermore, Inman, in a study of 86 tali, demonstrated that the trochlea of the talus "is a section of a frustum of a cone and not of a cylinder."[10] The apex of the cone is medial, with the conical angle of the frustum at 24° ± 6° (range, 10°-40°) (Fig. 10.16). In addition, Close and Inman made transverse saw marks across the trochlear surface of the talus along the frontal plane of the distal tibia throughout the range of plantar flexion and dorsiflexion of the ankle.[17] The markings were not parallel and converged toward a point 10.6 to 12.7 cm (4-5 in) medial to the ankle joint and the talar trochlea offered at any time to the bimalleolar fork not the transverse dimension but a larger and constant generating line of the truncated cone (Fig. 10.17). The potential play of the talus in plantar flexion is thus absent.

The functional implication of the segmental conical contour was correlated with the inescapable triplanar motion of the

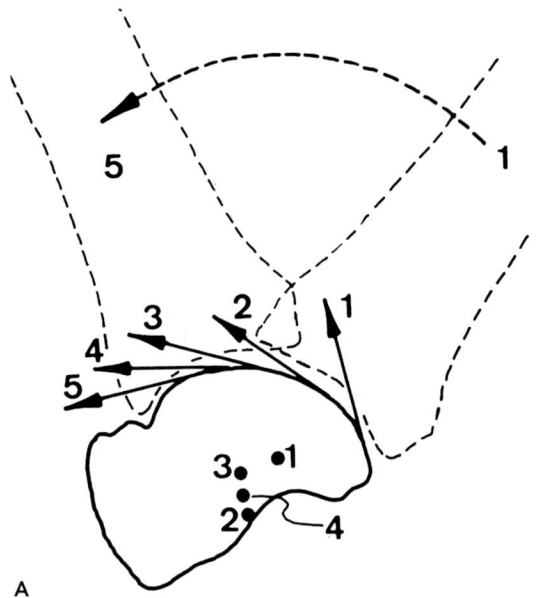

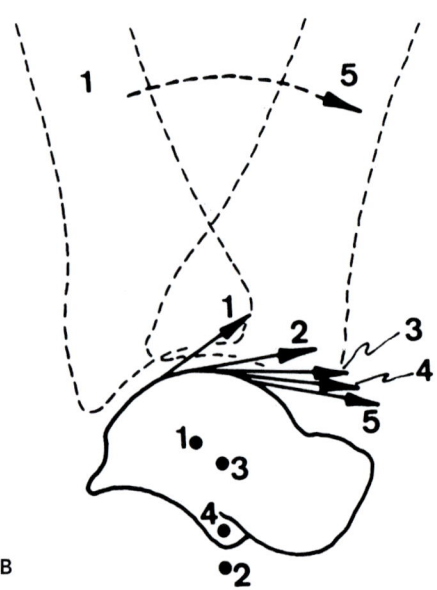

Figure 10.12 Instant centers of rotation and surface velocities from plantar flexion (*1*) to dorsiflexion (*5*) in the ankle. **(A)** Non–weight-bearing: the instant centers of rotation are located in the talus. The surface velocities indicate joint distraction at the beginning of motion, followed by sliding. **(B)** Weight-bearing: an instant center of rotation may be located below the talus. The surface velocities indicate also distraction, followed by sliding. Compression or jamming may occur in maximum dorsiflexion. (Reprinted from Sammarco JG, Burstein AH, Frankel VH. Biomechanics of the ankle: a kinematic study. *Orthop Clin North Am.* 1973;4[1]:75, with permission from Elsevier.)

TABLE 10.1 Reported Normal Ranges of Ankle Joint Motion		
	Range of Motion	
Author	Dorsiflexion (Extension)	Plantar Flexion
AAOS	18°	48
Bonin	10°-20°	25°-35
Weseley and coworkers	0°-10° (maximum, 23°)	26°-35° (minimum, 10°; maximum, 51°)
Sammarco and coworkers		
Weight-bearing	21° ± 7.21°	23° ± 8°
Non–weight-bearing	23° ± 7.5°	23° ± 9°
Boone and Azen (clinical measurements)	12.6° ± 4.4°	56.2° ± 6.1°

talus by Bremer.[19] Plantar flexion of the talus induces a functional varus or supination.

Barnett and Napier correlated the wedge contour of the talus with its potential for internal rotation.[11] During plantar flexion, the medial talar surface has a tendency to separate from the diverging medial malleolar surface, but this is neutralized by the synchronous internal rotation of the talus, which is possible only through the wedge contour of the talar trochlea, narrower posterolaterally. Furthermore, Barnett and Napier associated the degree of posterolateral wedging of the talar trochlea with the inclination of the plantar flexion axis of the ankle joint.[11] Increased inclination of this axis corresponded to marked wedging of the talus, and a minimum inclination corresponded to a minimum wedging. With a near horizontal plantar flexion axis, the talar medial and lateral surfaces were nearly parallel.

▶ **Mobility of the Fibula and Tibiofibular Syndesmosis**

Poirier and Charpy[20] described the tibiofibular mortise as elastic, accommodating the dimensions of the articular surface of the talus, and securing the contact between the articulating surfaces in all positions. Dorsiflexion of the foot presents the larger talar surface to the mortise. To accommodate, the fibula moves apart, the inferior tibioperoneal ligaments are tense, and the large synovial fringe located in the posterior cleft of the synostosis reenters the peroneotibial interline. On the contrary, in plantar flexion, the narrower posterior part of the talar surface is presented to the tibiofibular mortise. The fibula approaches the tibia. The inferior peroneotibial ligaments are relaxed and the synovial fringe is expulsed from the peroneotibial interval and appears in the external angle of the mortise.

During dorsiflexion at the ankle from the plantarflexed position, there is, as reported by Close, an increase in the internalleolar distance of approximately 1.5 mm (1-2 mm) and lateral rotation of the fibula in the horizontal plane, relative to the tibia, of 2.5°.[16] There is also an associated lateral rotation of the talus of 4° relative to the tibia (Fig. 10.18). Barnett and Napier correlated the mobility of the fibula at the proximal tibiofibular joint with the inclination of the dorsiflexion axis of the ankle

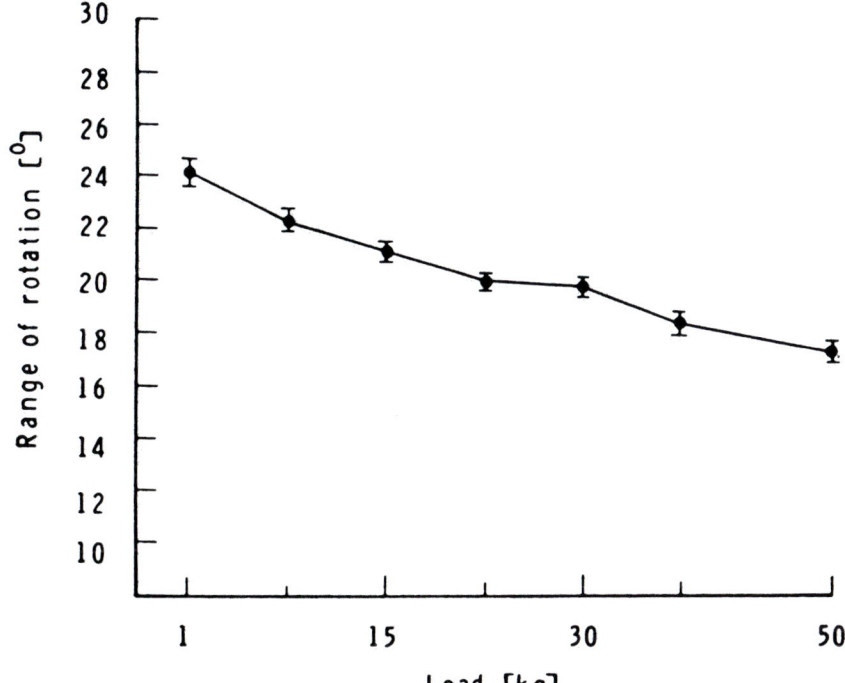

Figure 10.13 Mean range of horizontal talar medial rotation with a rotary torque of 3 N · m under variable degrees of vertical load. The horizontal talar rotation decreases with increased vertical load. (Republished with permission of British Editorial Society of Bone and Joint Surgery, from McCullough CJ, Burge PD. Rotary stability of the load-bearing ankle. An experimental study. *J Bone Joint Surg Br*. 1980;62[4]:460; permission conveyed through Copyright Clearance Center, Inc.)

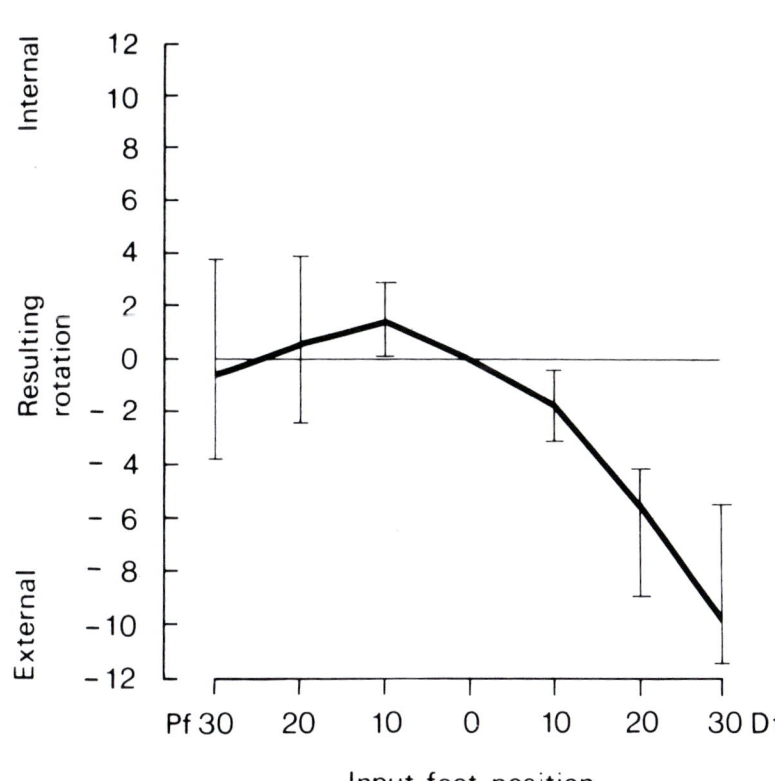

Figure 10.14 Horizontal rotation of the talus around the vertical axis at different dorsiflexion-plantar flexion input of the ankle-foot. (Lundberg A, Goldie I, Kalin BO, et al. Kinematics of the ankle/foot complex. Plantar flexion and dorsiflexion. *Foot Ankle*. 1989;9[4]:194. Copyright ©1989. Reprinted by Permission of SAGE Publications.)

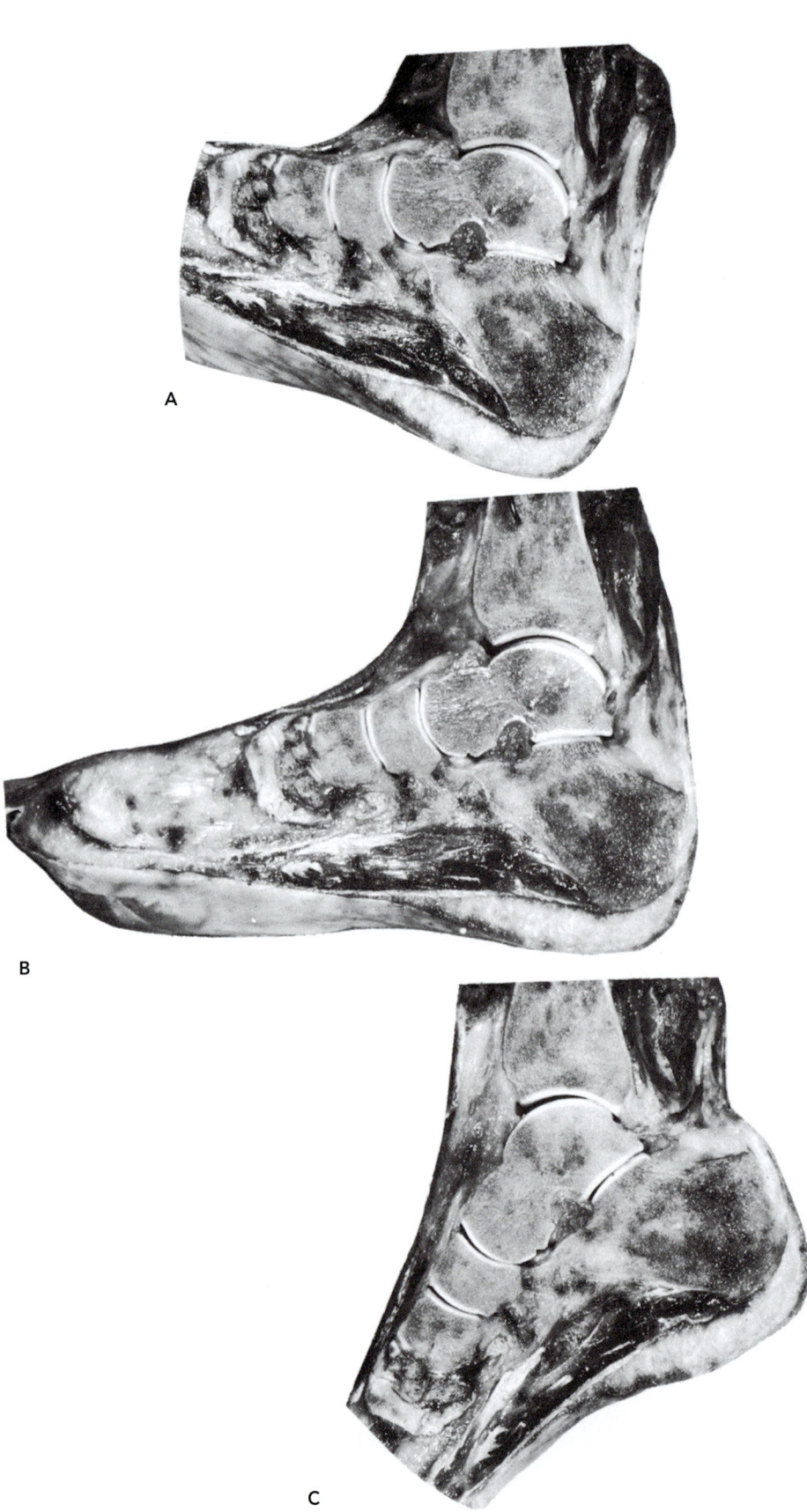

Figure 10.15 Sagittal cross section of the hindfoot, indicating that in (A) full dorsiflexion, (B) neutral position, and (C) full plantar flexion, the articular surface of the tibia covers two-thirds of the talar articular surface. At no time in plantar flexion is the narrower posterior third of the talus occupying the entire ankle mortise.

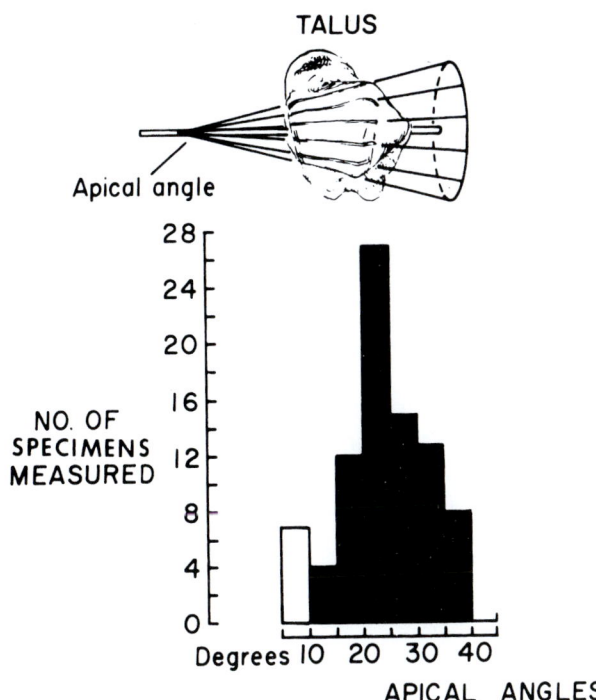

Figure 10.16 **Variations of the apical angles of the conical surface of the talar trochlea obtained by extending directions of saw cuts toward the medial side.** (From Inman TV. *The Joints of the Ankle*. Williams & Wilkins; 1976:23.)

joint.[11] In a study of 152 specimens, they classified the proximal tibiofibular joint into three types.

Type I (27%): There is a large, nearly circular, horizontal articular surface on the tibia, measuring more than 20 mm², with an inclination to the horizontal of less than 30°.

Type II (26%): The articular surface is moderately larger and elliptical and communicates frequently with the knee joint through the synovial bursa deep to the popliteus tendon.

Type III (28%): The articular surface is small (<15 mm²), irregular, and steeply inclined to the horizontal (an inclination angle of more than 30° to the horizontal).

The remaining 19% could not be classified.

A type I proximal articular surface of the fibula provided more mobility and corresponded to the maximally inclined dorsiflexion axis of the ankle joint. The minimally inclined axis correlated with the type III or the relatively immobile fibula.

Kärrholm and colleagues measured the fibular displacement at the ankle joint from plantar flexion to dorsiflexion in nine children and adolescents using roentgen stereophotogrammetric analysis with intraosseous embedded metal markers.[21] The distal fibular translation was measured along the three orthogonal coordinates. The total average lateral displacement of the distal fibula was 1.4 mm (0.5-2.4 mm) when the ankle moved from plantar flexion to dorsiflexion. The largest width of the

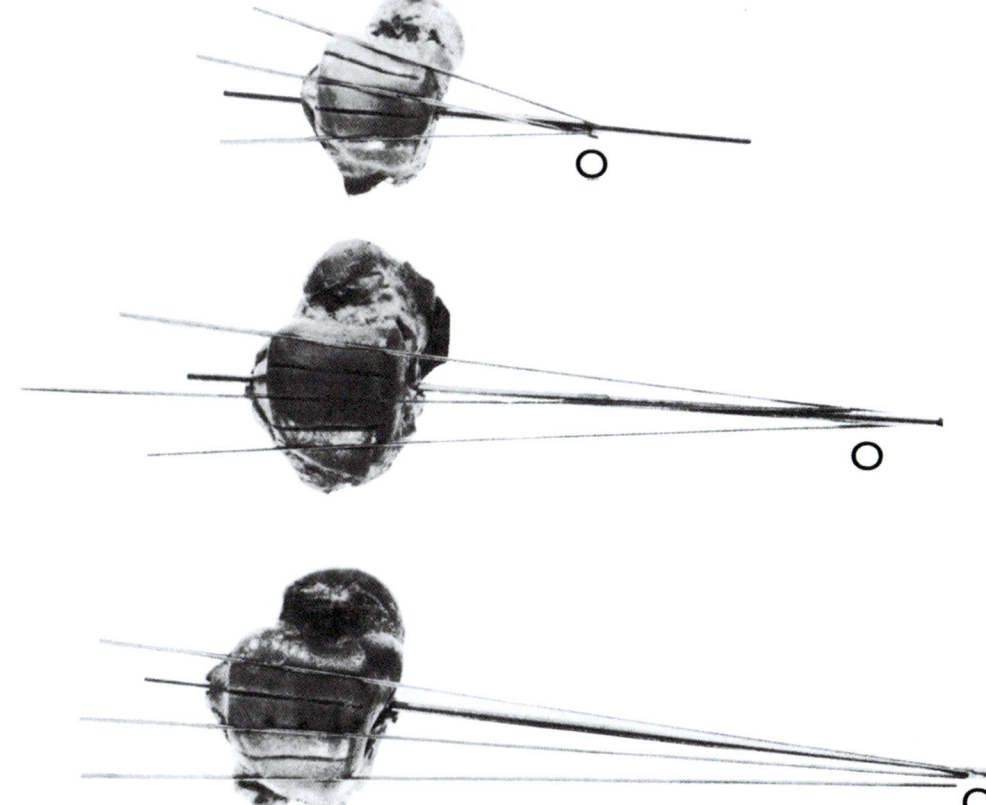

Figure 10.17 **The trochlear surface of the talus is a truncated cone.** The talus is carried from full dorsiflexion to full plantar flexion, and at each interval a saw cut is made on the trochlear surface along the anterior tibial articular margin. The serial saw cuts are not parallel but converge to the apex *O* of the cone, as demonstrated in the three tali. (From Inman TV. *The Joints of the Ankle*. Williams & Wilkins; 1976:21.)

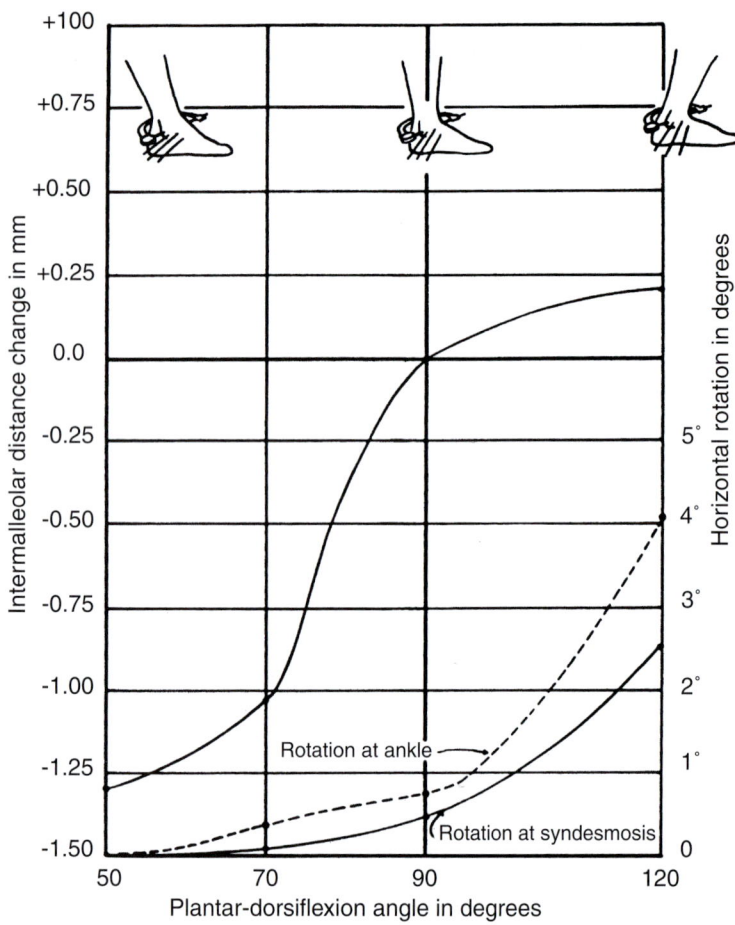

Figure 10.18 Rotation at the ankle and at the syndesmosis and the changes in the intermalleolar distance on dorsiflexion of the foot. (From Close JR. Some applications of the functional anatomy of the ankle joint. *J Bone Joint Surg Am.* 1956;38[1]:771.)

mortise was observed at maximum dorsiflexion of the ankle. Fibular translation occurred along the sagittal axis. The anterior translation (0.1 mm) from plantar flexion to neutral and the posterior translation (0.7 mm) from neutral to dorsiflexion were minimal. The translation along the vertical axis is also reported as a minimal (0.5 mm) distal displacement of the fibula during the same arc of motion. Most of the analyzed ankles demonstrated a posterolateral displacement of the distal fibula.

Weinert and coworkers described a downward and lateral motion of the fibula during the strike phase of running.[22] The dynamic study was performed with motion picture studies of athletes running barefoot on a football field. This was supplemented by a cineroentgenographic study of subjects running on an x-ray table. This dynamic fibular functional study was further expanded by Scranton and colleagues.[23] A distal shift of the fibula averaging 2.4 mm was measured radiographically in ten ankles with weight-bearing, with shift of the weight to the forefoot simulating initiation of push-off. The fibular descent was explained on the basis of the downward pull exerted by the flexors of the foot.

In 25 fresh frozen cadaver specimens, Xenos et al[24] investigated the role of the syndesmotic ligaments when the ankle was loaded with external rotation torque (5 N · m) with the foot held in neutral flexion. The syndesmotic ligaments were incrementally sectioned and direct measurements of anatomic diastasis were made.

A mean diastasis of 2.3 mm (range, 0.5-4.0 mm) occurred when the anterior tibiofibular ligament was sectioned. With the additional sectioning of the interosseous ligament, an additional increase of 2.2 mm in the mean diastasis was seen. With the additional sectioning of the posterior tibiofibular ligament, the total diastasis was 7.3 mm (range, 3.0-15.5 mm). The findings with regard to the degree of rotation paralleled those regarding diastasis. The mean external rotation increased 2.7° after the anterior tibiofibular ligament was cut. The mean total increase in rotation was 10.2° when all three ligaments were sectioned.

Beumer et al[25] analyzed the kinematics of the distal tibiofibular syndesmosis in 11 normal ankles using the radiostereometry technique. The mean age of the 11 volunteers was 50[26-59] years. "They all had tantalum markers implanted in the tibia, fibula and talus. Weight-bearing and combined 7.5 N · m external rotation moment on the foot caused external rotation of the fibula between 2 and 5°, medial translation between 0 and 0.25 mm and posterior displacement between 1.0 and 3.1 mm."

Hoefnagels et al[60] analyzed the biomechanical characteristics of the interosseous tibiofibular ligament and the anterior tibiofibular ligament in 12 pairs of ankles. The mounted bone-ligament preparations were subjected to elongation at 0.5 mm/s until rupture. The stiffness and failure loads were compared. The interosseous tibiofibular ligament was significantly stiffer

TABLE 10.2 Contact Areas in Intact Specimens			
		Average Area (cm²)	
Author	Neutral	Plantar Flexion	Dorsiflexion
Macko (1991)	5.22 ± 0.94[a]	3.81 ± 0.93 at (15°)[a]	5.40 ± 0.74 at (10°)[a]
Paar (1983)	4.15	4.15 at (10°)	3.63 at (10°)
Ramsey and Hamilton (1976)	4.40 ± 1.21[a]	3.69 at (20°)	
Kimizuka (1980)	4.83		
Libotte and colleagues (1982)	5.41	5.01 at (30°)	3.60 at (30°)

[a]Mean and standard deviation.

(234 ± 122 N/mm) than the anterior tibiofibular ligament (162 ± 64 N/mm). The mean failure mode of the interosseous tibiofibular ligament (822 ± 298 N) was significantly greater than that of the anterior tibiofibular ligament (625 ± 255 N). The interosseous tibiofibular ligament is suggested as an important stabilizer of the tibiofibular syndesmosis.

▶ Load-Bearing Characteristics of the Ankle Joint

The talar articular surface is in constant contact with the tibial plafond and the articular surfaces of the malleoli. The load-bearing surface of the ankle joint is 11 to 13 cm² and maximum contact area occurs at a position of the talus corresponding to 50% of the stance phase and averages 5.23 ± 0.6 cm².[61] The contact area of the talus in different positions of the ankle joint is as indicated in Table 10.2.

Lambert, in a strain-gauge study of five legs, demonstrated that, in the biostatic models, one sixth of the static load of the leg is carried by the fibula at the tibiofibular joint.[61] Ramsey and Hamilton, using powdered carbon black coating technique of the tibial and talar articular surfaces in 23 lower extremities, assessed the contact area on the talus with axial loading of 686 N (70 kg).[62] One millimeter of lateral displacement of the talus decreased the tibiotalar contact surface by 42%, thus potentially inducing a marked increase of the stress forces on the remaining smaller contact area, which in the clinical setup could possibly lead to traumatic arthritis.

Michelson et al[63] investigated the pressure distribution in the ankle joint under axial loading of 100 lb (220 N) in six above-knee lower extremity specimens. The feet were ranged from 30° of plantar flexion to 15° plantar flexion, neutral, 5°, 10°, and 20° of dorsiflexion. The intra-articular pressure was recorded with particular pressure-sensitive sensors. The data was routed to the collecting computer and analyzed.

The pressure increased at the fibulotalar articulation and at the medial malleolar-talar articulation from neutral position of the talus to 20° of dorsiflexion (Fig. 10.19). At the tibiotalar joint, the medial and lateral segments "exhibited different patterns of response to position of the ankle. On the medial side, there was a relatively constant force throughout plantar flexion, up to roughly 5 degrees of dorsiflexion. From there on, there was a rapid decrease in force. Laterally, tibiotalar forces gradually increased as the ankles moved from extreme plantar flexion to 5 degrees of dorsiflexion." With further dorsiflexion, the response to force flattened out (Figs. 10.19 to 10.22).

▶ Stability of the Ankle Joint

As specified by McCullough and Burge, the stability of the ankle is determined by passive and dynamic factors.[18] The passive stability depends on the contour of the articular surfaces, the integrity of the collateral ligaments, the integrity of the distal tibiofibular ligaments, the retinacular system around the ankle, and the crossing and attached tendon tunnels. The dynamic stability is conferred by gravity, muscle action, and the reaction between the foot and the ground.

The close pack or maximally stable position of the ankle is the dorsiflexed position.[64] In the non–weight-bearing position, the side-to-side stability of the ankle is provided mainly by the malleoli and the collateral ligaments, whereas the stability in the sagittal plane is ligament dependent. Posterolaterally and posteromedially, the peronei tendons, the tibialis posterior tendon, the flexor digitorum longus tendon, the flexor hallucis longus tendon, and their fibrous sheaths contribute to stability.

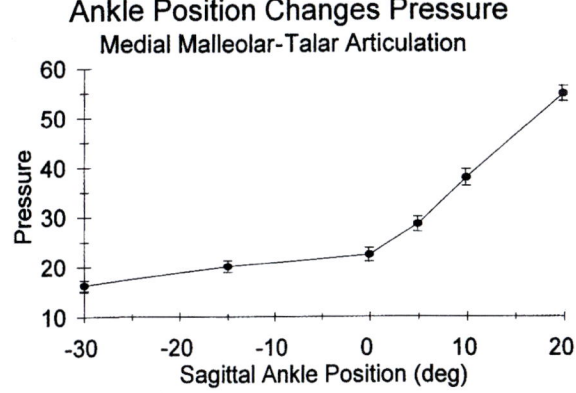

Figure 10.19 Change in force at the medial malleolar-talar articulation as a function of sagittal position of the ankle as measured by force transducers secured to the midpoint of the medial malleolar articular surface. The ankle specimen is axially loaded in neutral and cycled through a sagittal range of motion. (Michelson JD, Checcone M, Kuhn T, et al. Intra-articular load distribution in the human ankle joint during motion. *Foot Ankle Int*. 2001;3:226-233, Figure 5. Copyright ©2001. Reprinted by Permission of SAGE Publications.)

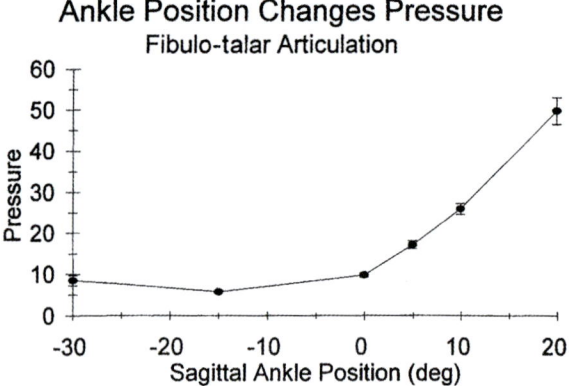

Figure 10.20 Change in force at the lateral malleolar-talar articulation as a function of sagittal position of the ankle as measured by force transducers secured to the midpoint of the lateral malleolar articular surface. The ankle specimen is axially loaded in neutral and then cycled through a sagittal range of motion. (Michelson JD, Checcone M, Kuhn T, et al. Intra-articular load distribution in the human ankle joint during motion. *Foot Ankle Int.* 2001;3: 226-233, Figure 6. Copyright ©2001. Reprinted by Permission of SAGE Publications.)

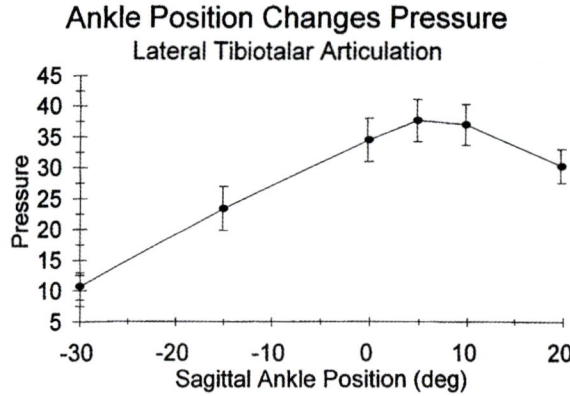

Figure 10.22 Change in force at the talar dome tibial plafond articulation as a function of sagittal position of the ankle as measured by force transducers secured to the midpoint of the articular surface of the lateral plafond. The ankle specimen is axially loaded in neutral and then is cycled through a sagittal range of motion. (Michelson JD, Checcone M, Kuhn T, et al. Intra-articular load distribution in the human ankle joint during motion. *Foot Ankle Int.* 2001;3:226-233, Figure 8. Copyright ©2001. Reprinted by Permission of SAGE Publications.)

Lateral Collateral Ligaments

Stabilizing Function Based on Anatomic Observation

With regard to the lateral collateral ligaments, Inman mentions that as they arise from the fibula close to the axis of ankle joint motion, "the normal flexion and extension movements of the ankle lead to little or no change in tension of these structures."[10] The average location of the axis of motion on the lateral side is 3 ± 2 mm distal and 8 ± 5 mm anterior to the tip of the lateral malleolus. The anteroinferior location of the axis does introduce appreciable tension in the ligaments unless the axis is specifically, in a given ankle, very close to the tip of the lateral malleolus. Based on dissected anatomic specimens prepared as models, valid observations can be made with regard to their function.

The *anterior talofibular ligament* is taut in plantar flexion and relaxed in dorsiflexion. It is a major ligament determining the anterior stability in tiptoe standing. In the acutely plantar flexed position, the ligament braces the talus and makes a marked turn around the anterolateral corner of the talar body (Fig. 10.23). It

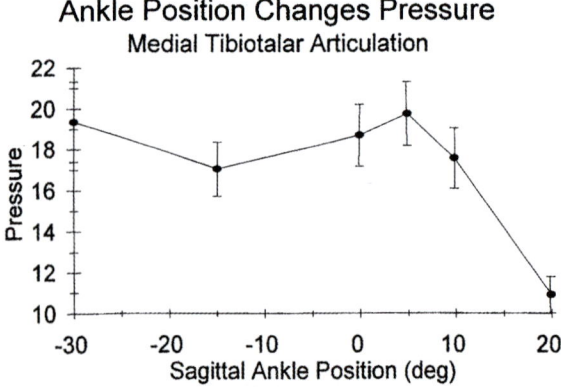

Figure 10.21 Change in force at the medial talar dome tibial plafond articulation as a function of sagittal position of the ankle as measured by force transducers secured to the midpoint of the articular surface of the medial plafond. The ankle specimen is axially loaded in neutral and cycled through a sagittal range of motion. (Michelson JD, Checcone M, Kuhn T, et al. Intra-articular load distribution in the human ankle joint during motion. *Foot Ankle Int.* 2001;3:226-233, Figure 7. Copyright ©2001. Reprinted by Permission of SAGE Publications.)

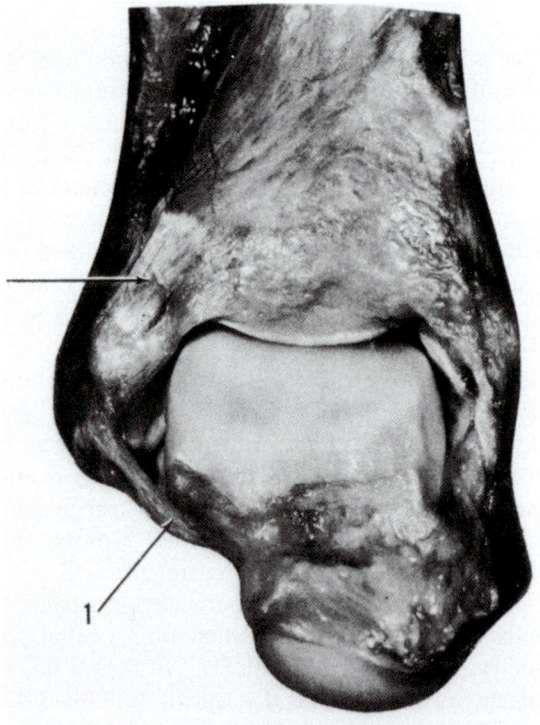

Figure 10.23 In marked plantar flexion, the anterior talofibular ligament (*1*) braces the talus and makes a turn around the anterolateral corner of the talar body.

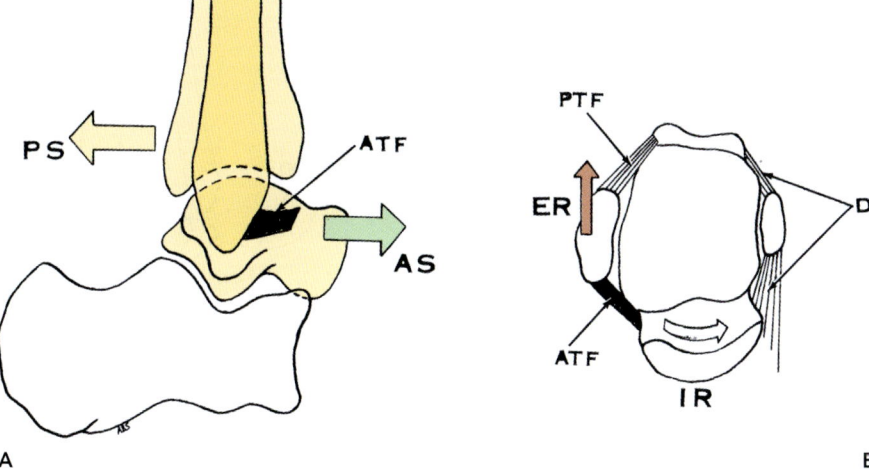

Figure 10.24 **Function of the anterior talofibular (ATF) ligament.** (A) ATF ligament limits the anterior shift of the talus or the posterior shift of the tibia-fibula. (B) ATF ligament limits the internal rotation of the talus or the external rotation of the fibula. (AS, anterior shift; D, deltoid ligament; ER, external rotation of the fibula; IR, internal rotation of the talus; PS, posterior shift; PTF, posterior talofibular ligament.)

limits the anterior shift and the medial rotation of the talus or the posterior shift of the tibia and the external rotation of the fibula (Fig. 10.24). This ligament also contributes in resisting the lateral talar tilt. According to DeVogel, when the anterior talofibular ligament is formed by two bands, the upper band is taut in plantar flexion but the lower band remains taut in all positions.[65]

The *posterior talofibular ligament* has increased tension in dorsiflexion and relaxes in plantar flexion. It braces the talus posteriorly. It limits the dorsiflexion on the foot and the posterior shift of the talus or the anterior displacement of the leg. This ligament is contributory in resisting the external rotation of the talus or the internal rotation of the fibula-tibia. It helps to transmit the internal rotation force of the leg to the talus (Fig. 10.25). Anatomically, the anterior fibers of the ligament are shorter than the posterior fibers. According to DeVogel, the anterior fibers remain taut throughout the entire arc of motion in the sagittal plane, whereas the posterior fibers are tense in dorsiflexion.[65]

The *calcaneofibular ligament* is the ligament of the ankle and of the subtalar joint. The tension in the ligament is affected by both joints. This ligament is taut in dorsiflexion and relaxed in plantar flexion (Fig. 10.26). However, in some specimens, the ligament is taut in plantar flexion and less tense in dorsiflexion (Fig. 10.27), whereas in others the tension in this ligament remains constant in all positions.

The subtalar position affects the tension in the ligament. Here also the results are variable as one observes different specimens. In the specimen of the hindfoot, illustrated in Figures 10.28 to 10.30, with varus position of the os calcis—lateral talar tubercle is high in the sinus tarsi—the calcaneofibular ligament is relatively relaxed. The anterior advancement of the calcaneus contributes to the relaxation of the ligament as its insertion shifts anteriorly. In the same specimen, in the valgus position—lateral talar tubercle low in the sinus tarsi—the os calcis shifts posteriorly relative to the talus and the calcaneofibular ligament is taut.

The variability of the tension in the calcaneofibular ligament may be explained on the basis of the insertional variability of the ligament. As demonstrated by Ruth, the ligament may be oblique, horizontal, vertical, or fan shaped (Fig. 10.31).[66] This has a direct bearing on the tension developed by this ligament during motion. When the calcaneofibular ligament is nearly horizontal, in valgus position of the heel, the distance between

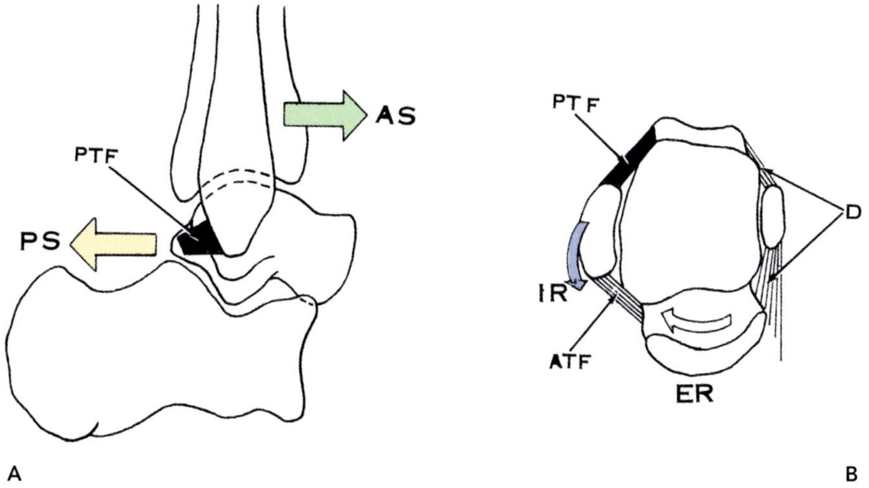

Figure 10.25 **Function of the posterior talofibular ligament (PTF).** (A) PTF limits the posterior shift of the talus or the anterior shift of the fibula-tibia. (B) PTF limits the external rotation of the talus or the internal rotation of the fibula. (AS, anterior shift of the tibia-fibula; ATF, anterior talofibular ligament; D, deltoid ligament; ER, external rotation of the talus; IR, internal rotation of the fibula; PS, posterior shift of the talus.)

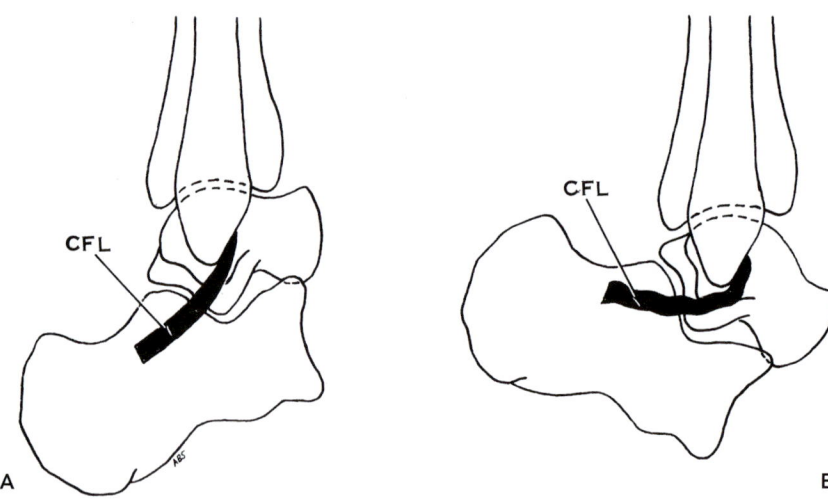

Figure 10.26 Tension in calcaneofibular ligament (*CFL*). (A) CFL taut in dorsiflexion of ankle. (B) CFL relaxed in plantar flexion of ankle.

the origin and the insertion increases; the distance decreases in varus (Fig. 10.32). The ligament is taut in valgus, less tense in varus. When the ligament is vertical in neutral, the distance between the origin and the insertion is increased in varus and decreased in valgus. The ligament is taut in varus and less tense in valgus (see Fig. 10.32). When the ligament has an intermediary obliquity, the ligament tension remains unchanged throughout the motion.

Inman stressed the coupling effect of the calcaneofibular ligament and the anterior talofibular ligament in preventing the talar tilt on the lateral side.[10] In dorsiflexion, the calcaneofibular ligament approaches the vertical position, acts as a true collateral ligament, of the ankle joint, and prevents the talar tilt of the talus. In plantar flexion, the anterior talofibular ligament is vertical and functions as a collateral ligament, stabilizing the talus laterally. The average angle between the two ligaments, measured in their projection on the sagittal plane, is 105° ± 24°.[10] The reciprocal arrangement of the two ligaments is efficient if the angle between the two ligaments is 90°. A horizontal calcaneofibular ligament does not provide the same stability.

The *peroneotalocalcaneal ligament* of Rouvière and Canela Lazaro is taut in dorsiflexion and relaxed in plantar flexion. It also limits the anterior displacement of the leg. Both authors have demonstrated that the section of the ligament appreciably increases the anterior displacement of the leg when the foot is stabilized on a table and weight is applied to the anteriorly rotating leg.

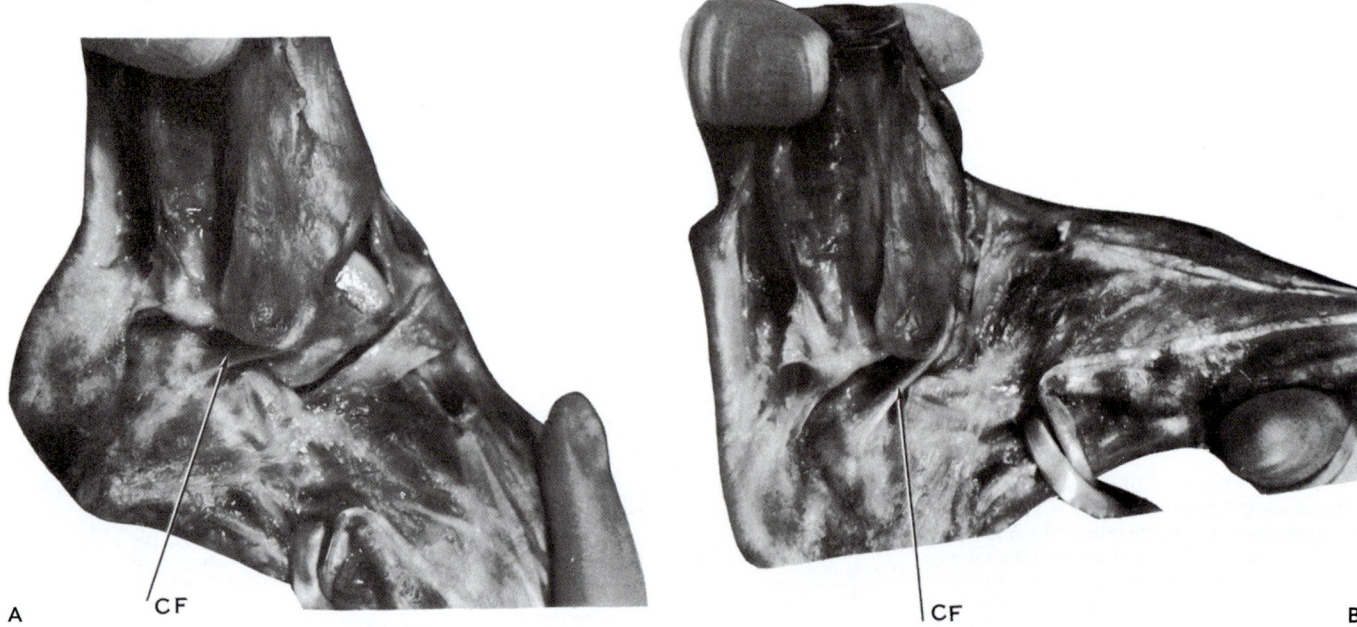

Figure 10.27 In this anatomic specimen of the ankle, the calcaneofibular ligament (*CFL*) is taut in plantar flexion (A) and less tense in dorsiflexion (B).

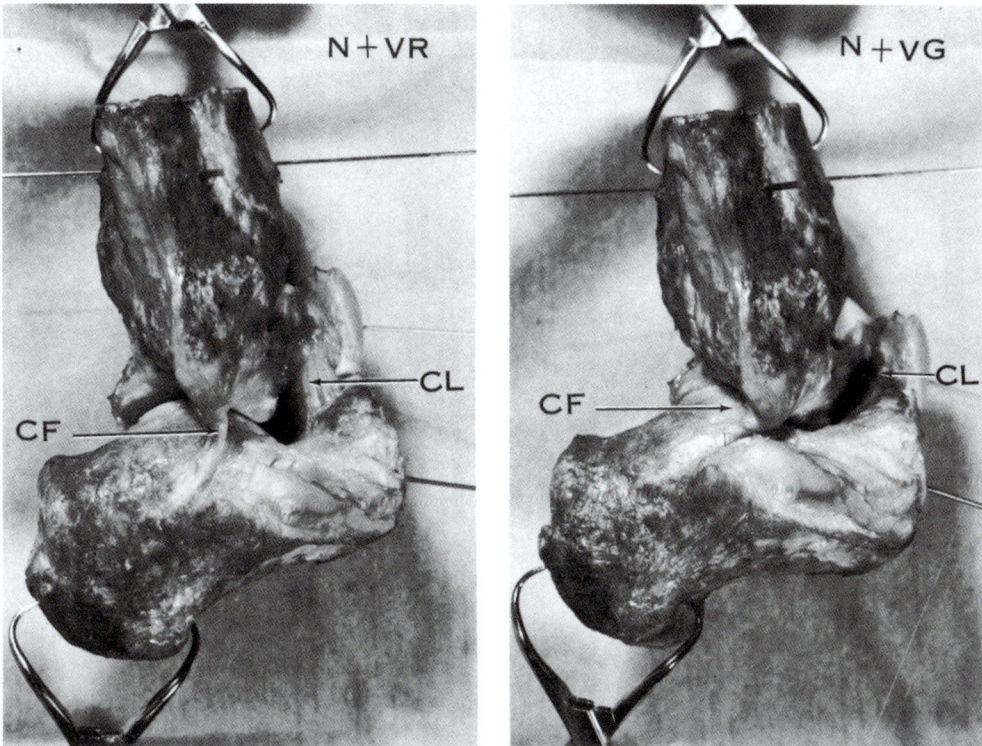

Figure 10.28 Hindfoot specimen, lateral view. The ankle is held in neutral position (*N*) and the os calcis is moved into varus (*VR*) or valgus (*VG*). In varus, the calcaneofibular ligament is relaxed and the cervical ligament is vertical and tense. In valgus, the calcaneofibular ligament is taut and the cervical ligament is oblique or horizontal but still tense. (*CFL*, calcaneofibular ligament; *CL*, cervical ligament.)

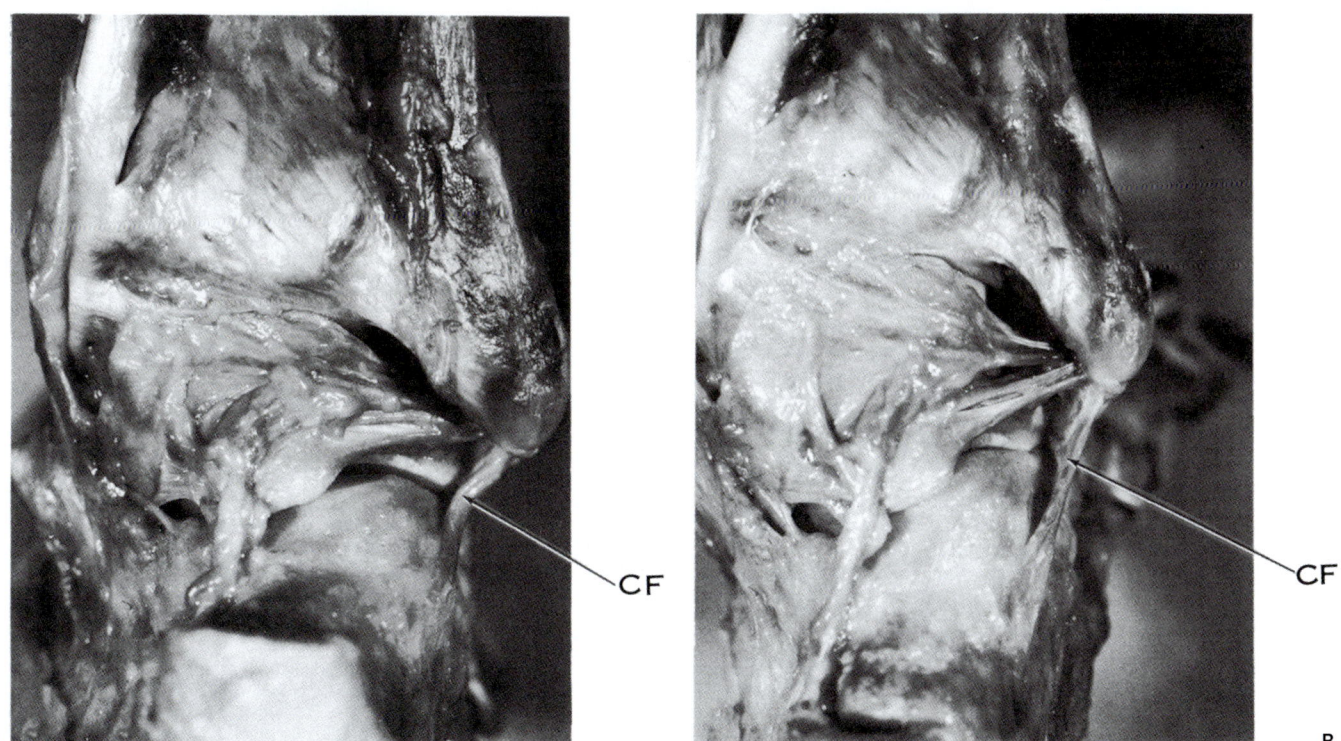

Figure 10.29 Hindfoot specimen, posterolateral view. The ankle is held in neutral. **(A)** The heel is in varus and the calcaneofibular ligament (*CFL*) is relaxed. **(B)** The heel is in valgus and the calcaneofibular ligament is taut.

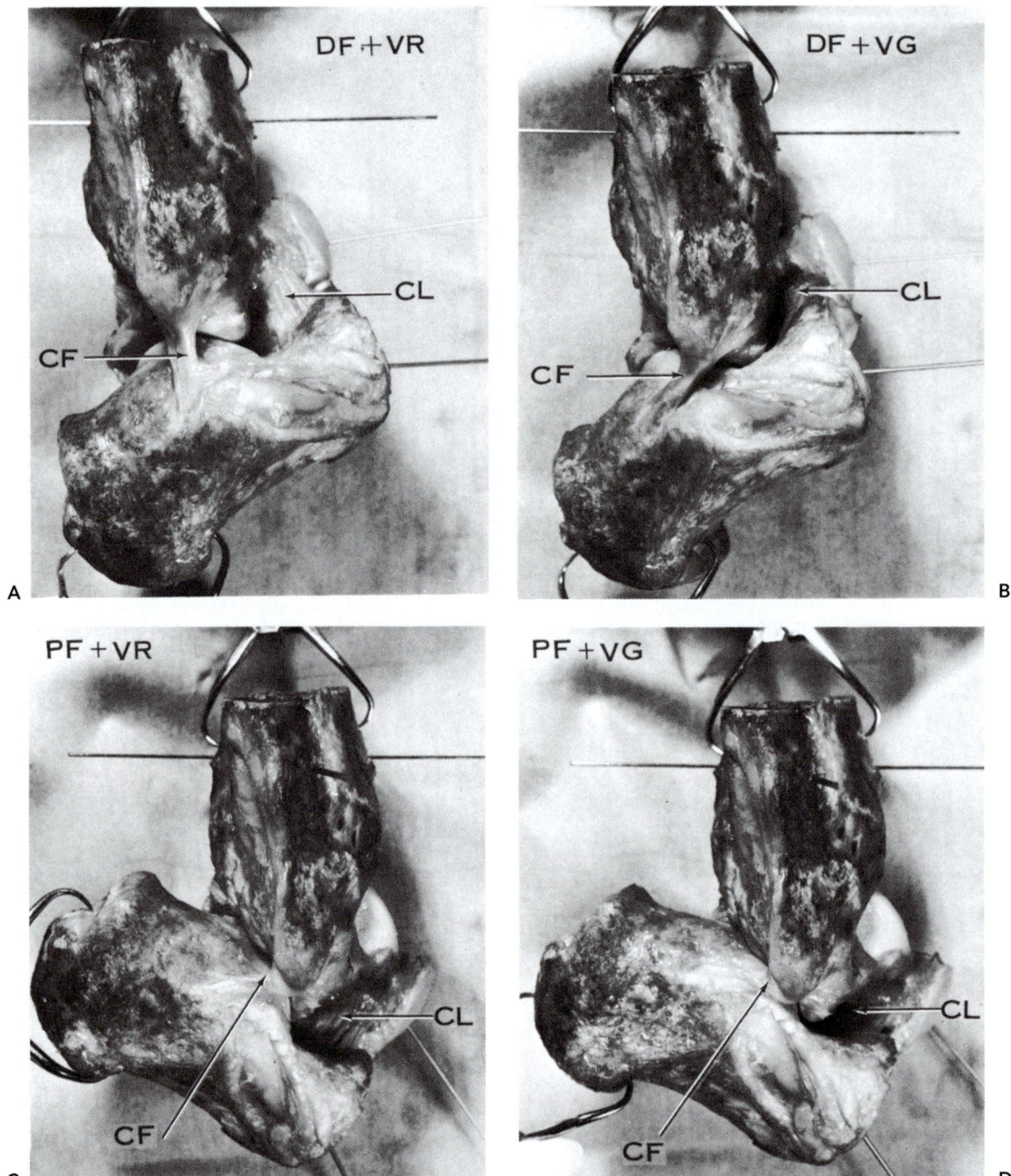

Figure 10.30 **Hindfoot specimen, lateral view, in dorsiflexion (*DF*) and plantar flexion (*PF*) combined with varus (*VR*) or valgus (*VG*) of the os calcis.** The dorsiflexion and plantar flexion are indicated by the Kirschner wires (K-wires) implanted in the talus and the os calcis. The valgus and varus are recognized by the relative position of the talus and os calcis: in varus the lateral talar process is away from the postero-lateral corner of the sinus tarsi, whereas in valgus the same process strikes or is very close to the sinus tarsi of the os calcis. **(A)** Combination of dorsiflexion and varus. **(B)** Combination of dorsiflexion and valgus. The calcaneofibular ligament is taut, more so in valgus. **(C)** Combination of plantar flexion and varus. **(D)** Combination of plantar flexion and valgus. In **C** and **D**, the calcaneofibular ligament is less taut than in **A** and **B**, yet slightly more tension is present in the ligament in valgus. The cervical ligament (*CL*) is nearly vertical and parallel to the calcaneofibular ligament in dorsiflexion of the ankle and varus of the heel. The cervical ligament is taut in both valgus and varus.

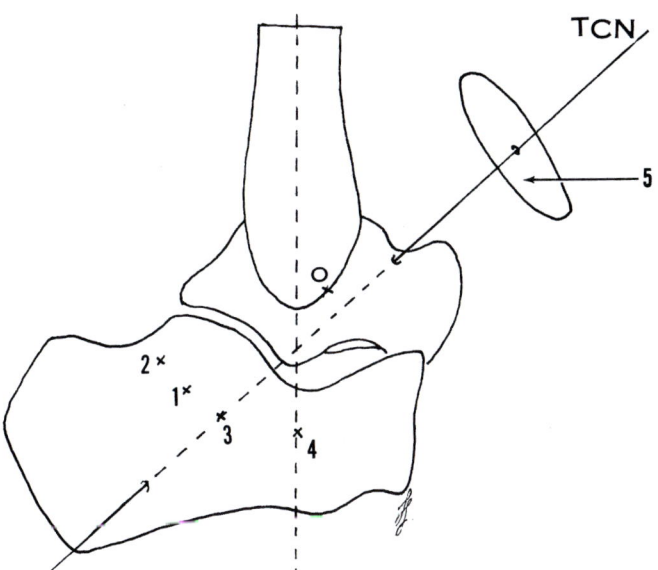

Figure 10.31 Hindfoot, lateral view. *O* indicates the origin of the calcaneofibular ligament and the numbers 1 to 4 the calcaneal insertion of the same ligament. The variable insertion determines the obliquity of the ligament; *1*, common insertion, oblique ligament; *2*, horizontal ligament; *3*, ligament located along the projection of the talocalcaneonavicular axis *(TCN)*; *4*, vertical ligament. The displacement of the insertional points *1* to *4* is along arcs of circles parallel to the circle *5*, which is perpendicular to the talocalcaneonavicular axis.

Strain Patterns in Lateral Collateral Ligaments

Renstrom and colleagues studied the strain patterns during motion, without load, of the anterior talofibular and calcaneofibular ligaments in five cadaveric ankles.[67] The foot was transfixed to a platform at the level of the metatarsal head and the os calcis and the motion of plantar flexion to dorsiflexion was carried out separately or in combination with internal-external rotation of the fixed foot or supination-pronation. In the transfixed foot, the latter motion is truly an inversion-eversion of the foot when both the heel and forefoot are moved forcefully in the same direction. The strain gauges were attached to the mid segment of the corresponding ligament.

In the anterior talofibular ligament, the strain increased 3.3% through the range of motion from 10° of dorsiflexion to 40° of plantar flexion. There was a slight increase in the strain in internal rotation and a decrease in strain of 1.9% in external rotation (Fig. 10.33).

The calcaneofibular ligament remained essentially isometric during the arc of plantar flexion-dorsiflexion at the ankle. The foot position affected the strain pattern in the ligament. External rotation, supination (truly inversion in the present setup), and supination-internal rotation significantly increased the strain in the calcaneofibular ligament relative to the neutral position (Fig. 10.34). The highest values were obtained in dorsiflexion and the strain values greatly diminished with progressive plantar flexion. The synergistic function of the anterior talofibular ligament and the calcaneofibular ligament was again confirmed. During the arc of extension-flexion, when one ligament is relaxed, the other is strained, and vice versa. This is similar to Inman's concept of coupling of the two ligaments.

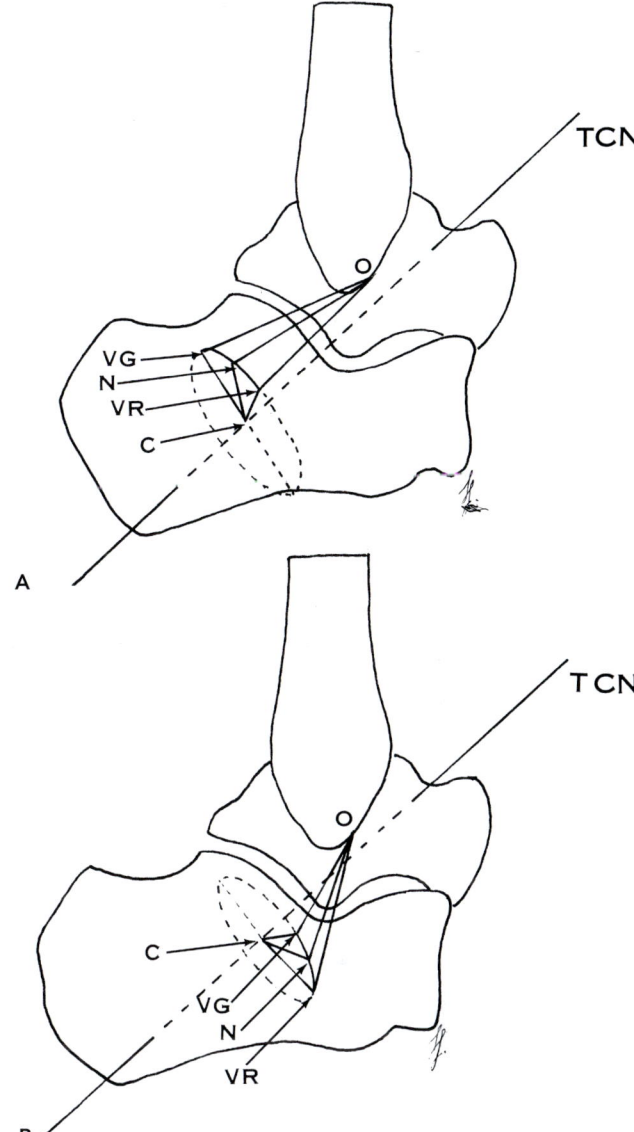

Figure 10.32 Calcaneofibular ligament with common insertion. **(A)** *O* indicates the origin of the ligament and *N* the insertional position in neutral. In valgus *(VG)* and varus *(VR)* the displacements occur along the circle *C*, which is perpendicular to the talocalcaneonavicular axis *(TCN)*. In valgus the distance from the origin to the insertion is longer and the calcaneofibular ligament is taut. In varus the distance is shorter and the ligament is more relaxed. **(B)** In the vertical type of calcaneofibular ligament, the distance between the origin of the ligament and its insertion is greater in varus and less in valgus. The ligament is taut in varus and relaxed in valgus.

Normal Talar Tilt

The instability of the ankle in the coronal plane (lateral talar tilt) and in the sagittal plane (anterior talar shift) is of great clinical significance and has been the subject of extensive investigation in defining the role of the components of the lateral collateral ligament.

Cox and Hewes, in a study of 404 ankles, tested 202 young adults between the ages of 17 and 20 years.[66] Manual supination force was applied to the hindfoot with the ankle in approximately 30° of plantar flexion. The measurement was

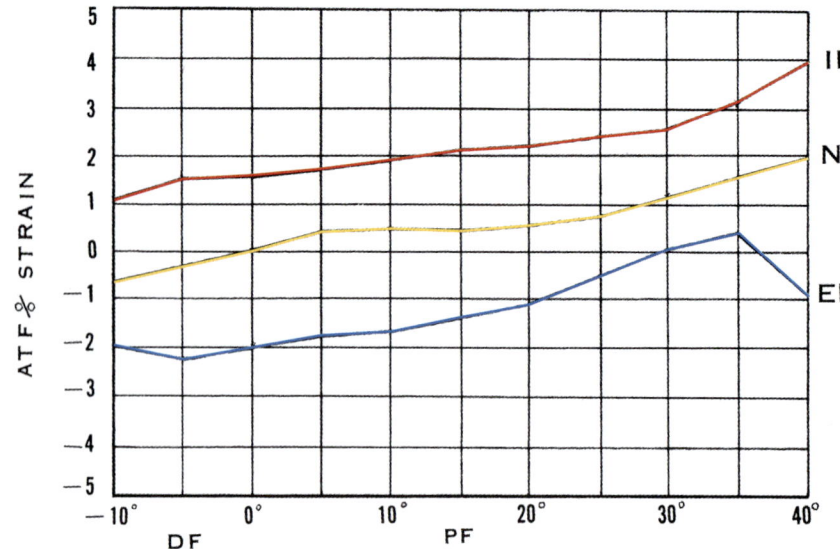

Figure 10.33 Percent strain in anterior talofibular ligament (*ATF*) with the foot in different degrees of plantar flexion, dorsiflexion—in neutral or combined with external-internal rotation of the foot. In the neutral position of the ankle, the internal rotation increases the strain, whereas the external rotation decreases the strain in the ligament. (Adapted from Renstrom P, Wertz M, Incavo S, et al. Strain in the lateral ligaments of the ankle. *Foot Ankle*. 1988;9[2]:62. Copyright ©1988. Reprinted by Permission of SAGE Publications)

roentgenographic. In this large group, 90.4% had no lateral talar tilt, 7.9% had a tilt between 1 and 5°, and 1.7% had a tilt greater than 5°. One ankle measured 17°, another 16°.

Rubin and Witten, in a roentgenographic study of 150 normal volunteers, found the lateral talar tilt to range from 0° to 23°.[68] However, 93% of the group had a talar tilt of 10° or less.

Glasgow and coworkers[26] consider a talar tilt of up to 6° as normal and, for Freeman,[27] a difference in talar tilt of 6° or more between the injured and the uninjured ankle is pathologic. The variations of the normal talar tilt are as indicated in Table 10.3.

Normal Anterior Talar Shift

Normally the talus may be displaced anteriorly when the leg is pressed backward and the heel is brought forward. Landeros and colleagues, in describing the anterior displacement of the talus or anterior drawer sign with manual force, consider the normal anterior talar shift to be 2.5 to 3 mm.[28] They also specify that the ankle is to be stressed with the leg-ankle at 90° and "because of the geometry of the bones, anterior displacement of the talus must be accompanied by caudad displacement of the talus as its dome rides forward under the anterior articular margin of the tibia."[28] They further mention that with plantar flexion of 30° or more, the anterior talar shift may not be present; this is probably due to the increased tension in the anterior talofibular ligament. Laurin and Mathieu studied the sagittal mobility of the normal ankle in 40 people ranging in age from 6 to 27 years.[29] The force applied on the leg, with the heel being supported on a rest, varied from 20 to 70 lb. The measurements were taken in neutral and equinus. In the neutral position, the anterior talar shift averaged 3.3 to 0.3 mm, and in equinus the

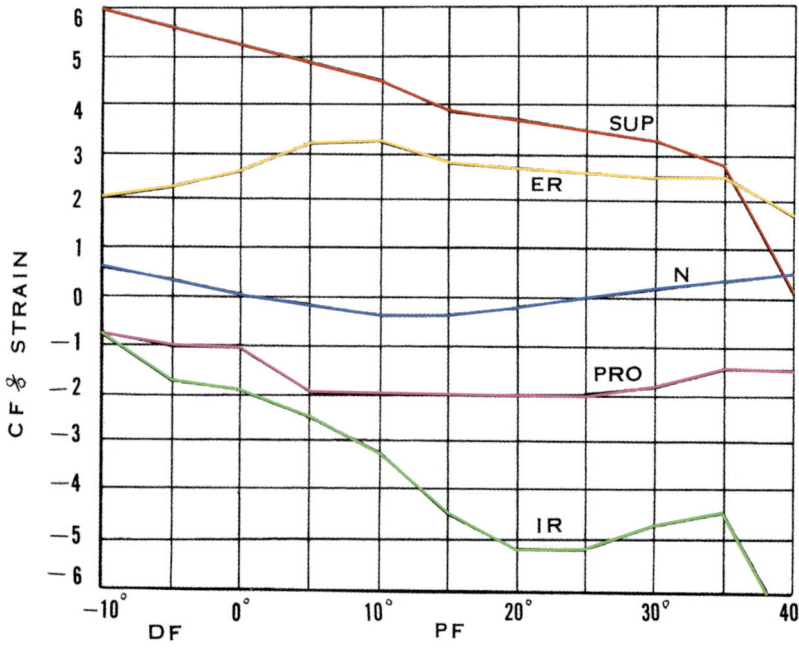

Figure 10.34 Percent strain in calcaneofibular ligament with the foot in different degrees of plantar flexion, dorsiflexion—in neutral or combined with supination-pronation or internal-external rotation of the foot. In neutral position of the ankle, the external rotation or the supination of the foot increases the strain of the ligament, whereas the pronation and the internal rotation decrease the strain. (*N*, neutral; *SUP*, supination; *PRO*, pronation; *IR*, internal rotation; *ER*, external rotation.) (Adapted from Renstrom P, Wertz M, Incavo S, et al. Strain in the lateral ligaments of the ankle. *Foot Ankle*. 1988;9[2]:62. Copyright ©1988. Reprinted by Permission of SAGE Publications.)

TABLE 10.3 Variations in Degree of Normal Talar Tilt	
Author and Method	Normal Talar Tilt
With manual force without anesthesia	
Duquennoy and coworkers	5° (0°-10°)
Cox and Hewes	0° (90.4%)
Glasgow and colleagues	>5°-17° (1.7%) up to 6°
Freeman	<6° between injured and uninjured
With a device without anesthesia	
Rubin and Witten	0°-23° with 93% ≤ 10%°
Sedlin	8° (0°-15°)
Laurin and St. Jacques	7° (0°-27°)
Ouellet and coworkers	5° (0°-27°)

average shift was less, measuring 1.3 to 0.2 mm. The methodology used affects the measurements (Table 10.4).

Experimental Studies of Anterior and Lateral Ankle Stability and Transverse Rotational Stability

The contribution of the components of the lateral collateral ligaments to the stability of the ankle in the frontal, sagittal, and transverse planes has been analyzed in experimental setups. The ligamentous components are transected in a sequential manner, the ankle is subjected to stress, and the displacement of the talus is assessed.

Glasgow and colleagues examined 20 cadaveric ankles.[26] Division of the anterior talofibular ligament allowed anterior subluxation and medial rotation of the talus. There was no lateral talar tilt with the varus stress except for a minimal degree at the extreme of plantar flexion. The transection of both the anterior talofibular and the calcaneofibular ligaments resulted in marked lateral tilt and anteromedial subluxation of the talus when the foot was plantigrade or in equinus. The isolated division of the calcaneofibular ligament resulted in a minor degree of lateral talar tilt when the foot was plantigrade and the anterior talar subluxation was absent (Fig. 10.35).

TABLE 10.4 Normal Anterior Talar Displacement	
Author and Method	Displacement
With manual force	
Landeros and colleagues	2.5-3 mm
Laurin and Mathieu	
In neutral	9.2 ± 0.7 mm
In equinus	6.1 ± 0.4 mm
With defined force	
Laurin and Mathieu	
In neutral	3.3-0.3 mm
In equinus	1.3-0.2 mm
Castaing and Delaplace	5-8 mm

Johnson and Markolf analyzed the supportive role of the anterior talofibular ligament in a quantitative manner.[30] Thirty fresh-frozen cadaver ankles were used in their investigation. Initially, the intact specimens were subjected to an increasing anteroposterior force of a maximum of ±100 N and an inversion-eversion or internal-external torque of a maximum of ±2 N · m applied on the talus. The displacements of the talus were measured in the three orthogonal planes and the same measurements were repeated after transection of the anterior talofibular ligament. After sectioning the anterior talofibular ligament, the anterior talar shift increased 93%, or 4.3 ± 2 mm, from 5.5 ± 1.7 mm in the dorsiflexed position (Fig. 10.36). In neutral position, the anterior shift increased 64%, or 3.7 ± 1.88 mm, from 6.6 ± 2.3 mm, and 39%, or 2.5 ± 1.6 mm, from 5.8 ± 1.8 mm in plantar flexion. With an inversion torque of 2 N · m, the lateral talar tilt increased 49%, or 5.2° ± 2.3°, from 12.6° ± 3.8° plantar flexion (Fig. 10.37). In the neutral ankle position, the initial lateral talar tilt of 9.6° ± 3.2° increased 2.8° ± 1.9°, or 35%, after transection of the ligament, and in dorsiflexion the initial tilt of 7.2° ± 2.5° increased 2.5° ± 1.5°, or 43%.

These findings demonstrated the occurrence of lateral talar tilt with the transection of the anterior talofibular ligament in all positions of the ankle, in contradiction to the previous studies indicating a lateral talar tilt only in extreme plantar flexion. These results "establish the structural importance of the anterior talo-fibular ligament in all positions of flexion for three modes of loading."[30]

With an internal rotational torque of 2 N · m, the internal rotation of the talus of 14.3° ± 5.1° increased 10.8° ± 6.1°, or 86%, in plantar flexion (Fig. 10.38). In the neutral position, the initial internal rotation of 13.8° ± 4.6° increased 7.7° ± 4.6°, or 62%, after transection of the ligament, and in dorsiflexion the increase was 5.7° ± 3.6°, or 62%, from the initial talar rotation of 10.2° ± 6.7°. In essence, the release of the anterior talofibular ligament increases the anteromedial shift of the talus and allows a lateral talar tilt.

McCullough and Burge analyzed the rotary stability of the load-bearing talus.[18] In eight intact cadaveric ankles held in plantigrade position, a horizontal torque of 3 N · m was applied to the talus. Weight-bearing was simulated by applying vertical loads ranging from 1 to 50 kg and the horizontal rotation of the talus was assessed. With the ligaments intact, under a load of 1 kg, the horizontal rotation of the talus was 24.1° and decreased 7.5° ± 1.5° in a linear fashion as the vertical load reached 50 kg (see Fig. 10.13). In three ankles with the division of the anterior talofibular ligament, the range of medial talar rotation at a load of 15 kg increased by 5.9° ± 1.9°, but the joint was stable to inversion stress. The progressive transection of the calcaneofibular and the posterior talofibular ligaments increased the medial talar rotation another 5.4° ± 1.9°. There was, however, a substantial decrease in the horizontal talar rotation under a vertical load of 50 kg (Fig. 10.39).

To simulate an external rotational injury of the ankle, a sequential division of the anterior two-thirds of the deltoid ligament, the anterior tibiofibular ligament, and the posterior talofibular ligaments was carried out and the stressed external rotation of the talus was measured. With a vertical load of 15 kg, there was a linear progressive increase of 20° in the talar rotation from 24° to 46°, or 83%. With vertical loading of 50 kg, the rotation decreased to 30° (Fig. 10.40).

In five ankles, the isolated transfixation of the inferior tibiofibular syndesmosis decreased the external talar rotation by 9.3° ± 1.3° at 15 kg and by a smaller amount at 50 kg (Fig. 10.41). McCullough and Burge also presented the interesting concept of the components of the collateral ligaments forming a ring resisting the horizontal rotation (external or internal) of the talus by tension in opposing pairs (Fig. 10.42).[18] They also specified that the range of horizontal rotation measured in their cadaveric ankles is greater than that in living subjects, because of the added dynamic stability provided by the muscles.

Rasmussen conducted a comprehensive study of the stability of the ankle in function of the supportive ligaments.[31] This anatomic pool consisted of 152 cadaveric ankles, mostly elderly. In a subgroup of 113 ankles, mobility pattern curves were determined with a pin inserted into the talus connected to torque and angle sensors registering the rotary movements in

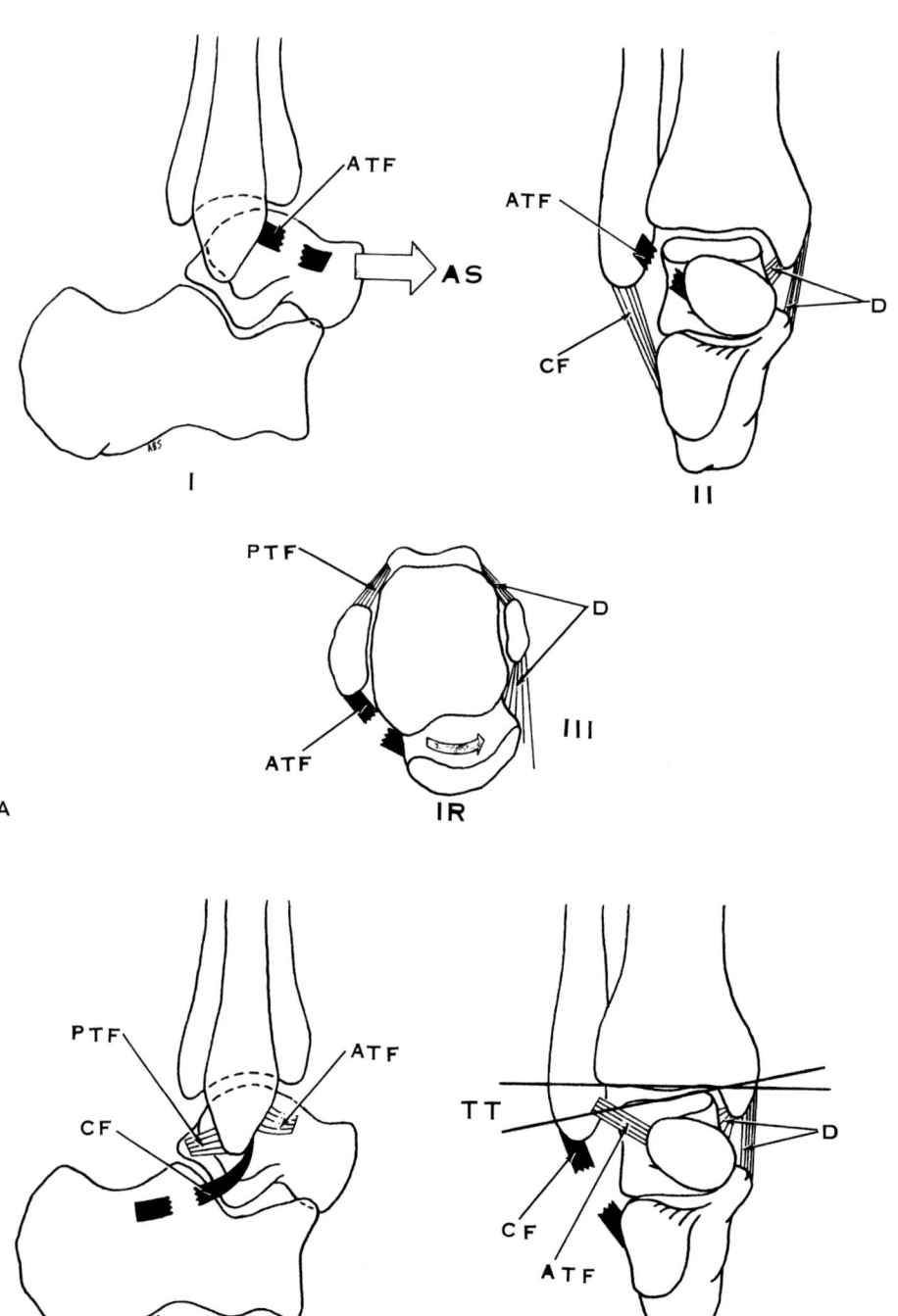

Figure 10.35 (A) The isolated tear of the anterior talofibular ligaments results in (*I*) anterior shift of the talus, (*II*) no lateral tilt of the talus with varus stress except for a minimal degree at the extreme of plantar flexion, (*III*) medial rotation of the talus. (B) The isolated transection of the calcaneofibular ligament results in (*I*) no anterior shift, (*II*) minor lateral talar tilt when the foot is plantar flexed. (C) Transection of the anterior talofibular and calcaneofibular ligaments results in (*I*) marked anterior shift of the talus, (*II*) lateral talar tilt, (*III*) internal rotation of the talus when the foot is plantar flexed. (*ATF*, anterior talofibular ligament; *CFL*, calcaneofibular ligament; *PTF*, posterior talofibular ligament; *IR*, internal rotation of talus.) (Data from Glasgow M, Jackson A, Jamieson AM. Instability of the ankle after injury to the lateral ligament. *J Bone Joint Surg Br*. 1980;62[2]:196.)

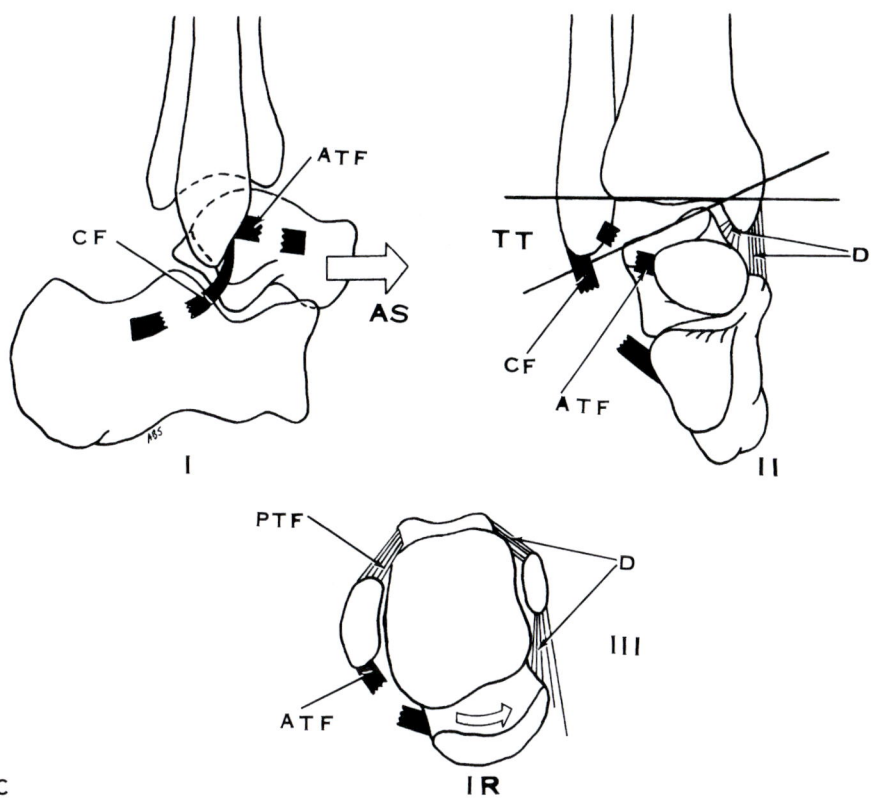

Figure 10.35 Cont'd

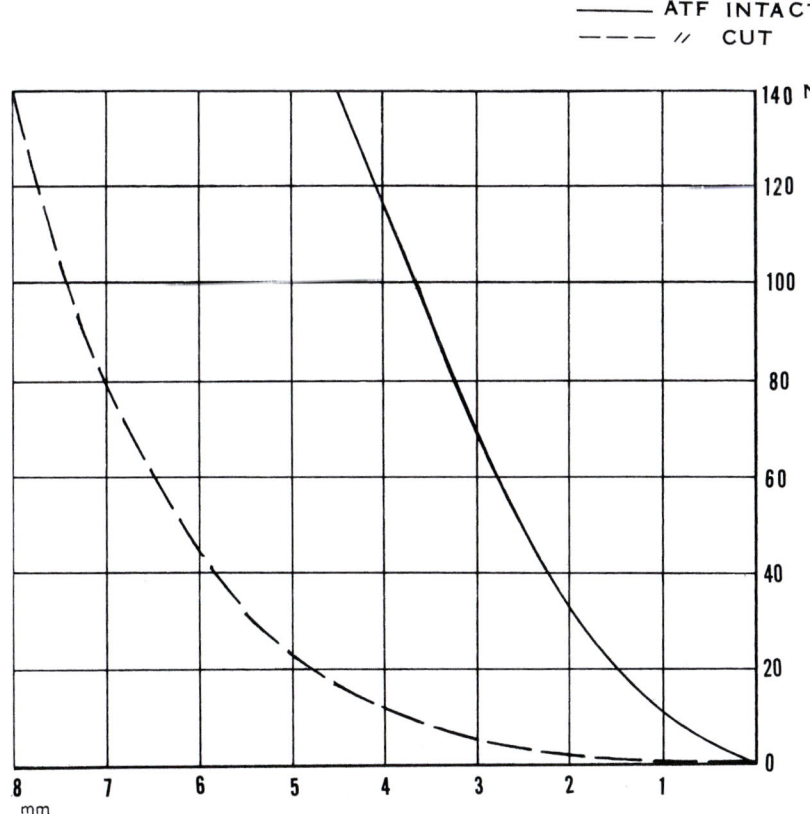

Figure 10.36 **Anterior shift of the talus before and after section of the anterior talofibular ligament in dorsiflexion with variable degree of force applied.** (*ATF*, anterior talofibular ligament; *ANT shift*, anterior displacement; *N*, Newton [force unit applied].) (Adapted from Johnson EE, Markolf KL. The contribution of the anterior talo-fibular ligament to ankle laxity. *J Bone Joint Surg Am.* 1983;65[1]:86.)

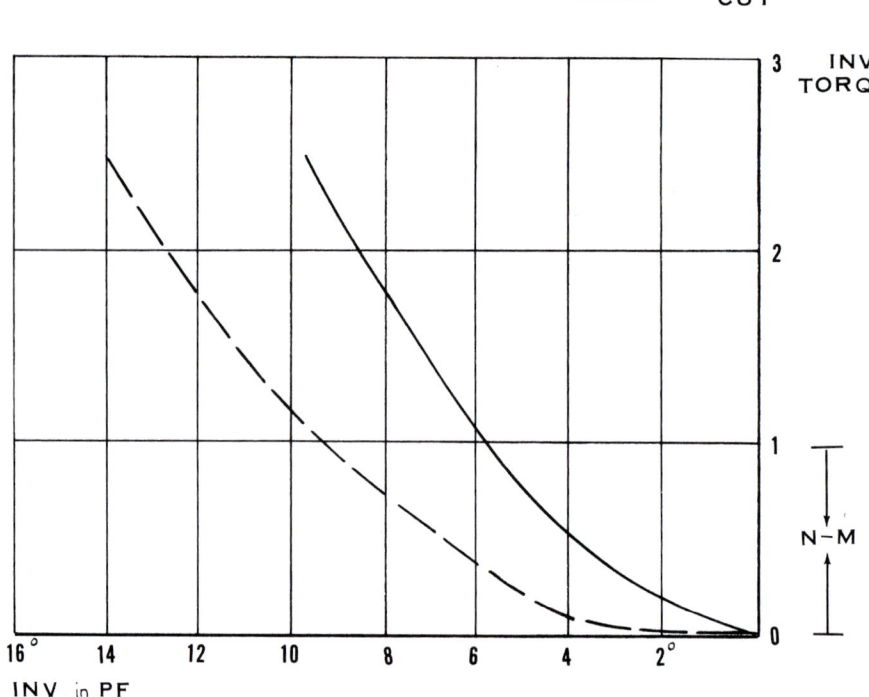

Figure 10.37 Inversion of the talus or lateral talar tilt in plantar flexion before and after section of the anterior talofibular ligament with variable inversion torque applied. (*ATF*, anterior talofibular ligament; *INV*, in *PF*, inversion or lateral tilt in plantar flexion; *INV torque*, inversion torque in Newton-meters.) (Adapted from Johnson EE, Markolf KL. The contribution of the anterior talo-fibular ligament to ankle laxity. *J Bone Joint Surg Am.* 1983;65[1]:86.)

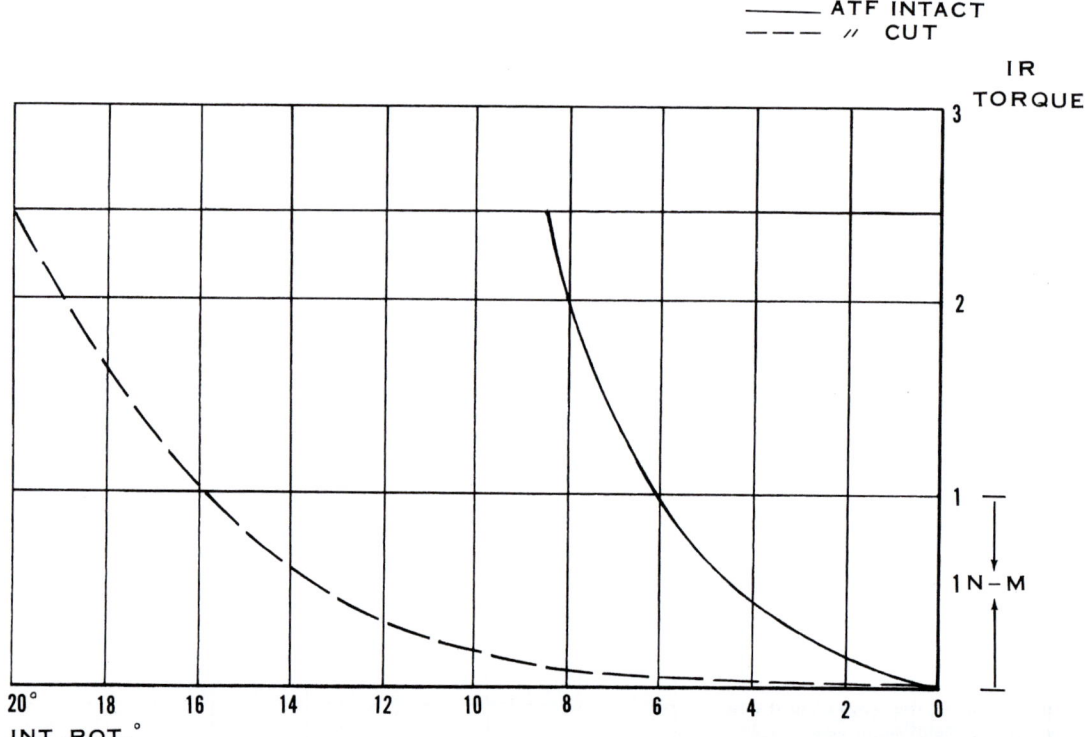

Figure 10.38 Internal rotation of the talus before and after section of the anterior talofibular ligament with variable internal rotation torque applied. (*ATF*, anterior talofibular ligament; *INT. ROT*, internal rotation of talus; *IR TORQUE*, internal rotational torque in Newton-meters.) (Adapted from Johnson EE, Markolf KL. The contribution of the anterior talo-fibular ligament to ankle laxity. *J Bone Joint Surg Am.* 1983;65[1]:86.)

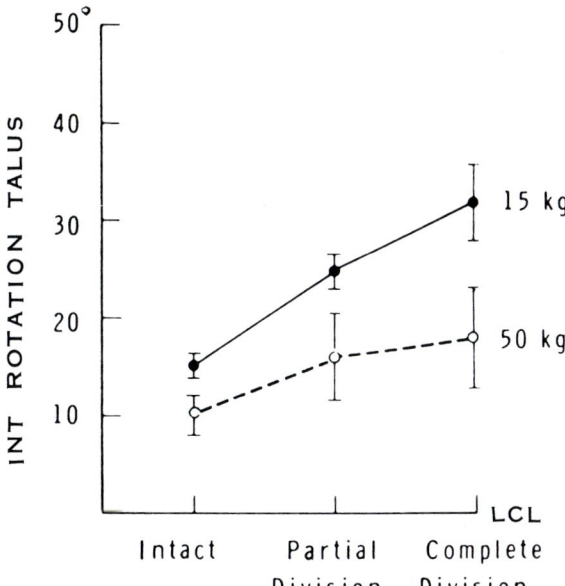

Figure 10.39 Mean range of medial talar rotation under vertical loading with lateral collateral ligament (*LCL*) intact, with partial division (section of the anterior talofibular ligament), and with complete division of the ligament (added section of the calcaneofibular and posterior talofibular ligaments). (Republished with permission of British Editorial Society of Bone and Joint Surgery, from McCullough CJ, Burge PD. Rotary stability of the load-bearing ankle. An experimental study. *J Bone Joint Surg Br*. 1980;62[4]:461; permission conveyed through Copyright Clearance Center, Inc.)

plantar flexion 36.89° ± 8.97°. In 50 ankles, the talar tilt or talar adduction was 5.58° ± 2.68°, and the reverse talar tilt or talar abduction measured 4.84° ± 1.96°. Internal rotation of the talus in 63 ankles was 8.60° ± 2.62°, and the external rotation was 8.21° ± 3.02°.

The mobility pattern was analyzed in 12 ankles in the frontal plane and another 12 ankles in the horizontal plane after transection of the anterior talofibular ligament. In the frontal plane, the talar tilt or adduction increased 4.83° ± 1.80°, mainly in plantar flexion. In the horizontal plane, the medial rotation of the talus increased 10° ± 3.59° (Figs. 10.43 and 10.44).

With transection of both the anterior talofibular ligament and the calcaneofibular ligament in nine ankles, the talar tilt or adduction increased 11.44° ± 6.15°, mostly in dorsiflexion and neutral. The medial rotation of the talus increased and the external rotation was unaffected also (see Figs. 10.43 and 10.44). Transection of the anterior talofibular ligament, the calcaneofibular ligament, and the entire posterior talofibular ligament resulted in marked instability. The lateral talar tilt was 45° to 60°, the horizontal talar medial rotation increased to more than 21°, and the talar external rotation increased by 10.67° ± 4.63° (see Figs. 10.43 and 10.44). The isolated transection of the calcaneofibular ligament in six ankles produced a negligible increase of 1.33° ± 1.37° in the lateral talar tilt, and the medial or lateral talar horizontal rotation was nearly unaffected.

Cass and coworkers investigated, in non–axially loaded configuration, the stability role of the components of the lateral collateral ligament in seven cadaveric ankles subjected to an inversion force.[32] The study was performed with intact ligaments and with serial transections of the same. The calcaneus remained transfixed to its reference grid. Quantitative triaxial measurements of the motion were made. In the intact specimens with an inversion force of 2 kg, there was 12.1° of adduction and 3.6°

the ankle simultaneously in two planes when affecting the talus by a torque of 1.5 N · m in different directions. The study was conducted with intact and with divided ligaments.

With intact ligaments, in 113 ankles, the dorsiflexion-plantar flexion was about 58°, with dorsiflexion 20.87° ± 7.53° and

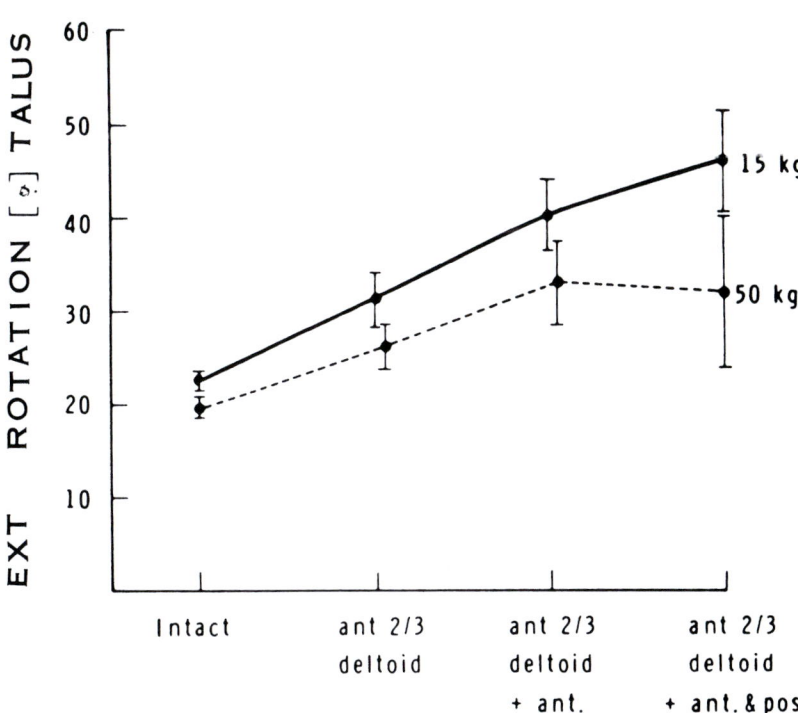

Figure 10.40 Mean range of external talar rotation under vertical loading with the ligaments intact and with sequential cuts of the anterior two thirds of the deltoid ligament and the anterior and posterior tibiofibular ligaments. (Republished with permission of British Editorial Society of Bone and Joint Surgery, from McCullough CJ, Burge PD. Rotary stability of the load-bearing ankle. An experimental study. *J Bone Joint Surg Br*. 1980;62[4]:461; permission conveyed through Copyright Clearance Center, Inc.)

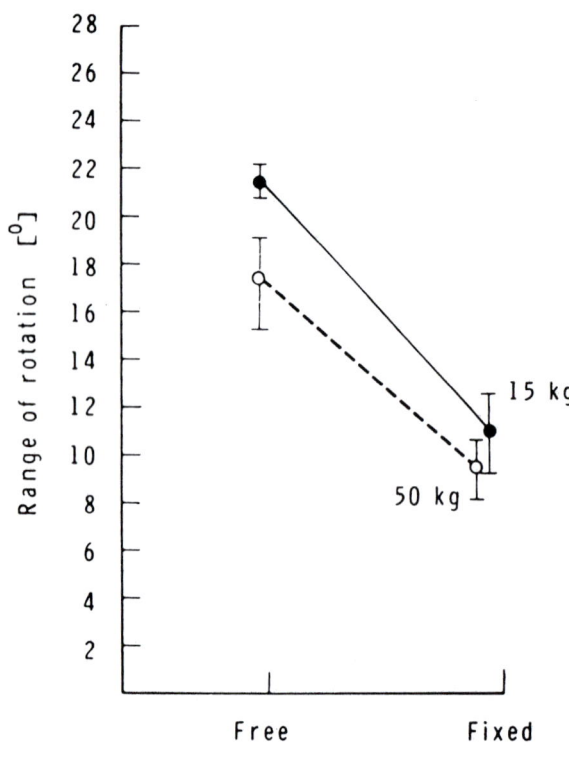

Figure 10.41 **Mean range of talar external rotation under vertical load with the inferior tibiofibular joint free or fixed.** (Republished with permission of British Editorial Society of Bone and Joint Surgery, from McCullough CJ, Burge PD. Rotary stability of the load-bearing ankle. An experimental study. J Bone Joint Surg Br. 1980;62[4]:402; permission conveyed through Copyright Clearance Center, Inc.)

of external rotation of the tibia relative to the talus. The tibial motion relative to the calcaneus was a mean maximum of 38° of adduction and 24° of external rotation. The sequential division of the three components of the lateral collateral ligament in an anteroposterior direction produced a gradual increase of the tibial adduction-external rotation. The isolated division of the calcaneofibular ligaments minimally affected these motions, with a 10% increase in adduction and a 3% increase in external rotation near 15° of plantar flexion, whereas that of the anterior talofibular ligament increased the tibial adduction by 30% and the external rotation by 8% at 30° of plantar flexion.

The combined division of these two ligaments produced instability near neutral position, with a tibial adduction increase of 41% and an external rotation increase of 65° (Fig. 10.45). Cass and colleagues stressed the importance of the coupling of the adduction-external rotation instability of the leg and attributed the sensation of "giving way" in the patients with unstable ankles during gait "to a sudden external rotation subluxation of the leg on the talus."[32] The normal mandatory external rotation of the leg with respect to the fixed foot when walking on level ground occurs at 15% to 20% of the stance phase and the external rotation of the tibia-fibula relative to the talus is resisted by the anterior talofibular ligament.[32] This ligament is an essential component of the supportive horizontal ligamentous ring (see Fig. 10.42). The external rotation of the leg places the ligament under tension and the excess may lead to its rupture.

Experimental Study of Posterior Ankle Stability

Harper investigated posterior ankle stability in six cadaveric ankles.[33] The posterior malleolus was ostetomized and the ankle was subjected to a posteriorly directed stress force, and the stability was assessed by lateral radiographs. The removed posterior malleolar fragment was increasingly larger, representing 30% to 40% and then 50% of the tibial articulating surface. No posterior talar subluxation was observed. In all six specimens, the medial malleolus was then ostetomized and the same posteriorly directed force applied manually, and no talar posterior shift was observed. By indirect proof, Harper concluded that the posterior talofibular ligament and the calcaneofibular ligaments "appeared to be the key structures providing posterior talar stability."

Mechanical Characteristics of the Lateral Collateral Ligaments

The tensile strength of the anterior talofibular ligament was investigated by St. Pierre and colleagues in 36 cadaver ankles.[34] The specimens consisted of the ligament attached to the lateral malleolus and to the talus. The average age of the cadavers was 64 years, with a range of 27 to 86 years. The tensile tests were conducted in pure tension to rupture or avulsion with the long

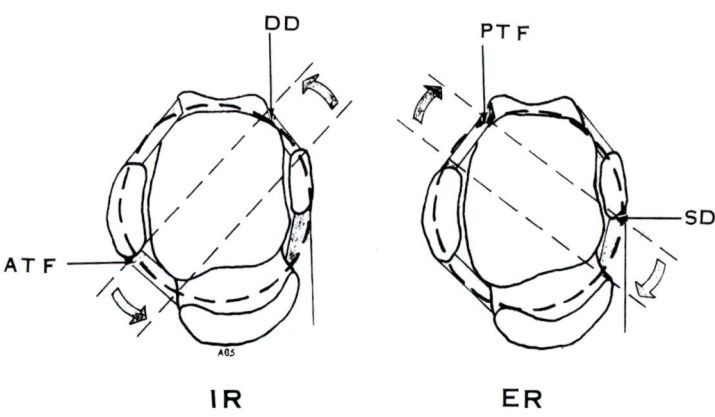

Figure 10.42 **The components of the collateral ligaments of the ankle forming a ring resisting the horizontal rotation of the talus by tension in opposing pairs.** Resisting the internal rotation (IR): the anterior talofibular ligament and the deep deltoid ligament. Resisting the external rotation (ER): the posterior talofibular ligament and the superficial deltoid ligament. (*ATF*, anterior talofibular ligament; *DD*, deep deltoid ligament; *PTF*, posterior talofibular ligament; *SD*, superficial deltoid ligament.)

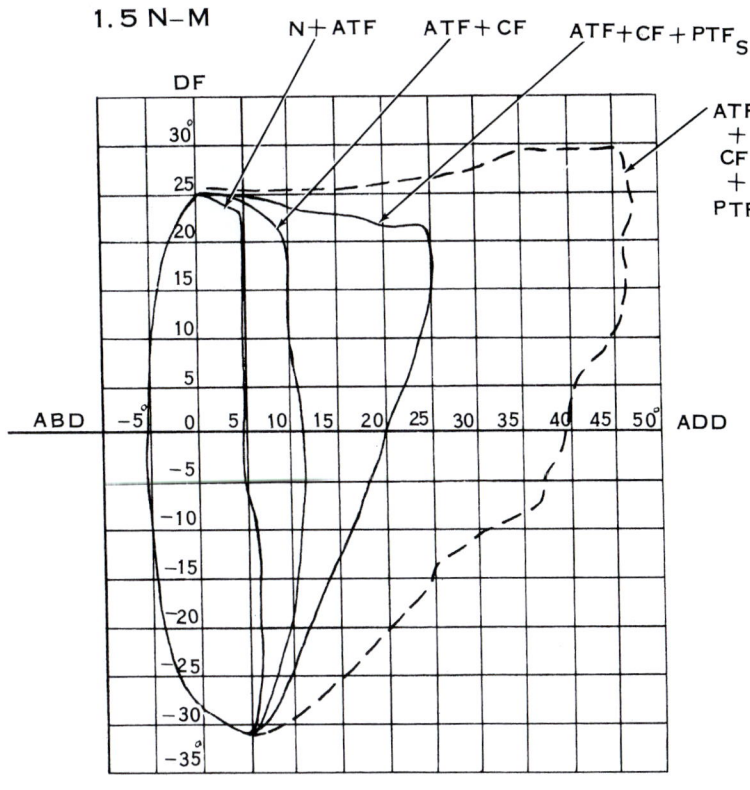

Figure 10.43 Mobility pattern in the sagittal and front planes after progressive section of the components of the lateral collateral ligament. The torque applied is 1.5 N m. (N, neutral; ATF, anterior talofibular ligament; CFL, calcaneofibular ligament; PTFS, posterior talofibular ligament short fibers; PTF, total posterior talofibular ligament; DF, dorsiflexion; PF, plantar flexion; ABD, abduction of talus; ADD, adduction of talus or lateral talar tilt.) (Adapted from Rasmussen O. Stability of the ankle joint: analysis of the function and traumatology of the ankle ligaments. *Acta Orthop Scand*. 1985;56[suppl 211]:34. Reproduced by permission of Taylor and Francis Group, LLC, a division of Informa plc.)

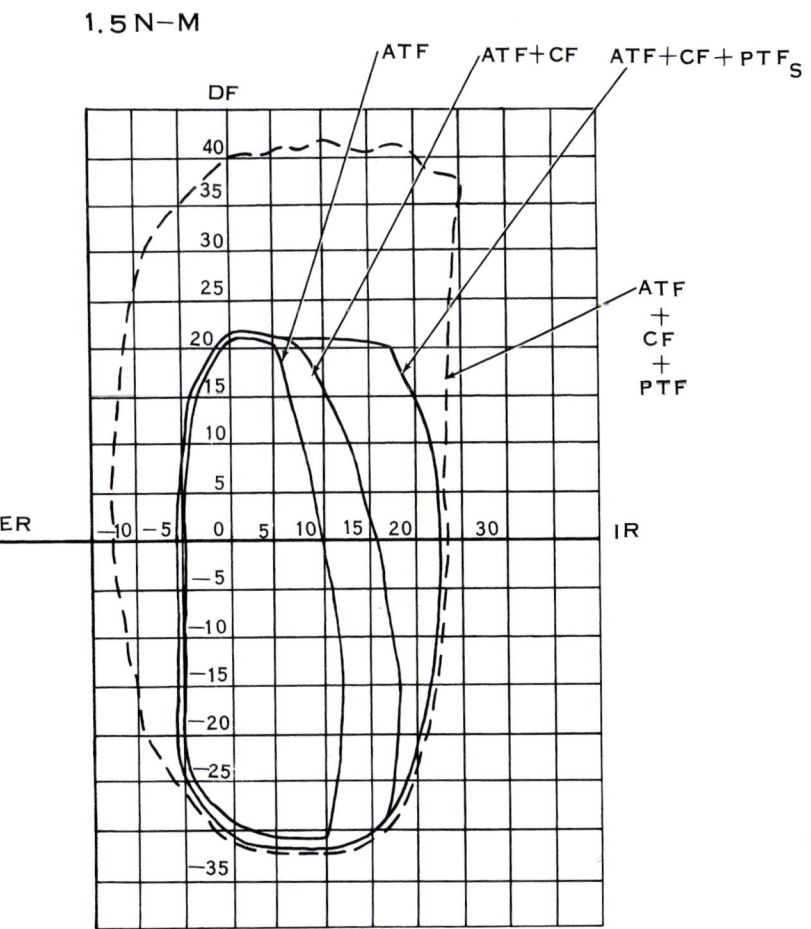

Figure 10.44 Mobility pattern in the sagittal and horizontal planes after progressive section of the components of the lateral collateral ligaments. The torque applied is 1.5 N · m. (ATF, anterior talofibular ligament; CFL, calcaneofibular ligament; PTFS, short fibers of posterior talofibular ligament; ER, external rotation; IR, internal rotation; DF, dorsiflexion; PF, plantar flexion.) (Adapted from Rasmussen O. Stability of the ankle joint: analysis of the function and traumatology of the ankle ligaments. *Acta Orthop Scand*. 1985;56[suppl 211]:34. Reproduced by permission of Taylor and Francis Group, LLC, a division of Informa plc.)

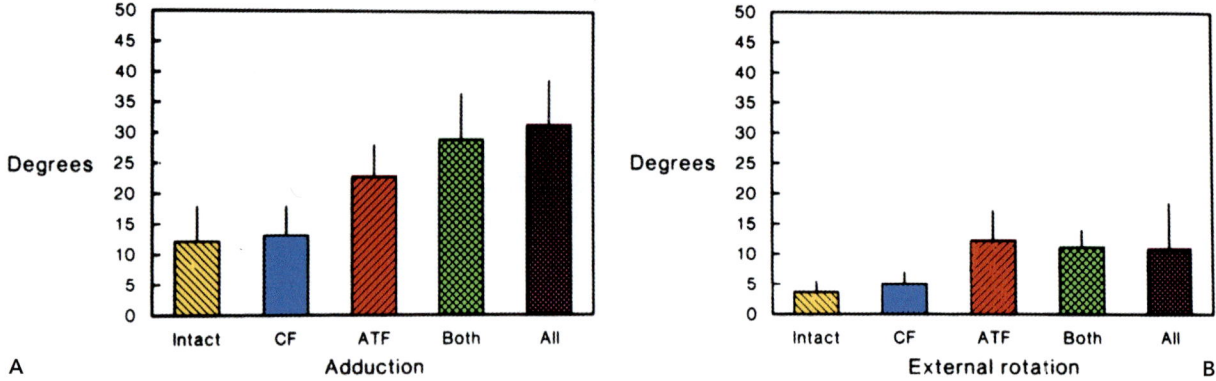

Figure 10.45 Mean maxima for adduction (A) and external rotation (B) of the tibia relative to the talus with the lateral collateral ligament intact and with sequential transection of its components. (*CFL*, calcaneofibular ligament; *ATF*, anterior talofibular ligament.) (Cass JR, Morrey BF, Chao EYS. Three-dimensional kinematics of ankle instability following serial sectioning of lateral collateral ligaments. *Foot Ankle*. 1984;5[3]:45. Copyright ©1984. Reprinted by Permission of SAGE Publications.)

axis of the anterior talofibular ligament nearly parallel to the axis of the lateral malleolus; the displacement rate was 12.5 cm/min. The tensile strength of the ligament to rupture had a mean value of 206 N (21 kg), ranging from 58 to 556 N (5.9-56.7 kg). In 50%, the failure was by bony avulsion from the talus and in 45% it was by mid substance failure. In 5%, the mode of failure was not clear, but none avulsed from the fibula.

Attarian and colleagues conducted a biomechanical study of the lateral collateral ligament and compared segments of tendon (peroneus brevis, split peroneus brevis, long extensor of the fourth toe).[35] Twenty cadaveric ankles provided the bone-ligament-bone specimen of the anterior talofibular and the calcaneofibular ligaments. The donor age ranged from 23 to 82 years, with a mean of 58 years. Load-deflection tests were conducted to the point of failure. Cyclic loading at physiologic deflections prior to testing was done to stabilize the specimens. The anterior talofibular ligament load to failure was 138.9 ± 23.5 N, and that of the calcaneofibular ligament was 345.7 ± 55.2 N. Comparatively, the tensile strength to rupture of the peroneus brevis tendon and of the split peroneus brevis tendon was nearly the same, 258.1 ± 63.5 N and 258.8 ± 110.6 N, respectively. The long extensor of the fourth toe ruptured at 130.1 ± 20.9 N.

Siegler and coworkers studied the tensile mechanical properties of the collateral ligaments of 20 ankles.[36] The average donor age was 67.8 ± 15.2 years, ranging from 33 to 85 years. The lateral collateral ligaments were prepared as bone-ligament-bone. In each experiment, the long axis of the tested ligament was aligned with the line of application of the tensile force. The specimen was initially subjected to 15 preconditioning cycles. The maximal tensile force was increased by 44.5 N until failure of the ligament by avulsion or rupture. Tension-ligament elongation curves were determined (Fig. 10.46) where the yield point-load represents the failure of some fibers of the ligament that is still intact and the ultimate load corresponds to the failure of the ligament.

The anterior talofibular ligament had a yield force of 222 N and an ultimate load of 231 N and elongated 0.246 cm on average. The failure occurred by bone avulsion in 58% and by rupture in 42%. The calcaneofibular ligament yield force was 289 N and failure occurred at an ultimate load of 307 N. The mode of failure was bone avulsion in 70% and substance rupture in 30%. The strongest of the lateral collateral ligaments was the posterior talofibular ligament, with a yield force of 400 N and an ultimate load of 418 N, and a mode of failure similar to that of the calcaneofibular ligament. These experiments were conducted with the tested ligament oriented near vertically, which corresponds to a position of plantar flexion for the anterior talofibular ligament and a position of dorsiflexion for the calcaneofibular and the posterior talofibular ligaments.

Deltoid Ligament

Anatomic Observations

Contrary to the lateral collateral ligament, the deltoid ligament is one ligament, in continuity, with some overlapping of its constitutional fibers. A division of this ligament into distinct anatomic separate entities is artificial and can be accomplished only by considering their insertional sites.

The ligament may be considered as being formed by two layers: superficial and deep. The superficial layer, delta shaped, extends from the anterior colliculus to insert on the talus, the navicular, the inferior calcaneonavicular ligament, the sustentaculum tali, and the posteromedial talar tubercle. The deep layer extends from the intercollicular groove and the inferior colliculus to the talar body as one or two strong bands.

The deep deltoid, the strongest component, prevents the lateral shift of the talus and limits the dorsiflexion of the ankle or the anterior rotation of the leg when the foot is stabilized. Its fibers are nearly horizontal in orientation and resist the external rotation of the leg relative to the talus or the internal rotation of the talus. It is an important component of the peritalar horizontal ligamentous ring (see Fig. 10.42). The talocalcaneal component of the superficial deltoid ligament limits the eversion of the calcaneus at the subtalar joint and contributes to the medial stability of the talus. The anterior tibiotalar ligament and the tibionavicular ligament restrict the plantar flexion of the foot

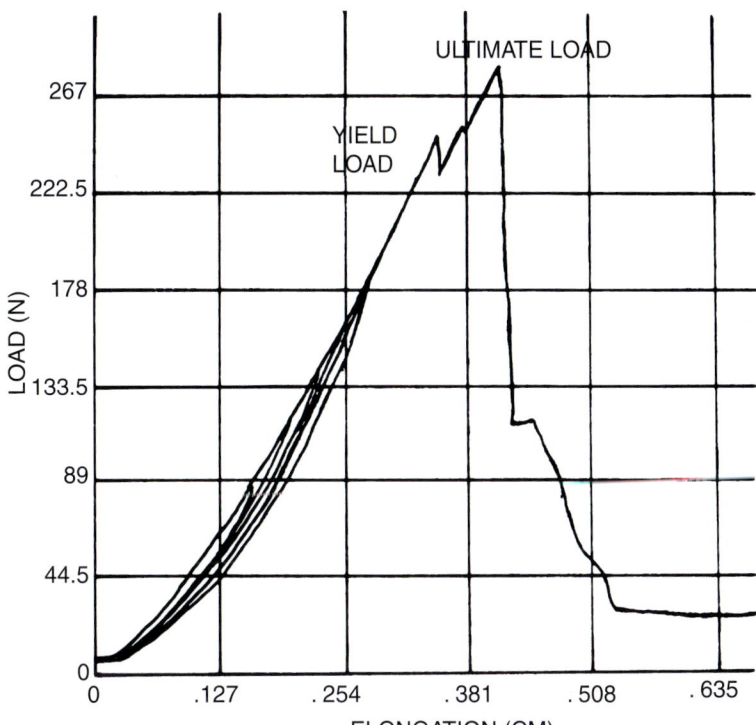

Figure 10.46 **Tension-elongation results obtained from a tensile test conducted on a lateral collateral ankle ligament prepared as bone-ligament-bone.** The yield point-load represents the failure of some fibers of the ligament, which is still intact. The ultimate load corresponds to the failure of the ligament. (*N*, Newton.) (Siegler S, et al. The mechanical characteristics of the collateral ligaments of the human ankle joint. *Foot Ankle*. 1988;3[5]:239. Copyright ©1988. Reprinted by Permission of SAGE Publications.)

and ankle. The former limits the external rotation of the talus in the ankle mortise and contributes to the transmission of the internal rotation of the tibia to the talus. The tibio-spring ligament fascicle or the superficial deltoid ligament provides the suspensory support to the inferior calcaneonavicular ligament against gravity and against the dynamic pressure exerted inferomedially by the talar head. The plantar segment of the tibialis posterior tendon supplements this support.

Experimental Investigation of the Role of the Deltoid Ligament

Close, in his experimental investigation, demonstrated the importance of the deep deltoid ligament in limiting the lateral talar shift (Fig. 10.47).[16] Harper defined the relative functional role of the superficial and deep components of the deltoid ligament and of the lateral malleolus in a study of 24 cadaveric ankles subjected to manual stressing.[37] The talar anterior and lateral shifts and the medial or valgus tilt were assessed. In the ankles, with transection of the anterior capsule, there was no talar lateral shift or medial tilt with stress. The anterior talar shift was limited to an average of 0.9 mm (range, 0-2.5 mm). With the lateral malleolus and its ligaments intact, transection of the superficial or the deep deltoid component resulted in no change in the talar lateral or anterior shift or in the medial tilt. The transection of both the superficial and deltoid ligaments resulted in a medial talar tilt or abduction of 14° (range, 13°-16°) but without associated increase of the talar anterior or lateral shift (Fig. 10.48).

With removal of the lateral malleolus and both components of the deltoid ligament intact, there was no talar medial tilt or abduction. However, the anterior talar shift increased an

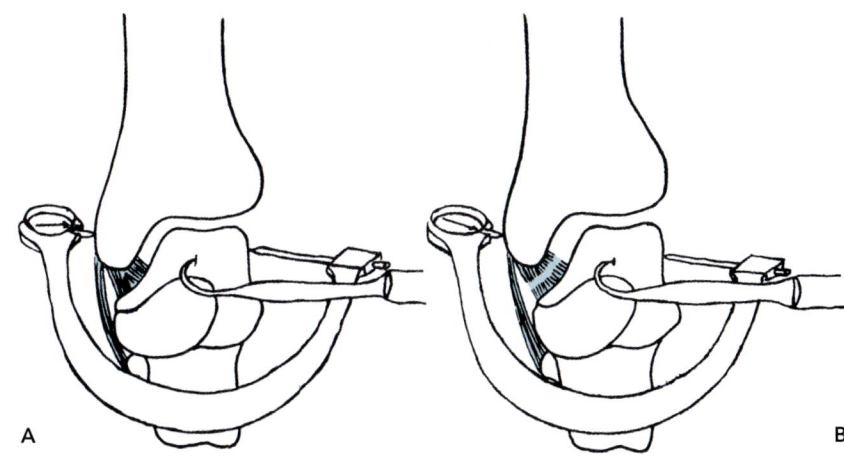

Figure 10.47 **Lateral displacement of the talus after excision of the fibula and after added transection of the deep component of the deltoid ligament.** **(A)** Talus laterally displaced 2.0 mm after removing fibula. **(B)** After sectioning the deep portion of the deltoid ligament 3.7 mm displacement of talus is possible. (From Close JR. Some applications of the functional anatomy of the ankle joint. *J Bone Joint Surg Am*. 1956;38[1]:766.)

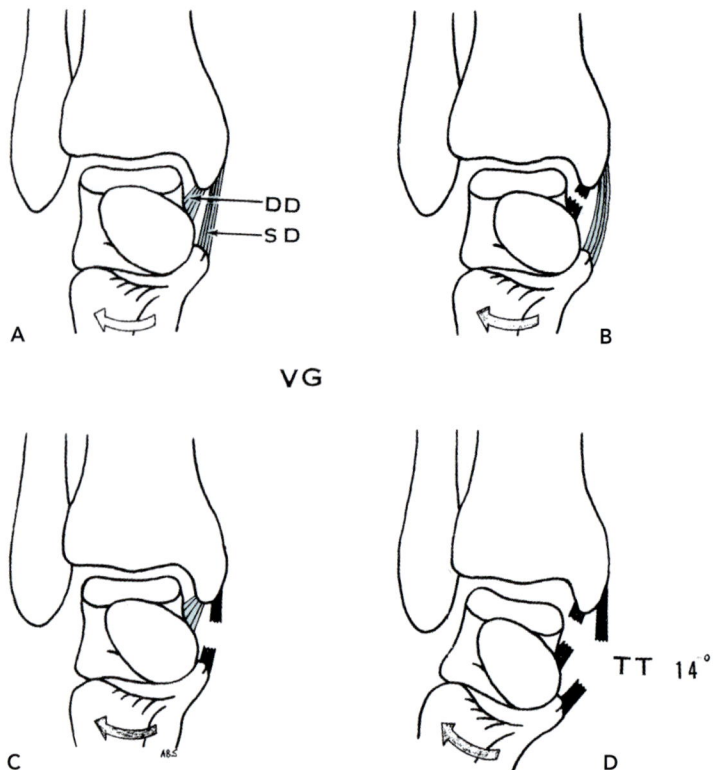

Figure 10.48 **Medial talar tilt or talar abduction with valgus stress applied.** (A) Superficial and deep deltoid components intact. (B) Transection of deep deltoid: no talar tilt. (C) Transection of superficial deltoid: no talar tilt. (D) Transection of both deltoid components: medial talar tilt. The lateral malleolus is intact. (*SD*, superficial deltoid ligament; *DD*, deep deltoid ligament; *TT*, medial talar tilt; *VG*, valgus stress.) (Data from Harper MC. Deltoid ligament: an anatomical evaluation of function. *Foot Ankle.* 1987;8[1]:19.)

average of 5.6 mm (range, 4-6 mm), and the lateral talar shift increased an average of 1.9 mm (range, 1.5-3 mm).

The transection of the superficial deltoid did not then affect the talar stability.

With the superficial deltoid remaining intact, the transection of the deep deltoid ligament would result in an increase in the anterior talar shift to 8 mm (range, 7-9 mm) and in the lateral talar shift to 3.8 mm (range, 3-4.5 mm) (Fig. 10.49). No medial or valgus tilting of the talus was possible. Harper concluded the following:

An anterior talar shift of 2.5 mm is possible in an ankle intact except for the anterior capsule.

The deltoid ligament is the primary restraint against the talar valgus tilt.

The lateral malleolus and its ligament are the primary restraints against the anterior and lateral talar shifts. The deep deltoid ligament is the secondary restraint against the lateral and anterior talar shifts.

Rasmussen investigated the contribution of the different components of the deltoid ligament by transection and experimental determination of the mobility pattern of the ankle.[31] For the sake of clarifying the findings, the anatomic interpretation used by Rasmussen is to be defined first.

The tibiocalcaneal ligament is considered the sole component of the superficial deltoid ligament. The anterior tibiotalar ligament is considered "the anterior portion of the deep layer of the deltoid ligament." The intermediate tibiotalar ligament and the posterior tibiotalar ligament are also components of the deep deltoid.

In our interpretation, although the last two are indeed deep components of the ligament, the anterior tibiotalar and tibionavicular ligaments are considered as superficial components. Furthermore, the tibio-spring ligament component, a superficial component of the deltoid ligament, has not been recognized in this investigation.

In 15 ankles, the transection of the tibiocalcaneal ligament increased the abduction of the talus or the medial tilt by $2.27° \pm 1.83°$. The talar mobility in the horizontal or the sagittal planes was not altered. In seven ankles, cutting of the tibiocalcaneal ligament and the anterior tibiotalar ligament minimally altered the above instability and plantar flexion did not increase. In four ankles, transection of the tibiocalcaneal ligament, the anterior talotibial ligament, and the intermediate talotibial ligament, which in our interpretation is equivalent to transection of most of the superficial deltoid ligament and of the anterior component of the deep deltoid ligament, resulted in an increase of $8.75° \pm 4.19°$ in talar abduction, most marked in plantar flexion. In the horizontal plane, the abnormal lateral rotation of the talus amounted to $2.40° \pm 1.52°$. In addition to the above components, transection of the posterior tibiotalar ligament or the major component of the deep deltoid ligament resulted in such a lax ankle medially that no mobility pattern could be plotted. Isolated cutting of the anterior tibiotalar ligament did not cause any instability.

Quiles and coworkers investigated the function of the components of the deltoid ligament in 35 ankles by measuring the distance between the origin and the insertion of the ligaments at rest, during flexion-extension at the ankle, and during

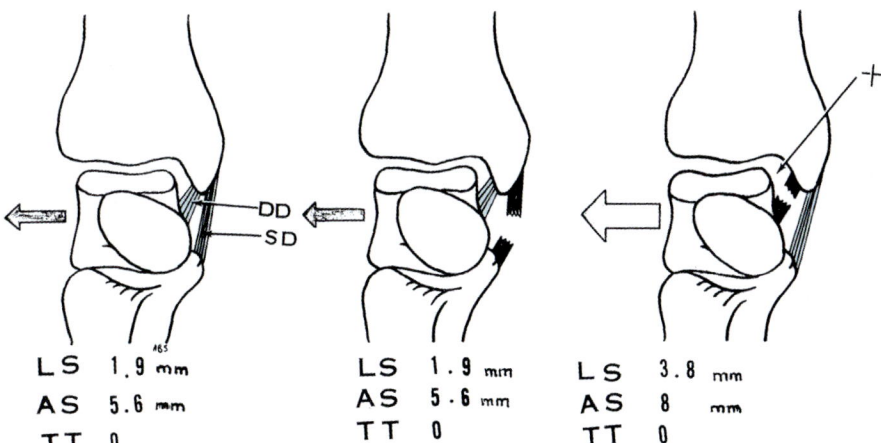

Figure 10.49 The lateral malleolus is excised. The talar lateral shift (*LS*), anterior shift (*AS*), and medial tilt (*TT*) are assessed with the components of the deltoid intact or with the transection of the superficial or the deep components of the deltoid ligament. The displacements are indicated in average millimeter values. (Data from Harper MC. Deltoid ligament: an anatomical evaluation of function. *Foot Ankle*. 1987;8[1]:19.)

abduction-pronation of the foot.[38] Pins were inserted at the attachment sites of the ligaments and the distances measured and plotted.

In plantar flexion, the calcaneotibial ligament and the posterior talotibial ligament relax, and the tibionavicular ligament is taut. In dorsiflexion, the reverse occurs. With abduction of the foot, the tibionavicular ligament is under tension and the posterior tibiotalar ligament is relaxed.

The transection of the posterior tibiotalar ligament affects the function of the other components, but the reverse does not occur. With complete transection of the deltoid, there was lateral displacement of the talus.

Mechanical Characteristics of the Deltoid Ligament

Siegler and colleagues investigated the tensile mechanical properties of the components of the deltoid ligament with the same anatomic pool of 20 ankles used to study the lateral collateral ligament.[36] Surprisingly, their investigation indicated an early failure of the tibiocalcaneal ligament at an ultimate load of 44.5 N, indicating a negligible support provided by this component. In their study, "it was discarded as a significant supporting structure of the ankle."

In reviewing the anatomic preparation of the different components of the deltoid ligament (specifically in Figures 1 and 2 in the article by Siegler and colleagues),[36] it appears to us that the tibiocalcaneal ligament has been "prepared" as an unusually narrow band, which is not the case in our anatomic dissections. This may account for the weak mechanical characteristics reported in this study.

The posterior tibiotalar ligament or major component of the deep deltoid ligament had superior mechanical properties with a yielding force of 405 N and an ultimate load of 467 N.

The mode of failure was avulsion in 60% and tear in 40%. This ligament thus could provide significant resistance to ankle dorsiflexion and to lateral or posterior shift of the talus. The tibio-spring ligament also manifested strong mechanical characteristics, with a yield force of 351 N and an ultimate load of 432 N. The mode of failure was avulsion in 31% and tear in 69%. Our interpretation of the potential function of this ligament has already been presented in the functional study of the deltoid ligament. The superficial tibionavicular ligament was the weakest, with a yield force of 107 N and an ultimate load of 120 N. The mode of failure was tearing in 100%.

▶ Stability of the Loaded Ankle

Stormont and coworkers studied the stability of the loaded ankle in 12 distal leg-midfoot specimens that were stabilized through the tibia and the calcaneus.[39] The specimen was equilibrated with the foot at 90° to the long axis of the tibia and tested with an axial load of 0 and 670 N (68 kg). Six specimens were subjected to internal and external rotational stress in unloaded and loaded conditions. The stability of the ankle with intact or divided ligament(s) was studied in 20° of plantar flexion, in neutral, and in 15° of dorsiflexion in two specimens each. The six remaining specimens were tested identically with inversion-eversion loads. The serial sectioning was performed in a sequential manner: posterior talofibular, calcaneofibular ligament, retinaculum, anterior joint capsule, anterior talofibular ligament, posterior capsule, deltoid ligament, lateral talocalcaneal ligament, and finally the tibiofibular syndesmosis. A torque ranging from 336 to 398 N · m was applied to determine the initial range of displacement.

Stormont and colleagues, by arbitrary convention, considered any structure providing more than 33% of the restraint to a specific displacement as a primary restraint, whereas a structure providing 10% to 33% of the restraint was considered a secondary restraint, and a structure providing less than 10% was considered an insignificant contributor to the stability of the joint.[39] In internal rotation of the foot on the leg with 20° of plantar flexion and without load, the anterior talofibular ligament provided 56% of resistance and the deltoid 30%; they are considered the two primary major restraints. Their restraining function was determined by the ankle position. In neutral, the deltoid provided 75% of the stability and the anterior talofibular ligament 17%; in dorsiflexion, the deltoid contributed 63% of the restraint and the anterior talofibular ligament 26%.

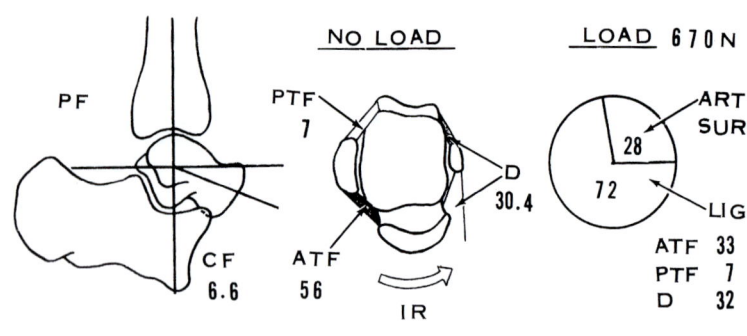
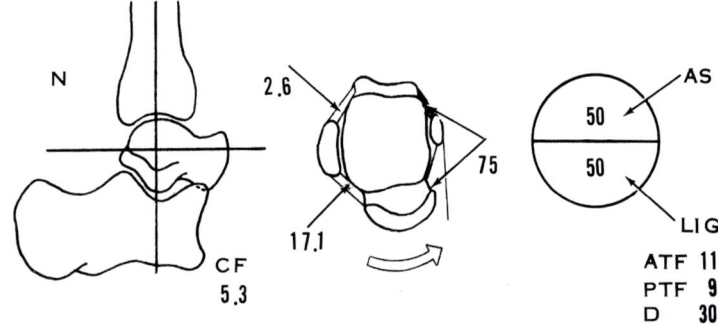
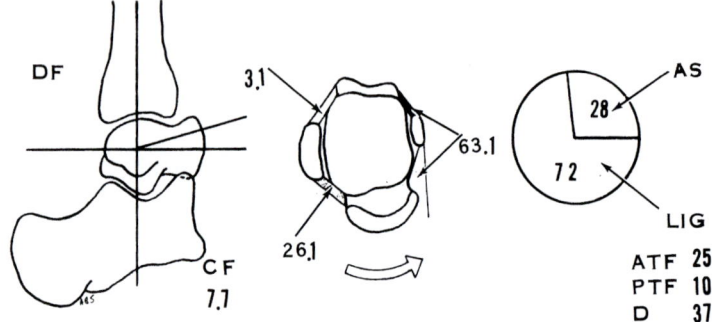

Figure 10.50 Stability of the ankle in internal rotation stress with and without vertical load of 670 N. Percentage of restraint to the internal rotation torque-displacement by each component of the collateral ligaments and the articular surfaces is presented in neutral, dorsiflexion, and plantar flexion positions of the ankle. (*AS*, articular surface; *ATF*, anterior talofibular ligament; *CFL*, calcaneofibular ligament; *D*, deltoid ligament; *IR*, internal rotation; *PTF*, posterior talofibular ligament.) (Data from Stormont DM, Morrey BF, Kai-nan AN, et al. Stability of the loaded ankle: relation between articular restraint and primary and secondary static restraints. *Am J Sports Med.* 1985;13[5]:295.)

The calcaneofibular ligament and the posterior talofibular ligaments were insignificant contributors (Fig. 10.50).

Under load, in neutral position, the articular surface provided 50% of the stability and the posterior talofibular ligament became a secondary constraint. In external rotation of the foot on the leg without load, the calcaneofibular ligament becomes a major contributor, averaging 65% to stability. The posterior talofibular ligament is a secondary restraint. This ligament provides no resistance in 15° of dorsiflexion. The deltoid ligament and the anterior talofibular ligament have secondary influences. With loading, the calcaneofibular restraint averages 43% and the posterior talofibular ligament 24%. The deltoid ligament now provides substantial support, averaging 20% except in neutral (3.2%), and the anterior talofibular ligament contributes an average of 17% to stability except in plantar flexion (5.3%). The articular surfaces under loading provide an average of 27% of stability (Fig. 10.51).

In inversion or varus stress, the lateral collateral ligament provided 87% of the resistance in the unloaded condition with the following average contribution from each component: anterior talofibular ligament, 27%; calcaneofibular ligament, 53%; posterior talofibular ligament, 11%, with only 5.6% contribution in plantar flexion. The deltoid ligament provided insignificant resistance in neutral and dorsiflexion and 11% in plantar flexion. In the loaded condition, no ligament contributed to stability, and the restraint was provided 100% by the articular surfaces. In eversion or valgus stress, the deltoid ligament provided 83% of the stability and the lateral collateral ligament 17% (Fig. 10.52). In the loaded mode, once again no ligament contributed to stability, and the resistance to the valgus stress was 100% articular. The study indicates that during inversion or eversion, "the ankle instability may occur during loading or unloading but not once the ankle is fully loaded."[39]

Chapter 10: Functional Anatomy of the Foot and Ankle 543

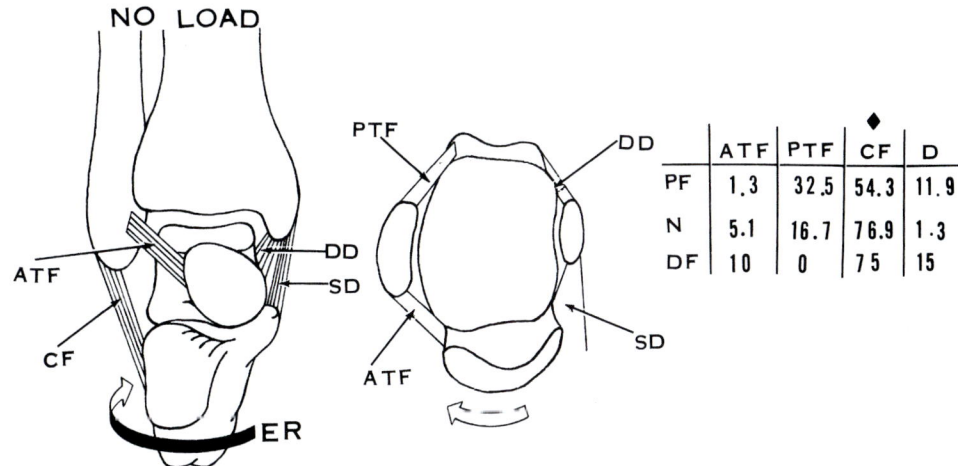
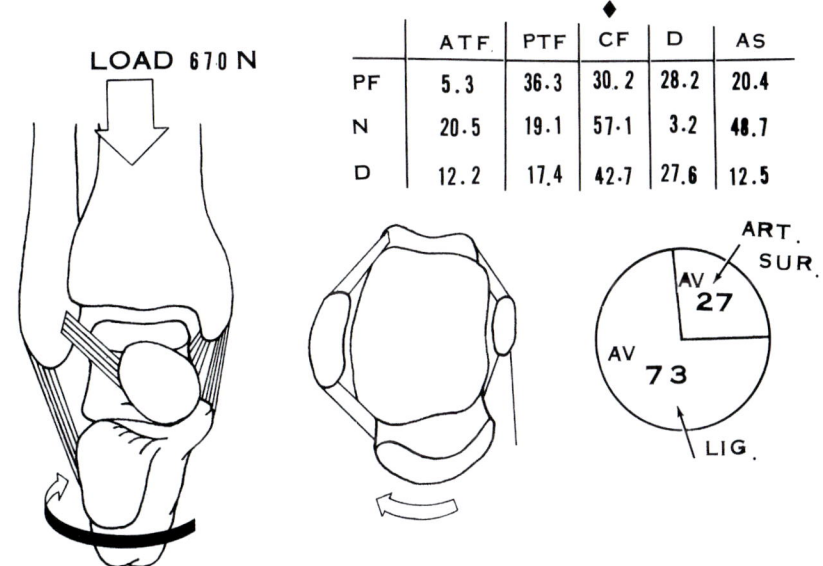

Figure 10.51 Stability of the ankle in external rotation stress with and without vertical load of 670 N. Percentage of restraint to the external rotation torque-displacement by each component of the collateral ligaments and the articular surfaces is presented in neutral, dorsiflexed, and plantar flexed positions of the ankle. The calcaneofibular ligament is a major restraining structure. (AS, articular surface; ATF, anterior talofibular ligament; AV, average contribution; CFL, calcaneofibular ligament; D, deltoid ligament; ER, external rotation; PTF, posterior talofibular ligament.) (Data from Stormont DM, Morrey BF, Kai-nan AN, et al. Stability of the loaded ankle: relation between articular restraint and primary and secondary static restraints. *Am J Sports Med.* 1985;13[5]:295.)

FUNCTIONAL SEGMENTAL ANALYTIC STUDY OF THE FOOT

▸ Subtalar or Talocalcaneal Joint Motion

Single Axis of Motion

The axis of the subtalar joint was studied by Manter,[40] Hicks,[12] Isman and Inman,[41] and Inman.[10] It is oblique, oriented upward, anteriorly and medially. It penetrates the posterolateral corner of the os calcis, passes perpendicular to the canalis tarsi, and pierces the superomedial aspect of the talar neck. Manter reported the angulation of the axis to have a 42° average inclination (range, 29°-47°) in the sagittal plane relative to the horizontal line and a 16° average medial deviation (range, 8°-24°) in the transverse plane relative to the long axis of the foot passing through the first interdigital space.[40] Inman provided measurements that are very similar: 42° ± 9° of inclination in the sagittal plane and 23° ± 11° of medial deviation in the horizontal plane relative to the axis of the foot passing through the second interdigital space (Fig. 10.53).[10]

The motion components at the subtalar joint can be determined from a simple vectorial analysis of the subtalar joint axis components, which are three: longitudinal, vertical, transverse. The greater longitudinal component generates supination-pronation, the vertical component generates abduction-adduction, and the lesser transverse component generates flexion-extension. Any instantaneous motion is a combination of the three simultaneously occurring motions. The axis of the talocalcaneal joint invariably generates two combination patterns of motion: pronation-abduction-extension and supination-adduction-flexion (Figs. 10.54 to 10.56). This basic motion of the calcaneus was clearly demonstrated in our specimens (Fig. 10.57) and was demonstrated by Farabeuf in anatomic models (Fig. 10.58).[42]

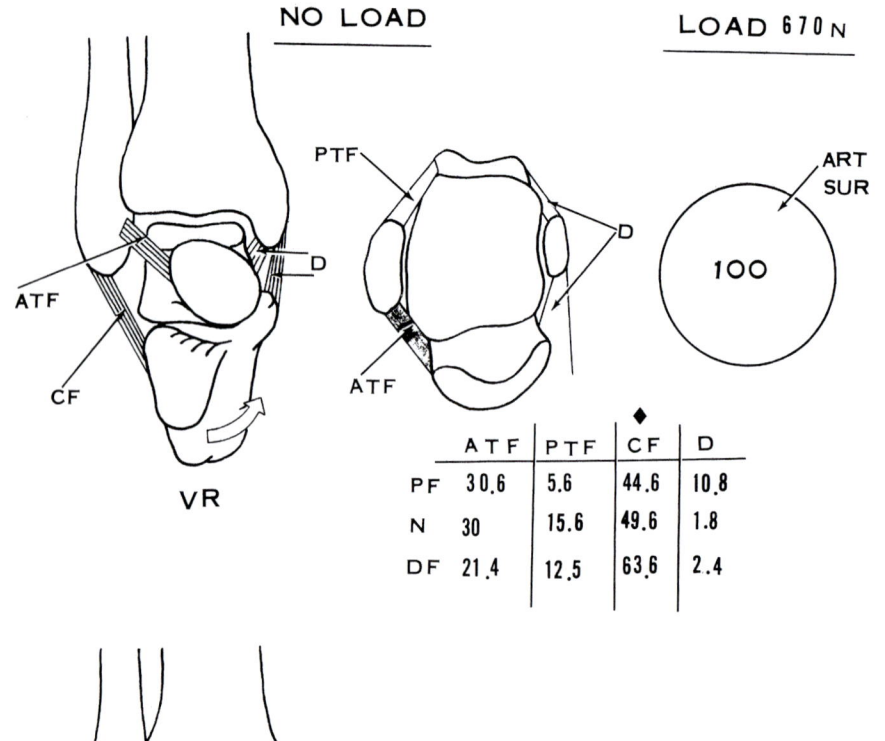

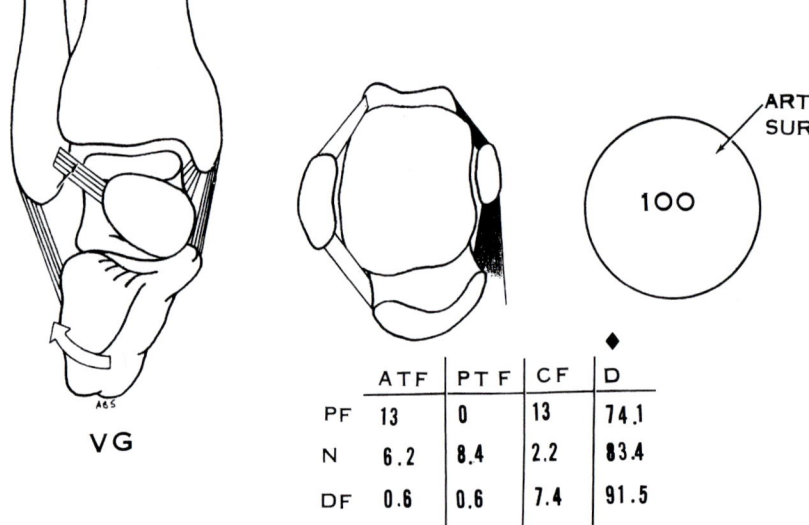

Figure 10.52 **Stability of the ankle in varus and valgus stress with and without vertical load of 670 N.** Percentage of restraint to the varus or valgus stress by each component of the collateral ligaments and the articular surfaces is presented in neutral, dorsiflexion, and plantar flexion of the ankle. The calcaneofibular ligament is a major restraining structure in varus stress, whereas the deltoid ligament is a major restraining structure in valgus stress of the ankle. Under vertical load, the stability is provided by only the articular surfaces. (Data from Stormont DM, Morrey BF, Kai-nan AN, et al. Stability of the loaded ankle: relation between articular restraint and primary and secondary static restraints. *Am J Sports Med.* 1985;13[5]:295.)

The turning in of the heel was termed endorotation of the calcaneus by Lewis and the reverse was termed exorotation.[43] For the clinician, exorotation of the calcaneus corresponds also to valgus of the heel and endorotation to varus.

Manter, in his study of the motion around the subtalar axis, recognized and measured a longitudinal displacement along the axis and described the motion at the subtalar joint as that of a screw.[40] He compared the posterior calcaneal surface to the helical surface of a screw. Serial sections of this calcaneal surface made perpendicular to the subtalar joint axis revealed spiral rather than circular arcs. He considered this surface as being an "oblique helicoid, or screw-shaped surface." He measured the helix angle of the posterior calcaneal surface by dropping a perpendicular line from a point on the axis to the articular surface (Fig. 10.59). The average helix angle was found to be 12°. In pronation, the calcaneus, being held fixed, the talus advances along the subtalar axis approximately 1.5 mm for each 10° of rotation at the joint. Van Langelaan measured also the helical motion at the subtalar joint.[3] The axial translation of the talus was 1.7 mm (range, 1-2.6 mm) in a posterolateral direction during the exorotation of the leg of 30°. Manter described the subtalar joint behavior "like a right-handed screw in the right foot and like a left-handed one in the left foot" (Fig. 10.60).[40] The calcaneus advances along the subtalar axis during

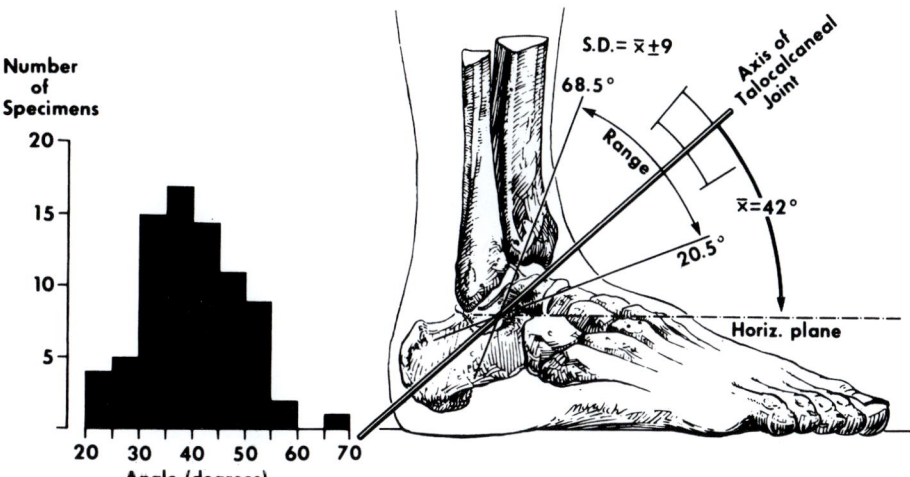

Figure 10.53 Variations in inclination of axis of subtalar joint as projected upon sagittal plane. The single observation of an angle of almost 70° was present in a markedly cavus foot. (From Inman TV. *The Joints of the Ankle*. Williams & Wilkins; 1976:37.)

supination-adduction-flexion or varus of the heel and retreats along the same axis during pronation-abduction-extension or valgus of the heel.

The subtalar range of motion is variable, as indicated in Table 10.5. For the clinician, 25° to 30° of inversion and 5° to 10° of eversion is a practical average range of motion. During the stance phase of the gait on even ground, the heel strikes with minimal inversion at the subtalar joint, followed by eversion ranging from 5° to 10° at 10% of the walking cycle. From there on, inversion occurs at the subtalar joint, reaching a maximum of 5° at 62% of the walking cycle.

Multiple Axes of Motion

Van Langelaan, in an x-ray photogrammetric study of ten cadaver leg-foot preparations with incorporated metal markers, determined the polyaxial helical nature of the tarsal—including subtalar—motions.[3] The extremities were loaded with 120 N of weight (12.24 kg) and subjected to 30° to 35° of external rotation, and the joint axes and motions were determined.

The subtalar motion was analyzed as being helical with continuous change in the position of the axes and thus forming a discrete bundle of axes (Fig. 10.61). A resultant single axis of the subtalar joint had an average angle of inclination of 41.4° (range, 27°-54.9°) relative to the horizontal plane and an average angle of deviation of 22.2° (range, 7°-35.8°). With 30° of external rotation of the leg, the talus rotated 23.6° (range, 15.5°-30°) in "abduction-eversion," corresponding to abduction-pronation-extension, and shifted along the subtalar axis in a posterolateral direction of 1.7 mm (range, 1-2.6 mm).

Motion and Stability

The motion at the subtalar joint is guided by the contour of the articular surfaces, their orientation, and the intrinsic and extrinsic ligaments.

The posterior calcaneal surface has been considered as a segment of a cone with the axis of the revolution of the surface directed anteromedially, intersecting the sustentaculum tali at nearly a right angle in the adult.[9] Manter considered the posterior calcaneal surface as an oblique helicoid or screw-shaped surface.[40] Inman demonstrated a screwlike behavior of the surface in 58% of 42 specimens and concluded that "the remarkable variation is the important factor."[10] Huson stressed the strong curvature of this surface medially, forming a bottleneck, whereas the lateral segment of the surface has a lesser curvature.[8]

The posterior talar articular surface is quadrilateral, usually rectangular medially and more or less oval laterally. The surface is strongly concave in the long axis and usually flat or minimally concave transversely. From a functional point of view, the posterior calcaneal articular surface may be considered as a male ovoid surface and the posterior talar articular surface as a female ovoid surface. The combined anterior and middle calcaneal surfaces form a female ovoid surface and the inferior articular surface of the talar head forms a male more or less flattened ovoid surface. MacConaill and Basmajian analyzed the motion components generated by the moving ovoid surfaces relative to each other.[64] A male ovoid surface moving on a female ovoid surface slides, rolls, and spins. The rolling is in a direction opposite to the sliding (Fig. 10.62). A female ovoid surface moving on a male ovoid surface slides, rolls or rocks, and spins. The rolling is in the direction of sliding (Fig. 10.63). The roll is a tilt that maintains the surface contact and the spin maximizes the congruency. Huson analyzed the spin at the posterior talocalcaneal joint.[8] Because of the differential of the curvatures of the articular surface—more curved medially and less curved laterally—a pure sliding creates more incongruency of the corresponding surfaces, whereas an associated spin minimizes the incongruency (Fig. 10.64). This interpretation is inclusive in the broader and more comprehensive analysis of the movement of ovoid surfaces presented by MacConaill and Basmajian.[64] If the ovoid surfaces are obliquely oriented with regard to the long axis of the foot, the generated motion will have two components. The associated spin creates the third motion component.

More specifically, the posterior calcaneal articular surface is oriented obliquely from posteromedial to anterolateral. Furthermore, the posterior segment is more dorsal and the

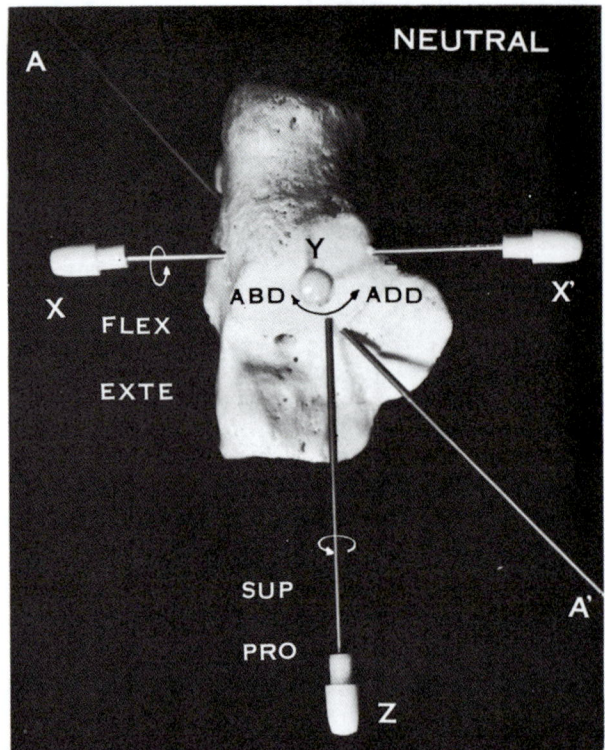
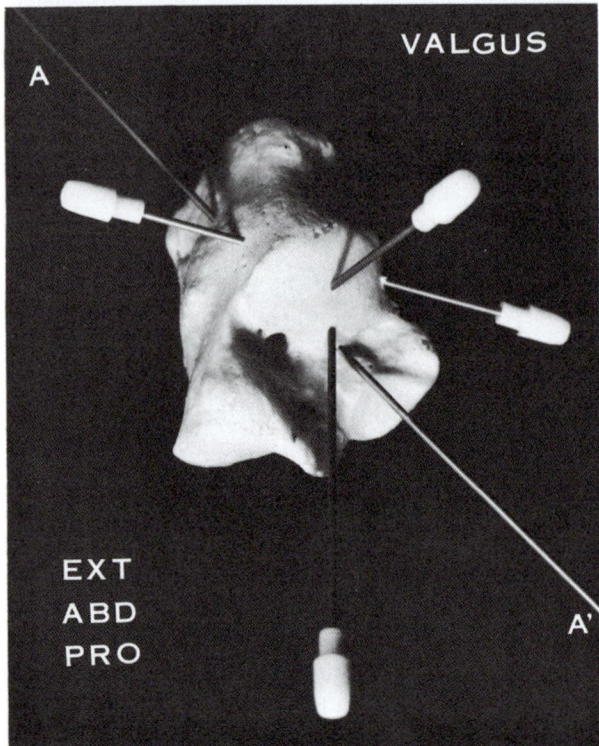
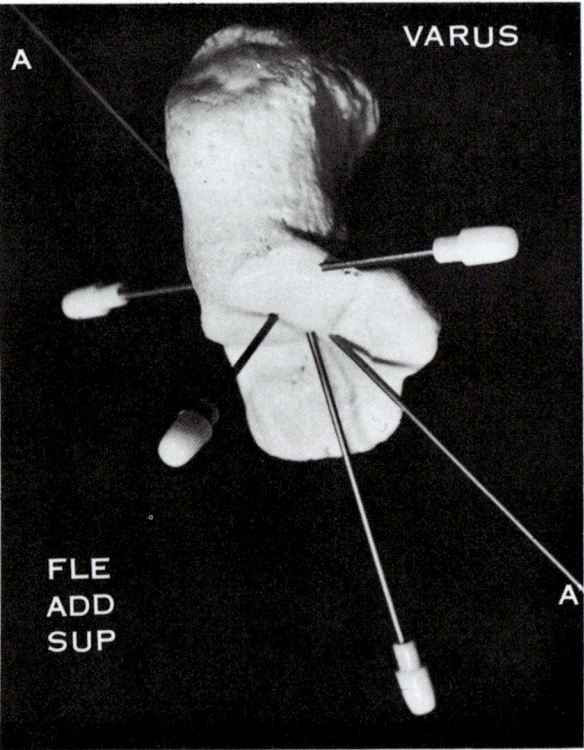

Figure 10.54 **The axis of the talocalcaneonavicular joint AA' as indicated passing through the os calcis in neutral position.** The axis *AA'* has three components: *XX'*, which generates flexion-extension (*FLEX-EXTE*); *Y*, which generates abduction-adduction (*ABD-ADD*); *Z*, which generates supination-pronation (*SUP-PRO*). In valgus position, the anterior aspect of the os calcis is simultaneously extended, abducted, and pronated. In varus position, the anterior aspect of the os calcis is simultaneously flexed, adducted, and supinated.

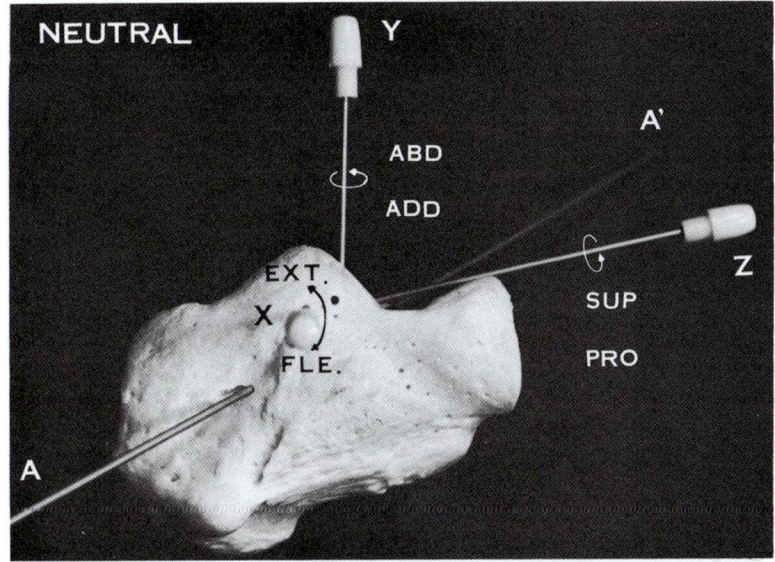
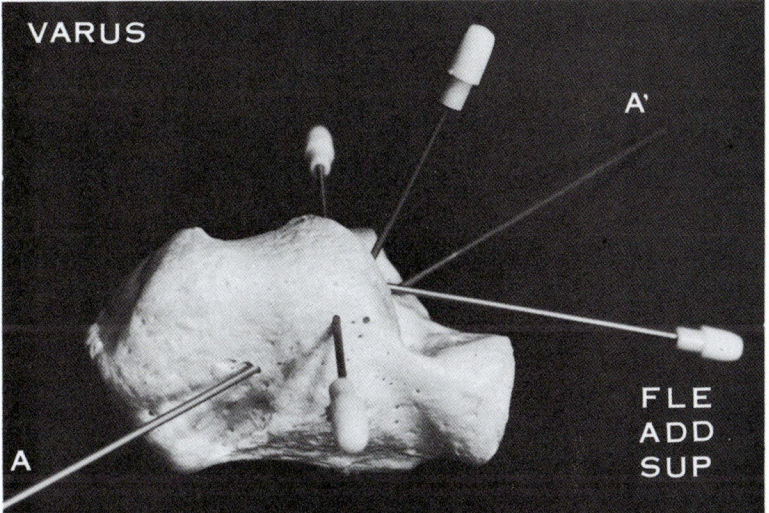
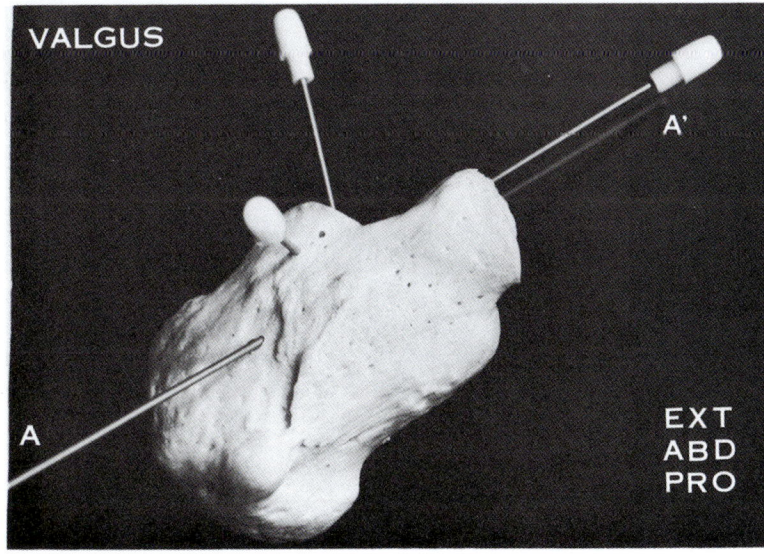

Figure 10.55 Axis of the talocalcaneonavicular joint *AA'* seen in lateral view with the secondary axes *X, Y,* and *Z*. The middle figure indicates the os calcis in varus and demonstrates the flexion (*FLE*) and supination (*SUP*) components. The bottom figure indicates the os calcis in valgus and demonstrates the components of extension (*EXT*) and pronation (*PRO*). (*ABD*, abduction; *ADD*, adduction.)

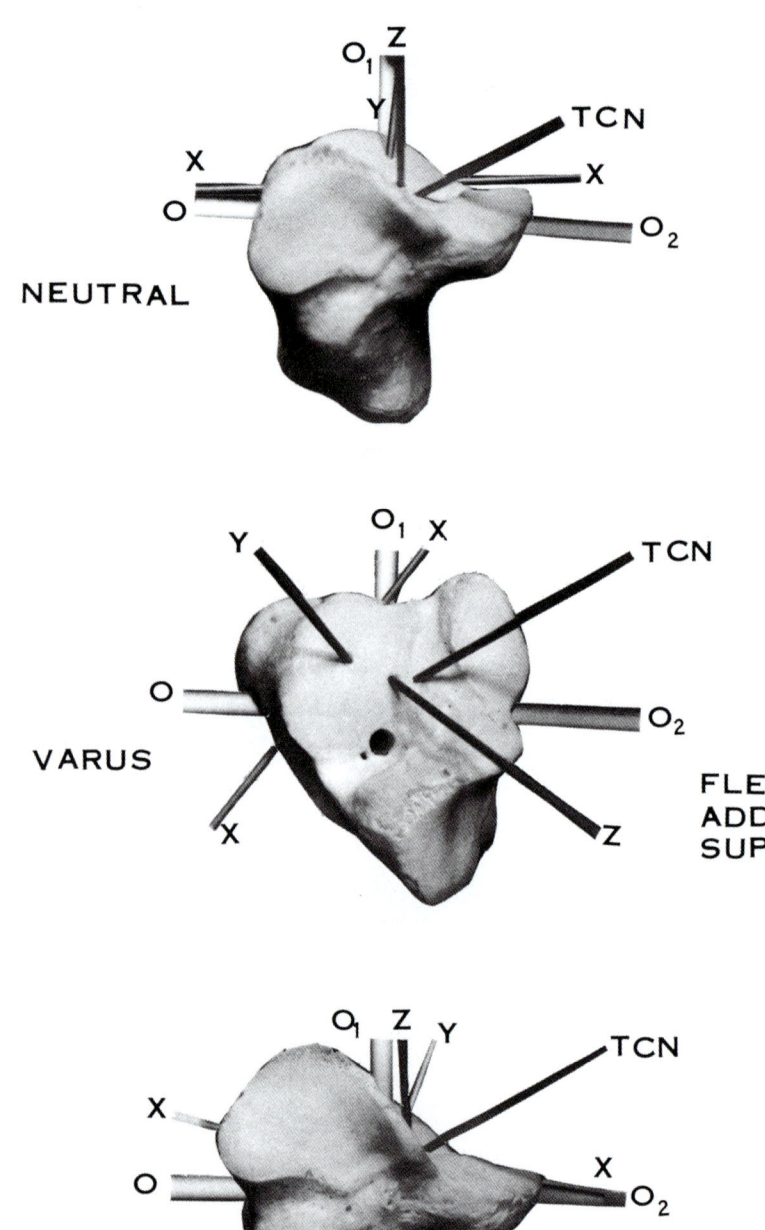

Figure 10.56 Frontal view of the os calcis. In varus of the heel, the anterior aspect of the os calcis is flexed (*FLE*), adducted (*ADD*), and supinated (*SUP*). In valgus of the heel, the anterior aspect of the os calcis is extended (*EXT*), abducted (*ABD*), and pronated (*PRO*). (*TCN*, talocalcaneo-navicular axis; *XX*, transverse axis of flexion-extension; *Y*, vertical axis of abduction-adduction; *Z*, longitudinal axis of supination-pronation; O, O_1, O_2, cruciform reference line.)

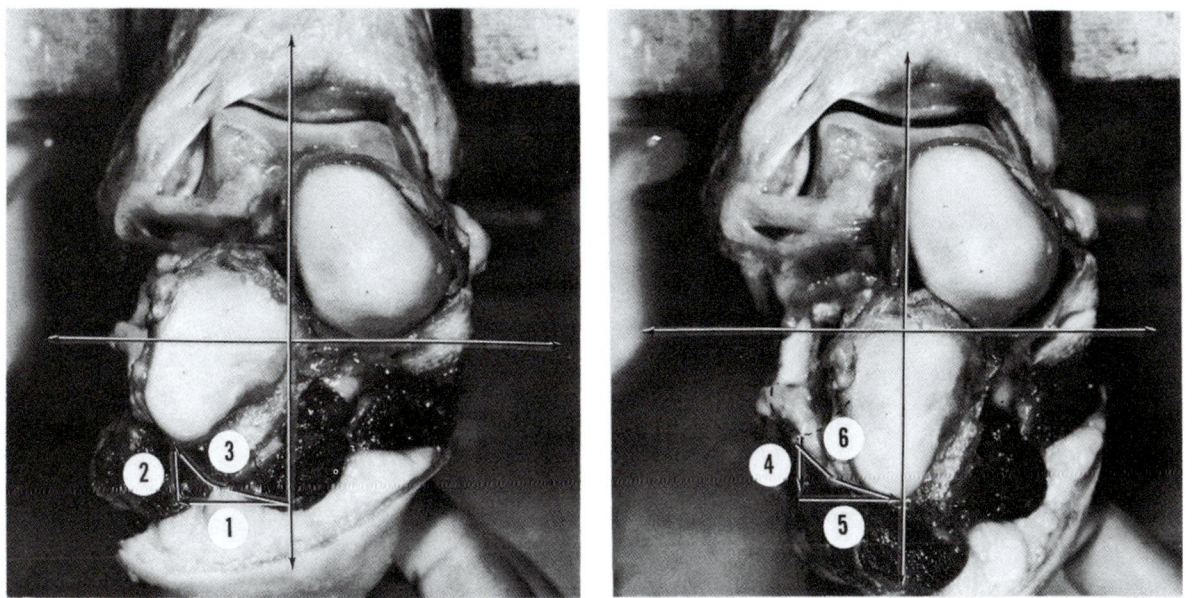

Figure 10.57 Anatomic model of the hindfoot. (A) Valgus position of the os calcis involving (*1*) abduction, (*2*) extension, and (*3*) pronation. **(B)** Varus position of the os calcis involving (*4*) flexion, (*5*) adduction, and (*6*) supination.

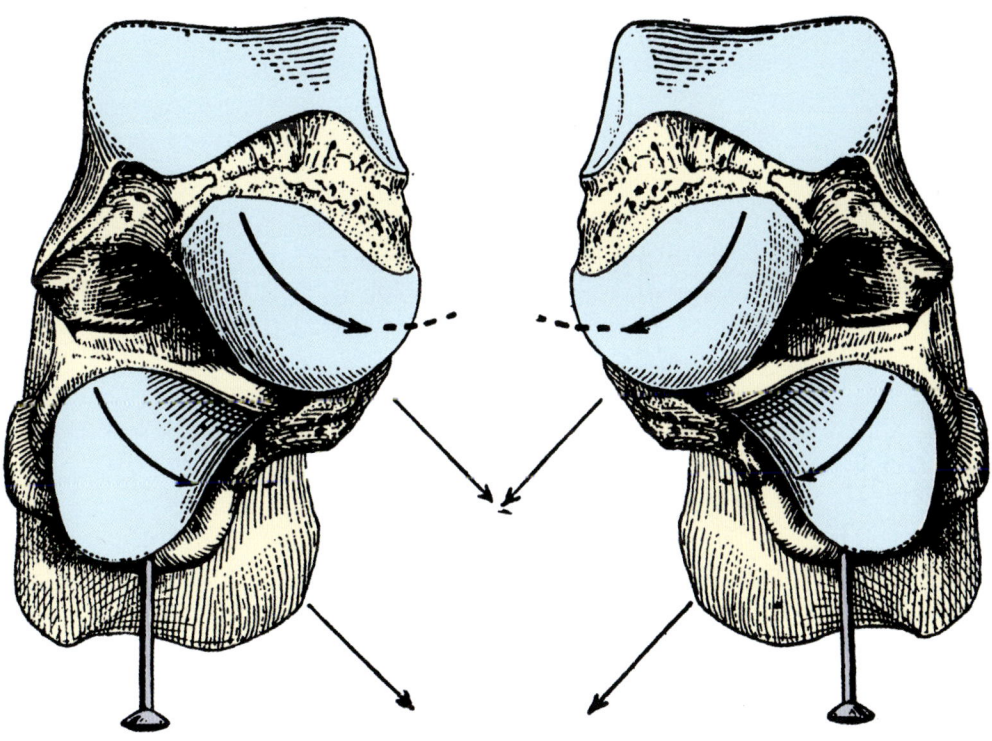

Figure 10.58 (A) Relationship of the talus and the calcaneus in the standing position as indicated by the vertical pin inserted in the calcaneus. The posterior calcaneal surface is covered by the external apophysis of the talus. The "condylar" surface of the talus is medial relative to the "trochlear" surface of the calcaneus. The long axis of the talar condylar surface is parallel to the long axis of the trochlear surface of the cuboid. Both axes (arrows) are directed inferiorly, medially, and posteriorly, and this allows an "oblique flexion inwards." **(B) The talus has remained unchanged.** The calcaneus is turned inward, as evidenced by the obliquity of the calcaneal pin. The long axes of the talar condylar and calcaneal trochlear surfaces are convergent. This corresponds to the "physiologic varus of flexion + adduction + supination," which results from the combined movements of the navicular on the talus, the cuboid on the calcaneus, and the calcaneus on the talus. (Adapted from Farabeuf LH. *Precis de Manuel Operatoire*. Maisson; 1889:827.)

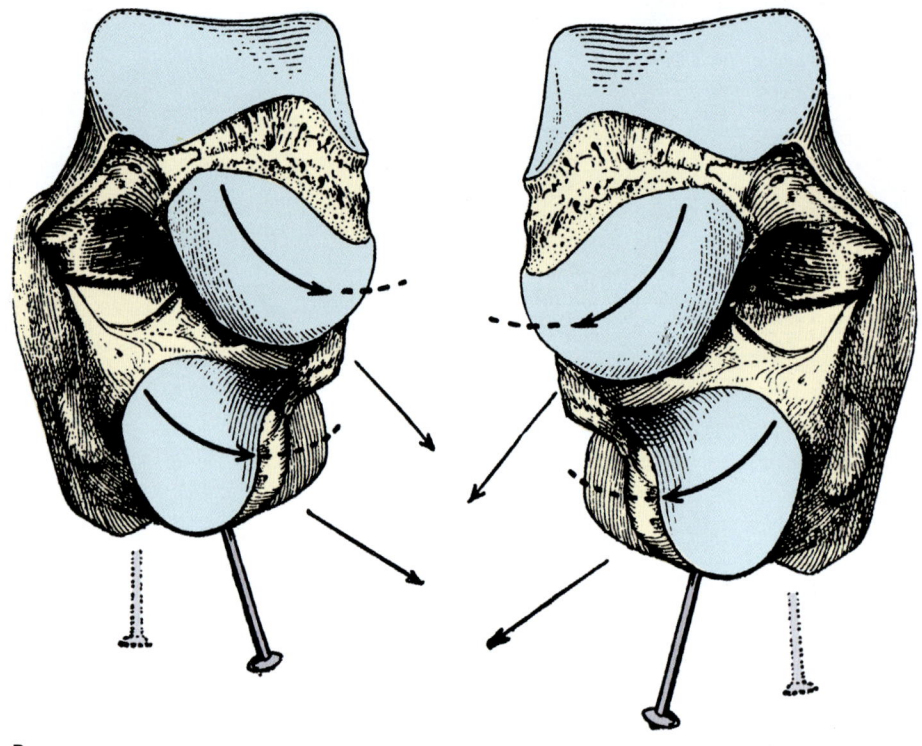

Figure 10.58 Cont'd

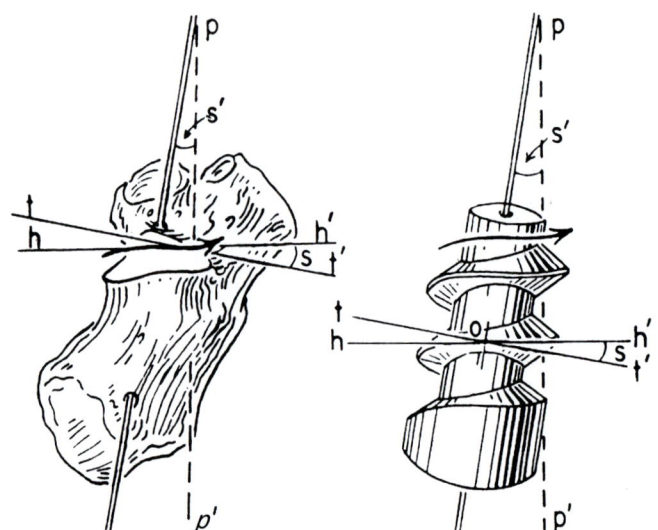

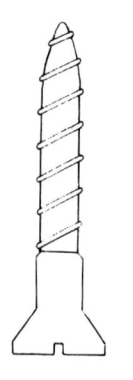

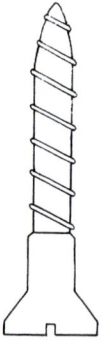

Figure 10.59 Comparison of the posterior calcaneal facet of the right subtalar joint with a right-hand screw. *Arrow* represents the path of a body following the screw. hh' is the horizontal plane in which motion is occurring. tt' is a plane perpendicular to the axis of the screw. s is the helix angle of the screw, equal to the angle s', which is obtained by dropping a perpendicular pp' from the axis. (From Manter JT. Movements of the subtalar and transverse tarsal joints. *Anat Rec*. 1941;80:402.)

R   L

Figure 10.60 Right-hand (R) and left-hand (L) screws.

TABLE 10.5 Reported Ranges of Subtalar Motion	
Author	Range of Motion
Manter (1941)	10°–15°
Hicks (1953)	24°
Close and colleagues (1967)	9.9°–28°
Inman (1976)	10°–65° (average, 40° 6 7°)
MacMaster (1976)	30° (25° inversion, 5° eversion)
American Medical Association (1988)	50° (30° inversion, 20° eversion)

anterior segment of the surface is more plantar. A female ovoid surface moving along this surface will naturally flex or extend and at the same time will supinate-pronate. Theoretically, a convex male surface oriented transversely will generate only the motion of flexion-extension, whereas such a surface oriented longitudinally will generate only the motion of supination-pronation. The oblique orientation of the posterior calcaneal surface will generate a combination of both flexion-extension and supination-pronation (Fig. 10.65). The inescapable spin creates the third motion component present at this joint: adduction-abduction. In "reading" into the contour and orientation of the posterior talocalcaneal joint, we can now clearly see that the generated motion is that of flexion-supination-adduction or extension-pronation-abduction. The talus and the calcaneus move in opposite directions to reach the end-position. In the clinician's "valgus" of the heel, the calcaneus moves in extension-pronation-abduction or the talus moves in flexion-supination-adduction. In "varus," the calcaneus is in flexion-supination-adduction and the talus moves in extension-pronation-abduction (Fig. 10.66).

The degree of orientation of the articular surfaces affects the amplitude of the motion components. The posterior calcaneal surface has an inclination angle with an average of 65°, a minimum of 55°, and a maximum of 75° relative to a line drawn along the superior surface of the calcaneal body. A larger inclination angle provides more flexion component to the motion (Fig. 10.67). The posterior talar articulating surface has a declination angle with an average of 37°, a minimum of 26°, and a maximum of 50° relative to the anterior trochlear line. A greater declination angle orients the surface in a longitudinal direction that will increase the flexion-extension component, whereas a smaller declination angle orients the surface more transversely and increases the supination-pronation component (Fig. 10.68).

MacConaill and Basmajian consider the subtalar joint as a bicondylar joint between the talus and the calcaneus, and the "rotation of one or the other of the mating bones can take place around an axis between the condyles."[64] This axis of motion is indeed located and passes through the canalis tarsi and the medial segment of the talocalcaneal interosseous ligament. Farabeuf stressed the rotational motion of the talus in a "tourniquet" fashion over the os calcis, or vice versa, taking place around a center located in the innermost part of the canalis tarsi through a twisting of the fibers of the interosseous ligament.[42] He clearly demonstrated this rotation on his diagram (Fig. 10.69).

The fibers of the talocalcaneal interosseous ligament are oriented upward, medially, and anteroposteriorly. The lateral fibers are longer and have more excursion laterally, whereas the shorter fibers on the inner side have less excursion. The cervical ligament originates on the calcaneal surface of the sinus tarsi and is oriented upward, anteriorly, and medially to insert on the talar neck. This arrangement of the ligaments promotes—as

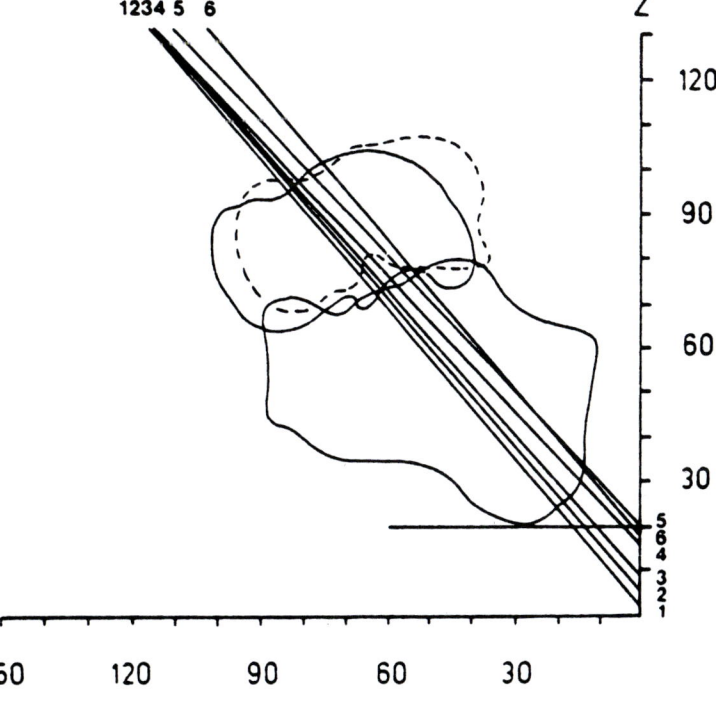

Figure 10.61 Relative talocalcaneal helical axes with 10° of talocalcaneal exorotation projected on sagittal plane. (Copyright © 1983. Van Langelaan EJ. A kinematical analysis of the tarsal joints; an X-ray photogrammetric study. *Acta Orthop Scand*. 1983;54[suppl 204]:147. Reproduced by permission of Taylor and Francis Group, LLC, a division of Informa plc.)

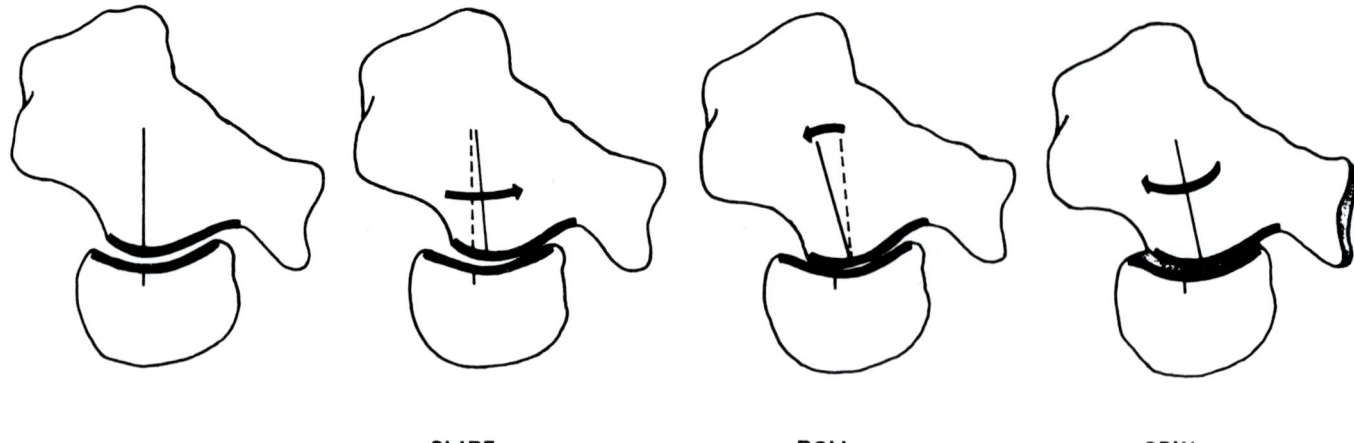

Figure 10.62 **A male ovoid surface (posterior calcaneal articular surface) moving on a female ovoid surface (posterior talar articular surface) slides, rolls, and spins.** The rolling is in a direction opposite to the sliding. The sliding advances the moving surface but creates a gap that is closed by the reverse rolling, and the maximum surface contact is achieved by the spinning of the moving surface.

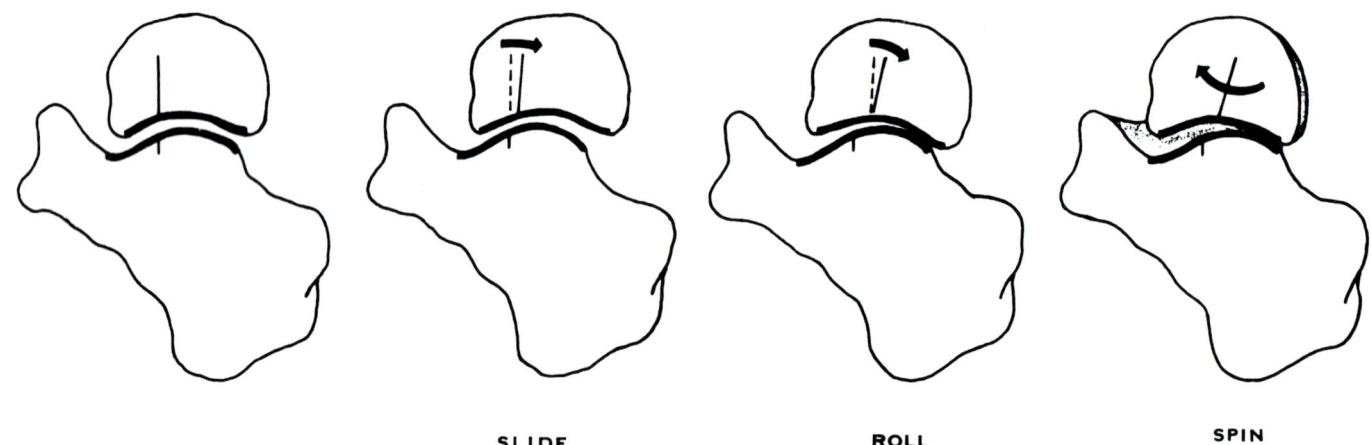

Figure 10.63 **A female ovoid surface moving on a male ovoid surface slides, rolls, and spins.** The rolling is in the direction of the sliding.

qualified by Huson—a "swinging motion" with a center of movement located along the short medial fibers of the ligament of the canalis tarsi.[8] The cervical ligament remains tight in both exorotation (valgus) and endorotation (varus) of the heel. The talocalcaneal interosseous ligament of the canalis tarsi and the cervical ligament may be considered as cruciate ligaments of the subtalar joint, as determined by their opposite orientation. The cervical ligaments and the calcaneofibular ligament have an approximate similar orientation.

The bony stability of the subtalar joint or close-pack position is achieved with exorotation or valgus of the calcaneus. In this position, there is maximum contact and near congruous fit at the posterior talocalcaneal joint. The talar lateral process descends and advances on the posterior calcaneal surface and the solid talar wedge or male V fits into the female V of the calcaneal surface.

With endorotation or varus of the calcaneus, the sustentaculum talus moves toward the posteromedial tubercle of the talus and considerably narrows the medial opening of the canalis tarsi.

The talar lateral process is now dorsal on the corresponding calcaneal surface. This anatomic relationship laterally allows the clinician to recognize the valgus or varus position of the hindfoot roentgenographically. The cervical ligament and the inferior extensor retinaculum limit the endorotation of the calcaneus.[44] The talocalcaneal interosseous ligament of the canalis tarsi remains tight during the endo- and exorotation of the calcaneus.[8,44] Smith, however, considers the talocalcaneal ligament of the canalis tarsi as limiting the exorotation or eversion of the calcaneus.

Tochigi et al[45] analyzed five fresh frozen cadaver lower extremities (ages 25-85 years) for the three-dimensional

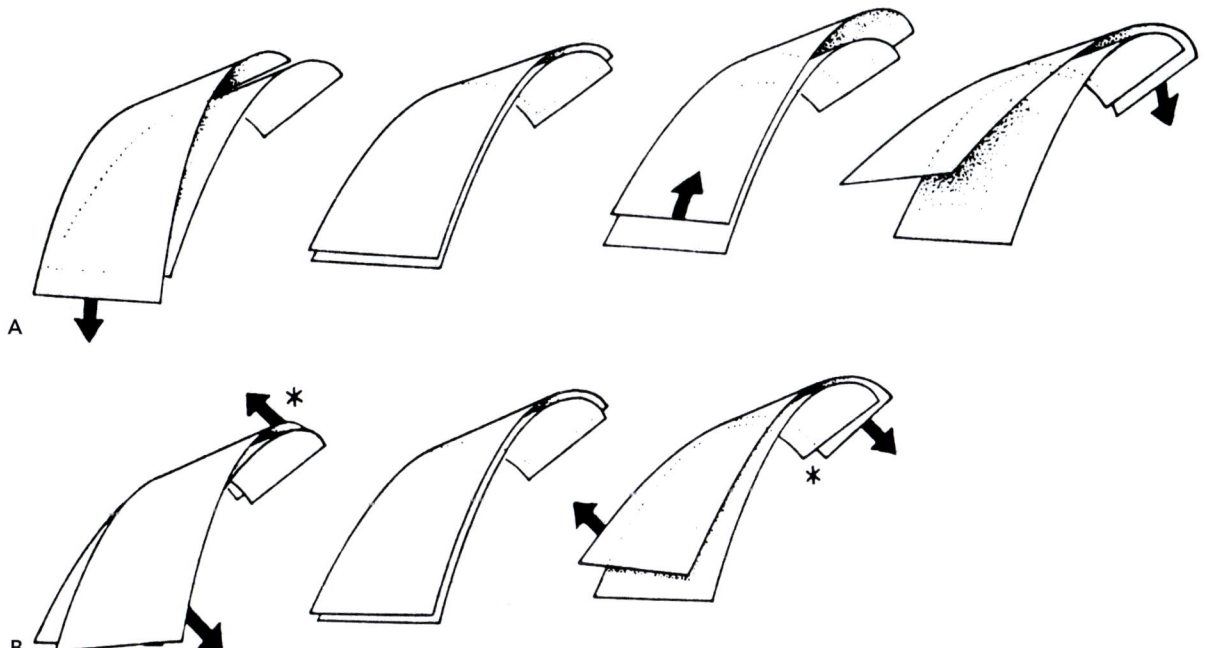

Figure 10.64 Diagrammatic representation of the posterior calcaneotalar articular surfaces. **(A)** The posterior calcaneal surface has "convex profiles lying in a medial, backward, and upward direction. The curvatures grow stronger in the same direction and in addition the profiles of the medial and anterior part of the facet, bordering on the canalis tarsi, are more curved than the lateral ones. Such surfaces in gliding over each other will show great discongruencies when they follow their strongest or weakest curvatures," as seen on the lower diagrams. **(B)** If this shift is simultaneously combined with a turn, the discongruencies are limited to a circumscribed part (indicated by the asterisk) of the articular surfaces. (From Huson A. *Anatomical and Functional Study of the Tarsal Joints*. Drukkerij, Luctor et Emergo; 1961:137.)

movement of the talus and calcaneus relative to the tibia under axial loading from 89.8 to 686 N. The induced talar and subtalar motions were triaxial. When the axial load was increased from 9.8 to 686 N, the maximum total ankle rotation averaged 3.5° ± 1.2° with plantar flexion 2.6° ± 1.1°, adduction 2.1° ± 1.0°, and negligible inversion 0.1° ± 0.7°. In the intact subtalar joint, under axial loading the induced motion was also triaxial. The total subtalar motion averaged 3.2° ± 1.3°, mostly eversion, with dorsiflexion 0.8° ± 0.9° and abduction 0.8° ± 1.0°.

The ankle rotation did not significantly change after isolated sectioning of the anterior talofibular ligament. After the combined sectioning of the interosseous talocalcaneal and anterior talofibular ligaments the maximum ankle joint

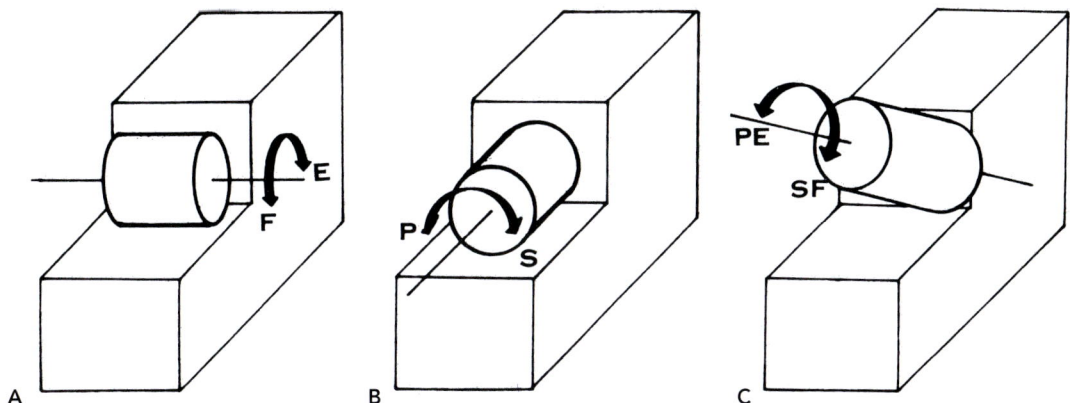

Figure 10.65 Convex male surface. (A) A convex male surface oriented transversely generates the motion of flexion (F) and extension (E). **(B)** A convex male surface oriented longitudinally generates the motion of pronation (P) and supination (S). **(C)** A convex male surface oriented obliquely—as indicated—generates a combination of pronation-extension (PE) and supination-flexion (SF).

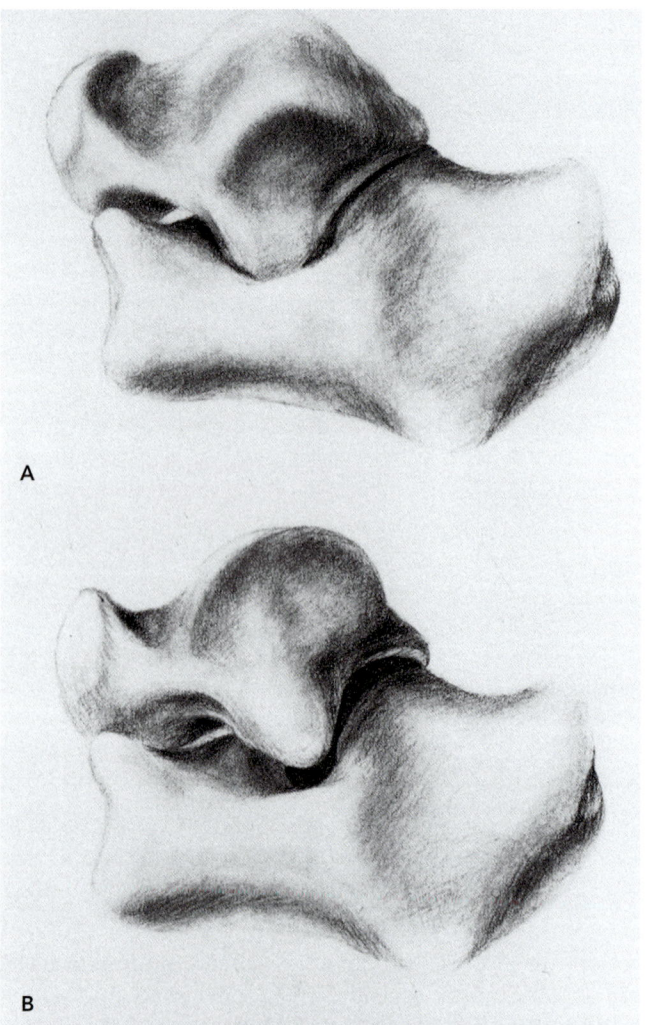

Figure 10.66 **Valgus and varus of the heel. (A)** Valgus of the heel. With the calcaneus being held fixed, the talus moves in flexion-supination-adduction. The lateral process of the talus is low and strikes Gissane angle of the calcaneus. If the talus is held in neutral, then the calcaneus is in extension-pronation-abduction. **(B)** Varus of the heel. With the calcaneus being held fixed, the talus moves in extension-pronation-abduction. The lateral process of the talus is high in position in the sinus tarsi. If the talus is held in neutral, then the calcaneus is in flexion-supination-adduction.

rotation averaged 5.2° ± 1°, whereas plantar flexion averaged 4.0° ± 0.9°, and adduction 3.3° ± 0.8°.

Tochigi et al[46] investigated the load-displacement characteristics of the subtalar joint in six cadaver specimens, using an axial distraction test and a transverse multidirectional drawer test. Cyclical loading (±60 N) was applied and load-displacement responses were collected before and after cutting the interosseous talocalcaneal ligament. The results confirmed the role of the interosseous talocalcaneal ligament in maintaining apposition at the subtalar joint suggesting that interosseous talocalcaneal ligament failure causes inversion instability of the subtalar joint. They also suggested the role of the interosseous talocalcaneal ligament in stabilizing the subtalar joint against drawer forces applied to the calcaneus from lateral to medial. The authors suggested examining a patient with possible subtalar instability with a drawer force applied "along the preferential axis roughly from the posterior aspect of the fibula to the central region of the medial malleolus."[46]

Fujii et al[47] assessed the mechanical characteristics of the ankle-hindfoot complex in 13 cadaver specimens mounted in a testing apparatus. A constant rotational force in the form of inversion-eversion, internal-external rotation was applied throughout the entire range of the ankle sagittal plane and the resulting calcaneotibial motion was measured.

With inversion force applied, the calcaneotibial inversion was greatest in maximal plantar flexion (mean 22.1° ± 6°) and gradually decreased with dorsiflexion. With eversion force applied, the calcaneotibial eversion gradually increased with increasing dorsiflexion to 12.7° ± 7.4°. With internal rotation force applied, calcaneotibial rotation increased from plantar flexion to neutral ankle position. With external rotation force applied, calcaneotibial external rotation from neutral to maximal dorsiflexion increased. Their conclusion was that "the ankle is less stable in plantar flexion when inversion and internal rotation forces are applied" and "the ankle was less stable in dorsiflexion when eversion and external rotational forces were applied."

Kjaersgaard-Andersen and colleagues determined experimentally the stabilizing effect of the ligamentous structures in the sinus and canalis tarsi at the subtalar joint.[48] In 20 cadaveric specimens, the total range of motion was measured at the subtalar joint and the subtalar-ankle joint complex.

A continuous movement was obtained by applying a constant torque and moment of 1.5 N · m. This resulted in a force transmission to the subtalar joint of 10 N (or 1.02 kg). The movement was recorded and computer analyzed in three planes. The study was conducted first in the intact specimens. In 10 specimens, the motion was assessed after transection of the cervical ligament. In another 10 specimens, the motion was assessed after transection of the talocalcaneal interosseous ligament of the canalis tarsi.

In the first 10 specimens, the median movement at the talocalcaneal joint was 15.5° in neutral. This small range of motion may be explained by the fact that the applied force was minimal (1 kg) and the specimens may have been obtained from an older age group. Lang and Wachsmuth have demonstrated indeed that with aging, the field of motion of the foot contracts in the transverse segment.[9]

After transection of the cervical ligament, the increase of motion was as follows:

- In the horizontal plane (internal-external rotation): 10%
- In the frontal plane (pronation-supination): 14%; this motion is termed adduction-abduction by the authors
- In the sagittal plane (dorsiflexion-plantar flexion): 20%

In the second group of 10 specimens, the median movement at the talocalcaneal joint with an intact ligament was 11.9° in neutral. After transection of the talocalcaneal ligament of the canalis tarsi, the increase in the range of motion was as follows:

- In the horizontal plane (internal-external rotation): 21%
- In the frontal plane (pronation-supination): 16%
- In the sagittal plane (dorsiflexion-plantar flexion): 57%, with 43% of the increase in dorsiflexion and 14% in plantar flexion

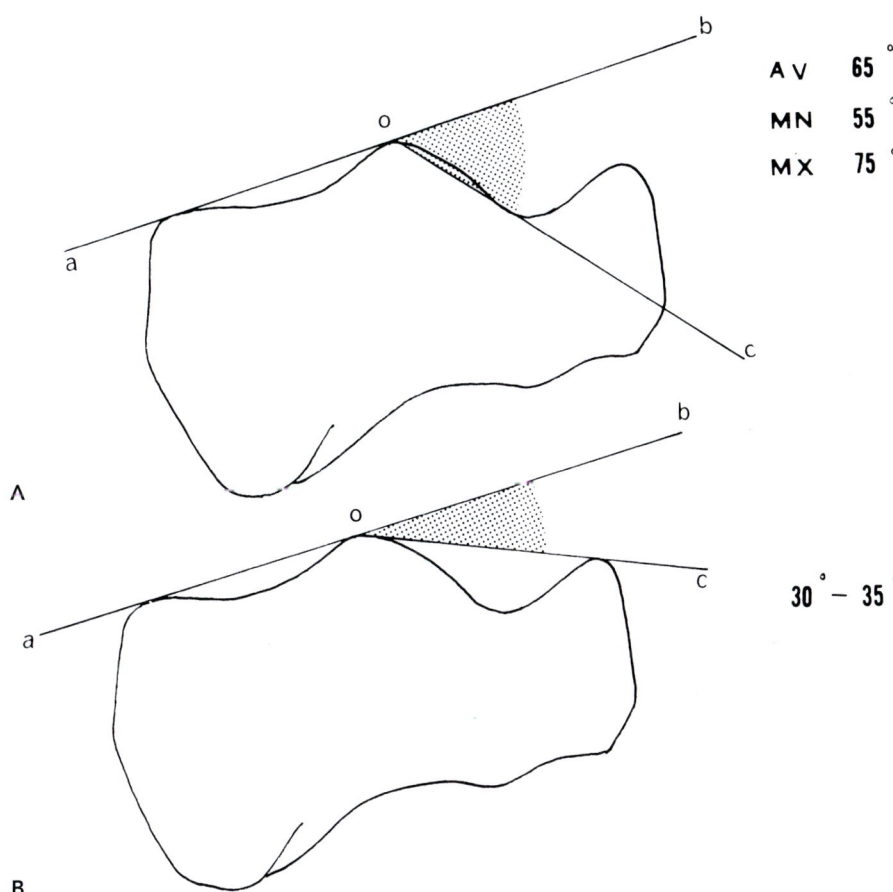

Figure 10.67 (A) Inclination angle of the posterior calcaneal surface. (B) Böhler angle.

This study is suggestive of the more important stabilizing role of the talocalcaneal ligament of the canalis tarsi limiting the exorotation or valgus of the calcaneus.

The stabilizing role of the ankle ligaments in subtalar motion was also investigated by Kjaersgaard-Andersen and colleagues in two different studies.[49,50]

The role of the tibiocalcaneal fascicle of the deltoid ligament was analyzed in ten cadaveric ankle-feet.[49] A torque or moment of 1.5 N · m was applied with an effective force of 10 N (1 kg) acting on the joint. Data were obtained from continuous movement curves and subjected to computer and statistical analysis. The motion was registered in three planes. After immobilization of the ankle joint with an external fixator, the talocalcaneal motion was assessed before and after transection of ligaments. The external fixator was removed, and the total range of motion was assessed again.

The median percentage of increase of motion at the subtalar joint after transection of the tibiocalcaneal fascicle of the deltoid ligament was as follows:

- In the horizontal plane (internal-external rotation): 12%, with 10% in external rotation and 2% in internal rotation.
- In the frontal plane (pronation-supination): 31%, with 30% in pronation and 1% in supination. This motion is termed abduction-adduction by the authors.
- In the sagittal plane (dorsiflexion-plantar flexion): 40%, with 30% plantar flexion and 10% dorsiflexion.

It is apparent that the transection of this ligament results in an increase in plantar flexion, pronation, and external rotation at the talocalcaneal joint.

The motion increased also at the combined tibiotalocalcaneal joint complex, mainly in pronation, external rotation, and

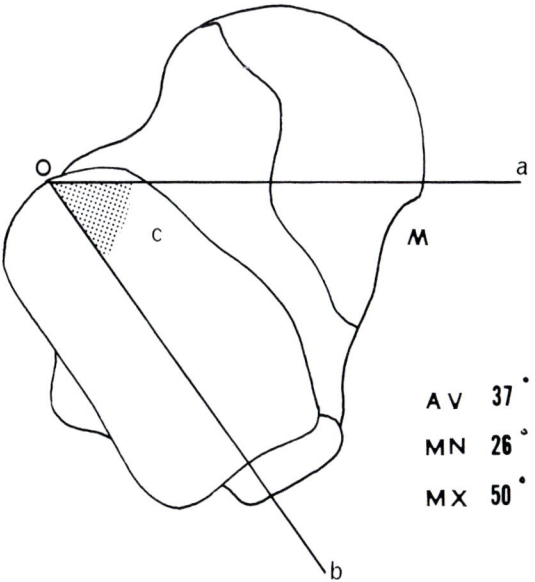

Figure 10.68 Declination angle of the posterior talar articular surface.

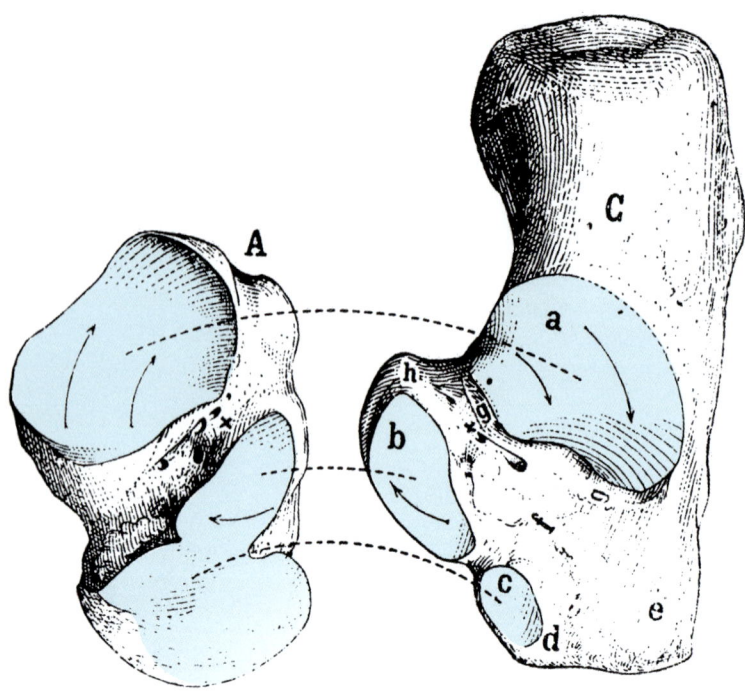

Figure 10.69 **The rotational motion of the talus over the calcaneus.** The arrows indicate the direction of rotation in a "tourniquet" fashion around the axis of rotation X located in the canalis tarsi. (*A*, talus; *C*, calcaneus; *a*, posterior calcaneal articular surface, cone shaped; *b*, sustentacular surface; *c*, anterior calcaneal surface; *d, e, f, g* refers to the non articular surfaces of the calcaneus.) (From Farabeuf LH. *Precis de Manuel Operatoire*. Maisson; 1889:818.)

plantar flexion, indicating the supportive role of the ligament at the ankle joint also.

Using the same methodology, Kjaersgaard-Andersen and colleagues analyzed the role of the calcaneofibular ligament with regard to the motion at the subtalar joint.[50] Ten cadaveric ankle-foot preparations were used. A torque or moment of 1.5 N · m was applied and the mobility of the talocalcaneal and tibiotalocalcaneal joint was assessed on the intact specimens and after sectioning the calcaneofibular ligament.

The motion in the frontal plane or supination (termed adduction by the authors) was assessed at different degrees of dorsiflexion-plantar flexion. After sectioning of the calcaneofibular ligament, the mean increment of supination at the combined tibiotalocalcaneal joint complex was 3° to 7°, increasing from the plantar-flexed position to maximum dorsiflexion (Fig. 10.70). The mean increment of supination at the subtalar joint was 3.1° to 4.6°, increasing from 5° of plantar flexion to 5° of dorsiflexion (Fig. 10.71). This study demonstrated the

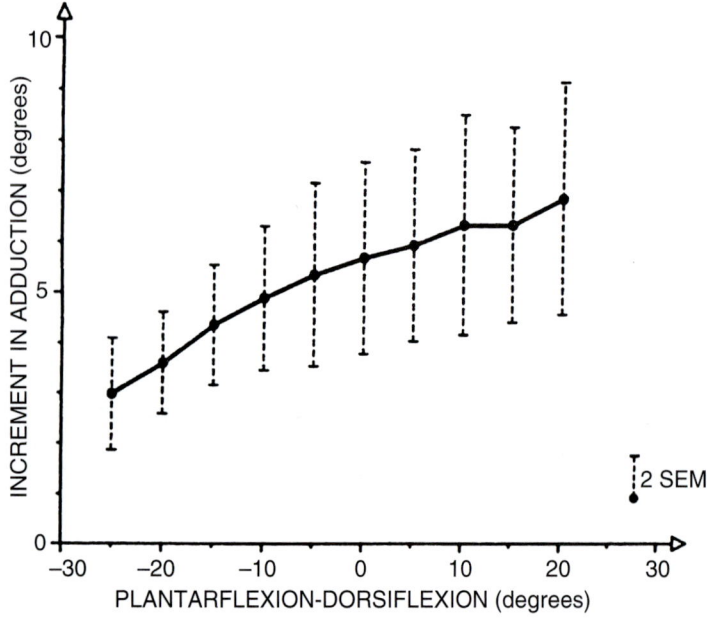

Figure 10.70 **Mean increments of adduction (or supination) at the tibiotalocalcaneal joint complex after section of the calcaneofibular ligament in 10 specimens.** (Kjaersgaard-Andersen P, Wethelund JO, Nielsen S. Lateral talocalcaneal instability following section of the calcaneo-fibular ligament: a kinesiologic study. *Foot Ankle*. 1987;7[6]:358. Copyright ©1987. Reprinted by Permission of SAGE Publications.)

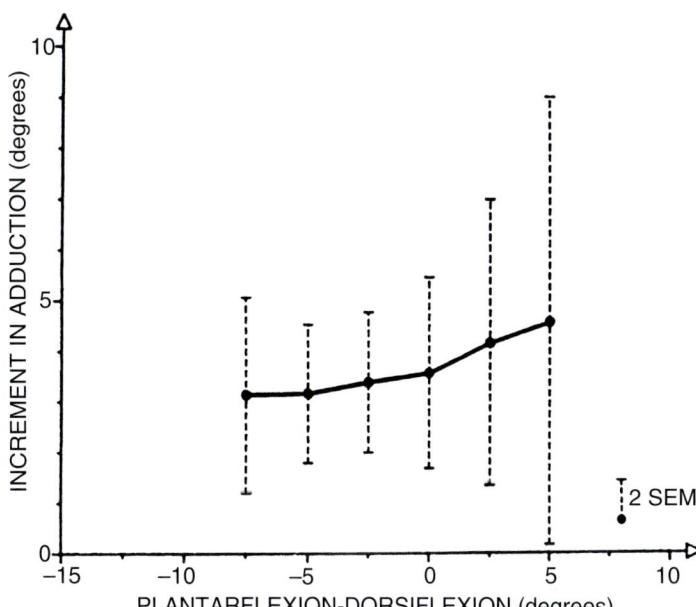

Figure 10.71 Mean increments of adduction (or supination) at the talocalcaneal joint after section of the calcaneofibular ligament in 10 specimens. (Kjaersgaard-Andersen P, Wethelund JO, Nielsen S. Lateral talocalcaneal instability following section of the calcaneo-fibular ligament: a kinesiologic study. *Foot Ankle*. 1987;7[6]:359. Copyright ©1987. Reprinted by Permission of SAGE Publications.)

importance of the calcaneofibular ligament in determining the lateral stability of the subtalar joint.

This finding is contrary to that of Cass and coworkers, who detected no influence of the calcaneofibular ligament on subtalar supination (author's adduction), which remained constant in plantar flexion or dorsiflexion.[32]

The variability of the orientation of the calcaneofibular ligament, as analyzed by Ruth, may contribute to the explanation of these functional discrepancies.[66] Furthermore, the functional implication of the variable anatomic relationship between the calcaneofibular ligament and the lateral talocalcaneal ligament was investigated by Trouilloud and colleagues in 26 ankles.[51] They divided their specimens into three types: A, B, and C. In type A (35%), a lateral talocalcaneal ligament blends with or reinforces intimately the calcaneofibular ligament and diverges from the latter at the talar or at the calcaneal insertion. In type B (23%), a distinct lateral talocalcaneal ligament is present just anterior to the calcaneofibular ligament. In type C (42%), the lateral talocalcaneal ligament is absent.

The transection of the calcaneofibular ligament in type B did not affect the subtalar or the talocalcaneonavicular motions, whereas in types A and C, it affected the subtalar motion, resulting in the author's interpretation of a talonavicular subluxation.

Martin et al[52] investigated the elongation behavior of calcaneofibular and cervical ligaments during inversion loads in nine cadaver specimens (ages range 63-81 years). Two methods of inversion assessment were used: manual and roentgenographic. Under inversion load with the calcaneofibular ligament intact the mean elongation of the cervical ligament was 0.58 ± 0.33 mm by manual measurement and 0.46 ± 0.23 mm by x-ray measurement. With the calcaneofibular ligament transected, under inversion load, the elongation of the cervical ligament was 0.88 ± 0.37 mm by manual measurement and 0.78 ± 0.37 mm by x-ray measurement. With the transection of the calcaneofibular ligament, the inversion range of motion increased 7.5° ± 2.75° manually and 7.7° ± 2.95° by x-ray measurement.

▶ Midtarsal Joint Motion: Calcaneocuboid, Talonavicular, and Cubonavicular

The midtarsal joint—transverse tarsal joint or Chopart joint—is formed by the calcaneocuboid and the talonavicular joints. A functional unit is formed by the cuboid and the navicular, which form an amphiarthrosis and move upon the anterior calcaneal surface and the talar head. Manter has described two axes to the midtarsal joint: longitudinal and transverse (Fig. 10.72).[40]

The longitudinal axis passes through the posterolateral aspect of the calcaneus and the beak of the cuboid, and is directed from posterolaterally to anteromedially. This axis slopes upward anteriorly 15° and is medially deviated 9°. With the calcaneus held fixed, the movement around this axis is that of pronation-supination, with some abduction associated with pronation and some adduction associated with supination. The motion around this axis is also helical, involving a screw-like action. The helix angle is 10°. The direction of the screw is opposite that of the subtalar joint. It is left-handed in the right foot and right-handed in the left foot (Fig. 10.73). The second axis of the midtarsal joint is quite steep and oblique. The inclination angle is 52°, and the declination or medial deviation is 57°. The motion generated is that of dorsiflexion-abduction or plantar flexion-adduction of the cubonavicular when the talus and the calcaneus are held fixed. No helical motion was detected along this axis.

Hicks also describes two axes to the midtarsal joint: oblique and longitudinal (Fig. 10.74).[12] The longitudinal axis is directed from the inferior aspect of the navicular to the posterolateral

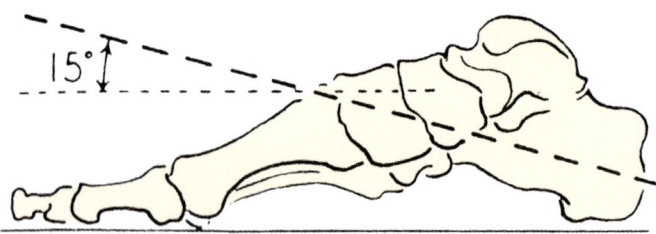

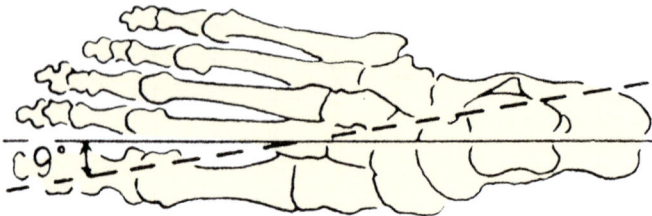

Figure 10.72 The longitudinal axis of the transverse tarsal joint projected in the sagittal and the horizontal planes of the foot. (Adapted from Manter JT. Movements of the subtalar and transverse tarsal joints. *Anat Rec.* 1941;80:407.)

aspect of the heel. It slopes upward anteriorly. The major motion occurring around this axis is pronation with slight abduction-extension and supination with slight adduction-flexion. The range of motion is 8°.

The oblique axis is directed from the superomedial aspect of the talar head to the inferolateral aspect of the heel. This axis generates the motion of pronation-abduction-extension and of supination-adduction-flexion. The range of motion is 22°.

▶ Calcaneocuboid Joint Motion

The anterior calcaneal surface is saddle shaped, convex transversely and concave vertically. A spiral-type groove is present, more accentuated medially. It is directed downward medially and posteriorly. The surface is oriented "from laterodistal to medioproximal"[3] (Fig. 10.75). At the medial end of the

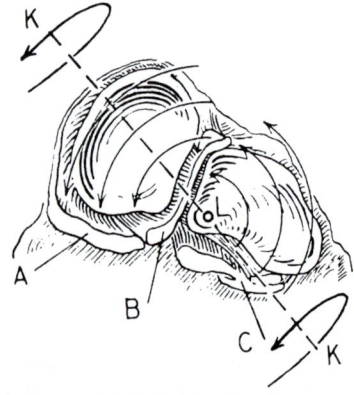

Figure 10.73 Posterior view of the right transverse tarsal joint shows the articular surfaces of the navicular and the cuboid. Light arrows indicate motion about a longitudinal axis *L*; heavy arrows indicate motion about an oblique axis *KK*. (*A*, plantar calcaneonavicular ligament; *B*, deep portion of the bifurcate ligament; *C*, long and short plantar ligaments.) (From Manter JT. Movements of the subtalar and transverse tarsal joints. *Anat Rec.* 1941;80:404.)

calcaneal groove is the calcaneal coronoid fossa, just in front of the sustentaculum tali. This fossa receives the beak of the cuboid. The superomedial corner of the articular surface makes a shelflike projection anteromedially. This beak or rostrum of the os calcis overhangs the cuboid.

The articular surface of the cuboid is also saddle shaped, concave transversely and convex vertically. The lateral segment of the articular surface may have a rather attenuated contour with more or less an element of flattening. The inferomedial end of the surface is prolonged by the beak of the cuboid, and this process (the pyramidal apophysis or coronoid of the cuboid) augments the concavity of the articular surface in the transverse direction and presents a strong convexity in the near vertical direction. The cuboid beak "undershoots" the calcaneal surface, supporting it in a bracketlike way.[53] The study of the contours and fit of the articular surfaces provides further basic information about the functioning of the joint. When one observes the calcaneocuboid joint from the dorsal aspect, it becomes evident that when the cuboid is held fixed, the endorotation of the calcaneus, or varus, results in an incongruous fit of the surfaces, whereas the exorotation of the calcaneus results in a congruous fit at the joint (Fig. 10.76). These two positions correspond to the loose-pack and close-pack positions of MacConaill and Basmajian. The exorotation of the calcaneus is a component of the untwisting of the lamina pedis, whereas the endorotation is a component of the twisting of the lamina pedis. When the calcaneus is held fixed, as seen from the medial aspect, pronation of the cuboid results in an incongruous fit, whereas supination of the cuboid results in a congruous fit (Fig. 10.77).

If the calcaneus is endorotated—in varus—a close fit is achieved with adduction-flexion-supination of the cuboid. The cuboid slides, rolls, and spins, and the cuboidal beak fits against the corresponding calcaneal surface, reaching the coronoid fossa. Further motion is blocked by the overhanging calcaneal surface (Fig. 10.78). In this congruous fit, the foot is not plantigrade. As described by Farabeuf, with the heel in varus, the forefoot is flexed, adducted, and supinated.[54] The lateral border of the foot is lowered, whereas the medial border is relatively elevated with an element of cupping of the plantar surface (Fig. 10.79).

The ligamentous stability of the joint is provided mainly by the short plantar or plantar calcaneocuboid ligament and dorsally by the calcaneocuboid component of the bifurcate ligament. Lewis has stressed the medial shift of the cuboid insertion of the plantar calcaneocuboid ligament, which determines the obliquity of the ligament, from proximolateral to distalmedial (Fig. 10.80).[43] This ligament is then tight with supination of the cuboid or exorotation (pronation or valgus) of the calcaneus (Fig. 10.81). This is a component of the untwisting of the lamina pedis. Lewis mentions the tensioning of the calcaneocuboid component of the bifurcated ligament with calcaneal exorotation.[43]

In 1960, Elftman presented an empirical interpretation of the axes of the calcaneocuboid joint and mentioned that "the eye of the connoisseur never has difficulty in recognizing both axes" of the joint.[55] His methodology was not experimental. The first axis of the calcaneocuboid joint lies within the

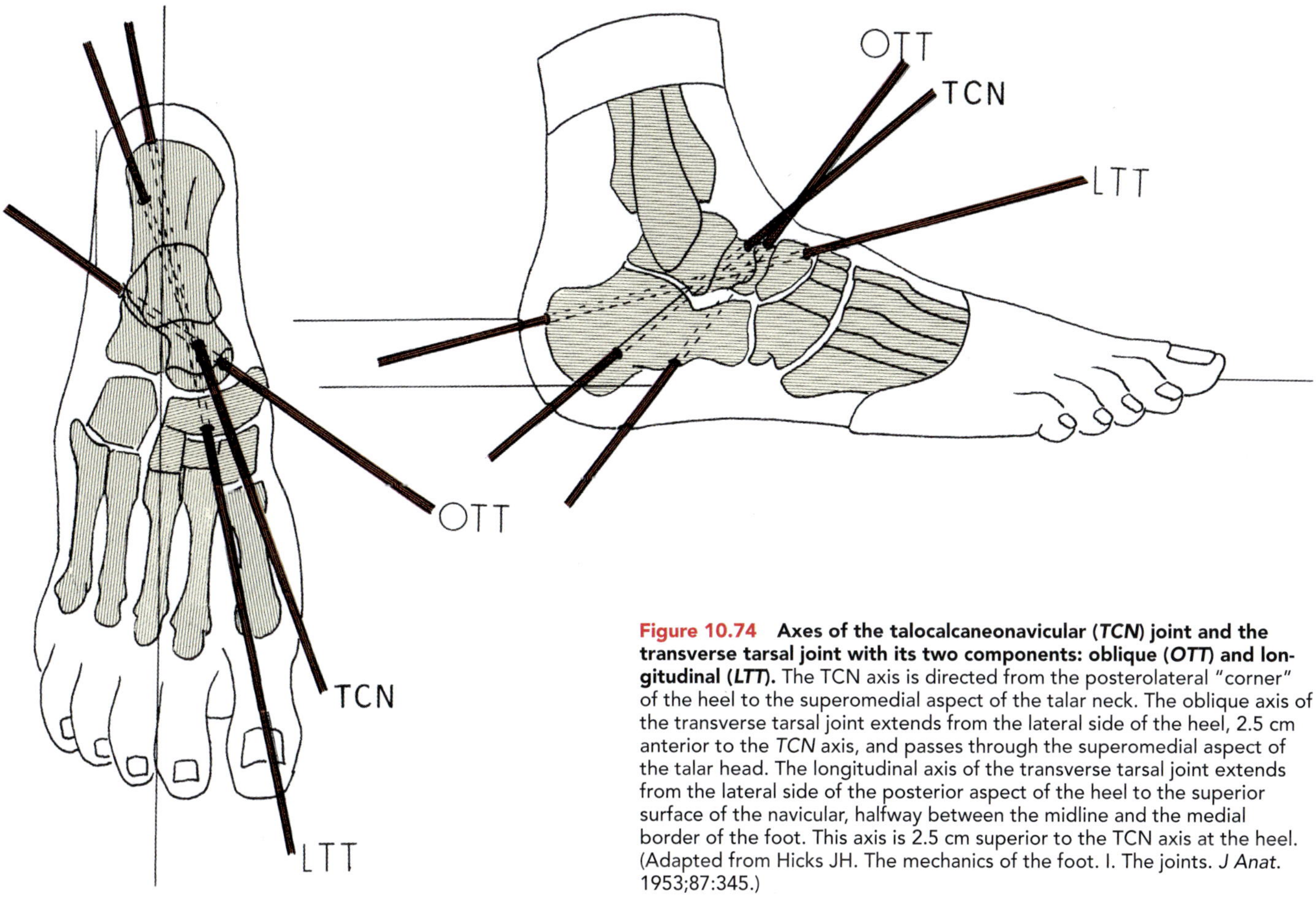

Figure 10.74 Axes of the talocalcaneonavicular (*TCN*) joint and the transverse tarsal joint with its two components: oblique (*OTT*) and longitudinal (*LTT*). The TCN axis is directed from the posterolateral "corner" of the heel to the superomedial aspect of the talar neck. The oblique axis of the transverse tarsal joint extends from the lateral side of the heel, 2.5 cm anterior to the *TCN* axis, and passes through the superomedial aspect of the talar head. The longitudinal axis of the transverse tarsal joint extends from the lateral side of the posterior aspect of the heel to the superior surface of the navicular, halfway between the midline and the medial border of the foot. This axis is 2.5 cm superior to the TCN axis at the heel. (Adapted from Hicks JH. The mechanics of the foot. I. The joints. *J Anat.* 1953;87:345.)

calcaneus and is determined by the convex component of the calcaneal surface. It is projected upward and passes through the head of the talus (Fig. 10.82). The second axis lies in the cuboid and is at a right angle to the first axis. This corresponds to the concavity of the calcaneal surface. The resultant of the two axes intersects the perpendicular line uniting both axes (Fig. 10.83). This instantaneous axis passes just below the sustentaculum tali and through the head of the talus. It closely approximates the oblique axis of the midtarsal joint as defined by Manter[40] and Hicks.[12]

Van Langelaan determined experimentally the calcaneocuboid axes during exorotation of the leg at 30° to 35°.[3] The inclination of the axis had a mean value of 51.9° (range, 43.3°-72°) and was directed from anterosuperior to posteroinferior (Fig. 10.84). The declination angle or deviation of the axis had a mean value of 2.7° (range, −15.5°-19.9°). The range of rotation at the calcaneocuboid joint was 15.8° (range, 8.8°-25.3°), with a translation of the cuboid along the axis having a mean value of 1.8 mm (range, 0.6-3.4 mm). This corresponded to the helical motion of the cuboid.

Leland et al[56] investigated the stability of the calcaneocuboid joint in the transverse plane to a lateral force of 2 Kp applied with a Telos machine in 25 volunteers (mean age, 33.3 years;

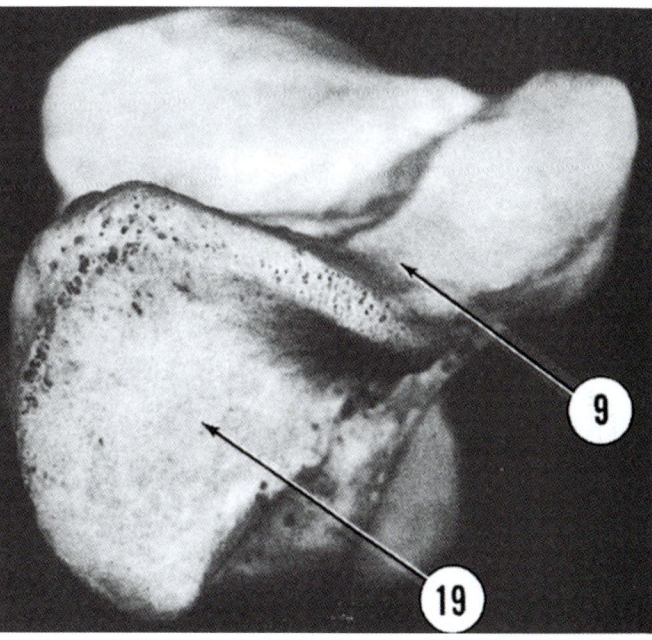

Figure 10.75 Anterior calcaneal articular surface (*19*) is convex transversely and concave vertically. It is directed downward, medially, and posteriorly in a spiral-groove manner. *9* denotes the calcanea coronoid fossa.

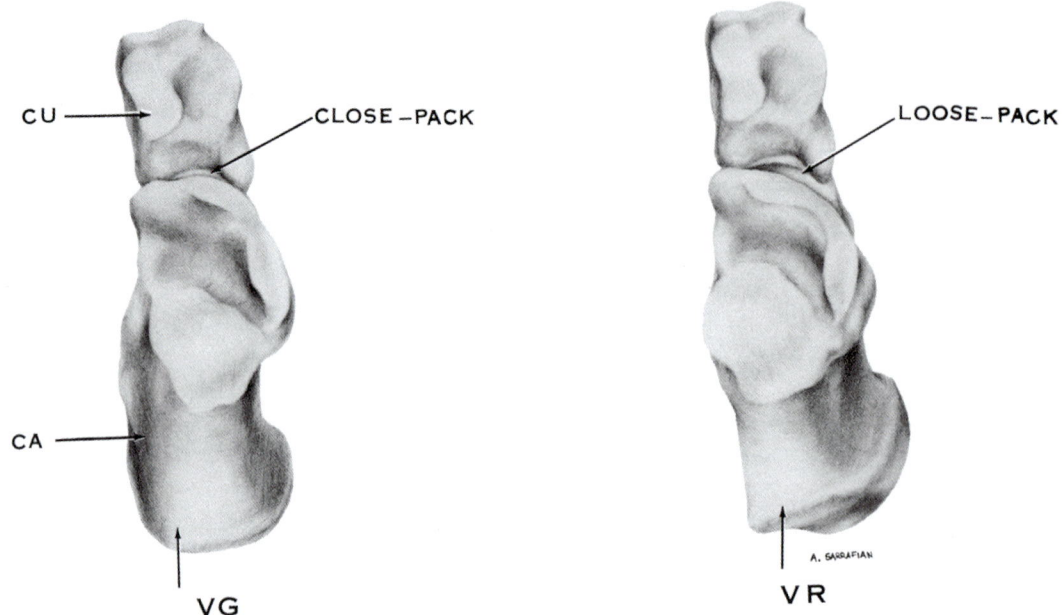

Figure 10.76 Calcaneocuboid joint stability. The cuboid is held fixed. The endorotation or varus of the calcaneus results in incongruous fit (loose-pack). The exorotation or valgus of the calcaneus results in congruous fit (close-pack). (*CA*, calcaneus; *CU*, cuboid; *VG*, valgus; *VR*, varus.)

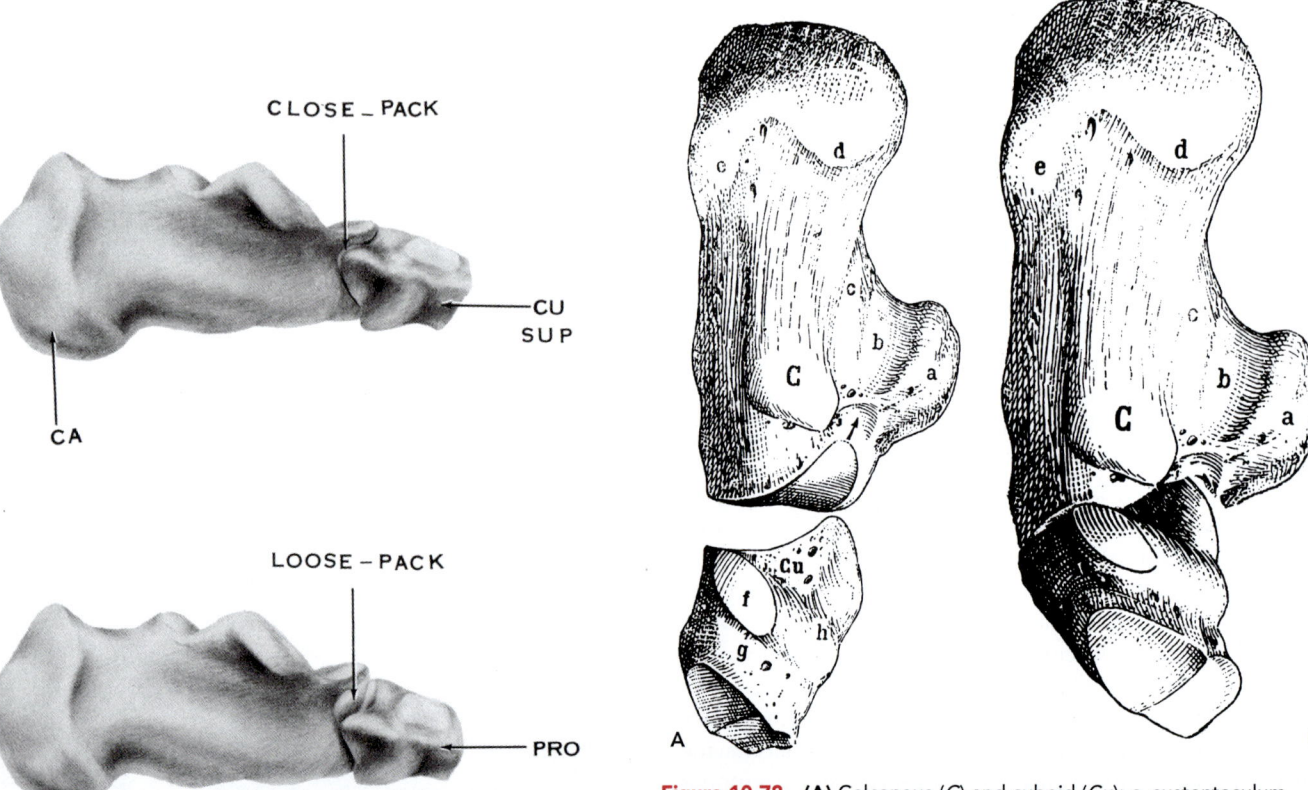

Figure 10.77 Calcaneocuboid stability. The calcaneus is held fixed. The cuboid pronation results in incongruous fit (loose-pack). The cuboid supination results in congruous fit (close-pack). (*CA*, calcaneus; *CU*, cuboid, *PRO*, pronation; *SUP*, supination.)

Figure 10.78 **(A)** Calcaneus (*C*) and cuboid (*Cu*); *a*, sustentaculum tali; *b*, groove of the flexor hallucis longus tendon. *Arrow* indicates the coronoid groove, which will receive the beak of the calcaneus. **(B)** The cuboid is in maximum flexion-adduction. The beak of the cuboid is directed into the coronoid fossa. (From Farabeuf LH. *Precis de Manuel Operatoire.* Maisson; 1889:821-822.)

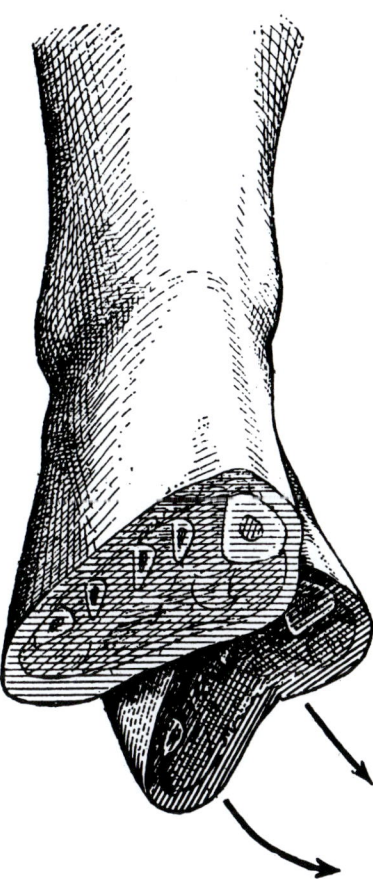

Figure 10.79 The forefoot is at rest above, corresponding to the standing position. Below, the forefoot is flexed and adducted and supinated. The lateral border of the foot is under the medial border, and the foot is rolled inward, as indicated by the curved arrow. (From Farabeuf LH. *Precis de Manuel Operatoire*. Maisson; 1889:828.)

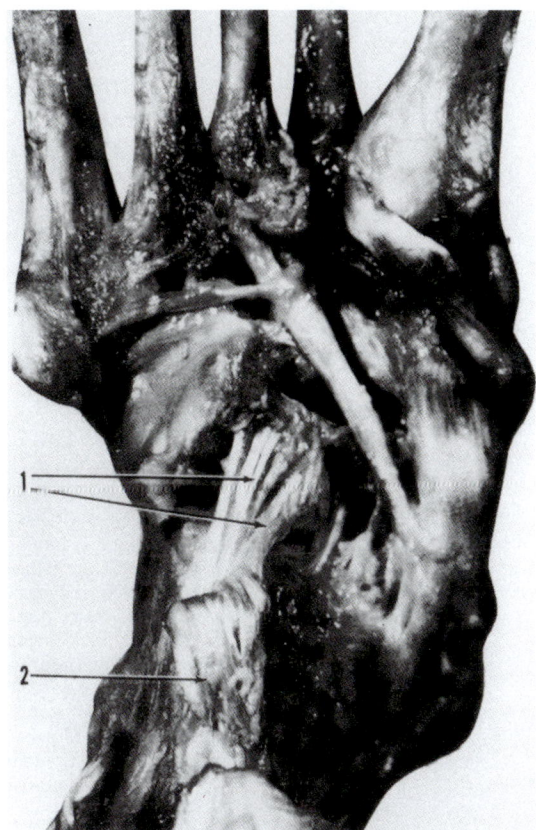

Figure 10.80 The plantar calcaneocuboid ligament (*1*) is directed from proximal-lateral to distal-medial. *2* is the calacneocuboid component off the bifurcate ligament which is more dorsal.

range, 23-54) and in five unembalmed cadaver lower legs. Roentgenograms were taken to assess the cubocalcaneal gap with or without stress.

In the volunteer's group, the mean calcaneocuboid gap for the unstressed feet was 3.9 mm and for the stressed feet it was 5.5 mm (Fig. 10.85).

In the cadaveric feet, the calcaneocuboid gap without stress was 4.1 mm and with mediolateral stress it was 5.1 mm. Transecting the dorsal calcaneocuboid ligaments increased the gap to 6.2 mm and further destabilization with added transection of the plantar calcaneocuboid ligament increased the roentgenographic gap to 7.2 mm (Fig. 10.86). This study was limited to the assessment of the stability of the calcaneocuboid joint in the transverse plane only.

▶ Talonavicular Joint Motion

The talar head is ellipsoid and convex in its greater and lesser curvatures. The surface is inclined and the long axis is oriented downward and inward. The motion generated by the surface is that of flexion-adduction-supination or extension-abduction-pronation (Fig. 10.87). The navicular articular surface is biconcave and frequently presents an inferior extension forming the beak of the navicular. It is smaller than the corresponding talar

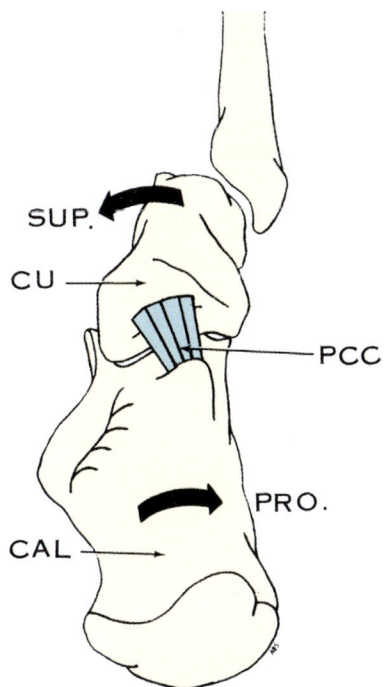

Figure 10.81 The plantar calcaneocuboid ligament (*PCC*) is tight with pronation (*PRO*) of the calcaneus (*CAL*) or supination (*SUP*) of the cuboid (*CU*).

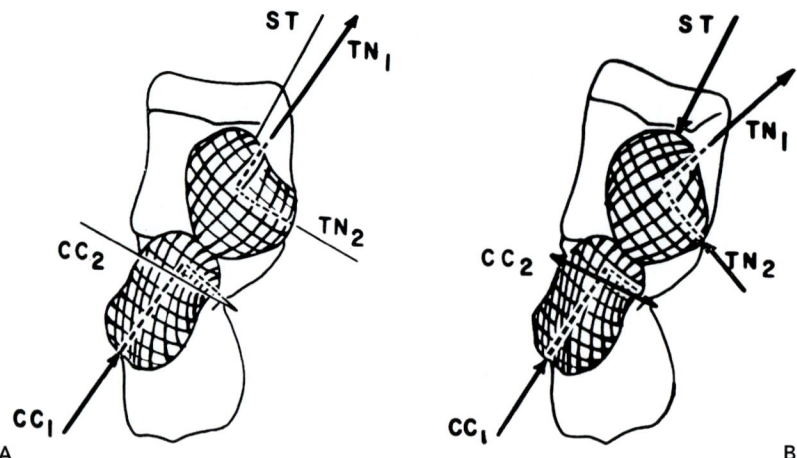

Figure 10.82 Axes of the transverse tarsal joint in pronation (A) and in supination (B). The axis of the convex curvature of the os calcis CC_1 at the calcaneocuboid joint is located in the os calcis and when projected upward passes through the head of the talus. The axis of the concave curvature of the same surface CC_2 is perpendicular to CC_1 and passes through the cuboid. The axis of the major convexity of the talar head TN_1 at the talonavicular joint and the axis of the lesser convexity of the same surface TN_2 are also perpendicular to each other. The major displacements are perpendicular to the axes CC_1 and TN_1. In full pronation **(A)**, the axes CC_1 and TN_2 coincide, "allowing free movement without involving other axes." The forefoot moves at the midtarsal joint freely without the need of motion between the talus and the os calcis. In supination, the CC_1, and TN_1 axes do not coincide and motion is required around the secondary axes CC_2 and TN_2 and around the subtalar joint axis ST, so that the resultant of CC_1 and CC_2 axes is identical to the combined resultant of TN_1-TN_2 and ST axes. In supination, the midtarsal joint motion requires associated motion at the subtalar joint between the talus and the os calcis; incongruity of the surfaces may otherwise result. (From Elftman H. The transverse tarsal joint and its control. *Clin Orthop Relat Res.* 1960;16:41.)

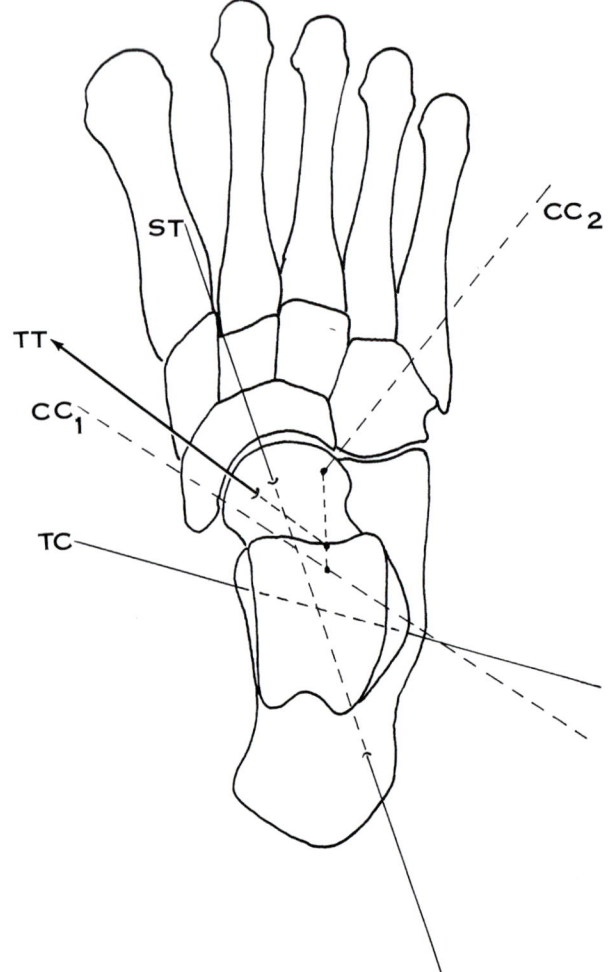

Figure 10.83 The transverse tarsal joint axis (TT) has an instantaneous variable position as the foot passes from a pronated to a supinated position. This TT axis passes through a line perpendicular to the major CC_1 and the minor CC_2 axes of the calcaneocuboid joint. (ST, subtalar joint axis; TC, talocrural joint axis.) (Redrawn from Elftman H. The transverse tarsal joint and its control. *Clin Orthop Relat Res.* 1960;16:41.)

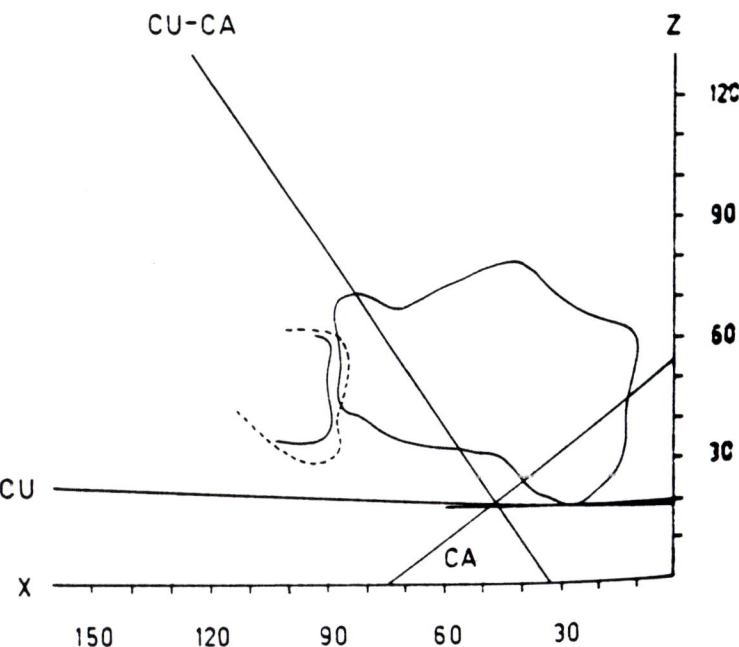

Figure 10.84 Projection of relative cuboid-calcaneal (*CU-CA*) helical axis with exorotation of the leg. (Copyright © 1983 Van Langelaan EJ. A kinematical analysis of the tarsal joints: an X-ray photogrammetric study. *Acta Orthop Scand.* 1983;54[suppl 204]:180. Reproduced by permission of Taylor and Francis Group, LLC, a division of Informa plc.)

head. The motion of the navicular over the talar head is that of a female ovoid surface over a male ovoid surface, and consequently the navicular surface slides, rolls, and spins and the rolling is in the same direction as the sliding.

The axis of surface revolution of the talar head at the talonavicular joint does not coincide with the subtalar axis. As demonstrated by Huson, when the talus is externally rotated (through abduction-pronation-extension) with the calcaneus, and the navicular and the cuboid are held fixed, a talonavicular subluxation results, evidenced by an inferomedial opening of the joint.[8] This is reduced by adduction-flexion-supination at the midtarsal joint (Fig. 10.88).

Elftman recognized empirically two axes of motion at the talonavicular joint corresponding to the greater and lesser curvatures of the talar head.[55] The two axes pass through the talar head and are perpendicular to each other (see Figs. 10.82 and 10.83).

Van Langelaan determined experimentally the talonavicular axes during exorotation of the leg at 30° to 35°.[3] The mean inclination angle of the axis was 38.5° (range, 27°-47.4°), and

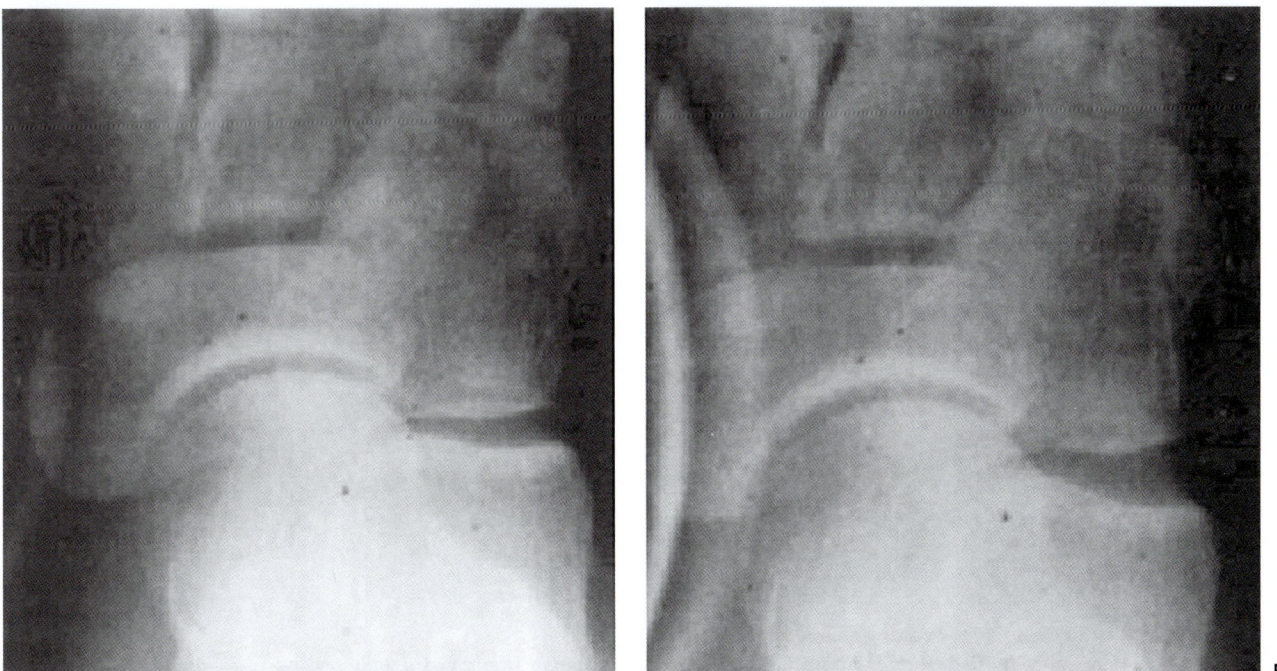

Figure 10.85 Clinical radiographs demonstrating unstressed (A) and stressed (B) calcaneocuboid joint in a normal individual. (Leland RH, Marymont JV, Trevino SG, Varner KE, Noble PC. Calcaneocuboid stability: a clinical and anatomic study. *Foot Ankle Int.* 2001;11:880-884, Figure 2. Copyright ©2001. Reprinted by Permission of SAGE Publications.)

the mean declination or deviation angle was 14.1° (range, 3.8°-21.4°) (Fig. 10.89). The talar rotation around the relative talonavicular axis had a mean value of 43.1° (range, 29.9°-50.7°), and an anterosuperior translation of the talus was present along the axis with a mean value of 1.2 mm (range, 0.4-1.9 mm). The motion is thus helical in nature.

▶ Cubonavicular Movements

A small articular surface is present on the medial surface of the cuboid for the navicular in 45% to 50% of the cases. A transversely oriented interosseous ligament is present between the two bones. It originates from a narrow vertical segment of the cuboid and inserts on the anteroinferior segment of the lateral

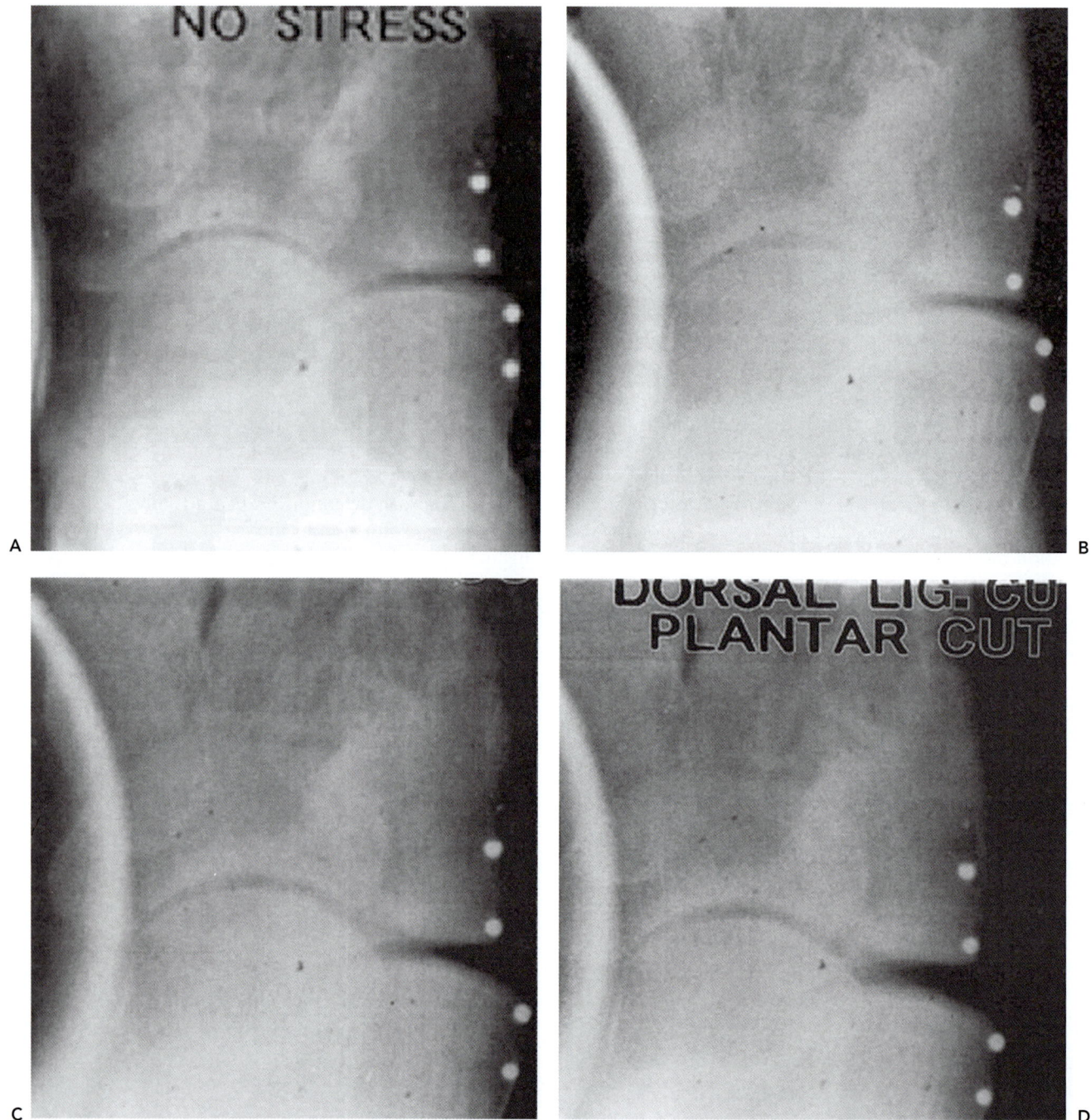

Figure 10.86 Cadaveric radiographs demonstrating calcaneocuboid laxity under (A) unstressed and (B) stressed conditions with unsectioned ligaments, (C) sectioned dorsal ligament, and (D) sectioned dorsal plus plantar ligament. (Leland RH, Marymont JV, Trevino SG, et al. Calcaneocuboid stability: a clinical and anatomic study. *Foot Ankle Int.* 2001;11:880-884, Figure 3. copyright ©2001. Reprinted by Permission of SAGE Publications.)

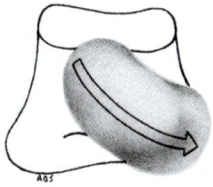
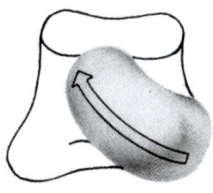

FLE-ADD-SUP   EXT-ABD-PRO

Figure 10.87 Motion generated at the articular surface of the talar head along with major axis. Combination of flexion-adduction-supination or extension-abduction-pronation.

end of the navicular. When the small articular surface is present, the interosseous fibers originate from above and below the articular surface. The two bones are further connected by a plantar and dorsal cubonavicular ligament transversely oriented (Figs. 10.90 and 10.91).

The dorsal cubonavicular ligament is triangular, and the apex originates from the dorsal aspect of the navicular and inserts on the dorsum of the cuboid in its distal half. The plantar cubonavicular ligament is a rectangular band. It originates from the inferior surface of the cuboid near its medial border and inserts on the inferior surface of the navicular.

Van Langelaan is the only author to provide objective data with regard to the motion between the navicular and the cuboid.[3] The relative movement between the two bones is that of "eversion of the cuboid in relation to the navicular," which means "inversion of the navicular." This results in a very slight flattening of the transverse arch.[2] The axis of motion runs "approximately in the longitudinal direction of the foot, virtually horizontally from antero-latero-superior to postero-medio-inferior" (Fig. 10.92). The mean inclination angle of the axis was 13.2° (range, 2.6°-25.2°) and the mean deviation or declination angle was 8.4° (range, 39.9°-7.1°). The mean range

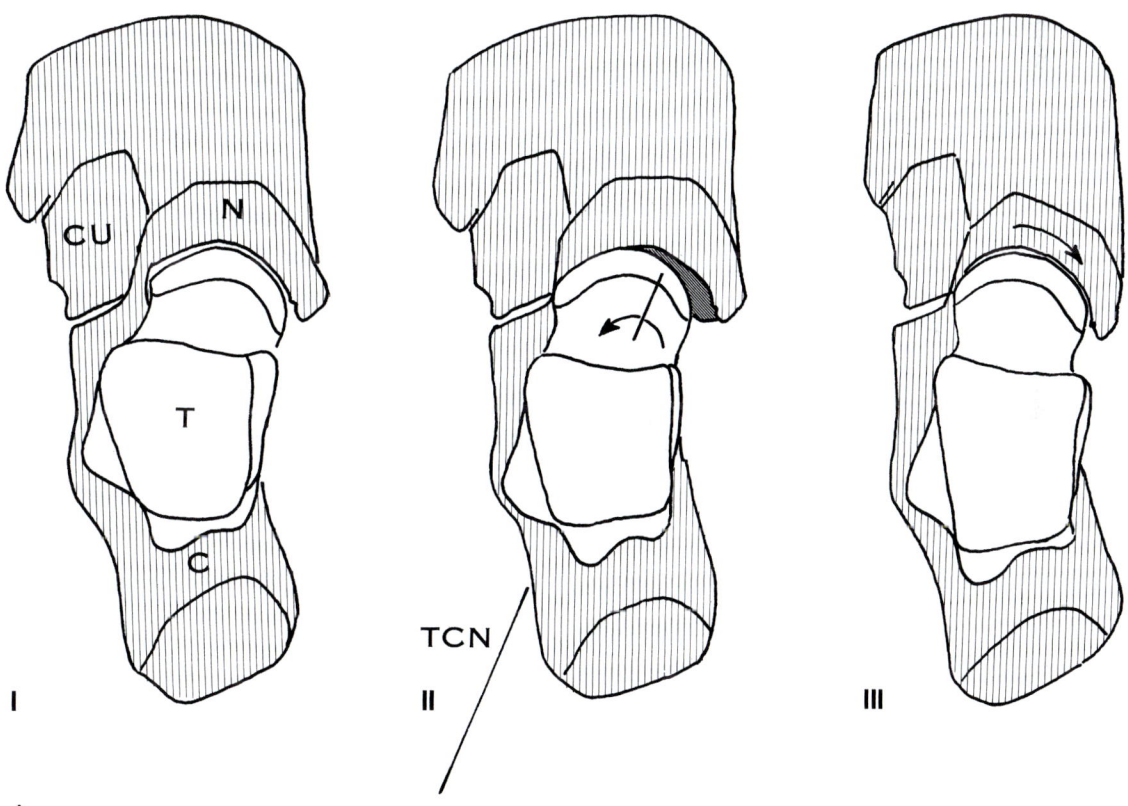

Figure 10.88 **(A)** (*I*) The relationship of the talus (*T*), navicular (*N*), cuboid (*CU*), and calcaneus (*C*) in the standing position. (*II*) The os calcis is held fixed experimentally and the talus is turned against the calcaneus around the talocalcaneonavicular axis (*TCN*) in pronation combined with abduction and extension. This is equivalent to a "supination" of the foot. If the navicular and the cuboid are prevented from rotating, a dislocation in the talonavicular joint is observed medially. This is due to the fact that the axis of the talocalcaneonavicular joint and the axis of the revolution of the articular surface of the talar head do not coincide. (*III*) The above dislocation is immediately reduced by the simultaneous motion of the navicular and the cuboid, which undergo an adduction-supination and some degree of flexion. (Diagrams after photographic documentation by Huson A. *Anatomical and Functional Study of the Tarsal Joints*. Drukkerij, Luctor et Emergo; 1961:134, 135.) **(B)** (*I*) The calcaneus is stabilized in neutral with a nail and the forefoot is in plantigrade position. (*II*) The forefoot is stabilized in neutral. The talus is exorotated, and this results in talonavicular subluxation at site *X*. (*III*) The subluxation is reduced by adduction-flexion-supination of the forefoot, as indicated by arrow. (Described by Huson.)

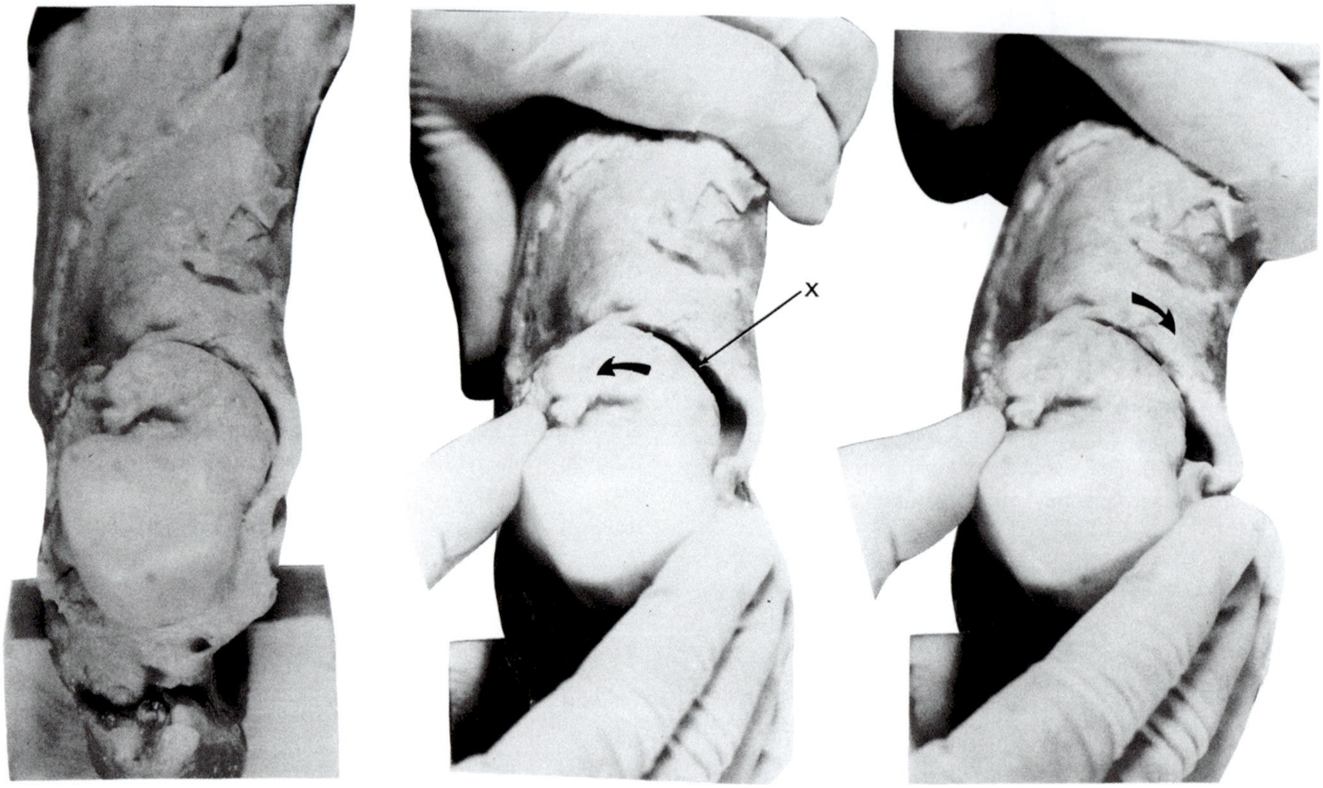

B I   II   III

Figure 10.88 (Continued)

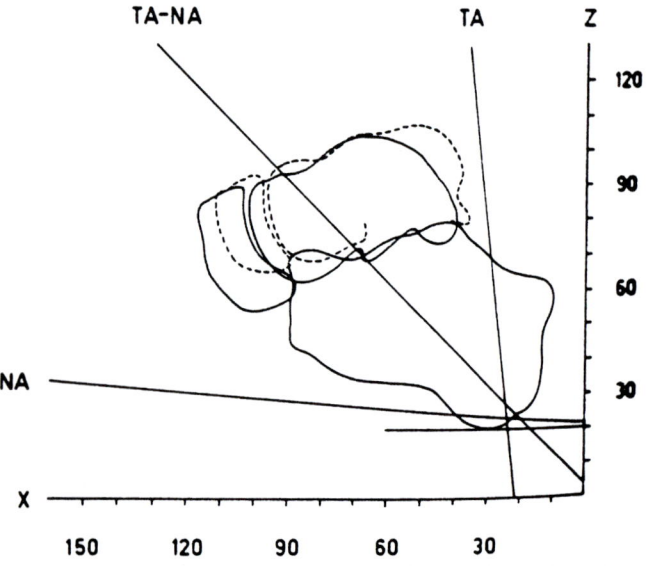

Figure 10.89 Projection of the relative talonavicular TA-NA helical axis during exorotation of the leg. (Copyright © 1983. Van Langelaan EJ. A kinematical analysis of the tarsal joints: an X-ray photogrammetric study. *Acta Orthop Scand*. 1983;54[suppl 204]:212. Reproduced by permission of Taylor and Francis Group, LLC, a division of Informa plc.)

of rotation of the cuboid was 6.8° (range, 3.9°-9.9°), with a translation along the axis having a mean of 0.9 mm (range, 0.4-1.6 mm). The cuboid moved in a posterior direction.

▶ Combined Midfoot-Forefoot Motion

The supination twist of the midfoot-forefoot is a counterclockwise rotation for the right foot, and the pronation is a clockwise rotation. This is a fundamental motion component determining the plantigrade position of the foot when the calcaneus is exorotated (valgus) or endorotated (varus) in response to tibiotalar loading in internal or external rotation.

Hicks analyzed in detail the anatomic and functional basis of the hindfoot-forefoot relationship in the plantigrade position.[12] Ouzounian and Shereff investigated in ten cadaveric specimens the motion contribution of the midtarsal joint, the naviculocuneiform joints, and the tarsometatarsal joints during supination-pronation twist of the midfoot-forefoot.[57] Reference pins were inserted in the corresponding bones and were used to trace the total motion relative to a fixed coordinate system. A three-space tracker was used to obtain the coordinates after replacing the localized metallic pins with

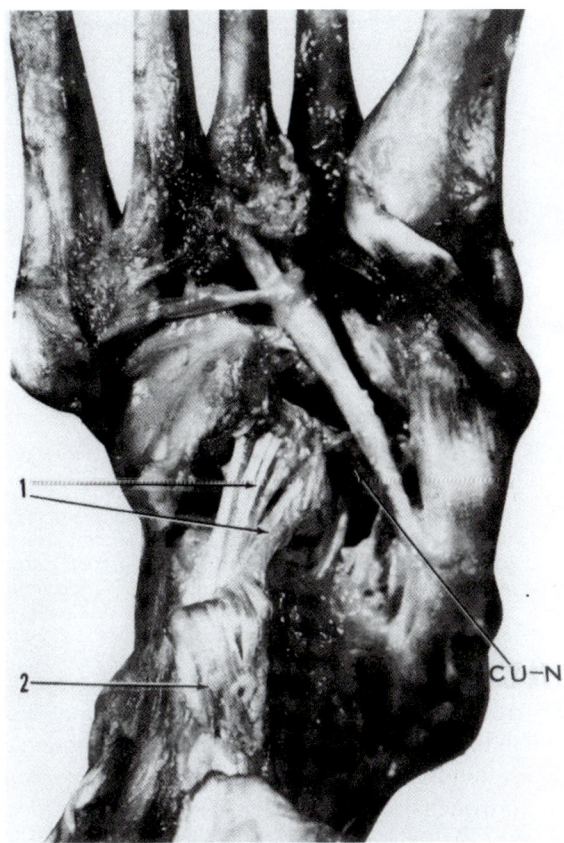

Figure 10.90 Plantar cubonavicular ligament (CU-N). *2* is the calcaneocuboid component off the bifurcate ligament which is more dorsal.

nonmetallic reference pins. Supination twist was simulated by applying a dorsolateral force at 45° on the first metatarsal and a plantar-medial force at 45° on the fifth metatarsal, thus creating a rotational couple. Pronation twist was simulated by applying a plantar-lateral force at 45° on the first metatarsal and a dorsomedial force at 45° on the fifth metatarsal. The segmental motion contribution of the joints to the supination-pronation was as follows:

Midtarsal Joint
  Talonavicular: 17.7° (range, 4.4°-33.8°)
  Calcaneocuboid: 7.3° (range, 2.3°-14.5°)
Naviculocuneiform
  Naviculo—medial cuneiform: 7.3° (range, 3.5°-9.9°)
  Naviculo—middle cuneiform: 3.5° (range, 2.9°-4.1°)
  Naviculo—lateral cuneiform: 2.1° (range, 0.2°-4.2°)
Tarsometatarsal
  Medial cuneiform—first metatarsal: 1.5° (range, 0°-2.6°)
  Middle cuneiform—second metatarsal: 1.2° (range, 0.5°-1.9°)
  Lateral cuneiform—third metatarsal: 2.6° (range, 0.1°-9.4°)
  Cuboid—fourth metatarsal: 11.1° (range, 5.5°-21.2°)
  Cuboid—fifth metatarsal: 9° (range, 3.5°-24.4°)

The same data read in a columnar fashion as a medial column formed by the talonavicular, naviculocuneiforms, and cuneiform-metatarsals 1 to 3 and a lateral column formed by the calcaneocuboid and the cubometatarsals 4 to 5 reveal a gradient of motion that decreases in a proximodistal direction in the medial column except for the lateral cuneiform-third metatarsal joint. In the lateral column, the motion increases from a proximodistal direction (Fig. 10.93).

The same authors investigated the sequential motion contribution when a dorsiflexion or plantar flexion force was applied to the first and fifth metatarsals, with the results as follows:

Midtarsal
  Talonavicular: 7° (range, 0.1°-14.9°)
  Calcaneocuboid: 2.3° (range, 0.1°-8.8°)
Naviculocuneiform
  Naviculo—medial cuneiform: 5° (range, 0.7°-8.7°)

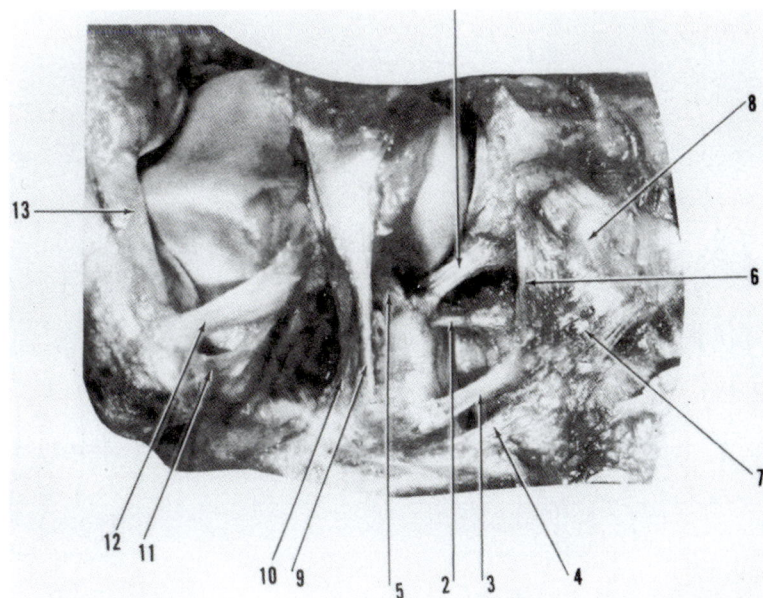

Figure 10.91 Dorsal cubonavicular ligament. (Lundberg A, Svensson OK, Bylund C, et al. Kinematics of the ankle/foot complex, part 2: pronation and supination. *Foot Ankle*. 1989;9(5):248. copyright ©1989. Reprinted by Permission of SAGE Publications.)

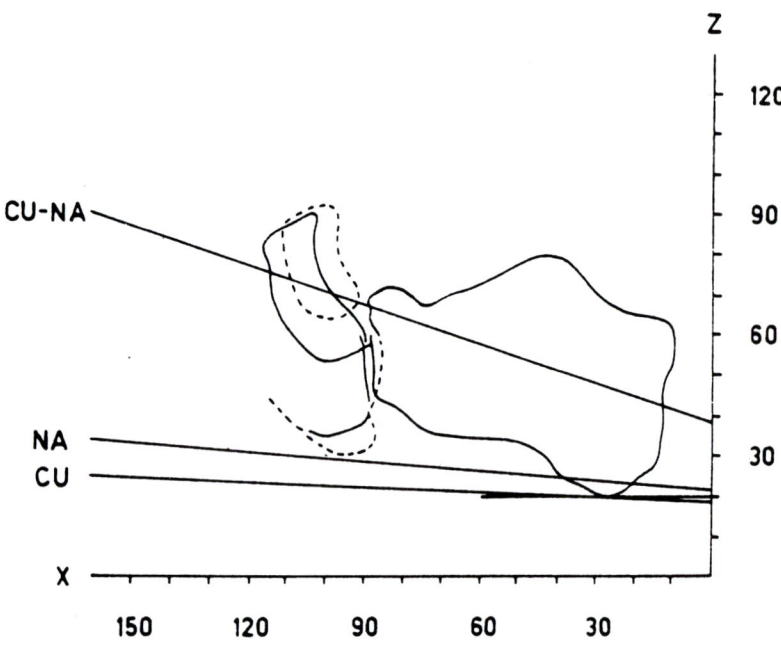

Figure 10.92 Projection of relative cuboid navicular *CU-NA* helical axis with external rotation of the leg. (Copyright © 1983. Van Langelaan EJ. A kinematical analysis of the tarsal joints: an X-ray photogrammetric study. *Acta Orthop Scand*. 1983;54[suppl 204]:221. Reproduced by permission of Taylor and Francis Group, LLC, a division of Informa plc.)

Naviculo—middle cuneiform: 5.2° (range, 1.1°-7.2°)
Naviculo—lateral cuneiform: 2.6° (range, 0.9°-5.2°)

Tarsometatarsals
Cuneo—first metatarsal: 3.5° (range, 1.9°-5.3°)
Cuneo—second metatarsal: 0.6° (range, 0.1°-1°)
Cuneo—third metatarsal: 1.6° (range, 0.1°-6.3°)
Cubo—fourth metatarsal: 9.6° (range, 4.8°-19.4°)
Cubo—fifth metatarsal: 10.2° (range, 1.1°-29.4°)

The decreasing motion gradient from a proximodistal direction is evident in the medial column, and an increasing motion gradient in a proximodistal direction is present in the lateral column.

Hicks provided functional data from one selected specimen.[12] During supination-pronation twist, the contribution of the first ray was 22° and that of the fifth ray was 10°.

Waninvenhaus and Pretterklieber analyzed the motion at the first tarsometatarsal joint in 100 specimens.[58] Biplane

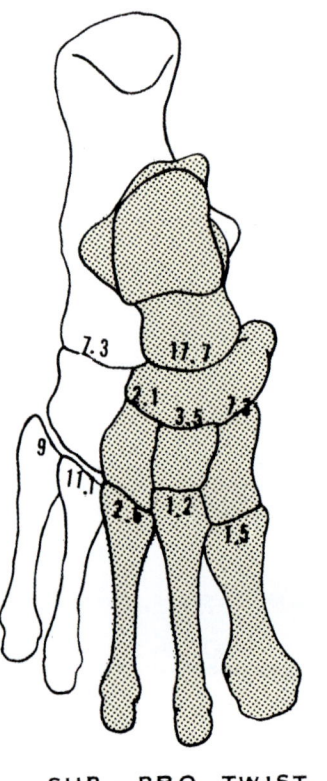
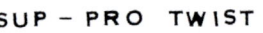

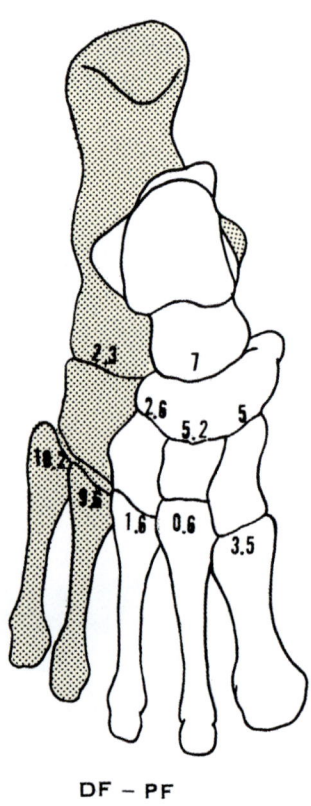

Figure 10.93 Contribution of the midtarsal joint, the naviculocuneiform joints, and the tarsometatarsal joints during supination-pronation twist and flexion-extension of the forefoot, expressed in degrees. (Data from Ouzounian TJ, Shereff MJ. In vitro determination of midfoot motion. *Foot Ankle*. 1989;10[3]:140-146.)

roentgenograms were taken, followed by manual side-to-side compression of the forefoot, in an attempt to approximate the first and second metatarsals. Transfixation of the metatarso$_1$-cuneiform$_1$ joint was achieved with two crossing Kirschner wires (K-wires). In each bone, two wires were inserted, transverse and perpendicular. The mobility of the joint was restored, and the motion was assessed by the angular deviation of the wires.

Congruous motion occurred at the metatarso$_1$-cuneiform$_1$ joint in the form of abduction of the first metatarsal in 11%. The average abduction was 4.4° (range, 3°-5°). Medial wedge opening occurred in 15% at the same joint, in 9% at the inter-cuneiform joint, and in 5% at the cuneo$_1$-navicular joint. Dorsiflexion of 4.3° (range, 3°-5°) was present in 9%. Supination (authors' eversion or external rotation) or pronation (authors' inversion or internal rotation) was negligible.

After dorsal shift of the first metatarsal, on average 2.6 mm (range, 0-6 mm), rotation was now possible in supination of 6.2° in 92% and pronation of 4.1° in 6%. Abduction of 5.89° (range, 2°-10°) was recorded in 51% and adduction of 5° (range, 2°-10°) in 30%. The authors found an intermetatarsal 1 to 2 joint in 53% of their specimens.

Romash and colleagues assessed roentgenographically the passive motion at the metatarso$_1$-cuneiform$_1$ joint in 118 subjects with bunions.[59] Weight-bearing x-rays were taken with and without side-to-side compression of the metatarsals through a tightly applied elastic bandage. Incongruous motion or medial wedge "book opening" with side-to-side compression was demonstrated at the metatarso$_1$-cuneiform$_1$ joint in 38%. Furthermore, the articular relationship of metatarsals 1 to 2 at their bases was assessed and classified into three types:

Type I (35%): no articular facet
Type II (38%): transition lateral facet present
Type III (27%): with well-developed lateral articular joint surface (Fig. 10.94)

Stress incongruous motion with medial wedge "book opening" was demonstrated in 27% in type I, 24% in type II, and 50% in type III. It thus became apparent that the presence of an articular surface M_1-M_2 limits the abduction of the first metatarsal. Stress narrowing of the M_1-M_2 angle without a medial wedge opening at the metatarso$_1$-cuneiform$_1$ joint does not, however, necessarily translate into range of abduction-adduction occurring at that joint, because wedge opening at the cuneo$_1$-navicular joint or at the intercuneiform level, which could affect the M_1-M_2 angle, could occur and was not assessed in this study. The fact that such an opening could occur was demonstrated by Waninvenhaus and Pretterklieber.[58]

▶ Tarsometatarsal Joint Stability and Contact Mechanics

The tarsometatarsal joint or Lisfranc joint is formed by three separate joint components:

Cuneo$_1$-M_1
Cuneo$_{2-3}$–M_2-M_3
Cubo-M_{4-5}

The stabilization of the joint complex is provided by the following ligaments:

Dorsal
　C_1M_1
　C_1M_2, C_2M_2, C_3M_2
　C_3M_3
　Cu-M_4, Cu-M_5
Plantar
　C_1M_1
　$C_1M_1M_2$
　No C_2M_2 ligament
　$C_3M_3M_4$ ligament inconstant
　Cu-M_4M5 often absent
　Long Cubo-M_5 (from crest of cuboid) is part of plantar ligament
Interosseous
　C_1M_2 (Lisfranc ligament)
　C_1C_2, C_2C_3, C_3Cu
　Second and third interosseous CM ligaments: very variable

Lisfranc ligament (first interosseous C_1-M_2) has been recognized by the anatomists as a major stabilizer of Lisfranc joint. Sappey has considered the plantar cuneo$_1$-metatarsal$_{2,3}$ ligament as a very strong ligament and key to the tarsometatarsal transverse arch.[13]

Lakin et al[69] investigated in six fresh cadaver lower extremity specimens the mechanical response of the tarsometatarsal joints to axial loading. The foot position varied from 10° of dorsiflexion to neutral, 30° of plantar flexion, 10° of inversion, and 10° of eversion. The axial loads corresponded to 0.5, 1.0, 1.5, and 2 times body weight. The tarsometatarsal joints investigated were the C_1-M_1, C_2-M_2, C_3-M_3, and Cu-M_4M_5. The contact mechanics (areas, pressures, and forces) were quantified using joint interposed film transducers. In the neutral position, the second and third tarsometatarsal joints "bore approximately 50% to 200% more of the load applied to the foot in neutral position." These two joints "demonstrated the largest increases (3.5 and 3.3 times, respectively) in contact force as a function of the applied load. The forces and areas across the second and third tarsometatarsal joints with the foot in neutral position were typically two to three times the forces and areas across the first and fourth/fifth tarsometatarsal joints. The second and third tarsometatarsal joints bore the majority of the force as the foot position changed in the sagittal and frontal planes. However, the first and fourth/fifth tarsometatarsal joints had a more active role in these foot positions than they did in neutral position. The forces borne by the first and fourth/fifth tarsometatarsal joints were comparable to each other, as were the forces borne by the second and third tarsometatarsal joints." The authors concluded that "the third tarsometatarsal joint bore the most force at virtually all loads and foot positions" and that "the second and third tarsometatarsal joints are stiffer and not as mobile and, because of this, are able to withstand large force amplitudes and maintain the anatomic congruity of the tarsometatarsal joint complex." They also attributed a key role to the mobility of the the first and fourth/fifth tarsometatarsal joints in handling force overloads emanating from radical changes in foot position or high loads.

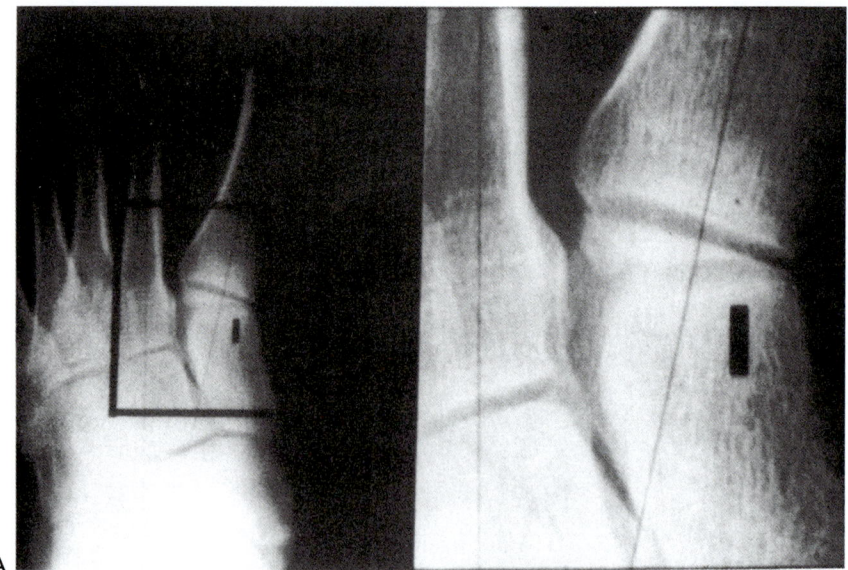
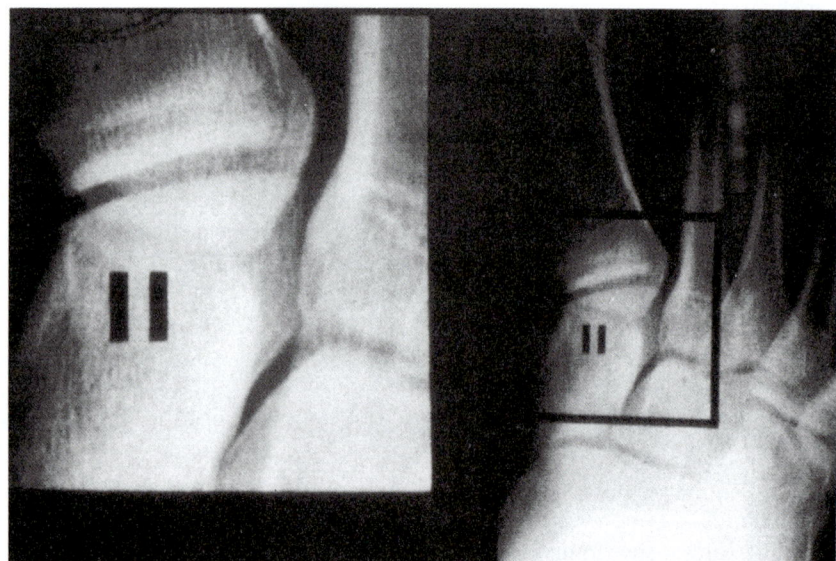
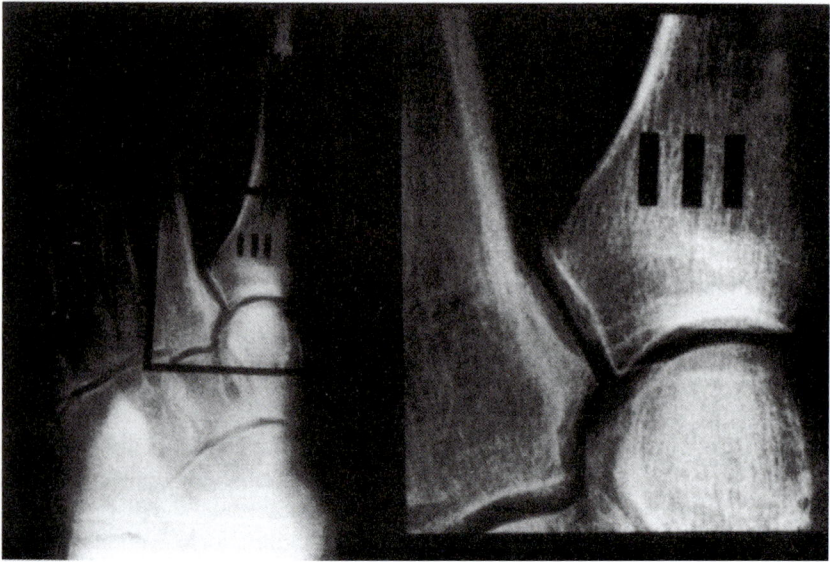

Figure 10.94 **(A)** Type I: No articular facet between M_1-M_2. **(B)** Type II: Articular facet between M_1-M_2. **(C)** Type III: Well-developed articular facet between M_1-M_2. (Romash MM, Fugate D, Yanklowit B, et al. Passive motion of the first metatarsal cuneiform joint: preoperative assessment. *Foot Ankle*. 1990;10[6]:293. Copyright ©1990. Reprinted by Permission of SAGE Publications.)

Sloan et al[70] conducted a study in 40 cadaver feet to analyze the mechanical properties of the ligaments—dorsal, interosseous, plantar—connecting the first cuneiform and the second metatarsal. The stiffness of the specimens was assessed in their experimental setup and the authors concluded that "the Lisfranc/plantar complex is stiffer and stronger than the dorsal ligament of the second tarsometatarsal joint and that the Lisfranc ligament is stronger than the plantar ligament."

Kaar et al[71] analyzed the Lisfranc joint displacement following sequential ligament sectioning. The purpose was to determine the specific ligament deficiency to reproduce a Lisfranc joint injury: transverse or longitudinal. Ten fresh frozen cadaver lower limbs were used. The specimens underwent sectioning of the interosseous C_1-M_2 (Lisfranc ligament) and were divided in two groups. The transverse group underwent sectioning of the plantar ligament between C_1 and M_2,M_3 on the plantar aspect of the C_2-M_2 joint whereas the longitudinal group underwent sectioning of the interosseous ligament between C_1 and C_2. Weight-bearing, adduction, and abduction stress x-rays were taken before and after each ligament was sectioned. Instability was defined as ≥2 mm of displacement. Transection of two ligaments was necessary to produce an instability pattern. Transection of the Lisfranc ligament supplemented by the transection of the plantar C_1–M_2M_3 ligament produced a transverse pattern of instability. Transection of Lisfranc ligament supplemented by the transection of the C_1-C_2 ligament produced a longitudinal pattern of instability. "Compared with weight-bearing radiographs, injury specific manual stress radiographs showed qualitatively greater displacement when used to evaluate both patterns of instability."[71]

Mizel[72] defined the role of the plantar M_1-C_1 ligament as a stabilizer of the first metatarsal in weight-bearing. The investigation was based on seven fresh below-knee amputation specimens. The specimen was mounted on a test stand with 5.5 kg dorsiflexion force applied to the distal first metatarsal. On testing, "no appreciable movement of the first metatarsal was noted until the ligament was cut. Dorsal displacement of the distal first metatarsal averaged 5.9 mm after sectioning of the ligament."[72]

▶ Metatarsophalangeal and Interphalangeal Angular Relationship and Motion

This inclination of the metatarsals relative to the horizontal ground level determines the neutral position at the metatarsophalangeal joint and it is of great clinical relevance in the understanding of the pathomechanics of metatarsalgia. The inclination of the first metatarsal is crucial in determining the position of the proximal phalanx in the arthrodesis of the metatarsophalangeal joint.

According to Viladot, referring to Fick, the inclination angle of the metatarsals has a gradient, being higher for the first metatarsal and lower for the fifth.[73]

The inclination angles are as follows:

First metatarsal: 18° to 25°
Second metatarsal: 15°
Third metatarsal: 10°
Fourth metatarsal: 8°
Fifth metatarsal: 5° (Fig. 10.95)

Johnson considers the inclination angle of the first metatarsal as being 15° relative to the horizontal plantar aspect of the foot.[74] Joseph analyzed the range of flexion-extension of the great toe in 50 men.[75] The neutral position is the angular relationship between the metatarsal and the phalanges in the standing plantigrade position. In this position the proximal phalanx is slightly dorsiflexed (average 16°) on the metatarsal and the distal phalanx is also dorsiflexed (average 11.6°) relative to the proximal phalanx. "In many cases, however, the distal phalanx is plantar flexed on the proximal"[75] (Fig. 10.96). The distribution of the neutral angles at both joints is as indicated in the histogram in Figure 10.97.

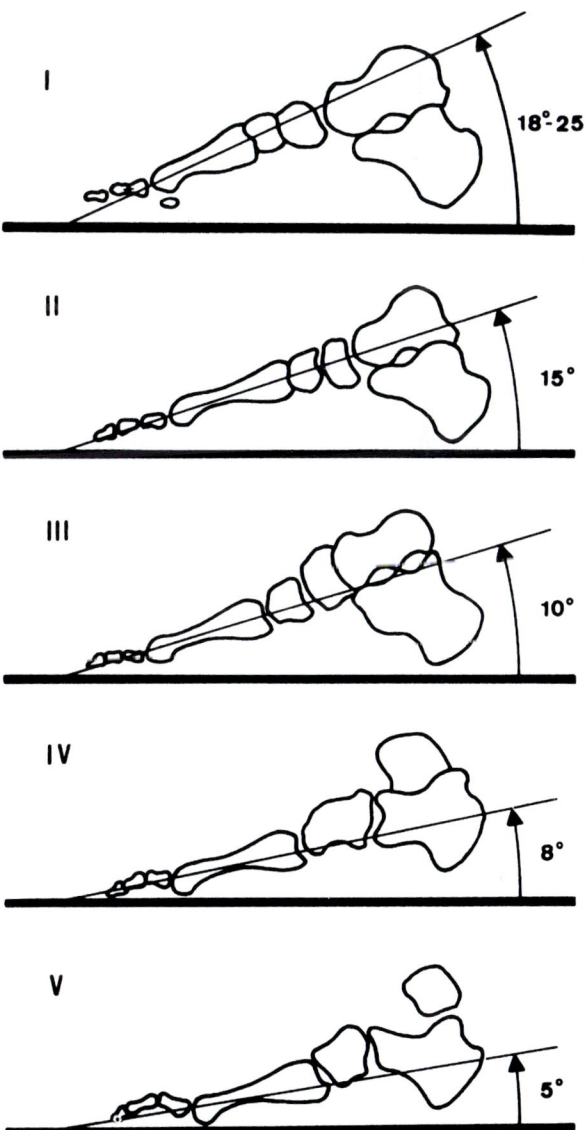

Figure 10.95 Inclination angles of the metatarsal shafts I to V relative to the ground. (From Viladot Perice A. *Patologia del Antepie.* Ediciones Toray; 1974:4.)

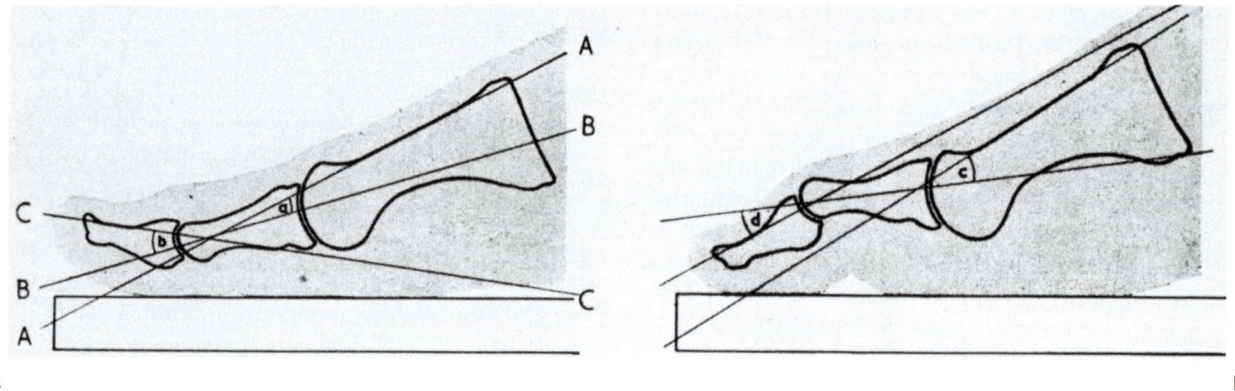

Figure 10.96 Metatarsophalangeal and interphalangeal joint axes in the "neutral position." **(A)** *a*, metatarsophalangeal (MP) angle of extension: 11°; *b*, interphalangeal (IP) angle of extension: 24°. **(B)** *c*, MP angle of extension: 25°; *d*, IP angle of flexion: 21°. (*AA*, axis of the first metatarsal; *BB*, axis of the proximal phalanx; *CC*, axis of the distal phalanx.) (Republished with permission of British Editorial Society of Bone and Joint Surgery, from Joseph J. Range of movement of the great toe in men. *J Bone Joint Surg Br.* 1954;36:451. Permission conveyed through Copyright Clearance Center, Inc.)

In the plantigrade weight-bearing position, the neutral position of the great toe in the transverse plane is of great clinical importance. Hardy and Chapman roentgenographically investigated this angular relationship in the hallux of 126 healthy adults.[76] The ages ranged from 16 to 65 years, with a large preponderance between the ages of 16 and 20 years. In these 252 ft, the normal degree of hallux valgus in the weight-bearing position was 15.7° in mean value, with a mode of 12° to 16° and a range of 0° to 36° (Fig. 10.98). In relation to the degree of hallucal valgus, the first intermetatarsal M_1-M_2 angle is of relevance for the clinician and measures 8.5° as a mean value with a mode of 8° to 9° and a range of 0° to 17° (Fig. 10.99). The plantar plate and its incorporated sesamoids move with the proximal phalanx of the hallux. The normal position of the tibial sesamoid has been standardized in relation to the long axis of the first metatarsal (Fig. 10.100), and in 90%, this sesamoid is in position 3 or less of displacement.

Steel and coworkers investigated radiographically 82 normal feet in 41 adults ranging in age from 40 to 60 years.[77] The normal metatarso$_1$-phalangeal$_1$ angle is 12° in the 50% distribution and ranges from 0° to 32°. The first intermetatarsal angle M_1-M_2 is 7° in the 50% distribution and ranges from 4° to 23°. The interphalangeal$_{1-2}$ angle of the hallux measures 14.5° as a mean value, with a range of 6° to 24°.

Wilkinson investigated the fibular or outward deflexion of the terminal phalanx of the interphalangeal joint of the hallux contributing to the normal hallux valgus posture.[78] The investigation was carried out radiographically on the feet of 30 young subjects—aged 18 to 21 years—and on the terminal phalanges from the great toes of 35 cadavers. The study was further supported by the anatomic study of great toes from 17 adults, 10 infants, and 6 fetuses. The fibular diaphyseal shift of the distal phalanx or valgus shift was found to be a normal feature and measured 14.7° on average, ranging from 8° to 23°. Wilkinson mentions "though the distal articular surface of the proximal phalanx is rarely placed exactly at right angles to the shaft of this bone, the deflexion is relatively small."[78] The same deviation was found in the histologic sections of fetal great toes and to the same degree as noted in the adult.

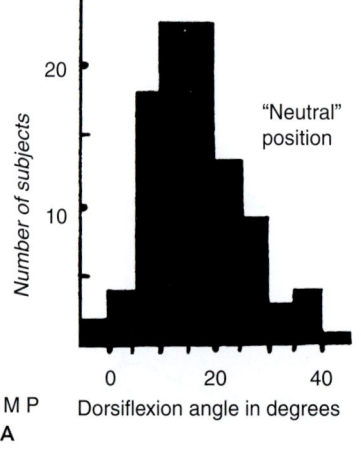
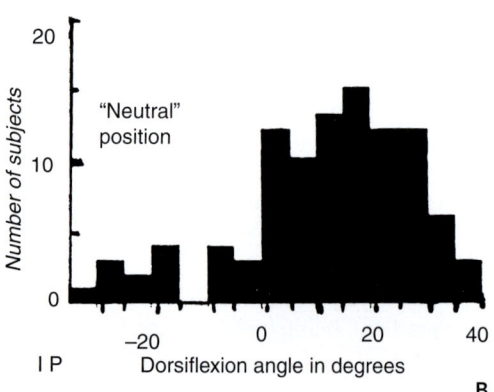

Figure 10.97 **(A)** Histogram of the angles of the metatarsophalangeal joints of the big toe in "neutral position." **(B)** Histogram of the interphalangeal angles of the big toe in the "neutral position." (Republished with permission of British Editorial Society of Bone and Joint Surgery, from Joseph J. Range of movement of the great toe in men. *J Bone Joint Surg Br.* 1954;36:452, 454. Permission conveyed through Copyright Clearance Center, Inc.)

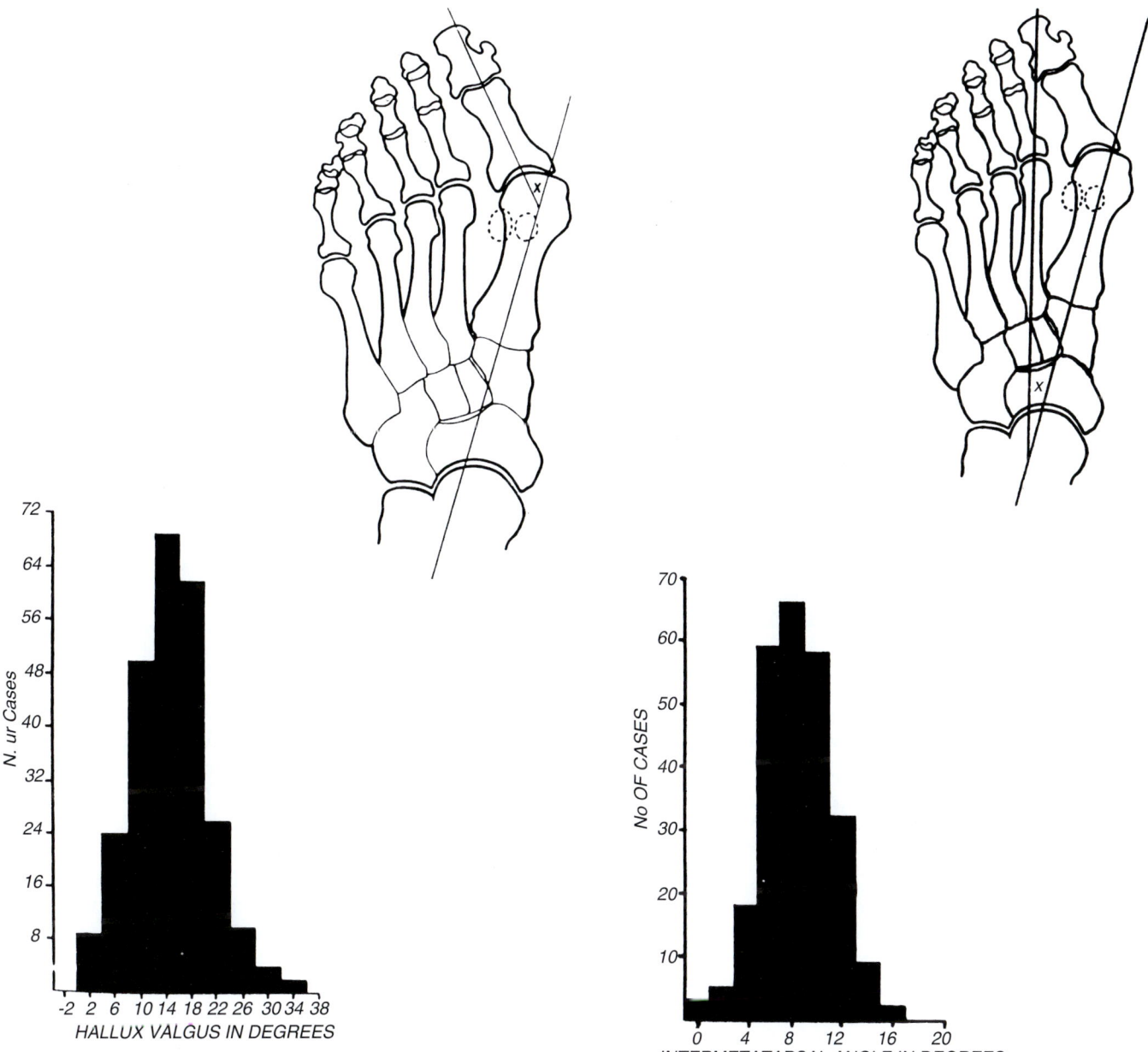

Figure 10.98 Histogram of radiographic measurements of hallux valgus angle x in control group of 84 persons. Age range from 16 to 65 years, with a large preponderance between the ages of 16 and 20 years, 62% female and 38% male. (Republished with permission of British Editorial Society of Bone and Joint Surgery, from Hardy RH, Chapman JCR. Observations on hallux valgus based on a controlled series. *J Bone Joint Surg Br.* 1951;33:381. Permission conveyed through Copyright Clearance Center, Inc.)

Figure 10.99 Histogram of radiographic intermetatarsal angle x measurements between the first and second metatarsal bones in control group as defined in Figure 10.92. (Republished with permission of British Editorial Society of Bone and Joint Surgery, from Hardy RH, Chapman JCR. Observations on hallux valgus based on a controlled series. *J Bone Joint Surg Br.* 1951;33:382. Permission conveyed through Copyright Clearance Center, Inc.)

Scheck roentgenographically investigated, in the weight-bearing position of the foot, the normal dorsiflexion posture of the proximal phalanx of the second toe at the metatarsophalangeal joint in 80 paired feet or 160 second toes.[79] The average dorsiflexion angle of the proximal phalanx of the second toe was 23.5° in the young male and female adults (age group 20-30 years) and 33° and 38° in the older male and female adults (age group 50-70 years). The range of motion of the great toe was assessed by Joseph as indicated in Table 10.6.[75] He has provided an accurate roentgenographic measurement. The actual range of movement was "expressed as the movement from the 'neutral' position" in the standing position. The motion of the proximal phalanx at the metatarsophalangeal joint was correctly measured relative to the long axis of the first metatarsal and not relative to the plantar surface or border of the foot. The average active dorsiflexion at the metatarsophalangeal joint is 50.6° and the added passive extension is 22.6°. The distribution of these motions is as indicated in the histograms in Figure 10.101. Analyzing the data, "it is found that the greater the angle of active dorsiflexion, the smaller the angle of additional passive dorsiflexion."[75] The motion at the interphalangeal joint of the large toe is also as indicated in Table 10.6. The average active dorsiflexion at the interphalangeal joint is 11.9°, and the added average passive extension is 19°.

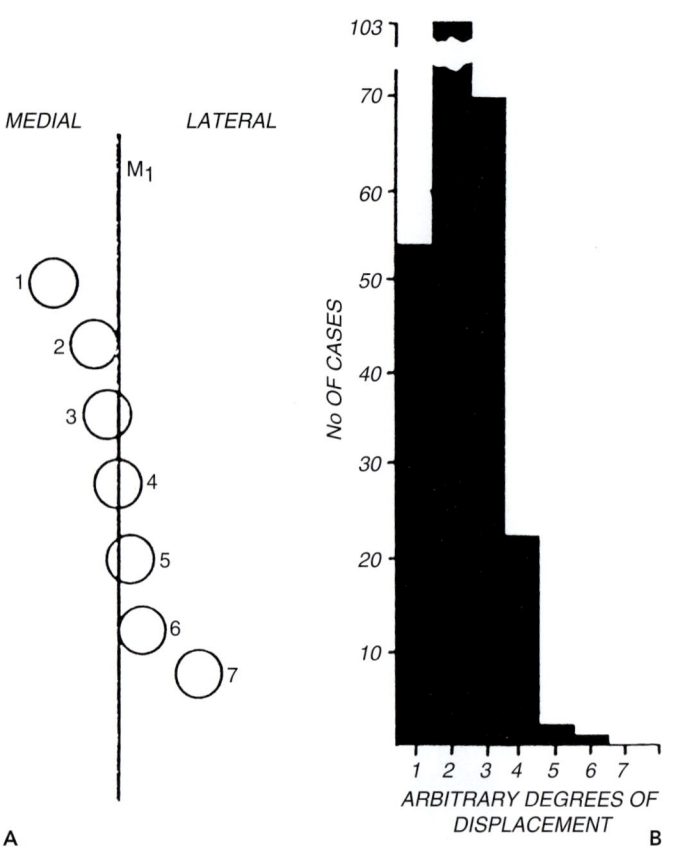
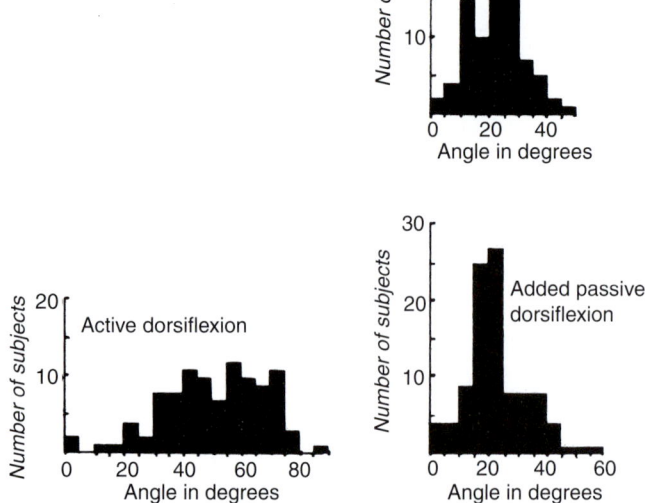

Figure 10.100 (A) Displacement of medial sesamoid of first metatarsophalangeal joint—seven positions in relation to the axis of the first metatarsal. (B) Histogram of distribution of sesamoid displacement in control group. (Republished with permission of British Editorial Society of Bone and Joint Surgery, from Hardy RH, Chapman JCR. Observations on hallux valgus based on a controlled series. *J Bone Joint Surg Br.* 1951;33:385. Permission conveyed through Copyright Clearance Center, Inc.)

Figure 10.101 Histogram of the hallucal metatarsophalangeal joint—active plantar flexion, active dorsiflexion, and added passive dorsiflexion. (Republished with permission of British Editorial Society of Bone and Joint Surgery, from Joseph J. Range of movement of the great toe in men. *J Bone Joint Surg Br.* 1954;36:452. Permission conveyed through Copyright Clearance Center, Inc.)

The average active flexion at the same joint is 46.1°. The distribution of these motions is as indicated in the histogram in Figure 10.102. Joseph indicates that "the range of plantar flexion at the metatarsophalangeal joint is small but dorsiflexion is much freer, whereas the opposite is the case at the interphalangeal joint."[75] Furthermore, as mentioned by Kelikian, a gradient of flexion-extension is present and "the flexion of the toes at the metatarsophalangeal joints gains greater range from the medial to the lateral border. The converse occurs in extension."[80]

Myerson and Shereff, in a study of ten normal cadaveric feet, measured with a goniometer the range of motion in the joints of the lesser toes.[81] The measurements were recorded to the nearest 5°. At the metatarsophalangeal joints, the extension decreased little and the flexion increased from the second to the fifth toe. At the proximal interphalangeal joints, the flexion decreased from the second to the fifth toe, whereas it was the same for all toes at the distal joint (Table 10.7).

Sammarco, in the study of the flexion-extension at the metatarsophalangeal joint of the hallux in normal weight-bearing conditions, located the instant velocity centers not within the metatarsal head but in variable positions.[82] The instant surface velocities corresponding to the velocity centers indicate a sliding motion at the joint from flexion throughout most of the arc except at the limit of extension where compression occurs (Fig. 10.103). In the transverse plane, the instant center of motion is located at the base of the first metatarsal and the surface-velocity vectors are of a tangential type to the distal articular surface and indicate a translation between the two bones (Fig. 10.104).[82] The range of abduction-adduction is small.

Shereff and colleagues analyzed also the instant centers of motion and the corresponding surface-velocity vectors of the metatarsophalangeal joint of the hallux in six fresh anatomic specimens.[83] The instant centers of rotation in the sagittal plane

TABLE 10.6 Range of Motion in Big Toe of 50 Adults[75]		
	Metatarsophalangeal Joint	Interphalangeal Joint
Normal standing angle	16° extension (from 5° flexion to 45° extension)	12° extension (from 35° flexion to 4° extension)
Active flexion	23° (3°-43°)	46° (0°-86°)
Active extension	51°	12°
Total extension (active + passive)	74° (40°-100°)	31° (6°-73°)

Data from Joseph J. Range of movement of the great toe in men. *J Bone Joint Surg Br.* 1954;36:450.

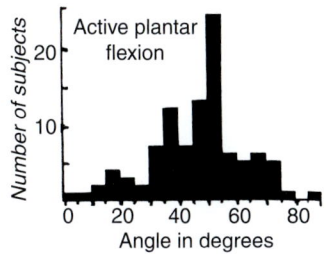

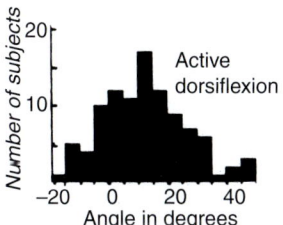 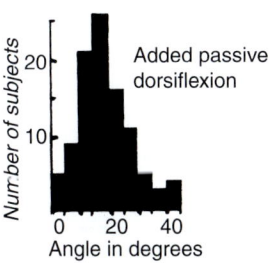

Figure 10.102 Histogram of hallucal interphalangeal joint—active plantar flexion, active dorsiflexion, and added passive dorsiflexion. (Republished with permission of British Editorial Society of Bone and Joint Surgery, from Joseph J. Range of movement of the great toe in men. *J Bone Joint Surg Br.* 1954;36:454. Permission conveyed through Copyright Clearance Center, Inc.)

second interdigital space (maximum, 72.5°; minimum, 53.5°) (Fig. 10.107).[41] The subsequent phase of the push-off occurs around a transverse axis passing through metatarsal heads 1 and 2.

THE FOOT AS A FUNCTIONAL UNIT

The foot is a flexible multisegmented system convertible through compression, torque, and instant remodeling into a rigid structure capable of bearing weight and of acting as an efficient lever arm for the purpose of propulsion.

In 1945, MacConaill presented and demonstrated anatomically and functionally the fundamental concept of the synarthrodial (*syn* = with, together) posture of synovial joints; "in this posture the synovial joints function as if they were synarthroses... In the synarthrodial position, the joint surfaces are maximally congruent, the chief ligaments are tense, and the joint is 'screwed home.' This is usually brought about by a stretch and a twist; that is, by movements which put the main ligaments of the system on the stretch accompanied or followed by a twisting of the osteofibrous mass about its long axis."[85] He called the synarthrodial posture the close-packed posture of the joint. MacConaill further presented a second important concept of considering the foot as an osteofibrous mass unit formed by the entire foot minus the talus.

This plantar skeleton with its ligaments was called the foot plate or lamina pedis. It is an anatomic and functional entity (Fig. 10.108).

The third concept of MacConaill was that of considering the foot plate or lamina pedis as a twisted plate.[85] The calcaneus or posterior segment is compressed sideways and the anterior segment or forefoot is compressed in a dorsoplantar direction. The connection of the two segments determines the twist of the lamina pedis and creates the two arches: longitudinal and transverse. This is clearly seen in the model representations in Figures 10.109 and 10.110.

Blechschmidt, while describing the connective tissue architectural pattern of the heel, recognized the torsion pattern of the foot and noted that "even the entire skeleton of the foot fits into the torsion of this whorl. Viewing a foot skeleton from the back, the skeletal rays are located frontally next to each other but in the back they lie over each other. This way they appear to be turned around each other so that the continuations of the rays overlap spirally. This is the same torsion as seen in the connective tissue whorl of the calcaneus padding."[86]

were located in the head of the first metatarsal and the surface-velocity vectors indicate a tangential sliding motion from maximum plantar flexion to about 40° of extension, followed by compression of the articular surfaces (Fig. 10.105).

The sesamoids at the metatarsophalangeal joint of the hallux form an anatomic and functional unit with the proximal phalanx. Shereff and coworkers, in the same study, measured an arc of motion of the medial sesamoid of 49° from flexion to full extension.[83] The absolute displacement of the sesamoids ranged from 10 to 12 mm. In flexion, the sesamoid bones lie near the head-neck junction and in extension they are carried distally by the proximal phalanx and tilt dorsally.[84] The instant velocity centers of the medial sesamoid bone of the hallux were also located in the metatarsal head during flexion-extension and the instant surface-velocity vectors indicated minor distraction early in plantar flexion followed by sliding in the remaining arc of extension (Fig. 10.106).

The toes work in unison. During gait, the initial phase of the push-off occurs around an oblique axis passing through the metatarsal heads 2 to 5. This determines the metatarsal break angle, which measures (according to Isman and Inman) 62° on average, relative to the mid axis of the foot passing through the

TABLE 10.7 Average Range of Motion of the Metatarsophalangeal and Interphalangeal Joints in Normal Toes before Dissection[a]				
	Second Toe	**Third Toe**	**Fourth Toe**	**Fifth Toe**
Metatarsophalangeal joint	25°-80°	25°-75°	30°-70°	35°-60°
Proximal interphalangeal joint	70°-0°	60°-0°	50°-0°	45°-0°
Distal interphalangeal joint	25°-0°	25°-0°	25°-0°	25°-0°

[a]Motion assessed as flexion to extension.
From Myerson MS, Shereff MJ. The pathologic anatomy of claw and hammer toes. *J Bone Joint Surg Am.* 1989;71(1):45.

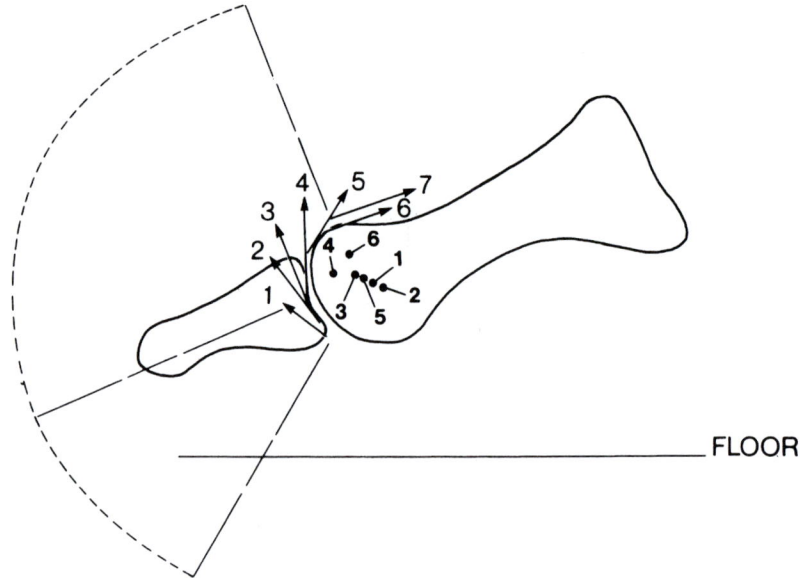

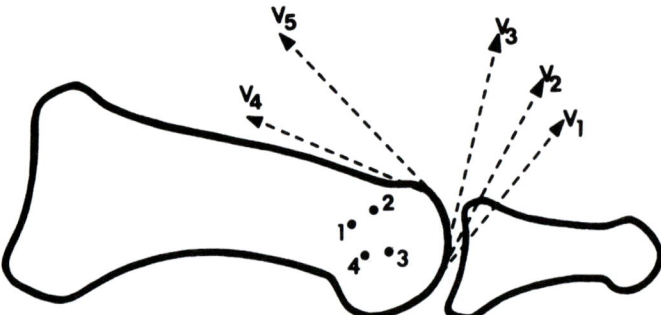

Figure 10.103 **Instant center of motion and surface velocity at the metatarsophalangeal joint of the big toe in the sagittal plane.** The numbered dots represent the instant centers, and the numbered arrows represent the corresponding surface velocities. The motion is of the sliding type except in the last stages of hyperextension, when compression occurs. (From Sammarco JG. Biomechanics of the foot. In: Frankel VH, Nordin M, eds. *Basic Biomechanics of the Skeletal System*. Lea & Febiger; 1980:203.)

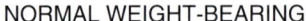

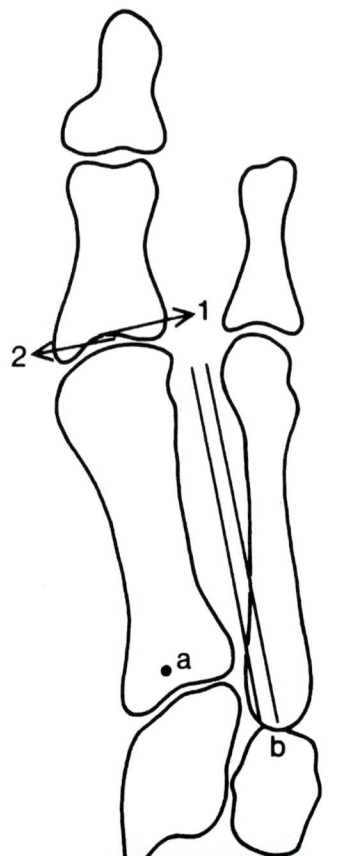

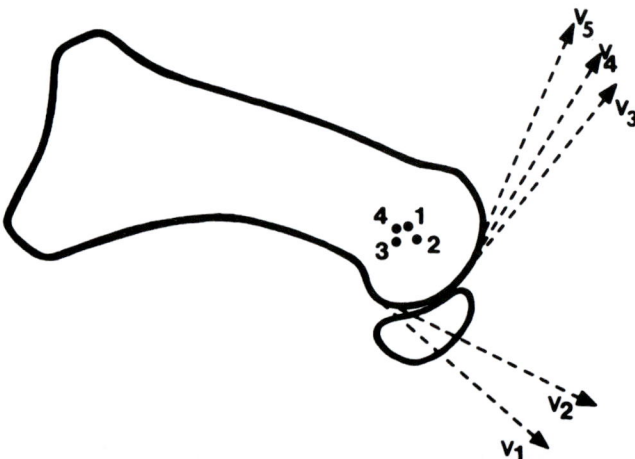

Figure 10.105 Typical instant centers of rotation and surface-velocity vectors plotted through the entire range of motion for the first metatarsophalangeal joint in normal specimens. *1, 2, 3, 4* represent the instant centers of motion. (From Shereff MJ, Bejjani FJ, Kummer FJ. Kinematics of the first metatarsophalangeal joint. *J Bone Joint Surg Am*. 1986;68[3]:394.)

Figure 10.104 **Instant centers for analysis of medial and lateral motion at the hallucal metatarsophalangeal joint lie far from the joint surface.** Sliding occurs at the joint surface (*1-2* surface velocity vector) even though the range of motion (abduction-adduction) is small (*b*). The instant center of rotation in the transverse plane is at the base of the 1st metatarsal (*a*). (From Sammarco JG. Biomechanics of the foot. In: Frankel VH, Nordin M, eds. *Basic Biomechanics of the Skeletal System*. Lea & Febiger; 1980:204.)

Figure 10.106 Typical instant centers of rotation and surface-velocity vectors of the articulation between the medial sesamoid of the hallux and the metatarsal head in normal specimens. *1, 2, 3, 4* represent the instant centers of motion. (From Shereff MJ, Bejjani FJ, Kummer FJ. Kinematics of the first metatarsophalangeal joint. *J Bone Joint Surg Am*. 1986;68[3]:395.)

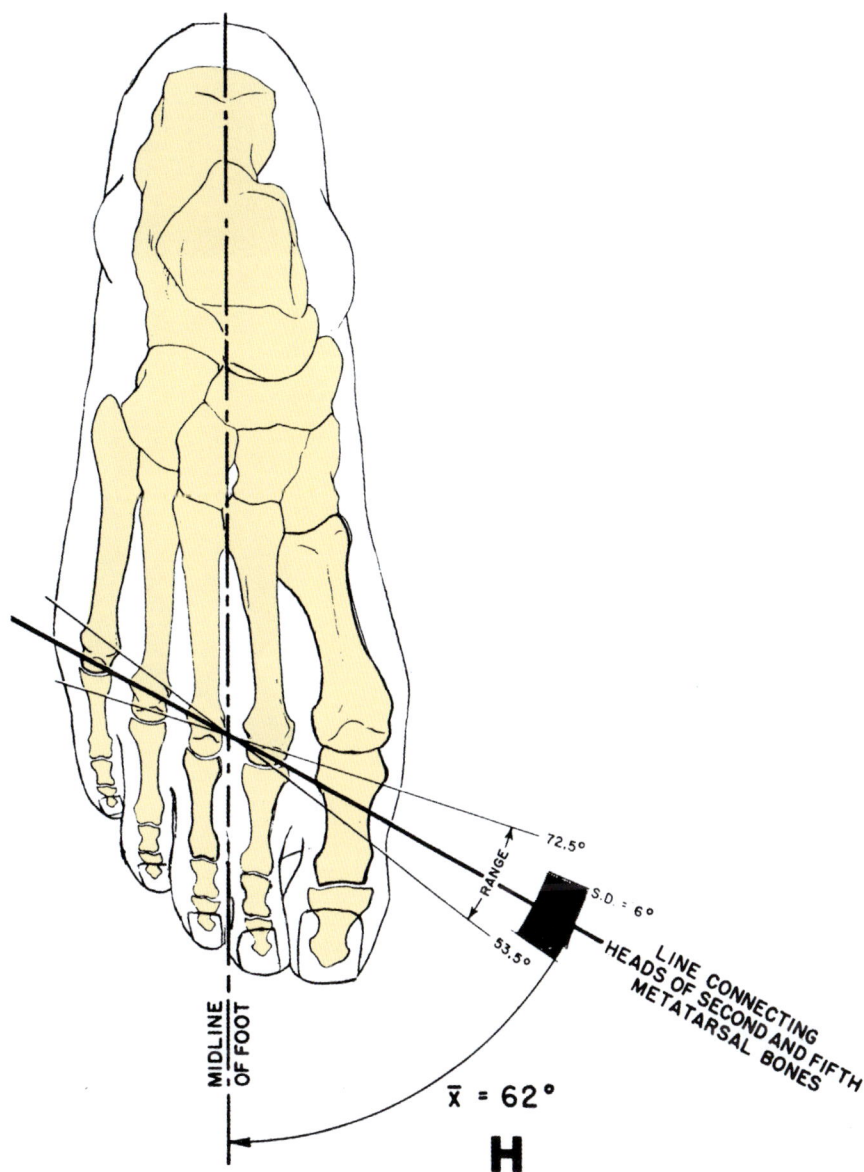

Figure 10.107 Metatarsal break angle (*H*) or angle between the line connecting the heads of the second and fifth metatarsals and the midline of the foot. This line represents also the oblique axis of the take-off in walking. (Adapted from Isman RE, Inman VT. *Anthropometric Studies of the Human Foot and Ankle.* Biomechanics Laboratory, University of California, 1968:26.)

The fourth concept of MacConaill is as follows: the synarthrodial posture or close-packed position is achieved with the untwisting or "supination" of the lamina pedis.[85] This untwisting involves supination of the forefoot and valgus or pronation or eversion of the heel. Lewis, to avoid the terminologic contradictions of using the term *pronation* in the "supination" of the lamina pedis, has introduced the term *exorotation of the calcaneus* in lieu of pronation or valgus of the heel.[43] The loose-packed position is reached with further twisting or "pronation of the lamina pedis." This involves pronation of the forefoot and supination or endorotation or varus or inversion of the heel. MacConaill's anatomic and functional demonstrations[85] have been supported by Hicks,[12] Lewis,[43] and Sarrafian.[87]

▶ Functional Remodeling of the Lamina Pedis Under Vertical Loading and Horizontal Rotation of the Leg

Vertical Loading and Internal Rotation of the Tibiotalar Column

In the standing weight-bearing position on even ground, the internal rotation of the tibiotalar unit induces instant remodeling of the foot plate. The talus is internally rotated (adducted), flexed, and supinated. The talar body is in its lower position relative to the calcaneus and the talar lateral process, forming a solid male V wedge, is in close contact with the corresponding female V contour of the calcaneus laterally at the junction of the

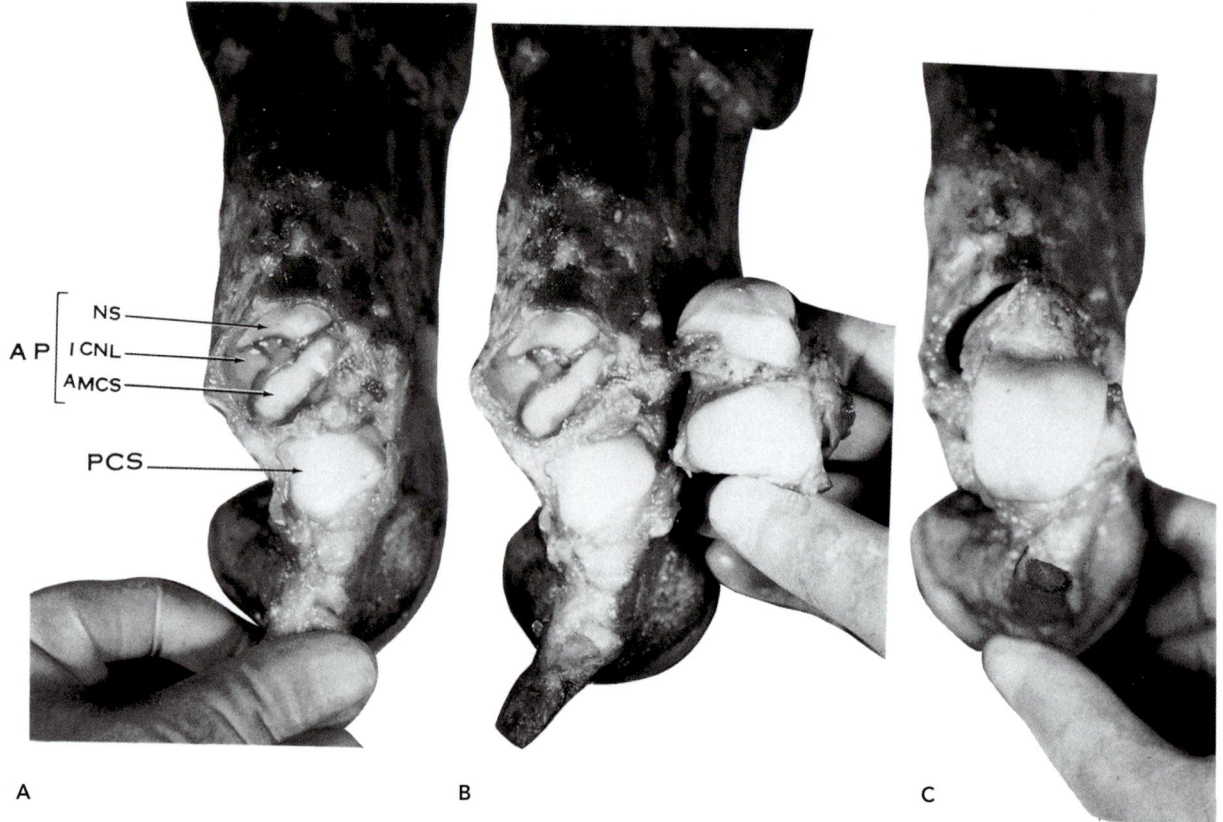

Figure 10.108 Lamina pedis. **(A)** Lamina pedis is the entire foot minus the talus. Acetabulum pedis (*AP*) is formed by the anterior and middle calcaneal surfaces (*AMCS*), the inferior calcaneonavicular ligament (*ICNL*), and the navicular surface (*NS*). (*PCS*, posterior calcaneal surface.) **(B)** Lamina pedis with juxtaposed talus. **(C)** Lamina pedis with talus in situ. The talus acts as an intercalated bone between the leg and the lamina pedis. It is the activator of the lamina pedis that responds as a unit.

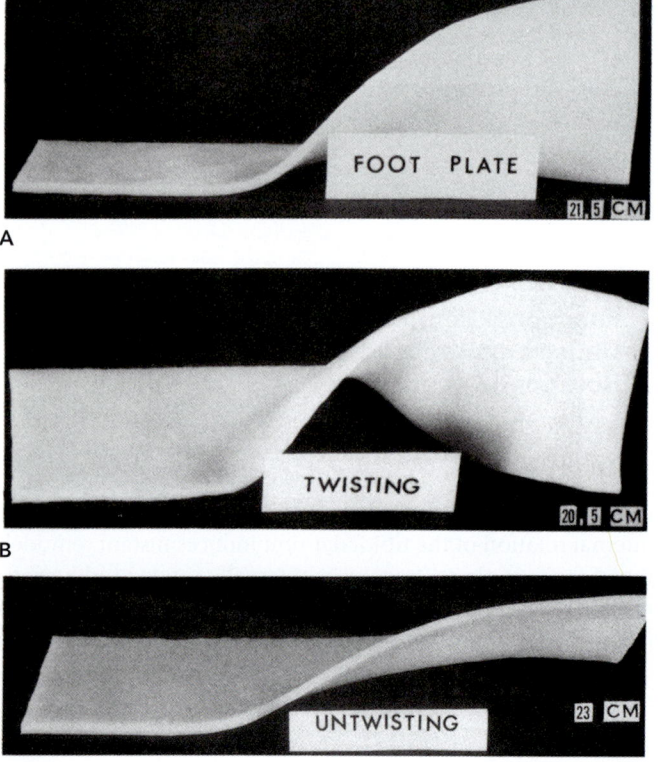

Figure 10.109 **(A)** A rectangular plate has been twisted as indicated. One end is perpendicular to the transverse plane, whereas the opposite end rests on the horizontal plane. The perpendicular or posterior segment is compressed sideways, whereas the anterior or transverse segment is compressed in the dorsoplantar direction. The transitional segment has two curves, inner longitudinal and transverse. The plate is in a plantigrade position and measures 21.5 cm. **(B)** The plate has been further twisted. The posterior segment is inclined inward (varus). The arches are higher. The anterior segment remains in the horizontal plane. The plate is in a plantigrade position; it is shorter and measures 20.5 cm. **(C)** The plate has been untwisted. The posterior segment is inclined outward (valgus). The arches are lower. The anterior segment remains in the horizontal plane. The plate is in a plantigrade position; it is longer and measures 23 cm. (Sarrafian SK. Functional characteristics of the foot and plantar aponeurosis under tibio-talar loading. *Foot Ankle*. 1987;8[1]:5. Copyright ©1987. Reprinted by Permission of SAGE Publications.)

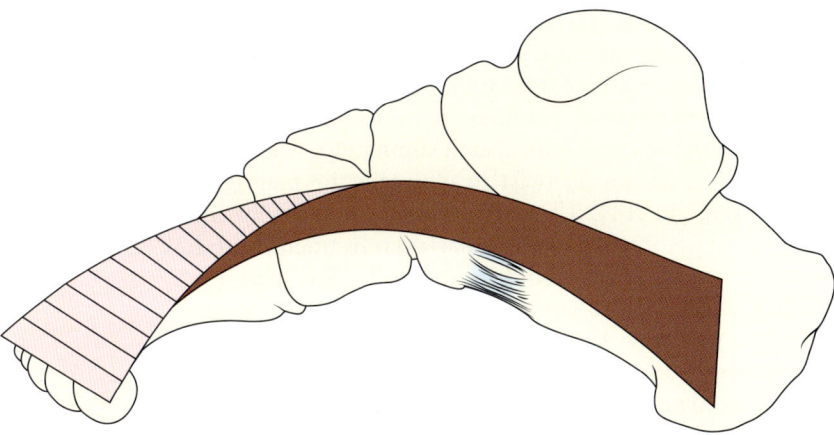

Figure 10.110 The lamina pedis.

sinus tarsi and the posterior calcaneal surface. The talar head compresses medially into the acetabulum pedis, which offers an increased capacity of volume.[88] The calcaneus is in exorotation (pronation, valgus, and eversion). The navicular and the cuboid are also in pronation, whereas the forefoot is in supination twist to maintain the plantigrade posture (Fig. 10.111). The inferior calcaneonavicular ligament and the superomedial calcaneonavicular ligament are under tension. The subtalar cervical ligament and the calcaneotalar interosseous ligament of the canalis tarsi are also under tension. In this position, the talus is in a synarthrodial position at the talocalcaneonavicular joint and is in the close-pack position. With the combination of exorotation or valgus of the hindfoot and supination of the forefoot, the lamina pedis is untwisted. As demonstrated by Lewis, in this position the short plantar calcaneocuboid ligament is also under tension because of its oblique disposition (calcaneal origin, proximolateral, and cuboidal insertion, distomedial) (Fig. 10.112).[43] The foot now has a lower medial longitudinal arch and is longer and wider. The lowering of the medial longitudinal arch further tenses the plantar ligaments and the plantar aponeurosis (Fig. 10.113). The foot is now less flexible, more rigid, and converted to a more efficient lever arm.

The integrated response of the tarsus to the vertical loading with torque supports Huson's concept of the tarsus being a closed kinematic chain.

Vertical Loading and External Rotation of the Tibiotalar Column

In the standing position on even ground, the external rotation of the tibiotalar column also induces an instant remodeling of the foot plate.

The talus is externally rotated or abducted, extended, and pronated. The talar body rides high on the posterior calcaneal surface and the talar head offers less volume to the acetabulum pedis, which once more adjusts its retention capacity. As

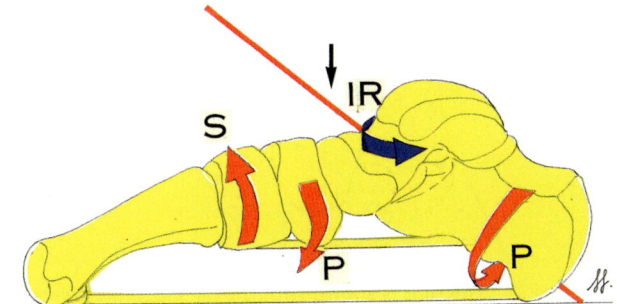

Figure 10.111 Internal rotation (*IR*) and vertical loading of the foot plate by the tibiotalar column. The foot plate is untwisted. The hindfoot is pronated (*P*) (valgus). The midfoot is pronated and the forefoot is supinated (*S*). Without the supination, the forefoot will be off the ground on the lateral side. (Sarrafian SK. Functional characteristics of the foot and plantar aponeurosis under tibio-talar loading. *Foot Ankle*. 1987;8[1]:15. Copyright ©1987. Reprinted by Permission of SAGE Publications.)

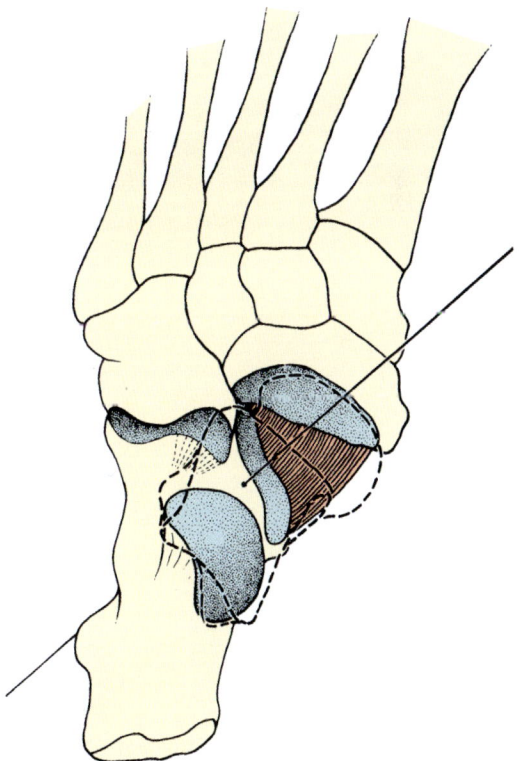

Figure 10.112 The foot plate is shown untwisted at the midtarsal joint and everted at the subtalar joint. The subtalar axis is shown, and the talus is indicated in the broken line superimposed on the lamina pedis. The plantar calcaneonavicular (spring) ligament is shown, and the plantar calcaneocuboid (short plantar) ligament is indicated in the broken line as though visualized through the foot; both ligaments are under tension. (Adapted from Lewis OJ. *Functional Morphology of the Evolving Hand and Foot*. Clarendon Press; 1989:247.)

described by Huson, the navicular is then flexed-adducted-supinated to overcome the slight talonavicular subluxation resulting from the external rotation of the talus.[8] The calcaneus is in endorotation (supination, varus, inversion). The navicular and the cuboid are also in supination, whereas the forefoot is in pronation twist to maintain the plantigrade posture (Fig. 10.114). The inferior calcaneonavicular ligament, the superomedial calcaneonavicular ligament, and the short plantar calcaneo-cuboid ligaments are less tense (Fig. 10.115). The untwisted lamina pedis is in a loose-pack position. The foot now has a higher medial longitudinal arch and is shorter and narrower. The plantar ligaments and the plantar aponeurosis are relaxed (Fig. 10.116). The foot is now more flexible.

Quantitative data with regard to the tarsal remodeling with vertical loading and exorotation of the tibiotalar column were provided by Ambagtsheer in 1978.[2] The data were based on the study of 10 leg-foot preparations. Pins were inserted in the corresponding bones and a triaxial photographic analysis was performed measuring the rotations of the tarsal bones.

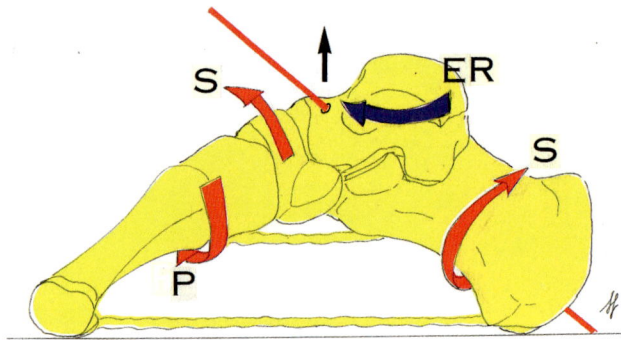

Figure 10.114 External rotation (*ER*) and vertical loading of the foot by the tibiotalar column. The foot plate is twisted. The hindfoot is supinated (*S*) (varus). The midfoot is supinated and the forefoot is pronated (*P*). Without the pronation, the forefoot will be off the ground on the medial side. (Sarrafian SK. Functional characteristics of the foot and plantar aponeurosis under tibio-talar loading. *Foot Ankle*. 1987;8[1]:13. Copyright ©1987. Reprinted by Permission of SAGE Publications.)

Exorotation of the talus induced a supinatory remodeling of the tarsus. From the neutral position to the maximum external rotation of the tibiotalar column (the medial border of the foot still remaining in contact with the supportive surface),

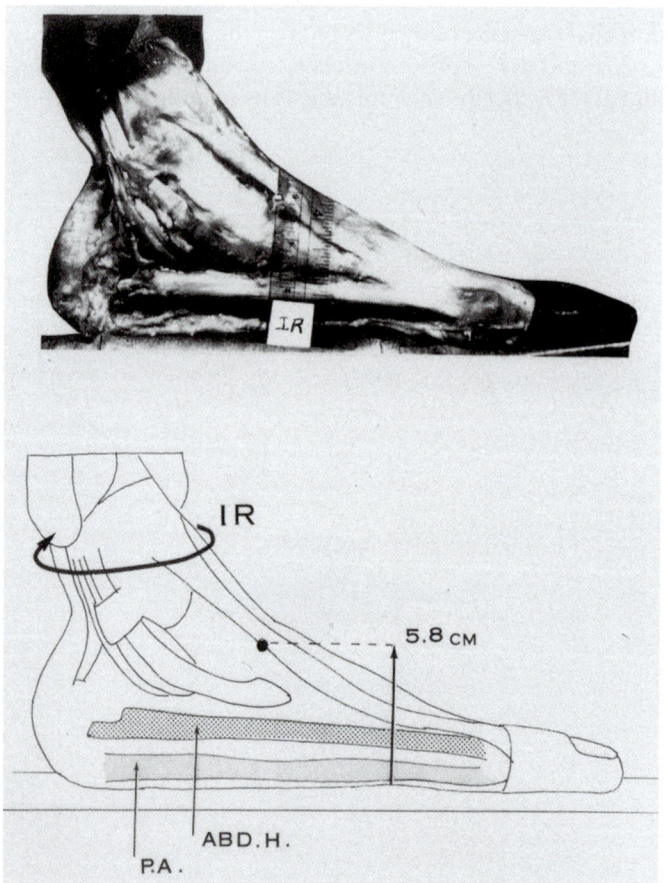

Figure 10.113 Anatomic preparation of the foot with the plantar structures in view. Internal rotation is applied to the tibiotalar column, and the foot is maintained in the plantigrade position. The height of the medial longitudinal arch measures 5.8 cm. It is low in comparison with a high-arch situation measuring 7 cm in the same specimen. The plantar aponeurosis (*P*) and the abductor hallucis muscle (*ABD H*) are seen under tension. They are not undulant. (Sarrafian SK. Functional characteristics of the foot and plantar aponeurosis under tibio-talar loading. *Foot Ankle*. 1987;8[1]:16. Copyright ©1987. Reprinted by Permission of SAGE Publications.)

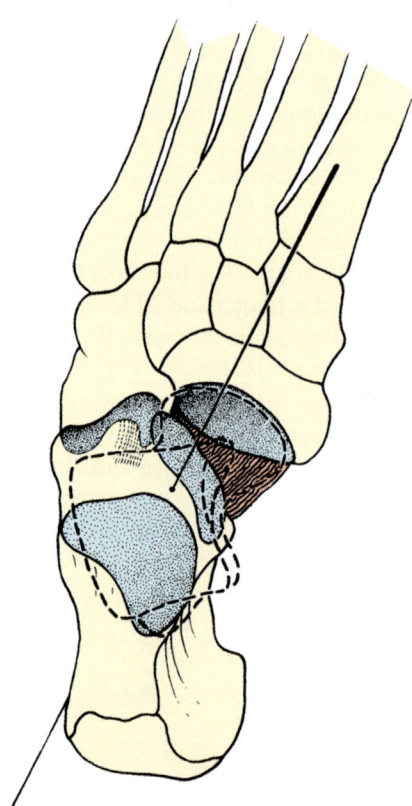

Figure 10.115 The foot is shown with the lamina pedis twisted at the midtarsal joint and inverted at the subtalar joint. The subtalar axis is shown and the talus is indicated in the broken line superimposed on the lamina pedis. The plantar calcaneonavicular (spring) ligament is shown and the plantar calcaneocuboid (short plantar) ligament is indicated in the broken line as though visualized through the foot; both ligaments are relaxed. (Adapted from Lewis OJ. *Functional Morphology of the Evolving Hand and Foot*. Clarendon Press; 1989:247.)

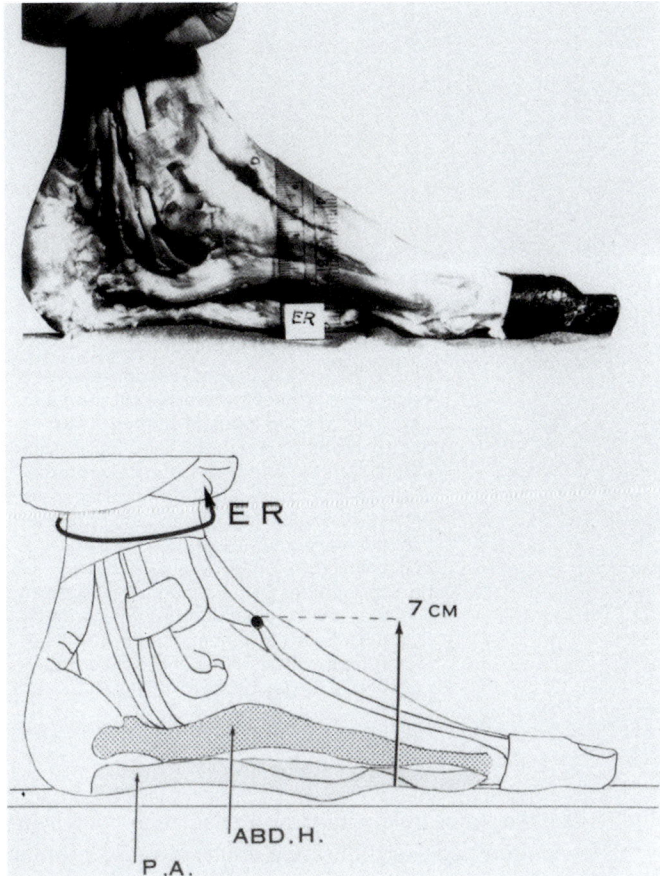

Figure 10.116 **Anatomic preparation of the foot with the plantar structures in view.** External rotation is applied to the tibiotalar column, and the foot is maintained in a plantigrade position. The height of the medial longitudinal arch measures 7 cm. It has increased as compared with a low-arch situation measuring 5.8 cm in the same specimen. The plantar aponeurosis (*PA*) and the abductor hallucis muscle (*ABD H*) are seen relaxed and undulant. (Sarrafian SK. Functional characteristics of the foot and plantar aponeurosis under tibio-talar loading. *Foot Ankle*. 1987;8[1]:14. Copyright ©1987. Reprinted by Permission of SAGE Publications.)

the talus exorotated 23° and the tarsus supinated with the following distribution:

- Calcaneus: 8°
- Navicular: 16°
- Cuboid: 14°

The remodeling of the foot-ankle with rotation of the leg was studied by Lundberg and colleagues in 1989.[7] In eight healthy volunteers, 0.8-mm tantalum marker beads were introduced into the tibia, talus, calcaneus, navicular, medial cuneiform, and first metatarsal bones. The subject was asked to externally rotate the weight-bearing leg from a 20° internally rotated position to 10° of external rotation with increments of 10°. The movements induced in the corresponding bones were analyzed by roentgen stereophotogrammetry, and the rotations occurring between these bones were calculated along the three axes—transverse, vertical, and longitudinal.

With exorotation of the leg from 0° to 10°, the calcaneus and the navicular are both supinated, internally rotated or adducted, and plantar flexed, the navicular more so at the navicular-talar joint.

At 10° of exorotation of the leg, the motions are as follows (Figs. 10.117 and 10.118):

Calcaneus at calcaneal-talar joint
Supination: 5.2° ± 2.7°
Internal rotation: 7.4° ± 3.3°
Plantar flexion: 6.4° ± 2.5°

Navicular at naviculotalar joint
Supination: 11.5° ± 3.1°
Internal rotation: 12° ± 5.7°
Plantar flexion: 7.8° ± 2.8°

During the same motion of 10° exorotation of the leg, the first cuneiform and the first metatarsal are pronated-plantar flexed, whereas the motion around the vertical axis is minimal.

At 10° of exorotation, the motions are as follows (Figs. 10.119 and 10.120):

First cuneiform at $cuneo_1$-navicular joint
Pronation: 3.9° ± 2.3°
Plantar flexion: 2° ± 1.9°
External rotation: 0.1° ± 0.7°

First metatarsal at $metatarso_1$-$cuneiform_1$ joint
Pronation: 1.6° ± 0.7°
Plantar flexion: 0.1° ± 0.4°
Internal rotation: 0.7° ± 1.6°

At 20° of internal rotation of the leg, the calcaneus and the navicular are both pronated, externally rotated or abducted, and dorsiflexed, and the range of motion is as follows (see Figs. 10.117 and 10.118):

Calcaneus at calcaneotalar joint
Pronation: 0.9° ± 1.3°
External rotation: 1.2° ± 1.1°
Dorsiflexion: 1.1° ± 1°

Navicular at naviculotalar joint
Pronation: 2.9° ± 2.4°
External rotation: 1.9° ± 1.3°
Dorsiflexion: 1.3° ± 1.1°

During the same 20° of internal rotation of the leg, the first cuneiform is in minimal pronation-dorsiflexion-external rotation, whereas the first metatarsal is supinated-externally rotated with the range of motion as follows (see Figs. 10.119 and 10.120):

First cuneiform at $cuneo_1$-navicular joint
Pronation: 0.4° ± 0.7°
External rotation: 0.3° ± 0.3°
Plantar flexion: 0.2° ± 0.5°

First metatarsal at $metatarso_1$-cuneiform joint
Supination: 0.8° ± 0.6°
External rotation: 2.2° ± 1°

The above experimental data obtained in vivo confirm Hicks' concept of hindfoot-forefoot remodeling secondary to the external and internal rotational input by the tibiotalar column. A minor interpretative adjustment is to be made in the response of the forefoot to the pronatory remodeling of the tarsus.

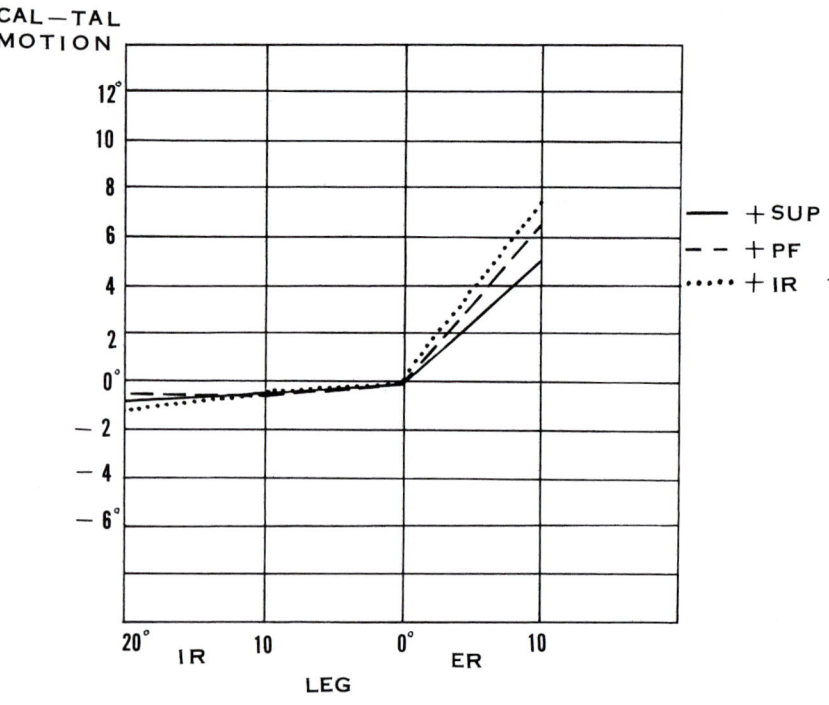

Figure 10.117 Calcaneal response at calcaneotalar joint to internal rotation and external rotation input of the leg. With external rotation input, the calcaneus is supinated, plantar flexed, and internally rotated. With internal rotation input, the calcaneus is pronated, dorsiflexed, and externally rotated. (*DF*, dorsiflexion; *ER*, external rotation; *IR*, internal rotation; *PF*, plantar flexion; *PRO*, pronation, SUP, supination.) (Data from and adapted from Lundberg A, Svensson OK, Bylund C, Selvik G. Kinematics of the ankle/foot complex. Part 3: Influence of leg rotations. Foot Ankle. 1989;9[6]:304-309.)

McElvenny and Caldwell had a brilliant clinical grasp of the relationship of the hindfoot with the forefoot and applied the concept to the understanding and surgical correction of a subgroup of flexible pes planus and pes cavus.[89] A pronation contracture of the forefoot on non–weight-bearing results in varus position of the hindfoot on weight-bearing. Similarly, a supination contracture of the forefoot on non–weight-bearing results in valgus position of the hindfoot on weight-bearing (Fig. 10.121). Using the same principle, Coleman and Chestnut advocated a test for assessment of hindfoot mobility in the cavovarus foot.[90]

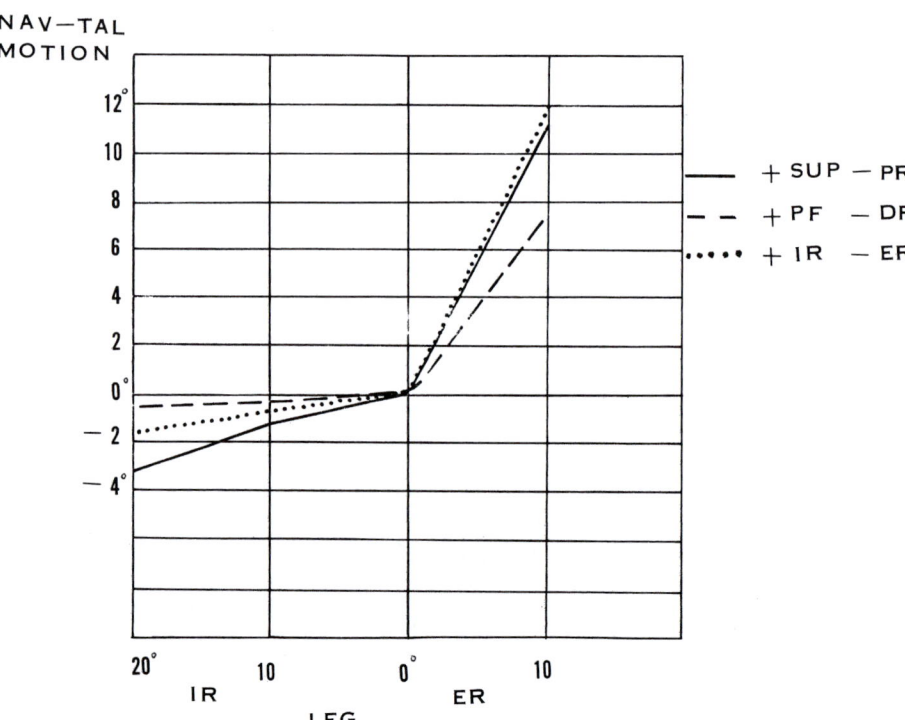

Figure 10.118 Navicular response at naviculotalar joint to internal rotation and external rotation input of the leg. With external rotation input, the navicular is supinated, plantar flexed, and internally rotated. With internal rotation input, the navicular is pronated, dorsiflexed, and externally rotated. (*DF*, dorsiflexion; *ER*, external rotation; *IR*, internal rotation; *PF*, plantar flexion; *PRO*, pronation; *SUP*, supination.) (Data from and adapted from Lundberg A, Svensson OK, Bylund C, Selvik G. Kinematics of the ankle/foot complex. Part 3: Influence of leg rotations. Foot Ankle. 1989;9[6]:304-309.)

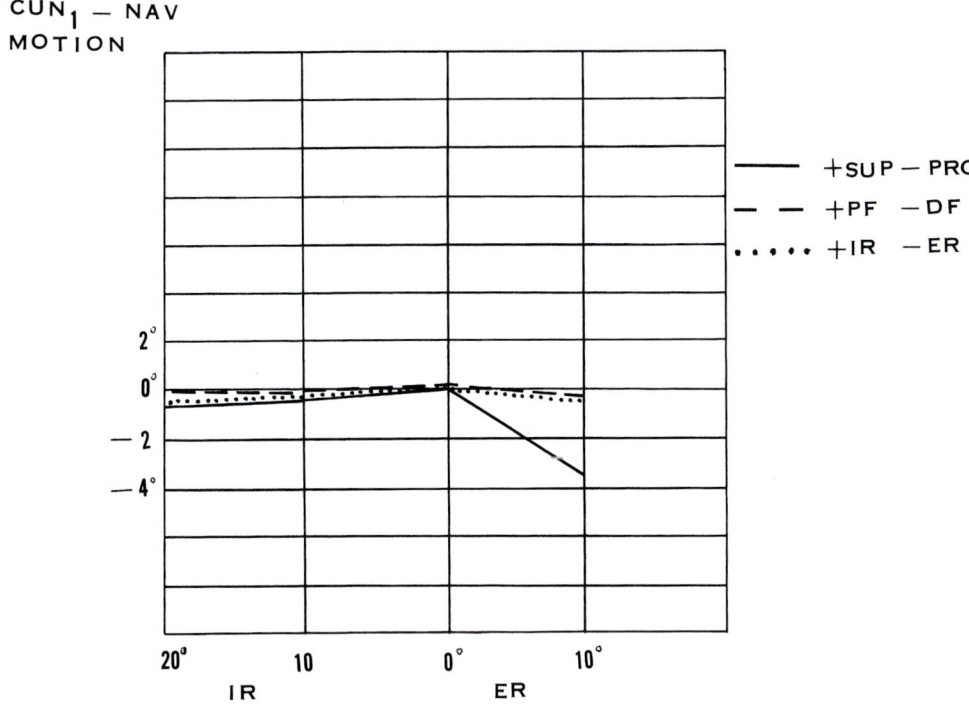

Figure 10.119 First cuneiform response at the cuneiform$_1$-navicular joint to internal and external rotational input of the leg. (DF, dorsiflexion; ER, external rotation; IR, internal rotation; PF, plantar flexion; PRO, pronation; SUP, supination.) (Data from and adapted from Lundberg A, Svensson OK, Bylund C, Selvik G. Kinematics of the ankle/foot complex. Part 3: Influence of leg rotations. Foot Ankle. 1989;9[6]:304-309.)

▶ **Functional Remodeling Under Tibial Loading With Pronation-Supination of the Foot Plate**

Pronation of the foot as a unit (eversion) or supination of the foot as a unit (inversion) occurs when standing on an inclined plane.

Olerud and Rosendahl analyzed the quantitative relationship between the supination-pronation of the entire foot and the horizontal rotation of the leg in an experimental setup using ten fresh cadaver legs-feet.[91] For each degree of supination of the foot, an average of 0.44° of outward rotation of the tibia was found. In these experiments, the metatarsal heads were transfixed to the rotating platform with screws.

Lundberg and coworkers, continuing their investigation in eight healthy subjects with the previously described methodology, analyzed the motion in the components of the ankle-foot

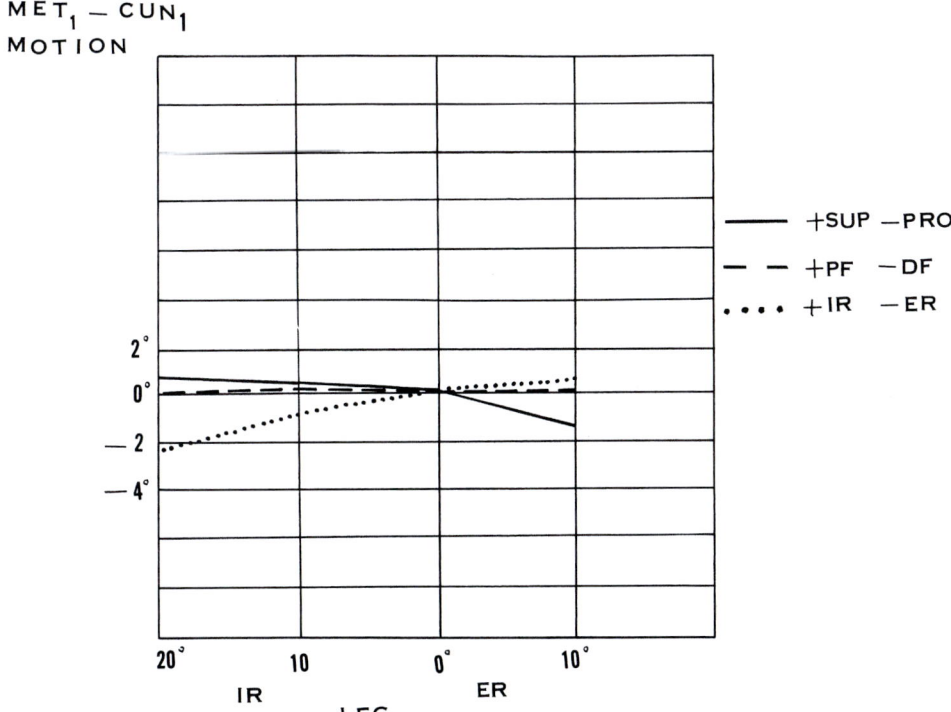

Figure 10.120 First metatarsal response at the metatarso$_1$-cuneiform$_1$ joint to internal rotation and external rotation input of the leg. (DF, dorsiflexion; ER, external rotation; IR, internal rotation; PF, plantar flexion; PRO, pronation; SUP, supination.) (Data from and adapted from Lundberg A, Svensson OK, Bylund C, et al. Kinematics of the ankle/foot complex. Part 3: Influence of leg rotations. Foot Ankle. 1989;9[6]:304-309.)

complex in response to the supination-pronation of the foot with weight-bearing.[6] The supportive platform was tilted from a neutral position to 10° and 20° of pronation and supination, and the triaxial motion analysis in the corresponding joint was carried out.

The results indicate that from 0° to 20° of supination, the calcaneus and the navicular are supinated, internally rotated or adducted, and plantar flexed, again the navicular more so at the navicular-talar joint. At 20° of supination, the motions are as follows (Figs. 10.122 and 10.123):

Calcaneus at calcaneotalar joint
Supination: 5.5° ± 2.9°
Internal rotation: 5.6° ± 2.1°
Plantar flexion: 5.1° ± 2.0°

Navicular at naviculotalar joint
Supination: 12.8° ± 3.5°
Internal rotation: 6.6° ± 2.3°
Plantar flexion: 4.4° ± 2.1°

The forefoot remodeling is minimal and more or less in the same direction as the hindfoot and midfoot. The motions are as follows (Figs. 10.124 and 10.125):

Cuneiform 1 at $cuneo_1$-navicular joint
Supination: 1° ± 1.3°
External rotation: 0.3° ± 0.5°
Dorsiflexion: 0.2° ± 0.7°

Metatarsal 1 at $metatarso_1$-$cuneiform_1$ joint
Supination: 1.3° ± 1.0°
Internal rotation: 0.3° ± 0.6°
Plantar flexion: 0.2° ± 0.3°

With the foot moving from 0° to 20° of pronation (eversion), the calcaneus and the navicular are pronated, externally rotated, and dorsiflexed, the navicular more so than the calcaneus. At 20° of pronation (eversion) of the foot, the motions are as follows (see Figs. 10.122 and 10.123):

Calcaneus at calcaneotalar joint
Pronation: 2.7° ± 3.2°
External rotation: 1.8° ± 1.9°
Dorsiflexion: 2.7° ± 2.2°

Navicular at naviculotalar joint
Pronation: 7.5° ± 5.5°
External rotation: 2.2° ± 3.0°
Dorsiflexion: 1.3° ± 2.0°

The forefoot remodeling is in the same direction along the longitudinal axis, with the motions as follows (see Figs. 10.124 and 10.125):

Cuneiform 1 at $cuneo_1$-navicular joint
Pronation: 3.5° ± 1.8°
Internal rotation: 0.2° ± 1.1°
Plantar flexion: 1.8° ± 1.9°

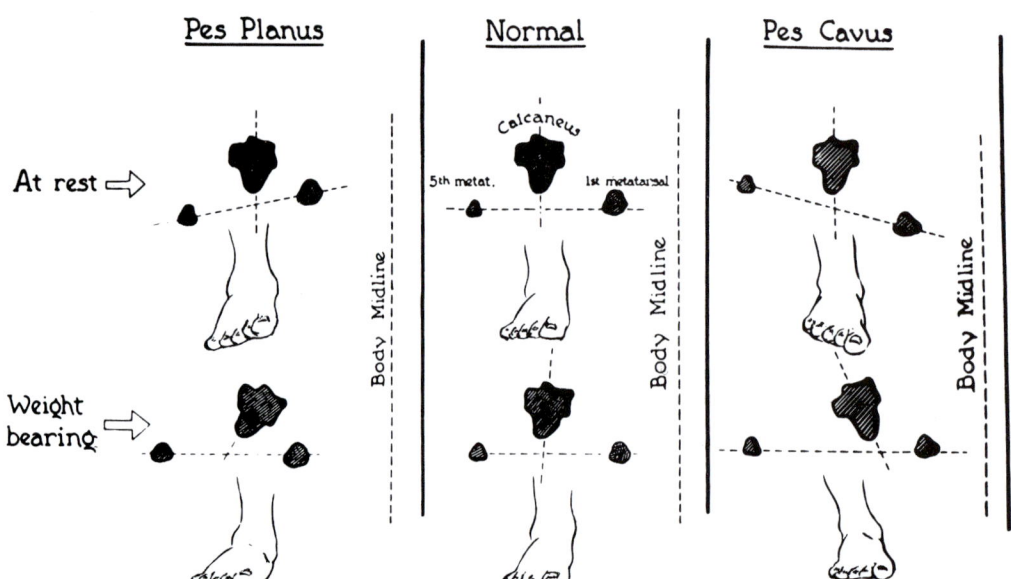

Figure 10.121 Relationship of the hindfoot and forefoot at rest and in weight-bearing in the normal foot, pes cavus, and pes planus. In the normal foot, at rest the heel is neutral and the forefoot transmetatarsal headline M_1 to M_5 is perpendicular to the vertical axis of the heel; on weight-bearing, the same relation of the hindfoot and forefoot is preserved. In pes cavus (flexible type), at rest when the heel is held in neutral, the forefoot is pronated; on weight-bearing, the heel moves into varus, carrying the forefoot into a horizontal plantigrade position. In pes planus (flexible type), at rest when the heel is held in neutral, the forefoot is supinated; on weight-bearing, the heel moves into valgus, carrying the forefoot into a horizontal plantigrade position. (Reprinted by permission from McElvenny RT, Caldwell GD. A new operation for correction of cavus foot: fusion of first metatarso-coneiform-navicular joints. *Clin Orthop Relat Res.* 1958;11:85.)

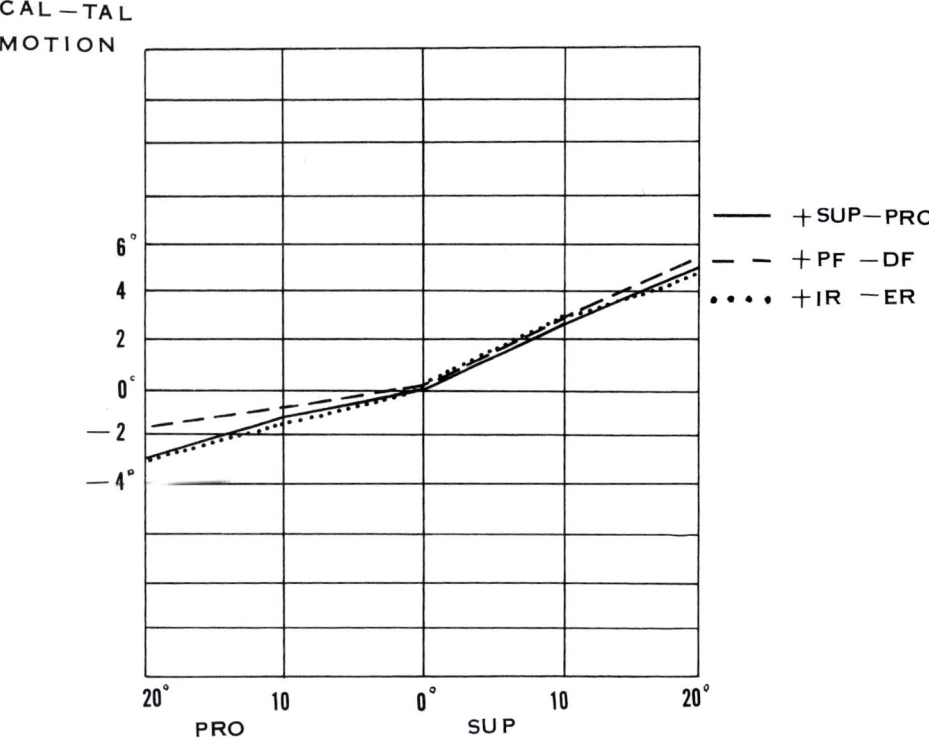

Figure 10.122 Calcaneal response at calcaneotalar joint to pronation and supination input of the foot. (*DF*, dorsiflexion; *ER*, external rotation; *IR*, internal rotation; *PF*, plantar flexion; *PRO*, pronation; *SUP*, supination.) (Data from and adapted from Lundberg A, Svensson OK, Bylund C, et al. Kinematics of the ankle/foot complex. Part 2: Pronation and supination. *Foot Ankle*. 1989;9[5]:248-253.)

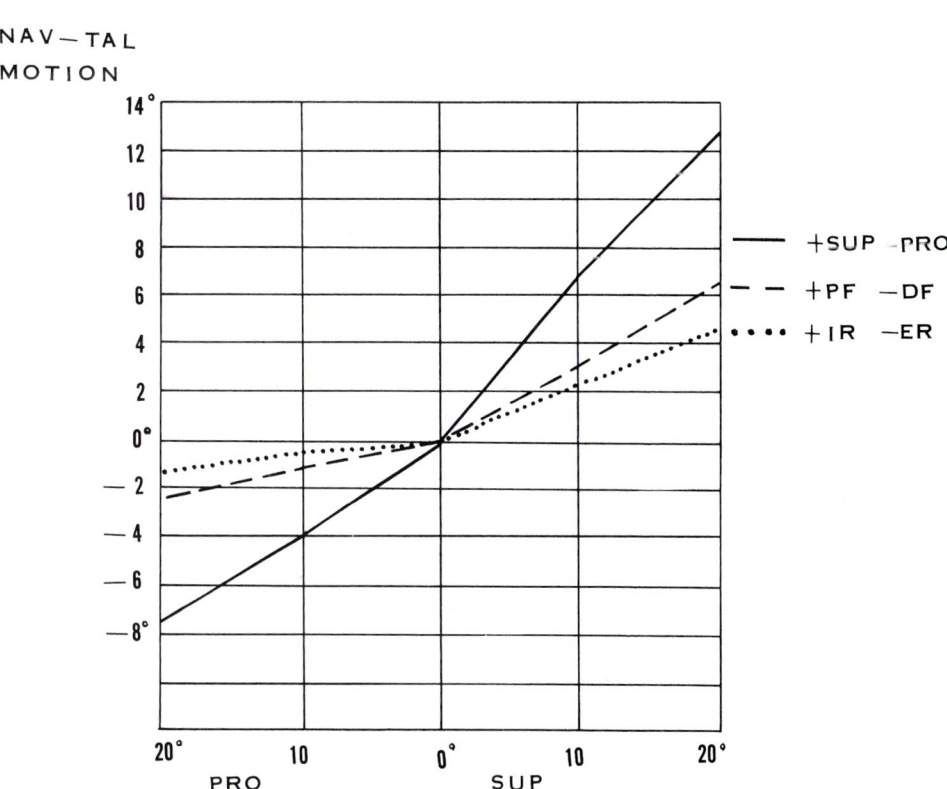

Figure 10.123 Navicular response at naviculotalar joint to pronation and supination input of the foot. (*DF*, dorsiflexion; *ER*, external rotation; *IR*, internal rotation; *PF*, plantar flexion; *PRO*, pronation; *SUP*, supination.) (Data from and adapted from Lundberg A, Svensson OK, Bylund C, et al. Kinematics of the ankle/foot complex. Part 2: Pronation and supination. *Foot Ankle*. 1989;9[5]:248-253.)

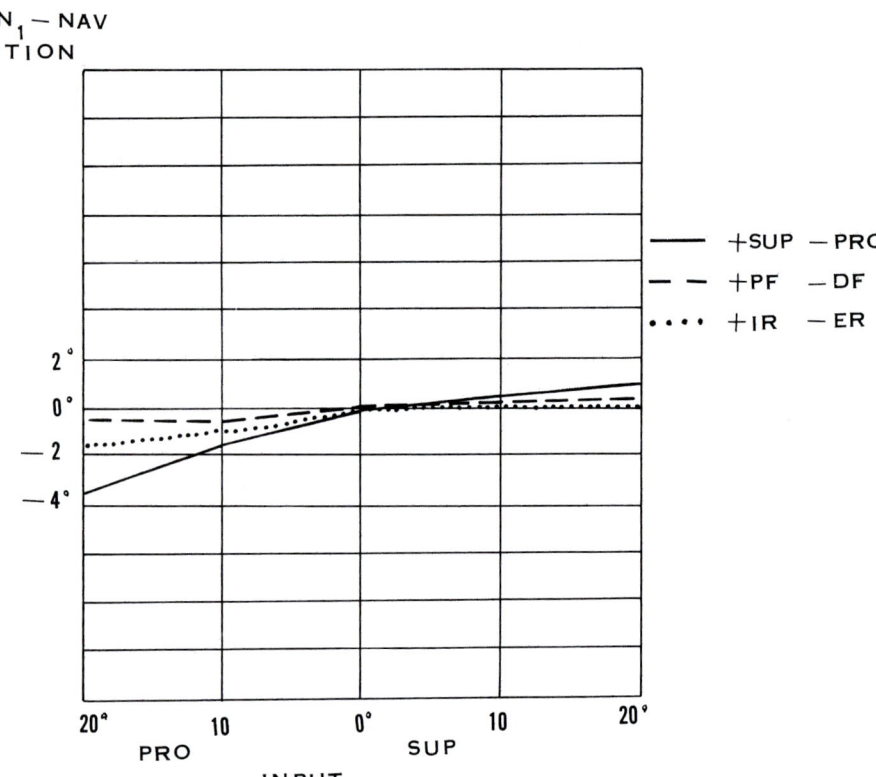

Figure 10.124 First cuneiform response at cuneiform$_1$-navicular joint to pronation and supination input of foot. (*DF*, dorsiflexion; *ER*, external rotation; *IR*, internal rotation; *PF*, plantar flexion; *PRO*, pronation; *SUP*, supination.) (Data from and adapted from Lundberg A, Svensson OK, Bylund C, et al. Kinematics of the ankle/foot complex. Part 2: Pronation and supination. *Foot Ankle.* 1989;9[5]:248-253.)

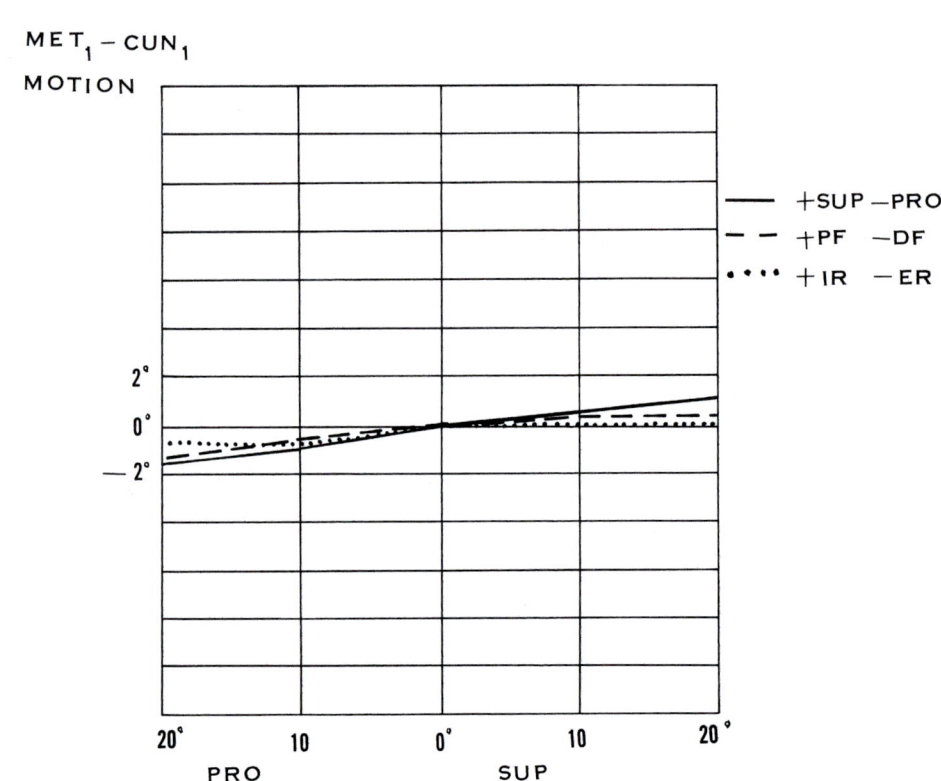

Figure 10.125 First metatarsal response at metatarso$_1$-cuneiform$_1$ joint to pronation and supination input of foot. (*DF*, dorsiflexion; *ER*, external rotation; *IR*, internal rotation; *PF*, plantar flexion; *PRO*, pronation; *SUP*, supination.) (Data from and adapted from Lundberg A, Svensson OK, Bylund C, et al. Kinematics of the ankle/foot complex. Part 2: Pronation and supination. *Foot Ankle.* 1989;9[5]:248-253.)

Metatarsal 1 at metatarso$_1$-cuneiform$_1$ joint

Pronation: 1.8° ± 1.5°
External rotation: 1.7° ± 1.1°
Plantar flexion: 0.6° ± 0.4°

During supination-pronation of the foot, the talus moves also at the ankle joint. At 20° of supination of the foot, the talar motion is as follows:

Supination: 0.4° ± 0.4°
External rotation: 2.4° ± 2.3°
Dorsiflexion: 1.1° ± 3.6°

At 20° of pronation, the talar motion is as follows:

Pronation: 0.9° ± 0.4°
Internal rotation: 0.6° ± 0.9°
Plantar flexion: 2.7° ± 1.4°

▶ Functional Remodeling Under Tibiotalar Loading During Plantar Flexion and Dorsiflexion at the Ankle Joint

The remodeling or the distribution of plantar flexion-dorsiflexion within the ankle-foot complex was also analyzed in vivo by Lundberg and colleagues in the eight volunteers described previously.[5]

The contribution and the triaxial motion of the talus at the talotibial joint were already analyzed. Remodeling of the lamina pedis occurs with minimal motion of the calcaneus and the forefoot, more so of the navicular at the talonavicular joint. From 30° of plantar flexion to the neutral position, the calcaneal motion at the calcaneotalar joint was limited.

From 0° to 30° of dorsiflexion, the calcaneal motion at the calcaneotalar joint is as follows:

Supination: 1.3° ± 1.6°
Internal rotation: 1.4° ± 1.5°
Plantar flexion: 1.8° ± 1.4°

From 0° to 30° of plantar flexion, the calcaneal motion is as follows:

Supination: 1.3° ± 1.7°
Internal rotation: 2.4° ± 1.3°
Plantar flexion: 2.2° ± 1.3°

The first ray (navicular-cuneiform$_1$-metatarsal$_1$) participates in the plantar flexion from 0° to 30° with, however, minimal contribution to dorsiflexion (Fig. 10.126).

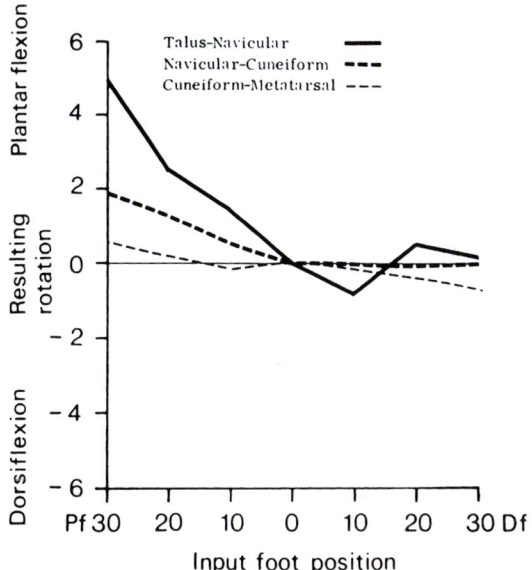

Figure 10.126 Dorsiflexion-plantar flexion input of the foot and resulting dorsiflexion-plantar flexion motion at the talonavicular, navicular-cuneiform, and cuneiform-metatarsal joints. (Lundberg A, Goldie I, Kalin BO, et al. Kinematics of the ankle/foot complex. Plantar flexion and dorsiflexion. *Foot Ankle.* 1989;9[4]:198. Copyright ©1989. Reprinted by Permission of SAGE Publications.)

During gait, the plantar flexors develop four times more energy than the dorsiflexors. The following motors are the plantar flexors with their work capacity expressed in meter kilograms, as presented by Lang and Wachsmuth: triceps surae, 16.4; flexor hallucis longus muscle, 0.9; flexor digitorum longus muscle, 0.4; tibialis posterior muscle, 0.4; peroneus longus muscle, 0.4; peroneus brevis muscle, 0.3 (total, 18.8).[9] Approximately nine-tenths of the plantar flexor energy is provided by the triceps surae.

Dorsiflexors

The tendons located anterior to the talocrural joint axis are the dorsiflexors of the ankle. With the foot fixed on the ground, they rotate the leg forward. The following muscle units are the dorsiflexors, with their work capacity expressed in meter kilograms: tibialis anterior muscle, 2.5; extensor digitorum longus muscle, 0.8; extensor hallucis longus muscle, 0.4; peroneus tertius muscle, 0.5 (total, 4.2).[9]

▶ Talocalcaneonavicular and Midtarsal Motors (see Fig. 10.127)

The axis of the talocalcaneonavicular joint and the oblique axis of the midtarsal joint are very close in orientation. The motors located on the medial aspect of the talocalcaneonavicular axis of motion are the invertors, whereas the motor units located on the lateral aspect of the same axis are the evertors (see Fig. 10.127). With the foot fixed on the ground, the evertors internally rotate the leg and the invertors rotate the leg externally.

ANKLE-FOOT MOTORS

▶ Ankle Motors (Fig. 10.127)

Plantar Flexors

The tendons located posterior to the talocrural joint axis of motion are the plantar flexors of the ankle. When the foot is fixed on the ground, the same motors rotate the leg posteriorly.

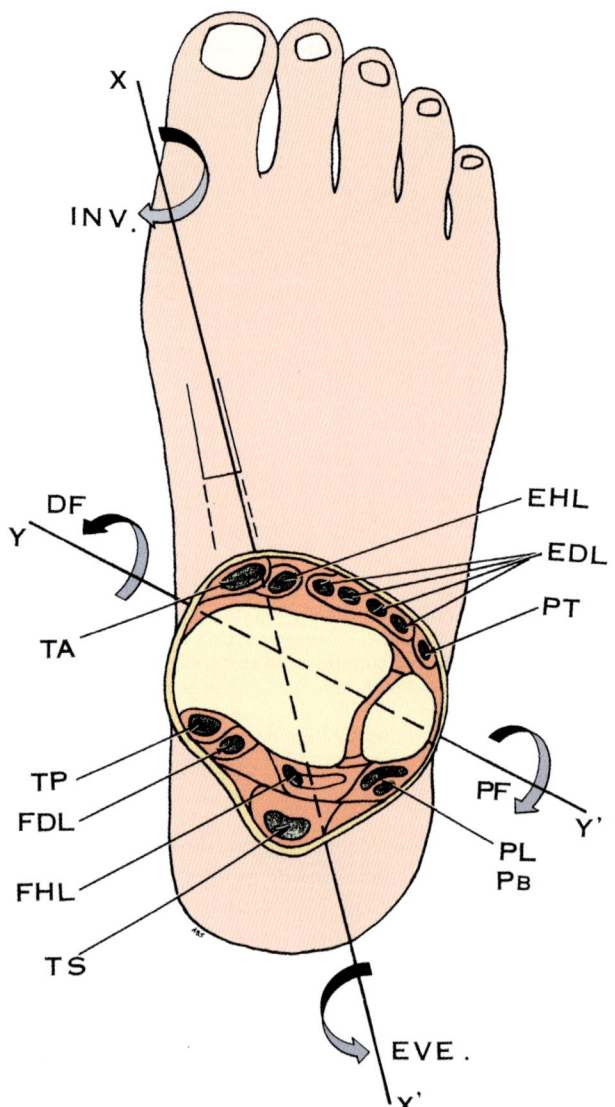

Figure 10.127 Motors of the ankle and the talocalcaneonavicular joint (*TCN*). (*XX'*, axis of motion of the TCN joint; *YY'*, axis of motion of the ankle joint; *INV*, inversion; *EVE*, eversion; *DF*, dorsiflexion; *PL*, plantar flexion.) *Invertors: TA*, tibialis anterior; *TP*, tibialis posterior; *FDL*, flexor digitorum longus; *FHL*, flexor hallucis longus; *TS*, triceps surae. *Evertors: PL*, peroneus longus; *PB*, peroneus brevis; *EHL*, extensor hallucis longus; *EDL*, extensor digitorum longus; *TA*, tibialis anterior; *PT*, peroneus tertius. *Plantar flexors:* TP, FDL, FHL, TS, PL, PB. *Dorsiflexors:* TA, EHL, EDL, PT.

Invertors

The following units are the invertors, with their work capacity expressed in meter kilograms, as presented by Lang and Wachsmuth: triceps surae, 4.8; tibialis posterior muscle 1.8; flexor digitorum longus muscle, 0.8; flexor hallucis longus muscle, 0.8; tibialis anterior muscle, 1.0 (total, 8.2).[9]

Evertors

The following motor units are the evertors, with their work capacity expressed in meter kilograms: peroneus longus muscle, 1.7; peroneus brevis muscle, 1.3; extensor digitorum longus muscle, 0.8; peroneus tertius muscle, 0.5; extensor hallucis longus muscle, 0.1; tibialis anterior muscle, 0.3 (total, 4.8).[9]

▶ **Toe Motors and Function**

The toes participate in weight-bearing, in giving hold against the ground, and in tensing the plantar aponeurosis and the plantar skin during the push-off phase of the walking cycle. The last two functions are more effective with the first and second toes. The long flexors of the toes also act as plantar flexors of the ankle and invertors of the talocalcaneonavicular joint, whereas the long extensors of the toes act as dorsiflexors of the ankle and evertors of the talocalcaneonavicular joint.

In 1889, Ellis stated that "the principal function of the toes is to give good foot-hold by active pressure against the ground so as to supplement the passive pressure of the body's weight. This is affected by the same means as that which, when the toes are free to move, moves them."[92] The long toe flexors act from their distal anatomic insertions and as such they act as joint-stabilizing muscles.[93]

During the walking cycle, the long toe flexors are in concentric contraction when the metatarsophalangeal joints are extending (30%-55% of the cycle) and act as stabilizers of the toes, invertors of the hindfoot, and plantar flexors of the ankle. The long toe extensors are in concentric contraction during the swing phase of gait and act as extensors of the metatarsophalangeal joints, evertors of the hindfoot, and dorsiflexors of the ankle.

Big Toe Motors

In the big toe in the non–weight-bearing position, the distal joint is extended by the extensor hallucis longus tendon through its wide insertion on the dorsum of the distal phalanx. The proximal phalanx is extended by the extensor digitorum brevis and by the transverse lamina of the extensor aponeurosis activated by the proximal pull of the extensor hallucis longus. This is the sling mechanism of extension described by Sarrafian and Topouzian.[94]

The centralization of the extensor hallucis longus tendon relative to the vertical axis passing through the metatarsal head is of prime importance. If the tendon shifts lateral to this axis—as in hallux valgus—it will act as an adductor of the hallux and will exert a medially directed force on the first metatarsal head, which may result in a varus deformity of the first metatarsal bone.

In the non–weight-bearing position, the distal phalanx is flexed by the flexor hallucis longus.

The flexion of the metatarsophalangeal joint is provided by the lateral head of the flexor hallucis brevis, the medial head of the flexor hallucis brevis, the adductor hallucis, the abductor hallucis, and the flexor hallucis longus.

It is apparent that the flexor or "pressor" power of the metatarsophalangeal joint is greater than the extensor power. Furthermore, the action of a tendon-muscle unit over a joint is measured by the moment developed by the motor unit relative to the axis of motion at the joint. The moment is measured by the product of the acting force and its perpendicular distance from the axis of rotation. The sesamoids in this sense not only have a weight-bearing function but also increase the perpendicular distance of the plantar intrinsic muscles from the axis of flexion-extension of the metatarsophalangeal joint and augment the flexion moment of the intrinsic muscles. Excision of the sesamoids will result in a decrease of the flexor moment or flexor power so essential at this joint.

The abductor of the big toe is the abductor hallucis, and the adductor hallucis provides the adduction. Balance between these two deviators is necessary to maintain the big toe in neutral position. In a hallux valgus deformity, the abductor hallucis shifts laterally and its abductor component is more in a plantar position. The muscle loses its abductor power and acts mainly as a flexor. The side motion is overtaken by the adductor hallucis.

In the plantigrade position, the proximal phalanx of the big toe is normally extended. The flexion of the distal phalanx is possible only if the proximal phalanx is further extended to create the necessary "room" for the flexion to occur. However, this is prevented by the powerful flexion-pressor pull of the intrinsic muscles, and, as stated by Ellis, the flexor hallucis longus "exerts all its influence on a straight great toe."[92] Excision of the sesamoids may result in a cock-up deformity of the big toe through weakening of the intrinsic muscles. Occasionally, the same deformity may be seen as a complication of a Keller excisional arthroplasty because the flexion power of the intrinsics is lessened by excision of the proximal third of the proximal phalanx.

Lesser Toe Motors

The lesser toes' functional units are as follows:

- The long extensors with the extensor digitorum brevis for toes 2 to 4
- The flexor digitorum longus with the flexor digitorum brevis for toes 2 to 5
- The plantar interossei for toes 3, 4, and 5
- The dorsal interossei for toes 2, 3, and 4
- The lumbricals for toes 2 to 5
- The abductor and the flexor digiti quinti
- The deep sagittal band attachment of the plantar aponeurosis acting on the proximal phalanx and the plantar plate

All tendons passing dorsal to the axes of motion act as extensors and all tendons passing plantar to the axes of motion act as flexors. The long extensor tendons pass dorsal to the axes of motion at the metatarsophalangeal and interphalangeal joint whereas the flexor digitorum longus tendons pass plantar to the same axes (Fig. 10.128). The extensor digitorum brevis tendon passes dorsal to the axis of motion at the metatarsophalangeal and proximal interphalangeal joint, whereas the flexor digitorum brevis passes plantar to the axes of the same two joints.

The plantar, dorsal interossei tendons and the lumbricals pass plantar to the axis of motion at the metatarsophalangeal joint. The lumbrical tendon and a few fibers of the interossei terminate dorsal to the axis of motion at the proximal interphalangeal joint and act through the lateral tendons on the terminal extensor tendon.

The long extensors and the extensor digitorum brevis are strongly attached to the plantar aspect of the proximal phalanx through the transverse portion of the extensor aponeurotic lamina. They have only a loose connection with the dorsal capsule or the dorsum of the proximal phalanx (Fig. 10.129).

Functionally, when traction is applied on a tendon, it will first act at its firm attachment site and then secondarily on the bridged joints. A pull applied on the long extensor tendon results in a hyperextension of the proximal phalanx at the metatarsophalangeal joint. The proximal phalanx is lifted into extension through the dorsal pull exerted by the proximal transverse segment of the dorsal extensor apparatus: the sling mechanism of extension (Fig. 10.130).[94] The proximal phalanx is extended, but the middle and distal phalanges remain slightly flexed (Fig. 10.131).

A pull exerted on the long flexor of the toe results initially in flexion of the distal interphalangeal joint with subsequent flexion at the proximal interphalangeal joint and finally at the metatarsophalangeal joint (Fig. 10.132). The flexor digitorum brevis first flexes the proximal interphalangeal joint and then the proximal phalanx (Fig. 10.133).

The combined pull on the long extensor, the extensor brevis on the dorsal side, and the long flexor, the flexor brevis on the

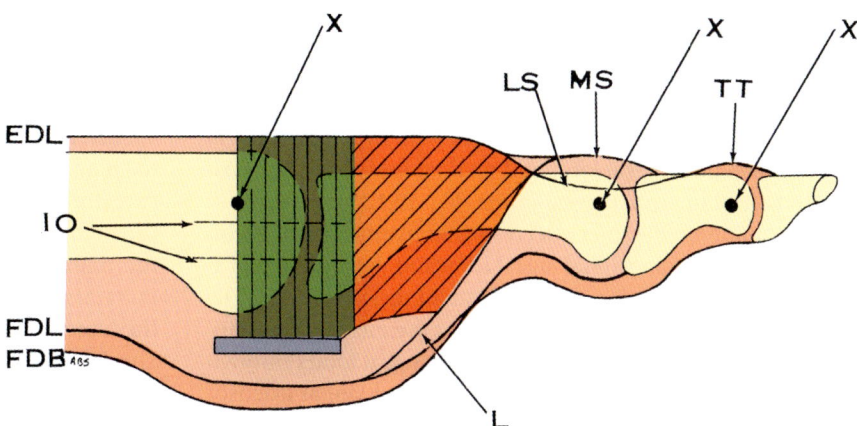

Figure 10.128 **Motors of a lesser toe.** X axes of motion at the metatarsophalangeal (MP) and interphalangeal (IP) joints. All motors passing dorsal to the axis of motion of a corresponding joint are extensors. All motors passing plantar to the axis of motion of a corresponding joint are flexors. Specifically, the interossei are flexors of the MP joint; the lumbrical is a flexor of the MP and the extensor of the IP joints. The extensor sling is delineated by vertical parallel lines and the extensor wing by oblique parallel lines. (*EDL*, extensor digitorum longus; *FDB*, flexor digitorum brevis; *FDL*, flexor digitorum longus; *IO*, interossei; *L*, luimbrical; *LS*, lateral slip; *MS*, middle slip; *TT*, terminal tendon.)

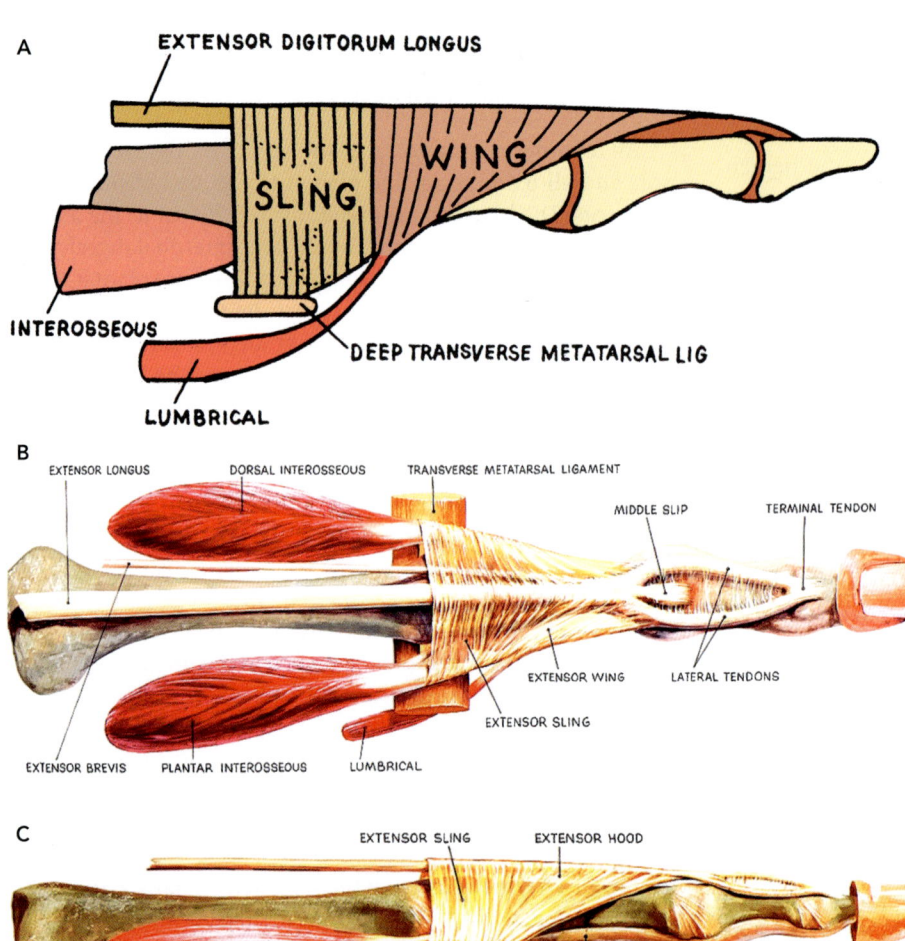

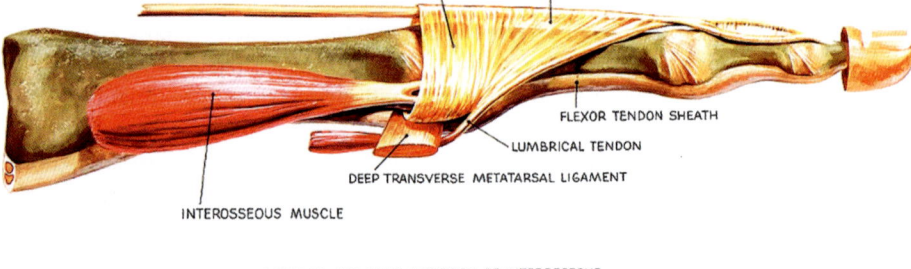

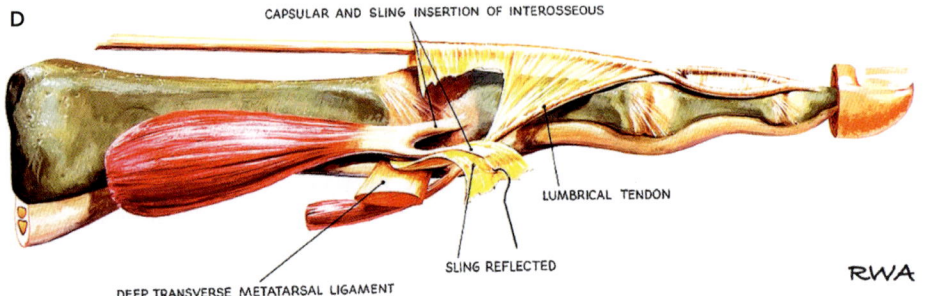

Figure 10.129 Lesser toe. **(A)** Extensor aponeurosis of a lesser toe. **(B)** Sling mechanism of extension of the metatarsophalangeal joint of the lesser toe. **(C)** Extensor mechanism of the lesser toe with the intact sling. **(D)** The resected sling showing the capsular and sling insertion of the interosseous. (**B-D** are the work of the renowned artist and illustrator Robert W. Addison. This project was presented at the 1968 American Academy of Orthopedic Surgeons in Chicago.)

plantar side, results in clawing of the toe with hyperextension at the metatarsophalangeal joint and marked flexion at the proximal and distal interphalangeal joints (Fig. 10.134).

The traction on the interossei results in plantar flexion stabilization at the metatarsophalangeal joint and weak extension at the proximal and distal interphalangeal joint (Fig. 10.135). The pull on the lumbrical results in flexion at the metatarsophalangeal joints and extension at the interphalangeal joints through its tendinous connection with the middle and lateral extensor slips (Fig. 10.136).

The increased tension in the plantar aponeurosis results in plantar flexion at the metatarsophalangeal joint. The coordinated plantar flexion at the metatarsophalangeal joint through the action of the interossei, the lumbricals, and the plantar aponeurosis prevents the hyperextension at the metatarsophalangeal joint, allowing the long extensor and the extensor brevis to extend the interphalangeal joints. The long flexor and the flexor brevis will then act as flexor-pressor of the toe unit at the metatarsophalangeal joint (Fig. 10.137).

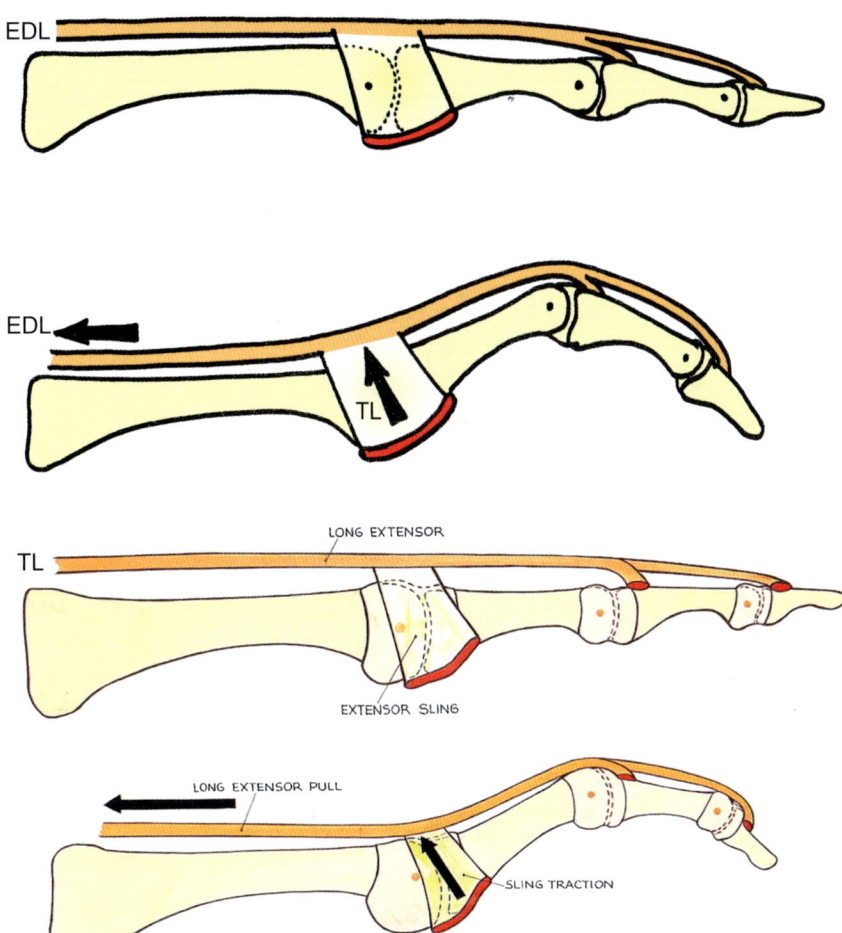

Figure 10.130 **(A)** Sling mechanism of extension of the metatarsophalangeal joint of the lesser toe. The pull of the extensor digitorum longus *A* is transmitted as traction to the transverse lamina *B*, which acts as a sling and lifts the proximal phalanx into extension. **(B)** The pull exerted by the long extensor results in hyperextension of the metatarsal phalangeal joint. The interphalangeal joints remain slightly flexed. Hyperextension at the metatarsal phalangeal joint of the lesser toes through the pull on the long extensors of the toes in a cadaver foot. (**A**, Redrawn after Sarrafian SK, Topouzian LK. Anatomy and physiology of the extensor apparatus of the toes. *J Bone Joint Surg Am.* 1969;51[4]:669. **B**, is the work of the renowned artist and illustrator Robert W. Addison. This project was presented at the 1968 American Academy of Orthopedic Surgeons in Chicago.)

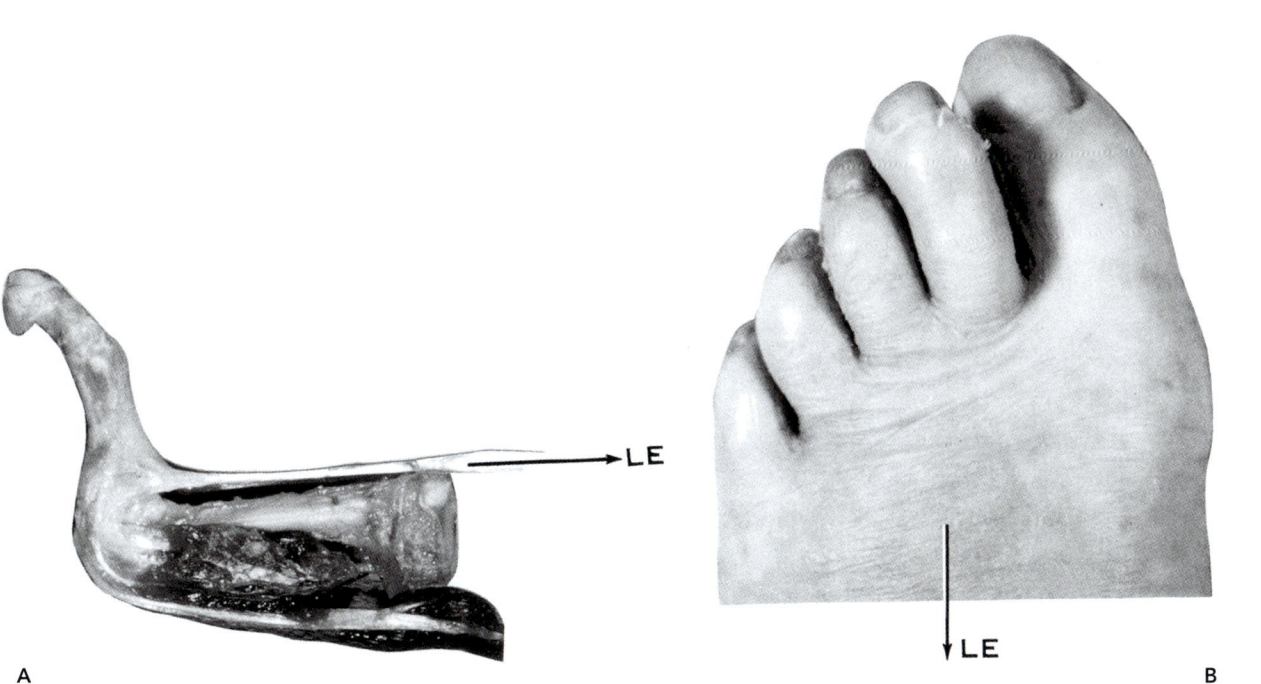

Figure 10.131 **(A)** The pull exerted by the long extensor (*LE*) results in hyperextension of the metatarsophalangeal joint. The interphalangeal joints remain slightly flexed. **(B)** Hyperextension at the metatarsophalangeal joints of the lesser toes through the pull on the long extensors of the toes (*LE*) in a cadaver foot.

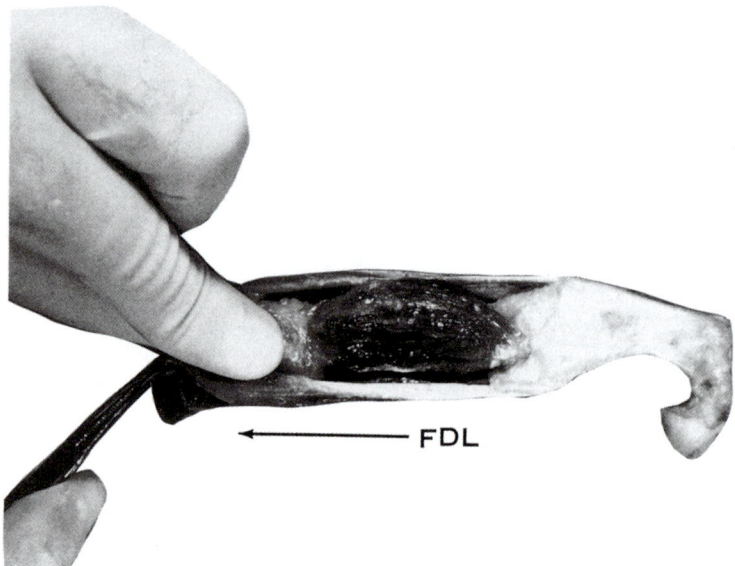

Figure 10.132 The pull exerted on the flexor digitorum longus (FDL) results in flexion of the interphalangeal joints and, to a lesser degree, the metatarsophalangeal joint.

In the plantigrade position, the pull of the long flexor and the flexor brevis of the toe may result in flexion of both interphalangeal joints combined with secondary further extension at the metatarsophalangeal joint from its initial position of extension. The pull of the intrinsic muscles and the tension of the plantar aponeurosis prevent excess hyperextension at the metatarsophalangeal joint. Furthermore, in the plantigrade position and under body weight, the flexor digitorum brevis may flex the proximal interphalangeal joint with the distal interphalangeal joint remaining in extension. In this position, both flexors then press the toes against the ground. As stated by Ellis, the lesser toes "grip the ground…by pressure of the undersurfaces of tips against the ground."[92]

Toes as Tensors of the Plantar Aponeurosis and of the Skin

The plantar aponeurosis of the foot is attached posteriorly to the os calcis and anteriorly to the proximal phalanges of the toes through the longitudinal septa (in the big toe the septa are

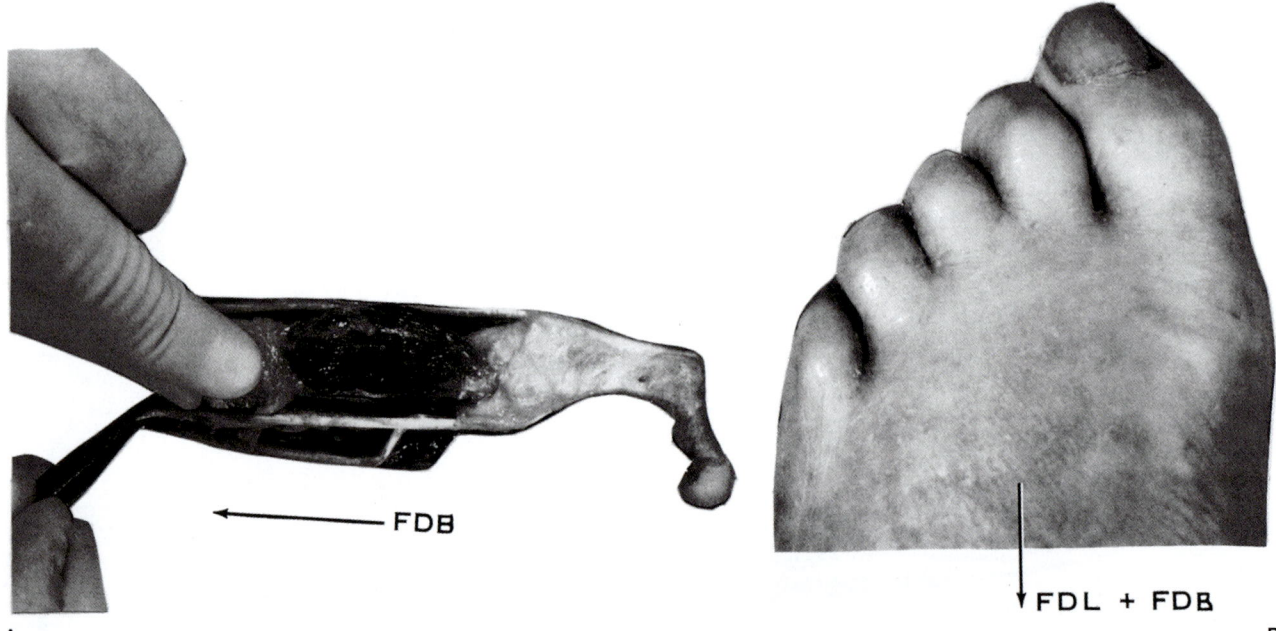

Figure 10.133 **(A)** The flexor digitorum brevis (FDB) flexes the proximal interphalangeal joint and, to a lesser degree, the metatarsophalangeal joint. **(B)** Combined pull on the flexor digitorum longus (FDL) and the flexor digitorum brevis (FDB) in a cadaver foot results in flexion of the interphalangeal joints and, to a lesser degree, the metatarsophalangeal joint.

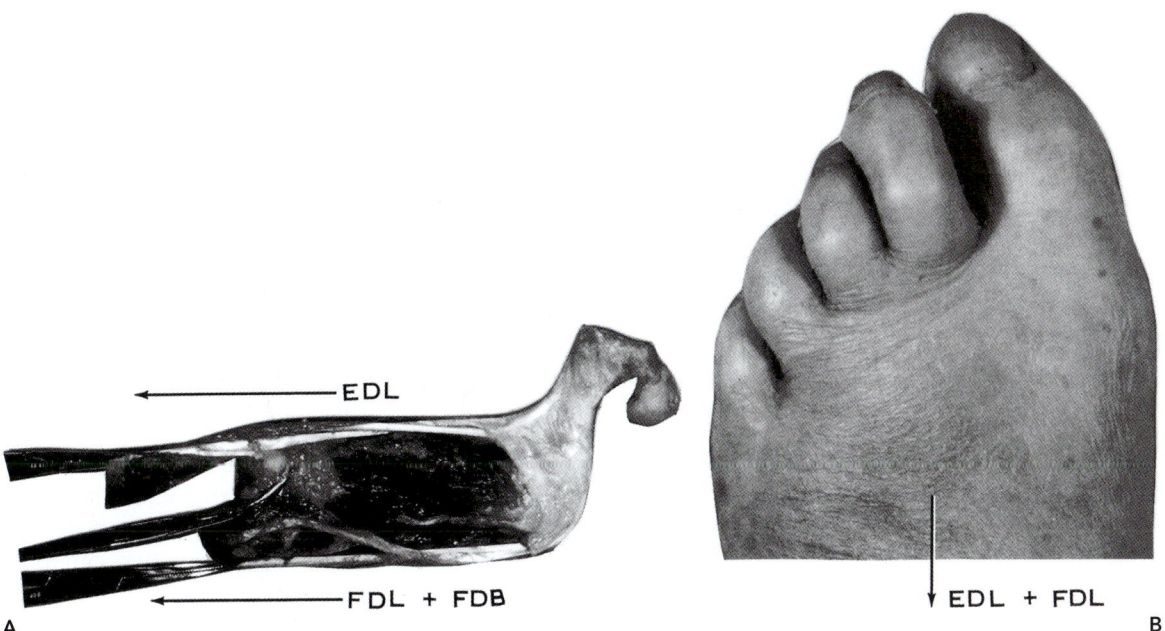

Figure 10.134 **(A)** Clawing of the toe produced by the simultaneous pull on the extensor digitorum longus (*EDL*), the flexor digitorum longus (*FDL*), and the flexor digitorum brevis (*FDB*). The clawed toe is hyperextended at the metatarsophalangeal joint and flexed at the interphalangeal joints. **(B)** Clawing of the lesser toes produced in a cadaver foot by the simultaneous pull on the extensor digitorum longus (*EDL*) and the flexor digitorum longus (*FDL*). The metatarsophalangeal joints are hyperextended and the interphalangeal joints flexed.

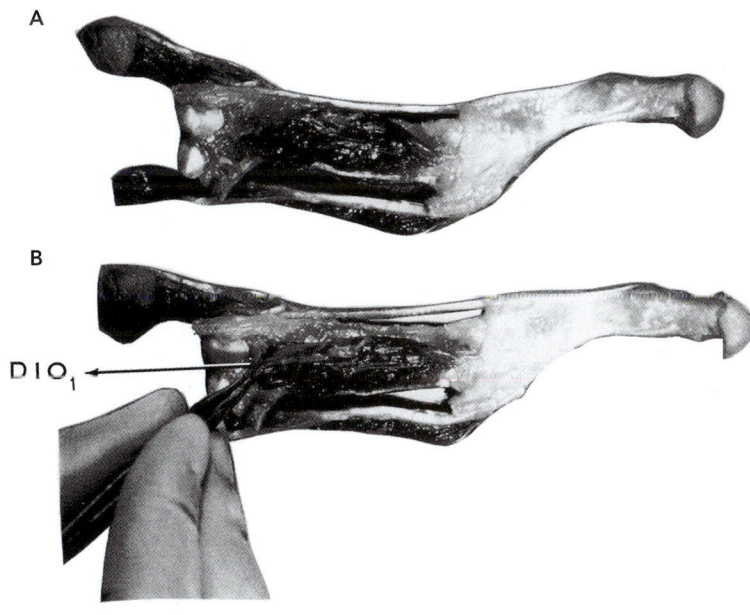

Figure 10.135 **Action of the first dorsal interosseous muscle of the second toe.** **(A)** Second toe at rest with hyperextension at the metatarsophalangeal joint. **(B)** Traction exerted on the first dorsal interosseous muscle decreases the hyperextension at the metatarsophalangeal joint through flexion. (*DIO₁*, first dorsal interosseous muscle.)

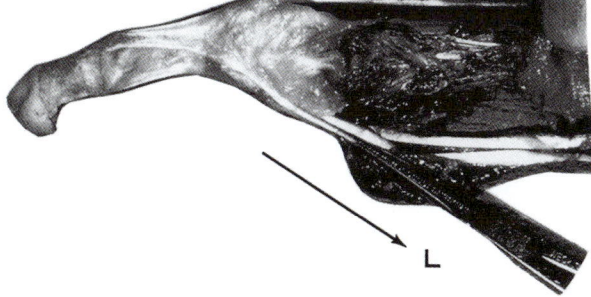

Figure 10.136 **Action of the lumbrical.** The pull exerted by the hemostat on the lumbrical tendon results in flexion of the metatarsophalangeal joint and extension of the interphalangeal joints.

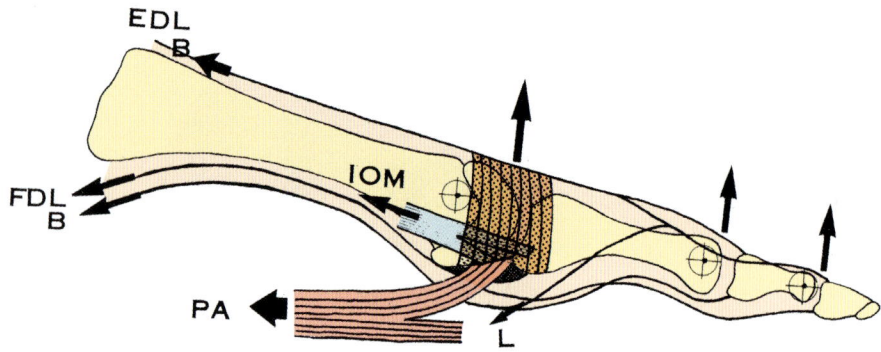

Figure 10.137 The straight lesser toe. The hyperextension at the metatarsophalangeal (MP) joint through the pull of the extensor digitorum longus (*EDL*) and brevis (*EDB*) is prevented by the flexion forces exerted at the same joint by the interossei muscles (*IOM*), the lumbrical (*L*), the plantar aponeurosis (*PA*), and the flexor digitorum longus (*FDL*) and brevis (*FDB*). The extension force exerted by the *EDL*, the *EDB*, and the *L* at the interphalangeal joints is counterbalanced by the *FDL*, with the *FDB* acting only at the proximal interphalangeal joint.

attached to the lateral and medial sesamoids), and it is attached to the skin of the ball of the foot through the vertical fibers and through the transverse lamellae of the natatory ligament farther distally.

Plantar Aponeurosis as Flexor of Metatarsophalangeal Joints

As described by Hicks, hyperextension of the toes at the metatarsophalangeal joints tenses the plantar aponeurosis, raises the longitudinal arch of the foot, inverts the hindfoot, and externally rotates the leg.[95]

This is the windlass mechanism; the metatarsal head is the drum of the windlass, the proximal phalanx is the handle, and the cable wound onto the drum is the plantar aponeurosis. The hyperextension of the toe winds the plantar aponeurosis around the metatarsal head. The calcaneus remains fixed, the forefoot flexes about 1 cm, and the longitudinal arch becomes shorter but higher through the increased tension in the plantar aponeurosis (Figs. 10.138 and 10.139). The windlass mechanism is more efficient with the big toe because the diameter of the drum is increased by the presence of the sesamoids. The first ray flexes an average of 10° and the lateral ray 5°. The windlass mechanism works also in reverse. As mentioned by Hicks, the lowering of the raised arch through the body weight or anterior shift of the leg unwinds the windlass, and the increased tension in the plantar aponeurosis flexes the toe at the metatarsophalangeal joint.[95] This is clearly demonstrated in the simple model in Figure 10.140.

Scheck demonstrated anatomically that the pull on the proximal segment of the transected plantar aponeurosis flexes the toe at the metatarsophalangeal joint.[79] He mentions that, historically, "In 1853, in an article on gait, Fick[96,97] noted that on weight-bearing the toes are plantar flexed by the tensing of the plantar aponeurosis."[79]

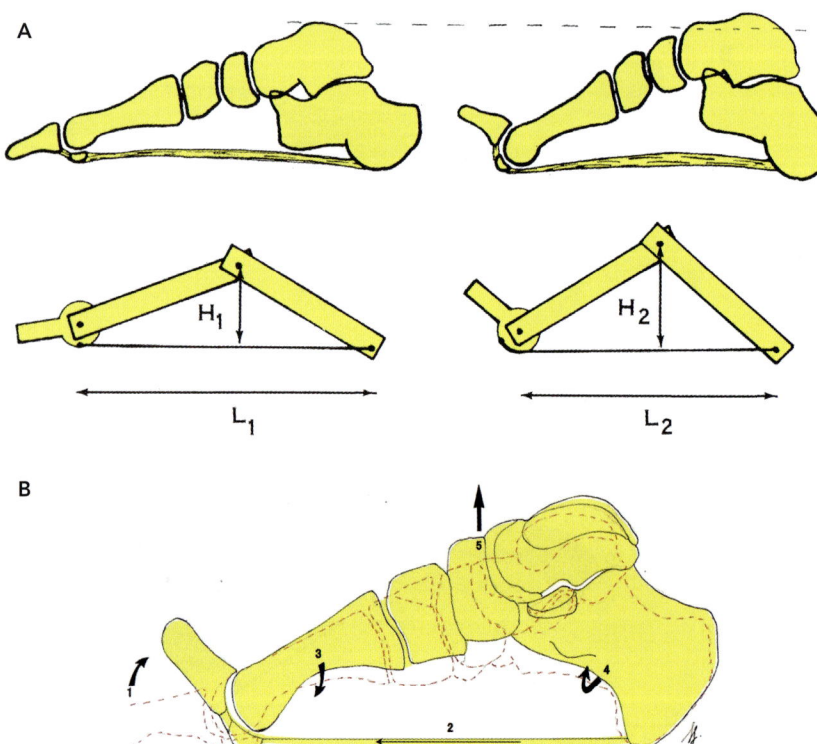

Figure 10.138 The "windlass." **(A)** The drum of the windlass is the head of the metatarsal, the handle is the proximal phalanx, and the cable wound onto the drum is the plantar aponeurosis through its attachment to the plantar pad of the metatarsophalangeal joint. The dorsiflexion of the toe winds the plantar aponeurosis around the metatarsal head. The initial length L_1 of the foot diminishes to L_2, and the initial height of the arch H_1 increases to H_2. **(B)** Dorsiflexion of the first toe (1) winds the plantar aponeurosis (2). Plantar flexion of the first metatarsal (3). Supination of the heel (4). High-arch position (5). (**A**, From Hicks JH. The three weight-bearing mechanisms of the foot. In: Evans FG, ed. *Biomechanical Studies of the Musculo-Skeletal System*. Charles C Thomas; 1961:176. **B**, Sarrafian SK. Functional characteristics of the foot and plantar aponeurosis under tibio-talar loading. *Foot Ankle*. 1987;8[1]:10. Copyright ©1987. Reprinted by Permission of SAGE Publications.)

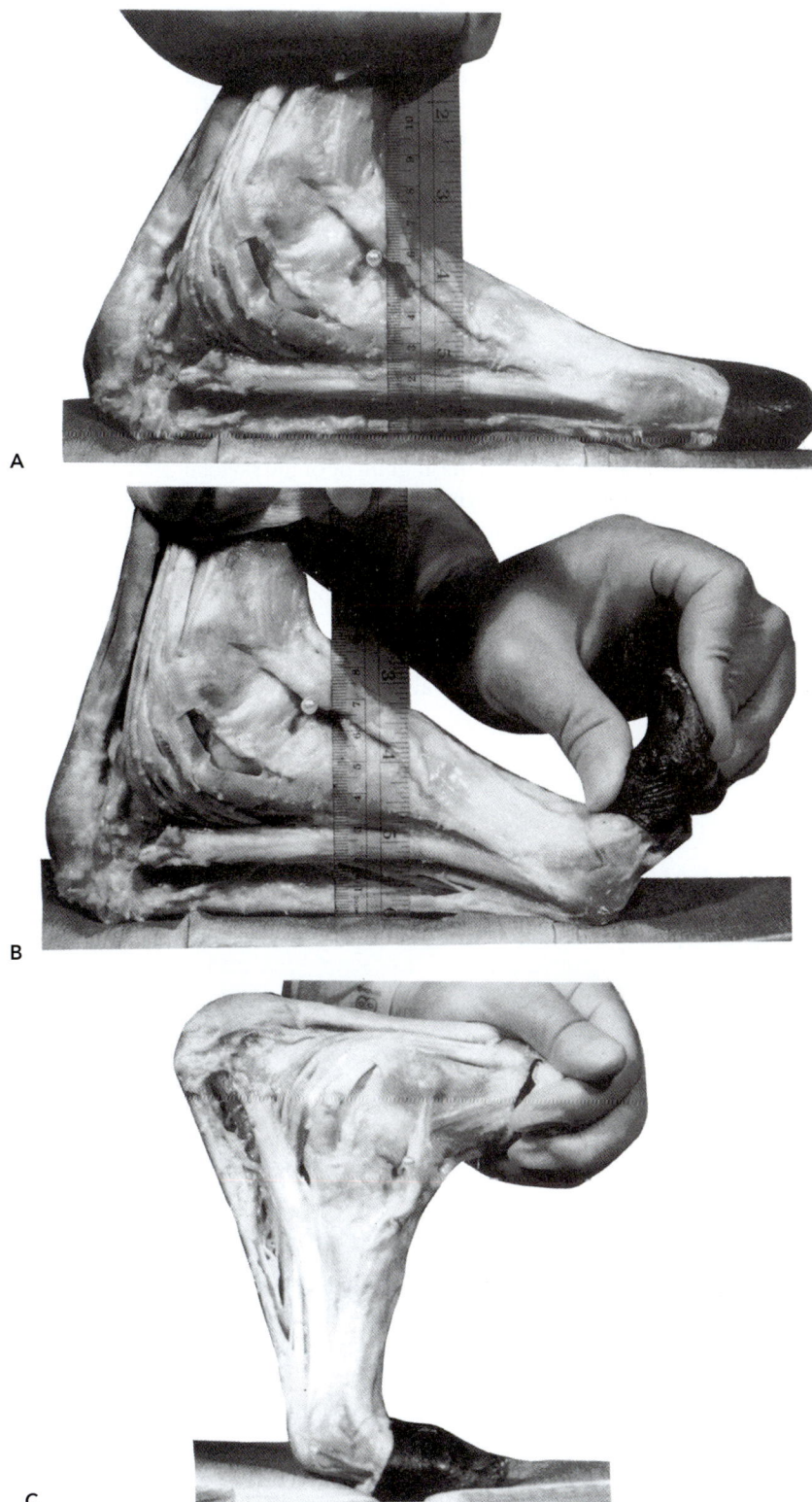

Figure 10.139 The tension in the plantar aponeurosis increases with: (A) the anterior flexion of the leg or relative dorsiflexion of the foot; (B) the hyperextension of the big toe or windlass mechanism of Hicks; (C) the heel off, the toes remaining hyperextended.

During the windlass mechanism, the effective shortening or displacement of the plantar aponeurosis is 10 mm for the first ray.[95] Bojsen-Møller reports an average displacement of 15 mm of the plantar aponeurosis for the first toe and 8 mm for the third toe.[98] Extension of the metatarsophalangeal joints of the toes also affects the tension of the skin on the ball of the foot; it is transformed from a soft pliable ball "into a firm pad that can resist tangential, or shear forces, and the skin mobility is greatly reduced."[98]

LOAD TRANSMISSION AND ARCHES OF THE FOOT

When defining the arches through the alignment of the skeletal elements, a major longitudinal arch is recognized medially—formed by the calcaneus, talus, navicular, cuneiforms 1, 2, and 3, and metatarsals 1, 2, and 3—and there is a minor lateral longitudinal arch formed by the calcaneus, cuboid, and metatarsals 4 and 5.

In the transverse direction, an arch or a niche is found in the mid segment of the foot. Distally, all five metatarsal heads bear weight, and a transverse arch is nonexistent. Structurally, in the sagittal plane, the foot skeleton is arranged in an arcuate fashion, taking support posteriorly through the os calcis and anteriorly through the metatarsal heads, and spanning the mid segment of the foot; the spanning is high medially and very low laterally. The arcuate units are five in number, fused posteriorly at the level of the os calcis and separated anteriorly through the corresponding metatarsal bones. Structurally, a weight-bearing arcuate structure may behave as an arch, a truss, or a curved beam.

An arch is a multisegmented arcuate structure, usually with a central wedge-shaped keystone and two "flanks" leading down from each side of the keystone, the flanks supported by fixed segments such as two columns or embankments. Without the fixed support at both ends, the arch collapses.

A truss is a variant of the arch (Fig. 10.141). The separation of both ends is prevented by a tie-rod at the base. The truss is triangular in arrangement, with sides formed by two struts and the base by the tie-rod. When load is applied at the apex, the struts are under compression and the tie-rod is under tension: bending is eliminated. A tie-rod mechanism is provided to the foot by the plantar aponeurosis (Fig. 10.142).

A curved beam is unisegmental. When loaded vertically in its mid segment, it generates compressive forces on the convex surface and tensile forces on the concave surface. An arch may behave like a convex beam if the multiple segments are bound together on the concave surface by connecting elements such as the strong ligaments seen in the foot (Figs. 10.143 and 10.144).

Lapidus considers the foot as a truss, with the talus and os calcis forming the posterior strut and the forefoot up to the metatarsal heads forming the anterior strut.[99] Both are subjected to compression. The plantar structures, mainly the plantar aponeurosis, are the tie-rod, "taking up the tension and eliminating bending."[99]

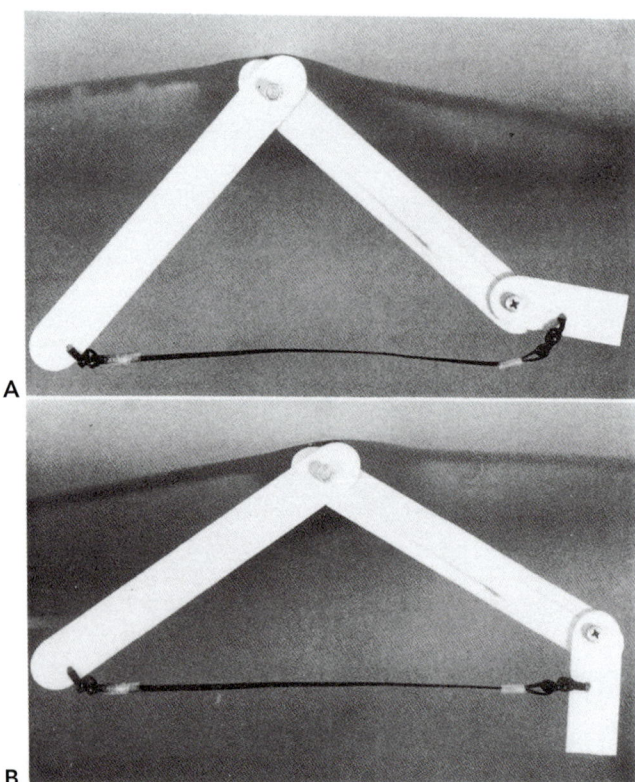

Figure 10.140 **The reversed windlass mechanism. (A)** A model representing the truss mechanism. The string represents the plantar aponeurosis connected to the hyperextended big toe at the metatarsophalangeal joint. **(B)** Lowering of the arch tenses the plantar aponeurosis, resulting in flexion of the big toe at the metatarsophalangeal joint. (Sarrafian SK. Functional characteristics of the foot and plantar aponeurosis under tibio-talar loading. *Foot Ankle*. 1987;8[1]:10. Copyright ©1987. Reprinted by Permission of SAGE Publications.)

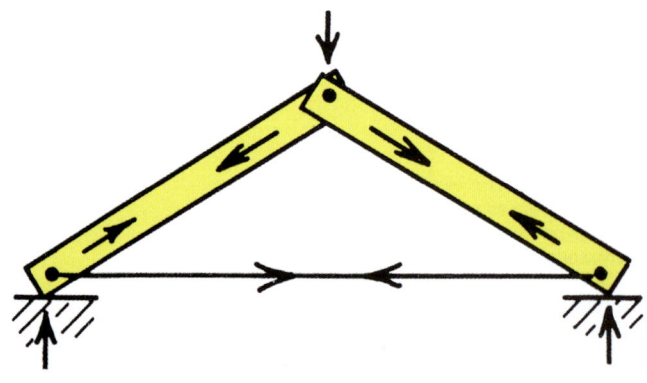

Figure 10.141 **A truss is a variant of an arch.** The two struts are connected at the base by a tie. When load is applied at the apex, the struts are under compression and the tie-rod under tension. Bending is eliminated. The three weight-bearing mechanisms of the foot. (Adapted from Hicks JH. The three weight-bearing mechanisms of the foot. In: Evans FG, ed. *Biomechanical Studies of the Musculo-Skeletal System*. Charles C Thomas; 1961:161-191.)

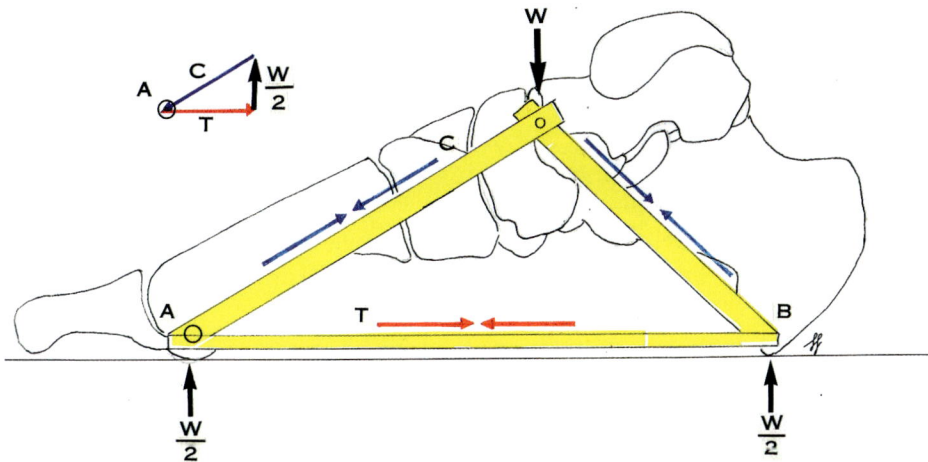

Figure 10.142 **The truss mechanism of the foot.** Under body weight (*W*), the struts are under compression (*C*) and the tie rod or plantar aponeurosis is under tension (*T*). Any joint, for example, point A, is in vectorial equilibrium, as indicated in the inset diagram. (Sarrafian SK. Functional characteristics of the foot and plantar aponeurosis under tibio-talar loading. *Foot Ankle*. 1987;8[1]:9. Copyright ©1987. Reprinted by Permission of SAGE Publications.)

▶ Internal Compressive Forces

Manter experimentally measured the compressive forces under static loading between the bones of seven cadaveric foot specimens.[100]

A downward thrust of 60 lb was exerted with a lever arm over the talar dome. The generated compressive forces between the joints of the lamina pedis were measured. A compressive force gradient was present from a proximal to a distal direction, and these forces were transmitted along the medial column (talonaviculocuneiforms-metatarsals 1-3) and the lateral column (calcaneocuboid-metatarsals 4-5) (Fig. 10.145). The longitudinal compression provides axial rigidity. Furthermore, a transverse compression was demonstrated between the cuboid and the three cuneiforms, further adding to the stability of the foot.

Indeed, a true keystone arch configuration is present only laterally as described by MacConaill and Basmajian: "the true arch of the foot, that part whose posterior pillar is the upward sloping calcaneus, whose key stone is the cuboid and whose anterior pillar is composed of the fourth and fifth metatarsals."[101] The transverse compression loads the keystone.

▶ Truss and Beam

Hicks, in an experimental study, demonstrated that, under weight-bearing conditions in the plantigrade position, the foot reacts as a truss and a beam.[102] The load on the foot tends to force the ends apart and "the tension in the tie therefore provides a measure of the arch-flattening effect."[102] In the plantigrade standing position, the flattening effect is resisted by both the truss and the beam mechanism. In the toe-standing position or the corresponding phase of walking, the truss mechanism takes over from the beam mechanism; this is caused by the windlass mechanism tightening the plantar aponeurosis. The bending strain on the beam diminishes, and in the extreme heel-raised position, the truss mechanism assumes the entire load.

From a quantitative point of view, Hicks expresses the tension in the tie or the arch-flattening effect as

$$t = W \frac{l}{L} \cdot \frac{P}{Q}$$

where t = tension in the tie or plantar aponeurosis, W = body weight, L = length of foot from heel to ball, l = distance of

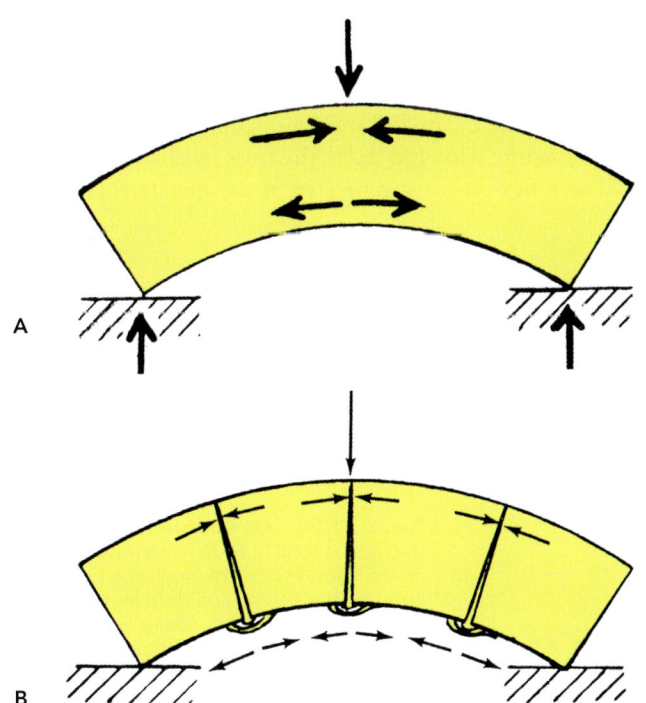

Figure 10.143 **(A)** A curved beam, when loaded vertically in its mid segment, generates compressive forces on the convex surface and tensile forces on the concave surface. **(B)** An arch may behave as a convex beam if the segmental components are bound on the concave surface by connecting elements such as strong ligaments, as seen on the plantar aspect of the foot. The ligaments are under tension. (From Hicks JH. The three weight-bearing mechanisms of the foot. In: Evans FG, ed. *Biomechanical Studies of the Musculo-Skeletal System*. Charles C Thomas; 1961:161-191.)

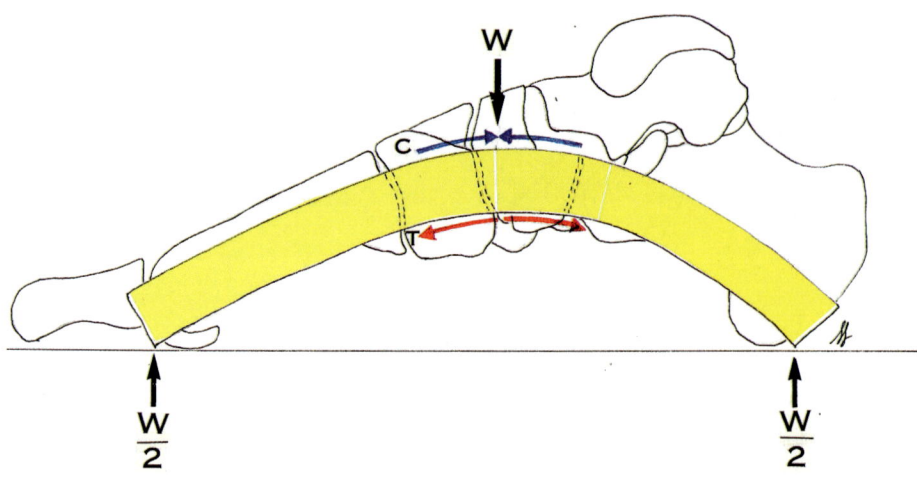

Figure 10.144 The multisegments of the foot bound strongly by the plantar ligaments form a structure similar to a beam. The central loading of the beam by the body weight (*W*) generates compressive forces (*C*) on the upper segment of the beam and tensile forces (*T*) on the lower segment. (Sarrafian SK. Functional characteristics of the foot and plantar aponeurosis under tibio-talar loading. *Foot Ankle*. 1987;8[1]:7. Copyright ©1987. Reprinted by Permission of SAGE Publications.)

line of weight anterior to the heel, and *P* and *Q* = constants related to the shape of the individual arch (height) (Fig. 10.146).[102,103]

It is apparent that the arch-flattening effect of the body weight is variable and is nil when *W* passes through the heel ($l = 0$, $t = 0$) and maximum when *W* passes through the ball of the foot (l = max, t = max). In other words, when one leans forward on the plantigrade foot and transfers the weight-bearing line anteriorly, there is more tendency to flatten the longitudinal arch, and subsequently more strain is exerted on the plantar structures and the plantar aponeurosis.

In the average foot, the ratio *P/Q* is 1.8. When *W* passes through the ball of the foot, *l/L* is equal to 1, and the flattening effect on the foot is 1.8 *W*, or nearly double the body weight. In the high-arch foot, *Q* is increased, *P/Q* is decreased, and the flattening strain is less on the foot, whereas in the flatfoot, *Q* is decreased and *P/Q* is increased, resulting in increased strain on the weight-bearing foot.

In the clinical setup, it can be demonstrated that when the body weight is shifted forward over the plantigrade foot, the tension in the plantar aponeurosis is increased, as demonstrated by the limited active hyperextension of the hallux (Fig. 10.147) or by the increased flexion force under the pad of the hallux, because one is then unable to slip a piece of paper under the big toe (Hicks test).[103] The increased flexion force under the big toe with anterior flexion of the leg is not due to an increased tension in the flexor hallucis longus. When one stands on the edge of a step with the metatarsophalangeal joint of the big toe free, anterior flexion of the leg brings forth flexion at the metatarsophalangeal joint without concomitant flexion at the interphalangeal joint. The interphalangeal joint is easily extended passively and the flexor hallucis longus is unloaded.[87]

In an experimental setup, Hicks has quantitated the contribution of the beam and truss mechanism in the foot under vertical loading with 100 lb.[102] The truss mechanism was measured as a flexion force generated at the metatarsophalangeal

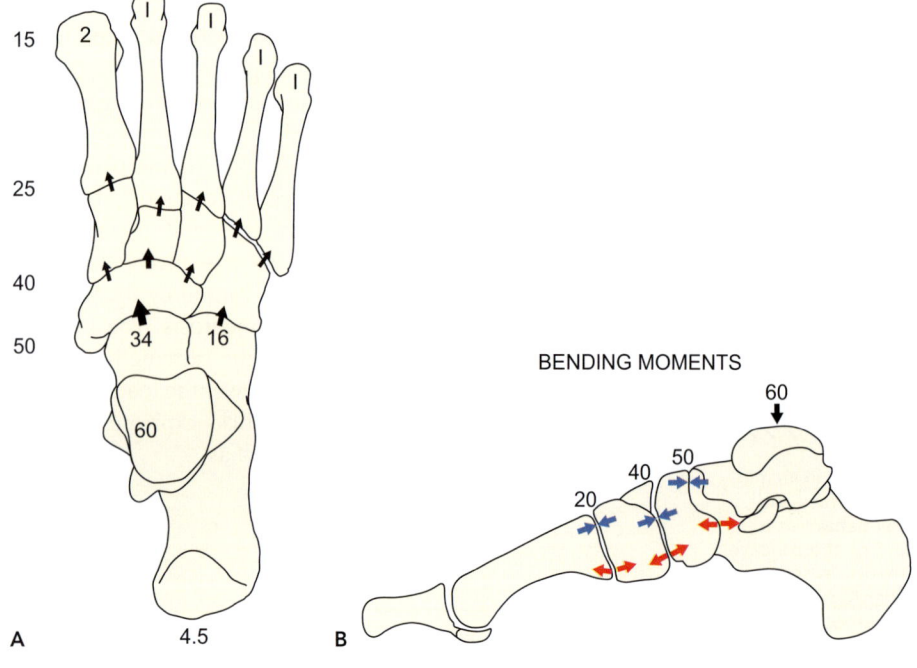

Figure 10.145 **(A)** Compressive forces in the foot. A total of 60 lb has been applied on the talus. The line of application passes between the second and third metatarsals. A gradient of compressive forces is generated. The load under the first metatarsal head is one half of the total load under the lesser metatarsal heads. With a 3- to 4-mm shift of the talar load, the force application line passes between the first and second metatarsals, and the load under the first metatarsal head is doubled, equaling the load under the lesser metatarsal heads. **(B) Bending moments of the medial column of the foot.** A total of 60 lb has been applied on the talus. Red arrows indicate the bending moments, while blue arrows indicate the compressive forces.

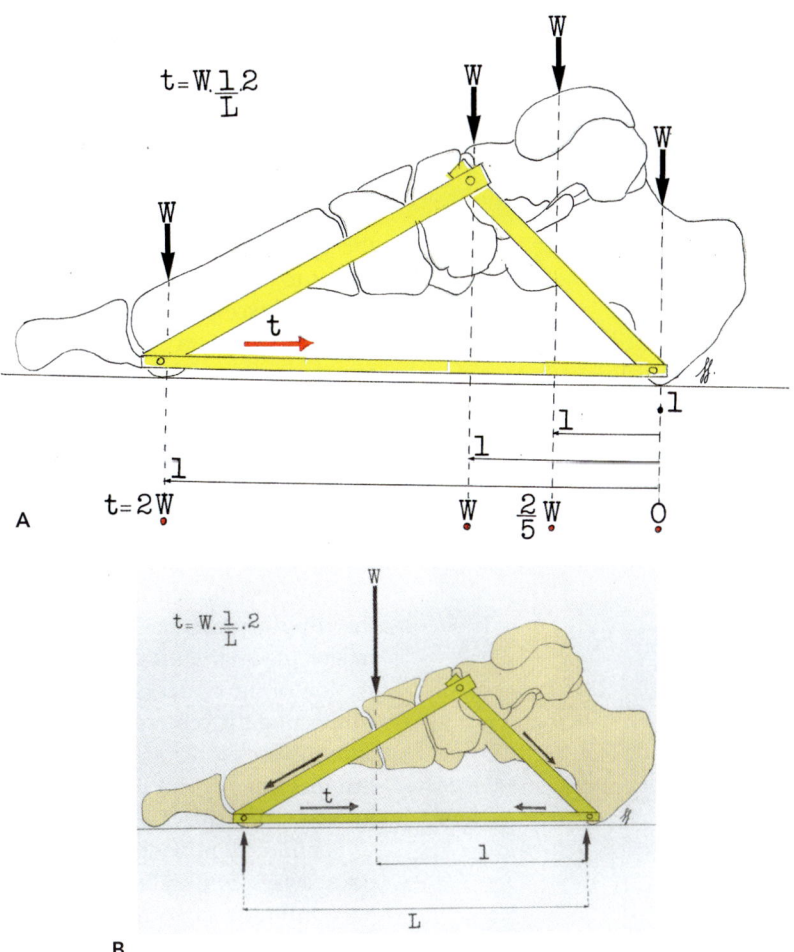

Figure 10.146 **(A)** Tension in the tie rod under the body weight (W) expressed by Hicks formula, where t = tension in plantar aponeurosis generated by the increased span of the truss (lowering of the arch); W = body weight; L = length of the foot measured from the heel to the metatarsal head; l = distance of the line of application of W measured forward from the heel. With W passing at the level of the heel, l = 0 and t = 0 and the plantar aponeurosis is relaxed. With W passing at the level of the metatarsal head, l = L and t = 2 W, the plantar aponeurosis is under maximum tension. The plantar pad of the toe is then firmly applied to the ground (reversed windlass mechanism). **(B)** The tension in the tie of the truss in the foot. The tension t represents the arch-flattening effect. When the load W is applied, the sum of the moments at point h is as follows:

$$\sum M_h = Wl - bL = 0$$
$$bL = Wl \quad (1)$$
$$\tan \theta = \frac{b}{t}$$
$$b = t \tan \theta \quad (2)$$

Replacing b in (1)

$$t \tan \theta \cdot L = Wl$$
$$t = W \cdot \frac{l}{L} \cdot \frac{1}{\tan \theta}$$
$$t = W \cdot \frac{l}{L} \cot \theta$$
$$t = W \cdot \frac{l}{L} \cdot \frac{P}{Q}$$

Q is the height of the arch of the foot. The higher the arch, the greater is Q and the lesser the tension t or flattening action. The lower the arch, the lesser is Q and the greater the tension t or flattening action. Obesity increases W and the tension t. (t, tension in tie; W, body weight; h, upward thrust from ground on the heel; b, upward thrust from ground on the ball of the foot; L, length of foot from heel to ball; l, distance of line of weight anterior to heel [varies from 0 to L]; P, Q, constants related to shape of individual arch [high or low arch]; θ, the inclination angle of the anterior strut of the foot.) (**A**, Sarrafian SK. Functional characteristics of the foot and plantar aponeurosis under tibio-talar loading. *Foot Ankle*. 1987;8[1]:12. Copyright ©1987. Reprinted by Permission of SAGE Publications. **B**, Diagram and equations after Hicks JH. The foot as a support. *Acta Anat*. 1955;25:34. By permission of S. Karger AG, Basel.)

joint through the tension in the plantar aponeurosis and the longitudinally bridging intrinsic muscles.

The beam mechanism was measured optically by the bend of the first metatarsal under load. With the foot intact, the vertical load of 100 lb was absorbed by the truss and beam mechanisms as follows:

Truss: 60 lb
Beam: 24 lb
Unaccounted: 16 lb

With the plantar aponeurosis transected, the distribution was as follows:

Truss: 13 lb
Beam: 55 lb
Unaccounted: 32 lb

With both the plantar aponeurosis and the abductor hallucis muscle transected, the values were as follows:

Truss: 6 lb
Beam: 81 lb
Unaccounted: 13 lb

As a corollary, an inefficient plantar aponeurosis transfers the load to the beam, which then relies on the plantar ligaments to fulfill its supportive action. Failure of these ligaments results in excessive bending stress with sagging of the arch in a mode of extension.

STANDING AND PRESSURE DISTRIBUTION UNDER THE BARE FEET

In the standing, comfortable position, the heels are in contact, the feet turned out. The gravity line pierces the base of the support near or slightly posterior to its geometric center. In the "normal attitude," Braune and Fischer locate the intersection of the center of gravity line at 4 cm anterior to the line connecting the centers of the ankle joints (Fig. 10.148).[104] This anterior location has been confirmed in the data review by Brunnstrom,[105] with the reported ranges of the distance as follows: 1 to 4.8 cm,[106] 3.6 to 6.7 cm,[107] and 4.92 to 5.65 cm.[108]

Stability is provided by the feet during standing, but the body sways continuously. The anteroposterior oscillation has an amplitude larger than lateral oscillation.[107,109] The sway in the anteroposterior direction may range from 9 mm minimum to 27 mm maximum,[106] and the center of pressure moves within an area of 4 cm².[103,105,106,108,110,111] The postural sway is influenced by both respiration and heart rate variability.[110] During the relaxed standing, the anteroposterior oscillations of the tibia on the talus are regulated by the soleus, tibialis posterior, and peroneus brevis, as evidenced by the electromyographic investigations on seven subjects.[112]

The very minor transverse sway seemed to be also modulated by the tibialis posterior and peroneus brevis.[112] The role of the muscles in the arch support was investigated electromyographically by Basmajian and Stecko in 20 subjects.[113] To eliminate any postural effect that the muscles might have on the leg and foot, the subjects were seated, and standing condition was simulated by applying a variable load through a lever arm onto the bent knee. With loads of 445 N (100 lb) to 890 N (200 lb) the muscle activity was negligible to slight (Fig. 10.149). Passive structures (ligaments and bones) provide the support to the arches. With a load of 1780 N (400 lb), the tibialis posterior demonstrated an average moderate activity, the tibialis anterior demonstrated an average less than slight activity, and the peroneus longus remained inactive. The flexor hallucis longus, the flexor digitorum brevis, and the abductor hallucis exhibited low levels of participation. The authors concluded that "in the standing-at-ease posture, muscle activity is not required and the muscles are inactive; however in positions in which excess stresses are applied, as in the take-off phase of gait, the muscles do react. Without any question, the first line of defense is

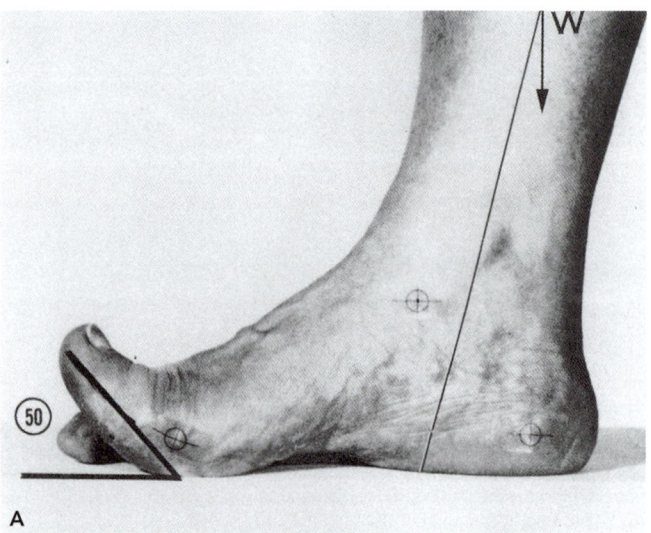
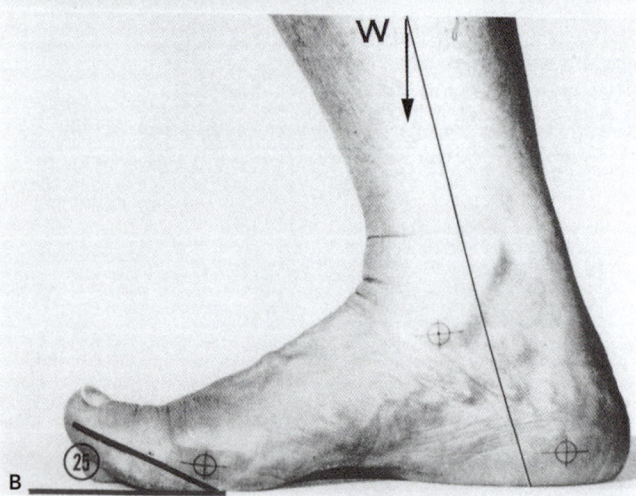

Figure 10.147 (A) When the body weight (W) passes at the level of the heel, the tension in the plantar aponeurosis is minimal and the active hyperextension at the metatarsophalangeal (MP) joint of the big toe is maximal—50° in this foot. The medial longitudinal arch is high. (B) With the body weight (W) passing in mid segment of the foot, the plantar aponeurosis is under tension and the active hyperextension at the MP joint is now limited to 25°. The medial longitudinal arch is lower. (Sarrafian SK. Functional characteristics of the foot and plantar aponeurosis under tibio-talar loading. Foot Ankle. 1987;8[1]:11. Copyright ©1987. Reprinted by Permission of SAGE Publications.)

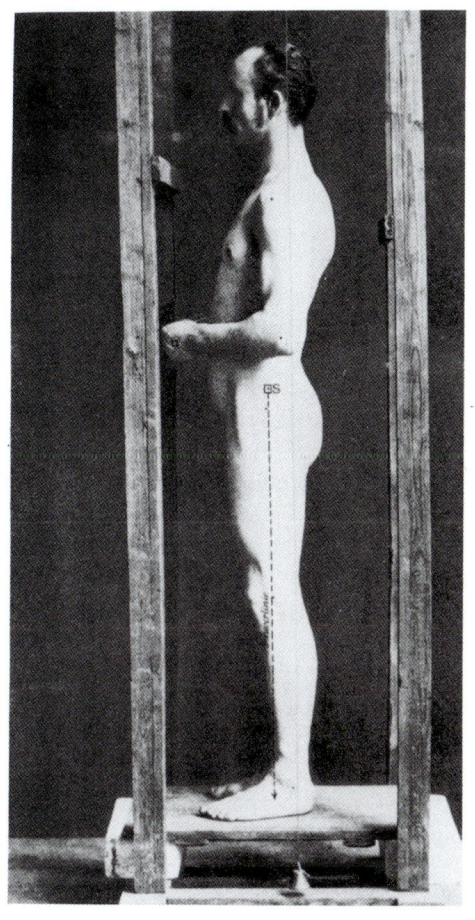 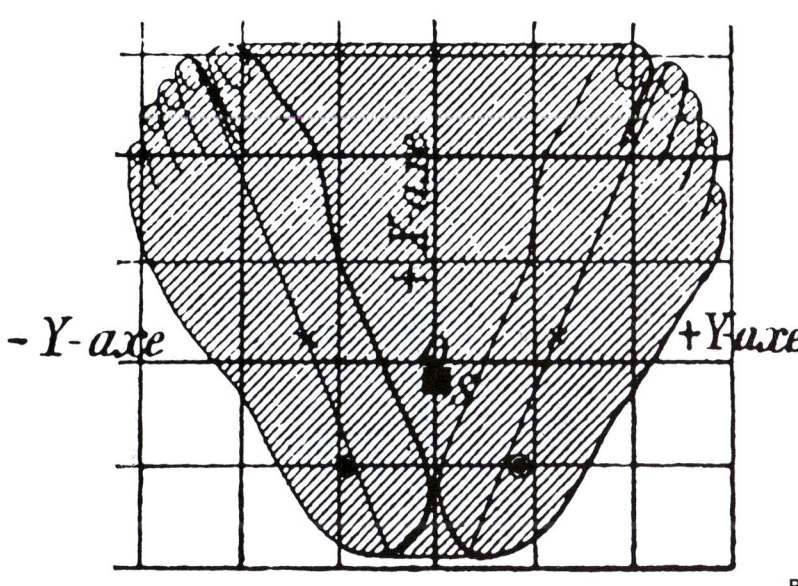

Figure 10.148 **(A)** Comfortable attitude, side view. Projection of the center of gravity ☐ S of the whole body. **(B)** Support area and its intersection ■ S by the line of gravity in comfortable attitude. The gravity line passes anterior to the line connecting the centers of the ankle joint. (Reprinted by permission from Braune W, Fischer O. *On the Center of Gravity of the Human Body*. Springer-Verlag; 1985:68.)

provided by the passive structures. During activity, the muscles would appear to contribute to the normal maintenance of the longitudinal arch."[113]

Cavanagh and colleagues investigated the plantar pressure distribution of 107 ft of 66 males and 41 females during barefoot standing using a capacitance mat.[114] Footprints were taken and "divided into 10 regions to enable analysis of the pressures in relation to the anatomical structures" (Fig. 10.150). The subjects stood up with even distribution of weight between the right and left foot. The peak pressure in a given region and the peak pressure for a given foot were reported. Furthermore, "the distribution of the entire contact force of one-half the body weight between the 10 anatomical regions was calculated." With the peak applied force of 0.5 × body weight, the mean peak pressure was 140 ± 30 kPa. The calculated average pressure was approximately 70 kPa. The regional distribution of the peak pressures is as indicated in Figure 10.151. The largest pressure was on the medial heel with 138.9 ± 31.4 kPa and the mean peak heel pressure was about 2.6 times greater than that in the forefoot. The mean pressure peak under the first metatarsal head was less (38.4 kPa) than the corresponding pressure under the second metatarsal head (51.8 kPa). The mean peak weight distribution was 60.5% on the heel, 7.8% in the midfoot, 28.1% in the forefoot, and 3.6% in the toes, which have a minor role bearing weight in standing (Fig. 10.152). The ratio of weight distribution for the metatarsal heads grouped as 1-2-3 to 5 is 1:1.5:2.5.

Cavanagh and coworkers further analyzed the metatarsal head pressure distribution along an oblique line approximating the first and fifth metatarsal head.[114] The peak pressure occurred at about 45% of the forefoot width as measured from the lateral border (Fig. 10.153). This negated the presence of a transverse functional arch, which would have been manifested by less pressure in the central segment.

Jones, in a study of weight-bearing in the standing position, demonstrated that the load distribution "is readily changed by a number of factors."[115] In the standing position, eversion brought about by abduction of the leg increases the load on metatarsals 2 to 5, whereas inversion brought about by adduction of the leg increases the load on the first metatarsal head. Dorsiflexion of the ankle increases the load on the first metatarsal head, and plantar flexion of the ankle shifts more weight onto metatarsals 2 to 5.

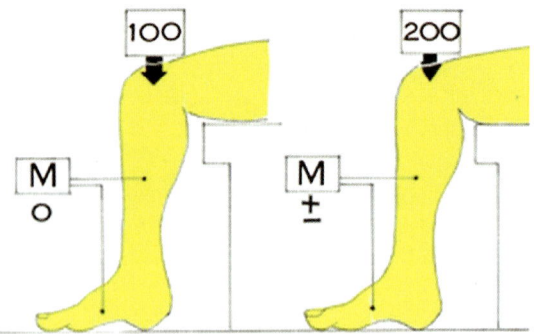

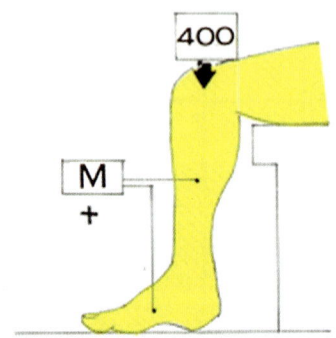

Figure 10.149 Role of muscles and ligamentous-skeletal frame in the support of the longitudinal arch of the foot. Subject is in sitting position with variable load applied over the knee, and the electrical activity of the leg-foot muscles is recorded. With a load of 100 lb, no myoelectrical activity is recorded. With 200 lb, a negligible to slight myoelectrical activity is recorded. With a 400-lb load, the tibialis posterior demonstrates an average moderate activity, the tibialis anterior an average less than slight activity, and the peroneus longus remain inactive. (Data from Basmajian JV, Stecko G. The roles of muscles in arch support of the feet: an electromyographic study. *J Bone Joint Surg Am.* 1963;45[6]:1184.)

▶ Orientation of Bony Trabeculae

Within the pedal skeletal framework, the transmission of the forces orients the bony trabeculae. The orientation of the trabeculae is not affected or interrupted by the presence of an articular interval, and a linear continuity is maintained throughout the skeletal frame. Two curved trabecular systems are initiated from the distal tibia (Fig. 10.154).[8,116-120] The anterior tibial trabecular system has a posterior concavity and is directed downward and posteriorly. It passes through the talus and terminates in the posterior segment of the os calcis in a fan-shaped pattern. The posterior tibial trabecular system is concave anteriorly, directed downward and anteriorly. It passes through the talus, the navicular, and the medial three metatarsals.

The architecture of cancellous bone was studied by Singh.[117] He defined a "type I made up entirely of fine rods anastomosing to form a meshwork" and "a type II with subtypes a, b, and c consisting of plates arranged parallel to each other." In type IIc, "the plates are separated by spaces traversed by rods that appear to hold the plates apart." Type III cancellous bone "is made up entirely of plates of varying size and shape that anastomose to form a meshwork" (Fig. 10.155).

Pal and Routal[118] investigated the architecture of the cancellous bone of the human talus in 25 specimens. The structure of the cancellous bone in the body of the talus consisted of thick plates that were arranged vertically, parallel to each other.

These fenestrated plates were almost oval in shape and occupied a major part of the body of the talus (Fig. 10.156). The cancellous bone of the neck "was present in the form of an irregularly arranged meshwork." The cancellous bone of the head "was made of thick, parallel running semiarched plates."

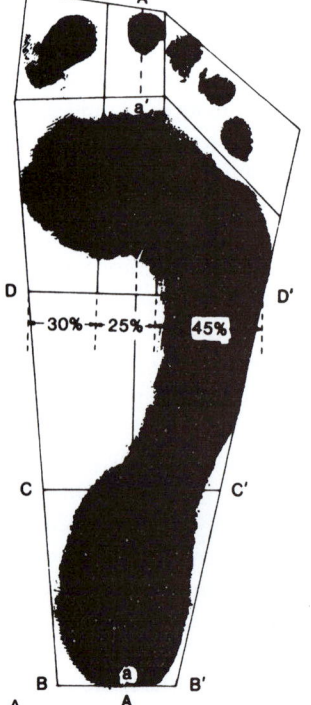
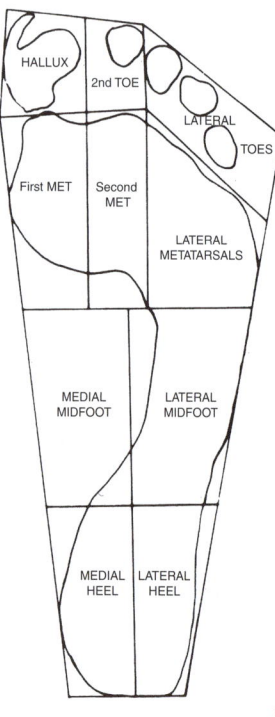

Figure 10.150 Regional division of the footprints for the study of the plantar pressure distribution during barefoot standing. **(A) The axis of the foot (AA') is drawn from the mid heel to the mid second toe print.** The axis length in the body of the foot (aa') is divided into three equal parts using lines perpendicular to the axis (BB', CC', and DD'). Tangents to the medial and lateral borders of the footprint are then drawn. By dividing the line DD' in the ratio of 0.45:0.25:0.30, the first, second, and lateral metatarsal head regions are defined. The toe regions are drawn by inspection. **(B)** The 10 anatomic regions that result from the regional division. (Cavanagh PR, Rodgers MM, Liboshi A, et al. Pressure distribution under symptom-free feet during barefoot standing. *Foot Ankle.* 1987;7[5]:265. Copyright ©1987. Reprinted by Permission of SAGE Publications.)

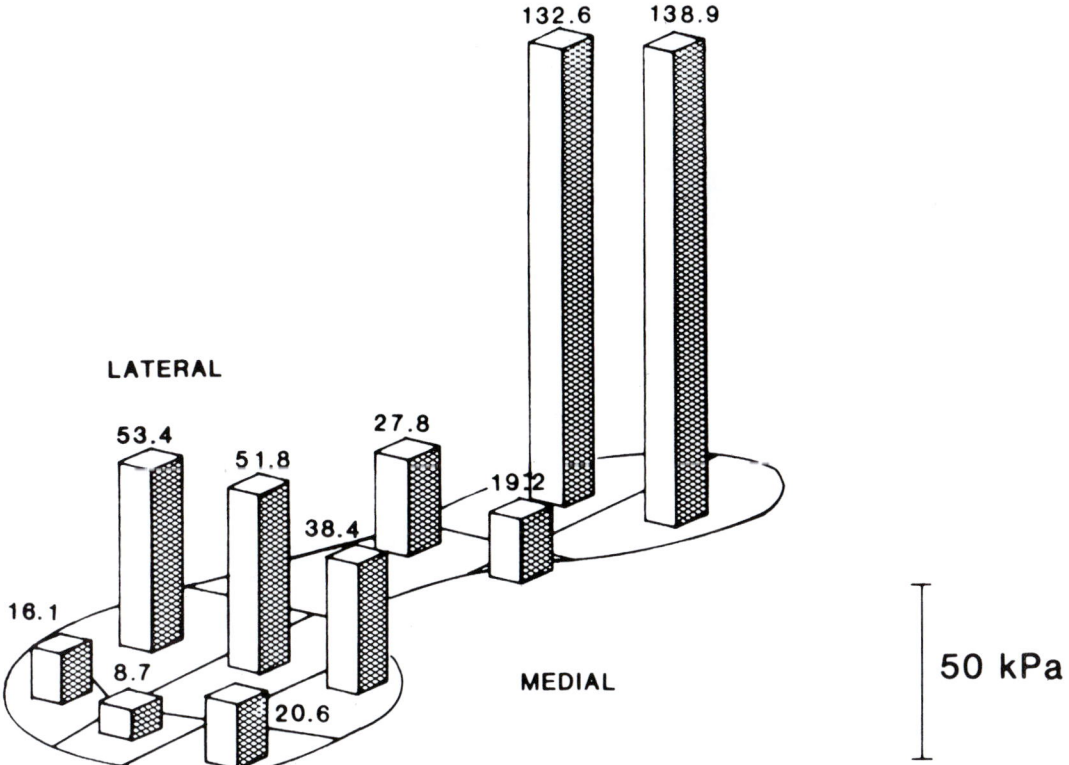

Figure 10.151 **Mean regional peak pressures (N = 107) during standing measured in kilopascals (kPa).** The ratio of peak rearfoot to peak forefoot pressures was approximately 2.6:1. (Cavanagh PR, Rodgers MM, Liboshi A, et al. Pressure distribution under symptom-free feet during barefoot standing. *Foot Ankle*. 1987;7[5]:267. Copyright ©1987. Reprinted by Permission of SAGE Publications.)

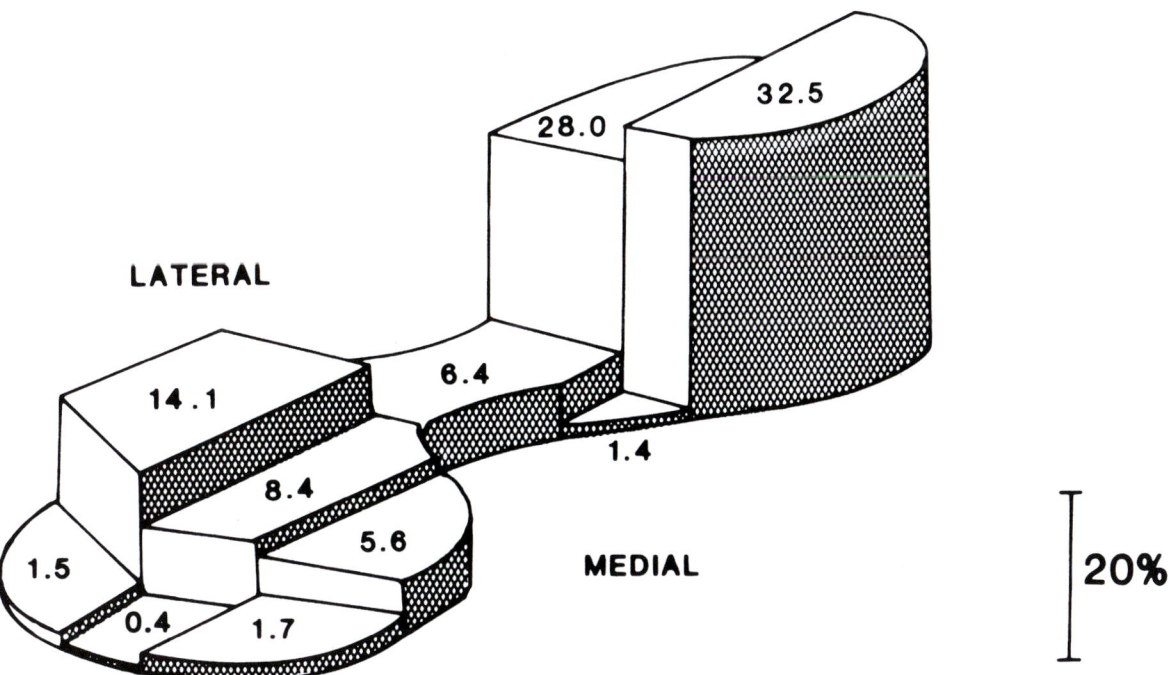

Figure 10.152 **Mean regional weight distribution (N = 107) expressed as a percentage of total load carried by the foot during standing.** Over 60% of the weight was distributed in the rearfoot and 28% in the ball. Note the importance of the lateral metatarsal heads and also that the toes have little involvement in the weight-bearing process. (Cavanagh PR, Rodgers MM, Liboshi A, et al. Pressure distribution under symptom-free feet during barefoot standing. *Foot Ankle*. 1987;7[5]:269. Copyright ©1987. Reprinted by Permission of SAGE Publications.)

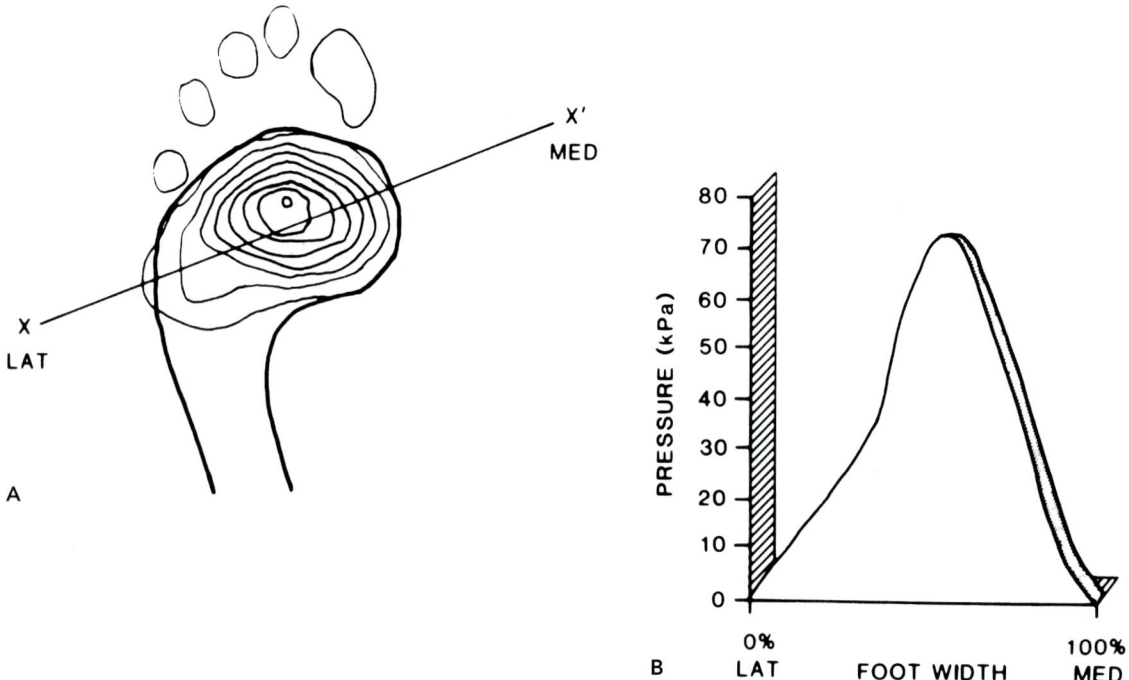

Figure 10.153 **Metatarsal head pressure distribution.** **(A)** A line (XX′) drawn on the contour plot between the approximate location of the first and fifth metatarsal heads. **(B)** The distribution of pressure along the metatarsal head line is determined from the contour plot and drawn as a slice of the forefoot distribution. The foot width is expressed as 100% to allow averaging among subjects. (Cavanagh PR, Rodgers MM, Liboshi A, et al. Pressure distribution under symptom-free feet during barefoot standing. *Foot Ankle.* 1987;7[5]:270. Copyright ©1987. Reprinted by Permission of SAGE Publications.)

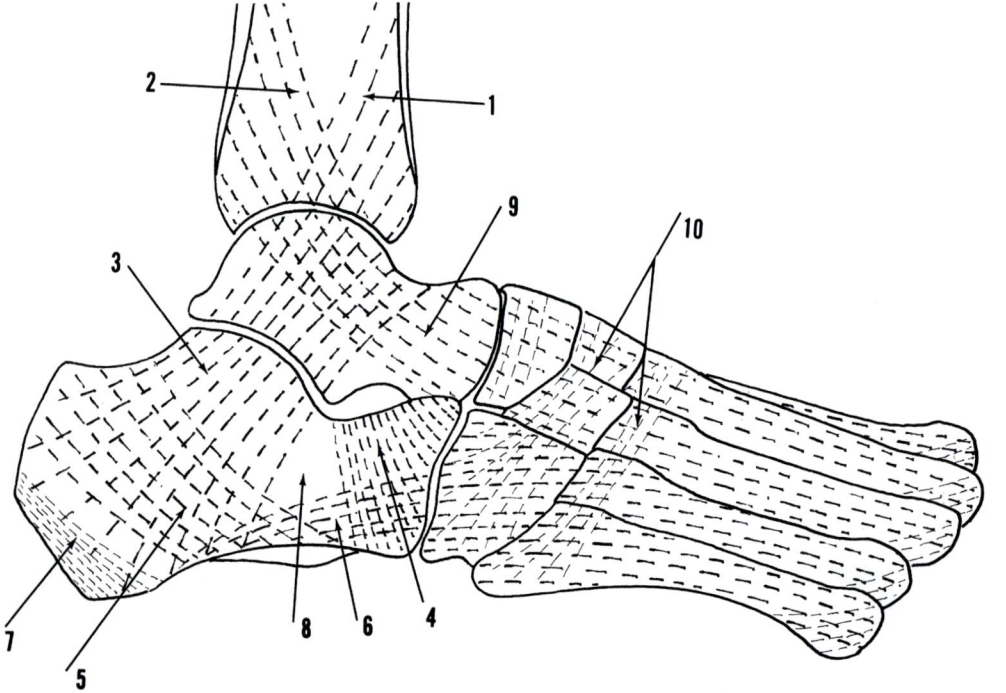

Figure 10.154 **Intraosseous trabecular patterns of the ankle and foot.** The anterior tibial trabecular pattern (*1*) is concave posteriorly and continues into the talus, forming the calcaneal thalamic system (*3*). The posterior tibial trabecular pattern (*2*) is concave anteriorly and continues through the talar body, neck, and head (*9*), the navicular, the cuneiforms, and the metatarsals 3 to 1. The calcaneal anterior apophyseal system (*4*) extends from the sinus tarsi to the cuboidal surface. The posterior (*5*) and anterior (*6*) plantar calcaneal systems delineate with the thalamic and anterior apophyseal systems a neutral zone (*8*) void of trabeculae and form a pseudocavity. The dense posterior calcaneal trabeculae (*7*) correspond to the insertion of the Achilles tendon. The anterior plantar calcaneal trabeculae continue through the cuboid and the metatarsals 4, 5. Midtarsal transverse trabeculae (*10*) cross the longitudinal system.

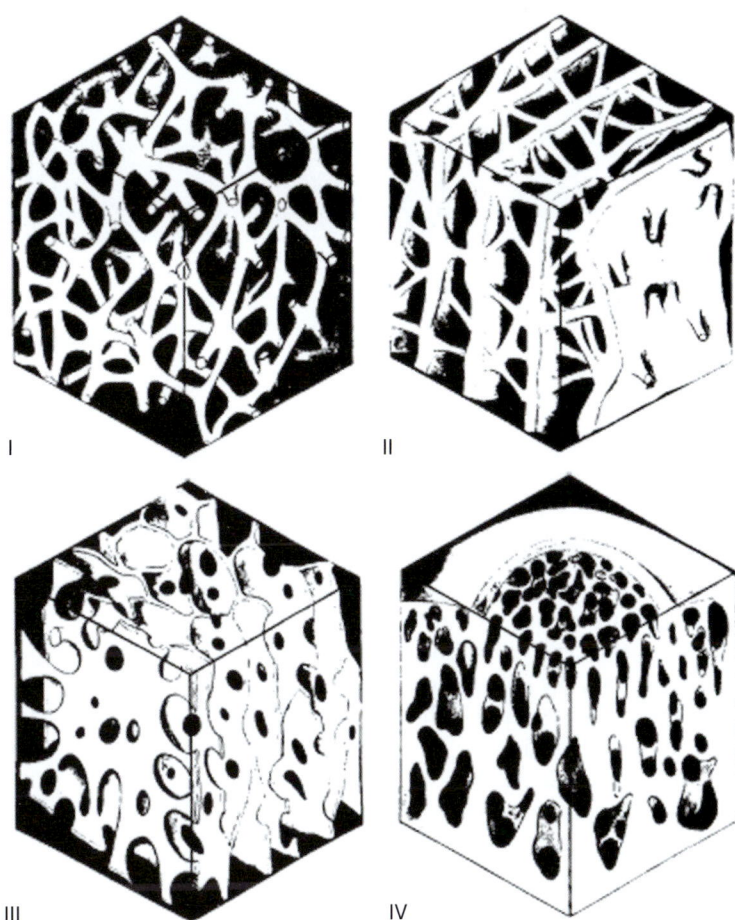

Figure 10.155 Cancellous bone types. Type I: made up entirely of fine rods anastomosing to form a meshwork. Type IIc: consisting of plates arranged parallel to each other. The plates are separated by spaces traversed by rods that appear to hold the plates apart. Type IIIb: Made up entirely of plates parallel to each other. The individual plates have numerous fenestrations. The plates bound longitudinal spaces and form a meshwork as seen from the top. They enclose tubular spaces, oriented parallel to each other. Type IIIc: solid mass of bone fenestrated by irregular spaces. (Republished with permission of John Wiley, from Singh I. The architecture of cancellous bone. *J Anat.* 1978;127[2]:307, Figures 1–4; permission conveyed through Copyright Clearance Center, Inc.)

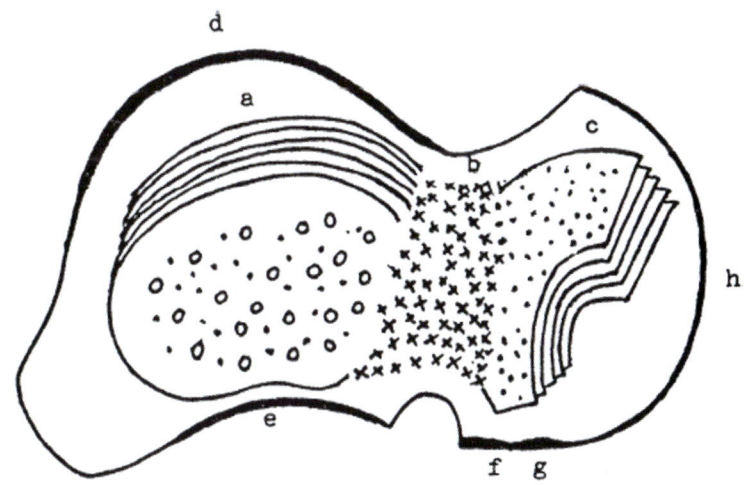

Figure 10.156 Diagrammatic representation of the trabecular architecture of the right talus as seen from the medial aspect. The body of the talus consists of vertical plates (a), the neck shows the trabecular meshwork of irregularly arranged plates (b), and head consists of semiarched plates (c). The proximal end of the horizontal limb of semiarched plates also extends into the distal half of the neck. The distal ends of the vertical and horizontal limbs of semiarched plates are shown with cut edges to demonstrate the semiarched nature. (From Pal GP, Routal RV. Architechture of the cancellous bone of the human talus. *Anat Rec.* 1998;252:190, Figure 8.)

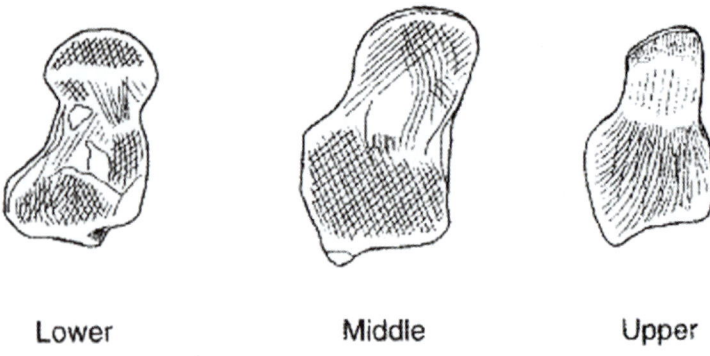

Figure 10.157 Horizontal axial sections of the talus: upper, middle, and lower indicating orientation and density of trabeculae. (Ebraheim NA, Sabry FF, Nadim Y. Internal architecture of the talus: implication for talar fracture. *Foot Ankle Int.* 1999;20[12]:794-796, Figure 1a. Copyright ©1999. Reprinted by Permission of SAGE Publications.)

These plates had two limbs: vertical and horizontal. Posteriorly the vertical plates were continuous with the trabecular meshwork of the neck and anteriorly extended up to the navicular area of the head (Fig. 10.156).

Ebraheim et al[119] investigated the internal architecture of the talus in 13 specimens through coronal, sagittal, and transverse section-slices of 0.5-mm thickness. In the transverse section, upper part, the trabeculae run in the long axis of the talus. These trabeculae are dense in the body of the talus and thin, less dense in the neck region.

In the transverse sections, midsegment, the head and the body portions have dense interlacing trabeculae. The neck region has few trabeculae.

In the lower transverse sections, the same trabecular pattern is identified in the head and the body. The neck trabeculae are more dense and longitudinal in orientation (Fig. 10.157).[4] The authors correlated the high level of talar neck fracture—50% of all talar fractures—with the small number of trabeculae in the neck of the talus.

Athavale et al[120] investigated the internal architecture of the talus in 50 specimens. They describe a regular arrangement of lamellae extending from the talar body, through the neck, reaching the head of the talus (Fig. 10.158).[5] More specifically, on a transverse-horizontal section of the talus, sagittal plates originate from the posteromedial aspect of the body, extend anteriorly through the neck, and continue as curved blades in the head.

The plates arising from the lateral part of the body are initially coronal in orientation. Those arising from the anterior third curve anteriorly, cross the neck, and terminate in the head as curved blades. The plates arising laterally from the posterior two-thirds curve posteriorly and run in the sagittal plane. These lateral plates are perpendicular to both the trochlear surface and to the lateral articular surface of the talus and "are suited to transmit forces to and from the tibia and fibula, respectively." The medially located sagittal plates can transmit forces to the posterior calcaneal facet and anteriorly to the middle and anterior calcaneal facets and to the navicular.

Within the os calcis, four trabecular systems are recognized: thalamic, anterior apophyseal, and plantar (posterior and anterior). The thalamic trabecular system is the continuation within the os calcis of the anterior tibial and talar trabecular system, as described above. The anterior apophyseal system is more or less vertical in direction. It originates from the floor of the sinus tarsi and terminates on the cuboid surface of the os calcis and the anterior segment of the plantar surface. The posterior plantar trabecular arrangement originates from the dorsal and posterior surfaces of the os calcis; the trabeculae are directed downward and anteriorly with an anterior concavity and terminate on the mid plantar aspect of the os calcis. The anterior plantar trabecular system originates from the inferior surface of the cuboidal surface of the os calcis; the trabeculae are directed downward and posteriorly with a plantar concavity and terminate also on the mid plantar segment of the bone. A fifth trabecular pattern may be recognized, corresponding to the insertion of the Achilles tendon. The four major calcaneal trabecular patterns delineate a triangular intertrabecular zone located under the lateral angle of the sinus tarsi and the anterolateral aspect of the posterior calcaneal surface.[121] This is the weaker segment of the os calcis, void of trabeculae, and forms a medullary pseudocavity. It yields easily and fractures under pressure exerted by the lateral wedge-shaped process of the talus (Figs. 10.159 and 10.160).[121,122] The plantar calcaneal trabecular system continues through the cuboid and the lateral two metatarsals. A transverse trabecular system is present in the midfoot and forms a cross pattern with the longitudinally oriented trabeculae.[9]

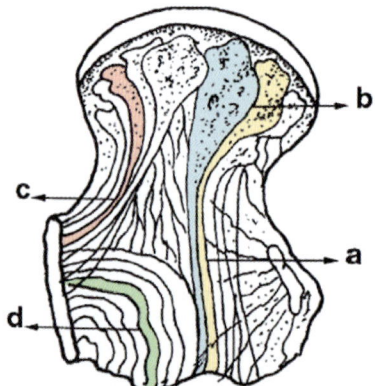

Figure 10.158 Schematic diagram showing horizontal section of left talus when viewed from superior aspect showing sagittal plates (a) in the medial part of body extending through the neck to continue as curved plates (b) in the head. Lamellae in the lateral part of body are initially coronal and then from the anterior one-third curve anteriorly (c) and from posterior two-third curve posteriorly (d) and run in the sagittal plane. (Athavale SA, Joshi SD, Joshi SS. Internal architecture of talus. *Foot Ankle Int.* 2008;1:82-86, Figure 7. Copyright ©2008. Reprinted by Permission of SAGE Publications.)

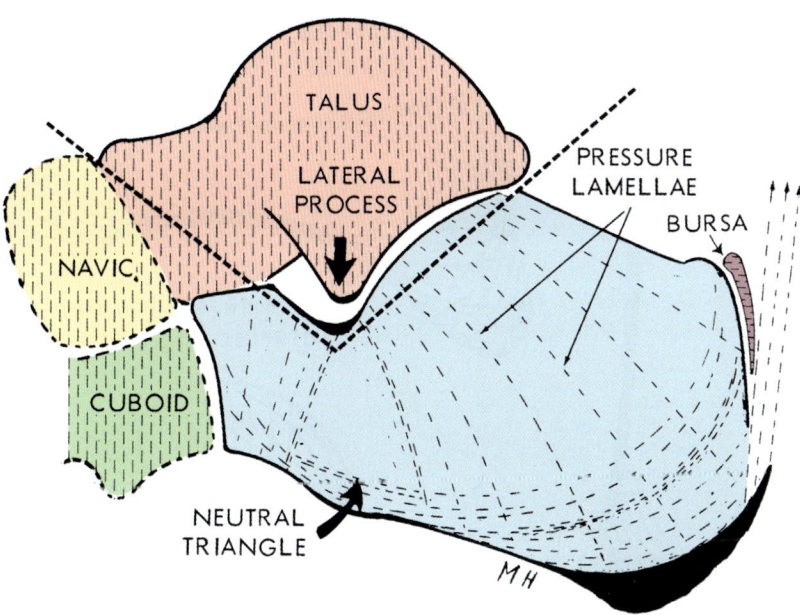

Figure 10.159 **The neutral triangle of the os calcis.** (Reprinted from Harty M. Anatomic considerations in injuries of the calcaneus. *Orthop Clin North Am.* 1973;4[1]:179, with permission from Elsevier.)

Viladot Perice[73] provides a detailed description of the osseous trabecular pattern in the metatarsals and the phalanges based on 136 osseous-section studies by Roig Puerta.[123]

The first metatarsal has three trabecular patterns: superior longitudinal, inferior longitudinal, and proximal transverse (Fig. 10.161). The superior longitudinal trabeculae originate in the upper segment of the epiphysis where they have a uniform distribution. They are curved with inferior concavity. No trabeculae are present in the diaphysis. In the distal metaphysis, the trabeculae fan out and are directed downward and medially with inferior concavity and interlace with the counterpart trabeculae directed externally.

The inferior longitudinal trabeculae originate proximally from the lower half of the epiphysis, interlace with the previous ones, and are more horizontal. These trabeculae condense in the diaphysis and fan out in the distal metaphysis, are directed upward and outward, and interlace with the previous trabecular system.

The transverse trabeculae in the proximal epiphysis cross the longitudinal trabeculae at nearly 90°. They fan out in the direction of the lateral facet corresponding to the second metatarsal. No transverse trabeculae are present in the distal epiphysis.

The second metatarsal, representative of the central metatarsals, also has three trabecular systems: superior longitudinal, inferior longitudinal, and transverse. The superior longitudinal trabeculae originate from the superior segment of the posterior surface and are grouped in internal, superior, and external trabeculae. They all coalesce with the dorsal cortex more precociously than in the first metatarsal. In the distal metaphysis, they fan out and are directed toward the inferior segment

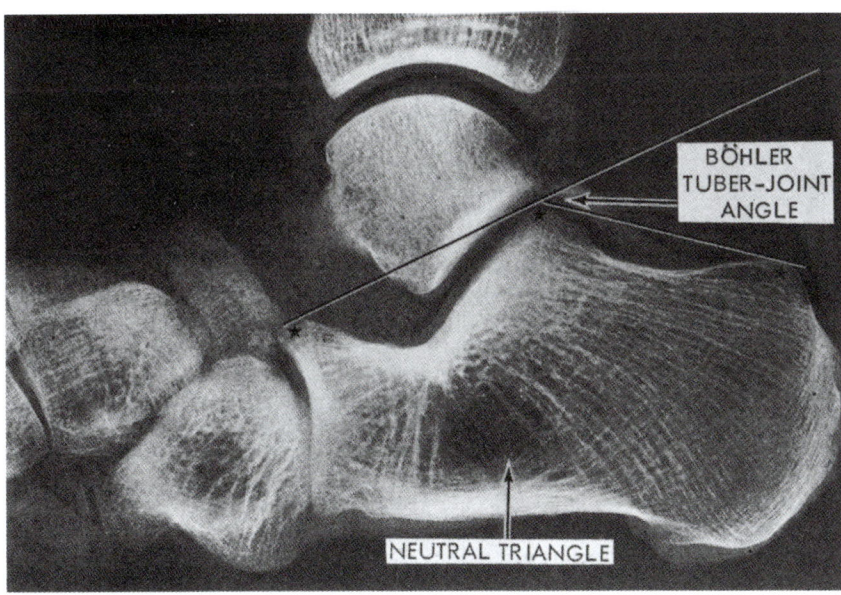

Figure 10.160 **Intracalcaneal trabecular pattern and the neutral triangle.** (Reprinted from Harty M. Anatomic considerations in injuries of the calcaneus. *Orthop Clin North Am.* 1973;4[1]:179, with permission from Elsevier.)

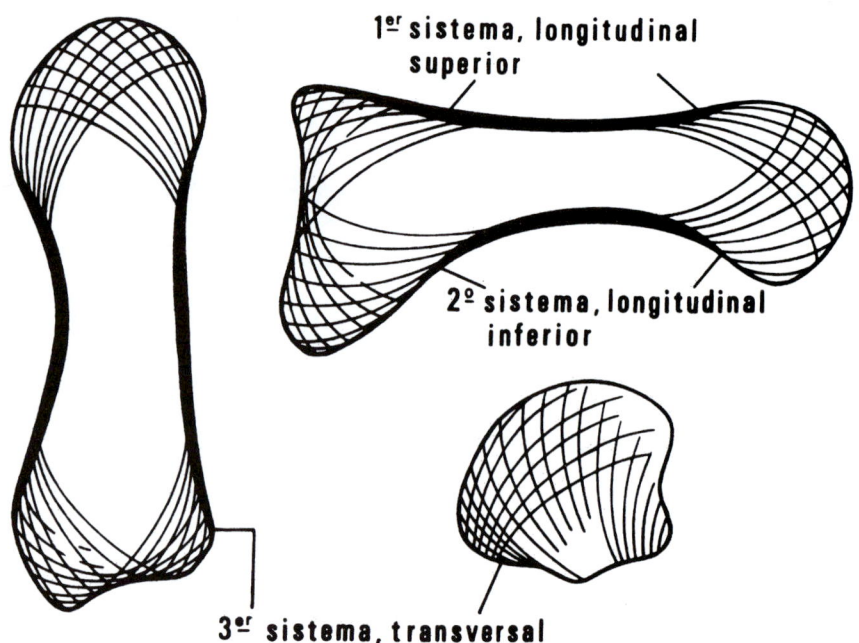

Figure 10.161 Trabecular pattern of the first metatarsal (longitudinal superior, longitudinal inferior, and transverse proximal). (From Viladot Perice A. *Patologia del Antepie*. Ediciones Toray; 1974:10.)

of the epiphysis, crisscrossing the ascending trabeculae (Fig. 10.162). The inferior longitudinal trabeculae originate from the inferior segment of the posterior surface and condense in the diaphyseal cortex. They fan out in the distal metaphysis and are directed toward the anterior and superior segment of the epiphysis, interlacing with the opposite group. The transverse trabeculae of the proximal epiphysis have a posterior convexity perpendicular to the longitudinal systems. They originate from the articular facets corresponding to the adjacent metatarsals. The internal transverse trabeculae are directed outward, whereas the external transverse trabeculae are directed inward, providing solidity to the metatarsal structure. This transverse system does not exit distally. The first and second trabecular systems of the fifth metatarsal have the same characteristics as the system of the other lesser metatarsals (Fig. 10.163). However, because of the presence of the apophysis, the trabeculae of the first system are more dense and abundant with a greater curvature, interweaving with the also abundant transverse trabeculae. The third transverse trabecular system originates from the articular surface corresponding to the fourth metatarsal, crosses the longitudinal systems at right angles, and curves toward the lateral surface.

In the proximal phalanx of the big toe, the trabecular pattern of the first and second systems is similar to that of the metatarsal. However, the trabeculae are less dense proximally, condense in the diaphysis, and fan out in the distal epiphysis. The third transverse trabecular system is much more developed than in the metatarsals. It originates not from the articular surface but

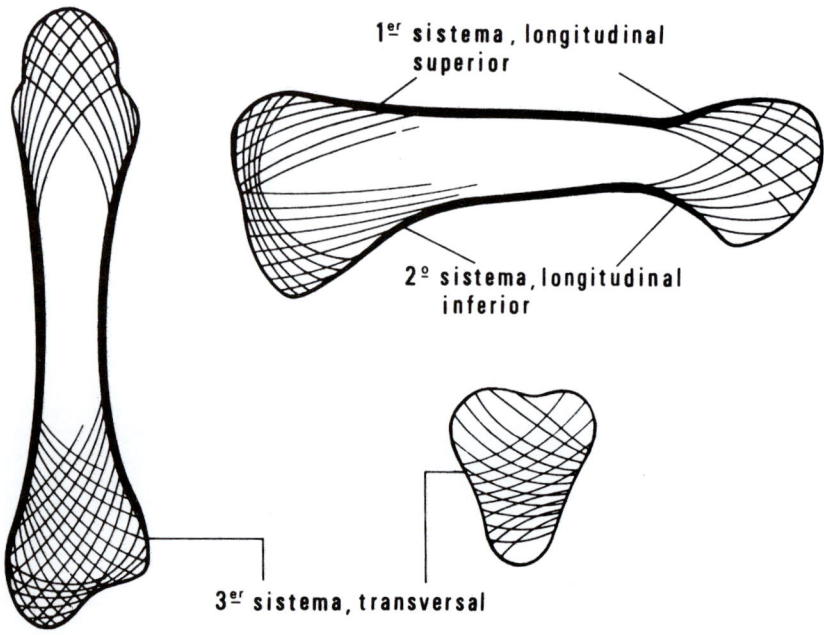

Figure 10.162 Trabecular pattern of the second metatarsal (longitudinal superior, longitudinal inferior, and transverse proximal). (From Viladot Perice A. *Patologia del Antepie*. Ediciones Toray; 1974:11.)

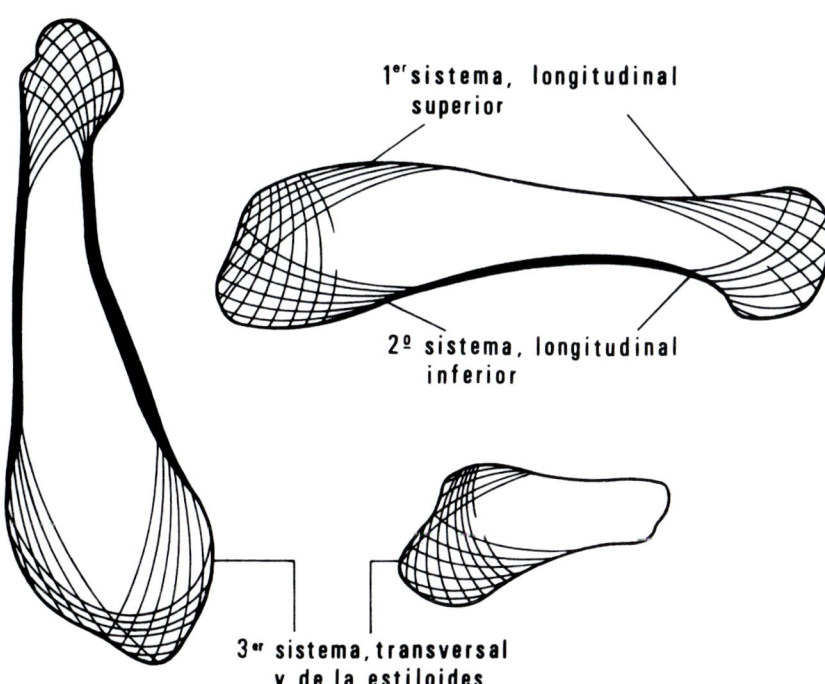

Figure 10.163 Trabecular pattern of the fifth metatarsal (longitudinal superior, longitudinal inferior, transverse proximal, and of the styloid process). (From Viladot Perice A. *Patologia del Antepie*. Ediciones Toray; 1974:12.)

from the cortex and presents a posterior concavity. It extends to the diaphysis and reaches the distal epiphysis, which extension does not occur in the metatarsals.

In the second phalanx of the big toe, the trabecular pattern is much less systematized; however, it is more structured than the trabecular pattern of the distal phalanges of the lesser toes. In the proximal phalanx of the lesser toes, the first and second trabecular systems are identifiable, and their diaphyseal condensations are similar to that of the metatarsals. The third transverse trabecular system is poorly represented and limited exclusively to the proximal epiphysis. In the middle phalanx of the lesser toes, the first and second trabecular systems are also distinguished. They converge into the diaphysis and immediately fan out distally to enlace their trabeculae in the distal epiphysis. The terminal phalanx is not given any functional significance.

LOCOMOTION: GAIT CYCLE

Walking is a bipedal form of locomotion resulting in a forward translation of the body. Constant maintenance of the body equilibrium is a prerequisite for the successful outcome of this transfer activity. For the body to be in equilibrium, the gravitational force or body weight, acting on the center of gravity, should pass through the supporting surface of the foot or through the support base defined by both feet joined anteriorly and posteriorly by a double tangent.[124] The foot contact surface may be complete or limited to the tip of the toes, and during locomotion the support base changes constantly in configuration and size. The leading lower extremity is placed on the ground, heel first, oriented in a forward diagonal direction and creating a restraining force. The body and its center of gravity move forward.

The gravity line passes sequentially through the support base and the single foot surface. The opposite foot is off the ground, and the implanted lower extremity is now oriented obliquely backward in a propulsion mode. As the gravity line passes forward beyond the supporting surface of the foot, the balance is lost but regained with the opposite heel touching the ground. "It is quite proper, therefore, to designate the human gait as a constant play between loss and recovery of the equilibrium."[125] The coordination involved in maintaining a constant relationship between the gravitational line and the supporting surface requires a high degree of neural control.

▶ General Description

Walking is a rhythmic motor activity. All body parts participate. There is an alternate forward placement of the feet and a synchronous shift of the body weight onto the supportive foot. As one foot supports, the other leg swings forward for preparation of the next support phase. Thus, it is convenient to distinguish a support phase and a swing phase in the gait cycle. The support phase starts with the heel-strike, terminates with the toe off, and occupies 62% of the cycle, whereas the swing phase, which terminates with the next heel-strike of the same foot, occupies 38% of the cycle.[126] A stride is the linear distance from heel-strike to heel-strike of the same foot (Figs. 10.164 and 10.165). Murray and colleagues reported the mean stride length in 60 normal men as 156.5 ± 14 cm and the mean stride width as 8.0 ± 3.5 cm.[127] The foot exorotation or foot angle formed by the long axis of the foot and the line of progression was 6.8° ± 5.6°. There was greater out-toeing in the older age group (60-65 years), which appears to increase the base of support.

The step length is the distance between successive points of foot-to-floor contact of alternate feet (see Fig. 10.165). The mean step length reported in 60 normal men was 78.4 ± 5.9 cm

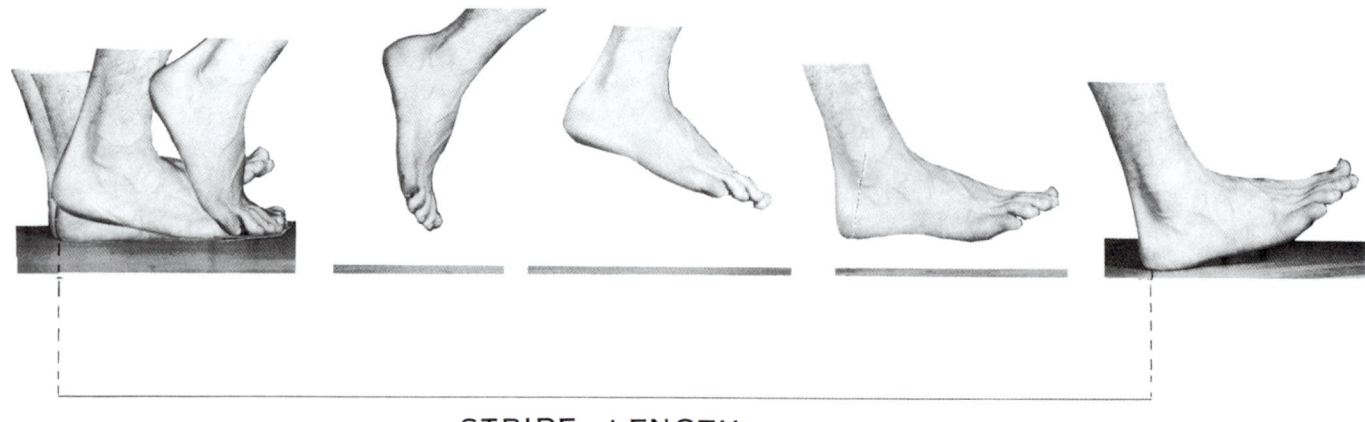

Figure 10.164 The stride is the linear distance from heel-strike to heel-strike of the same foot.

(left to right) and 78.1 ± 6.3 cm (right to left).[128] There are two steps in a stride. The cadence is the number of steps per minute. With a cadence of 112 steps per minute, the mean cycle duration is 1.02 ± 0.10 seconds.[128] "A step frequency of about 110 steps/min can be considered as typical, while step rates below 100 or above 120/min represent slow and fast gait. Comparable gait patterns for women are about 5 steps/min above these levels."[124] The walking velocity is the length of the stride, because the duration of the latter is nearly 1 second. The mean walking velocity is then 156.5 ±14 cm/s in the group of 60 men in the study by Murray and colleagues.[128]

In a study of five experienced joggers, Mann and Hagy report the locomotor velocities as follows: walking, 140 cm/s; jogging, 326 cm/s; running, 536 cm/s.[129] The increased velocity shortens the cycle time from 1 second for walking to 0.7 second for jogging and 0.6 second for running.[129] Furthermore, the number of strides per minute is increased from 58/min for walking to 84/min for jogging and to 100/min for running. This is accompanied by an increase of the stride length from 144 cm in walking to 231 cm in jogging to 322 cm in running.[129] The relationship between step rate/min or frequency and stride length is linear over the range of usual walking speeds of 70 steps/min to 130 steps/min and levels off at fast speeds toward a constant stride length (Fig. 10.166).[124]

Walking Cycle

One walking cycle—from heel-strike to heel-strike of the same foot—is divided into a support phase followed by a swing phase.[124-127,130] The support phase constitutes 62% of the cycle and the swing phase 38% (Figs. 10.167 to 10.169).[126]

Stance Phase

The stance phase is divided into an initial double support phase when both feet are on the ground lasting 12% of the cycle, followed by a single support phase lasting up to 50% of the cycle (Figs. 10.170 and 10.171). During the single support phase, the opposite leg is in the swing phase. The duration of the single support phase end of the opposite swing phase is 38% of the cycle. The single support phase is followed by a second double support phase lasting from 50% to 62% of the cycle, or duration of 12% of the cycle. At 50% of the cycle, the stance phase of the opposite leg is initiated through heel-strike.

On further analysis of the pedal relationship with the ground, at heel-strike the decelerating foot comes down and the heel cushion strikes the ground. A shock wave is generated, which travels in the lower extremity with impulses of up to 100 cycles per second in frequency.[131] After the heel-strike, the foot descends rapidly and its lateral border establishes contact with the ground, followed by the contact of the lateral and then the medial aspect of the ball of the foot. The contact occurs in all five toes at the same time or "by the first and fifth toes together with the ball, followed by a delayed contact of the second, third, and fourth toes."[132] The foot is now in the plantigrade or foot-flat position, which occurs as early as 7% of the walking cycle and continues until 34%. The mid stance is considered occurring at 25% of the cycle.

The foot keeps rolling upward and forward, diminishing progressively its surface contact. The heel rise or heel-off begins at 34% of the cycle and induces hyperextension at the metatarsophalangeal joints. At 62% of the cycle, the toes are off the ground; the swing phase is initiated.

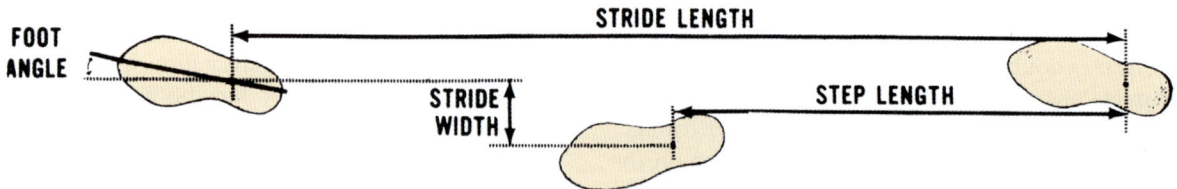

Figure 10.165 The step is the distance between successive points of foot-to-floor contact of alternate feet. There are two steps in a stride. (Adapted from Murray MP, Drought AB, Kory RC. Walking patterns of normal men. *J Bone Joint Surg Am.* 1964;46[2]:335.)

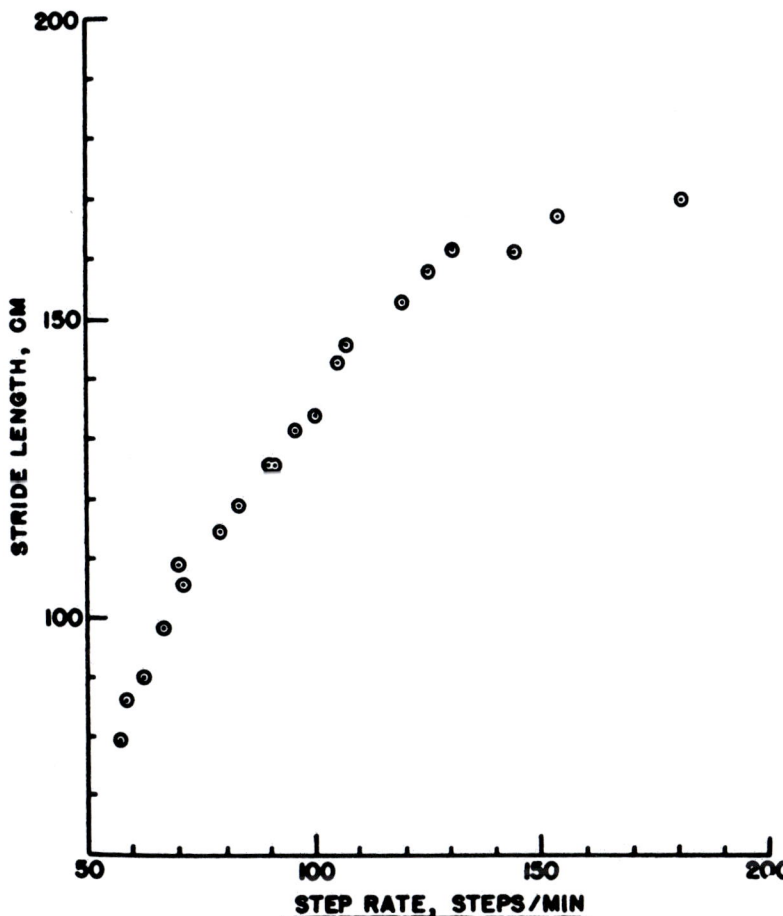

Figure 10.166 Relationship between stride length and step rate. Adult male walking over 43 m course. (Adapted from Inman VT, Ralston HJ, Todd F. *Human Walking.* Williams & Wilkins; 1981:23.)

Swing Phase

The swing phase (see Figs. 10.170 and 10.171) lasts 32% of the cycle and terminates with the ipsilateral heel-strike. The foot is accelerated and plantar flexed. In mid swing, it gradually dorsiflexes, thus clearing the toes from the ground. As the foot descends, it is decelerated and strikes the ground with the ankle at a right angle and the heel in minimal inversion. The walking cycle is completed.

In bipedal walking, there is an overlap of the standing periods during the double support phases. The stance phase is longer than the swing phase. In jogging and running, a period of double float is introduced, during which phase neither leg is in touch with the ground (Fig. 10.172).[125,129] There is an overlap now of the swinging phases: "the swinging of one leg begins while the other is still in the air."[125] Furthermore, in jogging and running, the swinging phase lasts longer than the support phase. The floating phase consumes 20% of the cycle time for jogging and 40% for running.[129]

▶ Kinematics

The kinematics of gait has been extensively analyzed by Braune and Fischer[133] and Inman and colleagues.[124] Further specific studies have been conducted by Levens and coworkers,[134] Saunders and colleagues,[135] Murray and colleagues,[128] Wright and colleagues,[133] Sutherland and Hagy,[136] and Mann and Hagy.[129] During walking, there is a coordinated movement of all the major parts of the body. The displacements occur in the three planes of space. The pelvis and the lower extremities move in phase, whereas the upper back, shoulders, and upper extremities move out of phase relative to the lower segments. When the pelvis rotates in one direction, carrying the lower extremities, the shoulder rotates in the opposite direction, carrying the upper extremities. The rotational transition occurs at the mid thoracic level, T7.[124] Movements of lesser magnitude occur simultaneously in the frontal plane.

▶ Center of Gravity

The body's center of gravity is intrapelvic, anterior to the second sacral vertebra, on the midline, at a distance from the ground corresponding to 55% of the total stature ±1.25% (Fig. 10.173A).[124,135-137] In normal walking, the center of gravity describes a low-amplitude sinusoidal curve in the sagittal plane of progress (Fig. 10.173B). The vertical oscillation or displacement of the center of gravity is 5 cm maximum at the usual speed of walking. During a cycle of two steps, two maxima occur at 25% and 75% of the cycle, which correspond to the middle of the single foot stance phase alternately. At 50% of the cycle, the center of gravity is at its lowest level (Fig. 10.174). At the maximum vertical displacement, the center of gravity is

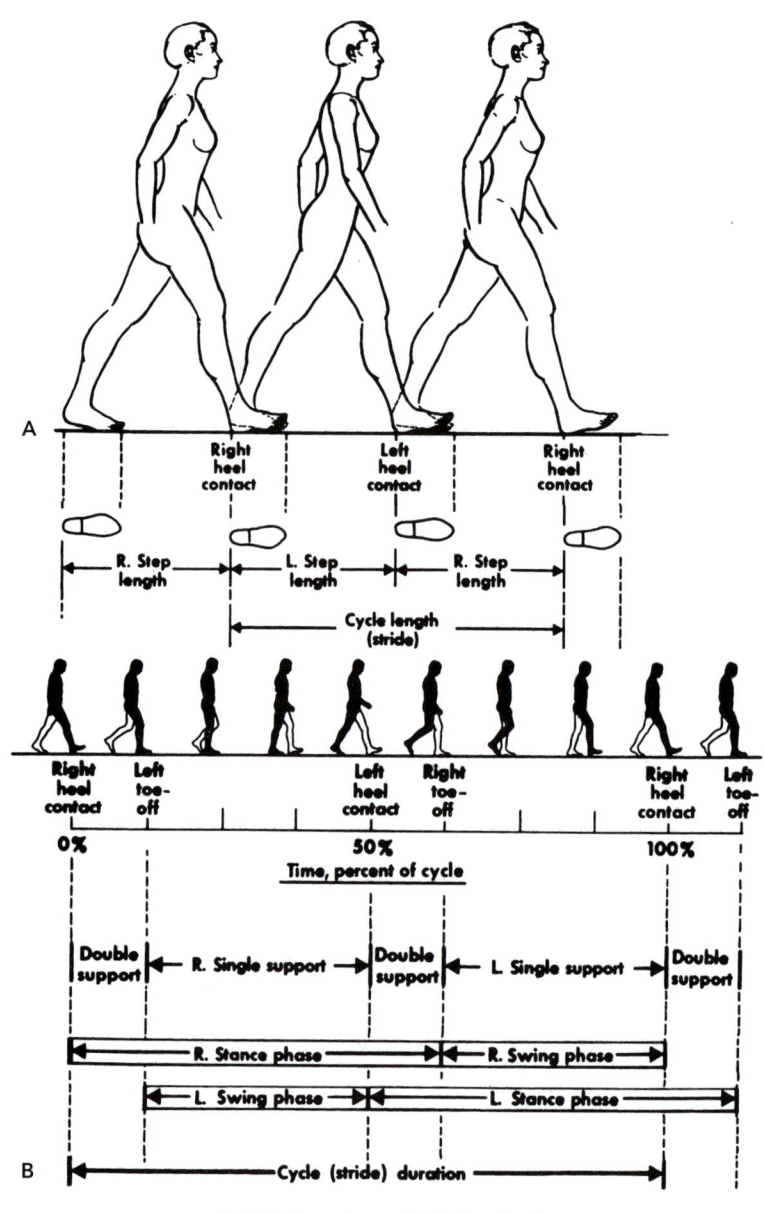

Figure 10.167 Distance and time dimensions of walking cycle. **(A)** Distance (length). **(B)** Time. (From Inman VT, Ralston HJ, Todd F. *Human Walking*. Williams & Wilkins; 1981:26.)

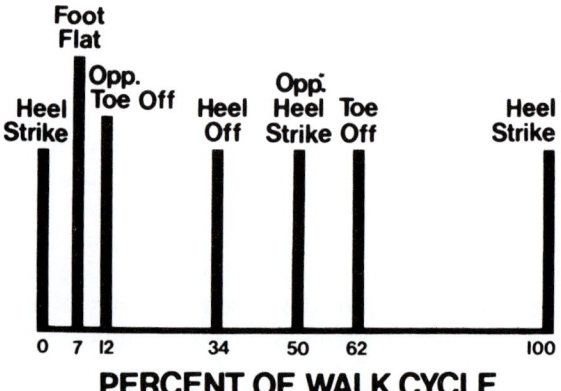

Figure 10.168 Events of the walking cycle. (Reprinted from Mann RA. Overview of foot and ankle biomechanics in disorders of the foot and ankle. In: Jahss MM, ed. *Medical and Surgical Management*. 2nd ed. WB Saunders; 1991:386.)

slightly lower than the corresponding center of gravity in the standing position; thus, a person is shorter while walking.

The center of gravity is also displaced laterally in the horizontal plane, describing a sinusoidal curve of displacement passing to the right and to the left alternately (Fig. 10.175), their maxima corresponding to the summits of the sinusoidal curve of the sagittal plane (see Fig. 10.174). Thus, when the center of gravity is maximally raised, it is also maximally shifted to the right or to the left. This lateral displacement is 4.5 cm, and the corresponding sinusoidal curve has half the frequency of the vertical curve.

▶ **Pelvic Motion and Transverse Segmental Rotations of the Lower Extremity**

The pelvis rotates alternately to the right and to the left in the horizontal plane during the forward progression of walking

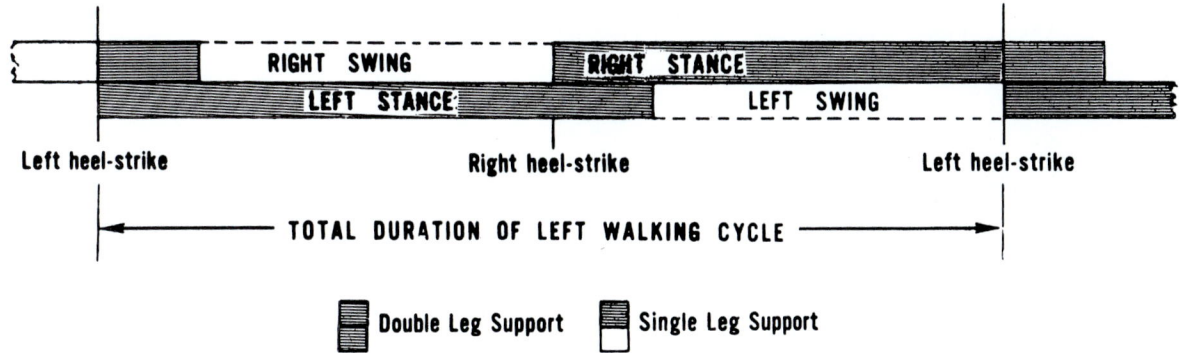

Figure 10.169 **Left walking cycle, showing the temporal relationships of stance, swing, double limb support, and single limb support.** (From Murray MP, Drought AB, Kory RC. Walking patterns of normal men. *J Bone Joint Surg Am.* 1964;46[2]:335.)

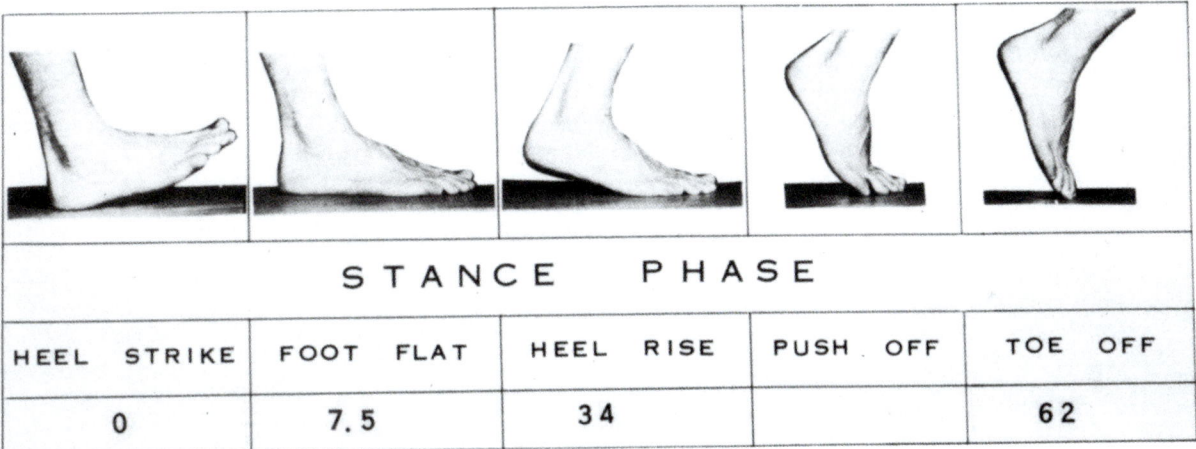

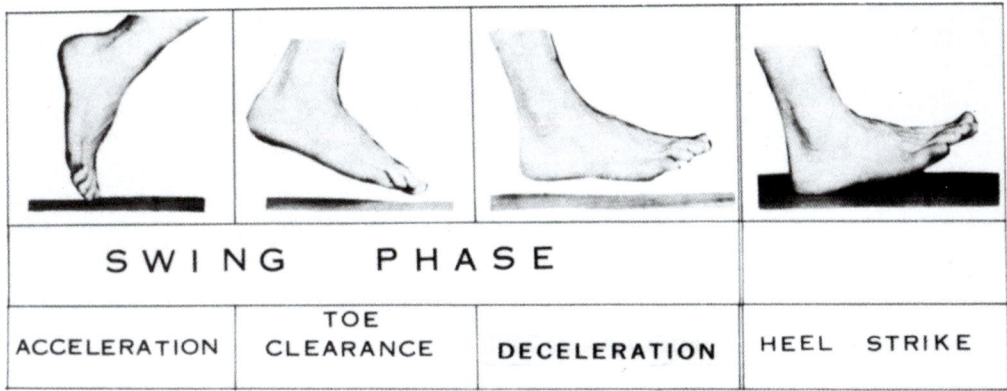

Figure 10.170 Walking cycle.

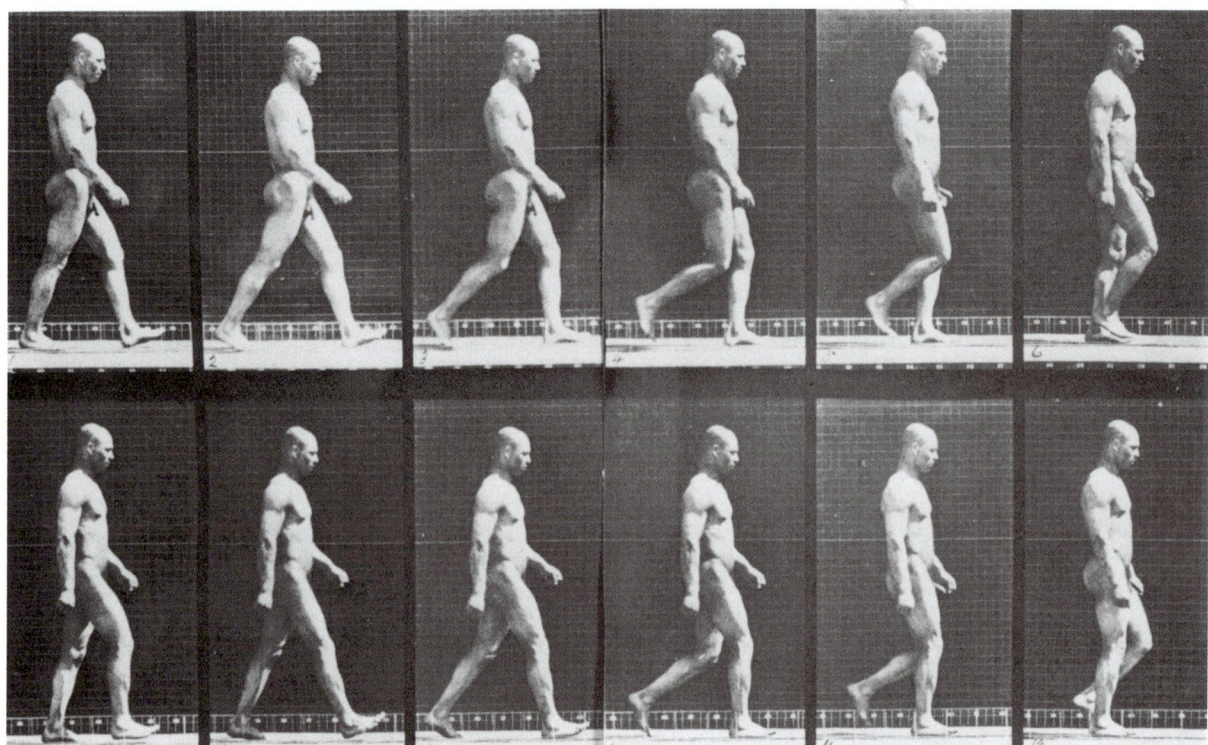

Figure 10.171 **Man walking.** (Republished with permission of Dover Publications, from Muybridge E. *The Human Figure in Motion*. Dover Publications; 1955. Permission conveyed through Copyright Clearance Center, Inc.)

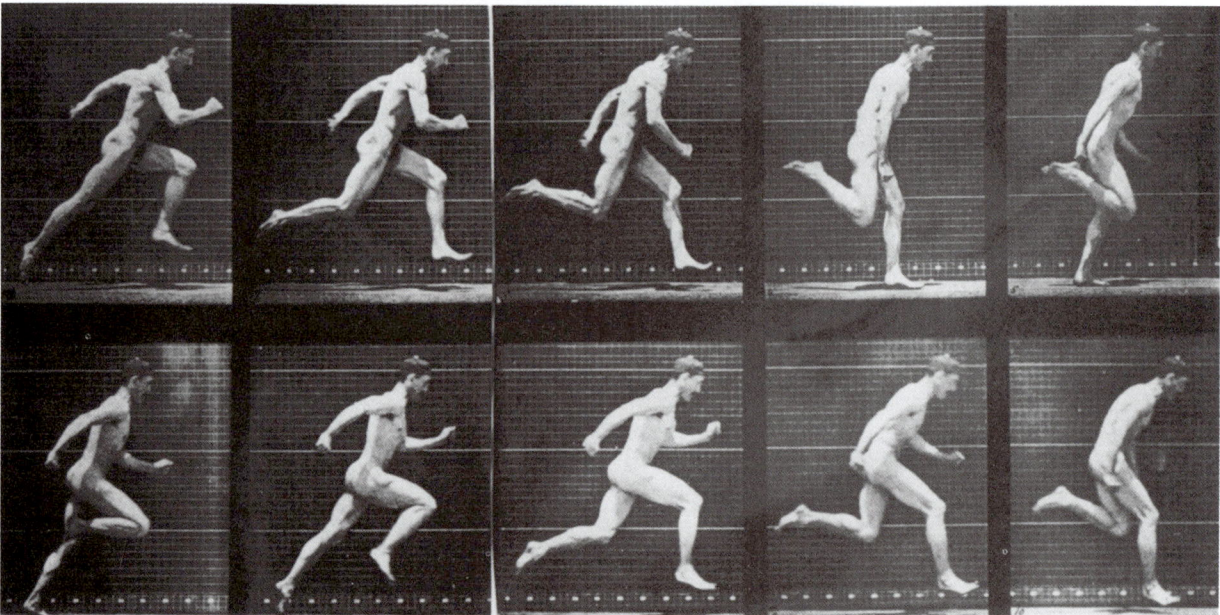

Figure 10.172 **Man running.** (Republished with permission of Dover Publications, from Muybridge E. *The Human Figure in Motion*. Dover Publications; 1955.)

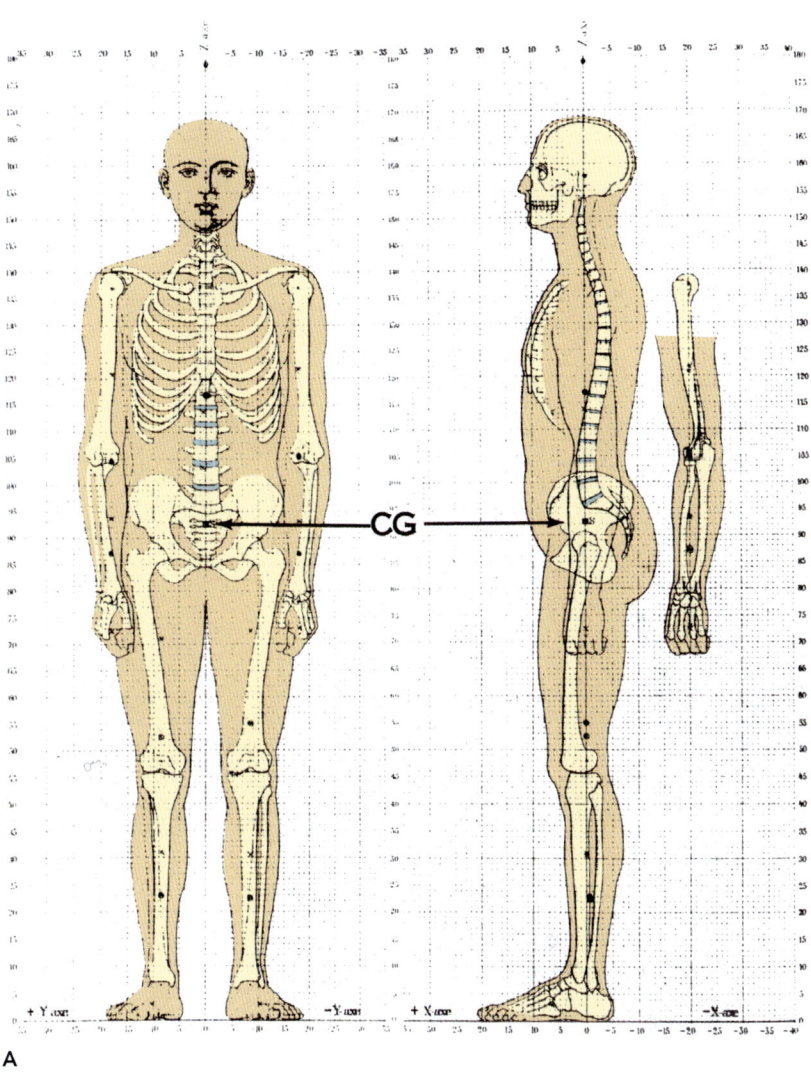
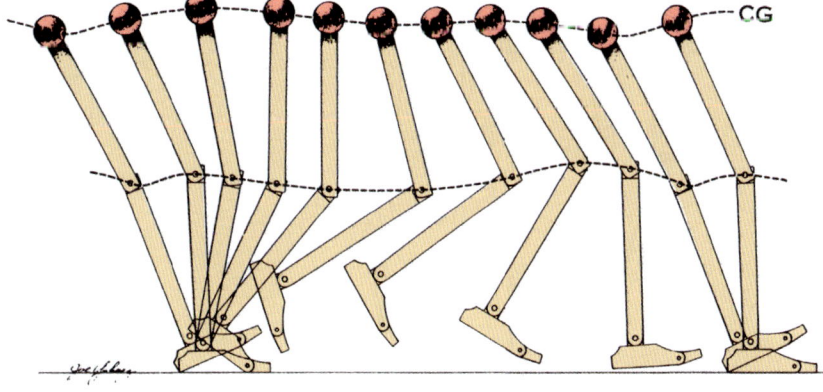

Figure 10.173 (A) Normal attitude of the human body and the center of gravity (*CG*). (B) Pathway of the center of gravity (*CG*) in walking at moderate speed. The path is sinusoidal in the sagittal plane of progress. (A, Adapted from Braune W, Fischer O. *On the Center of Gravity of the Human Body*. Springer-Verlag; 1985:26. B, Adapted from Saunders JB, Dec M, Inman VT, et al. The major determinants in normal and pathological gait. *J Bone Joint Surg Am*. 1953;35[3]:550.)

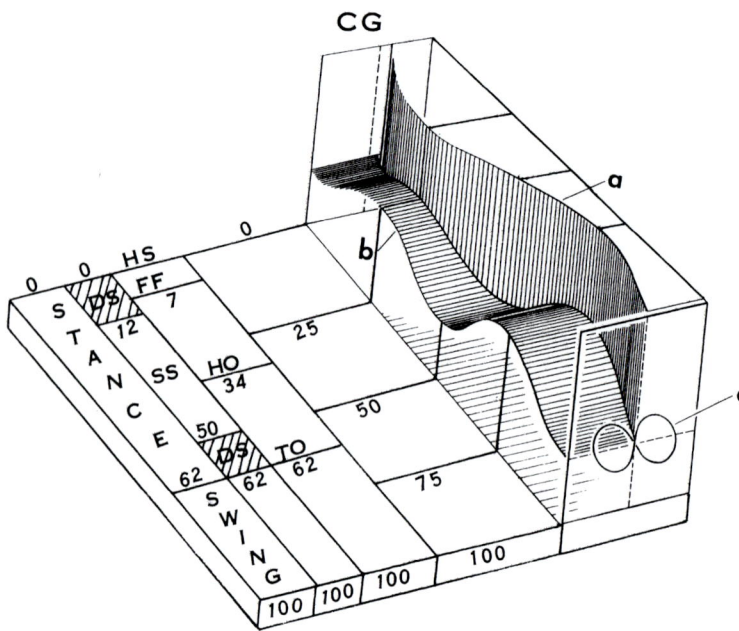

Figure 10.174 **The motion of the center of gravity (CG) during the gait cycle.** The displacement of the CG traces a sinusoidal curve *b* in the sagittal plane and a sinusoidal curve *a* in the transverse plane with a resultant curve *c*. In the sagittal plane, the maximum displacement of the CG occurs at 25% and 75% of the walking cycle, and the lowest point of the CG occurs at 50% of the cycle. (*DS*, double support; *HO*, heel-off; *HS*, heel-strike; *SS*, single support; *TO*, toe off.) The numbers indicate the percentage of the walking cycle.

(Fig. 10.176). Each transverse rotation is about 4° on either side, with a total of near 8°. The rotation occurs at each hip joint corresponding to the weight-bearing extremity. During the transverse pelvic rotation there is also an alternate pelvic tilt of an average of 45° on the side of the swinging lower extremity. This creates a relative adduction of the extremity in the swing phase. The pelvis shifts also laterally 4 to 5 cm toward and over the weight-bearing lower extremity to centralize the gravity line over the support foot surface. The physiologic femorotibial angle helps to maintain the feet surfaces closer during the forward progression, thus minimizing the obligatory lateral pelvic side-to-side shift.[124,134-136]

During the walking cycle, under weight-bearing, inward and outward rotations of the corresponding lower extremity segments occur.

Inward rotation occurs during the phase from minimal weight-bearing to full weight-bearing, and outward rotation occurs during the next phase from full weight-bearing to minimal weight-bearing.

There is a gradient to the transverse rotation, being minimum in the proximal segments and maximum distally.

The pelvis, the femur, and the tibia rotate inward from heel-strike to 17% of the walking cycle and then rotate externally from 17% of the cycle to toe-off. The total range of transverse rotation is as follows: pelvis average, 7.7° (range, 3°-13.3°); femur average, 15.3° (range, 8.6°-24.8°); tibia average, 19.3° (range, 13.4°-25.6°). Specifically, the transverse tibial rotation relative to the ground with the foot fixed on the floor is approximately 7° inward rotation from 7% to 17% of the walking cycle and approximately 8° outward rotation from 17% to 43% of the walking cycle. The transverse rotation of the femur relative to the pelvis is an average 8.4° (range, 4.9°-11.4°), and the rotation of the tibia relative to the femur is 8.7° (range, 4.1°-13.3°).

Distally, the transverse rotation is transmitted to and absorbed by the ankle-foot complex. The obliquity of the ankle joint axis in the coronal plane contributes, to a limited degree, to the absorption of the transverse rotation, because dorsiflexion or anterior flexion of the leg is accompanied by external

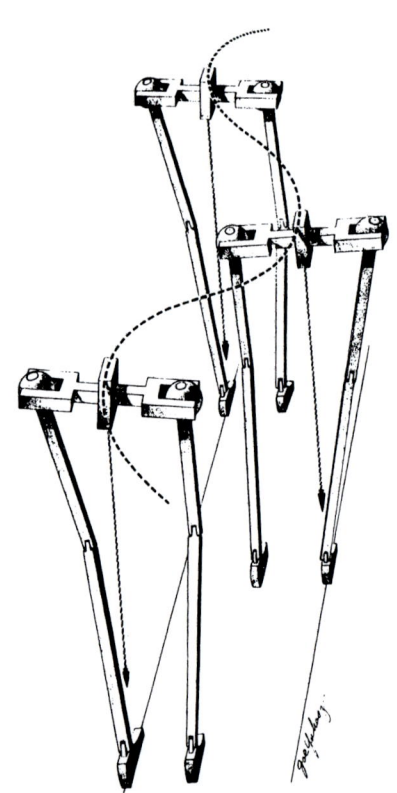

Figure 10.175 **Pathway of the center of gravity in the transverse plane during the walking cycle.** The pathway is sinusoidal. During each step, the body is displaced over the weight-bearing leg. With a wide walking phase (stride width), the amplitude is large. (From Saunders JB, Dec M, Inman VT, et al. The major determinants in normal and pathological gait. *J Bone Joint Surg Am*. 1953;35[3]:552.)

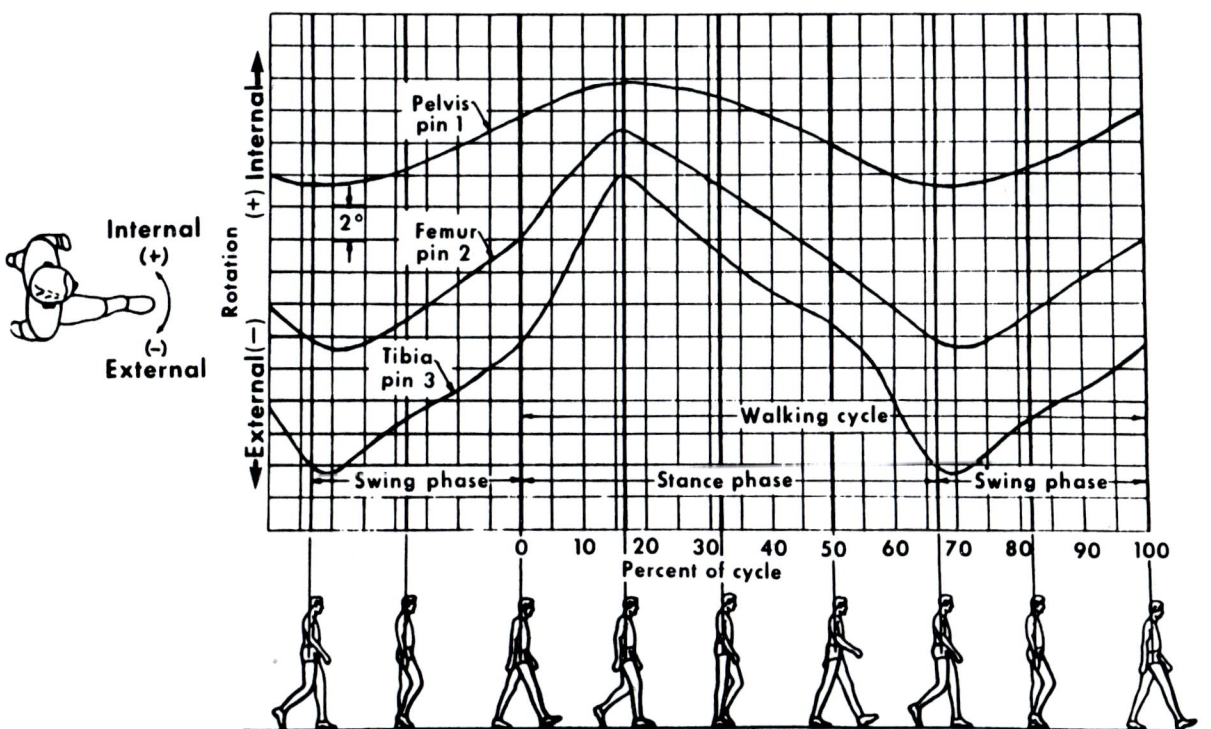

Figure 10.176 Rotations of pelvis, femur, and tibia in transverse plane: composite curves of 19 young male adults. (From Levens AS, et al. Transverse rotation of the segments of the lower extremity in locomotion. *J Bone Joint Surg Am.* 1948;30:802.)

rotation of the foot or a relative internal rotation of the leg. Conversely, with the plantar flexion of the foot or extension of the leg, there is a relative external rotation of the leg. The degree of rotation is in proportion to the obliquity of the ankle joint axis.

The next major or transmission conversion of the tibial transverse rotation occurs at the level of the subtalar joint, which has been qualified by Inman as a directional torque transmitter.[10] The obliquely oriented axis of the subtalar joint contributes in converting the transverse rotation of the leg into a triplane motion with a major component in the coronal plane in the form of supination-pronation at the subtalar joint. Internal rotation of the leg is associated with pronation or valgus or eversion of the heel, and external rotation of the leg is associated with supination or varus or inversion of the heel.

Wright and colleagues determined the contribution of the subtalar joint during the gait cycle (Fig. 10.177).[133] At heel-strike, the subtalar joint is slightly supinated (inversion), followed by pronation (eversion), which peaks at foot-flat and is maintained during the major portion of the stance phase. Just prior to heel-off (34% of the cycle), the subtalar joint is supinated (inversion) and reaches a maximum near 60% of the cycle. This is followed by a gradual pronation (eversion) at the subtalar joint, which brings the joint close to the neutral position during the swing phase. The motion at the subtalar joint during the stance phase of the walking cycle ranges from 5.9° to 6.9°.

According to Mann, the internal rotation of the lower extremity is initiated distally through the subtalar pronation under weight-bearing and is transmitted to the proximal joints.[126] The external rotation of the weight-bearing extremity is initiated proximally through the swinging opposite lower extremity, producing the external rotation of the pelvis of the stance leg. This external rotation is transmitted distally and is further enhanced by the obligatory external rotation of the leg through its anterior flexion during the stance phase. This external rotation is determined by the obliquity of the ankle joint axis. Additional external rotation of the leg occurs—as of heel rise—through the metatarsal break along the oblique axis oriented posterolaterally.

▶ Motion in the Sagittal Plane

At heel-strike, the hip is flexed, the knee is extended, and the ankle is in near neutral. Subsequently, during the stance phase the hip extends, whereas the knee flexes and then extends; the ankle plantar flexes, then dorsiflexes.[124,126,128,130,132,134] During the swing, the hip flexes and remains flexed (Fig. 10.178). The knee joint is also flexed initially, followed by further rapid flexion, which is followed in the last third of the walking cycle by extension of the knee. The ankle is initially plantar flexed during the swing phase, followed by dorsiflexion to neutral. The specific angular relationships at the hip-knee, ankle, and

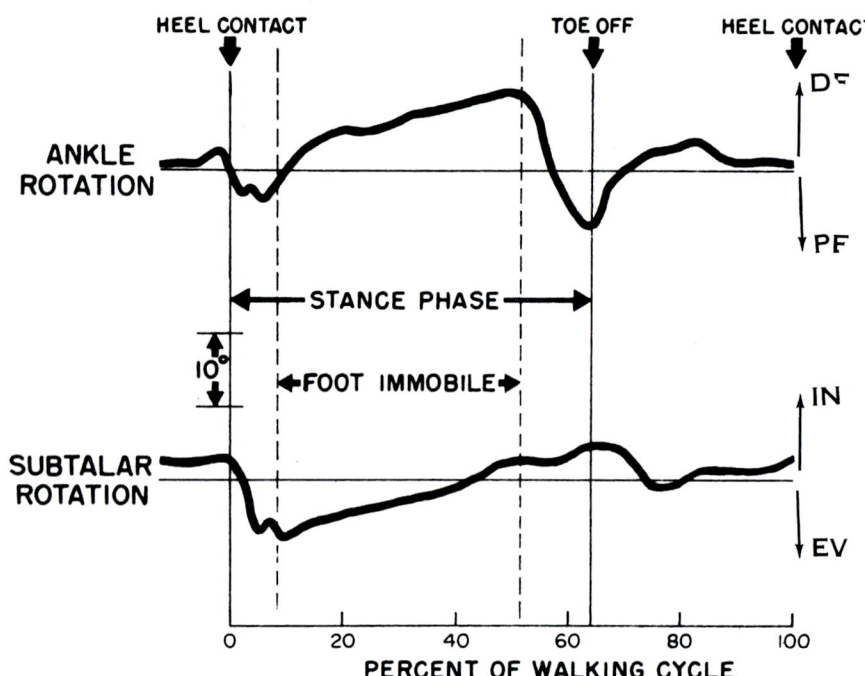

Figure 10.177 Ankle and subtalar rotations during normal walking. (From Wright DC, Desai SM, Henderson WH, et al. Action of the subtalar and ankle joint complex during the stance phase of walking. *J Bone Joint Surg Am.* 1964;46[2]:372.)

metatarsophalangeal joints in the sagittal plane are as follows in walking at average speed[130]:

Stance Phase
Heel-strike
  Hip: flexed 25° to 30°
  Knee: nearly extended
  Ankle: neutral or slightly plantar flexed
Foot-flat: 7.5% of cycle
  Hip: extension initiated; flexion reduced to 20° to 23°
  Knee: flexed 20°
  Ankle: plantar flexed (relative extension of leg)
Mid stance: 25% of cycle
  Hip: continues to extend; flexed 10°
  Knee: extends; flexion reduced to 10°
  Ankle: dorsiflexed 2° to 3° (relative flexion of leg)
Heel-off: 34% of cycle
  Hip: extended 10°
  Knee: further extended; flexion reduced to 2°
  Ankle: dorsiflexed 10° to 15° (relative flexion of leg)
Toe-off: 62% of cycle
  Hip: flexed 10°
  Knee: flexed 40°
  Ankle: plantar flexed 20°

Swing Phase
Acceleration
  Hip: flexed 30° to 50°
  Knee: flexed 65°
  Ankle: plantar flexed 22°
Mid swing
  Hip: flexed 25°
  Knee: flexed 65°
  Ankle: dorsiflexed to neutral for toe clearance

Deceleration
  Hip: flexed 25°
  Knee: extended to 0°
  Ankle: near neutral

▶ Function of the Toes

The toes are in contact with the ground during 75% of the stance phase of the walking cycle. This is initiated at foot-flat and lasts until toe-off.

Bojsen-Møller and Lamoreux analyzed the dorsiflexion of the toes in 21 young individuals with normal feet walking at a rate of approximately 100 steps per minute with a 65-cm length to the step.[98] At heel-strike, the great toe is dorsiflexed 20° to 30°. At foot-flat, the toes are in neutral position at the metatarsophalangeal joint. With rising of the heel, the push-off phase is initiated and the maximum dorsiflexion at the metatarsophalangeal joint is 50° to 60°.

During the unguligrade phase of the cycle, the relative dorsiflexion of the toes is undone, and at its conclusion, only the tip of the great toe and its nail have contact with the ground.

Bojsen-Møller describes the heel-rise and the push-off as taking place at the metatarsophalangeal joints around two primary axes, oblique and transverse (Fig. 10.179).[138] The heel-rise occurs first around the oblique axis, which passes through the metatarsophalangeal joints of the second through the fifth toes. This is followed by the push-off around the transverse axis passing through the metatarsophalangeal joints of the first and second toes. The resistance arm offered against the force-arm of the triceps surae during the push-off varies. This resistance arm is measured as the perpendicular distance from the primary oblique or transverse metatarsophalangeal axis to the secondary axis of the

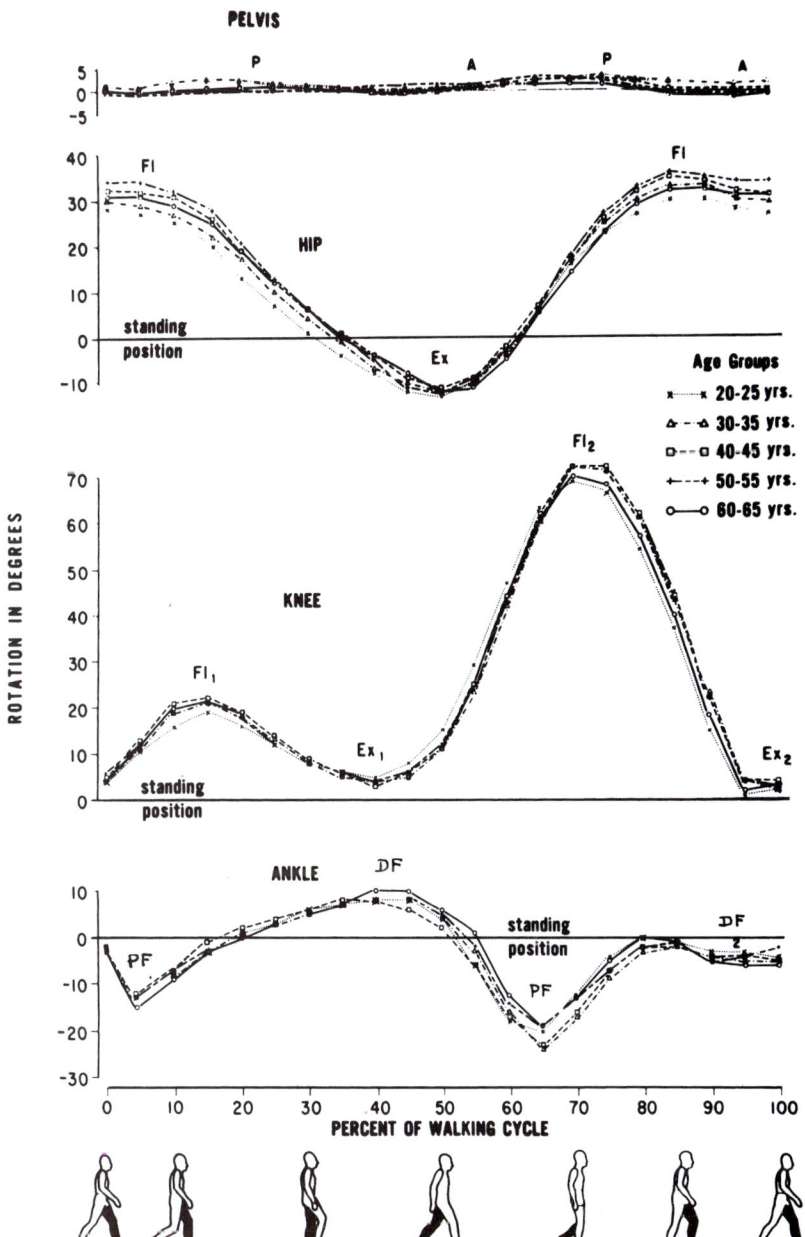

Figure 10.178 Motion in the sagittal plane during walking cycle. Mean patterns of sagittal rotation for five age groups, 12 men in each group, and two trials for each man. The zero reference positions are the angular positions of the respective targets in the standing position. (*A*, downward and forward movement of the anterior aspect of the pelvis; *DF*, dorsiflexion; *Ex*, extension; *Fl*, flexion; *P*, upward and backward movement of the anterior aspect of the pelvis; *PF*, plantar flexion.) (From Murray MP, Drought AB, Kory RC. Walking patterns of normal men. *J Bone Joint Surg Am.* 1964;46[2]:346.)

ankle joint complex (talocrural and subtalar). The mean ratio of the distances of the oblique and transverse axes at the metatarsophalangeal joints is 5/6. Thus, the resistance arm of the foot is 20% longer when the push-off is being performed along the transverse axis. "With the transverse axis, the leverage is further stepped up with the final advancement of the axis to the tip of the strong first toe while with the oblique axis the push-off continues more as a rollover of the ball of the foot."[138] Bojsen-Møller characterizes the motion around the oblique metatarsophalangeal joint axis as a low-gear motion (low speed, high power), and the motion around the transverse axis as a high-gear motion (high speed, low power).[132,138] The ratio between the gears is 5/6. The high gear is used for sprinting and the low gear for uphill walking with loads and in the first step of a sprint. The push-off starts with low gear and changes gradually into high gear.

▶ The Anatomic Basis of the Functional Remodeling and Stability of the Foot-Plate During Locomotion

The lamina pedis is axially loaded by the tibiotalar column in three ways: in neutral rotation, internal rotation, and external rotation.

The response of the lamina pedis to the rotational axial loading is as follows:

- With internal rotation: the heel is pronated (valgus posture) and the forefoot is supinated, resulting in a close-pack position, providing a firmer foot-plate for locomotion.
- With external rotation: the heel is inverted (varus posture) and the forefoot is pronated resulting in a loose-pack position.

These fundamental characteristics of the foot-plate have been defined by MacConaill who proposed then a clinical demonstration which is easily reproduced (Fig. 10.180). Sarrafian[87] demonstrated the same functional characteristics in the anatomic specimen setup subjected to the axial loading in internal and external rotation of the tibio-talar segment (see Figs. 10.113 and 10.116).

During locomotion, following heel-strike, the lateral aspect of the foot establishes contact with the ground, followed by foot-flat contact. The foot plate acquires firmness first in the lateral longitudinal column. As demonstrated by Manter,[100] on axial loading of the talus, the longitudinal compression of the five rays is accompanied by the transverse compression of the three cuneiforms and the cuboid. The compressed cuboid acts as the keystone of the lateral longitudinal arch whose posterior pillar is the calcaneus and the anterior pillar, the fifth and fourth metatarsals (Fig. 10.181). The lateral longitudinal column is firmly stabilized.

As locomotion progresses, the body weight is transferred toward the first ray through internal rotation axial loading and anterior flexion of the tibiotalar column. This results in the untwisting of the footplate with pronation of the heel and supination of the mid- and forefoot. The anterior flexion of the tibiotalar column activates the truss mechanism of the footplate. Concomitantly all essential plantar ligaments, the plantar aponeurosis, and the longitudinal intrinsic muscles are under tension.

Specifically in regard to the plantar ligaments, the inferior calcaneonavicular ligament through the pronation of the os calcis is under tension (see Fig. 10.112) and pulls the navicular against the talar head in a close-pack position. At the calcaneocuboid joint, the calcaneocuboid ligaments are also under tension and the joint is also in a close-pack position. As a result, the midtarsal joint is locked in a stable position.

At the level of the plantar aspect of the midfoot and forefoot, with the latter supinated, the following major ligaments are under tension (Fig. 10.182A, B).

- The strong plantar $cuneo_1$-M_2M_3 ligament; Sappey considers this ligament as the essential ligament stabilizing the transverse arch of the tarsus
- The plantar $cuneo_{2-3}$-navicular ligaments
- The plantar $cuneo_3$-M_3M_4 ligaments
- The plantar calcaneonavicular ligament and the calcaneocuboid ligament

All above result in providing a firm footplate lever arm.

At heel-off (34% of walking cycle), the stability is now provided by a combination of a passive and active mechanism. The passive mechanism is determined by the windlass mechanism of the big toe. The plantar aponeurosis is acting as a tie-rod and also inverts the os calcis (Fig. 10.183).

Dynamic stabilization is provided by the contraction of the peroneus longus and the tibialis posterior which are electromyographically in shortening contraction from heel-off to 45% of the walking cycle. Perez et al[139] described a locking mechanism of the first ray relative to the second ray (Fig. 10.184) through eversion of the C_1-M_1 unit and correlating this eversion action with the peroneus longus inserting on M_1-C_1.

The tibialis posterior tendon tarsometatarsal insertions are on cuneiforms C_1, C_2, and C_3, on cuboid, and on metatarsal bases M_2, M_3, M_4, and M_5 (Fig. 10.185).

At heel-off, the concomitant contraction of the tibialis posterior and peroneus longus, through their belt-tightening effect (see Fig. 10.185), lock the cubo-$cuneo_3$,$cuneo_2$, $cuneo_1$ into a rigid mass, maintaining the transverse arch and also locking the metatarsal bases against the firm tarsus. The footplate is thus transformed into an efficient firm lever arm that is then ready to leave the ground.

Van de Velde et al[140] investigated the tibiofemoral kinematics using an in vitro roboting system and in vivo combined dual fluoroscopic and magnetic resonance imaging technique. In regard to the normal tibiofemoral joint kinematics, they reported that at full extension, the healthy knee rotated

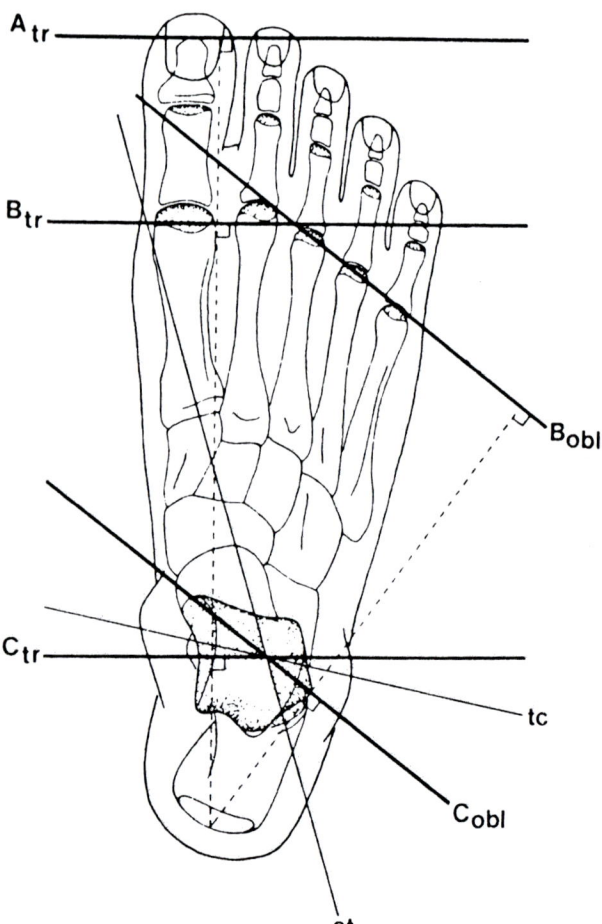

Figure 10.179 **Axes of the push-off.** The push-off is initiated along the oblique axis B_{obl} passing through the metatarsal heads 2 to 5 and continuing along the transverse axis B_{tr} passing through the metatarsal heads 1 and 2 and terminating along the distal transverse axis A_{tr} passing through the tip of the big toe. The dorsiflexion of the toes is accompanied by a motion of the ankle complex involving the axes of the talocrural (tc) and subtalar (st) joints, resulting in a secondary axis C_{obl} or C_{tr} that is parallel to the primary axes (B_{obl}, B_{tr}, or A_{tr}). The push-off along the oblique axis B_{obl} acts as a low-gear mechanism, whereas the push-off along the transverse axis B_{tr} acts as a high-gear mechanism of take-off. (Copyright © 1979 Bojsen-Møller F, Lamoreux L. Significance of free dorsiflexion of the toes in walking. *Acta Orthop Scand.* 1979;50[4]:471. Reproduced by permission of Taylor and Francis Group, LLC, a division of Informa plc.)

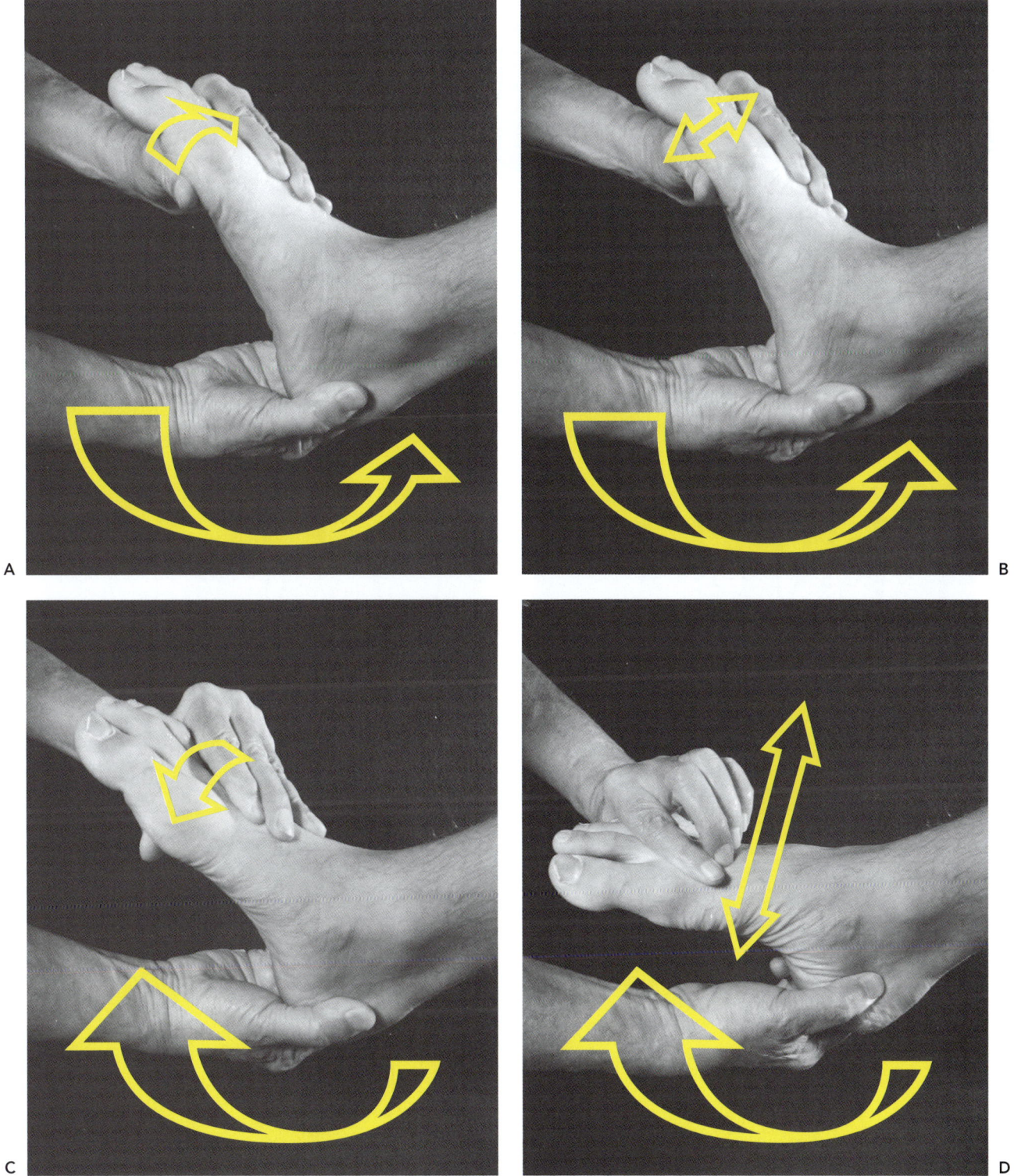

Figure 10.180 **(A)** Supination twist of the foot: the heel is in valgus; the forefoot is supinated. **(B)** In supination twist, the lamina pedis is more rigid. The forefoot flexion-extension is limited. **(C)** Pronation twist of the foot: the heel is in varus; the forefoot is pronated. **(D)** In pronation twist, the lamina pedis is flexible. The forefoot flexion-extension is much increased.

externally by 4.9° ± 7.2°, and at 30° of flexion of the knee, the tibia rotated internally by 3.6° ± 4.7°. Thereafter, the tibial internal rotation reached a maximum of 8.0° ± 4.5° at 90° of flexion.

Erdemir et al[141] investigated experimentally the dynamic loading of the plantar aponeurosis in walking simulation in seven cadaver feet. They used a gait simulator. The movements of the foot and the ground reaction forces during the stance

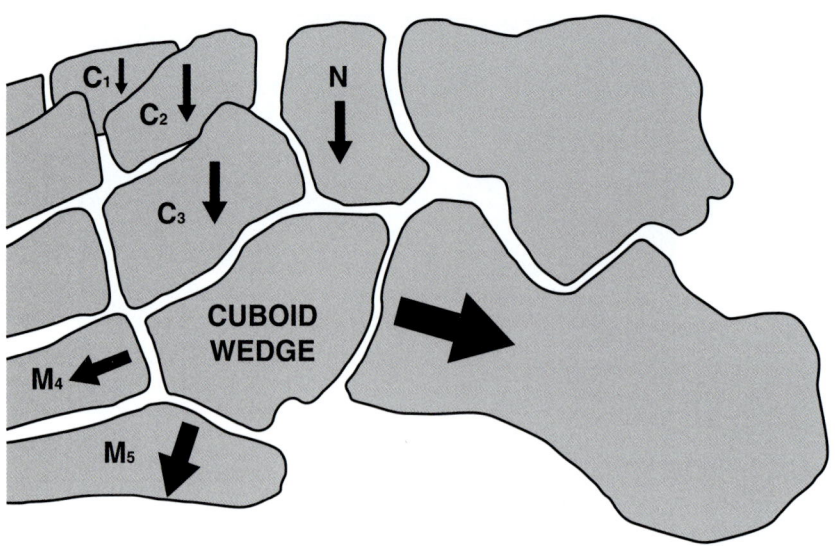

Figure 10.181 Cuboid. With the transverse compression of the three cuneiforms and the navicular, the cuboid, trapezoidal in contour, acts as a keystone of the lateral longitudinal arch whose posterior pillar is the calcaneus and the anterior pillar are the fifth and fourth metatarsal bases. The lateral longitudinal arch is stabilized.

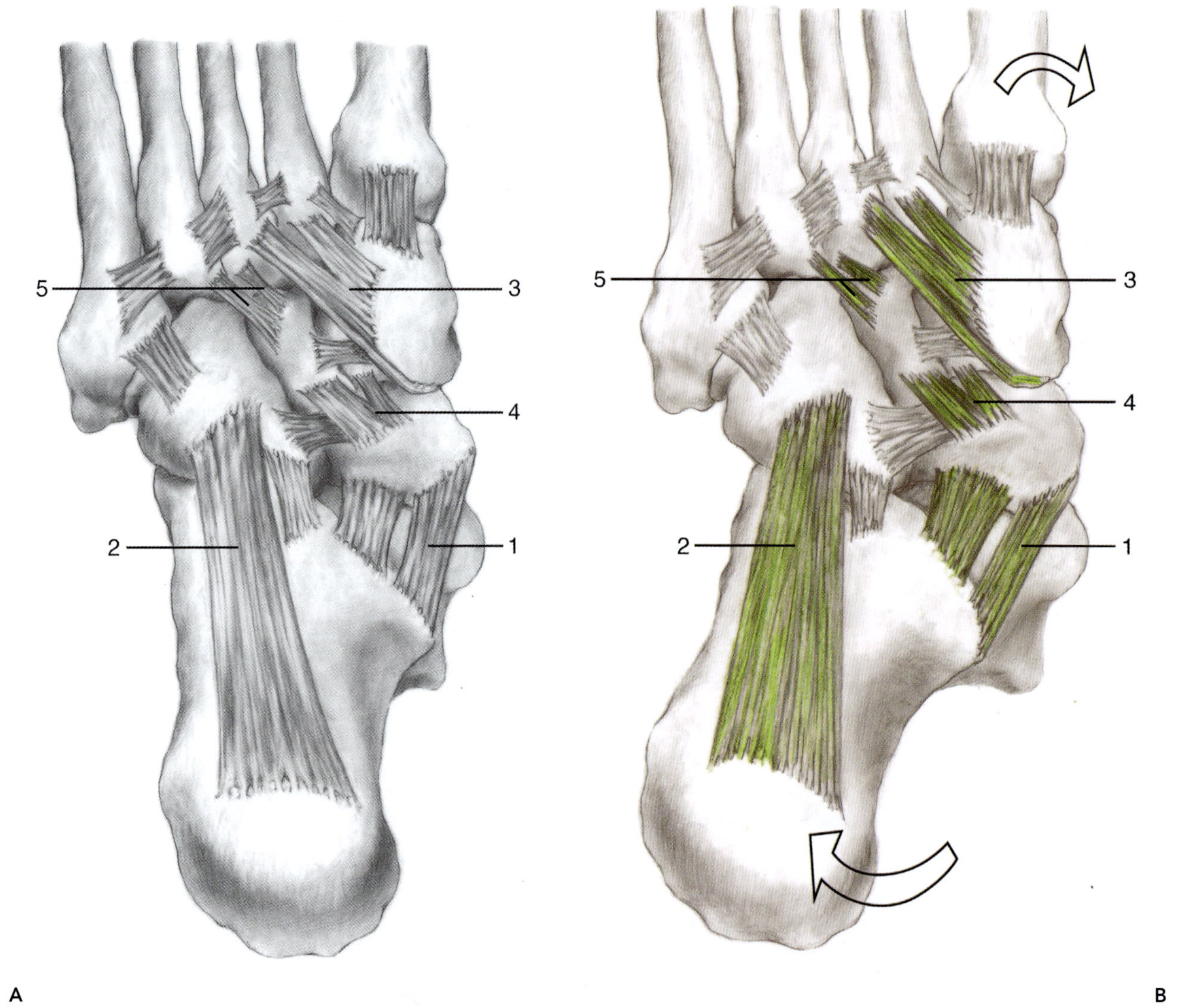

Figure 10.182 (A) Neutral posture sole of foot. (1, Inferior calcaneonavicular ligament; 2, inferior calcaneocuboid ligament; 3, plantar $cuneo_1$-$metatarsals_{2-3}$ ligament [ligament of Sappey]; 4, plantar naviculocuneiforms$_{2-3}$ ligament; 5, plantar $cuneo_3$-$metatarsals_{3-4}$ ligament.) (B) Supination twist of the foot plate with valgus of the calcaneus and supination twist of the forefoot. All above ligaments are under tension. The lamina pedis is rigid.

Chapter 10: Functional Anatomy of the Foot and Ankle 623

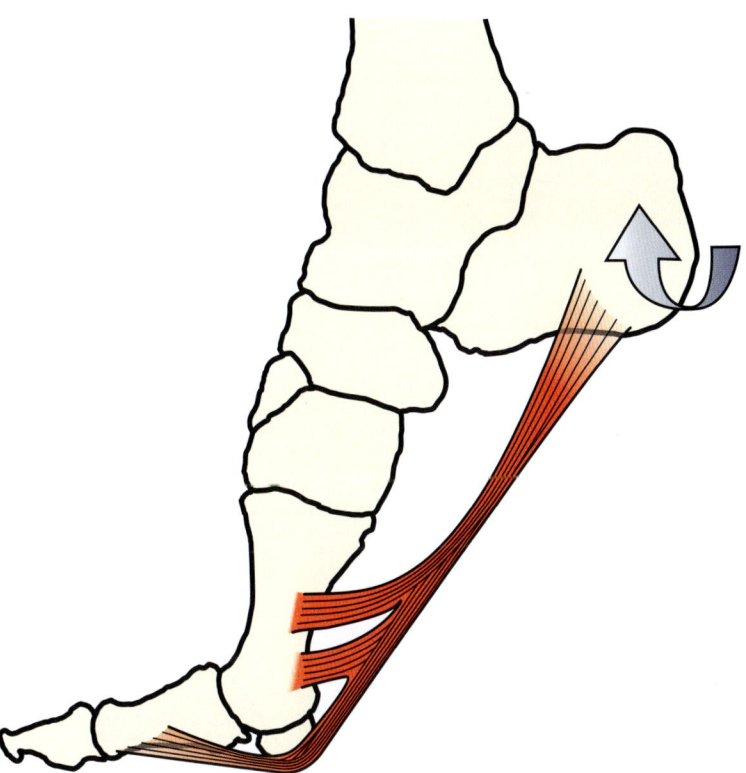

Figure 10.183 **At heel-off, the windlass mechanism of Hicks of the big toe is activated.** The plantar aponeurosis acts as a tie-rod and also inverts the heel.

phase were reproduced by prescribing the kinematics of the proximal part of the tibia and applying forces to the tendons of the extrinsic foot muscles. A fiberoptic cable was passed through the plantar aponeurosis perpendicular to its longitudinal axis for the purpose of measuring the force it carried. Ground reaction forces were measured by a force plate. "Plantar aponeurosis tension was relatively low at heel strike; gradually increased during midstance when both the heel and the forefoot were in contact with the ground; and peaked at approximately 80% of stance phase"[141] (Fig. 10.186). "Peak plantar aponeurosis forces during simulated walking were 538 + 139 N (0.96 ± 0.36 times estimated body weight)."[141]

Reeck et al[142] conducted a biomechanical investigation of the contributions of the talonavicular and talocalcaneal joints and the superomedial calcaneonavicular ligament in supporting the talus. Cadaver feet were mounted in a loading apparatus that applied axial forces through the tibia and fibula as well as the tensile loading of the tendons of extrinsic musculature. Eighteen specimens were tested in three selected positions of gait cycle: heel-strike, foot-flat, and near toe-off. In a series of 10 specimens, to study the contact characteristics of the bony support of the talus, the posterior and anteromedial facets of the talocalcaneal joint and the talonavicular joint-pressure sensitive films were placed between the articulating surfaces. In a second series of eight specimens, sensitive films were inserted between the talar head and the superomedial calcaneonavicular ligament. In stance position, the specimens were also tested without the posterior tibial tendon. The loading apparatus permitted nonvertical orientation of the tibia to allow foot dorsiflexion and plantar flexion, but still transmitting axial forces through it.

Each foot was tested in three positions: heel strike (5% of gait cycle), stance (30%), and near toe-off (45%). At these points in the gait cycle, the axial load has been determined to be 68% of body weight, 82% of body weight, and 110% of body weight, respectively (Fig. 10.187). Loads were applied for a period of 32 seconds for heel-strike, 48 seconds for stance, and 83 seconds for toe-off. For the calcaneonavicular ligament study, loads were applied for a period of 31, 45, and 75 seconds.

"The region of contact in the posterior facet spanned the medial side of the facet from anterior to posterior. The anteromedial facet contacts are as seemed to be localized in both the anterior and medial portion portion of the facets. Talonavicular contact varied, in some cases occurring around the rim of the articular surface and in others, within a smaller region and more centralized. Contact area on the facet articulating with the calcaneonavicular ligament was diffuse in pattern."[142] The contact area was (Fig. 10.188) largest in the posterior facet at the three gait positions and maximum at near toe-off position. The mean joint pressures (Fig. 10.189) were uniform but maximum near toe-off at the posterior facet. The total force transmission across each joint surface showed a pattern similar to the contact areas (Fig. 10.190). The force transmission gradient was maximum in the posterior calcaneal surface and then in decreasing fashion in the talonavicular joint, followed by the anterior calcaneal surface and minimum in the calcaneonavicular ligament. In general, increasing contact force was found across all articulations as the foot moved from heel-strike to toe-off. "With the foot in stance position, contact area and force decreased numerically across the calcaneonavicular ligament articulation without posterior tibial tendon tension; however, these differences were not significant."[142]

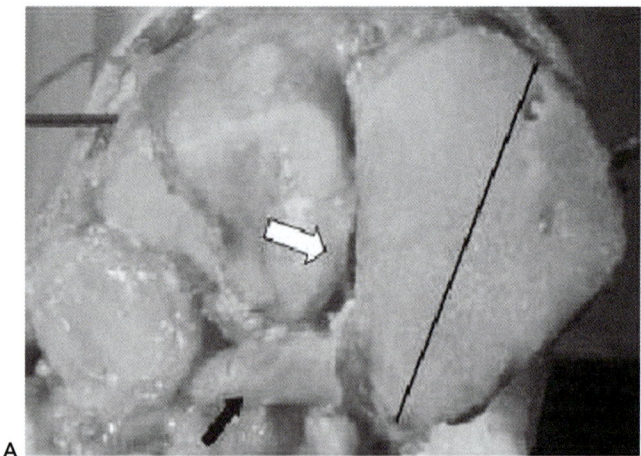
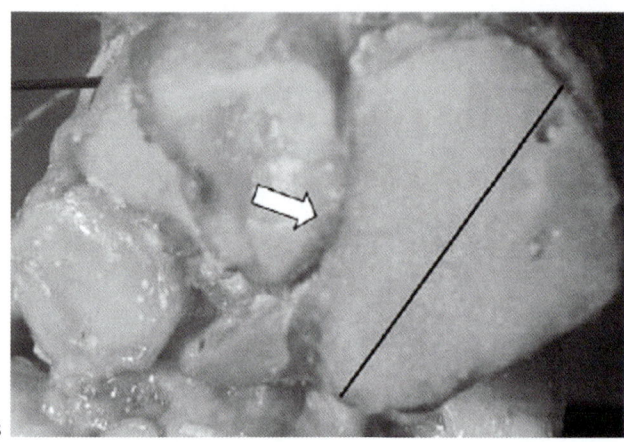

Figure 10.184 (A) Metatarsal bases with the first ray in neutral position. Increased space between the first and second rays. (B) First metatarsal ray is in an everted position. The space between the first and second rays is smaller. A close pack position is achieved. *White arrow* represent intermetatarsal space of first and second metatarsals base. *Black arrow* indicates insertion of PL. (Perez HR, Reber LK, Christensen JC. The effect of frontal plane position on the first ray motion: Forefoot locking mechanism. *Foot Ankle Int.* 2008;1:72-76, Figure 2. Copyright ©2008. Reprinted by Permission of SAGE Publications.)

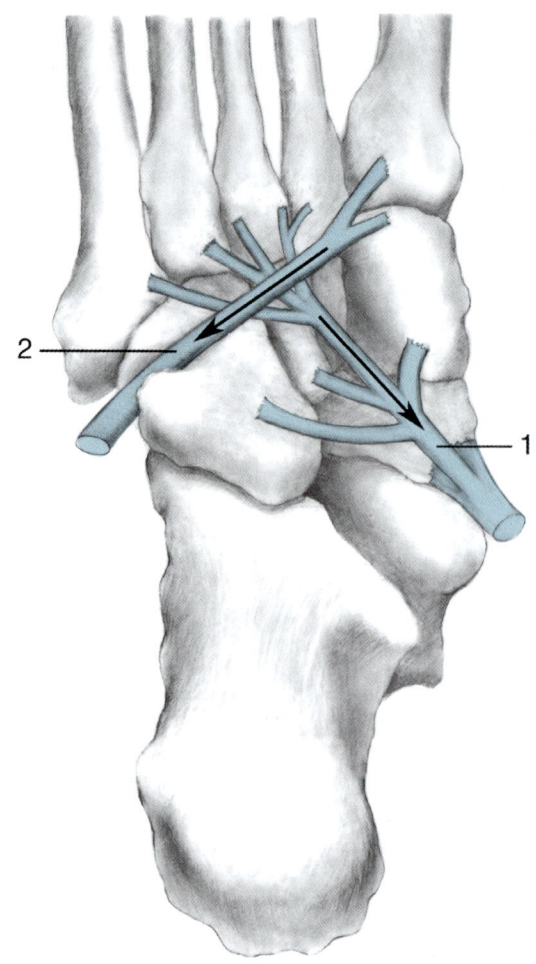

Figure 10.185 (*1*) Tarsometatarsals insertions of tibialis posterior tendon on cuneiforms, cuboid, and metatarsals$_{2,3,4,5}$. (*2*) Peroneus longus insertions on metatarsals$_{1,2}$. The concomitant contraction of tibialis posterior and peroneus longus locks the cubo-cuneo$_{1,2,3}$ into a rigid mass, providing stability to the tarsometatarsal complex.

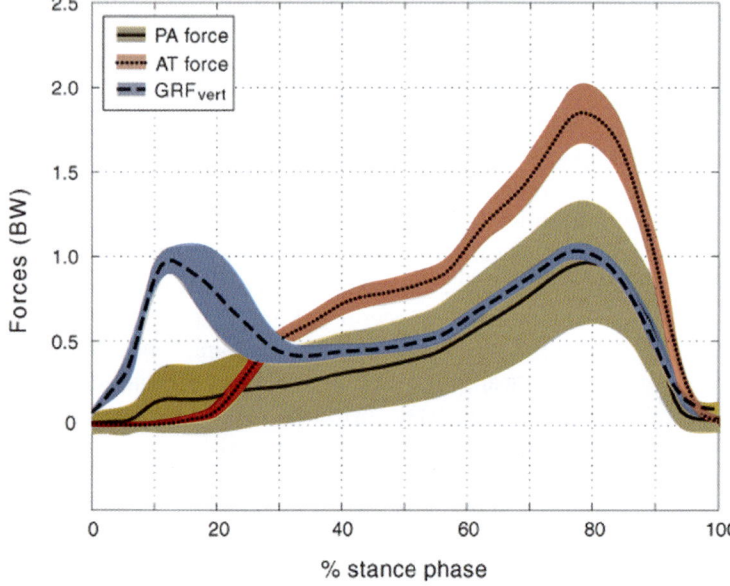

Figure 10.186 Mean plantar aponeurosis (*PA*) forces recorded by the fiberoptic transducer, Achilles tendon (*AT*) forces applied by the gait simulator, and ground reaction forces (*GRF*, vertical) recorded by the force plate, all normalized to estimated body weight (*BW*). Shading represents the standard deviation. Plantar aponeurosis tension gradually increased during stance phase, reaching peak values at the start of push-off. (Adapted from Erdemir A, Hamel AJ, Fauth AR, et al. Dynamic loading of the plantar aponeurosis in walking. *J Bone Joint Surg.* 2004;86A[3]:545-552, Figure 4.)

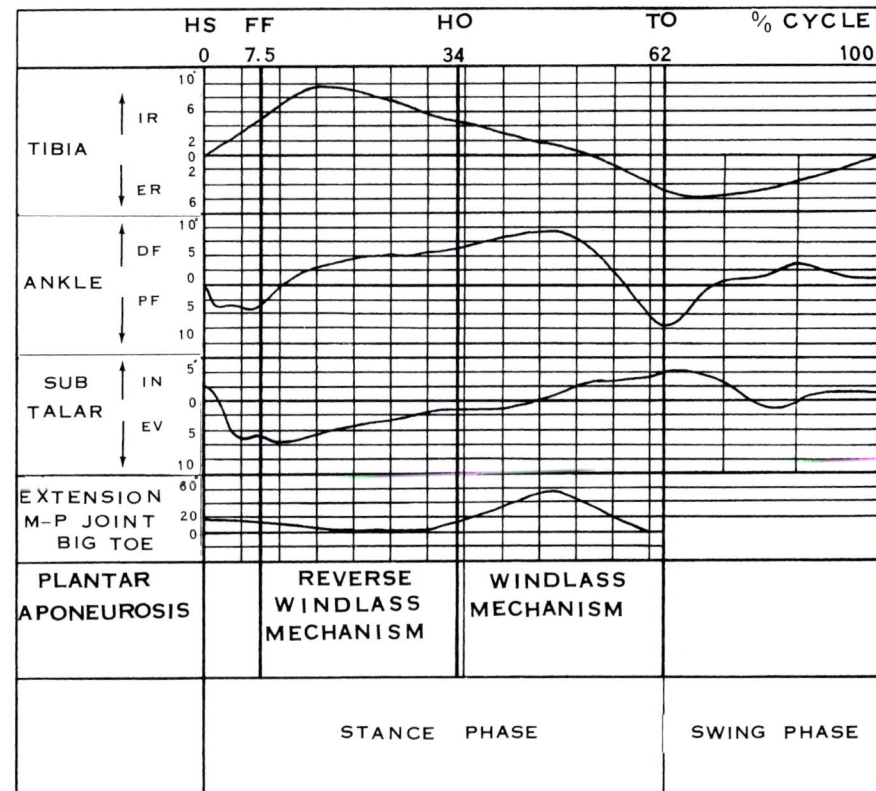

Figure 10.187 **Walking cycle.** (*DF*, dorsiflexion; *ER*, external rotation; *EV*, eversion; *FF*, foot flat; *HO*, heel-off; *IN*, inversion; *IR*, internal rotation; *PF*, plantar flexion; *TO*, toe off.)

Protective Loading of the Plantar Aponeurosis during Gait

During gait, the plantar aponeurosis is under protective tension mode when the corresponding lower extremity is in simultaneous extension at the hip, the knee, and the ankle.

The extension (dorsiflexion) at the ankle permits the anterior progression of the weight-bearing line relative to the heel, and this, in turn, increases the tension in the plantar aponeurosis which then prevents the failure of the longitudinal arch in flat-foot mode.

Observation of normal gait pattern in a natural setup will illustrate the relationship of the lower extremities and the functional status of their corresponding joints and deductively the protective tension in the plantar aponeurosis of the full weight-bearing foot. The mnemonic formula for the activation of the tension of the plantar aponeurosis is Triple-E or 3 E: simultaneous extension at the hip, the knee, and the ankle of the weight-bearing lower extremity (Figs. 10.191 and 10.192).

The correlation between a tight Achilles tendon and the development of flat foot has been analyzed and addressed by

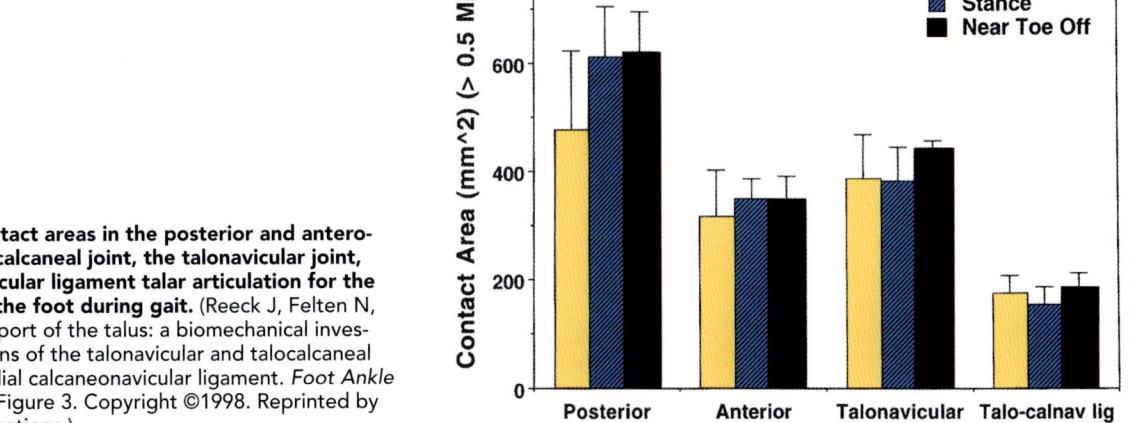

Figure 10.188 **Total contact areas in the posterior and anteromedial facets of the talocalcaneal joint, the talonavicular joint, and the talocalcaneonavicular ligament talar articulation for the three static positions of the foot during gait.** (Reeck J, Felten N, McCormack AP, et al. Support of the talus: a biomechanical investigation of the contributions of the talonavicular and talocalcaneal joints, and the superomedial calcaneonavicular ligament. *Foot Ankle Int.* 1998;19[10]:674-682, Figure 3. Copyright ©1998. Reprinted by Permission of SAGE Publications.)

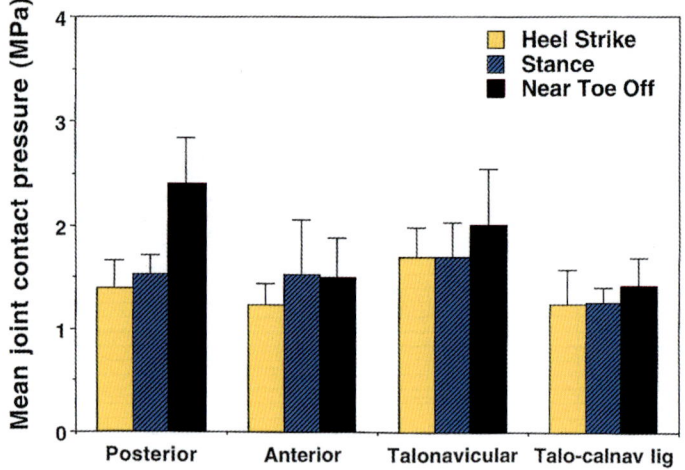

Figure 10.189 Mean contact pressures on the posterior and anteromedial facets of the talocalcaneal joint, the talonavicular joint, and the talocalcaneonavicular ligament talar articulation for the three static positions of the foot during gait. (Reeck J, Felten N, McCormack AP, et al. Support of the talus: a biomechanical investigation of the contributions of the talonavicular and talocalcaneal joints, and the superomedial calcaneonavicular ligament. *Foot Ankle Int*. 1998;19[10]:674-682, Figure 4. Copyright ©1998. Reprinted by Permission of SAGE Publications.)

Bohay, Anderson, and Gentchos.[143] Maskill et al[144] correlated similarly the contracture of the gastrocnemius with recalcitrant foot pain.

▶ Forces During Gait

Forces are imparted to the ground by the body in motion through the contact surface of the foot (Fig. 10.193). Ground reaction forces are generated that can be measured with force plates. These forces are the vertical force, the fore and aft shear, the medial and lateral shear forces, and the torque (Fig. 10.194). The progression of the center of pressure from the heel to the great toe is also determined. Pressure quantitation under specific areas of the foot during locomotion is provided by the use of a barograph with pressure-sensitive pads located in specific positions on the sole of the foot or by the use of pressure-sensitive walking surface material.

Vertical Forces

The transfer of the body weight to the weight-bearing leg generates sequential vertical ground reaction forces (Fig. 10.195).

At heel impact, an initial spike force is generated representing 80% of the body weight. At 12% of the walking cycle, the vertical force surpasses slightly the body weight and drops to 80% of the latter at 25% to 30% of the cycle when the center of gravity reaches a maximum vertical displacement. A second force peak occurs at 40% to 45% of the cycle, surpassing the body weight by 8% to 12%. This is followed by an abrupt drop of the force, which disappears at 62% of the cycle or at toe-off. The body weight has then been transferred to the opposite lower extremity (Fig. 10.196).[126,129,145]

The magnitude of the force varies with the speed of the gait. As reported by Mann, in slow walking the forces diminish and in rapid walking the forces increase.[126] In running, the vertical force increases to approximately two and one half to three times the body weight.

Fore and Aft Shear

Fore and aft shear forces have a lesser magnitude than the vertical forces with two maximums on the order of 10% of the body weight (see Fig. 10.196). The first spike occurs at heel-strike in the fore direction; the second peak occurs in the aft direction at 50% of the cycle and drops to 0 at toe-off.[126,129]

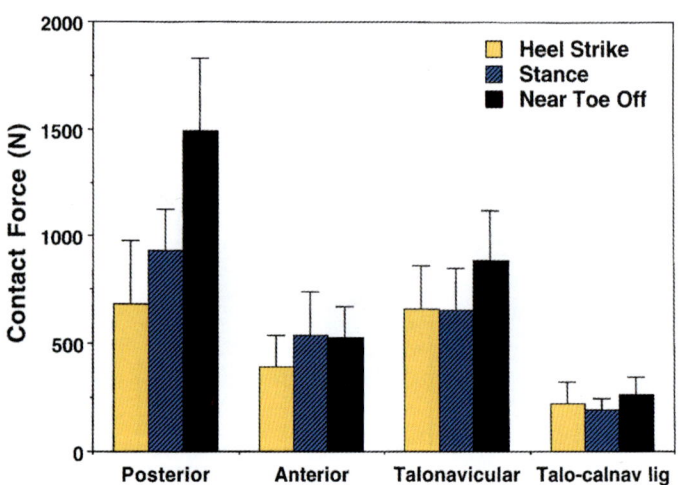

Figure 10.190 Total force across the posterior and anteromedial facets of the talocalcaneal joint, the talonavicular joint, and the talocalcaneonavicular ligament talar articulation for the three static positions of the foot during gait. (From Reeck J, Felten N, McCormack AP, et al. Support of the talus: a biomechanical investigation of the contributions of the talonavicular and talocalcaneal joints, and the superomedial calcaneonavicular ligament. *Foot Ankle Int*. 1998;19[10]:674-682, Figure 5. Copyright ©1998. Reprinted by Permission of SAGE Publications.)

Chapter 10: Functional Anatomy of the Foot and Ankle   627

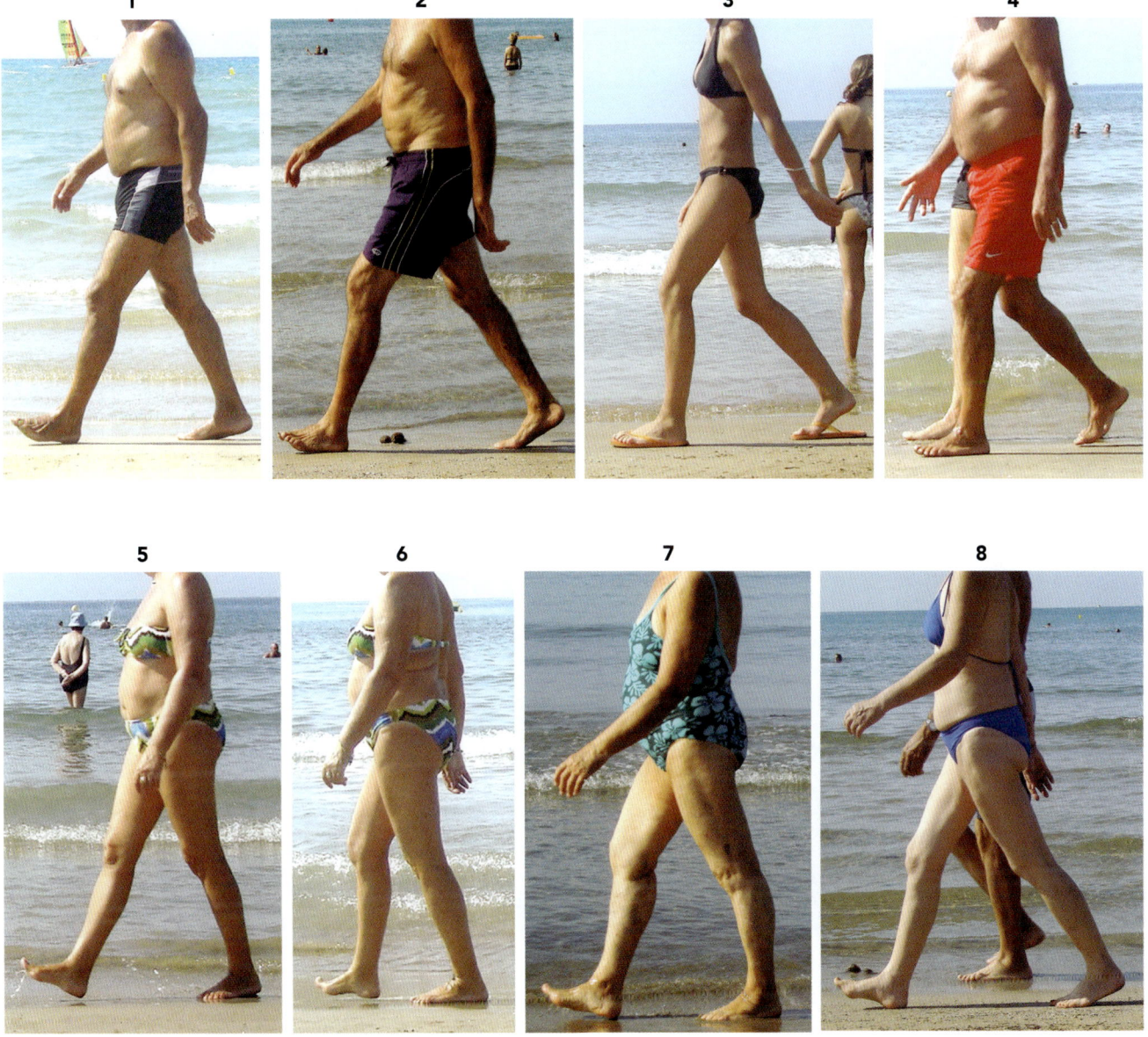

Figure 10.191 Composite of normal gait from right to left. Analysis of left lower extremity. *1*, Double support phase: hip flexed, knee flexed, ankle flexed, foot contact, foot with slight inversion; *2*, double support phase: hip flexed, knee flexed, ankle flexed, foot contact; *3*, double support phase: hip flexed, knee flexed, ankle neutral = no activation of plantar aponeurosis, foot flat; *4*, single support phase: hip flexed, knee flexed, ankle neutral = no activation of plantar aponeurosis; *5*, single support phase: hip extended, knee extended, ankle extended = activation of plantar aponeurosis; *6*, single support phase: hip extended, knee extended, ankle extended = activation of plantar aponeurosis; *7*, double support phase: hip extended, knee extended, ankle extended = activation of plantar aponeurosis; *8*, double support phase: hip extended, knee extended, ankle neutral. Activation of windlass mechanism.

Medial and Lateral Shear

Medial and lateral shear forces are also of a lesser magnitude than the vertical force, on the order of 10% of the body weight (see Fig. 10.196). At heel-strike, a medially directed shear force is present, followed by a lateral shear force, which remains until toe-off.

Torque[126,129]

Torque, created in response to the rotation of the tibia and measured in the horizontal plane against the ground, is internally directed at heel-strike and peaks at 15% of the walking cycle. It is followed by an external torque reaching

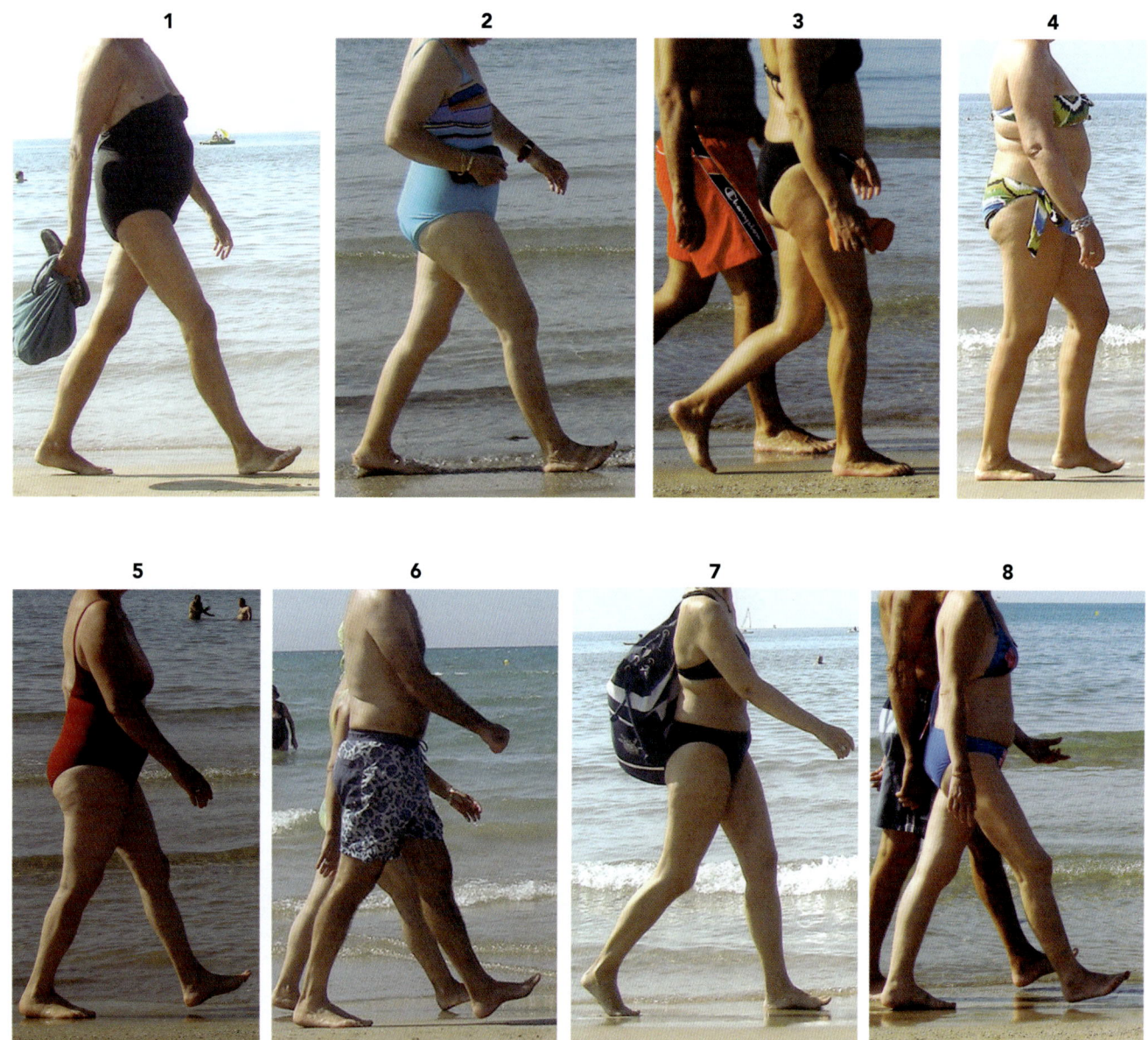

Figure 10.192 **Composite of normal gait from left to right.** Analysis of right lower extremity. *1*, Double support phase: hip flexed, knee flexed, ankle flexed, heel contact; *2*, double support phase: hip flexed, knee flexed, ankle flexed, foot contact in slight inversion; *3*, double support phase: hip flexed, knee flexed, ankle neutral, foot flat = no activation of plantar aponeurosis; background: *4*, single support phase: hip extended, knee extended, ankle extended = activation of plantar aponeurosis; *5*, single support phase: hip extended, knee extended, ankle extended = activation of plantar aponeurosis; *6*, single support phase hip extended, knee extended, ankle extended with marked tension in Achilles tendon = activation of plantar aponeurosis; *7*, double support phase: hip extended, knee flexed, ankle flexed = activation of windlass mechanism; *8*, contralateral single support phase: hip flexed, knee flexed, ankle flexed. Extremity in swing mode.

a maximum near 50% of the cycle and then drops to 0 at toe-off. The torque has a magnitude of 20 inch-pounds (see Fig. 10.196).

▶ Forces Acting at the Ankle Joint During Gait

Stauffer and coworkers have analyzed the compressive and tangential forces created in the stance phase at the level of the ankle joint.[15] The weight-bearing surface of the ankle joint is 11 to 13 cm^2 and the fibula bears and transmits to the talus one sixth of the load.[15,61] From heel-strike to foot-flat, the compressive forces exerted on the ankle increase gradually and reach a magnitude of about three times the body weight. A plateau level is reached until heel-off, followed by a second peak of compressive forces at 40% of the walking cycle, reaching nearly five times the body weight (Fig. 10.197).[15] The tangential forces

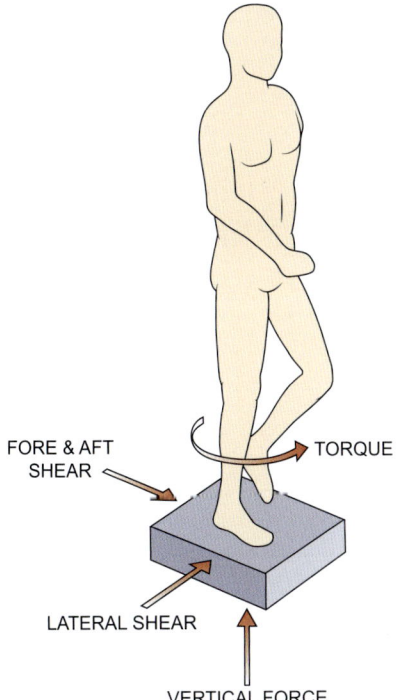

Figure 10.193 Forces imparted to the ground by the body in motion through the contact surface of the foot during gait.

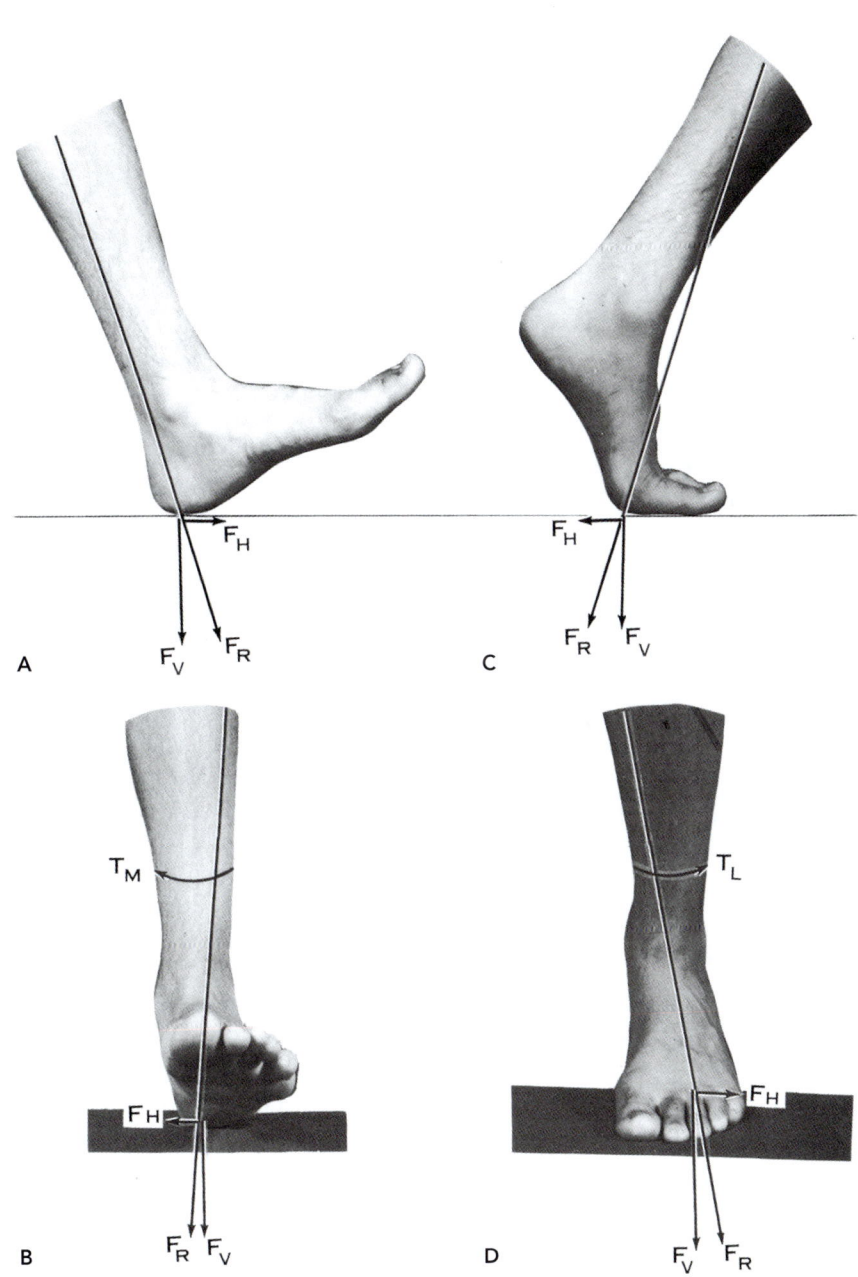

Figure 10.194 Forces during the stand phase of gait. **(A)** At heel-strike, the force exerted on the ground F_r has a vertical component F_v and a horizontal component F_H directed anteriorly. The ground reactions are opposite in direction. **(B)** At heel-strike, seen anteriorly, the force exerted has a medially directed shear, horizontal component F_H associated with a medially directed torque T_M. **(C)** At push-off, the force exerted on the ground F_R has a vertical component F_v and a horizontal component F_H directed posteriorly. **(D)** At push-off, seen anteriorly, the force exerted has a laterally directed shear, horizontal component F_H associated with lateral torque T_L.

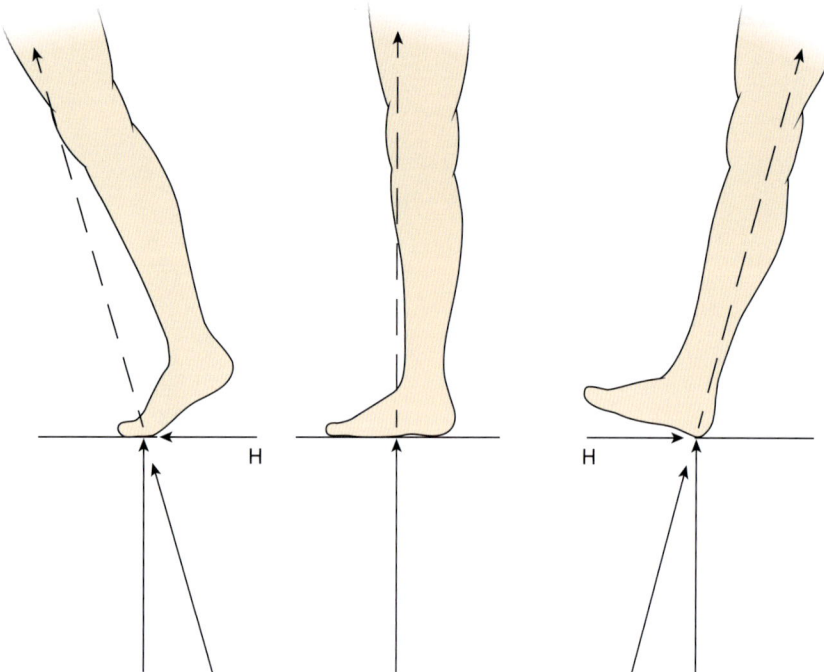

Figure 10.195 The transfer of the body weight during gait to the weight-bearing leg generates ground reaction (*FR*) with vertical (*V*) and horizontal (*H*) components.

created at the level of the ankle joint are biphasic: they are acting in the aft direction from heel-strike to foot-flat and in the fore direction during the push-off of the gait cycle.

The magnitude of the aft force is nearly 0.7% of the body weight and occurs between 35% and 40% of the walking cycle. The fore tangential force is of lesser magnitude, 0.3% of the body weight, and occurs between 50% and 55% of the walking cycle (Fig. 10.198).

▶ Load, Pressure Distribution, and Measurement Under the Foot During Gait

The dynamic pressure distribution under the foot has been extensively investigated. Elftman provided a limited but precise documentation of the distribution, magnitude, and direction of the forces under the foot in the stance phase of the walking cycle (Fig. 10.199).[146,147]

Hutton and colleagues analyzed the load distribution under the foot during gait using 12-channel vertical load sensors and recorders.[148-150] The progression of the load was documented at 5% intervals of the walking cycle. Longitudinal and transverse profiles of distribution were determined (Fig. 10.200). At 5% of the cycle, the load is concentrated on the heel. At 10% of the cycle, the forefoot participates in the load distribution, which gradually shifts to the forefoot. At 30% of the cycle, the heel leaves the ground and the load is concentrated on the forefoot; during the later part of foot contact, the toes carry about 30% of the total load at 50% of the cycle.[149] The pathway of the center of load has also been determined (Fig. 10.201). It progresses in a linear path axially, passing slightly on the medial aspect of the heel toward the medial aspect of the ball of the foot. The initial progression of the center of the load is rapid. From 30% to 50% of the cycle, two definite changes occur: the load transmission line shifts medially and the forward transmission of the load centers slows down; this results in clustering of the pressure centers on the medial aspect of the ball of the foot.

Subsequently, the load line passes between the first and second metatarsal heads and reaches the hallux at 57% of the walking cycle.

Betts and colleagues studied the peak pressures and the limits of normality under the foot over seven selected areas during walking: the heel, the five metatarsal heads, and the great toe.[151-153] The images produced by the pedograph were defined as pictures of pressure distribution and not load distribution. A normal pressure under the foot was defined—as a rough rule of thumb—not to exceed 10 kg/cm^2. The median values for metatarsal heads 1 to 3 were in the range of 3 to 4 kg/cm^2 and decreased laterally with a near peak value of 1 and 2 kg/cm^2 under the fifth metatarsal head. The first toe had the largest variability. The percentile curves of pressure distribution are as indicated in Figure 10.202.

Hughes and coworkers examined the weight-bearing function of the toes in 160 normal subjects with a pedobarograph.[154] The peak pressure and contact time for each toe were assessed. The toes were in contact with the ground for 75% of the stance phase of gait and exerted peak pressures similar to those of the metatarsal region. "The toes were not in contact with the ground for as long as the metatarsal heads but were down for longer than the heel and the base of the fifth metatarsal" (Fig. 10.203).[154] In 92% of subjects, all toes made contact with the ground and, in the remaining 8%, one or more toes—usually the fifth—did not make contact on one or both feet. The great toe reached the

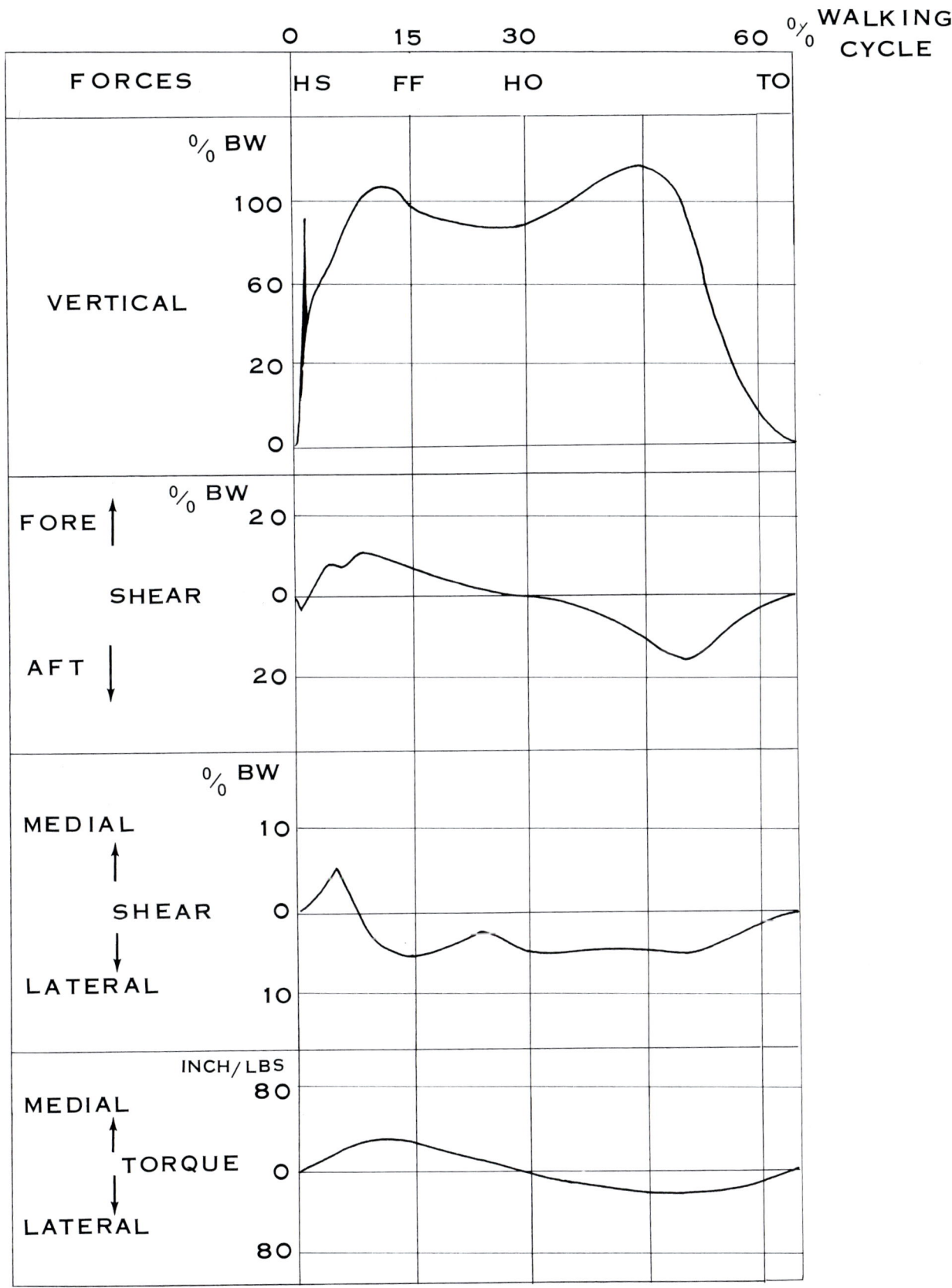

Figure 10.196 **Forces acting during the walking cycle.** (Adapted from Mann RA. Biomechanics. In: Jahss M, ed. *Disorders of the Foot*. Vol 1. WB Saunders; 1982:47, 49.)

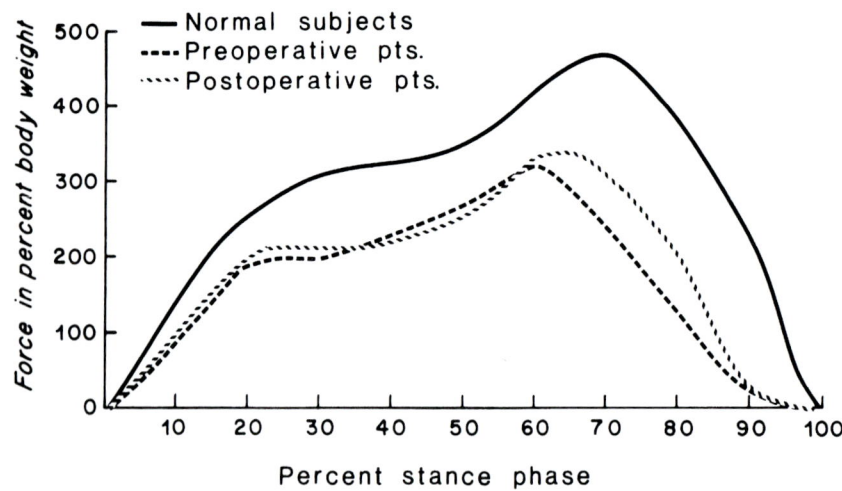

Figure 10.197 **Mean patterns of compressive forces at the ankle during the stance phase of the walking cycle.** The compressive forces across the ankle are three times the body weight at 20% to 30% of the stance phase and 4.5 to 5.5 times the body weight at 60% to 70% of the stance phase. (From Stauffer RN, Chao EYS, Brewster RC. Force and motion analysis of the normal, diseased and prosthetic ankle joint. *Clin Orthop Relat Res.* 1977;127:189.)

highest peak pressure of the whole foot, and the central metatarsals took more pressure than the lateral metatarsal heads. There was a gradual decrease of the median peak pressure from the great toe to the fifth toe (see Fig. 10.203).

The mean force as a percentage of the sum of the mean peak forces under all toes was calculated (Table 10.8). The force under the first toe was more than half of the total force under the toes, and the force under the lesser toes diminished from the second toe to the fifth toe.

It thus becomes evident "that the toes play an important part in increasing the weight-bearing area during walking."[154]

SHOCK-ABSORBING CHARACTERISTICS OF THE HEEL AND BALL OF THE FOOT

At heel impact during gait, a shock wave of up to 5 ms in duration is generated with a maximum frequency of 100 cycles per second (100 Hz) and the magnitude equals 80% of body weight.[131,155,156] This shock wave is propagated proximally through the segments of the lower extremity, the pelvis, the spine, and the skull. Walking creates peak forces just above the body weight, whereas running generates forces two to three times the body weight. For an individual weighing 68 kg (150 lb) walking 1 mile, the total force generated against the ground and to be absorbed by one foot is 63.5 tons, whereas in 1 mile of running it is 110 tons.[157,158] A force of this magnitude is to be dissipated and the associated vibrations are to be dampened in order to avoid injuries to the bones, the joints, the brain, and the vision.[159]

The heel pad and the ball of the foot are specifically constructed to function as efficient shock absorbers to attenuate the peaks of the dynamic forces and to dampen the vibrations. The shock-absorbing mechanism also includes the muscle lengthening under tension, the bony deformation, the joint motion, the intervertebral discs, and, to a lesser degree, the compression of the articular cartilage of the loaded joints in combination with the synovial fluid.[156]

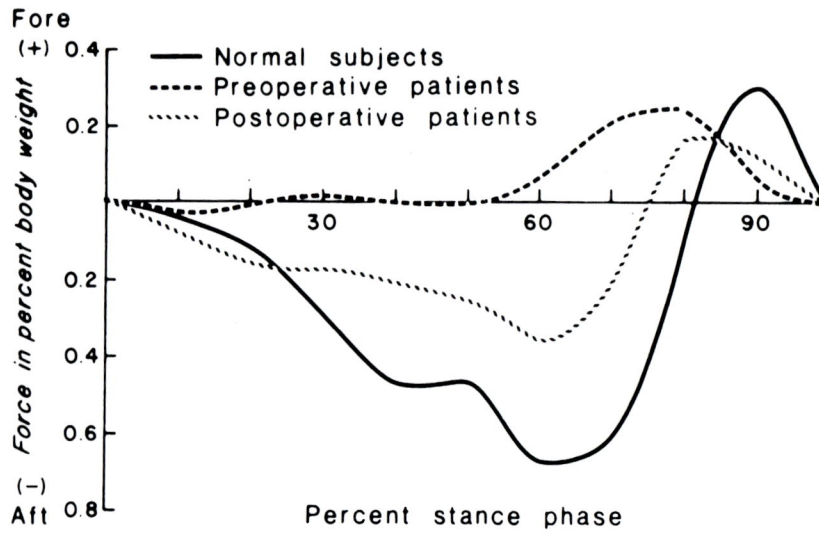

Figure 10.198 **Mean patterns of tangential forces at the ankle during the stance phase of the walking cycle.** The tangential forces are biphasic, directed in the aft direction during the heel-strike and foot-flat portions of the cycle and in the fore direction during the push-off. (From Stauffer RN, Chao EYS, Brewster RC. Force and motion analysis of the normal, diseased and prosthetic ankle joint. *Clin Orthop Relat Res.* 1977;127:189.)

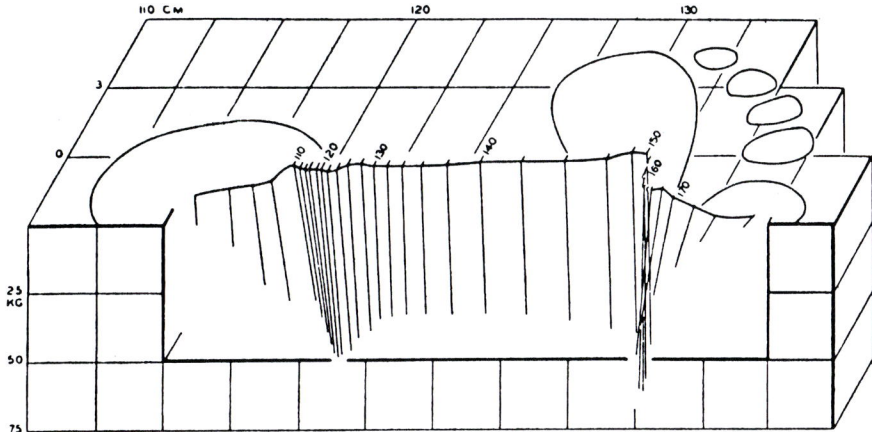

Figure 10.199 Distribution, magnitude, and direction of the forces under the foot in stance phase of the walking cycle. The point of application of the force is seen passing through the heel and the medial border of the foot. It reaches the ball of the foot at the level of the second metatarsal head, shifts medially toward the first metatarsal head, and progresses rapidly to the big toe. The curve of the magnitude of the forces is bimodal. As indicated, during the heel-strike, the forces are directed downward and anteriorly, become progressively vertical at mid stance, and are directed downward and posteriorly at push-off. (From Elftman H. Forces and energy changes in the leg during walking. *Am Physiol.* 1939;125:339.)

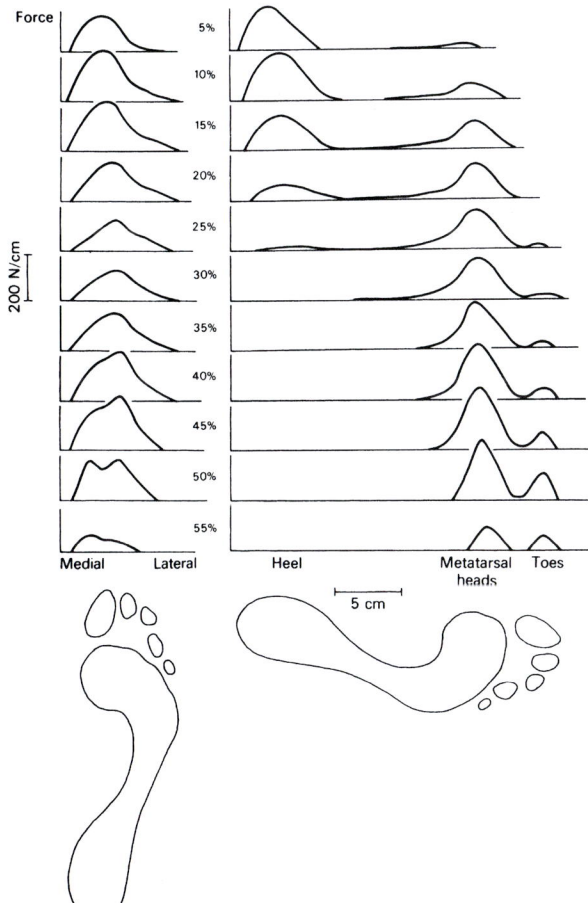

Figure 10.200 Distribution of load on a normal foot during walking. At heel-strike, the load is carried by the medial aspect of the heel. At 15%, the load is carried by the heel and the forefoot; the midfoot carries an insignificant load. At 30%, the load is over the ball of the foot, with participation of the toes. The forefoot load reaches a peak at 45% and gradually diminishes as the load is transferred more to the toes. (Republished with permission of John Wiley, from Hutton WC, Stott JRR, Stokes IAF. The mechanics of the foot. In: Klenerman L, ed. *The Foot and Its Disorders.* Blackwell Scientific Publications; 1976:40; permission conveyed through Copyright Clearance Center, Inc.)

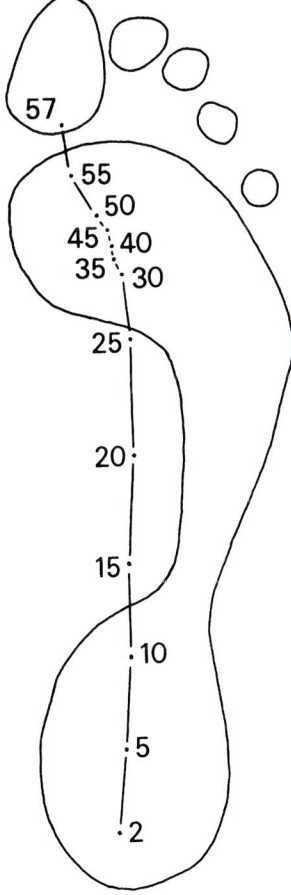

Figure 10.201 Progression of the center of load during the walking cycle. From heel-strike to heel-off, the progression of the center of load is rapid. It passes slightly on the medial aspect of the heel, along the medial border of the foot, and at 30% of the cycle it is over the medial aspect of the ball of the foot. From 30% to 50%, the progression slows and shifts further medially toward the first metatarsal head and then progresses rapidly along the plantar aspect of the big toe. (Republished with permission of John Wiley, from Hutton WC, Stott JRR, Stokes IAF. The mechanics of the foot. In: Klenerman L, ed. *The Foot and Its Disorders.* Blackwell Scientific Publications; 1976:41; permission conveyed through Copyright Clearance Center, Inc.)

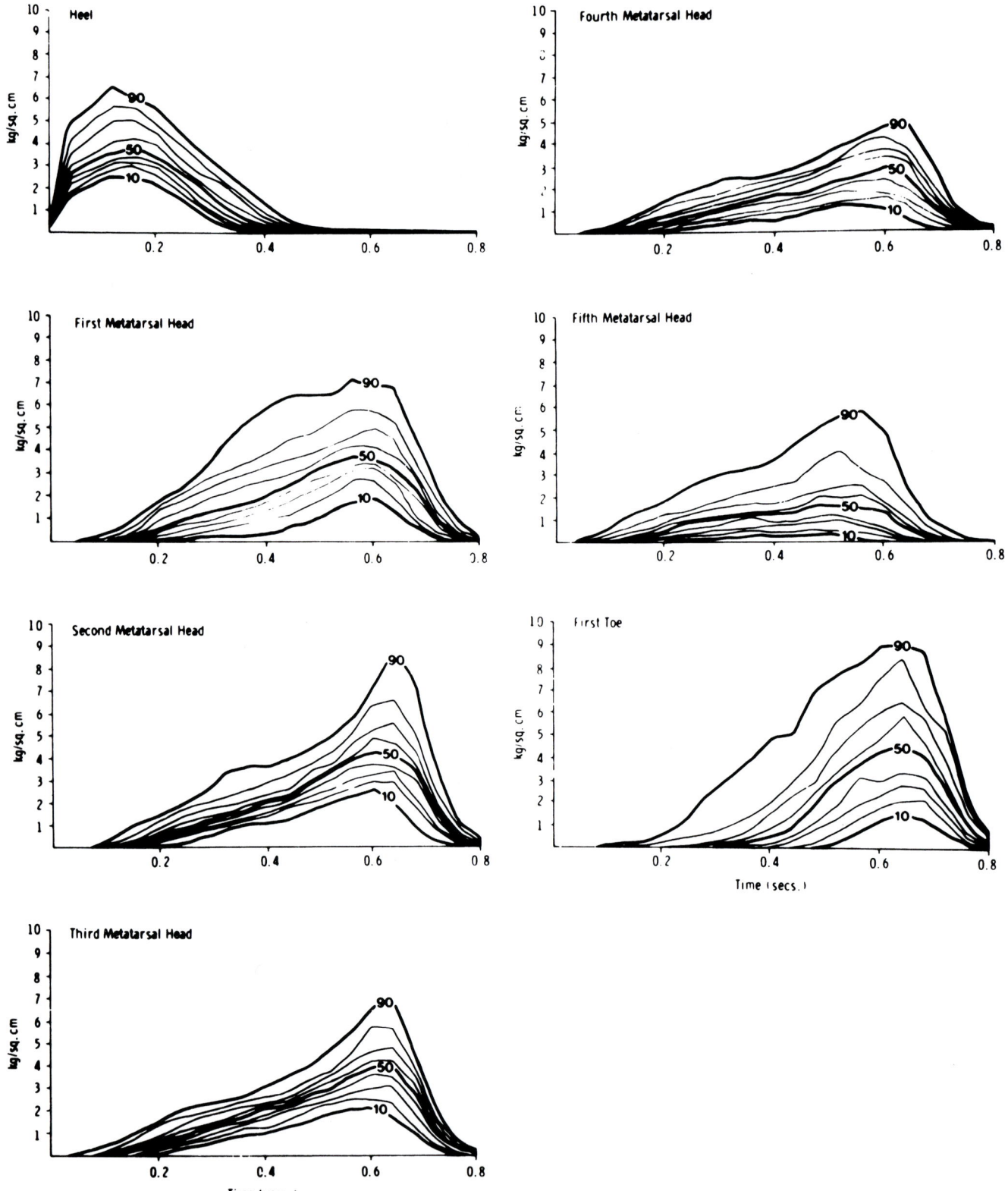

Figure 10.202 Percentile curves for the peak pressures during walking for the heel, the first toe, and the five metatarsal heads under the foot, obtained from control subjects. The time has been normalized to 0.8 seconds (1 kg/cm^2 = 98.1 kPa). (Republished with permission of IOP Publishing, from Betts RP, Franks CI, Duckworth T. Analysis of pressures and loads under the foot. Part 2: Quantification of the dynamic distribution. *J Clin Physiol Meas.* 1980;1:113-124; permission conveyed through Copyright Clearance Center, Inc.)

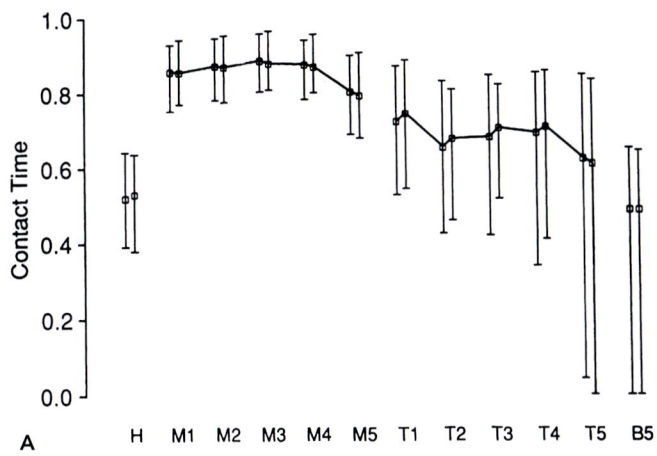

TABLE 10.8 Peak Force Under Toes During Walking				
	Left		Right	
Toe	Peak Force	Percent	Peak Force	Percent
Great	10.63	60.2	10.88	59.1
Second	2.42	13.7	2.61	14.2
Third	2.04	11.6	2.17	11.8
Fourth	1.58	8.9	1.66	9.0
Fifth	0.99	5.6	1.09	5.9
Sum	17.66	100.0	18.41	100.0

Republished with permission of British Editorial Society of Bone and Joint Surgery, from Hughes J, Clark P, Klenerman L. The importance of the toes in walking. *J Bone Joint Surg Br*. 1990;72(2):245; permission conveyed through Copyright Clearance Center, Inc.

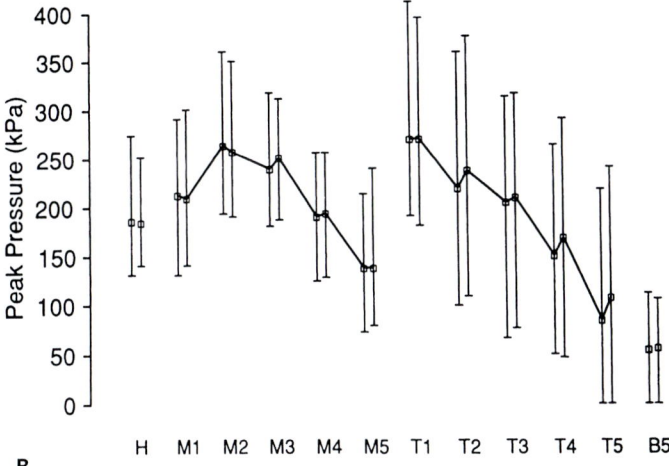

Figure 10.203 The median and 90% data interval (vertical bars) for: **(A)** contact time as a proportion of stance phase for left and right feet (left and right pairs of points); and **(B)** dynamic peak pressures for the left and right feet (left and right pairs of points) under the heel (*H*), the metatarsal heads (M_1-M_5), the toes (T_1-T_5), and the base of M_5 (*B5*). (kPa, kilopascal.) (Republished with permission of British Editorial Society of Bone and Joint Surgery, from Hughes J, Clark P, Klenerman L. The importance of the toes in walking. *J Bone Joint Surg Br*. 1990;72[2]:248. Permission conveyed through Copyright Clearance Center, Inc.)

▶ Heel Pad

The heel pad has an average thickness of 18 mm, with a range from 12 to 22 mm.[160-162] The skin (epidermis plus dermis) is of the thick type[163] with a mean epidermal thickness of 0.64 mm (comparatively, the mean epidermal thickness is 0.069 mm on the dorsum of the foot and 0.38 mm under the head of the first metatarsal).[164] The stratum corneum makes up 90% of the epidermal thickness. Large rete pege of the epidermis, measuring in length 0.23 mm, "the greatest of all sites studied,"[164] lock into the dermal papillae. The epidermal-dermal interface is "oriented in parallel rows seemingly to provide mechanical advantage in gripping the walking surface."[164]

Comprehensive studies of the heel pad architectural structure were made by Tietze,[165] Blechschmidt,[86] Kulms,[166] and Kimani,[167] and recently there has been further contribution by Jørgensen,[168] Jørgensen and colleagues,[169,170] and Bojsen-Møller and colleagues.[159]

The dermis of the heel plantar skin is divided into a superficial papillary dermis and a deep reticular dermis. The former contains numerous elastic fibers forming a subepidermal plexus and the latter forms a superficial connective tissue investing layer for the foot pad.[167]

The subcutis is divided by a fibrous layer or internal cup into a superficial stratum with microchambers and a deep stratum with macrochambers,[159,167] both retaining adipose tissue (Figs. 10.204 and 10.205). The microchambers are formed by dermal fibrous bands rich in elastic fibers, extending from the reticular dermis to the internal fibrous cup.[159,167] The microchambers lodge adipose tissue and the posterior extension of the plantar superficial venous network or the posterior segment of Lejars' "venous sole of the foot."[171] "The vascular system fits into the structure of the subcutis to such a large extent that it really serves as a picture of the topography of the connective tissue... their path demonstrates the main direction of the weaving connective tissue."[86]

Testut describes these veins as nearly all transversely oriented, sinuous, and prominent.[172] Each vein is retained in a true alveolar stroma, and this venous system is compared to an erectile tissue (Fig. 10.206). Functionally, with weight-bearing, "emptying of the vascular bed seems to add significantly to the compliance of the heel."[159] The cup ligament is formed from bundles of collagen fibers that run transversely and longitudinally,[167] and it is attached to the periosteal membrane of the tubercles of the calcaneus by septa. As described by Blechschmidt, the septa "near the sole of the foot...are almost transverse, while rising upward they experience a rotation, turning more and more in the direction of the plantar aponeurosis and with this converging toward the front medially. Finally this direction continues in the whorl which springs below and laterally from the calcaneus. Viewed from the above this whorl on the right foot turns to the right and on the left foot toward the left" (Fig. 10.207).[86]

The fibrous septa, rich in collagen fibers, form large sealed compartments retaining and preventing the outflow of fat. On sagittal and frontal cross sections, these macrochambers have a U-shaped appearance, whereas on the horizontal cross section they reveal the whorl spiral disposition of the septa (Fig. 10.208).[86,159] These primary chambers are "spirally twisted

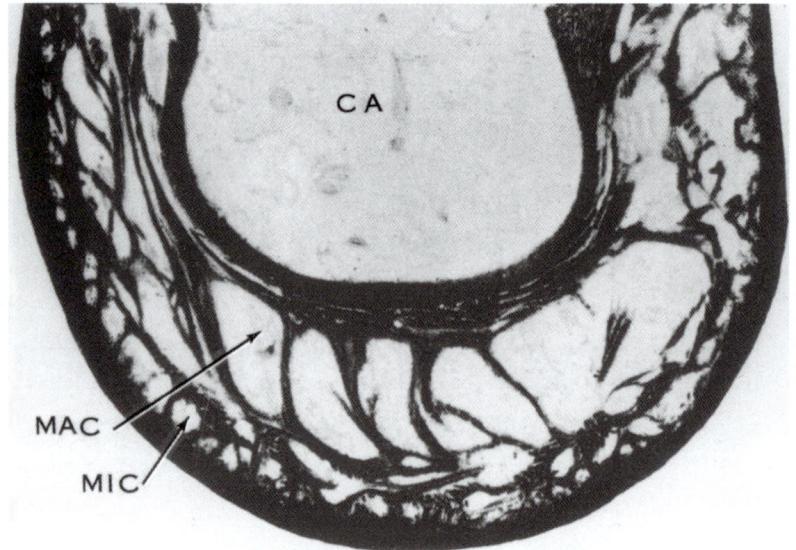

Figure 10.204 **Coronal section of the embryo heel demonstrating the curved fascial connections between the fascia of the calcaneus and the fibrous outer coat.** Macrochambers (*MAC*) and microchambers (*MIC*) are recognized. (*CA*, calcaneus.) (Blechschmidt E. The structure of the calcaneal padding, 1934. *Foot Ankle*. 1982;2[5]:269. Copyright ©1982. Reprinted by Permission of SAGE Publications.)

around each other"[86] and are subdivided into smaller compartments by delicate septa rich in elastic fibers.

The main septal system originates laterally at the calcaneus and is twisted medially and directed cranially. A smaller reversed septal system is also present, located below the major component. It is directed plantarward and forms, with the former, two curving groups crossing each other in opposite directions.[86] On weight-bearing, the calcaneus descends plantarward. The heel pad flattens and bulges laterally and upward. The heel chambers are not compressed, in spite of the shorter distance between the bone and the skin, and they turn around the tuberosity of the os calcis: they are deformed (Fig. 10.209). As stated by Blechschmidt, "the deformation of the entire padding is the sum of numerous individual deformations...without perceptible compressions."[86]

The individual deformation is provided by the major chambers. During locomotion, each chamber is subjected to compressive, shear, and torsional forces. The deformation of the major chambers and the flow of the enclosed adipose tissue contribute to the shock absorption.[86,159] The low viscosity of the retained specialized adipose tissue helps dissipate the energy, thus reinforcing the shock absorption.[173] The low viscosity of the heel fat pad is due to the high content of unsaturated fat.[173]

The structured and anchored rich collagen system provides mechanical stability to the heel pad, whereas the abundant elastic fibers of the subdermal plexus and the fine secondary septa of the large chambers provide tension modulation during the cyclic loading of locomotion. "Furthermore, the energy of recoil inherent in the elastic fiber system may facilitate the return of

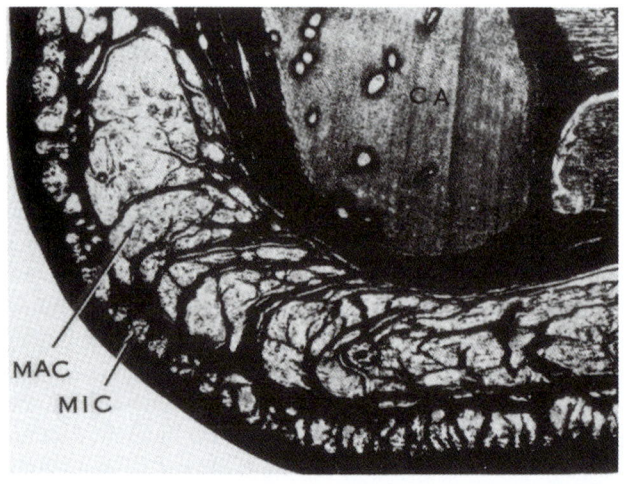 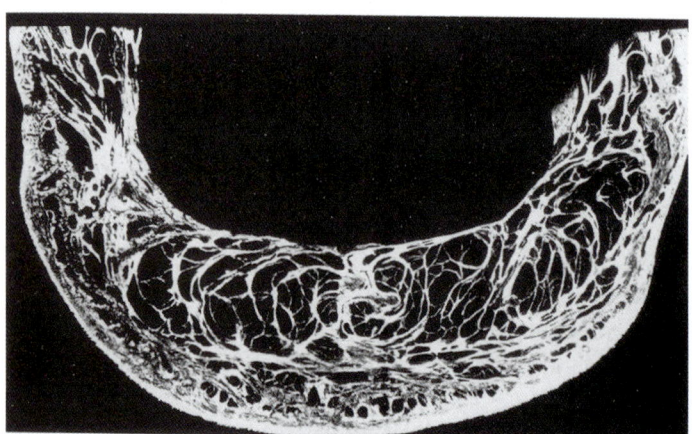

Figure 10.205 **(A)** Medial sagittal section of the heel in 6-month embryo. Macrochambers (*MAC*) and microchambers (*MIC*) are clearly seen with curved connections between the fascia of the calcaneus (*CA*) and the fibrous outer coat of the heel. **(B)** Coronal section through the heel of an adult. Macro- and microchambers are seen. The outer coat is fibrous, more collagenous. The fine interior architecture is elastic. (Blechschmidt E. The structure of the calcaneal padding, 1934. *Foot Ankle*. 1982;2[5]:268, 274. Copyright ©1982. Reprinted by Permission of SAGE Publications.)

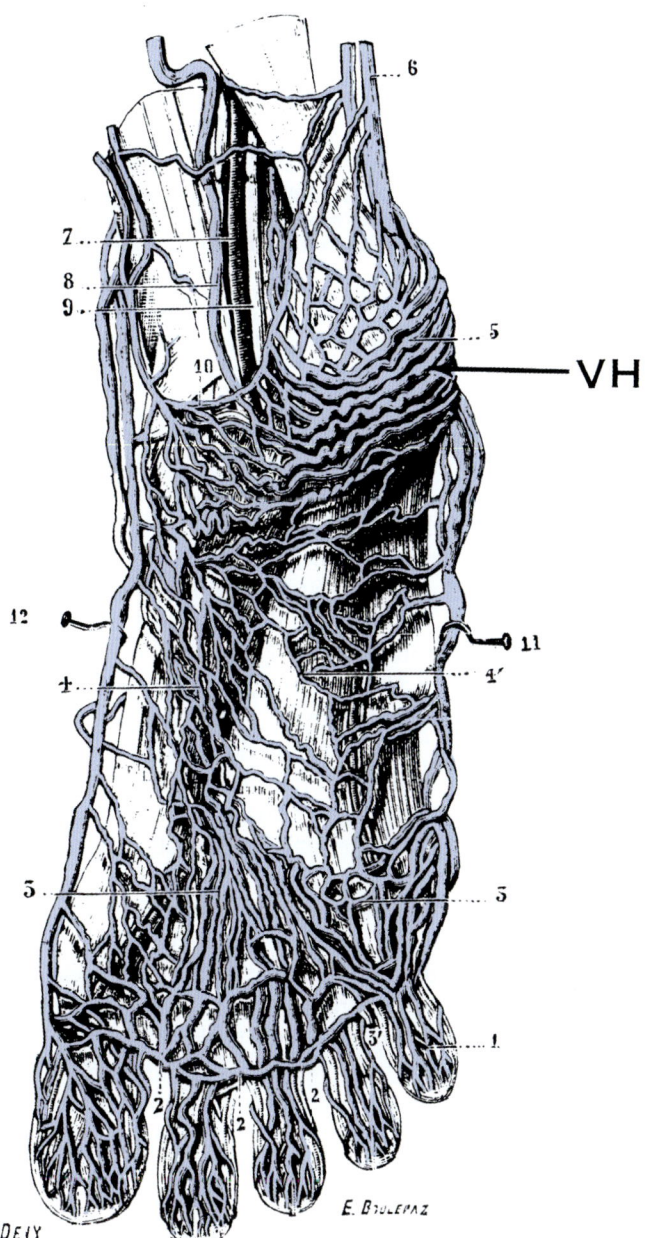

Figure 10.206 Transversely oriented veins of the heel (VH). Venous network of the sole of the foot (after a preparation of Lejars). (Adapted from Testut L. *Traité d'Anatomie Humaine, Tome II. Angeiologie-Système Nerveux Central.* Doin; 1921:339.)

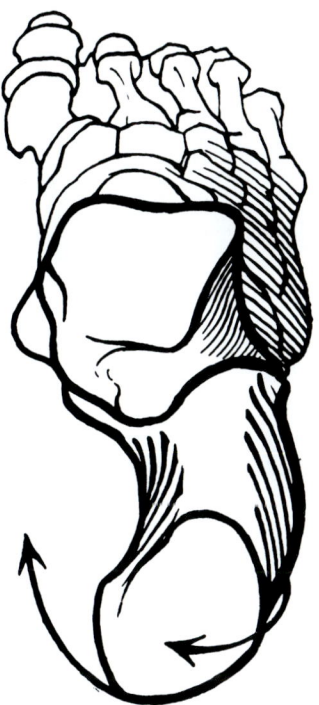

Figure 10.207 Scheme for the curvature and torsion of the whorls. They are in the same direction as the curvature and torsion of the calcaneus. (Blechschmidt E. The structure of the calcaneal padding, 1934. *Foot Ankle*. 1982;2[5]:271. Copyright ©1982. Reprinted by Permission of SAGE Publications.)

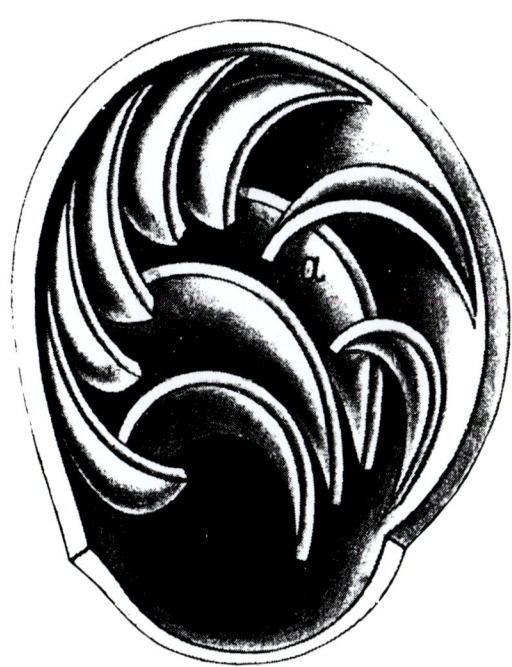

Figure 10.208 Construction of the padding of the heel and scheme for the function of the chambers. The padding is secured by the function of the "outer layer." (This operates in a fashion similar to that of the sole of the shoe.) (Blechschmidt E. The structure of the calcaneal padding, 1934. *Foot Ankle*. 1982;2[5]:282. Copyright ©1982. Reprinted by Permission of SAGE Publications.)

tissue components to their normal resting state when the foot leaves the ground to enter the swing phase."[167]

The shock absorbency of the heel pad has been tested experimentally by Jørgensen and Bojsen-Møller.[169] Ten human cadaver heel pads were subjected to drop test and exposed to impacts equivalent to heel-strike at fast walking. Compared to a viscoelastic polymer (Sorbothane) and to a common shock absorber in the shoe sole (ethylvinylacetate, or EVA), the heel pad shock absorbency "expressed as a ratio of the mean peak force reduction was found to be 1.13 and 2.09 times greater

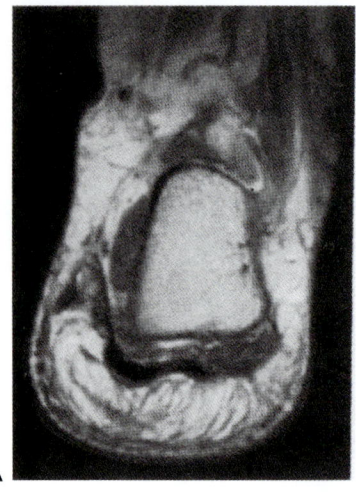 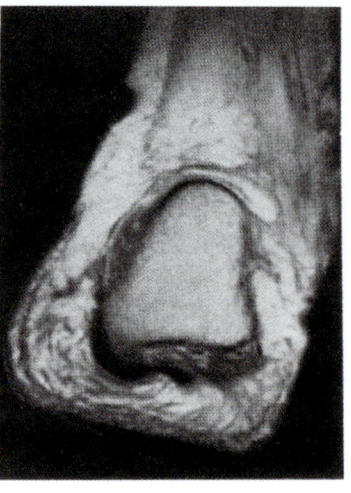

Figure 10.209 Coronal MRI sections through the mid calcaneus illustrating heel pad anatomy with non–weight-bearing and simulated weight-bearing. **(A)** Non–weight-bearing: Note the arch-shaped, elongated fat globules in the midline and the medial and lateral crescent-shaped globules. **(B)** Simulated weight-bearing: Note the compressed, flattened, central fat globules and the bending of the peripheral concentric globules, resulting in bulging of the medial and lateral walls of the heel pad. (Reprinted from Jahss MH, Kaye RA, Desai P, et al. Histology, histochemistry and biomechanics of the plantar fat pads in disorders of the foot and ankle. In: Jahss MM, ed. *Medical and Surgical Management*. 2nd ed. WB Saunders; 1991:2761.)

than that of the EVA foam and Sorbothane." The calculated vertical peak force output after impact force input was as follows:

Heel pad: 772 ± 95 N
Sorbothane: 1610 ± 48 N
EVA: 871 ± 17 N

with the ratios of the transmitted forces as

$$\frac{\text{Sorbothane}}{\text{heel pad}} = \frac{1610}{772} = 2.09$$

$$\frac{\text{EVA}}{\text{heel pad}} = \frac{871}{772} = 1.13$$

The transmitted force in the heel pads varied greatly, ranging from 533 to 1055 N.

In these experiments, the collision time was higher with the heel pad (13.9 ± 0.2 ms) and lower with Sorbothane (5.5 ± 0.1 ms) and EVA (8.8 ± 0.1 ms), indicating better energy dissipation provided by the heel pad (Fig. 10.210). The energy loss in the heel pad was 84%. This resulted in the suppression of any tendency of the heel to recoil at heel-strike, allowing the heel to stay longer on the ground and thus securing the grip. The energy is taken out as heat and as energy for the antigravitational return of the blood from the rich plantar venous network.

Injury to the heel may result in rupture of the fat-retaining compartments, allowing the fat to flow out when pressure is applied.[166,169,174] This decreases the shock absorbency of the heel, whereas the application of rigid external confinement to the heel augments it (Fig. 10.211). Jørgensen and coworkers devised a heel pad compressibility (HPC) device to quantify the heel pad shock absorbency in vitro and in vivo.[175] This was designed to examine the force/deformation characteristics of the heel pad through constant velocity compression and decompression of the stabilized heel. A force/deformation curve is established during compression of the heel pad. "During the compression, some of the energy is lost as heat; the rest is stored in the heel pad as elastic energy and is returned during decompression."[175] The magnitude of the energy loss between the energy input into the heel pad and the elastic energy output or return by the heel pad is an expression of shock absorbency.

The testing was performed on 200 heels of 100 normal subjects, 50 men and 50 women, with a mean age of 36 years (range, 17-84 years). The mean total deformation of the heel pad was 6.7 mm (range, 3.2-10.5 cm). A greater total deformation indicated a greater shock absorbency of the heel pad. The total deformation and thus shock absorbency decreased with age and was higher in men than in women. The heel pads with the lowest shock absorbency were the thinnest.

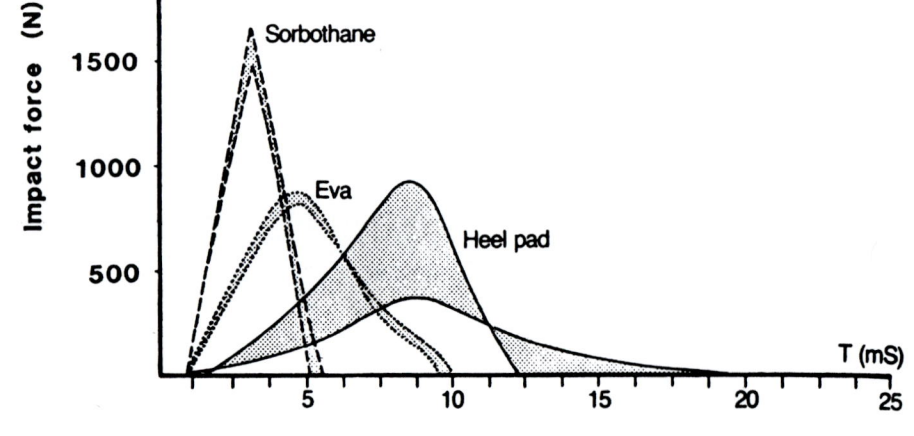

Figure 10.210 Individual variation in the heel pad shock absorbency. The mean heel pad shock absorbency was significantly better (lower impact force) than ethylvinylacetate (Eva) which in turn was significantly better than Sorbothane. (Jørgensen U, Bojsen-Møller F. The shock absorbency of factors in the shoe/heel interaction with special focus on the role of the heel pad. *Foot Ankle*. 1989;9[11]:296. Copyright ©1989. Reprinted by Permission of SAGE Publications.)

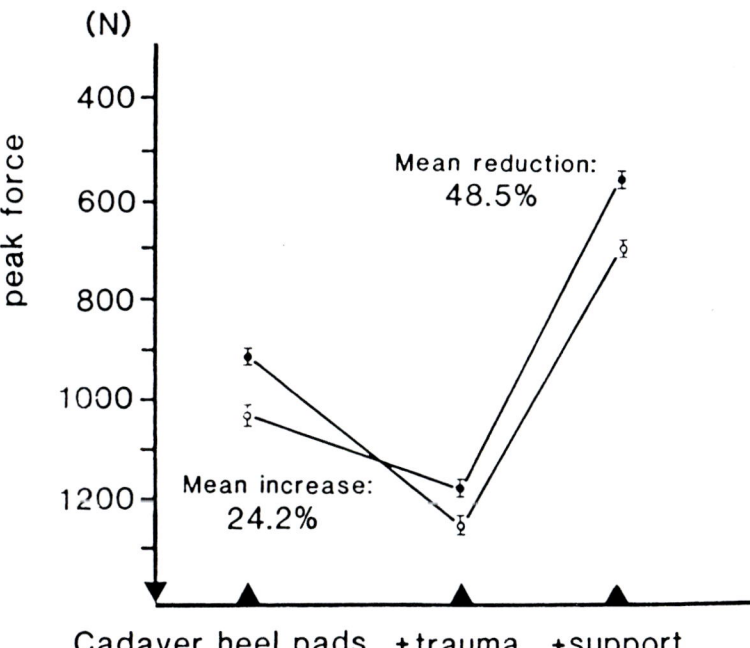

Figure 10.211 Trauma to heel pads reduced the shock absorbency significantly by increasing the peak force, whereas rigid external confinement reduced the peak force with a mean of 48.5%. (Jørgensen U, Bojsen-Møller F. The shock absorbency of factors in the shoe/heel interaction with special focus on the role of the heel pad. *Foot Ankle.* 1989;9[11]:296. Copyright ©1989. Reprinted by Permission of SAGE Publications.)

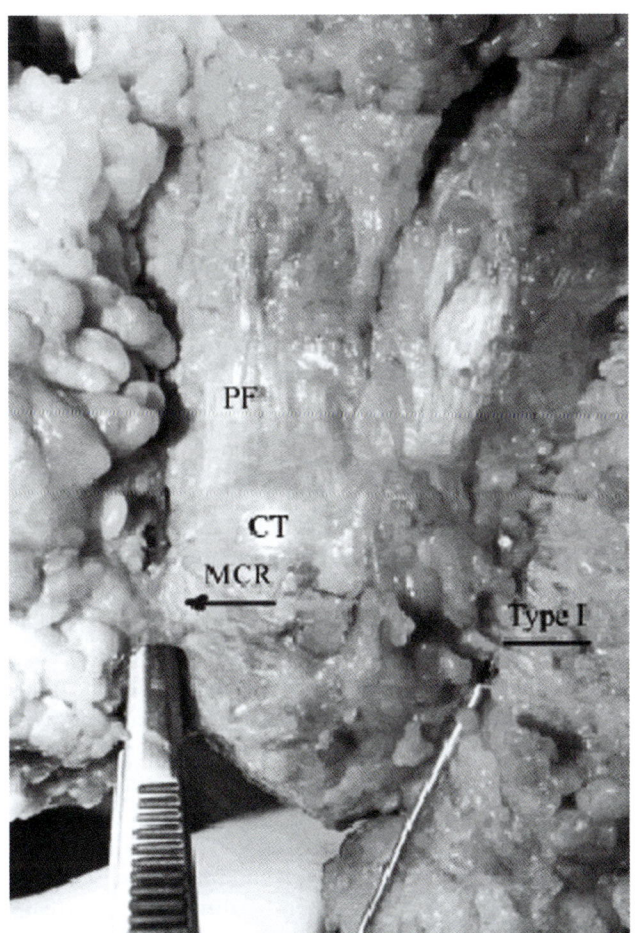

Figure 10.212 A plantar view of the hindfoot with the plan. (Snow SW, Bohne WHO. Observations on the fibrous retinacula of the heel pad. *Foot Ankle Int.* 2006;8:632-635, Fig. 6. Copyright ©2006. Reprinted by Permission of SAGE Publications.)

Jahss and colleagues made a histologic comparative study of three normal heel pads obtained from feet amputated for malignancy in patients 8, 17, and 18 years old and of five fresh specimens amputated in elderly patients because of vascular impairment.[176] The fat was quantitatively less in the senescent heel, but the striking feature was the presence of "more numerous, thicker and considerably fragmented" elastic fibers. This was considered a "hallmark of dermal degeneration." Both parameters may affect the shock-absorbency function of the heel pad during ambulation.

Snow and Bohne[177] investigated the anchoring of the heel pad in 10 adult cadaver feet. A longitudinal incision was made along the Achilles tendon and the plantar surface of the foot. The heel pad was reflected side-to-side exposing the calcaneal tuberosity. Anchoring "retinacular tethers of the heel pad" were observed and classified into two types: type 1, originating more from the plantar fascia and to a lesser degree from the calcaneus; and type 2 (fewer in occurrence), originating from both the medial and lateral sides of the calcaneus in two feet and only from the medial side in three feet. In 9 out of 10 specimens, a medial calcaneal retinaculum was identified, anchoring the heel pad, and originated from the medial process of the calcaneal tuberosity a few millimeters proximal to the origin of the plantar fascia and ranged from 5 to 25 mm in length and 4 to 8 mm in width (Fig. 10.212). The authors also observed that the peritenon of the Achilles tendon was continuous with the superficial fascia of the heel pad.

▶ Ball of the Foot: Forefoot Pad

During the stance phase of gait, the ball of the foot is subjected to compression, shear, and torque. Cushioning of the deep structures and stability of the skin are provided

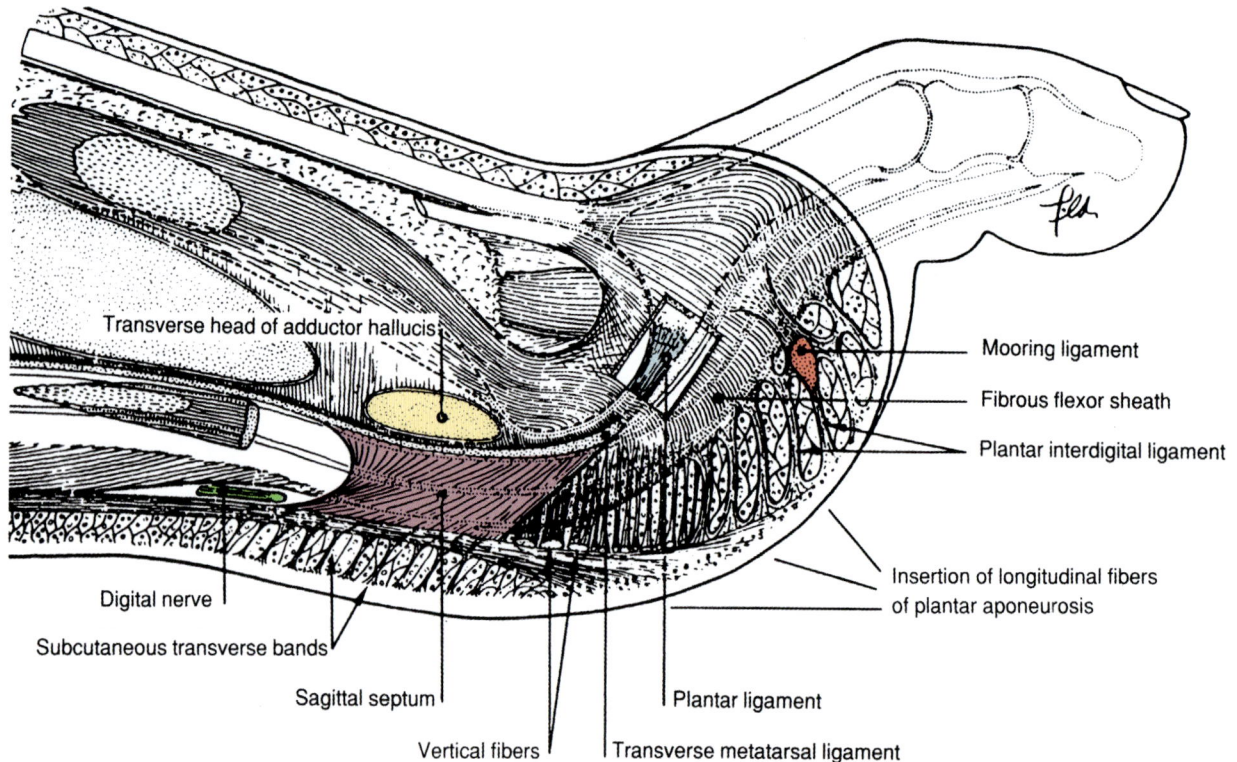

Figure 10.213 Drawing of a sagittal section through the second interstice showing the internal architecture of the three areas of the ball of the foot. The sagittal septum is attached to the proximal phalanx through the transverse metatarsal ligament and the plantar ligament of the joint. The vertical fibers and the lamellae of the plantar interdigital ligament are attached to the proximal phalanx through the fibrous flexor sheath. (Adapted from Bojsen-Møller F, Flagstad KE. Plantar aponeurosis and internal architecture of the ball of the foot. *J Anat.* 1976;121[3]:599.)

by a complex framework of connective tissue retaining the adipose tissue and providing attachment of the skin to the deep structures. A comprehensive description of their interrelationship has been provided by Bojsen-Møller and Flagstad,[178] expanding on the previous specific descriptions of Henkel[179] and Hicks.[95]

At the level of the ball of the foot, the superficial tracts of the plantar aponeurosis fan out and insert into the dermis, providing calcaneocutaneous attachment. The subcutaneous space, proximal to the aponeurotic insertion, is crossed by subtle transversely oriented connective tissue bands retaining adipose tissue. The subcutaneous space is converted into adipose tissue microchambers by additional vertical connective tissue bands, some of which arise from the sides of the digital flexor tendons' fibrous tunnel. Distally, the plantar digital ligament or natatory ligament with the transversely oriented band is attached vertically to the dermis and to the digital flexor tunnel. This provides the digitocutaneous anchorage reinforced by the mooring transverse digital ligaments (Fig. 10.213). Adipose tissue is retained between the transverse bands of the plantar interdigital ligament. The skin of the ball of the foot is thus anchored longitudinally, vertically, and transversely to the plantar aponeurosis and to the digital frame.

Proximal to each metatarsal head, the deep component of the plantar aponeurosis inserts onto the plantar plate and the deep transverse metatarsal ligament through two vertical septa. This is the anatomic basis of Hicks windlass mechanism. The hyperextension of the toes at the metatarsophalangeal joint tenses the plantar aponeurosis and subsequently stabilizes the skin of the ball of the foot. As mentioned by Bojsen-Møller, "In the relaxed state, the ball of the foot is a soft and pliable pad... however, with the toes extended and abducted, as during the push-off, the ball becomes tense and firm and no movement of the skin is allowed."[178] "This stiffening ensures that shear forces resulting from accelerations, decelerations or twists are not carried by the skin alone, but are conveniently taken up by the underlying connective tissue frame and transferred to the skeleton."[98]

Bojsen-Møller and Lamoreux, in an experimental setup, applied shear forces to the skin of the ball and central compartment of the foot and measured the skin displacement at 0° to 50° of hyperextension of the toes by increments of 10°.[98] At 0° of extension of the toes, there was a gradient of skin mobility from the central segment of the foot to the ball of the foot in a decreasing fashion. Furthermore, at the level of the ball of the foot, the medial plantar skin was more mobile

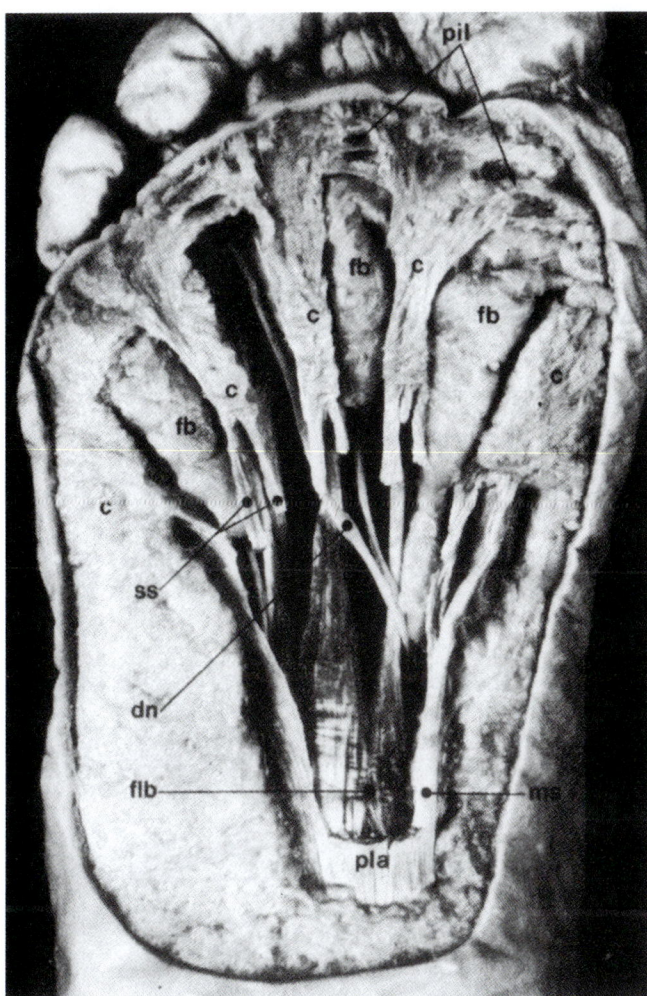

Figure 10.214 Dissected specimen of the sole of the foot. Five cushions (*c*) are located below the metatarsal heads with fat bodies (*fb*) between them. (*flb*, flexor digitorum brevis; *ms*, marginal septum; *pil*, plantar interdigital ligament; *pla*, plantar aponeurosis; *ss*, sagittal septa.) (From Bojsen-Møller F. Anatomy of the forefoot, normal and pathologic. *Clin Orthop Relat Res*. 1979;142:16.)

than the lateral. A large amount of dorsiflexion (35°-40°) of the toes was needed to achieve a 50% restriction of the skin displacement. It thus becomes apparent that a shoe with a rigid sole not allowing adequate hyperextension of the toes during gait interferes with the transmission of the shear tangential forces to the underlying deeper structures. The pressure absorption function of the ball of the foot is provided by the adipose tissue retained in specific locations by the connective tissue framework. In superficial locations are the subcutaneous microchambers proximally and the transverse chambers formed by the plantar interdigital bands distally. Deep in location are the five adipose cushions at the level of the metatarsal heads retained in the chambers formed by the flexor tendon sheath, the vertical connective tissue fibers, and the arcuate connective tissue fibers (Figs. 10.214 and 10.215). In between the metatarsal heads, plantar to the deep intermetatarsal ligaments, and covering the neurovascular bundles are the four large encapsulated "fat bodies" contributing to the shock-absorption mechanism.

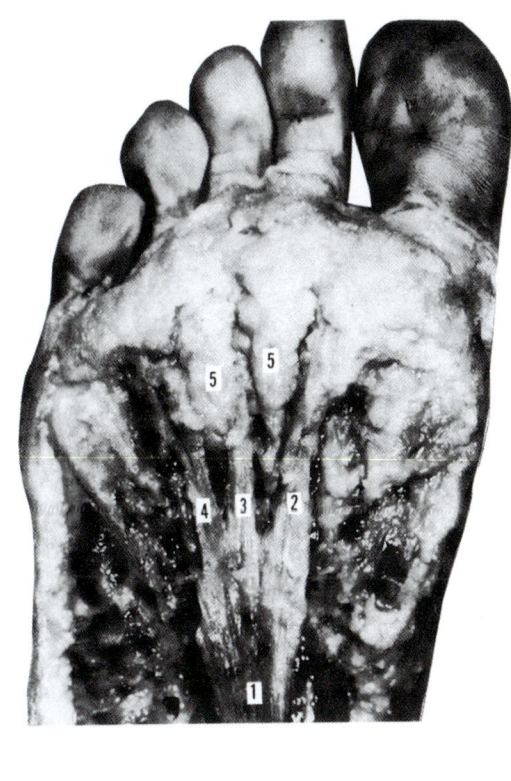

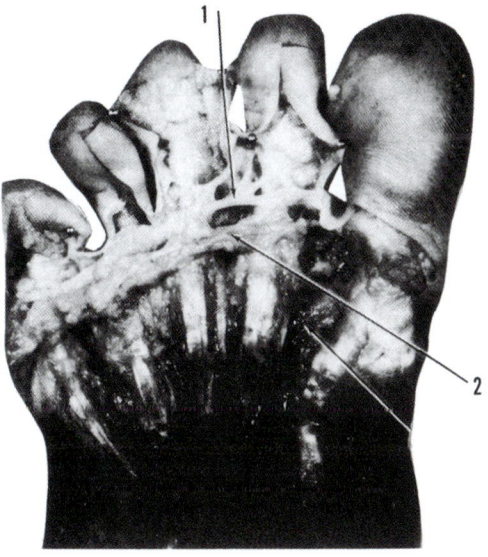

Figure 10.215 **(A)** The central segment of the plantar aponeurosis (*1*) with longitudinal bands (*2, 3, 4*) and fat bodies (*5*). **(B)** Retinacular natatory webbing ligaments (*1*) and transverse mooring ligament (*2*).

ELECTROMYOGRAPHIC ACTIVITIES DURING THE WALKING CYCLE

Electromyographically, the muscles acting on the foot-ankle complex may be grouped as follows (Fig. 10.216)[127,145,180-182]:

Anterior muscles: tibialis anterior, extensor digitorum longus, extensor hallucis longus

Posterior muscles: triceps surae, tibialis posterior, flexor digitorum longus, flexor hallucis longus, peroneus longus, peroneus brevis

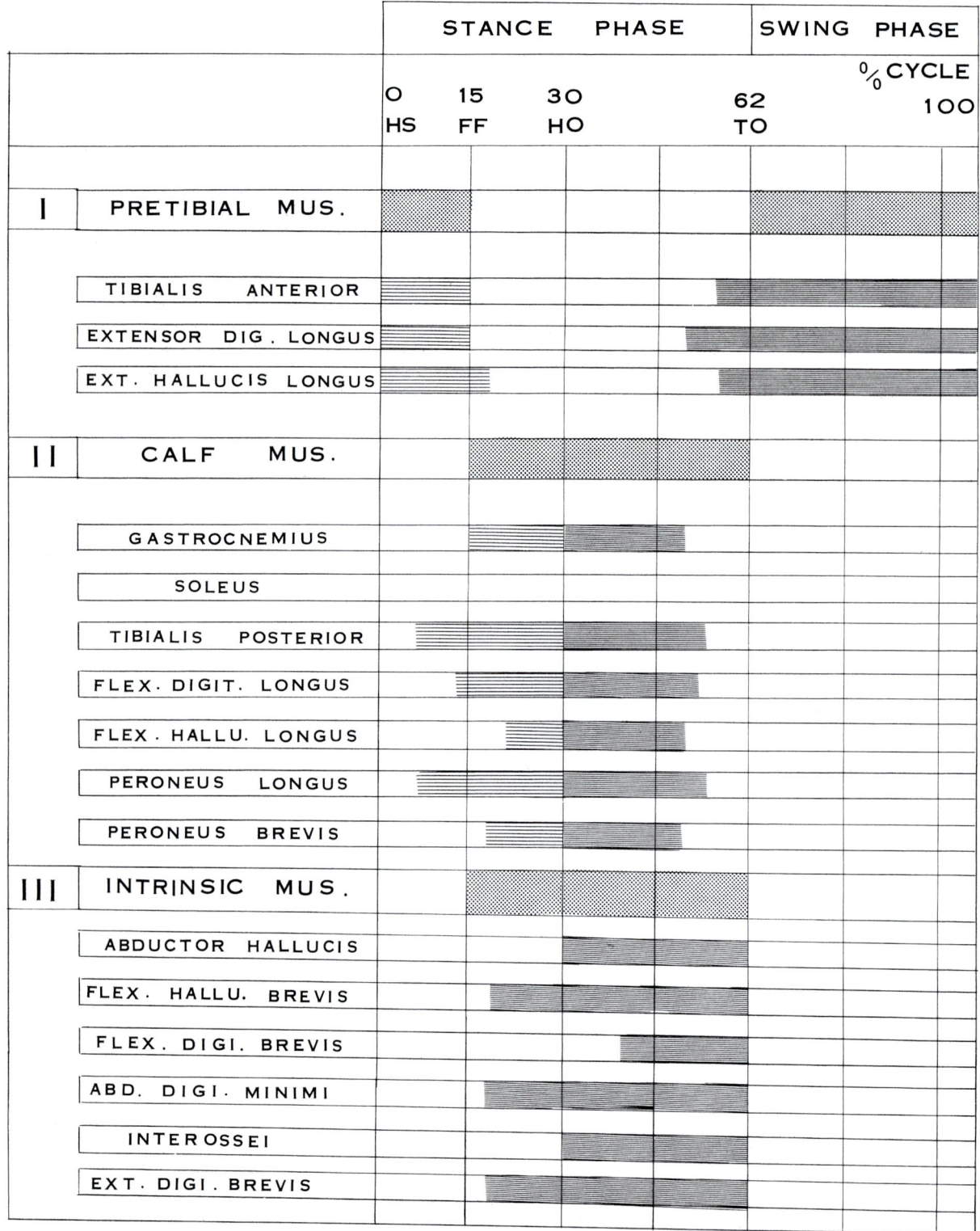

Figure 10.216 **Electromyography of the leg and foot muscle during the gait cycle.** Wider parallel lines indicate lengthening or eccentric contraction. Narrower parallel lines indicate shortening or concentric contraction. (*FF*, foot flat; *HO*, heel-off; *HS*, heel-strike; *TO*, toe-off.) (Data from Bowker JH, Hall CB. Normal human gait. In: *American Academy of Orthopedic Surgeons: Atlas of Orthotics: Biomechanical Principles and Application.* CV Mosby; 1975:141; and from Mann R, Inman VT. Phasic activity of intrinsic muscles of the foot. *J Bone Joint Surg Am.* 1964;46[3]:469.)

Intrinsic muscles: extensor digitorum brevis, flexor digitorum brevis, abductor hallucis, adductor hallucis, flexor hallucis brevis, abductor digiti minimi, interossei

The stance phase of the gait cycle may be divided into a single limb support and a double limb support. The latter occurs initially until 12% of the cycle and at the end of the support phase from 50% to 62%. The single support phase extends from 12% to 50% of the cycle.[128,145] The anterior muscle group is electrically active during the double support phases and the swing phase of the gait cycle. The posterior muscle group is electrically active during the single stance phase of the cycle.

The intrinsic muscles are inactive during the initial double support phase and early single support phase. They gradually increase their activity during the single support phase and remain active in the second double support phase.[183] More specifically, the anterior muscle group is active during the initial double support phase to control the plantar flexion, decelerate the foot, and prevent the foot from slapping the ground. The muscles undergo a lengthening or eccentric contraction. The second peak of activity of these muscles is related to the dorsiflexion of the foot to clear the toes from the ground. During the swing phase, the tibialis anterior muscle is responsible for the dorsiflexion of the accelerated foot. It undergoes a period of electric silence at mid swing as the foot is everting to allow adequate clearance; it increases its activity at deceleration and inverts the foot.[182] The contraction is of the concentric type.

The posterior muscle group is silent during the second double support phase of the cycle and the toe-off. During the first half of the single limb stance phase, the demands of propulsion and stability are minimum and the posterior muscle group activity is minimum. During the second half of the single limb stance phase, there is increasing forward velocity and precarious stability "created by the forward position of the body's center of gravity and the opposing swinging limb."[184] The posterior muscle group is active to restrain the forward movement of the tibia. This provides dynamic stability and "allows the body to lean farther forward beyond its base of support" to take a longer stride.[184] The contraction of the posterior muscles is initially of the lengthening type, followed by concentric contraction. It becomes apparent that it is the body forward momentum that causes the push-off or rolling phase, and the posterior muscles are not actively responsible for this phase of the gait cycle. The peroneus longus works in concert with the tibialis posterior and prevents excessive inversion of the foot and contributes to the maintenance of appropriate contact with the ground.[184]

The intrinsic muscles of the foot are considered to be invertors of the foot acting on the subtalar joint, and they contribute to the stabilization of the foot during propulsion. Their activity ceases at toe-off.[183]

REFERENCES

1. Huson A. Joints and movements of the foot: terminology and concepts. *Acta Morphol Neerl Scand.* 1987;25:117.
2. Ambagtsheer JBT. The function of the muscles of the lower leg in relation to movements of the tarsus: an experimental study in human subjects. *Acta Orthop Scand Suppl.* 1978;172:1-196.
3. Van Langelaan EJ. A kinematic analysis of the tarsal joints. An X-ray photogrammetric study. *Acta Orthop Scand Suppl.* 1983;204:1-269.
4. Benink RJ. The constraint mechanism of the human tarsus: a roentgenological experimental study. *Acta Orthop Scand Suppl.* 1985;215:1-135.
5. Lundberg A, Goldie I, Kalin BO, et al. Kinematics of the ankle/foot complex: plantar flexion and dorsi-flexion. *Foot Ankle.* 1989;9(4):194.
6. Lundberg A, Svensson OK, Bylund C, et al. Kinematics of the ankle/foot complex, part 2: pronation and supination. *Foot Ankle.* 1989;9(5):248.
7. Lundberg A, Svensson OK, Bylund C, et al. Kinematics of the ankle/foot complex, part 3: influence of leg rotations. *Foot Ankle.* 1989;9(6):304.
8. Huson A. *Ein Ontleedkundig-Functioneel Onderzoek van de Voetwortel.* Drukkerij; 1961.
9. Lang J, Wachsmuth W. *Praktische Anatomie: Ein Lehr und Hilfsbuch der Anatomischen Grundlagen Artztlichen Handelns*, Vol 1, Part 4. Springer-Verlag; 1972:370-376, 388-390.
10. Inman VT. *The Joints of the Ankle.* Williams & Wilkins; 1976:19-73.
11. Barnett CH, Napier JR. The axis of rotation at the ankle joint in man: its influence upon the form of the talus and the mobility of the fibula. *J Anat.* 1952;86:1.
12. Hicks JH. The mechanics of the foot. I: the joints. *J Anat.* 1953;87:345.
13. Lundberg A, Svensson OK, Nemeth G, et al. The axis of rotation of the ankle joint. *J Bone Joint Surg Br.* 1989;71(1):94.
14. Sammarco GJ, Burstein AH, Frankel VH. Biomechanics of the ankle: a kinematic study. *Orthop Clin North Am.* 1973;4(1):75.
15. Stauffer RN, Chao EYS, Brewster RC. Force and motion analysis of the normal, diseased and prosthetic ankle joint. *Clin Orthop Relat Res.* 1977;127:189.
16. Close JR. Some applications of the functional anatomy of the ankle joint. *J Bone Joint Surg Am.* 1956;38(1):761.
17. Close JR, Inman VT. *The Action of the Ankle Joint. Report to the Advisory Committee on Artificial Limbs, National Research Council.* Prosthetic Devices Research Project, Institute of Engineering Research, University of California; 1951. Series II, No. 22.
18. McCullough CJ, Burge PD. Rotary stability of the load-bearing ankle. An experimental study. *J Bone Joint Surg Br.* 1980;62(4):460.
19. Bremer SW. The unstable ankle mortise: functional ankle varus. *J Foot Surg.* 1985;24(5):313.
20. Poirier et Charpy. *Traite d'Anatomie Humaine Tome I Arthrologie.* Masson Ed; 1899:756.
21. Kärrholm J, Hansson LI, Selvik G. Mobility of the lateral malleolus: a roentgen stereo-photogrammetric analysis. *Acta Orthop Scand.* 1985;56:479.
22. Weinert CR Jr, McMaster JH, Ferguson RJ. Dynamic function of the human fibula. *Am J Anat.* 1973;138:145.
23. Scranton PE, McMaster JH, Kelly E. Dynamic fibular function: a new concept. *Clin Orthop Relat Res.* 1976;118:76.
24. Xenos JS, Hopkinson WJ, Mulligan ME, et al. The tibiofibular syndesmosis: evaluation of ligamentous structures, method of fixation, and radiographic assessment. *J Bone Joint Surg Am.* 1995;77:847-856.
25. Beumer A, Valstar ER, Garling EH, et al. Kinematics of the distal tibiofibular syndesmosis. Radiostereometry in 11 normal ankles. *Acta Orthop Scand.* 2003;74(3):337-343.
26. Glasgow M, Jackson A, Jamieson AM. Instability of the ankle after injury to the lateral ligament. *J Bone Joint Surg Br.* 1980;62(2):196.
27. Freeman MAR. Instability of the foot after injuries to the lateral ligament of the ankle. *J Bone Joint Surg Br.* 1965;47(4):669.
28. Landeros O, Frost HM, Higgins CC. Post-traumatic anterior ankle instability. *Clin Orthop Relat Res.* 1968;56:169.
29. Laurin C, Mathieu J. Sagittal mobility of the normal ankle. *Clin Orthop Relat Res.* 1975;108:99.
30. Johnson EE, Markolf KL. The contribution of the anterior talo-fibular ligament to ankle laxity. *J Bone Joint Surg Am.* 1983;65(1):81.
31. Rasmussen O. Stability of the ankle joint. Analysis of the function and traumatology of the ankle ligaments. *Acta Orthop Scand.* 1985;211:1-75.
32. Cass JR, Morrey BF, Chao EYS. Three-dimensional kinematics of ankle instability following serial sectioning of lateral collateral ligaments. *Foot Ankle.* 1984;5(3):142.
33. Harper MC. Posterior instability of the talus: anatomic evaluation. *Foot Ankle.* 1989;10(1):36.
34. Pierre RK St, Rosen J, Whitesides TE, et al. The tensile strength of the anterior talo-fibular ligament. *Foot Ankle.* 1983;4(2):83.

35. Attarian DE, McCrackin HJ, Devito DP, et al. A biomechanical study of human lateral ankle ligaments and autogenous reconstructive grafts. Am J Sports Med. 1985;13(6):377.
36. Siegler S, Block J, Schneck CD. The mechanical characteristics of the collateral ligaments of the human ankle joint. Foot Ankle. 1988;8(5):234.
37. Harper MC. Deltoid ligament: an anatomical evaluation of function. Foot Ankle. 1987;8(1):19.
38. Quiles M, Requena F, Gomez L, et al. Functional anatomy of the medial collateral ligament of the ankle joint. Foot Ankle. 1983;4(2):73.
39. Stormont DM, Morrey BF, Kai-nan AN, et al. Stability of the loaded ankle. Relation between articular restraint and primary and secondary static restraints. Am J Sports Med. 1985;13(5):295.
40. Manter JT. Movements of the subtalar and transverse tarsal joints. Anat Rec. 1941;80:397.
41. Isman RE, Inman VT. *Anthropometric Studies of the Human Foot and Ankle*. Technical Report. University of California, Berkeley, Biomechanics Laboratory; 1968.
42. Farabeuf LH. *Précis de Manuel Opératoire*. Masson; 1889:816-847.
43. Lewis OJ. *Functional Morphology of the Evolving Hand and Foot*. Clarendon Press; 1989:224.
44. Cahil DR. The anatomy and function of the contents of the human tarsal sinus and canal. Anat Rec. 1965;153:1.
45. Tochigi Y, Takahashi K, Yamagata M, et al. Influence of the interosseous talocalcaneal ligament injury on stability of the ankle-subtalar joint complex: a cadaveric experimental study. Foot Ankle Int. 2000;6:486-491.
46. Tochigi Y, Amendola A, Rudert MJ, et al. The role of the interosseous talocalcaneal ligament in subtalar joint stability. Foot Ankle Int. 2004;8:588-596.
47. Fujii T, Kitaoka HB, Luo ZP, et al. Analysis of ankle-hindfoot stability in multiple planes: an in vitro study. Foot Ankle Int. 2005;8:633-637.
48. Kjaersgaard-Andersen P, Wethelund J-O, Helmig P, et al. The stability effect of the ligamentous structures in the sinus and canalis tarsi on movements in the hindfoot. An experimental study. Am J Sports Med. 1988;16(5):512.
49. Kjaersgaard-Andersen P, Wethelund J-O, Helmig P, et al. Stabilizing effect of the tibio-calcaneal fascicle of the deltoid ligament on hindfoot joint movements: an experimental study. Foot Ankle. 1989;10(1):30.
50. Kjaersgaard-Andersen P, Wethelund J-O, Nielsen S. Lateral talocalcaneal instability following section of the calcaneo-fibular ligament: a kinesiologic study. Foot Ankle. 1987;7(6):355.
51. Trouilloud P, Dia A, Grammont P, et al. Variations du ligament calcanéo-fibulare (lig. calcaneo-fibulare). Application a la cinématique de la cheville. Bull Assoc Anat. 1988;72:31.
52. Martin LP, Wayne JS, Monahan TJ, et al. Elongation behavior of calcaneofibular and cervical ligaments during inversion loads applied in an open kinetic chain. Foot Ankle Int. 1998;19(4):232-239.
53. Manners-Smith T. A study of the cuboid and os peroneum in the primate foot. J Anat Physiol. 1908;42:399.
54. Farabeuf LH. *Précis de Manuel Opératoire*. Masson; 1889:836-847.
55. Elftman H. The transverse tarsal joint and its control. Clin Orthop Relat Res. 1960;16:41.
56. Leland RH, Marymont JV, Trevino SG, et al. Calcaneocuboid stability: a clinical and anatomical study. Foot Ankle Int. 2001;11:880-884.
57. Ouzounian TJ, Shereff MJ. In vitro determination of midfoot motion. Foot Ankle. 1989;10(3):140.
58. Waninvenhaus A, Pretterklieber M. First tarso-metatarsal joint: anatomical biomechanical study. Foot Ankle. 1989;9(4):153.
59. Romash MM, Fugate D, Yanklowit B. Passive motion of the first metatarsal cuneiform joint: preoperative assessment. Foot Ankle. 1990;10(6):293.
60. Hoefnagels EM, Waites MD, Wing ID, et al. Biomechanical comparison of the interosseous tibiofibular ligament and the anterior tibiofibular ligament. Foot Ankle Int. 2007;5:602-604.
61. Lambert KL. The weight-bearing function of the fibula: a strain gauge study. J Bone Joint Surg Am. 1971;53(3):507.
62. Ramsey PL, Hamilton W. Changes in tibio-talar area of contact caused by lateral talar shift. J Bone Joint Surg Am. 1976;58(3):356.
63. Michelson JD, Checcone M, Kuhn T, et al. Intra-articular load distribution in the human ankle joint during motion. Foot Ankle Int. 2003;3:226-233.
64. MacConaill MA, Basmajian JV. *Muscles and Movements: A Basis for Human Kinesiology*. Williams & Wilkins; 1969:78, 79.
65. DeVogel PL. *Enige functioneel-anatomische aspecten van ket bovenste spronggewricht*. Thesis; University of Leiden; 1970.
66. Ruth CJ. Surgical treatment of injuries of the fibular collateral ligament of the ankle. J Bone Joint Surg. 1961;43:229.
67. Renstrom P, Wertz M, Incavo S, et al. Strain in the lateral ligaments of the ankle. Foot Ankle. 1988;9(2):59.
68. Rubin G, Witten M. The talar tilt angle and the fibular collateral ligaments. J Bone Joint Surg Am. 1960;42:311.
69. Lakin RC, Degnore LT, Pienkowski D. Contact mechanics of normal tarsometatarsal joints. J Bone Joint Surg Am. 2001;83-A(4):520-528.
70. Sloan MC, Moorman CT, Miyamoto RG, et al. Ligamentous restrains of the second tarsometatarsal joint: a biomechanical evaluation. Foot Ankle Int. 2001;8:637-641.
71. Kaar S, Femino J, Morag Y. Lisfranc joint displacement following sequential ligament sectioning. J Bone Joint Surg Am. 2007;89:2225-2232.
72. Mizel MS. The role of the plantar first metatarsal first cuneiform ligament in weightbearing on the first metatarsal. Foot Ankle. 1993;14(14):82-84.
73. Viladot Perice A. *Patologia del Antepie*. Ediciones Toray, SA; 1974:4-14.
74. Johnson KA. *Surgery of the Foot and Ankle*. Raven Press; 1989:18.
75. Joseph J. Range of movement of the great toe in men. J Bone Joint Surg Br. 1954;36:450.
76. Hardy RH, Chapman JCR. Observations on hallux valgus based on a controlled series. J Bone Joint Surg Br. 1951;33:376.
77. Steel MW III, Johnson KA, DeWitz MA, et al. Radiographic measurements of the normal adult foot. Foot Ankle. 1980;1(3):154.
78. Wilkinson JL. The terminal phalanx of the great toe. J Anat. 1954;88:537.
79. Scheck M. Etiology of acquired hammer toe deformity. Clin Orthop Relat Res. 1977;123:63.
80. Kelikian H. The hallux. In: Jahss MH, ed. *Disorders of the Foot*. Vol 1. WB Saunders; 1982:540.
81. Myerson MS, Shereff MJ. The pathologic anatomy of claw and hammer toes. J Bone Joint Surg Am. 1989;71(1):45.
82. Sammarco JG. Biomechanics of the foot. In: Frankel VH, Nordin M, eds. *Basic Biomechanics of the Skeletal System*. Lea & Febiger; 1980:202-204.
83. Shereff MJ, Bejjani FJ, Kummer FJ. Kinematics of the first metatarsophalangeal joint. J Bone Joint Surg Am. 1986;68(3):392.
84. Jahss MH. Traumatic dislocations of the first metatarso-phalangeal joint. Foot Ankle. 1980;1:15.
85. MacConaill MA. The postural mechanism of the human foot. Proc R Ir Acad. 1945;50(14):265.
86. Blechschmidt E. The structure of the calcaneal padding. Foot Ankle. 1982;2(5):260.
87. Sarrafian SK. Functional characteristics of the foot and plantar aponeurosis under tibio-talar loading. Foot Ankle. 1987;8(1):4.
88. Barclay-Smith E. The astragalo-calcaneo-navicular joint. J Anat Physiol. 1896;30:390.
89. McElvenny RT, Caldwell GD. A new operation for correction of cavus foot: fusion of first metatarsal-cuneiform, navicular joints. Clin Orthop Relat Res. 1958;11:85.
90. Coleman SS, Chestnut WJ. A simple test for hindfoot flexibility in the cavo-varus foot. Clin Orthop Relat Res. 1977;123:60.
91. Olerud C, Rosendahl Y. Torsion transmitting properties of the hindfoot. Clin Orthop Relat Res. 1987;214:28.
92. Ellis TS. *The Human Foot: Its Form and Structure, Functions and Clothing*. Churchill; 1889:1-113.
93. MacConaill MA. Some anatomical factors affecting the stabilizing functions of muscles. Ir J Med Soc. 1946;6:160.
94. Sarrafian SK, Topouzian LK. Anatomy and physiology of the extensor apparatus of the toes. J Bone Joint Surg Am. 1969;51(4):669.
95. Hicks JH. The mechanics of the foot, II. The plantar aponeurosis and the arch. J Anat. 1954;88:25.
96. Fick L. Cited by R. Fick. *Handbuch der Anatomie und Mechanik der Gelenke, under Berücksichtigung der Bewegenden Muskeln, Part I*. Gustav Fischer; 1910:638.
97. Fick R. *Handbuch der Anatomie und Mechanik der Gelenke, under Berücksichtigung der Bewegenden Muskeln, Part I*. Gustav Fischer; 1910:638.
98. Bojsen-Møller F, Lamoreux L. Significance of free dorsiflexion of the toes in walking. Acta Orthop Scand. 1979;50(4):471.
99. Lapidus PW. Kinesiology and mechanical anatomy of the tarsal joints. Clin Orthop Relat Res. 1963;30:30.
100. Manter JT. Distribution of compression forces in the joints of the human. Anat Rec. 1946;96:313.

101. MacConaill MA, Basmajian JV. *Muscles and Movements: A Basis for Human Kinesiology*. Williams and Wilkins; 1969:245-246.
102. Hicks JH. The foot as a support. *Acta Anat*. 1955;25:34.
103. Hicks JH. The three weight-bearing mechanisms of the foot. In: Evans FG, ed. *Biomechanical Studies of the Musculo-Skeletal System*. Charles C Thomas; 1961:161-191.
104. Braune W, Fischer O. *On the Center of Gravity of the Human Body*. Maquet PGS, Furlong R (trans). Springer-Verlag; 1985:68.
105. Brunnstrom S. Center of gravity line in relation to ankle joint in erect standing. Application to posture training and artificial legs. *Phys Ther Rev*. 1954;34(3):109.
106. Hesser C. Var faller kroppens tyngdlinje i staende stallningar? *Svenska Lak Sallsk Handl*. 1918;44:133.
107. Basler A. Beitrage zur physiologie des Stehens. *Arbeits Physiol*. 1942-1943;12:104.
108. Hellebrandt FA, Braun GL. The influence of sex and age on the postural sway in man. *Am J Phys Anthropol*. 1939;24:347.
109. Hellebrandt FA, et al. The constancy of oscillographic stance patterns. *Phys Ther Rev*. 1942;22:17.
110. Takata K, Kakeno H, Watanabe Y. Time series analysis of postural sway and respiration using an autoregressive model. In: Matsui H, Kobayashi, eds. *Biomechanics*. Vol 8A. Human Kinetics Publishers; 1983:591.
111. Yamamoto T. Changes in postural stability with special reference to age. In: Morecki A, Fidelus K, Kedizor K, et al, eds. *Biomechanics*. Vol 7A. University Park Press; 1981:169.
112. Houtz SJ, Walsh FP. Electromyographic analysis of the function of the muscles acting on the ankle during weight-bearing with special reference to the triceps surae. *J Bone Joint Surg Am*. 1959;41(8):1469.
113. Basmajian JV, Stecko G. The roles of muscles in arch support of the foot: an electromyographic study. *J Bone Joint Surg Am*. 1963;45(6):1184.
114. Cavanagh PR, Rodgers MM, Liboshi A. Pressure distribution under symptom-free feet during barefoot standing. *Foot Ankle*. 1987;7(5):262.
115. Jones RL. The human foot: an experimental study of its mechanics and the role of its muscles and ligaments in the support of the arch. *Am J Anat*. 1941;68:1.
116. Testut L, Jacob O. *Traité d'Anatomie Topographique Avec Applications Médico-Chirurgicales*. Vol 2. Octave Doin; 1909:1110-1113.
117. Singh I. The architecture of cancellous bone. *J Anat*. 1978;127(2):305-310.
118. Pal GP, Routal RV. Architecture of the cancellous bone of the human talus. *Anat Rec*. 1998;252:185-193.
119. Ebraheim NA, Sabry FF, Nadim Y. Internal architecture of the talus: implication for the talar fracture. *Foot Ankle Int*. 1999;20(12):794-796.
120. Athavale SA, Joshi SD, Joshi SS. Internal architecture of the talus. *Foot Ankle Int*. 2008;1:82-86.
121. Paturet GL. *Traité d'Anatomie Humaine, Vol II. Membres Superieur et Inferieur*. Masson; 1951:603-604.
122. Harty M. Anatomic consideration in injuries of the calcaneus. *Orthop Clin North Am*. 1973;4(1):179.
123. Roig Puerta J. Nuevos metodos para la exploration complementaria del pie y estudio de la trabeculacion del astragalo. *Barcelona Quirurgia*. 1959;3:2.
124. Inman VT, Ralston HJ, Todd F. *Human Walking*. Williams & Wilkins; 1981:22.
125. Steindler A. *Kinesiology of the Human Body under Normal and Pathologic Conditions*. Charles C Thomas; 1970:631-664.
126. Mann RA. Overview of foot and ankle biomechanics. In: Jahss MH, ed. *Disorders of the Foot and Ankle. Medical and Surgical Management*. 2nd ed. WB Saunders; 1991:385-408.
127. Bowker HJ, Hall CB. Normal human gait. In: *American Academy of Orthotics. Biomechanical Principles and Application*. CV Mosby; 1975:133-143.
128. Murray MP, Drought AB, Kory RC. Walking patterns of normal men. *J Bone Joint Surg Am*. 1964;46(2):335.
129. Mann RA, Hagy JL. Running, Jogging and walking: a comparative electromyographic and biomechanical study in the foot and ankle. In: Bateman, Trott, eds. *American Orthopedic Foot Society*. BC Dekker; 1980:167-175.
130. Fryer C. *Normal Human Locomotion in Prosthetic-Orthotic Course*. Northwestern University Medical School; 1979.
131. Folman Y, Wask J, Voloshin A, et al. Cyclic impacts on heel strike: a possible biomechanical factor in etiology of degenerative disease of the human locomotor system. *Arch Orthop Trauma Surg*. 1986;104:363.
132. Bojsen-Møller F. Calcaneo-cuboid joint and stability of the longitudinal arch of the foot at high and low gear push-off. *J Anat*. 1979;129:165.
133. Wright DG, Desai SM, Henderson WH. Action of the subtalar and ankle joint complex during the stance phase of walking. *J Bone Joint Surg Am*. 1964;46(2):361.
134. Levens AS, Inman VT, Blosser JA. Transverse rotation of the segments of the lower extremity in locomotion. *J Bone Joint Surg Am*. 1948;30(4):859.
135. Saunders JB, Dec M, Inman VT, et al. The major determinants in normal and pathological gait. *J Bone Joint Surg Am*. 1953;35(3):543.
136. Sutherland DH, Hagy JL. Measurement of gait movements from motion picture film. *J Bone Joint Surg Am*. 1972;54(4):787.
137. Braune W, Fischer O. *The Human Gait*. Maquet P, Furlong R (trans). Springer-Verlag; 1987.
138. Bojsen-Møller F. The human foot—a two speed construction. In: Asmussen E, Jørgensen K, eds. *International Series of Biomechanics*. Vol 2A. University Park Press; 1978:261-266.
139. Perez HR, Reber LK, Christensen JC. The effect of frontal plane position on the first ray motion: forefoot locking mechanism. *Foot Ankle Int*. 2008;1:72-76.
140. Van de Velde SK, Gill TJ, Li G. Evaluation of kinematics of anterior cruciate ligament-deficient knees with use of advanced imaging techniques, three-dimensional modeling techniques, and robotics. *J Bone Joint Surg Am*. 2009;91(suppl 1):108-114.
141. Erdemir A, Hamel AJ, Fauth AR, et al. Dynamic loading of the plantar aponeurosis in walking. *J Bone Joint Surg Am*. 2004;86-A(3):546-552.
142. Reeck J, Felten N, McCormack AP, et al. Support of the talus: a biomechanical investigation of the contributions of the talonavicular and talocalcaneal joints, and the superomedial calcaneonavicular ligament. *Foot Ankle Int*. 1998;19:674-682.
143. Bohay DR, Anderson JG, Gentchos CE. Treatment of stage 2 posterior tendon dysfunction. In: Coetzee, Hurwitz, eds. *Arthritis and Arthroplasty*. Saunders; 2010:267.
144. Maskill JD, Bohay DR, Anderson JG. Gastrocnemius recession to treat isolated foot pain. *Foot Ankle Int*. 2010;1:19-23.
145. Mann RA, Baxter DE, Lutter LD. Running symposium. *Foot Ankle*. 1981;1(4):190.
146. Elftman H. A cinematic study of the distribution of pressure in the human foot. *Anat Rec*. 1934;59:481.
147. Elftman H. Forces and energy changes in the leg during walking. *Am J Physiol*. 1939;125:339.
148. Hutton WC, Stott JRR, Stokes IAF. The mechanics of the foot. In: Klenerman L, ed. *The Foot and Its Disorders*. Blackwell Scientific Publications; 1976:30-48.
149. Stott JRR, Hutton WC, Stokes IAF. Forces under the foot. *J Bone Joint Surg Br*. 1973;55:335.
150. Hutton WC, Dhanendran M. A study of the distribution of loads under the normal foot during walking. *Int Orthop*. 1979;3:153.
151. Betts RP, Franks CI, Duckworth T. Foot pressure studies: normal and pathologic gait analysis. In: Jahss MM, ed. *Disorders of the Foot and Ankle. Medical and Surgical Management*. 2nd ed. WB Saunders; 1991:484-519.
152. Betts RP, Franks CI, Duckworth T. Analysis of pressures and loads under the foot. Part 2: Quantification of the dynamic distribution. *Clin Phys Physiol Meas*. 1980;1:113.
153. Duckworth T, Betts RP, Franks CI, et al. The measurement of pressure under the foot. *Foot Ankle*. 1982;3:130.
154. Hughes J, Clark P, Klenerman L. The importance of the toes in walking. *J Bone Joint Surg Br*. 1990;72(2):245.
155. Munro M, Abernethy P, Paul I, et al. Peak dynamic force in human gait and its attenuation by the soft tissues (abstr). *Orthop Res Soc*. 1975;21:65.
156. Paul IL, Munro MB, Abernethy PJ, et al. Musculo-skeletal shock absorption: relative contribution of bone and soft tissues at various frequencies. *J Biomech*. 1978;2:237.
157. Cavanagh PR, LaFortune MA. Ground reaction forces in distance running. *J Biomech*. 1980;13:383.
158. Mann RA. Biomechanics of running. In: *AAOS Symposium on the Foot and Leg in Running Sports*. CV Mosby; 1982:30-44.
159. Bojsen-Møller F, Jørgensen U. The plantar soft tissues: functional anatomy and clinical applications. In: Jahss MM, ed. *Disorders of the Foot and Ankle: Medical and Surgical Management*. WB Saunders; 1991:532-540.
160. Steinbach HL, Russell W. Measurement of the heel pad as an aid to diagnosis of acromegaly. *Radiology*. 1964;82:418.

161. Gooding GAW, Stress RM, Graf PM, et al. Heel pad thickness: determination by high resolution ultrasonography. *J Ultrasound Med.* 1985;4:173.
162. Langfeldt B. Heel pad measurement. An aid to diagnosis of acromegaly. *Dan Med Bull.* 1968;15(2):40.
163. Ham AW. *Histology. The Integumentary Systems (The Skin and Its Appendages).* 2nd ed. JB Lippincott; 1953:438-443.
164. McCarthy DJ, Habowsky JE. Structural variability of the dermoepidermal interface of skin of the human foot as related to function. *J Am Podiatry Assoc.* 1975;65(5):450.
165. Tietze A. Concerning the architectural structure of the connective tissue in the human sole. *Foot Ankle.* 1982;2(5):252.
166. Kulms JG. Changes in elastic adipose tissue. *J Bone Joint Surg Am.* 1949;31(3):541.
167. Kimani JK. The structural and functional organization of the connective tissue in the human foot with reference to the histomorphology of the elastic fiber system. *Acta Morphol Neerl Scand.* 1984;22:313.
168. Jørgensen U. Achillodynia and loss of heel pad shock absorbency. *Am J Sports Med.* 1985;13(2):121.
169. Jørgensen U, Bojsen-Møller F. The shock absorbency of factors in the shoe/heel interaction with special focus on the role of the heel pad. *Foot Ankle.* 1989;9(11):294.
170. Jørgensen U, Ekstran J. The significance of heelpad confinement for the shock absorption at heel strike. *Int J Sports Med.* 1988;9:468.
171. Paturet G. *Traité d'Anatomie Humaine, Tome II. Membres Superieur et Inférieur.* Masson; 1951:1004-1005.
172. Testut L. *Traité d'Anatomie Humaine, Tome II. Angeiologie-Système Nerveux Central.* Doin; 1921:338-339.
173. Winter WG, Reiss OK. The plantar fat pads: anatomy and physiology of the heel pad. In: Jahss MH, ed. *Disorders of the Foot and Ankle. Medical and Surgical Management.* 2nd ed. WB Saunders; 1991:2745-2752.
174. Miller WE, Lichtblau PO. The smashed heel. *South Med J.* 1965;58:1229.
175. Jørgensen U, Larsen E, Varmarken JE. The HPC-device: a method to quantify the heel pad shock absorbency. *Foot Ankle.* 1989;10(2):93.
176. Jahss MH, Kaye RA, Desai P, et al. Histology, histochemistry and biomechanics of the plantar fat pads. In: Jahss MH, ed. *Disorders of the Foot and Ankle: Medical and Surgical Management.* 2nd ed. WB Saunders; 1991:2753-2762.
177. Snow SW, Bohne WHO. Observations on the fibrous retinacula of the heel pad. *Foot Ankle Int.* 2006;08:632-635.
178. Bojsen-Møller F, Flagstad KE. Plantar aponeurosis and internal architecture of the ball of the foot. *J Anat.* 1976;121(3):599.
179. Henkel A. Die aponeurosis plantaris. *Arch Anat Phys Anat.* 1913;113.
180. Mann RA. *Biomechanics of the foot.* In: American Academy of Orthopedic Surgeons. *Atlas of Orthotics: Biomechanical Principles and Application.* CV Mosby; 1975:257-266.
181. Eberhart JD, Inman VT, Bresler B. The principal elements in human locomotion. In: Klopsteg PE, Wilson PD, eds. *Human Limbs and Their Substitutes.* Hafner Publishing; 1968:437-471.
182. Gray EG, Basmajian JV. Electromyography and cinematography of the leg and foot ("normal" and flat) during walking. *Anat Rec.* 1968;161:1.
183. Mann R, Inman VT. Phasic activity of intrinsic muscles of the foot. *J Bone Joint Surg Am.* 1964;46(3):469.
184. Simon SR, Mann RA, Hagy JL, et al. Role of the posterior muscles in normal gait. *J Bone Joint Surg Am.* 1978;60(4):465.

II Applied Anatomy

Neuro Control of Stance and Gait

Shahan K. Sarrafian

11

Dedicated to Alice T. Lyon, MD "who preserved and restored my vision."

GRAVITY

Gravity prevails. Stance and gait are antigravitational activities. A skeleton held in upright position would collapse in flexion mode if unsupported (Fig. 11.1). Extensor muscles by spinal reflex motor contractions provide the initial extensor mode stability supplemented by the interaction of the cerebellovestibular system input. While standing, the center of gravity is located in front of the sacrum (Fig. 11.2).

In the standing position, the gravitational support surface is provided by a trapezoid surface defined by horizontal lines joining the heels posteriorly and the big toes anteriorly; the lateral borders of the feet enclose the supportive surface (Figs. 11.3 and 11.4). As indicated, the center of gravity, CG, projects at the intersection of the anterior/posterior axis of the support area, in midaxis, and the horizontal line, drawn at ⅔ on the posterio-anterior axis.

Based on this gravitation support diagram, we can sway along the posterio-anterior axis, more anteriorly (⅗) and less posteriorly (⅖), whereas the side-to-side sway is equal. During gait, we engage into a phase of alternate one for support base. Our equilibrium is more precarious on one foot as the center of gravity is to project alternately on a smaller surface. As indicated in Figure 11.5, the projector center of gravity of the body makes a sinusoidal displacement from stance-swing-stance phase.

The transfer of the body mass to the supporting foot, for example, the right, is accomplished by the facilitatory flexion-adduction of the corresponding left upper extremity (Fig. 11.6).

A ballerina performing "en pointe" posture has the exquisite motor skill of guiding the projection of the body mass or center of gravity to the tip of the supporting toes (Fig. 11.7).

As illustrated in Figures 11.8 and 11.9, during the stance on one lower extremity there is an asymmetric distribution of the body mass relative to the supporting extremity.

The body mass has the tendency to tilt laterally and anteriorly. The abnormal tilt of the body laterally and anteriorly is prevented by the simultaneous contraction of the gluteus medius and gluteus maximus muscles. During gait, the stance in equilibrium requires exquisite neuro control by input from the cerebellovestibular tracts. The balancing input from the corresponding upper extremity is provided by the rubrospinal tract receiving information from the cerebellum also (Fig. 11.10).

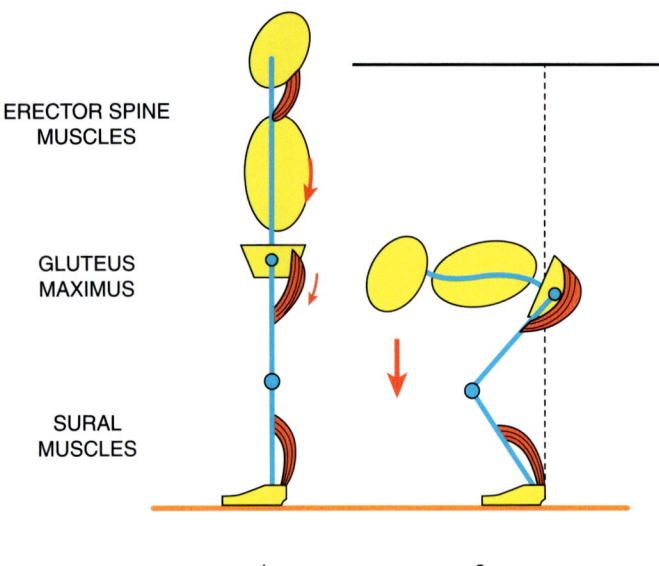

Figure 11.1 *1, Gravitational collapse is prevented by activation of extensor muscles of the head-neck, extensors of the spine, extensor of the hip by the gluteus maximus, and extension of the knee by the soleus muscle.* 2, The skeleton subjected to gravity collapses in flexion mode.

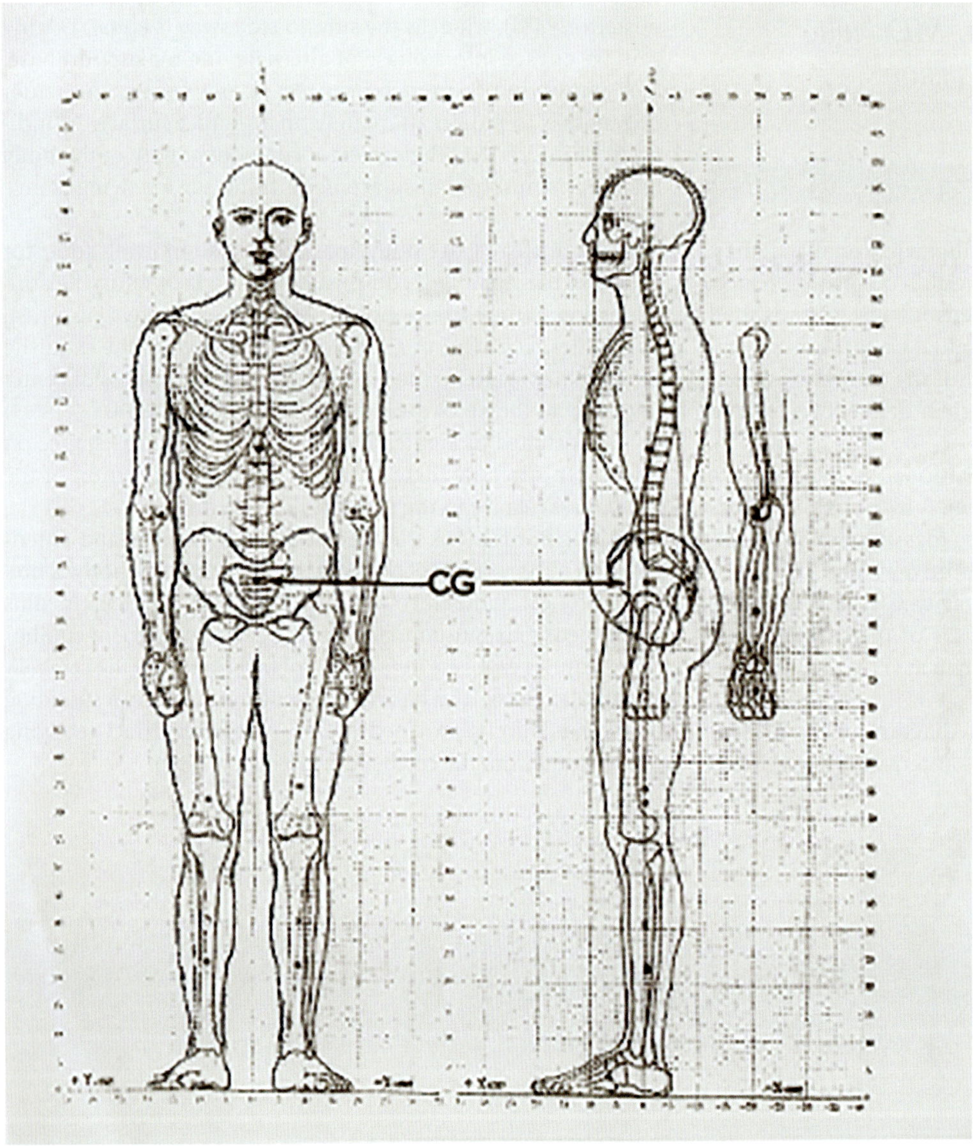

Figure 11.2 Location of the center of gravity (CG) of the human body. (With permission from D P E. On the centre of gravity of the human body by W. Braune and O. Fischer Springer-Verlag; 1985:96. DM 68. *Clin Biomech* (Bristol, Avon). 1986;1(1):59.)

Chapter 11: Neuro Control of Stance and Gait 649

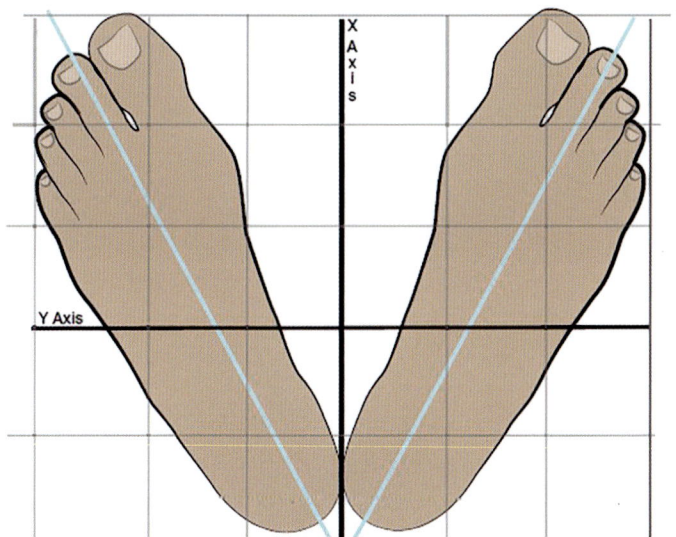

Figure 11.3 Gravitational body support is as indicated by the striated trapezoidal surface. The center of gravity (CG) is located at the transection of x-y axes.

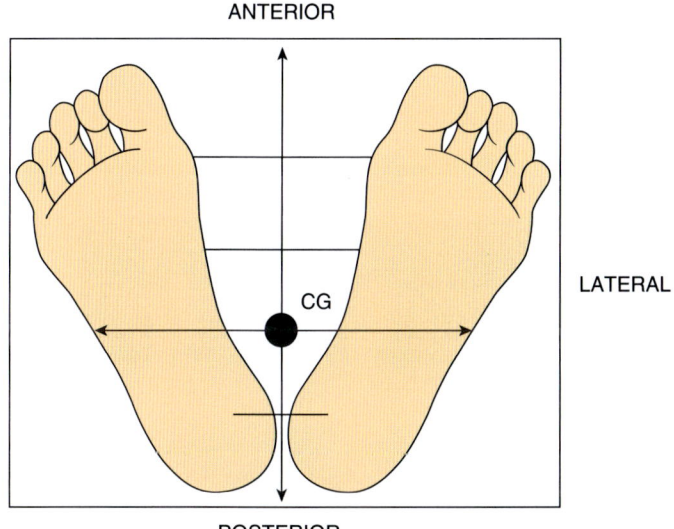

Figure 11.4 Amount of swing without losing equilibrium in the posterior-anterior and medial-lateral directions.

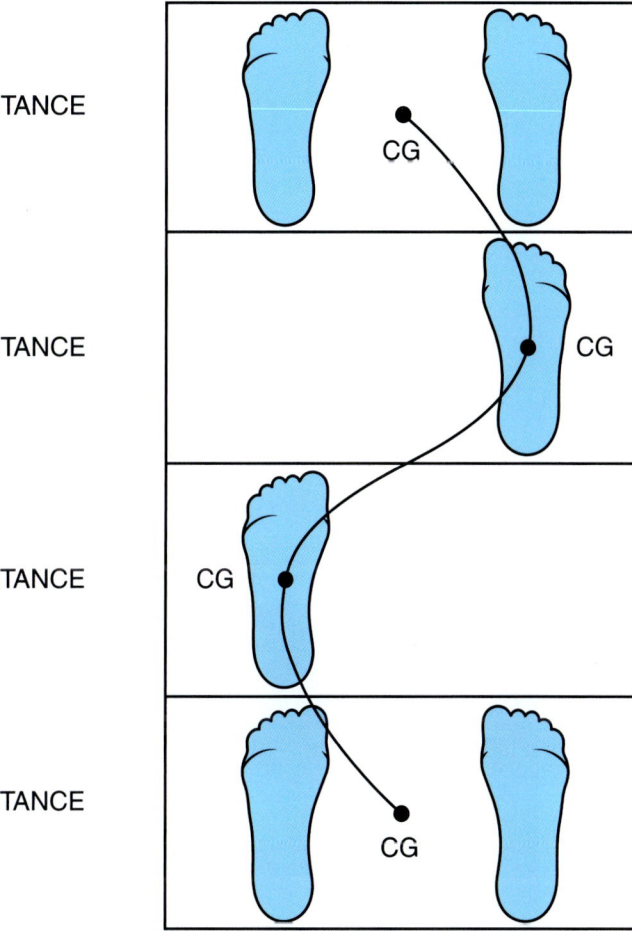

Figure 11.5 Sinusoidal displacement of the center of gravity (CG) in one swing-stand cycle.

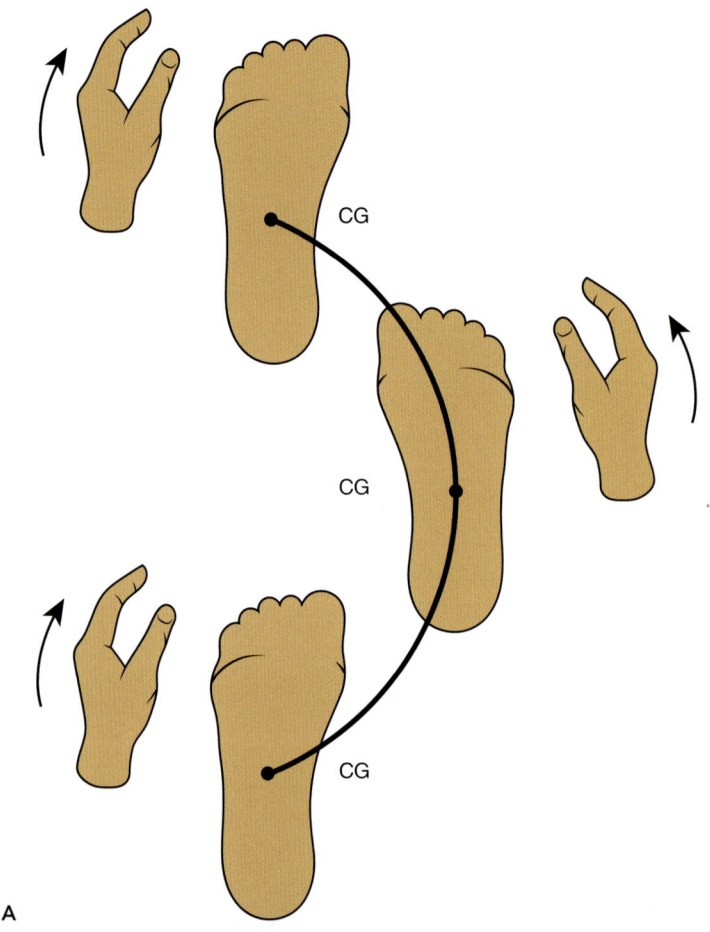

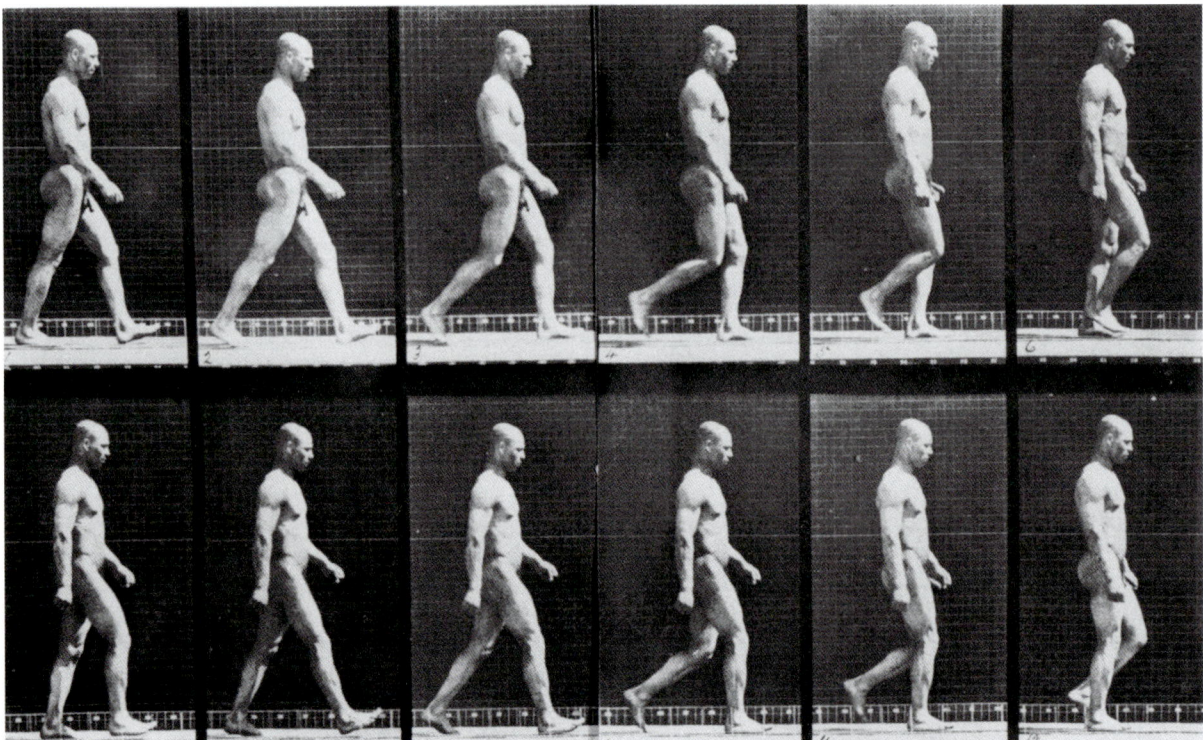

Figure 11.6 **(A) A stride has two steps component: the displacement of the center of gravity is sinusoidal and the upper extremity swings forward with opposite swinging forward foot and facilitates the transfer of the body mass forward. (B)** Man walking. (B, Republished with permission of Dover Publications, from Muybridge E. *The Human Figure in Motion*. Dover Publications; 1955. permission conveyed through Copyright Clearance Center, Inc.)

Chapter 11: Neuro Control of Stance and Gait   651

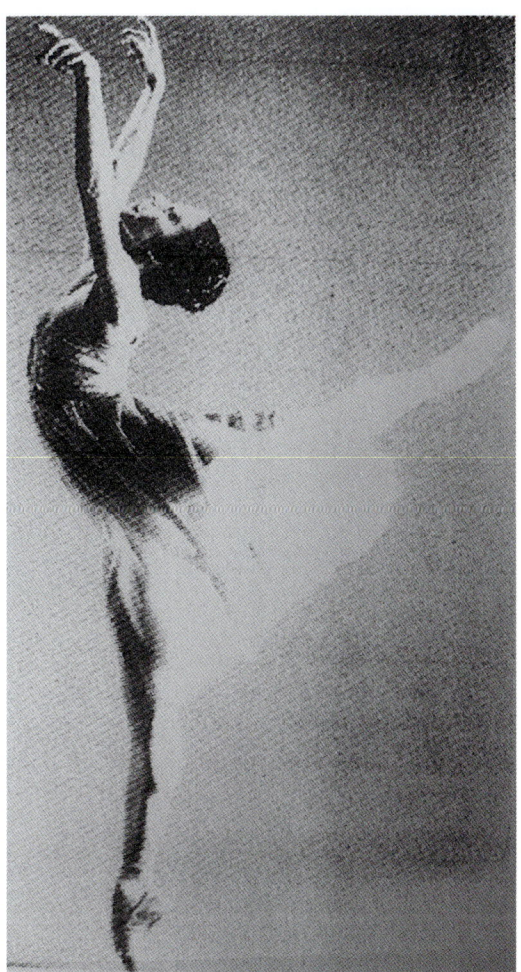

Figure 11.7 A ballerina achieves an "en pointe" by projecting the gravitational line on the supporting surface of the tips of the toes.

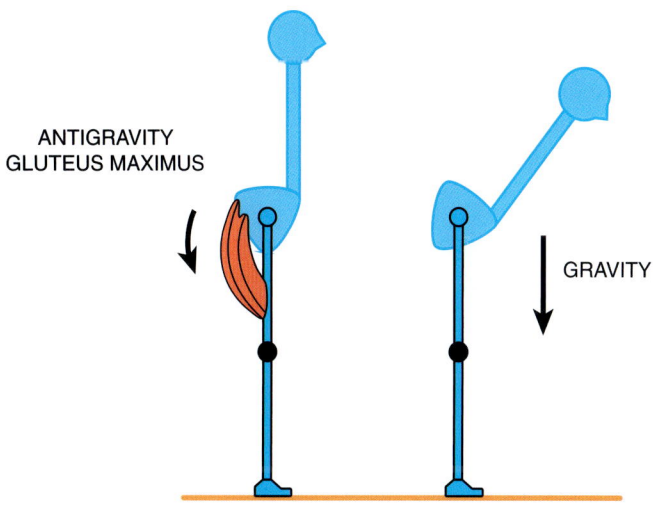

Figure 11.9 In the standing position, the body mass would tilt forward at the pelvis-hip joint. This tilt is prevented and erect position is maintained by the contraction of the gluteus maximums muscle.

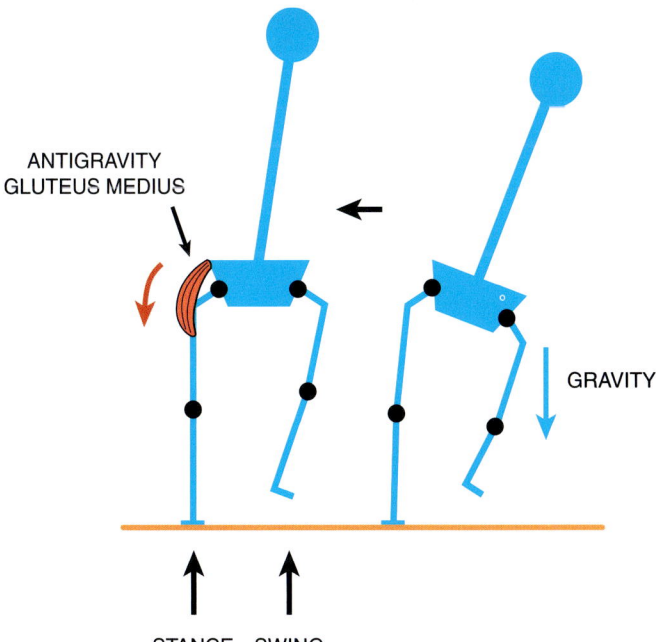

Figure 11.8 During walking, the pelvis trunk and swinging lower extremity tilt the body-pelvis to the nonsupported side. This is prevented by the contraction of the gluteus medius muscles on the stance side.

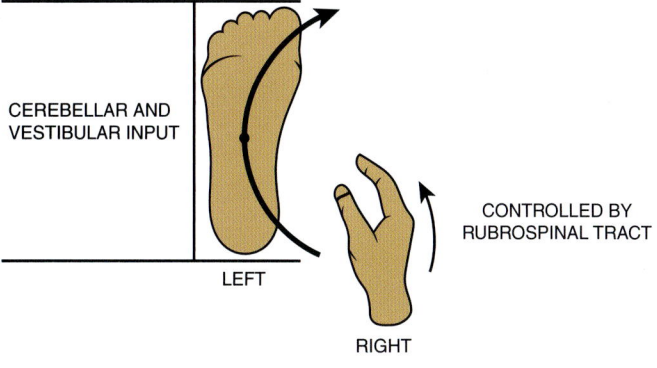

STANCE PHASE EQUILIBRIUM

Figure 11.10 Contribution to the projection of the center of gravity onto the foot surface of the stance phase by flexion-adduction of the opposite upper extremity. The projection of the center of gravity on one foot is determined by the neural input of the cerebellovestibular system. The contribution of the upper extremity is determined by the rubrospinal tracts which receive input from the cerebellum also.

FUNCTIONAL MOTOR UNIT

The spinal motor reflex loop is the fundamental component of ambulation. There are two types of sensors in the muscle-tendon unit triggering a reflex motor response. A stretch of the muscle stimulates the muscle spindle with resulting contraction of the muscle.

Contraction of the muscle stimulates the tendon Golgi sensor resulting in inhibition of the contracted muscle.

▶ Muscle Spindle[7,9]

As described by Enoka,[9] the muscle spindle is formed by up to 12 miniature skeletal muscle fibers that are enclosed in connective tissue capsule (Fig. 11.11). The muscle spindle fibers are referred to as intrafusal fibers. There are two types of intrafusal fibers based on the differences in the arrangement of the nuclei: chain fiber and bag fiber.

Each muscle spindle has a central nuclear bag area which is stretchable and is enlaced by sensory afferent nerve fibers Ia and II (Fig. 11.12). Afferent Ia stimulates the α motor neuron in the spinal cord and the afferent II stimulates the γ motor neuron. α motor neuron contracts the main muscle.

γ motor neuron contracts the polar muscles of the muscle spindle (Fig. 11.13).

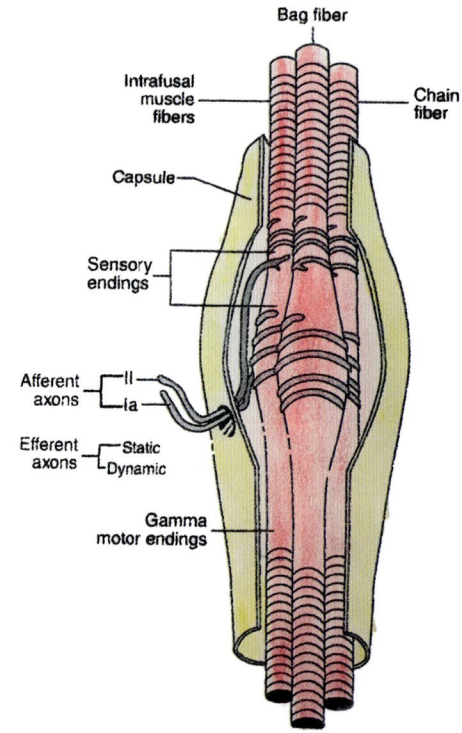

Figure 11.12 Stretch reflex motor loop components:
- Sensory afferent Ia fibers arising from the central nuclear bag area
- Sensory afferent II fibers arising from the peripheral chain areas
- γ motor fiber innervates the chain segment of the muscle spindle. (Reproduced with permission of Human Kinetics, Inc, from Enoka RM. *Neuromechanics of Human Movement.* 4th ed. Human Kinetics; 2008:259, Figure 7.4: permission conveyed through Copyright Clearance Center, Inc.)

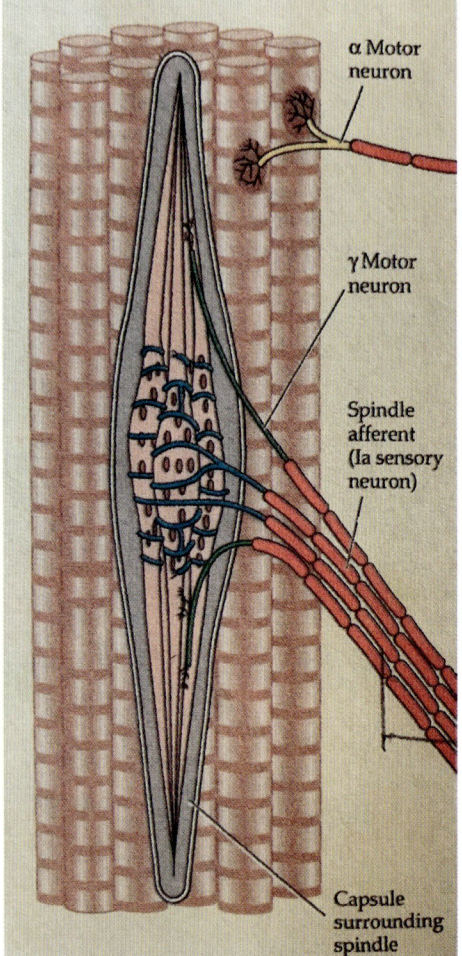

Figure 11.11 **Sensory afferents Ia arise from the cellular nuclear bag area.** Sensory afferents II arise from the peripheral chain area. Sensory inputs from Ia and II sensory afferents are essential components of the stretch reflex motor loop. (Purves D, Augustine GJ, Fitzpatrick D, et al, eds. *Neuroscience.* 3rd ed. Sinauer Associates; 2004:380, Figure 15.92, Reproduced with permission of the Oxford Publishing Limited through PLSclear.)

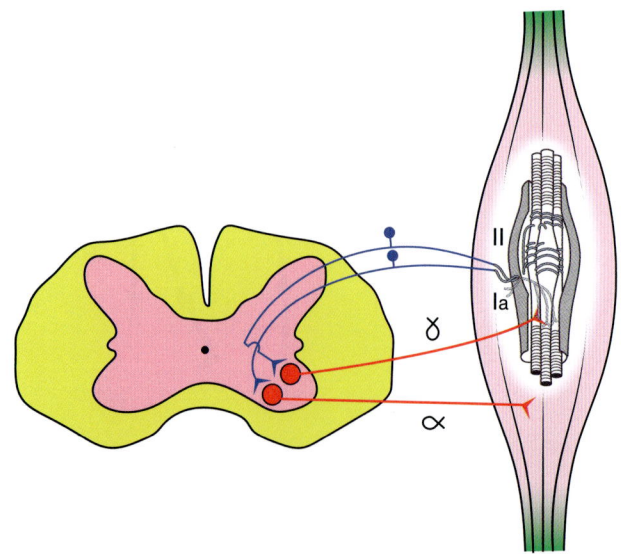

Figure 11.13 **Spinal reflex motor loop.** Stretch of the muscle results in the stimulation of afferents Ia and II of the muscle spindle. This results at the level of the spinal cord in the stimulation of the motor neurons α and γ. As a result the lengths of the muscle and muscle spindle are restored.

According to Enoka,[9] there are approximately 27,500 muscle spindles in the human body, 7.000 in each leg and the greatest part in the head and neck. The number of spindles in a single muscle varies from 6 to 1000 and their length varies from 2 to 6 mm and they are attached to intramuscular connective tissue.

▶ Golgi Tendon Organs[10,11]

Golgi tendon organs are slender encapsulated structures approximately 1 mm long and 0.1 mm in diameter located at the junction between skeletal fibers and tendon (Fig. 11.14). Each capsule encloses several braided collagen fibers connected in series to group of muscle fibers.

Each tendon organ is innervated by a single Ib axon that branches into many fine endings inside the capsule; these endings become intertwined with the collagen fascicles.

Stretching of the tendon organ straightens the collagen fibers, thus compressing the Ib nerve endings and causing them to fire.

The tendon organs are most sensitive to changes in muscle tension. Muscle contraction activates the Golgi tendon organ (Fig. 11.15). The tendon organs continuously measure the force of the contracting muscle.

The Ib axons from Golgi tendon organs contact inhibitory local circuit neurons in the spinal cord (called inhibitory interneurons) that synapse with the α motor neuron that innervate the muscle. There is also convergence onto Ib interneurons of joint afferent, cutaneous afferent, and descending channels.

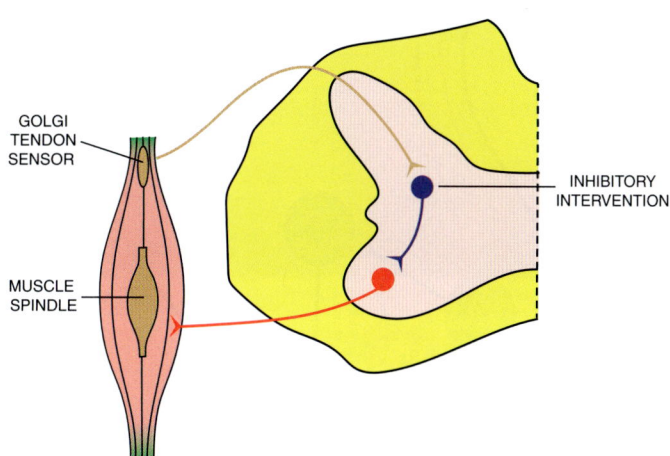

Figure 11.15 Contraction of the muscle stimulates the Golgi tendon organ which sends signals with the afferent Ib fibers to the inhibitory interneuron, inhibiting the α motor neuron. Muscle length is restored.

▶ Ia Inhibitory Interneuron[12]

As described by Pearson and Gordon,[35] the Ia inhibitory interneurons coordinate the muscles surrounding a joint. In the spinal stimulation by the muscle spindle, Ia efferent will stimulate, for example, the flexor muscle group but it will at the same time, through the intermediate inhibitory neuron, inhibit the α neuron corresponding to the extensor muscle on the same side (Fig. 11.16).

The Ia inhibitory interneurons involved in the stretch reflex are also used to coordinate muscle contraction during voluntary movements. The activity of spinal motor neuron is also regulated by another important class of inhibitory interneurons called the Renshaw cells (Fig. 11.17). Excited by collaterals of

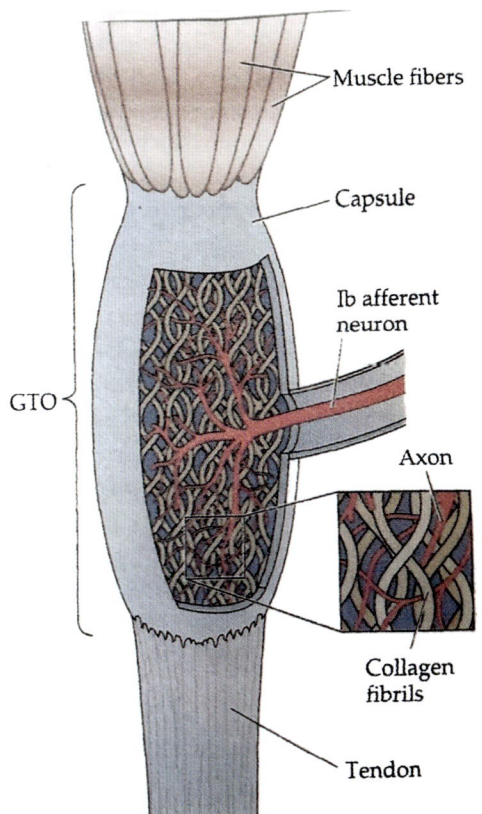

Figure 11.14 Golgi tendon organ. (Purves D, Augustine GJ, Fitzpatrick D, et al, eds. *Neuroscience*. 3rd ed. Sinauer Associates; 2004:383, Figure 15.11, Reproduced with permission of the Oxford Publishing Limited through PLSclear.)

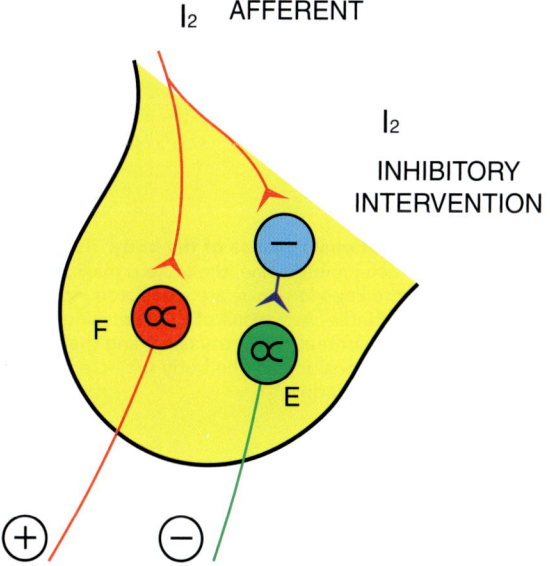

Figure 11.16 The stimulated Ia afferent stimulates at the levels of the anterior horn, for example, a flexor motor neuron α but at the same time stimulates an inhibitory extensor α neuron. This is essential for the maintenance of the flexion-extensor rhythmically during walking.

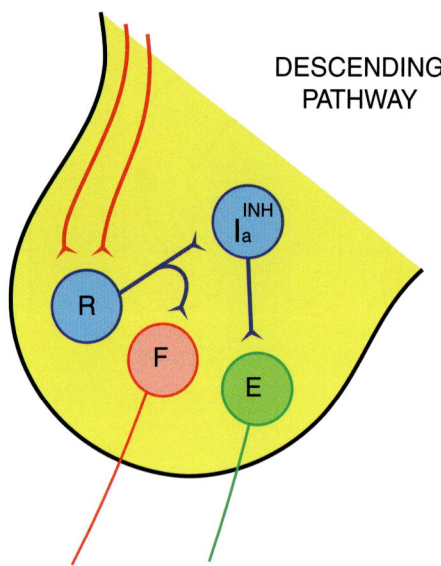

Figure 11.17 **The descending pathways stimulate the Renshaw cell which in turn stimulates the α flexor motor neuron and inhibits the corresponding α motor extensor neuron, thus determining flexor-extensor rhythmically of walking.** Desc. P, descending pathways; E, extensor motor neuron; F, flexor motor neuron; Ia inh, inhibitory interneuron; R, Renshaw cell.

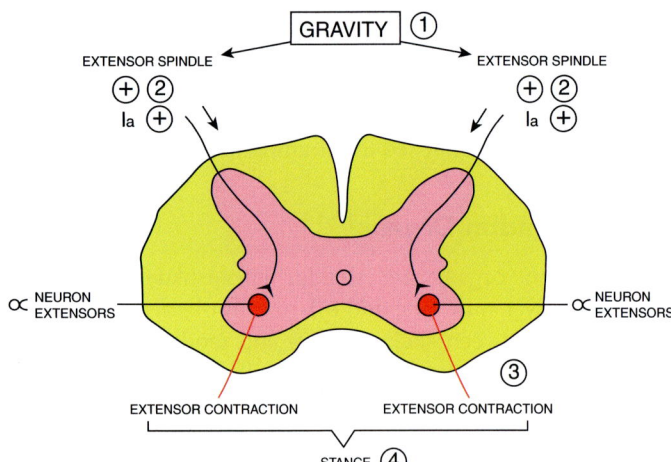

Figure 11.19 **The flexion mode stimulates the muscle spindles of the extensor muscle of the spine, the hips, and the knee resulting in the antigravity stance phase.**

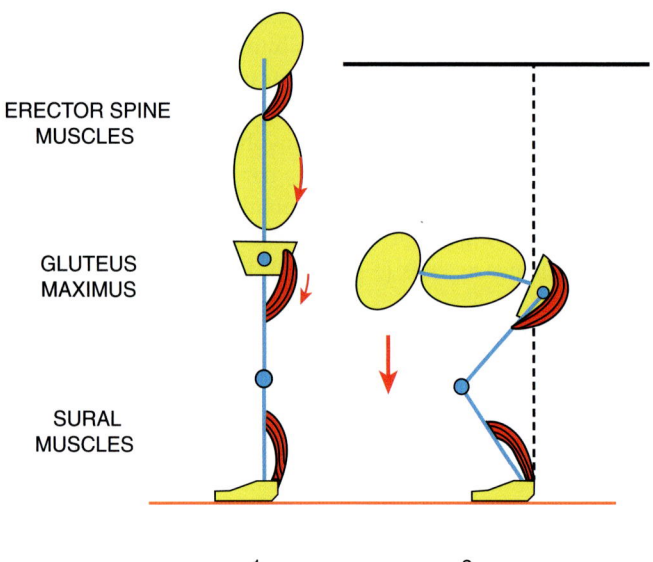

Figure 11.18 1, **Gravitational collapse of the body.** The extensors of the head-neck, thoraco-lumbar spine, the gluteus maximus at the hips, and the soles of the knee-leg-ankle are stimulated including their corresponding muscle spindle. As a result of the stretching of the muscle spindle, the extensor muscle contracts holding the body in the extensor, antigravitational position. 2, The body subjected to gravity would collapse in a flexion mode.

the axons of motor neurons, Renshaw cells make inhibitory synaptic connections with several populations of motor neurons, including the motor neurons that excite them and the Ia inhibitory interneurons.

The Renshaw cells receive significant synaptic input from the descending pathways.

As mentioned in the previous section, our body subjected to the force of gravity would collapse in the flexion mode.

The muscle spindles in the extensor of the spine, gluteus maximus, and soleus muscle are stretched and determine muscle contraction thus providing extension at the spine, hip, and ankle (Figs. 11.18 and 11.19).

Swing phase may be initiated by the stretch of the muscle spindle in the hip flexor during the hyperextension of the joint. Locomotion requires the simultaneous, alternate stimulation of α motor neurons of flexors and extensors in the spinal cord.

MODULATION OF MOTOR LOOP BY DESCENDING AND ASCENDING TRACTS

The spinal cord α, γ motor loop is regulated by the descending and the ascending tracts of the spinal cord providing the higher centers and peripheral neural input. These tracts in the spinal cord are represented in Figure 11.20.

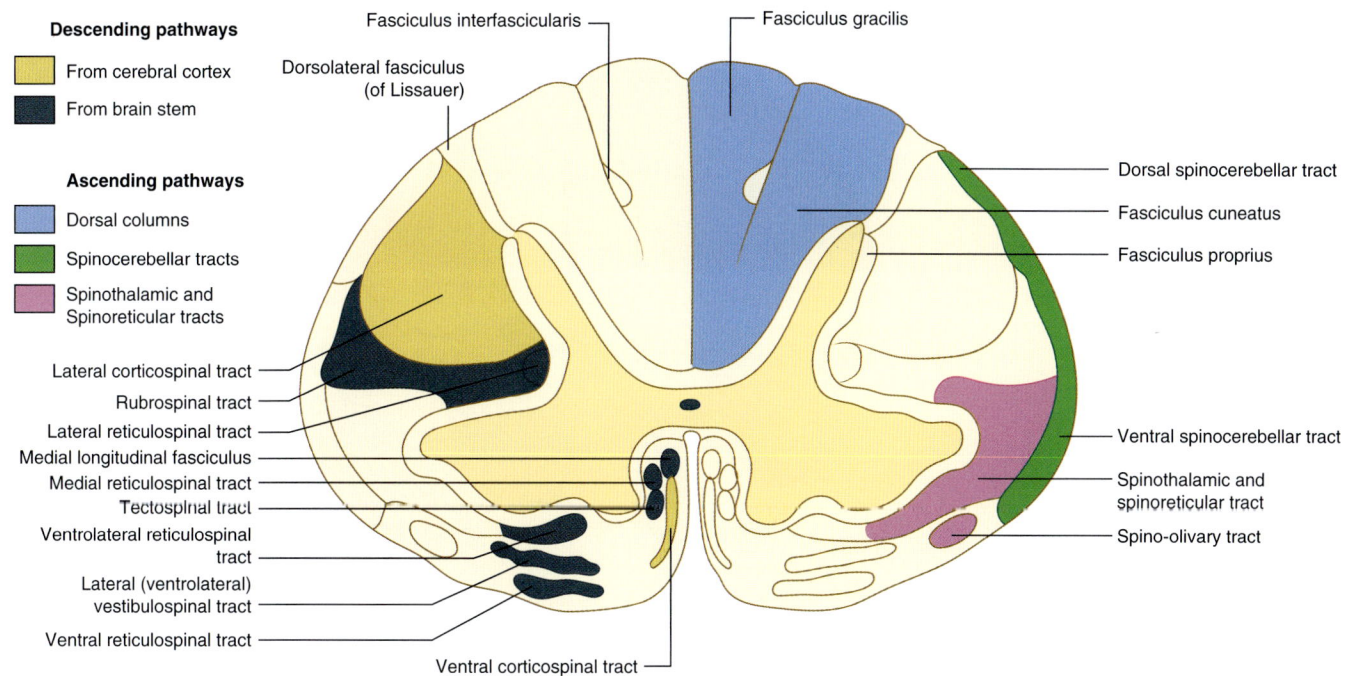

Figure 11.20 **Spinal cord tracts.** (Redrawn with permission of Elsevier, from *Gray's Anatomy: The Anatomical Basis of Clinical Practice*, 40th Edition in Spinal Cords. Susan Strandring (Ed.). Churchill Livingston; 2008, Figure 189; permission conveyed through Copyright Clearance Center, Inc.)

MODULATION OF GAIT

▶ Vision[13,14]

Vision in gait has a primordial role. Before walking, vision assesses the environment, the direction of walking, and the speed of walking and analyzes the possible obstacles that are to be avoided.

A comprehensive study of the control of gaze is provided by Goldberg and Walker,[13] and eye movements and sensory motor integration by Purves and associates.[14] As indicated in Figure 11.21, the eye projects the external image to the occipital cortex for further processing.

The retinal signal passes through the lateral geniculate body, the striate cortex, and expands dramatically into higher cortical areas.

Visual information extends from the occipital lobe to the parietal and frontal cortices. Visual areas in the parietal areas are concerned with motion, whereas visual areas in the temporal lobes are concerned with object recognition.[14] The eyes follow a target with 12 muscles, 6 for each (Fig. 11.22).

Six neuronal control systems keep the eyes on target[13]:

- Saccadic eye movements shift the fovea rapidly to a new visual target.
- Smooth-pursuit movements keep the image of a moving target on the fovea.
- Vergence movements move the eyes in opposite directions so that image is positioned on both foveas.
- Vestibulo-ocular reflexes hold images still on the retina during brief head movements.
- Optokinetic movements hold images stationary during sustained head rotation or translations.
- Saccades are ballistic eye movements that move the fovea from one fixation point to another. They scan the environment quickly.

Saccades to an unexpected stimulus normally take 200 ms to initiate and then 20 to 200 ms to process.[14] Six extra-ocular muscles control the eye movements rapidly to bring the fovea of 1.5 mm diameter to the external target (Fig. 11.22).

These muscles are controlled by cranial nerves III, IV, VI. This creates the most accurate muscular achievement in the body. The neural signals producing saccades are processed as follows: the ocular signal reaches the occipital visual cortex and is transmitted to the posterior parietal cortex, which sends the neural stimulus to the frontal eye field, which channels the visual information to the superior colliculus located in the upper segment of the midbrain. The signal is then transmitted from the superior colliculus to the mesencephalic and pontine reticular formation, which provide the neuromotor stimulation to the ocular motor nuclei resulting in saccadic eye motion (Fig. 11.23A).

The neuro pathway for the smooth pursuit eye movements extends similarly from the eye of the striate cortex and the neurosignal reaches the middle temporal and medial superior temporal areas and is channeled to the frontal eye field.

The frontal eye field sends the visual information to ocular motor nuclei via the dorsal pontine nuclei, and the vermis and the flocculus of the cerebellum, and the vestibular nuclei (Fig. 11.23B).

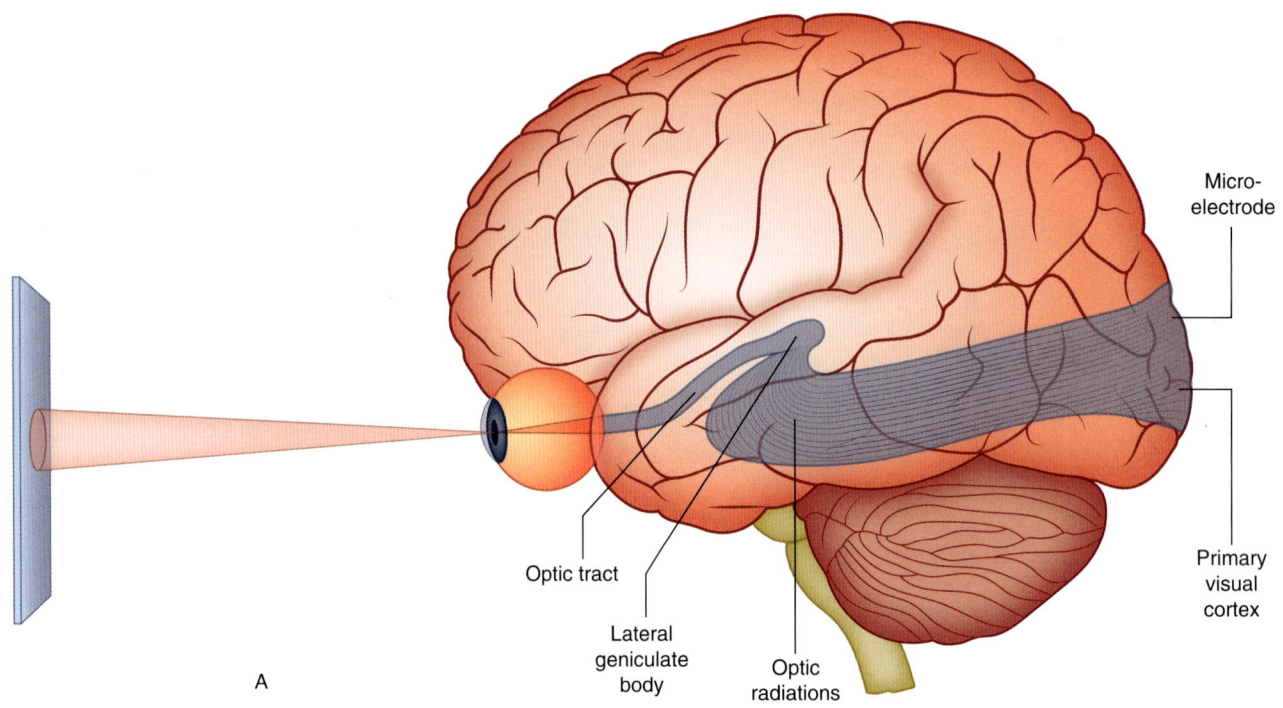
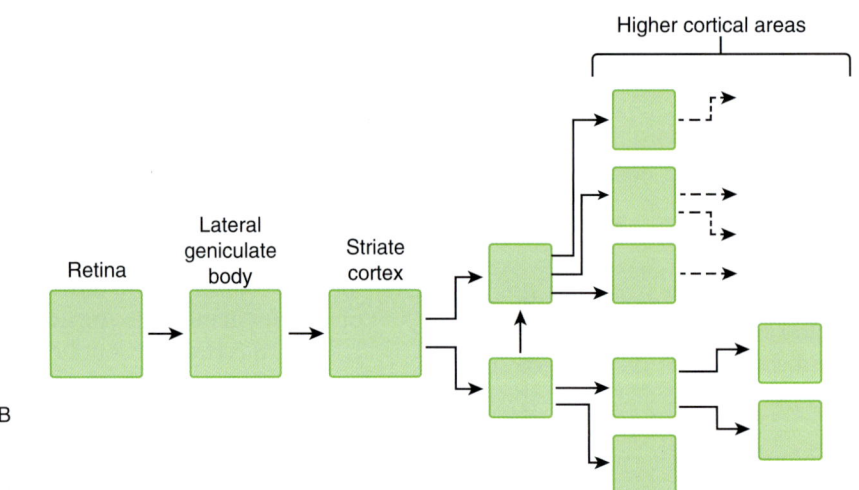

Figure 11.21 (A) Human brain with projection to the visual primary cortex pathway. (B) Visual pathway components. "Each structure as a box consists of millions of the cells aggregated into sheets. Each receives information from one or more structures at lower levels in the path and each sends the output to several structures at higher levels. The path has been traced only for four or five stages beyond the primary visual cortex."

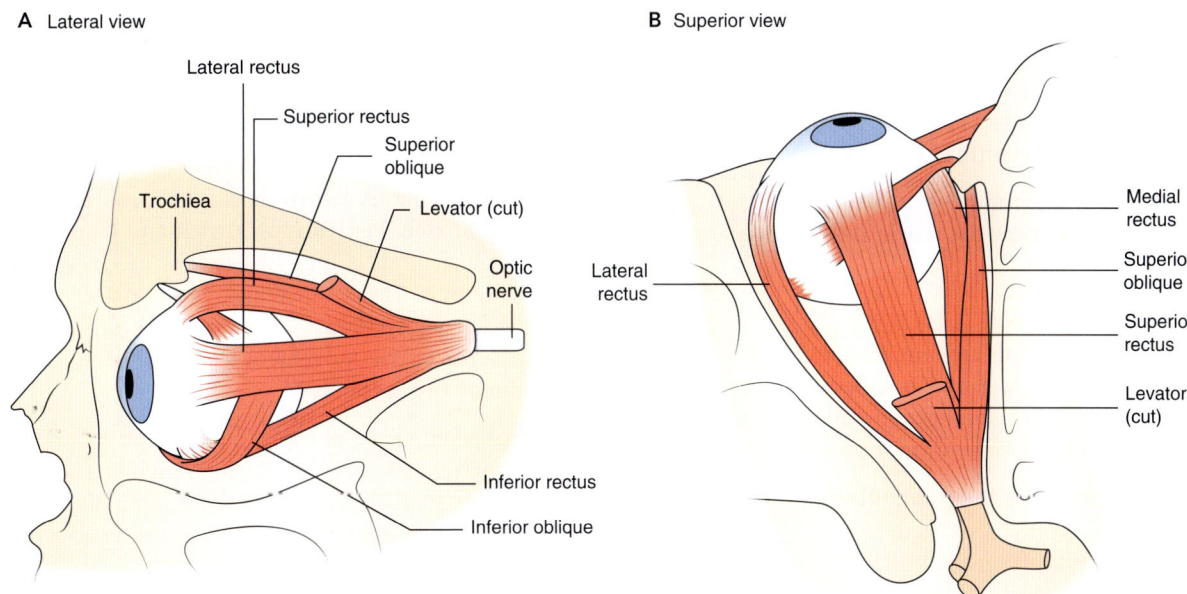

Figure 11.22 The origins and insertions of the extraocular muscles. (**A**) Lateral view of the left eye with the orbital wall cut away. Each rectus muscle inserts in front of the equator of the globe so that contraction rotates the cornea toward the muscle. Conversely, the oblique muscles insert behind the equator and contraction rotates the cornea away from the insertion. The superior oblique muscle passes through a bony pulley, the trochlea, before it inserts on the globe. The levator muscle of the upper eyelid raises the lid. (**B**) Superior view of the left eye and the roof of the orbit and the levator muscle cut away. The superior rectus passes over the superior oblique and inserts in front of the globe. (Redrawn with permission of Elsevier, from Goldberg ME, Walker MF. The control of gaze. In: Kandel ER, Schwartz JH, Jessell TM, eds. *Principles of Neural Science*. 2nd ed. Elsevier; 1985: Figure 39-4, p. 89; permission conveyed through Copyright Clearance Center, Inc.)

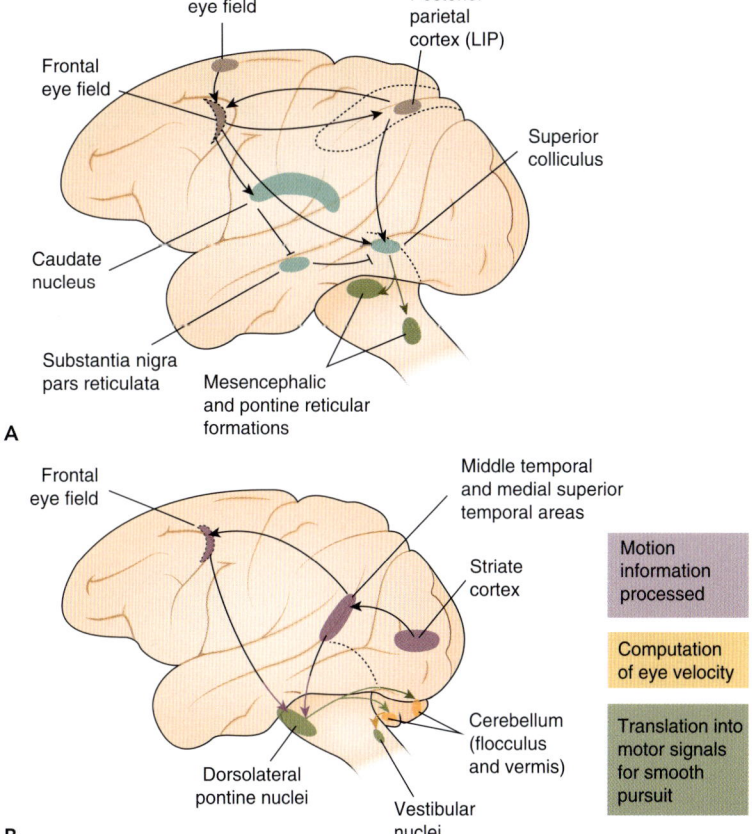

Figure 11.23 Cortical pathways for saccades. (**A**) In the monkey, the saccade generator in the brain stem receives a command from the superior colliculus. The colliculus receives direct, excitation projection from the frontal eye fields and the lateral intraparietal and inhibitory projection from the substantia nigra. The substantia nigra is suppressed by the caudate nucleus while in turn is excited by the eye fields. Thus the frontal eye fields directly excite the colliculus and indirectly release it from the suppression by the substantia nigra by exciting the caudate nucleus, which inhibits the substantia nigra. (**B**) Pathway for smooth pursuit eye movements in the monkey. The cerebral cortex processes information about motion in the visual field and sends it to the ocular motor neurons via the dorsal pontine nucleus, the vermis and flocculus of the cerebellum, and the lateral vestibular nuclei. The initiation signal for smooth pursuit may originate in part from the frontal eye field. (Redrawn with permission of Elsevier, from Goldberg ME, Walker MF. The control of gaze. In: Kandel ER, Schwartz JH, Jessell TM, eds. *Principles of Neural Science*. 2nd ed. Elsevier; 1985: Figure 39-10, p. 907; permission conveyed through Copyright Clearance Center, Inc.)

▶ The Vestibular System[15-17]

The vestibular system, membranous, is embedded in the intercranial petrous segment of the temporal bone. It is in continuity with the cochlea (Fig. 11.24).

The vestibular system is formed by five components:

- Three semicircular membranous canals
- Two spheroidal chambers: the utricle and the saccule

Semicircular Canals

The three semicircular canals are implanted on the utricle. One implantation site is enlarged and is called the ampulla. The utricle communicates with another spheroidal structure called the saccula. The vestibular nerve arises from five nerve roots:

- Three branches from the three ampullae of the semicircular canals.
- Two branches arising from the utricle and the saccule (Fig. 11.25).

Space is determined by three axes (Fig. 11.26):

$$x, y, z$$

Combination of two axes determines an oriented surface as follows:

- Horizontal surface determined by x, z axes
- Vertical surface, transverse, posterior determined by x, y axes
- Vertical lateral surface determined by z, y axes

The semilunar canals are located in the following surfaces of space:

- Posterior (x, y)
- Horizontal (x, z)
- Lateral (y, z)

The membranous labyrinth is filled with endolymph Na^+ poor and K^+ rich. Perilymph Na^+ rich and K^+ poor, similar to cerebrospinal fluid, is located between the membranous and bony labyrinth. The semicircular canals detect head rotation and angular acceleration.

The sensor of the movement is located in the ampulla. The components are as follows:

- Sensory epithelium or crista that contains hair cells.
- The hair bundles extend out of the crista into a gelatinous mass, the cupula, that bridges the width of the ampulla, forming a fluid barrier through which endolymph cannot circulate (Fig. 11.27).

The sensory hairs of the crista ampullaris or stereocilia increase in size to reach the highest cilia or kinocilia (Fig. 11.28A).

The sensory cells respond to the mechanical bending of the hairs. Bending the hairs from the smallest stereocilia toward the kinocilia stimulates the nerve cell. Bending the hairs from the kinocilia toward the smallest stereocilia hyperpolarizes the nerve cell, resulting in inhibitory activity (Fig. 11.28B). The hair cells are all oriented in the same direction in the same canal (Fig. 11.29).

The neurosignals are transmitted by the afferent fibers to the Scarpa bipolar ganglion which connects to the vestibular nuclei of the brain stem.

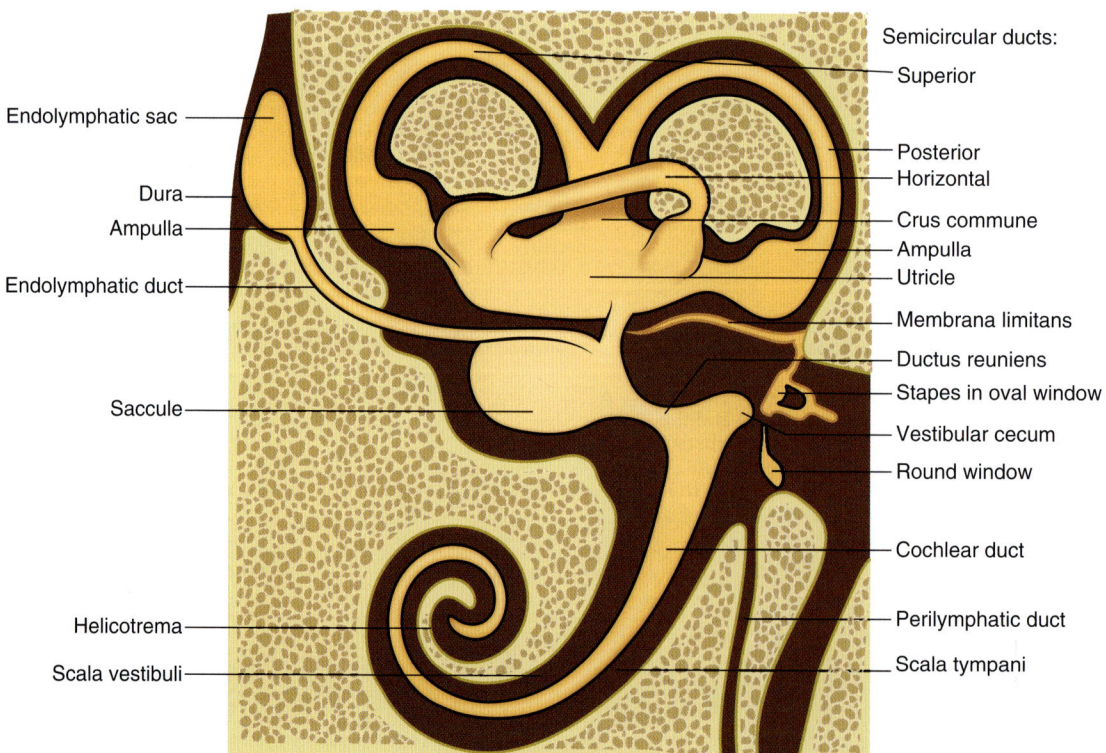

Figure 11.24 Intraosseous location of vestibular and cochlear apparatus. (Adapted with permission of Elsevier, from Kandel ER, Schwartz JH. *Principles of Neural Science*. 1st ed. Elsevier North-Holland; 1981, Figure 35, p. 407; permission conveyed through Copyright Clearance Center, Inc.)

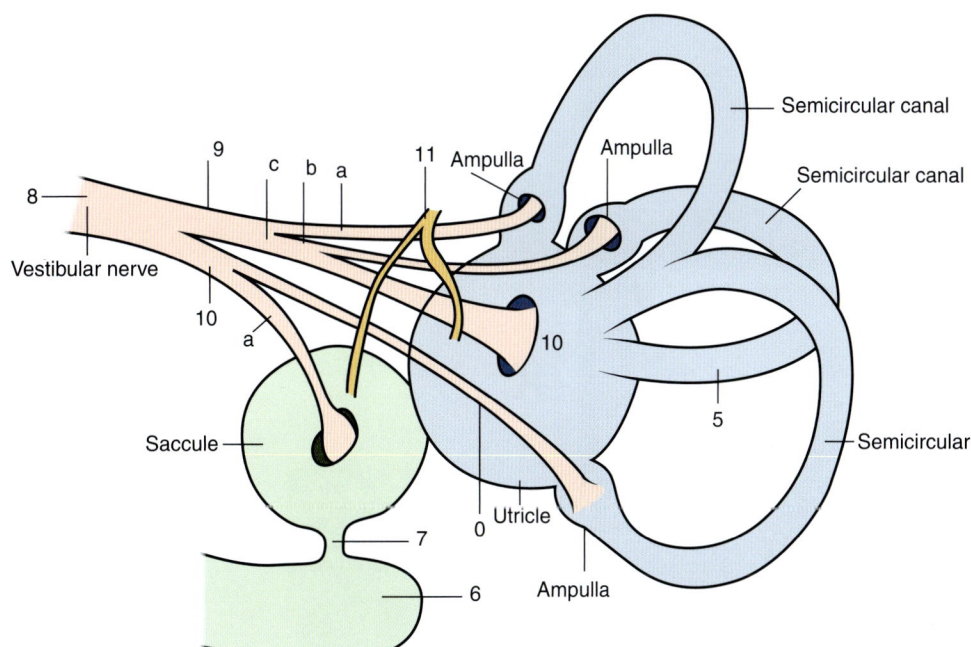

Figure 11.25 Anatomy of the vestibular system. (Reproduced with permission Testut L. *Traite d'Anatomie Humaine Livre II Arthrologie Tome.* Librairie Ovtave Doin; 1921:654.)

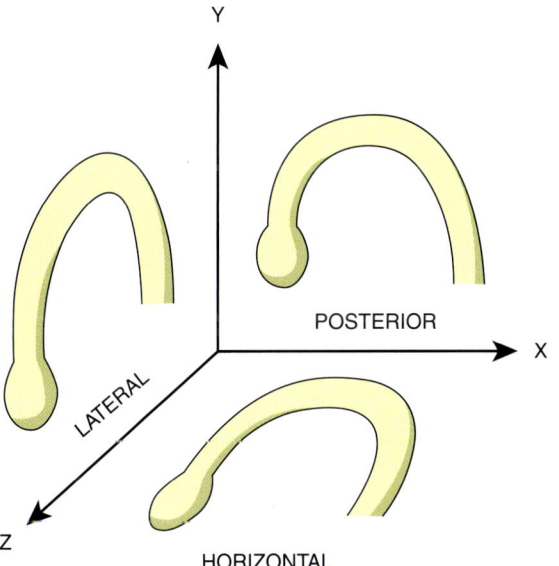

Figure 11.26 Location of the labyrinths in space according to x, y, z axes. Posterior labyrinth in posterior surface determined by x, y axes. Lateral labyrinth in lateral surface determined by y, z axes. Horizontal labyrinth in horizontal plane determined by x, z axes.

The Otolith Organs Utricle and Saccule

Gravity generates vertically oriented linear acceleration. The utricle and saccule detect the orientation of the head relative to gravity (Fig. 11.30). The striola is the directional line of alignment of the hair cells in the otolithic organs. In the utricle the kinocilia are directed toward the striola, whereas in the saccule they are directed away from the striola. A cross section of the utricle or saccule reveals its neurosensory arrangement.

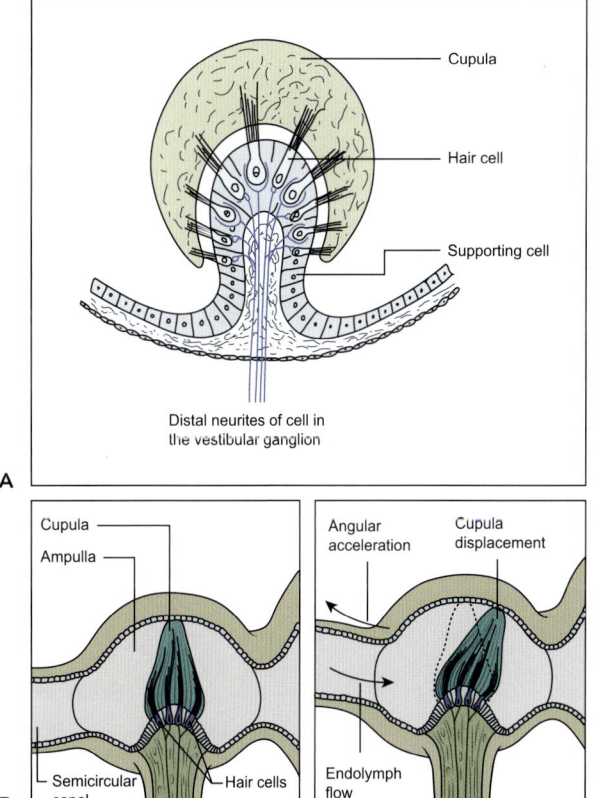

Figure 11.27 Anatomy of the crista ampullaris. Anatomy of the crista ampullaris. (**A**, Reprinted from Murray LB, Kiernan JA. *The Human Nervous System: An Anatomical Viewpoint.* 6th ed. Lippincott Williams & Wilkins; 1993:224, Figure 22-3. **B**, Purves D, Augustine GJ, Fitzpatrick D, et al, eds. *Neuroscience.* 3rd ed. Sinauer Associates; 2004:325; Figure 13.3, Reproduced with permission of the Oxford Publishing Limited through PLSclear.)

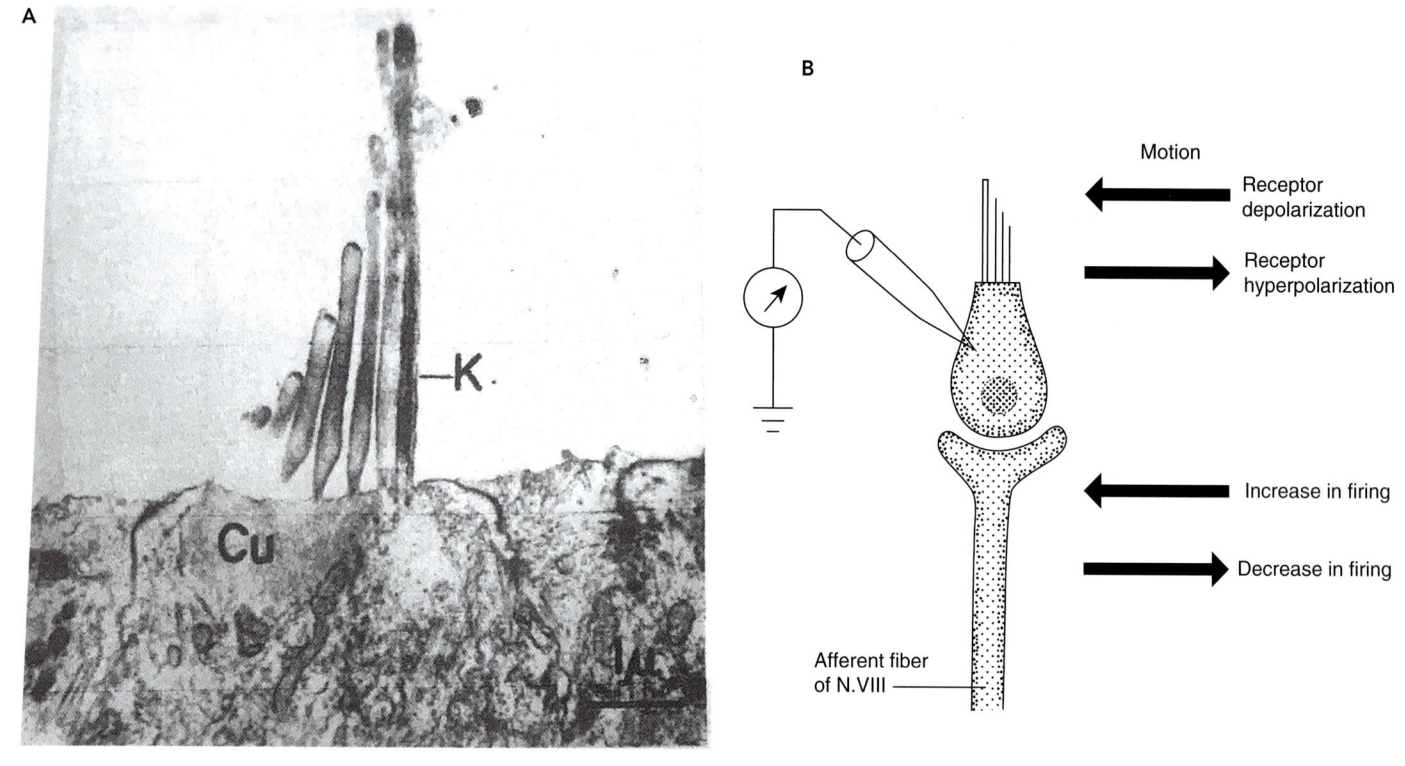

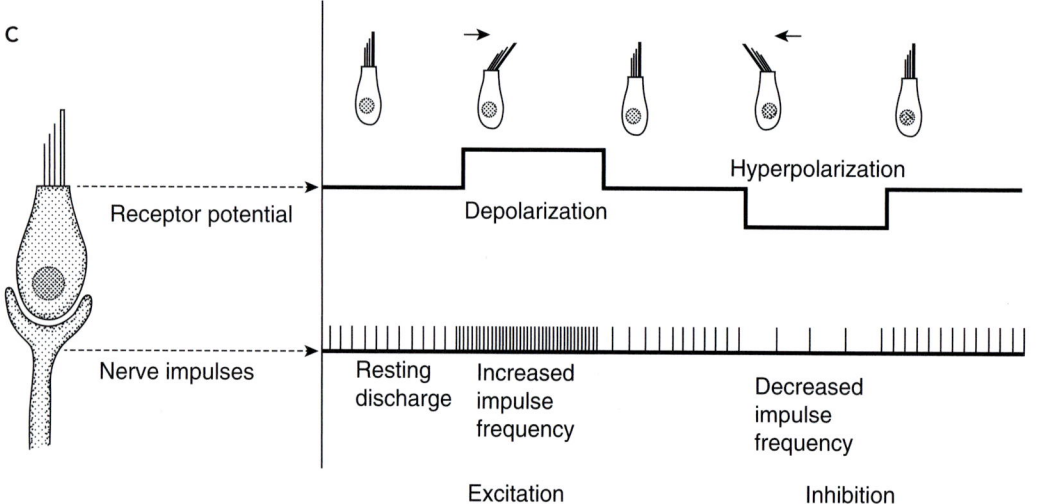

Figure 11.28 **Apical hairs of the hair cell.** (A) Transmission electron micrograph of the hair apical surface showing the stereocilia increasing in length toward the kinocilium (K). Directional selectivity of vestibular receptors to bending of the hairs. (B and C) Bending of the spinal hairs affects the polarization of the hair cells and firing rate of the eighth nerve afferent fibers. (Adapted from Kelly JP. Vestibular system. In: Kandel ER, Schwartz JH, eds. *Principles of Neural Science*. 1st ed. Elsevier North-Holland; 1981:407.)

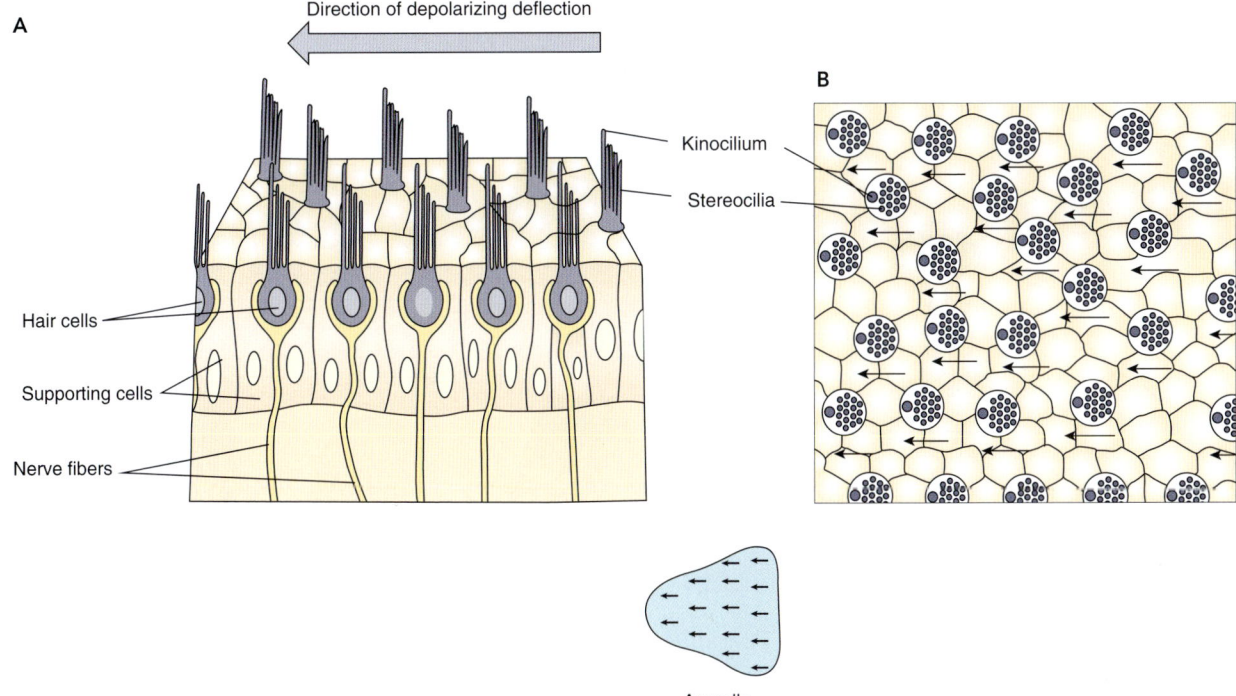

Figure 11.29 Anatomy and distribution of the hair cells in the crista ampullaris. (A) A cross-section of the hair cells shows the kinocilia of a group of hair cells are all located at the same side of the hair cells. The arrow indicates the direction of deflection that depolarizes the hair cell. (B) Top view. (Redrawn with permission from Purves D, Augustine GJ, Fitzpatrick D, et al, eds. *Neuroscience*. 3rd ed. Sinauer Associates; 2004:317, Figure 13.2, by permission of Oxford University Press.)

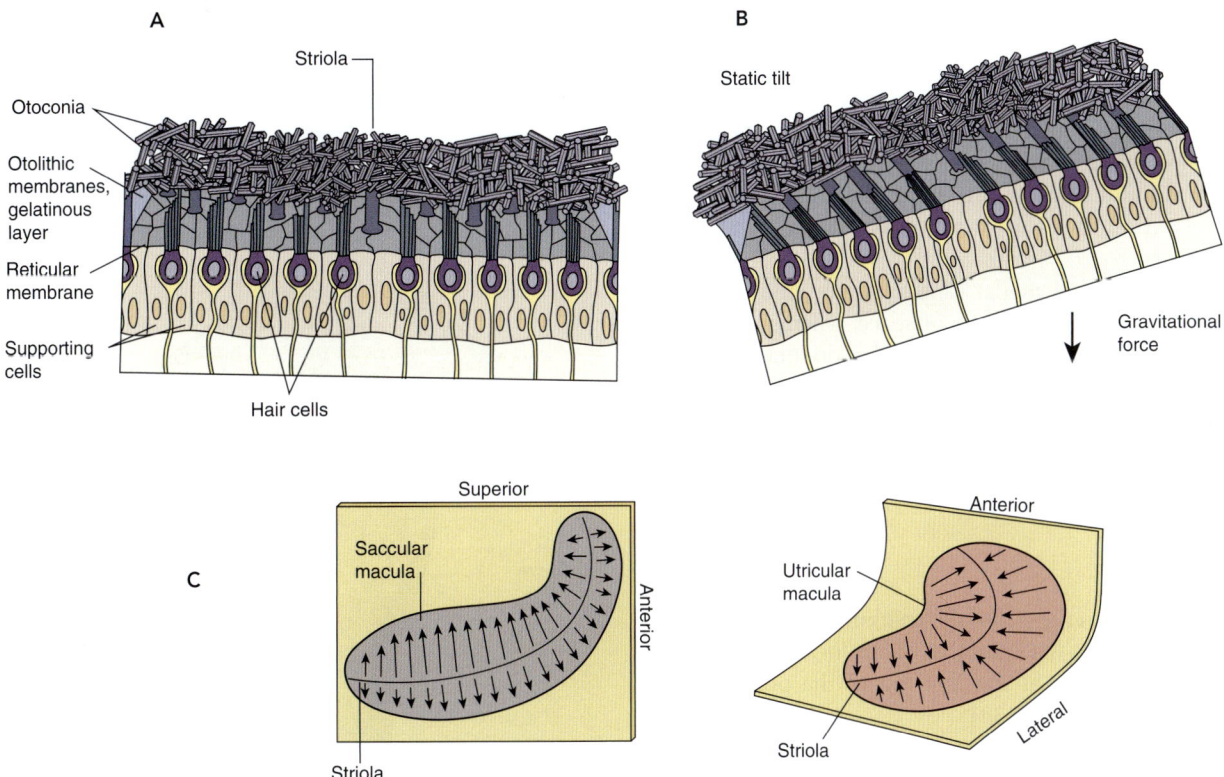

Figure 11.30 Cross section of the utricle and saccule. (A) Gravitational neurodetection in horizontal plane relative to gravity. No tilt of kinocilia. No signal preparation. (B) Tilt of the head or body results in an inclination of the otolith. Neurosignal is generated in neurocilia. (C) Orientation of the saccule and utricle relative to gravity. (Redrawn with permission from Purves D, Augustine GJ, Fitzpatrick D, et al, eds. *Neuroscience*. 3rd ed. Sinauer Associates; 2004:319, Figure 13.4, by permission of Oxford University Press.)

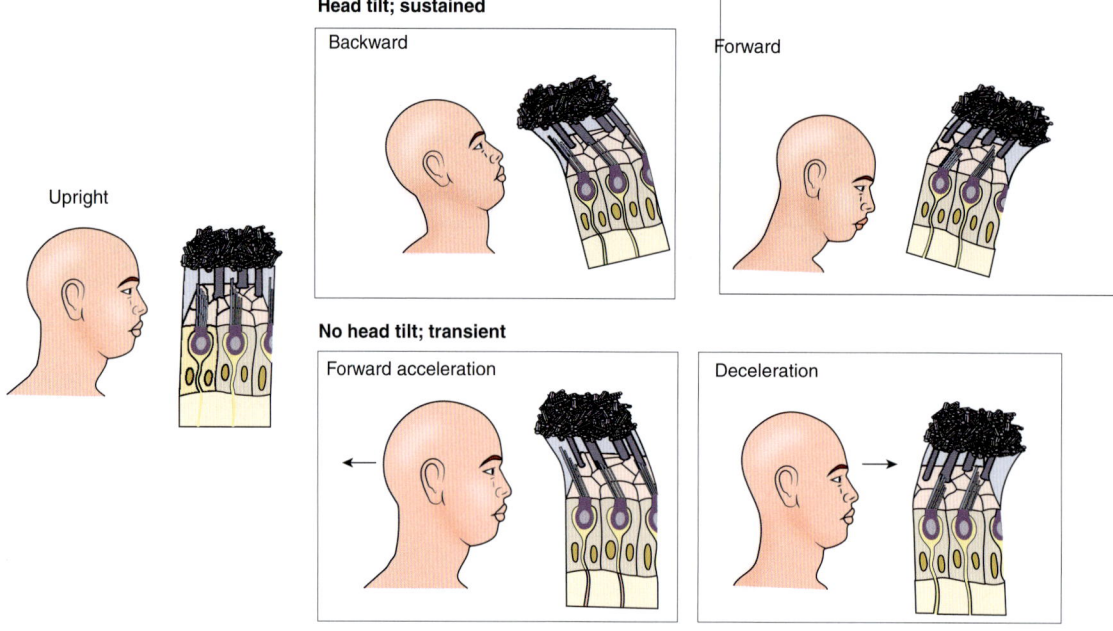

Figure 11.31 **The utricle and saccule detect head linear acceleration, deceleration, head tilt forward, backward, and sideways.** "Forces acting on the head and the resulting displacement of the otolithic membrane utricular macula. For each of the positions and accelerations due to transitional movement, some set of hair cells will be maximally excited, whereas another set maximally inhibited. Note that the head-tilt produces displacement similar to certain accelerations." (Redrawn with permission from Purves D, Augustine GJ, Fitzpatrick D, et al, eds. *Neuroscience*. 3rd ed. Sinauer Associates; 2004:322, Figure 13.5, by permission of Oxford University Press.)

Hair cells with their stereocilia and kinocilia are embedded in otolithic gelatinous layer by otoconia crystals. Their neuro cells are stabilized by supporting cells. A tilt of the head or of the body results in a significant tilt of the crystal layer of the otolithic organ. The corresponding tilt of the neurocilia cells generates the neurosignal which is transmitted to the vestibular nerve.

The utricle and saccula detect also head linear acceleration, deceleration, head tilt forward, backward, or sideways (Fig. 11.31).

In essence, the semicircular canals provide information in regard to the x, y, z components of space, whereas the utricle and saccule provide information on the orientation of the head-body in regard to gravity.

These spatial-gravitational signals are carried to the vestibular nerve which translates the signal to the corresponding neuromodulators.

Vestibular Nuclei

The vestibular nerve arises from the vestibular ganglion (Scarpa ganglion) and reaches the vestibular nuclei located on the floor of the fourth ventricle, at the junction of the pons and the medulla (Figs. 11.32 and 11.33).

As described by Kelly,[48] four distinct nuclei can be recognized in this complex:

1. The superior vestibular nucleus of Bechterew.
2. The lateral vestibular nucleus of Deiters.
3. The medial vestibular nucleus of Schwartz.
4. The inferior or descending vestibular nuclei of Roller.

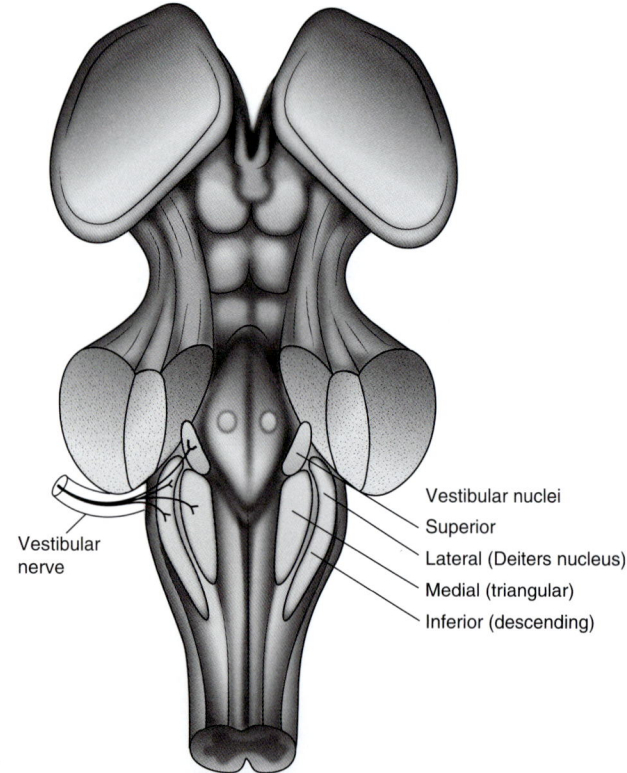

Figure 11.32 **Vestibular nerve reaching the vestibular nuclei located on the floor of the fourth ventricle at the junction of the pons and medulla.** Location of the vestibular nuclei in the brain stem: dorsal view. (Redrawn with permission from Kelly JP. In: Kandel ER, Schwartz JH. *Principles of Neural Science*. 1st ed. Elsevier North-Holland; 1981:414, Figure 35.1.)

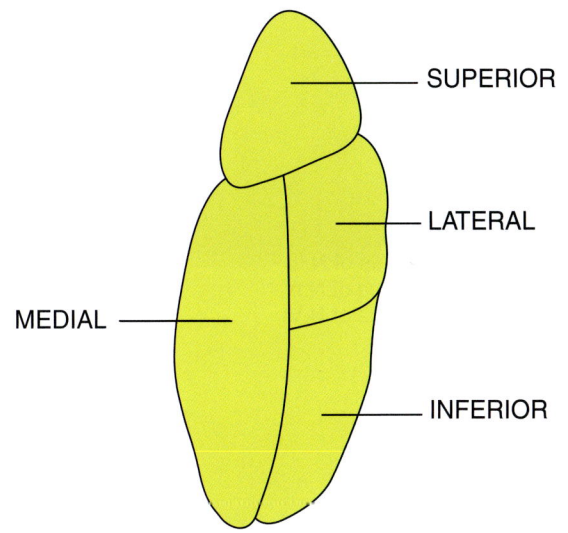

Figure 11.33 Vestibular nuclei.

As represented in Figure 11.34A, the vestibular nerve axons arising from the semicircular canals reach the superior and medial components of the vestibular nuclear complex. The axons from the utricle and the saccule end in the lateral vestibular nucleus.

The vestibular axons extend to the cerebellum through the mossy fibers and connect with the inhibitory Purkinje cells.

The lateral Deiters nucleus sends axons into the vestibulospinal tract, which terminates in the ipsilateral anterior horn of the spinal cord from cervical to lumbar level. This tract has a pronounced facilitatory effect on both alpha and gamma motor neurons to antigravity muscles. The neurons in the rostral part of Deiters nuclei respond selectively to tilting of the head. These neurons have a resting discharge which increases in response to tilt in one direction and decreases in response to tilt in the opposite direction. The magnitude of the response increases with increasing angle of the tilt.

A smaller number of rapidly adapting neurons respond whenever the angle of the body is changed.[48] Deiters nucleus receives input from the cerebellum's inhibitory Purkinje cells. It also receives spinal input (Fig. 11.34B).

The Medial and Superior Vestibular Nuclei

The medial and superior vestibular nuclei send their axons into the medial longitudinal fasciculus, a tract running to rostral parts in the brain stem just beneath the midline of the fourth ventricle[48] (Fig. 11.35).

Vestibulo-Ocular Reflex

As described in Figure 11.35 the vestibular nuclei connect in the brain stem with the following oculo motor nuclei:

- VI: Abducens
- IV: Trochlear
- III: Oculo-motor

The axonal connection is through the medial longitudinal fasciculus with the IV and III nuclei at the level of the inferior and superior colliculi. The vestibular-visual neural connector is essential for the functioning of the vestibulo-visual reflex (Fig. 11.36).

This reflex is helpful in avoiding an impact with an object while walking. Subject A sees an object in front of him while walking. He changes the direction of walking from A to B;

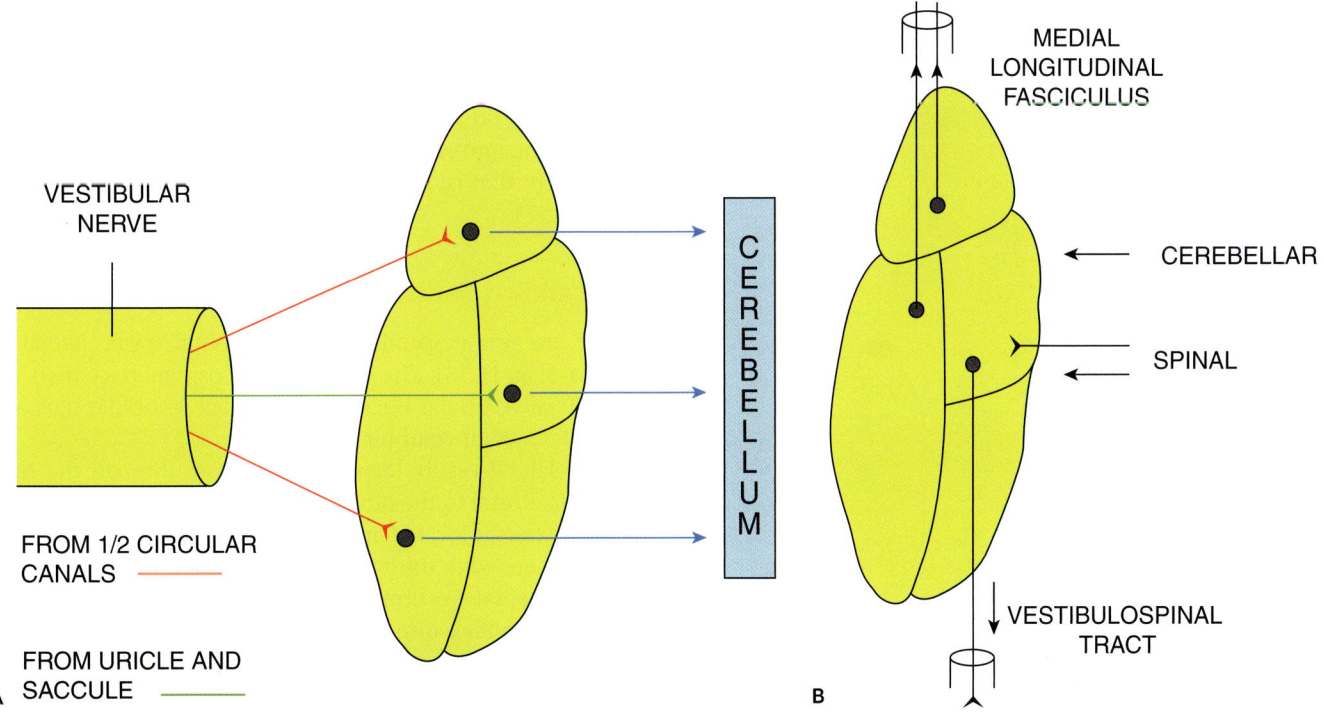

Figure 11.34 (A) Neuroinput from the vestibular nerve to the vestibular nuclei. (B) Input and output of superior, lateral, and medial vestibular nuclei.

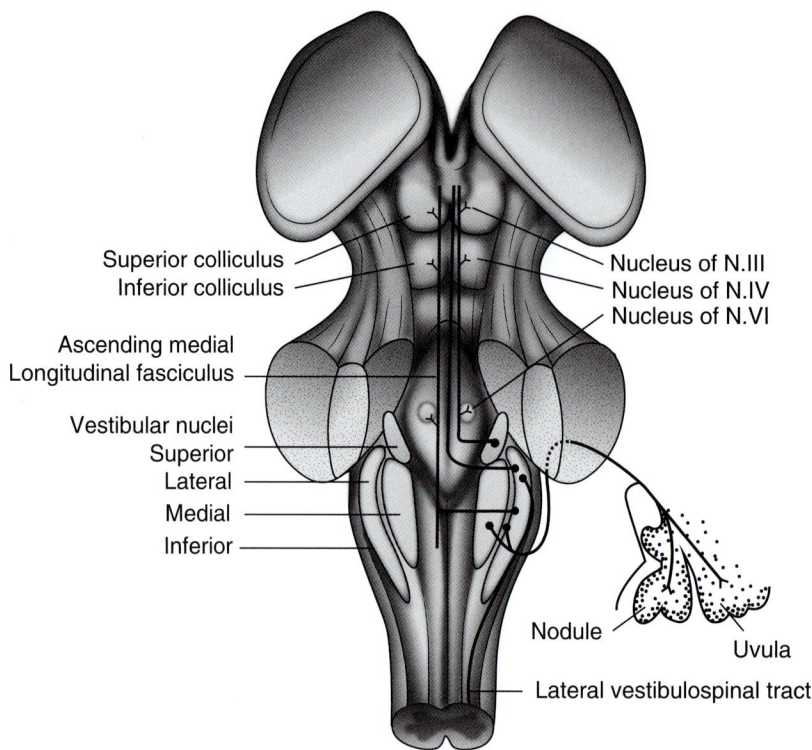

Figure 11.35 Location of the oculo-motor nuclei and the vestibular nuclei in the brain stem. (Redrawn with permission from Kelly JP. In: Kandel ER, Schwartz JH. *Principles of Neural Science*. 1st ed. Elsevier North-Holland; 1981:417, Figure 13.15.)

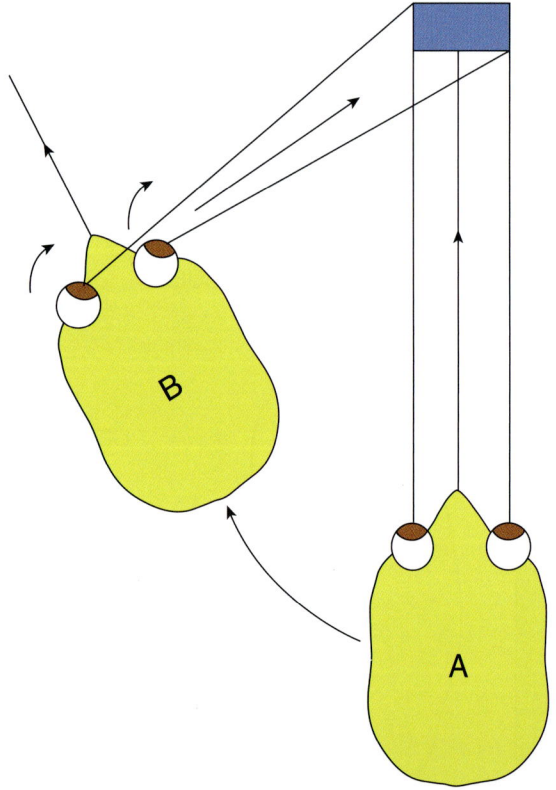

Figure 11.36 **Vestibulo-ocular reflex.** Subject A is walking and encounters a possible obstacle. The eyes are focused on the object. He changes directions by turning the head and the body to the left. The eyes however by a vestibular motor reflex remain now focused on the object on the right until clearance is established.

however, in position B the eyes still remain, by reflex, deviated to the right, focused on the obstacle, to avoid impact. This is accomplished by a reflex mechanism.

J. Kelly[48] gives the following description of the neuromechanism of the vestibular-visual reflex.

When the acceleration to the left first begins, the eyes undergo a slow deviation to the right, in a direction opposite to the motion of the head. This tends to keep the eyes fixed on a single point in space.

The eyes do not remain in this position; when they have reached the limit of their excursion, there is a rapid movement to the left, that is, in the direction of the angular acceleration (Fig. 11.37).

Descending Pathways From the Vestibular Nuclei

There are two descending vestibulospinal tracts: lateral and medial (Fig. 11.38). The lateral vestibulospinal tract arises from the lateral vestibular nucleus. The medial vestibular tract arises from the medial vestibular nucleus.

The lateral vestibulospinal tract passes through the rostral medulla, dorsal to the olivary nucleus. At the level of the spinal cord the tract is located anteriorly, penetrates the anterior horn, and connects with the α motor neuron.

The medial vestibulospinal, at the level of the rostral medulla, divides into two tracts forming the medial longitudinal fasciculus which passes anteromedially at the level of the spinal cord and terminates on the α motor neuron (Fig. 11.39).

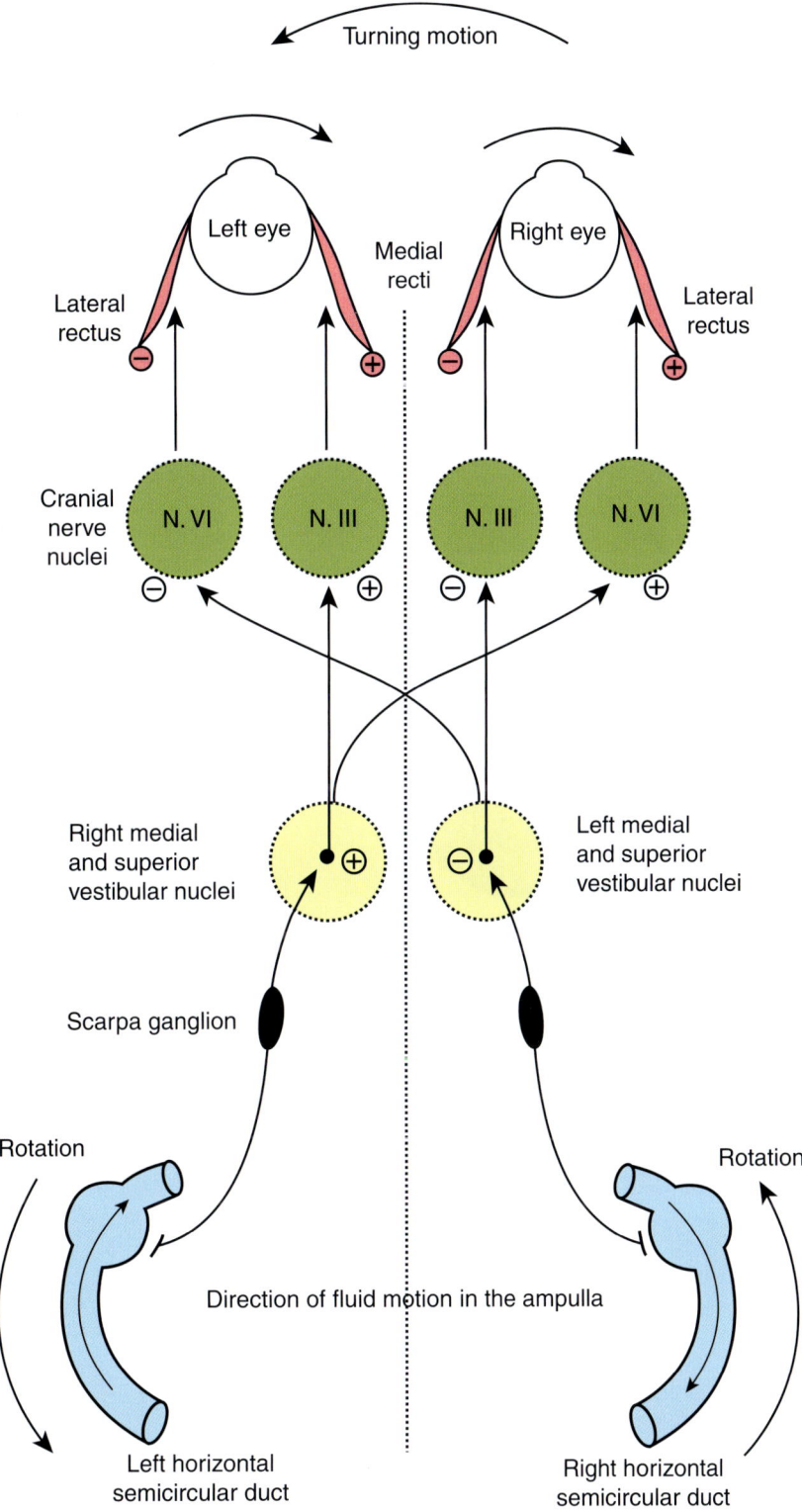

Figure 11.37 Schematic circuit diagram for the initial phase of the vestibulo-ocular reflex area. Increase (+) or decrease (−) in the rate of firing along a particular pathway is indicated. (Reproduced with permission from Kelly JP. Vestibular system. In: Kandel ER, Schwartz JH. *Principles of Neural Science*. 1st ed. Elsevier North-Holland; 1981:416, Figure 13.14.)

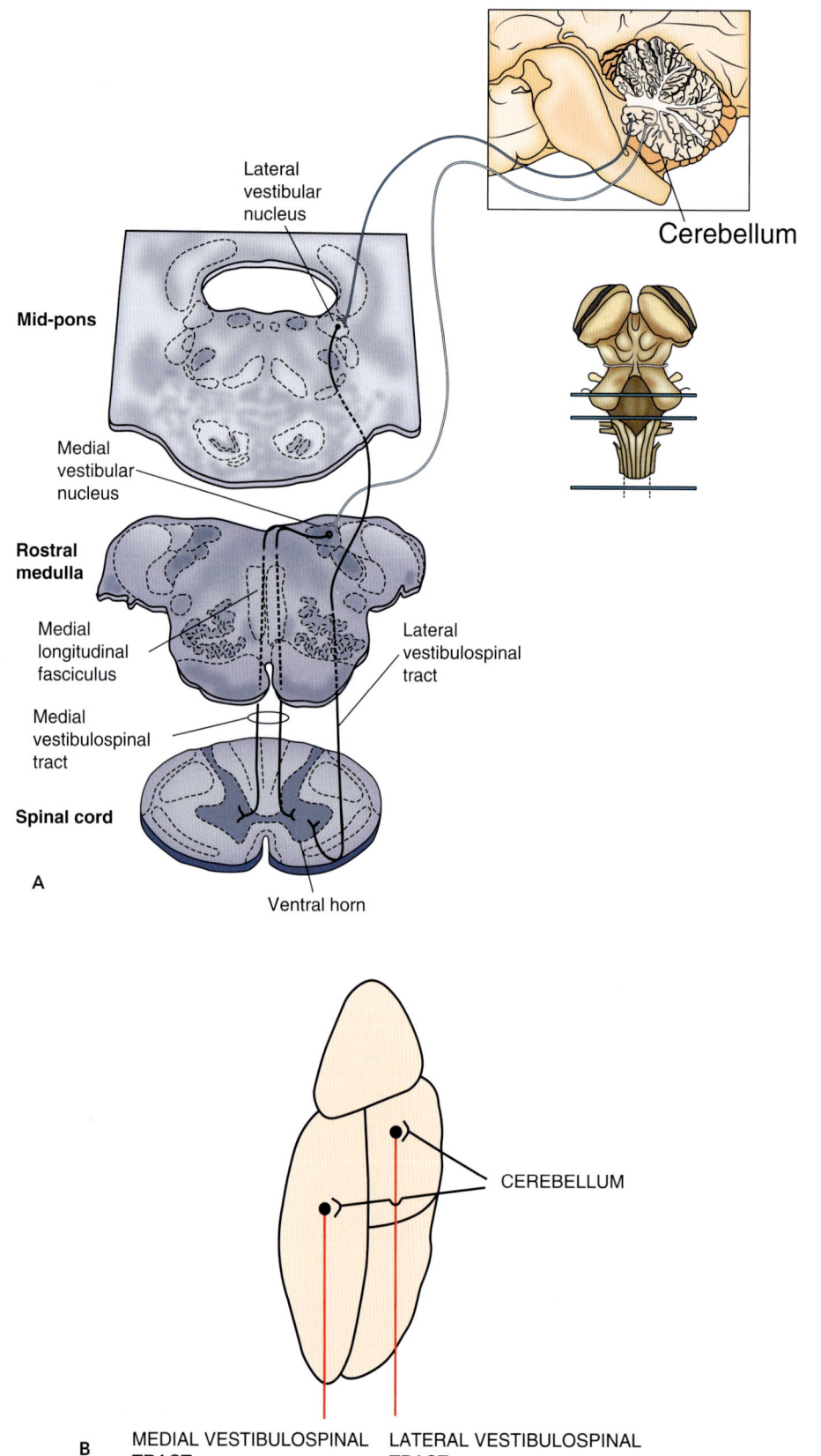

Figure 11.38 (A) **Vestibulospinal tracts lateral and medial.** (B) Lateral and medial vestibulospinal tracts receiving input from the cerebellum. (A, Redrawn with permission from Purves D, Augustine GJ, Fitzpatrick D, et al, eds. *Neuroscience*. 3rd ed. Sinauer Associates; 2004:331, Figure 13.11, by permission of Oxford University Press.)

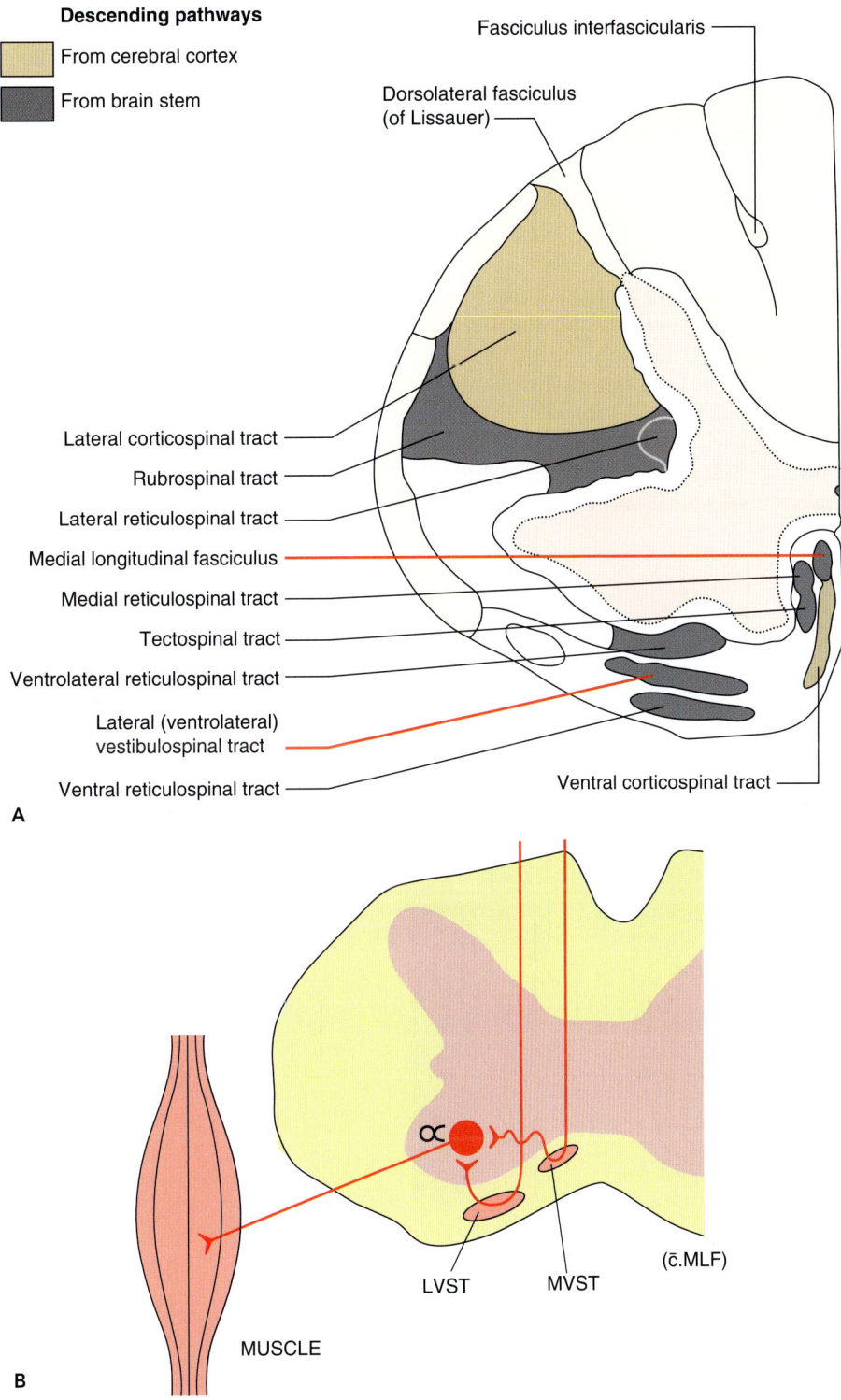

Figure 11.39 (A) Cross section of the spinal cord indicating the descending tracts and specifically the medial longitudinal fasciculus (MLF) and the lateral vestibulospinal tract (LVST). (B) LVST and medial vestibulospinal tract (MVST) descend with the MLF: innervating the α neurons. (A, Reproduced with permission of Elsevier, from *Gray's Anatomy: The Anatomical Basis of Clinical Practice*, 40th Edition. Susan Strandring (Ed.). Churchill Livingston; 2008, p. 262; Figure 18.9; permission conveyed through Copyright Clearance Center, Inc.)

As described in Purves,[38] descending projections from the vestibular nuclei are essential for posture adjustments of the head, mediated by the vestibulocervical reflex (VCR) and body, mediated by the vestibulospinal reflex (VSR). These postural reflexes are extremely fast, in part due to the small number of synapses interposed between the vestibular organs and the relevant motor neuron.

The anatomical substrate for VCR involves the medial vestibular nucleus, from which axons descend in the medial longitudinal fasciculus to reach the upper cervical levels of the spinal cord. This pathway regulates head position reflex activity of neck muscles in response to stimulation of the semicircular canals from rotational acceleration of the head.

For example, during a downward pitch of the body (eg, tripping) the superior canals are activated, and the head muscles reflexively pull the head up. The dorsal flexion of the head initiates other reflexes, such as forelimb extension and hindlimb flexion to stabilize the body and protect against a fall.

The VSR is mediated by a combination of pathways, including the lateral and medial vestibulospinal tract and the reticulospinal tract.

The input from the otolith organs projects mainly to the lateral vestibular nucleus, which in turn sends axons in the lateral vestibulospinal tract to the spinal cord.

These axons terminate monosynaptically on extensor neurons, and they disynaptically inhibit flexor motor neurons; the net result is a powerful excitatory influence on extension (antigravity) muscle.

When hair cells in the otolith organs are activated, signals reach the medial part of the ventral horn. By activating the ipsilateral pool of motor neurons innervating the exterior muscles in the trunk and limbs, this pathway mediates balance and the maintenance of upright posture.

Our vestibular apparatus provides pertinent information regarding our body relationship in regard to gravity both in stance and in walking (Fig. 11.40).

The body mass, at any instance, is to be projected on our pedal base support to prevent loss of balance. This instant correction is accomplished by the lateral input from otolith and the semicircular canals to medial vestibular nuclei in the brain stem.

Signals are then channeled to the cerebellar cortex which sends inhibitory cerebellar signals to the overactive deep cerebellar nuclei which transmit the neurosignals to the lateral and medial vestibular nuclei.

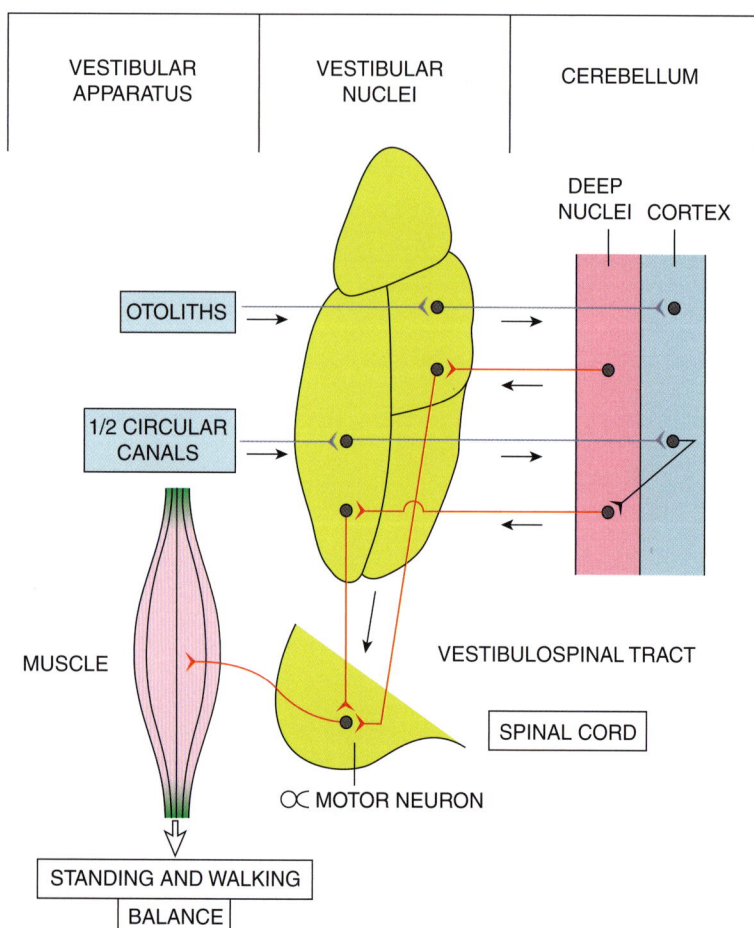

Figure 11.40 Flow chart indicating channeling of vestibular signals to the cerebellum resulting in corrective motor response.

These connect in the spinal cord with the corresponding αmotor neuron. The final corrective motor signal reaches the corresponding muscle. Balance is restored and fall is prevented in stance and in walking.

The superior and lateral vestibular nuclei send axons to the ventral posterior nucleus complex of the thalamus, which in turn projects to two cortical areas relevant to vestibular input (Fig. 11.41). One of these cortical targets is just posterior to the primary sensory cortex near the representation of the face; the other is at the transition between the somatic sensory cortex and the motor cortex (Brodmann area 3). Relevant cells respond to proprioceptive and visual stimuli as well as to vestibular stimuli. These cortical regions are involved in the perception of body orientation and extra personal space. Purves.[38]

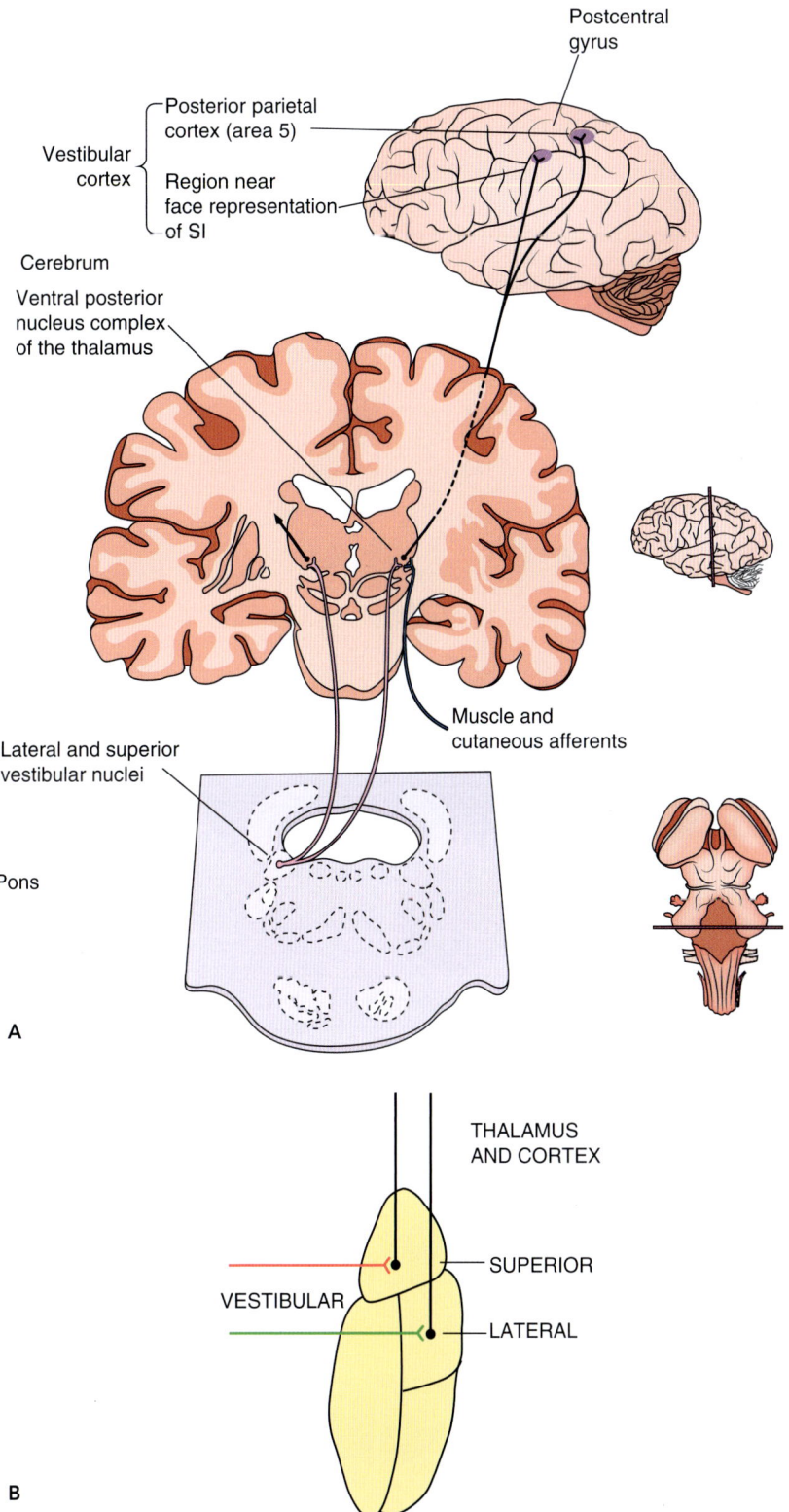

Figure 11.41 (A) Thalamus-cortical connections of the vestibular superior and lateral nuclei. (B) Vestibular input into the vestibular superior and lateral nuclei. (A, Redrawn with permission from Purves D, Augustine GJ, Fitzpatrick D, et al, eds. *Neuroscience*. 3rd ed. Sinauer Associates; 2004:334, Figure 13, by permission of Oxford University Press.)

THE CEREBELLUM[21-23]

The cerebellum controls:

- Posture
- Gait
- Planning and execution of movement

The cerebellum is located in the occipital cranial fossa and is attached anteriorly to the brain stem with two peduncles (Fig. 11.42).

▶ Cerebellar Hemispheres

The posterior surface of the cerebellum is divided transversely by fissures into foliac (Fig. 11.43).

Functionally the cerebellum is divided into two zones:

- Laterally the cerebrocerobellum
- Centrally the spinocerebellum

The vermis is the central segment of the spinocerebellum (Fig. 11.43). The cerebrocerebellum is an afferent receptor surface which channels the sensory signals to the cerebellar cortex and its major executor: the Purkinje cell layer. The afferents to the cerebrocerebellum are from the sensory association areas of the parietal lobe and motor association area of the frontal lobe[25] (Fig. 11.44A). The cortical fibers relay with pontine nuclei which extend their fibers to the cerebrocerebellum (Fig. 11.44B).

Planning and execution of the complex sequence of movements is controlled by the cerebrocerebellum. The central spinocerebellar is divided into central zone, the vermis, and two adjacent spinocerebellar zones (Fig. 11.45). It receives input directly from the spinal cord via the anterior and posterior spinocerebellar tracts and the peripheral somatosensory tracts via the olivary nucleus output.

The spinocerebellum is primarily concerned with the movements of the distal muscles involved with movement of the limbs in walking.[26]

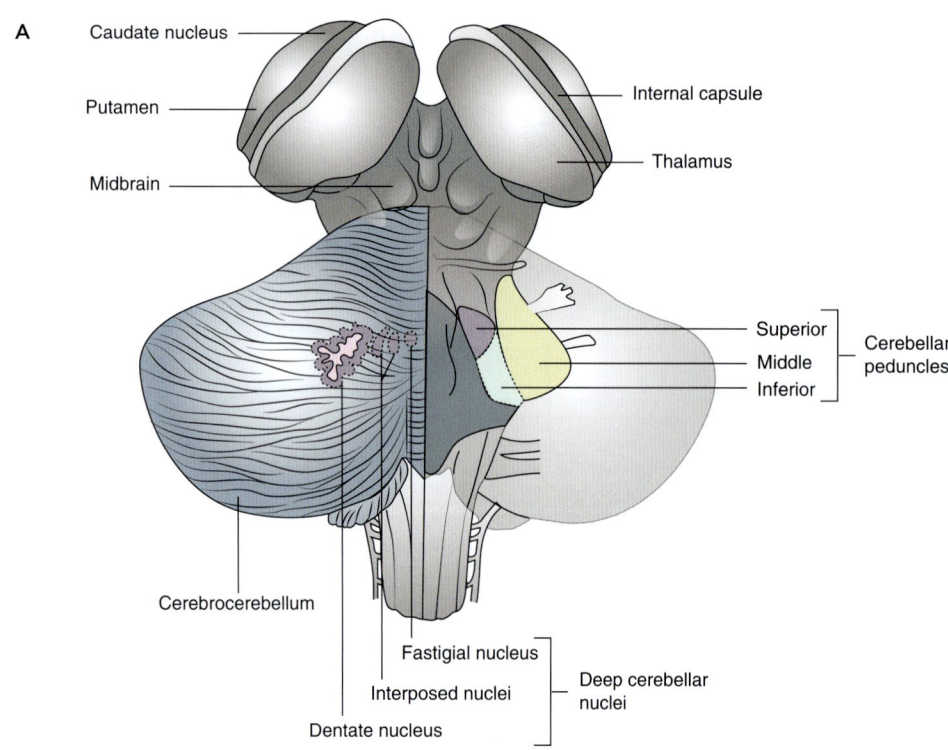

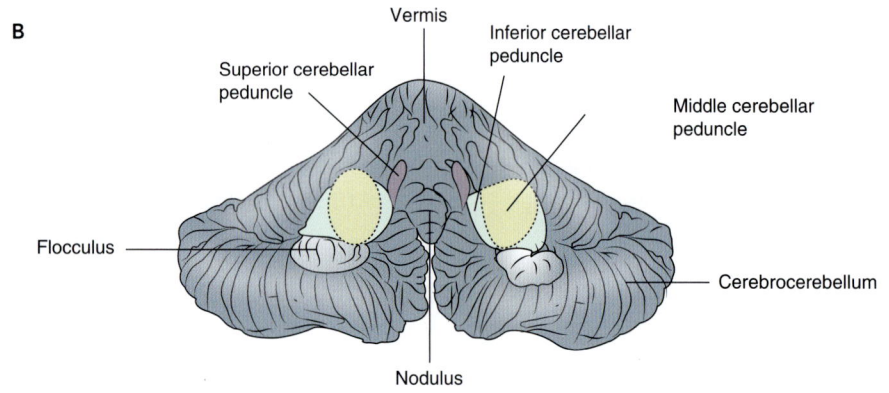

Figure 11.42 **(A) Dorsal view of left cerebellar hemisphere illustrating the location of the deep cerebellar nuclei.** The right hemisphere has been removed to show cerebellar peduncles. **(B)** Removal of the brain stem reveals the cerebellar peduncles on the anterior aspect of the inferior surface. (Redrawn with permission from Purves D, Augustine GJ, Fitzpatrick D, et al, eds. *Neuroscience*. 3rd ed. Sinauer Associates; 2004:436, Figure 18.1A, B, by permission of Oxford University Press.)

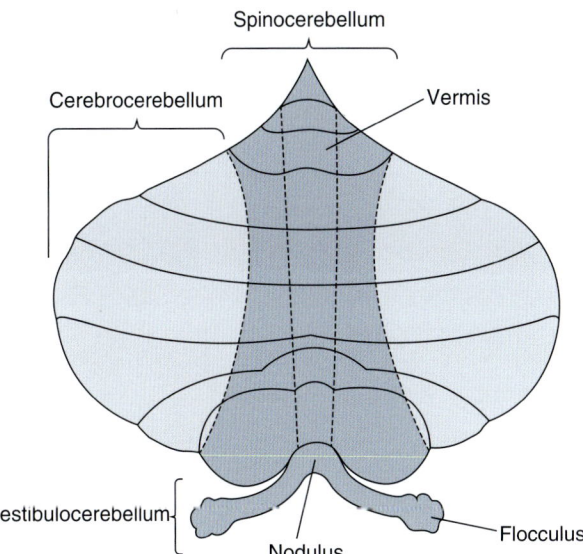

Figure 11.43 Flattened view of the cerebellar surface illustrating the three major subdivisions. (Redrawn with permission from Purves D, Augustine GJ, Fitzpatrick D, et al, eds. *Neuroscience*. 3rd ed. Sinauer Associates; 2004:436, Figure 18.1D, by permission of Oxford University Press.)

The vermis, or central segment of the spinocerebellum, is concerned with movements of proximal muscles and also regulates eye movements in response to vestibular input[26] (Fig. 11.45).

The vestibulocerebellum forms the caudal lobe of the cerebellum (Fig. 11.46) and includes the flocculus and the nodulus. It receives input from the vestibular nuclei of the brain stem and is primarily concerned with the regulation of movements underlying posture and equilibrium.[26]

▶ Cerebral Peduncles[27]

There are three cerebellar peduncles (Fig. 11.46):

- Superior
- Middle
- Inferior

The superior cerebellar peduncle is an efferent pathway. It gives rise to the following pathways to:

- Deep cerebellar nuclei
- Red nucleus
- Superior colliculus
- Thalamus
- Cerebral cortex: motor and premotor

The middle cerebellar peduncle is an afferent pathway to the cerebellum and gives rise to the following pathways from:

- The pontine nuclei
- Cerebral cortex
- Superior colliculus

The inferior cerebral peduncle is the smaller but most complex of the cerebellar peduncles containing multiple afferent and efferent pathways. The afferent fibers are from:

- Vestibular nuclei
- Spinal cord
- Brain stem tegmentum

The efferent fibers are to the:

- Vestibular nuclei
- The reticular formation

▶ Cerebellar Cortex and Circuits

The major cell of the cerebellar cortex is the Purkinje inhibitory GABAergic cell.

Excellent histologic preparation of the cell has been provided by the Spanish neurohistologist Ramon I Cajal (Fig. 11.47).

The Purkinje inhibitory cell receives input from the periphery by the mossy fibers and the climbing fibers. Contributions to the mossy fibers are the anterior and posterior spinocerebellar fibers and the cortico-pontocerebellar fibers and the vestibulocerebellar fibers.

The olivary nucleus in the medulla (Fig. 11.48) receives input from the posterior ascending sensory column and from the superior colliculus in the brain stem. The climbing tract to the cerebellum originates from the inferior olivary nucleus.

Functionally, the Purkinje cells inhibit the overactive deep cellular nuclei. In the animal model, transection of the Purkinje fibers to the deep cerebellar nuclei results in cerebral rigidity.

Destination and Function of Mossy Fibers[29,30]

One of the main components of the mossy fibers are the anterior and posterior spinocerebellar tracts (Fig. 11.49). An excellent description of the functional significance of these tracts has been presented by S. G. Lisberg and W. T. Tach.[30]

The dorsal spinal cerebellar tract conveys somatosensory information from muscle and joint receptors, providing the cerebellum with sensory feedback about the consequences of movement. This information flows whether the limbs are moved passively or voluntarily.

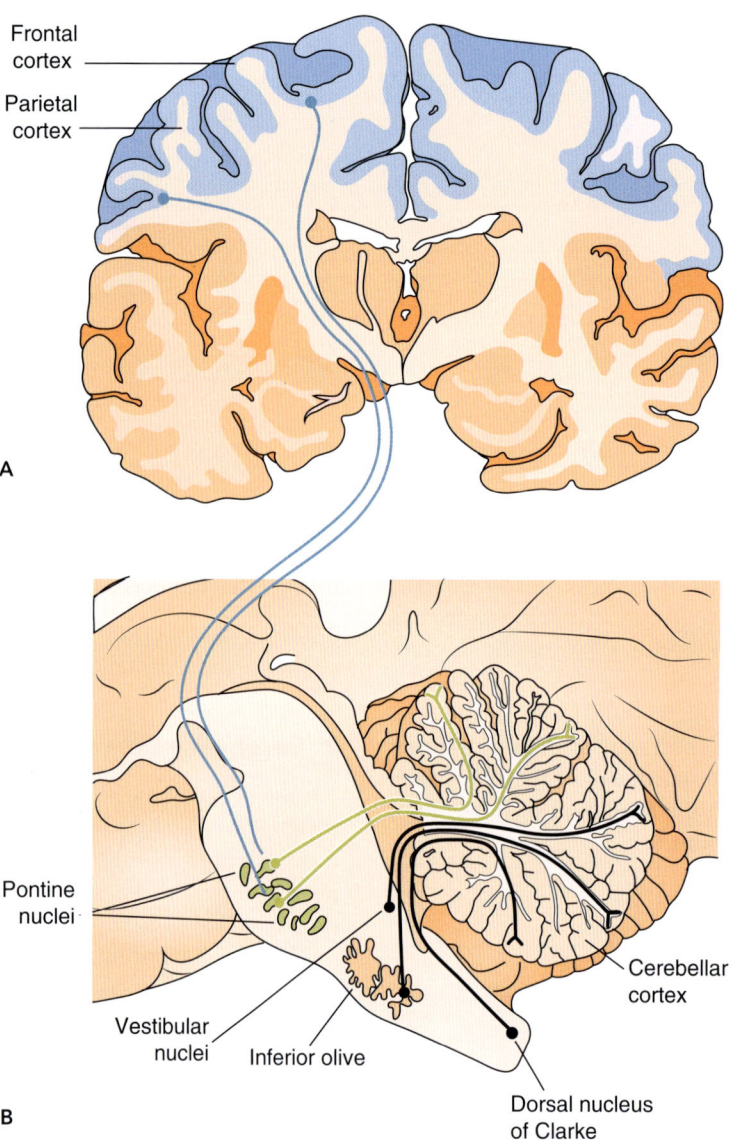

Figure 11.44 **(A) Region of the cerebral cortex that project to the cerebellum (shown in blue).** These cortical projections to the cerebellum are mainly from the sensory association cortex of the parietal lobe and motor association areas of the frontal lobe. **(B)** Idealized coronal and sagittal sections through the human brain stem and cerebellum, showing inputs to the cerebellum from the cortex, vestibular system, spinal cord, and brain stem. The cortical projections to the cerebellum are made via neurons in the pons. These pontine axons cross the midline within the pons and run to the cerebellum via the middle cerebellar peduncle. (Redrawn with permission from Purves D, Augustine GJ, Fitzpatrick D, et al, eds. *Neuroscience*. 3rd ed. Sinauer Associates; 2004, A. Figure 18.4, p. 439. B. Figure 18.3, p. 430, by permission of Oxford University Press.)

Chapter 11: Neuro Control of Stance and Gait 673

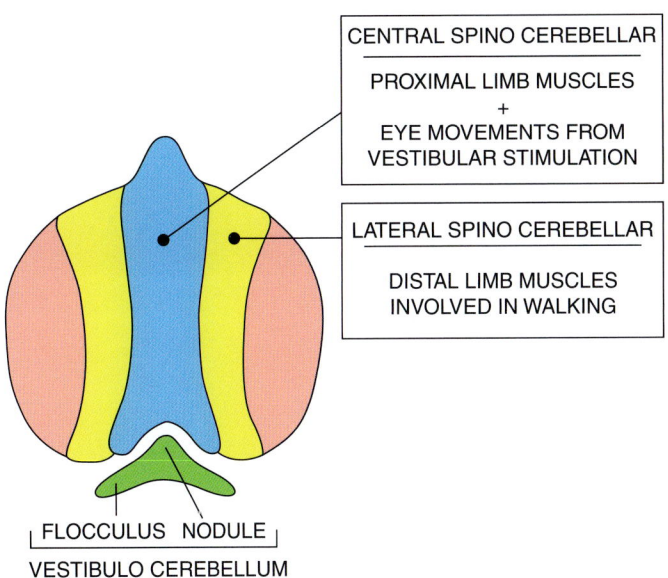

Figure 11.45 Functional subdivisions of the cerebellum.

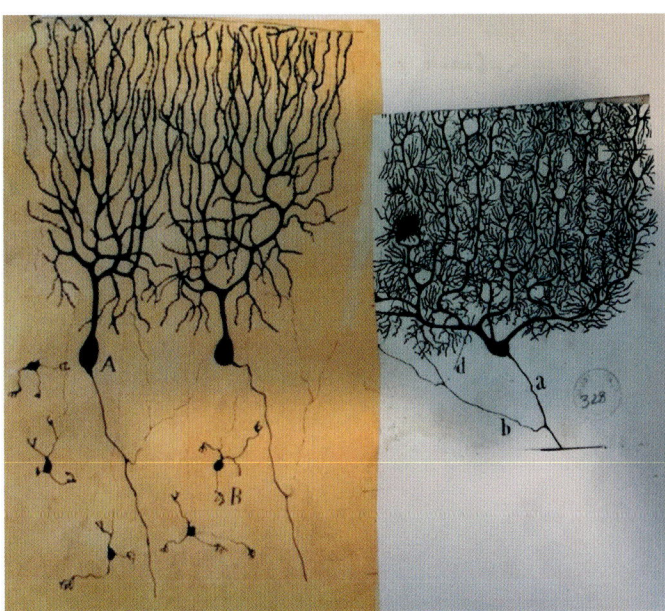

Figure 11.47 Neurologic preparations of Purkinje cells by Spanish neurohistologist Ramon I Cajal.

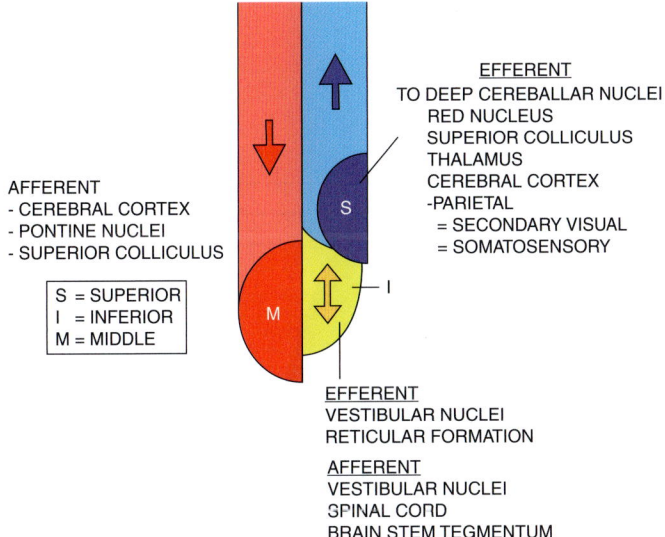

Figure 11.46 Cerebellar peduncular input-output.

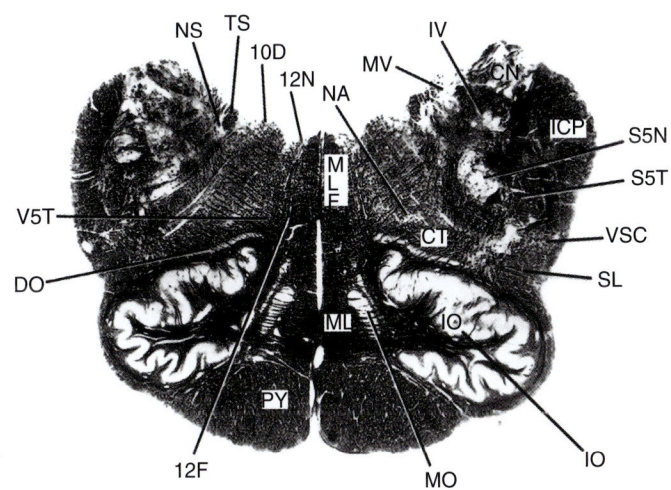

Figure 11.48 Cross-section of medulla.

In contrast, the ventral spinocerebellar tract is active only during active movements. Its cells of origin receive the same inputs as spinal motor neurons and interneurons, and it transmits an efferent copy or corollary discharge of spinal motor neuron activity that informs the cerebellum about the movement commands assembled at the spinal cord. The cerebellum is thought to compare this information on planned movement with the actual movement reported to the dorsal spinocerebellar tracts in order to determine whether the motor command must be modified to achieve the desired movement. The dorsal and ventral spinocerebellar tracts provide input from the hindlimbs.

The graphical representation is indicated in Figure 11.49. Mossy fibers (Figs. 11.50 and 11.51) synapse with granule cell in the granular layer of the cerebellar cortex. The granular cells give rise to parallel fibers which contribute and form T-shaped branches that relay information to the Purkinje cells which are stimulated.

Purkinje cell dendrites branch extensively in a plane at right angle to the trajectory of the parallel fibers and send a terminal axon connecting with the deep cerebellar nuclei.

▶ Climbing Fibers

Generated by the olivary nucleus of the medulla, the climbing fibers extend toward the apical region of the Purkinje cells and wrap their fibers around the Purkinje dendrites like vine tracts wrapping around trunk of a tree.

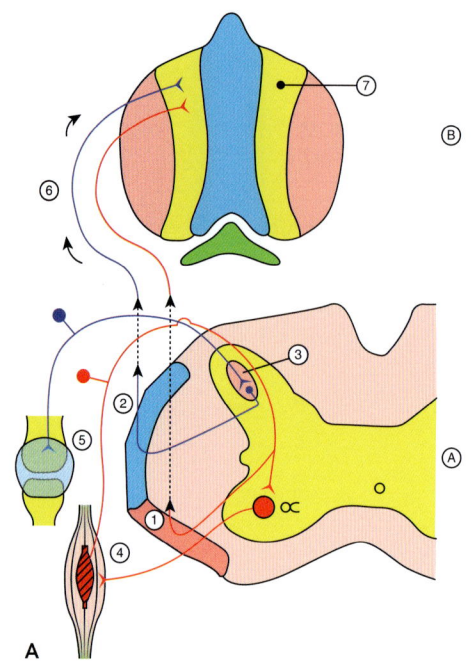

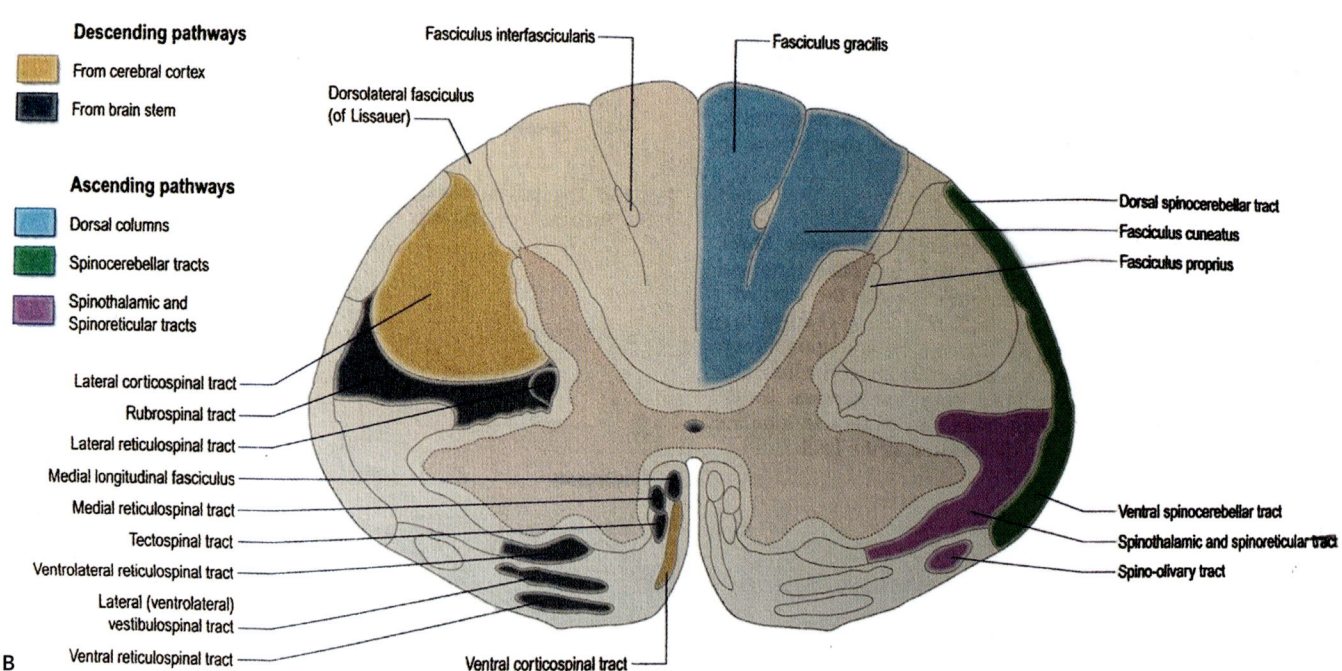

Figure 11.49 (A) Cerebellar input of anterior and posterior spinocerebellar tracts.

A, Spinal cord
B, Cerebellum
1, Anterior spinocerebellar tract
2, Posterior spinocerebellar tract
3, Nucleus dorsalis of Clark
4, Muscle spindle and muscle
5, Joint preceptors: capsule, ligaments
6, Mossy cerebellar fibers
7, Spinocerebellar division

(B) Cross section of spinal cord. The ascending tracts are shown on the left, and the descending tracts are shown on the right. (Reproduced with permission of Elsevier, from *Gray's Anatomy: The Anatomical Basis of Clinical Practice*, 40th Edition. Susan Strandring (Ed.). Churchill Livingston; 2008, Figure 18.9; permission conveyed through Copyright Clearance Center, Inc.)

Chapter 11: Neuro Control of Stance and Gait

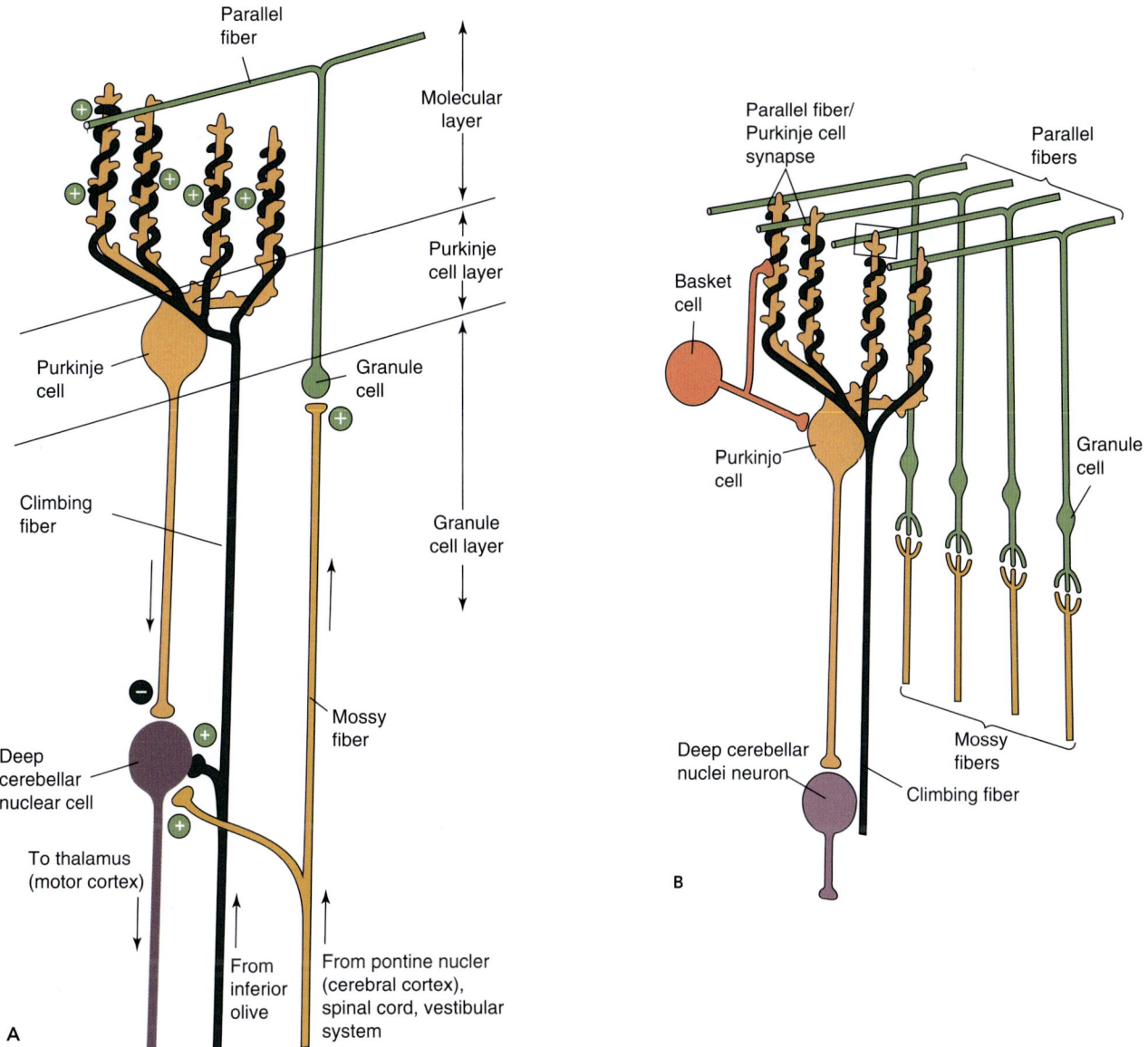

Figure 11.50 (A) Excitatory and inhibitory connections on the cerebellar cortex and deep cerebellar nuclei. The mossy fibers and the climbing fibers stimulate the Purkinje cell which inhibits the deep cerebellar nucleus. (B) Diagram showing convergent input onto the Purkinje cell from parallel fibers and local circuit neurons. (Redrawn with permission from Purves D, Augustine GJ, Fitzpatrick D, et al, eds. *Neuroscience*. 3rd ed. Sinauer Associates; 2004, Figure 18.9, p. 443. Figure 18.8, p. 442, by permission of Oxford University Press.)

The climbing fibers and the mossy fibers while coursing toward the cerebellar cortex extend excitatory branches to the adjacent cerebellar deep nucleus (Fig. 11.50).

▶ Deep Cerebellar Nuclei

The deep cerebellar nuclei are located at the level of the medulla, posterior to the IV ventricle (Fig. 11.52). The components of the cerebellar nuclei are the:

- Dentate nucleus
- Fastigious nucleus
- Embolliform nucleus
- Globose nuclei[2]

which represent one half of the pair of the deep cerebellar nuclei. The deep cerebellar nuclei are normally active. Their neuroactivity is inhibited by the Purkinje cells. The neuro output of the deep cerebellar nuclei is specific. The dentate nucleus receives its input from the cerebrocerebellum.

The emboli form and globose nuclei act as functional unit and receive their input from the spinocerebellum. The fastigial nucleus receives its input from the vestibulocerebellum (Fig. 11.53).

▶ Output of the Deep Cerebellar Nuclei

The neuro output from the deep cerebellar nuclei expresses the neuroefferent output of the cerebellum as a response of the corticocerebellar input, and the peripheral input from the vestibular system and from the spinocerebellar tracts (Fig. 11.54).

The dentate nucleus projects to the proximal pole (parvocellular) of the red nucleus and the connecting neurons

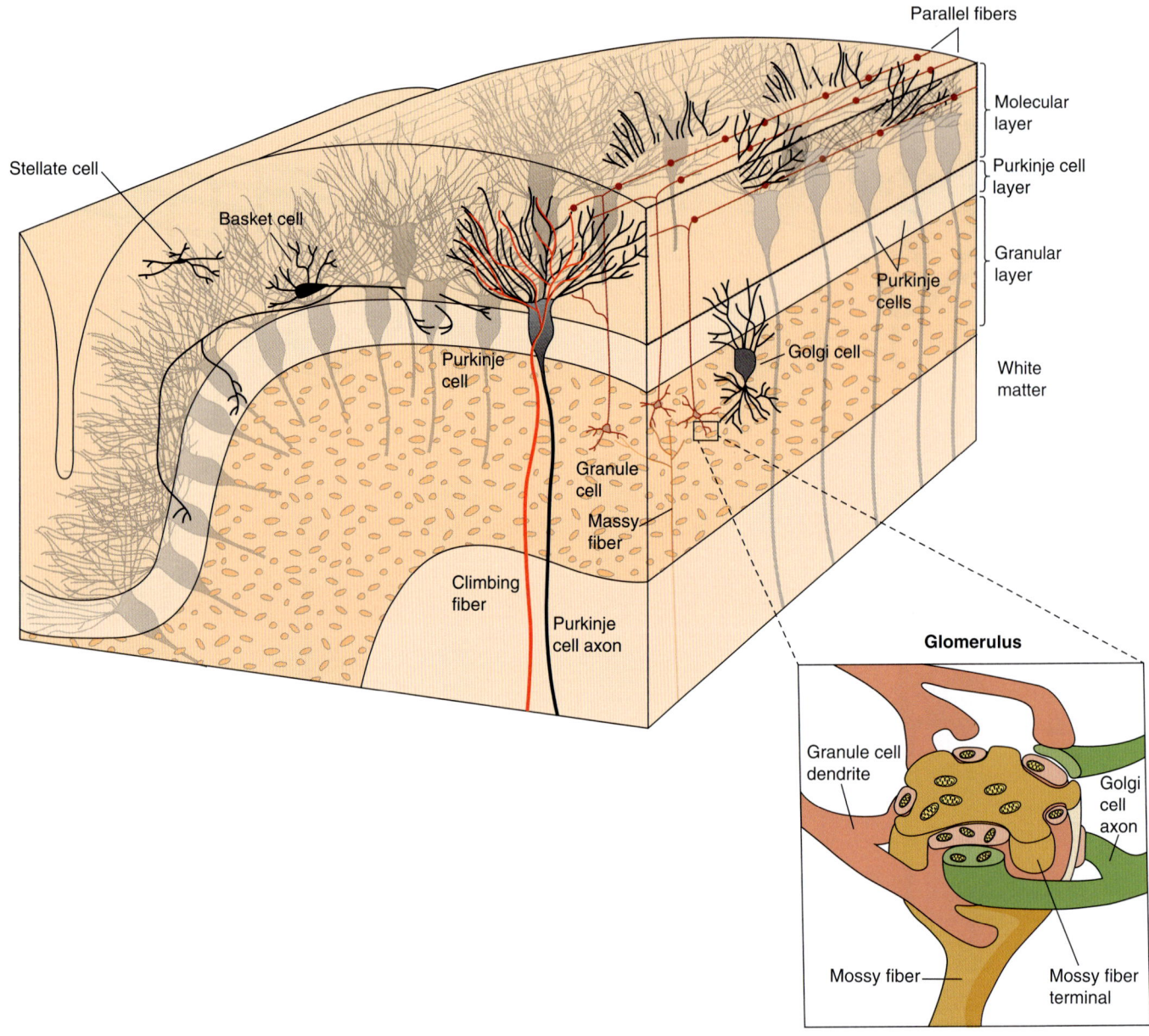

Figure 11.51 **The cerebellar cortex contains five types of neurons organized into three layers.** A vertical section of a single cerebellar folium illustrates the general organization of the cerebellar cortex. The detail of a cerebellar glomerulus in the granular is shown. A glomerulus is the synaptic complex formed by the bulbous axon terminal of a mossy fiber and the dendrites of several Golgi and granular cells. Mitochondria are present on all of the structures in the glomerulus consistent with their high metabolic activity. (Used with permission from The Cerebellar Cortex by Stephen A. Lisberg W. Thomas Tach. In: Kandel ER, Schwartz JH, Jessell TM, eds. *Principles of Neural Science*. 2nd ed. Elsevier; 1985:968, Figure 42.4.)

extend to the thalamus and primary motor cortex. The interposed nuclei make the connection with the lower pole (magnocellular) or the red nuclei which generates axons, extending to the spinal cord and forming the rubrospinal motor tract.

The fastigial nucleus extends to the lateral and medial vestibular tracts which extend into the spinal cord as the lateral and medial vestibulospinal tracts.

The fastigial nucleus also generates the connection with the spinal medial reticular tract.

Figure 11.55 summarizes the crucial role of the cerebellum as a modulator of motor function.

The cerebellar input for the final motor expression is from the following:

- Vestibular nerve
- Anterior and posterior spinocerebellar tracts
- Inferior olivary nucleus with sensory input from the periphery
- Further cerebral cortical input

The cerebellar output through the deep cerebellar nuclei is as follows:

- Lateral and medial vestibulospinal tracts
- Rubrospinal tract
- Reticular tract

Chapter 11: Neuro Control of Stance and Gait   677

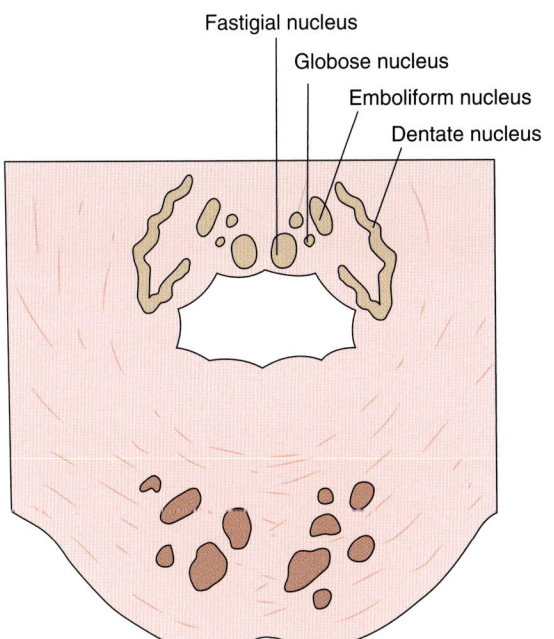

Figure 11.52 Central nuclei of the cerebellum. (Redrawn with permission from Barr ML, Kiernan JA. *The Human Nervous System: An Anatomical Viewpoint*. 5th ed. Lippincott Williams & Wilkins; 1988:158, Figure 10.9.)

Figure 11.53 Cerebellar cortical output to deep cerebellar nuclei.

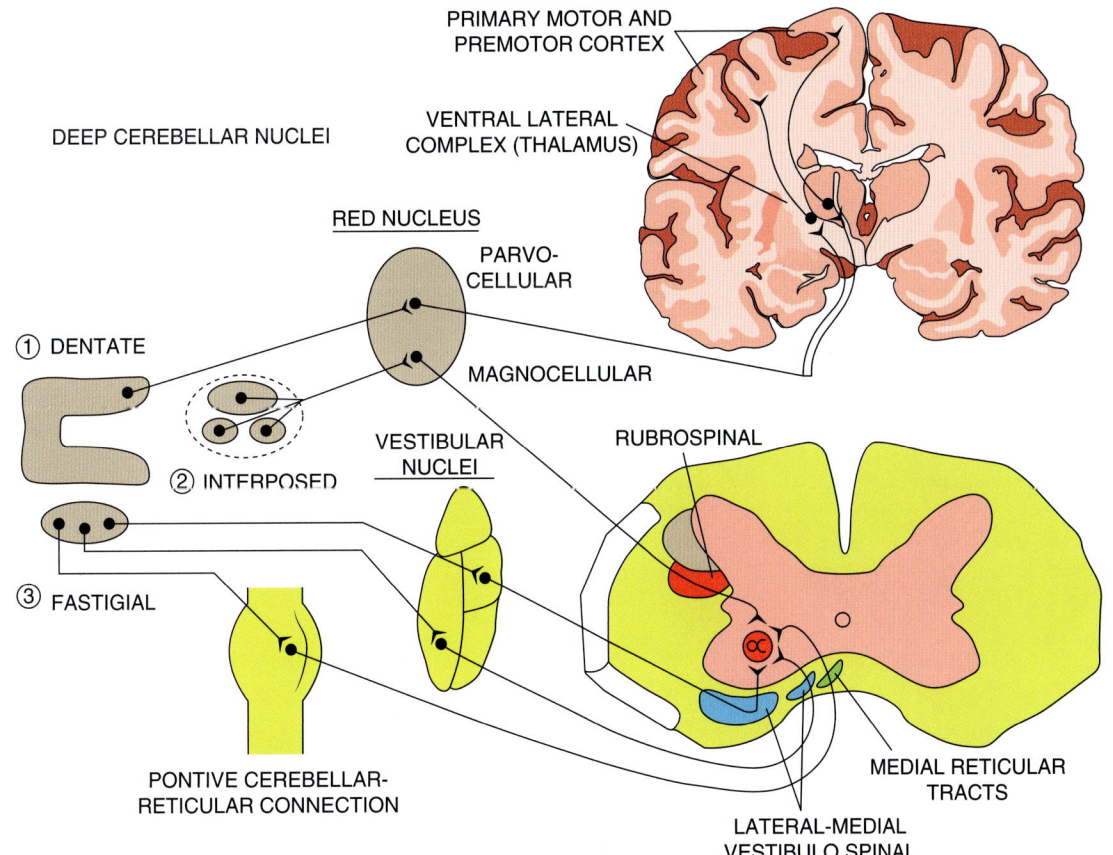

Figure 11.54 Cerebellar output.
1, Dentate nucleus to red nucleus (parvocellular) landing on the thalamus and primary and premotor cortex.
2, Interposed nuclei to red nucleus (magnocellular) and then to the rubrospinal tract of the spinal cord.
3, Fastigius nuclei
-To lateral and medial vestibulo-nuclei and terminal lateral and medial vestibulospinal tracts
-To pontine cerebelloreticular connection
-To spinal medial reticular tract.

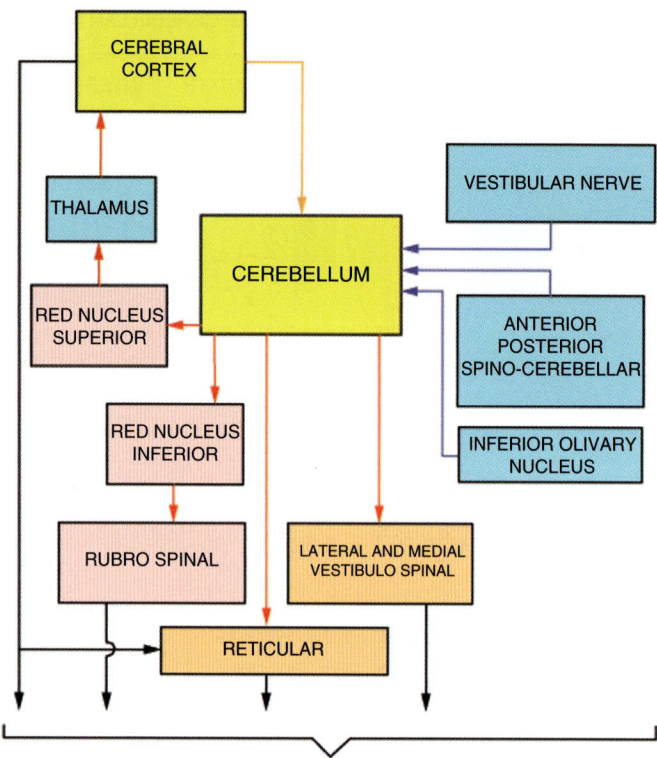

Figure 11.55 Modulators of spinal cord motor units.
-Reticular system
-Motor cerebral cortex
-Cerebellovestibular axis
-Rubrospinal tract.

The massive peripheral cerebellar input reaches the Purkinje cell layer which will appropriately inhibit (GABAergic) the constantly active deep cerebellar nuclei.

BASAL GANGLIA[31,32]

The basal ganglion is a major component of the cortico-cortical motor loop.

Its neurosignal is transmitted to the corticospinal motor tract which activates and modulates the alpha and gamma neuromotor loop.

The anatomy of the basal ganglion is best defined in a coronal section of the brain and the following are its components enclosed between the external and internal capsules:

- the putamen laterally
- the pallidum medially divide into a lateral and medial segments

The overall contour of the complex is triangular on the cross section (Figs. 11.56 and 11.57).

The caudate nucleus is an integral part of the basal ganglion and forms with the pallidum, the corpus striatum (Fig. 11.57A).

An excellent anatomical study by Barr demonstrates the integration of the caudate nucleus with the putamen. The caudate nucleus attaches to the putamen anteriorly; courses above, around, and inferior to the putamen; and terminates as the amygdaloid body (Fig. 11.57B).

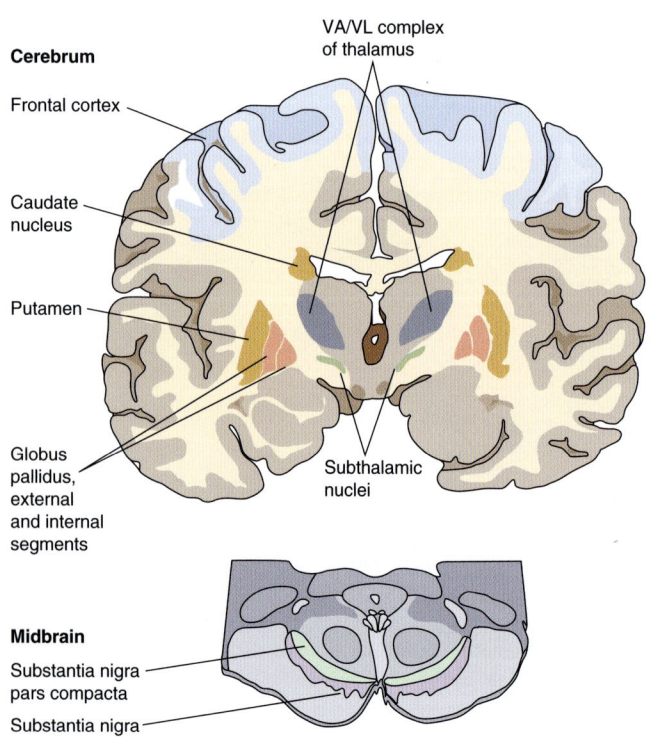

Figure 11.56 Cross section of the brain modulation of movement by basal ganglia. "Idealized cross section through the brain showing anatomical location of the structures involved in the basal ganglia pathway. Most of the structures are in the telencephalon although the substantia nigra is in the midbrain and the thalamus and subthalamic nuclei are in the diencephalon. The ventral anterior and ventral lateral thalamic nuclei (VA/VL complex) are the targets of the basal ganglia relaying the modulatory effects of the basal ganglion through motor neurons in the cortex." (Redrawn with permission from Purves D, Augustine GJ, Fitzpatrick D, et al, eds. *Neuroscience*. 3rd ed. Sinauer Associates; 2004:418, Figure 17.1B, by permission of Oxford University Press.)

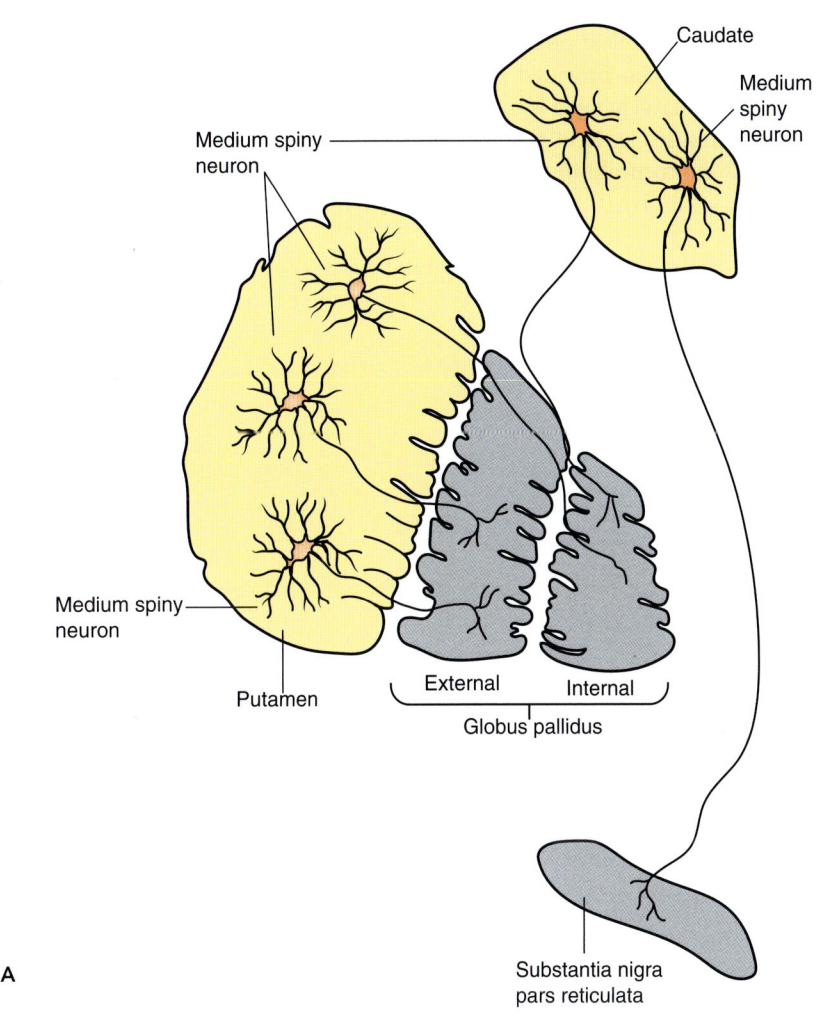
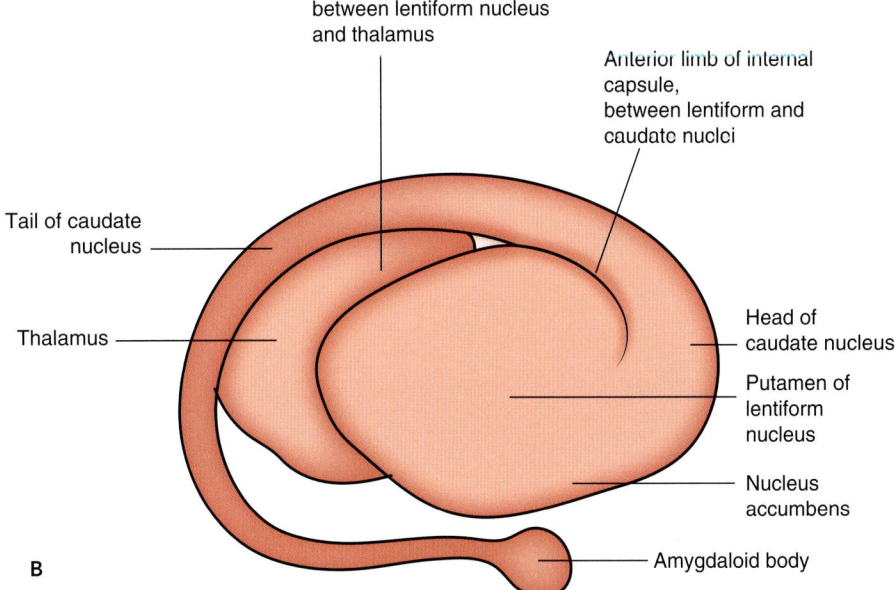

Figure 11.57 Modulation of movement by the basal ganglia. (A) Anatomy of the corpus striatum basal ganglia with the putamen laterally, external and internal globus pallidus medially. Functionally, the caudate nucleus and the substantia nigra of the midbrain are integrated with the basal ganglia. **(B)** Lateral aspect of the right corpus striatum showing the thalamus and amygdala. The globus pallidus and amygdala. The globus pallidus is concealed by the lateral putamen. (**A.** Redrawn with permission from Purves D, Augustine GJ, Fitzpatrick D, et al, eds. *Neuroscience*. 3rd ed. Sinauer Associates; 2004:420, Figure 17.3, by permission of Oxford University Press. **B.** Redrawn with permission from Murray LB, Kiernan JA. *The Human Nervous System: An Anatomical Viewpoint*. 6th ed. Lippincott Williams & Wilkins; 1993:224. Figure 12.)

The caudate nucleus also receives input from the cortical cortex and the substantia nigra pars compacta (Figs. 11.58 and 11.59).

Functionally, integral part of the basal ganglia is also the subthalamic nuclei. A clear presentation of the function of the basal ganglia has been provided by Purves et al.[32] The functional axis of the basal ganglia is formed by the triad: putamen-pallidum-thalamus (Fig. 11.60).

At rest with no cortical input only the pallidum is active and this activity is inhibitive (GABAergic). There is no input into the thalamus on the cerebral cortex.

When the cerebral cortex is active, the putamen is stimulated and the activity is excitatory (DOPAergic). This positive activity decreases the inhibitory activity of the pallidum. As a result, there is stimulation of the thalamus which then transmits the excitatory signals to the cerebral cortex. This creates functionally a cortico-basal ganglia-thalamo cortical loop. An excellent diagram of this cortico-cortical loop is presented by Wichman and Delong.[33]

As presented in Figure 11.61, the cortical input (in red) to the putamen (striatum) is followed by the modulating (in green) output of the pallidum-thalamus. The cerebral cortical areas providing the cortical input to the basal ganglia are as defined by Wichman and DeLong[33] in Figure 11.62.

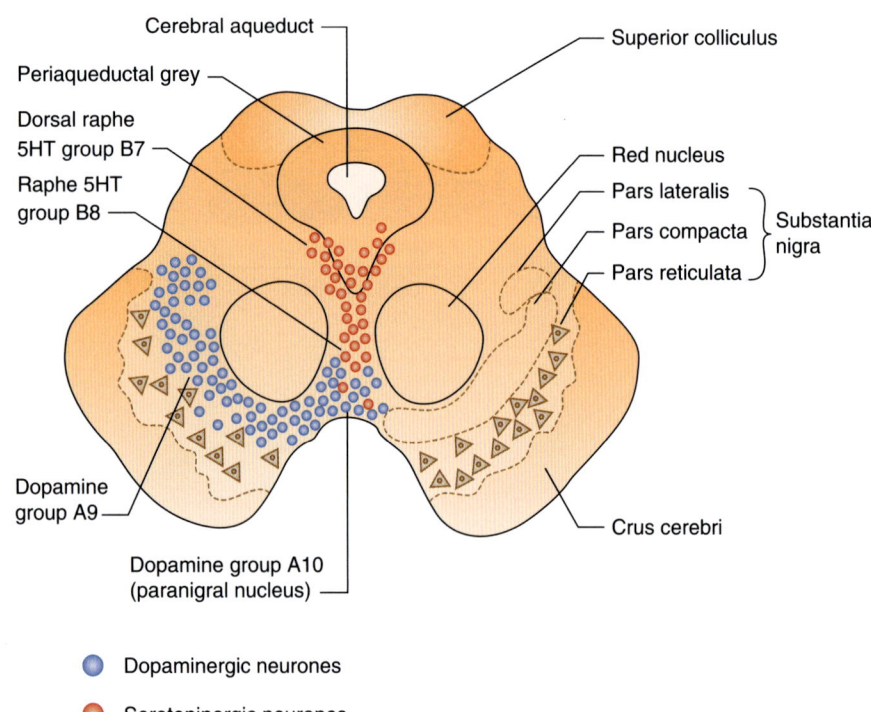

Figure 11.58 Transverse section through the midbrain to show the arrangement of dopaminergic cell group A9 and A10 in the substantial nigra (left) and serotoninergic cell groups B7 and B8 in the raphe.

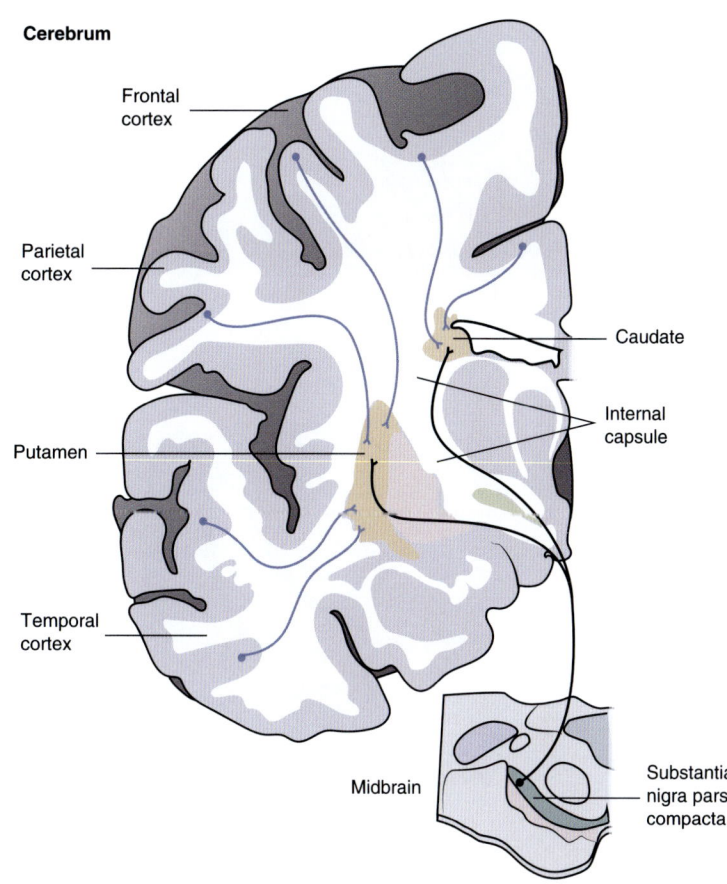

Figure 11.59 **Input from cerebral cortex and substantia nigra pars compacta.** (Redrawn with permission from Purves D, Augustine GJ, Fitzpatrick D, et al, eds. *Neuroscience*. 3rd ed. Sinauer Associates; 2004:419, Figure 17.2, by permission of Oxford University Press.)

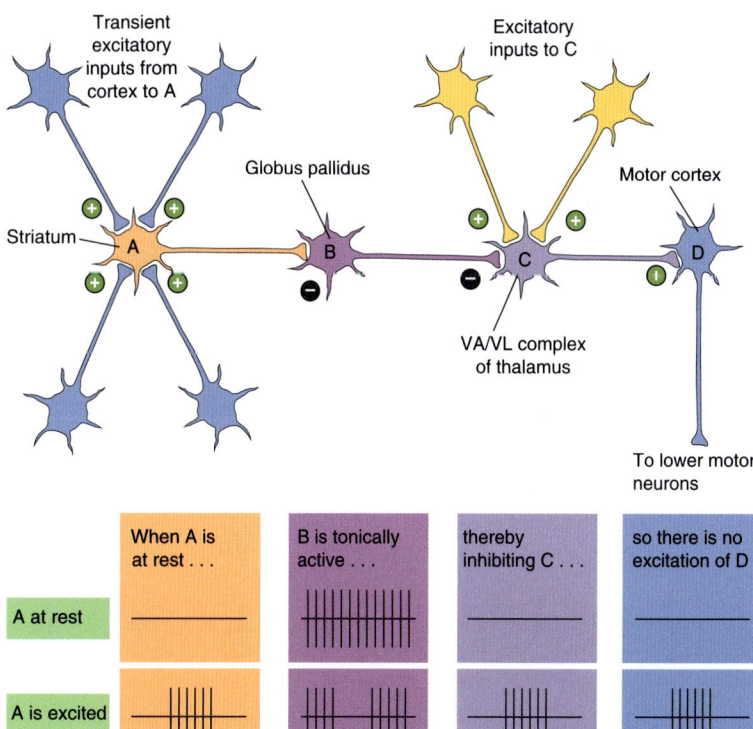

Figure 11.60 **Modulation of movement by basal ganglia.** A chain of nerve cells arranged in disinhibitory circuit. Top: Diagrams of the connections between two inhibitory neurons A and B and an excitatory neuron C. Bottom: Pattern of the action potential activity of cells A, B, and C at rest and when neuron A fires transiently as a result of its excitatory inputs. Such circuits are central to the gating operations of the basal ganglia. (Redrawn with permission from Purves D, Augustine GJ, Fitzpatrick D, et al, eds. *Neuroscience*. 3rd ed. Sinauer Associates; 2004:424, Figure 17.6, by permission of Oxford University Press.)

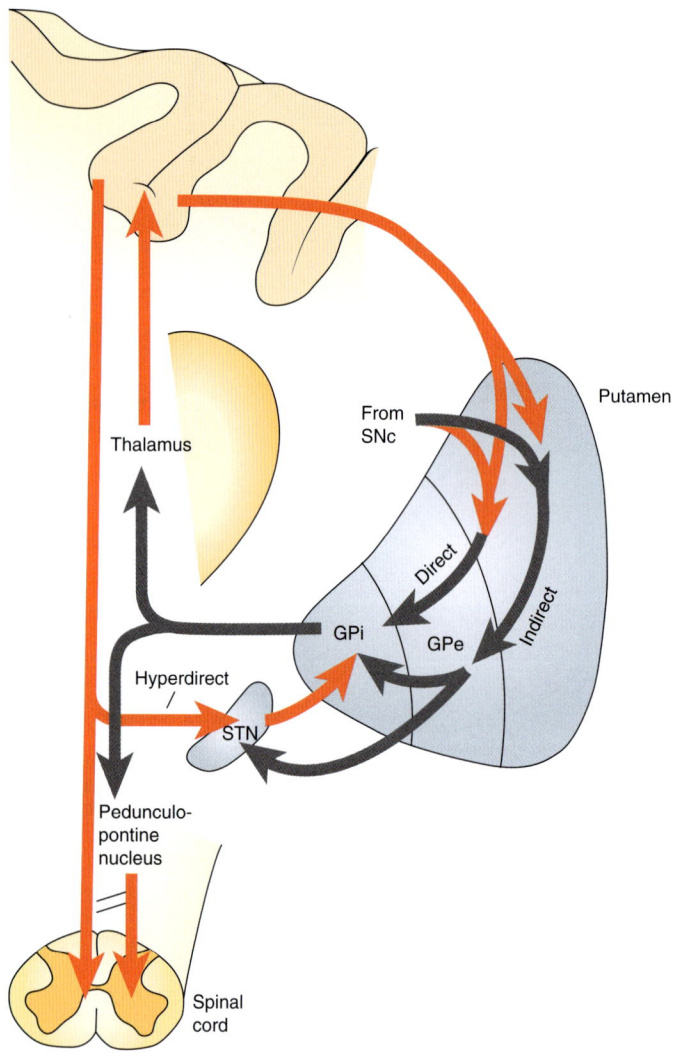

Figure 11.61 **Cortico-basal ganglia, thalamo cortical circuits, input resulting in corticospinal output.** (Redrawn with permission from Wichman T, DeLong MR. Basal Ganglia. In: Kandel ER, Schwartz JH, Jessell TM, eds. *Principles of Neural Science*. 2nd ed. Elsevier; 1985:984, Figure 43.2.)

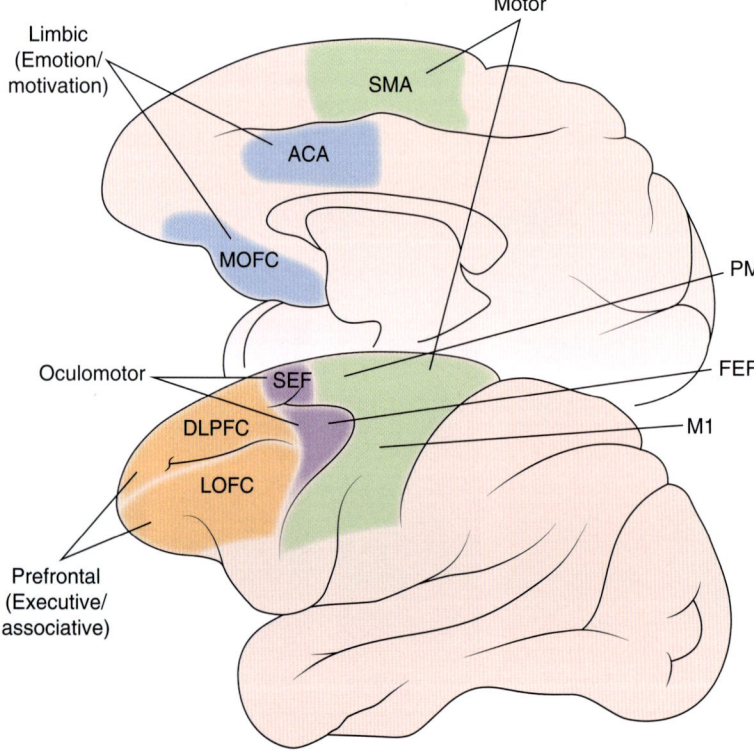

Figure 11.62 **Four cortical areas converge to the basal ganglia and thalamus.** ACA, anterior cingulate area; DLPFC, dorsolateral prefrontal cortex; LOFC, lateral orbitofrontal cortex; MOFC, medial orbitofrontal cortex; SEF, supplementary eye field; SMA, supplementary motor area. (Redrawn with permission from Wichman T, DeLong MR. Basal Ganglia. In: Kandel ER, Schwartz JH, Jessell TM, eds. *Principles of Neural Science*. 2nd ed. Elsevier; 1985:986, Figure 43.4.)

CEREBRAL MOTOR CORTEX[34-37]

Motor command for ambulation is provided by the cortical primary motor area 4 of Brodmann modulated by the cortical premotor area 6 and the parietal cortical association area (Fig. 11.63).

Penfield identified in motor area 4 the distribution of the body's motor units, based on electrical stimulation during surgery of specific cortical area (Fig. 11.64).

The motor and premotor areas are modulated by extensive input from the:

- Association cortices: frontal, parietal, temporal
- Basal ganglia and cerebellum via the thalamus
- Brain stem
- Association cortex of the contralateral hemisphere via corpus commissure forming the interhemispheric connections callosum and anterior (Fig. 11.65)

▶ Primary Motor Cortex

Structurally, as indicated in Figure 11.66, the neurons in the primary motor cortex are distributed over six layers. Pyramidal motor cells of layers 3 and 5 provide 70% of the axons of the motor corticospinal tract.

Remaining 30% of the motor tracts are provided by the premotor area. Functionally low intensity of current is necessary to elicit movements by electrical stimulation in this region. The low threshold for eliciting movements is an indication of a

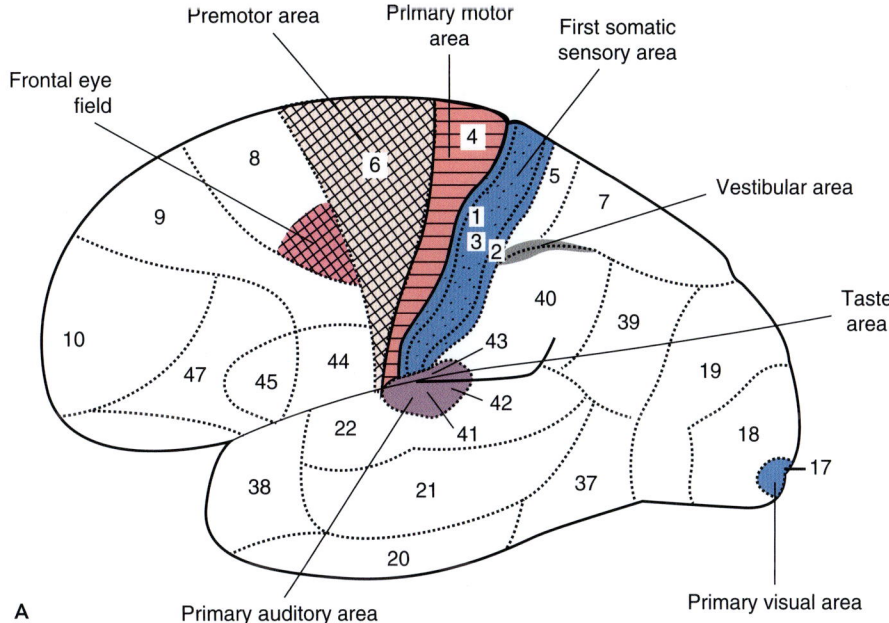

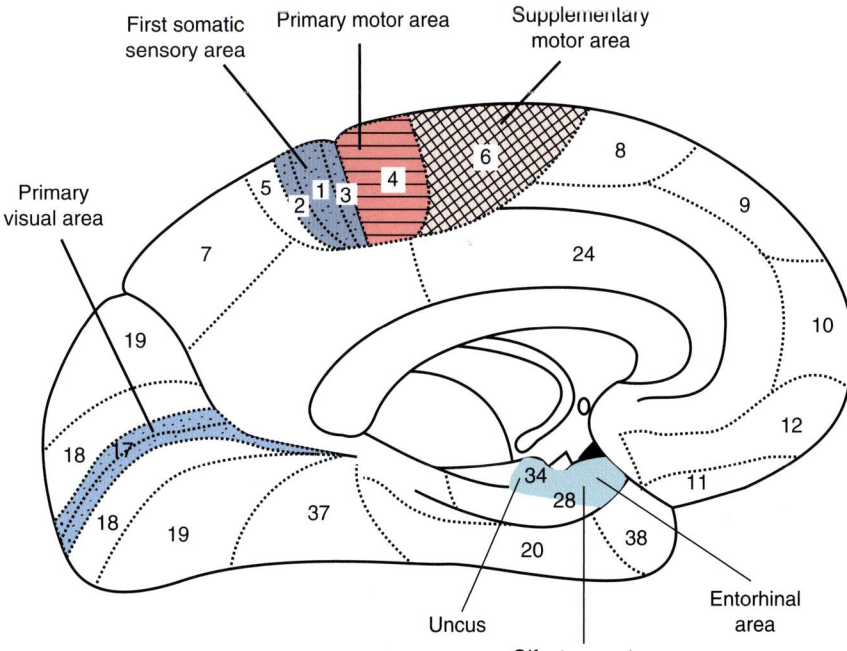

Figure 11.63 (A) Motor and primary sensory areas on the lateral surface of the left cerebral hemisphere. (B) Motor and primary sensory areas on the medial surface of the left cerebral hemisphere. Some of Brodmann's numbered areas, based on cytoarchitecture, are also shown. (Redrawn with permission from Murray LB, Kiernan JA. *The Human Nervous System: An Anatomical Viewpoint*, 6th ed. Lippincott Williams & Wilkins; 1993:257. Figure 15.1, 15.2, p. 256, p. 257.)

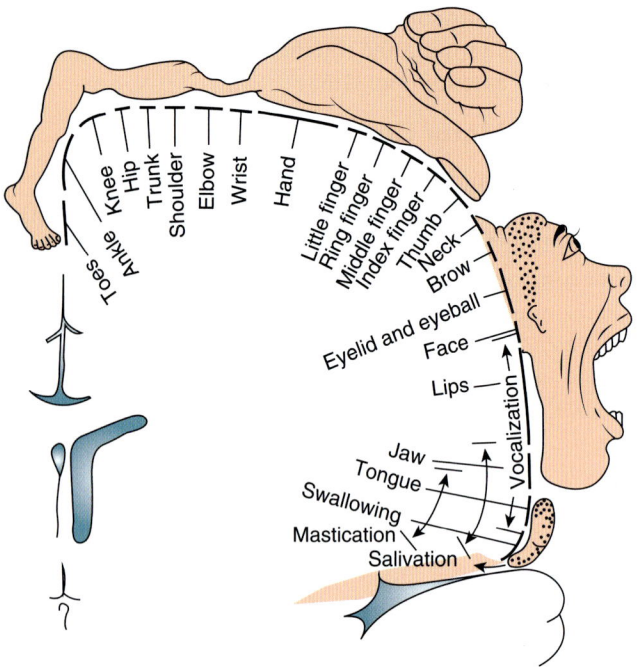

Figure 11.64 Penfield's representation of the different parts of the body in motor area 4. (Redrawn with permission from Guyton AC, Hall JE. *Textbook of Medical Physiology*. 10th ed. W.B. Saunders; 2000:685, Figure 55.2.)

Furthermore, it was demonstrated that the firing rate of the motor neurons determines the motor force generated and the neuronal activity of the primary motor cortex decreases as the direction of motion deviates from the preferred direction of the cortical neuron.[38]

Neuroexperiments showed that the activity of primary motoneurons is correlated not only with the magnitude but also with the direction of the force produced by muscles. Thus, some neurons show progressively less activity as the direction of movement deviates from the neuron's preferred direction.[38]

A single cortical motor neuron influences population of lower motor neurons in the spinal cord.[38] A number of different muscles are directly facilitated peripheral muscle by the discharge of a given upper motor neuron. This peripheral group is referred to as the muscle field of the upper motor neuron. These observations confirmed that single upper motor neuron contact several lower motor pools. Movements rather than individual muscles are encoded by the activity of the upper motor neurons in the cortex.

▶ **Premotor Cortex**[38]

Represented by Brodmann cortical area (Fig. 11.63), the premotor cortex has extensive reciprocal connections with the primary motor cortex. The premotor cortex uses information from other cortical regions to select movements appropriate to the context of the action.

As many as 65% of the lateral premotor cortex have responses that are linked in time to occurrence of movements; as in the primary motor area, many of these cells fire strongly in association with movements made in a specific direction.

The premotor neurons are also particularly involved in selection of movements based on external events.

relatively large and direct pathway from the primary area to the lower motor neurons of the brain stem and spinal cord.

More recent experiments indicate that organized movements rather than individual muscles are represented in the motor map.

A particular movement could be elicited by widely separated sites indicating that neurons' response is linked by local circuits to organize specific movements.

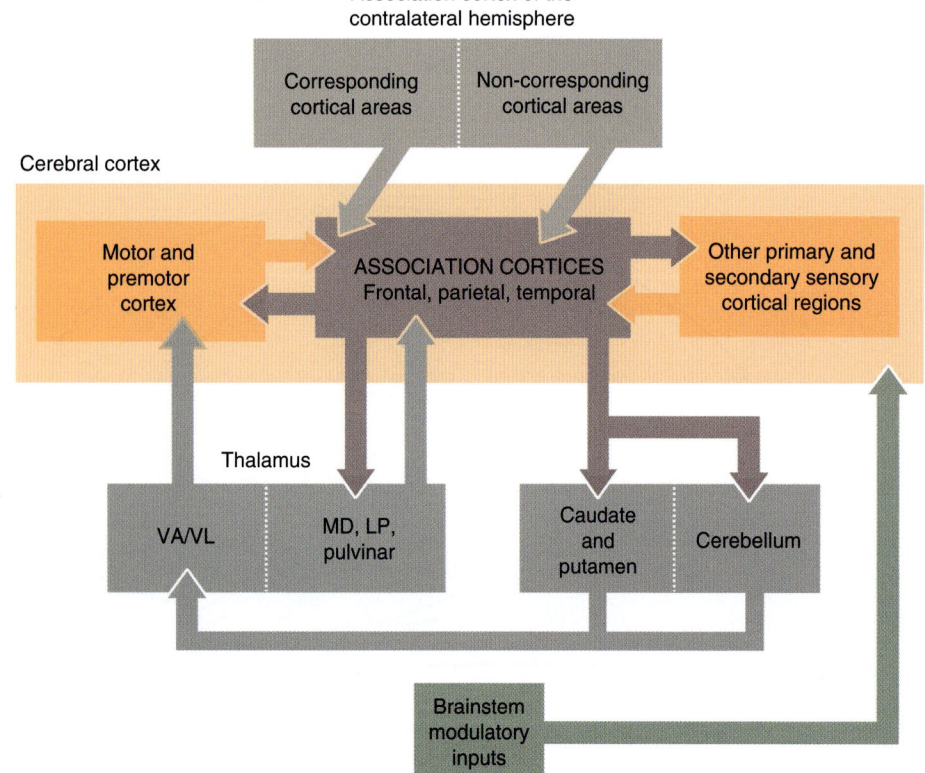

Figure 11.65 Connections of the association cortices. (Redrawn with permission from Purves D, Augustine GJ, Fitzpatrick D, et al, eds. *Neuroscience*. 3rd ed. Sinauer Associates; 2004:618, Figure 25.4, by permission of Oxford University Press.)

The medial premotor cortex mediates the selection of movements. However, this region appears to be specialized for initiating movement specified by inner rather than external cues.

The lateral and medial areas of the premotor cortex are involved in selecting a specific movement or sequence of movements from the repertoire of possible movements.

▶ Output of the Motor and Premotor Cortices

The distal axonal extensions from the motor cortices form two major tracts:

- Corticospinal
- Corticoreticular

The axons of the corticospinal tract pass through the internal capsule, between the basic ganglia and the thalamus. The axonal tract continues through the anterior midbrain, anterior pons, and at the level of the middle medulla the motor pyramidal tract extends a connection with the reticular nucleus tract (Fig. 11.67).

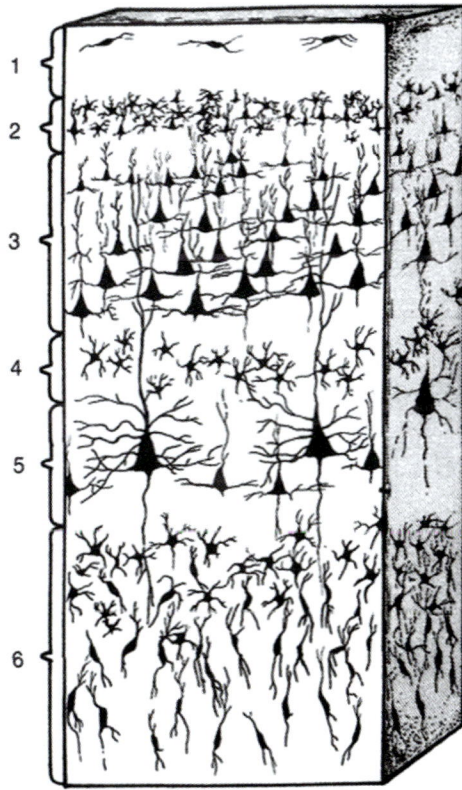

Figure 11.66 Cross section of the primary motor cortex Brodmann 4 with pyramidal cells in layers 3, 5. Cortical histology, as revealed by two staining methods.

Golgi method

1, Molecular layer
2, External granular layer
3, External pyramidal layer
4, Internal granular layer
5, Internal pyramidal layer
6, Multiform layer. (Reproduced with permission from Murray LB, Kiernan JA. *The Human Nervous System: An Anatomical Viewpoint*, 6th ed. Lippincott Williams & Wilkins; 1993:248, Figure 14.2.)

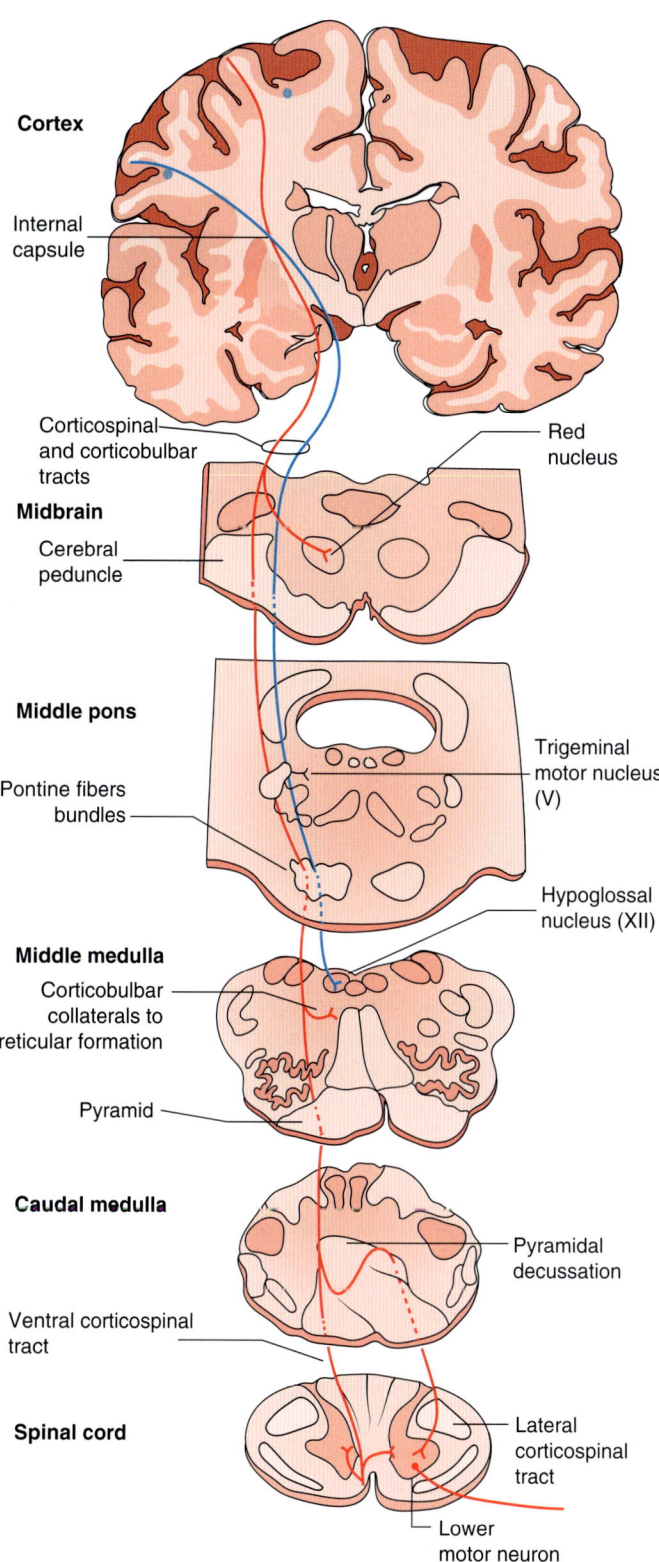

Figure 11.67 The corticospinal and corticobulbar tracts. Neurons in the motor cortex give rise to axons that travel throughout the internal capsule and coalesce on the ventral surface of the midbrain within the cerebral peduncle. These axons continue through the pons and come to lie on the ventral surface of medulla giving rise to the pyramids. Most of these pyramidal fibers cross in the caudal part of the medulla to form the lateral corticospinal tract on the spinal cord. These axons that do not cross form the ventral corticospinal tract. (Redrawn with permission from Purves D, Augustine GJ, Fitzpatrick D, et al, eds. *Neuroscience*. 3rd ed. Sinauer Associates; 2004:403, Figure 16.8, by permission of Oxford University Press.)

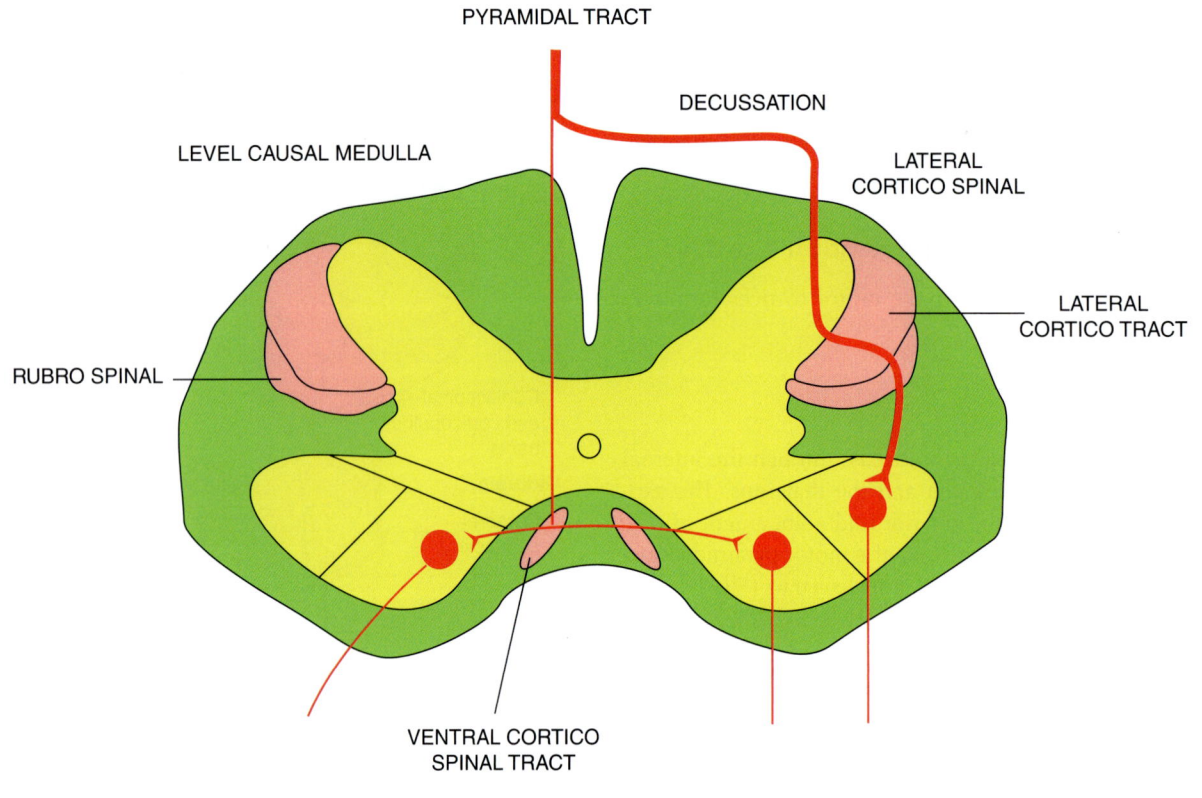

Figure 11.68 Pyramidal tract.

At the level of the medulla the axonal fibers are located anteriorly forming the medullary pyramids.

At the caudal medulla a major directional change occurs. Most of the corticospinal motor axons decussate, and pass to the opposite side forming the lateral corticospinal tract, whereas a smaller axonal group continues the straight tract and forms the ventral corticospinal tract (Fig. 11.67).

The axons of the ventral corticospinal tracts terminate bilaterally on the medial segment of the anterior horn and provide innervation to axial muscles and the proximal muscles.

The axons of the lateral corticospinal tract terminate in the later segment of the anterior horn and the intermediate zone (Fig. 11.68).

Topographically the neurons of the medial horn innervate the proximal and axial muscles, whereas the neurons of the lateral segment of the spinal horn innervate the distal muscles of the extremities (Fig. 11.69).

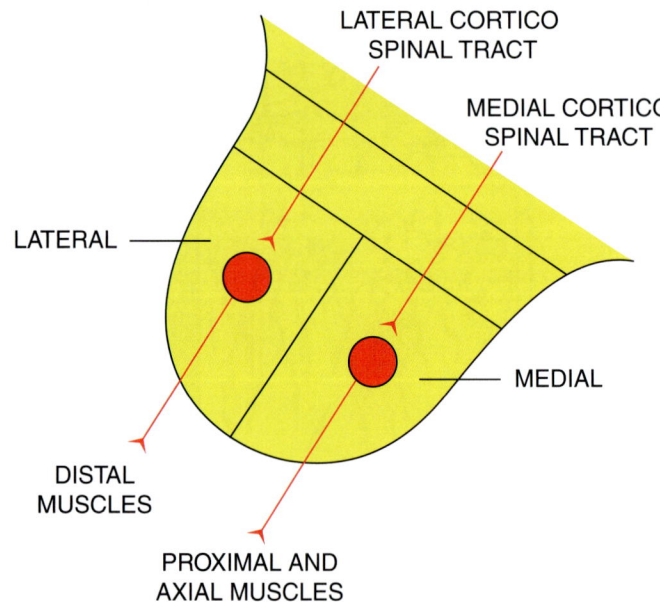

Figure 11.69 Spinal cord ventral horn.

RETICULOSPINAL MOTOR TRACT

Reticular formation is an automated motor tract extending from the brain stem to the spinal cord.

As described in Barr,[5] the reticular formation of the brain stem has a long phylogenetic history. The brains of primitive vertebrates consist in large part of neural tissue that is not well organized as nuclei and tracts; this diffuse arrangement of neurons is said to be "reticular" (forming a network). In the evolution of the mammalian brain, the rostral part developed preferentially, with additions to the thalamus and the appearance of neocortex. Fiber tracts were acquired to connect the spinal cord and the forebrain, and the tracts of necessity traverse the brain stem. Large nuclei, including the red nucleus, substantia nigra, and inferior olivary nucleus, also appeared or increased in size in the mammalian brain stem. The primitive reticular formation did not disappear; on the contrary, it persisted as an important component of the mammalian brain stem in those regions not completely occupied by tracts and nuclei.

The reticular formation is the recipient of data from most of the sensory systems and has efferent connections, direct or indirect, with all levels of the neuraxis. Constituting, in a sense, a central core of the brain, the reticular formation makes a significant contribution to several aspects of brain function, including a role in the arousal-sleep cycle. The reticular system of neurons is integrated into the motor system of the brain and spinal cord, and includes centers that regulate visceral functions. The primitive "reticular" characteristic is retained in the multi neuronal or polysynaptic nature of intrinsic pathways (Barr[5]).

The reticular system controls automatic motor rhythmic processes of respiration and cardiac rhythmic activity.

The peripheral motor integration of reticulospinal tract is as indicated in the motor flow chart of Figure 11.70.

Motor command is initiated by the primary motor and premotor cerebral cortices. The neurocommand is transmitted by the corticospinal neural tract to the α and γ motor neurons distally. Similarly, a neurocommand issued by the same cortical motor centers activates the reticular system targeting the same motor neurons.

▶ Anatomy of the Reticular Formation

At the level of the midbrain, the reticular formation originates as mesencephalic nuclear formations (Figs. 11.71 and 11.72). The bilateral tract continues distally as the caudal pontine and medullary reticular formation. The midbrain bilateral reticular tracts extend distally as cortico-reticulo-spinal tracts (Fig. 11.73).

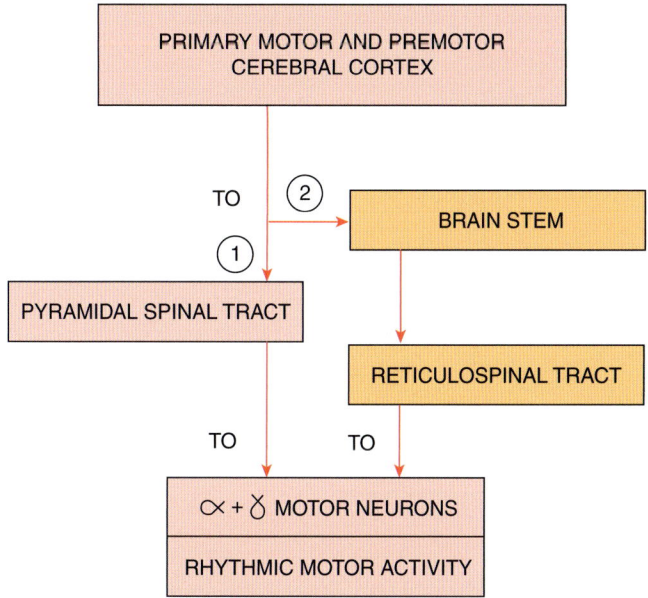

Figure 11.70 Reticulospinal and corticospinal motor tracts.

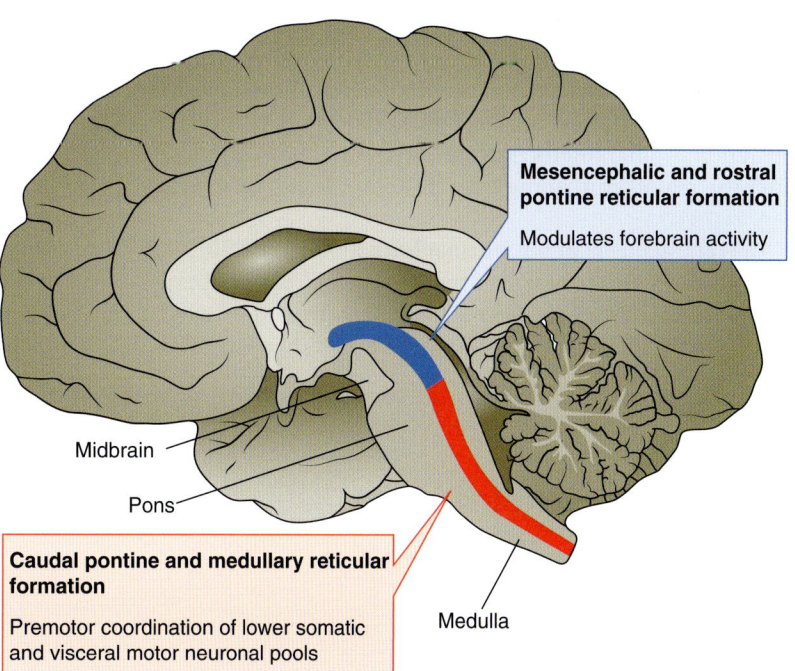

Figure 11.71 Reticular formation in the midbrain lateral view. Mid sagittal views of the brain showing the longitudinal extent of the reticular formation and highlighting the broad functional role performed by neuronal clusters in its rostral (*blue*) and caudal (*red*) sections. (Redrawn with permission from Purves D, Augustine GJ, Fitzpatrick D, et al, eds. *Neuroscience*. 3rd ed. Sinauer Associates; 2004:400, Figure 16.5, by permission of Oxford University Press.)

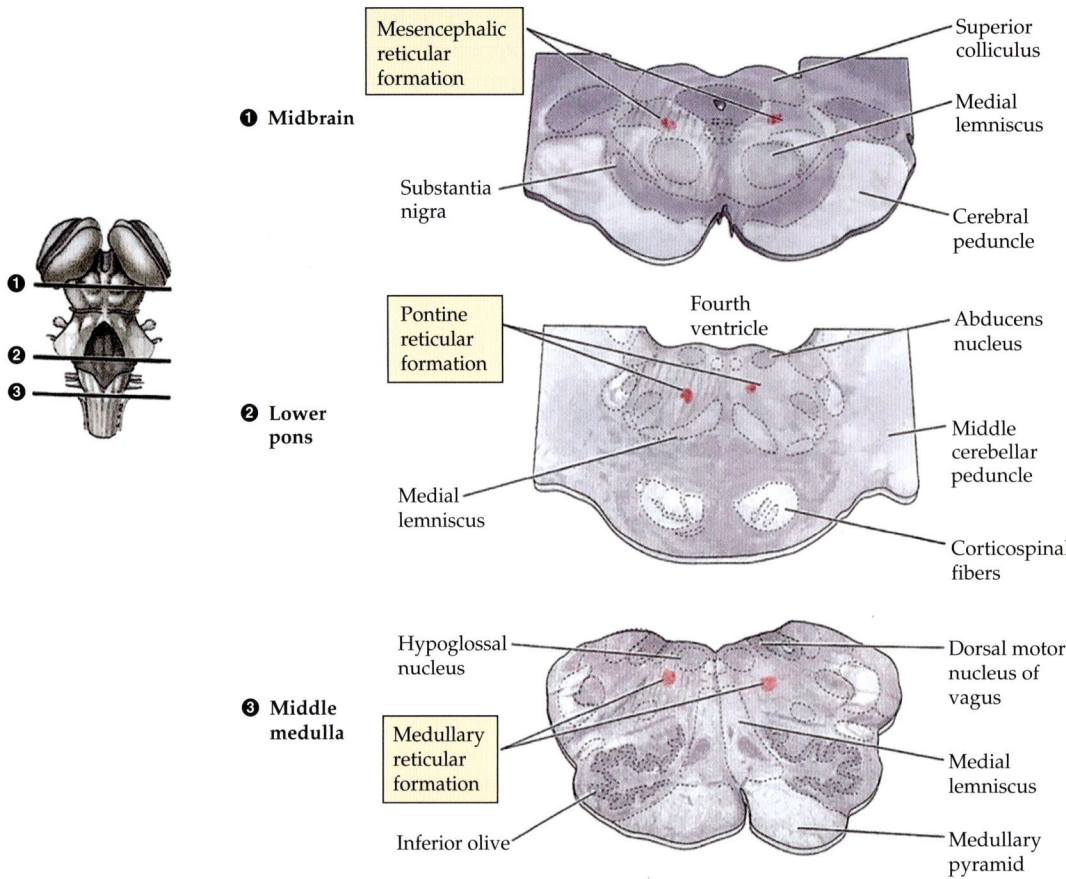

Figure 11.72 Locations of the reticular formation in the midbrain, lower pons, and middle medulla. (Reproduced with permission from Purves D, Augustine GJ, Fitzpatrick D, et al, eds. *Neuroscience*. 3rd ed. Sinauer Associates; 2004:400, Figure 16.4, by permission of Oxford University Press.)

At the level of the spinal cord, the reticular system forms the ventral reticulospinal tract, the ventrolateral reticulospinal tract, and medial reticulospinal tract (Fig. 11.74).

As described by Kierman,[6] many reticular fibers shift from the ventral into the lateral funiculus as they descend. The fibers of pontine and medullary origin do not occupy separate zones of white matter. Reticulospinal axons end bilaterally among spinal interneurons of the ventral horn and a few enter the region containing the cell bodies of motor neurons (Fig. 11.75).

The central nuclei of the reticular formation receive afferents from all the sensory system, from the premotor and supplementary motor areas of the cerebral cortex, from the fastigial nucleus of the vestibulocerebellum. and from other parts of the reticular formation.

Branching has been demonstrated also in the spinal cord so that a single reticulospinal neuronal axon may have terminations in cervical, thoracic, and lumbar segments.

This observation has led to the suggestion that the reticulospinal tracts control coordinated movements of muscles supplied from different segmental levels of the spinal cord, such as those of the upper and lower limbs in walking, running, and swimming.[6]

The functional motor roles of the reticulospinal tract are summarized in Figure 11.76.

The reticulospinal tract is a major modulator of the motor tract in conjunction to the vestibulo-spinal tract.

As we will review in the next section, the reticulospinal tract is the activator of the spinal automation center activating the spinal motor mechanism responsible for locomotion-walking.

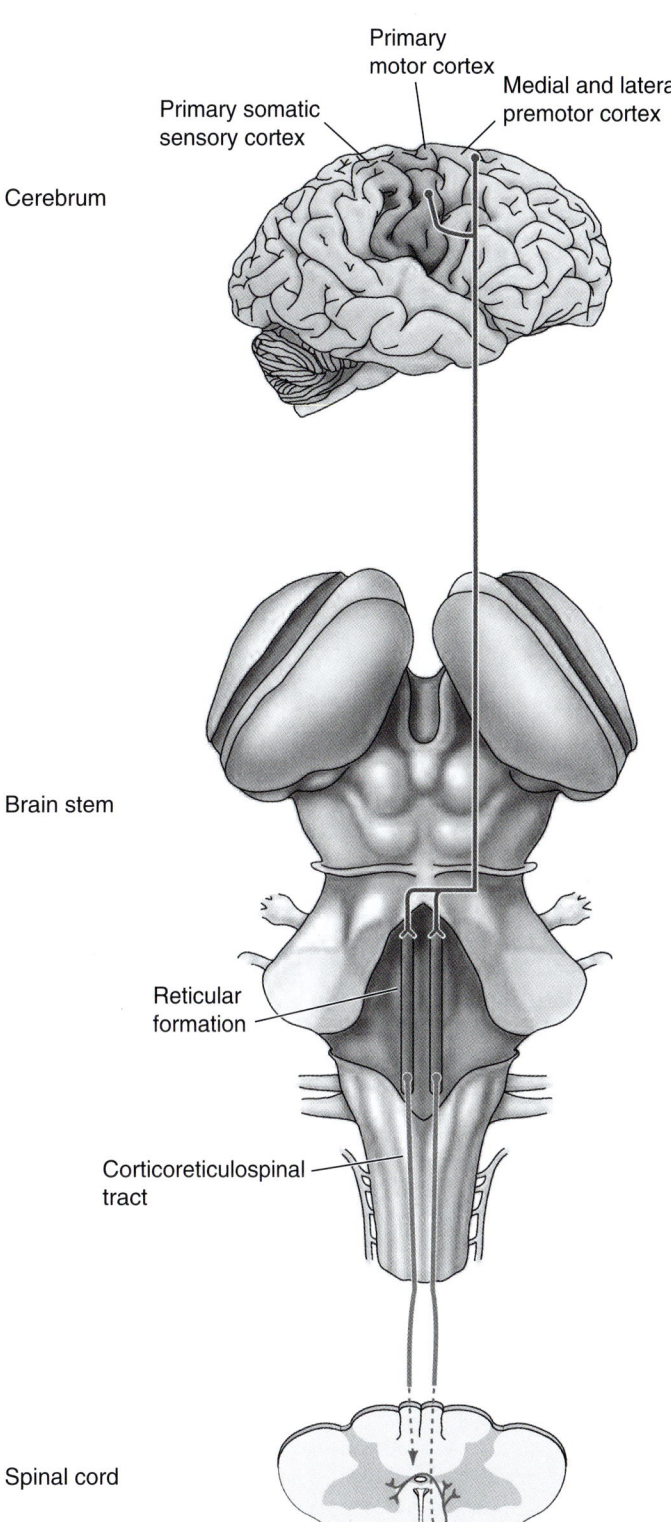

Figure 11.73 **Reticular formation extending as bilateral cortico-reticulo-spinal tracts.** (Reproduced with permission from Purves D, Augustine GJ, Fitzpatrick D, et al, eds. *Neuroscience*. 3rd ed. Sinauer Associates; 2004:396, Figure 16.3, by permission of Oxford University Press.)

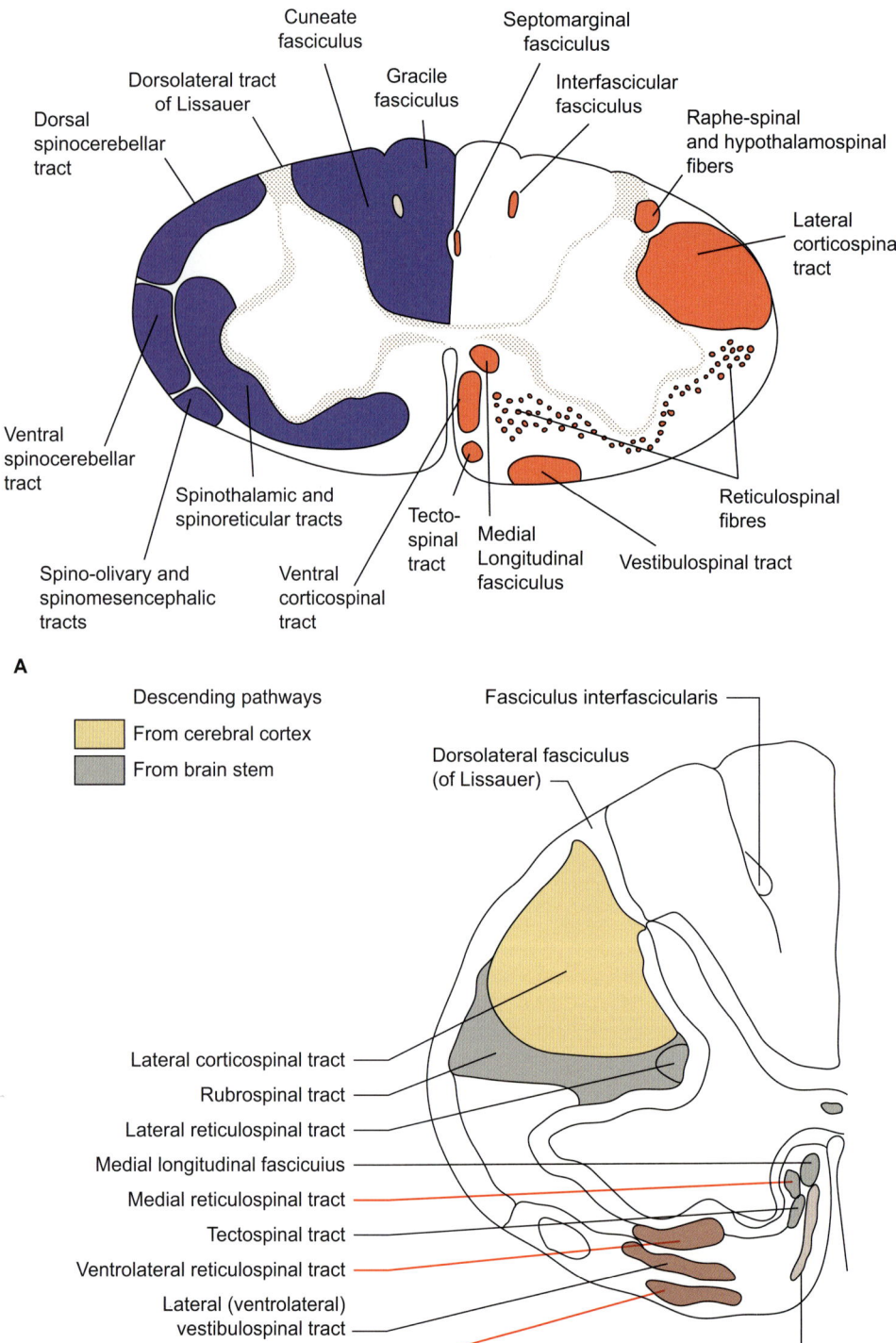

Figure 11.74 (A) Ventral reticulospinal and lateral reticulospinal tracts. (B) Spinal cross section. Spinal descending tracts. (A. Redrawn with permission from Murray LB, Kiernan JA. *The Human Nervous System: An Anatomical Viewpoint*. 6th ed. Lippincott Williams & Wilkins; 1993:75, Figures 5.9.)

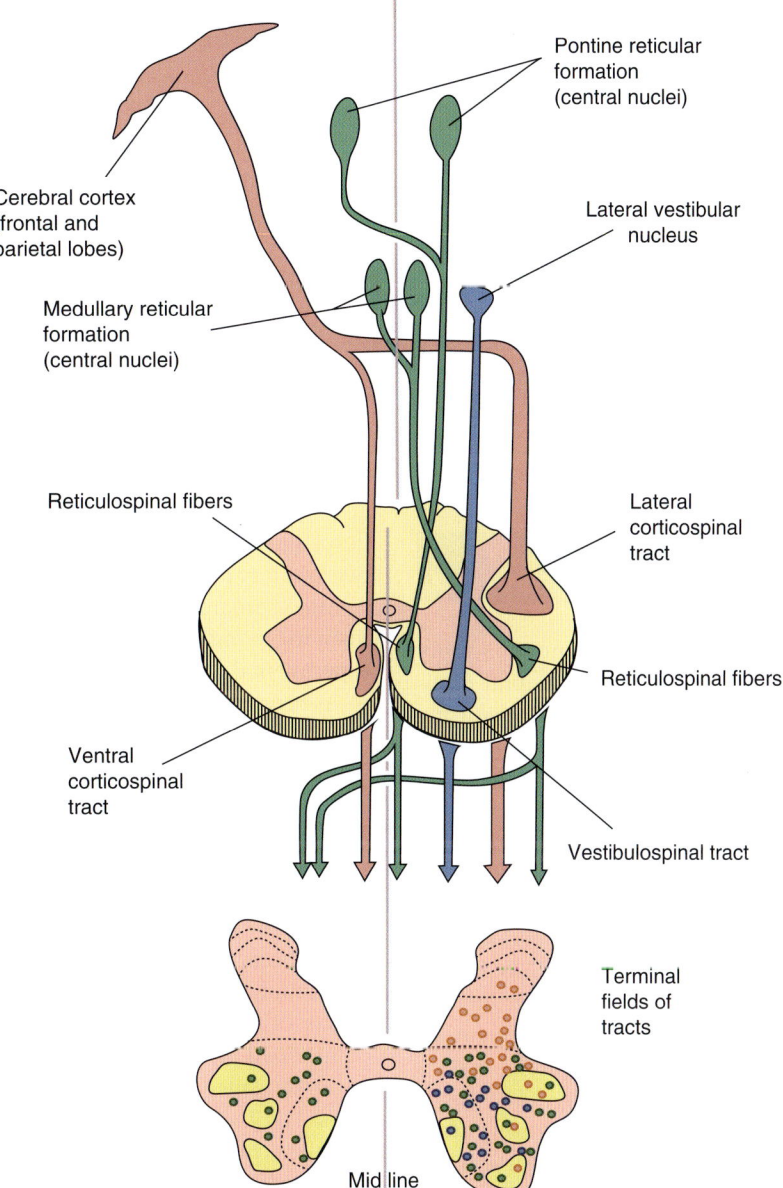

Figure 11.75 **Termination of spinoventral tracts into the anterior horn of gray matter connecting with the motor neurons.** Origins, courses, and terminal distributions of the major descending pathways concerned with the control of movement. The two reticulospinal tracts indicated in green in the diagram represent only part of a larger population of the reticulospinal fibers present through the ventral and ventrolateral funiculus of the spinal *white* matter. Corticospinal projections are *red* and the vestibulospinal tract is *blue*. Columns of cell bodies of spinal motor neurons are indicated in *yellow*. (Redrawn with permission from Murray LB, Kiernan JA. *The Human Nervous System: An Anatomical Viewpoint*. 6th ed. Lippincott Williams & Wilkins; 1993:379, Figure 23.2.)

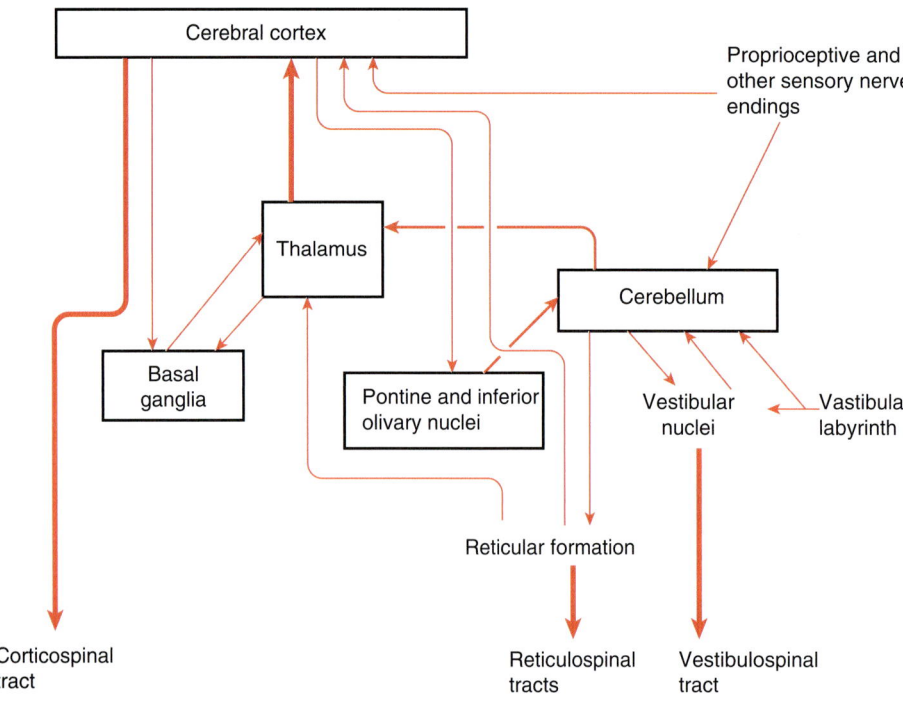

Figure 11.76 **Motor flow chart indicating importance of reticulo-spinal tract.** Drawing shows chain of command from sense organs and from cerebral cortex to motor neurons, with sites at which the activities of corticospinal and reticulospinal and vestibulospinal tracts can be modified by the basal ganglia and cerebellum. (Reproduced with permission from Murray LB, Kiernan JA. *The Human Nervous System: An Anatomical Viewpoint.* 6th ed. Lippincott Williams & Wilkins; 1993:381, Figure 23.3.)

NEURO CONTROL OF LOCOMOTION-WALKING[39,40]

Locomotion-walking is an alternate rhythmic motor activity of the extremities, initiated and terminated by cerebral cortical motor command. Locomotion is controlled automatically at relatively low levels of the central nervous system without intervention of higher centers.[41]

Neuroexperiments conducted mainly on cats provided the basic information for understanding of the neuromechanism of locomotion.

In 1896, Sherrington described his experiments. The transection of the brain stem in a cat between superior and inferior colliculi resulted in decerebrate rigidity. In 1898, Sherrington reported relieving the decerebrate rigidity by transecting the dorsal two roots of the corresponding spinal cord segment. In 1911, Thomas Graham Brown reported on a seminal experiment on a cat.

In the cat experimental model, after the transection of the spinal cord and dorsal spinal root of the distal segment, he recorded rhythmic motor activity in the tibialis anterior muscle and the gastrocnemius muscle (Fig. 11.77).

The unilateral motor activity was generated by the distal segment of the transected spinal cord. Thomas Graham Brown proposed a half-center spinal cord model to explain the alternate flexion-extension contraction.

Enoka[45] has provided a graphic representation of Graham's concept of half-model of the spinal cord (Fig. 11.78A). This model converts continuous input delivered by descending pathways into an alternating burst of action potential that is transmitted to muscle controlling the flexor-extensor rhythm regulated for locomotion. The half-model comprises reciprocal inhibition between neurons that project to motor neurons innervating flexor and extensor muscles and recurrent inhibition of the interneurons that produce reciprocal inhibition (Fig. 11.78A, B).

Major progress in our understanding of the neural mechanism triggering and controlling locomotion occurs with neuroexperimental work performed in the 1960s.

As reported by T. J. Crew,[40] in the mid-1960s a group of Russian scientists, M. L. Shik, F. V. Severin, and G. N. Orlowsky,[42] found that in decerebrate cats tonic electrical stimulation of the remaining brain stem caused animals to walk normally when placed on a treadmill (walking was unrelated to the pattern of electrical stimulation).

Furthermore, the gait of the animal depended on the strength of the stimulation and the treadmill speed. Weak stimulation produced walking, whereas progressively stronger stimulation produced trotting and finally galloping. The region of the brain stem that produced walking is rather circumscribed area of the mesencephalon which Orlowsky and coworker called the mesencephalic locomotion region (MLR) (Figs. 11.79 and 11.80).

As specified by K. G. Pearson and J. E. Gordon[39] the MLR is located in the rostral pons and makes connection with the medial reticular formation (MRF) in the caudal pons. The reticular axons descend in the ventrolateral region of the spinal cord, and signals that activate locomotion and control its speed are transmitted to the spinal cord by glutamatergic neurons with axons that travel in the ventral reticulospinal pathways.

The descending reticular axonal tracts connect at the level of the spinal cord with the neuronal motor network, thus forming the central pattern generator (CPG) (Fig. 11.81).

As described by K. G. Pearson and J. C. Gordon,[43] a CPG is a neuronal network within the central nervous system that is

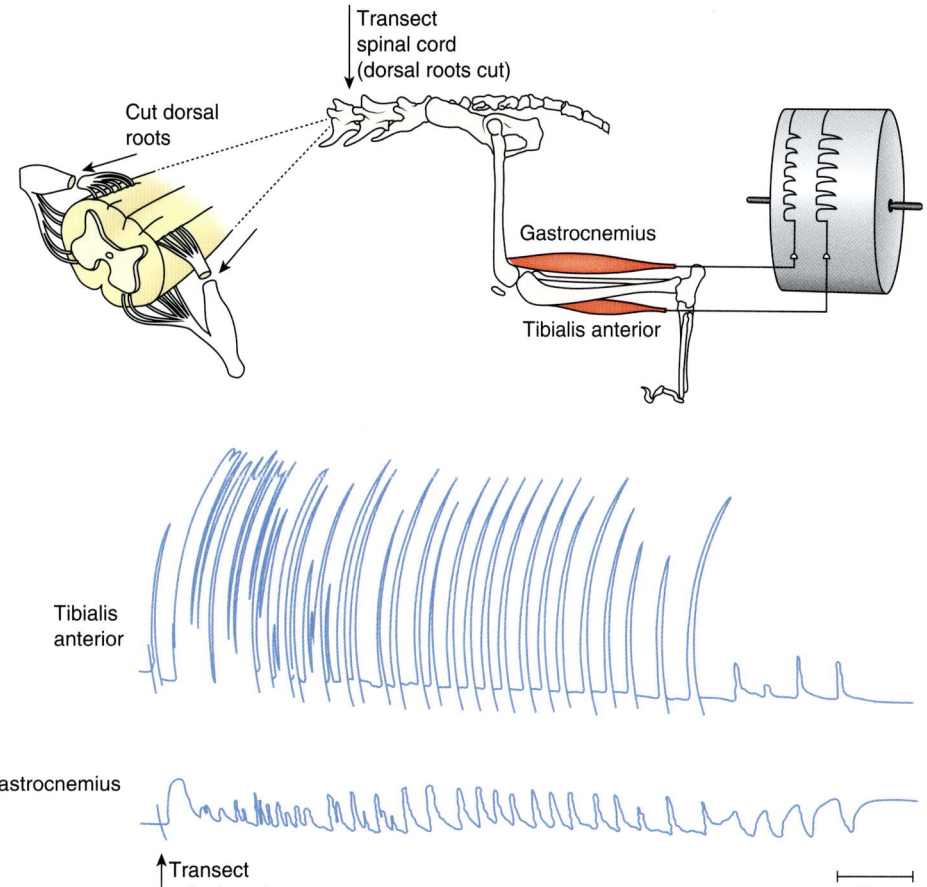

Figure 11.77 **1911 experiments of Thomas Graham Brown on cat.** Lower spinal cord is transected including the distal nerve roots. Spontaneous rhythmic activity is generated in the gastrocnemius and the tibialis anterior. (Redrawn with permission from Pearson KG, Gordon JE. Locomotion. In: Kandel ER, Schwartz JH, Jessell TM, eds. *Principles of Neural Science*. 2nd ed. Elsevier; 1985:817, Figure 36.)

capable of generating a rhythmic pattern of motor activity without phasic sensory input from peripheral receptors.

CPGs have been identified and analyzed in more than 50 rhythmic motor systems including those controlling such diverse behaviors as walking, swimming, feeding, respiration, and flying.[39]

The simplest CPG contain neurons that burst spontaneously. Such endogenous bursters can drive motor neurons and some motor neurons are themselves endogenous bursters. They are also found in the locomotor system. Locomotion, however, is an episodic behavior, so bursters in locomotion systems most are regulated. Two neurons that mutually inhibit each other can oscillate in alternating fashion if each neuron has property of post inhibitory rebound.[39]

As further described by K. G. Pearson and J. C. Gordon[39], compelling evidence for the existence of spinal rhythm-generating networks in humans comes from studies in development. Human infants make rhythmic stepping movements immediately after birth if held up and more over a horizontal surface. This suggests that some of the basic neuronal circuits for locomotion are innate.

A child stands up, in average at 1 year and proceeds to progressive walking naturally. The rhythmic pattern is automatic.

Dominici et al[46] reported on their comprehensive EMG studies on newborn infants, children, adolescents, and adults during their motor activities—spontaneous for newborns—and during walking (Fig. 11.82). The similarity of the EMG pattern indicates that locomotion is an automatic motor activity and inborn.

Basic stepping can occur in infants who lack located central hemispheres (anencephaly); their circuit must be below the brain stem, perhaps entirely within the spinal cord.

The CPG located in the spinal cord determines the automatic rhythmic contractions of flexor and extensor muscle. At present, the CPG represents Thomas Graham Brown's half-center model. The CPG is modulated by the neural input from the muscle and tendon afferents Ia, II, Ib inputs.

Enoka[45] presented a comprehensive diagram integrating the CPG in the spinal cord with the α motor neurons including the interneuronal pathways and the neuroinput from the extensor flexor muscles tendons through the muscle spindle afferents (Ia, II) and the Golgi tendon (Ib) (Fig. 11.83).

Three pathways reinforce the activation of the extensor muscles during the stance phase of walking:

- A monosynaptic excitation from Ia afferents (pathway 1 in Fig. 11.83)
- A disynaptic excitation from Ia and Ib afferents and the CPG to the extensor motor neurons (pathway 3 in Fig. 11.83)
- A polysynaptic excitation of the extensor half-center of the CPG by feedback from Ia and Ib afferents (pathway 4 in Fig. 11.83)

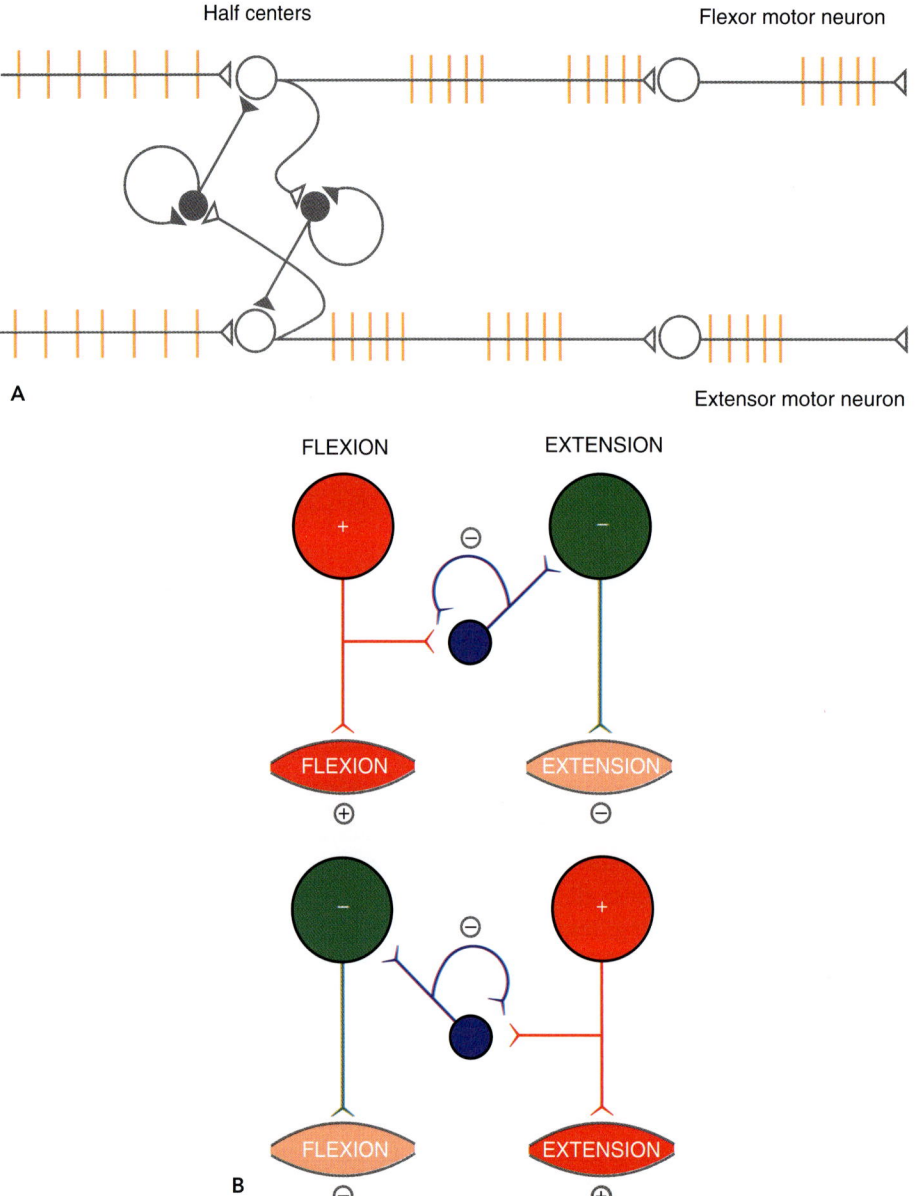

Figure 11.78 **(A) Graham Thomas Brown's half-center model of the spinal cord producing rhythmic activity of flexion and extension in the spinal cord.** The inhibitory neurons are presented as dark circles. **(B)** Diagrammatic representation of Thomas Graham Brown's model of the semi–spinal cord and interposed inhibitory—self-inhibited neuron explaining the alternate activity of the flexion and extensor motor neurons. **(A)** Flexion motor neuron stimulates the flexor muscle and the extension inhibitory interneuron which inhibits the extensor neuron followed by its own inhibition. **(B)** The extensor neuron is activated resulting in activation of the extensor muscle and inhibition of the flexor neuron. This mechanism determines the flexor-extensor rhythmicity in the hemi spinal cord.

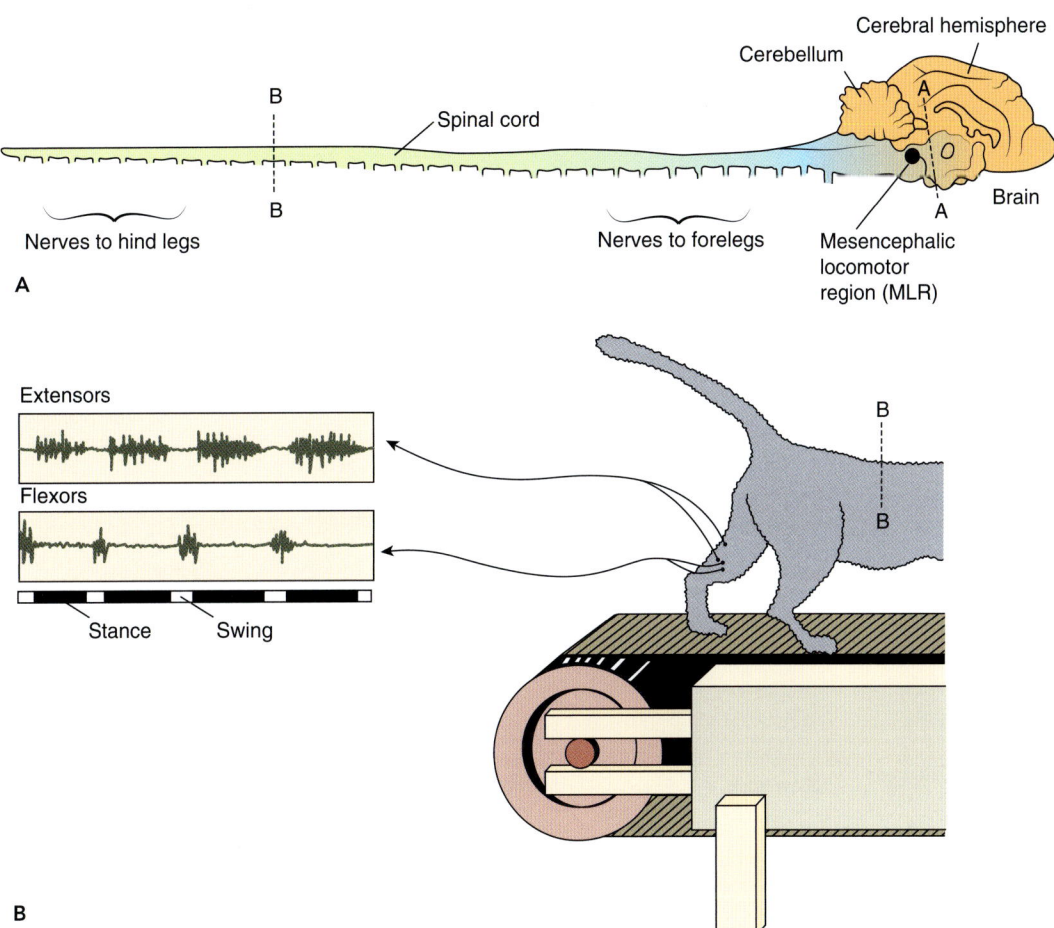

Figure 11.79 Spinal and supraspinal control of locomotion. (A) Spinal cord and lower brain stem of the cat isolated from cerebral hemisphere by transection at point A'-A. Locomotion can be produced in this preparation by electrical stimulation of the mesencephalic locomotor region (filled circle). Transection of the spinal cord at point B'-B isolates the hindlimb segments of the cord. The cats are still able to walk on the treadmill after recovery from surgery. **(B)** Locomotion of a cat transected at B'-B (as in part A) on a treadmill. Reciprocal bursts of electrical activity can be recorded from flexors during the swing phase and from extensors during the stance phase of walking. (**A.** Redrawn with permission from Crew TJ. Descending control of spinal circuits. In: Kandel ER, Schwartz JH, eds. *Principles of Neural Science.* 1st ed. Elsevier North-Holland; 1981:318.)

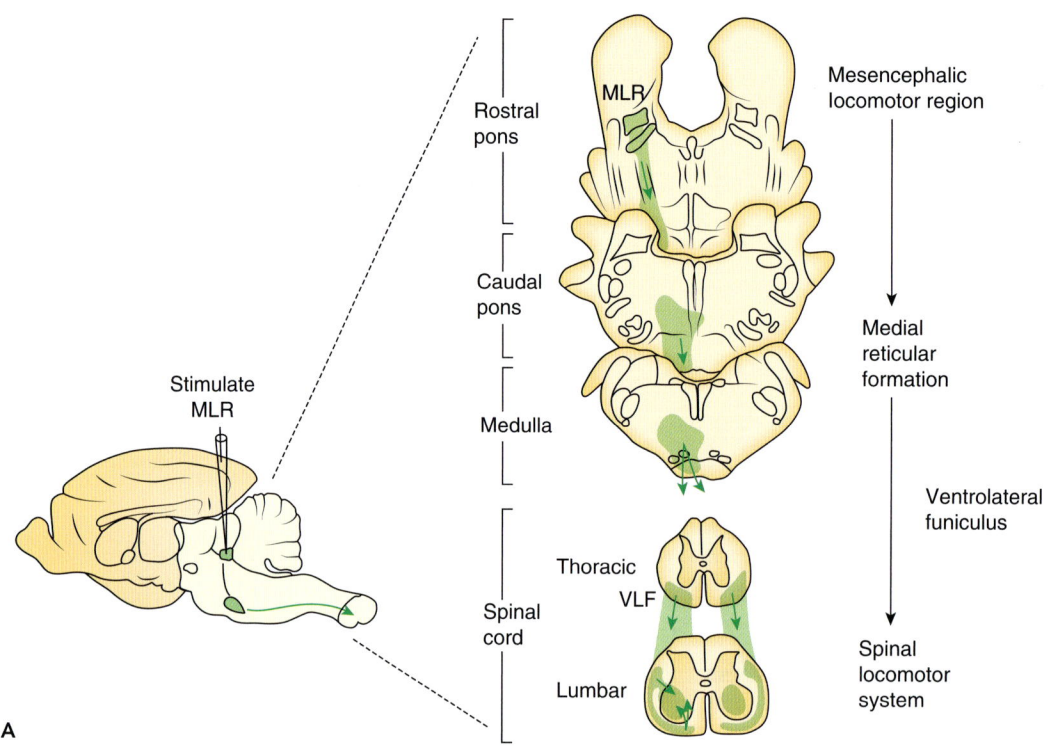

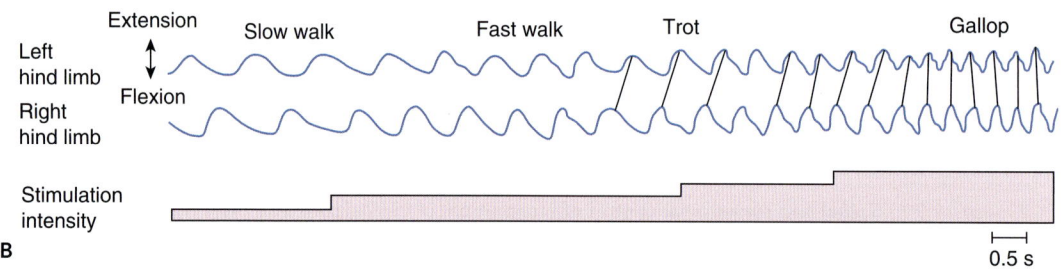

Figure 11.80 **The mesencephalic locomotor region (MLR) modifies stepping patterns. (A)** Stimulation of the MLR excites interneurons in the medial reticular formation whose axons descend in the ventrolateral formation (VLF) to the spinal locomotor system. **(B)** When the strength of stimulation of the mesencephalic locomotor region in a decerebrate cat walking on a treadmill is gradually increased, the gait and rate of stepping change from slow walking to trotting and finally to galloping. As the cat processes from trotting to galloping, the hindlimb shift from alternating to simultaneous flexion and extension. (Redrawn with permission from Pearson KG, Gordon JE. Locomotion. In: Kandel ER, Schwartz JH, Jessell TM, eds. *Principles of Neural Science*. 2nd ed. Elsevier; 1985:827, Figure 36.11.)

Chapter 11: Neuro Control of Stance and Gait   697

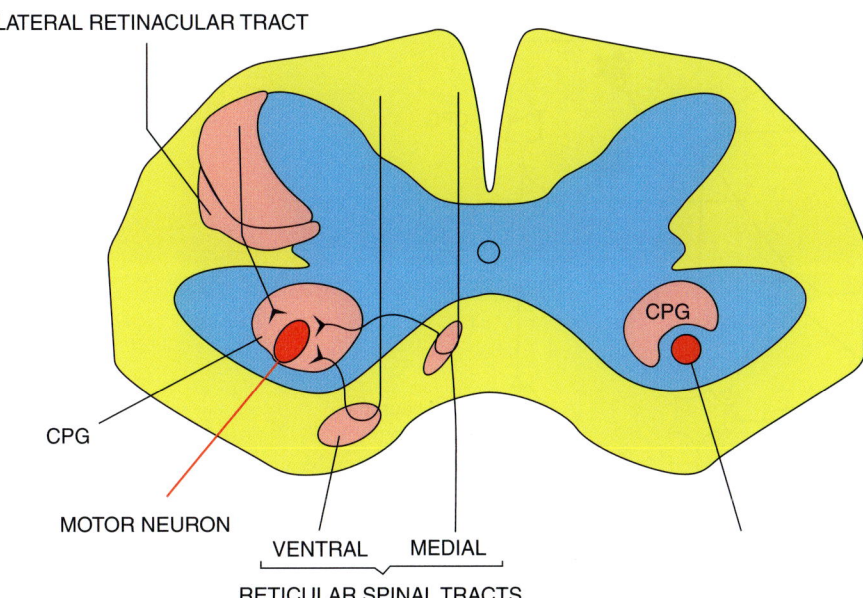

Figure 11.81 Central pattern generator (CPG) is a network that generates a rhythmic pattern of motor activity. It integrates the reticular motor system with cortical motor tract. Contributing to the CPG are the following reticulospinal tracts: lateral reticulospinal tract, anterior reticulospinal tract, and medial reticulospinal tract.

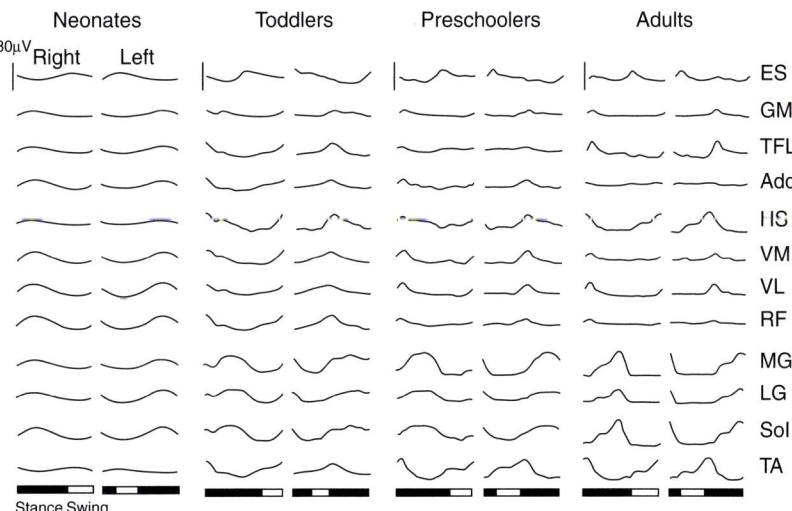

Figure 11.82 EMG pattern during walking or spontaneous in newborn. Recording EMG profiles and derived basic patterns. Ensemble—averaged (across all subjects of each group) EMG profiles during the step cycle, aligned with stance onset in the right leg. Shaded are the experimental data and black traces, the profiles reconstructed as weighted sum of the pattern extracted from the ensemble. ADD, adductor longus; ES, erector spinal; GM, gluteus maximus; HS, hamstrings; LG, gastrocnemius lateralis; MG, gastrocnemius medialis; RF, rector femoralis; SOL, soleus; TA, tibialis anterior; TFF, tensor fascial lata; VL, vastus lateralis; VM, vastus medialis.

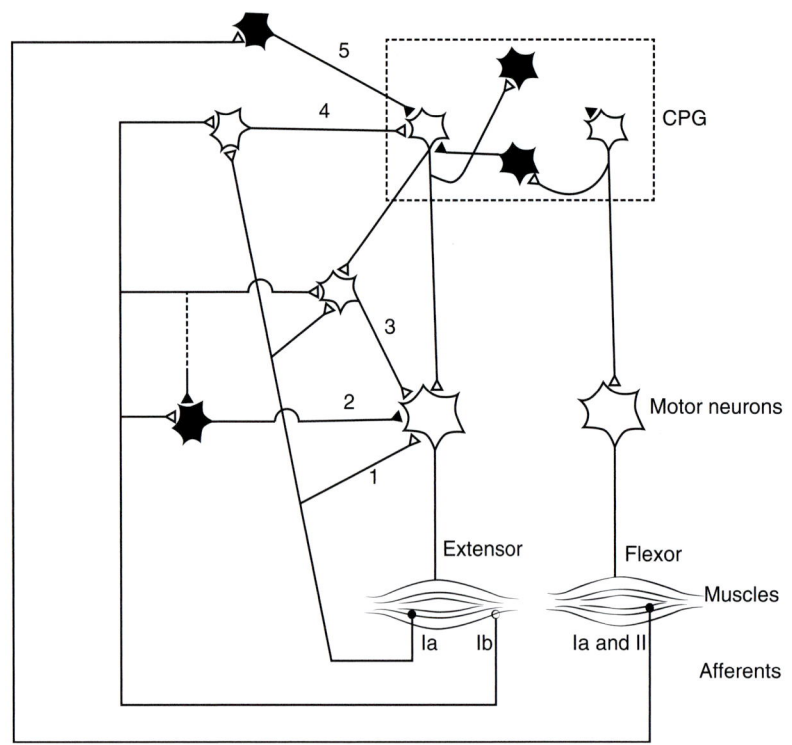

Figure 11.83 Some of the pathways from muscle spindles (Ia and Ib) and tendon organs (IIb) to motor neurons and locomotor CPG. (Redrawn with permission from Enoka RM. *Neuromechanics of Human Movement*. 4th ed. Human Kinetics; 2008:290, Figure 7.27.)

The reinforcement of muscle activity by group I afferents during the locomotor rhythm assists in accommodating changes in the surroundings, such as walking up an incline, walking backward, carrying a heavy load, and walking into a hard wind.

As specified by Enoka, in general, muscle afferents provide input that acts as on-off switch to set the range of motion about the involved joints. In contrast, cutaneous input is involved in determining the placement of the limbs during normal location or after a disturbance.

As indicated in Figure 11.83, during the walking cycle more extensor neuro tracts are involved than flexor neuro tracts. J. Stiefel attributed this discrepancy to the additional extensor activity necessary to project the center of gravity of the body onto the unilateral supporting foot surface.

Descending pathways involved in walking are presented in Figure 11.84.

The spinal cord locomotor complex is stimulated for walking by the MRF located in the caudal portion of the pons. The MRF is stimulated by the mesencephalic locomotor region (MLR) located in the rostral portion of the pons. The cerebellovestibular system is a powerful modulator of the MRF. The motor cortex with the basal ganglia are the modulators of the MRF. The basal ganglia are the only neurocenter with inhibitory, GABAergic influence of the mesencephalic locomotor center.

Supraspinal regulation of stepping can be divided into three functional systems. One activates the spinal locomotor system, initiates walking, and controls the overall speed of locomotion; another refines the motor pattern in response to feedback from the limbs; and the third visually guides limb movement[39,41] (Fig. 11.85).

Glutamatergic pathways are involved in initiating locomotor activity.[39] The cerebellum is a powerful neuromotor modulator. The posterior spinocerebellar tract is strongly activated by numerous leg proprioceptors and provides the cerebellum with detailed information about the mechanical status of the legs. In contrast, neurons in the anterior spinocerebellar tract are activated primarily by neurons in the CPG, providing the cerebellum with information about the status of the spinal locomotor network. The cerebellum compares achieved movements of the legs with intended movements. When the two types of information differ, representing an error, the cerebellum computes corrective signals and sends these to various brain stem nuclei.[39,41]

Humans, contrary to cats and dogs, with complete transection of the spinal cord do not walk. Some functional progress is achieved with specific physiotherapy in partial spinal cord injuries[39] (Fig. 11.86).

At the present we are still using Thomas Graham Brown's (1911) half-center model of the spinal cord to explain the alternate flexor-extensor neuronal activity in one half of the spinal cord.

Walking requires simultaneous alternate flexion-extension motor activity involving both sides of the spinal cord. Such neuronal model of the spinal cord is present in lampreys but still absent in the human.

As described (Fig. 11.87) by Purves[3] such bilateral neuromodulation exists in the spinal cord in the withdrawal reflex when stepping on a sharp object.

Much progress is still needed to explain the bilateral coordinated alternate neural activity of the spinal cord in walking.

Chapter 11: Neuro Control of Stance and Gait 699

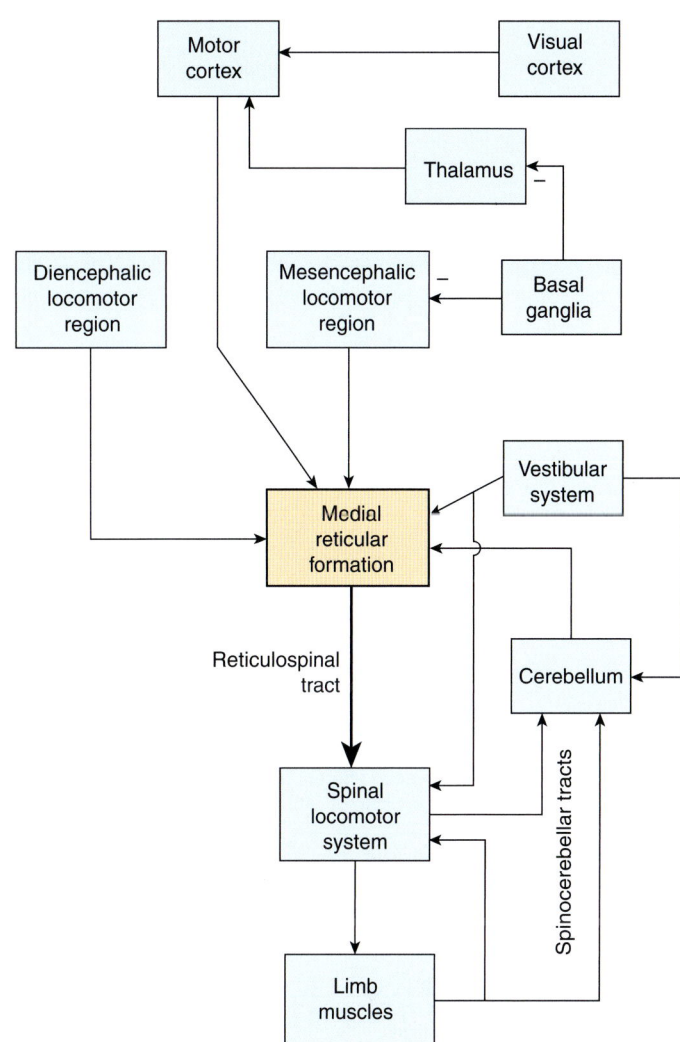

Figure 11.84 **Descending pathways influencing the motor output from the spinal locomotor system that includes the rhythm-producing CPG.** All connections are excitatory, except those within the basal ganglia to the mesencephalic locomotor region. Vestibulocerebellar connection added. (Redrawn with permission from Enoka RM. *Neuromechanics of Human Movement*. 4th ed. Human Kinetics; 2008:293, Figure 7.29.)

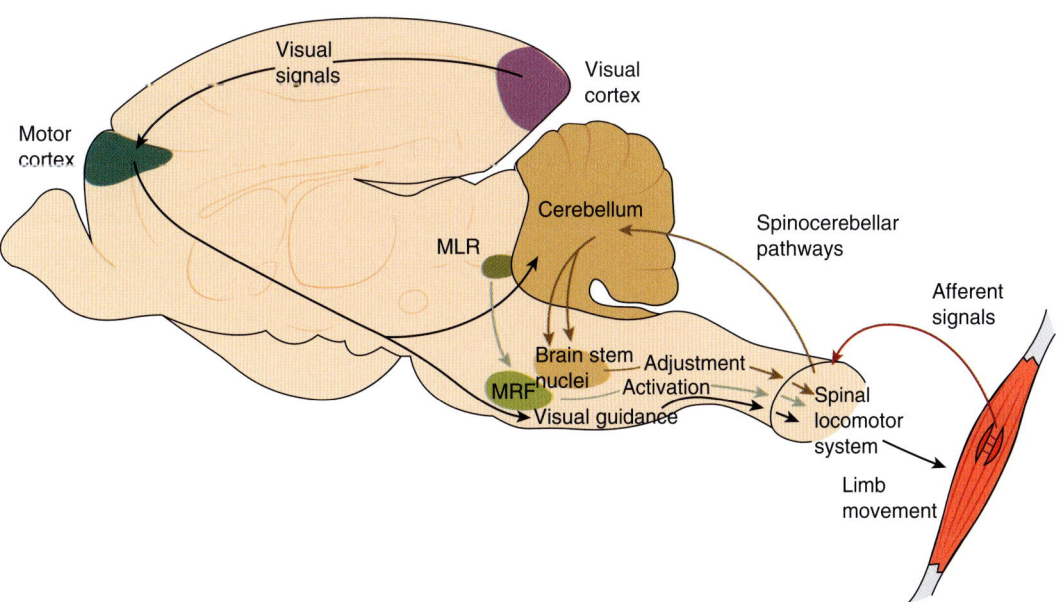

Figure 11.85 **The brain stem and motor cortex control locomotion.** The spinal locomotor system is activated by signals from the mesencephalic locomotor region (MLR) relied by neurons in the medial reticular formation (MRF). The cerebellum receives signals from both peripheral receptors and spinal central pattern generators and adjusts the locomotor pattern through connections in brain stem nuclei. Visual information conveyed to the motor cortex can also modify stepping movement. (Redrawn with permission from Pearson KG, Gordon JE. Locomotion. In: Kandel ER, Schwartz JH, Jessell TM, eds. *Principles of Neural Science*. 2nd ed. Elsevier; 1985:826, Figure 36.10.)

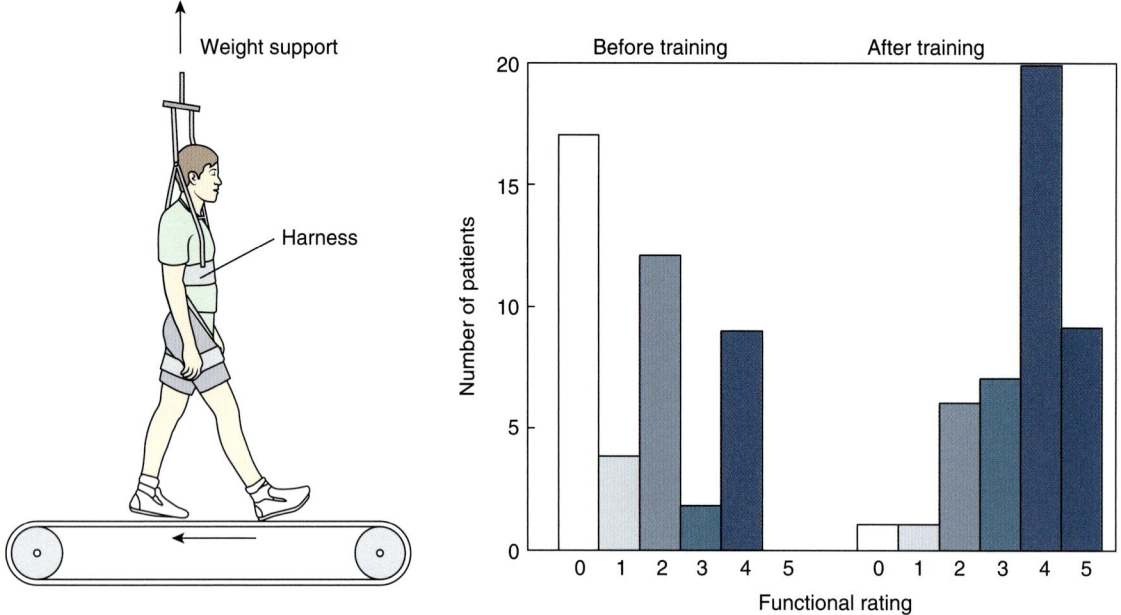

Figure 11.86 Improving walking after partial spinal cord injury. (Redrawn with permission from Pearson KG, Gordon JE. Locomotion. In: Kandel ER, Schwartz JH, Jessell TM, eds. *Principles of Neural Science*. 2nd ed. Elsevier; 1985:832, Figure 38.15.)

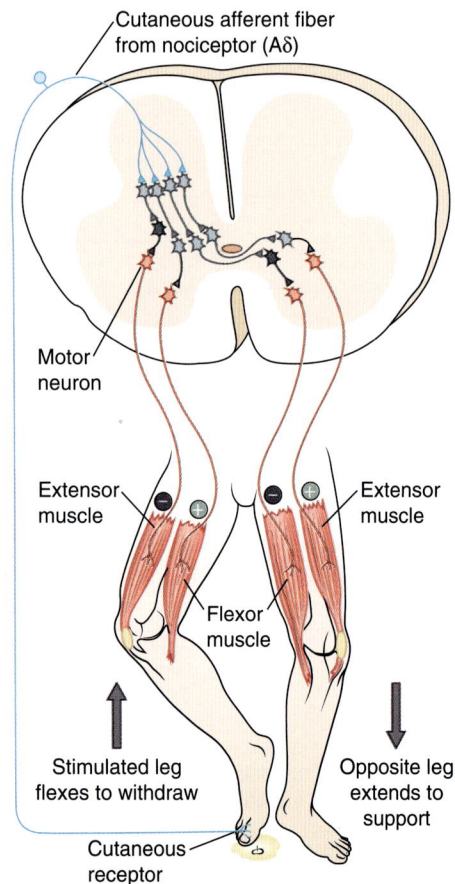

Figure 11.87 Stepping on a sharp object with the right foot results in activation of the right knee flexors and simultaneous extension of the left knee to maintain balance. Such a model of motor coordination at the level of the spinal cord in walking lacks at this time. (Redrawn with permission from Purves D, Augustine GJ, Fitzpatrick D, eds. *Neuroscience*. 3rd ed. Sinauer Associates; 2004, Figure 15.13, by permission of Oxford University Press.)

BIBLIOGRAPHY AND REFERENCES

1. Kandel ER, Schwartz JH. *Principles of Neural Science*. 1st ed. Elsevier North-Holland; 1981.
2. Kandel ER, Schwartz JH, Jessell TM, Siegelbaum SA, Hudspeth AJ. *Principles of Neural Science*. 5th ed. McGraw-Hill Professional; 2012.
3. Purves D, Augustine GJ, Fitzpatrick D, et al, eds. *Neuroscience*. 3rd ed. Sinauer Associates; 2004.
4. Enoka RM. *Neuromechanics of Human Movement*. 5th ed. Human Kinetics; 2015:290, Figure 7.27.
5. Barr ML. *The Human Nervous System*. 2nd ed. Harper & Row Limited; 1974:141.
6. Barr ML, Kiernan JA. *The Human Nervous System: An Anatomical Viewpoint*. 5th ed. Lippincott Williams & Wilkins; 1988:380-381.
7. Guyton AC, Hall JE. *Textbook of Medical Physiology*. 10th ed. W.B. Saunders; 2000.
8. Lower motor neuron circuits and motor control. In: Purves D, Augustine GJ, Fitzpatrick D, et al, eds. *Neuroscience*. 2nd ed. Sinauer Associates; 2001:379-386:chap 16.
9. Muscle spindle. In: Enoka RM, ed. *Neuromechanics of Human Movement*. 4th ed. Human Kinetics; 2008:257-259.
10. Pearson KG, Gordon JE. Golgi tendon organs. In: Kandel ER, Schwartz JH, Jessell TM, eds. *Principles of Neural Science*. 2nd ed. Elsevier; 1985:800.
11. Golgi tendon organs. In: Purves D, Augustine GJ, Fitzpatrick D, et al, eds. *Neuroscience*. 3rd ed. Sinauer Associates; 2004:386.
12. Pearson KG, Gordon J. Spinal reflexes. In: Kandel ER, Schwartz JH, Jessell TM, eds. *Principles of Neural Science*. 4th ed. McGraw-Hill; 2000:13-736.
13. Goldberg ME, Walker MF. The control of gaze. In: Kandel ER, Schwartz JH, Jessell TM, eds. *Principles of Neural Science*. 2nd ed. Elsevier; 1985:895-914.
14. Eye movements and sensory motor integration. In: Purves D, Augustine GJ, Fitzpatrick D, et al, eds. *Neuroscience*. 3rd ed. Sinauer Associates; 2004:453-457.
15. The vestibular system. In: Purves D, Augustine GJ, Fitzpatrick D, et al, eds. *Neuroscience*. 3rd ed. Sinauer Associates; 2004:315-334.
16. Kelly JP. The vestibular system. In: Kandel ER, Schwartz JH, Jessell TM, eds. *Principles of Neural Science*. 2nd ed. Elsevier; 1985:406-418.
17. Goldberg ME, Hudspeth AJ. The vestibular system. In: Kandel ER, Schwartz JH, Jessell TM, eds. *Principles of Neural Science*. 2nd ed. Elsevier; 1985:918-932.

18. Anatomy of the crista ampullaries. In: Purves D, Augustine GJ, Fitzpatrick D, et al, eds. *Neuroscience*. 3rd ed. Sinauer Associates; 2004:325, Figure 13.3A.
19. Kelly JP. Vestibular system. In: Kandel ER, Schwartz JH, Jessell TM, eds. *Principles of Neural Science*. 2nd ed. Elsevier; 1985:410, Figure 3.
20. The vestibular system. In: Purves D, Augustine GJ, Fitzpatrick D, et al, eds. *Neuroscience*. 3rd ed. Sinauer Associates; 2004:317-322, Figures 13.2 and 13.4.
21. The vestibular system. In: Purves D, Augustine GJ, Fitzpatrick D, et al, eds. *Neuroscience*. 3rd ed. Sinauer Associates; 2004:322, Figure 13.5.
22. Modulation of movement by the cerebellum. In: Purves D, Augustine GJ, Fitzpatrick D, et al, eds. *Neuroscience*. 3rd ed. Sinauer Associates; 2004:435, 449.
23. Ghez G, Fahn S. The cerebellum. In: Kandel ER, Schwartz JH. *Principles of Neural Science*. 1st ed. Elsevier North-Holland; 1981:23-34.
24. Lisberg SG, Thach WT. The cerebellum. In: Kandel ER, Schwartz JH, Jessell TM, eds. *Principles of Neural Science*. 2nd ed. Elsevier; 1985:960-979.
25. Modulation of movement by the cerebellum. In: Purves D, Augustine GJ, Fitzpatrick D, et al, eds. *Neuroscience*. 3rd ed. Sinauer Associates; 2004:439, 440.
26. Modulation of movement by the cerebellum. In: Purves D, Augustine GJ, Fitzpatrick D, et al, eds. *Neuroscience*. 3rd ed. Sinauer Associates; 2004:437.
27. Modulation of movement by the cerebellum. In: Purves D, Augustine GJ, Fitzpatrick D, et al, eds. *Neuroscience*. 3rd ed. Sinauer Associates; 2004:437-438.
28. Lisberg SG, Thach WT. The cerebellar cortex. In: Kandel ER, Schwartz JH, Jessell TM, eds. *Principles of Neural Science*. 2nd ed. Elsevier; 1985:968, Figure 42.4.
29. Circuits in cerebellum. In: Purves D, Augustine GJ, Fitzpatrick D, et al, eds. *Neuroscience*. 3rd ed. Sinauer Associates; 2004:441-443.
30. Lisberg SG, Thach WT. The cerebellum spino-cerebellar tract. In: Kandel ER, Schwartz JH, Jessell TM, eds. *Principles of Neural Science*. 2nd ed. Elsevier; 1985:970.
31. Upper motor control of the brain stem. In: Purves D, Augustine GJ, Fitzpatrick D, et al, eds. *Neuroscience*. 3rd ed. Sinauer Associates; 2004:393-397.
32. Modulation of movement by the basal ganglia. In: Purves D, Augustine GJ, Fitzpatric D, et al, eds. *Neuroscience*. 3rd ed. Sinauer Associates; 2004:417-432.
33. Wichman T, DeLong MR. The basal ganglia. In: Kandel ER, Schwartz JH, Jessell TM, eds. *Principles of Neural Science*. 2nd ed. Elsevier; 1985:982-997.
34. Upper motor control of the brain and spinal cord. In: Purves D, Augustine GJ, Fitzpatrick D, et al, eds. *Neuroscience*. 3rd ed. Sinauer Associates; 2004:392-415.
35. The association cortices. In: Purves D, Augustine GJ, Fitzpatrick D, et al, eds. *Neuroscience*. 3rd ed. Sinauer Associates; 2004:613-636.
36. Kalaska J, Rizzolatti G. Voluntary movement: the primary motor cortex. In: Kandel ER, Schwartz JH, Jessell TM, eds. *Principles of Neural Science*. 2nd ed. Elsevier; 1985:838-862.
37. Kalaska J, Rizzolatti G. Voluntary movement: the parietal and premotor cortex. In: Kandel ER, Schwartz JH, Jessell TM, eds. *Principles of Neural Science*. 2nd ed. Elsevier; 1985:866-891.
38. The premotor cortex. In: Purves D, Augustine GJ, Fitzpatrick D, et al, eds. *Neuroscience*. 3rd ed. Sinauer Associates; 2004:405-440.
39. Pearson KG, Gordon JE. Locomotion. In: Kandel ER, Schwartz JH, Jessell TM, eds. *Principles of Neural Science*. 2nd ed. Elsevier; 1985:812-833.
40. Carew TJ. Descending control of spinal cord. In: Kandel ER, Schwartz JH, eds. *Principles of Neural Science*. 1st ed. Elsevier North-Holland; 1981:313 320.
41. Pearson KG, Gordon J. Spinal reflexes. In: Kandel ER, Schwartz JH, Jessell TM, eds. *Principles of Neural Science*. 4th ed. McGraw-Hill; 2000:812.
42. Shik ML, Severin FV, Orlovskiĭ GN. Upravlenie khodʹboĭ i begom posredstvom elektricheskoĭ stimulatsii srednego mozga [Control of walking and running by means of electric stimulation of the midbrain]. *Biofizika*. 1966;11(4):659-666.
43. Pearson KG, Gordon JE. Locomotion. In: Kandel ER, Schwartz JH, Jessell TM, eds. *Principles of Neural Science*. 2nd ed. Elsevier; 1985:819.
44. Pearson KG, Gordon JE. Locomotion. In: Kandel ER, Schwartz JH, Jessell TM, eds. *Principles of Neural Science*. 2nd ed. Elsevier; 1985:829-831.
45. Locomotion. In: Enoka RM, ed. *Neuromechanics of Human Movement*. 4th ed. Human Kinetics; 2008:285-294.
46. Dominici N, Ivanenko YP, Cappellini G, et al. Locomotor primitives in newborn babies and their development. *Science*. 2011;334(6058):997-999.
47. Pearson KG, Gordon JE. Locomotion. In: Kandel ER, Schwartz JH, Jessell TM, eds. *Principles of Neural Science*. 2nd ed. Elsevier; 1985:821.
48. Kelly JP. The vestibular system. In: Kandel ER, Schwartz JH, Jessell TM, eds. *Principles of Neural Science*. 2nd ed. Elsevier; 1985:415.

Angiosomes of the Calf, Ankle, and Foot: Anatomy, Physiology, and Implications

Gregory A. Dumanian

It is an extremely useful concept to think of the body as a set of interconnected angiosomes. The term describes a unit of skin and underlying tissues (including fat, fascia, muscle, and bone) fed by a source artery and drained by a venous plexus. It is a valuable concept for surgeons because, despite some variability between individuals, there are distinctive patterns found in the human body. For the foot surgeon making incisions and raising skin flaps, the most relevant aspect of this concept is the physiology of how angiosomes react to injury with perturbed blood flow and possible necrosis of tissue. Understanding angiosome patterns of the leg and foot is critical for reconstructive surgeons who use them as a roadmap to increase dependability of tissue rearrangement and flap reconstruction.[1] For orthopedics, studies have shown that obeying the angiosome principle leads to improved wound healing rates and reduced amputation rates.[2,3] In vascular surgery, improvement in angiosome blood flow as picked up by single-photon emission computed tomography (SPECT)/CT has demonstrated freedom from amputation when the area of a foot wound demonstrates high response after revascularization.[4] Revascularization now can be minimally invasive, with targeting of angiosomes of the foot that are most in need of improved flow.[5]

This chapter focuses on the anatomy and physiology of the described angiosomes of the calf, ankle, and foot—using examples of flap elevation and flap reconstruction will be used to illustrate these concepts.

PHYSIOLOGY OF ANGIOSOMES AND CHOKE VESSELS

Taylor and Palmer first introduced the term "angiosome" over 2 decades ago in an elegant radiographic study on cadavers.[6] Since that time, a catalog of angiosomes throughout the human body has been developed, including detailed anatomic studies of angiosomes of the leg, foot, and ankle.[7-9] The angiosome is not simply defined by the blood vessel itself but, rather, the entire block of tissue supplied by its arborizations, which are in turn linked with the distal tributaries of neighboring angiosomes via choke vessels (Fig. 12.1). Choke vessels are small blood vessels that exist between choke vessels take time (days to weeks) to dilate and may not be able to sustain a neighboring angiosome in the face of acute vessel occlusion.

Through clinical experience, certain circumstances cause choke vessels to become more or less able to dilate and to support an adjacent vascular territory. Age is certainly a factor. For example, in the hand, there are two angiosomes based on the radial and ulnar arteries. In a large series of hands evaluated for blood flow using Allen's test, there was a significantly decreased ability of one blood vessel to perfuse the entire hand through the choke system with increasing age.[10] Tobacco smoke is another factor. Smoking impairs dilation of choke vessels[11]; this is why skin flap elevation should be minimized in patients that smoke tobacco.

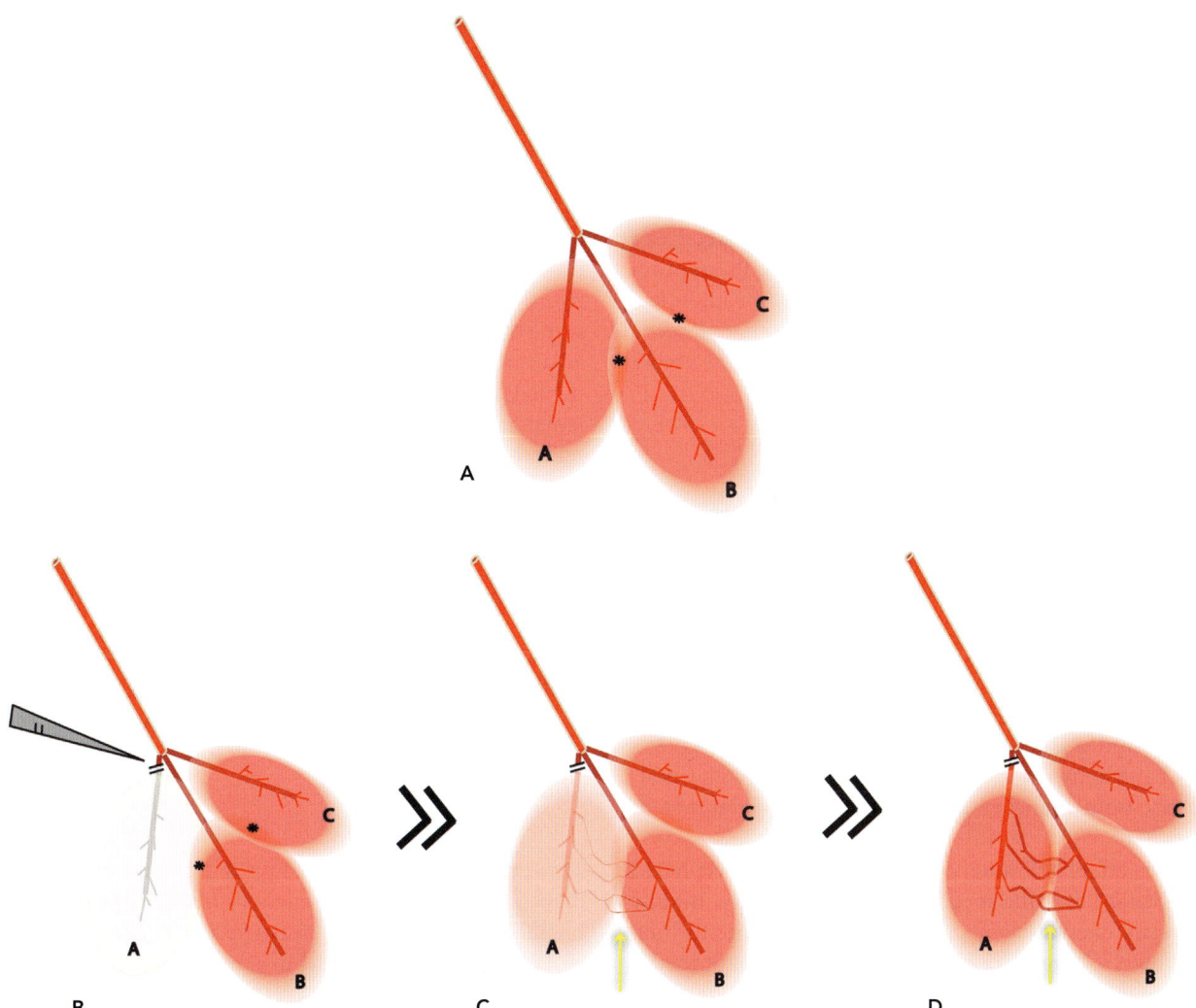

Figure 12.1 **(A)** Schematic of three angiosomes, interconnected by choke vessels (indicated with asterisk). **(B)** With damage to the source vessel, angiosome A becomes ischemic. **(C)** Choke vessels between angiosomes A and B open and some perfusion is reestablished to angiosome A. **(D)** With time, choke vessels dilate and normal perfusion is reestablished. Angiosome A now depends entirely on flow through angiosome B. Asterisk denotes a single angiosome supplied by a feeder vessel. A double hash line implies a division of the blood vessel supplying the angiosome.

SPECIFIC ANGIOSOMES OF THE CALF, ANKLE, AND FOOT

▶ Angiosomes of the Calf

As would be expected, the angiosomes of the leg, ankle, and foot mirror the named blood vessels contained within. The lower leg has five angiosome territories: popliteal, sural, anterior tibial, posterior tibial, and peroneal.[12] There are several clinically relevant details to highlight regarding calf angiosomes.

The Sural Angiosome in the Diabetic Patient

The medial and lateral sural arteries feed the medial and lateral gastrocnemius muscles and the overlying calf skin. The sural arteries originate from the popliteal artery, proximal to the characteristic level of injury from diabetes, and are typically patent despite tibioperoneal vascular disease in diabetics. In contrast, although the soleus receives some blood supply from the popliteal artery, the dominant supply comes from the peroneal and posterior tibial arteries, which are commonly diseased in diabetics. Therefore, the standard below-knee amputation is a transfer of the intact sural angiosome (including the medial and lateral gastrocnemius muscles and overlying skin) to cover the tibia and fibula after osteotomy. This is a clear example of how the knowledge of angiosomes can directly impact surgical outcomes.

The Peroneal Angiosome and Free Tissue Transfer

The peroneal angiosome can transfer the fibula, a swath of skin centered over and posterior to the fibula, and the posterior calf muscles such as the soleus and the flexor hallucis longus. This angiosome is quite well described and is the basis for the free fibula flap.

The Anterior Tibial and Posterior Tibial Angiosomes

The anterior tibial artery supplies the extensor muscles, a portion of the skin covering the tibia, and the anterolateral calf skin toward but not including the skin overlying the septum between the anterior and lateral compartments of the lower leg. The posterior tibial artery gives rise to a medial calf angiosome that supplies the tibia, deep flexor musculature, and overlying medial leg skin.

▶ Angiosomes of the Ankle

The anterior tibial artery is the primary vascular supply of the ankle although the peroneal and posterior tibial systems provide supplementary blood flow to the area.

The Anterior Tibial and Posterior Tibial Angiosomes of the Distal Tibia and Medial Ankle

The major blood vessel to the distal tibia and medial ankle is the medial metaphyseal artery and the anterior medial malleolar artery, both branches off of the anterior tibial system (Fig. 12.2).[13]

Branching off of the anterior tibial artery 3 cm cephalad to the tibiotalar joint, the medial metaphyseal artery initially travels directly laterally across the distal tibia, before turning 90° to follow the long axis of the tibia to supply the tibiotalar joint. The anterior medial malleolar artery branches off of the anterior tibial artery about at the level of the tibiotalar joint, courses medially underneath the tibialis anterior tendon, and divides into superficial and deep branches. The deep branch anastomoses with the medial metaphyseal artery, whereas the superficial branch supplies the medial malleolar skin. A less significant contribution to the medial malleolar blood flow is from the posterior medial malleolar artery off of the posterior tibial artery. The medial malleolar blood flow system illustrates three important points about angiosomes. First, there is significant variability between individuals and even between the two sides of the same individual. Second, the larger an angiosome becomes during embryonic development, the smaller the adjacent system will be (ie, the anterior medial malleolar and medial metaphyseal angiosomes vs the posterior medial malleolar angiosome). Finally, and perhaps most importantly, the human body is built with overcapacity and redundancy of its systems, as evidenced by:

- The existence of choke vessels (described previously) between the two vessel territories that can open, dilate, and allow the unimpeded flow of blood from one system to the other
- The presence of an alternate source vessel (the posterior medial malleolar artery in this example) that is capable, albeit not as effectively, of supplying the same area in the event of interruption of flow to the anterior tibial system

The Anterior Tibial and Peroneal Angiosomes of the Lateral Ankle

The lateral malleolus is supplied by the anterior lateral malleolar artery off of the anterior tibial artery and the posterior lateral branch of the peroneal artery. The anterior lateral malleolar artery originates within 7 mm either proximal or distal to the tibiotalar joint (average, 2 mm proximal) and travels on the surface of the tibia deep to the tendons. It subsequently

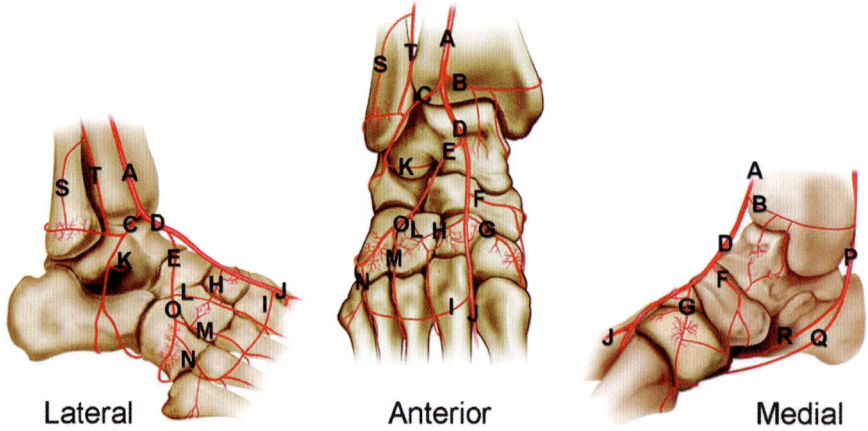

Figure 12.2 Diagram of the blood vessels of the foot and ankle. *A*, anterior tibial artery; *B*, anterior medial malleolar artery; *C*, anterior lateral malleolar artery; *D*, dorsalis pedis artery; *E*, proximal lateral tarsal artery; *F*, proximal medial tarsal artery; *G*, distal medial tarsal artery; *H*, distal lateral tarsal artery; *I*, arcuate artery; *J*, first dorsal metatarsal artery; *K*, artery of the sinus tarsi; *L*, longitudinal branch to second intermetatarsal space; *M*, longitudinal brand to third intermetatarsal space; *N*, longitudinal branch to fourth intermetatarsal space; *O*, transverse pedicle branch; *P*, posterior tibial artery; *Q*, medial plantar artery; *R*, lateral plantar artery; *S*, fibular metaphyseal artery; *T*, perforating peroneal artery. (From Gilbert BJ, Horst F, Nunley JA. Potential donor rotational bone grafts using vascular territories in the foot and ankle. *J Bone Joint Surg.* 2004;86-A:1857-1873. Used with permission.)

bifurcates, sending a transverse branch to anastomose with the perforating branch of the peroneal artery and a descending vertical branch that anastomoses with the branch to the sinus tarsi. The peroneal artery provides a redundancy of blood flow directly to the lateral malleolus through the fibular metaphyseal artery.

A patient with arthrogryposis with a nonhealing tibial fracture illustrates the anterior tibial angiosome. An arteriogram showed the anterior tibial artery to be occluded 15 cm above the ankle but the patient still to have flow to her foot via the posterior tibial artery. The scarred and ischemic anterior tibial angiosome had cellulitis, breakdown, and spontaneous exposure of the fracture site. Replacement of the soft tissues at the time of the instrumentation of the tibia was performed using a radial forearm free flap. As the anterior tibial artery was chronically occluded, the radial forearm soft tissue flap took its vascular supply from the posterior tibial system (Fig. 12.3).

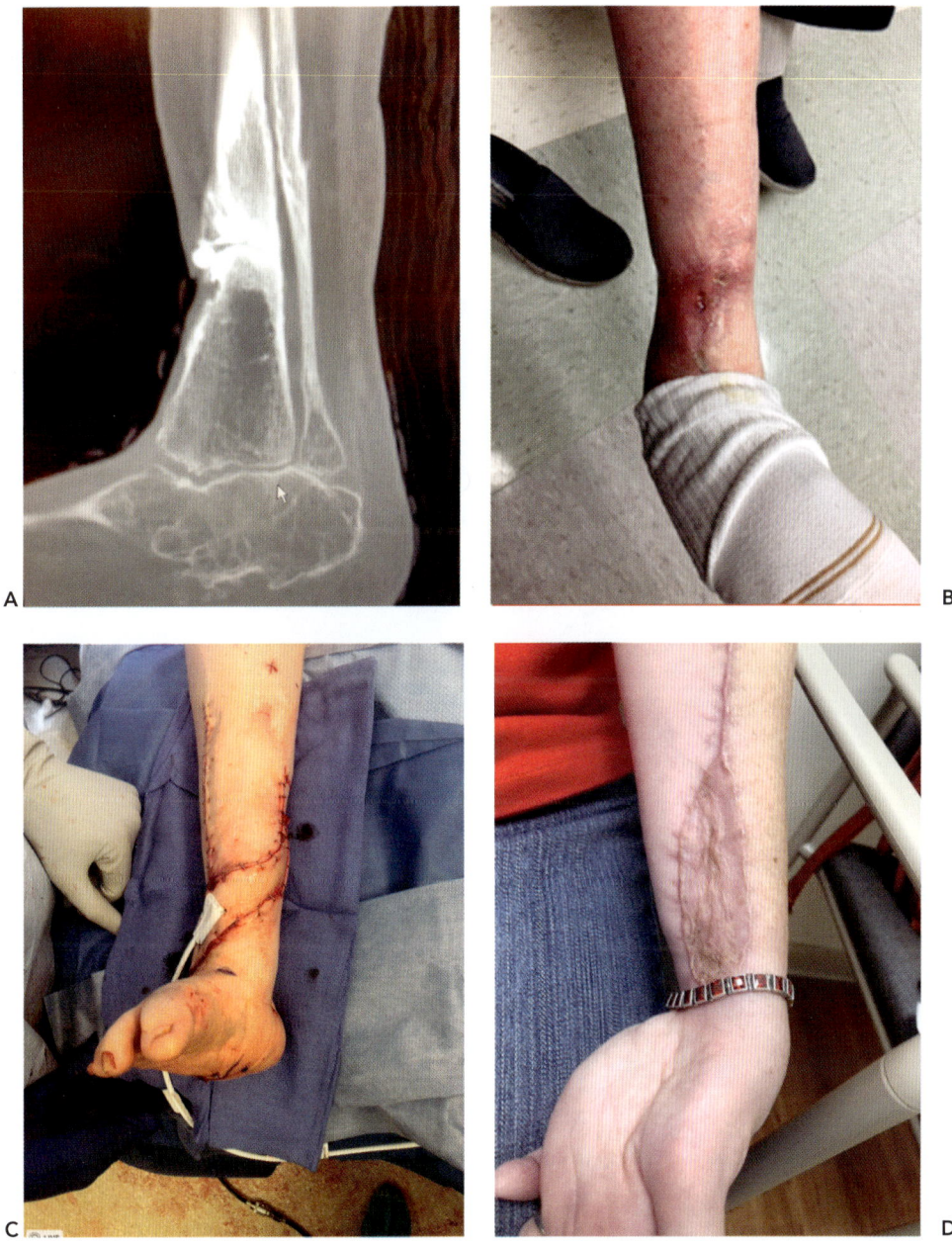

Figure 12.3 **(A)** Lateral x-ray of chronic nonunion of the right tibia. A lower extremity arteriogram showed the anterior tibialis artery to be chronically occluded. **(B)** Photograph of scarred anterior tibial angiosome at the ankle, with the tibial fracture sinus visible through the wound. **(C)** Radial forearm free flap performed at time of tibial rodding to resurface the anterior tibial angiosome and provide soft tissue cover to the healing fracture. **(D)** Radial forearm free flap donor site.

Angiosomes of the Foot

There are six angiosomes of the foot depicted in Figures 12.4 to 12.6. The heel (1) is supplied by two source arteries: the posterior tibial artery and peroneal artery. The medial and lateral sole (2, 3) is supplied by the posterior tibial artery. The dorsal foot (4) derives its flow from the anterior tibial artery and the peroneal artery provides flow to the anterolateral and posterolateral foot (5, 6). The great toe is encompassed by the angiosomes of both the medial sole and dorsal foot. Note that the heel and great toe are considered privileged because two different arteries overlap the same important area, much like the medial malleolus.

The Posterior Tibial and Peroneal Angiosomes of the Heel

The heel is supplied by parallel medial and lateral systems. Medially, the posterior tibial artery supplies the heel pad and calcaneus via the calcaneal branch of the posterior tibial artery (Fig. 12.7). This vessel branches off of the posterior tibial system within the tarsal tunnel. Laterally, paralleling the continuation of the sural nerve onto the foot is the calcaneal branch of the peroneal artery. The blood vessels of the heel travel in a mediolateral rather than in an axial direction. This was determined clinically in early reports of the optimal patterns of skin flap elevation to cover heel defects. The vessels also tend to travel around, rather than through, the tough plantar fascia overlying the calcaneus. This makes sense evolutionarily because vessels running directly through the heel fat pad would be subject to repeated occlusion from heel strike, unlike vessels remote from the direct line of force.

The Medial and Lateral Sole

As expected, there are two angiosomes of the plantar sole that are supplied by the two terminal branches of the posterior tibial artery, namely the medial and lateral plantar arteries. The bifurcation point is typically within the calcaneal canal.

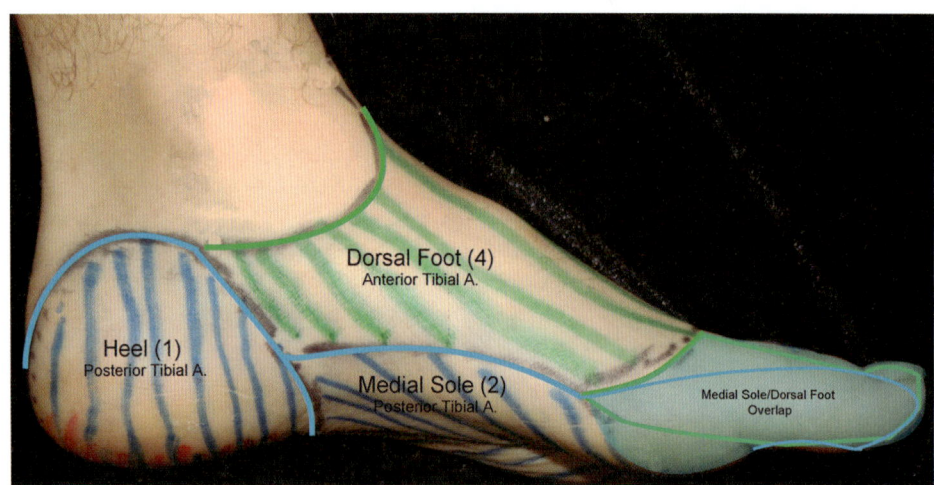

Figure 12.4 Medial view of the foot angiosomes.

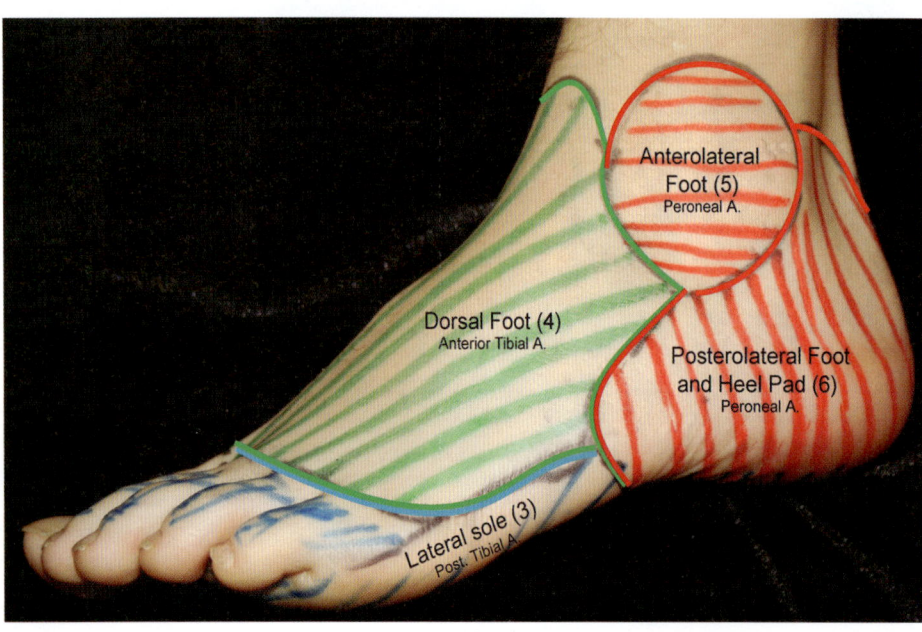

Figure 12.5 Lateral view of the foot angiosomes.

Chapter 12: Angiosomes of the Calf, Ankle, and Foot: Anatomy, Physiology, and Implications

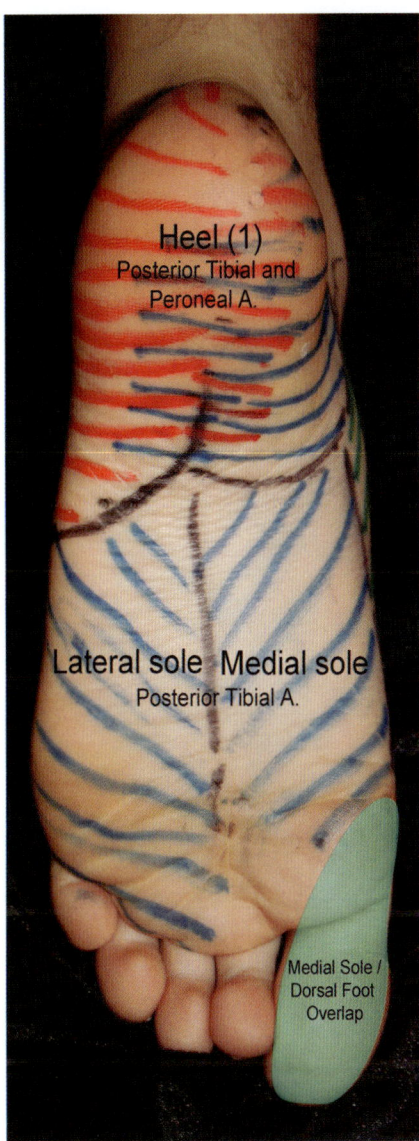

Figure 12.6 Plantar view of the foot angiosomes.

The Posterior Tibial Angiosome of the Medial Sole

At the level of the talonavicular joint, the medial plantar artery splits into deep and superficial branches. The deep branch is the basis for the medial plantar artery flap and travels deep to the abductor hallucis and adjacent to the medial intermuscular septum and the digital nerves. The superficial branch supplies the medial aspect of the navicular-cuneiform joint, along with skin perforators paralleling and superficial to the abductor hallucis. Anastomoses between the dorsalis pedis, first dorsal metatarsal artery, and the superficial branch of the medial plantar system exist in this instep area of the foot. Figure 12.8 illustrates the transposition of the medial plantar artery angiosome (posterior tibial angiosome of the medial sole) to cover the weight-bearing heel in a diabetic patient.

▶ The Posterior Tibial Angiosome of the Lateral Sole

The lateral plantar artery supplies the middle compartment of the foot, the flexor digitorum brevis, the deep plantar arch, the abductor digiti minimi, and the proper digital vessels to the lateral four toes.

The plantar sole is unusual in the repeated cycling of pressure across its surface. The perforating blood vessels in both the medial and lateral sole reach the subdermal plexus in a manner that can be explained by the constant pressure cycling. These perforating blood vessels exit the named plantar vessels at right angles and travel short distances directly outward radially toward the skin. This mimics the orientation of the blood supply to the heel and makes sense because short vessels are occluded for less time and have far less shear forces compared to longer, axially oriented blood vessels running along the surface of the sole.

The Anterior Tibial Angiosome of the Dorsal Foot

The dorsal foot angiosome is supplied typically by the dorsalis pedis artery and several consistent branches. However, in less than 10% of feet, a "peroneal magna" artery exists with an atretic dorsalis pedis, meaning that the peroneal artery is the main source of flow to the dorsal foot.

In terms of blood supply to the dorsal skin, there are several "hot spots" (areas with reliable perforators), as well as several "dead zones" (watershed areas). One hot spot is over the proximal lateral aspect of the foot. Here, the proximal lateral tarsal artery is important for its supply to the extensor digitorum brevis and the overlying skin. It has an overlap in territory with the terminal branch of the peroneal artery along the lateral side of the foot. The skin distal to the Lisfranc joint over the first dorsal metatarsal artery is another cutaneous zone with rich vascular input. Conversely, a dead zone exists between the extensor retinaculum and the area overlying the first and second metatarsals. The dorsalis pedis sends only two perforators to the skin in this zone. For this reason, widely undermined skin flaps on the dorsum of the foot that elevate the skin over the metatarsals and only preserve connections of the skin of the dorsum of the foot near the retinaculum

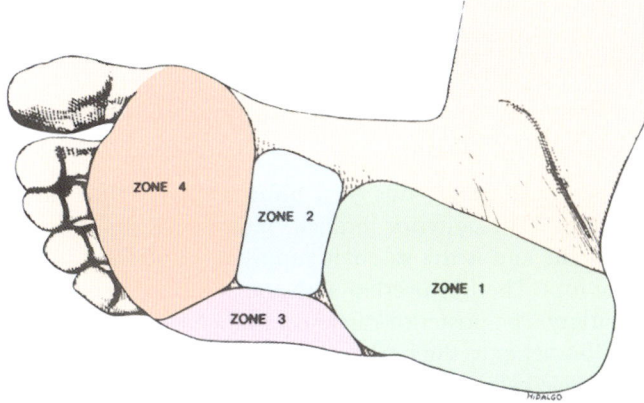

Figure 12.7 Arterial anatomy. Zone 1, the proximal plantar area; zone 2, the midplantar area; zone 3, the lateral foot; zone 4, the distal foot. (Adapted from Hidalgo DA, Shaw WW. Anatomic basis of plantar flap design. *Plast Reconstr Surg.* 1986;78[5]:627.)

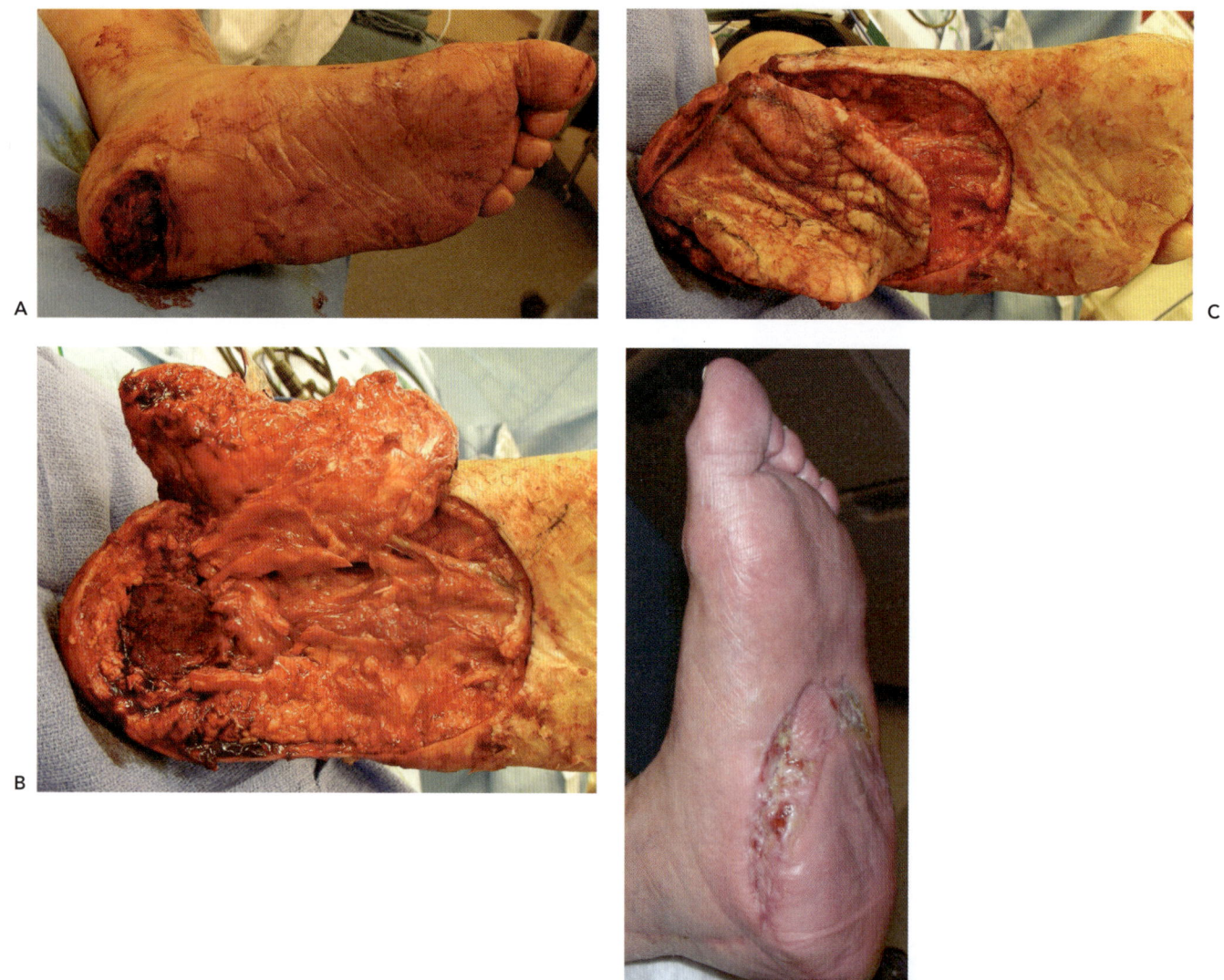

Figure 12.8 (A) Diabetic heel ulcer. (B) Proximally based medial plantar artery flap elevated to capture entire posterior tibial angiosome of the medial sole. The incisions border on the peroneal angiosome laterally. (C) Inset flap. (D) Healed flap.

can be unreliable and undergo necrosis. The following cases demonstrate the utility of understanding the anterior tibial angiosome of the dorsal foot.

Figure 12.9 represents the loss of soft tissue cover over a vascular bypass graft and illustrates the dead zone principle. A poorly planned random pattern skin incision over a bypass graft from the medial side of the foot had dehisced. The lateral tarsal artery was seen to be patent by arteriogram. A myocutaneous flap including the extensor digitorum brevis and the overlying skin perforators was transposed to cover the bypass graft.

Figure 12.10 represents the transfer of the entire dorsal foot angiosome for hand reconstruction. Although the entire dorsal foot angiosome did well, the proximal/lateral portion of the flap included the peroneal angiosome and that portion of the flap did not remain vascularized after the free flap transfer. This illustrates a very important concept about choke vessels. As described previously, although choke vessels may exist between two angiosomes, it often takes time for them to dilate to the size required to maintain adequate perfusion to an adjacent angiosome. In this instance, the demand on the yet undilated choke vessels outstripped their supply and the peroneal angiosome did not survive transfer.

The Peroneal Angiosome of the Posterolateral and Anterolateral Foot

The peroneal artery ends in a bifurcation near the lateral malleolus. The anterior branch pierces the interosseous membrane and is the vascular supply to the lateral dorsum of the foot. There is overlap with the anterior lateral malleolar artery. The posterior calcaneal branch sends four to five small branches to the heel and then travels parallel with the sural nerve before ending at the base of the fifth metatarsal. Retrograde flow and connections with small arteries that run along the sural nerve and lesser saphenous vein allow the performance of distally based sural neurocutaneous flaps (Fig. 12.11).

Chapter 12: Angiosomes of the Calf, Ankle, and Foot: Anatomy, Physiology, and Implications   709

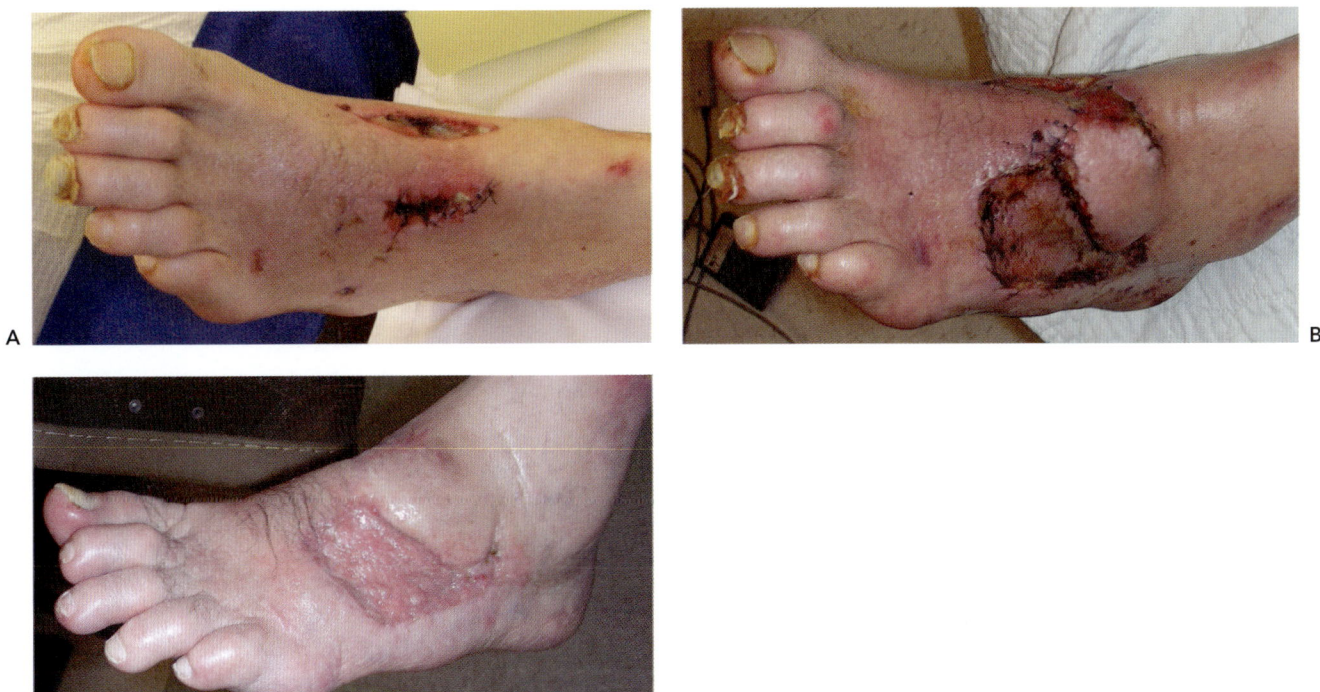

Figure 12.9 **(A)** Exposed bypass graft to the dorsalis pedis. A medial relaxing incision and reclosure by another surgical team had failed. **(B)** The myocutaneous extensor hallucis brevis flap based on an intact lateral tarsal artery angiosome (seen on closing arteriogram) elevated and transferred over the débrided surgical site. **(C)** Healed wound.

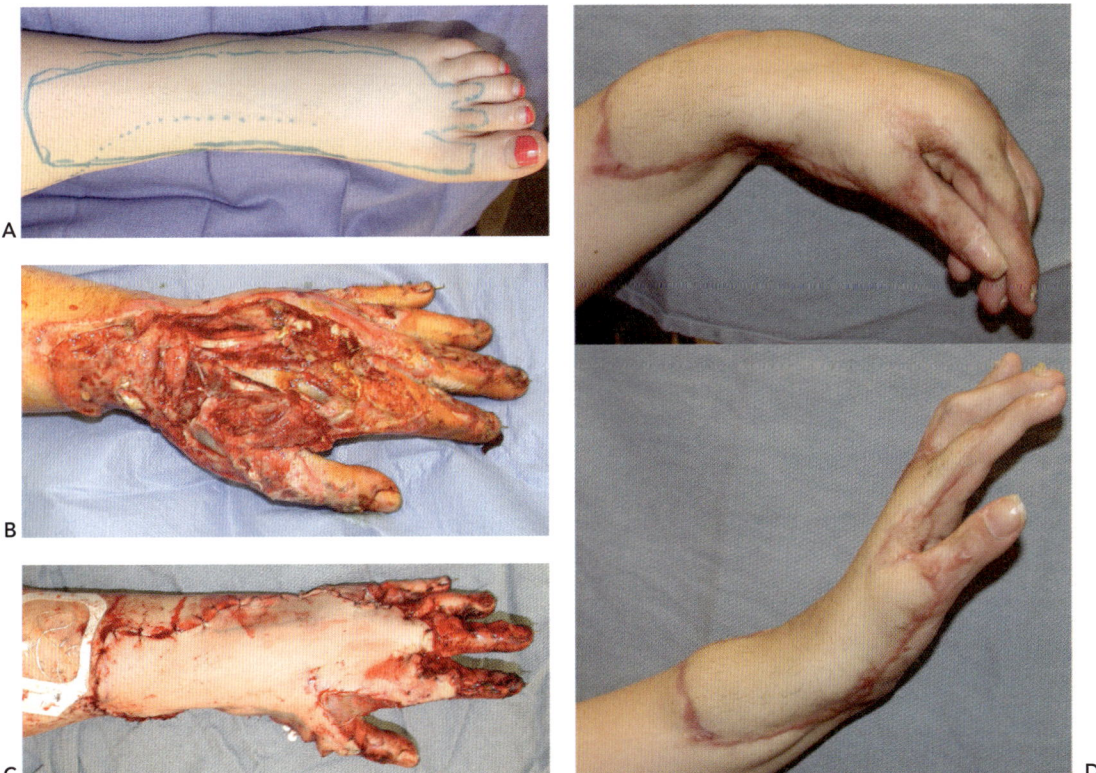

Figure 12.10 **(A)** Massive dorsalis pedis artery flap with edges outside the boundaries of the dorsalis pedis angiosome in a young paraplegic with a dorsal grinder injury of the hand. Wrist and finger extensors are all avulsed. **(B)** Dorsal hand wound. **(C)** Flap inset suffered some marginal edge necrosis on proximal border of flap that was due to the flap attempting to capture angiosome territory outside the primary area of the dorsalis pedis system. **(D)** Healed hand and movement.

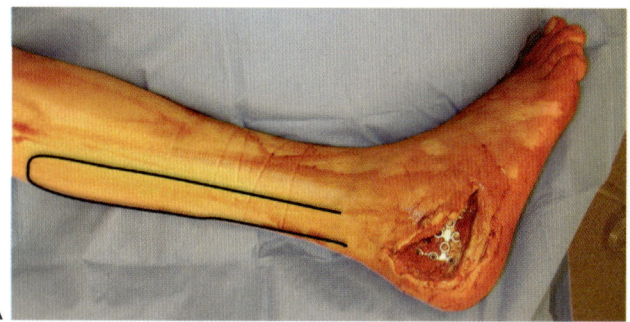
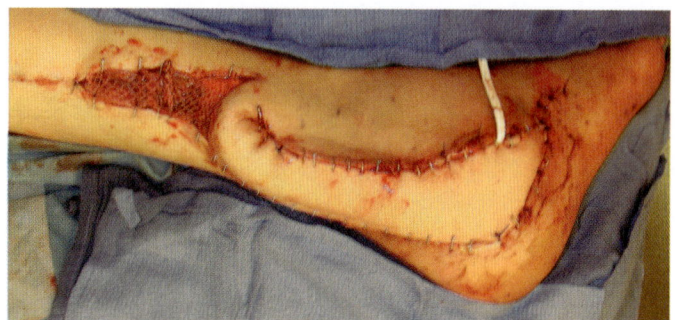
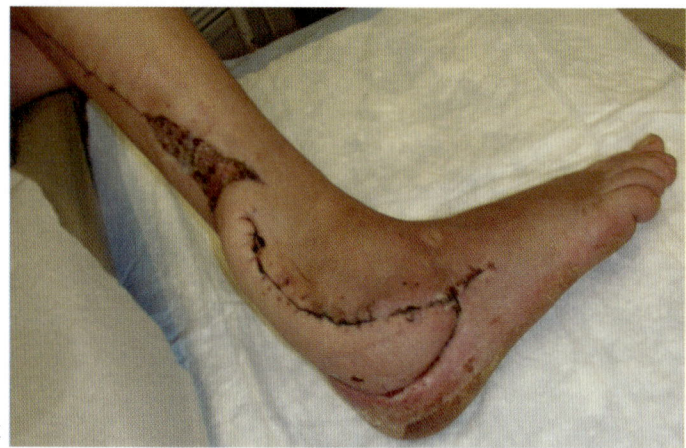

Figure 12.11 (A) Lateral calcaneal wound breakdown after open reduction and internal fixation of a calcaneal fracture. The sural flap is drawn encompassing the peroneal angiosome of the lower calf and the sural angiosome of the upper calf. (B) The flap is transposed. (C) Healed wound.

THE GREAT TOE

The dominant source of blood flow to the great toe is highly variable. There is communication between the plantar and dorsal angiosomes via the vertical descending branch of the dorsalis pedis. Protected from pressure and located between the first and second metatarsals, this conduit between the two angiosomes allows for great variability in the blood flow to the great toe and first web space area and the deep plantar arch. It has been determined that the dorsalis pedis system is more dominant than the plantar system in 80% of specimens. The first dorsal metatarsal artery emerges off of the dorsalis pedis distal to the takeoffs of the laterally directed arcuate artery and the vertical descending branch (directed to the plantar angiosomes). Emerging and traveling within the first intermetatarsal space, in 78% of feet the artery is located on the surface of the interosseous muscle and 22% of the time it is within the muscle to then travel more superficially toward the web space. The anatomy of the first dorsal metatarsal artery is critical to be understood before the elevation of toe and web space flaps. The web space is an area of interconnection and overlap in the angiosomes of the foot and both the plantar and dorsal circulations can be dominant. Figure 12.12 illustrates the transfer of the great toe angiosome in the replacement of a missing thumb. In this case, the dominant arterial supply was from the plantar circulation and the drainage was dorsal.

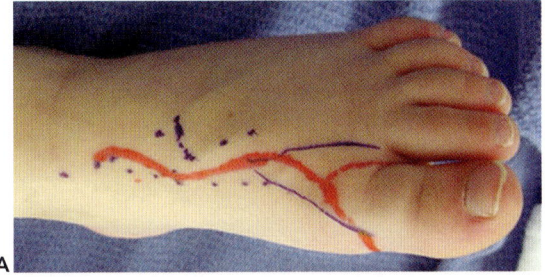
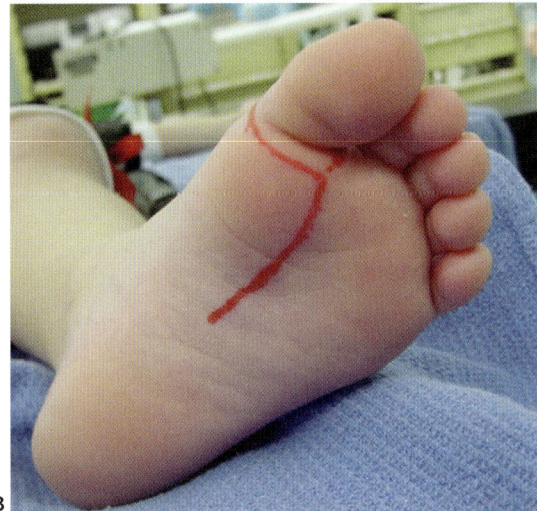
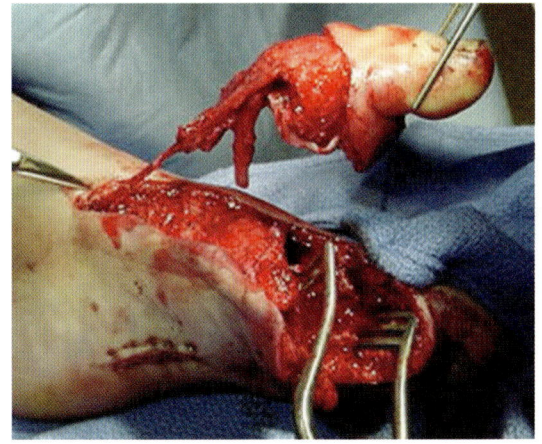

Figure 12.12 Toe-to-hand transfer. **(A)** Dorsal incisions planned. **(B)** Plantar incisions planned. **(C)** Dissected great toe angiosome.

FOOT AND ANKLE INCISIONS

There are many competing interests for planning incisions. The surgeon needs to anticipate the exposure needed. Minimizing skin flap elevation is important. Joints should not be crossed with perpendicular incisions in order to prevent scar contractures. The skin should be incised in the internervous plane in order to not divide small nerve endings with the complications of numbness and formation of painful neuromas. And, finally, the skin incision itself should not cause ischemia to the tissues. The first decision to be made is if any of the angiosomes of the foot are ischemic. In a well-vascularized foot, the best incisions are between angiosomes. These incisions tend to lie between the nerves and so the incisions make sense for two different reasons.

Figure 12.13 demonstrates the incision used to débride a heel pressure sore and the use of an abductor digiti minimi flap. The exposure was gained in this well-vascularized foot with an incision between the lateral sole angiosome and the posterolateral heel angiosome of the peroneal artery. Another excellent incision for the sole is in the midline, between the medial and lateral sole angiosomes. Again, this incision tends to be in the internervous plane.

Much more difficult to plan and perform is the incision in the patient with absent pulses. As previously described, chronic ischemia causes choke vessels to mature between angiosomes. A foot incision that divides these collaterals can create unexpected wound healing and tissue necrosis. The use of a Doppler ultrasound and the sequential occlusion of the inflow vessels are helpful in avoiding unexpected division of collateral flow. To perform this physical examination, the Doppler probe determines the presence or absence of pulsatile flow in the named large vessels of the foot—dorsalis pedis, posterior tibial, and peroneal. While listening with the probe to the flow of a vessel on the foot, the other arteries are sequentially compressed with a finger to ensure that the signal does not disappear. For example, if the signal on the dorsum of the foot disappears due to compression of the posterior tibial artery at the ankle, then the dorsal circulation is entirely due to collateral flow. In this instance, if an incision must be made on the dorsum of the foot, positions to avoid would be the instep, the lateral border of the foot, and the lateral malleolus. Instead, an incision in the middle of the angiosome should be made rather than between the dorsal foot angiosome and the sole/lateral foot angiosomes so that the fewest collaterals will be interrupted.

Understanding the angiosomes of the calf, ankle, and foot in health and disease markedly increases the ability of the foot surgeon to achieve a successful outcome.

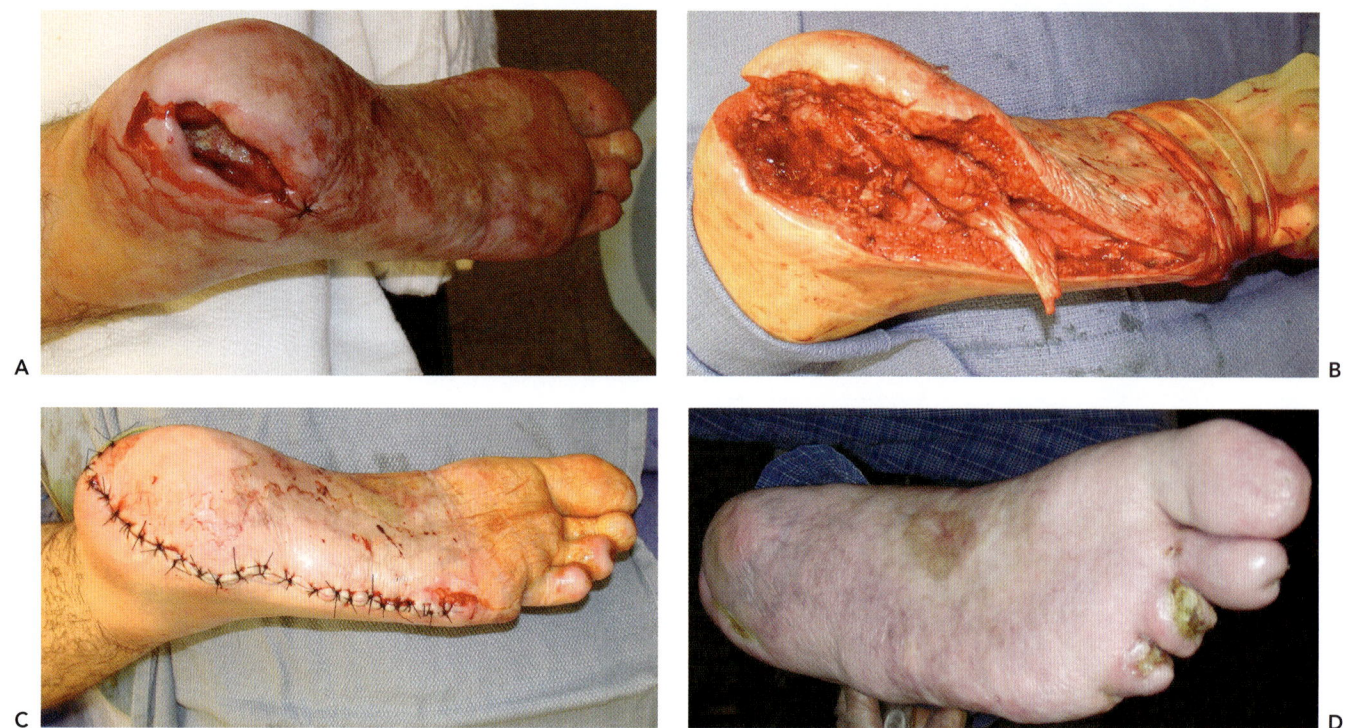

Figure 12.13 **(A)** Calcaneal osteomyelitis in a pressure sore induced heel ulcer. **(B)** Abductor digiti minimi flap placed after débridement. **(C)** Incision placed between the lateral plantar and the peroneal angiosomes. **(D)** Healed plantar incision. Patient regained ambulation.

REFERENCES

1. Schierle CF, Rawlani V, Galiano RD, et al. Improving outcomes of the distally based hemisoleus flap: principles of angiosomes in flap design. *Plast Reconstr Surg.* 2009;123(6):1748-1754.
2. Hammit MD, Hobgood ER, Tarquinio TA. Midline posterior approach to the ankle and hindfoot. *Foot Ankle Int.* 2006;27(9):711-715.
3. Neville RF, Attinger CE, Bulan EJ, et al. Revascularization of a specific angiosome for limb salvage: does the target artery matter? *Ann Vasc Surg.* 2009;23(3):367-373.
4. Chou TH, Alvelo JL, Janse S, et al. Prognostic value of radiotracer-based perfusion imaging in critical limb ischemia patients undergoing lower extremity revascularization. *JACC Cardiovasc Imaging.* 2021;14(8):1614-1624.
5. Ma J, Lai Z, Shao J, et al. Infrapopliteal endovascular intervention and the angiosome concept: intraoperative real-time assessment of foot regions' blood volume guides and improves direct revascularization. *Eur Radiol.* 2021;31(4):2144-2152.
6. Taylor GI, Palmer JH. The vascular territories (angiosomes) of the body: experimental study and clinical applications. *Br J Plast Surg.* 1987;40(2):113-141.
7. Taylor GI, Pan WR. Angiosomes of the leg: anatomic study and clinical implications. *Plast Reconstr Surg.* 1998;102(3):599-616.
8. Attinger C, Cooper P, Blume P. Vascular anatomy of the foot and ankle. *Oper Tech Plast Reconstr Surg.* 1997;4(4):183-198.
9. Oexeman S, Ward KL. Understanding the arterial anatomy and dermal perfusion of the lower extremity with clinical application. *Clin Podiatr Med Surg.* 2020;37(4):743-749.
10. Hosokawa K, Hata Y, Yano K, et al. Results of the Allen test on 2940 arms. *Ann Plast Surg.* 1990;24:149-151.
11. Booi D, Debats I, Boeckx W, et al. A study of perfusion of the distal free-TRAM flap using laser Doppler flowmetry. *J Plast Reconstr Aesthetic Surg.* 2008;61(3):282-288.
12. Attinger CE, Evans KK, Bulan E, et al. Angiosomes of the foot and ankle and clinical implications for limb salvage: reconstruction, incisions, and revascularization. *Plast Reconstr Surg.* 2006;117(suppl 7):261S-293S.
13. Gilbert BJ, Horst F, Nunley JA. Potential donor rotational bone grafts using vascular territories in the foot and ankle. *J Bone Joint Surg Am.* 2004;86-A(9):1857-1873.

Diagnostic Imaging Techniques of the Foot and Ankle

Imran M. Omar

Diagnostic imaging of the foot and ankle has made numerous advancements in the past 35 to 40 years and allows rapid, noninvasive, high-resolution depiction of anatomy and pathology. Technical advances in magnetic resonance imaging (MRI), including faster gradients, higher field strength magnets, and better coils; computed tomography, including the advent of helical and cone-beam acquisition and multidetector capabilities; and ultrasound, including higher frequency transducers, have allowed better understanding of foot and ankle pathology and associated findings. For example, high-frequency ultrasound is well suited to examine superficial structures commonly encountered in the musculoskeletal system like peripheral nerves, tendons, and ligaments, and visualization of structure during real-time scanning can be used to give physiologic or biomechanical information such as detecting abnormal tendon subluxation or ligament insufficiency during dynamic or stress maneuvers.[1]

Imaging of the foot and ankle is particularly challenging for several reasons. There are numerous small structures in close proximity with complex, nonlinear courses, such as the lateral ankle ligaments and intrinsic musculature, which can be difficult to distinguish without thorough understanding of the anatomy. Many of these structures are difficult to see without proper patient positioning, optimization of the plane of scanning to image the desired anatomy, or adjusting image acquisition parameters to obtain the highest possible resolution. Furthermore, patient positioning and imaging planes may not be standardized between institutions, which may cause differences in the appearance and orientation of structures. Therefore, imagers must be aware of the differences in the appearances of certain structures based on patient positioning in order to avoid misinterpretation.

Moreover, on cross-sectional imaging there is no consensus on nomenclature of standard orthogonal imaging planes, especially in the forefoot. In the hindfoot and ankle, the axial, sagittal, and coronal planes are contiguous with the lower extremity. However, in the forefoot, some imagers refer to the short axis as the axial plane, while others refer to it as the coronal plane. This may cause confusion when reported findings are communicated to others. Thus, it is important to describe suspected sites of pathology on several planes whenever possible.

Finally, ultrasound in particular is highly dependent on probe positioning and often relies on smaller field-of-view images than other imaging modalities. This makes sonographic images difficult to reproduce and may not allow the study interpreter to adequately place suspected pathology within an anatomic context.

However, with increasing utilization of diagnostic imaging in the foot and ankle, imagers and clinicians are becoming more aware of these considerations. This will help to mitigate the impact the issues may have and further improve the diagnostic capabilities of noninvasive imaging.

RADIOGRAPHY

Conventional radiography is the standard initial diagnostic imaging modality to assess the foot and ankle.[2] A number of factors allow radiography to serve as an excellent survey modality in the musculoskeletal system. First, this modality has excellent spatial resolution of osseous structures compared with CT and MRI, and offers strong contrast resolution to discriminate between bone, metal or calcification, fat and soft tissues. Therefore, it provides an excellent anatomic survey of the bones to help diagnose fractures, identify and characterize areas of periosteal reaction and osteolysis, and evaluate osseous alignment in order to suggest biomechanical alterations or sites of related injuries. Moreover, radiographs can depict areas of soft tissue swelling or calcifications, which often allows diagnosis of specific pathologies or limits the differential diagnosis to help guide further diagnostic testing.[2] Compared with cross-sectional imaging modalities, radiographs are relatively resistant to artifacts from metals, which can degrade other imaging studies and render them unable to be interpreted.[3] As a result, radiographs are helpful in assessing for orthopedic hardware alignment and potential complications such as fractures or loosening.

Additionally, radiographs can be obtained fairly quickly and inexpensively, which helps clinicians and imagers to quickly make decisions and initiate therapy in a timely manner. Furthermore, the images are reproducible, with most institutions obtaining standard views of the foot and ankle, including AP (Fig. 13.1), lateral (Fig. 13.2), mortise (Fig. 13.3), and possibly oblique images (Fig. 13.4) of the ankle, and AP (Fig. 13.5), lateral (Fig. 13.6), and oblique (Fig. 13.7) images of the foot. Additional standard radiographic protocols are available for bones that may be difficult to characterize on standard ankle or foot radiographs, such as the calcaneus (Figs. 13.8 and 13.9) and sesamoid bones (Figs. 13.10 and 13.11). The guidelines for obtaining many of these projections, including the descriptions for acquiring the standard views outlined in the figure legends in this chapter, have been established for many years, having been first compiled in the current standard text Merrill's *Atlas of Roentgenographic Positions* since 1949.[4,5] As such, diagnostic radiographs performed at one institution can also be interpreted by other institutions, and radiographs of the same body parts can be serially obtained, allowing radiographic follow-up and helping to guide longitudinal management of patients.

On the other hand, a few limitations of conventional radiography have necessitated the development of additional imaging modalities. While radiographs are very good for depicting osseous pathology, they are less helpful than cross-sectional techniques in evaluating soft tissue derangements.[3] Unless there is a significant fat component or calcification, the soft tissues often have similar attenuations, which may make discriminating soft tissue structures and pathology difficult.

Because radiographs are two-dimensional representations of three-dimensional structures, the images rely on proper patient and x-ray beam positioning to prevent superimposition of bones and other radiopaque structures. The perspective of anatomic structures and the way the structures are radiographically depicted change depending on the orientation of the x-ray beam with respect to the structures being imaged, a principle known as *parallax*.[6] Awareness of parallax is important in properly positioning patients, especially in foot and ankle imaging, since subtle alterations in the x-ray beam orientation can obscure areas of interest. For example, a true AP radiograph of the foot often distorts the appearance of the tarsometatarsal joint, while angulating the x-ray beam toward the heel by about

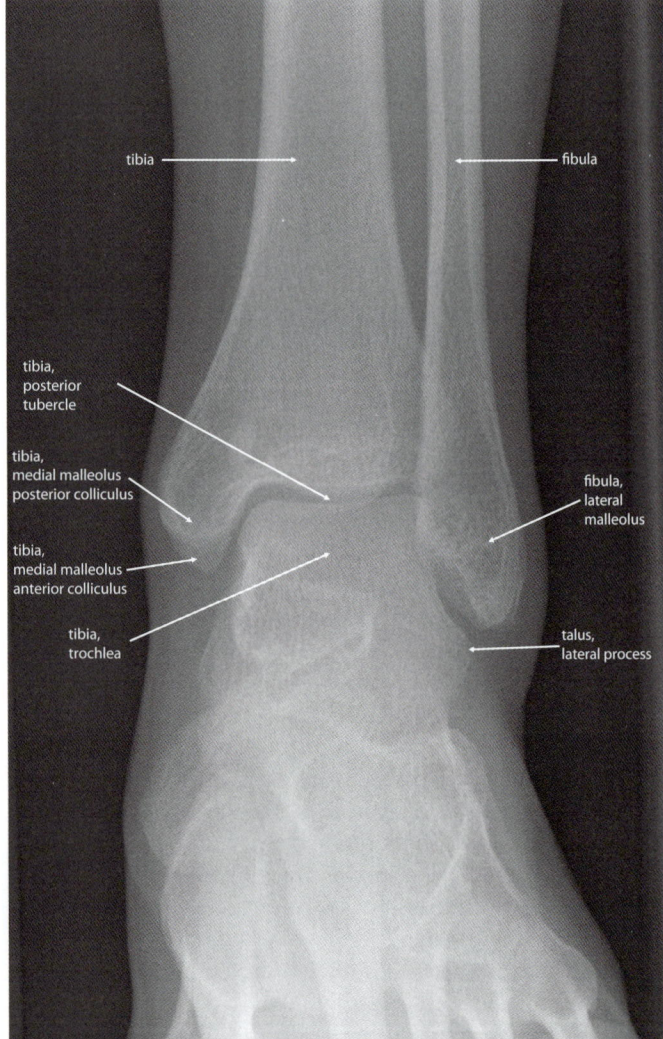

Figure 13.1 **AP ankle radiograph.** In a standard AP image of the ankle, the patient is imaged with the leg extended and the patient supine. The foot is positioned so its long axis is approximately perpendicular to the long axis of the lower extremity. The x-ray beam is centered between the malleoli at the tibiotalar joint. The image should include the distal third of the tibia and fibula to the proximal metatarsals. The talar dome is seen in profile. There is mild overlap of the lateral malleolus and the lateral talus while the medial tibiotalar joint is open. Weight-bearing views are also commonly performed. In this instance, the patient is erect on the platform with the heels abutting the image receptor (IR) and the toes directed forward. Both feet are often included on the same image for comparison.

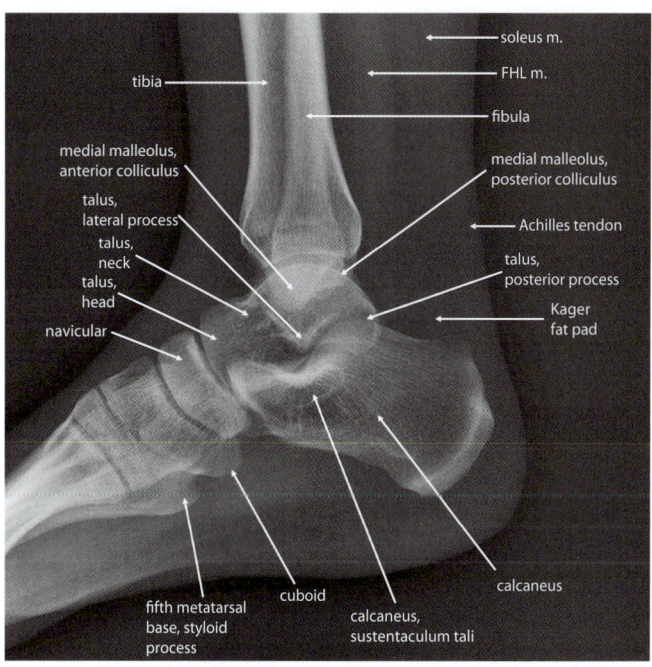

Figure 13.2 Lateral ankle radiograph. On the lateral radiograph either mediolateral (ML) or lateromedial (LM) images can be performed. In the ML image, the lateral margin of the foot is placed against the IR with the long axis of the IR parallel to the long axis of the lower extremity. As in the AP view, the foot is positioned so its long axis is approximately perpendicular to the long axis of the lower extremity. Alternatively, the LM view is performed with the medial portion of the foot against the IR. While the ML view is generally more comfortable, the LM view more commonly represents a true lateral of the foot and ankle in which there is greater superimposition of the metatarsals. The beam is centered about 2 cm above the inferior tip of the lateral malleolus. The standard image shows the medial and lateral margins of the talar dome in profile overlapping one another. The fibula should project over the posterior half of the tibia, the medial malleolus should be slightly anterior to the lateral malleolus, and the base of the fifth metatarsal should be visible.

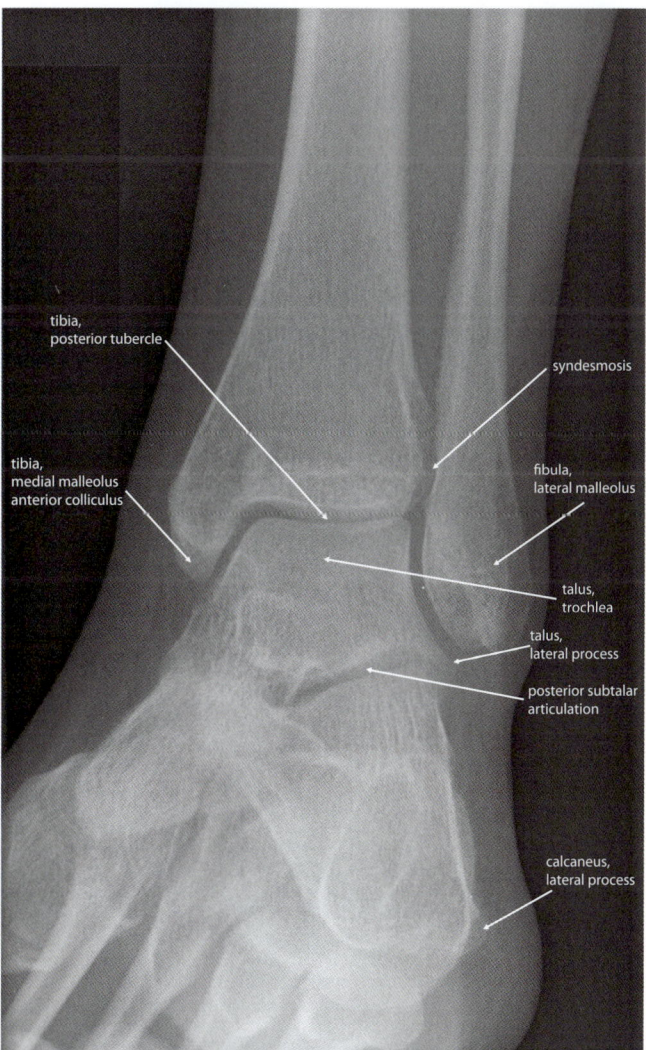

Figure 13.3 Mortise view. This view is more common than internal oblique ankle radiographs and is useful for examining the talar dome in profile. The patient is placed between 15° and 20° of internal rotation with the long axis of the foot perpendicular to the long axis of the calf. The x-ray beam is centered between the malleoli at the tibiotalar level. In this view, there is no overlap of the lateral malleolus and the lateral talus. However, there is mild overlap of the distal tibia and fibula. Normally, there is uniform joint space width along the tibiotalar and talofibular articulations measuring approximately 5 mm.

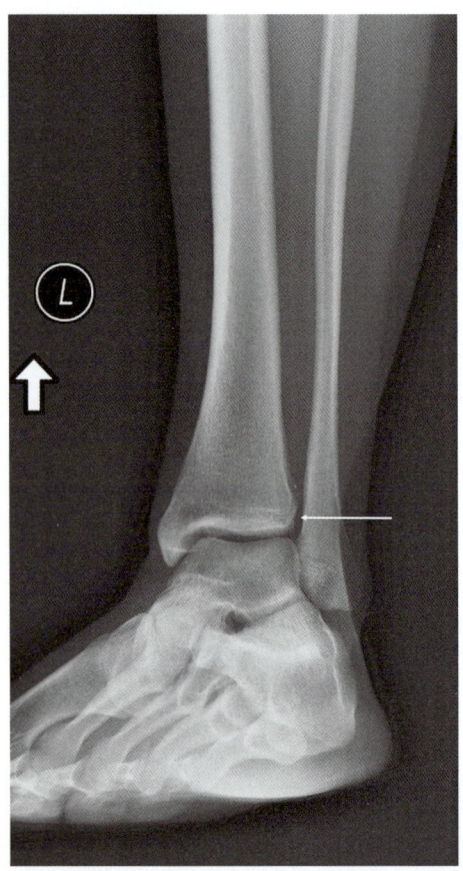

Figure 13.4 Oblique ankle radiograph. This view is usually performed to see the distal tibiofibular (syndesmosis) joint in profile (*white arrow*) and is obtained with the patient in approximately 35° to 45° of internal rotation. The patient is imaged with the foot in 10° to 15° of plantar flexion, which prevents overlap of the posterior calcaneus and lateral malleolus. The externally rotated oblique is less commonly obtained but may be useful in assessing the anterior tibial tubercle and the lateral malleolus.

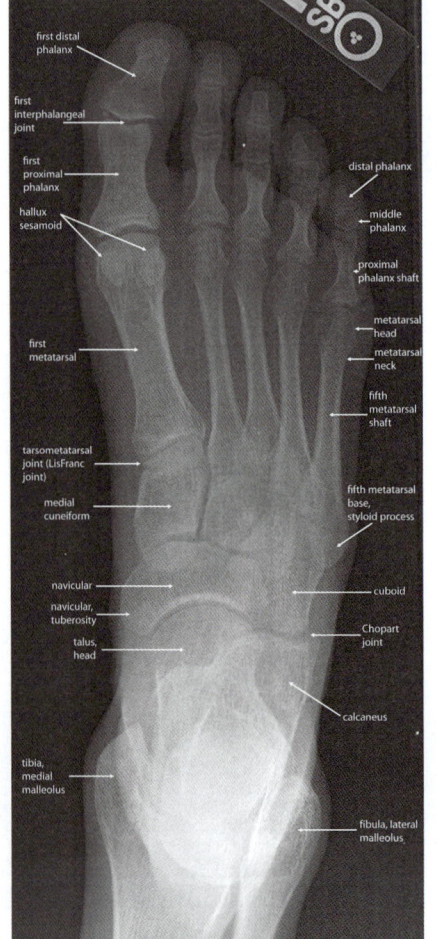

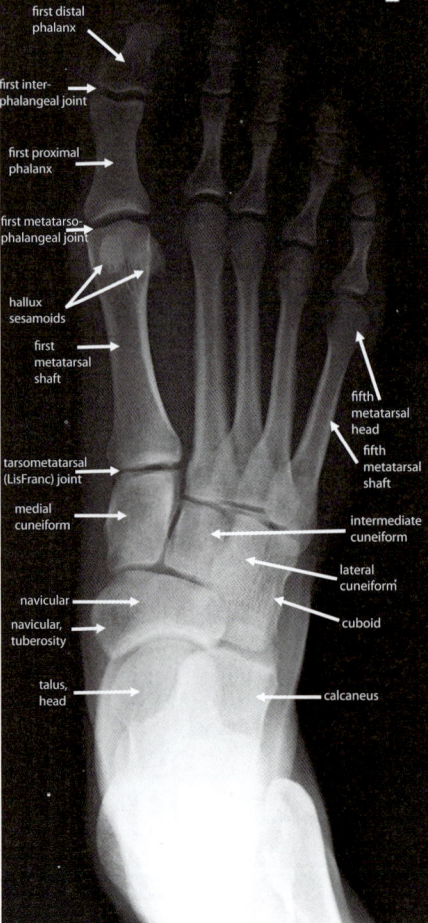

Figure 13.5 AP foot radiographs. The AP radiograph of the foot is obtained with the patient supine and the knee flexed so that the sole of the foot rests on the table. The x-ray beam is centered at the third metatarsal base. The beam may be perpendicular to the table (**A**) or may be angulated about 10° toward the heel (**B**) to view the tarsometatarsal joint in profile. This subtle difference is an example of how parallax affects the image. On the standard image, the articulation between the medial and intermediate cuneiforms is seen in profile; the second, third, and fourth metatarsal bones are evenly spaced; and the second through fifth metatarsal bases overlap.

A

B

Chapter 13: Diagnostic Imaging Techniques of the Foot and Ankle 717

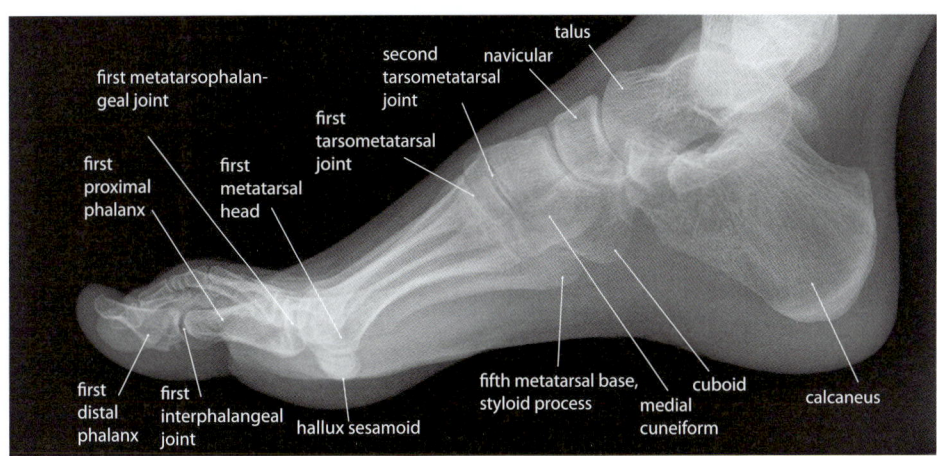

Figure 13.6 Lateral foot radiograph. As in the lateral ankle radiograph, the lateral foot radiograph can be performed in the ML or LM positions. The LM is usually less comfortable but more reliably produces a standard lateral image. The foot should be positioned so its long axis is perpendicular to the long axis of the calf, and the x-ray beam is directed at the third metatarsal base. In this view, the metatarsals are superimposed and the fibula projects over the posterior tibia. Because there may be slight distortion in the appearance of the subtalar and tibiotalar joints compared with a lateral ankle radiograph, the lateral foot radiograph should not substitute for a true lateral ankle radiograph.

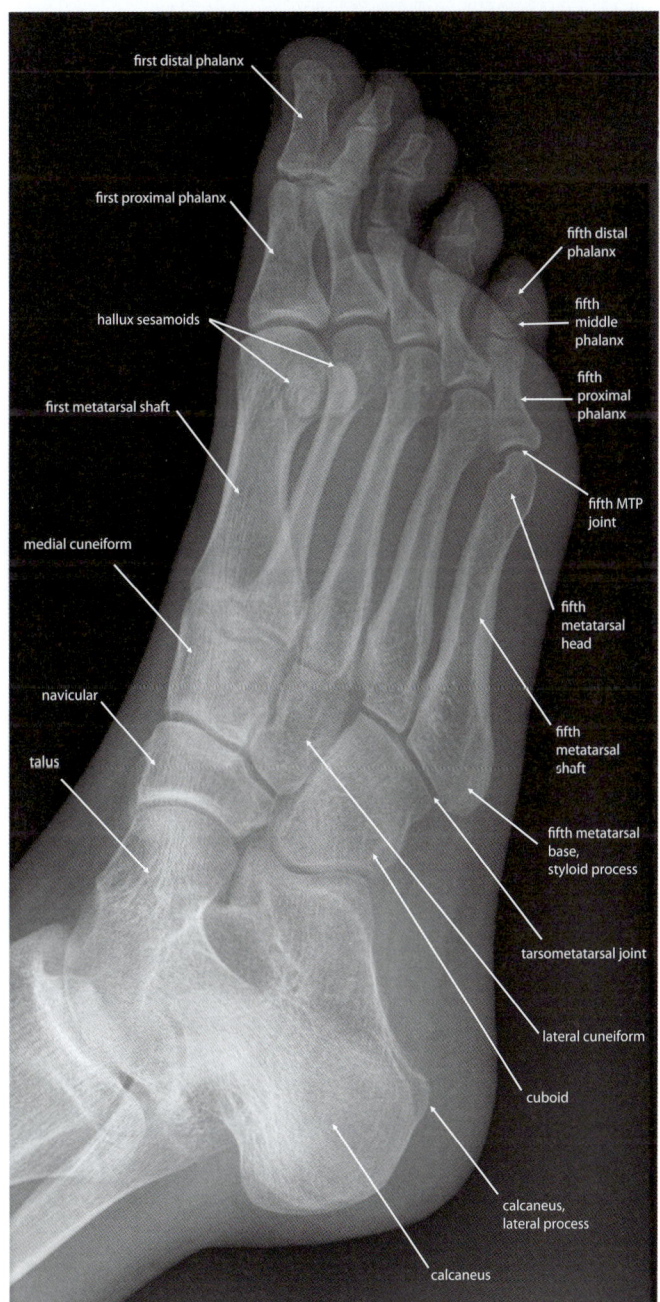

Figure 13.7 Internally rotated oblique radiograph. This view is best used to image the cubocalcaneal, cubocuneiform, and cubometatarsal joints, which are seen in profile. The patient is supine with the knee flexed and the plantar surface of the foot resting on the table. The thigh is then internally rotated to make a 30° angle opening laterally between the sole of the foot and the table. The x-ray beam should be centered at the third metatarsal base. On this image, the fifth metatarsal base is well seen and there is no overlap of the third, fourth, or fifth metatarsal bases. Occasionally, an externally rotated oblique may be performed with external rotation of the thigh that produces a 30° angle opening medially between the sole of the foot and the table. This view is better for looking at the medial and middle cuneiforms, first and second metatarsals, and navicular.

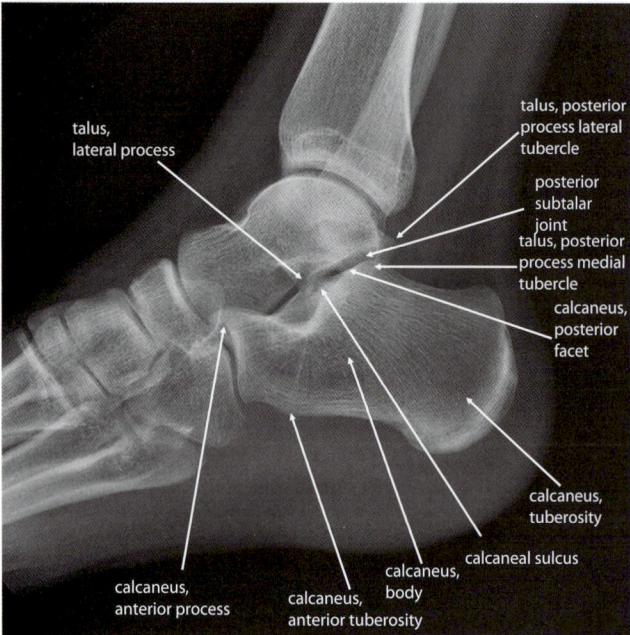

Figure 13.8 **Lateral calcaneus radiograph.** This is an ML view with the lateral aspect of the foot resting on the IR. The x-ray beam is centered on the central calcaneal body, approximately 2.5 cm distal to the medial malleolus. There should be no calcaneal rotation, the sustentaculum tali and lateral calcaneal tuberosity should be visible, and the subtalar joint should be seen in tangent.

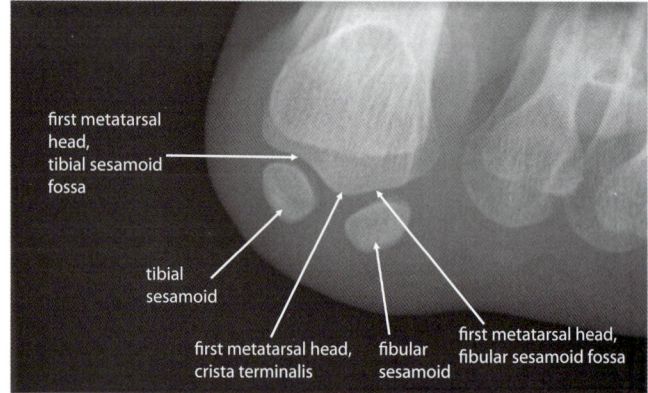

Figure 13.10 **Sesamoid tangential radiograph.** This view is used to see the sesamoid bones and hallux/sesamoid articulations in profile. It can be performed with the patient supine or prone and the great toe extended. Often a towel or strap is used to support the great toe in passive extension.

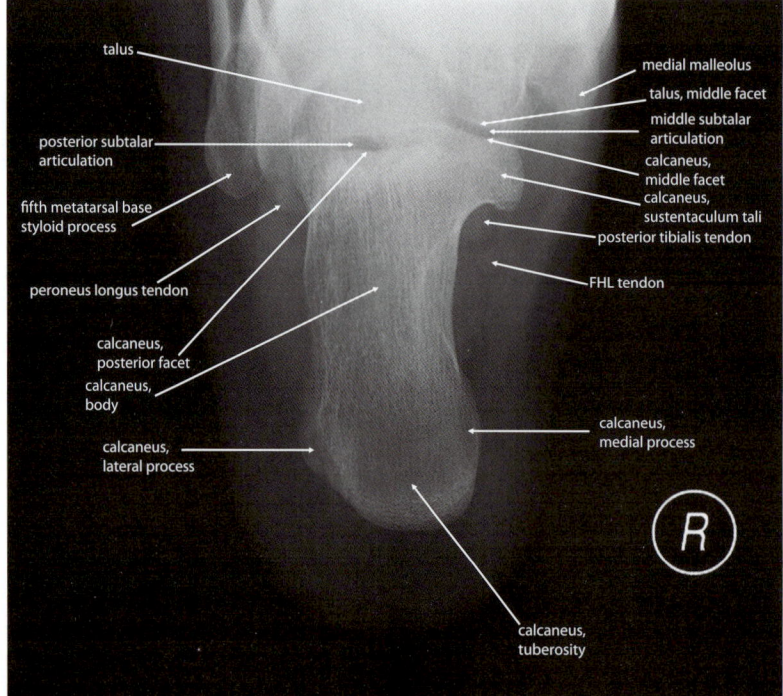

Figure 13.9 **Plantar-dorsal or dorsoplantar (axial) radiographs of the calcaneus.** These produce an AP image of the calcaneus and are helpful in seeing the posterior and middle subtalar joints in profile. The plantar-dorsal radiograph is obtained with the patient supine and the lower extremity extended. The foot is dorsiflexed so its long axis is perpendicular to the IR. The x-ray beam is then angled cephalad about 40° to the long axis of the foot and first penetrates the sole of the foot. The dorsoplantar view is performed with the patient prone and wedge or pillow placed under the distal calf. With the foot dorsiflexed to produce a 90° angle between the long axes of the foot and calf, the x-ray beam is directed caudally 40° to initially penetrate the posterior heel.

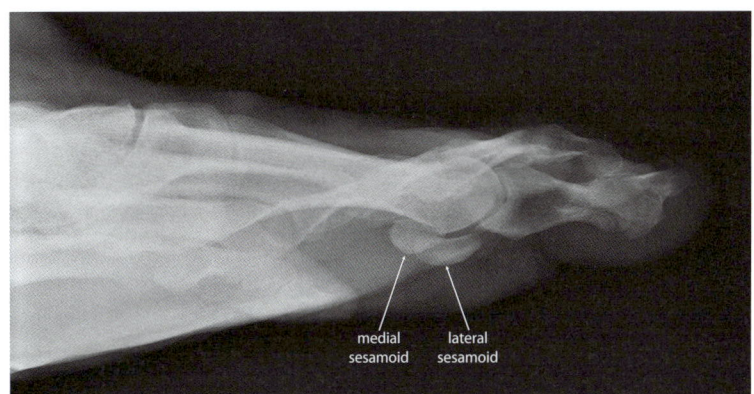

Figure 13.11 Causton sesamoid tangential radiograph. This oblique LM view of the sesamoid bones separates the bones and avoids significant overlap. With the patient in the LM position, the x-ray beam is angled 40° and directed toward the heel. The x-ray initially penetrates the lateral margin of the forefoot.

10° often shows the joint in profile and may help to better show subtle pathologies such as Lisfranc fracture-dislocations (see Fig. 13.5). In many instances, this overlap is unavoidable, and certain structures cannot be adequately assessed on standard projections. For example, on standard forefoot radiographs, the sesamoid bones overlap with one another or the metatarsal head, which may preclude their thorough assessment and require additional views, such as the Causton view or the sesamoid axial view[7] (see Figs. 13.11 and 13.12) for better radiographic evaluation.

Because of the complex anatomy of the foot and ankle and the importance of radiography on patient positioning with respect to the x-ray beam, a number of specialized views in which the x-ray beam is oblique to the standard orthogonal planes are effectively employed to help see structures that normally overlap on conventional views. Other techniques, including stress views, can help identify soft tissue injuries not normally seen on radiographs. Osseous alignment during stress can be objectively quantified and compared with the contralateral side, and can provide insight into abnormal foot and ankle biomechanics.[8] A common example of a stress view is a weight-bearing view that can detect flatfoot deformities or areas of joint space narrowing that may not be seen on non–weight-bearing views. AP stress views of the ankle can be performed with passive inversion to suggest lateral collateral ligamentous complex tears or insufficiency (Fig. 13.13A), or with laterally directed force either manually (Fig. 13.13B) or with gravity (Fig. 13.13C,D) to detect medial joint widening in the setting of deltoid ligament insufficiency and/or tibiofibular instability. Furthermore, a sagittal stress view of the ankle can show anterior talofibular ligament insufficiency (Fig. 13.13E,F).

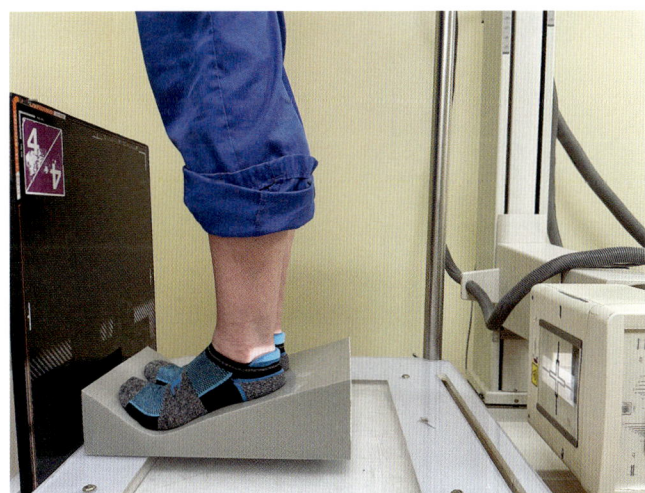
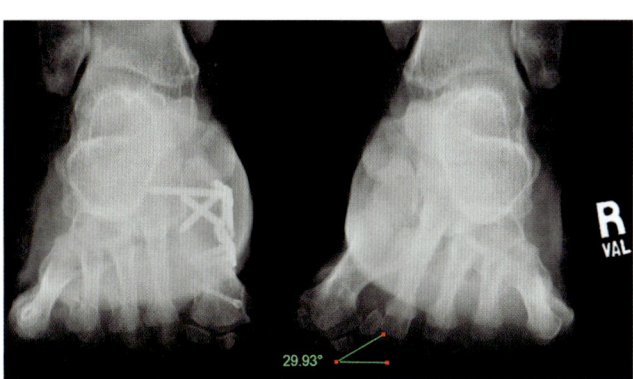

Figure 13.12 Sesamoid axial radiograph. This view is used to assess hallux-sesamoid alignment, particularly in the setting of hallux valgus. **(A)** The foot is placed on a specially created sponge with weight-bearing that puts the great toe in dorsiflexion, and the x-ray beam is directed anteriorly from the heel through the hallux/sesamoid articulation. **(B)** The horizontal short axis of the metatarsal head and the bi-sesamoid axis, which is a line connecting the sesamoid articular surfaces, should be parallel to the horizontal surface of the sponge. Any angle greater than 0 is considered abnormal. Additionally, each sesamoid bone should be centered in its fossa along the plantar surface of the metatarsal head. In this case, there is bilateral hallux/osteoarthritis, right greater than the left, and the right weight-bearing sesamoid is internally rotated by 30° while the left is rotated by less than 10°.

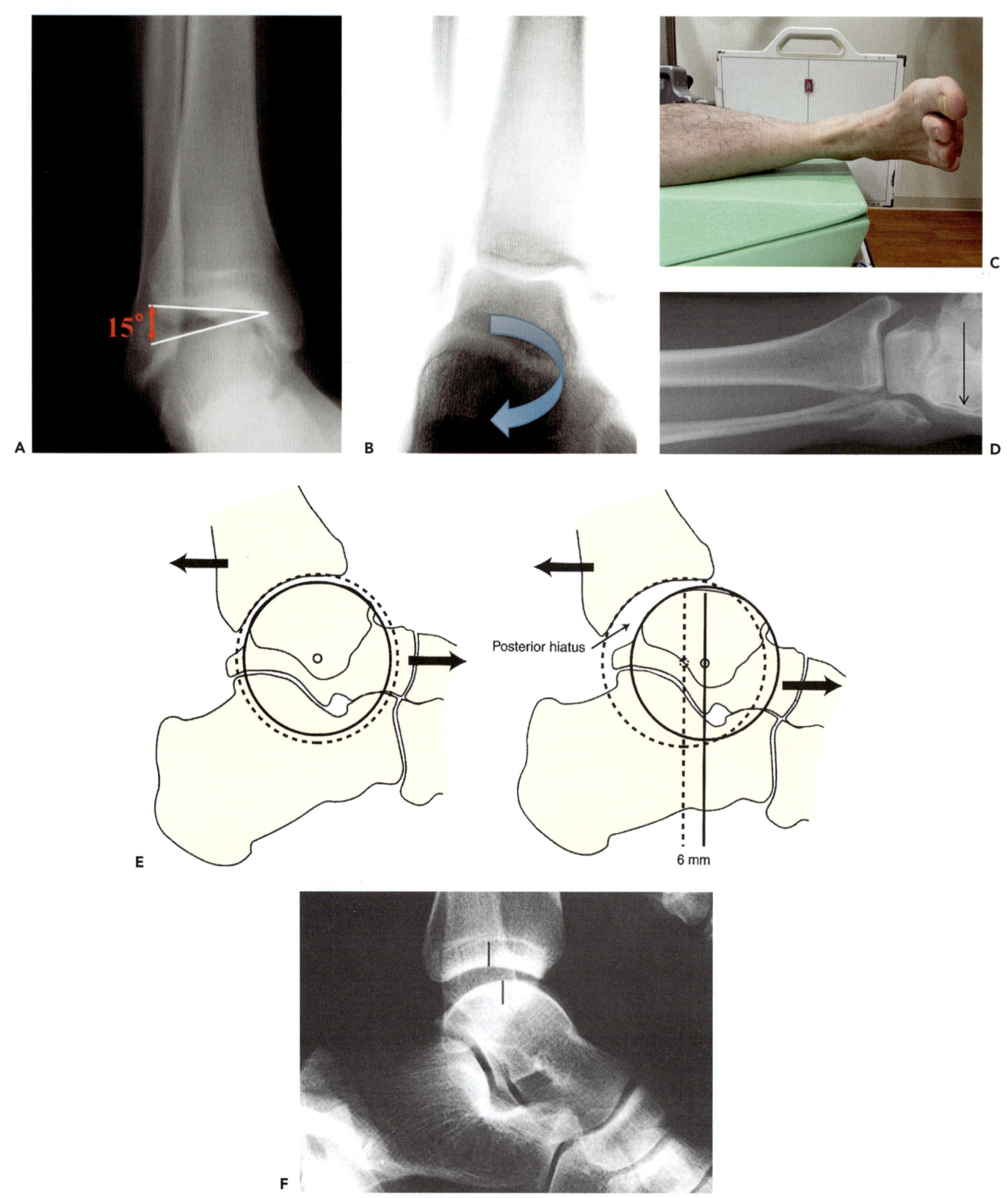

Figure 13.13 Stress radiographs of the ankle. (A) An AP ankle stress radiograph is helpful to assess the integrity of the medial and lateral ankle ligaments. The ankle is imaged in the AP projection with the distal calf immobilized and either inversion stress to test the lateral ligaments or eversion stress to test the medial ligaments is placed on the ankle. The study indicates ligament insufficiency if there is abnormal opening of the joint on the side of suspected ligament injury. However, there is great variability among normal people in the degree of opening during stress maneuvers, and it is frequently necessary to obtain a similar image of the asymptomatic contralateral side. One grading system measures the tilt angle between the tibial plafond and the talar dome. Angles less than 5° are considered normal. Angles between 5° and 15° are borderline abnormal; those between 15° and 25° are probably abnormal; and those angles greater than 25° are definitely abnormal. **(B)** A manual mortise abduction and external rotation radiograph shows widening of the medial tibiotalar joint space in the setting of deltoid ligament insufficiency. **(C)** A gravity mortise stress view is obtained by placing the patient in a decubitus position with the affected limb down on a sponge, which is as reliable as a manual stress view. **(D)** In this example, the gravity stress view shows medial tibiotalar joint widening, consistent with deltoid ligament insufficiency. **(E)** A schematic diagram of the sagittal stress view shows the normal relationship of the talar dome and the tibial plafond (*left*), which should be congruent and have parallel arcs of curvature. In patients with anterior talofibular insufficiency (*right*), the talar dome should shift anterior to the tibial plafond. **(F)** In this case, the sagittal stress view was performed with 20° of plantar flexion. The apex of the talar dome translates anteriorly more than 6 mm relative to the center of the tibial plafond, indicating anterior tibiotalar instability and anterior talofibular ligament insufficiency. Additionally, there is widening of the posterior tibiotalar joint space, called the posterior hiatal sign. (E, Republished with permission of McGraw Hill, from *Operative Treatment of the Foot and Ankle*. Kelikian A, ed. Appelton and Lange, Stamford, Conn 1999; permission conveyed through Copyright Clearance Center, Inc.)

COMPUTED TOMOGRAPHY

Like radiography, CT uses ionizing radiation for imaging. However, CT generates a regularly spaced stack of contiguous two-dimensional images generally oriented transverse to the long axis of the imaged structure. The complex anatomy of the foot and ankle and the differences in orientations of imaged structures on cross-sectional examinations from those seen in surgical dissection or conventional radiography make interpretation of cross-sectional studies challenging. As a result, adequate interpretation of these studies requires good understanding of the imaged anatomy. However, cross-sectional imaging techniques provide a noninvasive method to more clearly visualize complex anatomic relationships than radiography since they resolve the problem of overlapping structures that can prevent adequate radiographic visualization of structures. CT easily distinguishes bone and calcifications, metal, soft tissue, gas, and fat and is particularly useful in musculoskeletal imaging in the assessment of osseous pathology. In foot and ankle imaging, CT is most commonly used to detect radiographically occult fractures, or to characterize complex injuries such as calcaneal fractures for intra-articular fracture extension to the subtalar joint, articular surface incongruity, or intra-articular fracture fragments.[9] CT can also help to detect areas of osteolysis[10] or periosteal reactions that may indicate aggressive bone destruction, and soft tissue calcifications in processes like tophaceous gout or tumors with calcified matrix.[11] Tendons are well-seen on routine CT, and this modality can be useful in the foot and ankle to demonstrate the position of tendons with respect to fracture fragments, and to help determine whether there may be tendon impingement[8].

CT is also commonly used following surgery to determine osseous and hardware alignment and detect signs of orthopedic hardware failure. Metal often creates a "beam hardening" artifact, which produces dark streaks across the images adjacent to the metal and can prevent visualization of the margins of the metallic structure.[12,13] However, techniques like using thinner section collimation or maximizing the tube current and peak voltage, or using software corrections, can reduce the impact of this artifact and often allow CT to be useful for appraising the hardware and adjacent soft tissues.[12]

Modern CT scanners are very fast, often obtaining reproducible image sets with extended fields-of-view within seconds. To help clarify anatomy, the imaging data from these studies can be reconstructed in other cross-sectional planes either oriented to the long axis of the imaged body part or along other structures (Fig. 13.14). Alternatively, the data can be used to create three-dimensional renderings that can be helpful as an anatomic overview and guide interventional planning.[14] A recent application of using 3D modeling to help preoperative planning in the foot is to determine screw length, diameter, and placement to optimize the chances of healing and decrease the complication rate when fixing Jones fractures in the fifth metatarsal bone (Fig. 13.15).[15]

While intravenous iodinated contrast administration is not routinely performed, it is indicated in specific circumstances including depicting vascular anatomy,[16] detecting synovial proliferation and fluid collections, and characterizing soft tissue lesions for necrosis or cystic components. This is most commonly used in diagnosing and characterizing inflammatory arthropathies or infections and detecting fluid collections, such as abscesses.[17]

Two more recent advancements, dual energy CT (DECT) and cone-beam CT (CBCT), have increased the indications of CT in imaging of the foot and ankle. DECT uses two beams of ionizing radiation with differing and known energies rotating around the anatomy of interest. Each x-ray beam interacts with materials of differing atomic numbers, like calcium, iodine, and urate crystals, in predictable ways, and using x-ray beams of two different energies allows mapping of these materials on routine grayscale CT images.[18]

DECT of the foot and ankle has most commonly been used in detecting urate crystals in patients with known or suspected gout, and can help differentiate these patients from those with infections, which can have a similar clinical presentation in the acute phase (Fig. 13.16). DECT has also been used to detect areas of marrow abnormality, such as posttraumatic contusions or fractures, or intraosseous tumors, and may obviate the need for MRI in some patients. DECT techniques can also reduce the degree of metal artifact and allow improved assessment of the

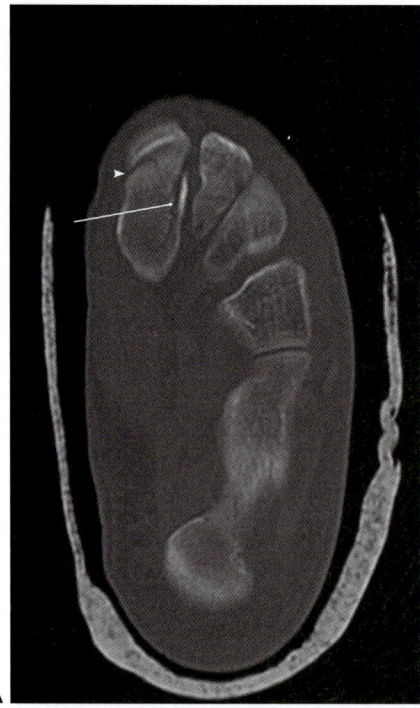
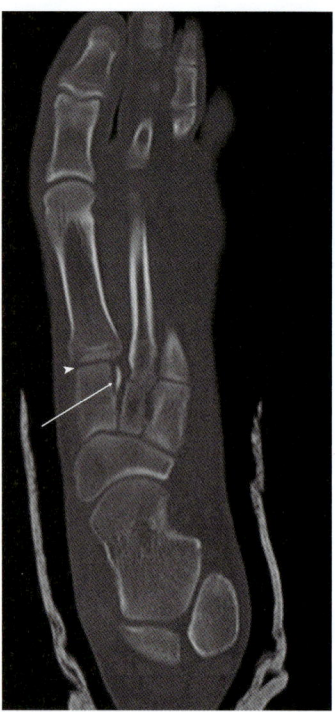
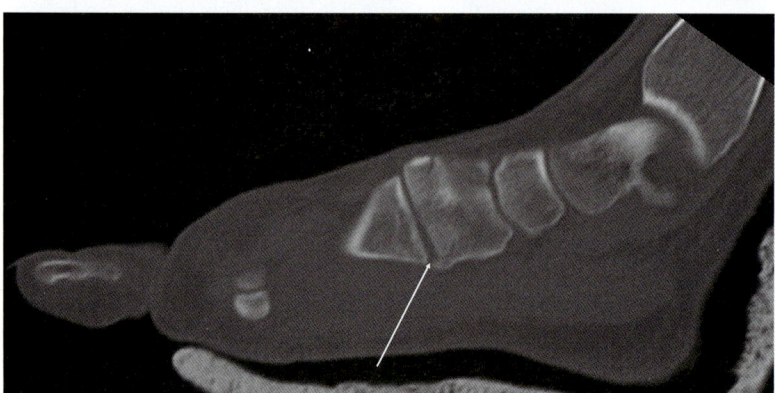

Figure 13.14 CT of hindfoot and midfoot showing the utility of multiplanar reformatted imaging. (A) Axial CT of the hindfoot and midfoot demonstrates a fracture of the lateral surface of the medial cuneiform (*arrow*) in the region of the Lisfranc ligament attachment. The *arrowhead* indicates the first tarsometatarsal joint. Since the patient was positioned with the ankle in plantar flexion, the anatomic relationships of the midfoot and the relationship of the fracture to the intercuneiform and tarsometatarsal joints are difficult to assess. Reformatted horizontal long-axis image of the foot **(B)** better depicts the fracture, while sagittal reformatted image **(C)** demonstrates 3 mm of distal medial cuneiform articular surface step-off at the tarsometatarsal joint that was difficult to perceive on the true axial images.

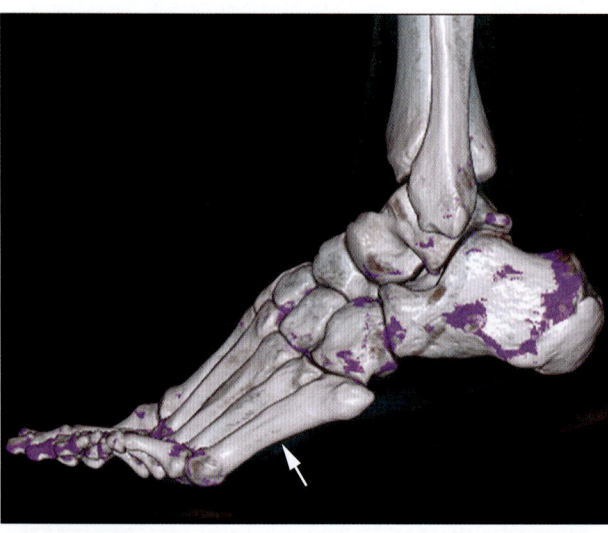

Figure 13.15 Sagittal lateral 3D reformatted image of the foot with attention to the fifth metatarsal shaft morphology. The image shows a gentle dorsal curvature of the fifth metatarsal shaft (*arrow*), which is a common anatomic variant. This curvature and medullary width should be considered when planning the trajectory, diameter, and length of a screw used for fifth metatarsal fracture fixation.

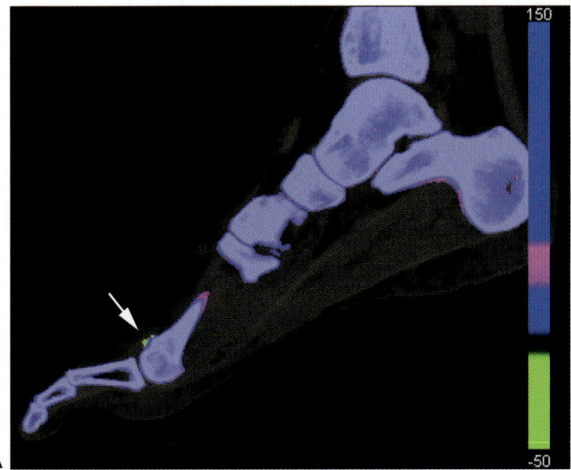 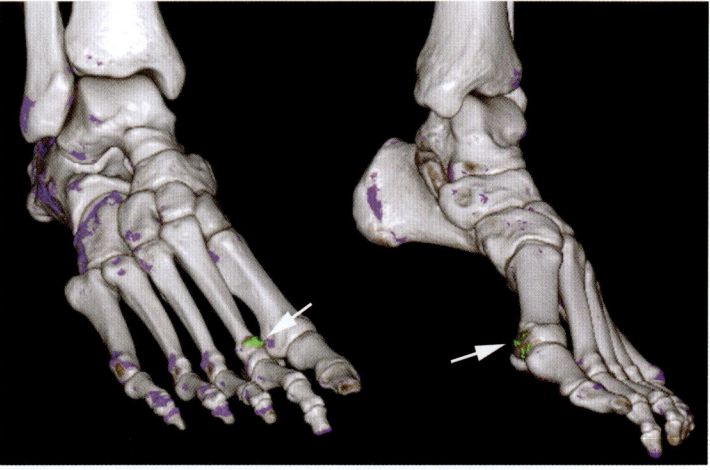

Figure 13.16 **Dual-energy CT gout protocol in a patient with right second metatarsophalangeal pain and swelling. (A)** Sagittal color map reformatted image demonstrates focal uric acid deposition dorsal to the right second metatarsal head (*arrow*), which is consistent with gout and was helpful clinically to differentiate the findings from infection. For this protocol, 2D color map images are able to discriminate certain materials of different anatomic numbers from one another. By convention, structures containing sufficient amounts of calcium, such as bone, are assigned blue or purple colors, while areas of uric acid deposition are mapped with a green color. **(B)** 3D reformatted image of the same patient was helpful in detecting other foci of uric acid that were clinically silent at the time of imaging. On this image, there was a second tophus along the left first metatarsal head (*arrow*), which was not previously noted to be clinically active.

bone and soft tissue adjacent to orthopedic implants. Finally, DECT can be helpful following the injection of intravenous contrast to map the deposition of the iodinated contrast agent, which may make enhancing areas more conspicuous or provide virtual noncontrast images without having to scan the patient before and after contrast administration.[19]

Since DECT requires specific scanners, some institutions may not offer this technique or may need to schedule patients on a DECT scanner if patients have appropriate indications. Furthermore, DECT may result in higher radiation dose to the patient. However, modern CT systems employ techniques, such as dose modulation, to greatly reduce radiation exposure, and the foot and ankle are thinner than other regions of the body, which allows lower energy x-ray beams to penetrate the tissues easily to decrease the radiation dose. Moreover, the extremities are not very radiosensitive and are sufficiently far from typically radiosensitive organs, such as the gonads, thyroid gland, and eyes, which helps to greatly limit radiation to these areas.[20]

CBCT uses an x-ray beam rotating around the anatomy of interest to produce a cylindrical volume of imaging data that is mathematically reconstructed so the data can be displayed as recognizable anatomy in the form of a planar image similar to a conventional radiograph (Fig. 13.17), a contiguous stack of cross-sectional images in any imaging plane, or 3D surface rendering.[21]

CBCT offers many advantages for foot ankle imaging, perhaps the biggest of which is the ability to perform weight-bearing studies. This provides a more physiologic assessment of bony alignment and may help foot and ankle surgeons diagnose cases of instability and plan more anatomically appropriate surgical corrections. The only other weight-bearing imaging modality commonly in clinical use is conventional radiography. However, as previously noted, conventional radiographs are subject to parallax, while the planar images obtained by cone-beam techniques do not suffer this distortion, and osseous alignment can be measured more accurately.[22] CBCT offers very high spatial resolution of bone, which provides exquisite trabecular and cortical detail. Moreover, current CBCT systems used in orthopedic clinical settings have much smaller footprints than conventional whole-body CT systems, and they are often self-shielded. Therefore, a CBCT device can be placed in a smaller location than a whole-body CT and does not require expensive shielding of the walls. Because the devices are self-shielded, there is no significant radiation to technologists or radiosensitive regions of the body. Finally, these systems are much less expensive than larger, whole-body systems.[21]

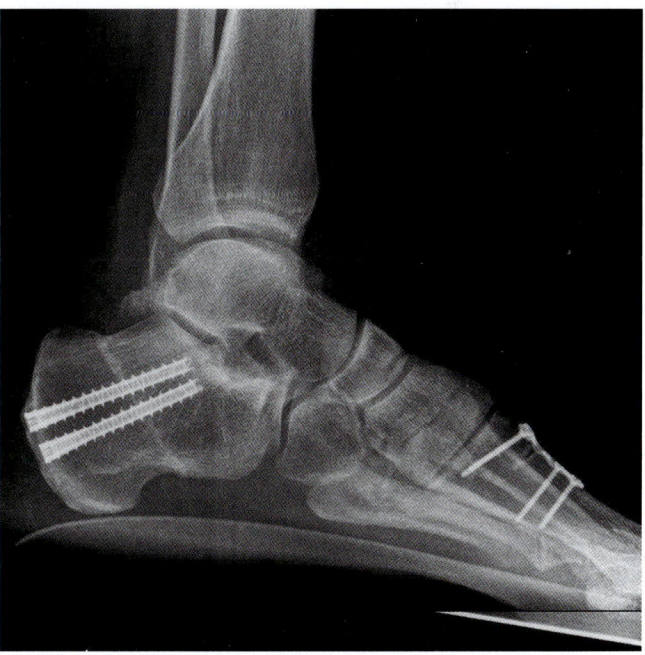

Figure 13.17 **Planar lateral image of the ankle and midfoot from a cone-beam CT acquisition.** The images from this technique are slightly grainier that conventional radiographs. However, they do not suffer from parallax, which helps to provide more accurate treatment planning.

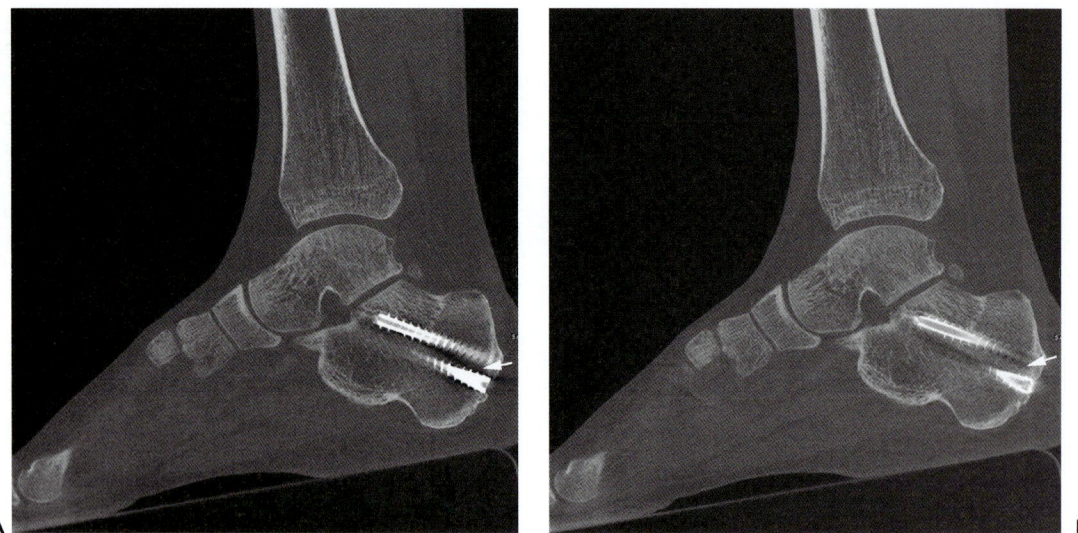

Figure 13.18 Cone-beam CT of the ankle with metal artifact reduction. (A) Sagittal reformatted image of the hindfoot without metal artifact reduction in a patient with calcaneal osteotomy shows degradation of image detail around the screws and particularly between them (*arrow*). **(B)** With metal artifact reduction, the trabecular detail is much better seen (*arrow*). Since the metal artifact reduction relies on a mathematical interpolation, both sets of images should be examined to give a more complete assessment of the bone and soft tissues around metal implants.

Similar to whole-body CT scanners, CBCT can produce 3D surface renderings of the bones and orthopedic hardware that are useful for surgical planning, and there are metal artifact reduction techniques that better visualize the bone and soft tissue surrounding metal implants to look for implant displacement and peri-hardware osteolysis (Fig. 13.18). Whole-body CT scanners often produce smoother, more visually pleasing renderings and metal artifact reduction; however, CBCT images are quite diagnostic.

On the other hand, CBCT has some important drawbacks to consider before deciding which type of CT scan a patient may need. The device's smaller footprint results in a smaller field-of-view that generally excludes a portion of an average-sized foot and ankle. As a result, suspected hindfoot pathology will not usually include the distal forefoot, and suspected forefoot pathology may not include the posterior calcaneus. Although the spatial resolution is exquisite for bone detail, there is substantial noise on the images that makes soft tissues look grainy and difficult to characterize (Fig. 13.19). To generate aesthetically pleasing 3D surface renderings, the cross-sectional images need to be acquired at submillimeter increments,

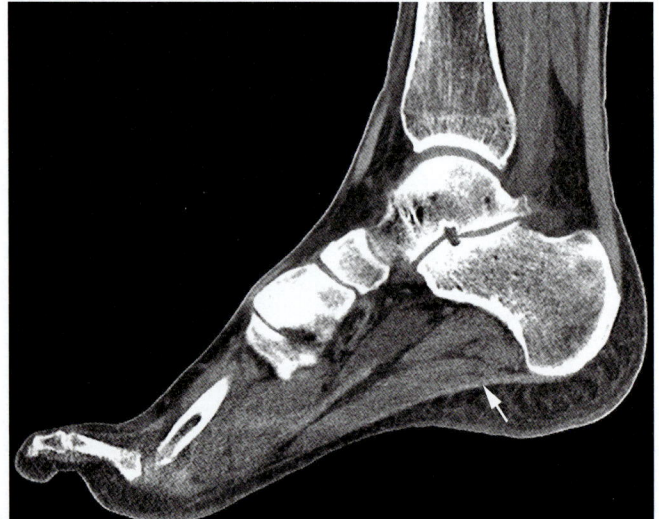
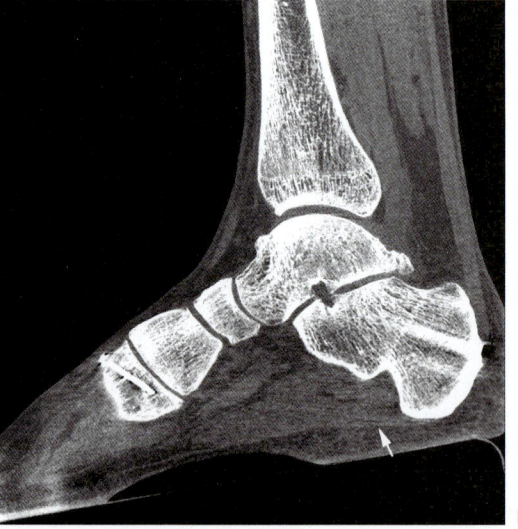

Figure 13.19 Comparison of whole-body CT and cone-beam CT in assessing the soft tissues. (A) Sagittal whole-body CT reformatted image is able to include the entire foot and ankle. The soft tissues appear smooth with sharp margination of the intermuscular fascial planes. Structures like the plantar fascia (*arrow*), ligaments, and tendons appear slightly hyperdense compared with skeletal muscle and fluid, which allows them to be better identified and characterized. **(B)** Sagittal cone-beam CT image of the hindfoot and midfoot at the same level has a smaller field-of-view that excludes the toes and some of the metatarsophalangeal joints. There is a noisy appearance of the soft tissues with decreased contrast resolution. As a result, the plantar fascia (*arrow*), ligaments, and tendons have a similar density to skeletal muscle, which may preclude adequate characterization.

which greatly increase the number of images to examine and can lead to fatigue for those viewing the studies. Finally, many measurements of the foot and ankle have been verified for weight-bearing conventional radiography. However, given the distortion noted on radiography, these measurements would need to be verified again for weight-bearing CBCT before they can be applied clinically.[23,24]

Based on the strengths and weakness of the CBCT, there are a number of common indications, including preoperative assessment of osteoarthritis and anatomic alignment, confirmation of fractures that may be suspected on radiography, assessment of fracture healing and estimation of the degree of bridging trabeculae, and assessment of orthopedic hardware alignment and complications, such as hardware fracture, loosening, or malalignment. Some centers have used CBCT to perform CT arthrography when characterizing articular cartilage loss or the stability of osteochondral defects. However, if CT assessment of soft tissue structures, such as tendons, ligaments, or muscle, is needed, a whole-body CT scanner may be a better choice.[21,22]

MAGNETIC RESONANCE IMAGING

After obtaining initial radiographs, MRI is often the test of choice to further image the foot and ankle. In the ankle, MRI is most commonly indicated when assessing the tendons and ligaments,[25,26] neurovascular structures such as within the tarsal tunnel, plantar fascia,[27] and the osseous structures to look for radiographically occult fractures,[28] detect findings of ankle impingement syndromes,[29] and characterize osteochondral injuries of the talar dome.[30] Within the forefoot, the most common MRI indications include evaluation for signs of infection,[31] detection of stress fractures[32] and Morton neuromas,[33] and assessment of plantar plate injuries or other causes of metatarsalgia.[34] MRI has much better contrast resolution when compared with other imaging modalities and allows discrimination of subtle changes in signal that often indicates pathology.[35] While CT is useful for looking for cortical disruption, areas of osteolysis or subtle calcification, abnormalities affecting the marrow like fractures and contusions, neoplasms, and inflammation may only be seen on MRI.[36] MRI also can give better insight into the chemical composition of structures such as determining lipid[37,38] or fluid content.[39] This can noninvasively provide specificity to many diagnoses and help direct appropriate management.

MRI serves as an excellent survey of anatomy and pathology because it can include large fields-of-view. This distinguishes MRI from diagnostic ultrasound, which currently uses focused imaging to examine specific structures. Furthermore, ultrasound relies on high-frequency transducers to generate high spatial resolution images of near-field structures like tendons and ligaments. Unlike ultrasound in which the use of lower frequency transducers to adequately penetrate deep structures significantly decreases spatial resolution, MRI is able to generate diagnostic images of deep musculoskeletal structures in most patients. Additionally, the ultrasound beam does not effectively penetrate bone and has little utility in assessing internal bone pathology. On the other hand, MRI is commonly used to look at the internal structure of bone like the marrow cavity. Finally, MRI can reproducibly generate images of the foot and ankle in standard orthogonal planes, in addition to obtaining images in nonstandard planes that may better show anatomy and pathology. Even though specific pulse sequences may differ from one institution to another, MRI protocols are routinely uniform within an institution, which improves standardization of interpretation. Meanwhile, ultrasound currently has greater operator-dependence and relies on sonographers to obtain images that best depict pathology and to give anatomic reference points.

▶ Pulse Sequences

Most MRI protocols employ a combination of high spatial resolution sequences and fluid-sensitive sequences. High spatial resolution sequences include non–fat-suppressed T1-weighted or proton density sequences (Fig. 13.20A,C) and allow discrimination of small structures from one another with excellent edge definition of these structures. T1-weighted sequences are relatively insensitive to fluid, which appears low in signal, but are useful for assessing edge detail of bones and trabecular injury. Proton density sequences are intermediate in weighting with fluid appearing higher in signal than skeletal muscle but not to the same degree as in more heavily fluid sensitive pulse sequences.[36] Both of these sequences use low echo times (TE) during image acquisition, making them susceptible to an artifact called magic angle. In this phenomenon, structures like ligaments and tendons that have a parallel fiber arrangement and are oriented at 55° to the axis of the magnetic field may exhibit intermediate signal on pulse sequences with low or intermediate TE (≤25 ms) like T1-weighted and proton density techniques. This is especially important in the musculoskeletal system and commonly seen in foot and ankle imaging where a number of tendons, such as the peroneal tendons, have a curvilinear course and often demonstrate focal signal alterations due to artifact that can be misinterpreted as tendinopathy.[40]

Fluid sensitive sequences include short tau inversion recovery (STIR) or fat-suppressed T2-weighted sequences (Fig. 13.20B) and are useful since most pathologies, including fluid collections, soft tissue edema, and marrow signal abnormalities, are high in signal on these sequences. The exquisite contrast resolution of MRI used in conjunction with techniques that suppress the signal from fat in the subcutaneous tissues or within the yellow marrow allows otherwise subtle signal alteration to become more visible (Fig. 13.21). Current T2-weighted fat-suppressed techniques identify frequencies associated with fat and selectively suppress them (frequency-selective fat suppression). The STIR sequence is a T1-weighted technique in which the T1 signal mainly seen in fat and yellow marrow is inverted, effectively suppressing fat.[41] The TE is also elevated which introduces T2-weighting to the image and causes fluid and edema to appear high in signal intensity. Thus, this sequence appears similar to a T2-weight fat-suppressed image.

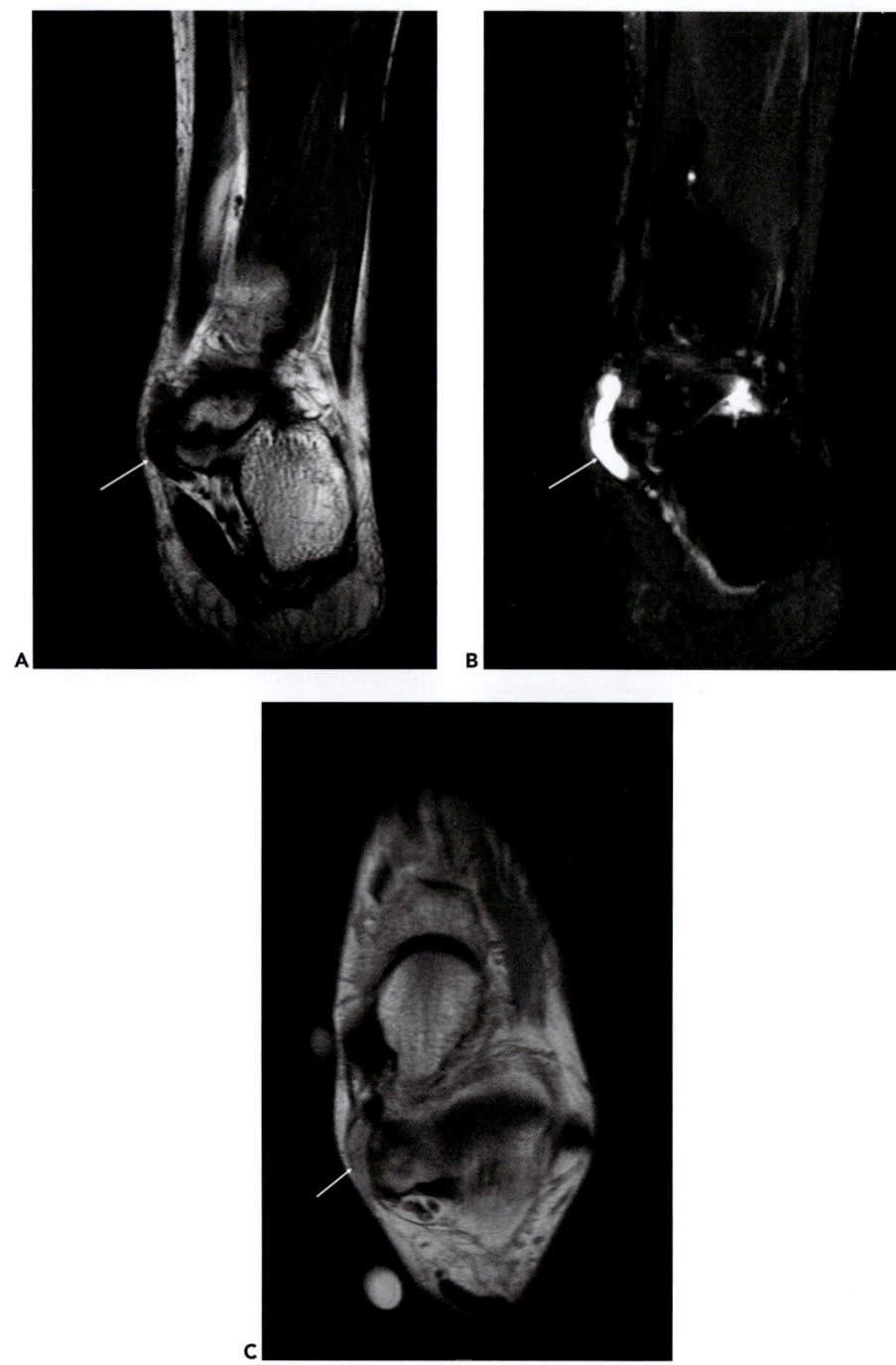

Figure 13.20 **Standard appearance of pulse sequences commonly used in musculoskeletal imaging.** **(A)** Coronal T1-weighted non–fat-suppressed (NFS) image of the hindfoot at the level of the posterior subtalar joint shows adipose and yellow marrow as high signal, bright structures. The skeletal muscle is intermediate in signal, while the fluid within a medial ganglion cyst arising from the posterior subtalar joint is lower in signal intensity to skeletal muscle. **(B)** Coronal T2-weighted fat-suppressed (FS) image of the hindfoot at a similar level shows darkening of the fat and yellow marrow related to frequency-selective fat suppression. The fluid in the ganglion cyst is much brighter than skeletal muscle, which is intermediate in signal intensity. **(C)** Axial NFS proton density of the hindfoot through the ganglion cyst shows sharp anatomic detail. The fluid within the ganglion cyst is brighter than the extensor digitorum brevis skeletal muscle but slightly darker than the adjacent subcutaneous fat. However, the differences are much less conspicuous than on fat-suppressed images, and the lesion could be missed on initial interpretation without comparing to the T2-weighted FS sequence.

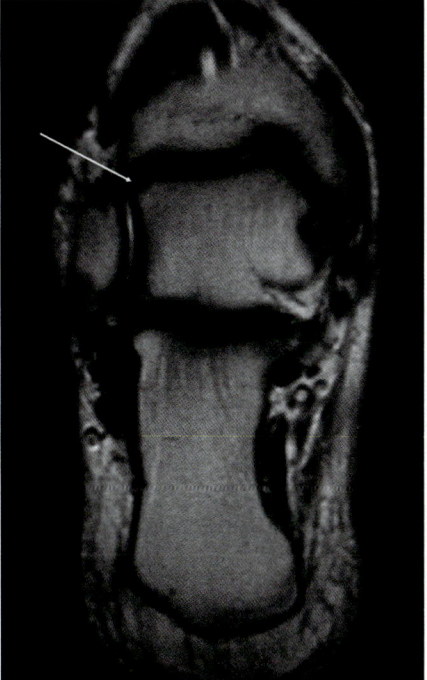 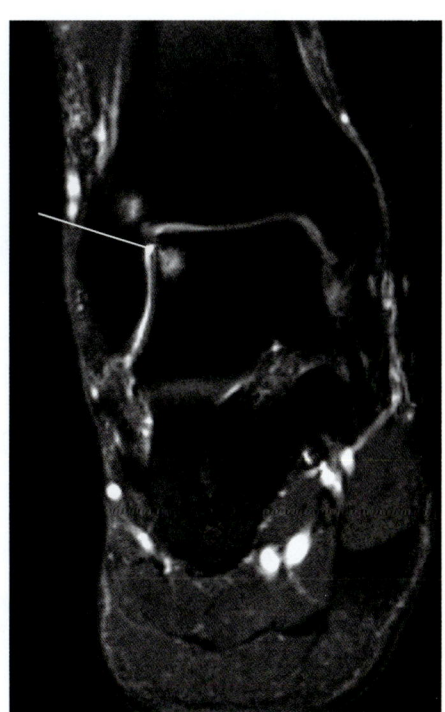

Figure 13.21 Effect of fat suppression on fluid-sensitive sequences. (A) Coronal oblique T2-weighted non–fat-suppressed image of the hindfoot in a 25-year-old woman shows subtle cortical irregularity (arrow) along the lateral talar dome indicating an osteochondral lesion. (B) Coronal T2-weighted fat-suppressed image of the hindfoot at a similar level shows focal marrow signal abnormality (arrow) in this area not seen on the non–fat-suppressed sequence, which makes the lesion more conspicuous.

While similar in appearance, T2-weighted and STIR sequences have important differences that may influence when they are used. The T2-weighted fat-suppressed sequence has a higher signal-to-noise ratio (SNR), and the extra signal can be used to achieve better spatial resolution. However, it is more susceptible to magnetic field inhomogeneity and commonly produces inhomogeneous fat suppression.[41] Furthermore, complete failure of the frequency-selective fat-suppression may actually cause water suppression where fluid and edema appear dark and fat appears bright. This may obscure areas of edema or other signal abnormalities and prevent accurate diagnosis of pathology. This inhomogeneity is often seen with imaging structures that have complex morphology, such as the foot and ankle. On the other hand, the STIR sequence generally has robust, uniform fat suppression and is more sensitive in detecting fluid and marrow signal abnormalities. However, its generally poorer spatial resolution may limit its use in the foot and ankle because it may not adequately characterize a number of small but important structures (Fig. 13.22). Although both sequences are among the longer sequences routinely used in current musculoskeletal MRI protocols, STIR sequences tend to be longer, which may impact patient comfort and limit the number of studies that can be performed per day. Many institutions have used a combined approach in which a STIR sequence is used in one plane as a survey view, and T2-weighted fat-suppressed sequences are used in other planes. Using this method, the T2-weighted images can be used to examine the anatomy and look for areas of possible marrow edema, while the STIR sequence can be used to confirm areas of high T2 signal. If these areas persist on STIR images, they are likely real; while if they are not seen on the STIR images, they are likely related to inhomogeneity of the fat suppression.

As the spatial resolution and ability of MRI scanners to detect subtle alterations in the composition of material improve, hyaline cartilage imaging is becoming more widely indicated. MRI has long been used to diagnose or characterize osteochondral lesions predominantly of the talar dome. A number of pulse sequences have been used to assess hyaline cartilage in an effort to identify cartilage disease before the underlying subchondral bone becomes affected. Pulse sequences designed to evaluate the morphology of cartilage should have both high spatial resolution to be able to identify subtle chondral surface defects and contrast resolution to perceive changes in the cartilage infrastructure like chondral edema or blistering.[42] The most common sequences currently used include high-resolution T2-weighted or proton density fast spin echo techniques in which the cartilage appears intermediate in signal between fluid, which is bright, and the underlying bone marrow, which is dark, and gradient echo techniques in which the cartilage often appears brighter than skeletal muscle. Like spin echo or fast spin echo sequences, which are more commonly used in musculoskeletal imaging, gradient echo sequences can either be T1-weighted or T2-weighted depending on the sequence parameters. Using these techniques, one can obtain very thin section, high-resolution imaging of the imaged anatomy. However, they tend to have poorer soft tissue contrast than equivalent spin echo sequences (Fig. 13.23). Furthermore, gradient echo sequences are susceptible to signal voids from metal and calcification, which limits their utility in examining bone pathology or in studying postoperative patients.[43] In addition to these morphologic cartilage techniques, several newer sequences, including delayed gadolinium-enhanced MRI of cartilage (dGEMRIC) which helps to show local glycosaminoglycan content, T1 rho mapping which indicates proteoglycan content, and T2

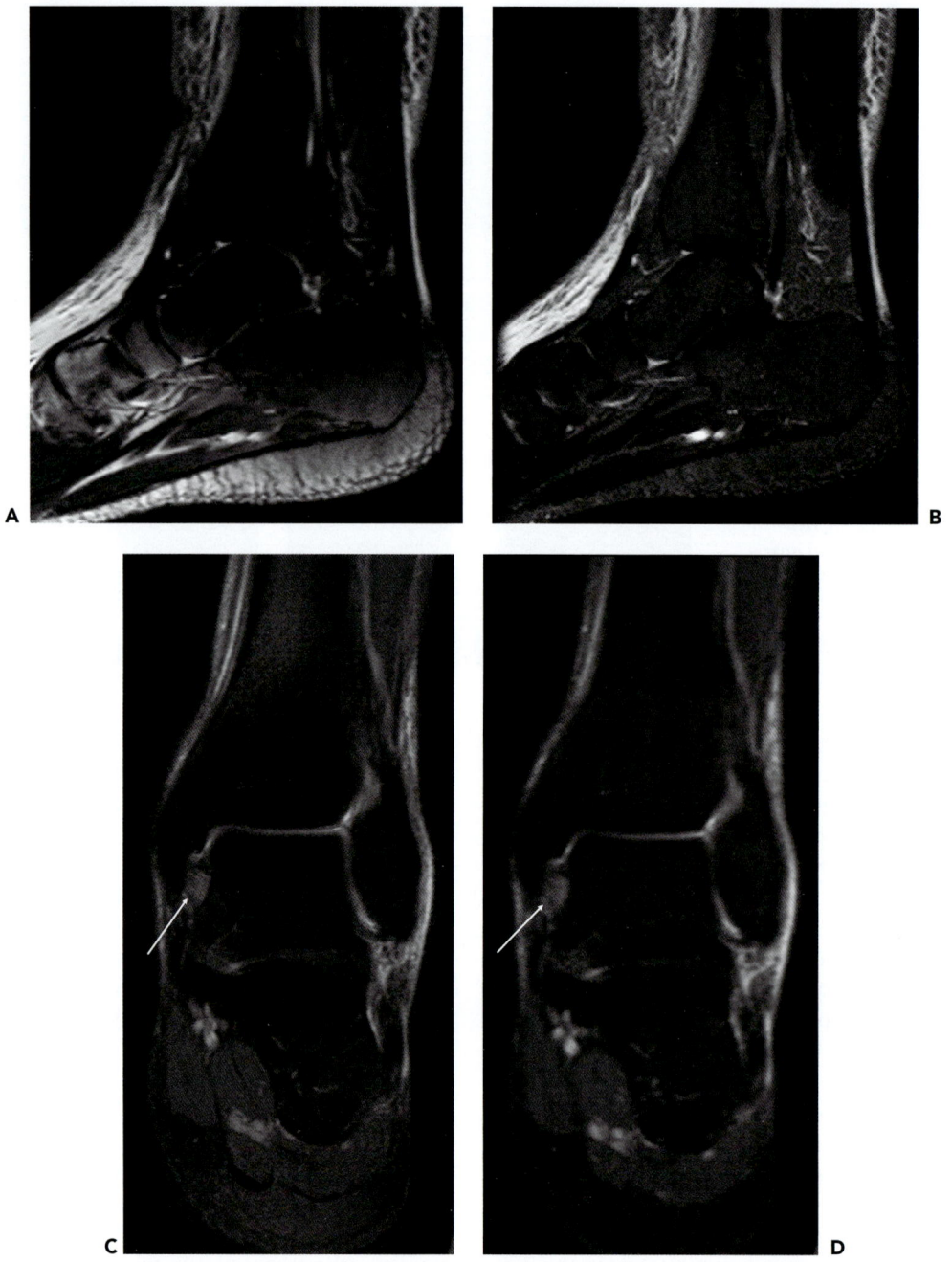

Figure 13.22 **Difference between T2-weighted FS and STIR images. (A)** Sagittal T2-weighted FS image of the ankle shows good spatial resolution of the anatomic structures. However, there is inhomogeneous fat-suppression along the distal and plantar aspect of the midfoot. Without adequate fat-suppression, soft tissue or marrow pathology in this region could be missed. **(B)** Sagittal STIR image of the hindfoot at a similar level shows uniform fat suppression. No marrow or soft tissue edema is seen. However, the STIR images have poorer signal-to-noise ratio and consequently have poorer spatial resolution. Both T2-weighted and STIR sequences show marked dorsal subcutaneous edema. **(C)** However, the corresponding T2-weighted FS image shows much sharper edge detail. For example, the edges of the fibers of the deltoid ligament (*arrows*) are more clearly defined than on the corresponding STIR image. **(D)** Coronal STIR image again shows homogeneous fat-suppression.

mapping which shows water content, have been used to analyze the composition of hyaline cartilage and predict areas of chondral degeneration or injury.[44]

T1-weighted pulse sequences are also useful in musculoskeletal imaging to detect gadolinium chelate contrast media that are commonly administered intravenously or intra-articularly during MR arthrography. The T1-shortening effect of gadolinium-based contrast agents causes them to become conspicuous on T1-weighted sequences. These techniques are performed in conjunction with fat-suppression techniques to make the gadolinium contrast agent even more evident (Fig. 13.24). When administered intravenously, contrast media help to detect areas

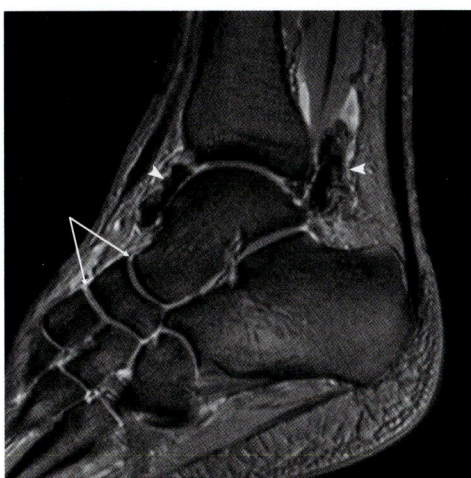

Figure 13.23 Gradient echo imaging in a patient with pigmented villonodular synovitis (PVNS). A sagittal T2-weighted FS gradient echo image in a 43-year-old woman with ankle pain and swelling shows lobulated low-signal-intensity soft tissue surrounding the tibiotalar joint anteriorly and posteriorly (*arrowheads*). Although gradient echo images often cause markedly accentuated signal voids in the region of metal and calcium (called blooming), which limits its usefulness in the musculoskeletal system, the presence of blooming associated with the periarticular soft tissue is characteristic of PVNS, and a diagnosis can be made with direct tissue sampling. Additionally, the soft tissue contrast resolution is not as great as in typical spin echo sequences (as seen in the figure), which may also limit the ability to detect subtle signal abnormalities. Although the sequence is not optimized to evaluate articular cartilage, the intertarsal and tibiotalar cartilage is well seen (*arrows*) with similar signal intensity to the skeletal muscle. The cartilage is conspicuous adjacent to the subchondral bone.

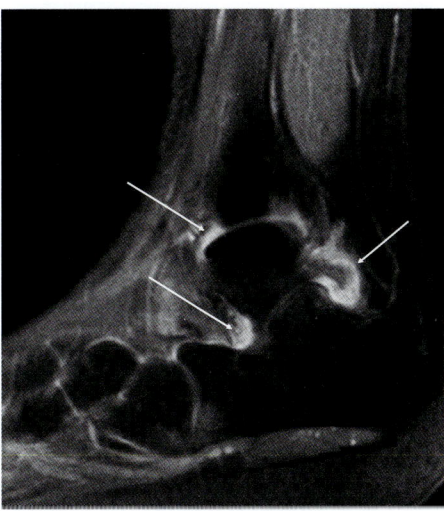

Figure 13.24 Postcontrast T1-weighted FS image. Sagittal T1-weighted FS image of the ankle and hindfoot in a 35-year-old woman shows enhancing synovial proliferation around the tibiotalar and subtalar joints (*arrows*) in a patient with previously undiagnosed rheumatoid arthritis. The enhancement helps to identify the degree of involvement, additional sites of disease, and developing erosions. It can also be helpful to assess disease activity following therapy.

of inflammation or hyperemia, such as in infections or inflammatory arthropathies. They can also be helpful to characterize whether a lesion is solid or cystic or determine the extent of intralesional necrosis.[45,46]

▶ Patient Position

Proper patient positioning for MRI is critical in the foot and ankle. Many centers image the patient while supine in a neutral position, including between 20° and 30° of external rotation. The foot may be imaged with its long axis at a right angle to the long axis of the lower extremity, or with about 15° to 20° of plantar flexion. Some authors have reported several benefits from imaging the patient with mild plantar flexion. These include reduction of magic angle phenomenon, better delineation of the plane between the peroneal tendons at the lateral malleolar level, and improved visualization of the calcaneofibular ligament.[40,47] On the other hand, plantar flexion may make assessment of the Achilles tendon more difficult. Although supine patient positioning is more common, some centers may place the patient prone and plantarflex the ankle to a greater degree. This limits the magic angle effect and improves imaging of the midfoot and forefoot[48,49] but also can prevent adequate assessment of some of the hindfoot structures such as the Achilles tendon.[50] Thus, the patient position should be modified based on patient symptoms and the clinical concerns whenever possible.

The foot should be centered within the bore of the magnet when possible since this area provides the study the highest SNR and spatial resolution. Once in the coil the foot should be comfortably immobilized to try to prevent motion, which can degrade imaging. It is also important to select an appropriate coil targeted to the body part of interest. Coils are devices that transmit radiofrequency (RF) pulses used to excite sections of the body prior to imaging, and receive and amplify RF pulses generated by the body in response to the excitation pulse. The RF pulses detected by coils provide the information MRI scanners need to produce images. The amplification process improves/increases the SNR and consequently the spatial resolution. Thus, coils that are well-contoured for a specific body part have a dramatic impact on the appearance of the images.

▶ MRI Techniques

The foot and ankle can be divided into three parts for the purposes of imaging: the forefoot, midfoot, and hindfoot/ankle. Since many of the common foot and ankle pathologies sent for MRI either involve the forefoot or hindfoot, and since the midfoot is frequently included on forefoot or hindfoot imaging, only forefoot and hindfoot protocols may be routinely necessary.[51] Specialized midfoot protocols can be prescribed if the clinical interest is limited to the midfoot.[52] In designing routine hindfoot and forefoot protocols, it is important to limit the field-of-view to the body part being examined. For example, the hindfoot field-of-view should be about 12 to 14 cm, while the forefoot should be about 8 to 12 cm depending on the size of the patient.[53] The smaller field-of-view improves spatial resolution, while larger field-of-view imaging may be useful as an overall survey to better visualize anatomy and anatomic alignment. In addition, larger field-of-view images can be used as an adjunct to extend coverage to additional areas of suspected pathology that may be incompletely characterized on initial small field-of-view images. Imaging of the entire foot and ankle is uncommon in many musculoskeletal radiology practices and may be reserved for the assessment of inflammatory arthropathy or infections, when detailed characterization of small structures like tendons, ligaments, and articular cartilage is unnecessary.

Most MRI protocols image the foot and ankle in three standard orthogonal planes: axial, coronal, and sagittal (see Appendix). In the forefoot, the coronal and axial planes are carried on from the rest of the lower extremity. Therefore, the coronal plane is equivalent to the short axis of the forefoot, while the axial plane is equivalent to the horizontal long axis. However, some institutions may commonly refer to the horizontal long axis of the forefoot as the coronal plane and the short axis of the forefoot as the axial plane, causing confusion.[53-55] The terms *short axis* and *horizontal long axis* can be used to refer to the coronal and axial planes, respectively, in order to avoid confusion. It is important to prescribe the planes of imaging according to the axes of the foot and ankle rather than the long axis of the calf or the magnetic field. This will help to standardize depiction of foot and ankle anatomy and may make certain structures more easily seen.

Some structures are particularly well seen in specific planes, and it is important to have a checklist of structures to be assessed on each plane in order to perform a thorough interpretation. In the ankle, the axial images depict most structures in cross-section, including the tendons and many ligaments. The coronal images are better to look at the insertions of some of the tendons, including the posterior tibialis and peroneal tendons and the distal portions of the flexor hallucis longus and flexor digitorum longus tendons, as well as the plantar fascia, deltoid and spring ligaments. Because the calcaneofibular ligament is oblique to the standard axial and coronal planes, both planes should be used to adequately assess this structure. Alternatively, an oblique sequence can be performed along the long axis of the ligament. However, obtaining this may increase scanning times. The sagittal sequence is useful as an overview of the ankle, providing information about osseous alignment and to look for fluid collections such as tibiotalar or subtalar joint effusions or bursal fluid around the Achilles tendon. It is also helpful to see the Achilles tendon and plantar fascia in long axis.[55]

In the forefoot, the coronal images depict many of the most important structures, such as the flexor and extensor tendons, the intrinsic foot musculature, the hallux sesamoid complex, digital neurovascular bundles to diagnose Morton neuromas, and plantar plates, in cross-section. The axial images are useful in examining the osseous alignment, collateral ligaments of the metatarsophalangeal and interphalangeal joints, and the Lisfranc ligament. The sagittal images are also used to examine osseous alignment, to look for stress reaction or stress fractures particularly in the metatarsals, and to see the plantar plates in long axis.[55]

ARTHROGRAPHY

With the advent of cross-sectional imaging techniques, arthrography has become increasingly indicated to evaluate specific conditions in the ankle. Direct arthrography of the ankle is a two-step imaging modality in which a contrast medium is percutaneously instilled into the tibiotalar joint generally through an anterior or anteromedial approach with fluoroscopic or possibly sonographic guidance.[56] This causes joint capsular distension and increased intra-articular pressure, which force contrast into ligamentous, capsular, or chondral defects. Since some processes, such as arthrofibrosis, affect the distensibility of the joint capsule, the degree of capsular distensibility can also be assessed during the procedure. The patient is then imaged either by MRI or by CT (Fig. 13.25), preferably within 30 minutes of injection to evaluate the position of the contrast. Contrast extravasation in unexpected locations can suggest particular pathologies.

Unfortunately, there are several disadvantages to arthrography that may prevent this technique from being more widely used. First, it converts a noninvasive cross-sectional examination into an invasive procedure and exposes the patients to the risks involved with intra-articular or intravenous needle placement. These include infection, bleeding, and injury to nearby structures such as blood vessels and nerves. These risks are minimized by using aseptic technique and approaching

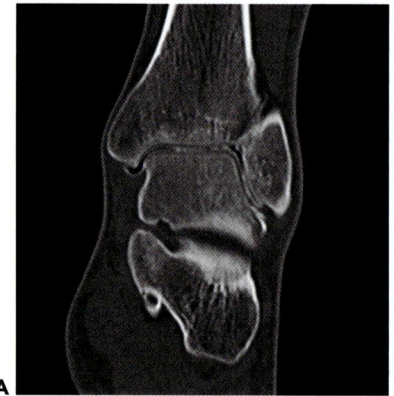

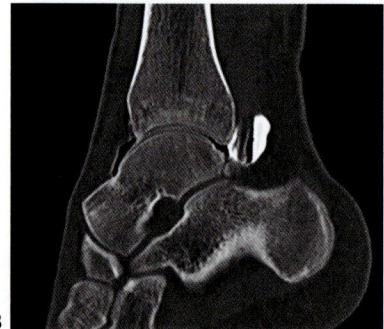

Figure 13.25 Single-contrast CT arthrography. Coronal (**A**) and sagittal (**B**) reformatted CT images of the hindfoot following intra-articular iodinated contrast administration outline the intra-articular structures and show a smooth surface of the hyaline cartilage.

the joint medial to the dorsalis pedis artery. In addition, while most patients tolerate this procedure well, placement of the needle and capsular distension often lead to greater patient discomfort. Furthermore, when fluoroscopy is used, the patient is also briefly subjected to ionizing radiation. As a result, the patient should be appropriately shielded prior to the procedure and care should be taken to limit the time of radiation exposure as much as possible. Finally, arthrography increases the time and expense of imaging, factors that may cause this technique to remain primarily as a problem-solving modality.[56]

In the foot and ankle, arthrography is most commonly performed on the tibiotalar joint and improves the sensitivity and accuracy of detecting a number of pathologic entities. Ligament tears are often better seen on arthrography since the contrast in the distended joint capsule outlines ligament tears as it extravasates through the defect. Osteochondral injuries particularly involving the talar dome can be diagnosed and characterized with this technique since hyaline cartilage irregularities are better visualized as the contrast outlines the cartilage surface. Furthermore, contrast undermining an osteochondral fragment has been shown as a reliable sign of an unstable fragment. Intra-articular contrast helps to outline the capsular surface to detect intra-articular bodies, focal synovitis, or other intra-articular processes such as synovial osteochondromatosis, pigmented villonodular synovitis, or arthrofibrosis. Finally, arthrography can help diagnose ankle impingement syndromes, especially if the physical examination is inconclusive. These processes are often associated with focal synovitis in specific locations and may be seen in association with osteophytes, articular cartilage loss, or marrow edema. When using CT, ankle arthrography can be performed either as a single-contrast or as a double-contrast technique depending on the indication. If ligament injury is suspected, a single-contrast technique is preferable. However, if there is clinical concern for articular cartilage loss, a double-contrast technique in which a small amount of gas is injected into the joint following iodinated contrast infusion can be performed and followed by CT.[57] The double-contrast technique is not appropriate for MRI since susceptibility from the intra-articular gas would obscure adjacent tissues including articular cartilage and preclude their assessment. Arthrography for other foot and ankle joints is much less common although forefoot arthrography involving the metatarsophalangeal joints can be useful in assessing capsular integrity.[58]

While direct arthrography is much more common than indirect arthrography, indirect arthrography has both benefits and drawbacks that may influence its use. When this technique is used in the foot and ankle, intravenous contrast is administered after which the patient performs light exercise for 5 to 10 minutes prior to performing either CT or MRI. During this time, diffusion of contrast from the synovium causes intra-articular contrast accumulation. Because the contrast is administered systemically, it travels anywhere there is blood flow rather than discriminatorily entering the joint. Thus, many structures like granulation tissue, synovium, and blood vessels will enhance, making interpretation difficult. On the other hand, the enhancement can provide physiologic information regarding the degree of blood flow that may not be evident on routine cross-sectional studies. Unlike direct arthrography, in which one of the major benefits is capsular distension, the joint capsule is not distended in indirect arthrography, which may decrease the sensitivity for detecting ligament and chondral injury. Lastly, a preexisting joint effusion may increase the intra-articular pressure, prevent adequate contrast diffusion into the joint, and limit the effectiveness of the technique.[59,60]

Indirect arthrography can be indicated in patients who have undergone direct arthrography but are discovered during the subsequent MRI to have incomplete joint distension. In this situation, indirect arthrography, which may allow enough intra-articular contrast to be visible to obtain a diagnostic study, can be performed rather than taking the patient off the MRI scanner and rescheduling the study.

RADIONUCLIDE BONE SCINTIGRAPHY

Unlike most other imaging modalities used to evaluate the musculoskeletal system, radionuclide bone scintigraphy, or bone scanning, provides a unique physiologic assessment of areas of bone metabolism and can be used to acquire whole-body images. This is performed by intravenously injecting a radiopharmaceutical, a combination of a gamma radiation–emitting radioisotope tagged to a ligand that has an affinity for accumulating in bone, and detecting the gamma rays with a gamma camera. The most commonly used radioisotope in bone scintigraphy is technicium-99m (^{99m}Tc), while diphosphonates, such as methylene diphosphonate (MDP), are excellent radioligands used in bone scanning due to their avidity for bone. ^{99m}Tc-MDP has excellent contrast between its target and background, providing improved spatial resolution compared with many other radiotracers. The patient is usually imaged between 2 and 3 hours following radiotracer injection. The degree of uptake depends on a number of factors, including blood flow, capillary permeability, intraosseous pressure, osteoblast metabolism, and rate of extraction.[61]

Bone scintigraphy is very sensitive in detecting areas of rapid bone turnover and can image the whole body at a relatively low cost. As such, it is often used to survey the bones for systemic processes like metastases (Fig. 13.26). However, the radiopharmaceutical can accumulate at any site where there is bone turnover and is not specific for particular processes. Therefore, the imaging of many conditions, including neoplasm, infection, and trauma, can have similar appearances.[62] One must view these studies in light of accurate and thorough clinical history to avoid misinterpretation. In addition, radionuclide bone scintigraphy has poorer spatial resolution compared with other imaging techniques, which may limit the ability to assign an accurate location to an area of increased radiotracer uptake.

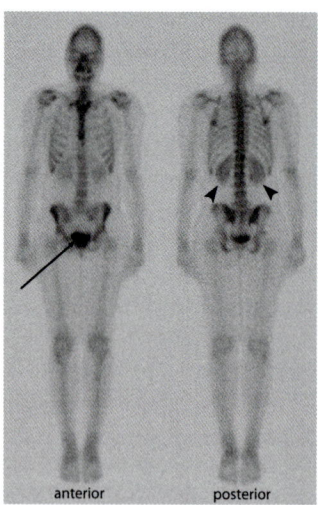

Figure 13.26 **Whole-body radionuclide bone scintigraphy.** Normal anterior (*left*) and posterior (*right*) views of the entire body show radiopharmaceutical (^{99m}Tc-MDP) osseous uptake, particularly in the axial skeleton. The spatial resolution of nuclear studies is poorer than other imaging modalities, although this technique can distinguish many individual bones such as the ribs to help in localizing lesions. There is excellent target-to-background ratio and little accumulation of the radiotracer in the soft tissues, which make the skeletal structures more conspicuous. The radiopharmaceutical is primarily excreted by the urinary tract. As a result, there is accumulation of the compound in the kidneys (*arrowheads*) and urinary bladder (*arrows*), which are also seen.

Imaging can be performed by several methods. The most well-established method is planar imaging, which is similar to conventional radiography because it creates two-dimensional images of three-dimensional objects. As a result, many structures can overlap one another and prevent estimation of depth. Imaging is either obtained of the whole body or with multiple spot images involving areas of interest. Because of their lower spatial resolution, these studies often need to be interpreted along with existing cross-sectional studies or be performed using one of the newer, CT-based techniques, such as single-photon emission computed tomography (SPECT) or a SPECT/CT fusion study, which aid in lesion localization. SPECT utilizes cross-sectional imaging to provide higher spatial resolution and improve the ability to detect and localize areas of abnormal radiopharmaceutical uptake.[63] Most recently, SPECT/CT fusion technology has allowed better localization and characterization of lesions by merging the physiologic data acquired through SPECT and the anatomic information obtained in CT imaging.[64]

In addition to the single-phase bone scan performed between 2 and 3 hours after injection, a three-phase bone scan is a common technique usually used to evaluate areas of inflammation. This technique takes advantage of the partial dependence of radiopharmaceutical accumulation on blood flow and capillary permeability to generate maps of regional hyperemia and inflammation. It does so by obtaining rapid serial images every 2 to 5 seconds soon after injection (flow phase), which detects perfusion, then a 5-minute delayed image (blood pool phase), which detects capillary permeability, and finally the standard 2- to 3-hour delayed images used to look for bone metabolism.

This procedure is most often used to differentiate soft tissue infections, in which there is often increased uptake on the first two phases only, and osteomyelitis, which shows uptake on the first two phases that persists on delayed images.[65]

APPENDIX: MRI ATLAS OF THE ANKLE/HINDFOOT AND FOREFOOT

This section contains an MRI atlas of the foot and ankle using high-resolution images performed on a 3-Tesla MRI. Many of the most commonly encountered structures are labeled whenever possible. It is divided into ankle/hindfoot and forefoot, and each body part is shown in the three standard orthogonal planes. In the ankle, the planes are sagittal, axial, and coronal, and the planes of section are continuous with those used in the calf. In the forefoot, the sagittal plane refers to the vertical long axis plane of the foot and has a similar orientation to the sagittal plane in the ankle/hindfoot. However, different authors refer to the short axis plane of the forefoot as the axial or transverse and the horizontal long axis plane as the coronal plane, while others continue the planes of reference from the ankle/hindfoot and refer to the short axis plane as coronal and the horizontal long axis plane as axial or transverse. Some authors have replaced the use of axial or coronal in describing the plane of section in the forefoot with the terms *short axis* and *horizontal long axis*. For purposes of this text, the short axis of the forefoot will be referred to as *coronal* or *short axis*, while the horizontal long axis images will be referred to as *axial* or *horizontal long axis*.

List of abbreviations:

ADQ: abductor digiti quinti (also called abductor digiti minimi)
AT: anterior tibialis
EDB: extensor digitorum brevis
EDL: extensor digitorum longus
EHB: extensor hallucis brevis
EHL: extensor hallucis longus
FDB: flexor digitorum brevis
FDL: flexor digitorum longus
FDM: flexor digiti minimi
FHB: flexor hallucis brevis
FHL: flexor hallucis longus
n: nerve

SECTION 1. ANKLE/HINDFOOT

▶ Set 1. Sagittal Proton Density Non–Fat-Saturated Images of the Ankle/Hindfoot

Contiguous images are shown sequentially from lateral to medial, extending from the calf to the midfoot. This plane provides an anatomic survey of the bones and joints as well as long-axis imaging of the Achilles tendon and plantar fascia.

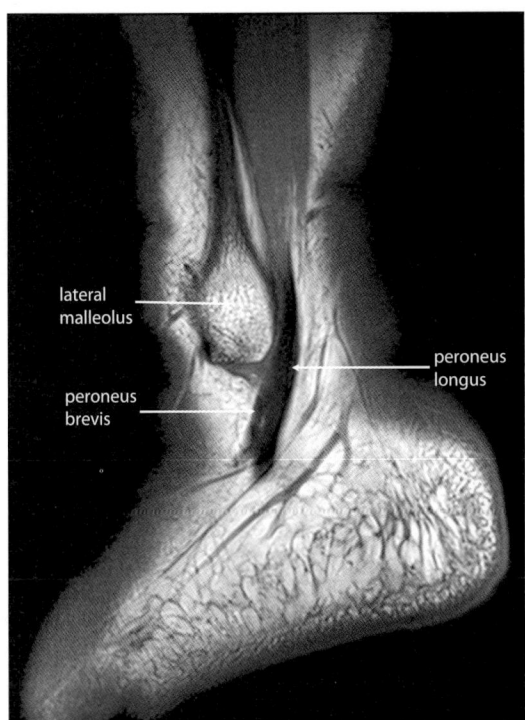
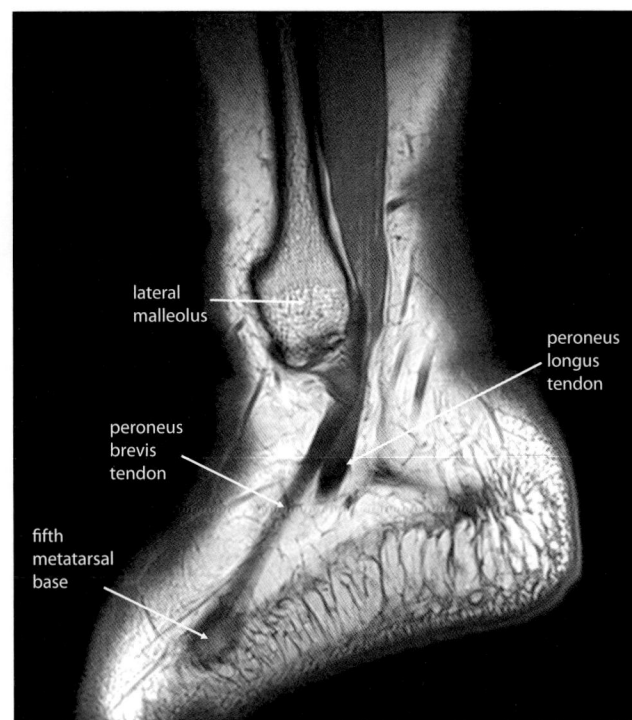
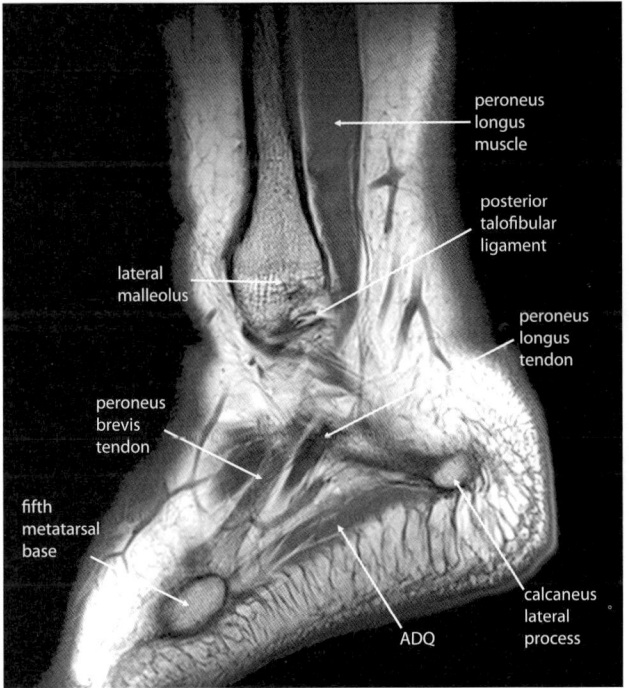
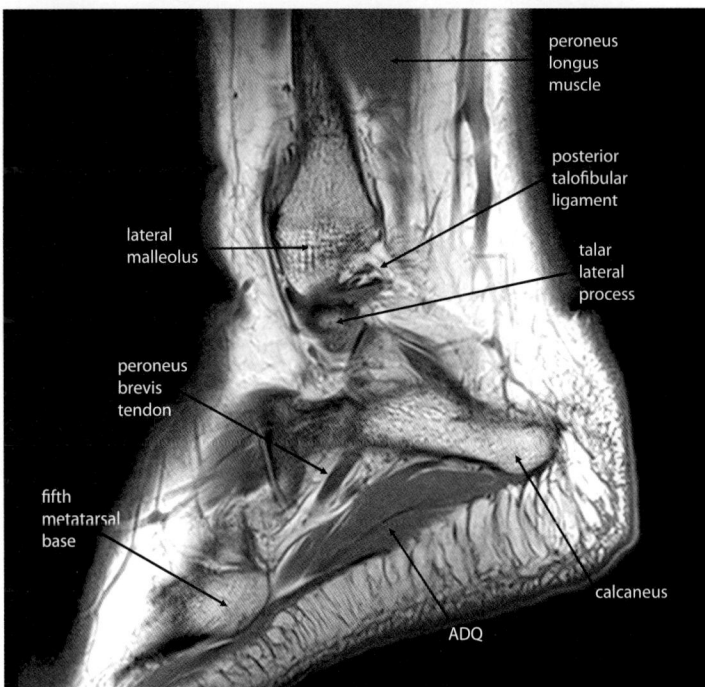

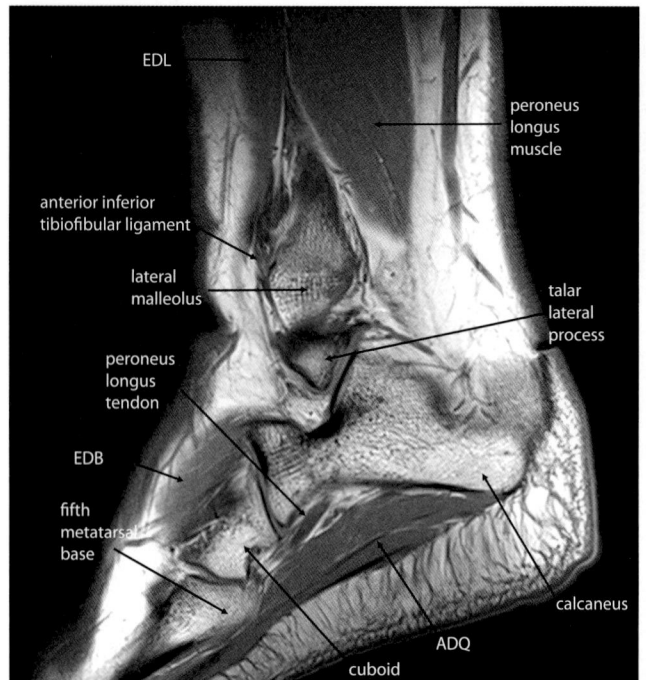
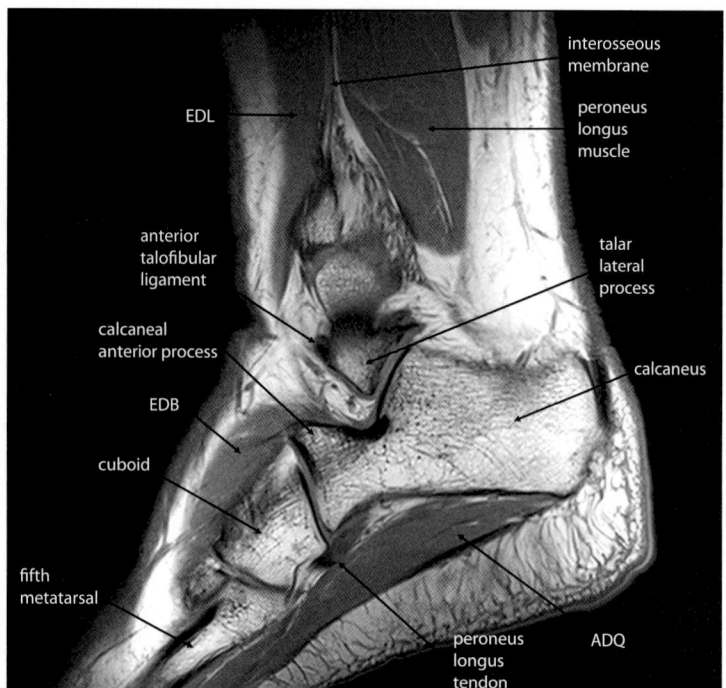
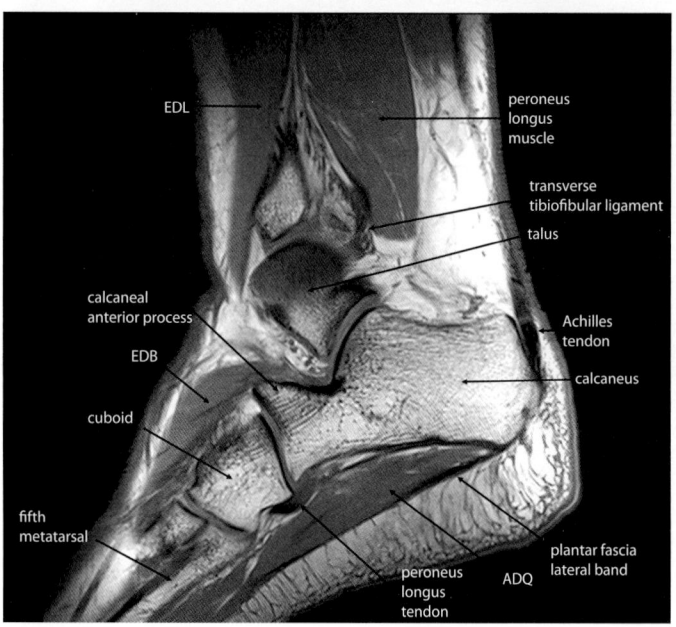
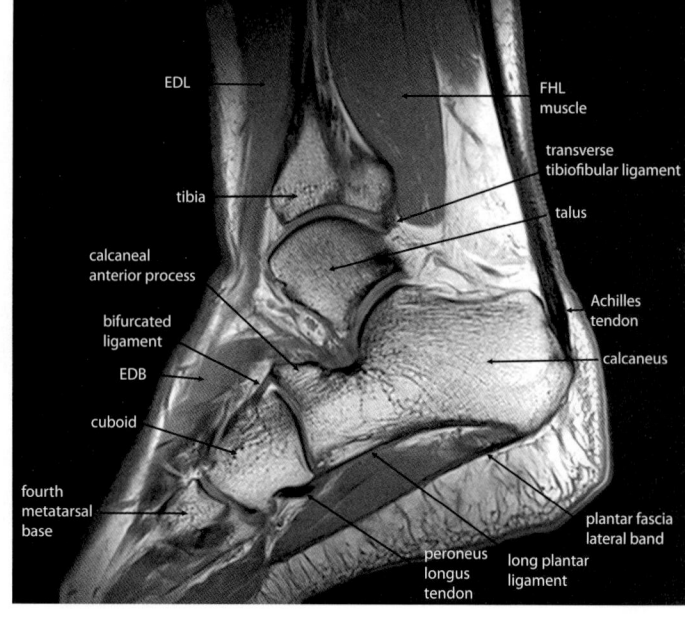

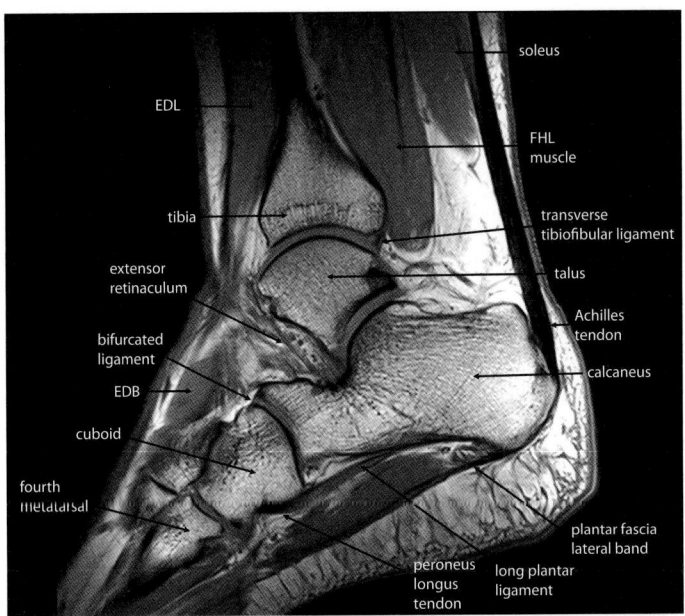
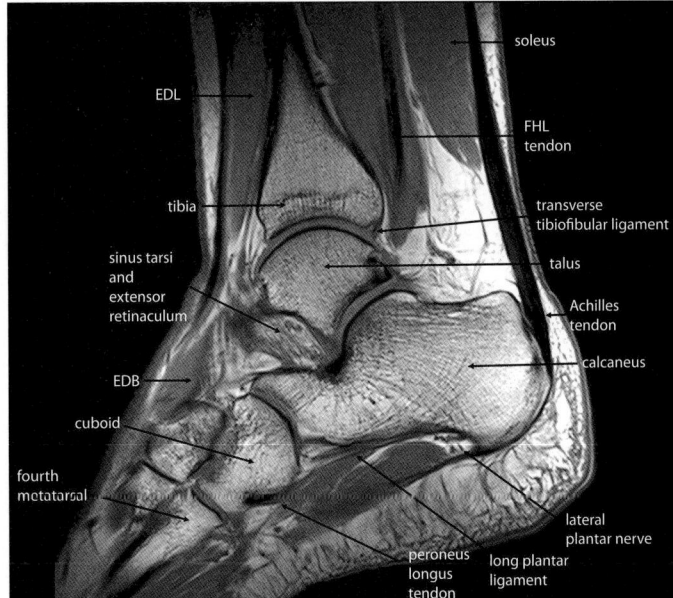
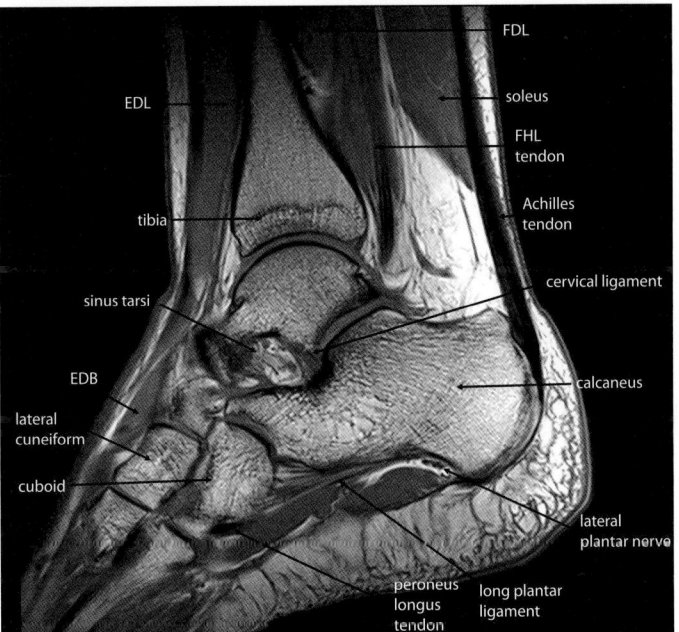
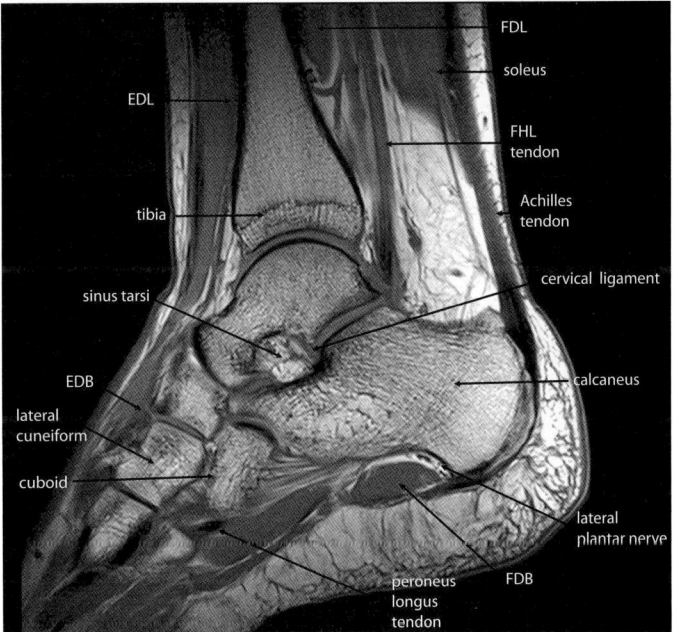

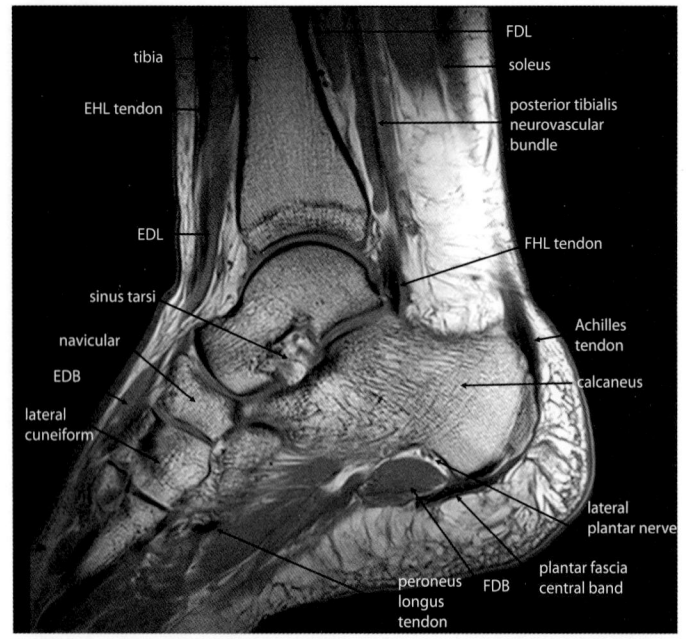
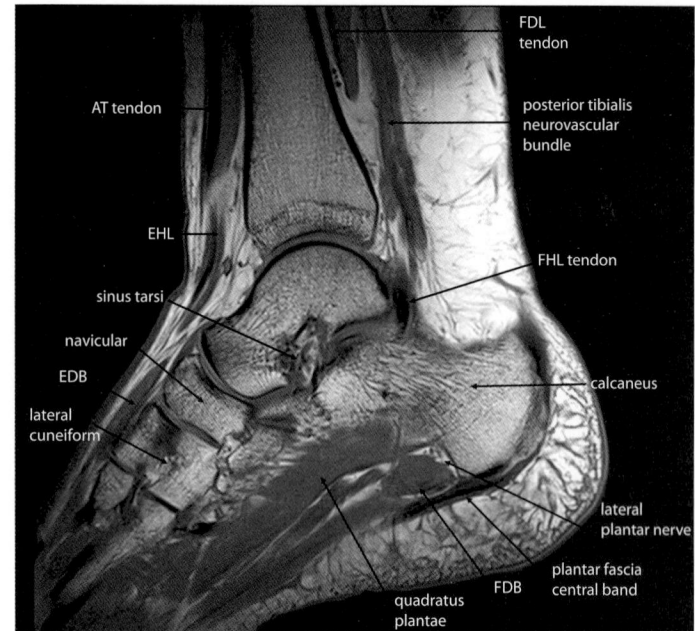
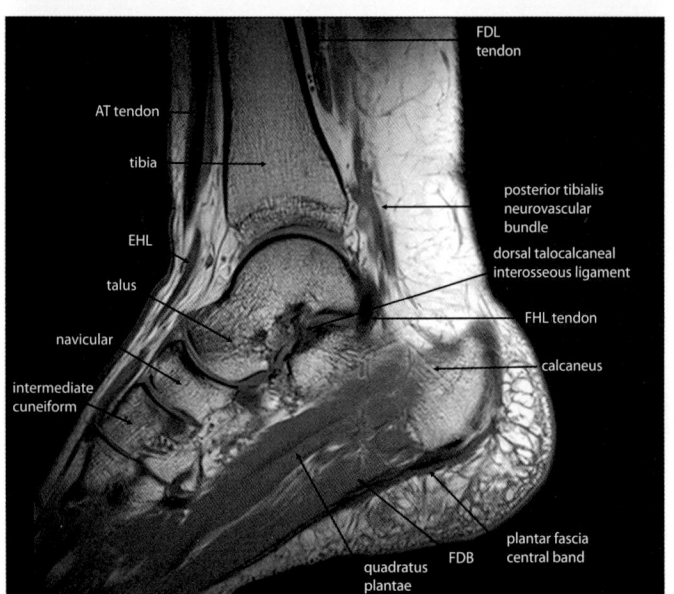
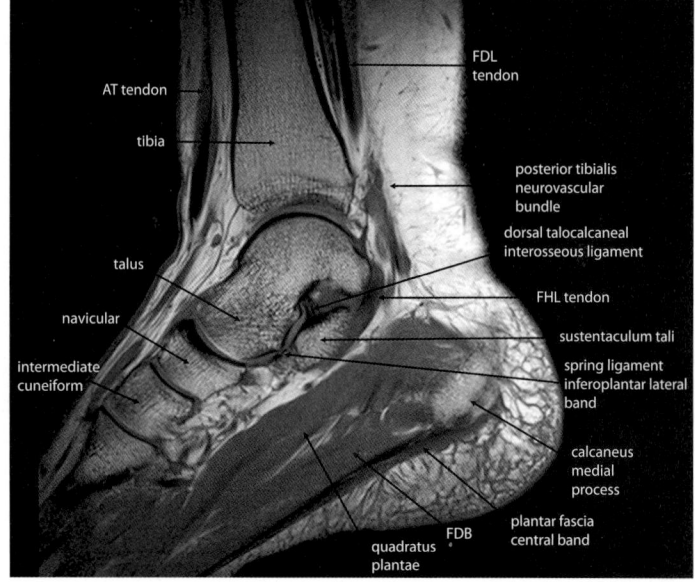

Chapter 13: Diagnostic Imaging Techniques of the Foot and Ankle

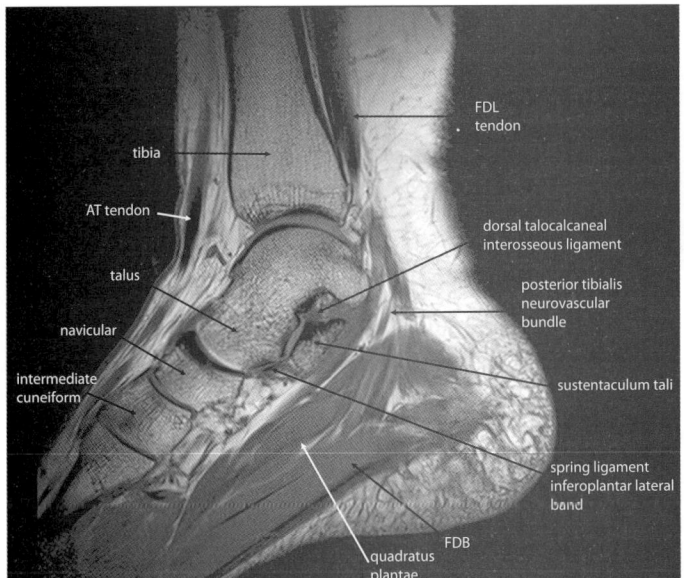
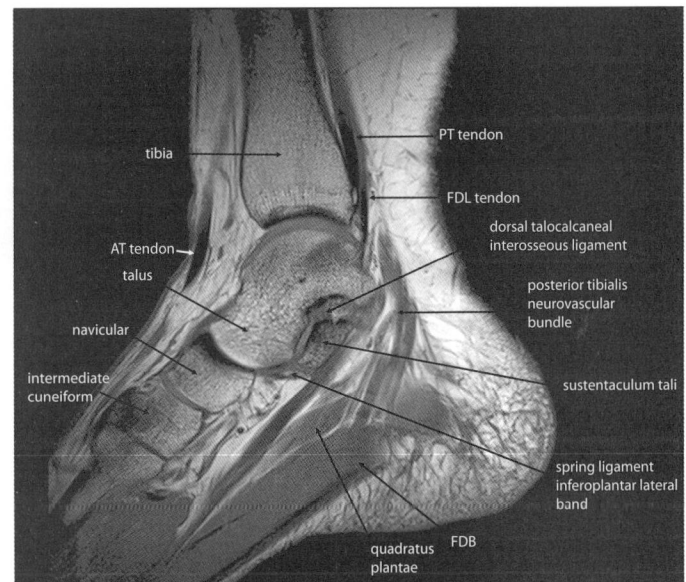
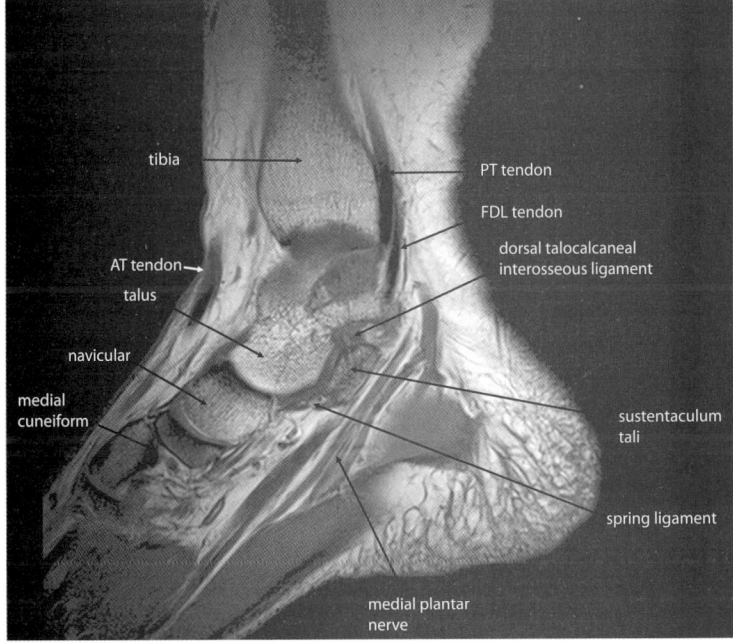
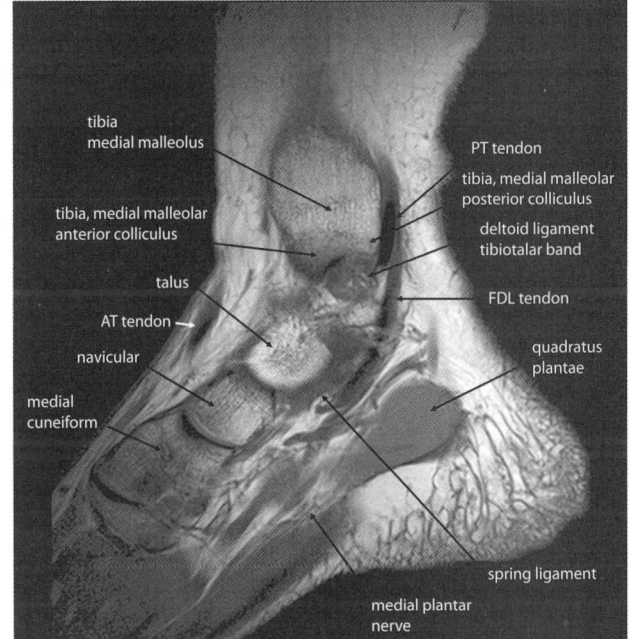

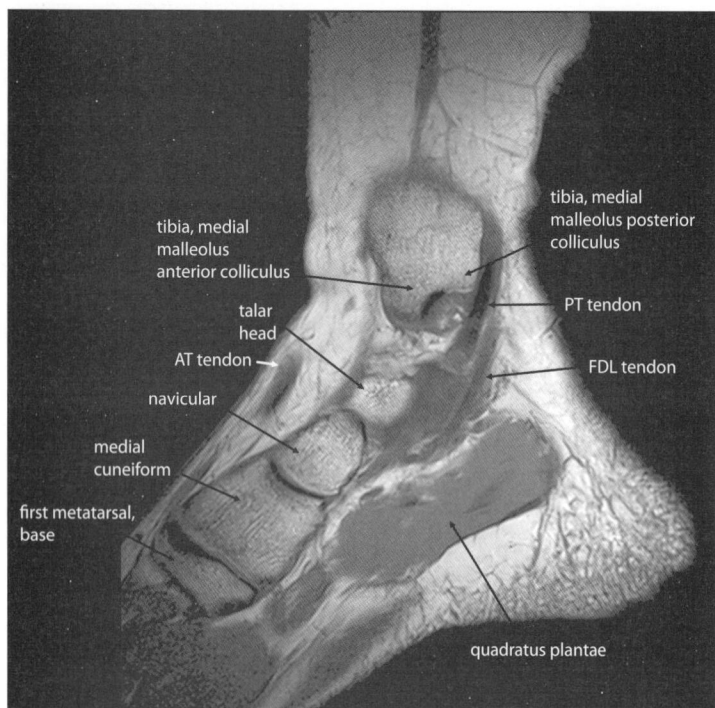
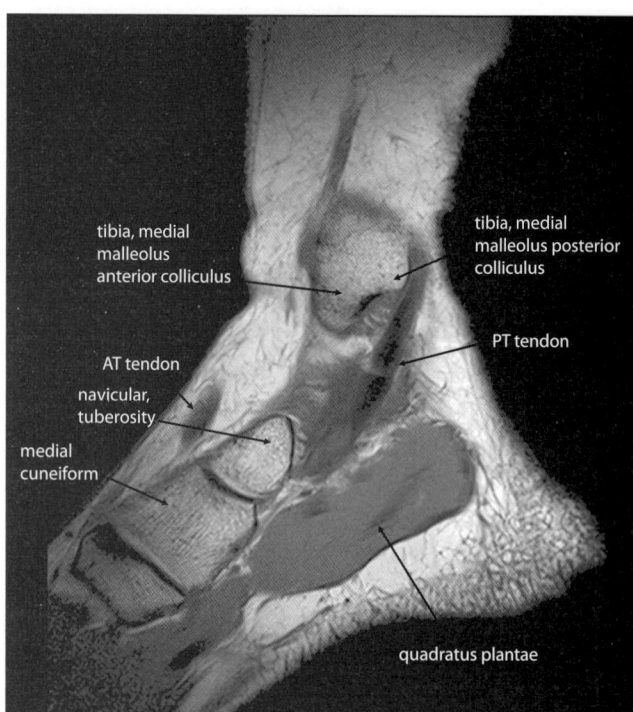

▶ Set 2. Coronal Proton Density Fat-Saturated Images of the Ankle/Hindfoot

Contiguous images are shown sequentially from posterior to anterior, extending from the calf to the midfoot. This plane often best depicts the talar dome to evaluate for osteochondral injuries and shows the deltoid and spring ligaments, along with the distal portions of the peroneus longus and brevis, flexor hallucis, and flexor digitorum longus tendons well.

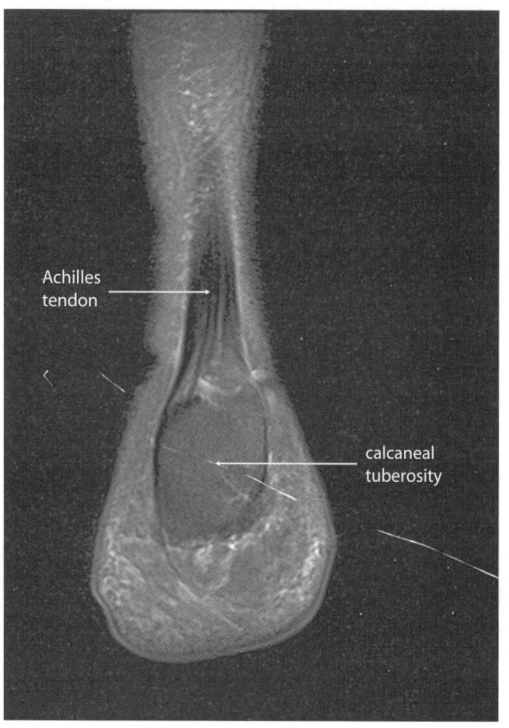
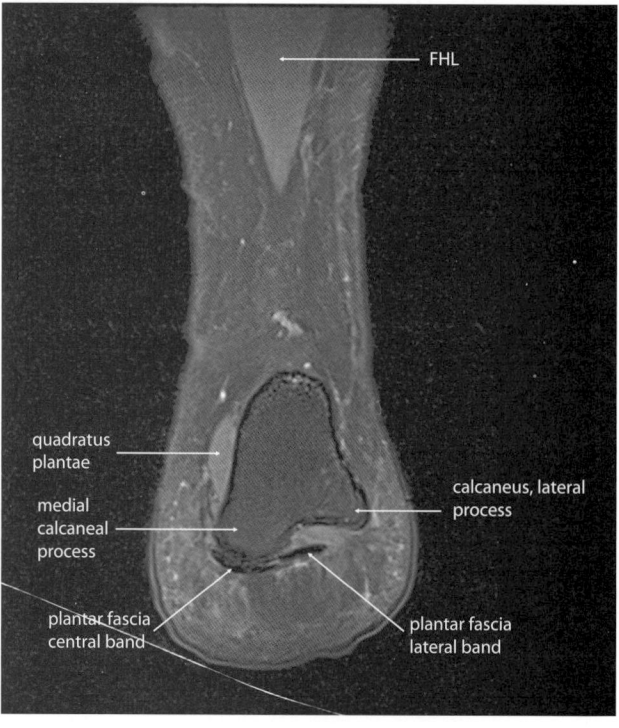

Chapter 13: Diagnostic Imaging Techniques of the Foot and Ankle 739

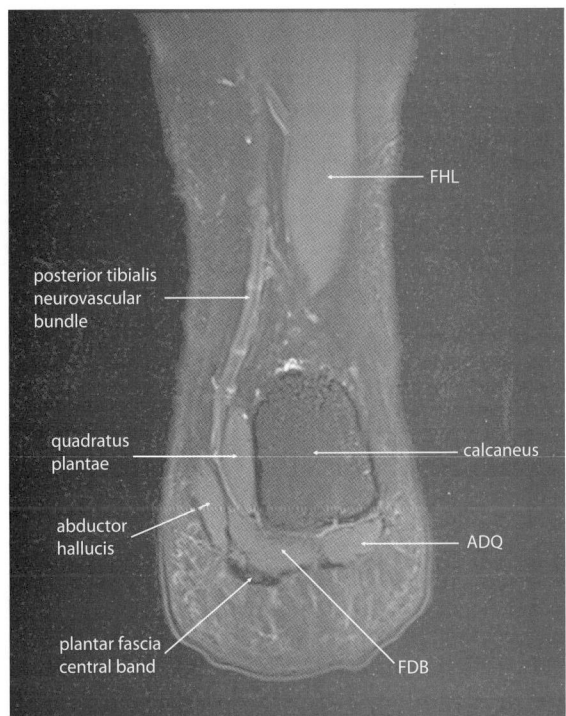
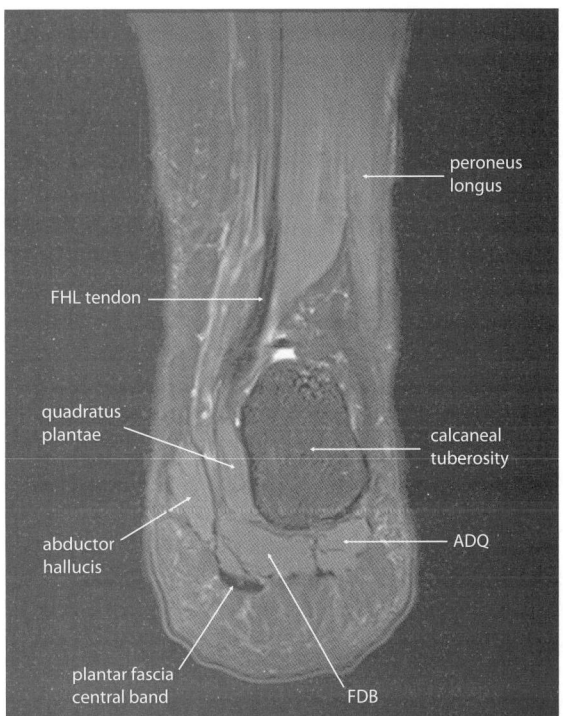
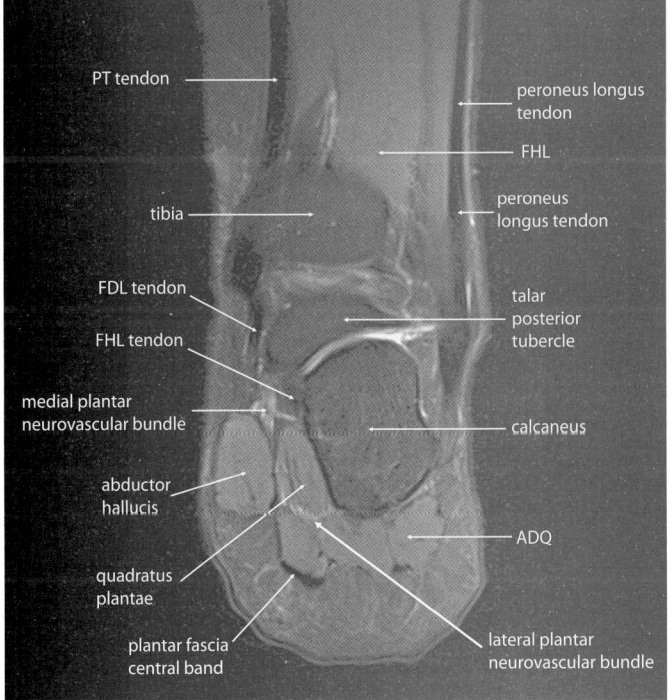
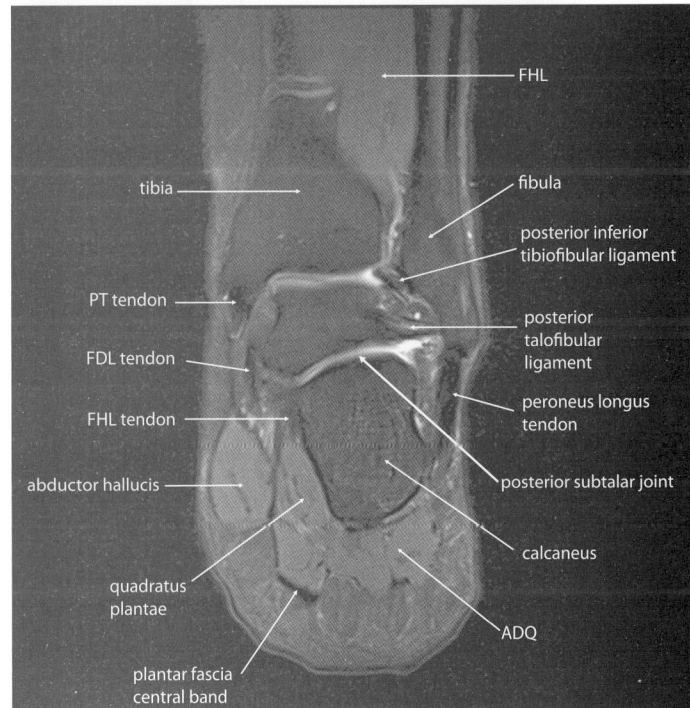

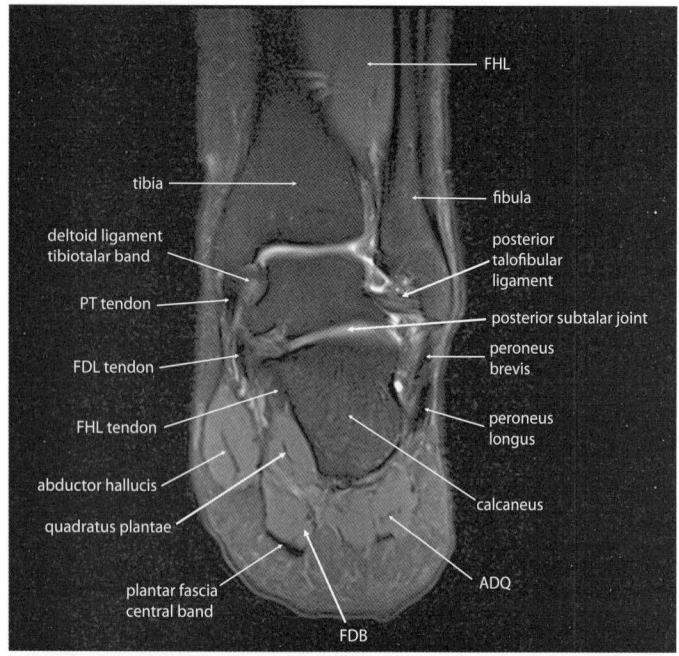
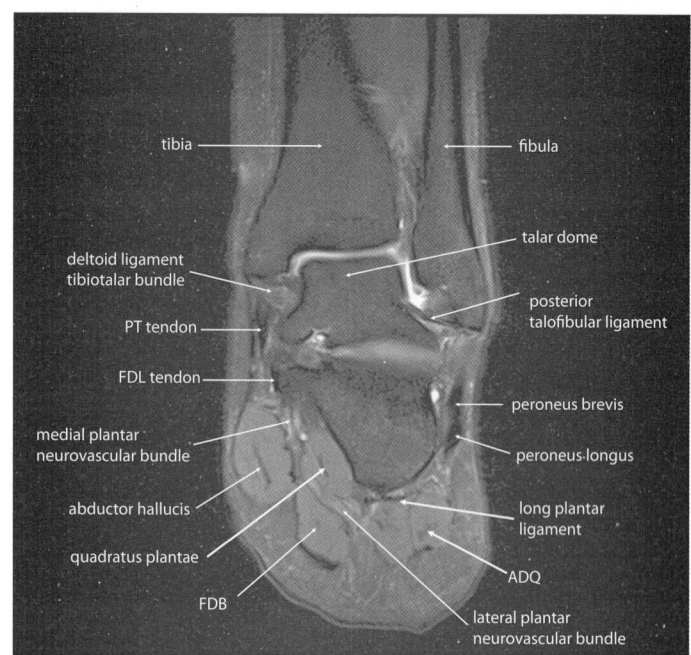
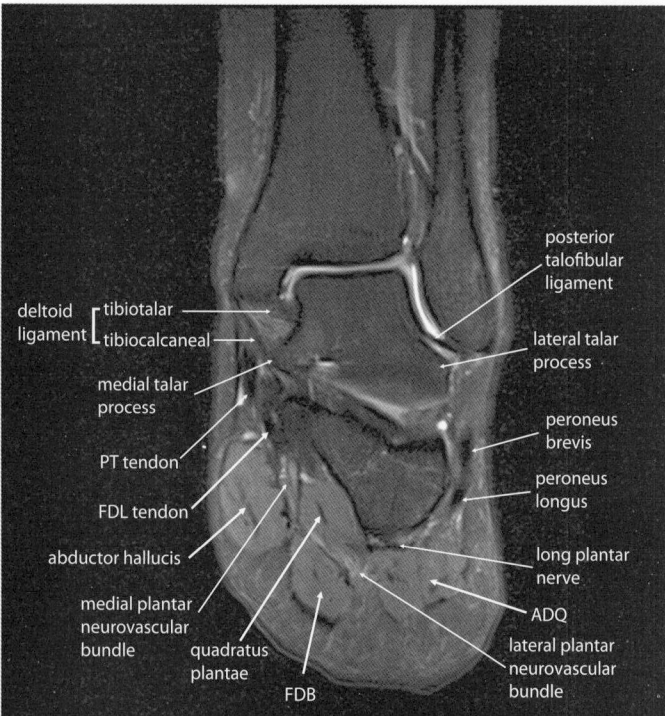
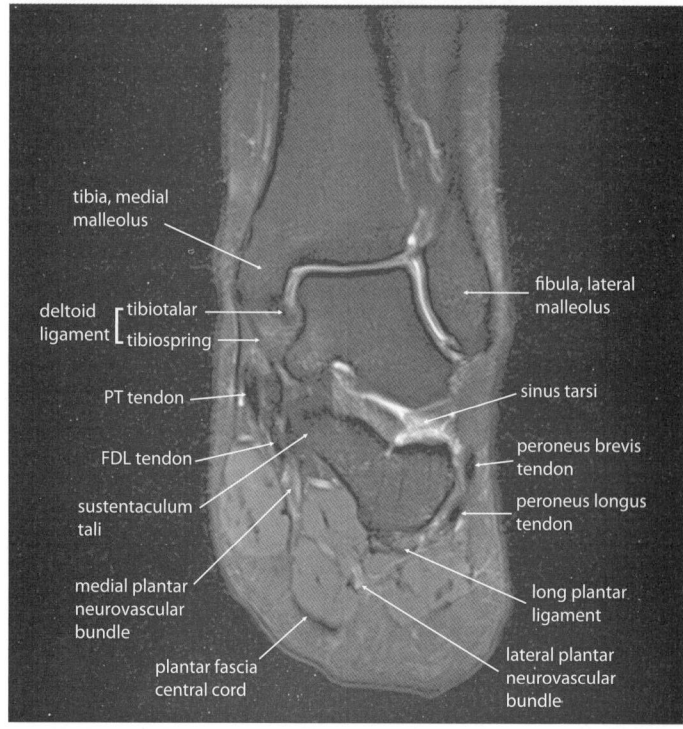

Chapter 13: Diagnostic Imaging Techniques of the Foot and Ankle   741

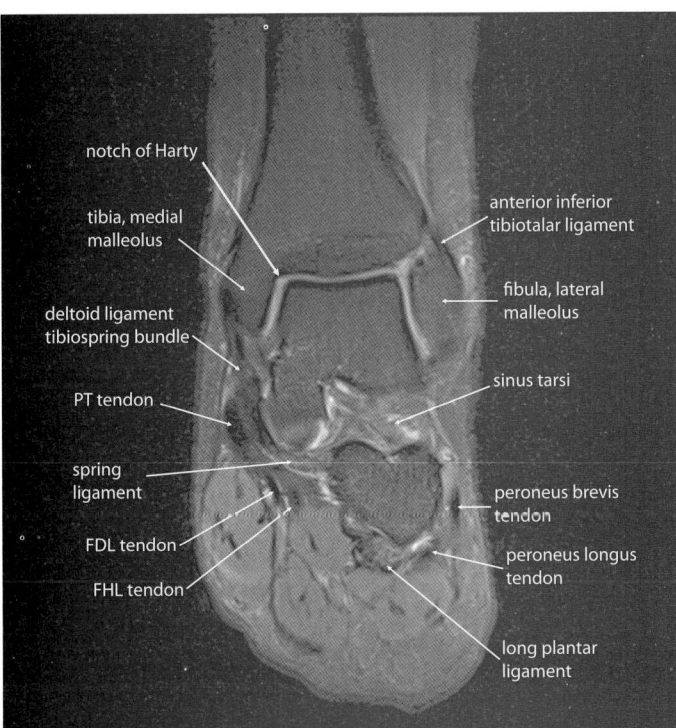
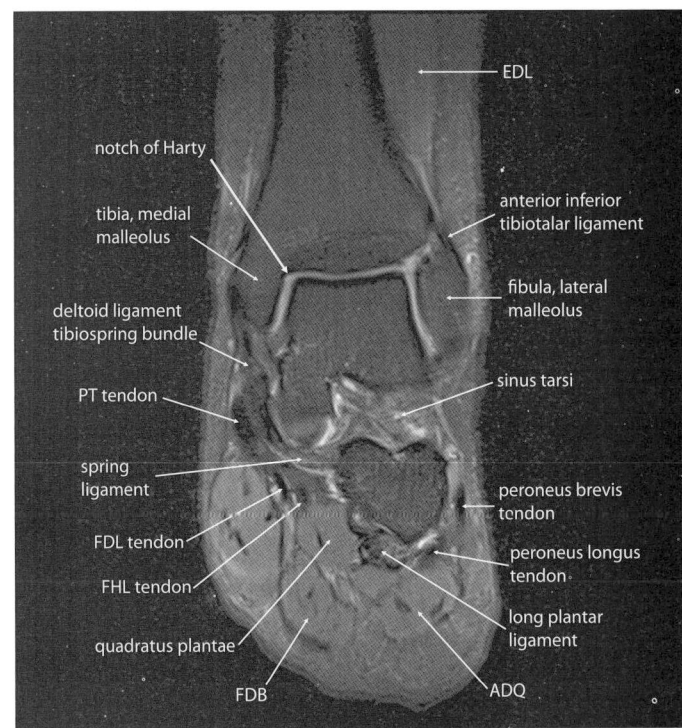
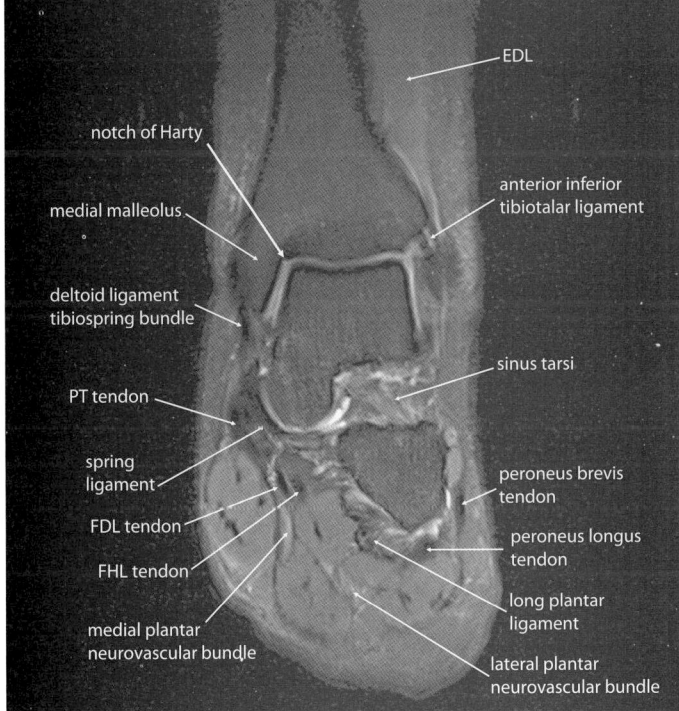
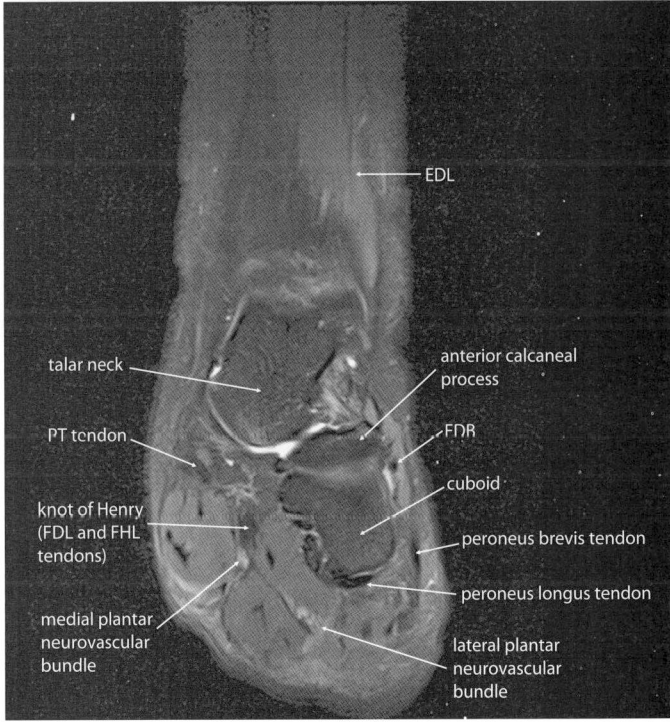

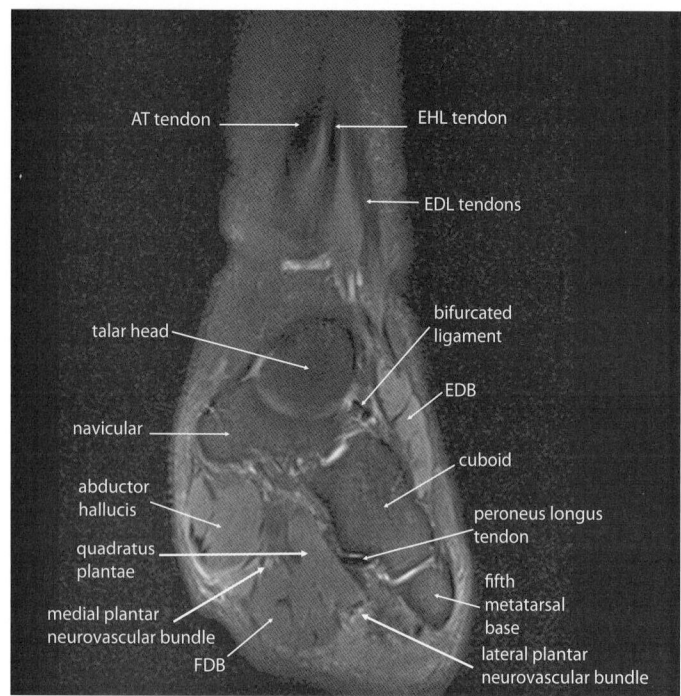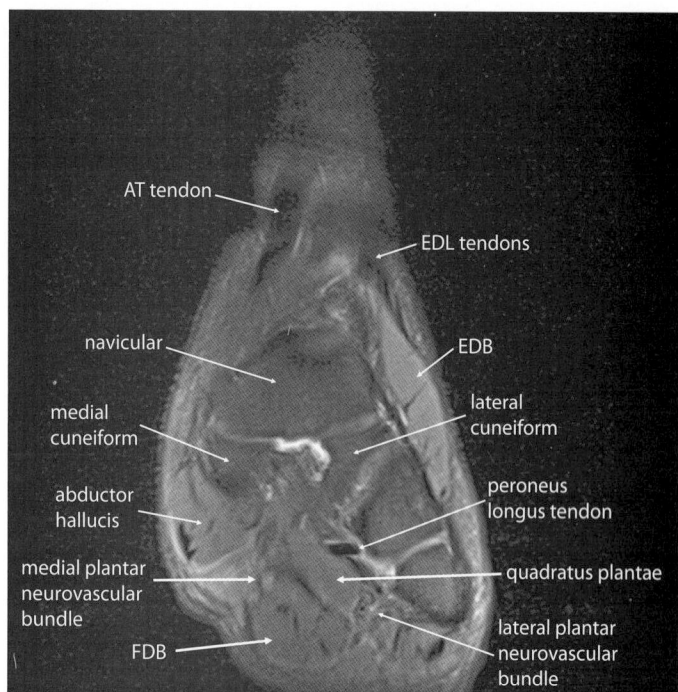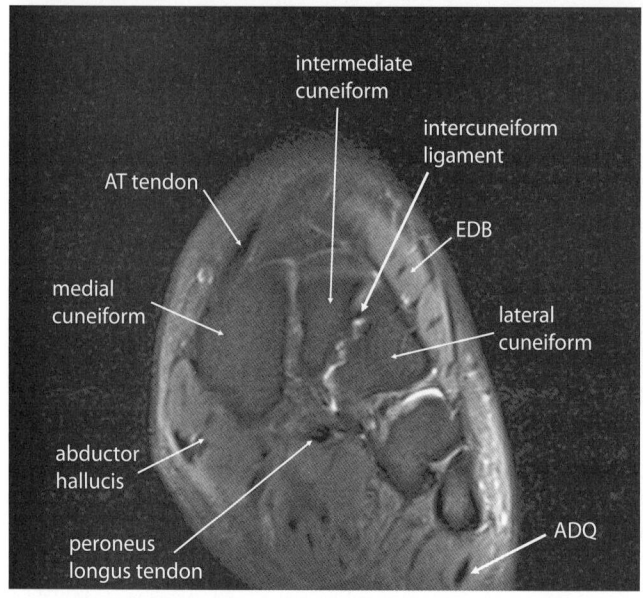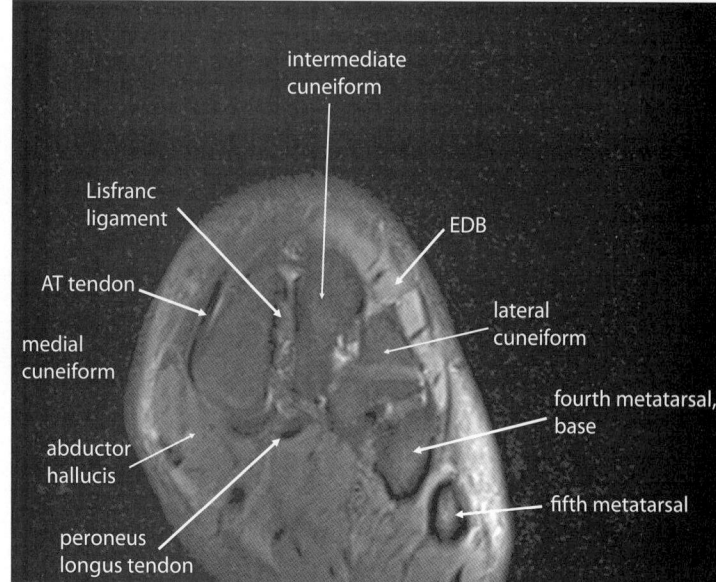

▶ Set 3. Axial Proton Density Non–Fat-Saturated Images of the Ankle/Hindfoot

Contiguous images are shown sequentially from anterior to posterior, extending from the calf to the midfoot. This plane shows most the ankle ligaments and tendons in cross-section and should be included in any hindfoot protocol in order to best detect and localize pathology. Structures in the midfoot, such as the Lisfranc ligament, are also often well seen on these images.

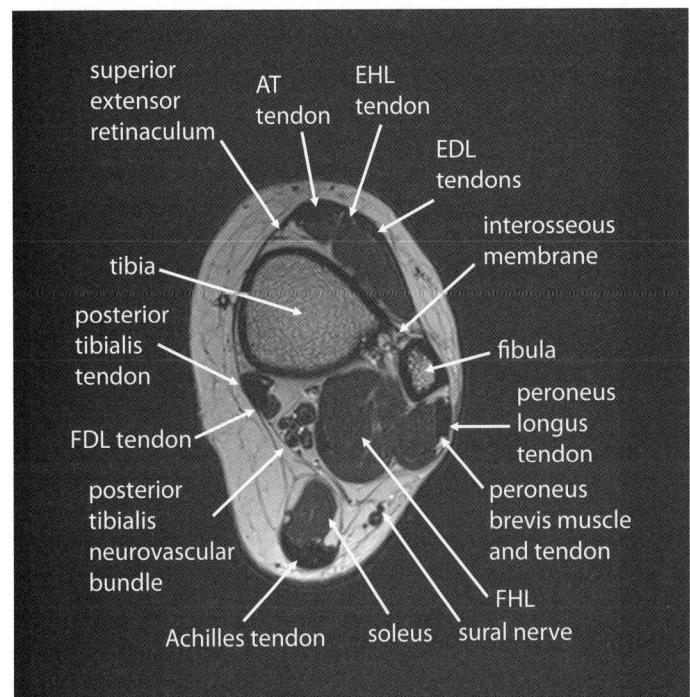
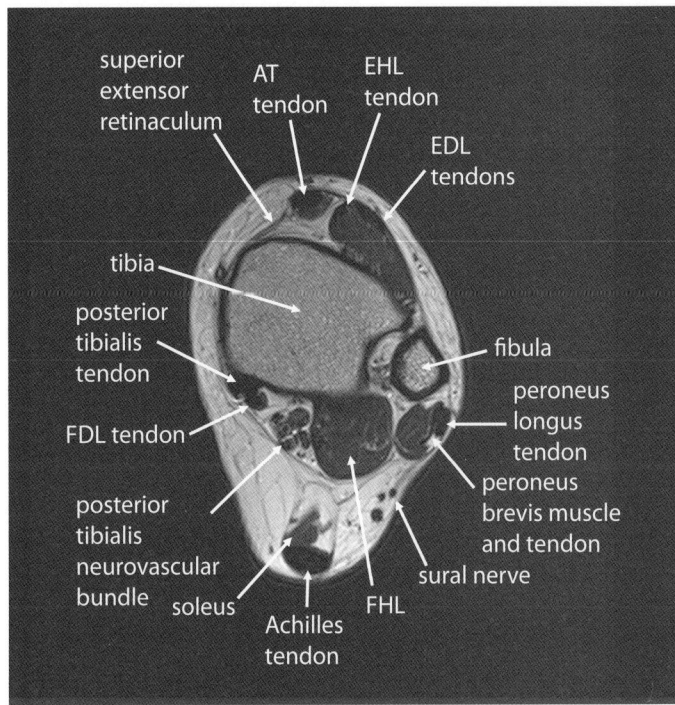
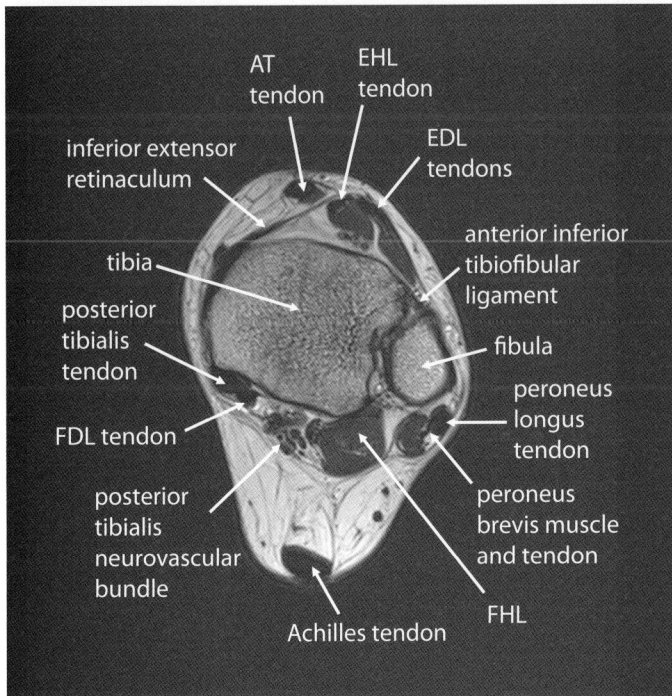
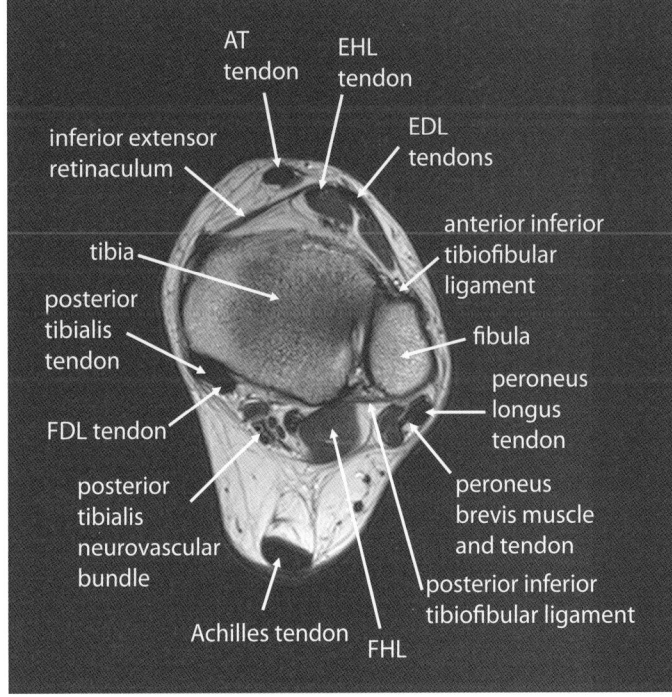

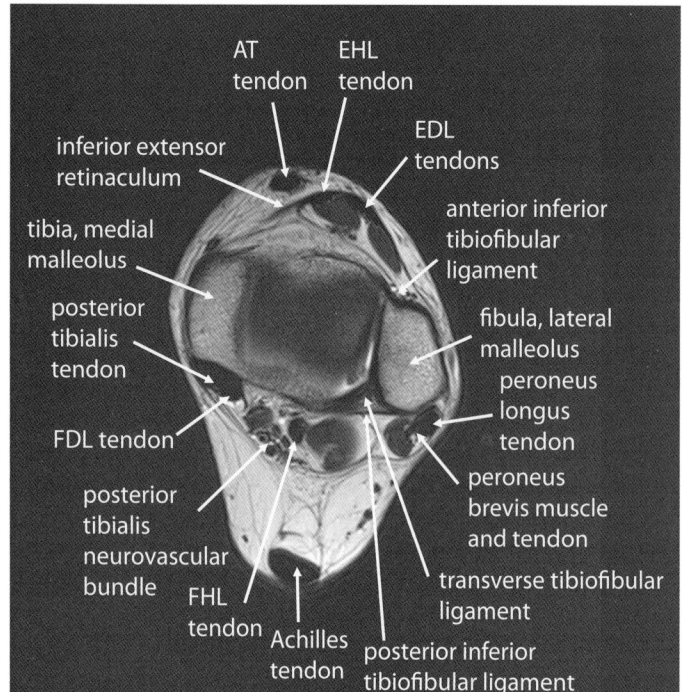
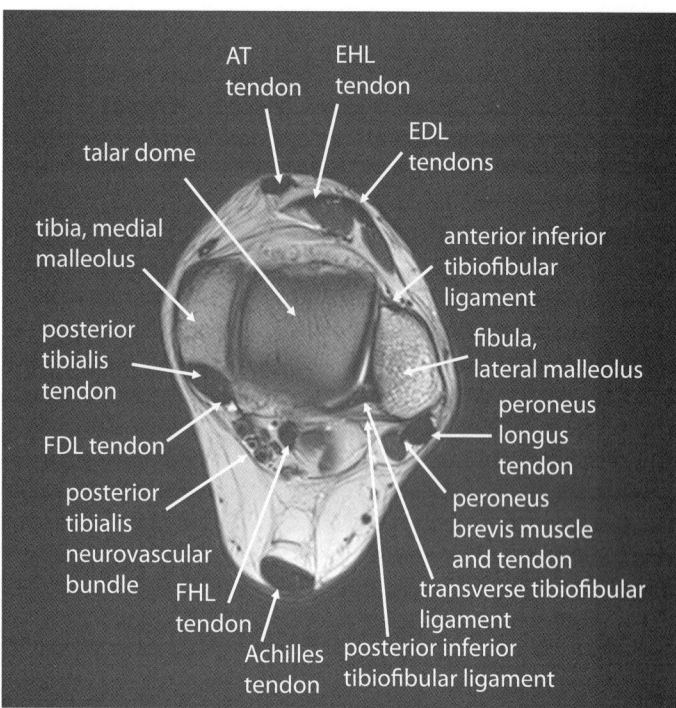
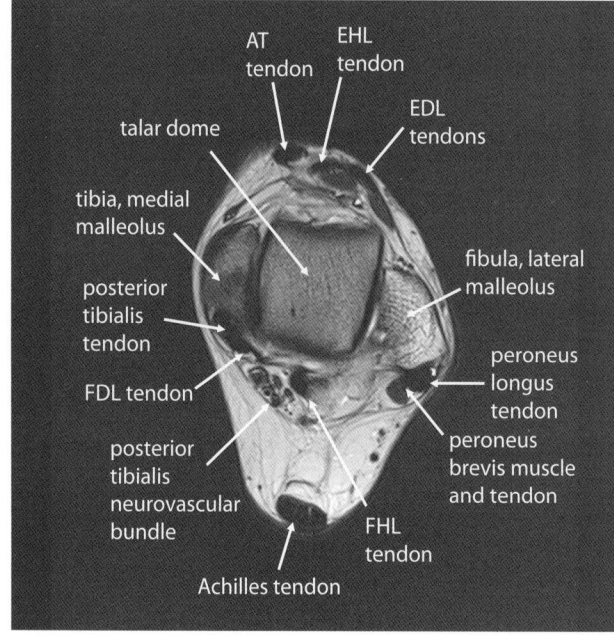
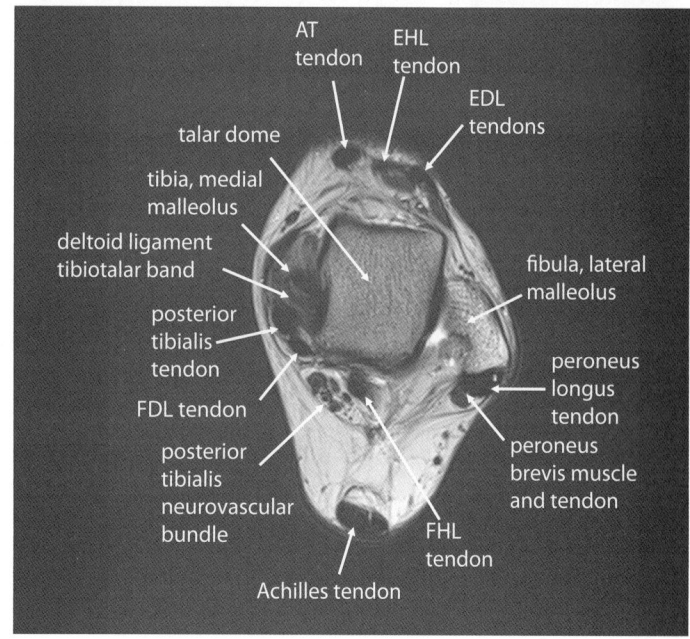

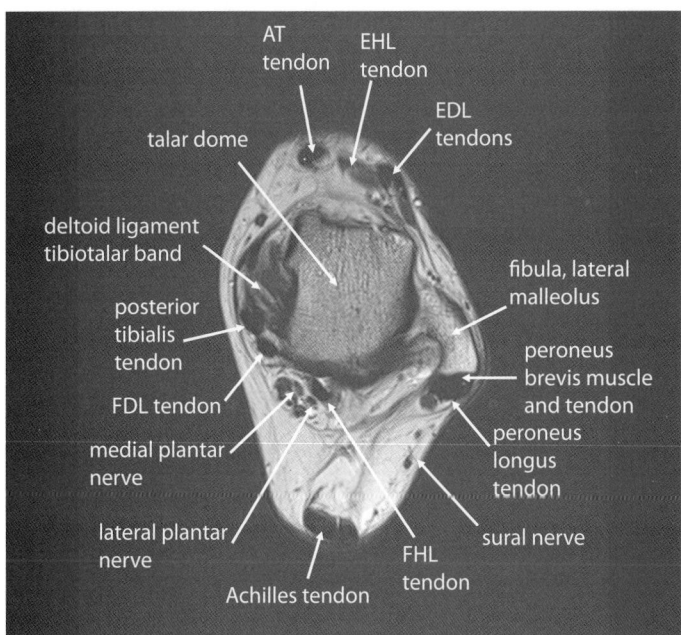
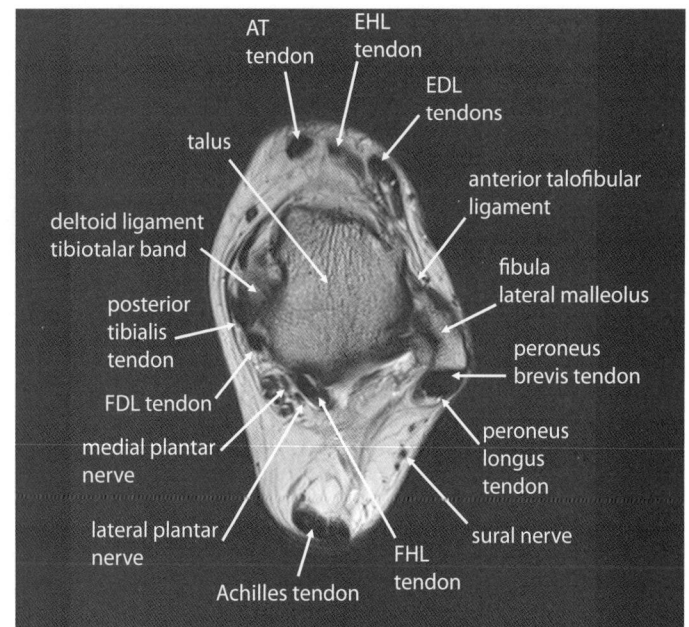
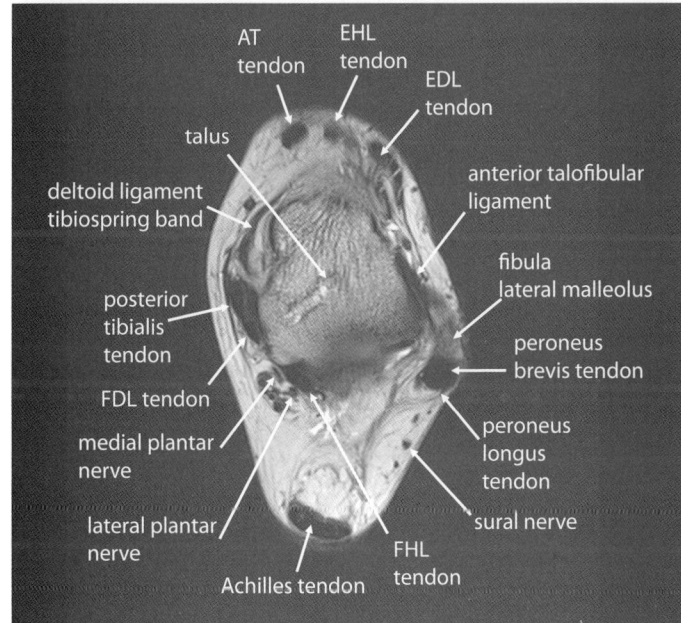
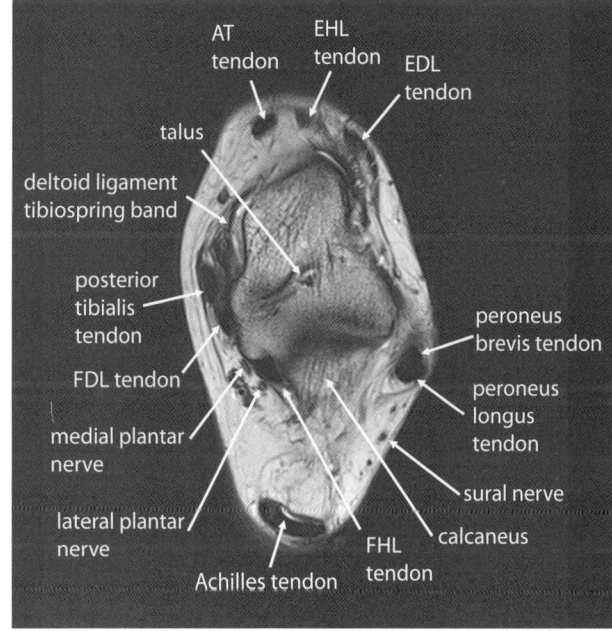

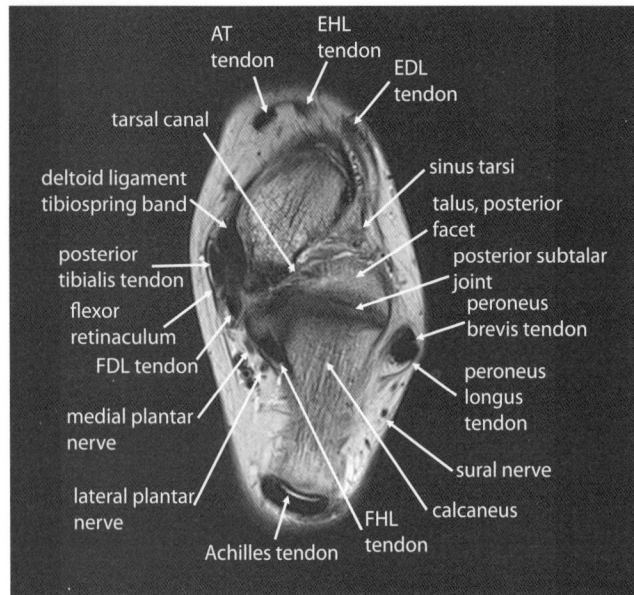
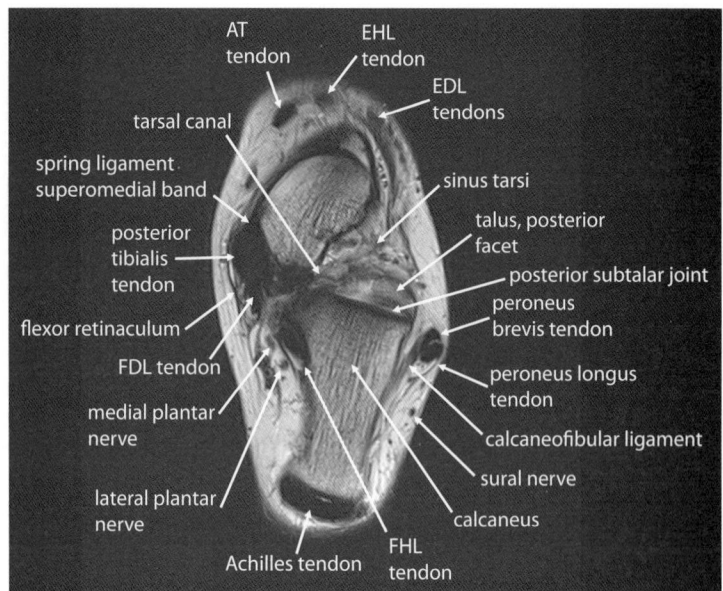
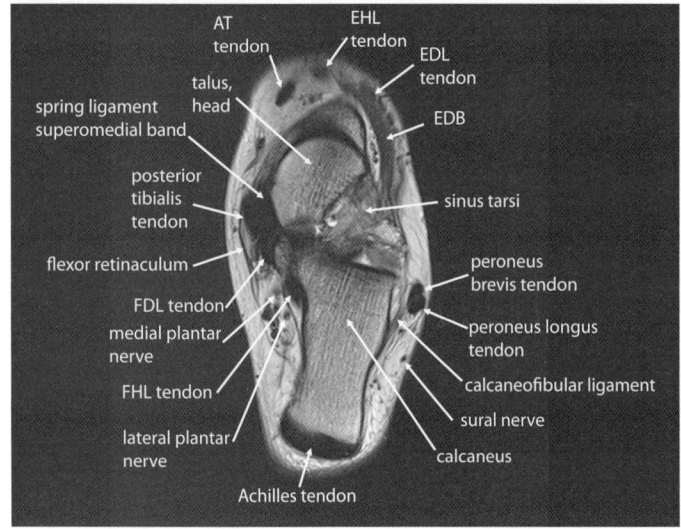
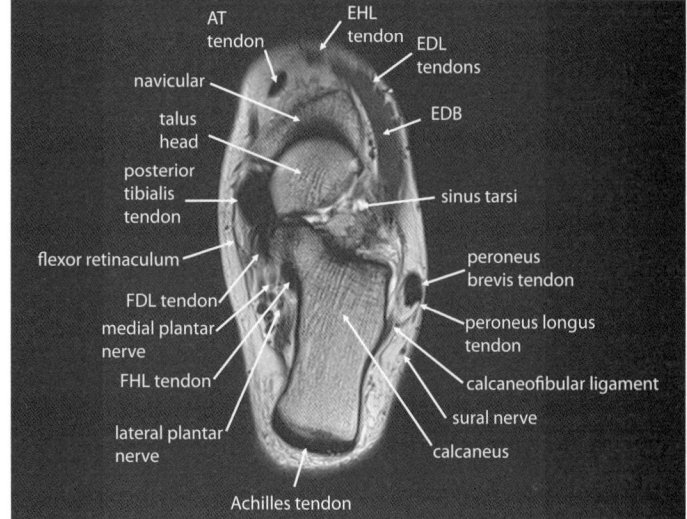

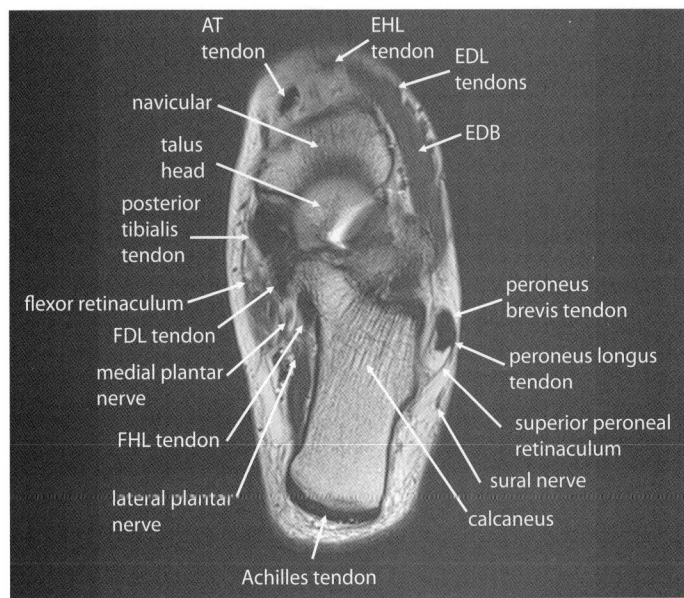
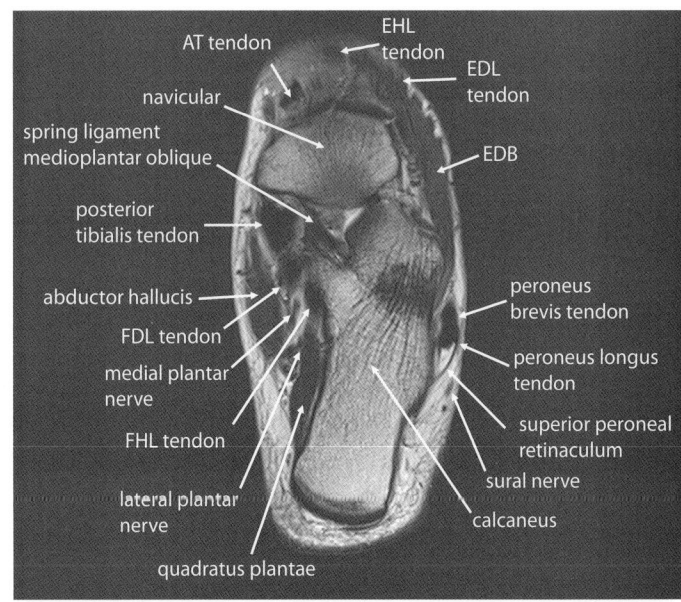
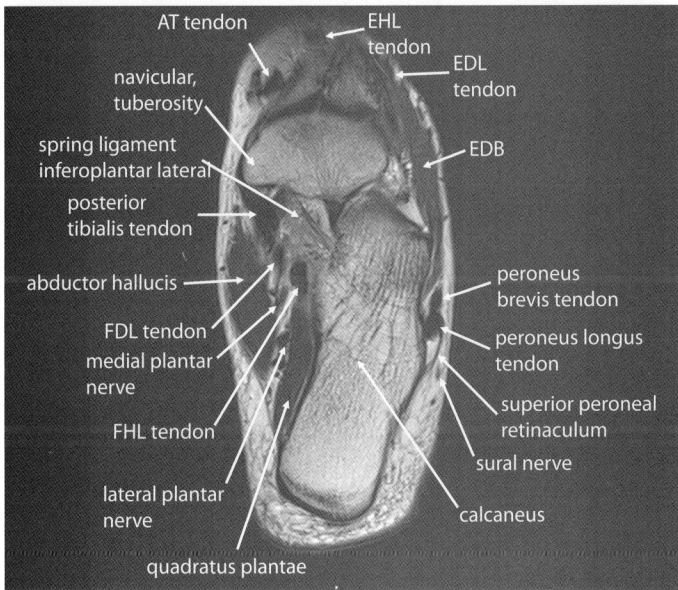
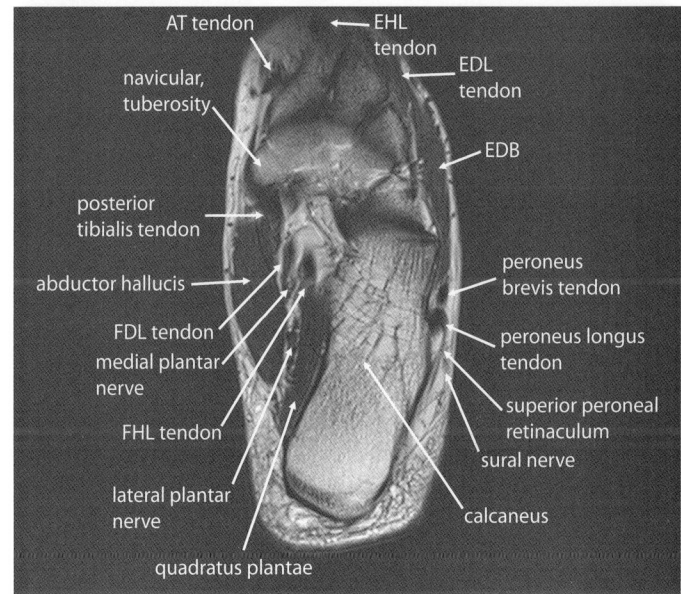

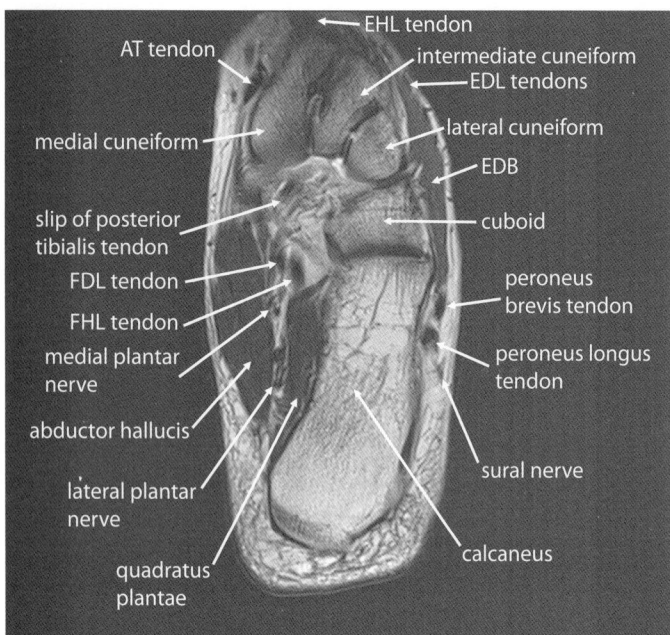
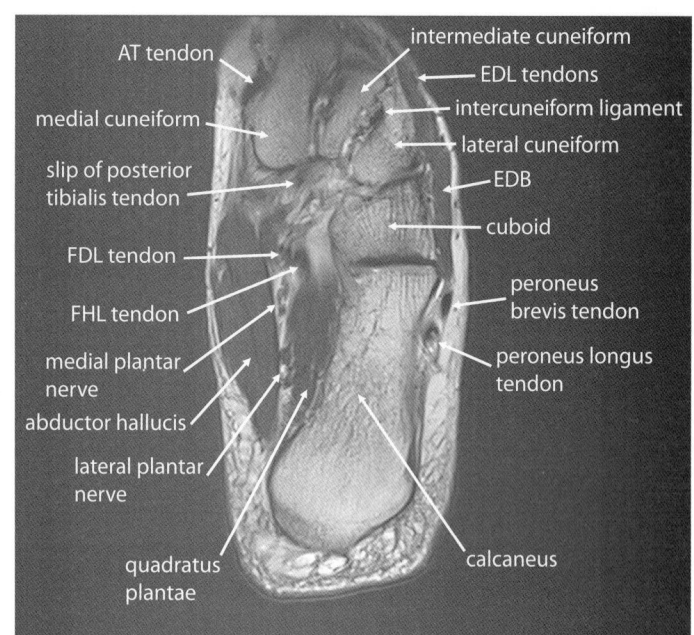
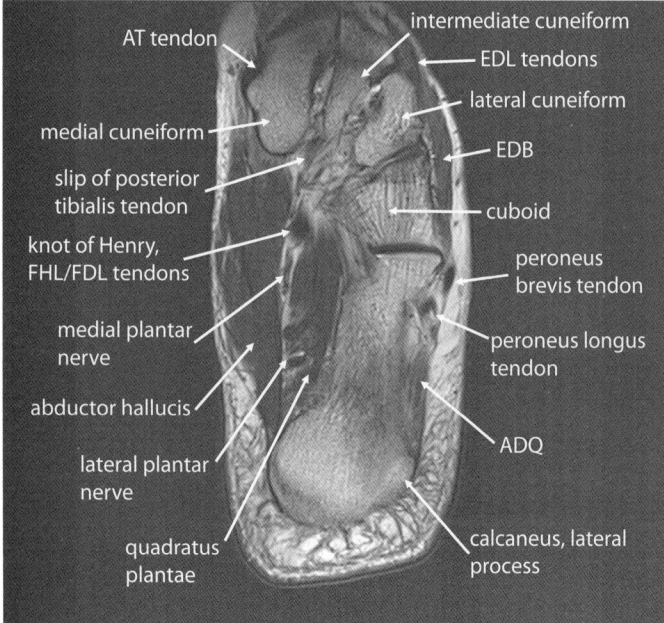
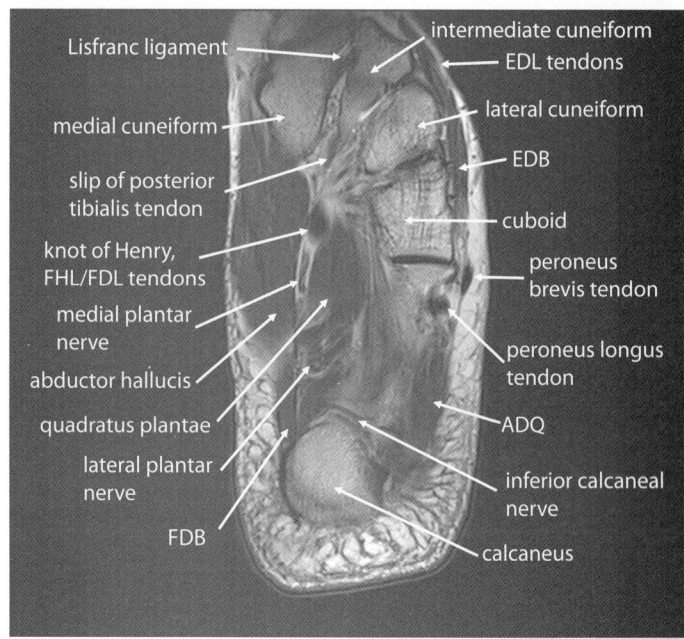

Chapter 13: Diagnostic Imaging Techniques of the Foot and Ankle   749

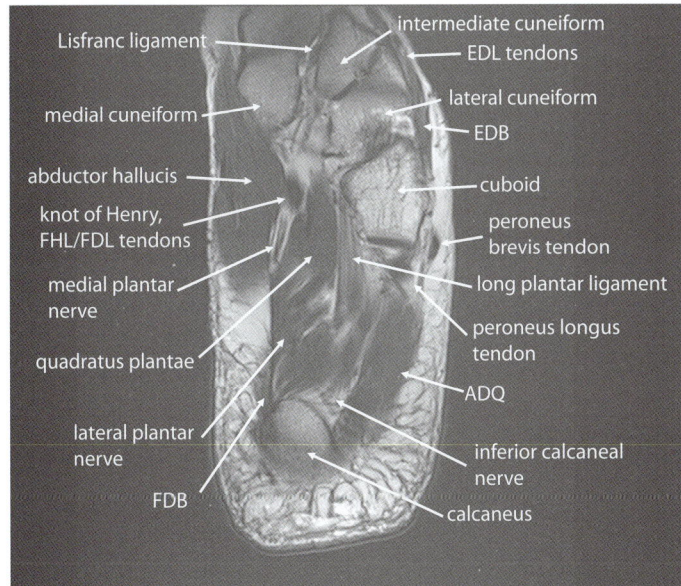
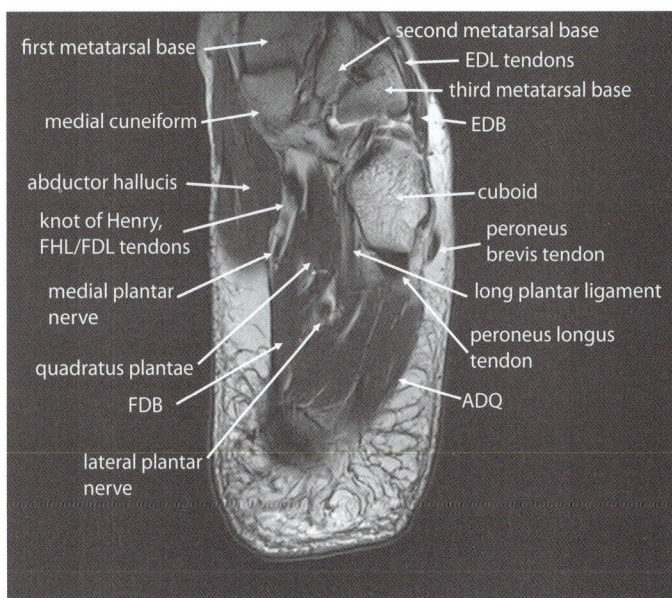

SECTION 2. FOREFOOT

▶ Set 1. Sagittal Proton Density Non–Fat-Saturated Images of the Forefoot

Contiguous images are shown sequentially from medial to lateral, extending from the talonavicular joint to the tips of the toes. This plane provides an anatomic survey of the bones and joints as well as long-axis imaging of the tendons and plantar plates.

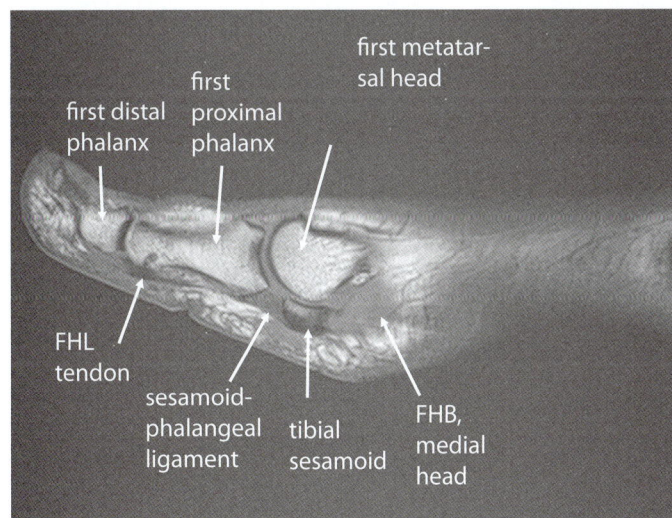
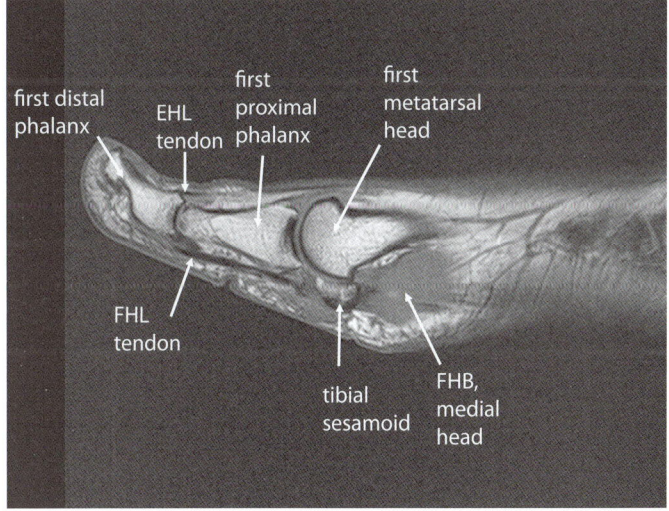

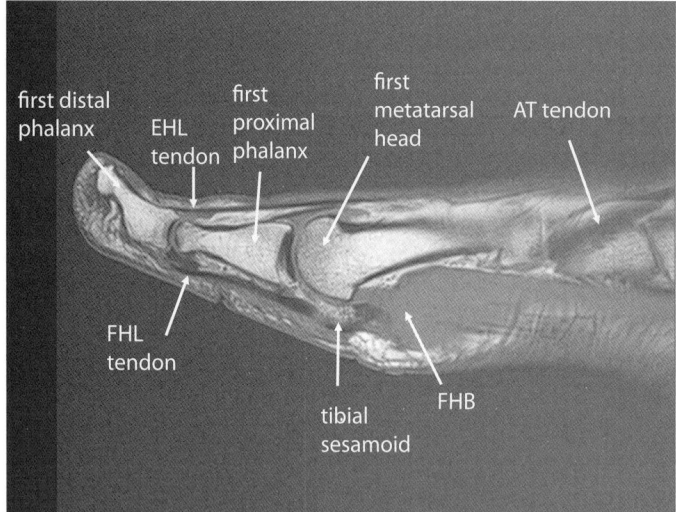
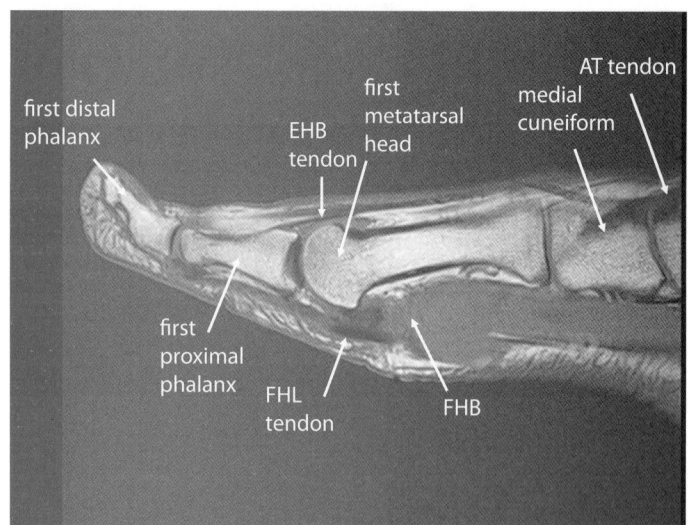
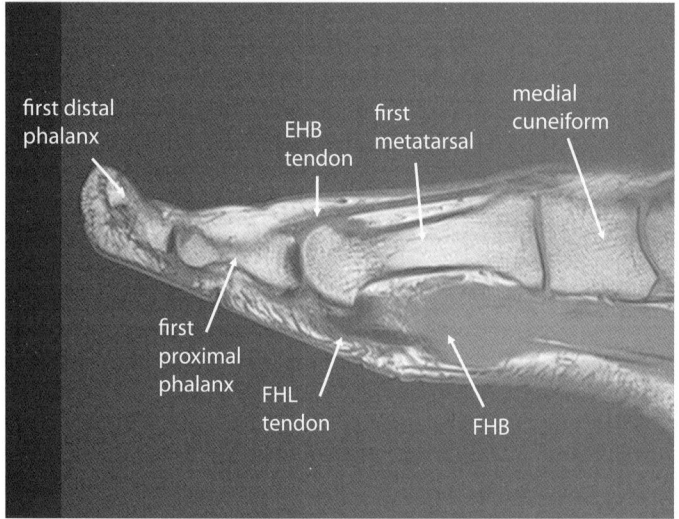
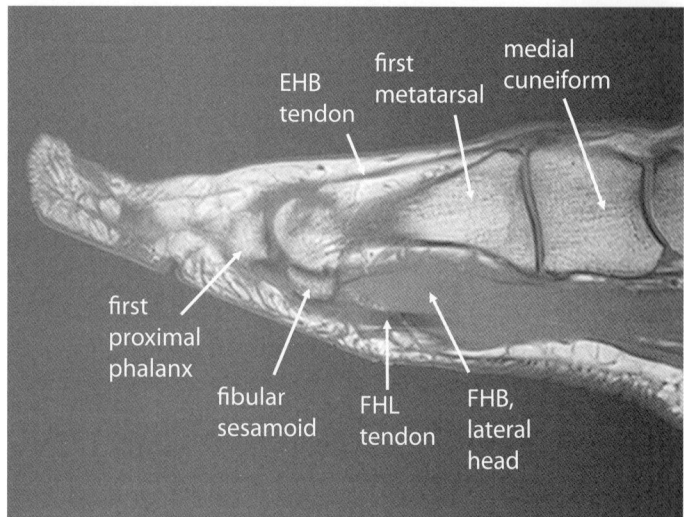

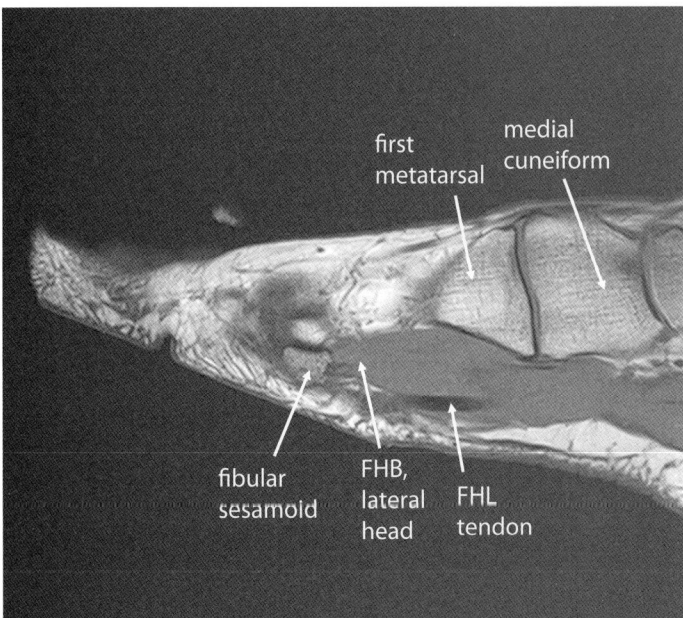
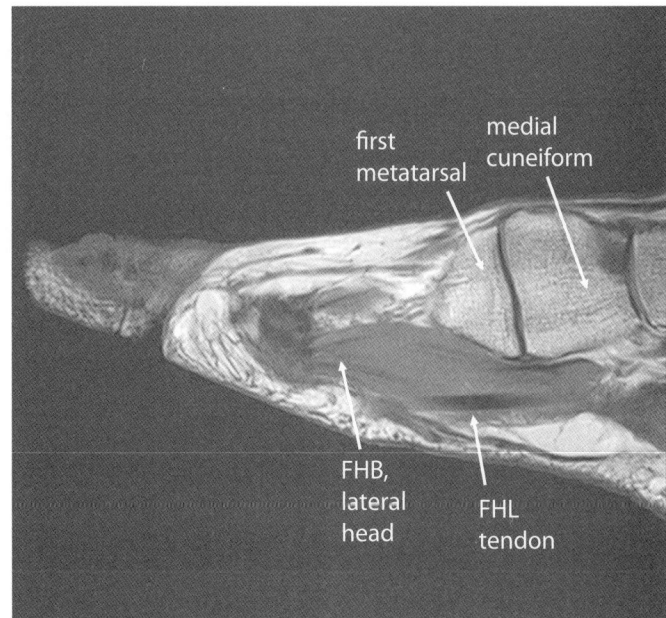
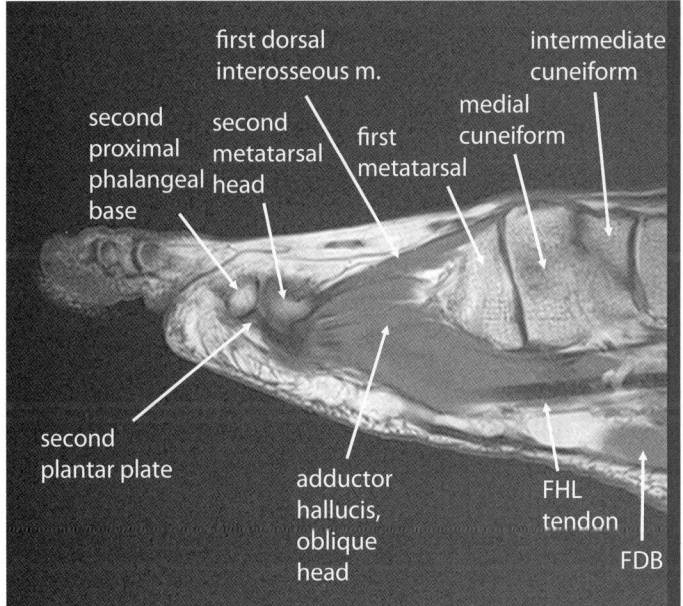
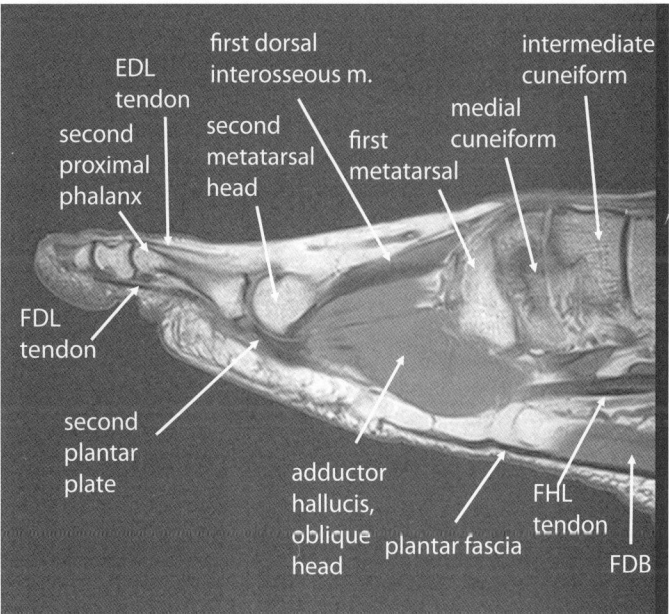

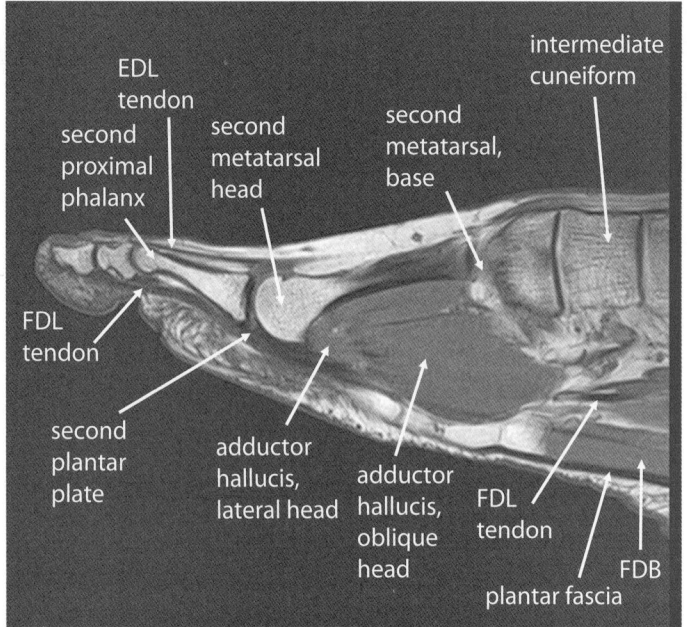
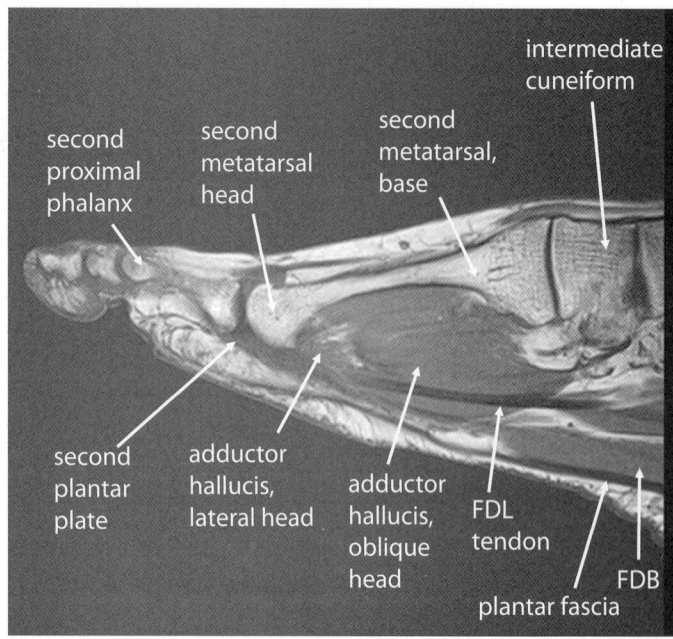
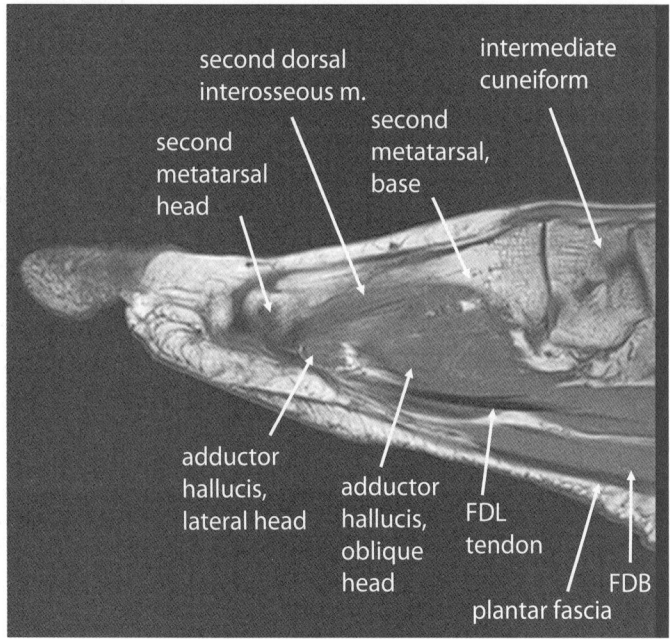
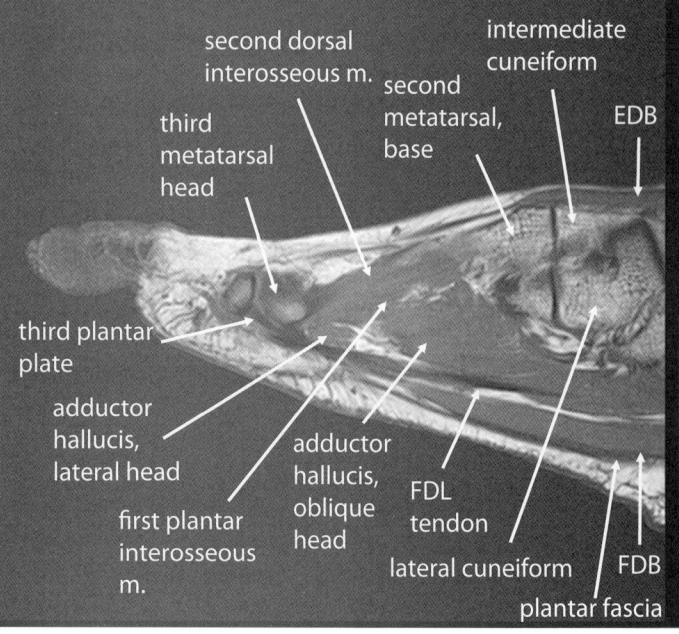

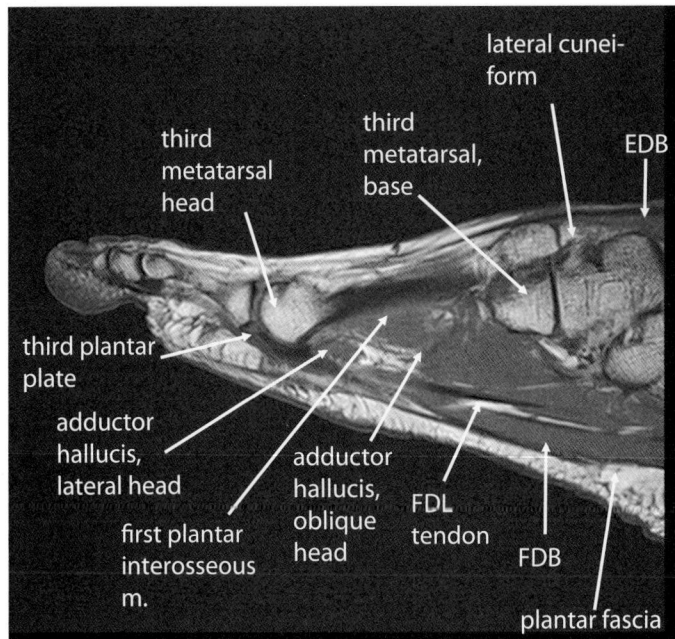
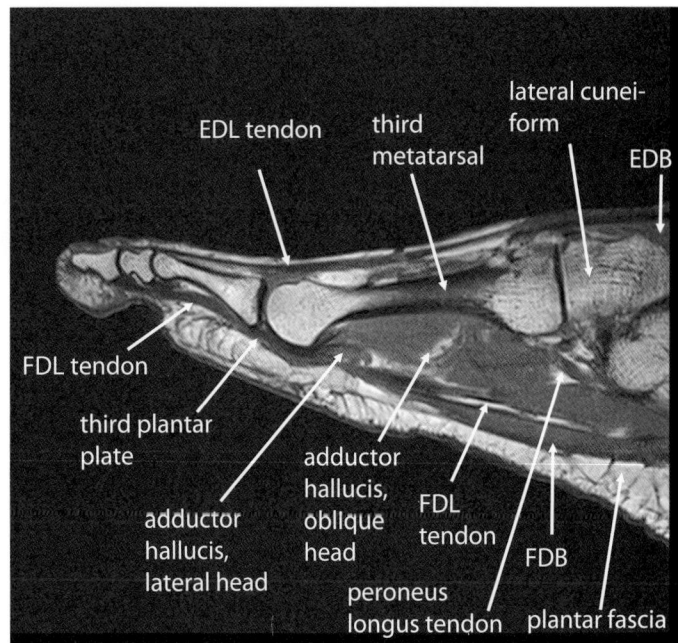
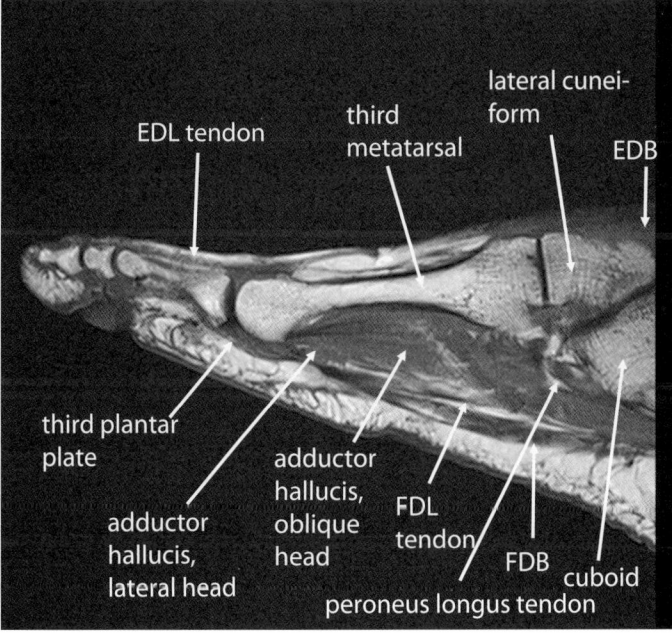
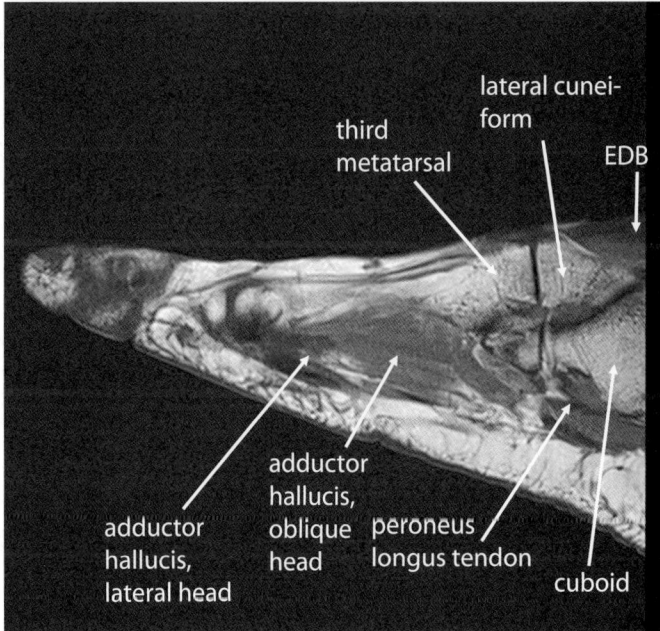

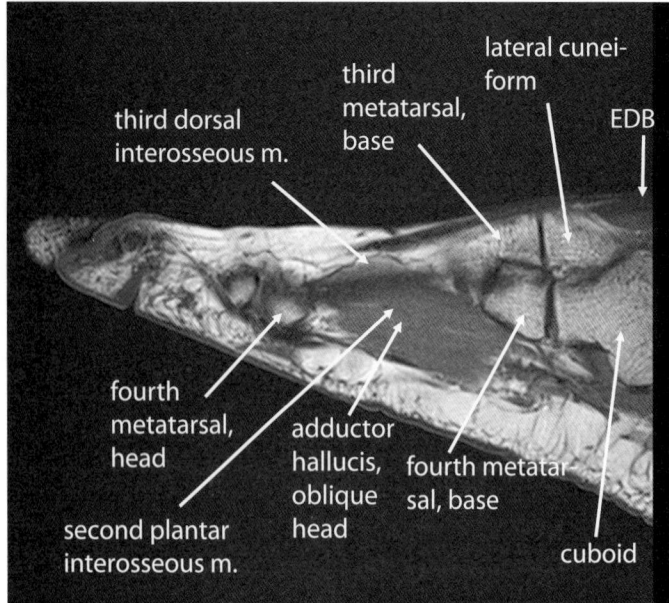
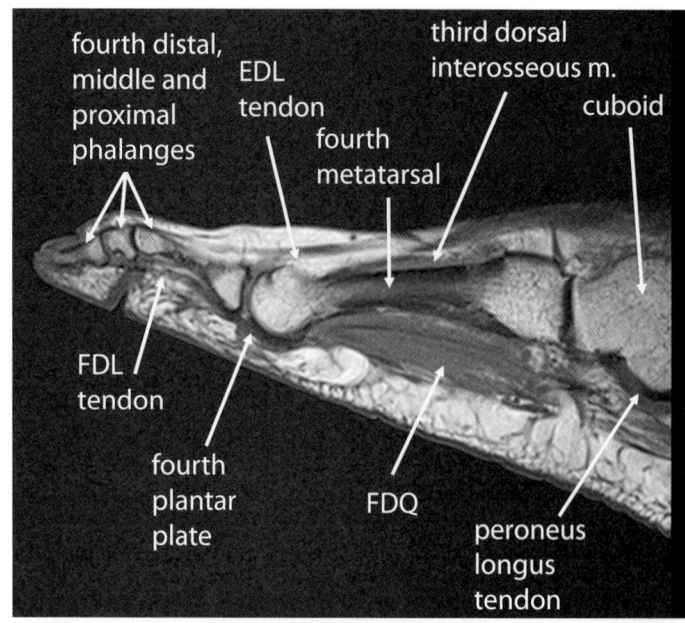
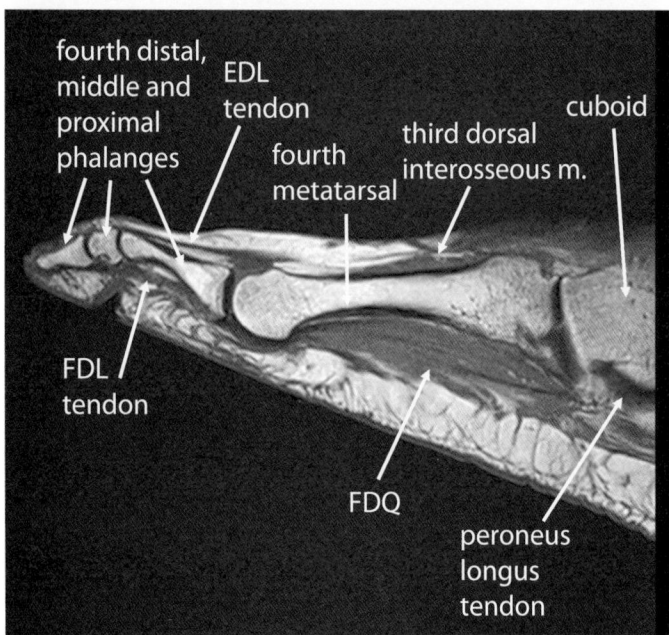
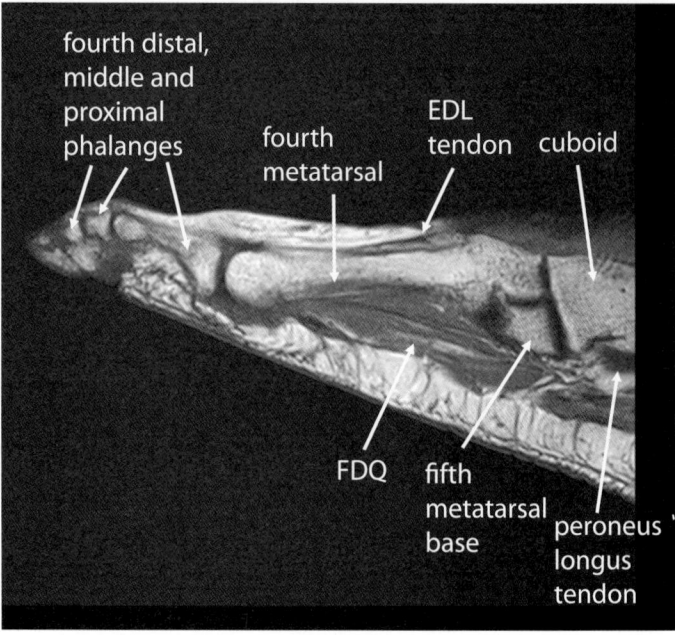

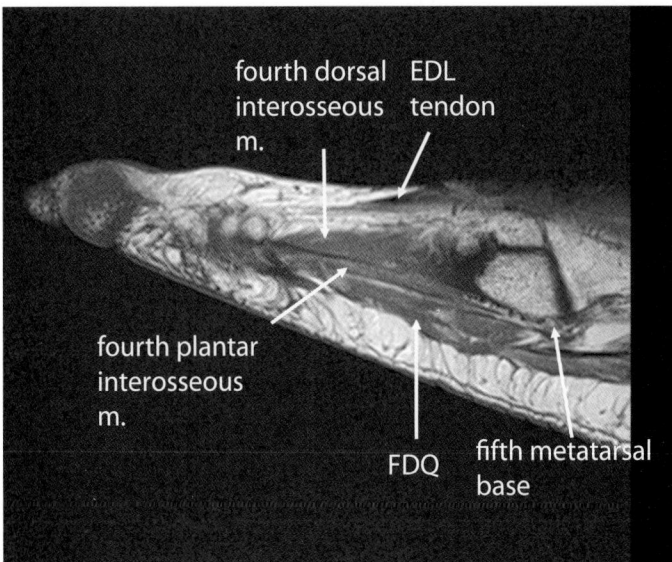
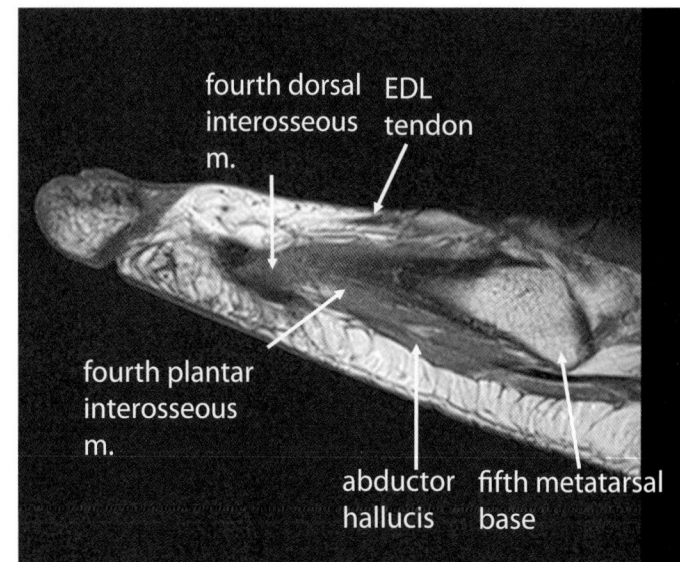
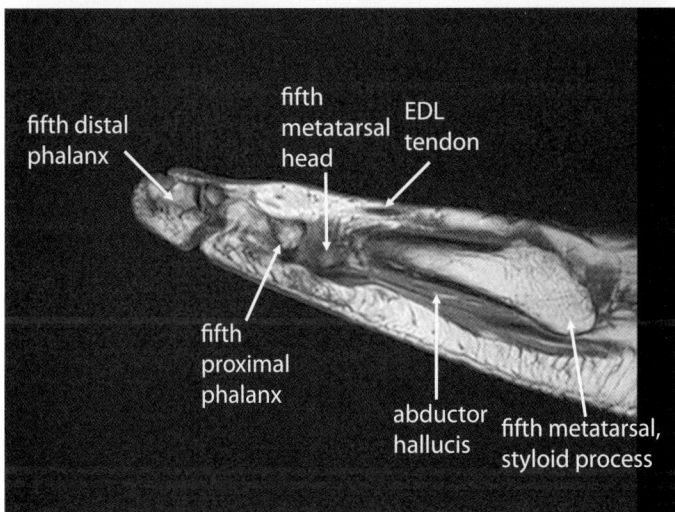
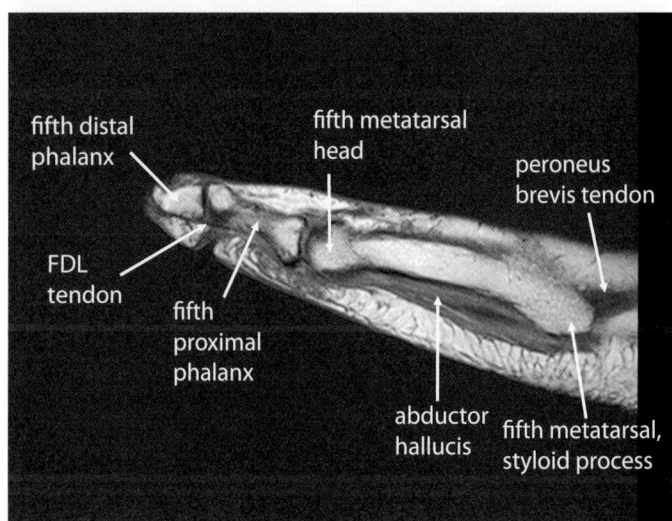

▶ Set 2. Horizontal Long Axis (Axial) Proton Density Non–Fat-Saturated Images of the Forefoot

Contiguous images are shown sequentially from dorsal to plantar, extending from the midtarsal region to the tips of the toes. Structures in the midfoot, such as the Lisfranc ligament, are also often well seen on these images. This imaging plane shows many of the muscles and metatarsals in long axis and is useful in detecting metatarsal fractures and metatarsophalangeal collateral ligament injuries.

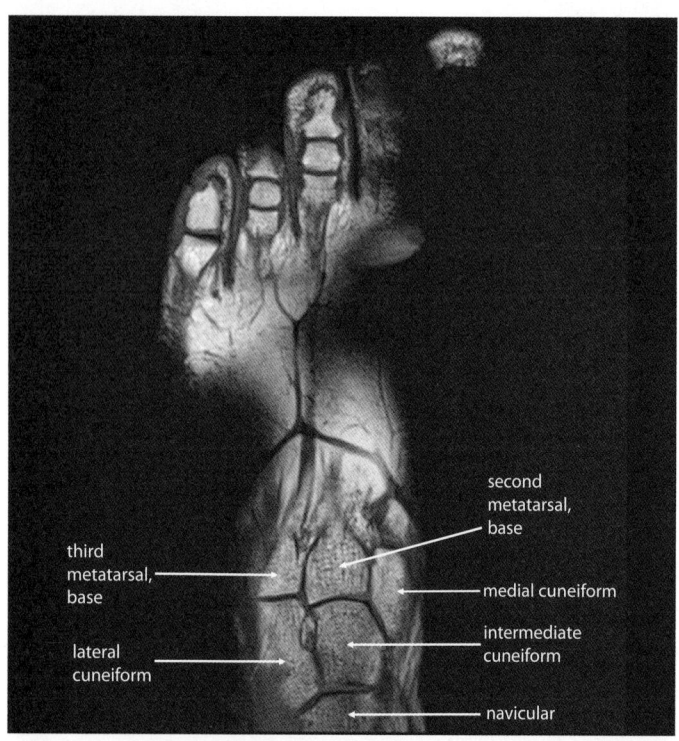
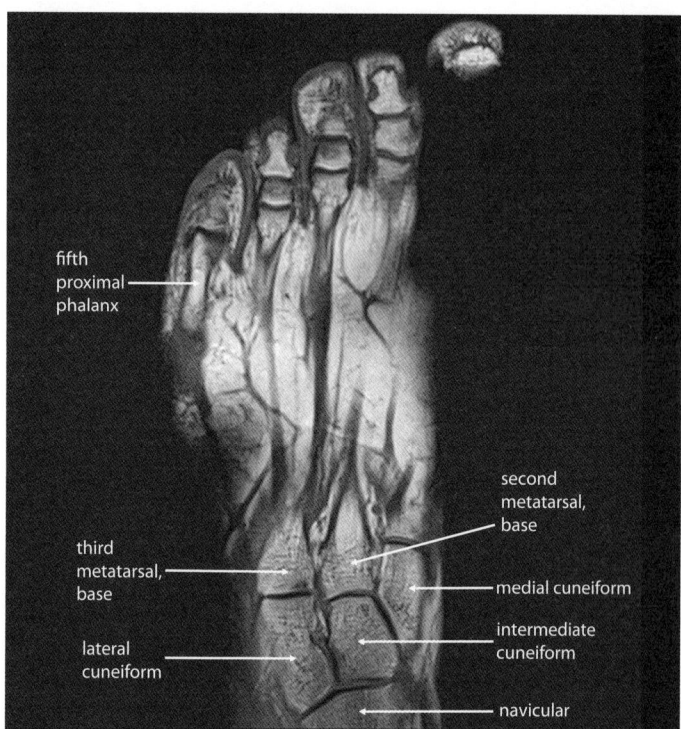
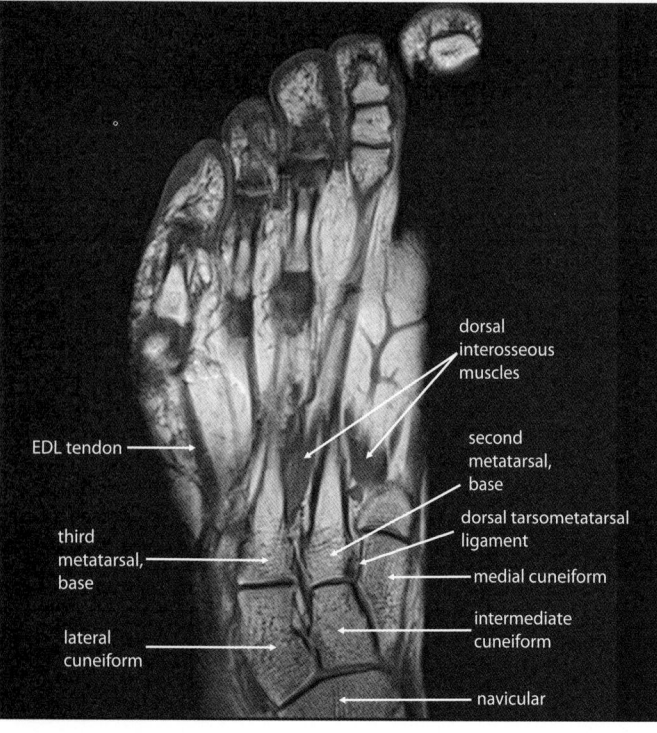
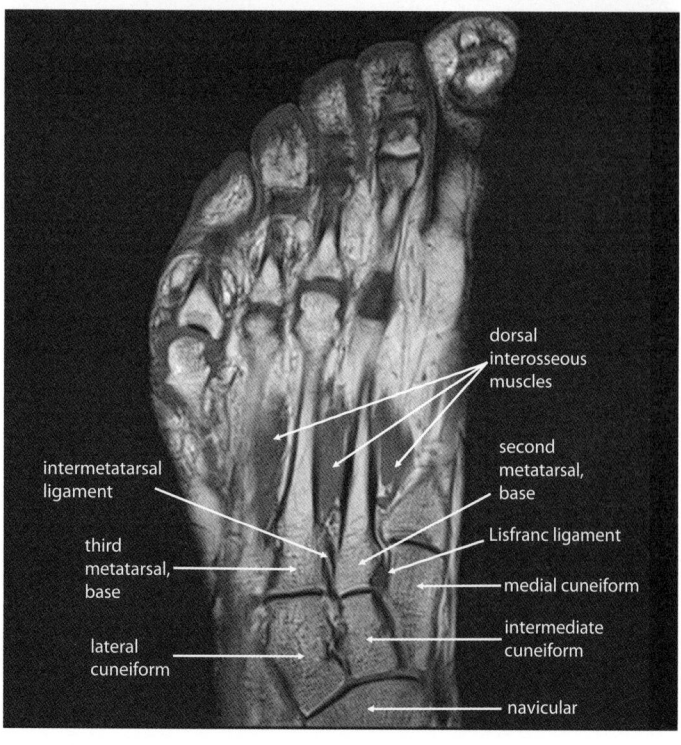

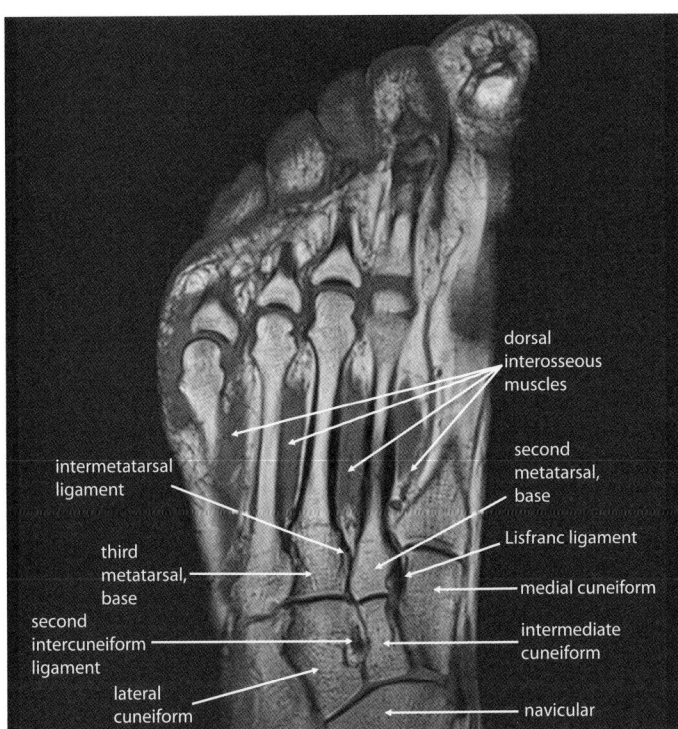
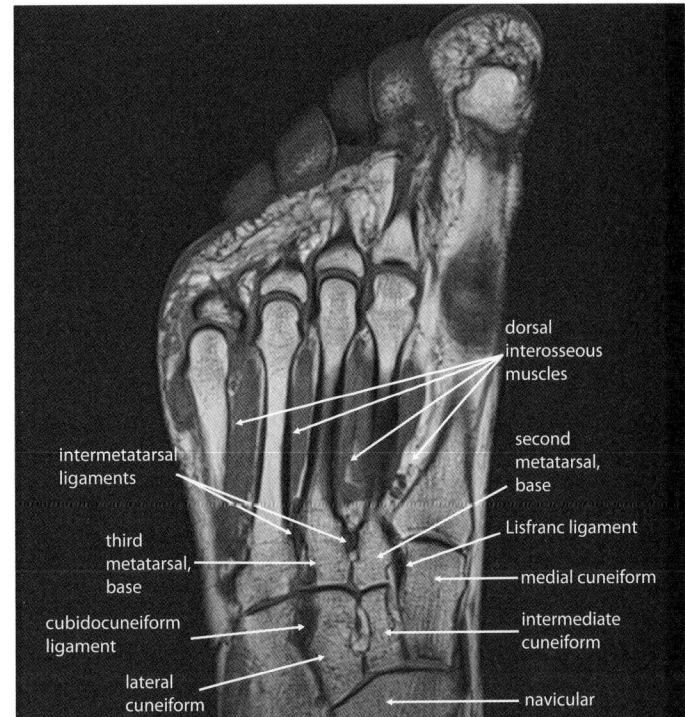
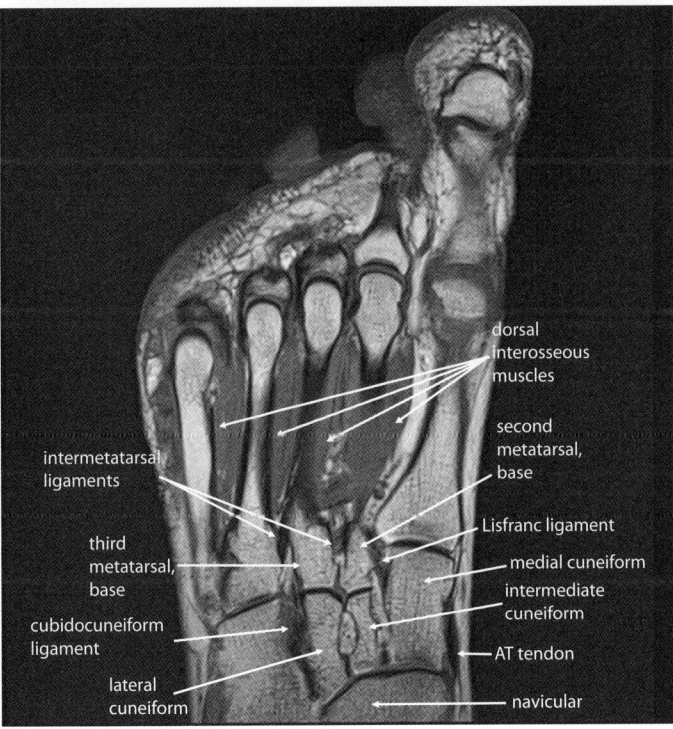
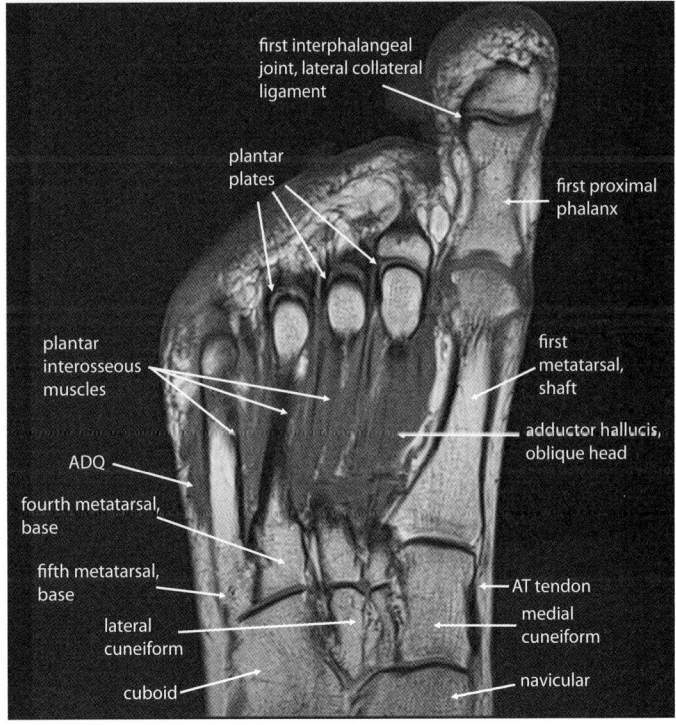

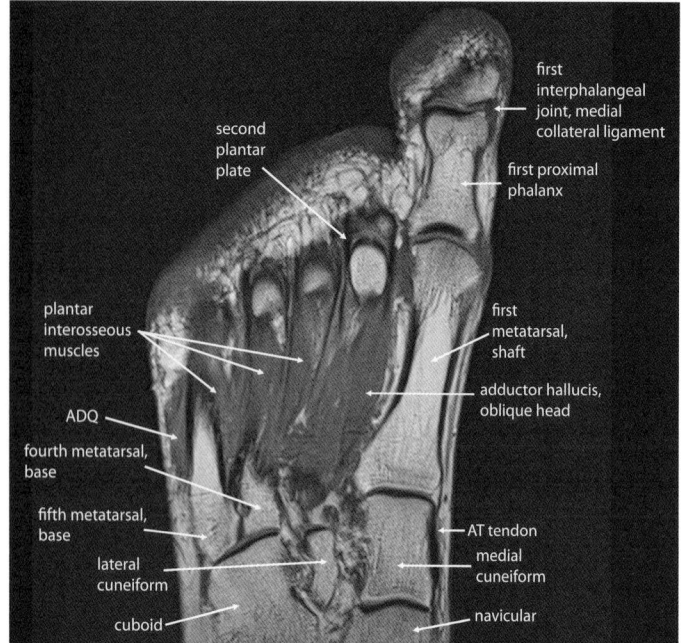
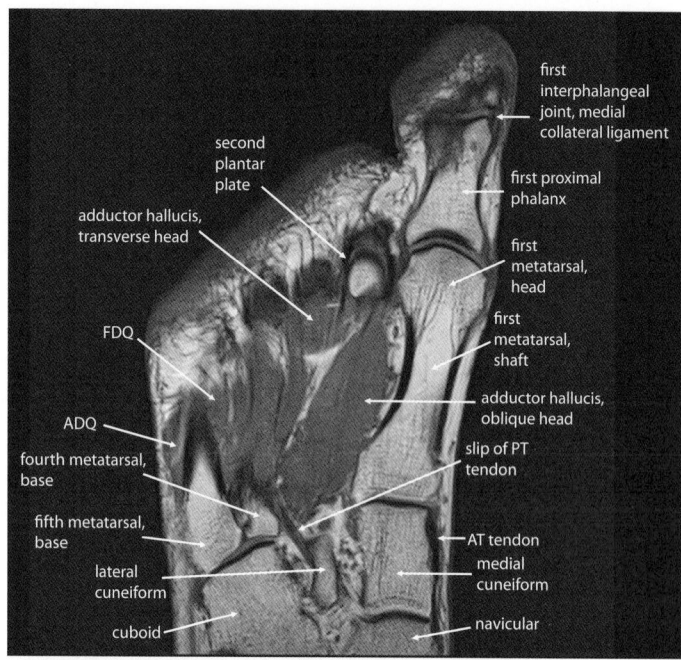
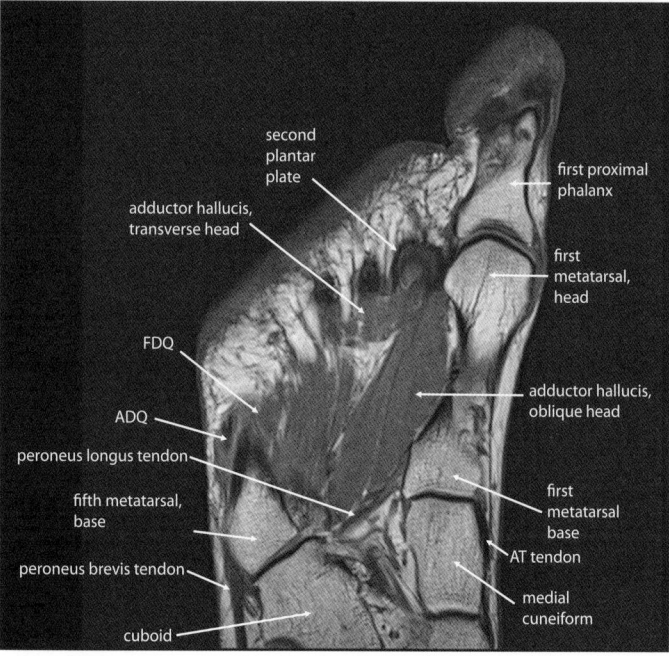
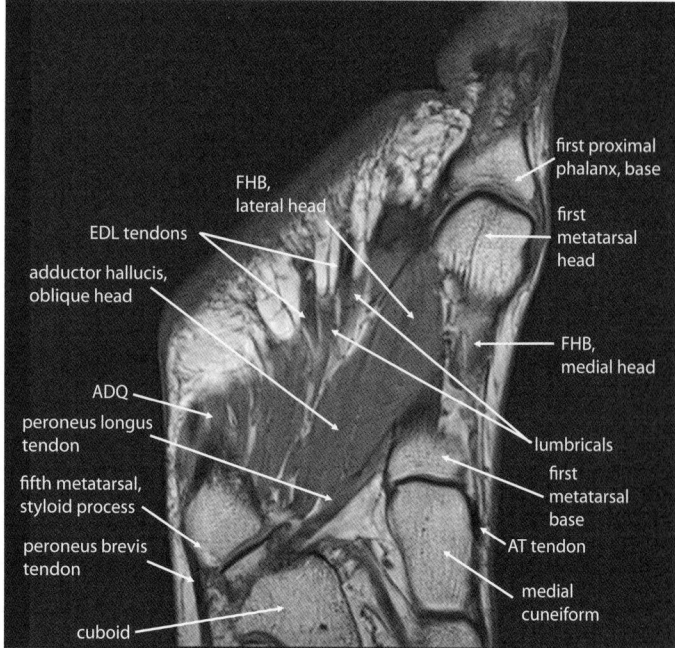

Chapter 13: Diagnostic Imaging Techniques of the Foot and Ankle 759

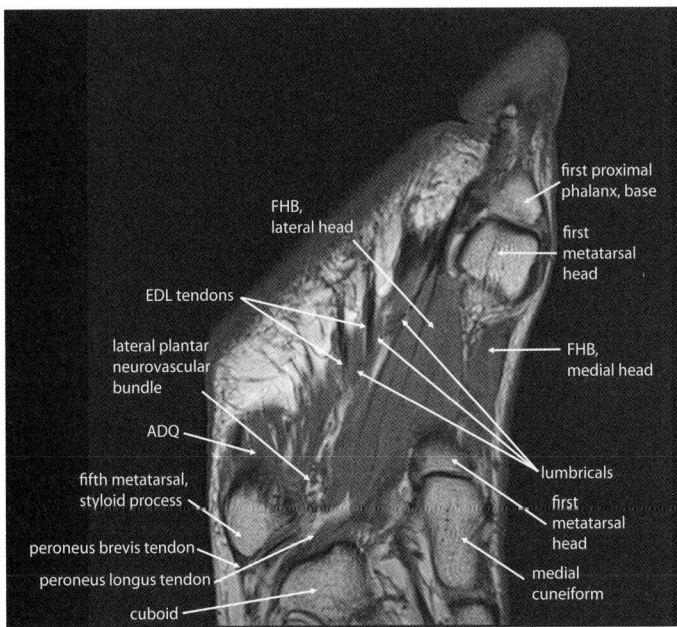
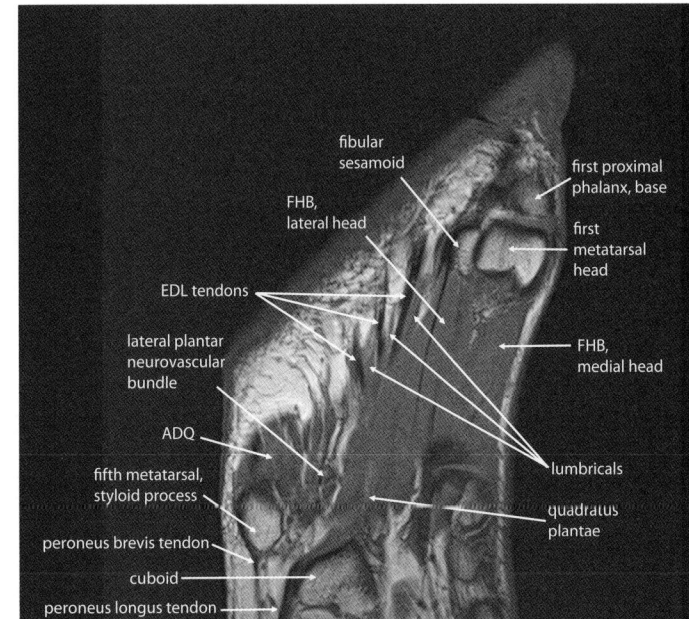
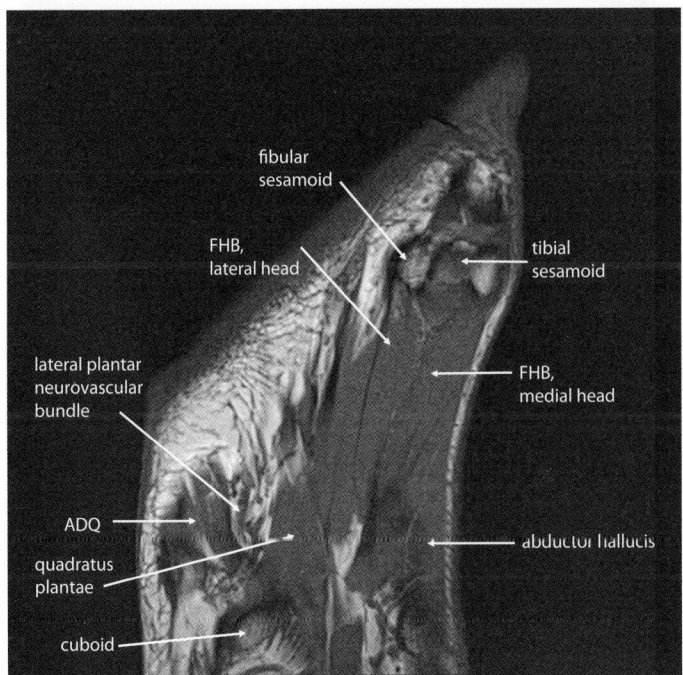
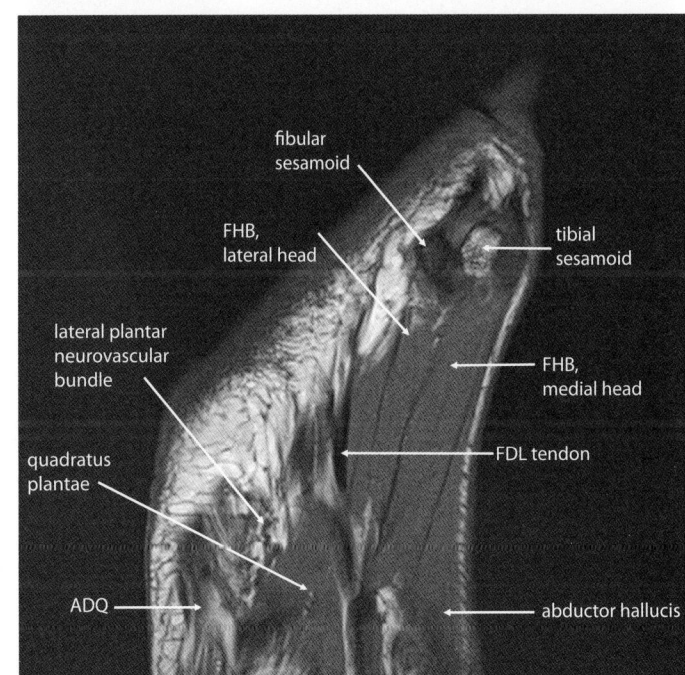

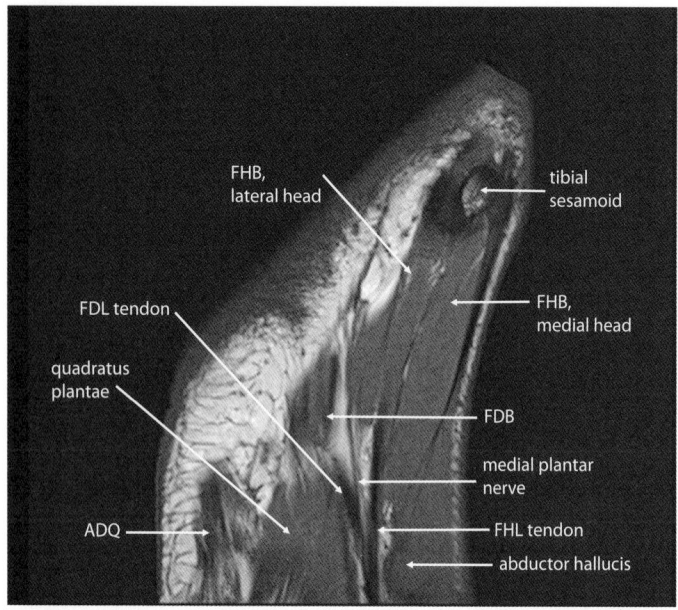
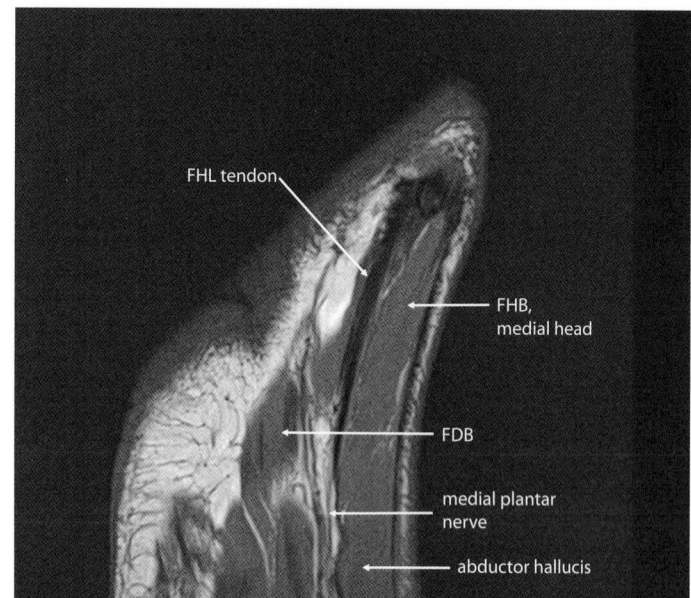
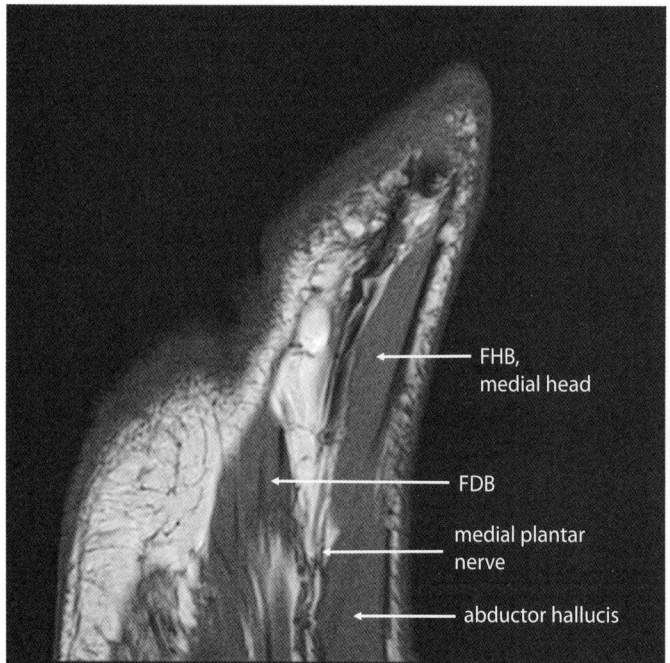
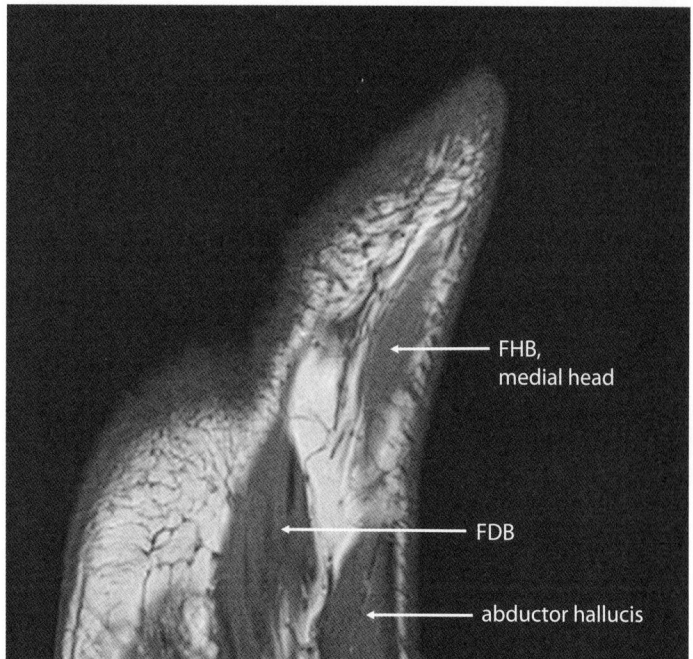

▶ Set 3. Short Axis (Coronal) Proton Density Fat-Saturated Images of the Forefoot

Contiguous images are shown sequentially from posterior to anterior, extending from the midtarsal region to the tips of the toes. This plane shows most the forefoot structures like tendons and muscles in cross-section and should be included in any hindfoot protocol to best detect and localize pathology. It is also helpful in examining the hallux sesamoid complex or injuries to the lesser metatarsophalangeal plantar plates, as well as the digital neurovascular bundles. Structures in the midfoot, such as the Lisfranc ligament, are also often well seen on these images.

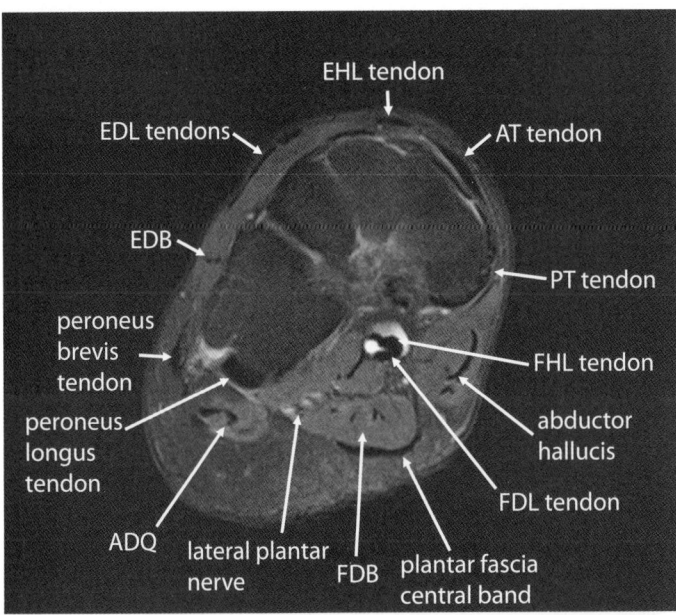
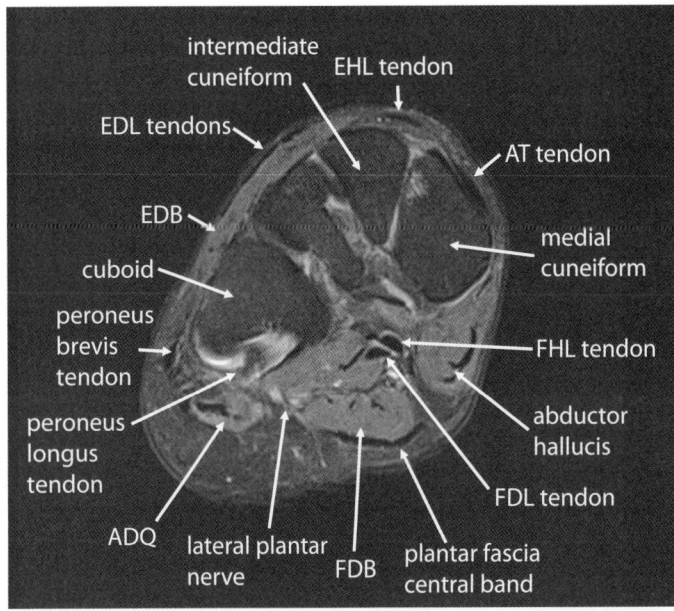
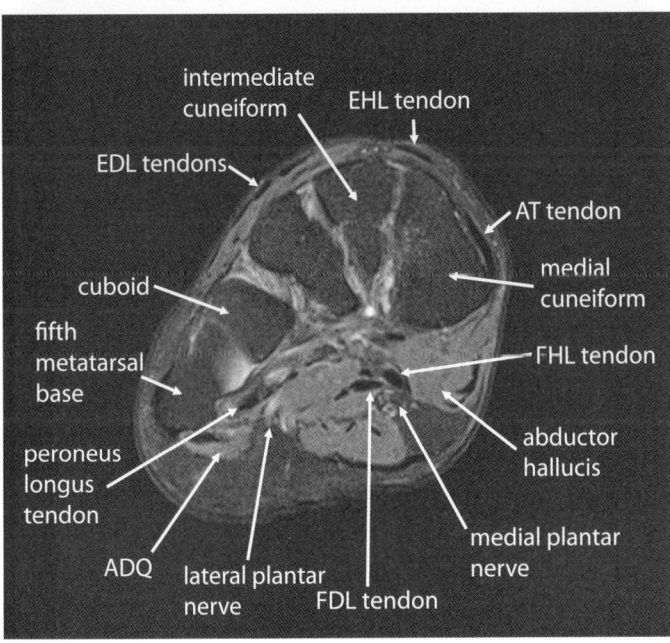
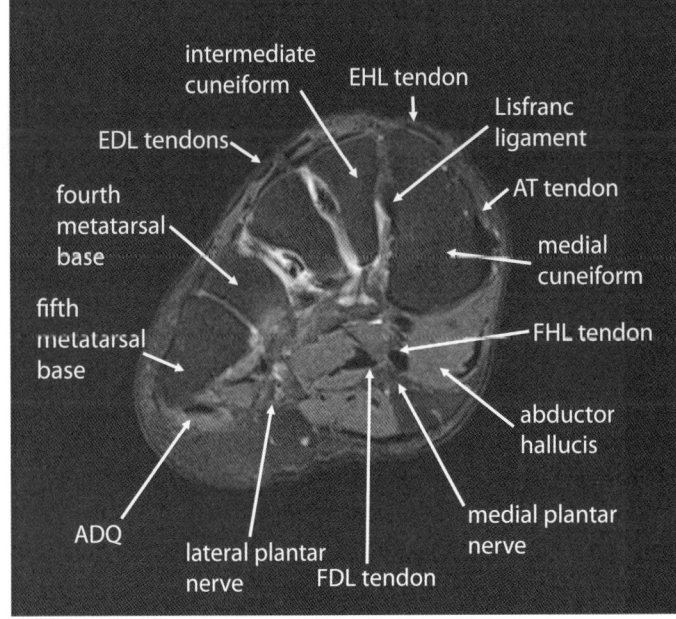

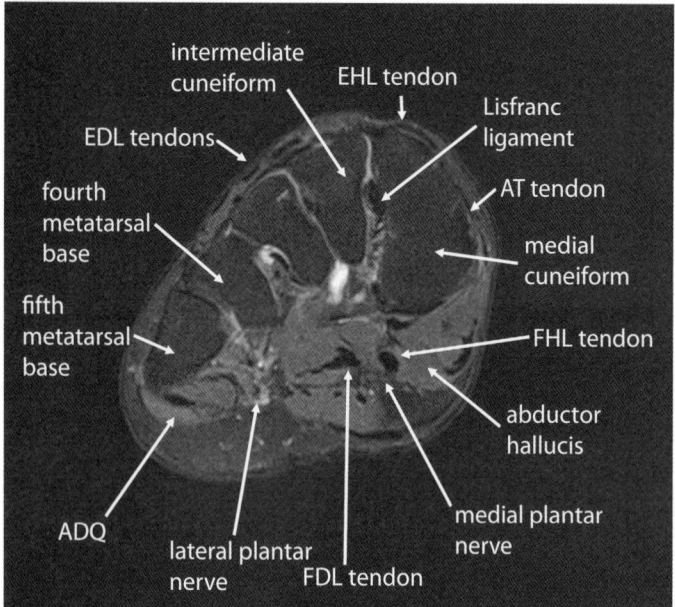
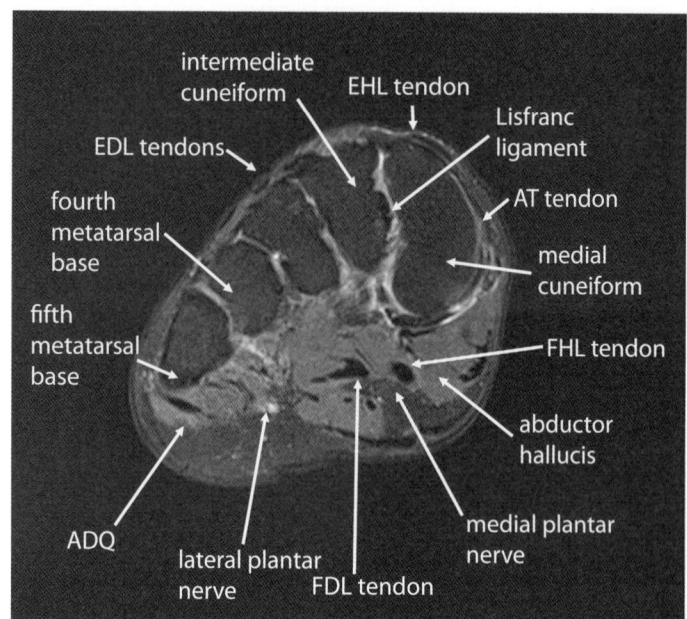
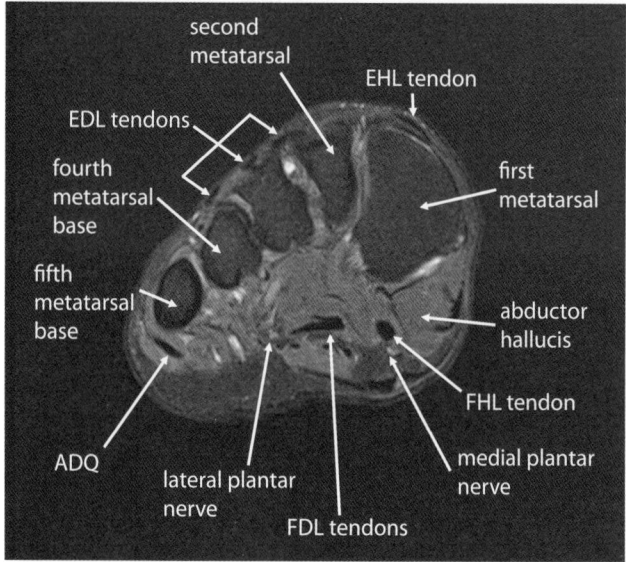
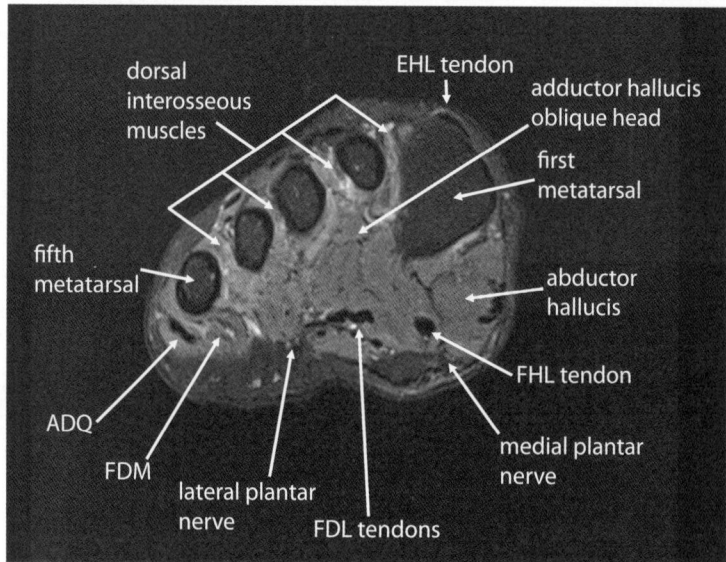

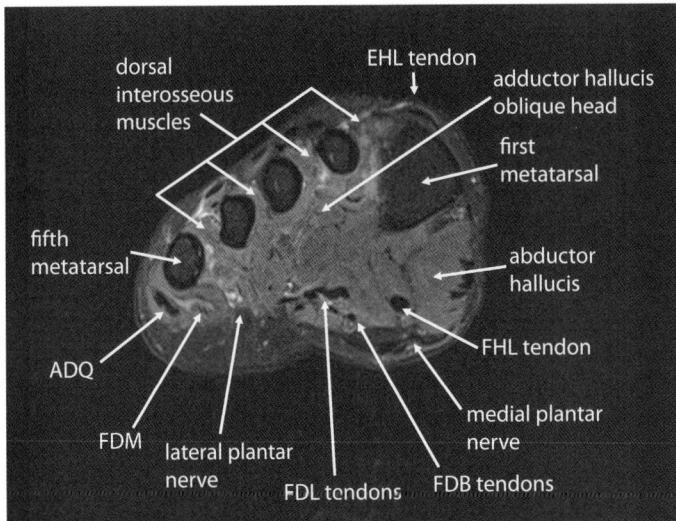
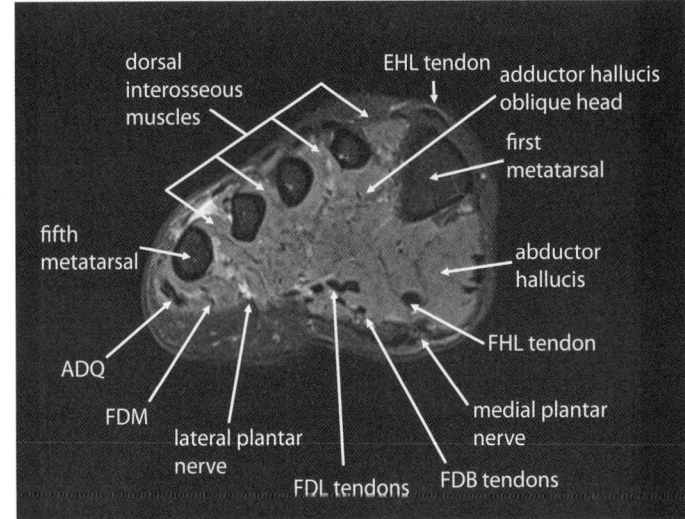
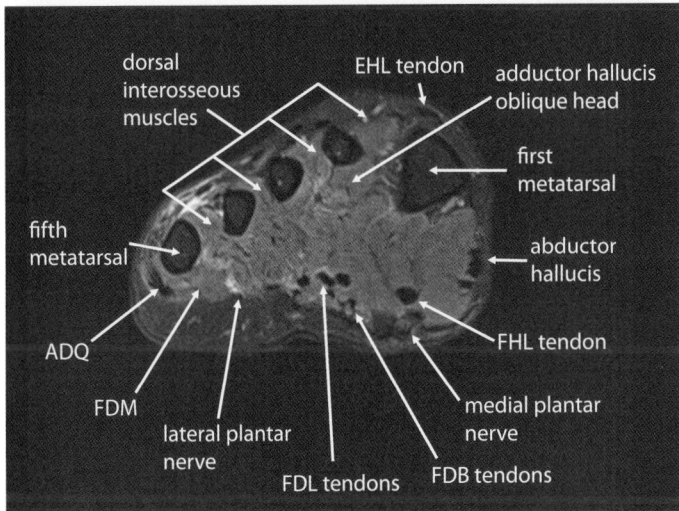
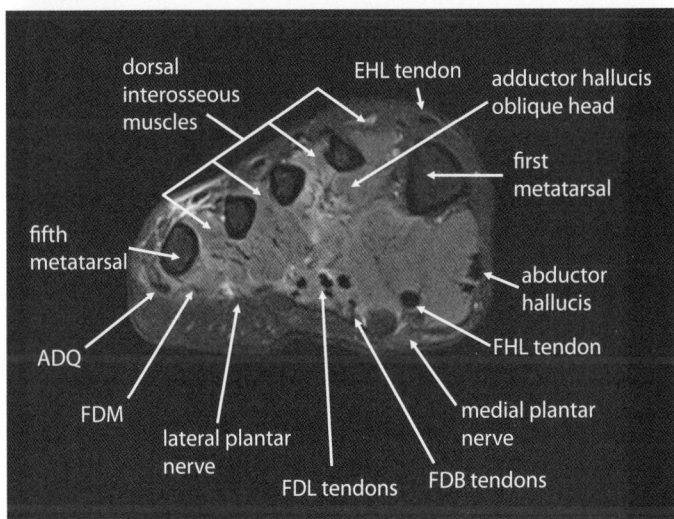

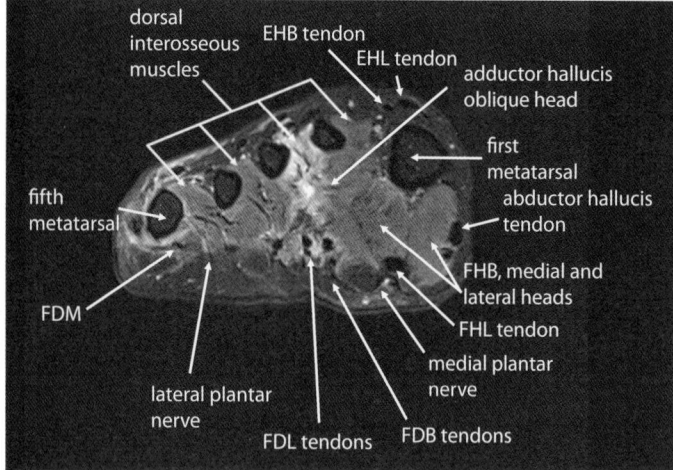
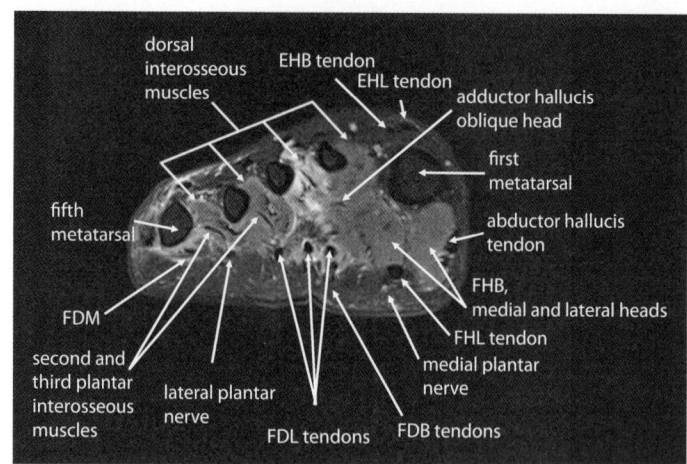
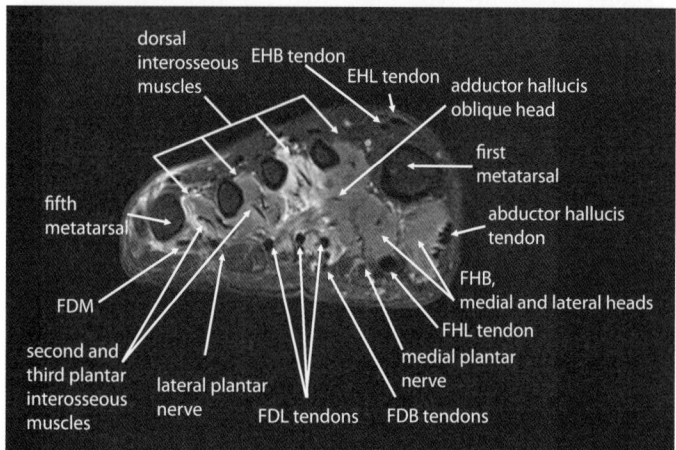
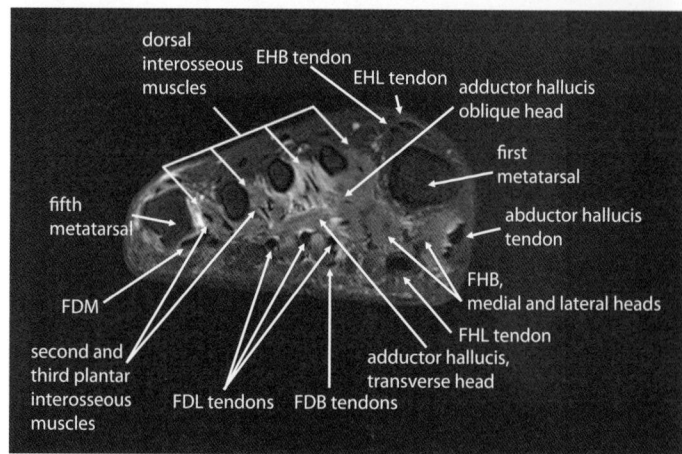

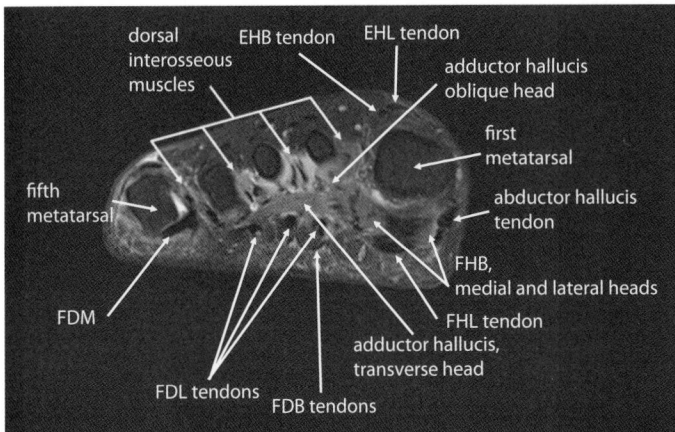
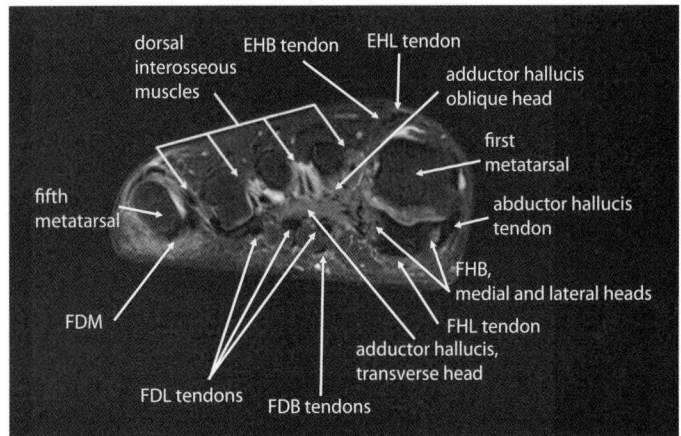
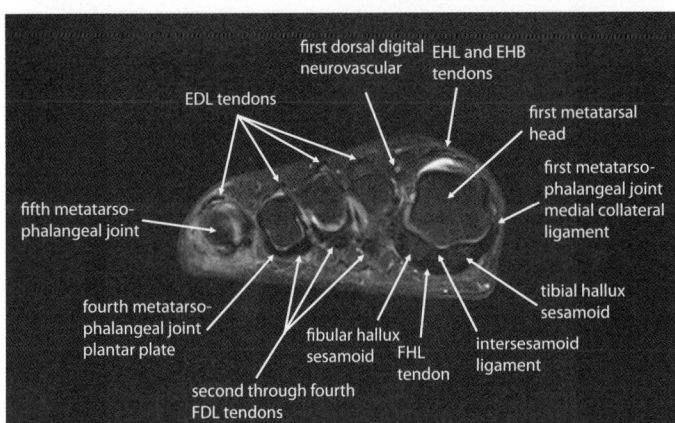
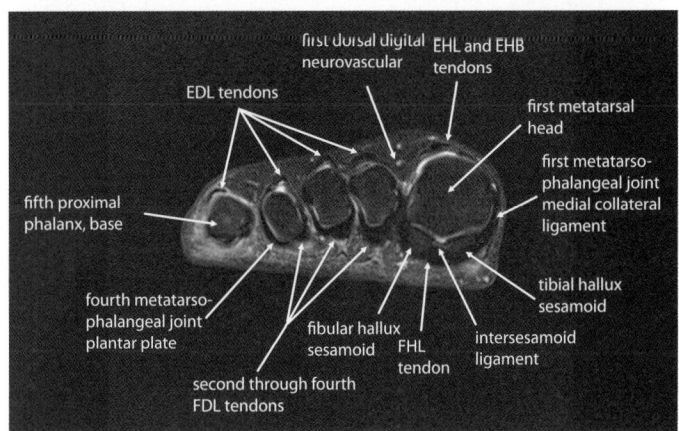

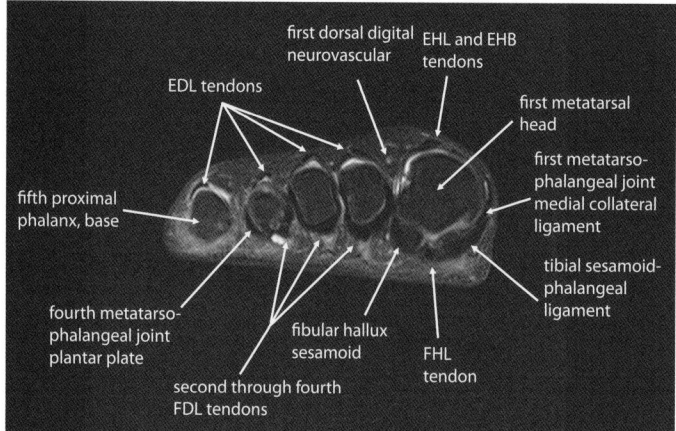
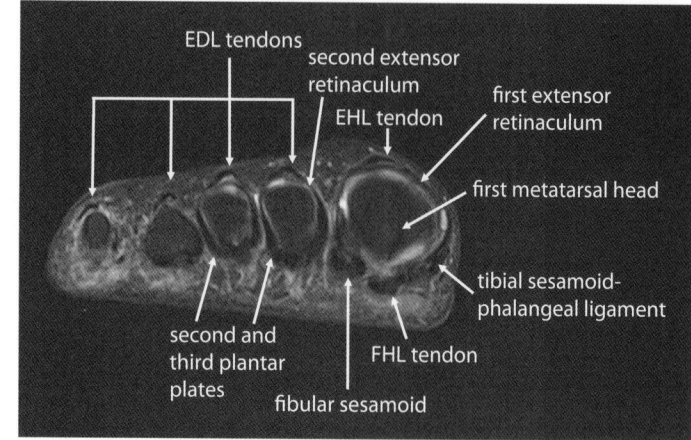
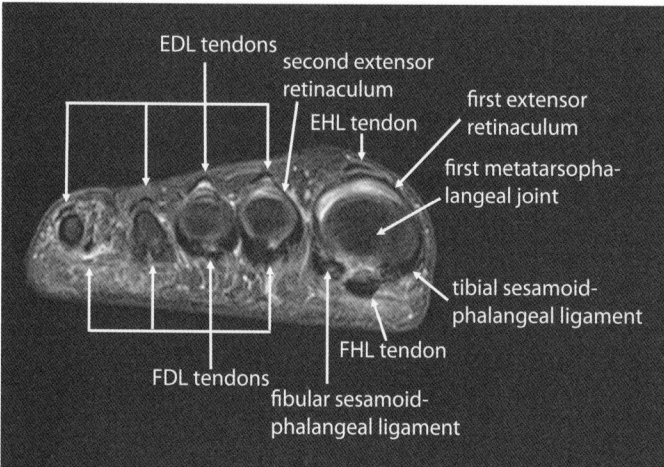
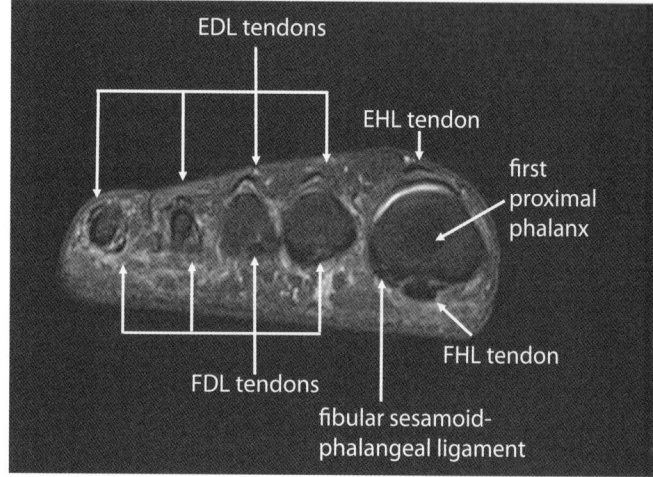

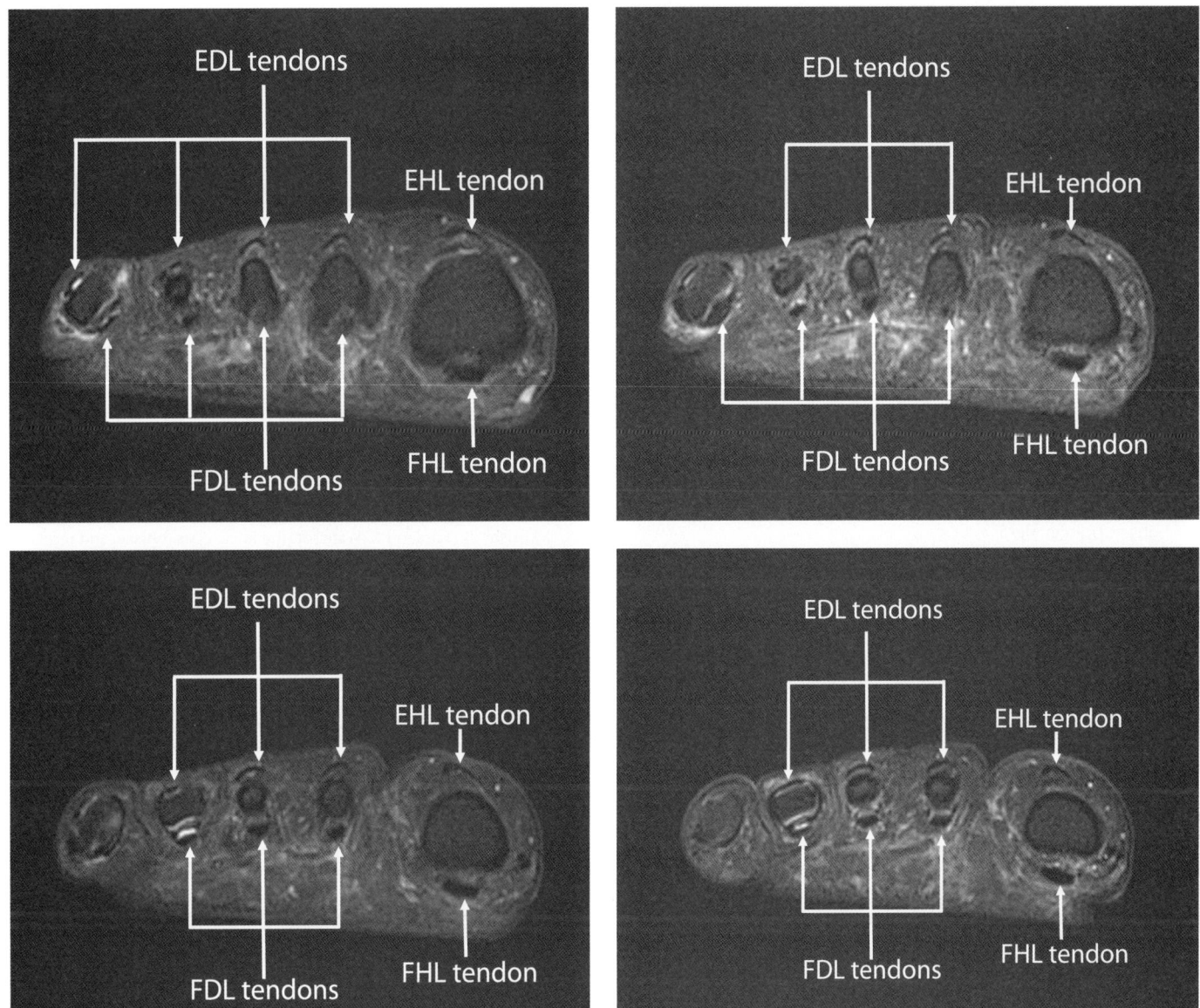

REFERENCES

1. Jacobson JA. Musculoskeletal ultrasound: focused impact on MRI. *AJR Am J Roentgenol*. 2009;193(3):619-627.
2. Renner JB. Conventional radiography in musculoskeletal imaging. *Radiol Clin North Am*. 2009;47(3):357-372.
3. Eustace S, Shah B, Mason M. Imaging orthopedic hardware with an emphasis on hip prostheses. *Orthop Clin North Am*. 1998;29(1):67-84.
4. Merrill V. *Atlas of Roentgenographic Positions*. CV Mosby; 1949.
5. Ballinger PW, Frank ED. *Merrill's Atlas of Radiographic Positions and Radiologic Procedures*. 10th ed. Mosby; 2003.
6. Daffner RH. Visual illusions in the interpretation of the radiographic image. *Curr Probl Diagn Radiol*. 1989;18(2):62-87.
7. Christman RA, ed. *Foot and Ankle Radiology*. 2nd ed. Lippincott Williams & Wilkins; 2015.
8. Senall JA, Kile TA. Stress radiography. *Foot Ankle Clin*. 2000;5(1):165-184.
9. Daftary A, Haims AH, Baumgaertner MR. Fractures of the calcaneus: a review with emphasis on CT. *Radiographics*. 2005;25(5):1215-1226.
10. Naudie DD, Rorabeck CH. Sources of osteolysis around total knee arthroplasty: wear of the bearing surface. *Instr Course Lect*. 2004;53:251-259.
11. Fayad LM, Bluemke DA, Fishman EK. Musculoskeletal imaging with computed tomography and magnetic resonance imaging: when is computed tomography the study of choice? *Curr Probl Diagn Radiol*. 2005;34(6):220-237.
12. Barrett JF, Keat N. Artifacts in CT: recognition and avoidance. *Radiographics*. 2004;24(6):1679-1691.
13. Young SW, Muller HH, Marshall WH. Computed tomography: beam hardening and environmental density artifact. *Radiology*. 1983;148(1):279-283.
14. Rydberg J, Buckwalter KA, Caldemeyer KS, et al. Multisection CT: scanning techniques and clinical applications. *Radiographics*. 2000;20(6):1787-1806.
15. Ochenjele G, Ho B, Switaj PJ, et al. Radiographic study of the fifth metatarsal for optimal intramedullary screw fixation of Jones fracture. *Foot Ankle Int*. 2015;36(3):293-301.
16. Fishman EK, Horton KM, Johnson PT. Multidetector CT and three-dimensional CT angiography for suspected vascular trauma of the extremities. *Radiographics*. 2008;28(3):653-665.
17. Kothari NA, Pelchovitz DJ, Meyer JS. Imaging of musculoskeletal infections. *Radiol Clin North Am*. 2001;39(4):653-671.
18. Goo HW, Goo JM. Dual-energy CT: new horizon in medical imaging. *Korean J Radiol*. 2017;18(4):555-569.
19. Cicero G, Ascenti G, Albrecht MH, et al. Extra-abdominal dual-energy CT applications: a comprehensive overview. *Radiol Med*. 2020;125(4):384-397.
20. Mallinson PI, Coupal TM, McLaughlin PD, et al. Dual-energy CT for the musculoskeletal system. *Radiology*. 2016;281(3):690-707.
21. Posadzy M, Desimpel J, Vanhoenacker F. Cone beam CT of the musculoskeletal system: clinical applications. *Insights Imaging*. 2018;9(1):35-45.
22. Lintz F, de Cesar Netto C, Barg A, et al; Weight Bearing CT International Study Group. Weight-bearing cone beam CT scans in the foot and ankle. *EFORT Open Rev*. 2018;3(5):278-286.
23. Pilania K, Jankharia B, Monoot P. Role of the weight-bearing cone-beam CT in evaluation of flatfoot deformity. *Indian J Radiol Imaging*. 2019;29(4):364-371.
24. de Cesar Netto C, Shakoor D, Roberts L, et al; Weight Bearing CT International Study Group. Hindfoot alignment of adult acquired flatfoot deformity: a comparison of clinical assessment and weightbearing cone beam CT examinations. *Foot Ankle Surg*. 2019;25(6):790-797.
25. Kong A, Cassumbhoy R, Subramaniam RM. Magnetic resonance imaging of ankle tendons and ligaments: part I—anatomy. *Australas Radiol*. 2007;51(4):315-323.
26. Bencardino JT, Rosenberg ZS, Serrano LF. MR imaging features of diseases of the peroneal tendons. *Magn Reson Imaging Clin N Am*. 2001;9(3):493-505.
27. Yu JS. Pathologic and post-operative conditions of the plantar fascia: review of MR imaging appearances. *Skeletal Radiol*. 2000;29(9):491-501.
28. Muthukumar T, Butt SH, Cassar-Pullicino VN. Stress fractures and related disorders in foot and ankle: plain films, scintigraphy, CT, and MR Imaging. *Semin Musculoskelet Radiol*. 2005;9(3):210-226.
29. Hopper MA, Robinson P. Ankle impingement syndromes. *Radiol Clin North Am*. 2008;46(6):957-971.
30. Schachter AK, Chen AL, Reddy PD, Tejwani NC. Osteochondral lesions of the talus. *J Am Acad Orthop Surg*. 2005;13(3):152-158.
31. Lalam RK, Cassar-Pullicino VN, Tins BJ. Magnetic resonance imaging of appendicular musculoskeletal infection. *Top Magn Reson Imaging*. 2007;18(3):177-191.
32. Ashman CJ, Klecker RJ, Yu JS. Forefoot pain involving the metatarsal region: differential diagnosis with MR imaging. *Radiographics*. 2001;21(6):1425-1440.
33. Bancroft LW, Peterson JJ, Kransdorf MJ. Imaging of soft tissue lesions of the foot and ankle. *Radiol Clin North Am*. 2008;46(6):1093-1103.
34. Gregg JM, Schneider T, Marks P. MR imaging and ultrasound of metatarsalgia: the lesser metatarsals. *Radiol Clin North Am*. 2008;46(6):1061-1078.
35. Bencardino JT, Rosenberg ZS. MR imaging and CT in the assessment of osseous abnormalities of the ankle and foot. *Magn Reson Imaging Clin N Am*. 2001;9(3):567-578.
36. Weishaupt D, Schweitzer ME. MR imaging of the foot and ankle: patterns of bone marrow signal abnormalities. *Eur Radiol*. 2002;12(2):416-426.
37. Murphey MD, Carroll JF, Flemming DJ, et al. From the archives of the AFIP: benign musculoskeletal lipomatous lesions. *Radiographics*. 2004;24(5):1433–1466.
38. Disler DG, McCauley TR, Ratner LM, et al. In-phase and out-of-phase MR imaging of bone marrow: prediction of neoplasia based on the detection of coexistent fat and water. *AJR Am J Roentgenol*. 1997;169(5):1439-1447.
39. Morrison JL, Kaplan PA. Water on the knee: cysts, bursae, and recesses. *Magn Reson Imaging Clin N Am*. 2000;8(2):349-370.
40. Wang XT, Rosenberg ZS, Mechlin MB, Schweitzer ME. Normal variants and diseases of the peroneal tendons and superior peroneal retinaculum: MR imaging features. *Radiographics*. 2005;25(3):587-602.
41. Hilfiker P, Zanetti M, Debatin JF, et al. Fast spin-echo inversion-recovery imaging versus fast T2-weighted spin-echo imaging in bone marrow abnormalities. *Invest Radiol*. 1995;30(2):110-114.
42. Gold GE, Chen CA, Koo S, et al. Recent advances in MRI of articular cartilage. *AJR Am J Roentgenol*. 2009;193(3):628-638.
43. Link TM, Stahl R, Woertler K. Cartilage imaging: motivation, techniques, current and future significance. *Eur Radiol*. 2007;17(5):1135-1146.
44. Koff MF, Potter HG. Noncontrast MR techniques and imaging of cartilage. *Radiol Clin North Am*. 2009;47(3):495-504.
45. Towers JD. The use of intravenous contrast in MRI of extremity infection. *Semin Ultrasound CT MR*. 1997;18(4):269-275.
46. Kransdorf MJ, Murphey MD. The use of gadolinium in the MR evaluation of soft tissue tumors. *Semin Ultrasound CT MR*. 1997;18(4):251-268.
47. Bencardino JT, Rosenberg ZS. Normal variants and pitfalls in MR imaging of the ankle and foot. *Magn Reson Imaging Clin N Am*. 2001;9(3):447-463.
48. Berquist TH. Magnetic resonance techniques in musculoskeletal diseases. *Rheum Dis Clin North Am*. 1991;17(3):599-615.
49. Weishaupt D, Treiber K, Kundert HP, et al. Morton neuroma: MR imaging in prone, supine, and upright weight-bearing body positions. *Radiology*. 2003;226(3):849-856.
50. Berquist TH. Foot, ankle, and calf. In: Berquist TH ed. *MRI of the Musculoskeletal System*. 5th ed. Lippincott Williams & Wilkins; 2006:431.
51. Mink JH. Tendons. In: Deusch AL, et al, eds. *MRI of the Foot and Ankle*. Raven Press; 1992:135.
52. Ting AY, Morrison WB, Kavanagh EC. MR imaging of midfoot injury. *Magn Reson Imaging Clin N Am*. 2008;16(1):105-115.
53. Ankle and foot. In: Resnick D, Kang HS, Pretterkleiber ML, eds. *Internal Derangements of the Joint*. 2nd ed. Saunders; 2007:2038.
54. Foot. In: Manaster BJ, Andrews CL, Crim J, et al, eds. *Diagnostic and Surgical Anatomy: Musculoskeletal*. Amirsys; 2006.
55. Stoller DW, Ferkel RD, Li AE, et al. The ankle and foot. In Stoller DW, ed. *Magnetic Resonance Imaging in Orthopaedics and Sports Medicine*. Vol 1, 3rd ed. Lippincott Williams & Wilkins; 2007:733-1050.
56. Cerezal L, Llopis E, Canga A, Rolón A. MR arthrography of the ankle: indications and technique. *Radiol Clin North Am*. 2008;46(6):973-994.
57. El-Khoury GY, Alliman KJ, Lundberg HJ, et al. Cartilage thickness in cadaveric ankles: measurement with double-contrast multi-detector row CT arthrography versus MR imaging. *Radiology*. 2004;233(3):768-773.
58. Powless SH, Elze ME. Metatarsophalangeal joint capsule tears: an analysis by arthrography, a new classification system and surgical management. *J Foot Ankle Surg*. 2001;40(6):374-389.

59. Bergin D, Schweitzer ME. Indirect magnetic resonance arthrography. *Skeletal Radiol.* 2003;32(10):551-558.
60. Morrison WB. Indirect MR arthrography: concepts and controversies. *Semin Musculoskelet Radiol.* 2005;9(2):125-134.
61. Gnanasegaran G, Cook G, Adamson K, Fogelman I. Patterns, variants, artifacts, and pitfalls in conventional radionuclide bone imaging and SPECT/CT. *Semin Nucl Med.* 2009;39(6):380-395.
62. Love C, Din AS, Tomas MB, et al. Radionuclide bone imaging: an illustrative review. *Radiographics.* 2003;23(2):341-358.
63. Horger M, Bares R. The role of single-photon emission computed tomography/computed tomography in benign and malignant bone disease. *Semin Nucl Med.* 2006;36(4):286-294.
64. Vijayanathan S, Butt S, Gnanasegaran G, Groves AM. Advantages and limitations of imaging the musculoskeletal system by conventional radiological, radionuclide, and hybrid modalities. *Semin Nucl Med.* 2009;39(6):357-368.
65. Palestro CJ, Love C. Radionuclide imaging of musculoskeletal infection: conventional agents. *Semin Musculoskelet Radiol.* 2007;11(4):335-352.

Ultrasound Anatomy of the Ankle and Foot

Thomas Grant

Musculoskeletal ultrasound (US) is a rapidly evolving technique that is gaining popularity for the evaluation and treatment of joint and soft-tissue diseases. A clear understanding of normal US anatomy is required to prevent misdiagnosis and ensure optimal patient care. The advantages of US include its unsurpassed depiction of normal and pathologic anatomy, accessibility, and multiplanar capability. Selective use of high-frequency transducers and optimization of sonographic parameters improve visualization of normal and pathological tissue. Comparison with the contralateral anatomical structures and dynamic scanning are invaluable in aiding learning and interpretation of normal and pathologic features.

Advances in technology with higher frequency transducers, power and color Doppler, superb microvascular imaging (SMI), and extended field-of-view functions have facilitated the progressive development of US (Fig. 14.1).[1-3] US offers a cost-effective alternative for imaging musculoskeletal disorders in many situations.

The major soft tissues of the ankle and foot are predominantly superficial and can be assessed with a high-frequency linear transducer. The in-plane spatial resolution and minimal slice thickness using these probes are far superior to those achieved with clinical MRI protocols. The small footprint probes are particularly useful to maintain constant uniform contact between the probe and skin. Active or passive movement can be used for dynamic evaluation of all tendons for tears, abnormal movement due to subluxation, and adhesive tenosynovitis.[4] Color or power Doppler imaging should be used if synovitis or a tendon abnormality is suspected. SMI is a new Doppler technique that depicts slow flow better than conventional Doppler imaging (Fig. 14.2).

GENERAL ULTRASOUND APPEARANCE

▶ Tendons

Tendons are better visualized with US than with MRI. Tendons consist of bundles of linearly arranged fibrils of type I collagen with a supporting matrix. The fibrils are oriented in a direction specific to the forces applied from the interaction between a tendon and its muscle and skeletal attachment.[5,6] When the US beam is perpendicular to the tendon, the energy of the beam is reflected back to the transducer, resulting in a fibrillar pattern of alternating hyperechoic and hypoechoic lines (Fig. 14.3). The fibrillar pattern is unique to tendons. If the beam loses this perpendicular orientation, the tendon will appear hypoechoic, simulating tendinopathy. This phenomenon is known as anisotropy and can be avoided by keeping the beam perpendicular to the tendon.

▶ Ligaments

Ligaments also contain longitudinally arranged parallel fibers of type I collagen.[7] However, their architecture is not as fibrillar (Fig. 14.4). Although anisotropy is observed, it is not a prominent imaging feature, but it can be used to find ligaments and distinguish them from surrounding connective tissue. Like tendons, ligaments must be imaged longitudinally and transversely.

▶ Nerves

Peripheral nerves, as small as 1 mm in diameter, can be identified using commercially available 24-MHz multifrequency transducers. Nerves are composed of multiple axons that are bundled together in neuronal fascicles. The fascicles are held together by loose connective tissue, the epineurium.[8,9] Normal peripheral nerves typically appear as echogenic fascicular structures and tend to be slightly less echogenic than tendons or ligaments. In a longitudinal plane, a nerve and tendon often look alike. Therefore, transverse imaging is the best method to visualize a nerve using US (Fig. 14.5).

▶ Capsule and Fascia

Capsular tissue and fascia appear hyperechoic.

▶ Cortical Bone

Cortical bone is hyperechoic, reflecting the insonating beam and producing a black acoustic shadow, hence precluding visualization of the osseous medulla.

Chapter 14: Ultrasound Anatomy of the Ankle and Foot   771

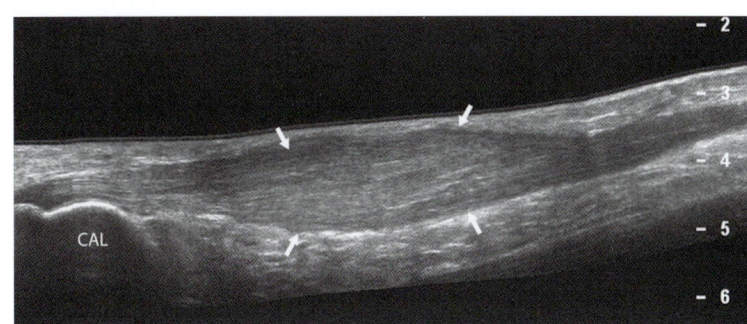

Figure 14.1 **Extended field-of-view image shows tendinopathy at the critical zone of the Achilles tendon.** Ultrasound demonstrates thickening and hypoechoic appearance of the tendon (*arrows*). Note the normal distal Achilles tendon adjacent to the calcaneous (*CAL*).

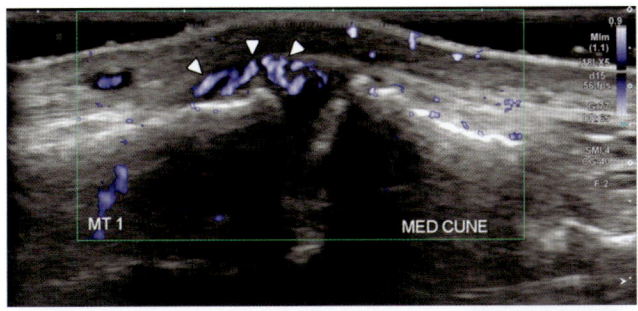

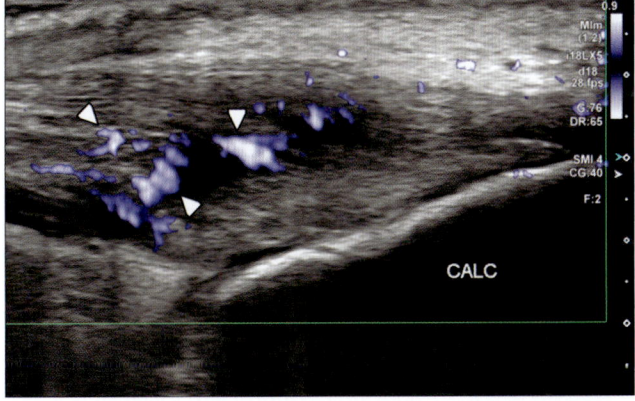

Figure 14.2 **Superb microvascular Doppler imaging.** **(A)** Rheumatoid arthritis with inflammatory synovitis at the dorsum of the medial cuneiform-first metatarsal joint space (*arrowheads*). **(B)** Neovascularity in a patient with insertional tendinosis of the Achilles tendon (*arrowheads*).

▶ **Articular Cartilage**

Hyaline articular cartilage is anechoic and homogenous and best seen on the dorsal aspect of the foot.

▶ **Muscle**

Muscle, like tendons and ligaments, has an organized structure. The epimysium is identified as an echogenic envelope surrounding the muscle belly, whereas the perimysium envelopes the muscular fascicles and is seen as short echogenic lines or dots on a hypoechoic background[5] (Fig. 14.6).

▶ **Fluid and Synovium**

Bland uncomplicated fluid and synovium appear uniformly anechoic. Posterior acoustic enhancement, the absence of vascularity on Doppler imaging, and the swirling movement of debris on intermittent pressure with the probe may differentiate simple fluid from synovium.

▶ **Normal Ultrasound Anatomy of the Ankle**

The ankle is the most frequently injured major joint in the body. It is also involved by degenerative and rheumatology-related diseases. US has become increasingly important imaging modality in the assessment and diagnosis of tendons, muscles, ligaments, nerves, and the soft tissues.[10-12] However,

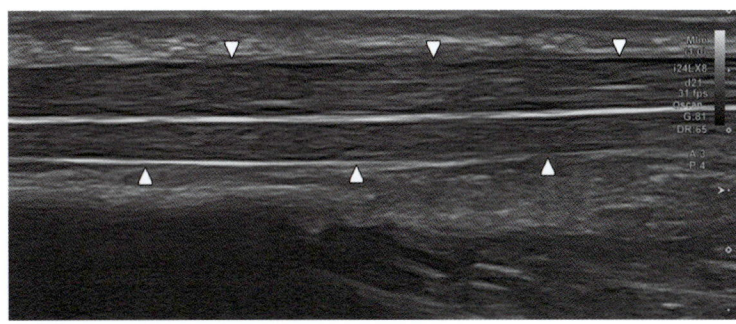

Figure 14.3 Normal ultrasound fibrillar appearance of the peroneal tendons (*arrowheads*).

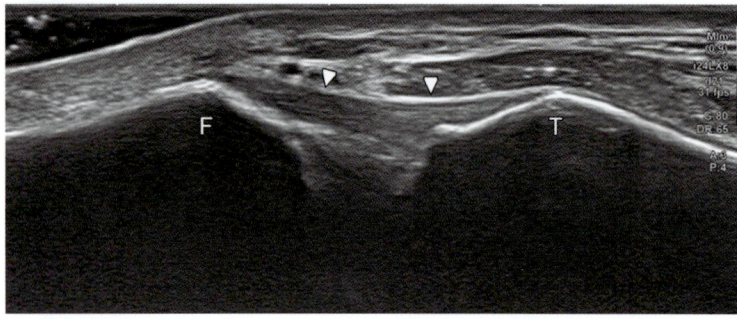

Figure 14.4 Normal ultrasound appearance of anterior tibiofibular ligament (*arrowheads*) between the tibia (*T*) and fibula (*F*).

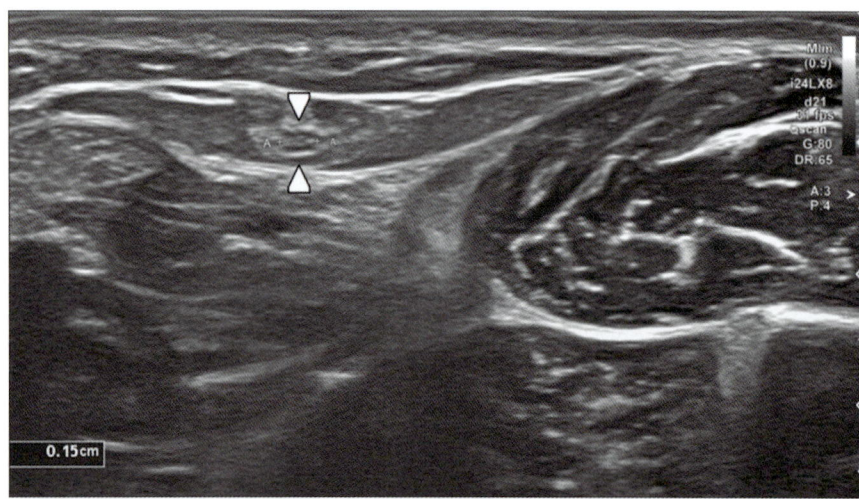

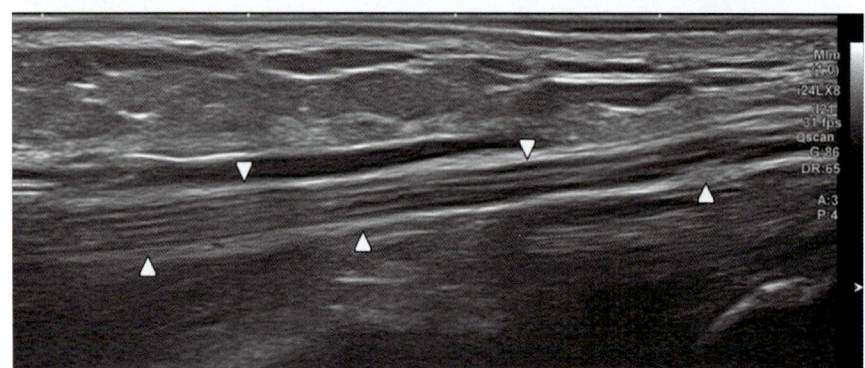

Figure 14.5 Normal ultrasound appearance of superficial peroneal nerve (A) and tibial nerve (B) at the ankle.

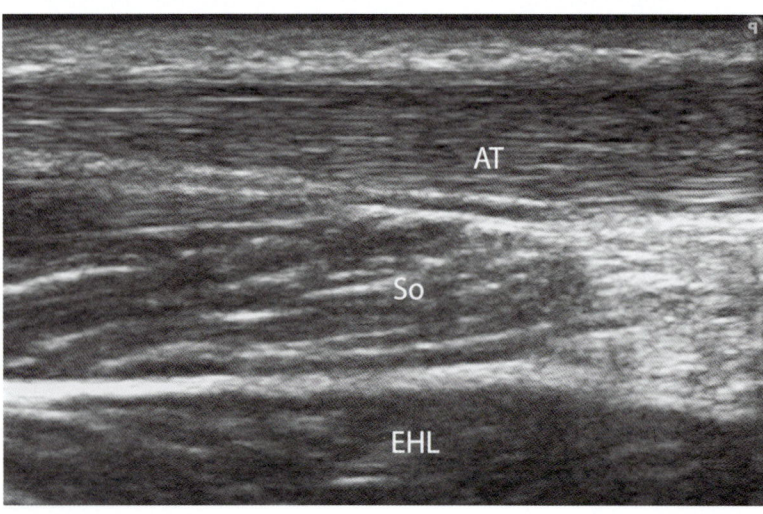

Figure 14.6 Transverse ultrasound image of the normal soleus (*SO*) muscle and extensor hallucis longus (*EHL*) muscle anterior to the Achilles tendon (*AT*).

radiographs of the ankle should be obtained to evaluate for bone lesions that can be overlooked or not visualized using US.

▶ Anterior Ankle

The tibialis anterior (TA), extensor hallucis longus (EHL) and extensor digitorum longus (EDL), the anterior tibial artery, the deep peroneal nerve, and a portion of the tibial talar joint can be assessed with US[13] (Fig. 14.7A).

The TA is the widest of the tendons and attaches to the anterior and inferior medial cuneiform and first metatarsal (Fig. 14.7B). The EHL and EDL lie adjacent to each other in the ankle and fuse with the extensor hood. The anterior tibial artery lies lateral the EHL tendon. It is assessed by visualizing its pulsatility or with Doppler imaging. The deep peroneal nerve runs adjacent to artery (Fig. 14.7C).

Due to acoustic shadowing from the overlying bone, only the anterior capsule of the joint is imaged. The articular cartilage of the talar dome is approximately 2 mm in thickness. Joint effusions and synovial thickening distend the joint. A joint effusion can be distinguished from synovial thickening by applying transducer pressure since fluid is readily compressible.

▶ Lateral Ankle

The lateral tendons, including the anterior talofibular and the calcaneofibular ligaments, can reliably be depicted with US[14] (Fig. 14.8). The anterior talofibular ligament appears as straight

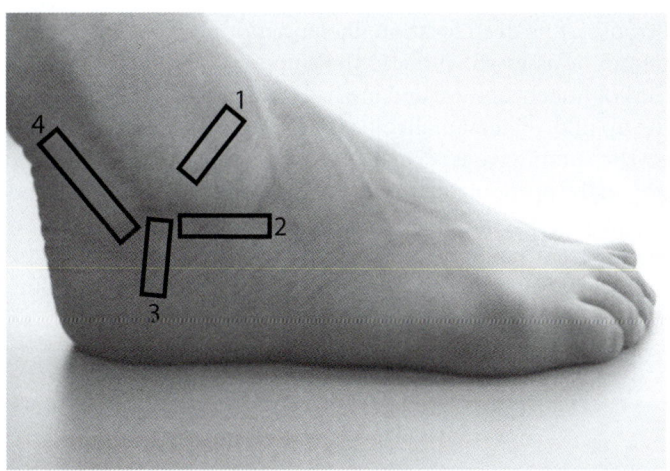

Figure 14.8 Diagram of the locations of the anterior tibiofibular ligament (*1*), anterior talofibular ligament (*2*), calcaneofibular ligament (*3*), and peroneal tendons (*4*).

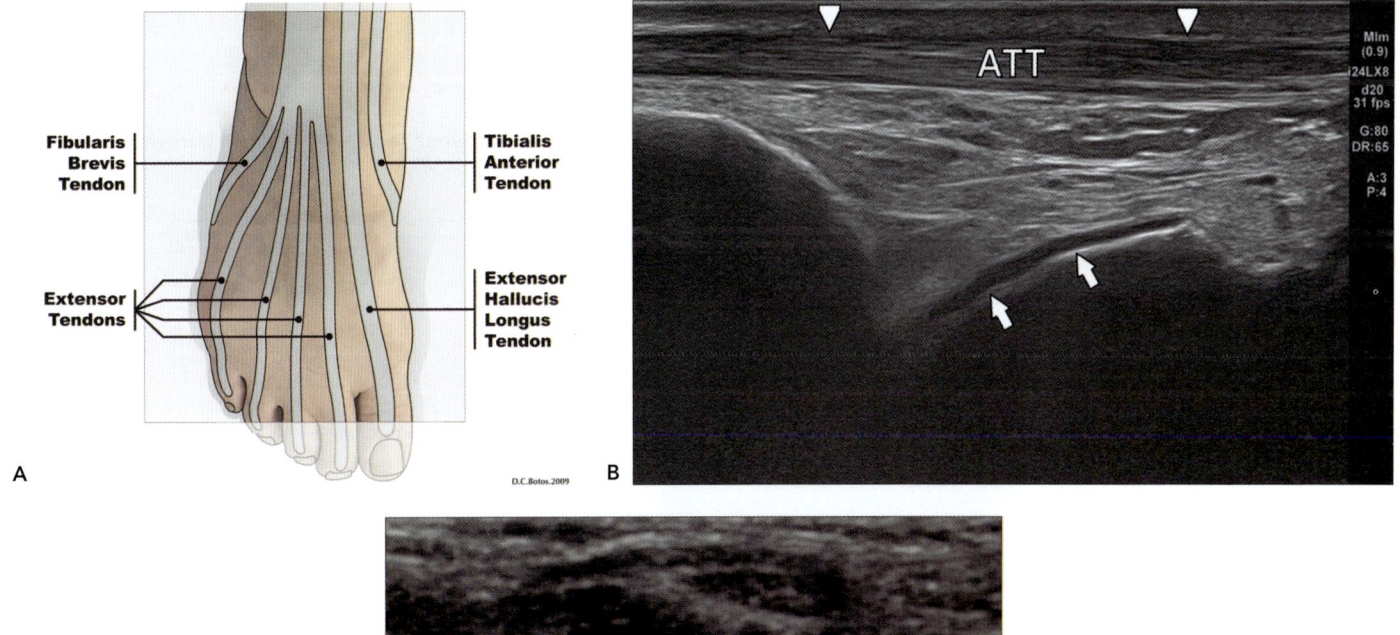

Figure 14.7 (**A**) Schematic drawing of the tendons of the dorsal ankle and foot. (**B**) Normal ultrasound appearance of tibiotalar joint with the anterior tibial tendon (*arrowheads*) and articular cartilage (*arrows*). (**C**) Dorsalis pedis artery (*arrow*) adjacent to the deep peroneal nerve (*arrowhead*).

fibrillar band connecting the anterior aspect of the tip of the lateral malleolus with the talar neck superficial to the joint line (Fig. 14.9). The caudal part of the calcaneofibular ligament is 2 to 3 mm thick and is visualized as a cordlike fibrillar structure, which overlies the lateral aspect of the calcaneus, whereas its cranial part courses deep to the peroneal tendons (Fig. 14.10). Because of its deep location, the posterior talofibular ligament cannot be assessed with US. The anterior tibiofibular ligament runs obliquely upward and medially from the anterior aspect of the tip of the lateral malleolus (see Fig. 14.4).

The sural nerve is a cutaneous nerve, providing only sensation to the posterolateral aspect of the distal third of the leg and the lateral aspect of the foot, heel, and ankle. The sural nerve is located between the Achilles and peroneal tendons and can be injured by penetrating trauma or damage during surgery to the lateral ankle. US can differentiate an injured nerve in continuity from a severed nerve[15] (Fig. 14.11).

US allows an accurate evaluation of the peroneal tendons in their supramalleolar, retromalleolar, and inframalleolar portions[16] (see Figs. 14.3 and 14.12A,B). In the supramalleolar region, the peroneus longus tendon courses lateral to the peroneus brevis muscle. As the peroneus brevis muscle approaches the lateral malleolus, it continues in a long tendon, which has a flattened curvilinear appearance, and is located anteromedial and then superior to the peroneus longus tendon. In the inframalleolar region, the peroneal tendons appear as oval diverging structures, which are separated by the peroneal tubercle of the calcaneus (Fig. 14.12C). The peroneus brevis tendon passes superior to the tubercle, whereas the peroneus longus is located inferior to it. The peroneal tendons have a common

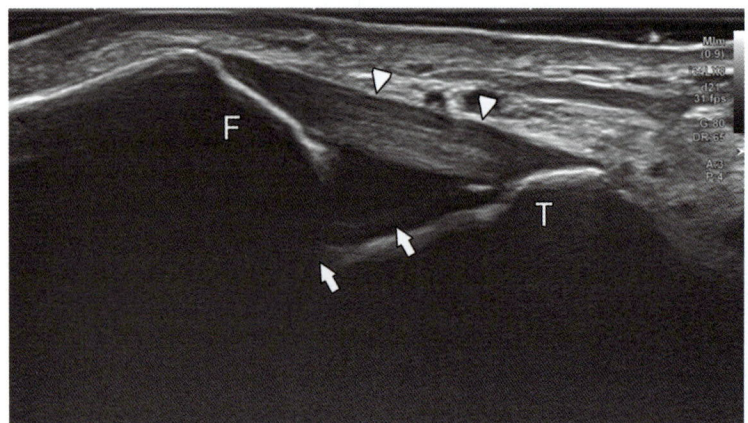

Figure 14.9 Anterior talofibular ligament (*arrows*) running between the fibula (*F*) and talus (*T*).

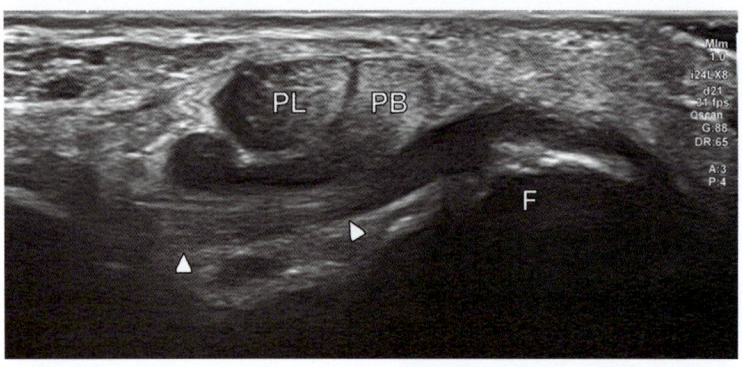

Figure 14.10 Calcaneofibular ligament (*arrowheads*) located deep to the peroneal tendon. (*F*, fibula; *PB*, peroneus brevis; *PL*, peroneus longus.)

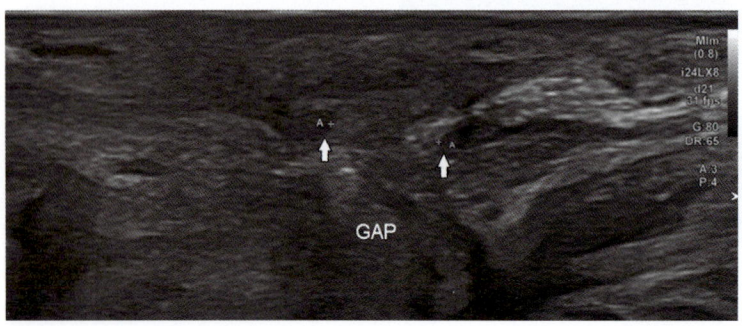

Figure 14.11 Lacerated sural nerve at the ankle (*arrows*) with a 2-mm gap between the proximal and distal stumps.

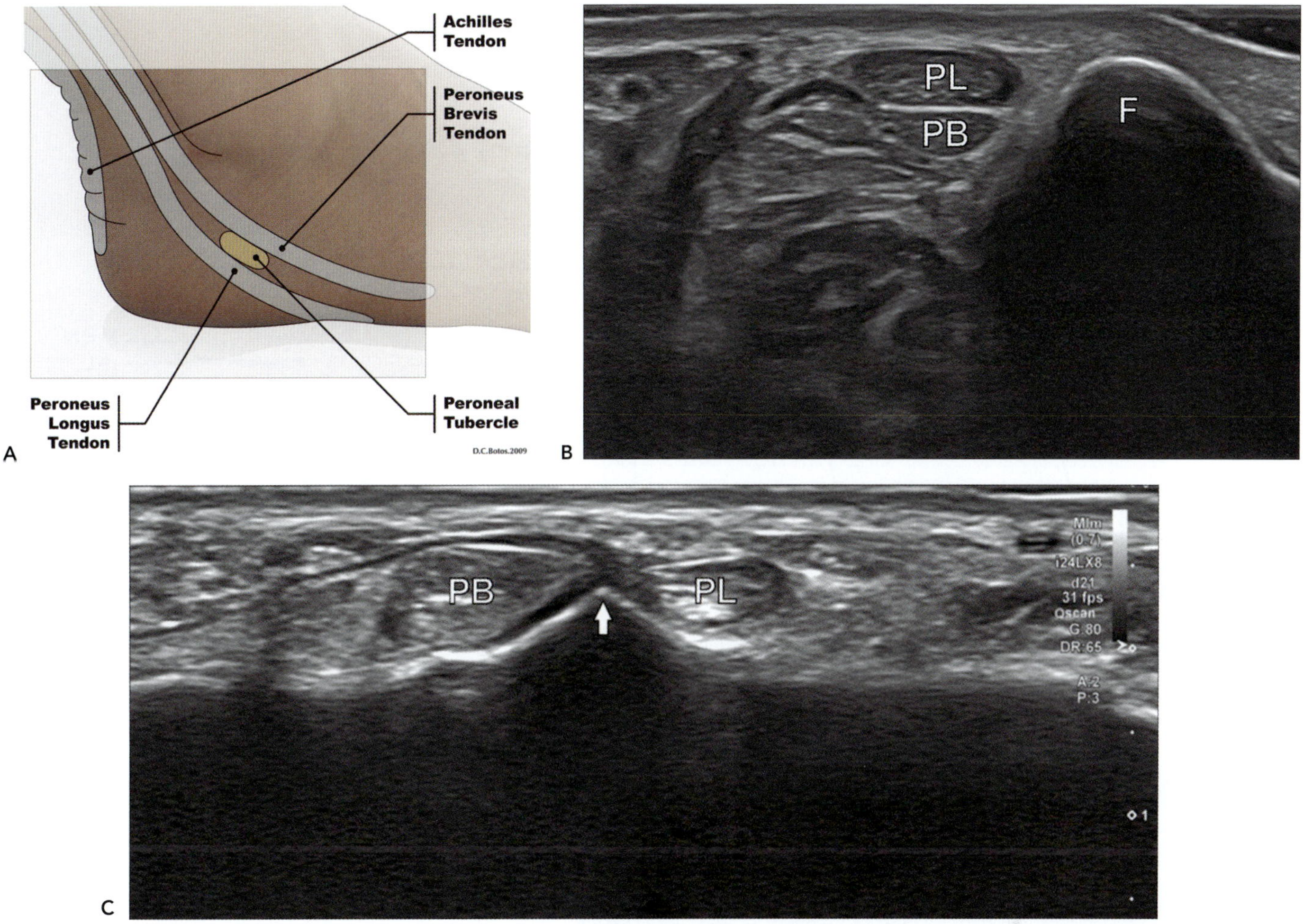

Figure 14.12 Peroneal tendons. **(A)** Diagram of the location of the peroneal tendons. **(B)** Peroneus longus (*PL*) and brevis tendons (*PB*) adjacent to the lateral malleolus (*F*). **(C)** PL and PB separated by the peroneal tubercle of the calcaneus (*arrow*).

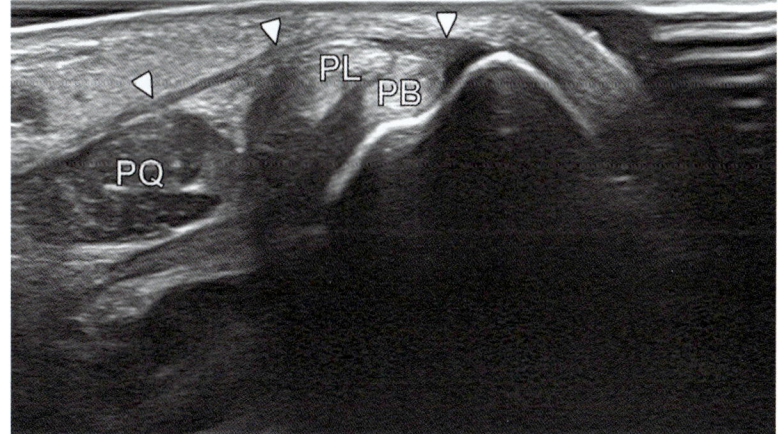

Figure 14.13 The peroneus quartus muscle (*PQ*) lies adjacent to the peroneus longus (*PL*) and peroneus brevis (*PB*) tendons. The thin superior peroneal retinaculum (*arrowheads*) overlies the peroneal tendons and inserts into the fibula cortex.

synovial sheath that splits at the peroneal tubercle to surround the diverging tendons. The superior peroneal retinaculum can be appreciated as thin laminar band that overlies the peroneal tendons and insert into the bone cortex of the fibula and calcaneus. A tear of the retinaculum can lead to dislocation of the peroneal tendons. The peroneus quartus muscle is an accessory muscle that shares the same anatomic space with the other peroneal tendons[17] (Fig. 14.13). It can be symptomatic, requiring surgical resection.

▶ **Medial Ankle**

The medial ligamentous complex of the ankle, commonly referred to as the deltoid ligament, is best imaged using coronal

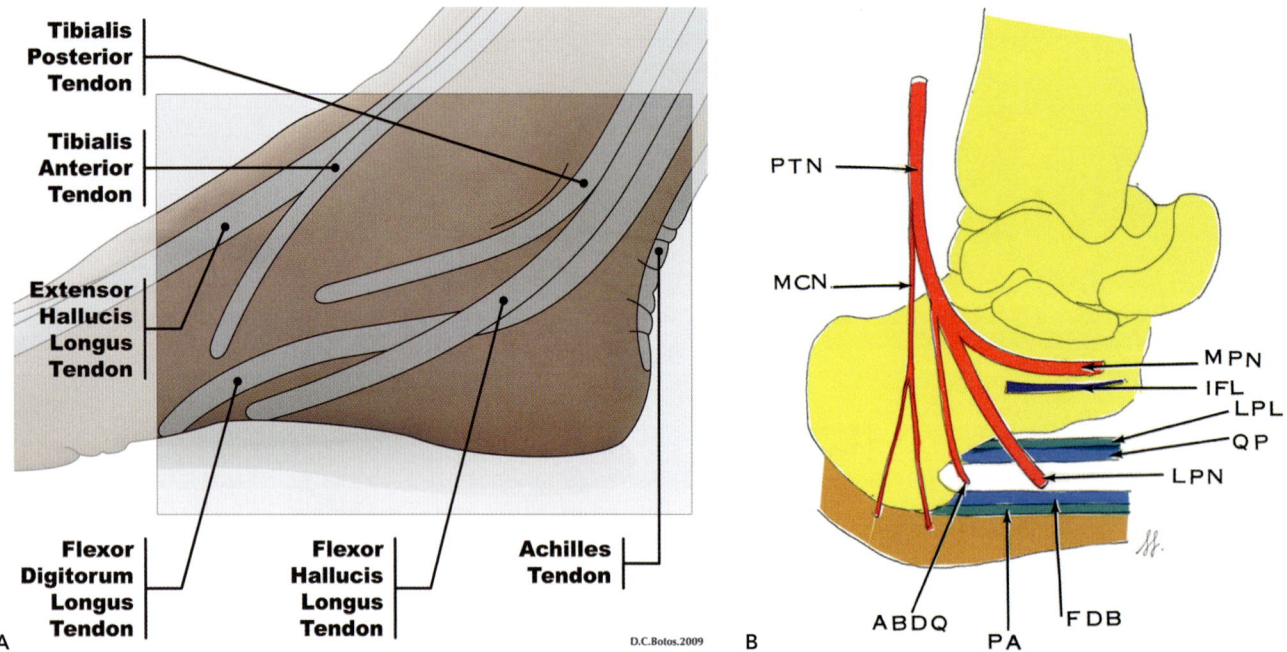

Figure 14.14 (A) Diagram of the medial ankle tendons. (B) Drawing of a left tarsal tunnel depicting the posterior tibial nerve (*PTN*), medial calcaneal nerve (*MCN*) branch to the abductor digiti quinti (*ABDQ*), terminal branches of the PTN, the medial plantar nerve (*MPN*) and the lateral plantar nerve (*LPN*), plantar aponeurosis (*PA*), flexor digitorum brevis (*FDB*), longitudinal plantar ligament (*LPL*), and interfascicular lamina (*IFL*).

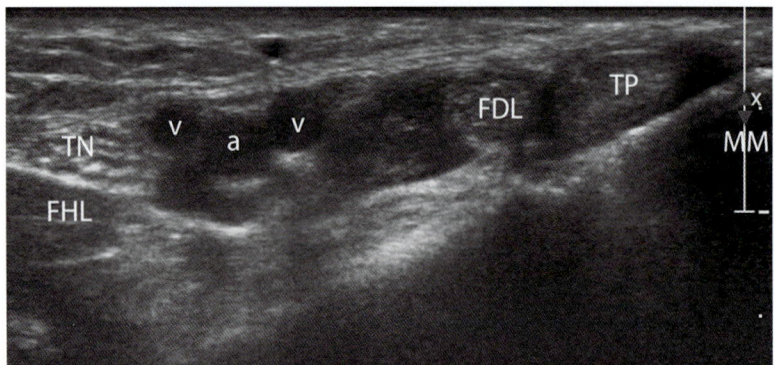

Figure 14.15 Normal anatomy of the medial ankle. Medial malleolus (*MM*), tibialis posterior tendon (*TP*), flexor digitorum longus tendon (*FDL*), tibial artery (*a*) and veins (*v*), tibial nerve (*TN*), and the flexor hallucis longus tendon (*FHL*).

scans. Because of its marked obliquity, the tibiotalar component appears as a hypoechoic thick structure bridging the medial malleolus and the posteromedial surface of the talus. Often, it exhibits an inhomogeneous striated appearance that can be correlated with areas of fatty tissue interspersed between the ligamentous fibers. US imaging is of limited utility in detecting deltoid ligament pathology.

The tibialis posterior, flexor digitorum longus, and flexor hallucis longus tendons are examined by means of short-axis and long-axis scans obtained in the supra- and inframalleolar region (Figs. 14.14A and 14.15). The tibialis posterior tendon lies in a shallow bony groove on the posterolateral aspect of the medial malleolus covered by the flexor retinaculum.[18,19] Just before its insertion on the tubercle of the navicular, the tendon fans out and often appears thickened and hypoechoic. The tibialis posterior tendon may contain the accessory navicular, a sesamoid bone that appears as a curvilinear hyperechoic structure (Fig. 14.16). This accessory bone can be located within the tendon at a variable distance from the dorsomedial aspect of the navicular bone (type I) or is joined to the navicular by a synchondrosis (type II). In the latter case, part of the tibialis posterior tendon can insert onto this ossicle rather than normally onto the navicular bone. The flexor digitorum longus tendon is located just posterior and slightly lateral to the tibialis posterior. The inframalleolar region of the flexor digitorum longus tendon passes over the medial surface of the sustentaculum tali. The inframalleolar portion of the flexor hallucis longus tendon can be visualized underneath the sustentaculum tali.

With high-resolution transducers, US can delineate the complex anatomy of the tarsal tunnel and is able to image the entire course of the tibial nerve and its branches at the medial ankle. The tibial nerve and its two terminal branches the medial and lateral plantar nerves lie posterior to the flexor digitorum longus and superficial to the flexor hallucis longus tendons, in

Figure 14.16 The distal tibialis posterior tendon (*arrowheads*) contains a type I accessory navicular bone (*arrows*).

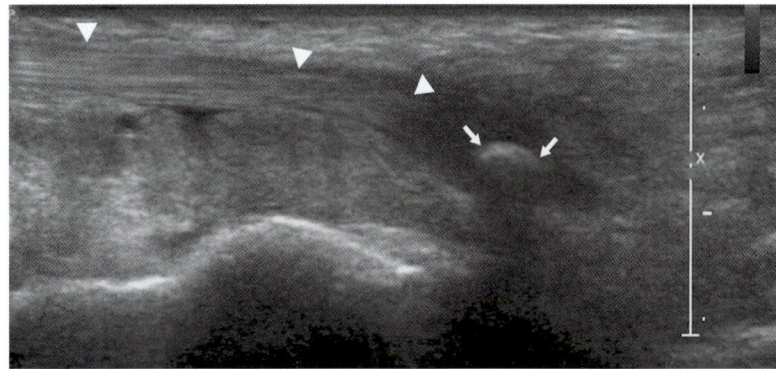

Figure 14.17 Large ganglion cyst (*GC*) compressing the tibial nerve (*arrowhead*) in the tarsal tunnel.

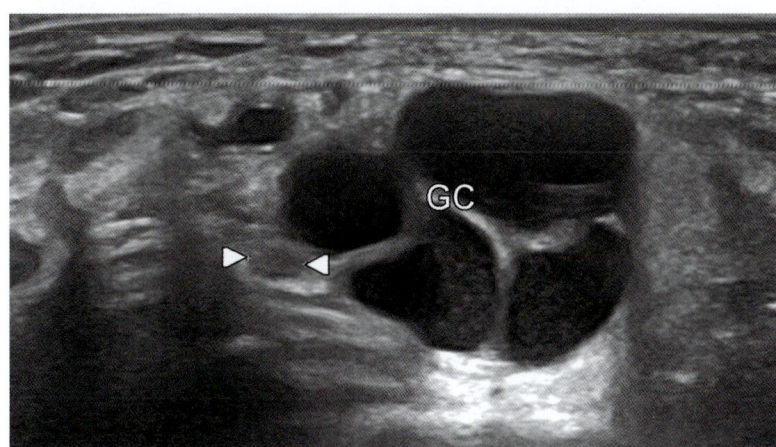

Figure 14.18 Normal fibrillar appearance of the Achilles tendon (*arrows*). Note the 1 cm attachment to the calcaneus (*CAL*). (*B*, retrocalcaneal bursa; *KF*, Kager fat.)

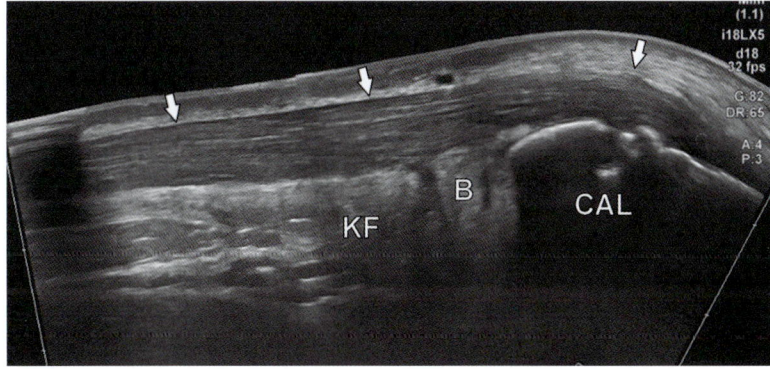

close proximity to the posterior tibial artery and veins (see Fig. 14.14B). Identification of the posterior tibial vessels with color Doppler imaging may be a useful landmark to identify the position of the nerve, which is typically located deep and slightly posterior to them (see Figs. 14.15 and 14.17).

▶ **Posterior Ankle**

The Achilles tendon is examined from its myotendinous junction to its calcaneal insertion.[20] On long-axis scans, the anterior and posterior boundaries of the normal Achilles tendon lie parallel below the soleus insertion. Occasionally, the convergent contributions from the lateral and medial heads of gastrocnemius and the soleus can be visualized proximally as a central thickened echo due to the union of respective peritendinous envelopes. The Achilles insertion on the calcaneus is approximately 1 cm long (Fig. 14.18). Close by on the medial aspect of the Achilles tendon, the plantaris tendon can be identified on transverse scans as a small oval hypoechoic structure. It is visualized better at the medial edge of the myotendinous junction of the Achilles tendon and can then be followed upward in the leg along the aponeurosis of the soleus and the medial head of the gastrocnemius. Accessory muscles can be detected with US. The accessory soleus presents as a space-occupying mass with characteristics identical to normal muscle located at the anteromedial side of the Achilles tendon.

Two bursae lie close to the insertion of the Achilles tendon on the calcaneus: the retro-Achilles bursa and the retrocalcaneal bursa. The retro-Achilles bursa is positioned between the skin and the Achilles tendon, whereas the retrocalcaneal bursa lies

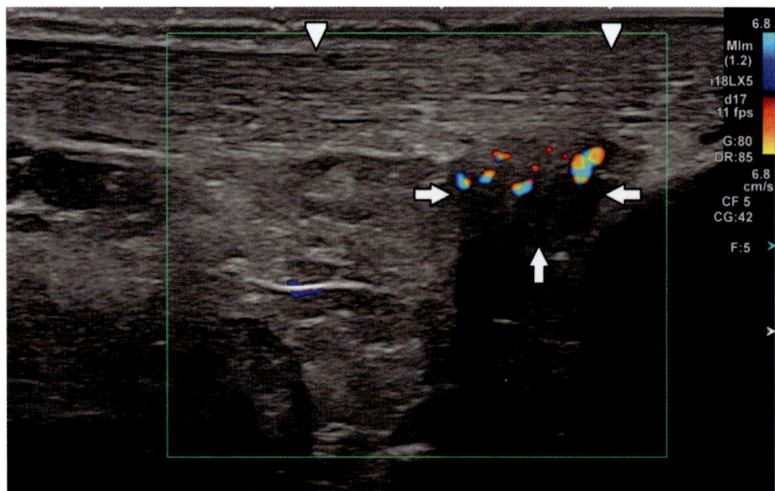

Figure 14.19 Color Doppler flow in a patient with retrocalcaneal bursitis (*arrows*). Achilles tendon indicated by *arrowheads*.

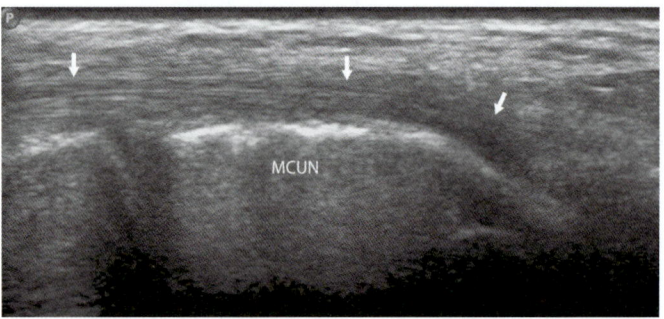

Figure 14.20 The distal tibialis posterior (*arrows*) tendon inserts on the navicular bone (*N*).

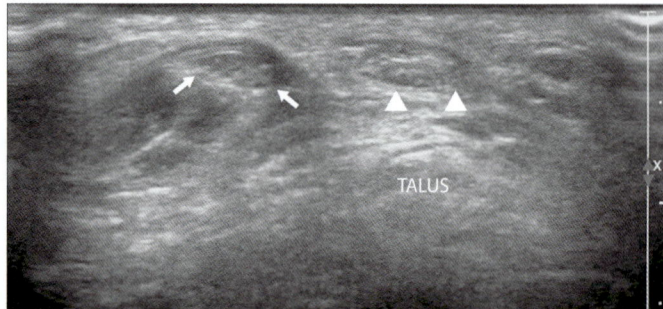

Figure 14.21 Transverse image of the tibialis anterior (*arrowheads*) and extensor hallucis longus tendons (*arrows*) anterior to the talus.

between the Achilles tendon insertion and the posterosuperior angle of the calcaneus. Normally, the retro-Achilles bursa is normally imperceptible with US. The retrocalcaneal bursa can be demonstrated as a comma-shaped hypoechoic structure or with abnormal Doppler flow secondary to bursitis (Fig. 14.19). Deep to the Achilles tendon, the Kager fat pad appears as a soft-tissue space filled with fat lobules.

▶ Dorsal Foot

Transverse US imaging planes are the best suited to identify the superficial long tendons as they course over the dorsum of the foot.[13] The most medial tendon is the tibialis anterior, which gradually tapers as it runs toward the medial border of the foot to insert on the anteromedial aspect of the medial cuneiform and the base of the first metatarsal (Fig. 14.20). In a more medial position, the extensor hallucis longus tendon is found as a thin tendon and can more easily be detected during passive flexion and extension movements of the great toe (Fig. 14.21). The four diverging slips of the extensor digitorum longus muscle for the lesser toes can be detected in a more lateral position (see Fig. 14.7A).

Occasionally, the peroneus tertius tendon can be appreciated as an accessory fifth lateral slip of the extensor digitorum longus directed toward the base of the fifth metatarsal. The extensor tendons can be imaged up to their distal insertion on the phalanges. The dorsalis pedis artery and the medial branch of the deep peroneal nerve can be detected over the anterior ankle using transverse planes and then followed down to reach the metatarsal region (see Fig. 14.7C). Sagittal US images over the ankle joint allow detection of the dorsal aspect of the tarsals, metatarsals, phalanges, and joint spaces.

▶ Plantar Foot

Sagittal US imaging obtained over the ankle images the preinsertional portion of the plantar fascia.[21] This appears as a distinct thick hyperechoic fibrillar band, somewhat similar to a tendon, running parallel to the skin of the sole (Fig. 14.22). Distally the fascia becomes progressively thinner and superficial as it proceeds toward the forefoot. The strong central cord of the plantar fascia lies over the surface of the thick muscle belly of the flexor digitorum brevis. In normal states, it is approximately 3 to 4 mm thick. More laterally, the thinner external part of the plantar fascia overlies the abductor digiti minimi muscle. The medial cord of the aponeurosis, which is located inferior to the abductor hallucis muscle, appears as the thinnest portion.

The abductor hallucis muscle is imaged from its posterior origin through to its distal insertion by means of coronal and oblique transverse planes. In a deeper location, the second muscle layer containing the quadratus plantae muscle,

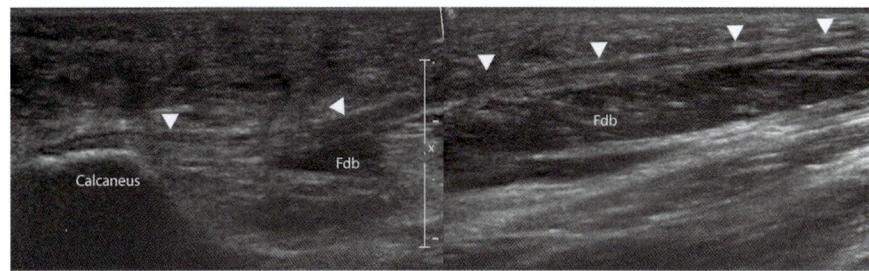

Figure 14.22 **Central cord of the plantar fascia (*arrowheads*).** (*Fdb*, flexor digitorum brevis muscle.)

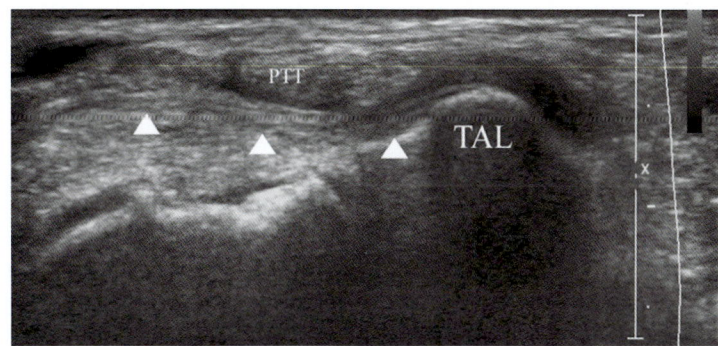

Figure 14.23 **Spring ligament (*arrowheads*) deep to the tibialis posterior tendon (*PTT*).** Note the attachment of the ligament to the sustentaculum tali (*TAL*).

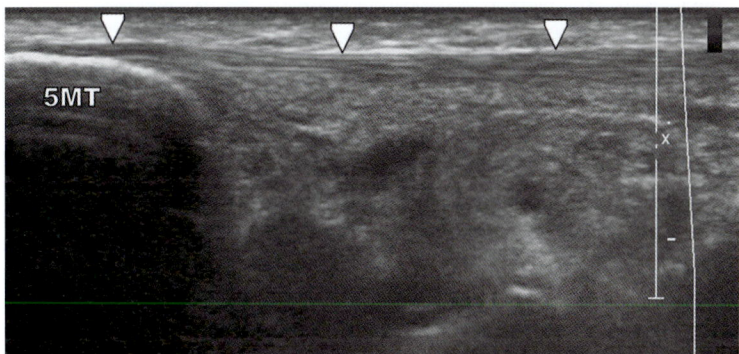

Figure 14.24 **Distal peroneus brevis tendon (*arrowheads*) inserting into the base of the fifth metatarsal (*5MT*).**

the lumbricals, and the tendons of the flexor hallucis longus and flexor digitorum longus is visualized. The sustentaculum tali is identified as a large bony prominence of the medial aspect of the calcaneus. It represents a useful landmark to identify the flexor digitorum longus tendon, which passes superficial to it, and the flexor hallucis longus tendon, which travels along its undersurface. Due to problems of access, US has intrinsic difficulties assessing the entire spring ligament, which courses from the sustentaculum tali to the navicular tubercle. However, the superior medial portion of the spring ligament, which has the greatest contribution of stability to the longitudinal arch of the foot, can be imaged[22] (Fig. 14.23).

More distally, in the sole, the flexor hallucis longus crosses the tendon of the flexor digitorum longus, to which it is connected by a thin fibrous slip. The medial and lateral plantar neurovascular bundles course in close relationship with the long flexors.

The peroneus brevis tendon inserts at the base of the fifth metatarsal (Fig. 14.24). The peroneus longus assumes an oblique course as it approaches the cuboid (Fig. 14.25). Using a plantar approach, the peroneus longus tendon runs obliquely across the sole to insert into the first metatarsal.

Transverse US images obtained over the metatarsophalangeal joint of the great toe show two sesamoids as paired oval

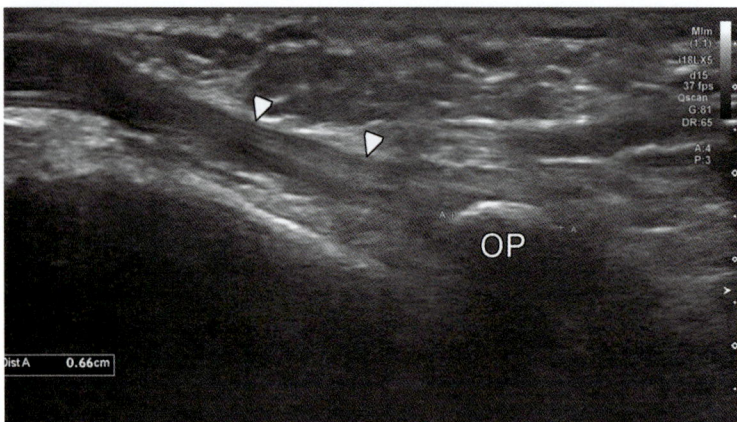

Figure 14.25 The peroneus longus tendon (*arrowheads*) adjacent to the lateral aspect of the cuboid. An os peroneum is present (*OP*).

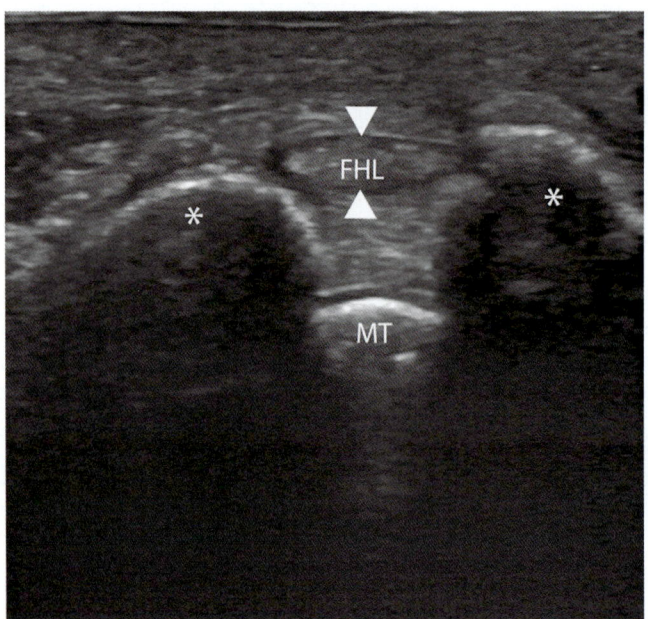

Figure 14.26 Transverse view of the plantar aspect of the first metatarsal head (*MT*), showing the two sesamoids (*asterisks*), flexor hallucis longus (*FHL*) tendon, and tendon sheath (*arrowheads*).

hyperechoic structures with posterior acoustic showing. The flexor hallucis longus tendon is held in between them. In this position the tendon is protected during the step-off phase of walking. At US examination, a bipartite sesamoid appears as a bony complex formed by two distinct ossicles invested by a cortical layer (Fig. 14.26). Typically, bipartite sesamoids have a larger size and exhibit rounded borders: this latter sign may aid in distinguishing an anatomic variant from an acute fracture. The plantar plate and cartilage of the lesser metatarsal-phalangeal joints are depicted using longitudinal imaging[23] (Fig. 14.27).

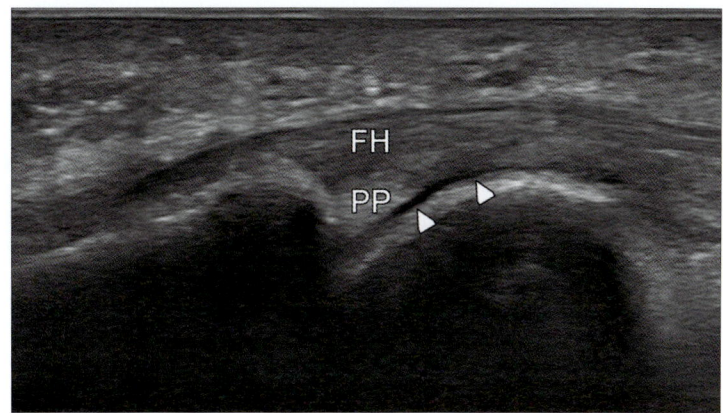

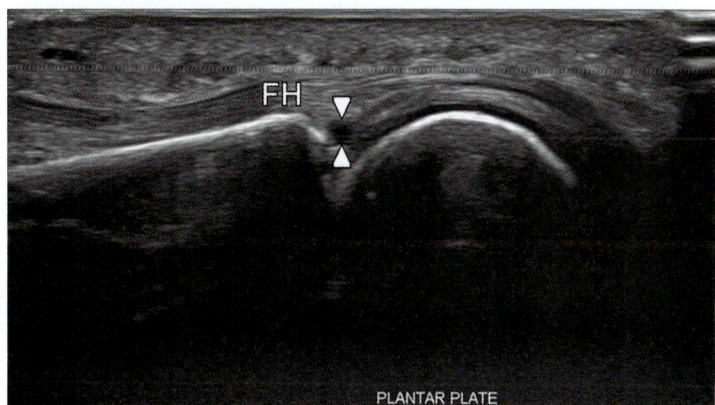

Figure 14.27 **(A)** Sagittal plantar view of the second metatarsal-phalangeal joint showing proximal phalanx (*PP*), metatarsal head (*MT*), flexor hallucis longus tendon (*FH*), plantar plate (*PP2*), and articular cartilage (*arrowheads*). **(B)** Partial plantar plate tear (*arrow*).

REFERENCES

1. Newman JS, Adler RS, Bude RO, et al. Detection of soft-tissue hyperemia: value of power Doppler sonography. *AJR Am J Roentgenol*. 1994;163:385-389.
2. Gittu S, Messina C, Chianoa V, et al. Superb microvascular imaging (SMI) in the evaluation of musculoskeletal disorders: a systemic review. *Radiol Med*. 2020;125(5):481-490.
3. Barberie JE, Wong JD, Cooperberg PL, et al. Extended field-of-view sonography in musculoskeletal disorders. *AJR Am J Roentgenol*. 1998;171:751-757.
4. Neustadter J, Raikin SM, Nazarian LN. Dynamic sonographic evaluation of peroneal tendon subluxation. *AJR Am J Roentgenol*. 2004;183:985-988.
5. Fornage BBD. *Ultrasonography of Muscles and Tendons: Examination and Technique and Atlas of Normal Anatomy of the Extremities*. Springer-Verlag; 1988.
6. Martinoli C, Derchi LE, Pastorino C, et al. Analysis of echotexture of tendons with US. *Radiology*. 1993;186:839-843.
7. van Holsbeeck MT, Introcaso JH. *Sonography of ligaments*. In: *Musculoskeletal Ultrasound*. Mosby; 2001:171-192.
8. Silvestri E, Martinoli C, Derchi LE, et al. Echotexture of peripheral nerves: correlation between US and histological findings and criteria to differentiate tendons. *Radiology*. 1995;197:291-296.
9. Martinoli C, Bianchi S, Dahmane M, et al. Ultrasound of tendons and nerves. *Eur Radiol*. 2002;12(1):44-55.
10. Rawool NM, Nazarian LN. Ultrasound of the ankle and foot. *Semin Ultrasound CT MRI*. 2000;21:275-284.
11. Williams A, Davies MS. Foot and ankle. In: Standring S, ed. *Gray's Anatomy: the Anatomical Basis of Medicine and Surgery*. 39th ed. Elsevier Churchill Livingstone; 2005.
12. Fessell DP, Vanderschueren GM, Jacobson JA, et al. Ultrasound of the ankle: technique, anatomy and diagnosis of pathologic conditions. *Radiographics*. 1998;18:325-340.
13. Fessell DP, Jamadar DA, Jacobson JA, et al. Sonography of dorsal ankle and foot abnormalities. *AJR Am J Roentgenol*. 2003;181:1573-1581.
14. Peetrons P, Creteur V, Bacq C. Sonography of ankle ligaments. *J Clin Ultrasound*. 2004;32:491-499.
15. Popieluszko P, Mizia E, Henry BM, et al. The surgical anatomy of the sural nerve: an ultrasound study. *Clin Anat*. 2018;31(4):450-455.
16. Grant TH, Kelikian AS, Jereb SE, McCarthy RJ. Ultrasound diagnosis of peroneal tendon tears a surgical correlation. *J Bone Joint Surg Am*. 2005;87(8):1788-1794.
17. Cheung YY, Rosenberg ZS, Ramsinghani R, et al. Peroneus quartus muscle: MR imaging features. *Radiology*. 1997;202:745-750.
18. Cheung Y, Rosenberg ZS, Magee T, et al. Normal anatomy and pathologic conditions of ankle tendons: current imaging techniques. *Radiographics*. 1992;12:429-444.
19. Jain NB, Omar I, Kelikian AS, et al. Prevalence of and factors associated with posterior tibial tendon pathology on sonographic. *PM R*. 2011;3:998-1004.
20. Hartgerink P, Fessell D, Jacobson J, et al. Full-versus partial-thickness Achilles tendon tears: sonographic accuracy and characterization in 26 cases with surgical correlation. *Radiology*. 2001;220:406-412.
21. Gibbon WW, Long G. Ultrasound of the plantar aponeurosis (fascia). *Skeletal Radiol*. 1999;28(1):21-26.
22. Harish S, Jan E, Finlay K, et al. Sonography of the superomedial part of the spring ligament complex of the foot: a study of cadavers and asymptomatic volunteers. *Skeletal Radiol*. 2006;36(3):221-228.
23. Gregg M, Siberstein T, Schneider JB, et al. Sonography of plantar plates in cadavers: correlation with MRI and histology. *AJR Am J Roentgenol*. 2006;186(4):948-955.

Arthroscopy of the Talocrural and Subtalar Joints

Armen S. Kelikian

The advent of arthroscopic surgery has opened a new window to in vivo anatomy. Correlations with topographic anatomy with regard to normal landmarks—relative to portal sites as well as joint access and structures at risk—are paramount to the arthroscopist's visualization. Knowledge of normal intra-articular anatomy and its variations allow one to address pathologic conditions. Watanabe first introduced ankle arthroscopy in 1970 and subsequently published a series of 28 ankles.[1] Guhl and, subsequently, Yates and Grana expanded visualization via invasive and noninvasive distraction apparatuses.[2,3] Ferkel published a classic text *Arthroscopic Surgery, The Foot and Ankle* in 1996.[4] Recently, van Dijk expanded techniques to the posterior approaches of the ankle, subtalar, and retrocalcaneal bursa as well as endoscopy of the peroneal, posterior tibial, and flexor hallucis longus tendons.[5]

ANATOMIC LANDMARKS

Osseous landmarks are the lateral and medial malleoli. The ankle joint is subtended by points 1 cm proximal to the medial malleolar tip and 2 cm proximal to the tip of the lateral malleolar (Fig. 15.1). The cross-section of the ankle at 1 cm from the tip of the medial malleolus (Fig. 15.2) demonstrates the following relationships: anteriorly from medial to lateral the saphenous vein and nerve over the medial malleolus.

The tibialis anterior tendon is at the junction of the medial malleolus with the tibial plafond. The extensor hallucis longus tendon is anterior to the medial aspect of the tibial plafond and the extensor digitorum longus tendons correspond to the lateral aspect of the tibial plafond and to the tibiofibular synovial fringe. The dorsalis pedal vessels (anterior tibial vessels) and the deep peroneal nerves are lateral and deep to the extensor hallucis longus tendon. These relationships are also well represented in the dissection of the ankle anteriorly (Fig. 15.3). The superficial peroneal nerve has already divided into its terminal branches—intermediate and medial dorsal cutaneous nerve at an average of 6.5 cm proximal to the tip of the lateral malleolus. The intermediate dorsal cutaneous nerve crosses over the tibiofibular syndesmosis, crosses obliquely the fifth and fourth extensor digitorum longus tendons, and courses over the third intermetatarsal space (Fig. 15.4). This nerve can be visualized and palpated with plantar flexion and inversion of the foot. The saphenous nerve crosses the medial malleolus anteriorly. Posteriorly on the cross-sectional study of the ankle, the tibialis posterior tendon is posterior to the medial malleolus and the peronei are posterior to the lateral malleolus. The posterior peroneal vessels are posterior to the tibiofibular syndesmosis. The Achilles tendon is central and medial; posterior to the tibial plafond are the flexor hallucis tendon and the posterior neurovascular bundle (Fig. 15.5). The short saphenous vein and sural nerve are in the interval between the peronei tendons and the Achilles tendon (Fig. 15.6).

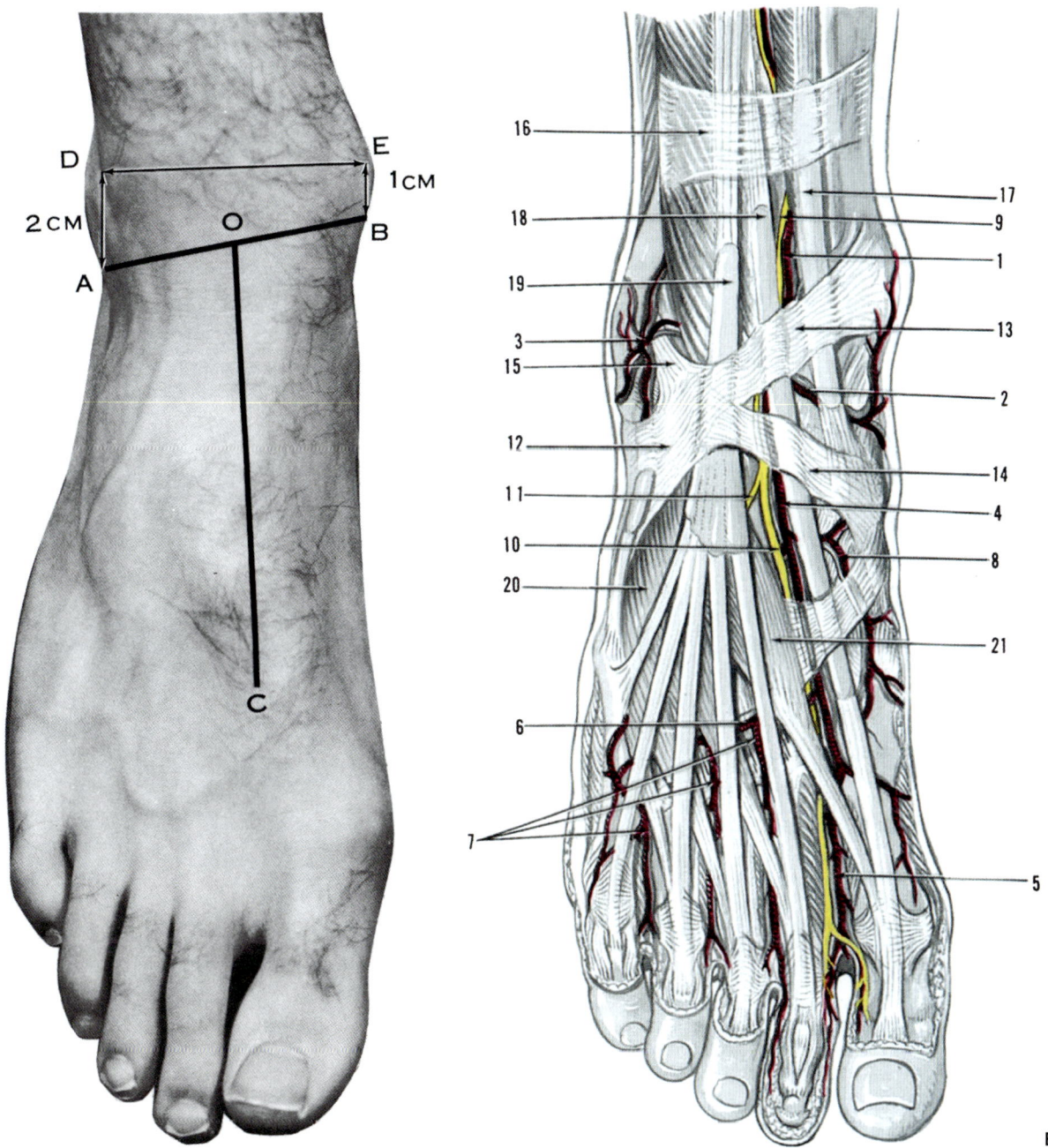

Figure 15.1 **(A) The dorsal vascular axis.** The bimalleolar axis of the ankle is indicated by the line *AB*. Point *O* is the middle of line *AB*. Point *C* is the proximal end of the first intermetatarsal space. Line *OC* indicates the direction and location of the dorsalis pedis artery. Line *DE* indicates the location of the talo-tibial articular interline. It is 2 cm proximal to the tip of the lateral malleolus and 1 cm proximal to the tip of the medial malleolus. **(B) First layer of the dorsum of the foot and ankle.** (*1*, Anterior tibial artery; *2*, anterior medial malleolar artery; *3*, anterior lateral malleolar artery; *4*, dorsalis pedis artery; *5*, first dorsal metatarsal artery; *6*, arcuate artery; *7*, dorsal metatarsal arteries 2, 3, 4; *8*, medial tarsal artery; *9, 10*, deep peroneal nerve; *11*, motor nerve branch to extensor digitorum brevis; *12*, inferior extensor retinaculum; *13*, superomedial band of inferior extensor retinaculum; *14*, inferomedial band of inferior extensor retinaculum; *15*, superolateral band of inferior extensor retinaculum; *16*, superior extensor retinaculum; *17*, tibialis anterior tendon; *18*, extensor hallucis longus tendon; *19*, extensor digitorum longus tendon; *20*, extensor digitorum brevis muscle to toes 2, 3, 4; *21*, extensor hallucis brevis muscle.)

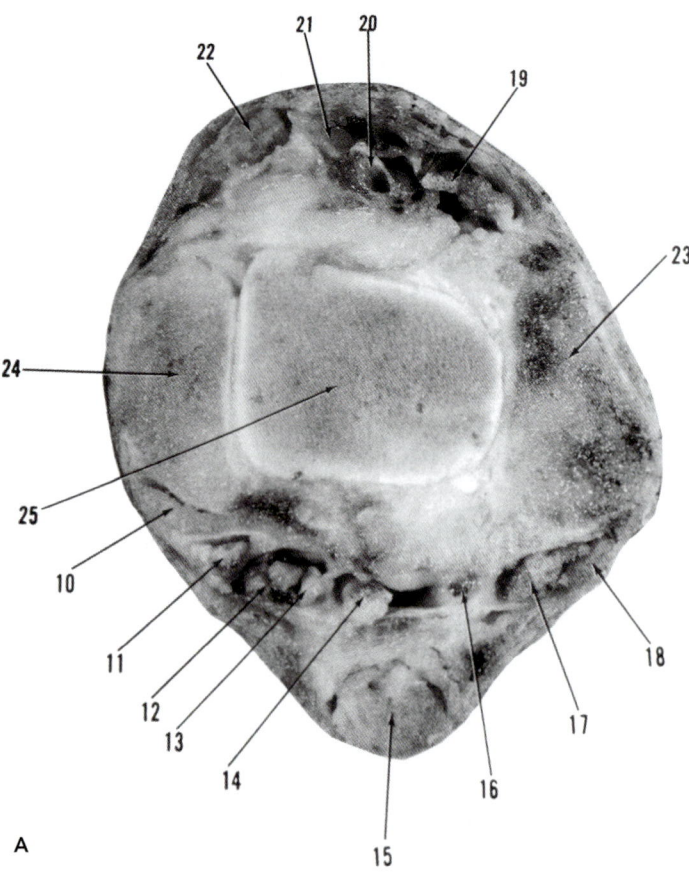
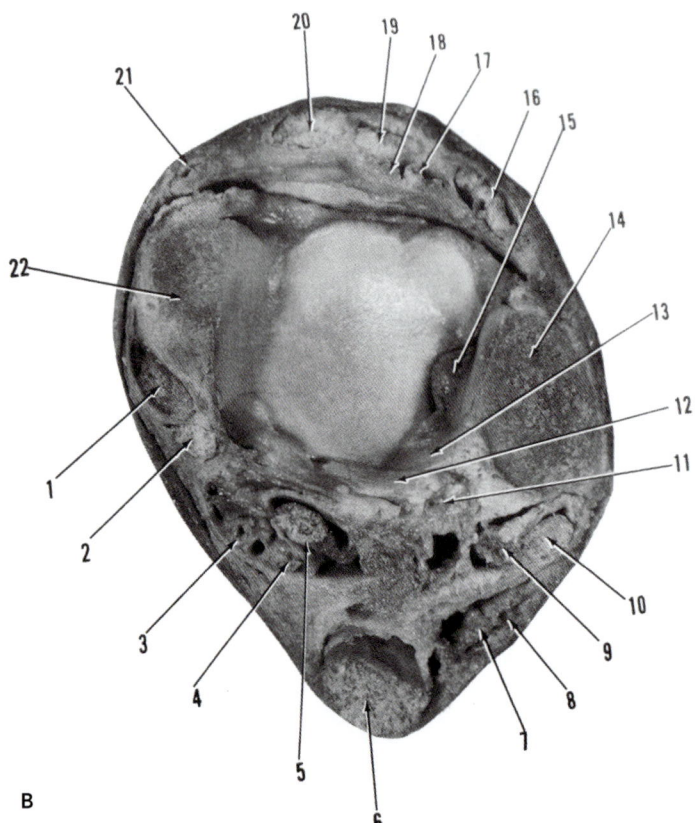
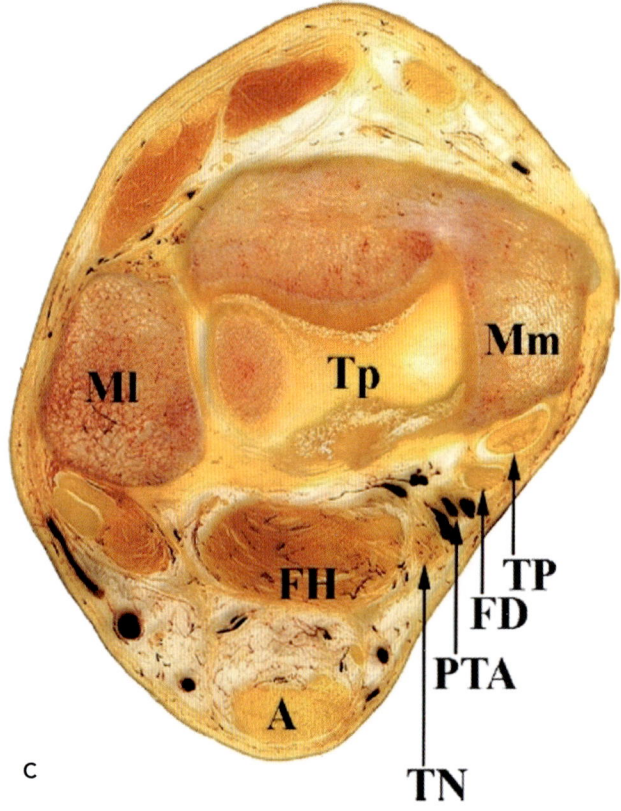

Figure 15.2 **(A) Cross-section of the ankle at 1 cm proximal to the tip of the medial malleolus.** Distal surface section. (*1*, Tunnel of tibialis anterior tendon; *2*, superomedial band of inferior extensor retinaculum determining tunnel of extensor hallucis longus tendon and anterior tibial neurovascular bundle; *3*, tunnel of extensor digitorum longus; *4*, tunnel of peronei; *5*, tunnel of Achilles tendon; *6*, tunnel of flexor hallucis longus tendon; *7*, tunnel of posterior tibial neurovascular bundle; *8*, tunnel of flexor digitorum longus tendon; *9*, tunnel of tibialis posterior tendon; *10*, tibialis posterior tendon; *11*, flexor digitorum longus tendon; *12*, posterior tibial vessels; *13*, posterior tibial nerve; *14*, flexor hallucis longus tendon; *15*, Achilles tendon; *16*, posterior peroneal vessels; *17*, peroneus brevis tendon; *18*, peroneus longus tendon; *19*, extensor digitorum longus; *20*, anterior tibial neurovascular bundle; *21*, extensor hallucis longus tendon; *22*, tibialis anterior tendon; *23*, lateral malleolus; *24*, medial malleolus; *25*, talus.) **(B) Cross-section of ankle at 1 cm proximal to tip of medial malleolus.** Distal surface section of nonsequential specimen. Talar dome removed. (*1*, Tibialis posterior tendon and tunnel; *2*, flexor digitorum longus tendon and tunnel; *3*, posterior tibial vessels and tunnel; *4*, posterior tibial nerve and tunnel; *5*, flexor hallucis longus tendon and tunnel; *6*, Achilles tendon and tunnel; *7*, sural nerve; *8*, short saphenous nerve; *9*, peroneus brevis tendon, frayed, and tunnel; *10*, peroneus longus tendon and tunnel; *11*, posterior peroneal vessels; *12, 13*, posterior tibiofibular ligaments; *14*, lateral malleolus; *15*, synovial fringe of tibiofibular syndesmosis; *16*, extensor digitorum longus tendons and tunnel; *17*, anterior tibial vessels; *18*, anterior tibial nerve; *19*, extensor hallucis tendon and tunnel; *20*, tibialis anterior tendon and tunnel; *21*, greater saphenous vein; *22*, medial malleolus.) **(C) Cross-section photograph of flexor digitorum longus (*FD*) tendon, posterior tibial tendon (*TP*), posterior tibial nerve (*TN*), flexor hallucis longus tendon (*FH*), and posterior tibial artery (*PTA*).** (Reprinted from Sora MC, Jilavu R, Grübl A, et al. The posteromedial neurovascular bundle of the ankle: an anatomic study of plastinated cross sections. *Arthroscopy.* 2008;24[3]:260, with permission from Elsevier.)

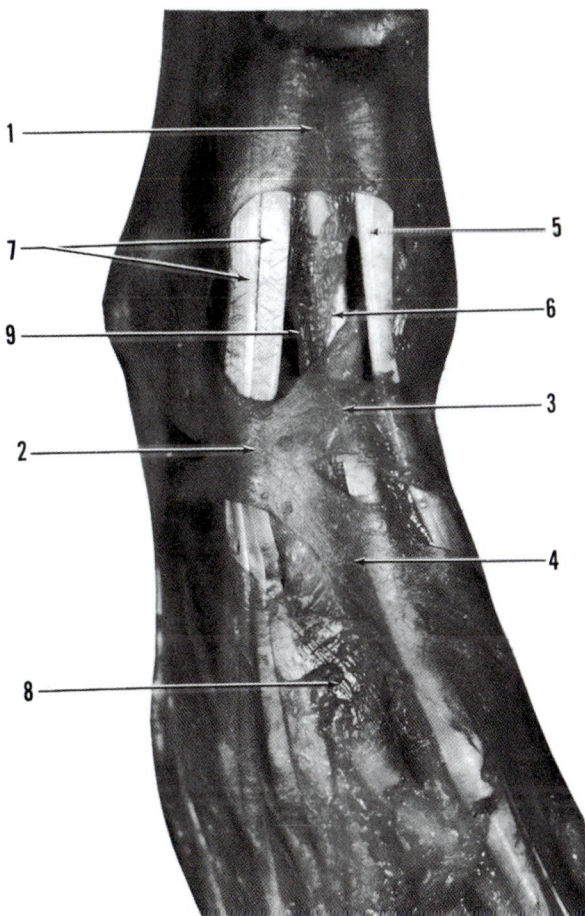

Figure 15.3 Dorsum of the ankle and foot. (*1*, Superior extensor retinaculum; *2*, stem of inferior extensor retinaculum; *3*, superomedial band of interior extensor retinaculum; *4*, inferomedial band of inferior extensor retinaculum; *5*, tibialis anterior tendon; *6*, extensor hallucis longus tendon; *7*, extensor digitorum longus tendons; *8*, extensor digitorum brevis muscle; *9*, neurovascular bundle—deep peroneal nerve and dorsalis pedis artery.)

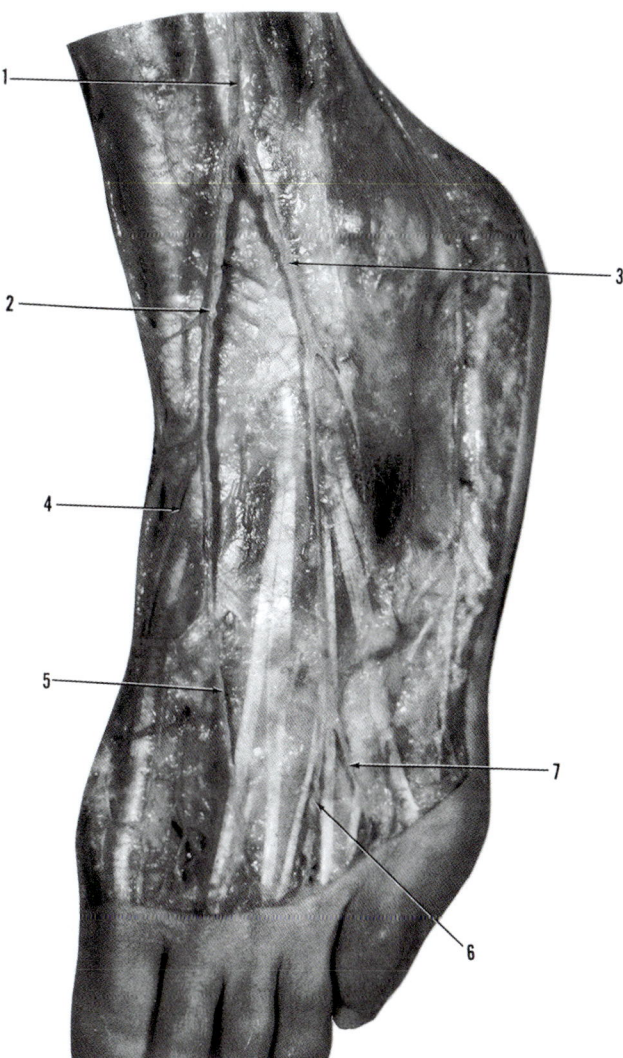

Figure 15.4 Superficial peroneal nerve (*1*) dividing into the intermediate dorsal cutaneous nerve (*3*) and the medial dorsal cutaneous nerve (*2*). The latter subdivides into the dorsomedial cutaneous nerve of the big toe (*4*) and the common digital nerve to the second web space (*5*). The intermediate dorsal nerve (*3*) supplies the dorsal cutaneous nerve of the third (*6*) and fourth (*7*) web spaces.

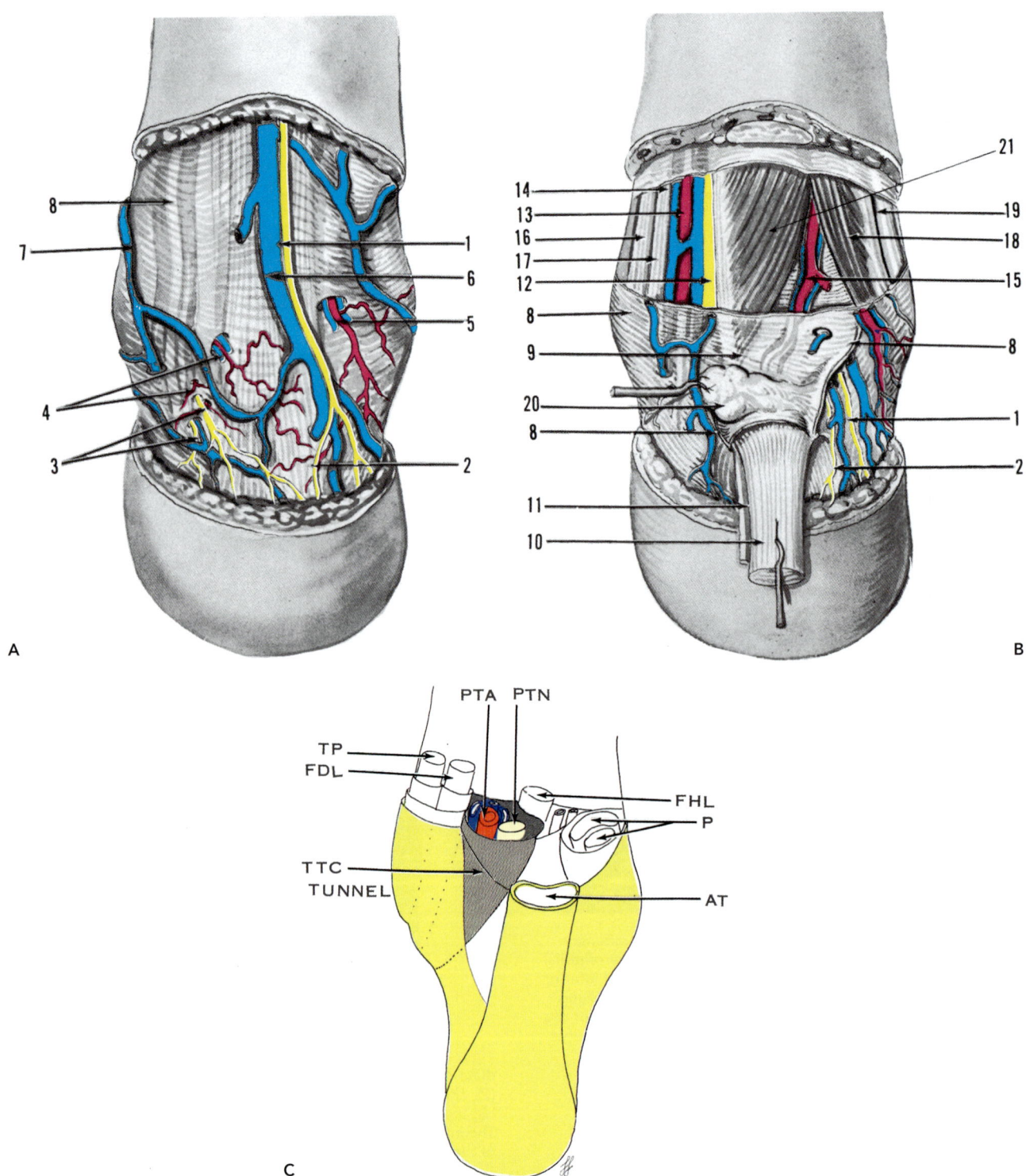

Figure 15.5 Posterior aspect of the ankle. (A) Superficial aspect. (B) Deep aspect. (1, Sural nerve; 2, lateral calcaneal nerve, posterior branch; 3, medial calcaneal and posteromedial nerve branches of posterior tibial nerve; 4, posteromedial and medial calcaneal arteries, branch of posterior tibial artery; 5, lateral calcaneal artery, branch of posterior peroneal artery; 6, lesser saphenous vein; 7, posterior medial malleolar vein; 8, superficial aponeurosis cruris, which splits and invests Achilles tendon [10] and plantaris tendon [11]; 9, deep aponeurosis cruris; 12, posterior tibial nerve; 13, posterior tibial artery; 14, posterior tibial vein; 15, posterior peroneal artery and veins; 16, tibialis posterior tendon; 17, flexor digitorum longus tendon; 18, peroneus brevis muscle–tendon; 19, peroneus longus tendon; 20, pre-Achilles tendon fat pad located in "safe zone" between superficial and deep aponeuroses cruris; 21, flexor hallucis longus.) (C) Posterior aspect of the ankle. (AT, Achilles tendon; FDL, flexor digitorum longus tendon; FHL, flexor hallucis longus; PTA, posterior tibial artery (red) and vein (blue); PTN, posterior tibial nerve (light yellow); TCC, tibiotalocalcaneal; TP, posterior tibial tendon. Peroneal tendons: the brevis is anterior to the longus (P).)

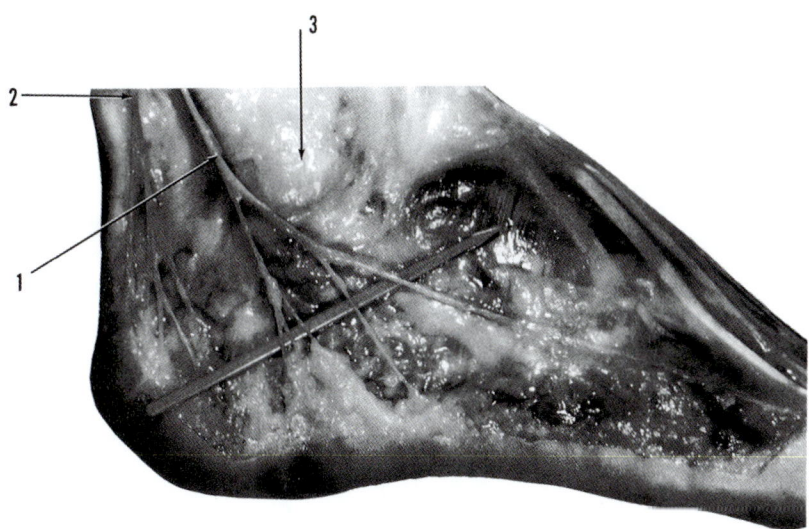

Figure 15.6 **Sural nerve** (*1*) dividing into lateral branches to the heel and the lateral border of the foot; lateral calcaneal nerve (*2*) dividing into multiple branches, lateral malleolar fat pad (*3*).

ANKLE ARTHROSCOPIC PORTALS

Arthroscopic portals in the foot and ankle rely on access, visualization, structures at risk, and cross-sectional anatomy. They provide a window to normal and abnormal anatomy. These portals are anteromedial, anterolateral, accessory anterolateral, accessory anteromedial, and posterolateral. The anterior medial portal is at the joint line, 1 cm proximal to the tip of the medial malleolus, and just medial to the anterior tibial tendon with the ankle dorsiflexed and distracted. The mean distension volume of the ankle joint is 20 mL (range 16-30 mL).[6] The anterior capsule insertion on the tibia is between 6 and 8 mm from the joint line proximally and about 8 to 10 mm distally from the talar articular surface according to Testut.[7] The anterolateral portal is at the same level and just lateral to the peroneus tertius tendon. The lateral portal can be determined by transilluminating the skin to visualize and avoid the superficial peroneal nerve. An accessory anterior portal can be used between the extensor hallucis longus and tibialis anticus tendons[8] (Fig. 15.7). The accessory anteromedial portal is 1 cm below the anterior edge of the anterior colliculus, whereas the accessory anterolateral portal is 1 cm anterior to the lateral malleolus[4] (Fig. 15.7). The posterolateral portal is just lateral to the lateral border of the Achilles tendon and between 12 and 25 mm proximal to the tip of the fibula[4] (Fig. 15.7). The posteromedial portal is medial to the Achilles tendon and directed toward the posterolateral canola away from the posterior neurovascular structures. This technique has been popularized by van Dijk.[5,9] Another utility portal also used for subtalar arthroscopy is the anterolateral, which is 2 cm anterior and 1 cm distal to the fibular tip.[4]

▶ Anterior Arthroscopy Portals

Numerous anatomic studies have shown the incisional hazards relative to the neurovascular structures that envelop the region of the ankle and subtalar joints. A Feiwell and Frey study found a 10% incidence of injury to the superficial peroneal nerve via the anterolateral portal, whereas the anterocentral portal (which has since then been abandoned) approached a 30% rate.[10-12] Anatomic variations such as a laterally situated anterior tibial artery in 5.5% of specimens according to Huber (see Chapter 7) and its transmalleolar branches further illustrates the value of regional anatomy for the arthroscopists[13] (Fig. 15.8). The medial and lateral transmalleolar arteries' distances from the joint line vary with ankle flexion and extension. The lateral transmalleolar branch distance from the joint line increases from 2.47 to 6.41 mm, whereas the medial branch distance goes from 1.58 to 4.73 mm with plantar flexion in 18 cadaveric dissection.[14]

Intra-articular Anatomy

The anteromedial portal affords excellent visualization in the anteroposterior direction because of the medially situated groove in the tibial plafond or notch of Harty.[15] It is the first portal established after saline insufflation. Again it is made at the level of the ankle joint line 1 cm above the medial malleolar tip in the soft spot just medial to the anterior tibial tendon. The saphenous nerve and vein have a safe zone 10 and 7.4 mm away or medial to this portal.[10] The cross sectional anatomy illustrates these structures (see Fig. 15.2).

The eight-point anterior and six-point central examinations are shown in Figure 15.9.[4] The anterolateral portal gives additional viewing when portals are changed. Once the anteromedial portal is employed, a spinal needle lateral to the peroneus tertius and intermediate branch of the superficial peroneal nerve is introduced. The lateral gutter can be well visualized with a 30-degree arthroscope. The posterolateral examination is made by introducing the spinal needle in the soft spot with triangular borders consisting of the superior calcaneal border inferiorly, the Achilles tendon posteriorly, and the peronei anteriorly (Fig. 15.7). The soft portion of the capsule or cul-de-sac just medial and below the transverse ligament (but lateral to the FHL) is penetrated. The deep deltoid, medial gutter, the articular surfaces, and posterolateral corner are inspected to complete the 21-point examination (Fig. 15.9).

When viewing the articular surface of the talus, the central depression just medial to this on the articular surface of the tibia is the notch of Harty (Fig. 15.10). There are three fascicles

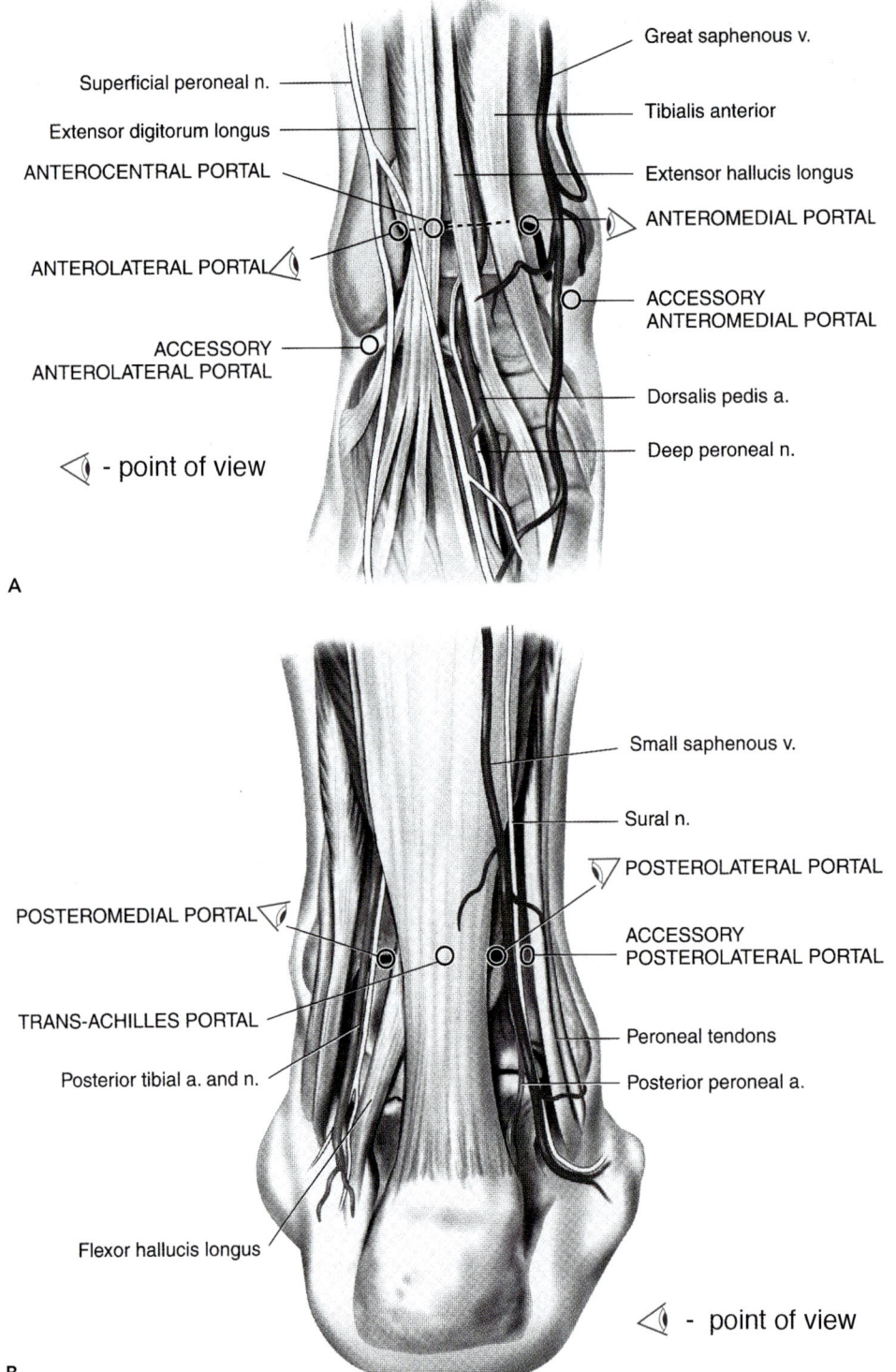

Figure 15.7 **Arthroscopy portals and examination.** (A) Anterior portals: anteromedial and anterolateral are the utility portals. (B) Posterior portals: posterolateral for increased visualization of posterior pathology. (C) Anteromedial portal 1 cm proximal to the medial malleolus and just medial to the anterior tibial tendon. (D) Right ankle of the intermediate branch of the superficial peroneal nerve whose topography is mapped out. It is next to the anterolateral portal (refer to Fig. 15.7A). (E) Posterolateral portal (refer to Fig. 15.7B). (F) Arthroscope from anteromedial portal with spinal needle in posterior lateral portal.

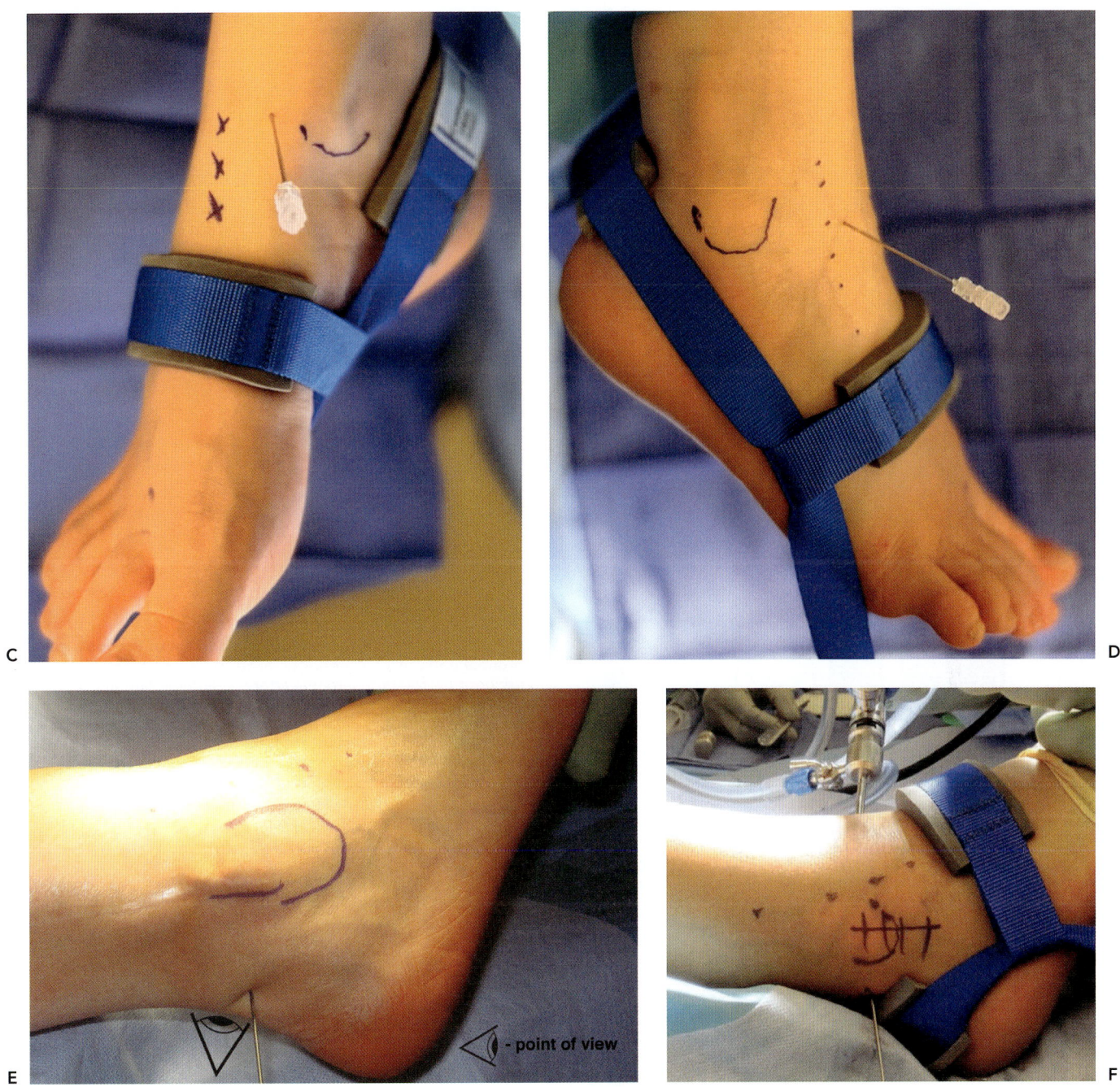

Figure 15.7 Cont'd

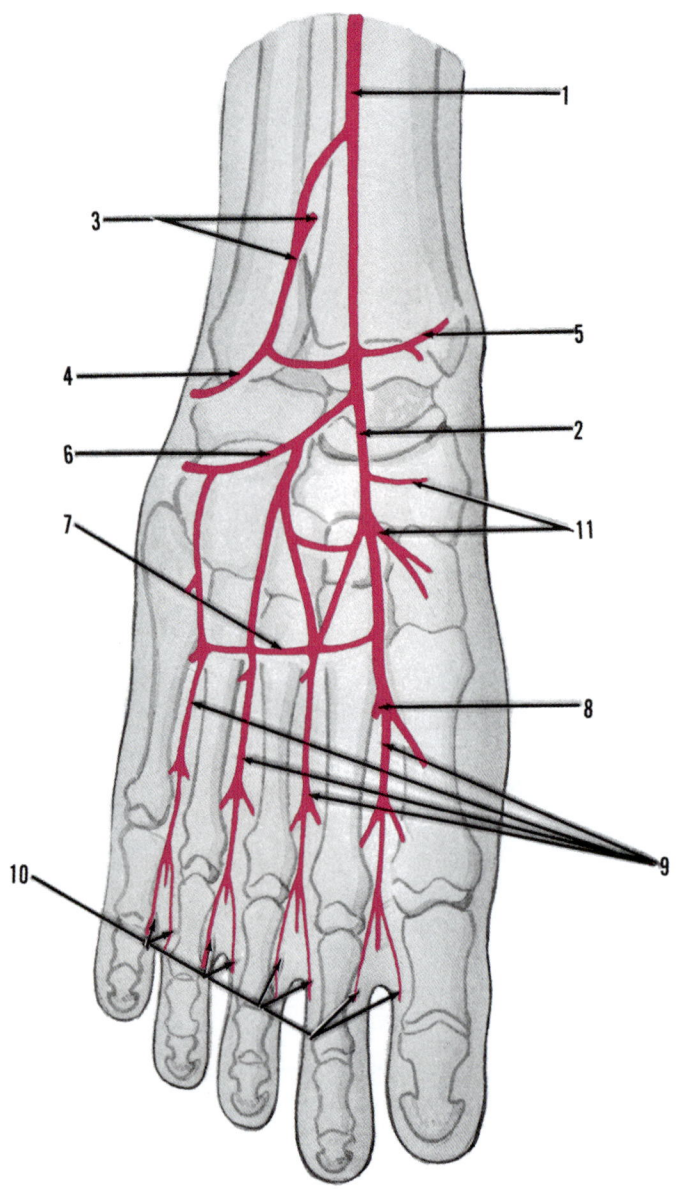

Figure 15.8 The arterial network of the dorsum of the foot, general or potential pattern. (*1*, Anterior tibial artery; *2*, dorsalis pedis artery; *3*, anterior or perforating peroneal artery; *4*, anterior lateral malleolar artery; *5*, anterior medial malleolar artery; *6*, lateral tarsal artery; *7*, arcuate artery; *8*, first proximal perforating artery; *9*, dorsal metatarsal arteries; *10*, dorsal digital arteries; *11*, medial tarsal arteries.) (From Huber JF. The arterial network supplying the dorsum of the foot. *Anat Rec.* 1941;80:373. By permission of Alan R. Liss, Publisher.)

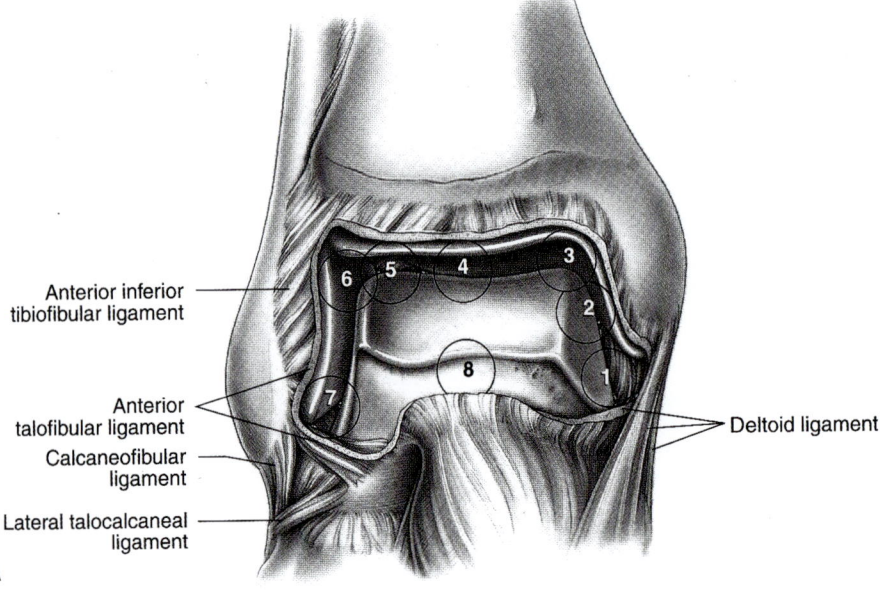

Figure 15.9 **(A)** Anterior eight-point examination, **(B)** central six-point examination, and **(C)** posterior seven-point examination. (Republished with permission of McGraw Hill, from Kelikian A, ed. *Operative Treatment of the Foot and Ankle*. McGraw-Hill; 1999. Chapter 19; permission conveyed through Copyright Clearance Center, Inc.)

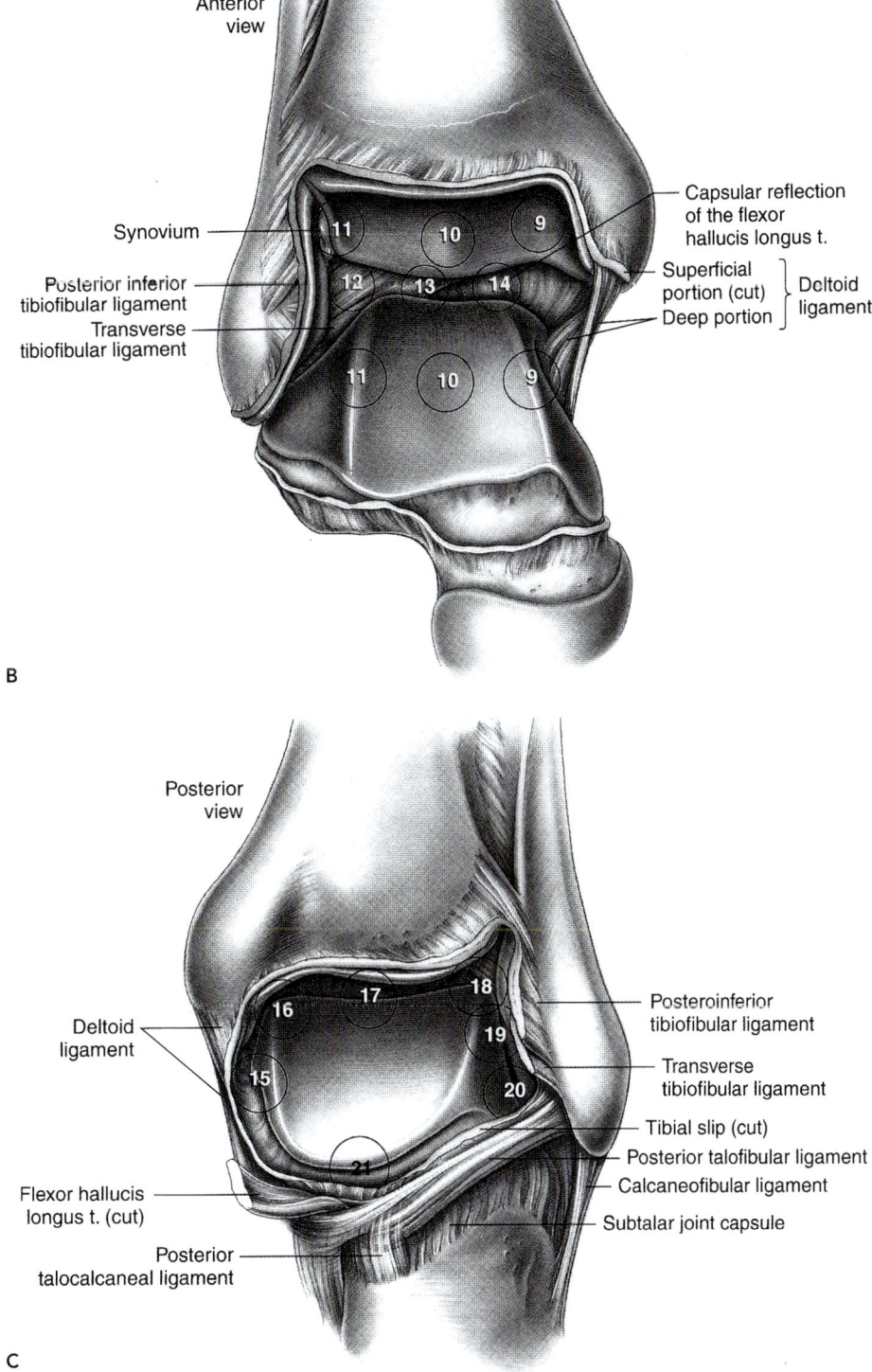

Figure 15.9 Cont'd

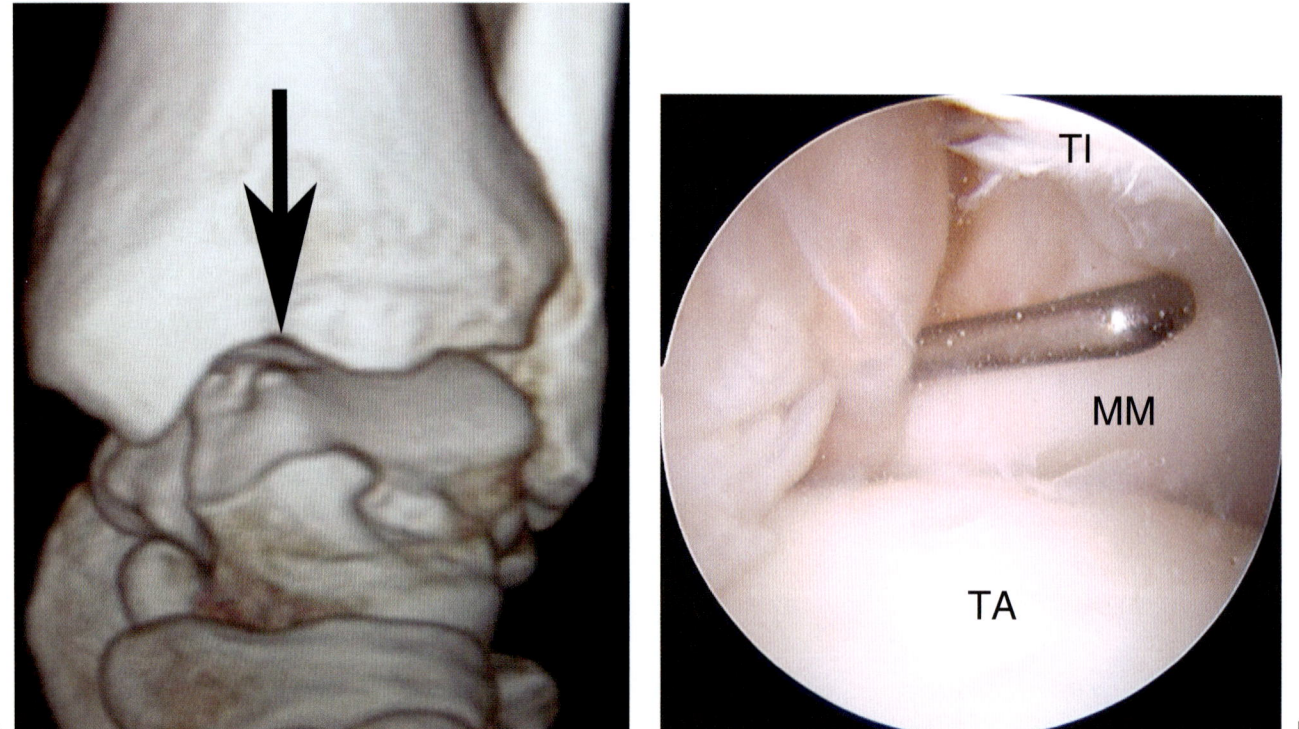

Figure 15.10 Groove of Harty. (A) Coronal reconstruction on CAT scan of a left ankle with the bold arrow depicting the groove of Harty in the medial tibial plafond. (B) Left ankle viewed from anterolateral portal with probe on groove of Harty in tibial plafond: talus (*TA*), medial malleolus (*MM*), and tibia (*TI*).

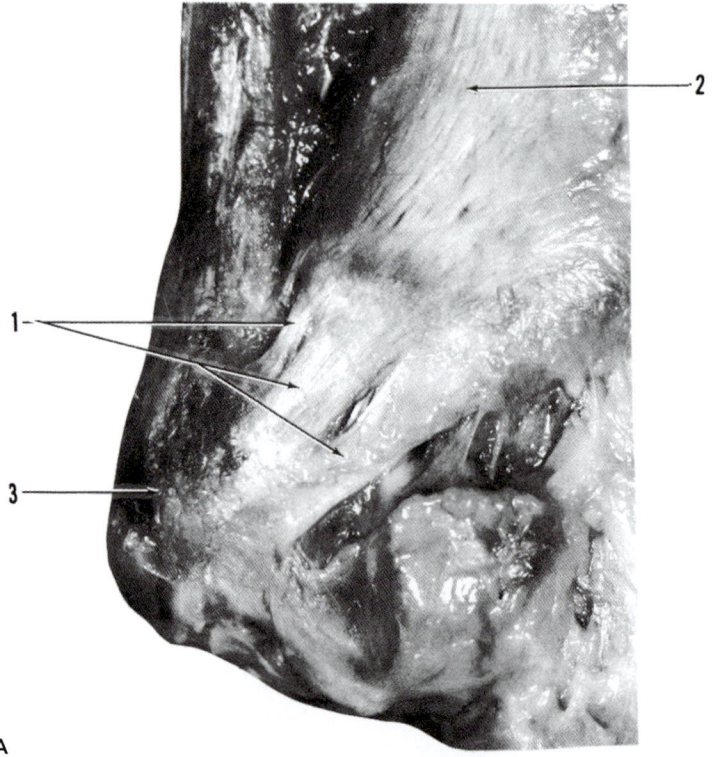

Figure 15.11 Anterior inferior tibiofibular ligament. (A) Dissection depicting the multiple fascicles of the anterior inferior tibiofibular ligament. (*1*, anterior tibiofibular ligament with three fascicles; *2*, tibia; *3*, lateral malleolus.) (B) Right ankle showing anterolateral talar dome viewed from anteromedial portal (see Fig. 15.7A): capsule (*CA*) and talus (*TA*). (C) Right ankle; *arrow* shows anterior inferior tibiofibular ligament. (D) Anteromedial portal of right ankle showing anterior tibia (*TI*), fibula (*F*), and talus (*TA*); *arrow* on anterior inferior tibiofibular ligament. (E) Right ankle viewing the tibiofibular syndesmosis with probe in tibiofibular cul-de-sac: tibia (*TI*), fibula (*F*), and talus (*TA*).

whose most distal component can be implicated as a cause of dorsiflexion impingement as described by Basset et al[16,17] (Fig. 15.11A). A distal fascicle has been identified in 21% of cases by Ray et al.[18] Nikolopoulos visualized the fascicle in up to 90% of impingement cases.[19] The anterior capsule and anterior talar dome is seen first when viewed from the anteromedial portal (see Fig. 15.11B). Laterally, one then encounters the anterior inferior tibiofibular ligament (see Fig. 15.11C, D). The lateral malleolar articular surface is visualized next in the eight-point examination as described by Ferkel and Scranton.[20] The interosseous ligament forms the proximal roof of the tibiofibular syndesmosis and is recessed 6 mm (see Fig. 15.11E). This can be probed but not visualized. The synovial fringe from this articulation is seen. With dorsiflexion of the ankle, the examiner will see the space or cul-de-sac between the transverse ligament and the distal ligaments increase; also, the synovial fringe will retract. Looking in the posterolateral corner, the posterior tibiofibular ligaments' deep component or transverse ligament is encountered. By virtue of its attachment from the malleolar fossa of the fibula to the posterior cartilaginous rim of the tibia, it is analogous to the labrum of the shoulder. The superficial component of this ligament cannot be seen from the anterior portal according to Golano et al.[21] There is discussion that an inferior slip of the deep ligament is a separate fascicle and referred to

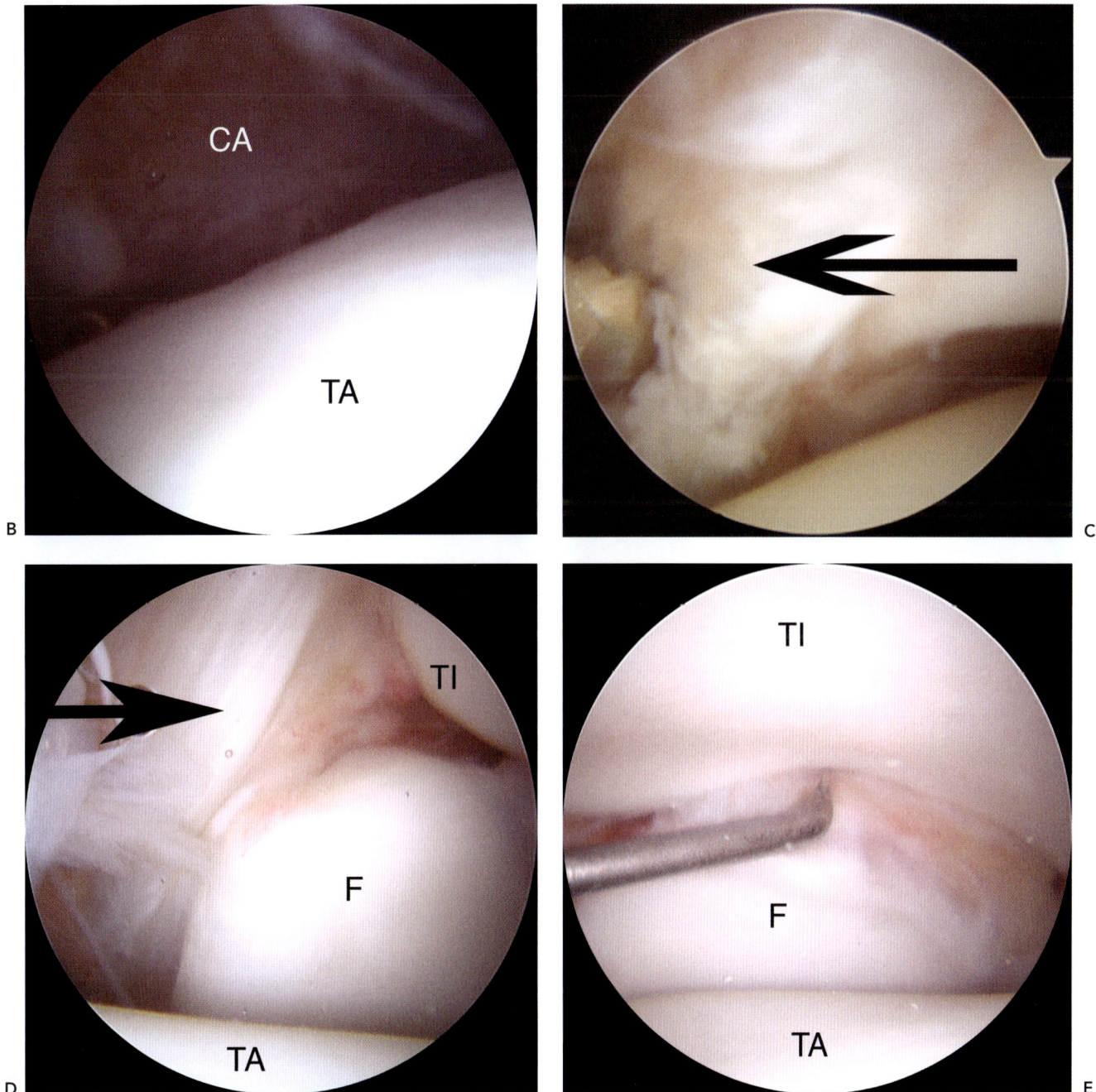

Figure 15.11 Cont'd

as the posterior intermalleolar ligament by Paturet.[21-23] It lies above the posterior talofibular ligament (Fig. 15.12). Others contend it represents the tibial slip of the posterior talofibular ligament, which is intracapsular but extrasynovial.[4] This triangle or soft spot allows for posterolateral portal placement (see Figs. 15.7E and 15.12C, D). Medial to the transverse ligament is the capsular reflection of the flexor hallucis longus tendon, which is directed from proximal lateral to distal medial as it is visualized. Medially, one can view the deep deltoid with a 30- or 70-degree arthroscope. The cartilaginous articulation between the talus and malleolar, as well as the deltoid, is best seen with a 70-degree arthroscope (see Fig. 15.13A). The deep deltoid fibers are visualized directed from the medial malleolar to the trochlear surface of the talus (Fig. 15.13B, C). Ferkel calls this area 1

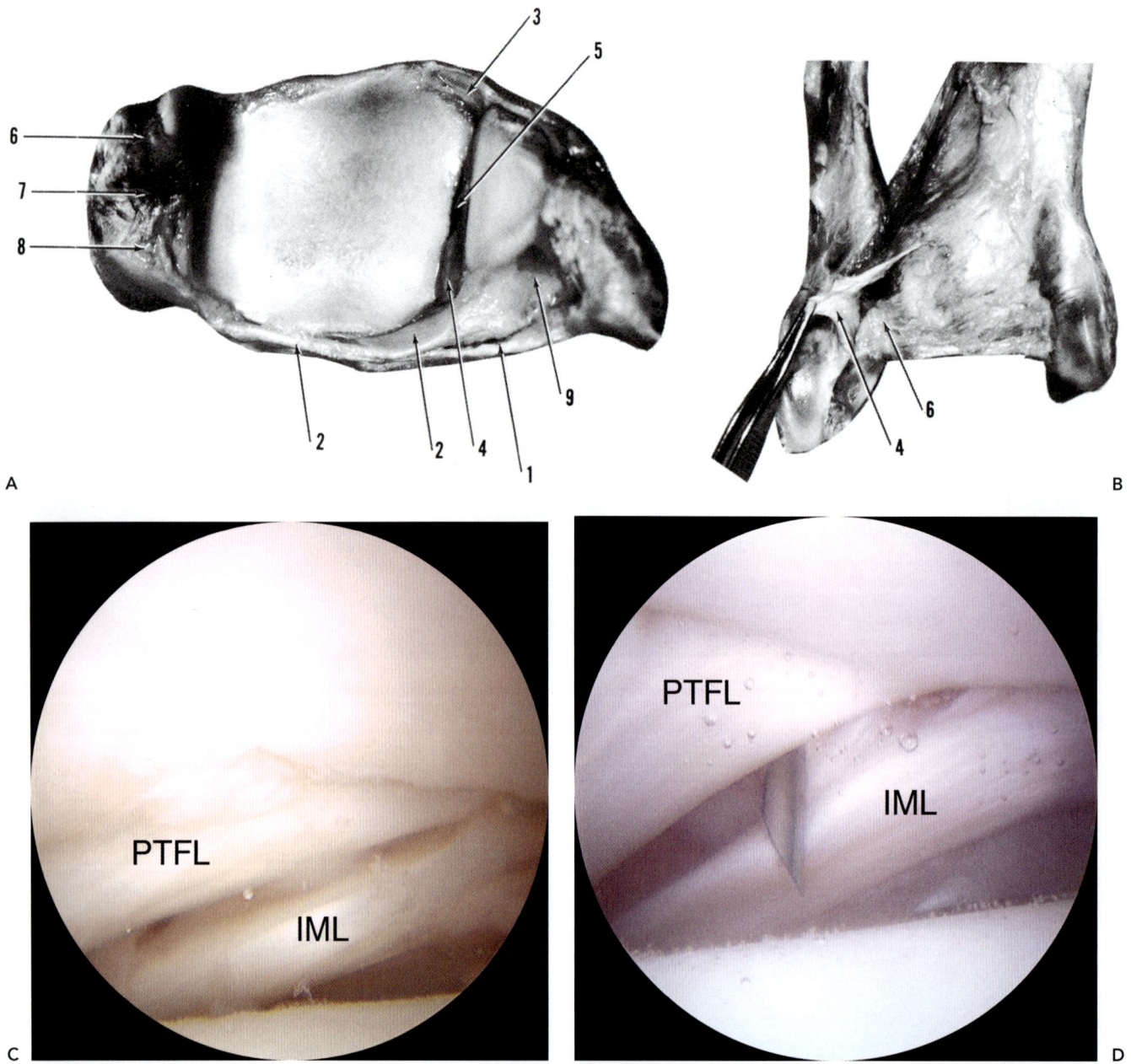

Figure 15.12 (A) Left ankle posteroanterior dissection showing posterior tibiofibular ligament viewed from axial plane. (1, Posterior tibiofibular ligament, superficial layer; 2, posterior tibiofibular ligament, deep layer; 3, anterior tibiofibular ligament; 4, synovial fringe of the tibiofibular recess; 5, tibiofibular recess; 6, anterior colliculus; 7, intercollicular groove; 8, posterior colliculus; 9, digital fossa of the lateral malleolus.) (B) Posterior tibiofibular ligament. (4, Partially detached posterior tibiofibular ligament, superficial layer; 6, posterior tibiofibular ligament, deep layer, posterior aspect.) (C) Right ankle viewed from anteromedial portal showing both fascicles of the posterior tibiofibular ligament (*PTFL*) and intermalleolar ligament (*IML*). (D) Needle placed through posterolateral portal entering above the intermalleolar ligament (*IML*).

in his 21-point diagnostic ankle examination[4] (see Fig. 15.9A). Going superior to zone 3—where the medial talar dome articulates with the distal tibia—there is the medial notch of Harty, which allows posterior passage with arthroscopic instrumentation and thus visualization posteriorly (see Fig. 15.10). The central concavity or groove of the talar body is appreciated.

Laterally, the plafond and talofibular articulation below the anterior inferior tibiofibular ligament is seen. The lateral gutter lies below this and, with a 70-degree arthroscope, the capsular reflection of the anterior talofibular ligament is present as well as the lateral process of the talus (Fig. 15.14C).

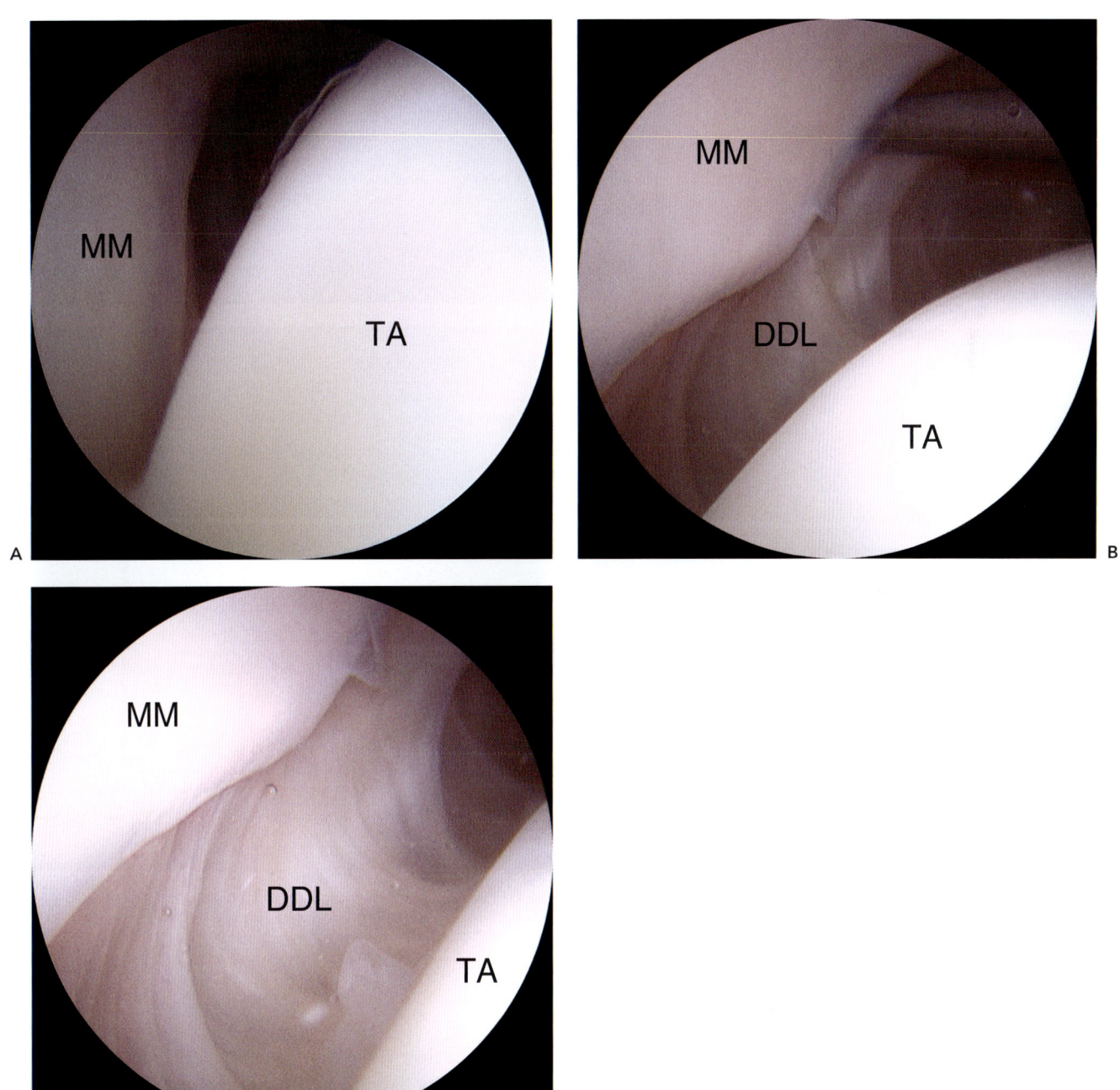

Figure 15.13 Left ankle. **(A)** View from anterolateral portal showing talar dome and medial malleolus: talus (*TA*) and medial malleolus (*MM*). **(B)** View from anterolateral portal: talus (*TA*), medial malleolus (*MM*), and deep deltoid or ibiotalar ligament (*DDL*). **(C)** View from anteromedial portal with deep deltoid ligament (*DDL*) between malleolus (*MM*) and talus (*TA*).

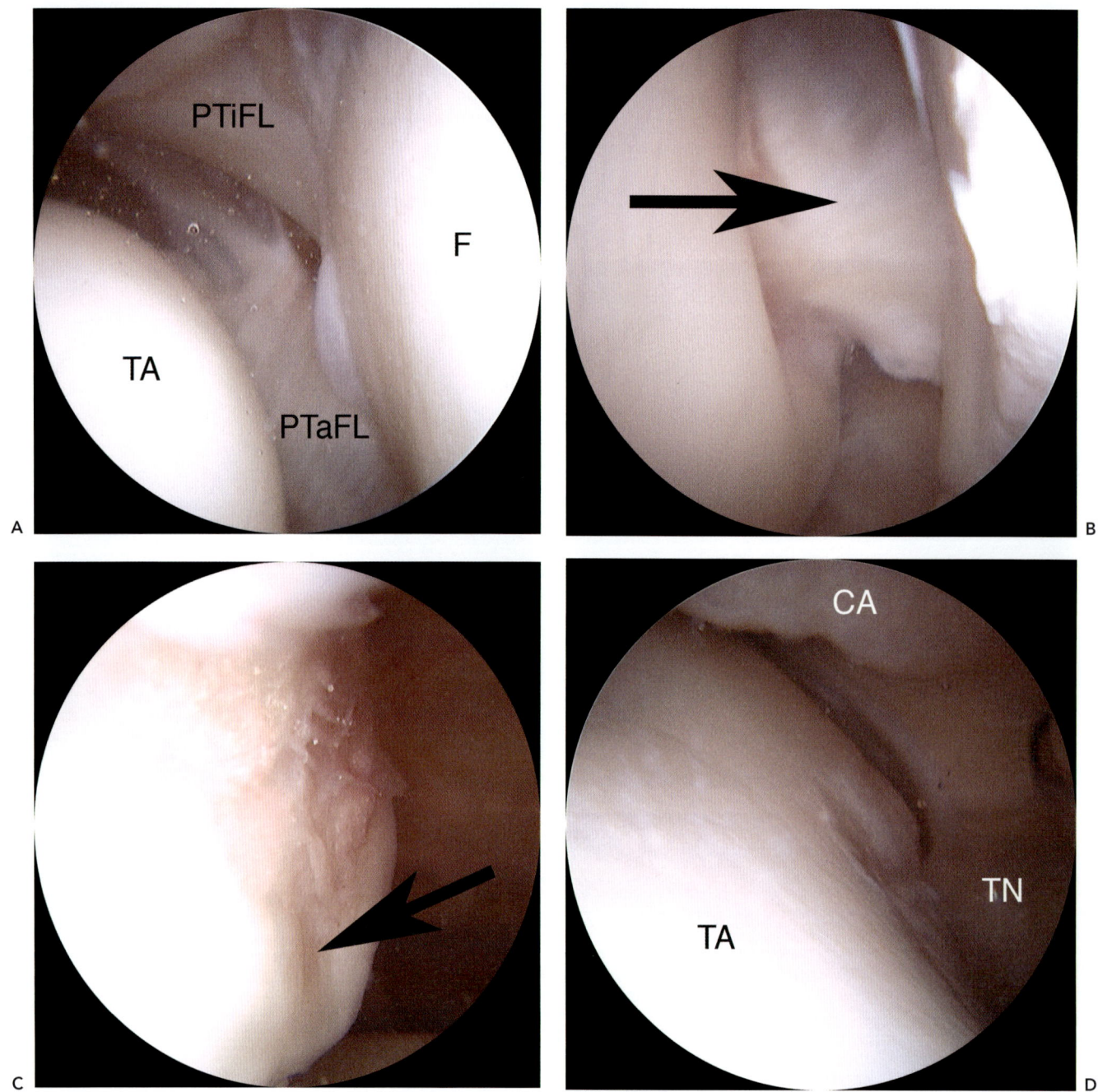

Figure 15.14 Left ankle. **(A)** Anterolateral talus and fibula (*F*) viewed from anterolateral portal (see Fig. 15.7A); the posterior tibiofibular ligament is seen above the posterior talofibular ligament. **(B)** *Arrow* shows posterior talofibular ligament from anterolateral portal. **(C)** *Arrow* on the lateral talar process viewed from anterolateral portal. **(D)** Anteromedial talar dome (*TA*), neck (*TN*), and *arrow* on the anterior capsule (*CA*).

SUBTALAR JOINT

Diagnostic subtalar arthroscopy was first described in 1985.[24] Numerous publications with regard to portals, pathologies, and therapeutic approaches have followed.[4,5,9,25,26] The subtalar joint is divided into anterior and posterior articulations separated by the tarsal canal. The talocalcaneal navicular joints occupy the anterior portion, whereas the talocalcaneal joint constitutes the posterior portion (Fig. 15.15). Knowledge of topographic landmarks in this complex and compact region is paramount. The sinus tarsi and its soft spot are easily palpated 2 cm anterior and 1 cm proximal to the tip of the fibula. A middle portal can be made over the sinus tarsi 1 cm anterior to the tip of the fibula. An accessory anterolateral portal can be made just anterior and superior to the anterolateral portal. The peroneal tendons are visualized and palpated at the fibular tip as well. Although hard to visualize, the sural nerve is 2 cm posterior and inferior to this landmark (see Fig. 15.6). The Achilles tendon insertion, medial malleolar, and tarsal tunnel are palpated and marked.

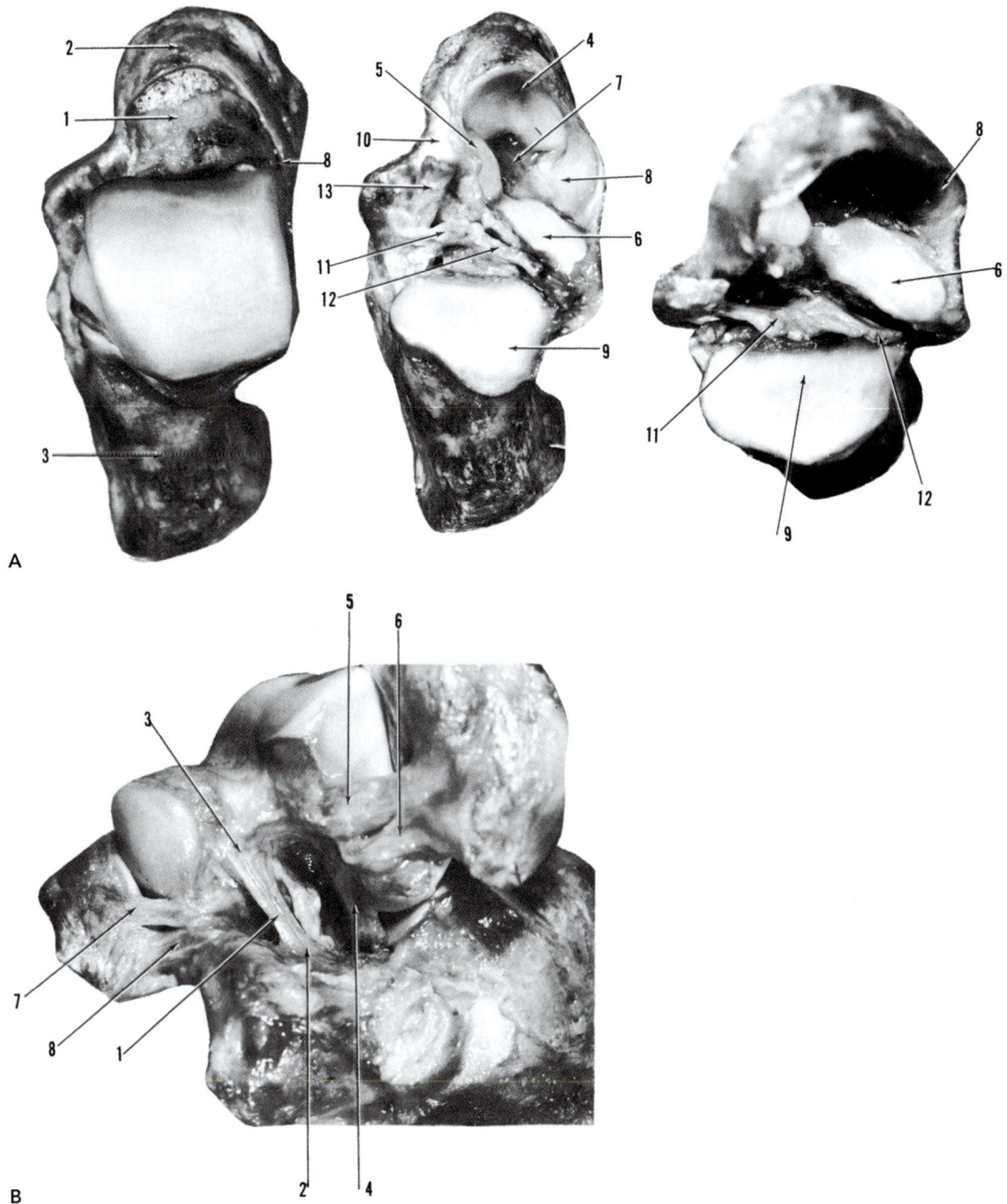

Figure 15.15 **Anatomy of the subtalar complex. (A)** Talocalcaneonavicular complex. (1, Talus; 2, navicular; 3, os calcis; 4, articular surface of the navicular for talar head; 5, anterior calcaneal surface; 6, middle calcaneal surface; 7, inferior calcaneonavicular ligament; 8, superomedial calcaneonavicular ligament; 9, posterior calcaneal surface; 10, lateral calcaneonavicular ligament; 11, medial root of inferior extensor retinaculum blending with interosseous talocalcaneal ligament [12] of the canalis tarsi; 13, cervical ligament.) **(B)** Lateral view of sinus tarsi. (1, Cervical ligament; 2, origin of 1 from sinus tarsi; 3, insertion of 1 on talar neck; 4, capsule of posterior talocalcaneal joint; 5, 6, anterior talofibular ligaments; 7, 8, lateral calcaneonavicular ligaments.) **(C)** Dorsal view of mid tarsus and ankle joint. (1, Lateral calcaneonavicular ligament; 2, medial calcaneocuboid ligament; 3, dorsolateral calcaneocuboid ligament; 4, lateral calcaneocuboid ligament; 5, cervical ligament; 6, dorsal cubonavicular ligament; 7, dorsal cuneo3 cuboid ligament; 8, dorsal navicularcuneo$_3$ ligament; 9, 10, intermediate and medial roots of interior extensor retinaculum; 11, 12, anterior talofibular ligaments; 13, anterior tibiofibular ligament). **(D)** Insertion sites in the sinus tarsi and canalis tarsi. (1, Lateral calcaneonavicular ligament; 2, medial calcaneocuboid ligament; 3, dorsolateral calcaneocuboid ligament; 4, extensor digitorum brevis muscle; 5, lateral root of inferior extensor retinaculum; 6, intermediate root of inferior extensor retinaculum; 7, 8, medial roots of inferior extensor retinaculum; 9, interosseous talocalcaneal ligament of canalis tarsi; 10, cervical ligament; 11, capsular ligament of anterior aspect of posterior talocalcaneal joint; 12, tunnel of peronei; 13, sinus tarsi; 14, canalis tarsi; 15, foramina of calcaneal antrum; 16, anterior and middle calcaneal articular surfaces; 17, posterior calcaneal articular surface.) **(E)** Anatomic preparation of canalis tarsi. Posterior half of talus is removed through an oblique osteotomy. (1, Talocalcaneal interosseous ligament of canalis tarsi; 2, anterior capsular ligament of posterior talocalcaneal joint; 3, insertion of lateral root of inferior extensor retinaculum on inferior peroneal retinaculum; 4, intermediate root of inferior extensor retinaculum; 5, 6, medial roots of inferior extensor retinaculum; 7, talus; 8, os calcis.)

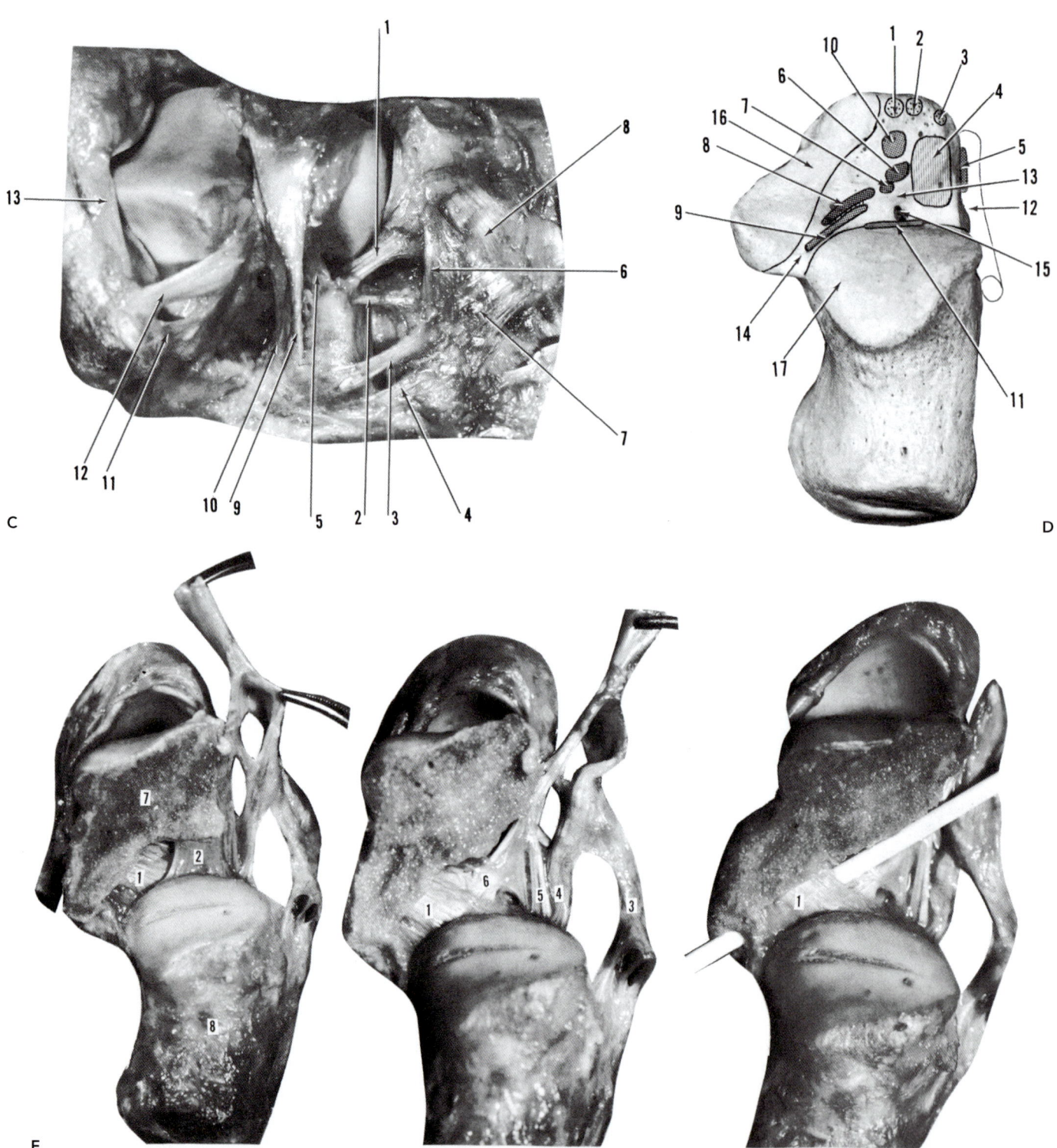

Figure 15.15 Cont'd

▶ Arthroscopic Portals

The anterolateral is via the soft spot described previously. The posterolateral portal is distal to that of the talocrural joint by about 7 mm or 5 mm proximal to the fibular tip and just lateral to the Achilles tendon. A line can be drawn from the lateral border of the insertion of the Achilles to the tip of the fibula and parallel to the sole of the foot with the ankle in neutral dorsiflexion (see Fig. 15.16B). The sural nerve can be within 4 mm of this portal as shown in anatomic dissections of structures at risk.[27,28] Just proximal to this line and juxtaposed to the Achilles insertion is this portal. A posteromedial portal is at the same level but on the medial border of the Achilles. It is directed away from the posterior neurovascular bundle and at an angle of 90° relative to the posterolateral portal.[26] Anatomic studies by Sitler and others have shown this portal to be 1 cm posterior to the neurovascular bundle (Fig. 15.17).[26,29-32]

Intra-articular Anatomy

The anterolateral portal visualizes the anterior one-third of the posterior facet of the subtalar joint. The interosseous talocalcaneal ligament is a landmark and reference point (see Fig. 15.16C). When rotating the arthroscope, the sinus tarsi floor as

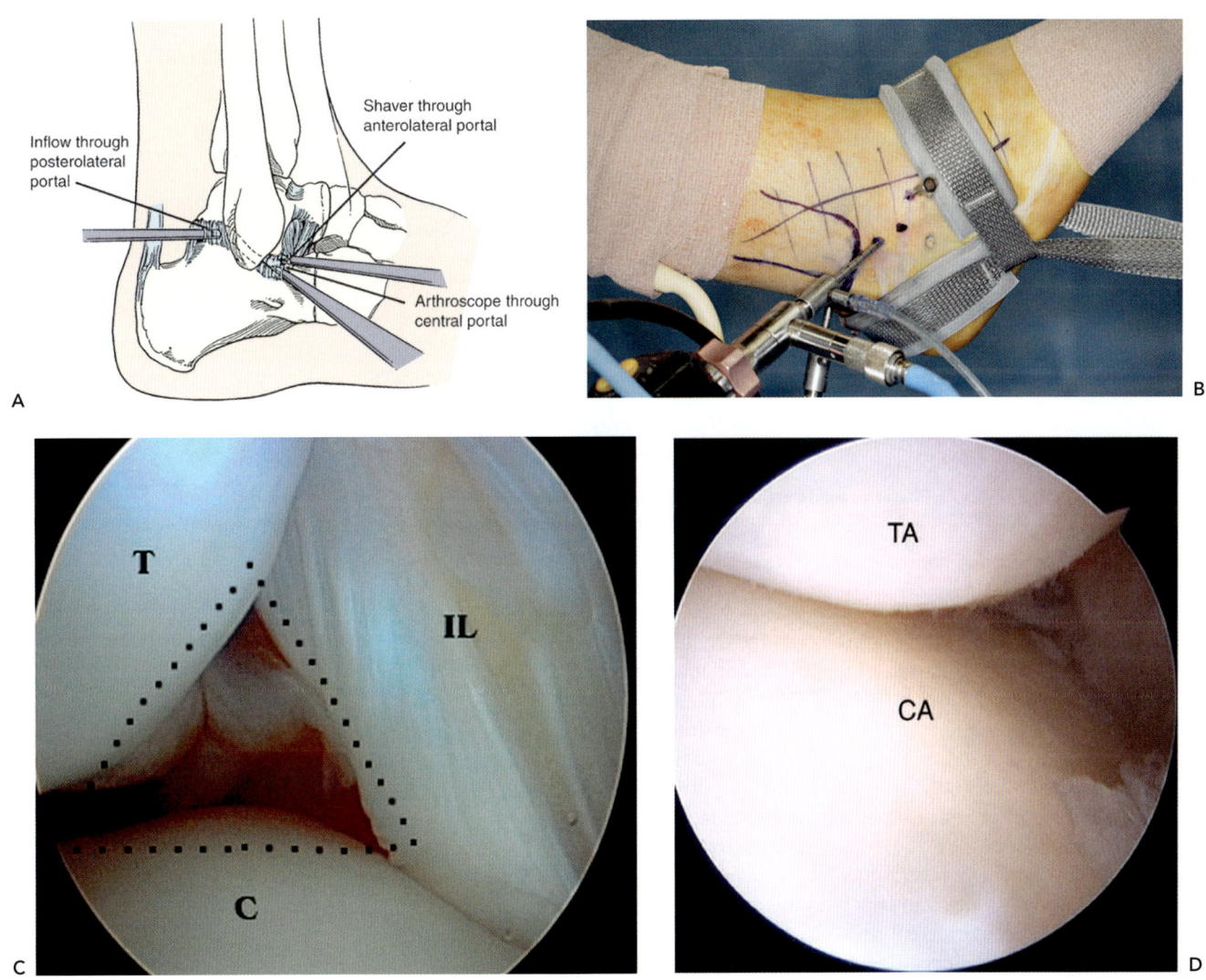

Figure 15.16 Subtalar arthroscopy. (A) Soft spot in the posterolateral corner of left ankle (see Fig. 15.7B) is where the inflow is established. Then the central portal is made. (B) Anterolateral portal is made after visualizing a spinal needle with the arthroscope in the central portal. (C) The subtalar triangle is formed by the interosseous ligament (IL), talus (T), and calcaneus (C) of the right subtalar joint viewed from central portal. (D) Anterior aspect of right talocalcaneal joint as seen from anterolateral portal. (TA, talus; CA, calcaneus.) (A–C, from Ferkel RD. Foot and Ankle Arthroscopy. 2nd ed. Wolters Kluwer; 2017, with permission.)

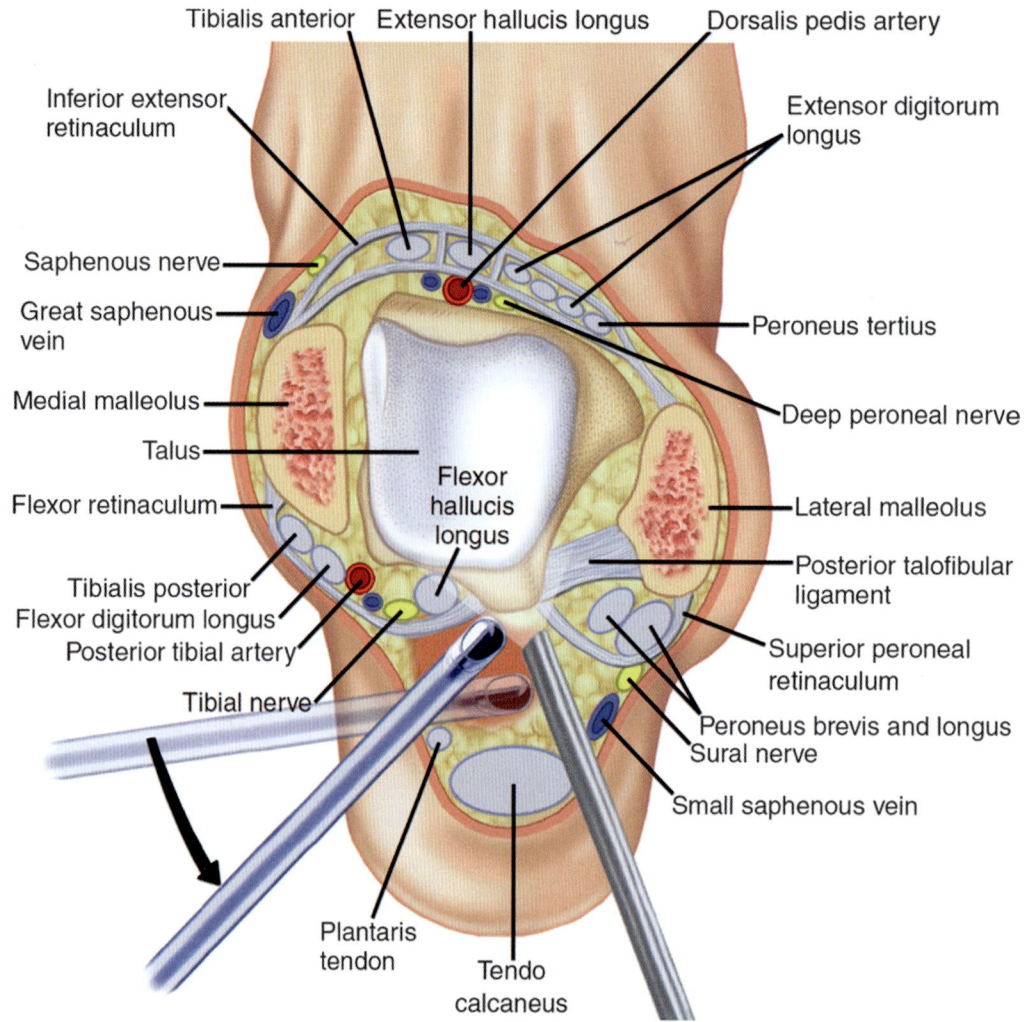

Figure 15.17 **Posterior ankle arthroscopy in the prone position.** The arthroscope is inserted through the posterolateral portal, and instruments are inserted through the posteromedial portal, lateral to the flexor hallucis longus. (From Johnson D, Amendola A, Alan Barber F, Field LD, Richmond JC, Sgaglione D. *Operative Arthroscopy*. 4th ed. Wolters Kluwer; 2012, with permission.)

well as the anterior process of the calcaneus can be visualized. From this portal, when rotating posteriorly, the articulation of the talocalcaneal joint and then the lateral gutter which represents the reflections of the lateral talocalcaneal and calcaneofibular ligaments can be seen (see Fig. 15.16D).

Via the posterolateral portal and beginning lateral, the gutter and then the posterior portions of the posterior facet are examined. This portal can be moved proximally to further visualize the ankle joint. The posteromedial recess and articulation are seen more medially. Van Dijk uses the two posterior portals—that is, the posteromedial and posterolateral[5,9,26,31] (Fig. 15.18A). The flexor hallucis longus tendon is the medial landmark (see Figs. 15.2B and 15.18B, C). The posterior aspect of the subtalar joint can be seen. With manual traction on the heel, the ankle joint can be entered after removing the joint capsule, and the posterior talar domes as well as the posterior tibiofibular ligaments are further visualized. Medially, the deep deltoid is visualized.

TENDOSCOPY

Tendoscopy, although extra-articular, provides a close up and dynamic anatomic assessment of certain tendons and pathologic entities. Achilles portals are just medial and lateral to the tendon. The pathologic condition dictates the craniocephalic position of the portal. The retrocalcaneal space, posterior calcaneal tuberosity, and bursar can be seen distally (Fig. 15.18D). The peroneal tendon portal is 2.5 cm above and below the tip of the fibula and directly over the sheath (Fig. 15.19A). The superior peroneal retinacular and peroneal groove is seen[29,30] (see Fig. 15.19B, C). Dynamically, subluxation and dislocation can be assessed. When viewing inferiorly, the longus and brevis tendons can be seen in their respective tunnels (see Fig. 15.19D, E). The posterior tibial tendon can be viewed in a similar manner via an inframalleolar portal medially (see Fig. 15.19F).

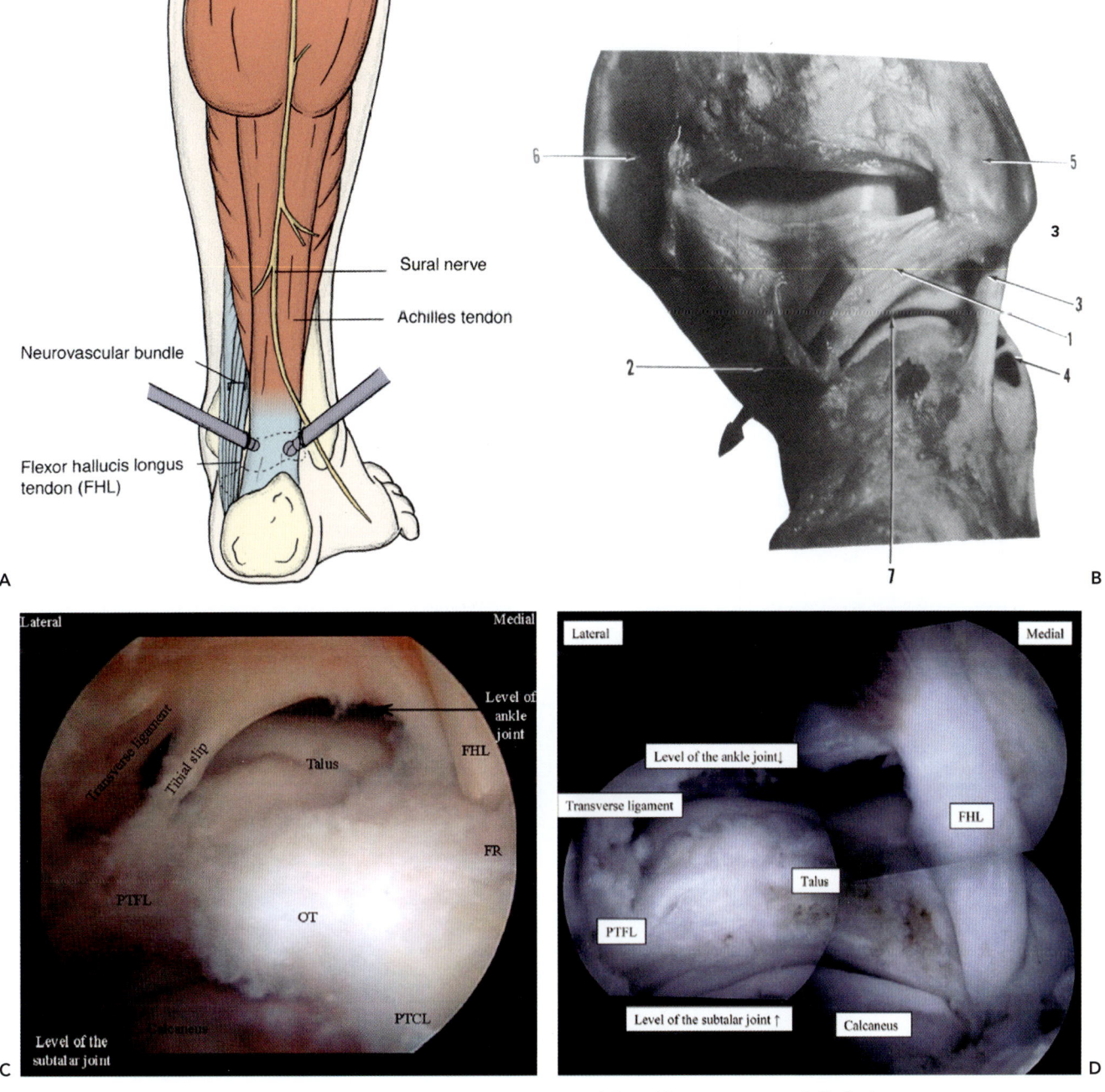

Figure 15.18 **(A)** Posterior portals. **(B)** Posterior aspect of the ankle. (*1*, Posterior talofibular ligament; *2*, fibrous tunnel of the flexor hallucis longus tendon; *3*, calcaneofibular ligament; *4*, inferior peroneal retinaculum; *5*, sulcus of the peronei tendons on posterior surface of the lateral malleolus; *6*, sulcus of tibialis posterior tendon on posterior aspect of the medial malleolus; *7*, posterior calcaneal articular interline.) **(C)** Posterior endoscopic view of the left ankle. The on trigonum (*OT*) is shown with the flexor hallucis longus tendon (*FHL*) in the upper right corner. On the medial side, the flexor retinaculum (*FR*) is attached to the OT. In the bottom right corner, the posterior talocalcaneal ligament (*PTCL*) is attached to the OT and, on the lateral side, the posterior talofibular ligament (*PTFL*) runs between the OT and the fibula. **(D)** Endoscopic view of the posterior ankle and subtalar joints separated by the posterior talar process. The flexor hallucis longus (*FHL*) tendon can be seen on the right after removal of the OT. (**C, D,** From Scholten PE, van Dijk CN, Krips R. Hindfoot endoscopy for posterior ankle impingement. *J Bone Joint Surg Am.* 2008;90-A[12]:2665-2672.)

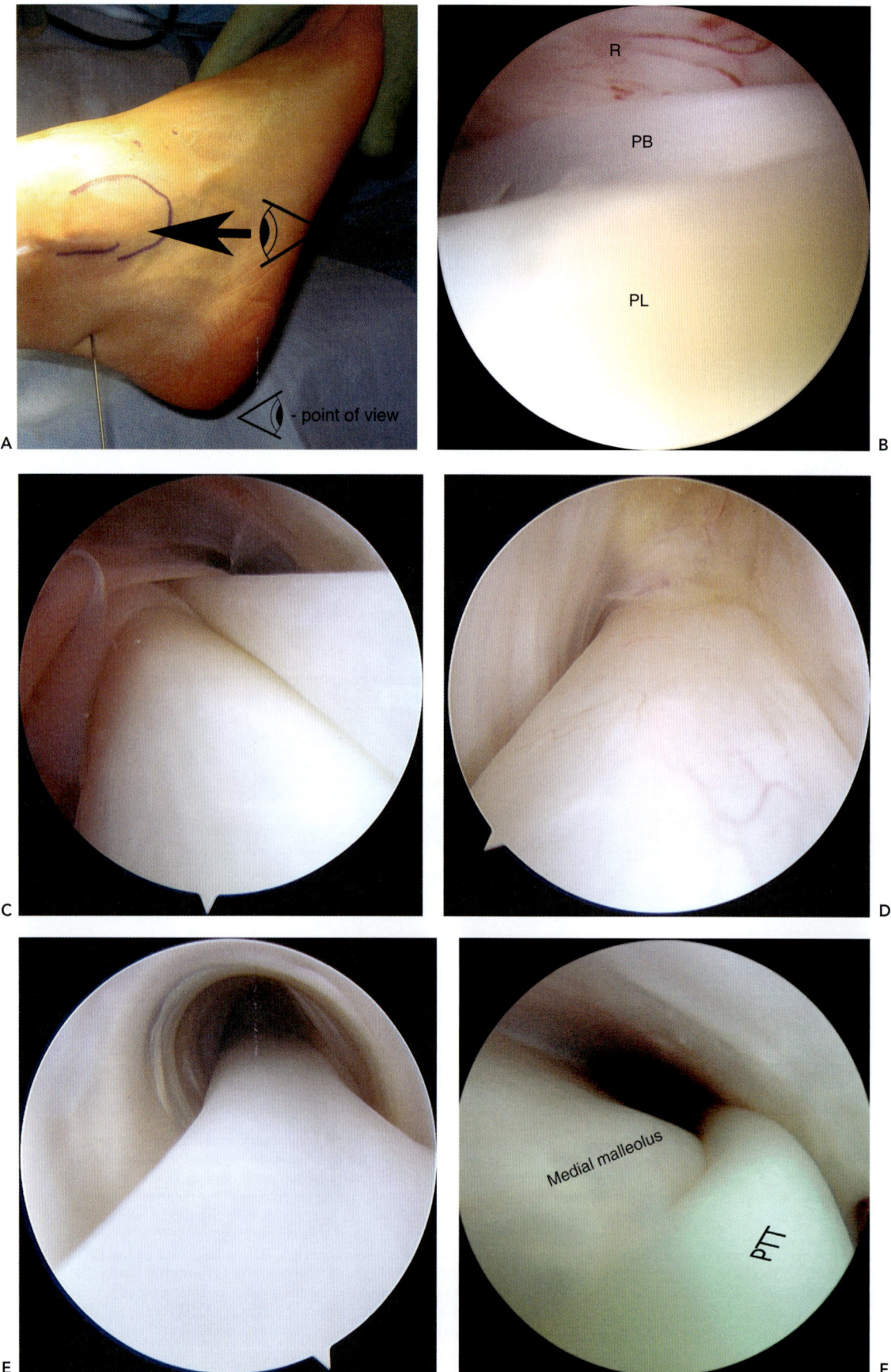

Figure 15.19 Peroneal endoscopy. (A) Right ankle showing inframalleolar portal. (B) Right ankle viewing retinaculum superior with peroneals (*PB*, *PL*) in foreground. (C) Peroneal longus to left and brevis to right. (D) Inferior tunnel of right peroneus brevis. (E) Inferior tunnel of right peroneus longus. (F) Right ankle view of a superior view of the posterior tibial tendon just inferior to the medial malleolus.

REFERENCES

1. Watanabe M, Takeda S, Ikeuchi H. *Atlas of Arthroscopy*. 2nd ed. Igkui-Schoin; 1969.
2. Guhl JF. *Ankle Arthroscopy: Pathological and Surgical Techniques*. Slack; 1988.
3. Yates CK, Grana WA. A simple distraction technique for ankle arthroscopy. *Arthroscopy*. 1988;4:103.
4. Ferkel RD. *Foot and Ankle Arthroscopy*. 2nd ed. Wolters Kluwer; 2017.
5. Scholten PE, Sierevelt IN, van Dijk CN. Hindfoot endoscopy for posterior ankle impingement. *J Bone Joint Surg*. 2008;90-A(12):2665-2672.
6. Draeger RW, Singh B, Pavekh SG. Quantifying normal ankle volume: an anatomic study. *Indian J Orthop*. 2009;43:72-75.
7. Testut L, Laterjet A. *Traite' d'Anatomic Humaine Livre. Tome II Arthrologic*. Libraire Octave Dain; 1921:634.
8. Buckingham RA, Winson IG, Kelly AJ. An anatomical study of a new portal for ankle arthroscopy. *J Bone Joint Surg Br*. 1997;79B(4):650-652.
9. Beimers L, Frey C, van Dijk CN. Arthroscopy of the posterior subtalar joint. *Foot Ankle Clin*. 2006;11(2):360-390.
10. Feiwell LA, Frey C. Anatomical study of arthroscopic portal sites of the ankle. *Foot Ankle*. 1993;14:142-147.
11. Takao M, Curio Y, Shu N. Anatomic basics of ankle arthroscopy: study of superficial and beep peroneal nerves around anterolateral and anterocentral approach. *Surg Radiol Anat*. 1998;20:317-320.
12. Saito A, Kikachi S. Anatomical relations between ankle arthroscopic portal sites and superficial peroneal and saphenous nerves. *Foot Ankle*. 1998;19:748-752.
13. Huber JF. The arterial network supplying the dorsum of the foot. *Anat Rec*. 1941;80:373-391.
14. Basarir K, Esmer AF, Truccar E, et al. Medial and lateral arteries in ankle arthroscopy: a cadaver study. *J Foot Ankle Surg*. 2007;46(3):181-184.
15. Harty M. Ankle arthroscopy, anatomical features. *Orthopedics*. 1985;8:1538-1560.
16. Bassett FH III, Glass HS, Billys JB, et al. Talar impingement by the anteroinferior tibiofibular ligament: a cause of chronic pain of the ankle after inversion sprain. *J Bone Joint Surg Am*. 1990;72:55-59.
17. Akseki D, Pinar H, Bozhurt M, et al. The distal fascicle of the anteroinferior tibiofibular ligament as a cause of anterolateral ankle impingement: the results of arthroscopic resection. *Acta Orthop Scand*. 1999;70:478-482.
18. Ray RG, Kriz BM. Anterior inferior tibiofibular ligament: variations and relationship to the talus. *J Am Podiatr Med Assoc*. 1991;81:479-485.
19. Nikolopoulus CE, Triskos AI, Sourmelis S, et al. The accessory anteroinferior tibiofibular ligament as a cause of talar impingement: a cadaveric study. *J Sports Med*. 2004;32:389-395.
20. Ferkel RD, Scranton PE Jr. Arthroscopy of the ankle and foot. *J Bone Joint Surg*. 1993;75-A(8):1233-1242.
21. Golano P, Vega J, Perez-Carro L, et al. Ankle anatomy for the arthroscopist. Part I: the portals. *Foot Ankle Clin*. 2006;11:254-273.
22. Golano P, Vega J, Perez-Carro L, et al. Ankle anatomy for the arthroscopist. Part II: role of the ankle ligaments in soft tissue impingement. *Foot Ankle Clin*. 2006;11:274-296.
23. Paturet G. *Traite' d'Anatomie Humaine Tome III; Articulation de Cou-de-Pied*. Maison et Co; 1951:704.
24. Parisien JS, Vangeness T. Arthroscopy of the subtalar joint: an experimental approach. *Arthroscopy*. 1985;1:53.
25. Parisien JS. Arthroscopy of the posterior subtalar joint. In: Jahss MH, ed. *Disorders of the Foot and Ankle*. WB Saunders; 1991:230.
26. Van Dijk CN. Hindfoot endoscopy. *Foot Ankle Clin*. 2006;11:391-414.
27. Tryfonidisi M, Whitefield CG, Charalambous CP, et al. The distance between the sural nerve and ideal lateral portal placement in lateral subtalar arthroscopy: a cadaveric study. *Foot Ankle Int*. 2008;29(8):842-844.
28. Sitler DF, Amendola A, Bialey C, et al. Posterior ankle arthroscopy: an anatomic study. *J Bone Joint Surg*. 2002;84-A(5):763-769.
29. Mekhail AO, Heck BE, Ehraheim NA, et al. Arthroscopy of the subtalar joint: establishing a medial portal. *Foot Ankle Int*. 1995;16(7):427-432.
30. Lipoi F, Lughi M, Baccarani G. Posterior arthroscopic approach to the ankle: an anatomical study. *Arthroscopy*. 2003;19(1):162-167.
31. Frey C, Gasser S, Feder K. Arthroscopy of the subtalar joint. *Foot Ankle Int*. 1994;15(8):424-428.
32. Johnson D, Amendola A, et al. *Operative Arthroscopy*. 4th ed. Wolters Kluwer; 2012.

Index

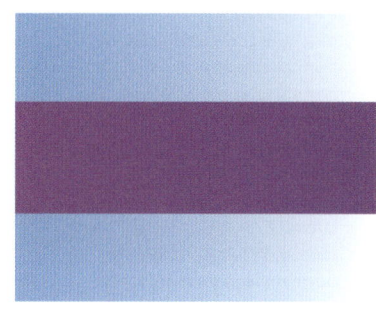

Note: Page numbers followed by "*f*" indicate figures and "*t*" indicate tables.

A

Abductor digiti minimi, 276, 278*f*, 343
　flap, débridement, 711, 712*f*
Abductor hallucis muscle/tendon, 260–261, 266*f*–268*f*, 343, 509
Accessory bones, 98
　os calcaneus secundarius, 99–100, 105*f*
　os cuboides secundarium, 100, 106*f*
　os cuneo$_1$ metatarsale$_1$ plantare, 101, 107*f*
　os intercuneiforme, 100, 107*f*
　os intermetatarseum, 99, 103*f*–104*f*
　os subfibulare, 103
　os subtibiale, 103
　os sustentaculi, 99, 105*f*
　os talonaviculare dorsale, 100
　os tibiale, 98–99, 100*f*–101*f*
　os trigonum, 98, 99*f*
　os vesalianum, 101–103, 107*f*
Accessory soleus muscle, 252–253
Acetabulum pedis, ligaments
　bifurcate, 190–195
　inferior calcaneonavicular, 190
　lateral calcaneonavicular, 190–195
　superomedial calcaneonavicular, 188, 196*f*
Achilles (calcaneal) tendon, 290–291, 290*f*, 290*t*
　blood supply of, 363–364
Adductor compartment, 446
Adductor hallucis muscle/tendon, 158, 160*f*, 273*f*, 509
　muscle bellies, 274
　oblique head of, 268, 273*f*–274*f*
　transverse head of, 268–269, 274–276
　variations of
　　oblique adductor, 269
　　transverse adductor, 269–274
Adipose mantle, 487, 488*f*
Anastomosis, 351
Angiosomes
　of ankle, 711, 712*f*
　　anterior, posterior tibial, of distal tibia and medial ankle, 704, 704*f*
　　anterior tibial, peroneal angiosomes of lateral ankle, 704–705, 705*f*
　of calf, 703
　　anterior tibial, 704
　　peroneal, free tissue transfer and, 703–704
　　posterior tibial, 704
　　sural angiosome, diabetic patient, 703
　of foot, 706, 706*f*–707*f*
　　posterior tibial, peroneal angiosomes of heel, 706, 707*f*
　great toe, 710, 711*f*
　incisions, foot and ankle, 711, 712*f*
　of medial and lateral sole, 706
　　anterior tibial, dorsal foot, 707–708, 709*f*
　　peroneal angiosome, posterolateral and anterolateral foot, 708, 711*f*
　　posterior tibial, 707, 708*f*
　physiology of, 702, 703*f*
Ankle
　angiosomes of, 704–705, 704*f*–705*f*
　anterior aspect
　　dorsal aponeurosis, 459–460, 461*f*–462*f*
　　dorsal fascial spaces/contents, 460–465, 463*f*–465*f*
　　skin and subcutaneous layer, 454–455, 456*f*
　　superficial nerves, 455–458, 459*f*–460*f*
　　superficial veins, 455, 457*f*–458*f*
　　surface anatomy, 452–454, 455*f*
　anterior (dorsal) aspect of, muscles of, 222–232
　arthroscopic portals, 787, 788*f*–789*f*
　　anterior, 787, 790*f*
　　intraarticular anatomy, 790*f*–796*f*, 793–795
　axis of motion
　　multiple, 512–513, 514*f*–518*f*
　　single, 512, 512*f*–513*f*
　gait, forces acting and, 628, 630, 632*f*
　incisions, 711, 712*f*
　lateral aspect of, muscles of, 232–244
　lateral ligament of
　　anterior talofibular ligament (ATFL), 166–169, 168*f*–169*f*
　　calcaneofibular ligament, 169–173, 170*f*–173*f*
　　fibulotalocalcaneal ligament, 174–175, 178*f*–180*f*
　　posterior talofibular ligament, 173–174, 174*f*–177*f*
　load-bearing characteristics of, 523, 523*f*–524*f*
　loaded, stability of, 541–542, 542*f*–544*f*
　medial aspect of, muscles of, 244–290
　mobility of fibula and, 518, 521–523, 522*f*
　motors of
　　dorsiflexors and, 587
　　plantarflexors and, 587
　posterolateral aspect, 466
　　deep aponeurosis, 468, 468*f*
　　skin, 466, 466*f*–467*f*
　　subcutaneous layer, 466, 466*f*–467*f*
　　superficial aponeurosis, 467
　　superficial nerves, 466, 466*f*–467*f*
　　superficial posterolateral compartment, 467
　　superficial veins, 466, 466*f*–467*f*
　　superior peroneal tunnel, 468, 469*f*
　range of motion, 513, 517–518, 518*f*, 519*f*–521*f*
　stability, deltoid ligament
　　anatomic observations, 536*f*, 538–539
　　experimental investigation, role of, 539–541, 539*f*–541*f*
　　mechanical characteristics of, 541
　stability, lateral collateral ligaments, 523–524
　　experimental studies, anterior and lateral, transverse rotational stability and, 531–532, 532*f*–537*f*, 535–536
　　experimental studies, posterior, 536

Ankle—*continued*
  mechanical characteristics of, 536, 538, 539*f*
  normal anterior talar shift, 530–531, 531*t*
  normal talar tilt, 529–530, 531*t*
  stabilizing function, anatomic observation, 524–526, 524*f*–529*f*
  strain patterns, 529, 530*f*
  ultrasound (US) anatomy
    anterior, 773, 773*f*
    lateral, 773–775, 773*f*–775*f*
    medial, 775–777, 776*f*–775*f*
    normal ultrasound anatomy of, 771, 773
    posterior, 777–778, 777*f*–778*f*
Anterior talofibular ligament (ATFL), 166–169, 168*f*–169*f*
Aponeurosis
  dorsal, 126–130, 128*f*–130*f*
  peroneal
    inferior peroneal tunnel and retinaculum, 131, 132*f*
    intermediary peroneal tunnel, 131
    superior peroneal retinaculum, 130–131
    superior peroneal tunnel, 130, 131*f*
  plantar, 143, 147*f*
    central component, 143–153, 148*f*–153*f*
    flexor, metatarsophalangeal joints, 594, 594*f*–596*f*, 596
    peroneal/lateral component, 153, 154*f*
    protective loading of, during gait, 625–626, 627*f*–628*f*
    tibial/medial component, 153
    toes as tensors of, 592, 594
    windlass, 594*f*–596*f*
Arches
  arch-flattening effect and, 597–598, 599*f*
  beam variant of, 597–598, 597*f*, 600
  load transmission and, 596, 596*f*–598*f*
    internal compressive forces and, 597, 598*f*
    truss and beam and, 597–598, 599*f*–600*f*, 600
  longitudinal, 596, 600*f*
  transverse, 596
  truss variant of, 597–598, 599*f*–600*f*, 600
Arcuate artery, 316–317
Arteries. *See also specific arteries*
  arcuate artery, 316–317
  cutaneous arterial supply, of foot and ankle
    dorsum of, 341–342
    malleolar skin, 342
    planta pedis, 342–343
  dorsal, of foot and ankle, 304–307, 305*t*, 307*f*–310*f*
  osseous, of foot and ankle
    big toe, sesamoids of, 362–363, 364*f*
    calcaneus, 351
    cuboid, 355
    cuneiforms, 355
    metatarsals. *See* Metatarsals
    navicular, 354–355, 356*f*–358*f*
    phalanges, 361–362, 363*f*
    talus, 347, 347*f*–348*f*
    tibia and fibula, distal end of, 343–347, 345*f*–346*f*
  posterior/plantar arterial network
    deep plantar arch, 334, 335*t*, 336*f*
    lateral plantar artery, 334, 335*f*
    medial plantar artery, 330–333, 332*f*–335*f*
    plantar metatarsal arteries, 335–339, 335*f*–339*f*
    posterior tibial artery, 328–330, 329*f*–331*f*
  prenatal development, fetal phase, 30–32, 30*f*–32*f*
  superficial muscles, of sole and dorsum of foot, 343
Arthrography, 730–731, 730*f*
Arthroscopy
  anatomical landmarks, 782, 783*f*–787*f*
  ankle portals, 787, 788*f*–789*f*
    anterior, 787, 790*f*–796*f*, 793–795
  subtalar joint, 796, 797*f*–798*f*
    portals, 799–800, 799*f*–801*f*
  tendoscopy, 800, 802*f*
Articular cartilage, ultrasound (US) anatomy, 771

B

Basal ganglia, neuro control, 678, 678*f*–682*f*, 680
Beam, 597–598, 599*f*–600*f*, 600
Bifurcate ligament (ligament of Chopart; V ligament), 190–195
Bipartition
  bipartite navicular, 114–115
  bipartite first cuneiform, 114, 114*f*
Boehler's angle, 551, 555*f*
Bone(s)
  accessory, 98
    os calcaneus secundarius, 99–100, 105*f*
    os cuboides secundarium, 100, 106*f*
    os cuneo$_1$ metatarsale$_1$ plantare, 101, 107*f*
    os intercuneiforme, 100, 107*f*
    os intermetatarseum, 99, 103*f*–104*f*
    os subfibulare, 103
    os subtibiale, 103
    os sustentaculi, 99, 105*f*
    os talonaviculare dorsale, 100
    os tibiale, 98–99, 100*f*–101*f*
    os trigonum, 98, 99*f*
    os vesalianum, 101–103, 107*f*
  prenatal development, 8–9
    cartilaginous stage, 9–11, 9*f*–10*f*
    fetal phase. *See* Fetal phase
    mesenchymal stage, 9, 9*f*
    osseous stage, 11, 11*f*–12*f*
    stages, 9–11
  trabeculae, orientation of, 602, 604*f*–609*f*, 606–609
Bursae, synovial, 299
  intermetatarsophalangeal, 301–303
  subcutaneous, 300
  subfascial, 300–301

C

Cadence, 610
Calcaneal nerve, lateral, 387*f*
Calcaneal tunnel. *See* Tibiotalocalcaneal tunnel
Calcaneocuboid coalition, 108–109
Calcaneocuboid joint, motion of, 558–559, 559*f*–564*f*, 561
Calcaneocuboid ligament
  dorsolateral, 202–203
  inferior, 203–205, 203*f*–205*f*
  medial, 202
Calcaneocubonavicular cuneiforms, 438
Calcaneofibular ligament, 169–173, 170*f*–173*f*
Calcaneonavicular coalition, 108, 108*f*–109*f*
Calcaneonavicular ligament(s)
  bifurcate ligament, 190–195
  inferior, 190
  lateral, 190–195
  superomedial, 188, 196*f*
Calcaneus, 59, 59*f*–60*f*, 351
  anterior, 66
  inferior, 63
  lateral, 64–65, 64*f*–65*f*, 351
  medial, 65–66, 66*f*, 351–353
  plantar, 353
  posterior, 66, 353–354, 353*f*–354*f*
  superior, 59, 61*f*, 351
    anterior third, 60–63, 62*f*, 63*f*
    middle third, 60, 62*f*, 62*t*
    posterior third, 59

Calf, angiosomes of, 703
　anterior tibial, 704
　peroneal, free tissue transfer and, 703–704
　posterior tibial, 704
　sural angiosome, diabetic patient, 703
Capsule, ultrasound (US) anatomy, 770
Caro quadrata of Sylvius. See Quadratus plantae muscle
Cartilage-covered gliding facet, 64
Cartilaginous stage, 9–11, 9f–10f
Central compartment, 490–498, 490f–499f
Central intermediary compartment, 442
Cerebellar cortex and circuits, 671, 673, 673f–674f
Cerebellar hemispheres, 670–671, 671f–673f
Cerebellum, 670, 670f
　cerebellar cortex and circuits, 671, 673, 673f–674f
　cerebellar hemispheres, 670–671, 671f–673f
　cerebral peduncles, 671, 673f
　climbing fibers, 673, 675, 675f
　deep cerebellar nuclei, 675–676, 677f–678f
Cerebral motor cortex, 683, 683f–684f
　output of, 685–686, 685f–686f
　premotor, 684–685
　primary, 683–684, 685f
Cerebral peduncles, 671, 673f
Cervical ligament, 195–197, 198f–199f, 551–557
　subtalar, 579
Choke vessels, 702, 703f
Chopart, ligament (bifurcate ligament; V ligament), 190–195
Climbing fibers, 673, 675, 675f
Coalition
　calcaneocuboid, 108–109
　calcaneonavicular, 108, 108f–109f
　cubonavicular, 110, 110f
　cuneo$_2$-metatarsal$_2$, 111
　cuneo$_3$-metatarsal$_3$, 111, 111f
　cuneonavicular, 110–111
　intercuneiform$_{2,3}$, 111, 111f
　interphalangeal, 111–114, 112f–113f
　multiple, massive, and associated coalitions, 114
　talocalcaneal, 105–108, 107f
　talonavicular, 108, 110f
Coleman block test, 582
Compartments, 120f, 490
　anterior, distal leg-ankle, 119
　dorsal aponeurosis and dorsal compartments, of foot, 126–130, 128f–130f
　　peroneal tunnels and retinaculum, 130–131
　inferior extensor retinaculum, 121f–124f
　　oblique inferomedial band, 124–126
　　oblique superolateral band, 126
　　oblique superomedial band, 124, 127f–128f
　　stem/frondiform ligament, 122–124, 125f
　organization of, 120f
　plantar, 153, 155f
　　adductor hallucis, 158, 160f
　　central segment of, 157, 157f
　　flexor digitorum brevis, 157, 158f
　　intermediary central compartment, 158, 158f
　　osteoaponeurotic plantar canal, 156, 156f
　　proximal segment of, 158, 159f
　　right foot, 153, 155f
　　superficial central compartment of, 157, 157f
　　upper and lower calcaneal chambers, 155, 155f
　plantar aponeurosis, 143, 147f
　　central component, 143–153, 148f–153f
　　peroneal/lateral component, 153, 154f
　　tibial/medial component, 153
　superior extensor retinaculum, 119–122, 121f
　tibiotalocalcaneal tunnel, 131

　lower talocalcaneal (tarsal) tunnel, 133–143, 135f–143f
　upper tibiotalar tunnel, 132–133, 133f–135f
Computed tomography (CT), 721, 723–725, 722f–724f
Cortical bone, ultrasound (US) anatomy, 770
Crista laterali, 63
Cross-sectional anatomy, 430, 431f
　coronal sections, of tarsus and forefoot and, 432, 438, 441–443, 443f–454f, 446, 448, 451
　distal leg and ankle, transverse cross-sections of, 430–432, 432f–438f
　oblique sections, hindfoot-tarsus and, 432, 438, 439f–442f, 441–443, 446, 448, 451
Cuboid, 67f, 355
　anterior, 70
　dorsal, 67, 68f–69f
　keystone, 620, 622f
　lateral border, 70
　medial, 70
　plantar, 67–70
　posterior, 70
Cubonavicular coalition, 110, 110f
Cubonavicular joint, motion of, 564–566, 567f–568f
Cubonavicular ligaments, 205
　dorsal, 205
　medial, 205
　plantar, 205
Cuneiform(s), 73, 355
　first, 73–75, 74f
　second, 75–77, 76f
　third, 77
Cuneo$_3$-cuboid ligaments, 207
Cuneo$_2$-metatarsal$_2$ coalition, 111
Cuneo$_3$-metatarsal$_3$ coalition, 111, 111f
Cuneonavicular coalition, 110–111
Cuneo$_1$-navicular joint
　exorotation of leg and, 581
　pronation of foot plate and, 584
　supination of foot plate and, 587
Cuneonavicular ligament(s), 205–207, 206f–207f
　dorsal, 207
　medial, 207
　plantar, 207
Cutaneous innervation, of foot, 423–424
Cutaneous nerve
　peroneal
　　deep, 394–405, 395f–406f
　　superficial, 391–394, 392f–394f
　saphenous, 423
　sural, 383–391, 384f–392f, 385t, 388t–389t, 391t
　tibial, posterior, 405–422, 407f–423f

D

Deep aponeurosis, 468, 468f
Deep cerebellar nuclei, 675–676, 677f–678f
Deep plantar arch, 334, 335t, 336f
Deltoid (medial) ligament
　ankle stability and
　　anatomic observations, 534f, 538–539
　　experimental investigation, role of, 539–541, 539f–541f
　　mechanical characteristics of, 541
　deep layer of
　　anterior tibiotalar fascicle, capsule, fat pad and, 179–188
　　deep anterior tibiotalar ligament, 179
　　deep posterior tibiotalar ligament, 179
Diagnostic imaging techniques
　arthrography, 730–731, 730f
　computed tomography (CT), 721–725, 722f–724f
　magnetic resonance imaging (MRI), 725
　　patient position, 729

Diagnostic imaging techniques—*continued*
    pulse sequences, 725–729, 726f–729f
    techniques, 729–730
  magnetic resonance imaging (MRI) atlas, 732
    ankle/hindfoot, 732–749
    forefoot, 749–767
  radiography, 713–719, 714f–720f
  radionuclide bone scintigraphy, 731–732, 732f
Digital arteries
  dorsal, 323, 325t
  plantar, of lesser toes, 339–341, 340f–341f
Digital formula, morphogenesis of feet, prenatal, 5–7, 6f
Distal metatarsal articular angle (DMAA), 90
Distal tibia, 33, 35f
Distal tibiofibular complex, 165
  ankle, lateral ligament of
    anterior talofibular ligament (ATFL), 166–169, 168f–169f
    calcaneofibular ligament, 169–173, 170f–173f
    fibulotalocalcaneal ligament, 174–175, 178f–180f
    posterior talofibular ligament, 173–174, 174f–177f
  anterior superficial tibiotalar fascicle and tibionavicular fascicle, 177, 190f
  calcaneonavicular joint, acetabulum pedis ligaments
    bifurcate ligament, 190–195
    inferior calcaneonavicular ligament, 190
    lateral calcaneonavicular ligament, 190–195
    superomedial calcaneonavicular ligament, 188, 196f
  deltoid (medial) ligament, 175, 181f–189f
Dorsal cubonavicular ligament, 72
Dorsal digital arteries, 323, 325t
Dorsalis pedis artery, 307–308
  caliber, 311–312
  variations, 308–311, 310f–313f
Dorsal venous network, 376
Dorsiflexors, 587

E

Electromyographic activities, walking cycle and, 641, 642f, 643
Eminentia retrotrochlearis, 64
Epiphyseal closures, 33
Extensor digitorum brevis muscle/tendon, 63, 229, 232f, 343, 462–463
  additional musculotendinous units, 230–231, 233f
  muscle cuneo-naviculo-fascialis, 232
  synovial tendon sheath of, 294
  variations of insertion and origin, 231–232
Extensor digitorum longus muscle/tendon, 228f, 462
  additional slips, 229
  bifid tendons, 229
  individual muscles, 228
  synovial tendon sheath of, 296–298
  transverse, quadrilateral lamina, extensor sling, 227
  triangular lamina, 228
  variations, 228
Extensor hallucis longus muscle, 223
  synovial tendon sheath of, 294
  variations, 226f
    accessory tendon, 225
Extensor retinaculum
  inferior, 121f–124f
    oblique inferomedial band, 124–126
    oblique superolateral band, 126
    oblique superomedial band, 124, 127f–128f
    stem/frondiform ligament, 122–124, 125f
  superior, 119–122, 121f

F

Facies articularis navicularis, 58
Facies articularis talaris anterior, 60
Facies articularis talaris media, 60
Facies externa accessoria, 60
Fascia, ultrasound (US) anatomy, 770
Femur, rotation, walking cycle, 616, 617f
Fetal phase
  arteries, 30–32, 30f–32f
  bones, 15–19, 16f–19f
  embryonic/early fetal phase, 11–14, 13f–15f
  joints, 19–20, 21f
  ligaments and tendon sheaths, 20–26, 22f–26f
  muscles and nerves, 27–30, 27f–29f
Fibrous flexor tunnels, 448
Fibula. *See also* Malleolus
  distal, 39f
    lateral surface, 38
    medial surface, 38, 40f
  lateral malleolus, 41f–42f
    lateral surface, 40
    medial surface, 40
    posterior surface, 40–42
  mobility of, 518, 521–523, 522f
Fibulotalocalcaneal ligament, 174–175, 178f–180f, 468
Fifth metatarsal
  base, 86–87, 87f
  shaft, 89–90, 90f
First metatarsal, 359–360, 359f, 361f–363f
  base, 79f–82f, 80–81
  head, 90
  shaft, 89
Flexor accessorius muscle. *See* Quadratus plantae muscle
Flexor digiti minimi brevis muscle, 276–277
Flexor digitorum brevis muscle, 258f, 343
  variations of insertion, 257
  variations of origin, 257
Flexor digitorum longus muscle, 142, 247, 438
  attachment, 250f
  long accessory of long flexors, 253–256, 255f–256f
  peroneocalcaneus internus muscle, 250–252, 252f–253f
  synovial tendon sheath of, 296–298
  tendinous connections, 249–250, 251f
  tibiocalcaneus internus, 252–253
Flexor hallucis brevis muscle/tendon, 261–268, 271f–272f
Flexor hallucis longus muscle/tendon, 142, 247–256
  blood supply of, 365–366, 368f
Flexor retinaculum, 470f, 471
Fluid, ultrasound (US) anatomy, 771
Foot. *See also specific joints*
  angiosomes of, 706, 706f–707f
  anterior aspect
    dorsal aponeurosis, 459–460, 461f–462f
    dorsal fascial spaces/contents, 460–465, 463f–465f
    skin and subcutaneous layer, 454–455, 456f
    superficial nerves, 455–458, 459f–460f
    superficial veins, 455, 457f–458f
    surface anatomy, 452–454, 455f
  ball of
    big toe, 504–508, 505f–507f
    contents, 501–504, 502f–504f
    plantar aponeurosis, 501–504, 502f–504f
    skin, 501
    subcompartments, 501–504, 502f–504f
    surface anatomy, 501
  bare, standing and pressure distribution, 600–602, 601f–604f
    bony trabeculae orientation, 602, 604f–609f, 606–609
  calcaneocuboid joint motion, 558–559, 559f–564f, 561
  combined midfoot-forefoot motion, 566–569, 568f
    midtarsal joint, 567
    naviculocuneiform, 567–568
    tarsometatarsal, 567–568

cubonavicular movements and, 564–566, 567f–568f
cutaneous innervation of, 423–424
dorsal aponeurosis, 126–130, 128f–130f
dorsal aspect of, arteries of, 304–307, 307f–310f
as functional unit, 575, 577, 578f–579f
   functional remodeling under tibial loading, pronation-supination of foot plate and, 583–584, 585f–586f, 587
   functional remodeling under tibiotalar loading, plantar flexion and dorsiflexion at ankle joint, 587, 587f
   vertical loading, external rotation of tibiotalar column, 577, 579–582, 579f–584f
incisions, 711, 712f
lateral aspect of, muscles of, 232–244
load transmission, arches and, 596–598, 596f–598f, 600
   internal compressive forces and, 597, 598f
   truss and beam and, 597–598, 599f–600f, 600
medial aspect of, muscles of, 244–290
metatarsophalangeal, interphalangeal angular relationship, motion and, 571–575, 571f–576f, 574t–575t
midtarsal joint motion, 557–558, 558f–559f
posterolateral aspect, 466
   deep aponeurosis, 468, 468f
   skin, 466, 466f–467f
   subcutaneous layer, 466, 466f–467f
   superficial aponeurosis, 467
   superficial nerves, 466, 466f–467f
   superficial posterolateral compartment, 467
   superficial veins, 466, 466f–467f
   superior peroneal tunnel, 468, 469f
shock-absorbing characteristics of, 632
   forefoot pad and, 639–641, 640f–641f
   heel pad, 635–639, 636f–639f
sole of
   adipose mantle, 487, 488f
   angiosomes, 707, 708f
   central compartment, 490–498, 490f–499f
   compartments, 490
   intermuscular septa, 490
   lateral compartment, 498–500
   medial compartment, 500–501
   muscles of, lateral aspect, 232–244
   muscles of, medial aspect, 244–290
   plantar aponeurosis, 488–490, 488f–489f
   skin, 483
   subcutaneous tissue, 483–487, 484f–486f
   superficial vessels/nerves, 483–487, 484f–486f
   surface anatomy, 483, 483f
subtalar, talocalcaneal joint motion
   motion and stability, 545, 551–557, 552f–557f
   multiple axes of motion, 545, 551f
   single axis of motion, 543–545, 545f–550f
talonavicular joint motion, 561, 563–564, 565f–566f
tarsometatarsal joint stability, contact mechanics and, 569, 571
ultrasound (US) anatomy
   dorsal, 778, 778f
   plantar, 778–780, 778f–781f
Foot-plate (lamina pedis)
gait cycle and, 619–623, 621f–626f
   plantar aponeurosis, protective loading of, 625–626, 627f–628f
Forefoot
magnetic resonance imaging (MRI) atlas
   horizontal long axis (axial) proton density non–fat-saturated images, 756–760
   sagittal proton density non–fat-saturated images, 749–755
   short axis (coronal) proton density fat-saturated images, 761–767
pad, shock-absorbing characteristics of, 639–641, 640f–641f
Fourth metatarsal
base, 83–85, 86f
shaft, 89
Functional anatomy. *See also* Ankle; Foot
axis of motion and, 511
field of motion and, 511–512, 511f
terminology, of motion, 509, 510f
Functional motor unit, 652
Golgi tendon organs, 653, 653f
Ia inhibitory interneuron, 653–654, 653f–654f
muscle spindle, 652–653, 653f

G

Gait cycle, 609
center of gravity, 611–612, 615f–616f
description of, 609–610, 610f–611f
   stance phase, 610, 613f–614f
   swing phase, 611, 614f
   walking cycle, 610, 612f–613f
foot-plate and, 619–621, 621f–626f, 623
   plantar aponeurosis, protective loading of, 625–626, 627f–628f
forces during, 626, 629f
   at ankle, 628, 630, 632f
   fore and aft shear, 626, 631f
   load, pressure distribution, measurement under foot, 630, 632, 633f–635f
   medial and lateral shear, 627, 631f
   normal pressure, 627f–628f
   torque, 627, 631f
   vertical, 626, 630f–631f
kinematics and, 611
pelvic motion, transverse segmental rotations of lower extremity and, 612, 616–617, 617f–618f
sagittal plane, motion in, 617–618, 619f
   stance phase, 618
   swing phase, 618
toes, function of, 618–619, 620f
Gait, modulation
vestibular system, 658, 658f
vision, 655, 656f–657f
Golgi tendon organs, functional motor unit, 653, 653f
Gravity, center of, 611–612, 615f–616f
center of, 611–612, 615f–616f
neuro control, 647, 648f–651f
Growth, foot
morphogenesis of feet, prenatal, 7–8, 8f
postnatal development, 32–33, 33f

H

Hallux valgus, 509
Heel, shock-absorbing characteristics of, 635–639, 636f–639f
Hindfoot, magnetic resonance imaging (MRI) atlas
axial proton density non–fat-saturated images, 743–749
coronal proton density fat-saturated images, 738–742
sagittal proton density non–fat-saturated images, 732–738

I

Ia inhibitory interneuron, functional motor unit, 653–654, 653f–654f
Incisions, foot and ankle, 711, 712f
Inferior tibiofibular joint
anterior tibiofibular ligament, 162, 163f
interosseous ligament, 162–165, 166f–167f
posterior tibiofibular ligament, 162, 164f–165f
Intercuneiform$_{2,3}$ coalition, 111, 111f
Intercuneiform ligaments, 207
Intermetatarsal ligaments, 211
Intermetatarsophalangeal bursae, 301–303, 302f
Intermuscular septa, 490
Interosseous ligament, 162–165, 166f–167f, 209–211, 210f–213f. *See also specific ligaments*
Interosseous membrane, 165, 167f

Interphalangeal coalition, 111–114, 112f–113f
Interphalangeal joints
  angular relationships, motion and, 571–575, 571f–577f, 574t–575t
  ligaments
    of big toe, 219
    of lesser toes, 214
  sesamoids, 97

J

Jogging velocity, 610

L

Lamina pedis, 575, 578f
  close pack, 575, 577
  foot plate, 619
  twisted plate, 575
  twist supination, 621f
Lateral compartment, 498–500
Lateral intermuscular septum, 490
Lateral malleolus, 41f–42f
  lateral surface, 40
  medial surface, 40
  posterior surface, 40–42
Lateral metaphyseal artery, 346–347
Lateral plantar artery, 334, 335f
Lateral surface, 351
Lateral tarsal arteries, 312, 313f
  distal, 314–315
  proximal, 312–314, 314f–315f
Leg, exorotation of, 581, 583f
Lesser metatarsals, 356–359, 360f
Lisfranc's joint, synovial compartments, 211–214, 214f
Ligament(s). *See also specific ligaments*
  anterior superficial tibiotalar fascicle, tibionavicular fascicle and, 177
    deltoid ligament, deep layer of, 179–188, 194f
    superficial posterior tibiotalar ligament, 177–179, 193f
    tibiocalcaneal ligament, 177, 192f
    tibioligamentous fascicle, 177, 192f
  calcaneocuboid
    dorsolateral, 202–203
    inferior, 203–205, 203f–205f
    medial, 202
  calcaneonavicular joint, acetabulum pedis ligaments
    bifurcate, 190–195
    inferior calcaneonavicular, 190
    lateral calcaneonavicular, 190–195
    superomedial calcaneonavicular, 188, 196f
  cuneo$_3$-cuboid ligaments, 207
  cuneonavicular ligaments, 205–207
  inferior tibiofibular joint
    anterior tibiofibular, 162, 163f
    interosseous, 162–165, 166f–167f
    posterior tibiofibular, 162, 164f–165f
  intercuneiform, 207
  intermetatarsal, 211
  interphalangeal joint
    of big toe, 219
    of lesser toes, 214
  lateral, of ankle
    anterior talofibular ligament (ATFL), 166–169, 168f–169f
    calcaneofibular ligament, 169–173, 170f–173f
    fibulotalocalcaneal ligament, 174–175, 178f–180f
    posterior talofibular ligament, 173–174, 174f–177f
  medial/deltoid ligament, 175, 181f–189f
  metatarsophalangeal
    of big toe, 219, 220f
    of lesser toes, 214
  morphologic development

arteries, fetal phase, 30–32, 30f–32f
bones, fetal phase, 15–19, 16f–19f
embryonic/early fetal phase, 11–14, 13f–15f
joints, fetal phase, 19–20, 21f
ligaments and tendon sheaths, fetal phase, 20–26, 22f–26f
muscles and nerves, fetal phase, 27–30, 27f–29f
  talocalcaneonavicular joints, 195
    cervical ligament, 195–197, 198f–199f
    lateral talocalcaneal ligament, 201
    medial talocalcaneal ligament, 201, 201f
    posterior talocalcaneal ligament, 201
    talonavicular ligament, 202, 202f
    tarsal canal, 197–201, 200f
  tarsometatarsal joint, 207, 208f
    dorsal, 209
    interosseous, 209–211, 210f–213f
    plantar, 209
  ultrasound (US) anatomy, 770, 772f
Lisfranc's joint, 569
Lisfranc's ligament (cuneo$_1$-metatarsal$_2$ ligament), interosseous, 569
Locomotion-walking, 692–693, 693f–700f, 698
Long accessory muscle of long flexors, 253–256, 255f–256f
Lower calcaneal chamber, 480
Lymphatics
  foot, deep, 381
  foot, superficial, 379–381, 380f
    sole, 379–381
    toes, 379
  joints, 381

M

Magnetic resonance imaging (MRI), 725, 732
  ankle/hindfoot, 732–749
    axial proton density non–fat-saturated images, 743–749
    coronal proton density fat-saturated images, 738–742
    sagittal proton density non–fat-saturated images, 732–738
  forefoot, 749–767
    horizontal long axis (axial) proton density non–fat-saturated images, 755–760
    sagittal proton density non–fat-saturated images, 749–755
    short axis (coronal) proton density fat-saturated images, 761–767
  patient position, 729
  pulse sequences, 725–729, 726f–729f
  techniques, 729–730
Malleolar artery
  anterior lateral, 327–328, 327t
  anterior medial, 326–327, 327t
Malleolus
  lateral, 41f–42f
    lateral surface, 40
    medial surface, 40
    posterior surface, 40–42
  medial, 46, 47f
Medial calcaneal nerves, surgical anatomy of, 477–481, 478f–482f
Medial compartment, 500–501
Medial metaphyseal artery, 345–346
Medial perforating veins, 455
Medial plantar artery, 330–333, 332f–335f
Medial plantar neurovascular bundle, 438
Medial surface, 351–353
Medial tarsal arteries, 326
  distal, 316–317, 316f
  proximal, 315–316
Metaphyseal artery
  lateral, 346–347
  medial, 345–346
Metatarsals, 36, 77–80, 79f
  base

fifth metatarsal, 86–87, 87f, 89f
first metatarsal, 79f–82f, 80–81
fourth metatarsal, 83–85, 86f
second metatarsal, 83, 84f
third metatarsal, 83, 85f
first metatarsal, 359–360, 359f, 361f–363f
head
  first metatarsal, 90
  lesser metatarsals, 90
lesser metatarsals, 356–359, 360f
shaft
  fifth metatarsal, 89–90, 90f
  first metatarsal, 89
  fourth metatarsal, 89
  second metatarsal, 89
  third metatarsal, 89
Metatarsal arteries
  dorsal
    first, 319 320, 320f
    first, variations of, 320–323, 321f
    second to fourth, 323
  plantar, 335–339, 335f, 337f–339f, 340t
    first, 317–319
    first, variations of, 323
Metatarsal formula, morphogenesis of feet, prenatal, 36
Metatarso$_1$-cuneiform$_1$ joint
  exorotation of leg and, 581–582, 583f
  pronation of foot plate and, 583–584
  supination of foot plate and, 584, 587
Metatarsophalangeal joint
  angular relationships, motion and, 571–575, 571f–577f, 574t–575t
  articular surface, 97
  nonarticular surface, 95
  plantar aponeurosis, flexor of, 594, 594f–596f, 596
  sesamoids, 94, 95f–96f
Metatarsophalangeal ligament
  of big toe, 219, 220f
  of lesser toes, 214
Metatarsus primus varus, 509
Midfoot-forefoot motion, 566–569, 568f
Midtarsal joints. *See also* Cubonavicular joint, motion of; Motion and; Talonavicular joint
  motion of, 557–558, 558f–559f
Morphologic development, skeletal elements
  arteries, 30–32, 30f–32f
  bones, 15–19, 16f–19f
  embryonic/early fetal phase, 11–14, 13f–15f
  joints, 19–20, 21f
  ligaments and tendon sheaths, 20–26, 22f–26f
  muscles and nerves, 27–30, 27f–29f
Motion. *See also specific joints*
  axis of, 511
  field of, 511–512, 511f
  terminology of, 509, 510f, 511
Motor loop modulation, descending and ascending tracts, 654, 655f
Motors, 587–588
  ankle
    dorsiflexors and, 587
    plantar flexors and, 587, 588f
  evertors, 588
  invertors, 588
  talocalcaneonavicular joints, 587–588
    evertors, 588
    invertors, 588
  toes
    big toe and, 588–589
    lesser toes and, 589–590, 589f–594f
Muscle(s). *See also specific muscles*

anterior aspect, ankle and dorsum of foot, 222–232
big toe, intrinsic, 260–276
calcaneal and plantaris tendons and, 290–291
fifth toe, intrinsic, 276–277
lateral aspect, of ankle, foot, sole, 232–244
lesser toes, intrinsic, 278–290
medial aspect, of ankle, foot, sole, 244–290
Muscle cuneo-naviculo-fascialis, 232
Muscle spindle, functional motor unit, 652–653, 653f
Musculus tensor fasciae dorsalis pedis, 223
Musculus tibioastragalus anticus of Gruber, 222–223, 225f
Musculus tibiofascialis anticus of Macalister, 223

N

Natatory ligament, 501, 640
Navicular, 354–355, 356f–358f
Naviculare secundarium, 73
Naviculotalar joint
  exorotation of leg and, 581, 583f
  pronation of foot plate and, 584
  supination of foot plate and, 587
Nerve(s)
  of ankle, 424–427, 425f–428f
  of joints, 424–427, 425f–428f
  peroneal
    deep, 394–405, 395f–406f
    superficial, 391–394, 392f–394f
  saphenous, 423
  sural, 383–391, 384f–392f, 385t, 388t–389t, 391t
  ultrasound (US) anatomy, 770, 772f
  tibial, posterior, 405–422, 407f–423f
  vascular anatomy, tarsal tunnel, 370–371, 371f–372f
Neuro control
  basal ganglia, 678f–682f, 680
  cerebellum, 670, 670f
    cerebellar cortex and circuits, 671, 673, 673f–674f
    cerebellar hemispheres, 670–671, 671f–673f
    cerebral peduncles, 671, 673f
    climbing fibers, 673, 675, 675f
    deep cerebellar nuclei, 675–676, 677f–678f
  cerebral motor cortex, 683, 683f–684f
    output of, 685–686, 685f–686f
    premotor, 684–685
    primary, 683–684, 685f
  functional motor unit, 652
    Golgi tendon organs, 653, 653f
    Ia inhibitory interneuron, 653–654, 653f–654f
    muscle spindle, 652–653, 653f
  gait modulation
    vestibular system, 658, 658f
    vision, 655, 656f–657f
  gravity, 647, 648f–651f
  locomotion-walking, 692–693, 693f–700f, 698
  motor loop modulation, descending and ascending tracts, 654, 655f
  reticulospinal motor tract, 687, 687f
    anatomy of, 687–688, 687f–692f
Neurovascular tunnel, 473–474

O

Oblique inferomedial band, 124–126
Oblique superolateral band, 126
Oblique superomedial band, 124, 127f–128f
Oblique talocalcaneal band, 123
Opponens digiti quinti muscle, 277
Os calcaneus secundarius, 99–100, 105f
Os calcis, 36
  medial surface of, 66
Os cuboides secundarium, 100, 106f

Os cuneo₁ metatarsale₁ plantare, 101, 107f
Os intercuneiforme, 100, 107f
Os intermetatarseum, 99, 103f–104f
Osseous stage, 11, 11f–12f
Ossification centers, primary and secondary, postnatal development, 33, 34f, 35t
Os subfibulare, 103
Os subtibiale, 103
Os sustentaculi, 99, 105f
Os talonaviculare dorsale, 100
Os tibiale, 98–99, 100f–101f
Os trigonum, 53, 54f, 98, 99f
Os vesalianum, 101–103, 107f

P

Pelvic motion, during gait cycle, 612, 616–617, 617f–618f
Perforating arteries
    anterior, 323–325, 325f
    posterior, 323
Peroneal artery
    perforating branch of, 328
    posterior, 341
Peroneal nerve
    deep, 394–405, 395f–406f
    superficial (musculocutaneous nerve), 391–394, 392f–394f
Peroneal sulcus, 42
Peroneal tendons, blood supply of, 367–368, 370f
Peroneal tunnel
    inferior, 131, 132f
    intermediary, 131
    superior, 130, 131f
Peroneocalcaneus internus muscle, 250–252
Peroneus brevis muscle, 40
    lateral peronei variations, 236, 239f
        peroneocalcaneal type, 240, 241f
        peroneus digiti quinti, 238–239
        peroneus quartus, 242f–244f
    synovial tendon sheath of, 294–295, 296f–297f
Peroneus brevis tendon, 65
Peroneus longus muscle, 40, 232, 236f–237f
    insertion, 233, 238f
    synovial tendon sheath of, 294–295, 296f–297f
    tendon of, 235f
Peroneus longus tendon, 441
Peroneus tertius muscle
    absence of, 232
    insertional variations of, 232
Peroneus tertius tendon, 462
Phalangeal apparatus, proximal, ligaments of, big toe, 214–219, 217f–219f
Phalanges, 361–362, 363f
    large toe, 92f
        distal phalanx, 91
        proximal phalanx, 90–91
    lesser toes, 93f
        distal phalanx, 93
        middle phalanx, 93
        proximal phalanx, 91
Plantar aponeurosis, 143, 147f, 488–490, 488f–489f, 592, 594, 594f–596f, 596
    central component, 143–153, 148f–153f
    peroneal/lateral component, 153, 154f
    tibial/medial component, 153
Plantar artery
    deep plantar arch, 334, 335t, 336f
    lateral, 334, 335f
    medial, 330
        deep branch, 332–333, 334f
        superficial branch, 332, 332f–333f
Plantar flexors, 587, 588f

Plantaris tendon, 290–291, 290f, 290t
Plantar metatarsal arteries, 335–339, 335f–339f
Plantar surface, 353
Plantar venous network
    deep, 377–379
    superficial, 377
Plantar/walking pads, 7, 7f
Posterior surface, 353–354, 353f–354f
Posterior talofibular ligament, 173–174, 174f–177f
Posterior tibial artery, 328–330, 329f–331f, 476
Posterolateral tubercle, 52
Postnatal development
    epiphyseal closures, 33
    normal foot growth
        epiphyseal closures, 33
        growth of, 32–33, 33f
        primary and secondary ossification centers, 33, 34f, 35t
    ossification centers, primary and secondary, 33, 34f, 35t
    structural changes
        distal tibia, 33, 35f
        metatarsals, 36
        os calcis, 36
        talus, 33–36
Prenatal development
    morphogenesis, of feet, 1, 2f–3f
        digital formula, 5–7, 6f
        foot growth, 7–8, 8f
        horizons/stages of development, 1–5, 2f–4f
        metatarsal formula, 7
        plantar/walking pads, 7, 7f
    skeleton, 8–9
        cartilaginous stage, 9–11, 9f–10f
        mesenchymal stage, 9, 9f
        osseous stage, 11, 11f–12f
        stages, 9–11
    skeleton, morphologic study of
        arteries, fetal phase, 30–32, 30f–32f
        bones, fetal phase, 15–19, 16f–19f
        embryonic/early fetal phase, 11–14, 13f–15f
        joints, fetal phase, 19–20, 21f
        ligaments and tendon sheaths, fetal phase, 20–26, 22f–26f
        muscles and nerves, fetal phase, 27–30, 27f–29f
Pronation, 509
Proximal metatarsal M₁ articular angle (PMAA), 81
Pulse sequences, 725–729, 726f–729f
Pyramidal apophysis (coronoid of cuboid), 558

Q

Quadratus plantae muscle, 257–260, 263f–265f

R

Radiography, 713–719, 714f–720f
Radionuclide bone scintigraphy, 731–732, 732f
Reticulospinal motor tract, 687, 687f
    anatomy of, 687–688, 687f–692f
Richet tunnel. *See* Tibiotalocalcaneal tunnel
Running velocity, 610

S

Saphenous nerve, 423, 458
Scaphoid (os naviculare), 70, 71f–72f
    anterior surface, 71, 72f
    dorsal surface, 71–72
    lateral end, 73
    medial end, 73
    plantar surface, 72
    posterior surface, 70, 72f

Second metatarsal
  base, 83, 84*f*
  shaft, 89
Septal system, of heel pad, 636
Sesamoid(s), 93, 94*f*
  articular surfaces, 448
  big toe, 95*f*
    interphalangeal joint, 97
    metatarsophalangeal joint, 94–97
  lesser toes, 97
  peroneus longus tendon, 97, 98*f*
  tibialis anterior tendon, 98
  tibialis posterior tendon, 98
Shear
  fore and aft, gait cycle, 626, 631*f*
  medial and lateral, gait cycle, 627
Sinus tarsi
  anterolateral segment of, 63
  arteries of, 325–326, 326*f*
  lateral border of, 64
Skin
  arterial supply to
    to dorsum of foot and ankle, 341–342, 342*f*
    malleolar skin, 342
    planta pedis, 342–343, 343*f*–344*f*
  of heel pad, 635–639, 636*f*–639*f*
  innervation, 487
Spring ligament (inferior calcaneonavicular ligament), 190
Squatting facets, tibia, lower end, 46, 46*t*
Stance phase, of walking cycle, 610, 613*f*–614*f*
Stem (frondiform) ligament, 122–124, 125*f*. *See also* Extensor retinaculum
Subcutaneous bursae, 300
Subfascial bursae, 300
  group I, 301
  group II, 301
Superficial posterior tibiotalar ligament, 177–179, 193*f*
Superficial aponeurosis, 467
Superficial nerves, 466, 466*f*–467*f*
Superficial posterior compartment, 431
Superficial vessels/nerves, 483–487, 484*f*–486*f*
Superior extensor retinaculum, 119–122, 121*f*
Superomedial calcaneonavicular ligament, 72, 188, 196*f*
Supination, 509
Sural nerve, 383–391, 384*f*–392*f*, 385*t*, 388*t*–389*t*, 391*t*, 484
Sustentaculum tali, 65, 244, 245*f*
  posterior border of, 65
  width and length of, 66
Swing phase, of walking cycle, 611, 614*f*
Synarthrodial, 575
Synovial bursae, 299
  intermetatarsophalangeal, 301–303
  subcutaneous, 300
  subfascial, 300–301
Synovial tendon sheaths, 294
  extensor digitorum brevis, 294
  extensor digitorum longus, 294
  extensor hallucis longus, 294
  flexor digitorum longus, 296–298
  flexor hallucis longus, 299
  peroneus longus and peroneus brevis, 294–295, 296*f*–297*f*
  tibialis anterior, 294, 295*f*–296*f*
  tibialis posterior, 296, 297*f*–298*f*
Synovium, ultrasound (US) anatomy, 771

T

Talar shift, anterior, lateral collateral ligaments and, 530–531, 531*t*
Talar tilt, lateral collateral ligaments and, 529–530, 531*t*
Talocalcaneal coalition, 53, 105–108, 107*f*
Talocalcaneal joint
  arthroscopy, 796, 797*f*–798*f*
    portals, 799–800, 799*f*–801*f*
  motion of
    motion and stability and, 545, 551–557, 552*f*–557*f*
    multiple axes of, 545, 551*f*
    single axis of, 543–545, 545*f*–550*f*
Talocalcaneal ligament, lateral, 51
Talocalcaneal tunnel, lower (tarsal tunnel), 133
  anatomic preparation, 133, 135*f*
  calcaneal canal, 141*f*
  distal talus-calcaneus, 143*f*
  distal tibia, talus, and lateral malleolus, 136, 138*f*
  flexor retinaculum, 133, 136*f*–137*f*
  sustentaculum tali, 142*f*
  talus, calcaneus, and distal malleoli, 136, 138*f*
  tibiotalocalcaneal tunnel, 139*f*
Talocalcaneonavicular joints, ligaments, 195
  cervical ligament, 195–197, 198*f*–199*f*
  lateral talocalcaneal ligament, 201
  medial talocalcaneal ligament, 201, 201*f*
  posterior talocalcaneal ligament, 201
  talonavicular ligament, 202, 202*f*
  tarsal canal, 197–201, 200*f*
Talonavicular coalition, 108, 110*f*
Talonavicular joint, motion and, 561, 563–564, 565*f*–566*f*
Talonavicular ligament, 202, 202*f*
Taloscaphoid capsule, 72
Talotibial joint, plantar flexion and dorsiflexion at ankle joint, 587
Talotibial ligament, 541
Talus, 33–36, 46, 347, 347*f*–348*f*
  anastomosis, 351
  body, 50*f*
    inferior surface, 53–55, 57*f*
    lateral surface, 49–51, 52*f*
    medial surface, 51–52
    posterior surface, 52–53, 53*f*–56*f*
    superior surface, 48–49, 51*t*
  declination angle, 48, 48*f*, 48*t*
  head, 58, 58*f*–59*f*
  inclination angle, 48*f*, 48*t*
  intraosseous territory, 347–349, 349*f*
  neck, 57*f*
    inferior surface, 56, 57*f*–58*f*
    lateral surface, 56
    medial surface, 58
    superior surface, 55–56
  variations, 350
Tarsal arteries
  lateral, 312, 313*f*
    distal, 314–315
    proximal, 312–314, 314*f*–315*f*
  medial, 326
    distal, 316–317, 316*f*
    proximal, 315–316
Tarsal canal (canalis tarsi) ligament of, 197–201, 200*f*
Tarsal tunnel. *See* Tibiotalocalcaneal tunnel
Tarsometatarsal (Lisfranc's) joint
  joint stability, contact mechanics and, 569, 571
  midfoot-forefoot motion and, 566–569
Tarsometatarsal joint ligaments, 207, 208*f*
  dorsal, 209
  interosseous, 209–211, 210*f*–213*f*
  plantar, 209
Tarsus, remodeling of, 581
Tendon(s). *See also specific tendons*
  bifid, of extensor digitorum longus muscle, 229
Tendon sheaths, synovial, 294–299

Tendons
    ultrasound (US) anatomy, 770, 771*f*
    vascular anatomy of, 363–365, 365*f*–367*f*
Tendoscopy, 800, 802*f*
Tenosynovial compartments, 462
Third metatarsal
    base, 83, 85*f*
    shaft, 89
Tibia
    distal, 33, 35*f*, 343–347, 345*f*–346*f*
        lateral metaphyseal artery, 346–347
        medial metaphyseal artery, 345–346
    loading, pronation-supination of foot plate, functional remodeling, 583–584, 585*f*, 587
    lower end of, 43*f*. *See also* Malleolus
        anterior surface, 44–46, 46*t*
        inferior surface, 44, 44*f*–45*f*
        lateral surface, 46
        medial malleolus, 46, 47*f*
        medial surface, 46
        posterior surface, 46
    rotation, walking cycle, 616
Tibial artery
    anterior, 704–705, 705*f*
    posterior, 328–330, 329*f*–331*f*
Tibial distal metaphysis, 431
Tibialis anterior muscle, 223*f*
    synovial tendon sheath of, 294, 295*f*–296*f*
    variations of, 224*f*
        bifurcation, 222
        extensions of attachment, 222
        loss of attachment, 222
        musculus tensor fasciae dorsalis pedis, 223
        musculus tibioastragalus anticus of Gruber, 222–223, 225*f*
        musculus tibiofascialis anticus of Macalister, 223
Tibialis anterior tendon, blood supply of, 366–367, 368*f*–369*f*
Tibialis posterior muscle, synovial tendon sheath of, 296, 297*f*–298*f*
Tibialis posterior tendon, 245*f*–250*f*, 246–247
    blood supply of, 364–365
Tibial nerve, posterior, 405–410, 407*f*–415*f*
    deep branch, 422
    plantar, lateral, 416–421, 417*f*–422*f*
    plantar, media, 410–416, 416*f*
    superficial branch, 421–423
Tibiocalcaneal ligament, 177, 192*f*, 540–541
Tibiocalcaneus internus muscle, 252–253
Tibiofibular ligament
    anterior, 162, 163*f*
    posterior, 162, 164*f*–165*f*
Tibioligamentous fascicle, 177, 192*f*
Tibionavicular fascicle, 177
    deltoid ligament, deep layer of, 179–188, 194*f*
    superficial posterior tibiotalar ligament, 177–179, 193*f*
    tibiocalcaneal ligament, 177, 192*f*
    tibioligamentous fascicle, 177, 192*f*
Tibionavicular ligament, 540–541
Tibiotalar column, vertical loading
    external rotation of, 579–582, 580*f*–584*f*
    internal rotation of, 577, 579, 579*f*–580*f*
Tibiotalar fascicle, anterior
    capsule, fat pad and, 179–188
    superficial, 177
        deltoid ligament, deep layer of, 179–188, 194*f*
        superficial posterior tibiotalar ligament, 177–179, 193*f*
        tibiocalcaneal ligament, 177, 192*f*
        tibioligamentous fascicle, 177, 192*f*
Tibiotalar joint, 587, 587*f*
Tibiotalar tunnel, upper, 132–133, 133*f*–135*f*
Tibiotalocalcaneal tunnel, 131, 469–471, 471, 471*f*–472*f*
    lower talocalcaneal (tarsal) tunnel, 133–143, 135*f*–143*f*
    talocalcaneal tunnel, 473–476, 475*f*–478*f*
    tibiotalar compartment, 471–473, 472*f*–474*f*
    upper tibiotalar tunnel, 132–133, 133*f*–135*f*
Toe, big
    angiosomes of, 710, 711*f*
    arterial supply of, 317–319, 317*f*–318*f*
    ball of foot
        big toe, 504–508, 505*f*–507*f*
        contents, 501–504, 502*f*–504*f*
        plantar aponeurosis, 501–504, 502*f*–504*f*
        skin, 501
        subcompartments, 501–504, 502*f*–504*f*
        surface anatomy, 501
    first dorsal metatarsal artery, 317–319, 318*f*
    first plantar metatarsal artery, 317–319, 319*f*
    interphalangeal joint, 219
        sesamoid, 97
    intrinsic muscles of, 260, 266*f*
        abductor hallucis, 260–261, 266*f*–268*f*
        adductor hallucis, 268–276
        flexor hallucis brevis, 261–268, 271*f*–272*f*
    lymphatics, 379
    metatarsophalangeal joint
        ligaments, 219, 220*f*
        sesamoids, 94–97
    motors, 588
    sesamoids of, 362–363, 364*f*
        flexor hallucis longus tendon, blood supply of, 365–366, 368*f*
        nerves vascular anatomy, tarsal tunnel, 370–371, 371*f*–372*f*
        peroneal tendons, blood supply of, 367–368, 370*f*
        tendons, vascular anatomy of, 363–365, 365*f*–367*f*
        tibialis anterior tendon, blood supply of, 366–367, 368*f*–369*f*
Toes, fifth
    intrinsic muscles of, 276
        abductor digiti minimi, 276, 278*f*
        flexor digiti minimi brevis, 276–277
        opponens digiti quinti, 277
Toes, lesser, 93*f*
    distal phalanx, 93
    interphalangeal joint, 214
    intrinsic muscles of, 278, 278*f*–279*f*
        dorsal interossei, 278–279, 280*f*–281*f*
        interossei, 279–290, 283*f*–288*f*
        lumbricals, 279, 283*f*, 290
        plantar interossei, 279, 280*f*–281*f*
    metatarsophalangeal ligaments, 214
    middle phalanx, 93
    motors, 589–590, 589*f*–594*f*
    plantar digital arteries of, 339–341, 340*f*–341*f*
    proximal phalanx, 91
    sesamoid, 97
    tensors, plantar aponeurosis, skin and, 592, 594
    walking cycle, function of, 618–619, 620*f*
Topographic anatomy
    anterior aspect, ankle and dorsum of foot
        dorsal aponeurosis, 459–460, 461*f*–462*f*
        dorsal fascial spaces/contents, 460–465, 463*f*–465*f*
        skin and subcutaneous layer, 454–455, 456*f*
        superficial nerves, 455–458, 459*f*–460*f*
        superficial veins, 455, 457*f*–458*f*
        surface anatomy, 452–454, 455*f*
    ball of foot, big toe
        big toe, 504–508, 505*f*–507*f*
        contents, 501–504, 502*f*–504*f*
        plantar aponeurosis, 501–504, 502*f*–504*f*
        skin, 501

subcompartments, 501–504, 502f–504f
surface anatomy, 501
medial calcaneal nerves, surgical anatomy of, 477–481, 478f–482f
posterolateral aspect, ankle and dorsum of foot, 466
  deep aponeurosis, 468, 468f
  skin, 466, 466f–467f
  subcutaneous layer, 466, 466f–467f
  superficial aponeurosis, 467
  superficial nerves, 466, 466f–467f
  superficial posterolateral compartment, 467
  superficial veins, 466, 466f–467f
  superior peroneal tunnel, 468, 469f
posteromedial aspect, ankle and tibiotalocalcaneal tunnel
  deep aponeurosis, 469–471
  flexor retinaculum, 470f, 471
  skin, 468–469
  subcutaneous layer, 468–469
  superficial veins/nerves, 468–471
  surface anatomy, 468
  tibiotalocalcaneal tunnel, 469–471, 471, 471f–472f
sole of foot
  adipose mantle, 487, 488f
  central compartment, 490–498, 490f–499f
  compartments, 490
  intermuscular septa, 490
  lateral compartment, 498–500
  medial compartment, 500–501
  plantar aponeurosis, 488–490, 488f–489f
  skin, 483
  subcutaneous tissue, 483–487, 484f–486f
  superficial vessels/nerves, 483–487, 484f–486f
  surface anatomy, 483, 483f
tibiotalocalcaneal neurovascular tunnel, surgical anatomy of, 477–481, 478f–482f
Torque, during gait cycle, 627–628, 631f
Triangular lamina, 228
Triaxial orthogonal, 509
Trigonal process, 53, 53f
Truss, 597–598, 599f–600f, 600
Tuberculum ligamenti calcaneofibularis, 65
Tuberositas ossis cuboidei, 68

U

Ultrasound (US) anatomy, 770, 771f
  ankle
    anterior, 773, 773f
    lateral, 773–775, 773f–775f
    medial, 775–777, 776f–775f
    normal ultrasound anatomy of, 771, 773
    posterior, 777–778, 777f–778f
  articular cartilage, 771
  capsule, 770
  cortical bone, 770
  fascia, 770
  fluid, 771
  foot
    dorsal, 778, 778f
    plantar, 778–780, 778f–781f
  ligaments, 770, 772f
  muscle, 771, 772f
  nerves, 770, 772f
  synovium, 771
  tendons, 770, 771f
Upper calcaneal chamber, 480
Ursus americanus, 236

V

Valgus, 509
Varus, 509
Vascular foramina, 56
Veins. *See also specific veins*
  blood flow, in foot, direction of, 379
  dorsal, of foot, 371, 373f
    deep dorsal venous network, 376
    greater and lesser saphenous veins, 371–376, 374f–378f
    superficial, 371
    superficial dorsal venous networks, 371
  plantar, of foot
    deep plantar venous network, 377–379
    superficial plantar venous network, 377
Vestibular system, gait modulation, 658, 658f
  descending pathways, 664, 666f–669f, 668–669
  medial and superior vestibular nuclei, 663, 664f
  otolith organs utricle and saccule, 659, 661f–662f, 662
  semicircular canals, 658, 659f–661f
  vestibular nuclei, 662–663, 662f–663f
  vestibulo-ocular reflex, 663–664, 664f–665f
V ligament (bifurcate ligament; ligament of Chopart), 190–195

W

Walking cycle, 610, 612f–613f
  electromyographic activities during, 641, 642f, 643
  stance phase of, 610, 613f–614f
  swing phase of, 611, 614f
  toes, function of, 618–619, 620f
Web space, first, arterial supply of, 319–320, 320f
  dorsomedial hallucal artery variations, 323
  first dorsal metatarsal artery variations, 320–323, 321f
  first plantar metatarsal artery variations, 323
  tibial plantar hallucal artery variations, 323, 324f